CLINICAL BRAIN IMAGING

Normal Structure and Functional Anatomy

CLINICAL BRAIN IMAGING

Normal Structure and Functional Anatomy

L. ANNE HAYMAN, M.D.
Professor of Radiology,
Director of MRI Research Laboratory,
Baylor College of Medicine;
Director of Clinical Neuroradiology,
The Ben Taub Hospital,
Houston, Texas

with VINCENT C. HINCK, M.D.
Emeritus Professor of Radiology,
Baylor College of Medicine,
Houston, Texas

with 798 *illustrations*

Mosby Year Book

St. Louis Baltimore Boston Chicago London Philadelphia Sydney Toronto

Mosby Year Book

Dedicated to Publishing Excellence

Editor: Anne Patterson
Developmental Editor: Maura Leib
Project Manager: Karen Edwards
Production Editor: Cynthia Miller
Designer: Gail Morey Hudson

Printed in the United States of America

Mosby–Year Book, Inc.
11830 Westline Industrial Drive, St. Louis, Missouri 63146

Library of Congress Cataloging in Publication Data

Hayman, L. Anne.
Clinical brain imaging : normal structure and functional anatomy / L. Anne Hayman ; with Vincent C. Hinck.
p. cm.
Includes bibliographical references and index.
ISBN 0-8151-4180-7
1. Brain—Imaging—Atlases. 2. Brain—Anatomy. 3. Brain—Imaging. I. Hinck, Vincent C. II. Title.
[DNLM: 1. Brain—anatomy & histology. 2. Brain—anatomy & histology—atlases. 3. Diagnostic Imaging. 4. Diagnostic Imaging—atlases. WL 17 H4223c]
QM455.H38 1992
611'.81—dc20
DNLM/DLC 92-12742
for Library of Congress CIP

92 93 94 95 96 CL/MY 9 8 7 6 5 4 3 2 1

CONTRIBUTORS

STEPHEN ALAN BERMAN, M.D., Ph.D.
Instructor,
Department of Neurology,
Harvard University;
Spinal Cord Injury Service,
West Roxbury VA Hospital,
Boston, Massachusetts

RICHARD A. BRONEN, M.D.
Assistant Professor,
Department of Diagnostic Radiology,
Yale University School of Medicine,
New Haven, Connecticut

R. NICK BRYAN, M.D., Ph.D.
Professor,
Department of Radiology,
The Johns Hopkins School of Medicine,
Baltimore, Maryland

EDWARD C. CALLAWAY, M.D.
Chief, Radiology Services,
Department of Radiology,
Sheppard Technical Training Hospital,
Witchita Falls, Texas

DALE A. CHARLETTA, M.D.
Department of Radiology,
Rush-Presbyterian, St. Luke's Medical Center,
Chicago, Illinois

ERIC COURCHESNE, Ph.D.
Professor,
Department of Neuroscience,
University of California, San Diego,
LaJolla, California;
Director,
Neuropyschology Research Laboratory,
Children's Hospital and Research Center,
San Diego, California

DAVID A. FEINBERG, M.D., Ph.D.
Radiologist,
New York University Medical School,
New York, New York

JOHN M. GUNDZIK, M.D.
Radiologist,
University of New Mexico Hospital,
Albuquerque, New Mexico

L. ANNE HAYMAN, M.D.
Professor of Radiology,
Director of MRI Research Laboratory,
Baylor College of Medicine;
Director of Clinical Neuroradiology,
The Ben Taub Hospital,
Houston, Texas

VINCENT C. HINCK, M.D.
Emeritus Professor of Radiology,
Baylor College of Medicine,
Houston, Texas

WILLIAM L. HIRSCH, M.D.
Assistant Professor of Radiology,
Department of Radiology,
Division of Neuroradiology,
University of Pittsburgh;
Staff Radiologist,
Department of Radiology,
Presbyterian-University Hospital,
Pittsburgh, Pennsylvania

NIRANJAN G. IYER, M.D.
Resident Physician,
Department of Internal Medicine,
St. Francis Hospital,
Evanston, Illinois

J. RANDY JINKINS, M.D.
Director of Neuroradiology,
Department of Radiology,
University of Texas Health Science Center,
San Antonio, Texas

JOEL B. KIRKPATRICK, M.D.
Professor,
Department of Pathology,
Baylor College of Medicine;
Attending Physician,
Department of Pathology,
The Methodist Hospital,
Houston, Texas

TODD ELLISON LANIER, M.D.
Radiologist,
University of California,
San Diego Medical Center,
San Diego, California

ROBERT B. LUFKIN, M.D.
Associate Professor of Radiology,
Director, Neurosciences Imaging,
Department of Radiology,
University of California, Los Angeles School of Medicine,
Los Angeles, California

MICHEL E. MAWAD, M.D.
Director of Neuroradiology,
Department of Radiology,
Baylor College of Medicine;
Department of Radiology,
The Methodist Hospital,
Houston, Texas

CRAIG B. McARDLE, M.D.
Staff Radiologist,
Department of Radiology,
Methodist Medical Center,
Dallas, Texas

JOHN J. PAGANI, M.D.
Radiologist,
Department of Radiology,
AMI Park Plaza Hospital,
Houston, Texas

MARK J. PFLEGER, M.D.
Clinical Assistant Neuroradiology Fellow,
Department of Radiology,
Massachussetts General Hospital,
Harvard Medical School,
Boston, Massachussetts

GARY A. PRESS, M.D.
Director of Magnetic Resonance,
Department of Radiology,
Kaiser Permanente Hospital,
San Diego, California

RONALD QUISLING, M.D.
Professor of Radiology,
Chief of Neuroradiology,
Department of Radiology,
University of Florida,
Gainesville, Florida

LOREN A. ROLAK, M.D.
Associate Professor of Clinical Neurology,
Department of Neurology,
Baylor College of Medicine;
Assistant Chief of Neurology,
Houston Veteran's Affairs Medical Center,
Houston, Texas

YOGESH P. SHAH, M.D.
Assistant Professor,
Department of Diagnostic Radiology,
Baylor College of Medicine,
Houston, Texas

REED A. SHANKWILER, M.D.
Neuroradiology Fellow,
Department of Radiology,
Baylor College of Medicine;
Department of Neuroradiology,
The Methodist Hospital,
Houston, Texas

ERIC M. SPICKLER, M.D.
Department of Diagnostic Radiology,
Division of Neuroradiology,
Henry Ford Hospital,
University of Michigan,
Detroit, Michigan

SUSAN WHEELER WEATHERS, M.D.
Assistant Professor,
Department of Radiology,
Baylor College of Medicine,
Houston, Texas

JULIE WENDT, M.D.
Department of Radiology,
Baylor College of Medicine,
Houston, Texas

RICHARD ERNEST WENDT, III, Ph.D.
Assistant Professor,
Department of Radiology,
Baylor College of Medicine,
Houston, Texas

JOHN W. WRIGHT, M.D.
Radiologist,
Cheyenne Radiology Group,
Cheyenne, Wyoming,

Foreword

In preparation for this foreword, I have reviewed the page proofs of this book with considerable enthusiasm for I find in it a fresh approach to the presentation of the brain and of the imaging approaches for visualization of the anatomy and certain pathological conditions of the brain by cross-sectional imaging methods: computed tomography, magnetic resonance imaging, and ultrasound. In addition, two chapters dealing with angiographic anatomy and diagrams of the type of displacements of blood vessels by intracranial masses are included.

What is striking about this text is that Dr. Hayman and her co-authors have understood the need for knowledge of structural brain anatomy in depth for anyone who deals with cross-sectional images that we encounter on a daily basis in the practice of clinical neuroradiology. In the past, we became experts in the cerebral spinal fluid spaces, the ventricles, and the subarachnoid cisterns, because these were the only aspects that were visualized by pneumoencephalography. Thus, we needed to have knowledge in depth of the outer surface of the brain in its supra and infra tentorial portions and of the inner cavities of the brain, the ventricular system. Today, however, that knowledge is insufficient. In addition to the gross surface anatomy, we need to know the actual structure of all of the portions of the brain, the brain stem, and the cerebellum, including the specific nuclei and the relationship of the various tracts and bundles to them and to the outer surface of the structures. Also we need to know the location of the nuclei of the cranial nerves as well as the paths of these nerves in and outside their point of origin. These aspects are all exhaustively covered in this text with numerous illustrations in all types of cross-sectional images.

In addition to the vascular chapters mentioned above, the text includes a chapter on the neurosecretory regions of the brain, most of which can be seen by gadolinium enhanced MR images because they do not possess a blood brain barrier. The text is completed with a chapter on the pituitary gland and the suprasellar regions.

Undoubtedly, this book will become a popular one among radiologists and neuroradiologists and among all of those interested in imaging of the central nervous system. It is replete with important cross-sectional anatomical information that we see in our daily practice and in addition contains the needed correlated imaging provided by computed tomography and magnetic resonance imaging side by side with the anatomical and pathological considerations.

Juan M. Taveras, M.D.

Preface

To interpret brain images well, clinicians must have at their disposal a wealth of relevant medical information. They should know what portion of the brain is to be imaged for evaluation of a specific symptom complex; which imaging modality will best serve in the pertinent area; normal appearances; and which anatomic terms precisely describe the location of the lesion *per se,* as well as the distortions of neighboring structures caused thereby.

Because of the sheer complexity of the central nervous system, one can scarcely hope to store all of this knowledge in memory. Regrettably, it is often very inconvenient and time consuming to retrieve it from standard textbooks of radiology, anatomy, and neurology. In response to a perceived need, the present book has been structured so that, during clinical interpretation of brain images, this information will be more readily available.

The anatomy of the neonatal brain, adult brain, cerebellum and vermis, cerebrospinal fluid spaces, and cerebral vessels is organized in an atlas format in **Chapters 1, 3, 6, 9, 11,** and **13.** The serial figures in these chapters are labeled with familiar radiographic terminology, and the level of each image is identified. All anatomic labels are indexed in these chapters so that the reader can quickly locate the illustration that depicts an unfamiliar structure. Companion chapters follow these atlases. They succinctly summarize and reference the recent literature concerning the normal appearance, clinically important functions, and pertinent information on the development and/or aging of each region.

Additional chapters provide easy access to information needed in specific clinical situations. For example, **Chapter 8** simplifies the imaging of patients with cranial nerve symptoms by diagraming the cisternal, nuclear, and central projections of each cranial nerve. Only the important clinical symptoms caused by lesions at each juncture along the pathway are described, but a table that comprehensively lists the functions of each nerve is provided. The cranial nerve syndromes are summarized in yet another table for consultation.

Questions regarding size and configuration of the ventricles and cisternal spaces are addressed in **Chapter 12.** The interpretation of a conventional or magnetic resonance arteriogram after discovery of a mass lesion by an axial imaging technique is addressed in **Chapter 15.** By consulting the diagrams provided, the reader can locate the lesion that most closely simulates the case at hand and then determine the vessel displacements that can be anticipated.

The problem of deciding if a lesion identified by an imaging technique is the cause of the patient's symptoms is addressed in **Chapter 16,** which uses a set of coronal and axial brain diagrams to provide an anatomic-functional correlation. The reader can also, after finding a lesion on CT or MR, choose the brain diagram that corresponds to the abnormal level and identify the specific arterial branch(es) that supply that area. This information can also be used to interpret the lateral projection of the arterial phase of a conventional or magnetic resonance angiogram.

In summary, this book contains material concerning brain anatomy and function that has been gathered from a wide range of clinical papers and anatomic atlases. The information is so organized that it can be used as a convenient, yet detailed, reference source in the clinical environment. However, it can also be used as a textbook to provide the student with a practical, current, detailed core of information on the functional and neuroanatomic imaging of the normal brain.

L. Anne Hayman

NOTE: We have made every effort to correctly cite the dosages of drugs throughout this text. However, the clinician should verify the correct dosage and route of administration by consulting the manufacturer's literature.

Acknowledgments

We are grateful for the help provided by the following individuals: **John J. Pagani, M.D.** provided almost all of the magnetic resonance images used in this book. He was assisted at the AMI Park Plaza Hospital by **Les Smith, R.T.** and **Jerry Mayes, R.T.** **David Gee** atended to all of the medical photography. **Patricia Stevenson, R.T.** and the technical staff at The Ben Taub Hospital provided virtually all of the computed tomographic images for this text. **Jackie Bogan** of the Baylor College of Medicine, Magnetic Resonance Center typed the manuscript (and its many revisions). **Niranjan Iyer, M.D.** proofread and critiqued the chapters. **Mohamed Hallem** of the Armed Forces Institute of Pathology provided access to the Yakovlev Brain Collection. **Cindy Miller** at Mosby–Year Book, Inc., was an invaluable resource in organizing the layout and the many indexes in this text.

Contents

CHAPTER 1

L. Anne Hayman
Yogesh P. Shah
Niranjan G. Iyer

Atlas of Neonatal Brain

◆

This chapter describes the anatomy of the neonatal brain. Before examining the atlas images, the reader may find it helpful to study the developmental events that result in the formation of a normal neonatal brain.

Figures 1-1, 1-2, and 1-3 are axial slices of the fetal brain at 16, 22, and 29 to 30 weeks of gestation, respectively.[1] These slices demonstrate the growth of the frontal, parietal, and temporal opercular gray matter over the insular cortex and the formation of the cortical gyral pattern. The dramatic maturation of the fetal brain that occurs from 30 weeks to 42 weeks can be visualized by comparing Figure 1-3 with the axial computed tomographic (CT) scans of a term infant shown in Figure 1-4. The earliest developmental changes that occur before 16 weeks are seen in Figure 1-5, *A* and *B*, which shows the serial maturation of the surface anatomy of the fetal brain in medial and lateral views. These serial views illustrate the posterior growth of the hemispheres, which causes them to fold over the third ventricle and thalami. Subsequent expansion of the cerebral hemispheres results in the formation of the temporal lobes. This process is described in detail in Chapter 4.

Recent advances in sonographic equipment and magnetic resonance imaging (MRI) have permitted the imaging clinician to visualize virtually all of the intracranial neuroanatomy in the premature and term infant. However, the potential usefulness of these techniques cannot be explored until a commensurate increase occurs in neuroanatomic knowledge. This chapter provides this information as a series of consecutive neonatal brain images that are matched with clinical ultrasound images in Figures 1-6 to 1-15 and magnetic resonance (MR) images in Figures 1-16 to 1-24. These images give the reader quick access to the standard nomenclature of clinically important structures. The labeled brain structures in this chapter are indexed so that unfamiliar terms mentioned in the following chapters can be easily located.

Almost all the brain sections used for this chapter were obtained from specimens in the collection of Dr. Paul Yakolev at the Armed Forces Institute of Pathology. They were taken at selected intervals from formalin-fixed neonatal brain sections. The reader should note that fixation has artificially enlarged the ventricles, sulci, and fissures in these slices. The stain used to process these brain slices highlights myelin and the vessels within and around the brain. The distance from base slice (0 mm) is indicated on each anatomic illustration in Figures 1-16 to 1-24. These distances reflect the in vivo distance between brain slices. The level and angle of the anatomic, ultrasound, and MR illustrations are indicated on small companion diagrams. Because it is not possible to match the anatomic sections exactly with the ultrasound and MR planes, the reader may find an area of interest in the anatomic images immediately before and/or after the related plane of interest.

Because of space considerations, it was not possible to label all the cisternal, sulcal, gyral, and cerebellar structures in the illustrations used for this chapter. These structures closely resemble those of the adult brain and are labeled in detail in subsequent atlas Chapters 3, 9, and 11. The neonatal brain structures that have a unique appearance because of active myelination are labeled in this chapter. Many excellent references were consulted to aid in identifying these structures.[1-13]

The following techniques were used to obtain the ultrasound images. An Acuson Ultrasound Instrument with a 5 MHz transducer was adjusted to the appropriately placed focal zones. All of the anatomic sections shown were produced by angling the transducer through the anterior fontanelle. The ultrasound examination was standardized by obtaining 10 images (Figures 1-6 to 1-15). Boxes 1-1 and 1-2 list the abbreviations used to designate cerebral gyri and cerebellar folia, respectively, in Figures 1-6 to 1-15.

DEVELOPMENTAL ANATOMY

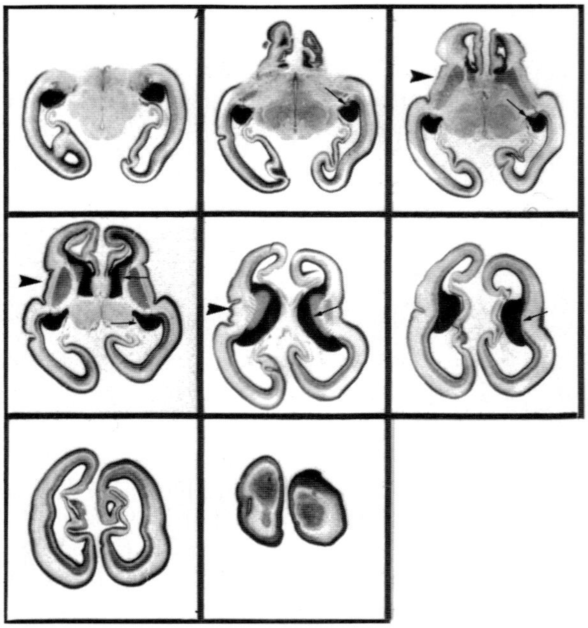

Figure 1-1 Fetus, 16 weeks of gestation. Serial, axial, stained brain slices from base to vertex. Note relatively small size of cerebral hemispheres compared with the brainstem and the very thin cortical layer of cells. A prominent subependymal germinal matrix can be seen as a symmetric, thick, dark area immediately adjacent to the large lateral ventricles (*arrows*). Note absence of a gyral pattern and the shallow sylvian fissures (*arrowheads*). (Reproduced with permission from Larroche JC: J *Neuroradiol* 8:93-108, 1981.)

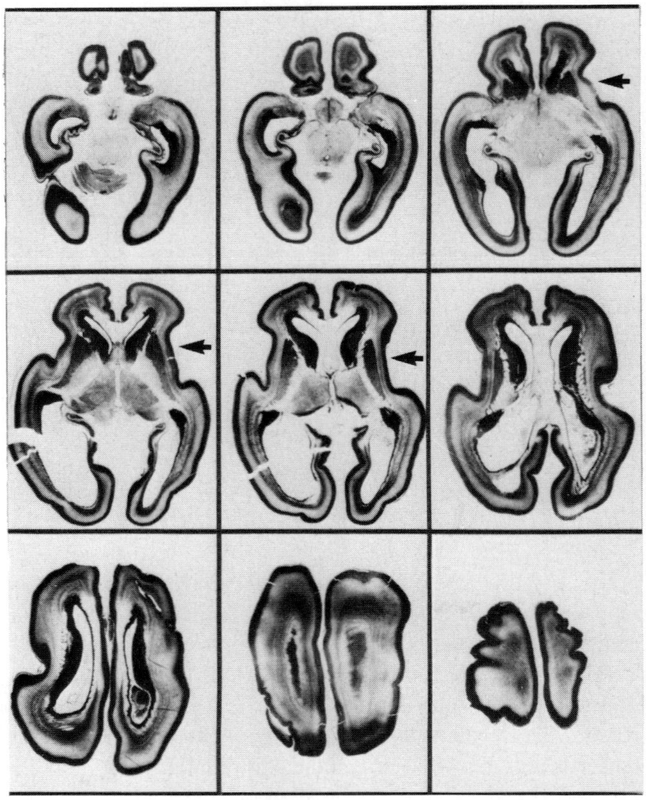

Figure 1-2 Fetus, 22 weeks of gestation. Serial, axial, stained brain slices from base to vertex. Note the disproportionate growth of the cerebral hemispheres compared with the brainstem. Sylvian fissures (*arrows*) have deepened compared with Figure 1-1. Note that the large ventricles and the thick germinal matrix persist. (Reproduced with permission from Larroche JC: J *Neuroradiol* 8:93-108, 1981.)

Figures 1-16 to 1-24 show the myelination pattern of the newborn brain in anatomic sections and on MR images. Myelinated areas are demonstrated as zones of *hypointensity* on long TR/long TE (T2-weighted) scans and zones of *hyperintensity* on short TR/short TE (T1-weighted) scans (TR, repetition time; TE, echo delay time). These axial MR images were obtained from a normal living infant at the 40th week of gestation. Two scan sequences are shown for each level; both the long TR/TE (2500/160) and the short TR/TE (800/20) scans were obtained on a 1.5 T (Tesla) General Electric Signa unit using an extremity coil. An 18 cm field of view was used to obtain 4 mm scans separated by a 2 mm gap. One average was obtained with a 256 × 198 matrix.

References

1. Larroche JC: Morphological criteria of central nervous system development in the human fetus, *J Neuroradiol* 8:93-108, 1981.
2. Pernkopf E: *Atlas of topographical and applied human anatomy,* Baltimore-Munich, 1980, Urban and Schwarzenberg.
3. Matsui T, Hirano A: *An atlas of the human brain for computed tomography,* Tokyo, 1978, Igaku-Shoin.
4. Barkovich AJ: *Contemporary neuroimaging, vol I, Pediatric neuroimaging,* New York, 1990, Raven.
5. Salmon G, Raynaud C, Regis J, Rumeau L: *Magnetic resonance imaging of the pediatric brain: an anatomic atlas,* New York, 1990, Raven.
6. Rorke LB, Riggs HE: *Myelination of the brain in the newborn,* Philadelphia, 1969, JB Lippincott.
7. Feess-Higgins A, Larroche JC: *Development of the human foetal brain: an anatomical atlas,* Paris, 1987, INSERM.
8. Roberts MP, Hanaway J, Morest DK: *Atlas of the human brain in section,* ed 2, Philadelphia, 1987, Lea & Febiger.

DEVELOPMENTAL ANATOMY

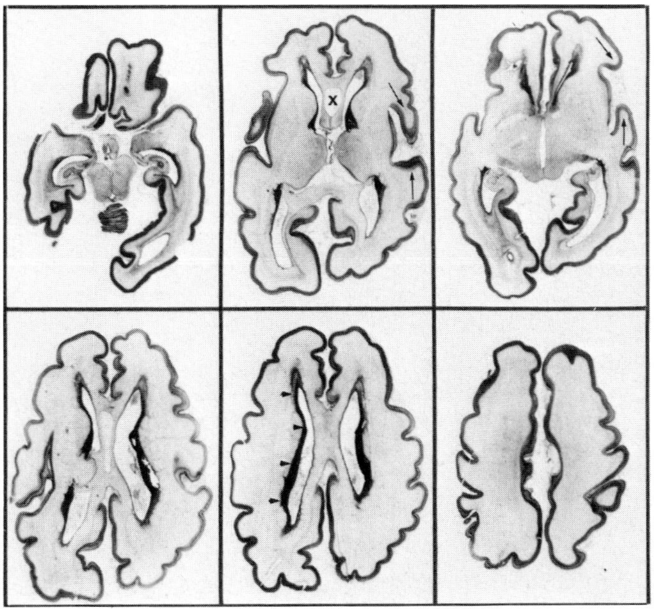

Figure 1-3 Fetus, 29 to 30 weeks of gestation. Serial, axial, stained brain slices from base to vertex. Note the cortical gyral pattern and gradual growth of the frontal and temporal cortices over the insula (*arrows*). Large ventricles, a cavum septi pellucidi (X), and germinal matrix (*arrowheads*) persist. (Reproduced with permission from Larroche JC: J *Neuroradiol* 8:93-108, 1981.)

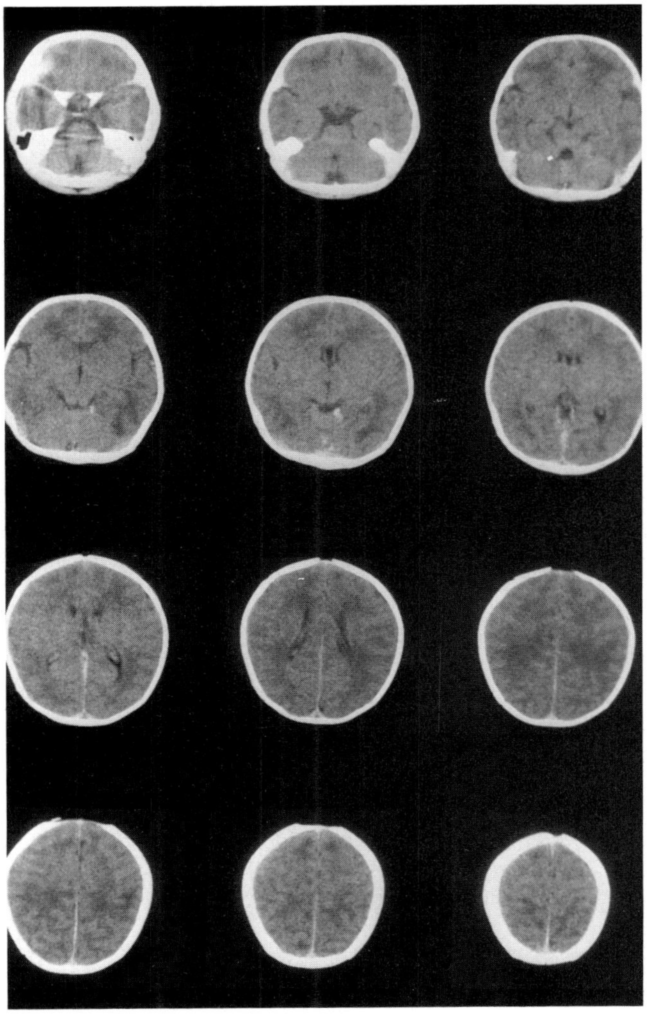

Figure 1-4 Normal newborn infant. Serial axial CT scans from base to vertex. Individual structures are labeled on axial MR scans in Figures 1-16 to 1-24. The poorly defined hypodense regions normally present in the centrum semiovale of the hemispheres do not correlate with myelination. These may represent variations in glial cell density or lipid content.

9. Yakovlev PI, Lecours AR: The myelogenetic cycles of regional maturation of the brain. In *Regional development of the brain in early life*, Philadelphia, 1967, FA Davis.
10. Naidich TP, Yousefzadeh DK, Gusnard DA, Naidich JB: Sonography of the internal capsule and basal ganglia in infants. Part II. Localization of pathologic processes in the sagittal section through the caudothalamic groove, *Radiology* 161:615-621, 1986.
11. Yousefzadeh DK, Naidich TP: US anatomy of the posterior fossa in children: correlation with brain sections, *Radiology* 156:353-361, 1985.
12. Naidich TP, Gusnard DA, Yousefzadeh DK: Sonography of the internal capsule and basal ganglia in infants. 1. Coronal sections, *AJNR* 6:909-917, 1985.
13. Naidich TP, Yousefzadeh DK, Gusnard DA: The neonatal head. II. Sonography of the normal neonatal head, *Neuroradiology* 28:408-427, 1986.

DEVELOPMENTAL ANATOMY

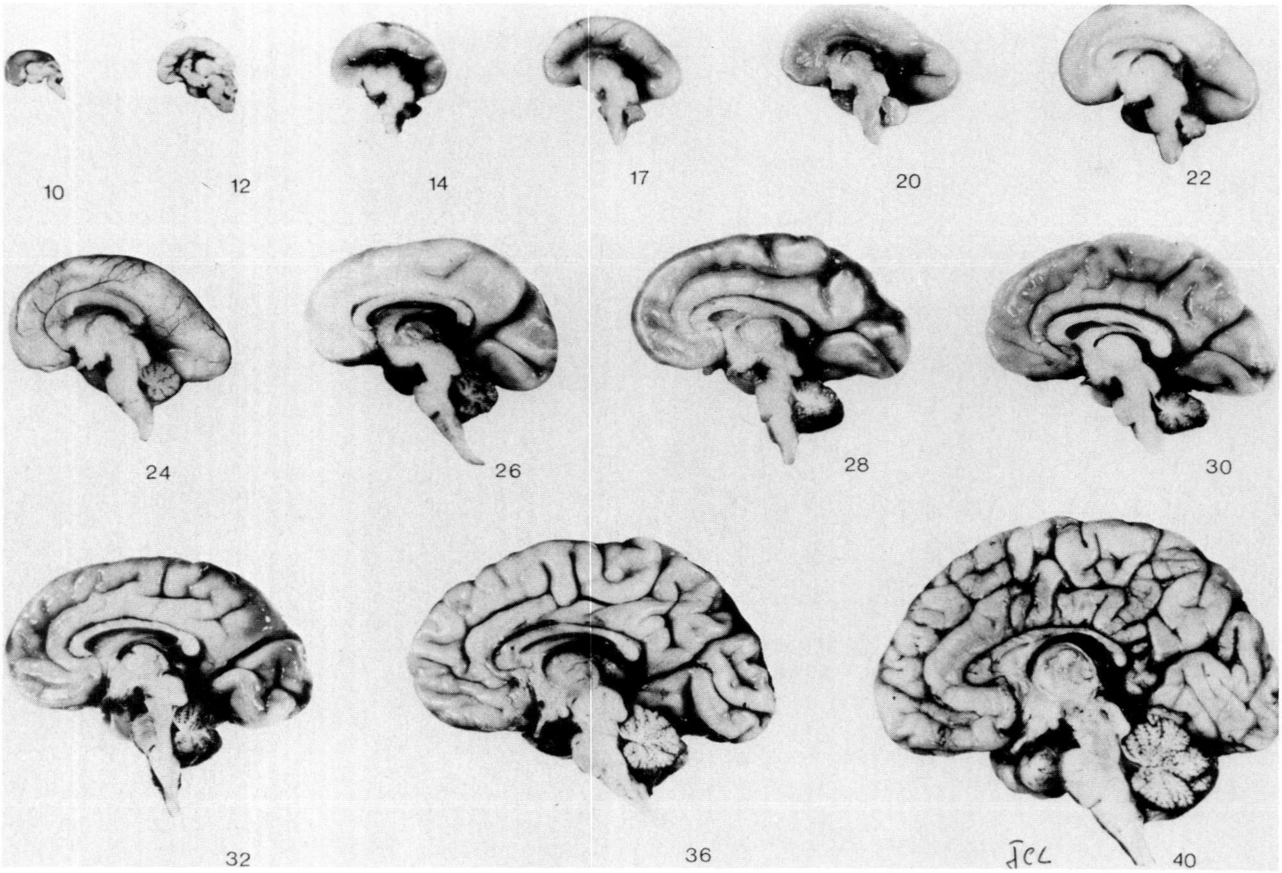

Figure 1-5 Serial views of the fetal brain surfaces from the 10th through the 40th weeks of gestation. **A,** Medial views show the progressive caudal growth of the corpus callosum and the relative increase in size of the cerebellar hemispheres.

BOX 1-1

Key for Identifying Neonatal Cerebral Gyri (Figures 1-6 to 1-15)

1. Cingulate gyrus
2. Superior frontal gyrus
3. Middle frontal gyrus
4. Inferior frontal gyrus
5. Frontal operculum
6. Insula
7. Orbital gyri
8. Rectal gyrus
9. Superior temporal gyrus
10. Middle temporal gyrus
11. Inferior temporal gyrus
12. Fusiform (lateral occipitotemporal) gyrus
13. Hippocampal gyrus
14. Parietal operculum
15. Transverse temporal gyrus
16. Supramarginal gyrus
17. Paracentral gyrus
18. Precuneus
19. Cuneus
20. Lingual gyrus
21. Uncus
22. Precentral gyrus
23. Postcentral gyrus

DEVELOPMENTAL ANATOMY

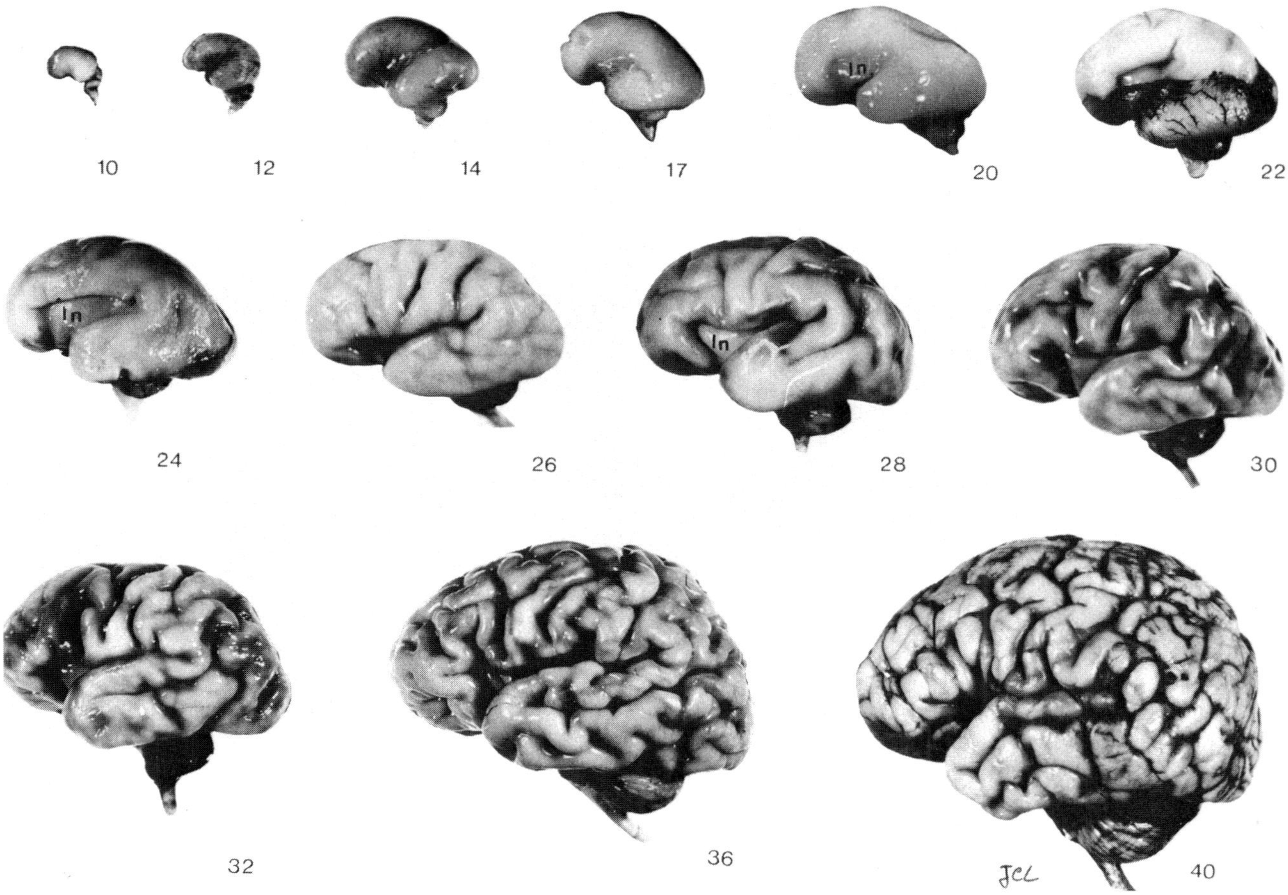

Figure 1-5, cont'd. B, Lateral views show the growth of the frontal, parietal, and temporal cortices over the insula (see weeks 20, 24, and 28). Both serial views show the development of the cortical gyral pattern. (Reproduced with permission from Larroche JC: J *Neuroradiol* 8:93-108, 1981.)

BOX 1-2

Key for Identifying Cerebellar Folia (Figures 1-6 to 1-15)

ce	Central lobule
cu	Culmen
d	Declive
f	Folium
l	Lingula
n	Nodule (nodulus)
p	Pyramis
t	Tuber
u	Uvula

CORONAL ULTRASOUND—ANATOMIC CORRELATIONS

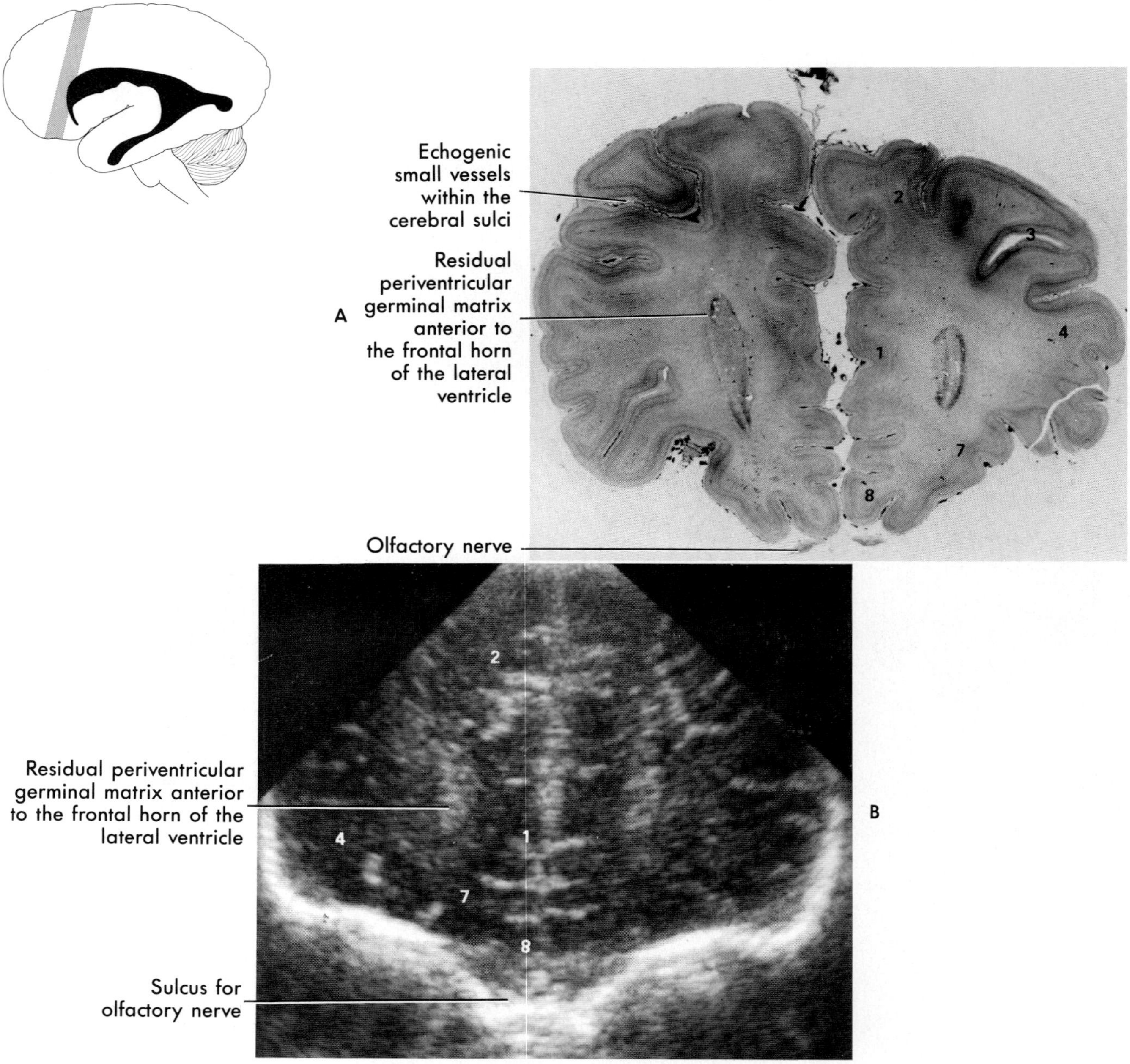

Figure 1-6 **A** and **B,** Coronal scan plane through anterior cranial fossa. 1, Cingulate gyrus; 2, superior frontal gyrus 4, inferior frontal gyrus; 7, orbital gyri; 8, rectal gyrus.

CORONAL ULTRASOUND—ANATOMIC CORRELATIONS

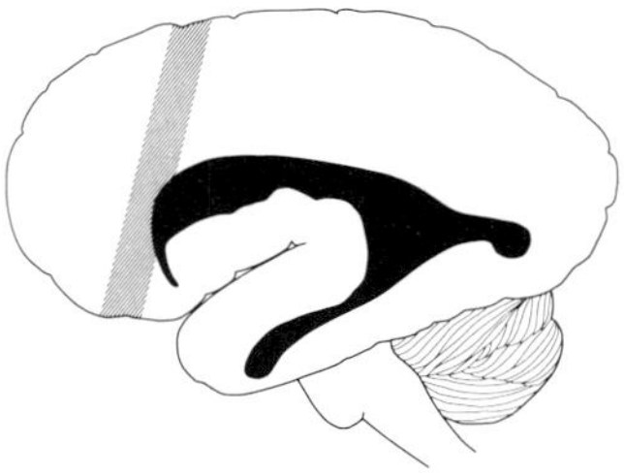

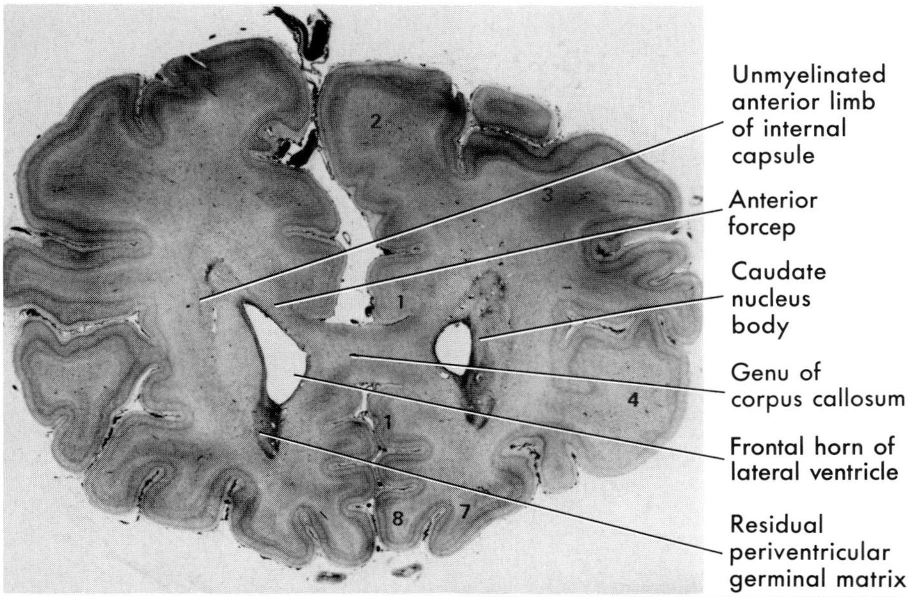

C

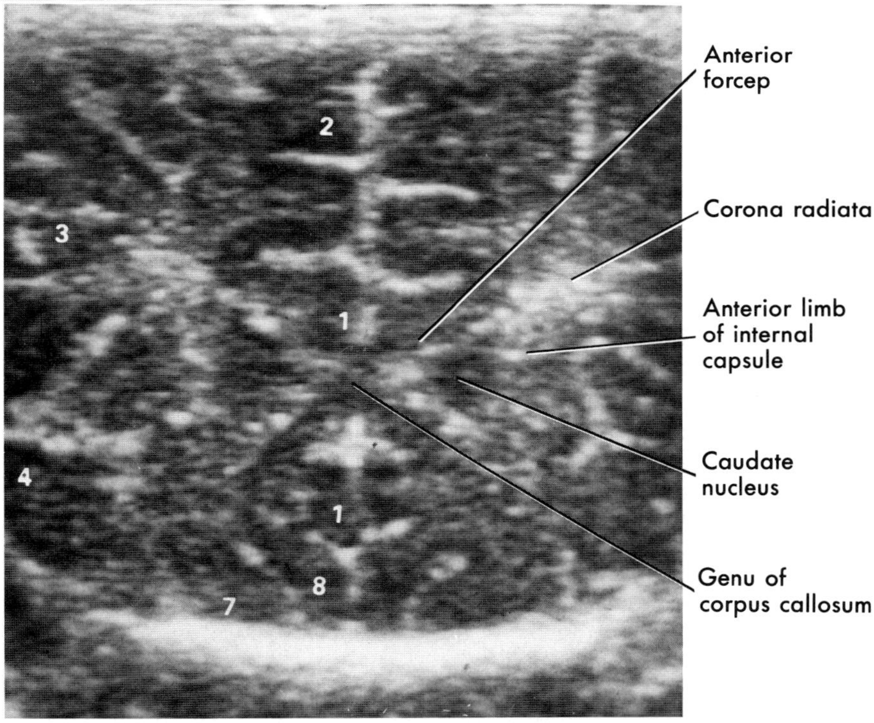

D

Figure 1-6, cont'd **C** and **D,** Coronal scan plane through anterior cranial fossa. 1, Cingulate gyrus; 2, superior frontal gyrus; 3, middle frontal gyrus; 4, inferior frontal gyrus; 7, orbital gyri; 8, rectal gyrus.

CORONAL ULTRASOUND—ANATOMIC CORRELATIONS

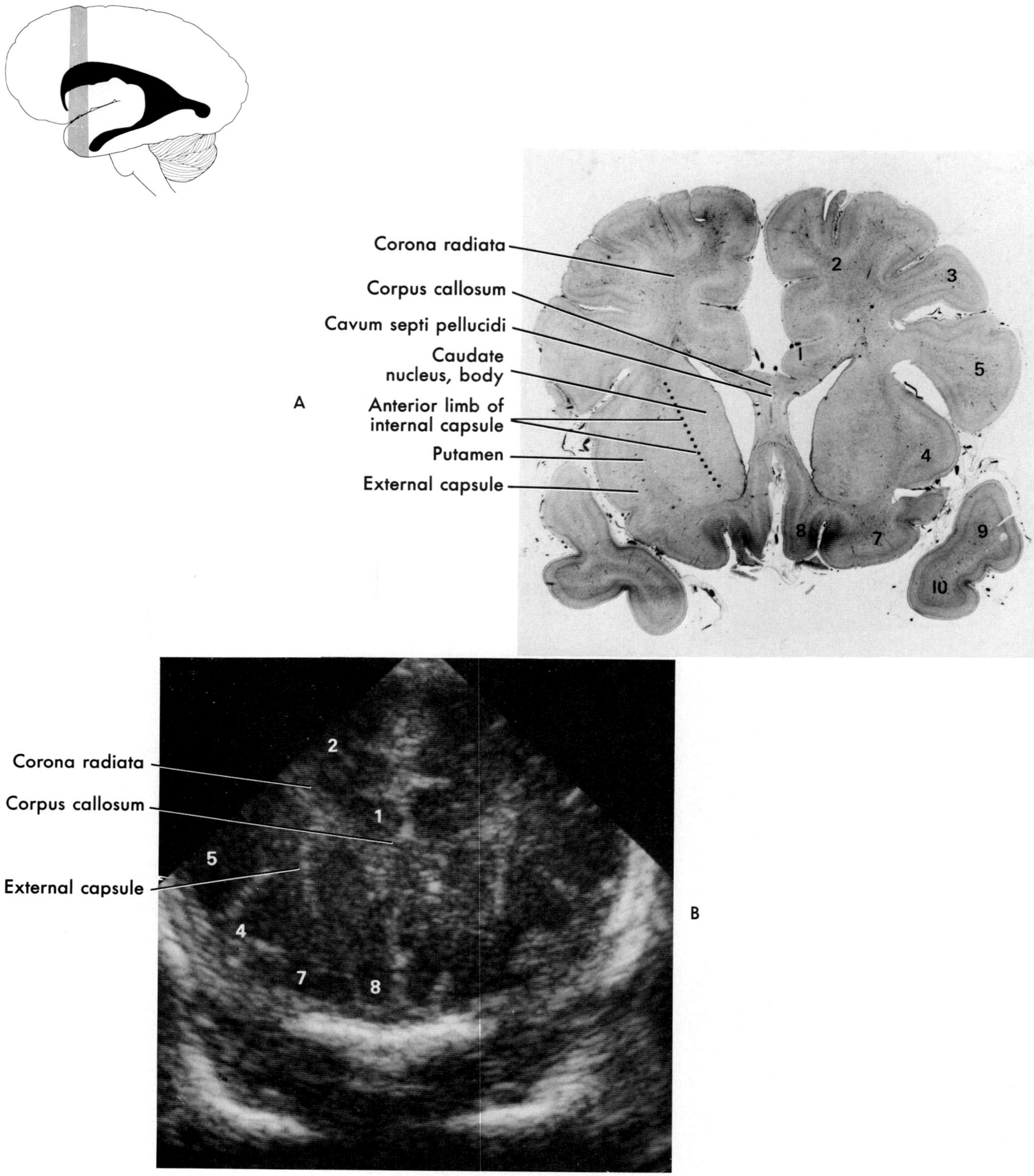

Figure 1-7 **A** and **B**, Coronal scan plane through internal carotid artery bifurcation. 1, Cingulate gyrus; 2, superior frontal gyrus; 3, middle frontal gyrus; 4, inferior frontal gyrus; 5, frontal operculum; 7, orbital gyri; 8, rectal gyrus; 9, superior temporal gyrus; 10, middle temporal gyrus.

CORONAL ULTRASOUND—ANATOMIC CORRELATIONS

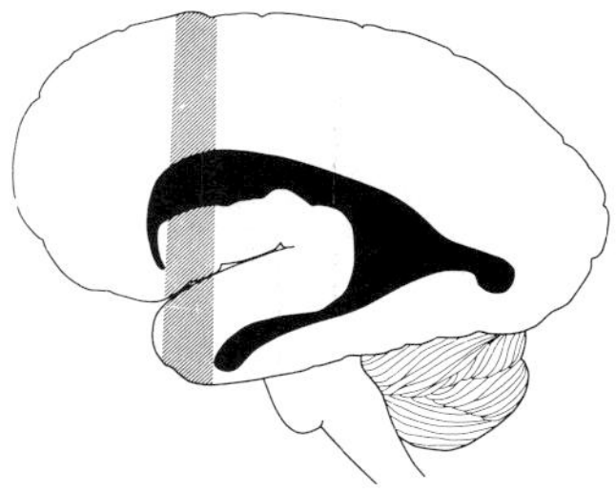

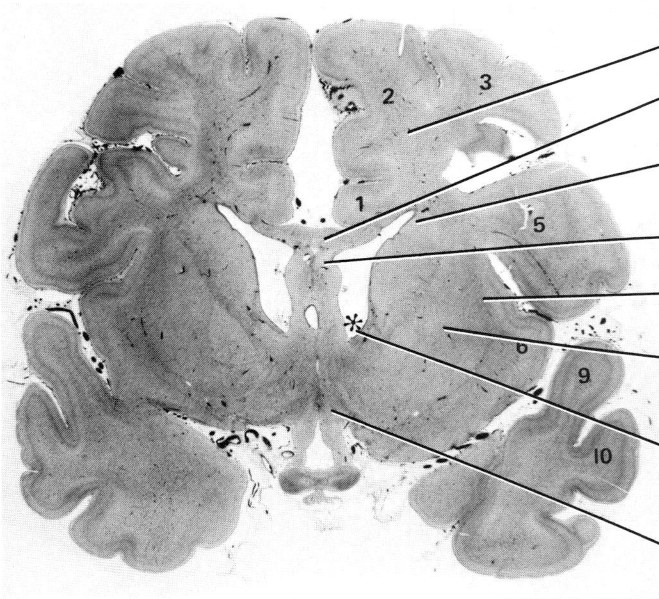

C

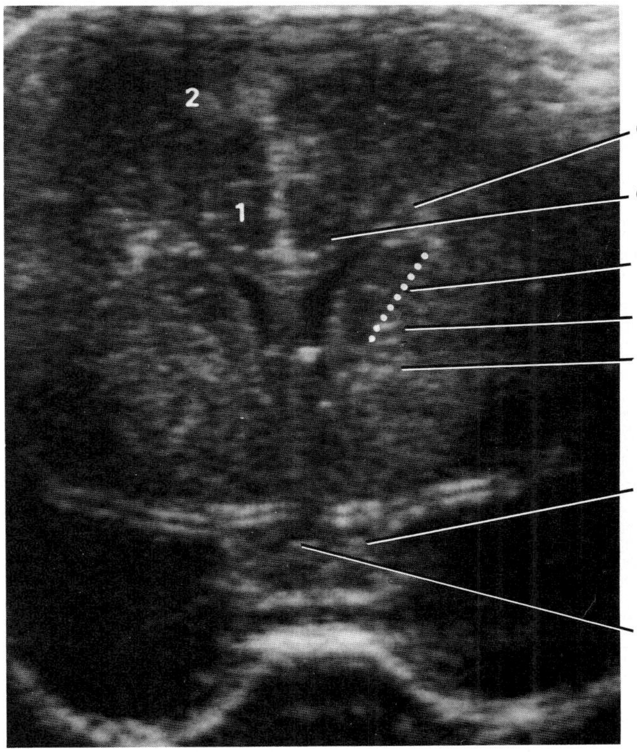

D

Figure 1-7, cont'd. **C** and **D**, Coronal scan plane through internal carotid artery bifurcation. 1, Cingulate gyrus; 2, superior frontal gyrus; 3, middle frontal gyrus; 5, frontal operculum; 6, insula; 9, superior temporal gyrus; 10, middle temporal gyrus.

CORONAL ULTRASOUND—ANATOMIC CORRELATIONS

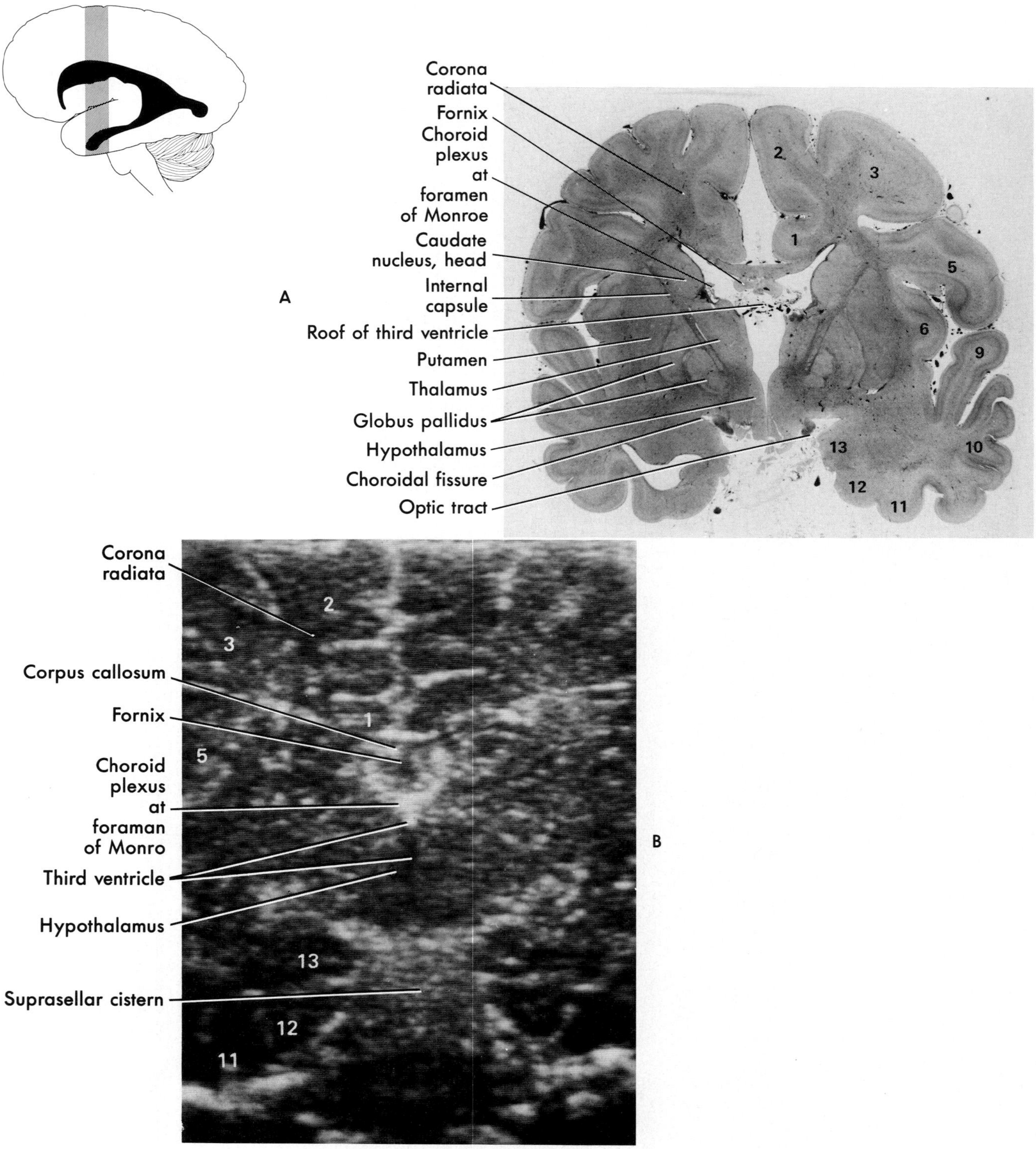

Figure 1-8 **A** and **B**, Angled coronal scan plane through interpeduncular cistern. 1, Cingulate gyrus; 2, superior frontal gyrus; 3, middle frontal gyrus; 5, frontal operculum; 6, insula; 9, superior temporal gyrus; 10, middle temporal gyrus; 11, inferior temporal gyrus; 12, fusiform gyrus; 13, hippocampal gyrus.

CORONAL ULTRASOUND—ANATOMIC CORRELATIONS

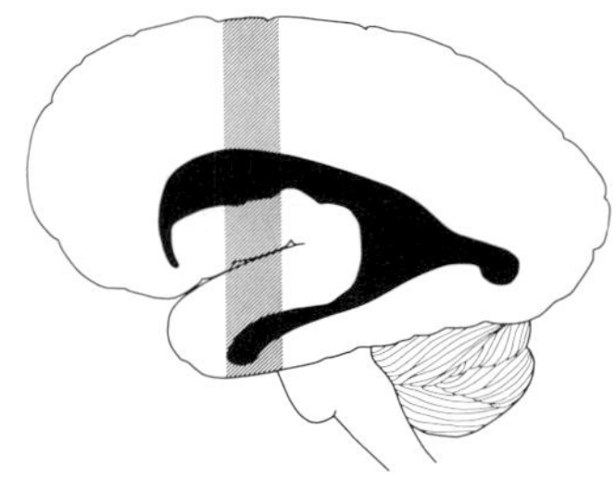

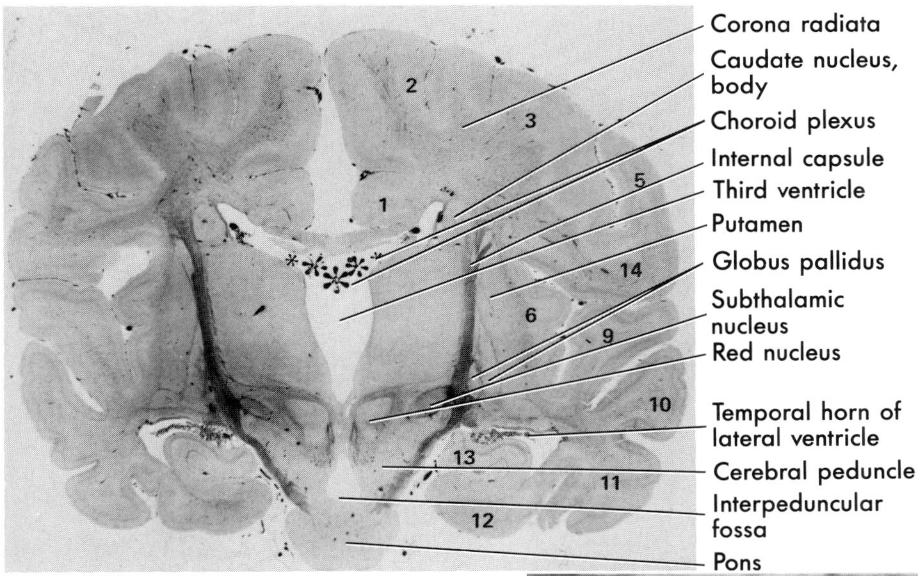

C

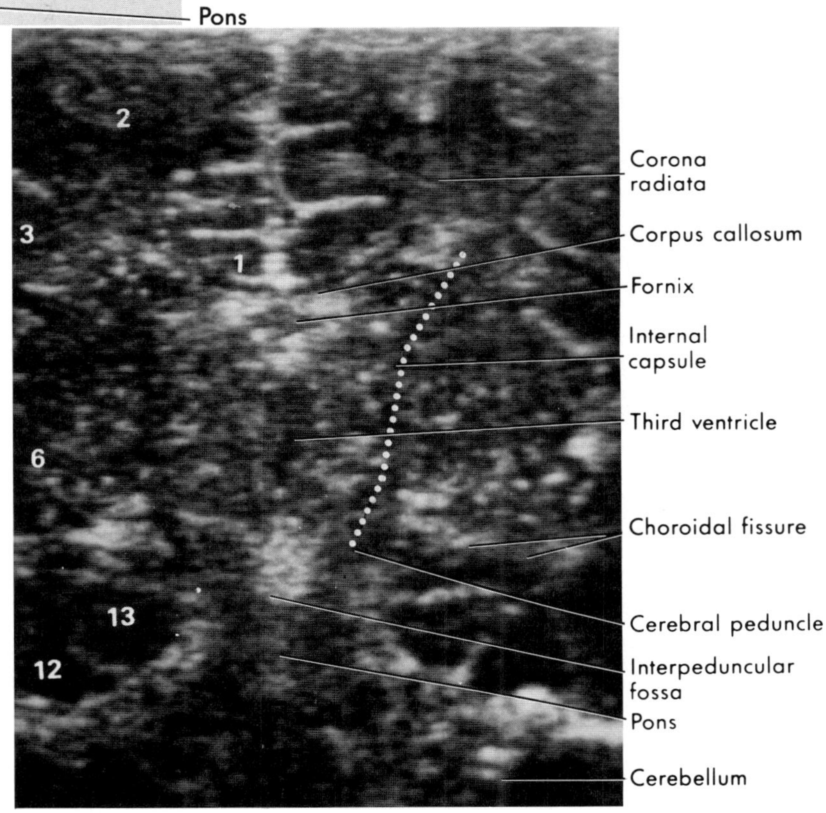

D

Figure 1-8, cont'd. **C** and **D**, Angled coronal scan plane through interpeduncular cistern. 1, Cingulate gyrus; 2, superior frontal gyrus; 3, middle frontal gyrus; 5, frontal operculum; 6, insula; 9, superior temporal gyrus; 10, middle temporal gyrus; 11, inferior temporal gyrus; 12, fusiform gyrus; 13, hippocampal gyrus; 14, parietal operculum.

CORONAL ULTRASOUND—ANATOMIC CORRELATIONS

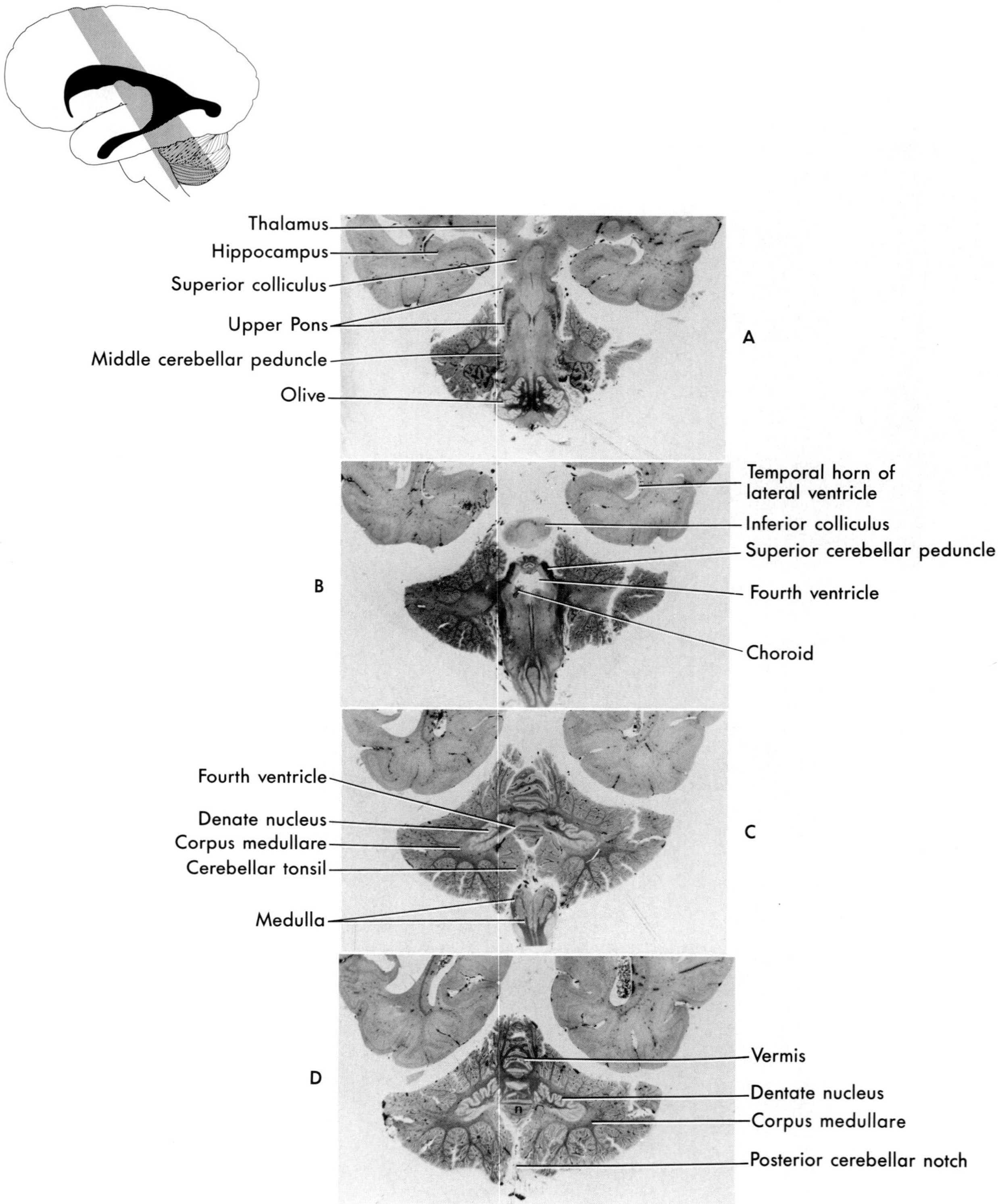

Figure 1-9 **A** to **D**, Angled coronal scan plane through fourth ventricle and quadrigeminal plate cistern.

CORONAL ULTRASOUND—ANATOMIC CORRELATIONS

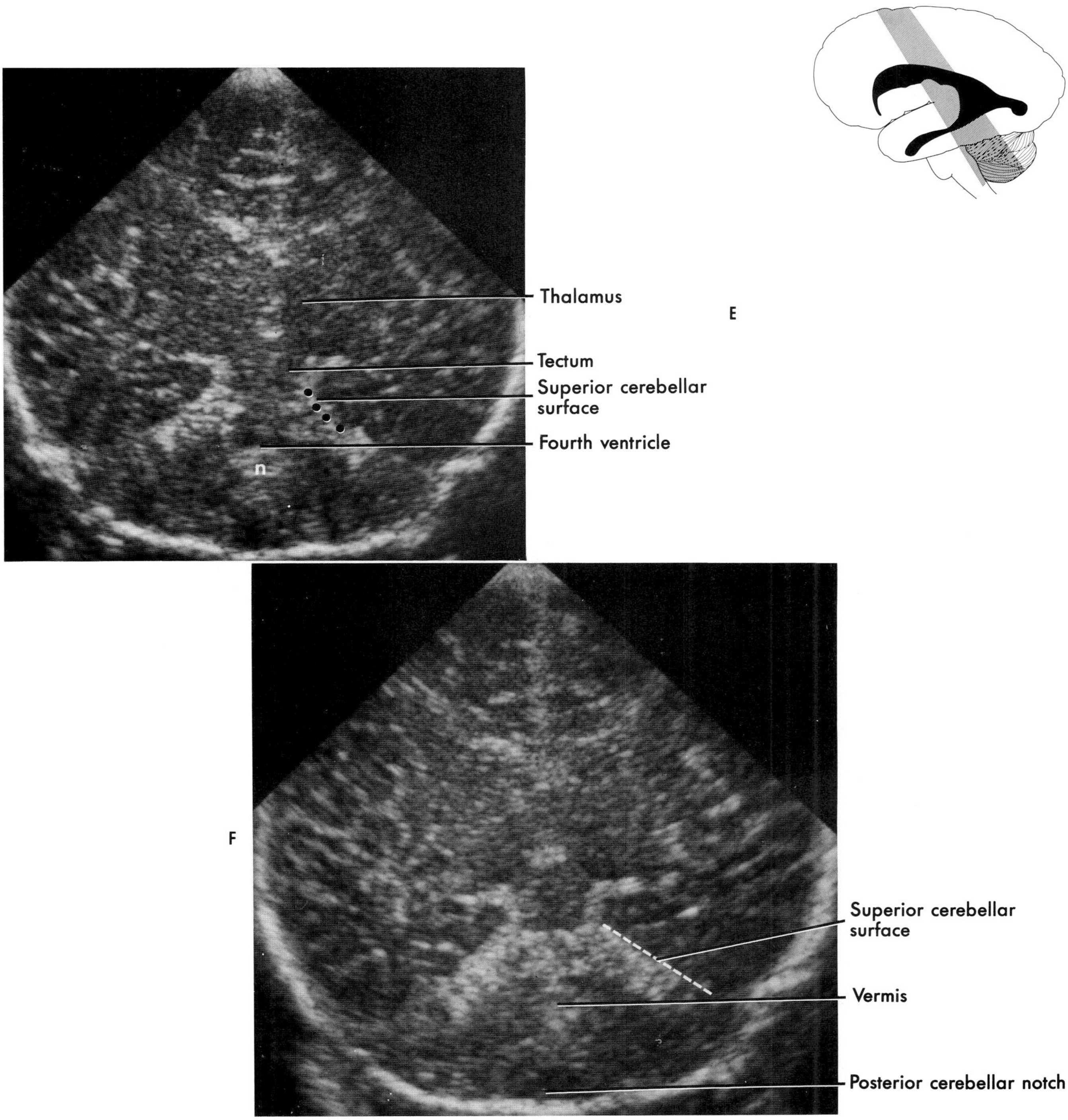

Figure 1-9, cont'd. **E** and **F**, Angled coronal scan plane through fourth ventricle and quadrigeminal plate cistern. *n*, Nodule.

CORONAL ULTRASOUND—ANATOMIC CORRELATIONS

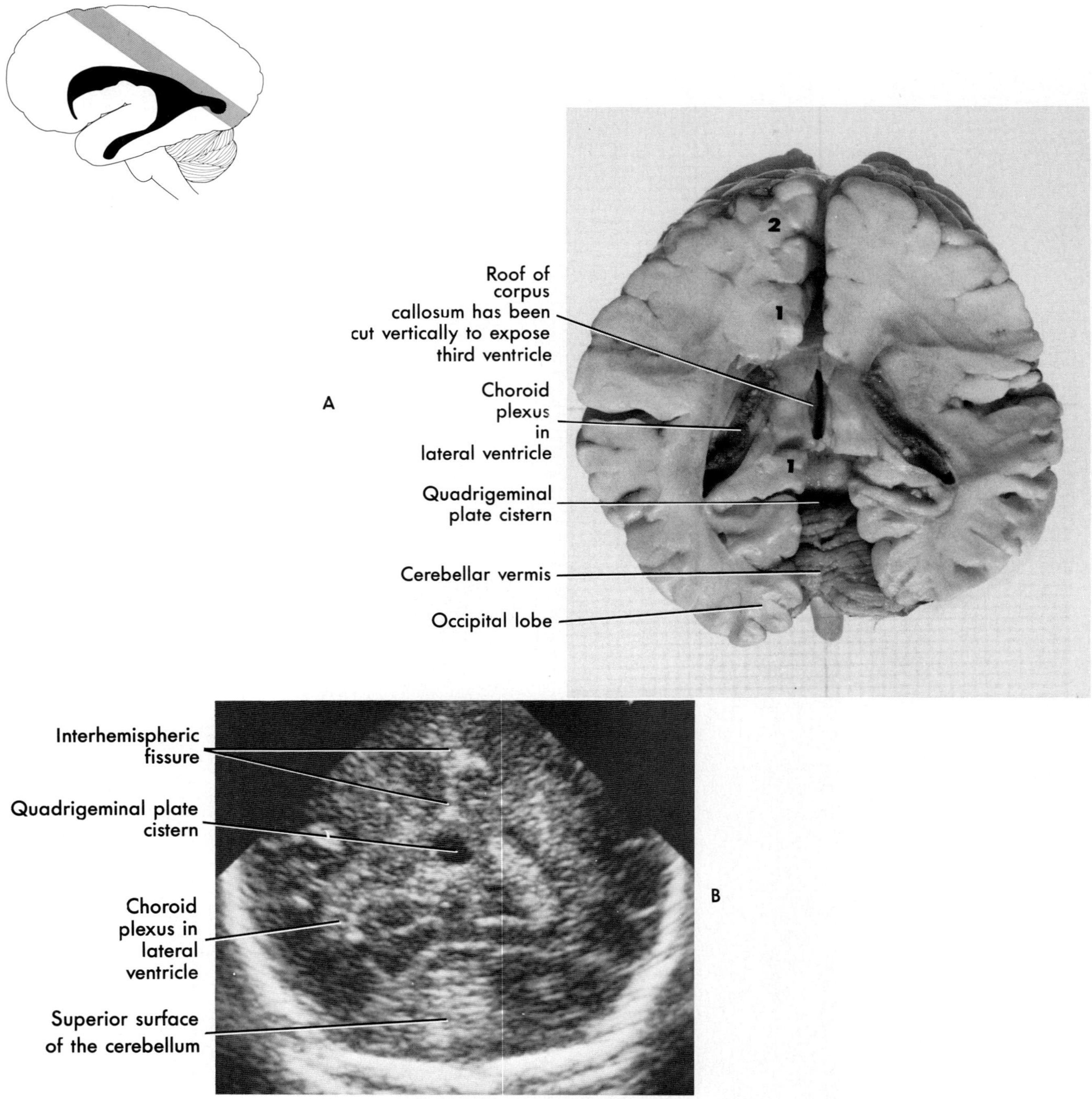

Figure 1-10 **A** and **B,** Inclined axial scan plane through glomus of choroid plexus. 1, Cingulate gyrus; 2, superior frontal gyrus.

CORONAL ULTRASOUND—ANATOMIC CORRELATIONS

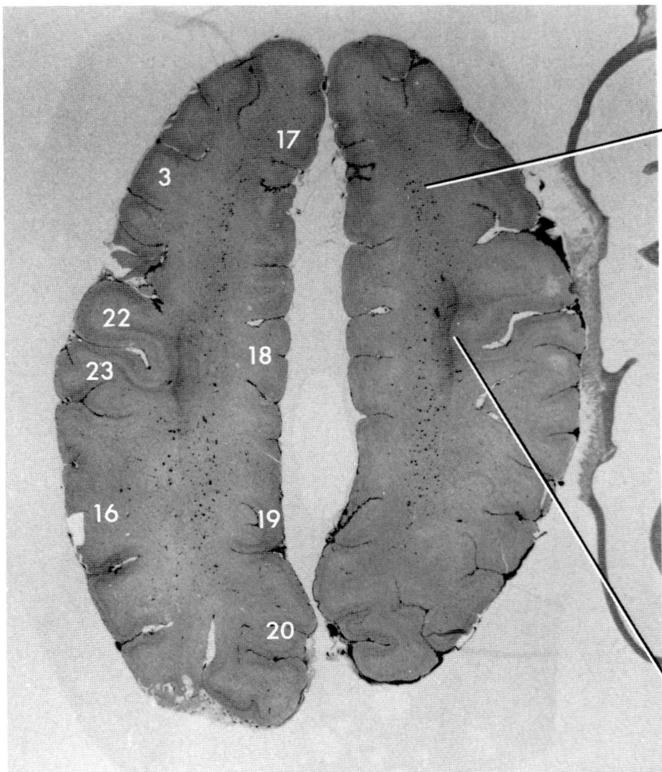

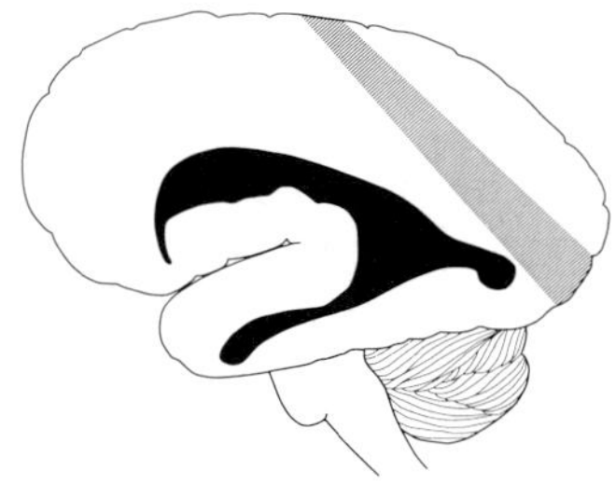

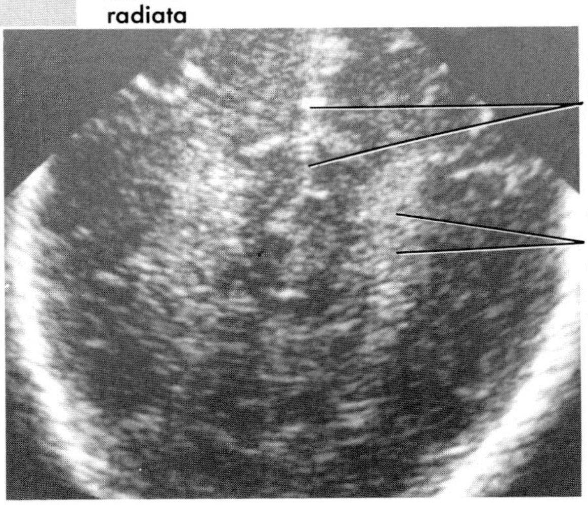

Figure 1-11 **A** and **B**, Axial scan plane superior to body of lateral ventricles. 3, Middle frontal gyrus; 16, supramarginal gyrus; 17, paracentral gyrus; 18, precuneus; 19, cuneus; 20, lingual gyrus; 22, precentral gyrus; 23, postcentral gyrus.

SAGITTAL ULTRASOUND—ANATOMIC CORRELATIONS

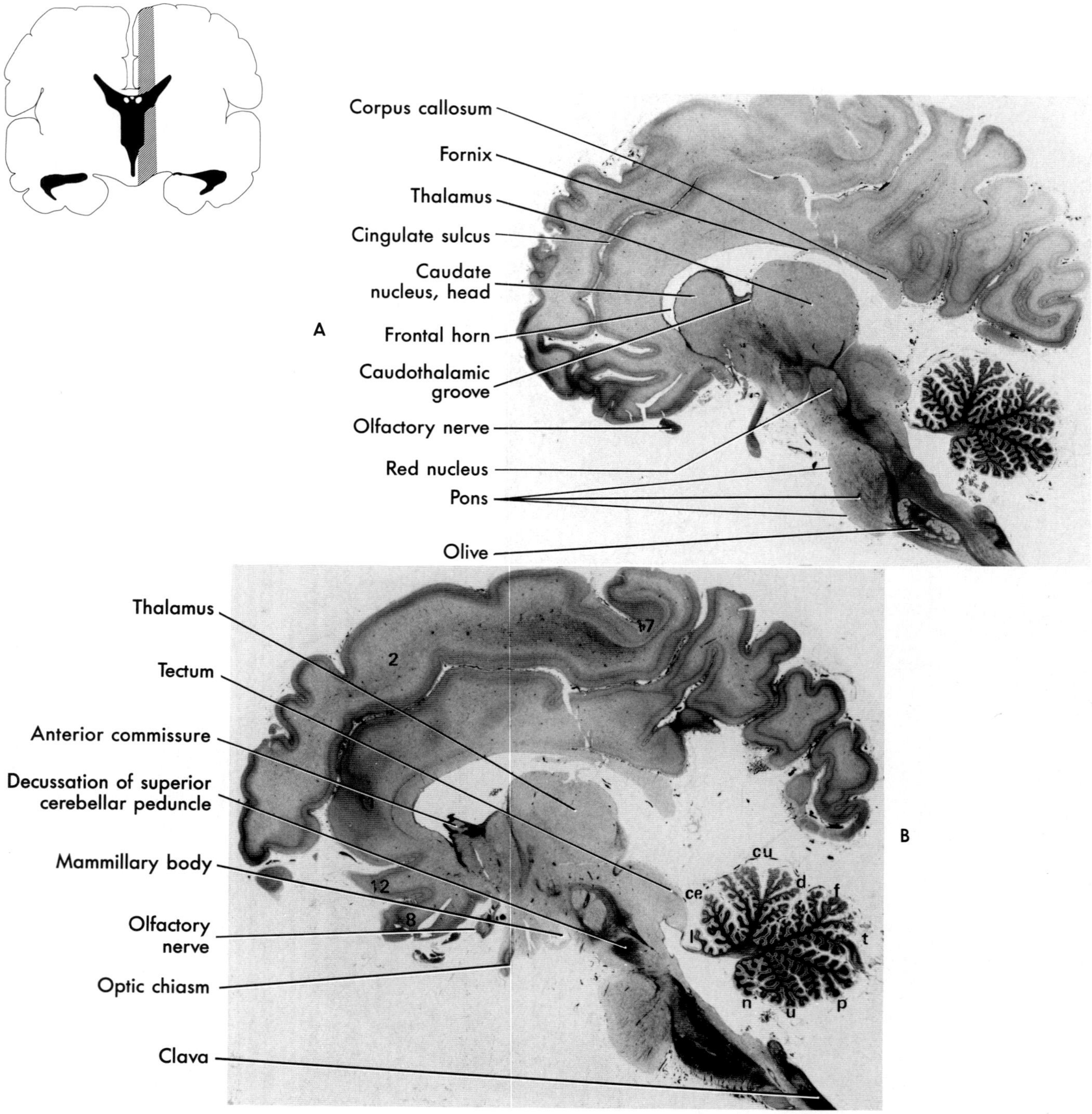

Figure 1-12 **A** and **B**, Midline sagittal scan plane. *ce*, Central lobule; *cu*, culmen; *d*,declive; *f*, folium; *l*, lingula; *n*, nodule; *p*, pyramis; *t*, tuber; *u*, uvula; 2, superior frontal gyrus; 17 paracentral gyrus.

SAGITTAL ULTRASOUND—ANATOMIC CORRELATIONS

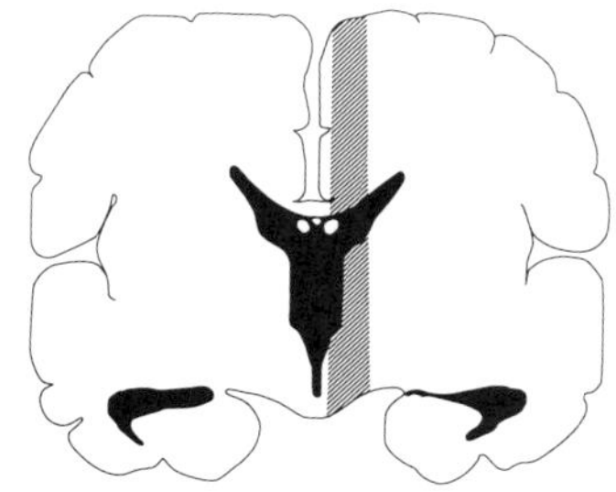

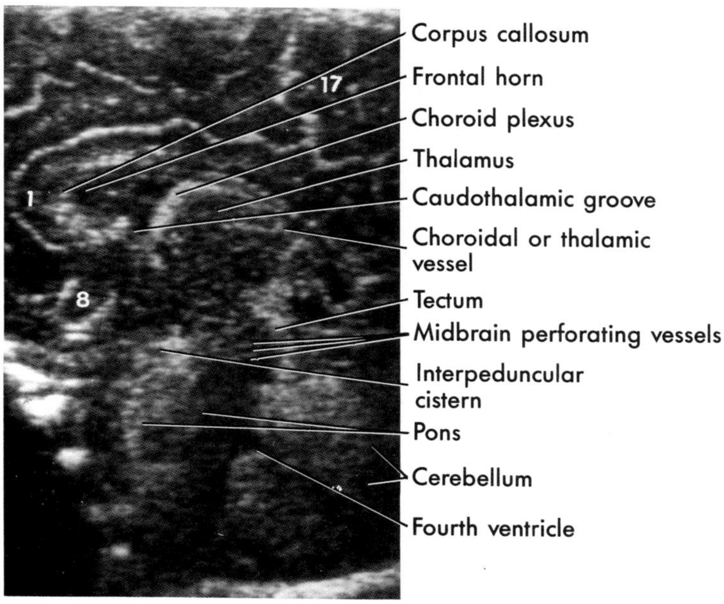

C

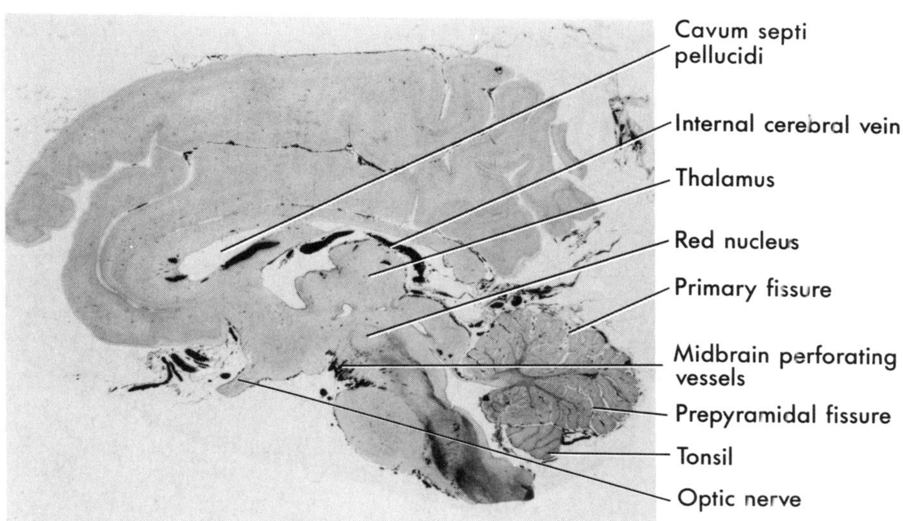

D

cont'd. **C** and **D,** Midline sagittal scan plane. 1, Cingulate gyrus; 8, rectal gyrus; 17, para-

SAGITTAL ULTRASOUND—ANATOMIC CORRELATIONS

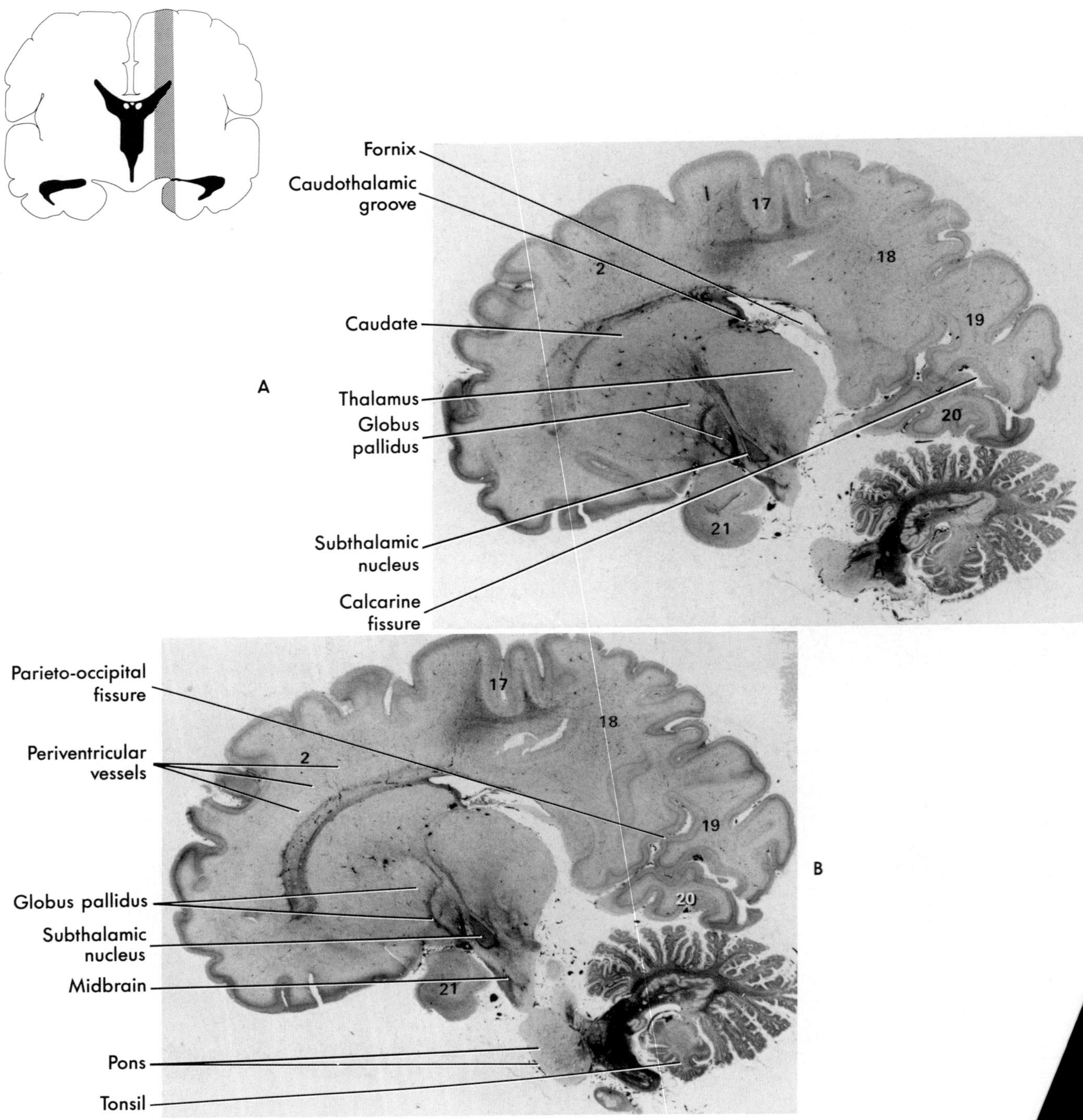

Figure 1-13 **A** and **B**, Parasagittal scan plane through uncus. 2, Superior frontal gyrus; 17, paracentral gyrus; 18, precuneus; 19, cuneus; 20, lingual gyrus; 21, uncus.

SAGITTAL ULTRASOUND—ANATOMIC CORRELATIONS

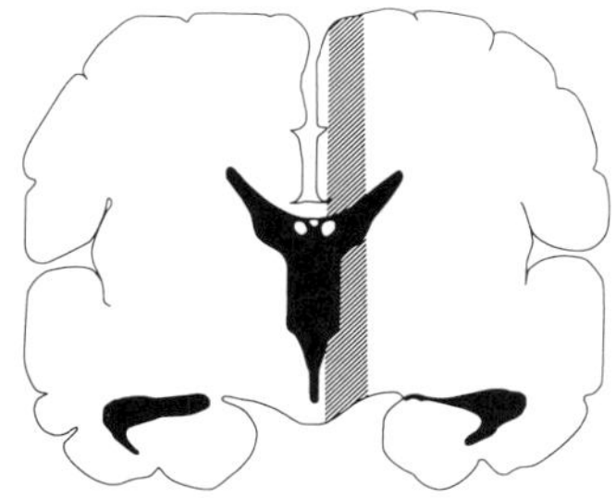

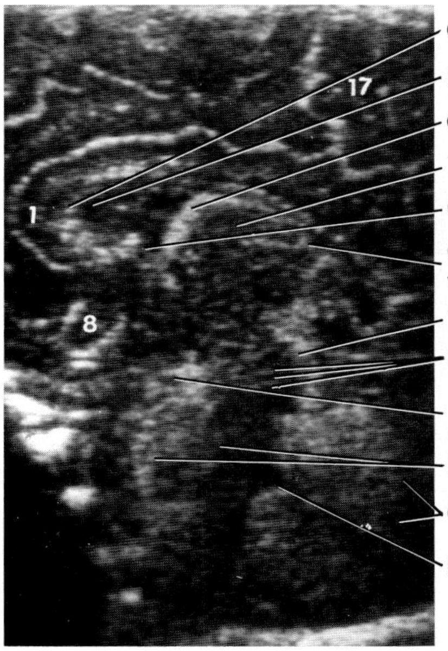

C

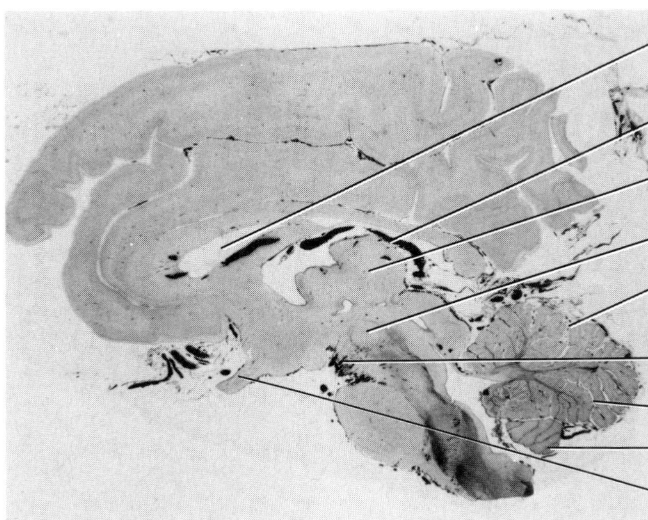

D

Figure 1-12, cont'd. **C** and **D**, Midline sagittal scan plane. 1, Cingulate gyrus; 8, rectal gyrus; 17, paracentral gyrus.

SAGITTAL ULTRASOUND—ANATOMIC CORRELATIONS

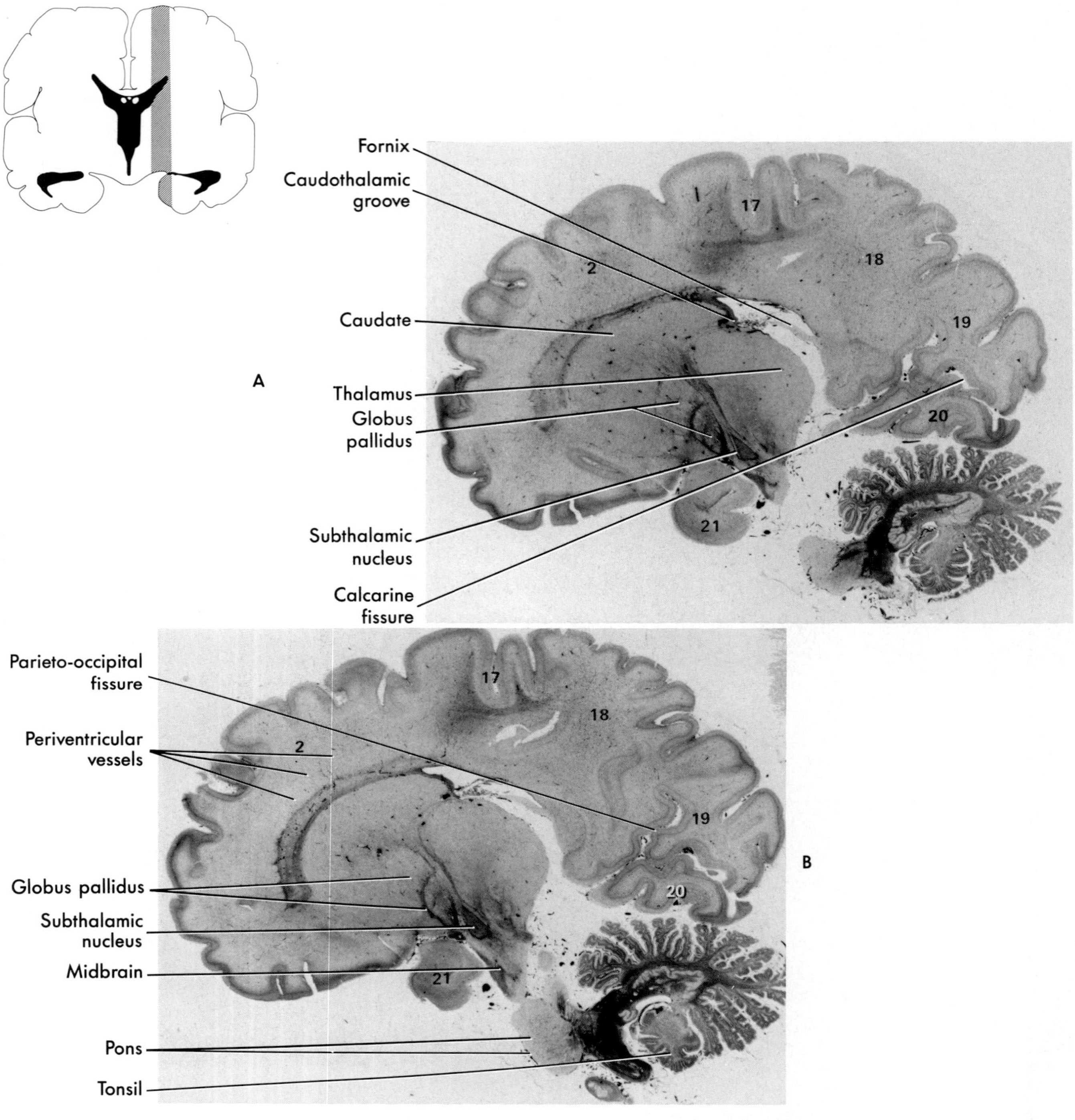

Figure 1-13 **A** and **B**, Parasagittal scan plane through uncus. 2, Superior frontal gyrus; 17, paracentral gyrus; 18, precuneus; 19, cuneus; 20, lingual gyrus; 21, uncus.

SAGITTAL ULTRASOUND—ANATOMIC CORRELATIONS

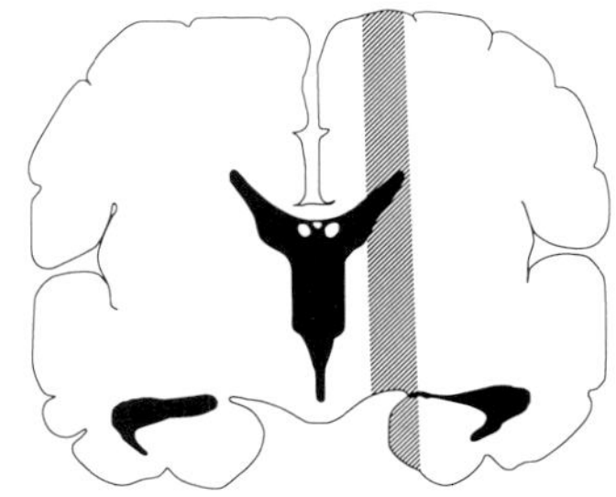

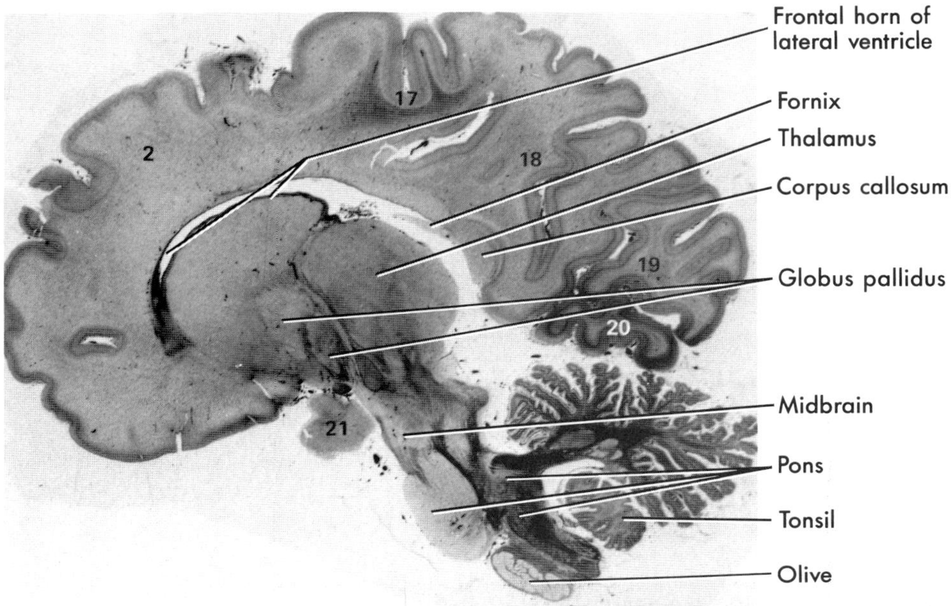

C

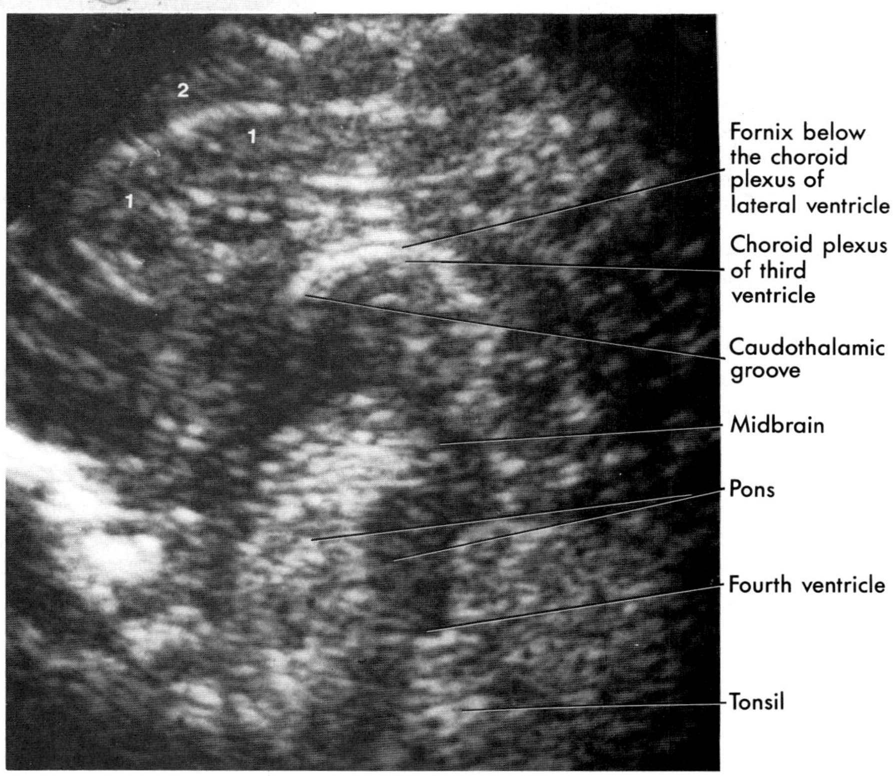

D

Figure 1-13, cont'd. **C** and **D**, Parasagittal scan plane through uncus. 1, Cingulate gyrus; 2, superior frontal gyrus; 17, paracentral gyrus; 18, precuneus; 19, cuneus; 20, lingual gyrus; 21, uncus.

SAGITTAL ULTRASOUND—ANATOMIC CORRELATIONS

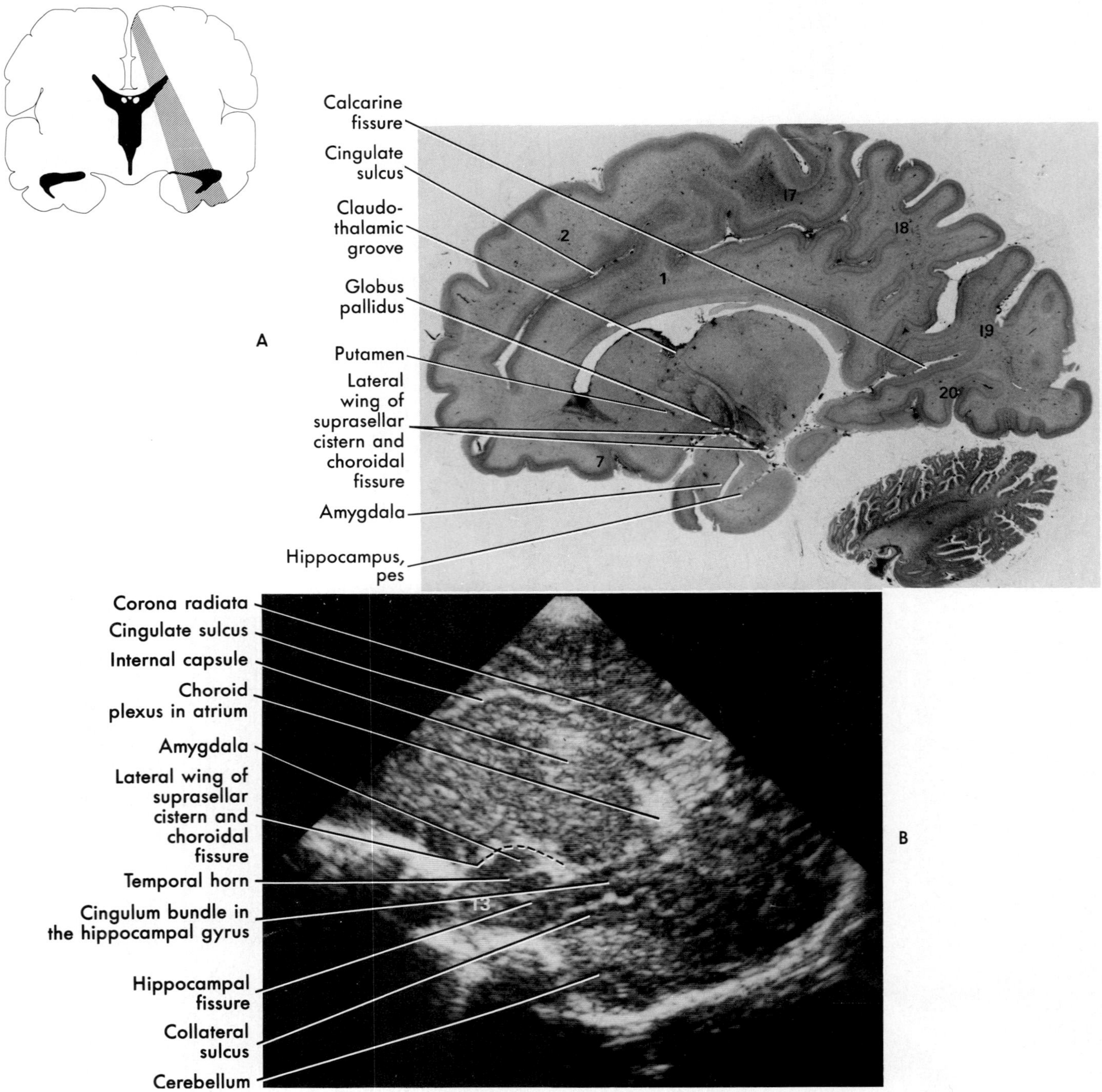

Figure 1-14 **A** and **B,** Angled parasagittal scan plane through caudothalamic groove. 1, Cingulate gyrus; 2, superior frontal gyrus; 13, hippocampal gyrus; 18, precuneus; 19, cuneus; 20, lingual gyrus.

SAGITTAL ULTRASOUND—ANATOMIC CORRELATIONS

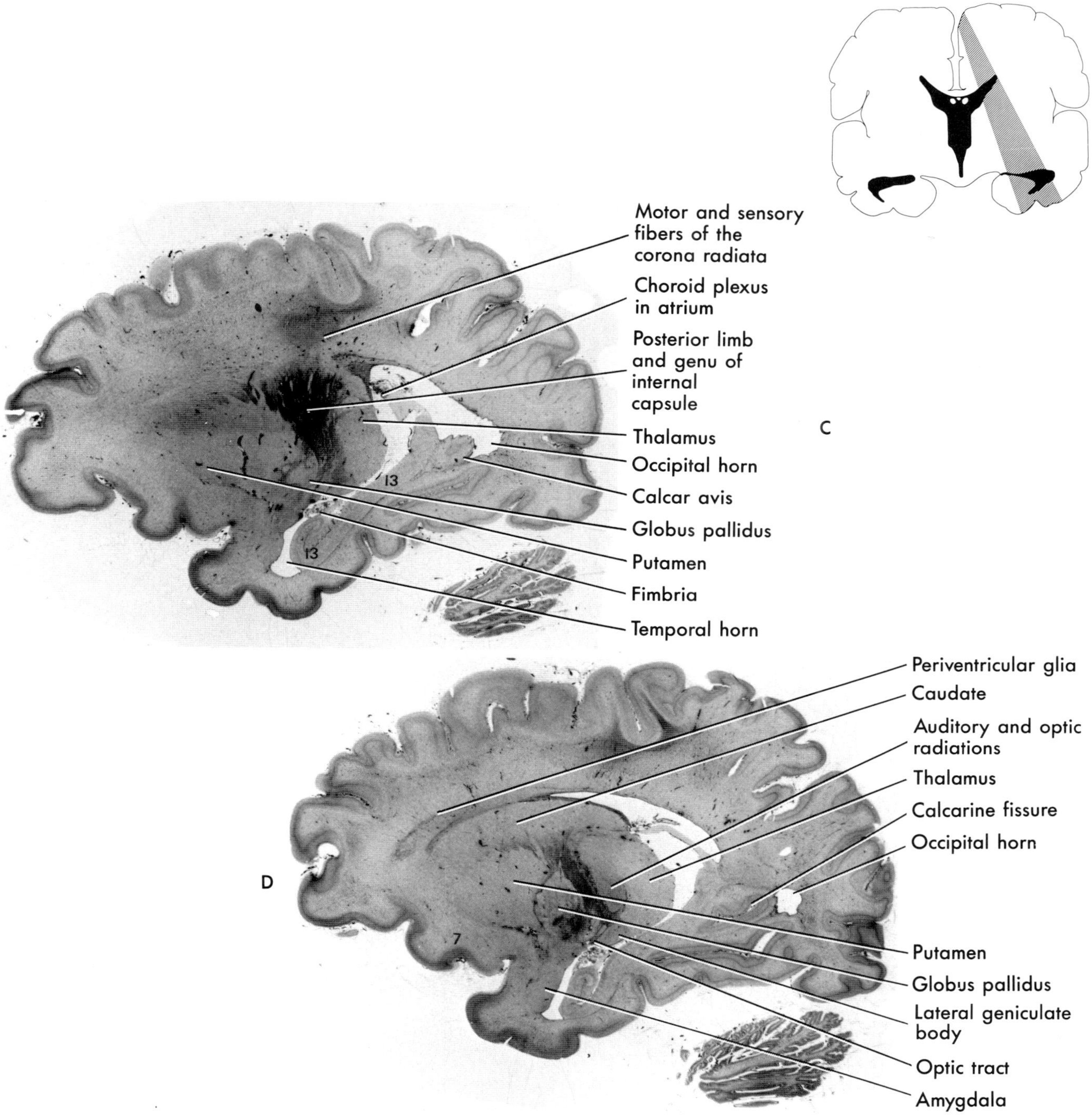

Figure 1-14, cont'd. **C** and **D**, Angled parasagittal scan plane through cavdothalamic groove. 13, Hippocampal gyrus.

SAGITTAL ULTRASOUND—ANATOMIC CORRELATIONS

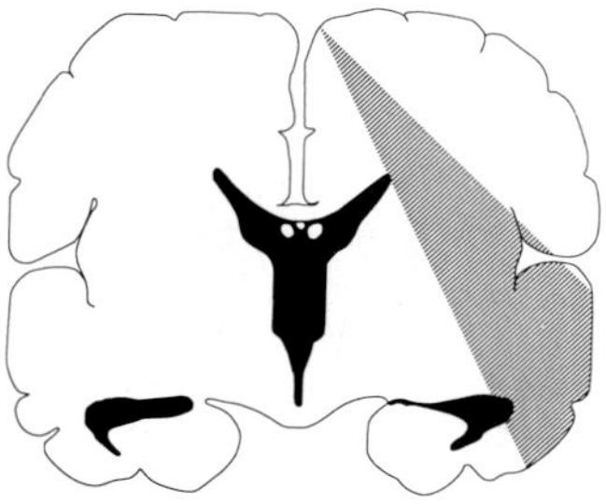

A

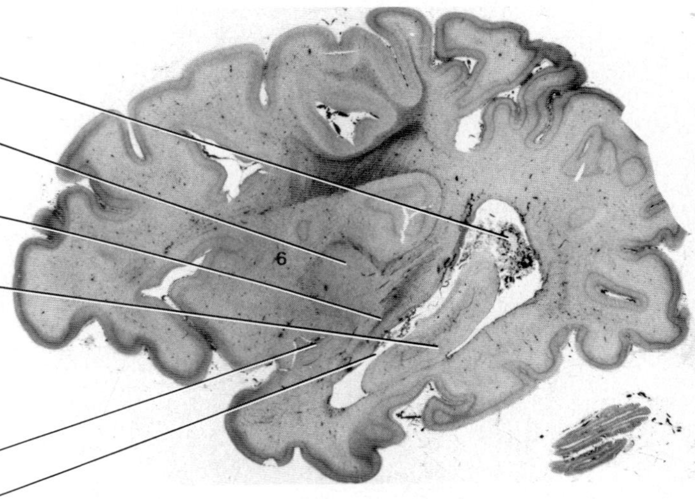

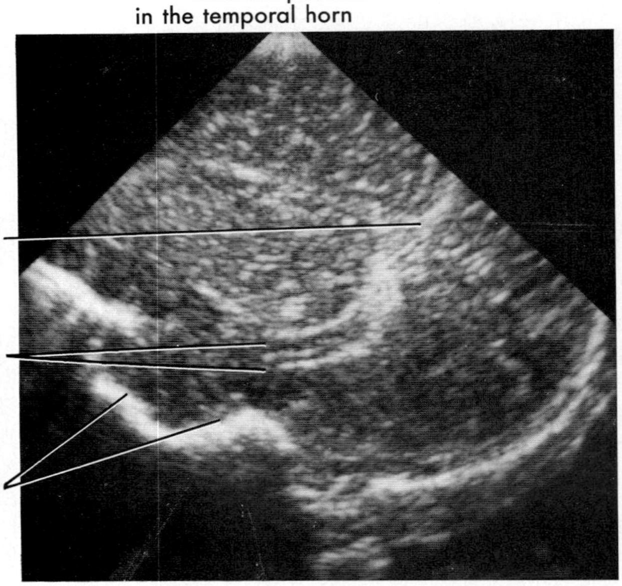

B

Figure 1-15 **A** and **B**, Angled parasagittal scan plane lateral to temporal horn.

SAGITTAL ULTRASOUND—ANATOMIC CORRELATIONS

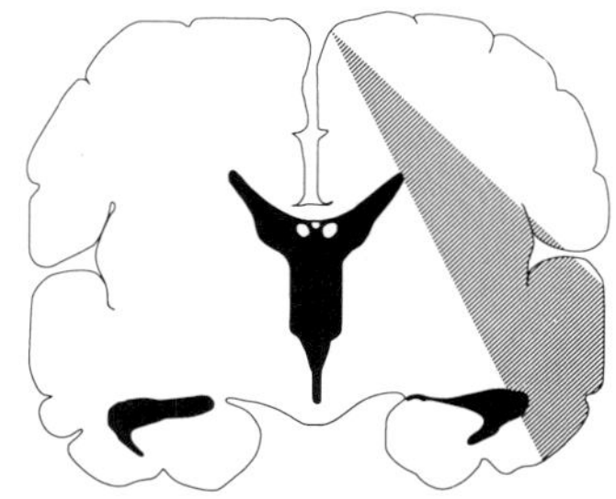

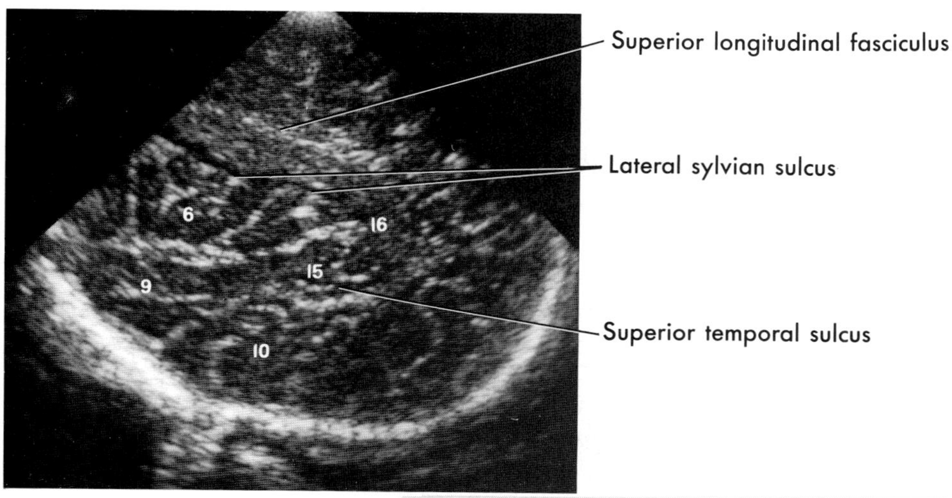

C

D

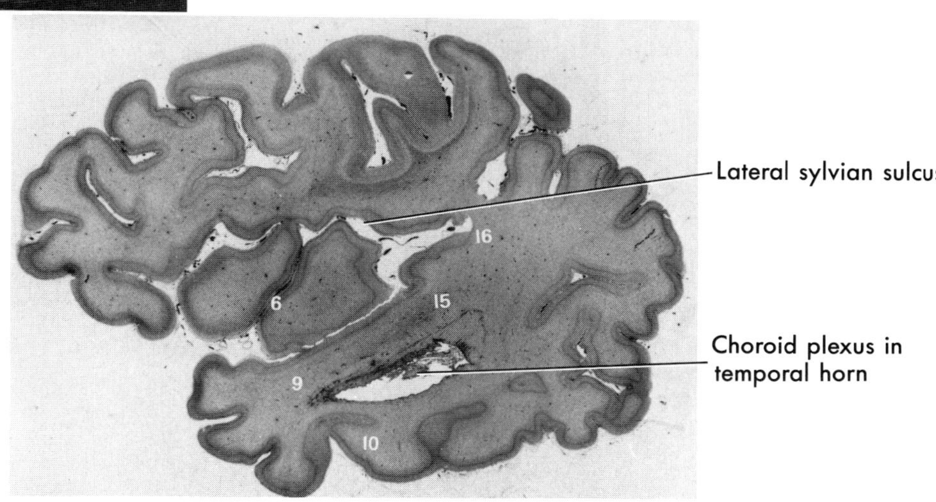

Figure 1-15, cont'd. **C** and **D,** Angled parasagittal scan plane lateral to temporal horn. 6, Insula; 9, superior temporal gyrus; 10, middle temporal gyrus; 15, transverse temporal gyrus; 16, supramarginal gyrus.

AXIAL MAGNETIC RESONANCE—ANATOMIC CORRELATIONS

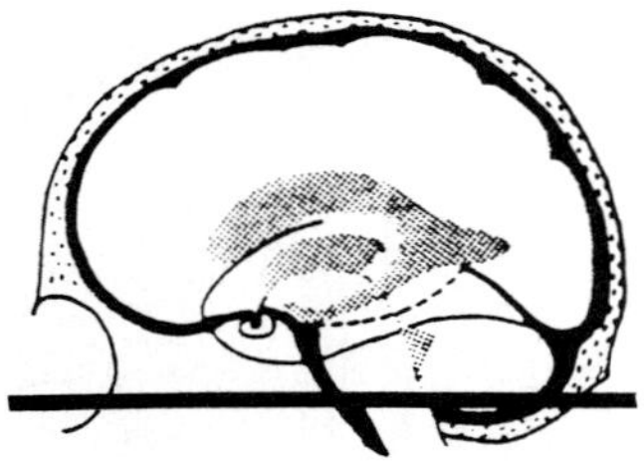

A

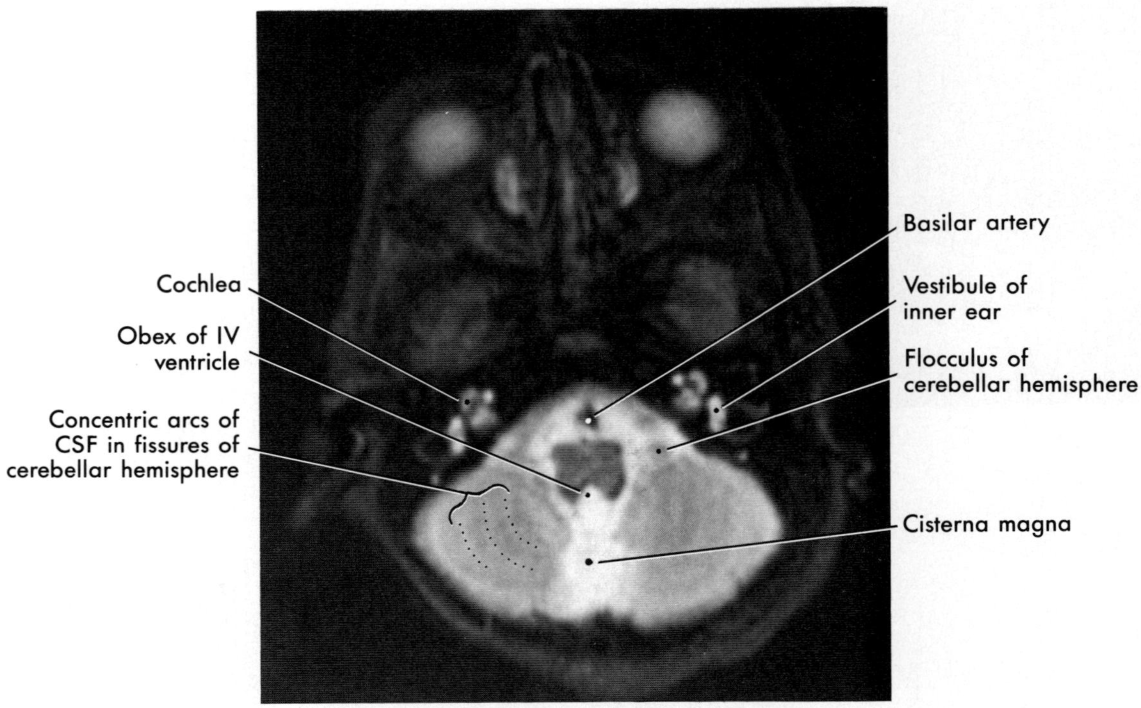

Figure 1-16 **A,** Axial scan plane through medulla of a 40-week-old infant (1.5T, 2500/160).

AXIAL MAGNETIC RESONANCE—ANATOMIC CORRELATIONS

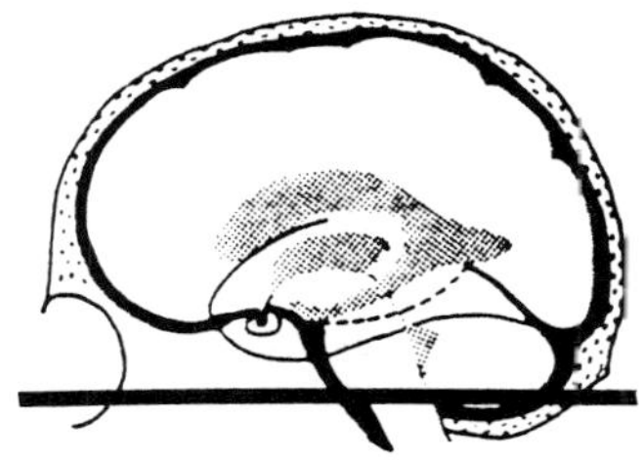

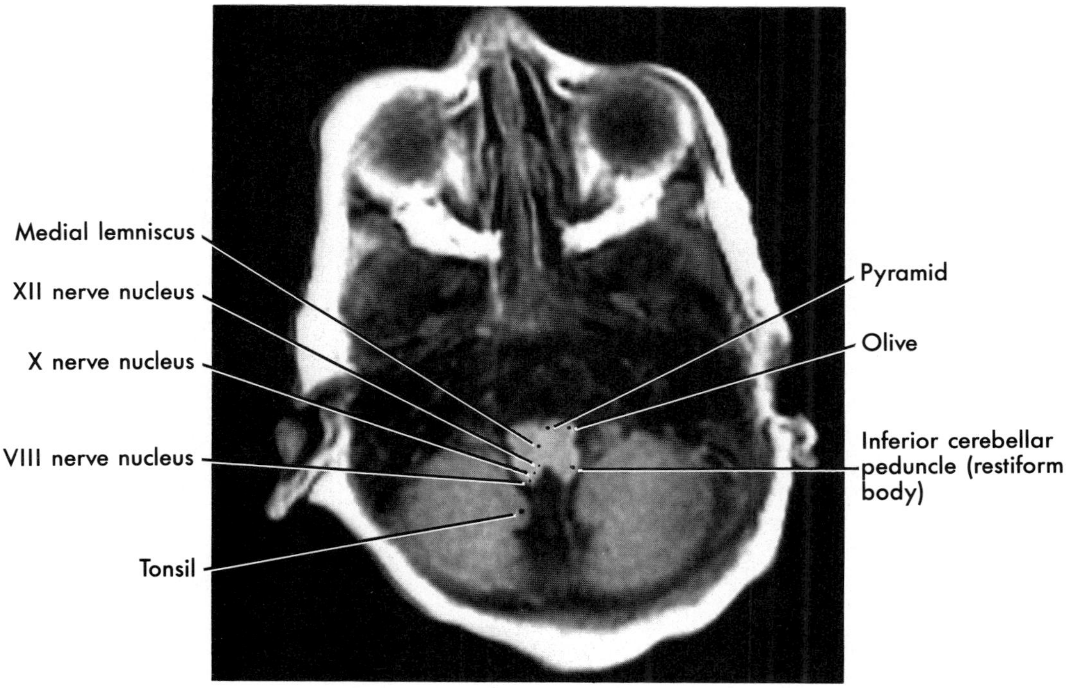

B

Figure 1-16, cont'd. **B,** Axial scan plane through medulla of a 40-week-old infant (1.5T, 800/20).

AXIAL MAGNETIC RESONANCE—ANATOMIC CORRELATIONS

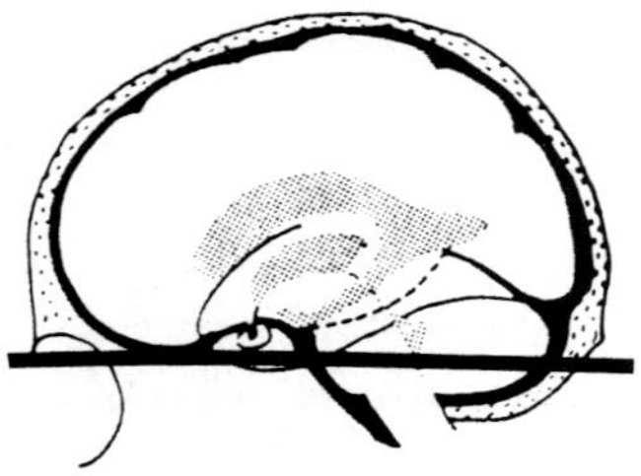

0 mm

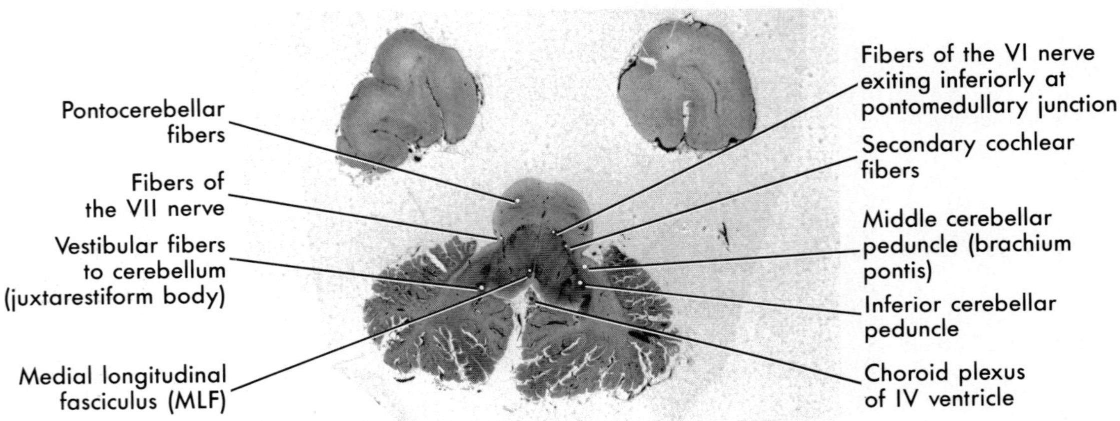

Figure 1-17 **A,** Axial anatomic plane through lower pons of a 40-week-old infant.

AXIAL MAGNETIC RESONANCE—ANATOMIC CORRELATIONS

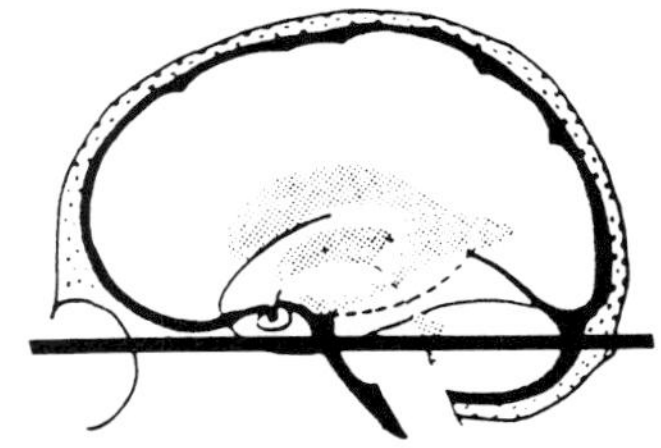

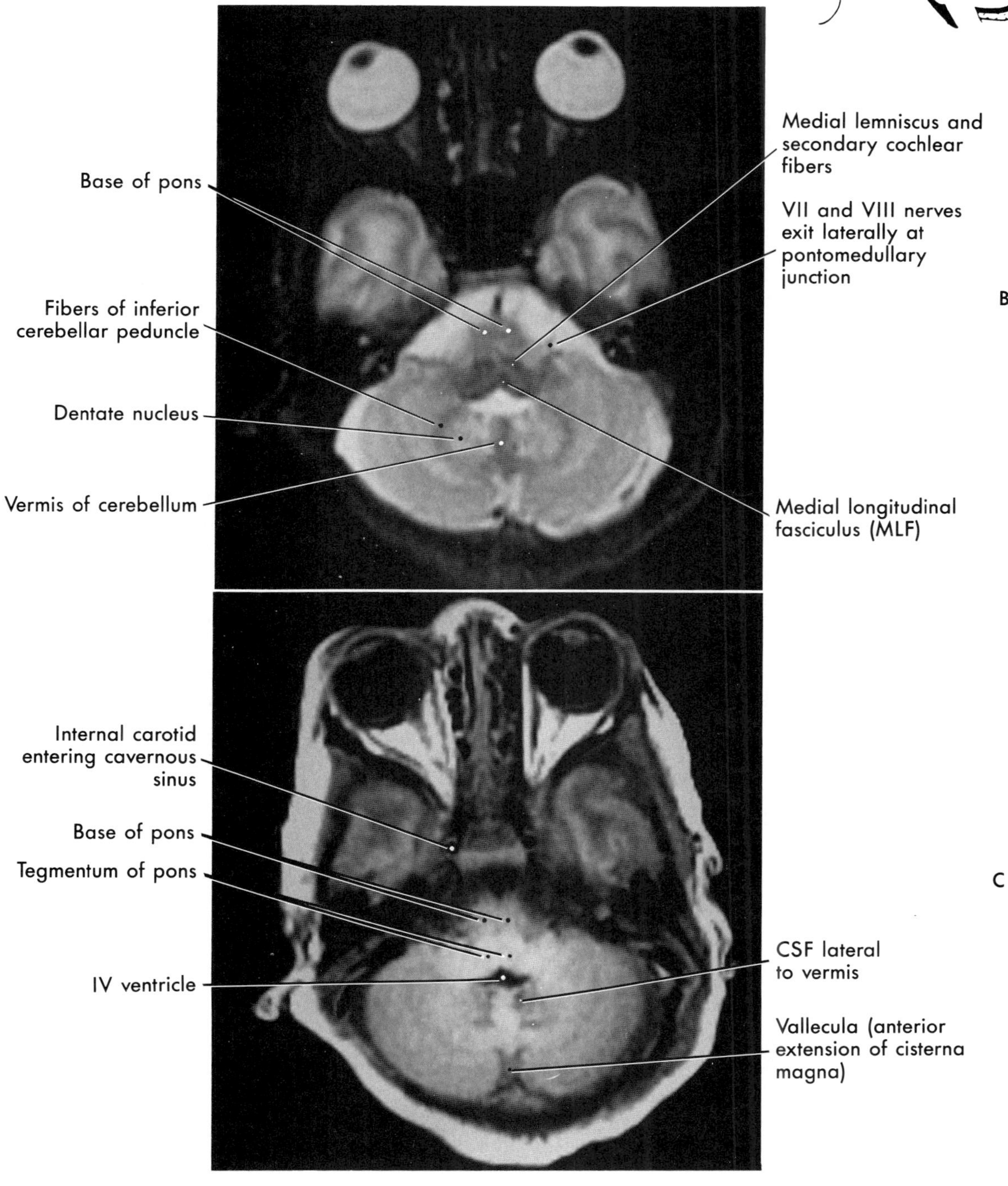

Figure 1-17, cont'd. **B** and **C**, Axial anatomic plane through lower pons of a 40-week-old infant (**B**, 1.5 T, 2500/160; **C**, 1.5 T, 800/20).

AXIAL MAGNETIC RESONANCE—ANATOMIC CORRELATIONS

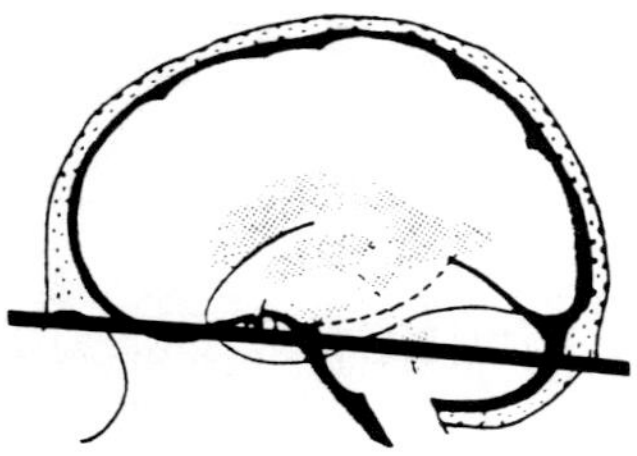

2 mm

A

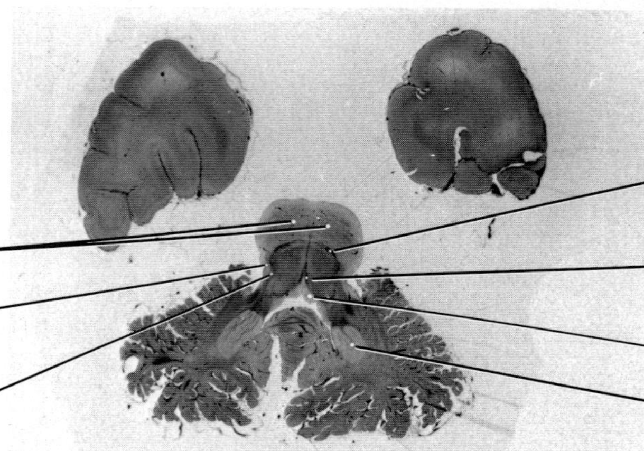

Figure 1-18 **A,** Axial anatomic plane through upper pons of a 40-week-old infant.

AXIAL MAGNETIC RESONANCE—ANATOMIC CORRELATIONS

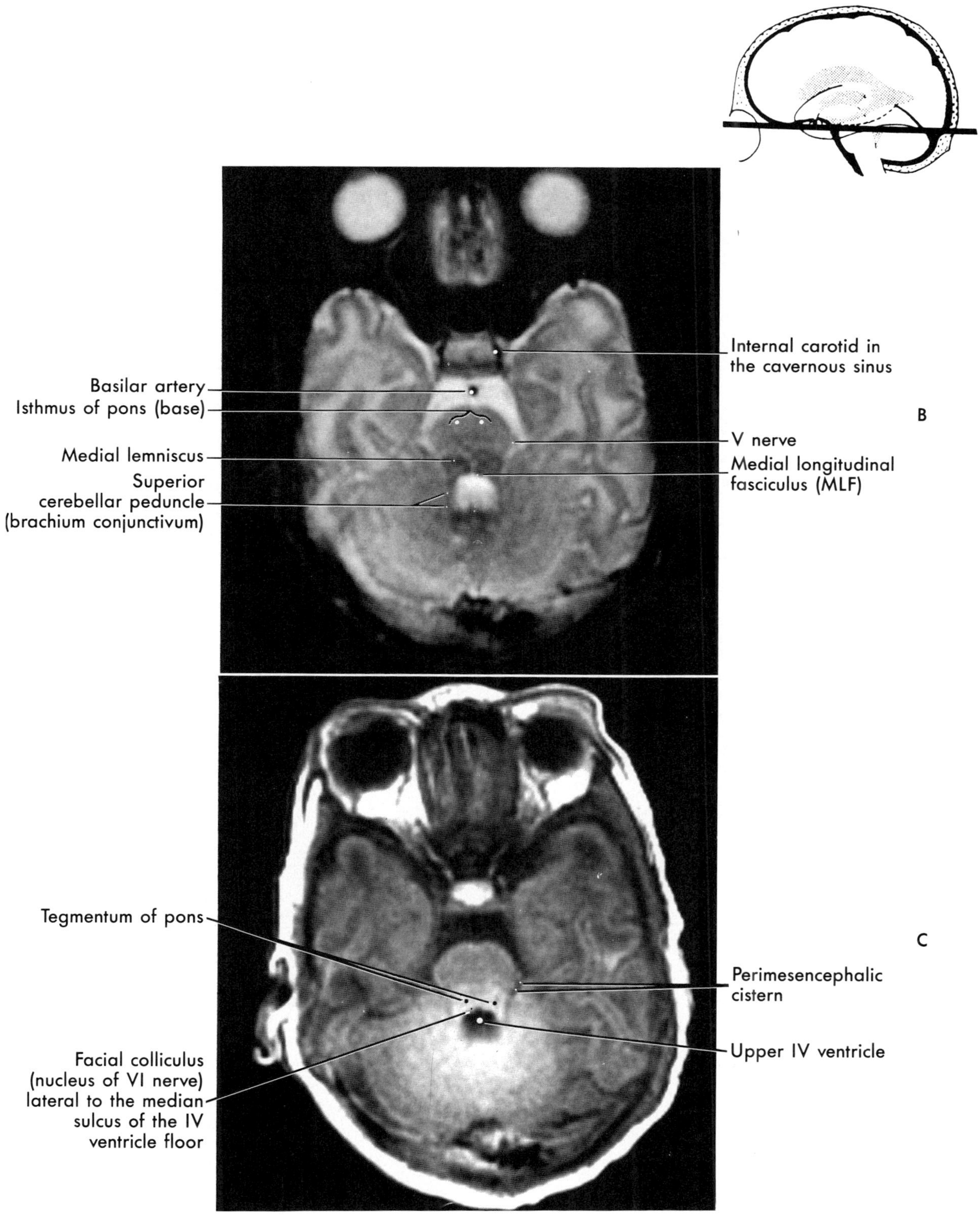

Figure 1-18, cont'd. **B** and **C**, Axial anatomic plane through upper pons of a 40-week-old infant (**B**, 1.5T, 2500/160; **C**, 1.5 T, 800/20).

AXIAL MAGNETIC RESONANCE—ANATOMIC CORRELATIONS

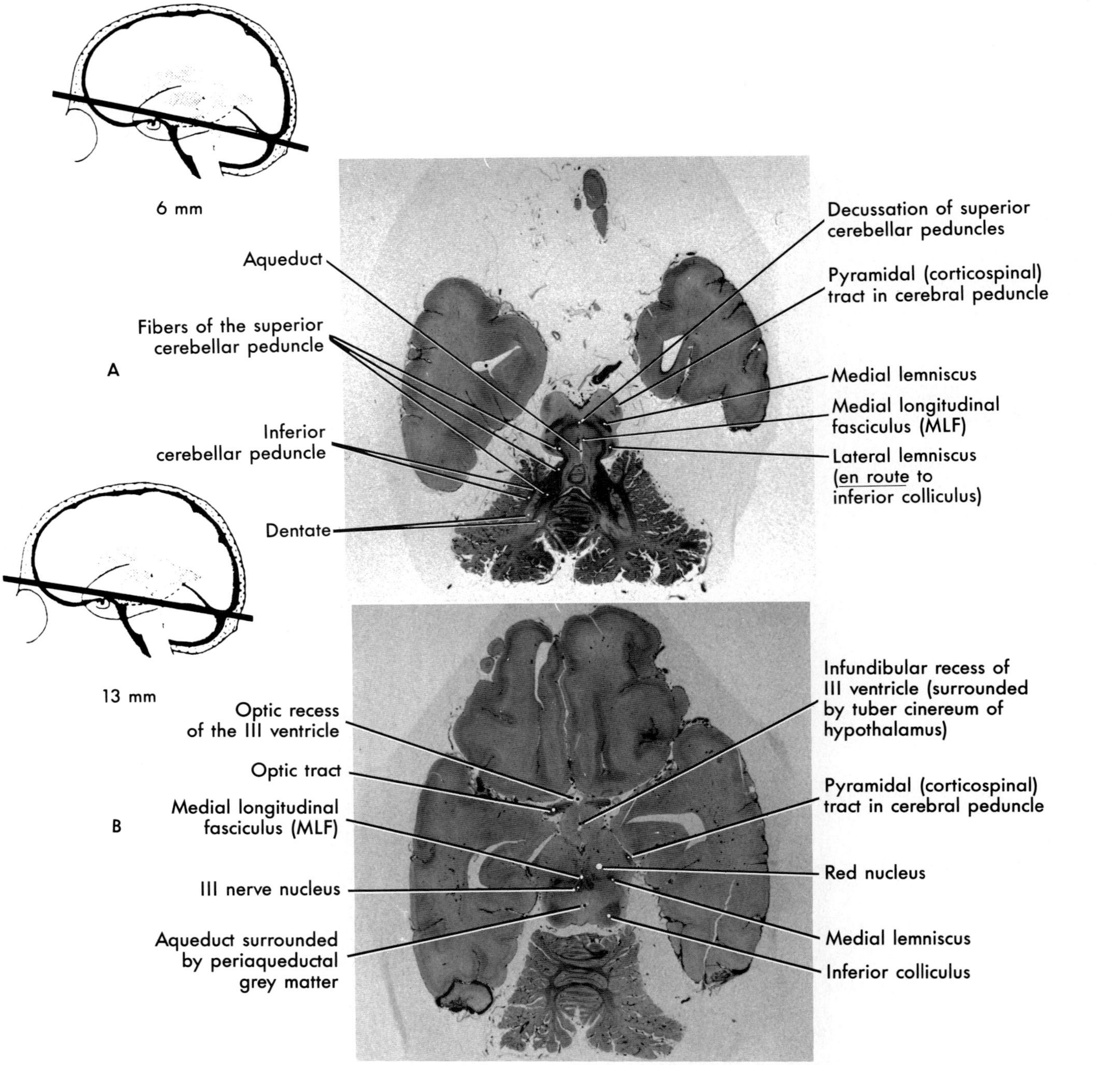

Figure 1-19 **A** and **B**, Axial anatomic plane through midbrain of a 40-week-old infant.

AXIAL MAGNETIC RESONANCE—ANATOMIC CORRELATIONS

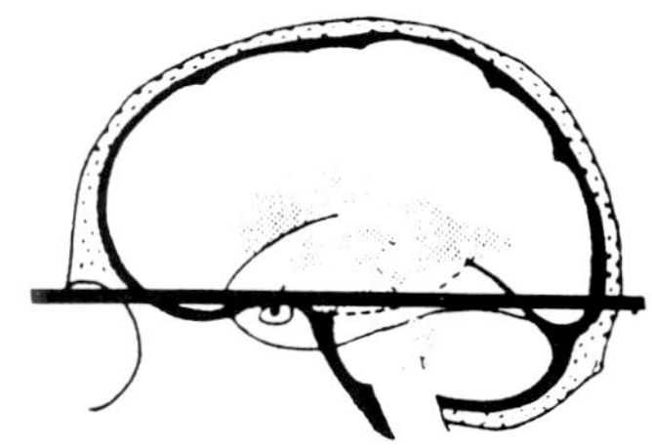

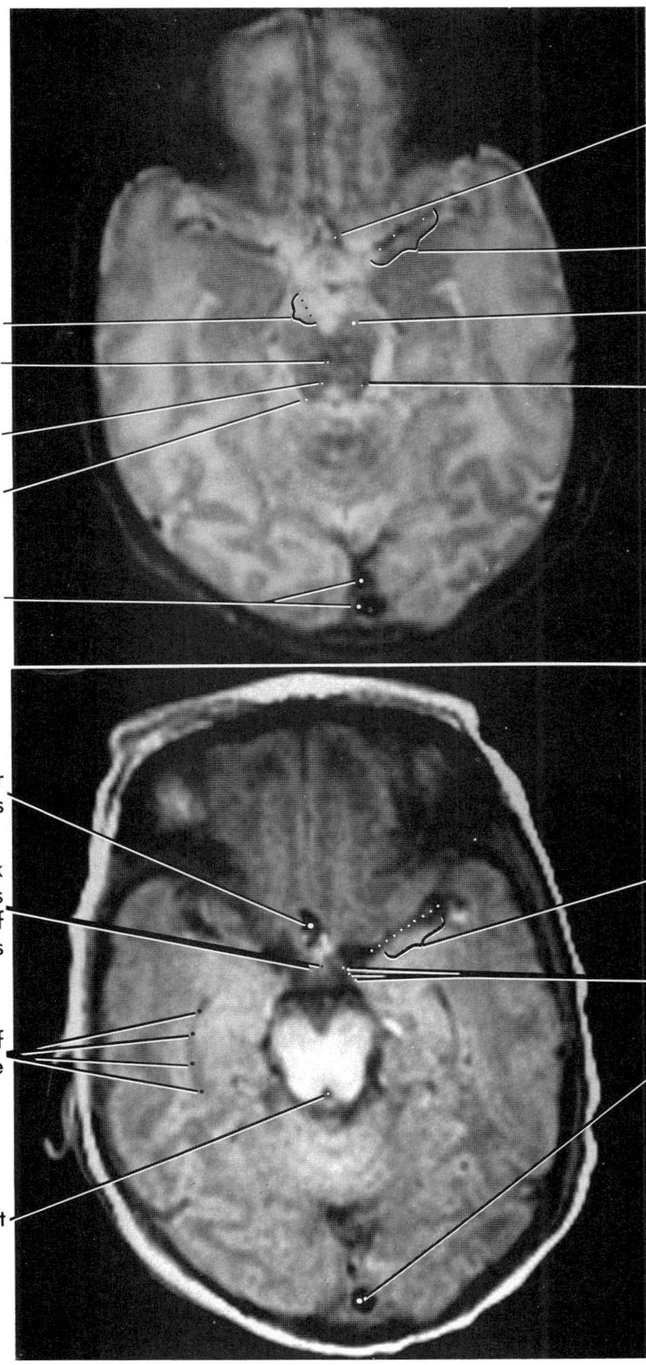

Figure 1-19, cont'd. **C** and **D**, Axial anatomic plane through midbrain of a 40-week-old infant (**C**, 1.5 T, 2500/160; **D**, 1.5 T, 800/20).

AXIAL MAGNETIC RESONANCE—ANATOMIC CORRELATIONS

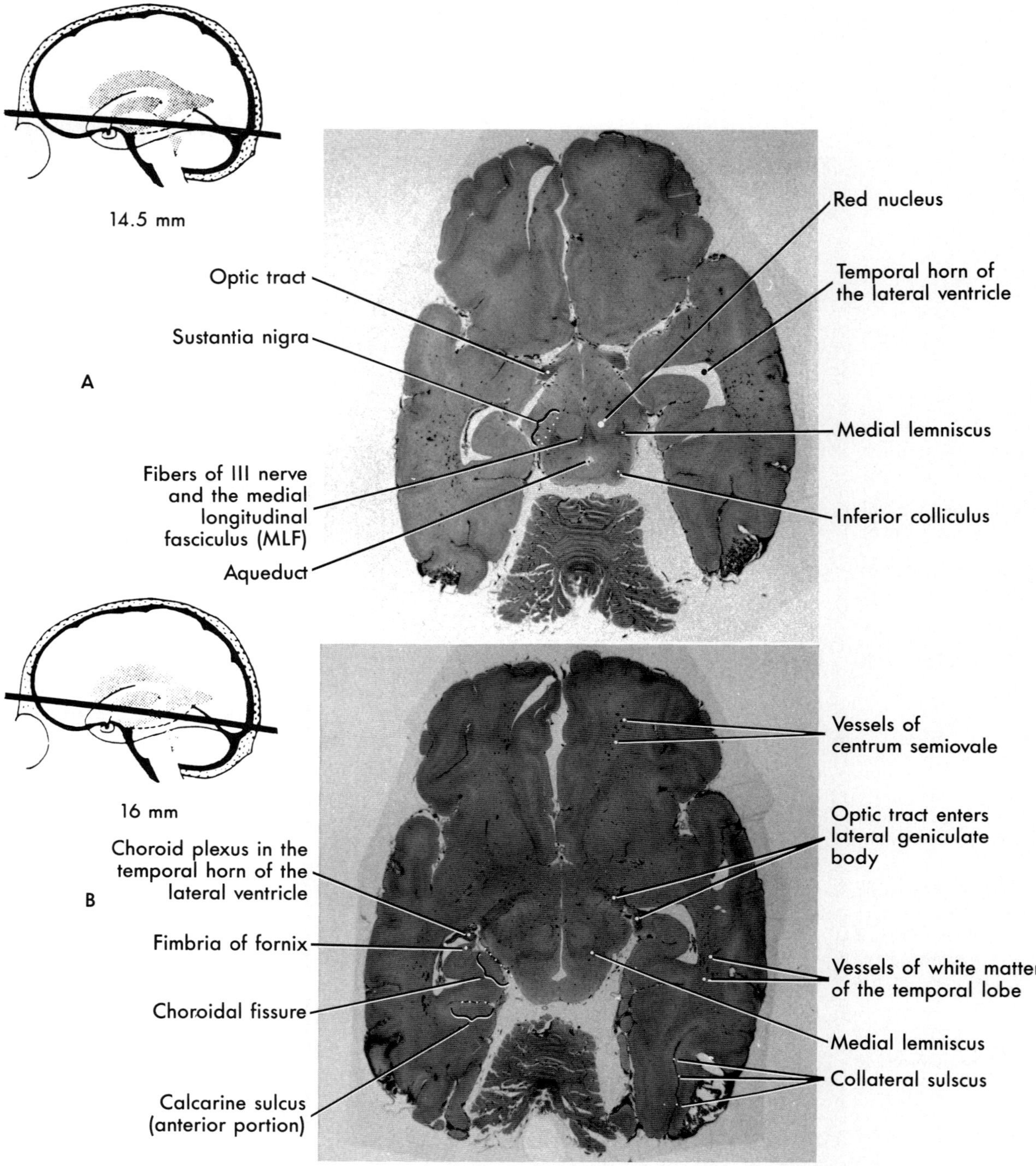

Figure 1-20 **A** and **B**, Axial anatomic plane through uppermost midbrain of a 40-week-old infant.

AXIAL MAGNETIC RESONANCE—ANATOMIC CORRELATIONS

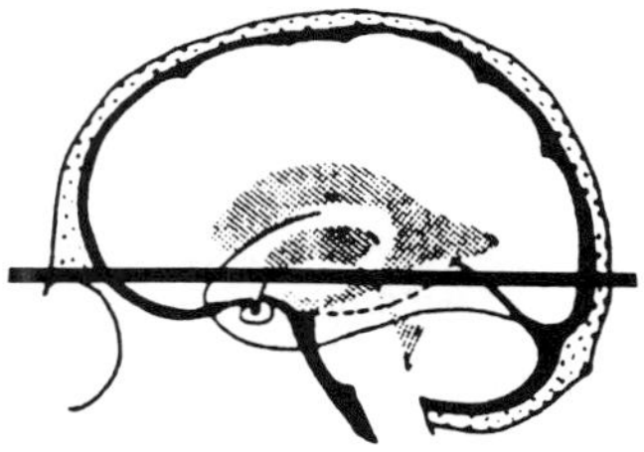

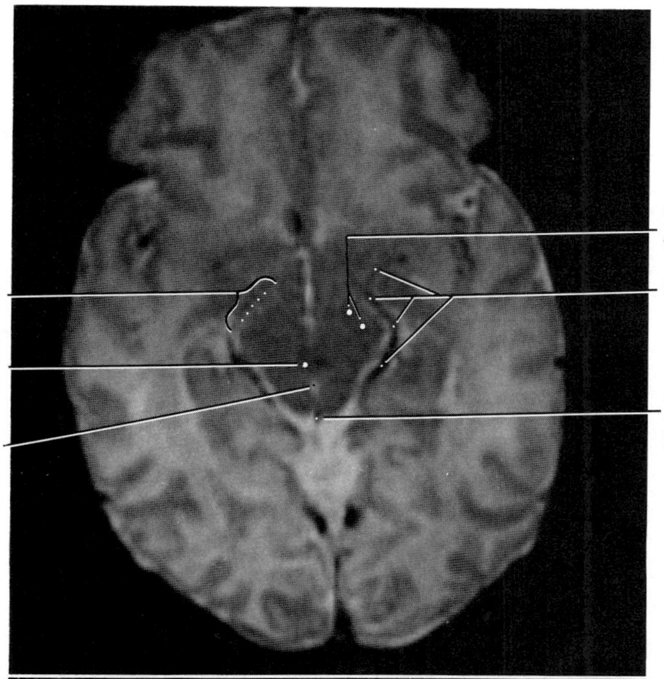

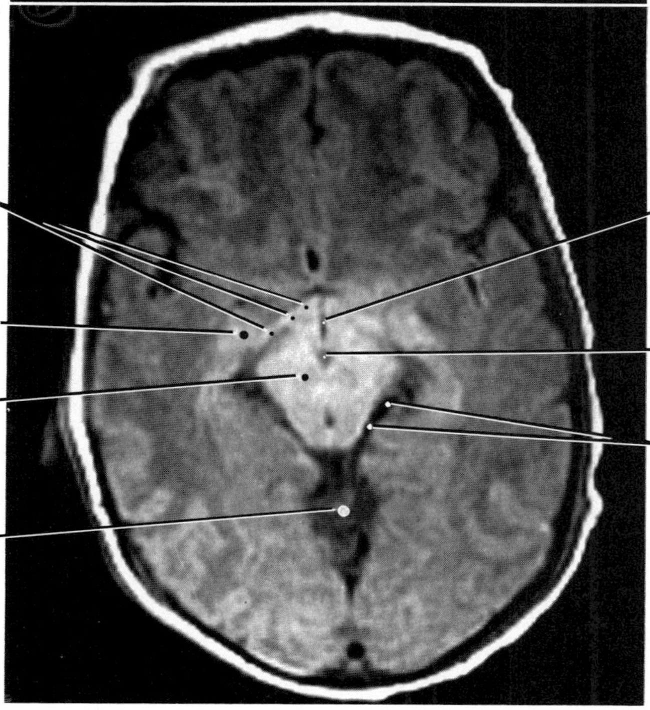

Figure 1-20, cont'd. **C** and **D**, Axial anatomic plane through uppermost midbrain of a 40-week-old infant (**C**, 1.5 T, 2500/160; **D**, 1.5 T, 800/20).

AXIAL MAGNETIC RESONANCE—ANATOMIC CORRELATIONS

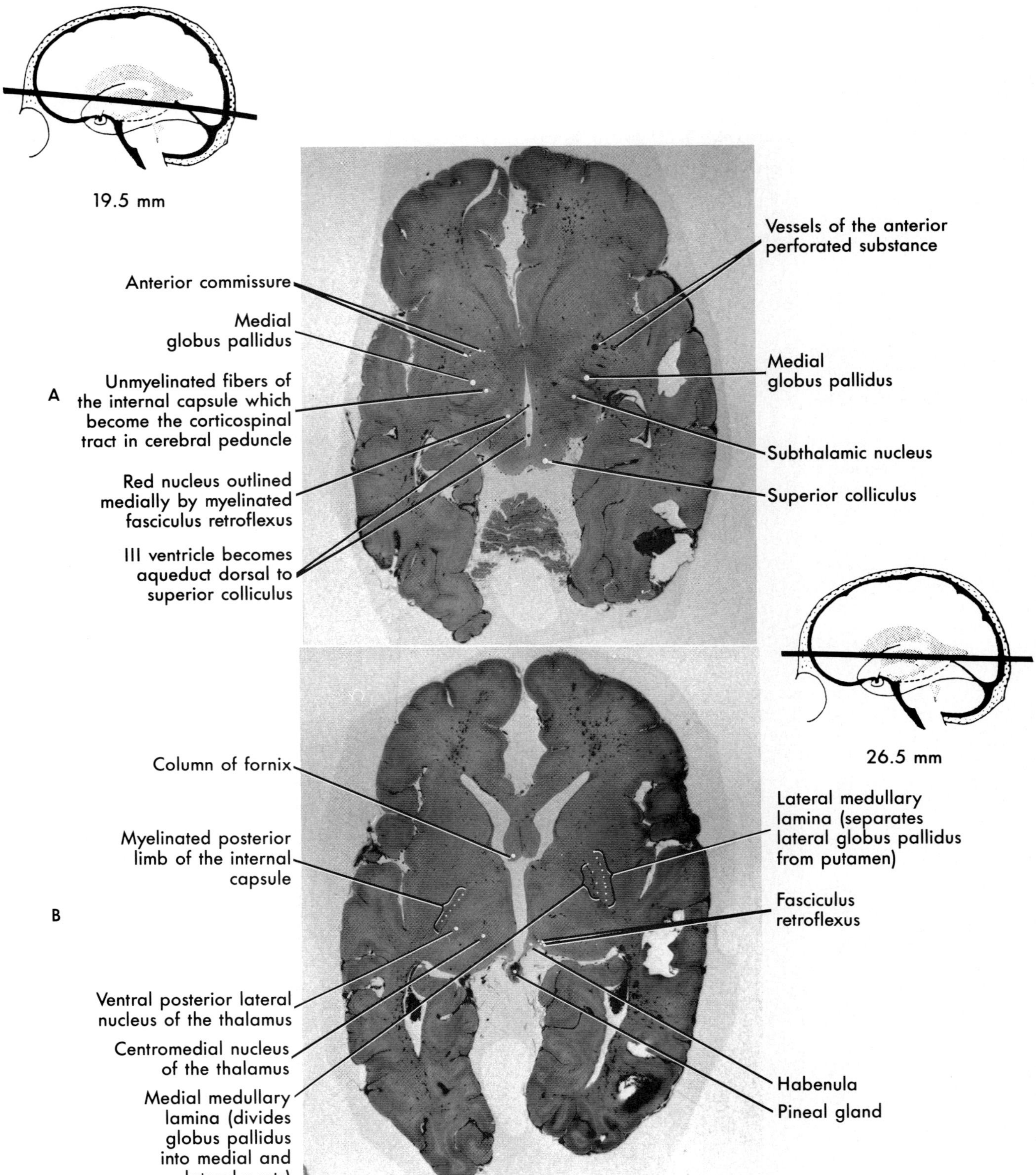

Figure 1-21 **A** and **B**, Axial anatomic plane through third ventricle of a 40-week-old infant.

AXIAL MAGNETIC RESONANCE—ANATOMIC CORRELATIONS

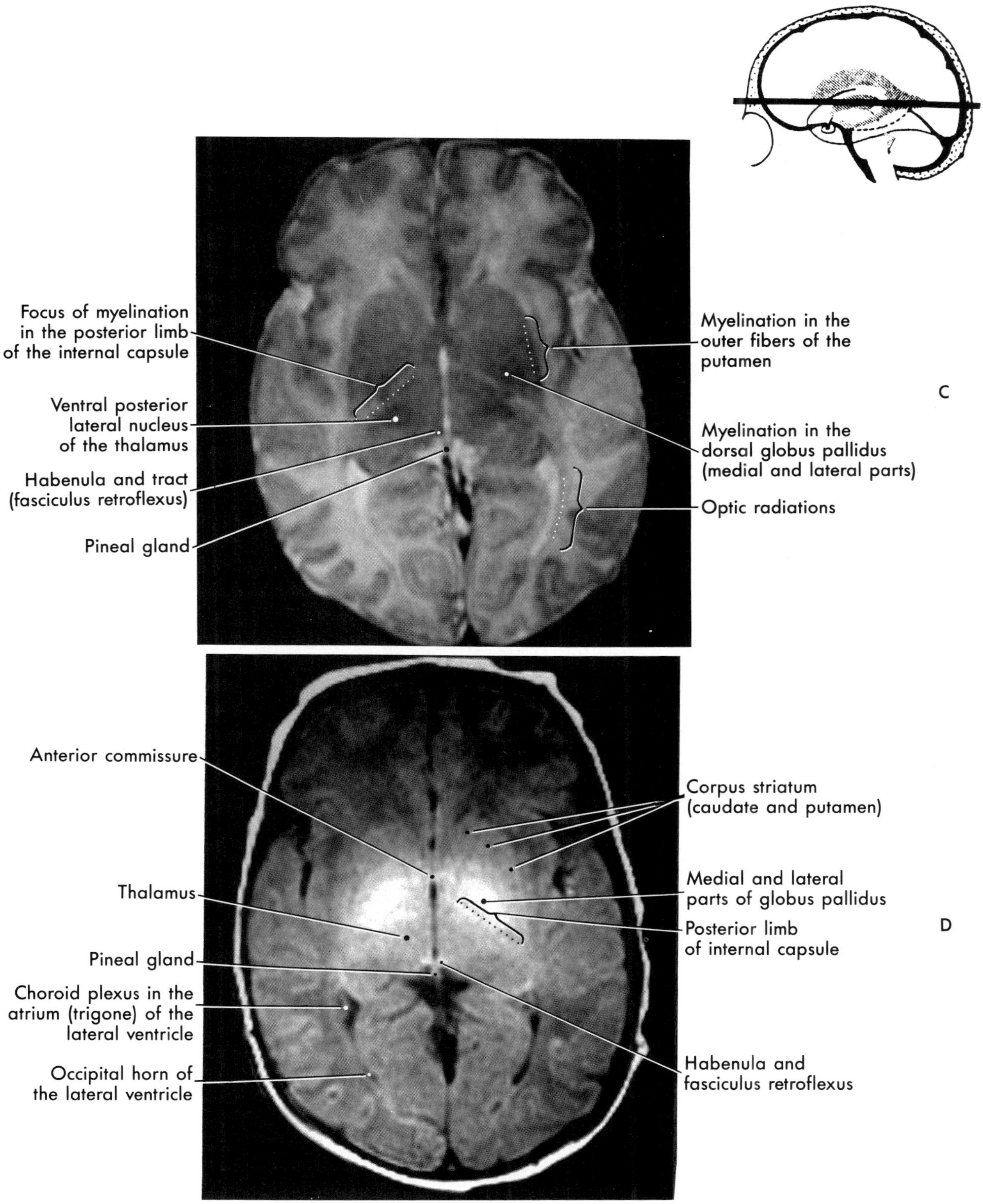

Figure 1-21, cont'd. **C** and **D**, Axial anatomic plane through third ventricle of a 40-week-old infant (**C**, 1.5 T, 2500/160; **D**, 1.5 T, 800/20).

AXIAL MAGNETIC RESONANCE—ANATOMIC CORRELATIONS

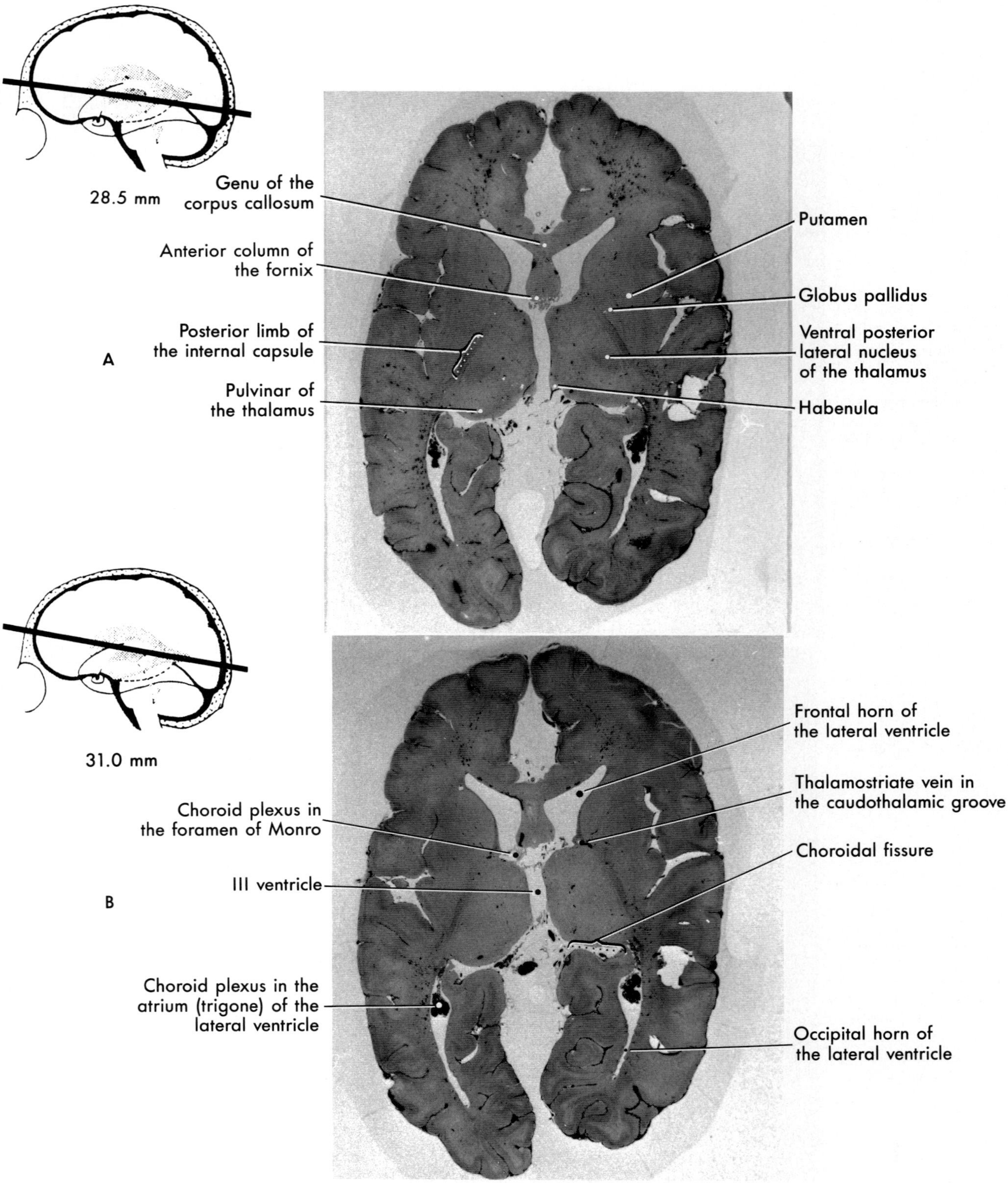

Figure 1-22 **A** and **B**, Axial anatomic plane through inferior aspect of foramen of Monro of a 40-week-old infant.

AXIAL MAGNETIC RESONANCE—ANATOMIC CORRELATIONS

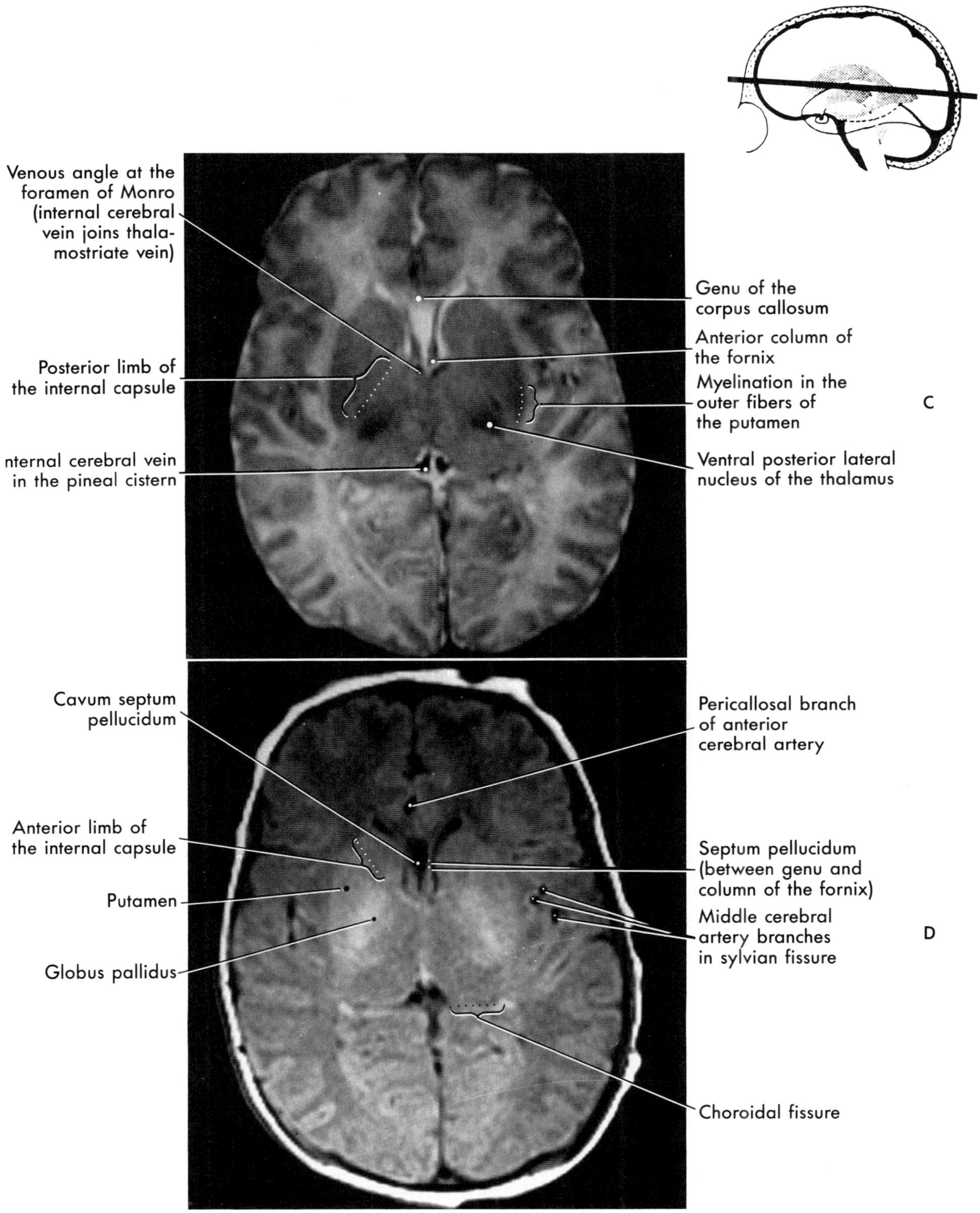

Figure 1-22, cont'd. **C** and **D**, Axial anatomic plane through inferior aspect of foramen of Monro of a 40-week-old infant (**C**, 1.5 T, 2500/160; **D**, 1.5 T, 800/20).

AXIAL MAGNETIC RESONANCE—ANATOMIC CORRELATIONS

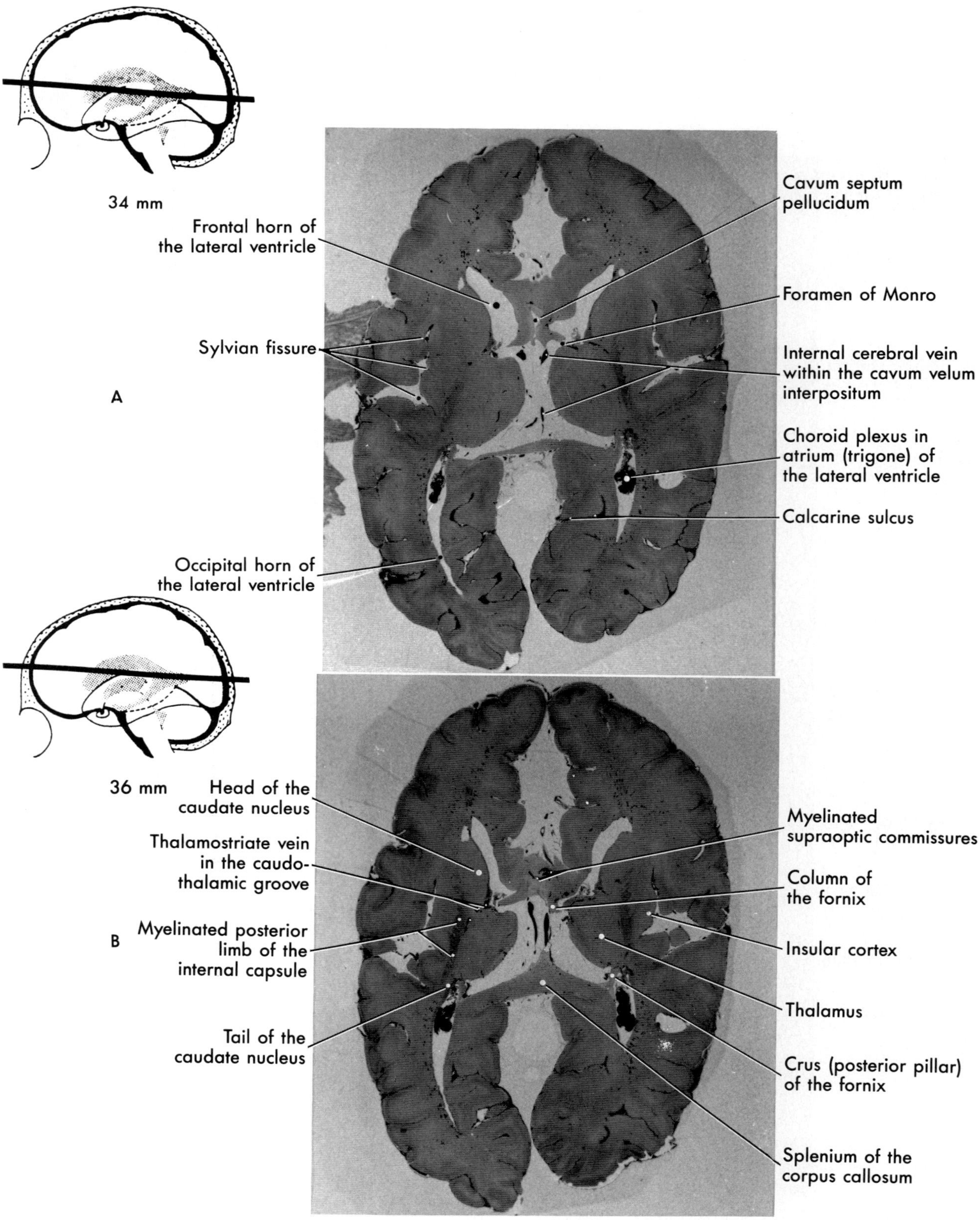

Figure 1-23 **A** and **B**, Axial anatomic plane through superior aspect of foramen of Monro of a 40-week-old infant.

AXIAL MAGNETIC RESONANCE—ANATOMIC CORRELATIONS

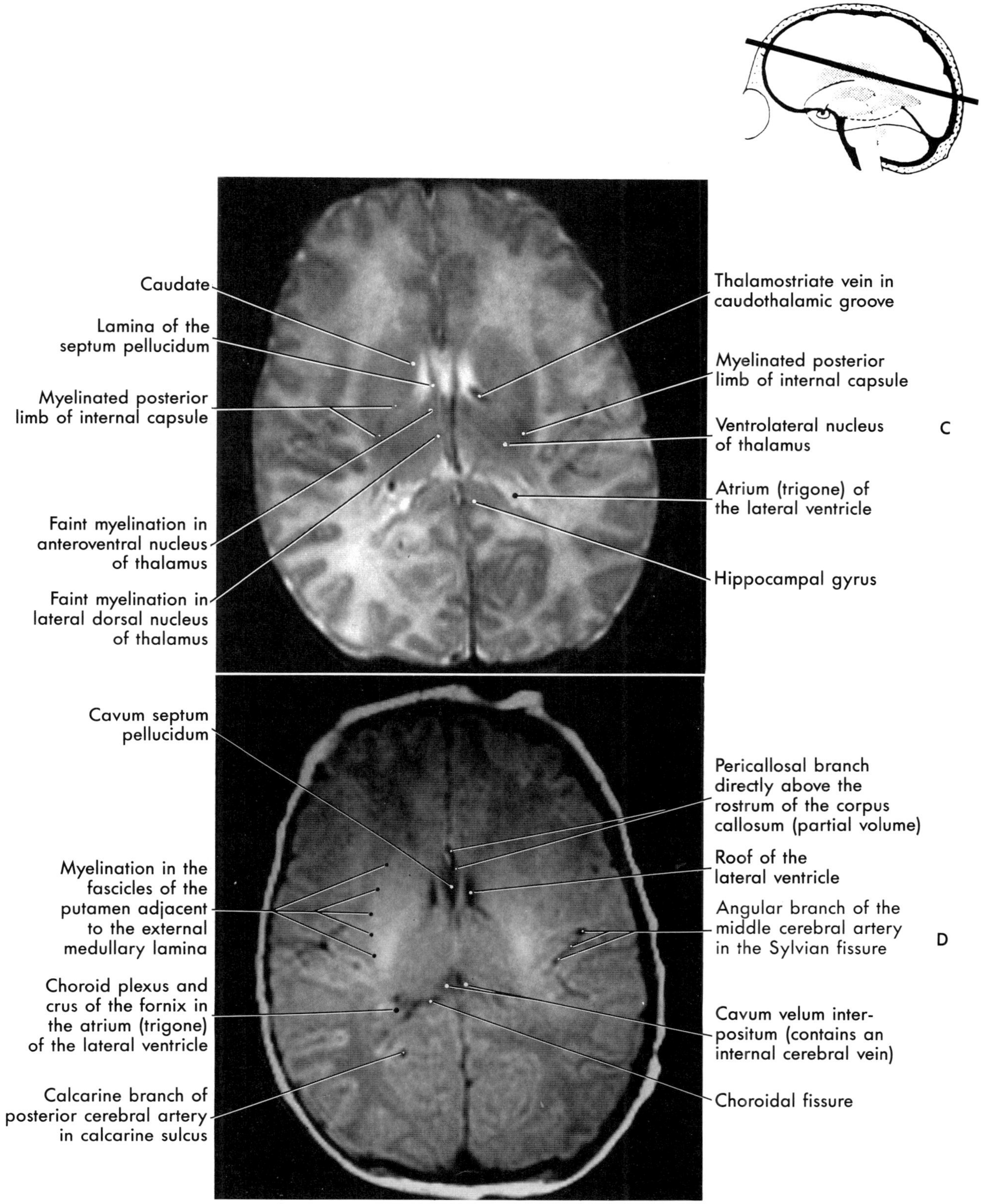

Figure 1-23, cont'd. **C** and **D**, Axial anatomic plane through superior aspect of foramen of Monro of a 40-week-old infant (**C**, 1.5 T, 2500/160; **D**, 1.5 T, 800/20).

AXIAL MAGNETIC RESONANCE—ANATOMIC CORRELATIONS

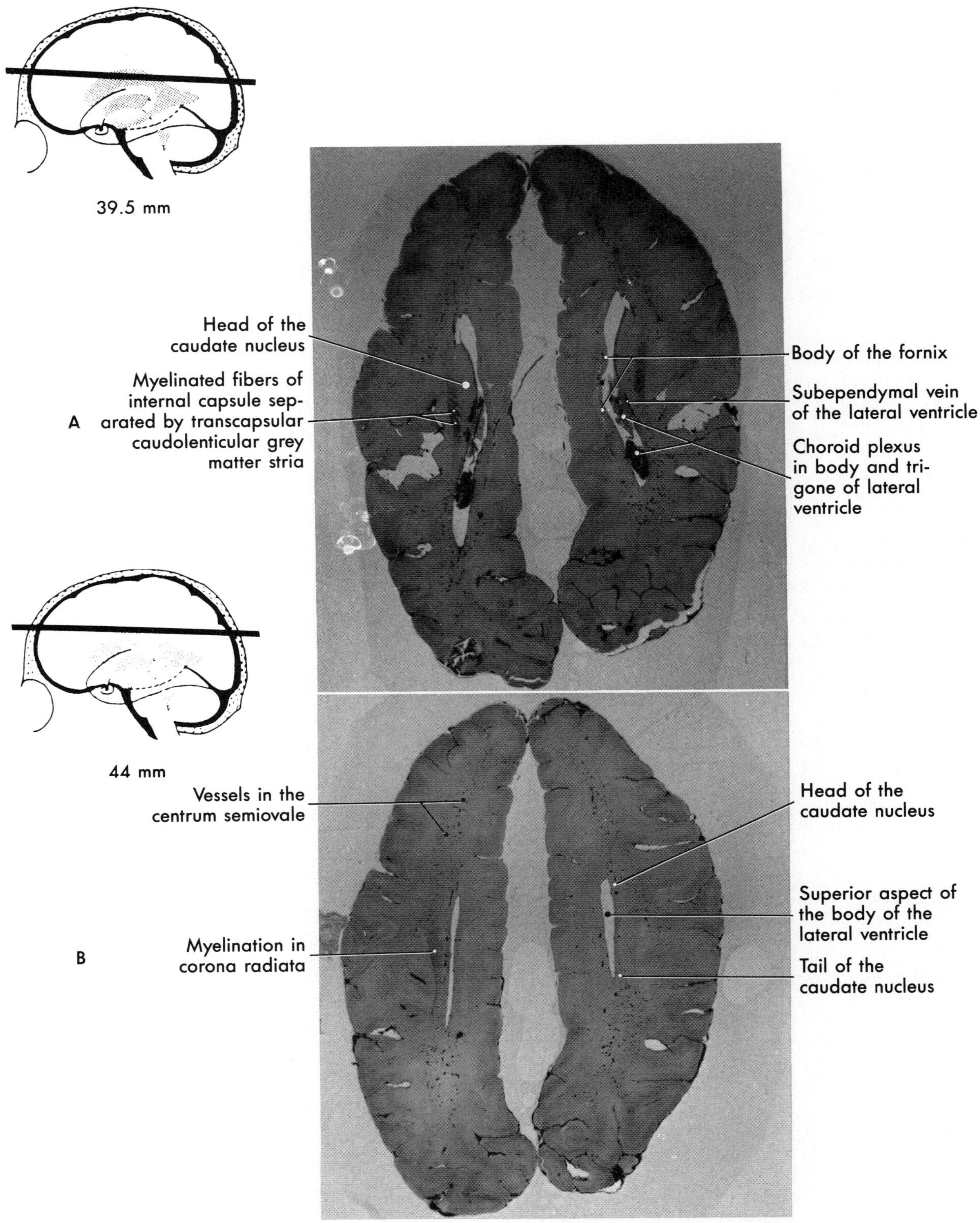

Figure 1-24 **A** and **B**, Axial anatomic plane through roofs of lateral ventricles of a 40-week-old infant.

AXIAL MAGNETIC RESONANCE—ANATOMIC CORRELATIONS

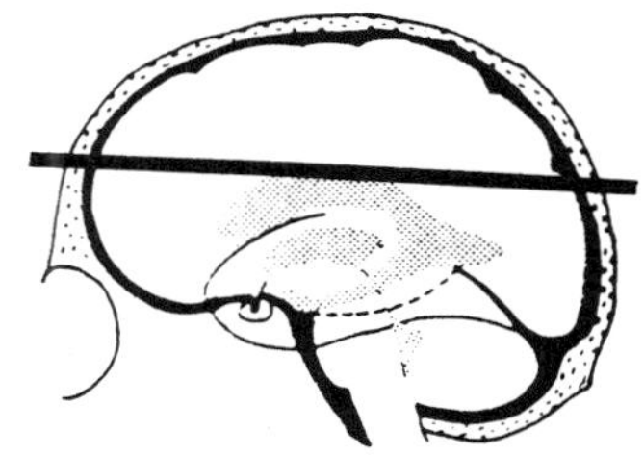

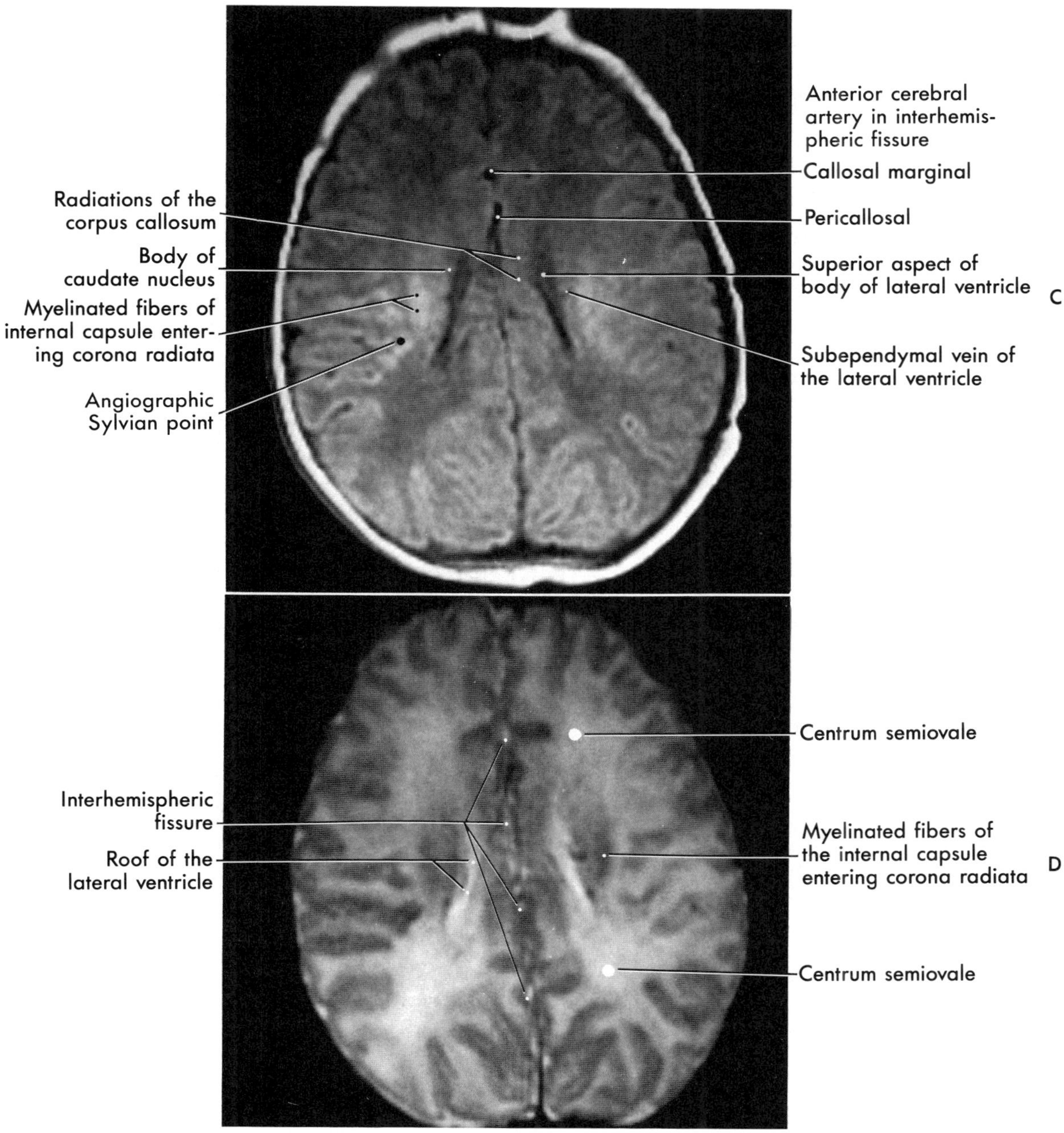

Figure 1-24, cont'd. **C** and **D**, Axial anatomic plane through roofs of lateral ventricles of a 40-week-old infant (**C**, 1.5 T, 2500/160; **D**, 1.5 T, 800/20).

INDEX TO THE ILLUSTRATIONS

Entries refer to figures in which the specific structures are labeled.

CHAPTER 2

L. Anne Hayman
Craig B. McArdle
Yogesh P. Shah

Neonatal Brain

IMAGING TECHNIQUES

Four imaging modalities can be used to examine the neonatal brain: ultrasound, computed tomography (CT), magnetic resonance imaging (MRI), and, rarely, arteriography. Portable ultrasound is most often employed because it avoids the problems associated with transporting, sedating, and monitoring infants. Also, ultrasound is relatively inexpensive and has the advantage of providing duplex Doppler capability. However, ultrasound is limited because it depends greatly on the size of the anterior fontanelle, through which the ultrasound images must be obtained. In addition, echogenic regions on ultrasound must be interpreted with care, since they may represent normal tissue, edema, infarction, or hemorrhage.

Unlike ultrasound, CT and MRI can specifically identify hemorrhage in the neonatal brain and can examine all regions of the brain, not being limited by size and location of the anterior fontanelle. Although sonography can accurately estimate the size of a hemorrhage, CT and MRI are better at defining its extent. However, small hemorrhages, which are sometimes isointense with surrounding brain parenchyma on CT, may be detected by ultrasound.[1]

When superior brain detail is needed, MRI is preferable to CT because MRI (1) is not hindered by the CT beam hardening artifacts created by bone, (2) provides improved gray-white matter contrast, and (3) can be reconstructed in various planes according to need. On the other hand, MRI of the neonatal brain is inferior to CT in detecting intracranial calcifications. These have diagnostic significance in congenital and infectious disease processes. Physiologic calcifications are not normally present in the neonatal brain.

The CT scan is usually chosen for neonatal brain evaluation because it is easier to monitor vital signs during the examination. The magnetic field around the medium or high field strength MR units destroys or significantly distorts the information produced by most vital signs monitors when they are placed near the bore of the magnet. Conversely, the radiofrequency of the vital signs monitors can interfere with the MR scanner's function and create artifacts, thereby degrading the images.[2,3] Specialized monitoring equipment has been developed[4] and purchased by institutions with a large infant population. In most hospital settings, however, "monitor friendly," ultralow field strength MRI or CT is used to examine infants evaluated initially by ultrasound.

Although complete CT examinations of the infant brain can be obtained in less than 5 minutes, MR scans usually require approximately 30 to 40 minutes. Thus MRI cannot be performed on infants without effective sedation. Infants, as with adults, should be kept from eating for at least 4 hours before sedation. The upper airway of a pediatric patient should be examined before sedation for conditions that could predispose to subsequent asphyxia. For sedation, chloral hydrate can be administered orally (50 to 100 mg/kg body weight) 30 minutes before the MR scan.[4] Alternatively, *a*tropine, *m*eperidine, *p*romethazine, and *s*ecobarbital (AMPS) can be given intramuscularly approximately 1 hour before scanning.[5] Ten percent of patients will require supplementary intravenous (IV) sedation. Pentobarbital (Nembutal, 2 to 6 mg/kg IV) may be given to patients in whom chloral hydrate has failed to produce sedation.[6] Using the previous measures, almost 90% of pediatric patients can be examined without general anesthesia. The use of sedation, rather than anesthesia, does not reduce the need for availability of resuscitative equipment and personnel trained in its use.[5]

Intraarterial and IV digital cerebral angiography of infants also requires sedation and immobilization of the head, but the latter can generally be achieved by simply taping across the forehead to either side of the table top. Some commercially available head clamps used for this purpose have caused reversible deformity in the skull. Therefore, if such apparatus is to be employed, newer, fully spongy models with larger contact surfaces are preferable.[7] The use of a nonionic contrast medium eliminates the "burning" sensation associated with injection of ionic media. Nonionic media should reduce the incidence of head movement that occurs as a result of contrast injection.

The optimum imaging protocols for ultrasound, CT, and MR examinations are outlined in the following sections.

Ultrasound

Echogenicity of an intracranial structure depends on the presence of an abrupt interface between neighboring structures, as when structures interface with cerebrospinal fluid (CSF). Ultrasound clearly images the walls of the ventricles, vessels and nerves within fissures and cisterns, frond-like interdigitations of the ventricular choroid plexus, as well as the falx and tentorium, because all of these structures have at least one interface with CSF. Other anatomic boundaries are represented on ultrasound by various shades of gray.[8]

A real-time sector ultrasound scanner is ideally suited for neonatal brain imaging because only a small window (i.e., the anterior fontanelle) is available in infants. The selection of transducer frequency and focal length should be optimized according to the area of interest in each examination. A 5.0 MHz transducer with medium focal length is generally satisfactory for an overview of the brain in most infants. In larger infants a lower-frequency transducer may be necessary to ensure adequate penetration. For the evaluation of the superficial cortex and subarachnoid space over the convexity, a 7.5 to 10.0 MHz transducer or gel pad may also be necessary. The examination can be recorded on videotape, but hard-copy images are necessary for quickly comparing serial scans. Computerized sonography with variable dynamic range, preprocessing and postprocessing capability, and multiple focal zones has remarkably improved resolution of sonographic images.[9,10]

The standard ultrasound examination is performed through the anterior fontanelle and, only rarely, through the posterior fontanelle or transcranially through the temporal bone.

Computed Tomography

The use of dynamic scan sequences reduces the time required to perform a CT scan of an infant, thereby minimizing the problems of monitoring the vital signs and maintaining body temperature during examination. Modern CT scanners can complete an infant brain examination in less than 3 minutes. To optimize brain contrast, the field of view (FOV) should be reduced and the milliamperes (mA) decreased compared with the adult setting. The smaller head diameter and skull thickness in infants, compared with the adult brain, cause an artifactual lowering of the measured CT brain attenuation values.[11] These factors may also cause the artifactual, thin, hyperdense rim immediately beneath the skull, which occasionally appears in images of normal infants examined with even the most advanced CT equipment.

Magnetic Resonance

The higher water content of neonatal brain tissue requires the use of modified adult pulse sequences for MRI. Table 2-1 demonstrates a protocol that can be used for neonatal imaging with a 1.5 T (Tesla) General Electric Signa system. Although not essential, the coronal plane does help to examine pathology in and around the ventricles. Note that the neonatal brain requires a more T2-weighted pulse sequence than the adult brain. The first echo delay time (TE) should be 80 msec. This produces a CSF signal that is less intense than white matter signal, thus facilitating hemorrhage identification. The same hemorrhage is much more difficult to see with the second echo (160 msec) because CSF is virtually isointense with the hemorrhage. However, the longer TE creates an improved gray-white matter discriminability.

With a 0.6 T Technicare unit, a protocol using a T2-weighted spin-echo (SE) sequence with TR/TE of 2000/120,240 msec and two excitations and a T1-weighted SE sequence with TR/TE of 600-800/32 and four excitations has been recommended (TR, repetition time).[4] It should be noted that both T1- and T2-weighted sequences are necessary to visualize hemorrhage in neonates. Therefore a neonatal study is not complete until a T2-weighted sequence is obtained. In the perinatal and postnatal periods, brain water content decreases because myelin is forming in the brain. Concomitantly, a change occurs in gray-white matter contrast on MRI, which is most likely related to decreasing water rather than increasing lipid from myelin. Furthermore, the contrast between myelinated and unmyelinated white matter lessens beyond the neonatal period. Although T1-weighted SE pulse sequences will visualize myelin, T1 weighting is related to age and brain water content. Therefore, SE sequences do not have the gray-white matter differentiation, which can be created by only inversion recovery (IR) sequences. For these reasons the SE sequence is most useful up to about 45 weeks after conception, and IR scanning is preferred thereafter (Table 2-2).

To evaluate developmental delay, one should obtain a T1-weighted SE sagittal image (as with the neonate), followed by an IR axial image with a 256 × 196 or 256 matrix to reduce truncation artifact. This is followed by a T2-

◆ **TABLE 2-1** Neonatal MR Protocol at 1.5 Tesla (Signa, Software 4.5)*

Plane	Pulsing sequence	TR	TE	NEX	Matrix	Time (min:sec)
Sagittal	SE	500	10	1	192	1:42
Axial	SE	600-700	10	1	192	2:03-2:23
Axial	SE	3000	80,160	1	128†	7:00
Coronal	SE	600-700	10	1	192	2:03-2:23

*Field of-view, 14 to 16 cm; slice, 5 mm/1 mm gap; extremity coil.
†Flow compensation, variable bandwidth.
SE, Spin echo; TR, repetition time; TE, echo delay time; NEX, number of excitations.

◆ **TABLE 2-2** Inversion Recovery MR Parameters Relative to Age at 1.5 Tesla*

Age	TR	TI	TE
Neonate-3 months	2500	1200	20
3 months-1 year	2500	1000	20
Over 1 year	2500	800	20

Reproduced with permission from McArdle, CB: *Diagn Imaging* 9(11):272-278, 1987.
*Field of view, 16 to 20 cm; slice, 5 mm/2.5 mm gap; extremity coil; time (min:sec), 11:03 (one excitation, 256 matrix).
TR, Repetition time; TI, inversion recovery time; TE, echo delay time.

weighted SE axial series and, time permitting, an IR coronal sequence with a 256 × 128 matrix. The T2-weighted sequence is helpful in establishing the presence of earlier intracerebral hemorrhage.

In infants and young children, use of a T2-weighted SE sequence with TR/TE of 2000/20,80 (useful in adults) will result in poor gray-white matter differentiation. For infants through 1 year of age, an SE 2500-3000/80,160 sequence is recommended. From 1 to 3 years of age, an SE 2000-2500/60,120 sequence should be used. These parameters apply at 1.5 T; at lower field strengths, more T2 weighting with longer TEs is preferred.

The increased signal-to-noise ratio (SNR) afforded by a small, cylindrical coil can decrease scan time to half of that needed with the adult head coil. An extremity coil with a transmit-receive design and measuring 17 cm in diameter is ideal. After 1 year of age, the child's head is usually so large that a head coil becomes necessary.

Angiography

Conventional

In infants, cerebral angiography is reserved for situations in which direct visualization of intracranial vasculature is mandatory. Selective femorocerebral catheterization usually necessitates use of general anesthesia. Nonionic contrast medium has been recommended for these procedures, although clinical trials have not been performed in infants. Digital subtraction angiography techniques allow the contrast medium to be diluted without altering visualization of the intracerebral vessels. A no. 3 French, preformed angiographic catheter (Cook) with curve DHNI can be used to select the carotid or vertebral vessels.

The risks to brain and femoral vessels discussed next relate to the pediatric population, since we found no report on complications in the neonatal population. A prospective study investigated the neurologic complication rate from pediatric angiography (mean age, 8 years) in 1581 consecutive patients in whom 3731 vessels were injected. The rate of procedure-related embolization was 0.9% of all patients and 0.4% of all vessels studied by a group of experienced pediatric angiographers. This is comparable to the rate reported in adults.[12] However, the complications were considerably less severe in the pediatric age-group measurably because (1) the use of general anesthesia with hyperventilation increases the oxygen tension of the brain and thereby partially protects this tissue; (2) better collateral cerebral circulation exists naturally in children; and (3) the emboli are probably composed of fibrin clots that form in or on the distal part of catheter, rather than composed of atheromatous plaque fragments as in adults.

The induction of any neurologic complications in children and the high complication rate from femoral arterial punctures have prompted some to use intravenous digital subtraction angiography (IDSA) in infants and children.[13]

Intravenous Digital Subtraction Angiography (DSA)

The advent of IDSA has enabled the imaging clinician to visualize intracerebral vessels after IV injection of contrast medium. This technique appears to result in lower morbidity than conventional angiography, and multiple reports describe its usefulness in a wide spectrum of abnormalities.[13-18] However, IDSA is not used widely in pediatric neuroradiology centers.

If IDSA is performed, straight catheters with side holes are less painful to insert and cause less damage to the vein than pigtail catheters. The largest catheter that can be placed in the vena cava of a newborn subject is generally a no. 3 French.[13,14] If smaller catheters are used, the rate of delivery of contrast bolus will be slower and the image quality of the IDSA compromised. Flow rates of 6 to 15 ml/sec of sodium and meglumine diatrizoate (Renografin-60) have been employed in the infant. The total dose of this contrast agent should not exceed 3 to 4 ml/kg.[14] Images should be obtained in frontal and Towne projections because IDSA normally opacifies all the cerebral arteries simultaneously. Lateral and oblique views are difficult to interpret because of overlapping of vessels.

NORMAL ANATOMY

Rapid developmental changes occur in the fetal brain during the last 15 weeks of gestation.[19] Thus it should not be surprising that many features of the brain in an infant born prematurely (at approximately the 32nd week of gestation and weighing 1500 g) are significantly different from those found in a term infant's brain at 38 to 42 weeks of gestation (see Chapter 1).

These differences can be seen on gross inspection of the brain and relate to the differences of the cerebral vasculature and dural cranial attachments, as well as to the degree of white matter myelination found in preterm and term infants. Each of these features is discussed separately in the following sections.

We should note at this point that all the published in vivo normative data on premature infants are suspect. Virtually all the infants referred to in the relevant literature have experienced perinatal hypoxia and have been subjected to imaging study because they had symptoms suggesting central nervous system damage!

Cisterns and Ventricles

All newborn infants have a CSF-filled cavum between the two layers of the septum pellucidum. This cavity forms when the decussation bed of the corpus callosum degenerates (see Chapter 5). The cavum usually disappears during the first 2 years of life but is found at autopsy in 20% and on in vivo imaging studies in 2% of normal adults (see Chapter 12).[20]

The extracerebral CSF space may appear widened on MR images in normal infants from 29 to 42 weeks of gestation. The subarachnoid space posterior to the parietal lobes can be particularly large, especially in premature infants.[21] The sulci of the left hemisphere are normally wider and deeper. However, the subarachnoid space around the right hemisphere may appear prominent because that hemisphere is normally smaller than the left in the developing brain.[22]

The rolandic and calcarine fissures are formed between 24 and 26 weeks of gestation. Shortly thereafter, the superior temporal and the precentral and postcentral gyri form. The remainder of the brain rapidly develops a gyral pattern from 30 to 32 weeks of gestation. The cortex that overlies the relatively flat gyri and shallow sulci of the preterm infant (32 weeks of gestation) is little more than a thin layer of tissue. The sylvian fissure is merely an indentation of the lateral aspect of the cerebral hemisphere. The temporal, parietal, and frontal cortex do not yet overlie the insular cortex. Once the infant brain reaches term (38 to 42 weeks of gestation), the ratio of gray to white matter increases. By this time the sylvian fissure and the cortical gyri and sulci are beginning to resemble the adult configuration[23] (see Chapter 1).

The orientation of the sylvian fissures in the neonatal brain is significantly different from that of the adult. These differences in gross morphology cause the characteristic differences in location of intracranial vessels when angiograms of neonatal brains are compared with those of adults (Figure 2-1). High-resolution CT studies have shown that the extraventricular CSF spaces vary in appearance in children under 2 years of age. These spaces may appear enlarged if compared with those of children from age 3 years to young adulthood, in whom the sulci can barely be identified. This cisternal enlargement may be associated with what appears to be a slightly enlarged ventricular system in neurologically normal children.[23]

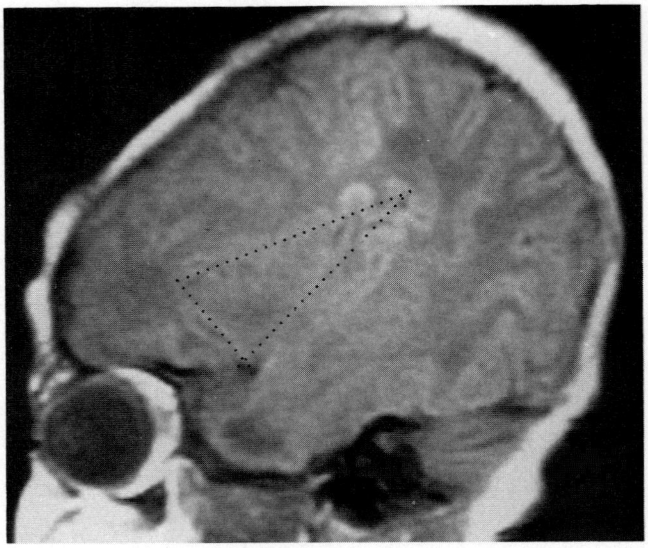

Figure 2-1 Sagittal MR image (TR/TE, 600/40) in a normal term infant. Note the normal "elevation" of the posterior portion of the sylvian triangle (*black dots*). The position of the normal adult sylvian triangle is shown in Chapters 3 and 11.

The normally large ventricular cavities found in the immature brain gradually decrease in size during intrauterine development.[24,25] Therefore, in premature infants, the ventricles are expected to be relatively large. The ventricles become mere slits at term, although some may show mild enlargement of the occipital horns. The variations in ventricular shape that occur in one sixth of adult brains from fusion or "coaptation" of the lateral and medial ventricular walls in the frontal and occipital horns are notably absent in newborns.[26]

Various CT studies have attempted to define the normal ventricular dimensions of the newborn brain.[21, 27-30] Figure 2-2 demonstrates the ratios (indices) between the ventricular lumen diameters and the internal diameter of the skull. Table 2-3 tabulates these bifrontal, bicaudate, and bioccipital indices and demonstrates that no significant difference exists between premature neonates born before or after 32 weeks of gestation.[28] The bifrontal index gradually declines from 29 to 42 weeks after conception.[21] Absolute measurements of the diameter of the lateral, third, and fourth ventricles have been reported for the first year of life (see Tables 2-4 to 2-6).[27]

◆ **TABLE 2-3** Cerebroventricular Indices of Normal CT Scans in Premature Infants

Index gestational age (weeks)	Range	Mean	Standard deviation
Bifrontal			
<32 (*n* = 15)	0.19-0.35	0.28	0.05
>32 (*n* = 16)	0.19-0.36	0.28	0.05
Bicaudate			
<32 (*n* = 15)	0.07-0.15	0.10	0.02
>32 (*n* = 16)	0.06-0.17	0.11	0.03
Bioccipital			
<32 (*n* = 11)	0.12-0.27	0.19	0.05
>32 (*n* = 16)	0.12-0.28	0.17	0.04

Reproduced with permission from Lorrencic M, Schmutzer L: AJNR 4:683-684, 1983.

◆ **TABLE 2-4** CT Evaluation of Lateral Ventricle Size in First Year of Life

	1-30 Days	2-6 Months	7-12 Months
Range of A plus B*	20-41 mm	31-51 mm	25-56 mm
Mean value	31.00	40.00	41.00
Median	33.00	41.00	42.00
Standard deviation	4.80	5.80	8.60
Standard error	1.05	1.09	1.54

Reproduced with permission from Naheedy MH, Strand RD, Gilles FH. J *Comput Assist Tomogr* 6(1):51-53, 1982.
*See Figure 2-2.

◆ **TABLE 2-5** CT Evaluation of Third Ventricle Size (Maximum Transverse Diameter) in First Year of Life

	1-30 Days	2-6 Months	7-12 Months
Range of diameter	2-6 mm	4-6 mm	4-8 mm
Mean value	4.00	5.00	5.40
Median	4.00	5.00	5.00
Standard deviation	0.77	0.60	1.40
Standard error	0.17	0.11	0.25

Reproduced with permission from Naheedy NH, Strand RD, Gilles FH: J *Comput Assist Tomogr* 6(1):51-53, 1982.

◆ **TABLE 2-6** CT Evaluation of Fourth Ventricle Size (Maximum Transverse Diameter) in First 18 Months of Life

	1-30 Days	2-6 Months	7-18 Months
Range of diameter	4-10 mm	5-13 mm	7-18 mm
Mean value	7.70	10.60	10.80
Median	8.00	11.00	11.00
Standard deviation	2.80	2.10	2.80
Standard error	0.84	0.51	0.61

Reproduced with permission from Naheedy NH, Strand RD, Gilles FH: J *Comput Assist Tomogr* 6(1):51-53, 1982.

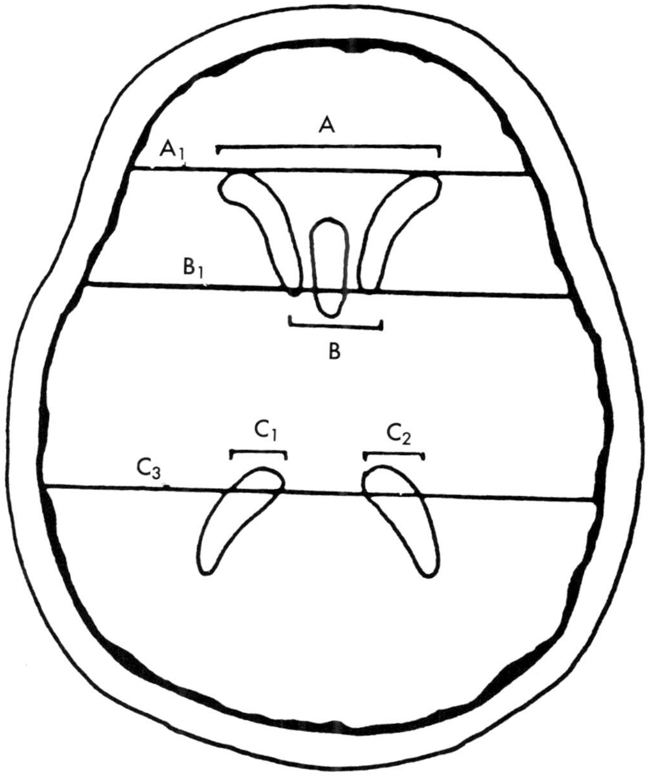

Figure 2-2 Schematic axial CT image of a premature brain. The distance between the lateral walls of the frontal horns (A) divided by the internal diameter of the skull at this level (A1) yields the *bifrontal index*. The distance between the lateral walls of the frontal horns at the foramen of Monro (B) divided by the internal diameter of the skull at this level (B1) yields the *bicaudate index*. The sum of the distance between the medial and lateral walls of the atria of the ventricles divided by the internal diameter of the skull at this level yields the *bioccipital index*. See Table 2-3 for normal values. (Reproduced with permission from Lovrencic MV, Schmutzer L: AJNR 4:683-684, 1983.)

White Matter

Myelination

Much normal variability exists in the rate of myelin formation in the brain. Generally, at 29 weeks of gestation, virtually no myelin is present except in the brainstem and cerebellar peduncles (see Chapter 1). Between 29 and 36 weeks, myelin formation has progressed from the brainstem to the posterior limb of the internal capsule. Myelin should be seen in the corona radiata adjacent to the lateral ventricles by 37 weeks of gestation and in the centrum semiovale cephalad to the lateral ventricles in the brain at term (42 weeks of gestation).[32] Further myelination of the white matter proceeds irregularly, and most myelin formation is not complete until early childhood.[23] Myelination of cortical association fibers actually continues until age 30 years. Details concerning myelination in specific regions of the brain can be found in the references cited in Chapter 1.

The neonatal brain is 88% to 97% water. The formation of myelin causes a reduction in total water content of brain tissue because myelin is relatively hydrophobic (having a water content of only 40%). Eventually, myelin accounts for more than one half of the dry weight of white matter.[33] It has been established that myelination alters the appearance of brain images obtained by CT and MRI. On CT examination the unmyelinated cerebral hemispheric white matter is significantly more hypointense (relative to adjacent gray matter) than myelinated adult white matter. CT studies of the neonatal brain have documented a progressively increasing signal intensity in white matter during the first months of life caused by myelin formation. These white matter changes were identified by comparing them with the CT signal from adjacent gray matter, which remains constant over this time frame.[33]

On MR scans, changes in both T1 and T2 relaxation times occur as myelination progresses.[34-38] Normal brain water can conceal cerebral infarction on MR scans in the newborn. On low field strength instruments (0.35 T), calculated T1 values for white matter drop from 1600 msec at birth to 580 msec at 1 year of age. A decrease in the T1 relaxation time of brain water has been postulated to reflect the increase in concentration of myelin components, especially protein, cholesterol, and glycolipids.[35] This T1 shortening is most apparent in the first 6 months of life and may explain why T1-weighted sequences are preferred for evaluation of myelination at this time.

T2 values of 90 msec at birth fall to 57 msec at 1 year of age. A decrease in T2 relaxation time is believed to reflect a decrease in brain water that accompanies further development of hydrophobic myelin.[35] Myelin maturation is most apparent after 6 months and accounts for the improved visualization of myelination with T2-weighted sequences, as opposed to T1-weighted sequences, after 6 months of life. The ages at which myelination becomes apparent in different regions of the brain on T1- and T2-weighted images have been reported.[32,35] These variations can be helpful in evaluating delayed myelination.

After the first year of life, the values for white matter slowly drop until they approximate the adult range at 11 to 14 years of age. These values cause the short TR/short TE MR scans of the neonatal brain to show unmyelinated white matter as low signal intensity relative to gray matter. These values also cause long TR/long TE scans to show unmyelinated white matter as isointense or hyperintense to gray matter. This pattern is the reverse of that seen in the adult brain using comparable scanning techniques. The neonatal pattern on MRI gradually changes to an adult pattern by 8 to 10 months as myelination decreases the water content of the white matter.

Although it seems intuitively obvious that delays in myelination will correlate with impaired neurologic functioning, the data to support this hypothesis are difficult to evaluate because of the wide individual patterns of myelination.[40] Preliminary studies suggest that the rate of myelin formation may be useful in identifying children who will experience developmental delay in neurologic performance.[34-37] The myelination pattern on MR images lags several weeks behind histologic measures of myelination, presumably because MRI is a less sensitive means for detecting the presence of myelin.

Water Content

The water content of the neonatal white matter is normally much higher than levels found in the adult brain. This is presumably the cause of the nonspecific periventricular hypodensities that have been noted in 58% to 100% of newborn CT scans.[24,25,41] They should not be interpreted as pathology, since poor correlation existed between these hypointense zones on CT and ischemic damage at autopsy. This occurs presumably because these zones can obscure and also mimic ischemic changes in the white matter on both MR and CT examinations.

Germinal Matrix

The lateral ventricles are completely surrounded by an extensive, highly vascular zone of glioblastic cells, most prominent along the caudothalamic groove and above the head of the caudate nucleus (see Chapter 1). These delicate capillaries and immature vessels receive their blood supply from the recurrent artery of Heubner and the anterior and posterior choroidal arteries. By 32 weeks of gestation, this zone has regressed and can no longer be identified on CT scans as a halo of hyperintense signal surrounding the lateral ventricles.[42] Remnants of germinal matrix may persist and may even be visualized in full-term infants. These are generally symmetric and are seen along the caudothalamic groove (see Chapter 1). They should not be mistaken for subependymal hemorrhages.[24,25] MR scans do not visualize the germinal matrix.

Dura Mater

On CT scans of the "normal" premature infant, only parts of the falx are visible. In term infants the superior aspect of the falx along the superior sagittal sinus is nearly always visible, but the anterior and posterior ends are inconsistently visualized.[42] On enhanced MR images, the dura is poorly seen, even in adults; therefore, dural prominence on MRI, especially in preterm infants, may indicate the presence of intradural hemorrhage. Autopsy series report idiopathic intradural hemorrhage in 48% of preterm infants.[24,25] These hemorrhages may be caused by compression of the preterm infant skull when it contacts the rigid cervix during delivery. Others have noted that the immature falx of the preterm infant has a looser arrangement of connective tissue than that of the term infant and that this may predispose to hemorrhage. Since intradural hemorrhage can also be seen in fetuses who died before birth, hypoxia must also account for some of these lesions.[24,25] Al-

◆ **TABLE 2-7** Mean Head Areas and Normal Ranges as Measured by CT

Age	Mean head area (cm^2) (range)*	Age	Mean head area (cm^2) (range)*
MONTHS		**YEARS**	
1	80.1 (66.8-93.3)	3	172.9 (155.2-190.2)
2	99.5 (86.3-112.8)	4	179.6 (162.1-197.1)
3	111.0 (97.8-124.3)	5	184.9 (167.4-202.4)
4	119.1 (105.8-132.3)	6	189.4 (171.9-206.9)
5	125.3 (112.1-138.6)	7	193.0 (175.5-210.5)
6	130.4 (117.2-143.7)	8	196.2 (178.7-213.8)
7	134.8 (121.5-148.0)	9	199.0 (181.5-216.5)
8	138.6 (125.3-151.9)	10	201.6 (184.1-219.1)
9	141.9 (128.7-155.1)	11	203.8 (186.5-221.3)
10	144.9 (131.6-158.1)	12	205.9 (188.4-223.4)
11	147.5 (134.3-160.8)	13	207.8 (190.5-225.5)
12	149.9 (136.7-163.2)	14	209.7 (191.6-226.6)
13	152.2 (138.9-165.4)	15	211.2 (193.7-228.7)
14	154.3 (141.0-167.6)	16	212.8 (195.3-230.3)
15	156.2 (134.8-169.5)	17	214.3 (196.8-231.8)
16	158.0 (144.8-171.3)	18	216.8 (199.3-234.3)
17	159.7 (146.4-173.0)		
18	161.3 (148.0-174.5)		
19	162.9 (149.6-176.1)		
20	164.3 (151.0-177.5)		
21	165.6 (152.4-178.9)		
22	167.0 (153.8-180.3)		
23	168.3 (155.0-181.5)		
24	169.5 (156.2-182.7)		

Reproduced with permission from Hahn FJ, Chu WK, Cheung JY: AJNR 6:537-538, 1984.
*Range reflects the 90% of the population closest to the mean.

though ultrasound consistently detects the dura, it cannot detect intradural hemorrhage. Fortunately, intradural hemorrhage has little clinical significance.

NORMAL GROWTH

The growth of the infant skull and brain have been well documented by head circumference measurements.[43] These measurements can be made on CT scans by having the computer calculate a region of interest (ROI) for the entire head (including the subcutaneous scalp) at the scan level that shows the maximum cranial diameter (i.e., the level in which the frontal horns are most prominent). Table 2-7 shows the values obtained with this technique; the most rapid brain growth occurs during the first 12 months of age.[44] Generalized retardation in brain growth causes characteristic abnormalities in the skull, in addition to the decrease in cranial circumference. These abnormalities include an increase in the width of the diploic space, small or prematurely closed sutures, a backward slope to the forehead, and loss of or reduction in the normal convolutional markings in the skull.

REFERENCES

1. London DA, Carroll BA, Enzmann DR: Sonography of ventricular size and germinal matrix hemorrhage in premature infants, *AJNR* 1:295-300, 1980.
2. McArdle CB, Nicholas DA, Richardson CJ, et al: Monitoring of the neonate undergoing MR imaging: technical considerations, *Radiology* 156:223-226, 1986.
3. McArdle CB: MR: monitoring of the neonate, *RSNA Today Videomagazine* 1(1):1986.
4. McArdle CB: MRI helps detect injury in neonatal infant brain, *Diagn Imaging* 9(11):272-278, 1987.
5. Thompson JR, Schneider S, Ashwal S, et al: The choice of sedation for computed tomography in children: a prospective evaluation, *Radiology* 143:475-479, 1982.
6. Strain JD, Campbell JB, Harvey LA, et al: IV Nembutal: safe sedation for children undergoing CT: *AJNR* 9:955-959, 1988.
7. Rosenblum J, Yousetzadeh DK, Ramilo JL: Skull radiography in infants: potential hazards of the use of head clamp, *Radiology* 161:367-368, 1986.
8. Pigadas A, Thompson JR, Grube GL: Normal infant brain anatomy: correlated real-time sonograms and brain specimens, *AJNR* 2:339-344, 1981.
9. Naidich TP, Gusnard DA, Yousefzadeh DK: Sonography of the internal capsule and basal ganglia in infants. 1. Coronal sections, *AJNR* 6:909-917, 1985.
10. Yousefzadeh DK, Naidich TP: US anatomy of the posterior fossa in children: correlation with brain sections, *Radiology* 156:353-361, 1985.

11. Thompson JR, Triolo PJ, Moore RJ, et al: CT scanning phantom for normalization of infant brain attenuation, *AJNR* 5:167-170, 1984.
12. Pettersson H, Fitz CR, Harwood-Nash DCF, et al: Iatrogenic embolization: complication of pediatric cerebral angiography, *AJNR* 2:357-361, 1981.
13. Faerber EN: Cerebral digital subtraction angiography. In *Digital subtraction imaging in infants and children,* Mount Kisco, NY, 1989, Futura.
14. Faerber EN, Giska LAB, Swartz JD, et al: Digital subtraction angiography in pediatric cerebrovascular occlusive disease, *Radiology* 152:391-394, 1984.
15. Lee BCP, Voorhies TM, Ehrlich ME, et al: Digital intravenous cerebral angiography in neonates, *AJNR* 5:281-286, 1984.
16. Wagner ML, Singleton EB, Egan ME: Digital subtraction angiography in children, *AJR* 140:127-133, 1983.
17. Capitanio MA, Faerber EN, Gainey MA, et al: Digital subtraction angiography and its application in children, *Pediatr Clin North Am* 32:S1449-S1460, 1985.
18. Mueller DL, Amundson GM, Wesenberg RL, et al: The application of IV digital subtraction angiography to cranial disease in children, *AJNR* 7:669-674, 1986.
19. Flodmark O, Becker LE, Harwood-Nash DC, et al: Correlation between computed tomography and autopsy in premature and full-term neonates that have suffered perinatal asphyxia, *Radiology* 137:93-103, 1980.
20. Sarwar M: The septum pellucidum: normal and abnormal, *AJNR* 10:989-1005, 1989.
21. McArdle CB, Richardson CJ, Nicholas DA, et al: Developmental features of the neonatal brain: MR imaging. II. Ventricular size and extracerebral space, *Radiology* 162:230-234, 1987.
22. Laffont J: Embryologie du cerveau (embryology of the brain), *J Neuroradiol* 9:5-14, 1982.
23. Harwood-Nash DC, Flodmark O: Diagnostic imaging of the neonatal brain: review and protocol, *AJNR* 3:103-105, 1982.
24. Ludwig B, Becker K, Rutter G, et al: Postmortem CT and autopsy in perinatal intracranial hemorrhage, *AJNR* 4:27-36, 1983.
25. Ludwig B, Brand M, Brockerhoff P: Postpartum CT examination of the heads of full term infants, *Neuroradiology* 20:145-154, 1980.
26. Friede RL: *Developmental neuropathology,* Berlin, 1989, Springer-Verlag.
27. Naheedy MH, Strand RD, Gilles FH: Evaluation of cerebral ventricles by computed tomography in the first year of life, *J Comput Assist Tomogr* 6(1):51-53, 1982.
28. Lovrencic M, Schmutzer L: CT measurement of the normal ventricular system in premature infants, *AJNR* 4:683-684, 1983.
29. Pedersen H, Gyldensted M: Measurement of the normal ventricular system and supratentorial subarachnoid space in children with computed tomography, *Neuroradiology* 17:231-237, 1979.
30. Goodwin LS, Hellmann J, Vannucci RC, Maisels J: Ventricular dimensions of the brain in premature and full-term infants, *Arch Neurol* 38:447-449, 1981.
31. Kleinman PK, Zito JL, Davidson RI, Raptopoulos V: The subarachnoid spaces in children: normal variations in size, *Radiology* 147:455-457, 1983.
32. McArdle CB, Richardson CJ, Nicholas DA, et al: Developmental features of the neonatal brain: MR imaging. I. Gray-white matter differentiation and myelination, *Radiology* 162:223-229, 1987.
33. Brant-Zawadzki M, Enzmann DR: Using computed tomography of the brain to correlate low white-matter attenuation with early gestational age in neonates, *Radiology* 139:105-108, 1981.
34. Dietrich RB, Bradley WG, Zaragoza EJ IV, et al: MR evaluation of early myelination patterns in normal and developmentally delayed infants, *AJNR* 9:69-76, 1988.
35. Barkovich AJ, Kjos BO, Jackson DE Jr, et al: Normal maturation of the neonatal and infant brain: MR imaging at 1.5 T, *Radiology* 166:173-180, 1988.
36. Stricker T, Martin E, Boesch C: Development of the human cerebellum observed with high-field-strength MR imaging, *Radiology* 177:431-435, 1990.
37. Martin E, Boesch C, Zuerrer M, et al: MR imaging of brain maturation in normal and developmentally handicapped children, *J Comput Assist Tomogr* 14(5):685-692, 1990.
38. Valk J, van der Knapp MS: *Magnetic resonance of myelin, myelination, and myelin disorders,* New York, 1989, Springer-Verlag.
39. Moore JB, Parker CP, Smith RJ, et al: Concealment of neonatal cerebral infarction on MRI by normal brain water, *Pediatr Radiol* 17:314-315, 1987.
40. Gilles FH, Leviton A, Dooling EC: *The developing human brain: growth and epidemiologic neuropathology,* Boston, 1983, John Wright/PSG.
41. Albright L, Fellows R: Sequential CT scanning after neonatal intracerebral hemorrhage *AJNR* 2:133-137, 1981.
42. Picard L, Claudon M, Roland J, et al: Cerebral computed tomography in premature infants, with an attempt at staging developmental features, *J Comput Assist Tomogr* 4(4):435-444, 1980.
43. Nellhaus G: Head circumference from birth to eighteen years, *Pediatrics* 41:106-114, 1968.
44. Hahn FJ, Chu WK, Cheung JY: CT measurements of cranial growth: alternative measurement method, *AJNR* 6:537-538, 1984.

CHAPTER 3

L. Anne Hayman
Mark J. Pfleger
John J. Pagani
Joel B. Kirkpatrick

Atlas of the Adult Brain

This chapter is designed to provide consecutive brain images that can be matched to clinical axial, coronal, or sagittal images, thereby giving the reader quick access to the nomenclature of clinically important regions. The chapter is indexed so that unfamiliar structures mentioned in subsequent chapters can be quickly found in the axial, coronal, and sagittal planes.

The magnetic resonance (MR) scans in this chapter are correlated with myelin-stained, normal, whole-brain, histologic sections. The MR images with a long repetition time/echo delay time (TR/TE, 2000/80) were obtained on a 1.5 Tesla (T) General Electric Signa unit. A 24 cm field of view was used to obtain 5 mm contiguous scans with two averages. The axial and coronal MR sequences used in this section were each obtained from a normal volunteer. The sagittal sequence, however, was obtained from a normal cadaver (without formalin fixation). Artifacts are present because of air bubbles within the cerebrospinal fluid (CSF) spaces in these cadaver MR scans.

The brain sections were obtained from the collection of Dr. Paul Yakolev at the Armed Forces Institute of Pathology. They were taken at selected intervals in the axial, coronal, and sagittal planes of the formalin-fixed brain specimens. On the *anatomic* illustrations the distance from the base slice (0 mm) is indicated. These distances reflect the in vivo distance between the brain slices. The level and angle of both the anatomic and the MR illustrations are indicated on adjacent, small schematic diagrams. Because it is not possible to match the anatomic sections exactly with the MR scan plane, the reader should study the anatomic sections that are paired with the MR scans immediately before and after each scan level. It should be noted that fixation has artificially enlarged the ventricles, sulci, and fissures in these brain slices.

Anatomic structures of clinical significance in imaging are labeled on both the MR images and the brain sections. This information was garnered from diverse sources.[1-8]

REFERENCES

1. Curnes JT, Burger PC, Djang WT, et al: MR imaging of compact white matter pathways, *AJNR* 9:1061-1068, 1988.
2. Naidich TP, Daniels DL, Peck P, et al: Anterior commissure: anatomic-MR correlation and use as a landmark in three orthogonal planes, *Radiology* 158:421-429, 1986.
3. Daniels DL, Haughton VM, Naidich TP: *Cranial and spinal magnetic resonance imaging: an atlas and guide,* New York, 1987, Raven.
4. Pernkopt E: *Atlas of topographical and applied human anatomy,* Baltimore-Munich, 1980, Urban and Schwarzenberg.
5. Matsui T, Hirano A: *An atlas of the human brain for computed tomography.* Tokyo, 1978, Igaku-Shoin.
6. DeArmond SJ, Fusco MM, Dewey MM: *Structure of the human brain,* ed 3, New York, 1989, Oxford University.
7. Roberts M, Hanaway J, Morset DK: *Atlas of the human brain in section,* Philadelphia, 1987, Lea & Febiger.
8. Riley HA: *An atlas of the basal ganglia, brainstem and spinal cord,* Baltimore, 1943, Williams & Wilkins.

CORONAL IMAGES

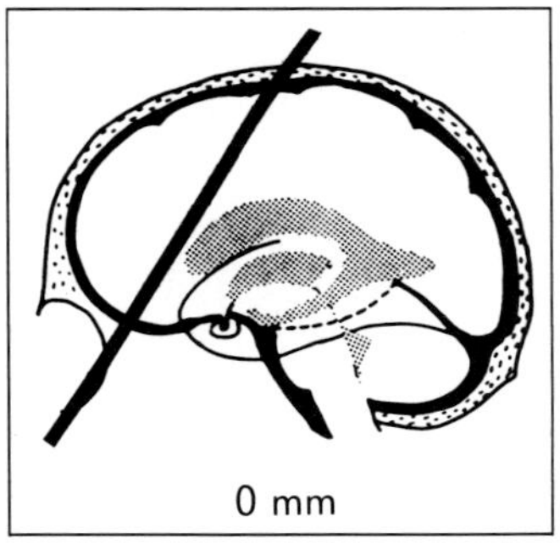

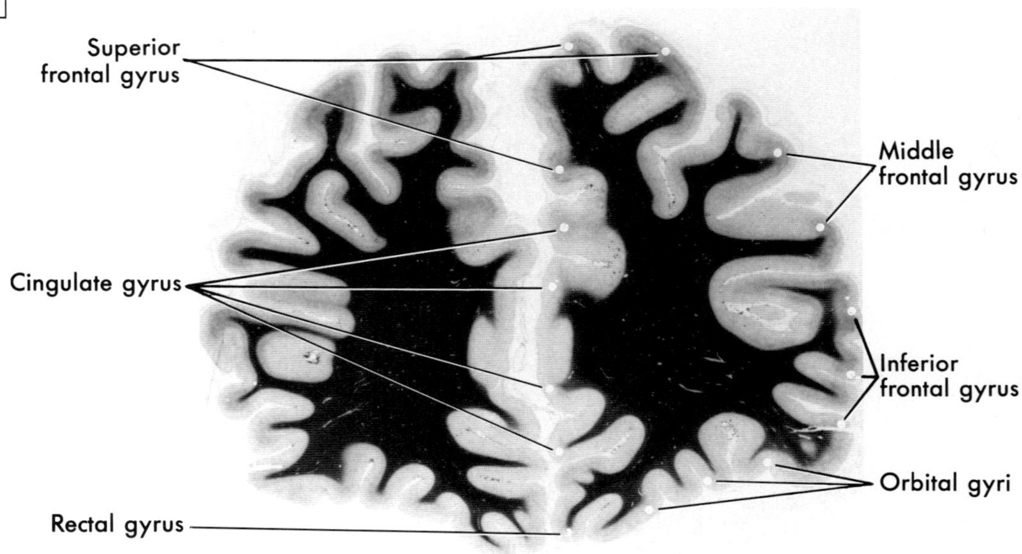

Figure 3-1

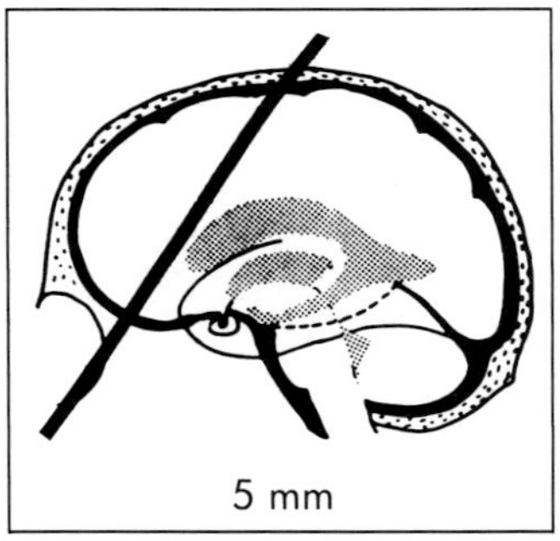

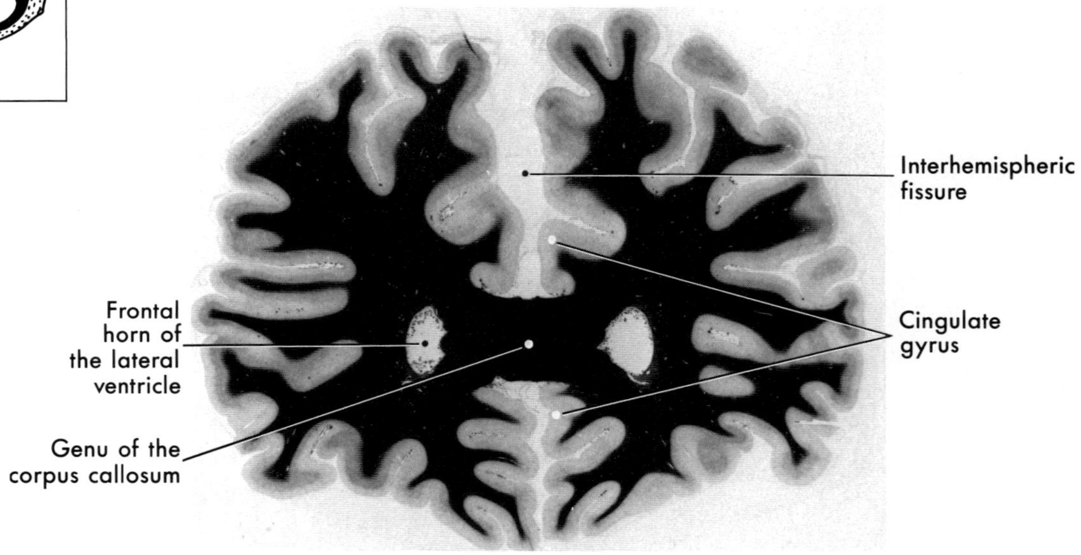

Figure 3-2

CORONAL IMAGES

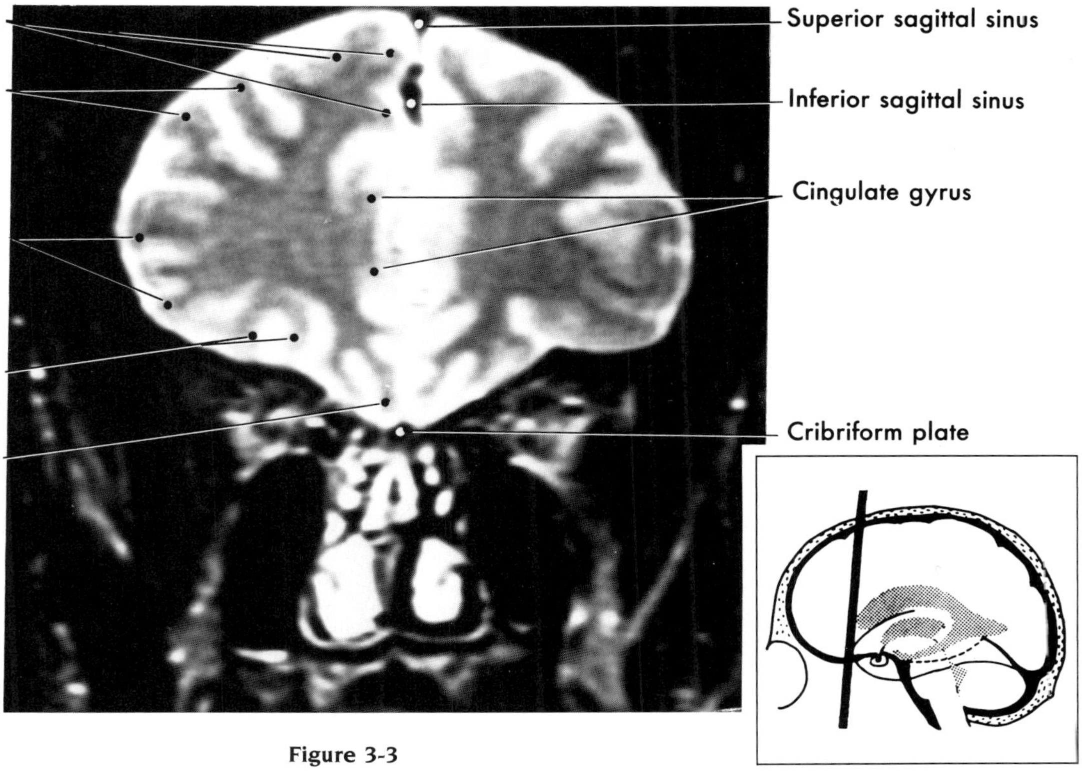

Figure 3-3

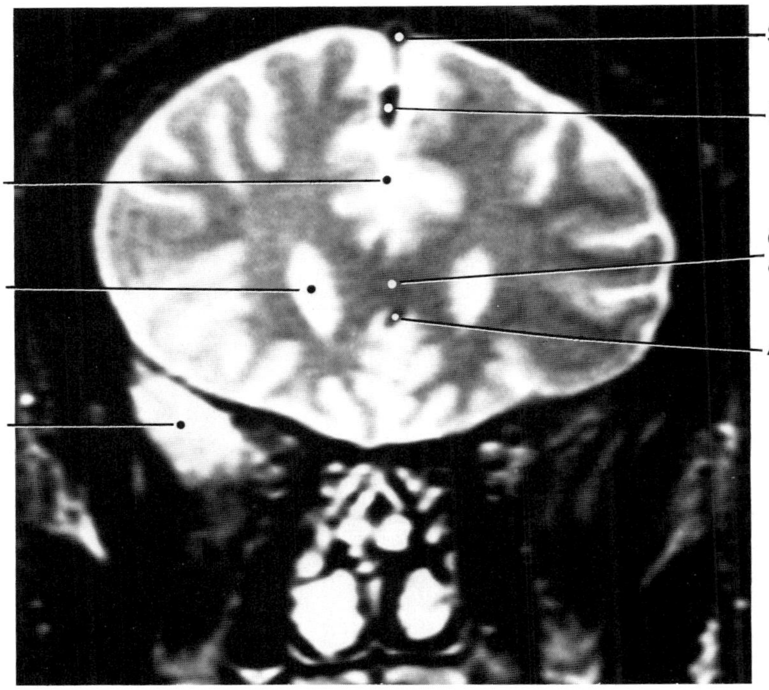

Figure 3-4

CORONAL IMAGES

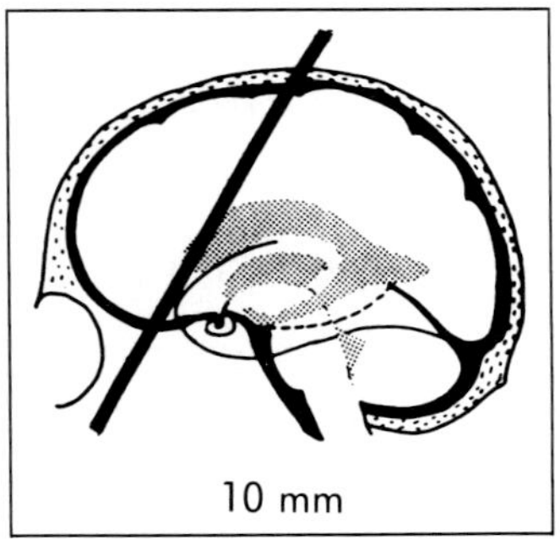

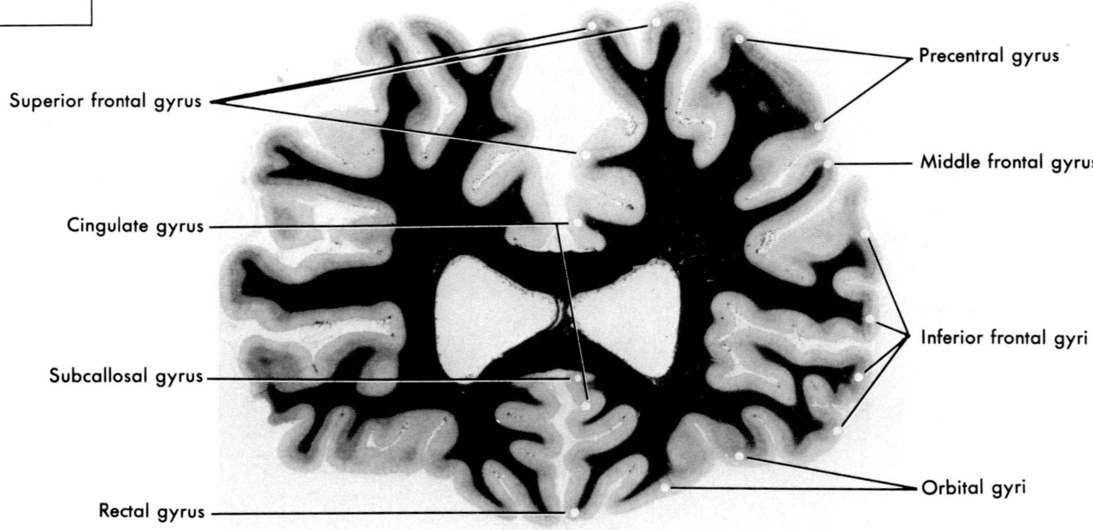

Figure 3-5

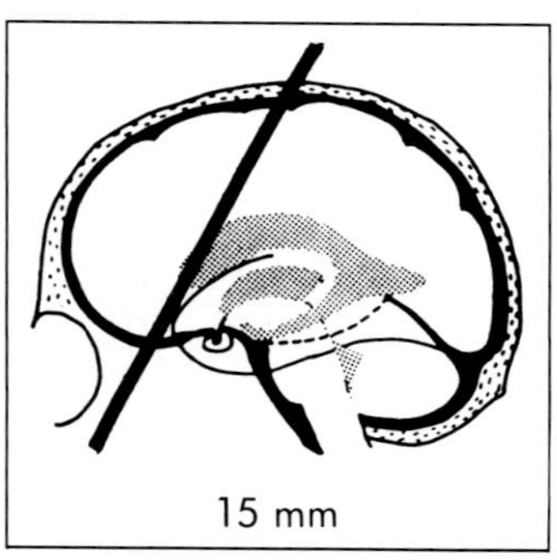

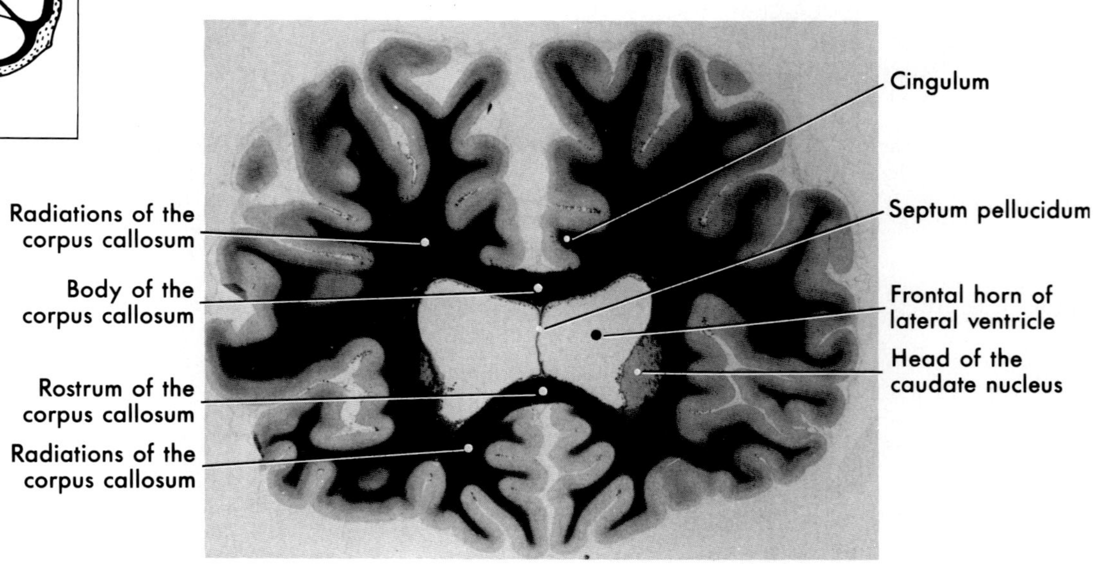

Figure 3-6

CORONAL IMAGES

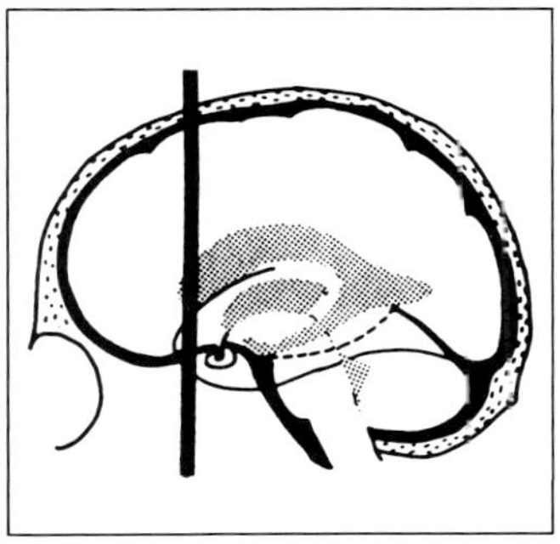

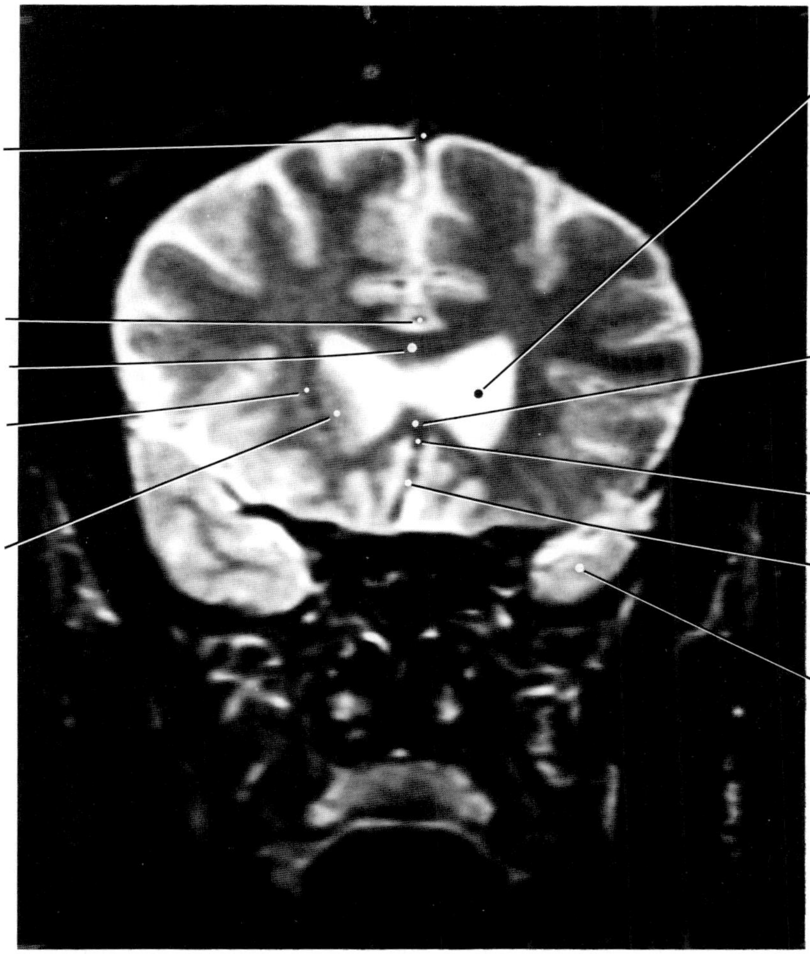

Figure 3-7

CORONAL IMAGES

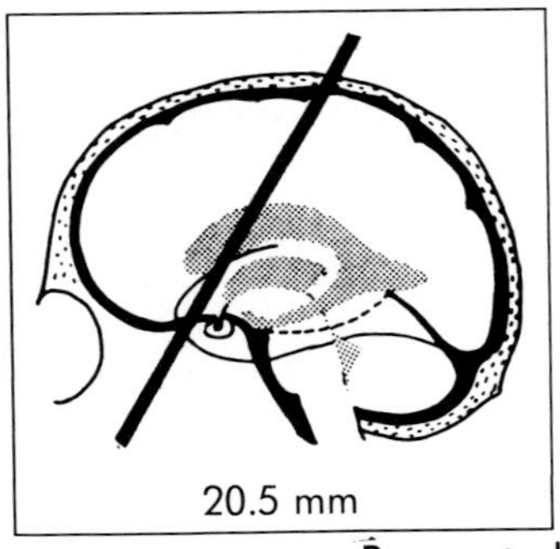

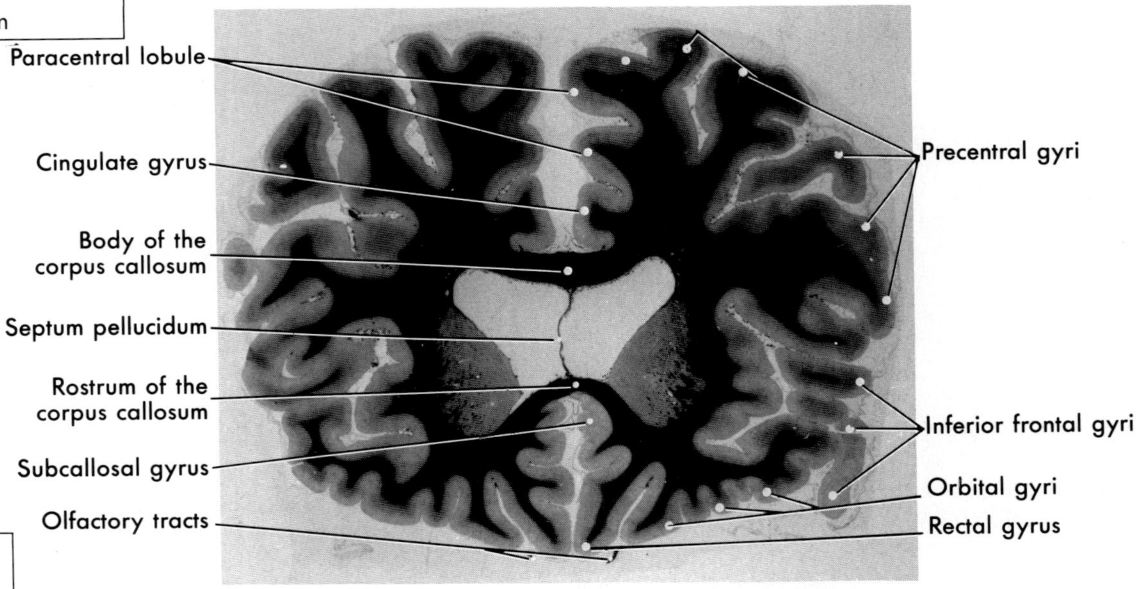

Figure 3-8

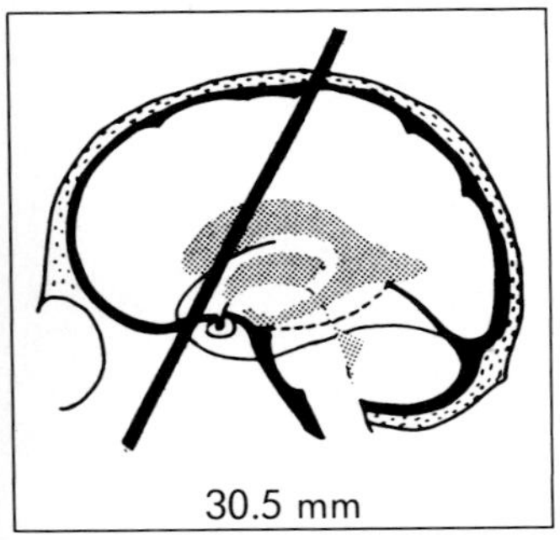

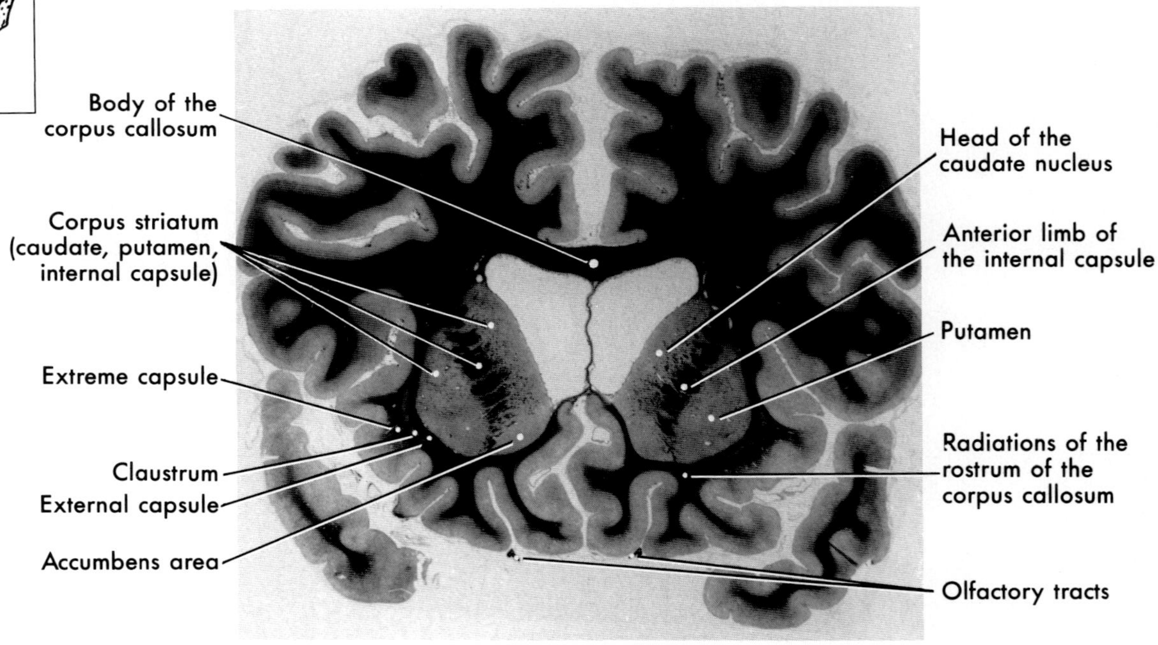

Figure 3-9

CORONAL IMAGES

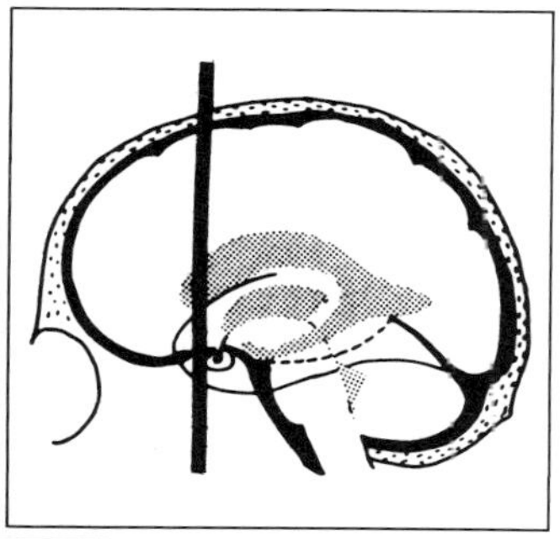

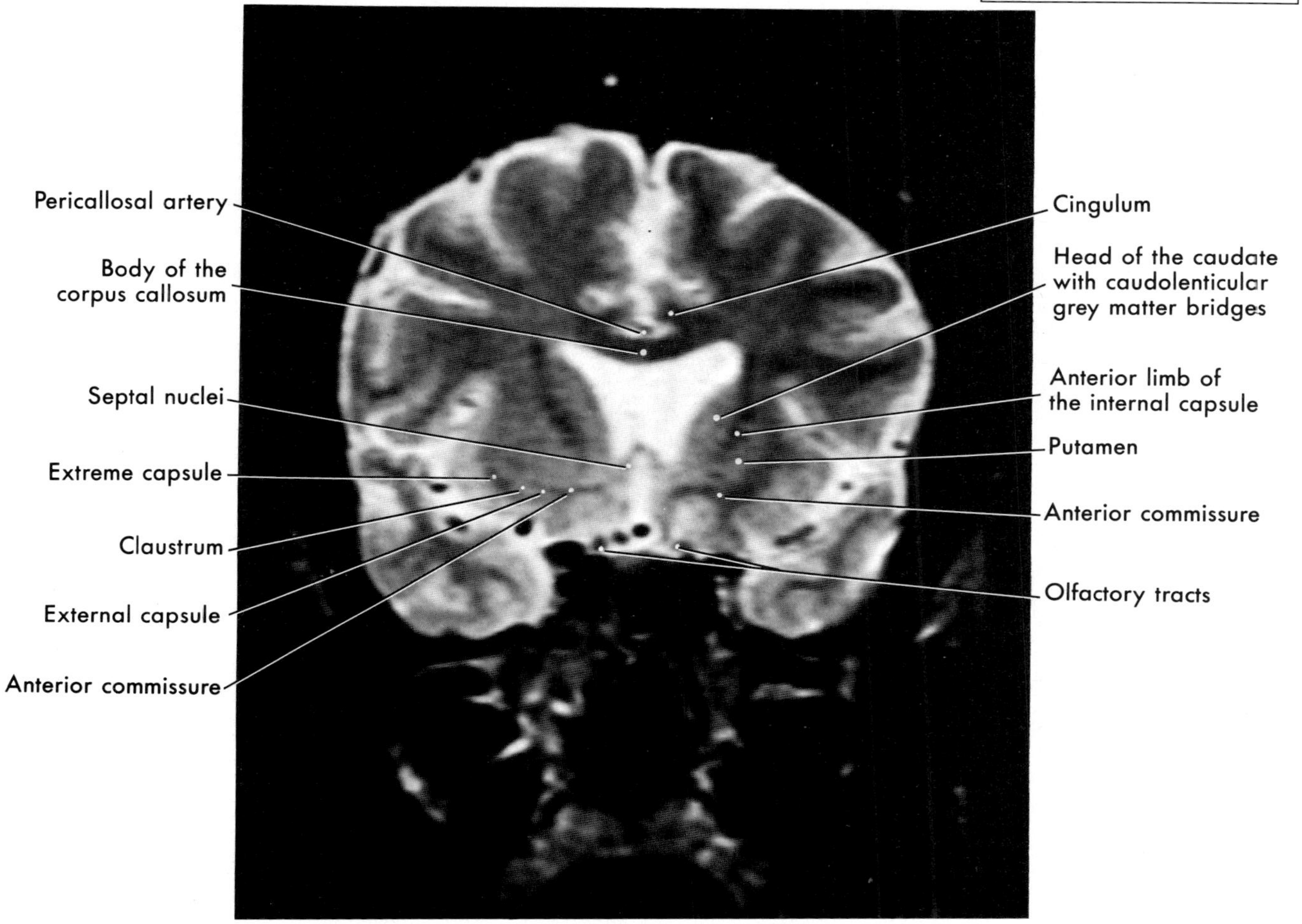

Figure 3-10

CORONAL IMAGES

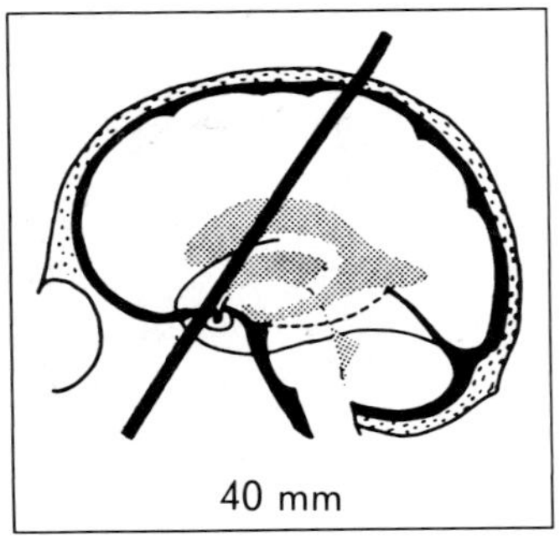

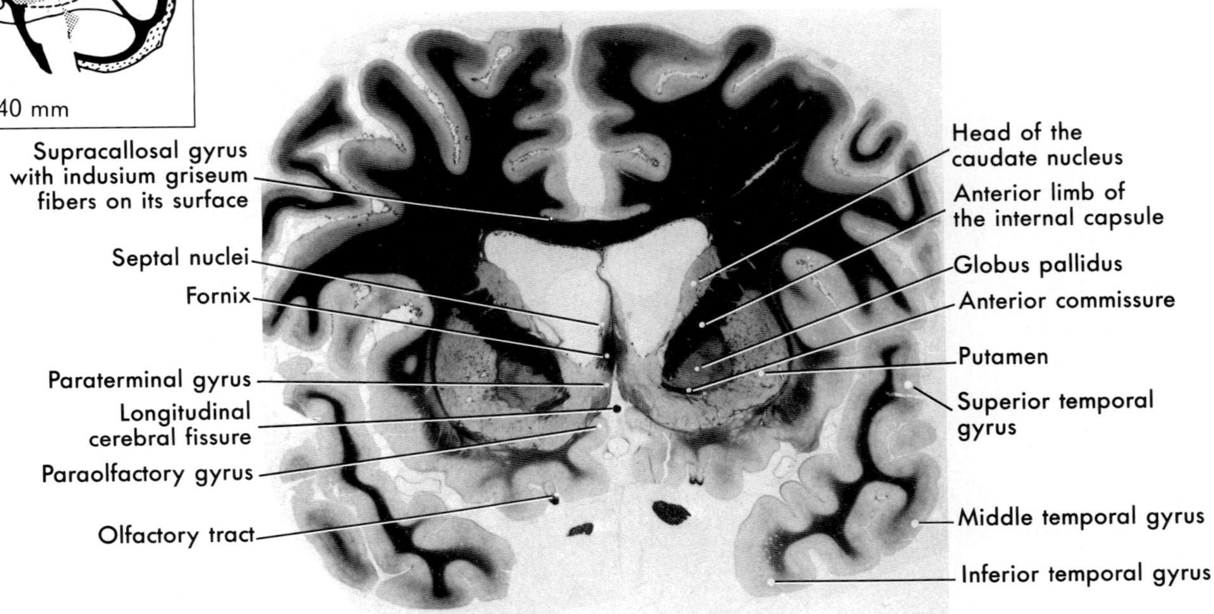

Figure 3-11

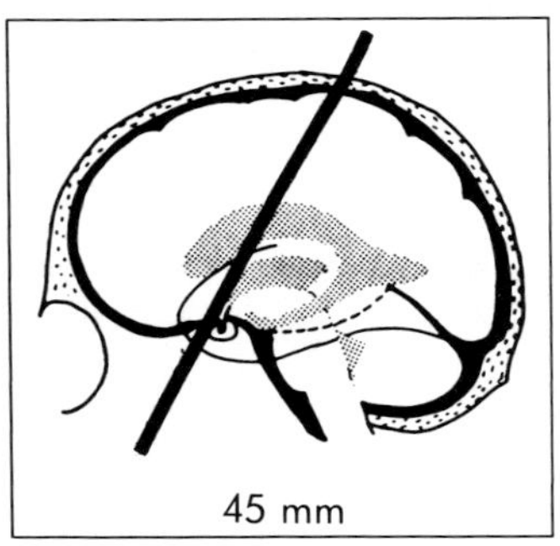

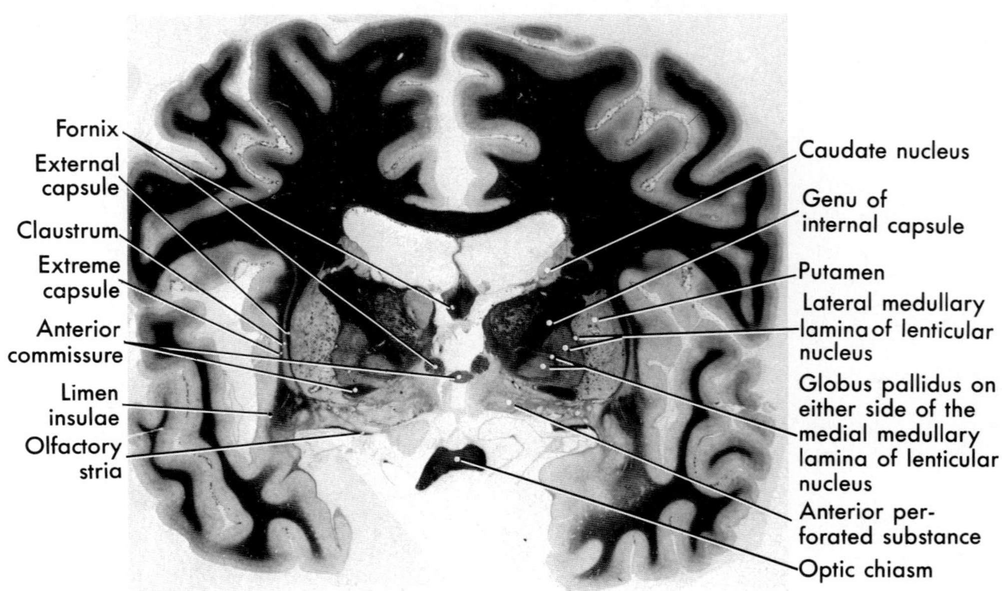

Figure 3-12

CORONAL IMAGES

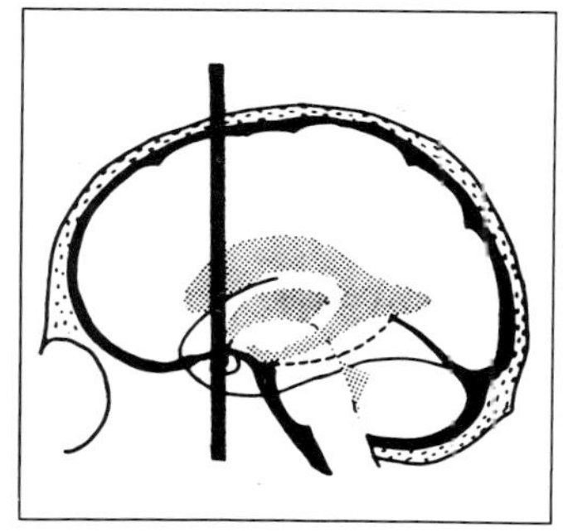

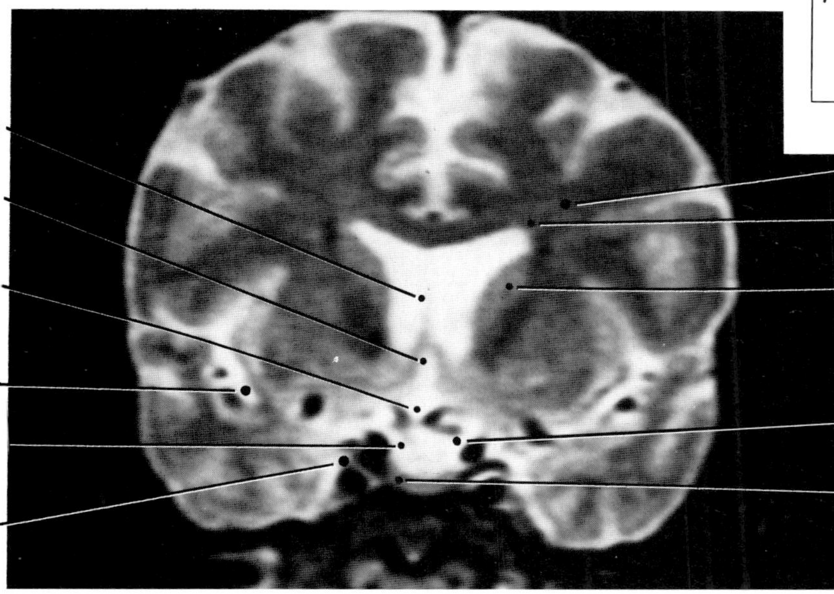

Figure 3-13

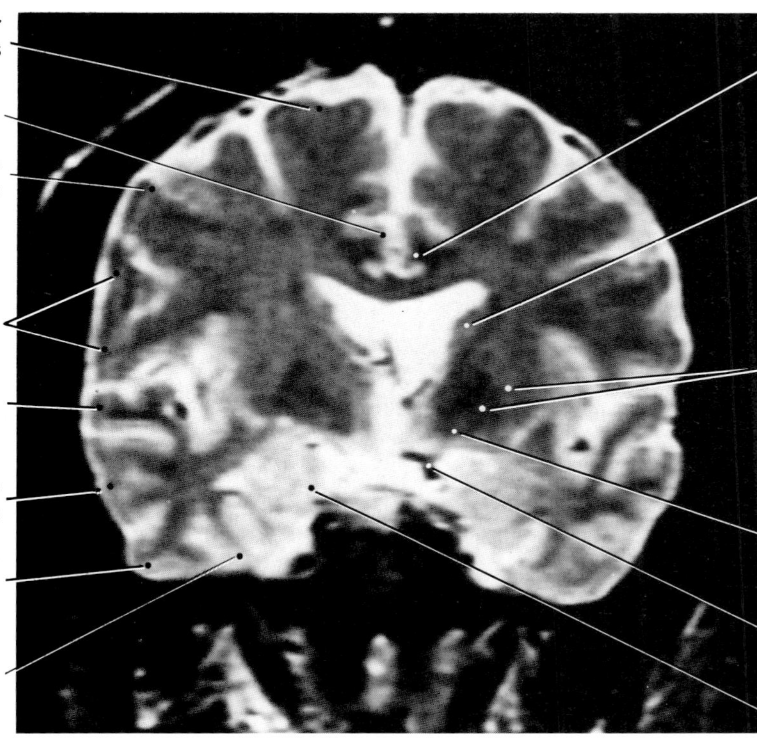

Figure 3-14

CORONAL IMAGES

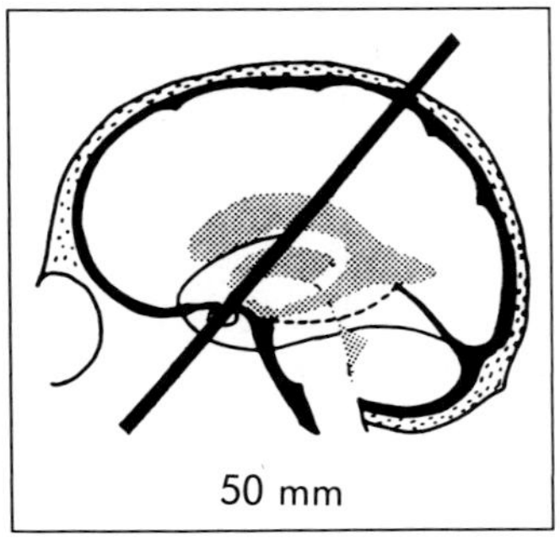

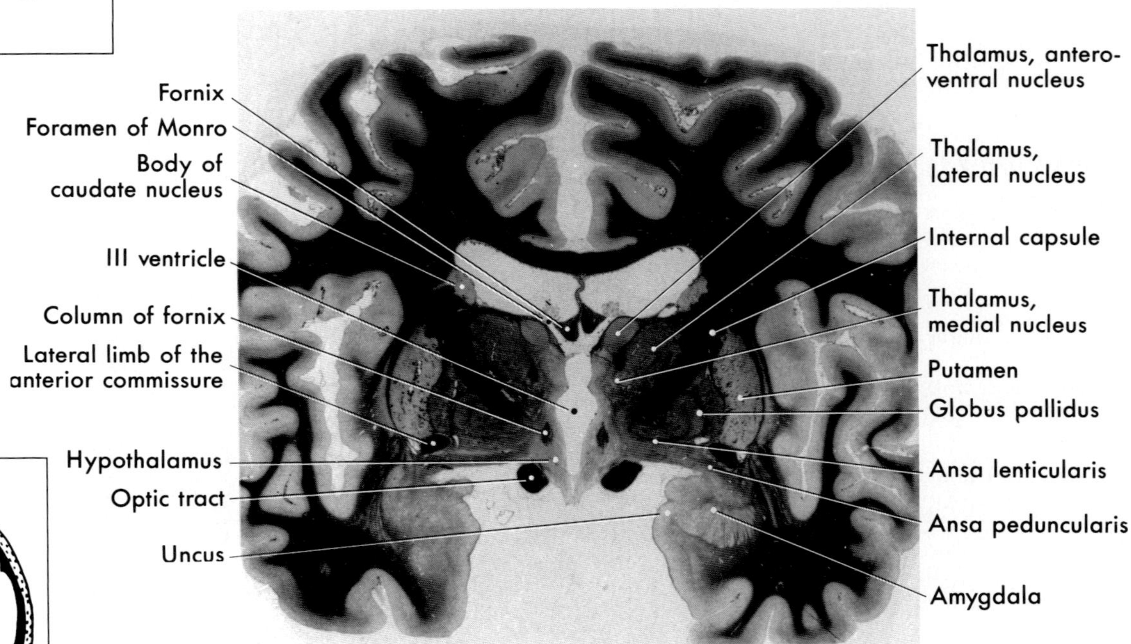

Figure 3-15

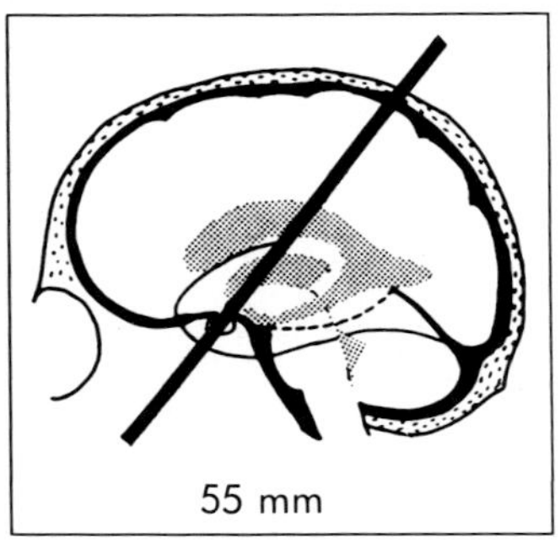

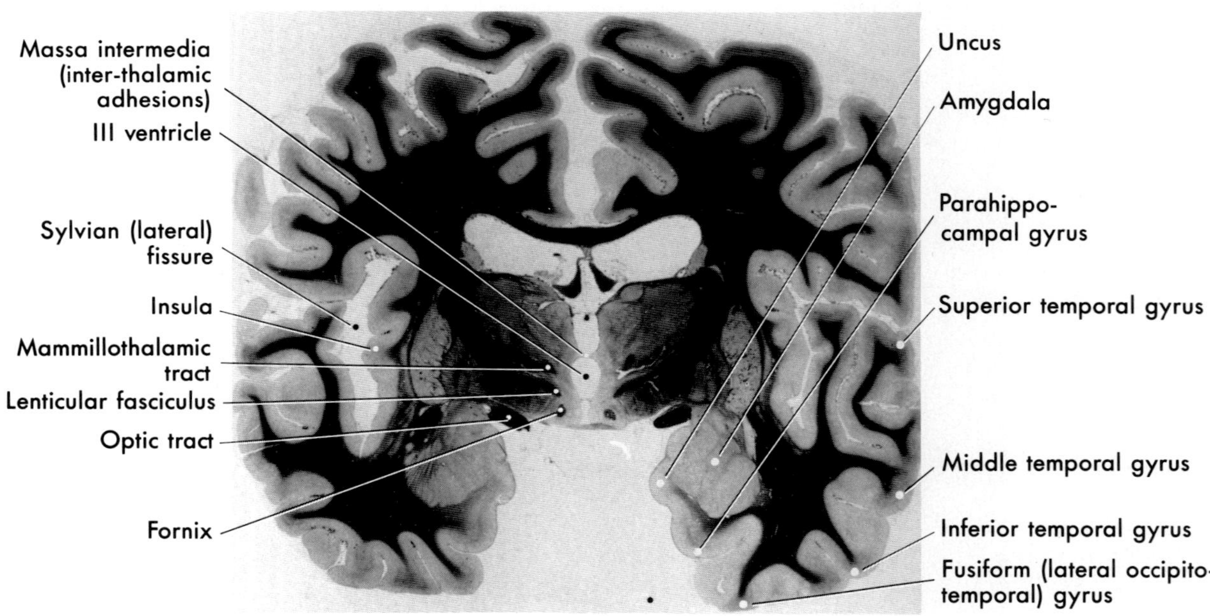

Figure 3-16

CORONAL IMAGES

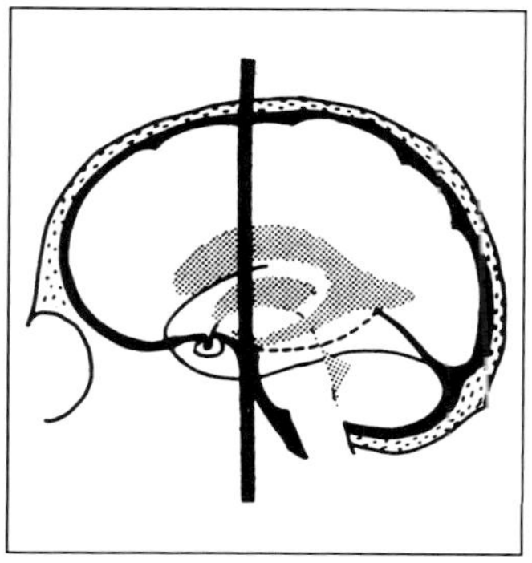

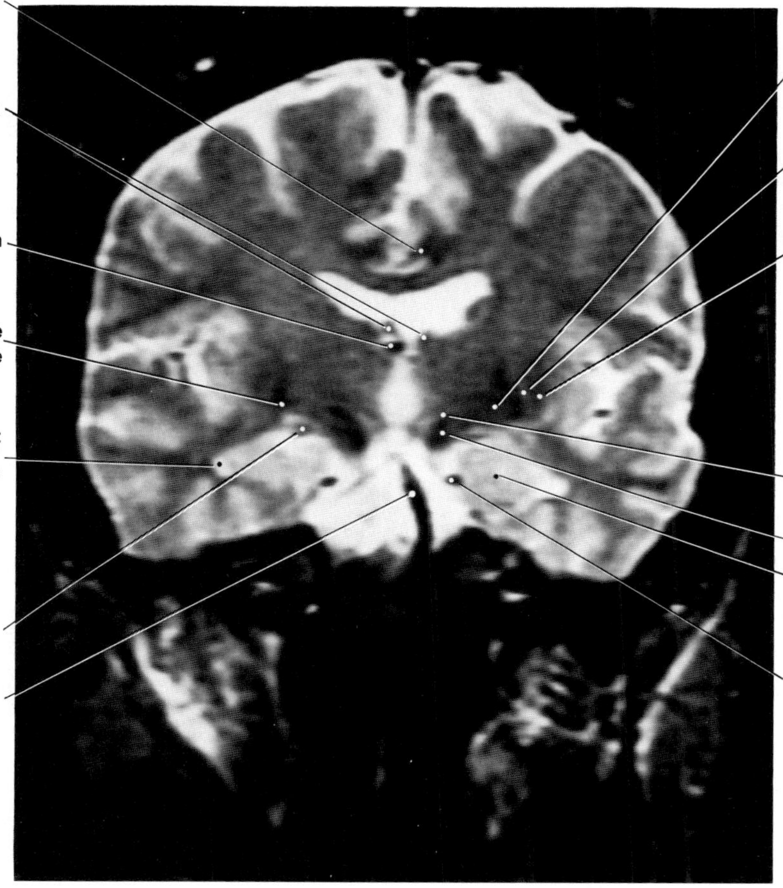

Figure 3-17

CORONAL IMAGES

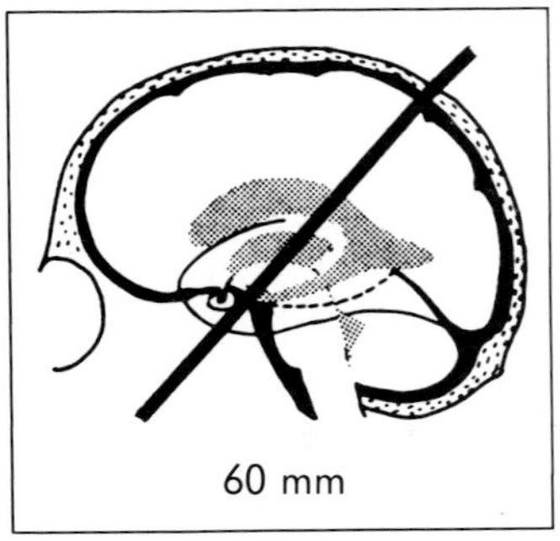

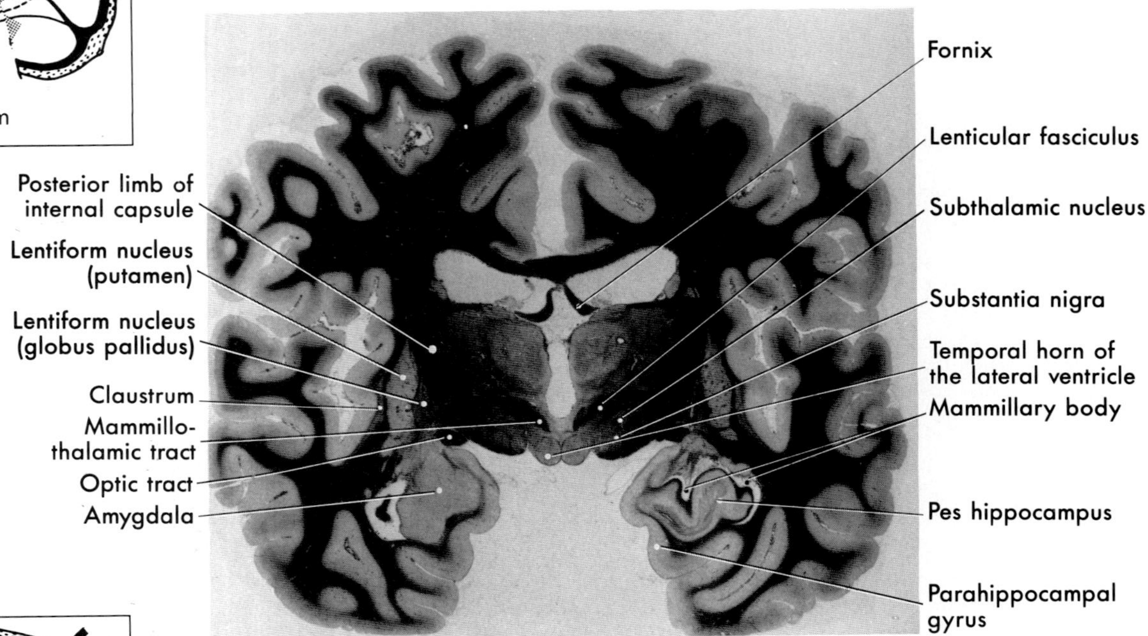

Figure 3-18

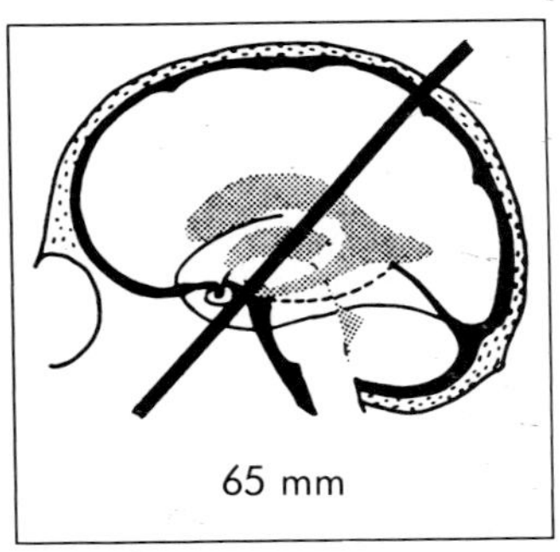

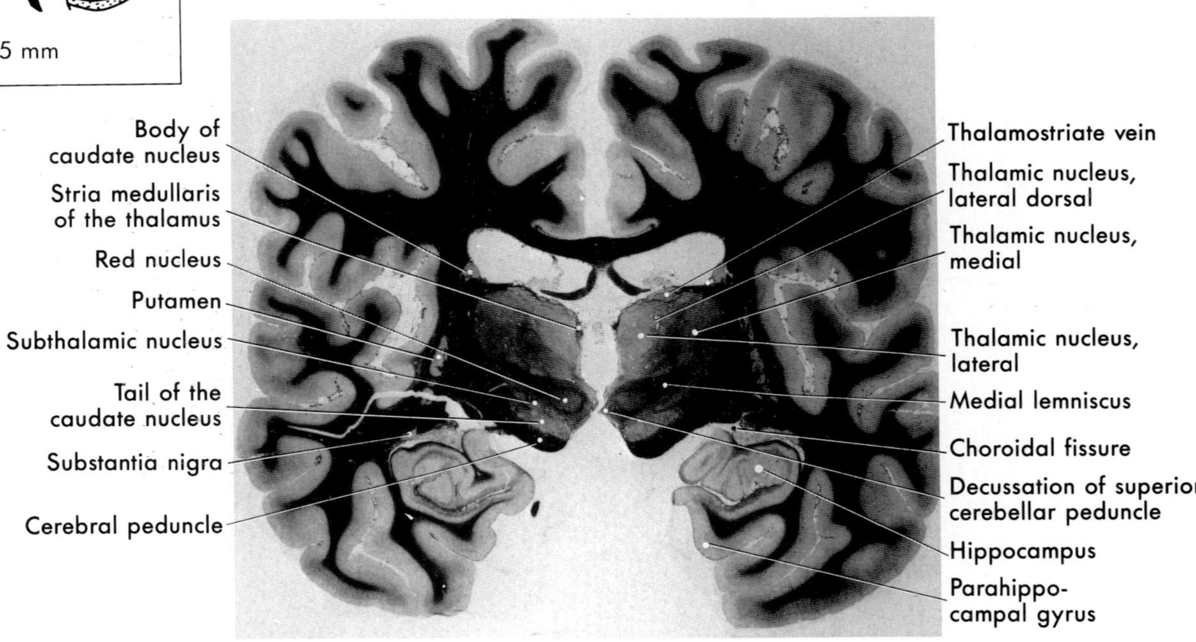

Figure 3-19

CORONAL IMAGES

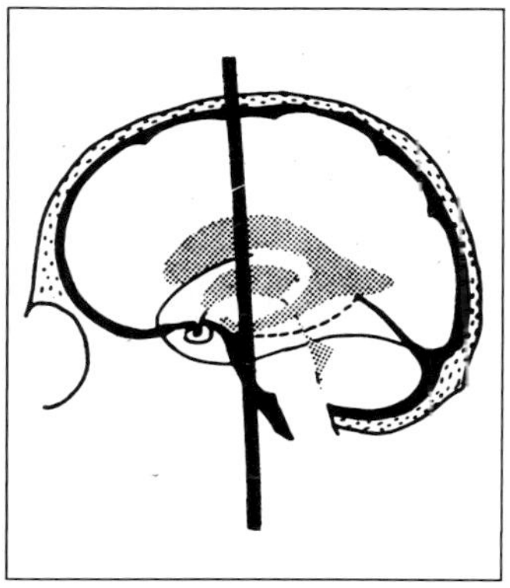

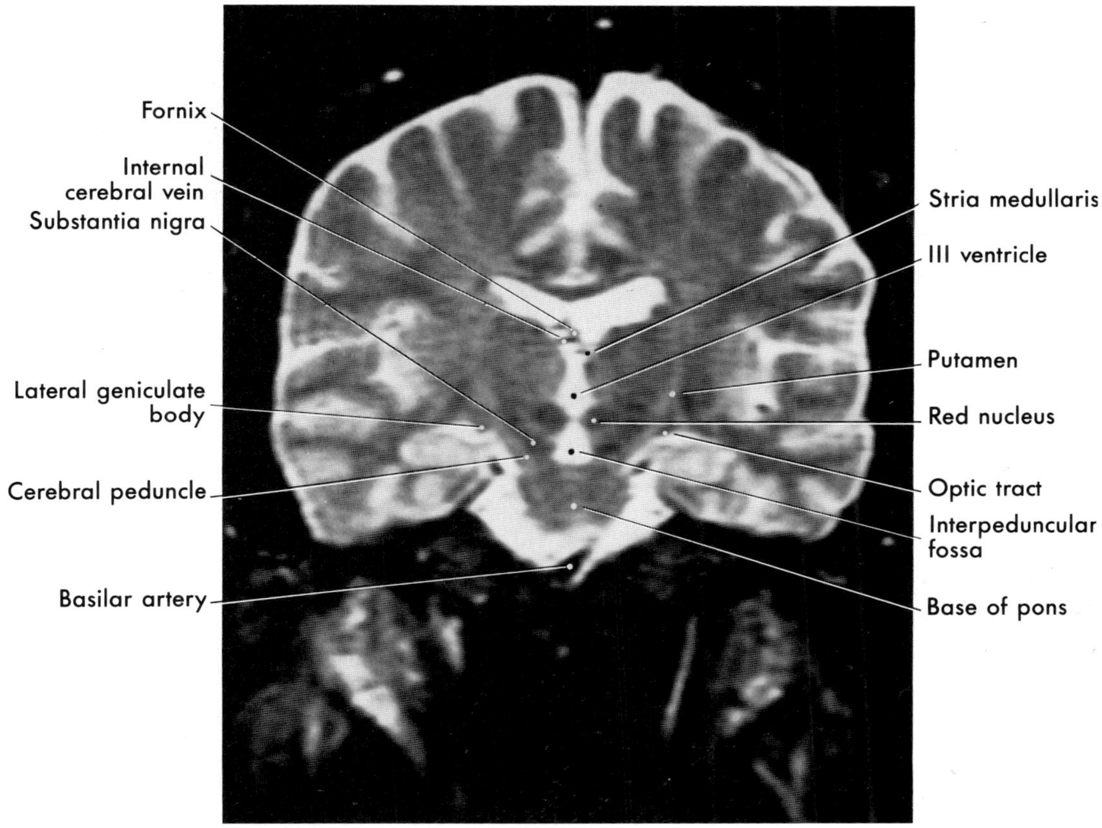

Figure 3-20

CORONAL IMAGES

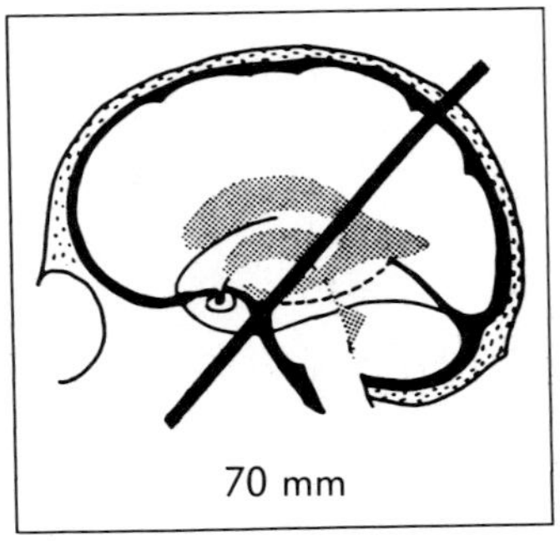

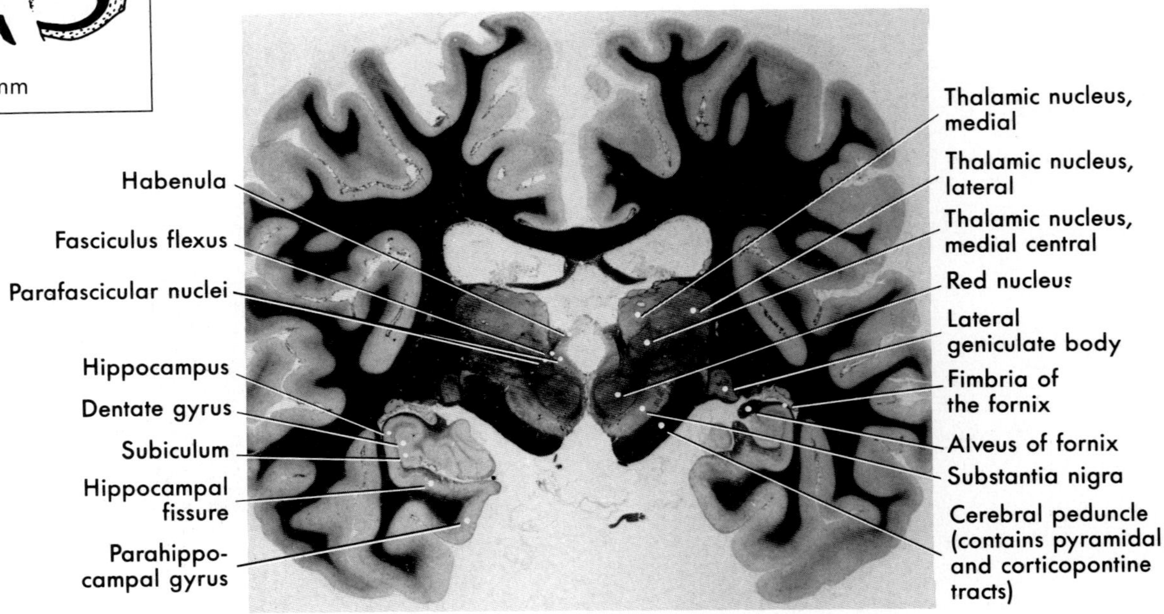

Figure 3-21

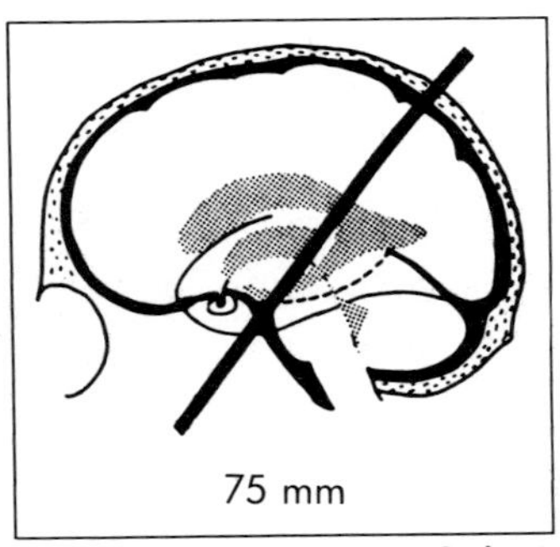

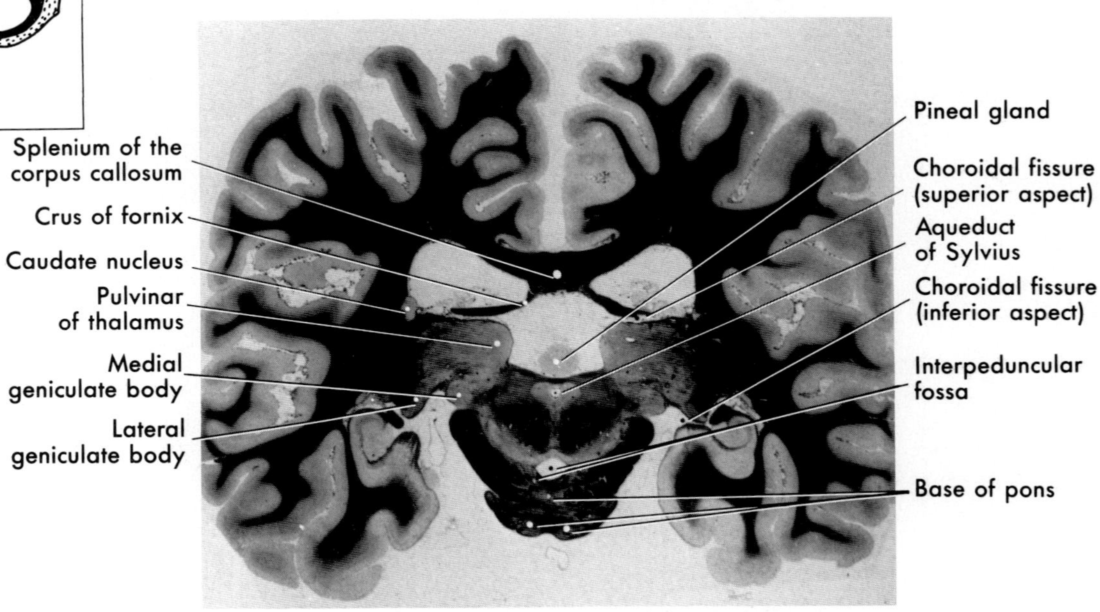

Figure 3-22

CORONAL IMAGES

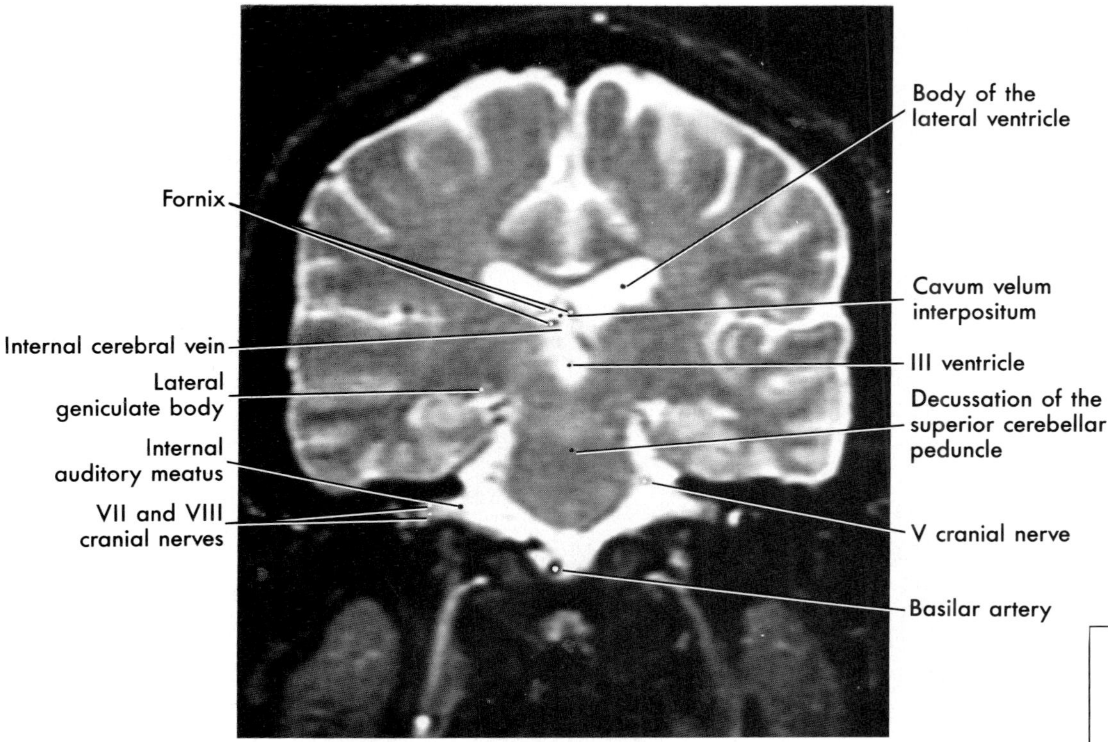

Figure 3-23

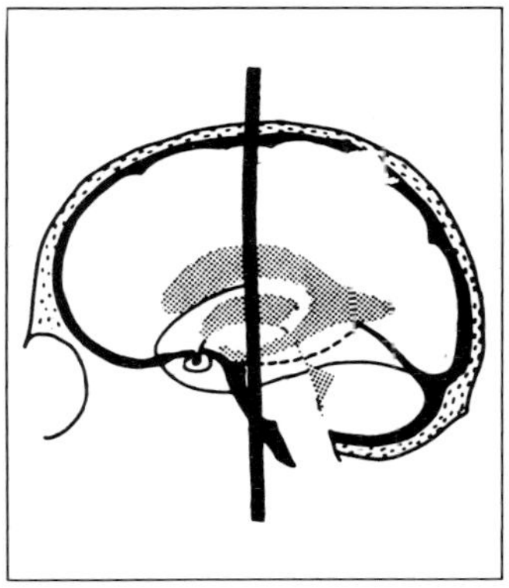

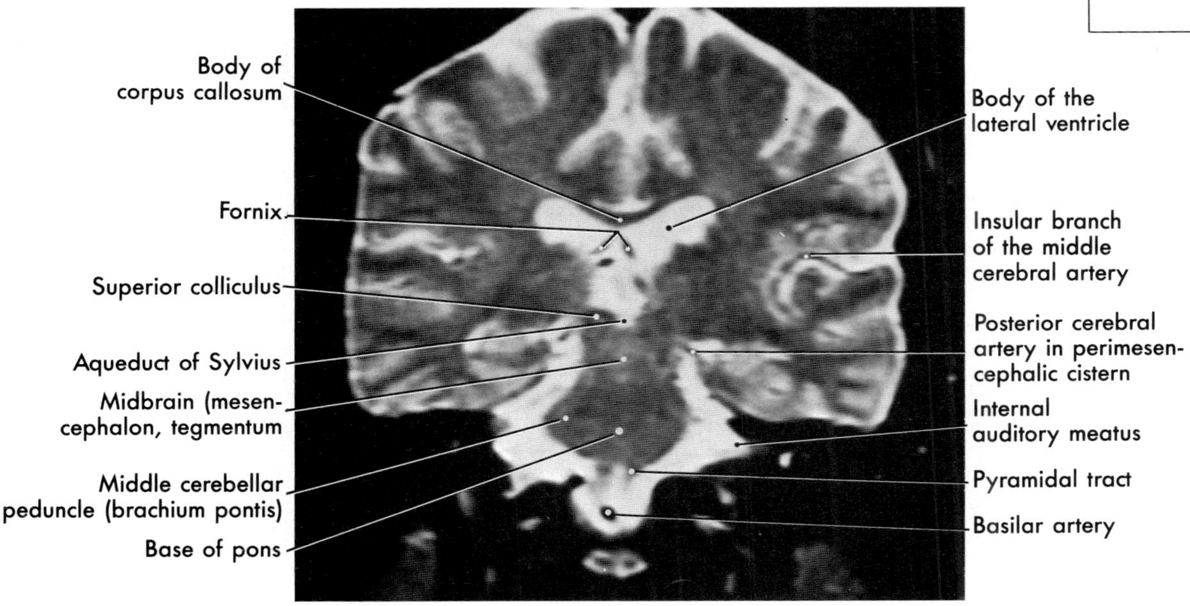

Figure 3-24

CORONAL IMAGES

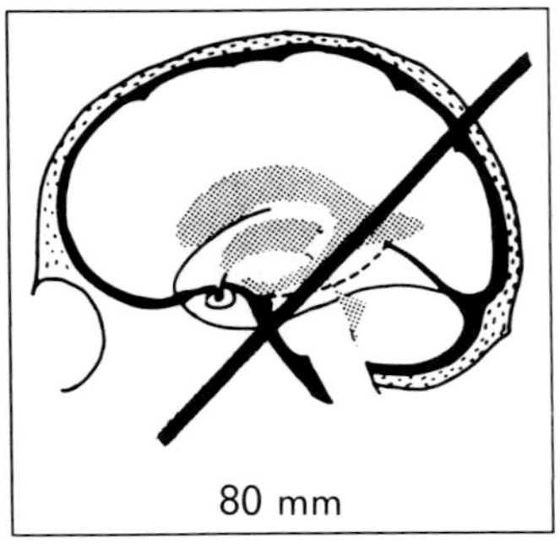

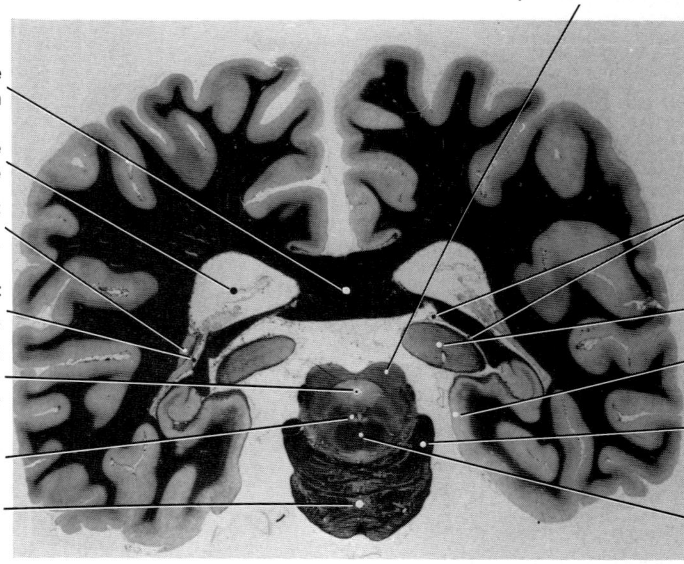

Figure 3-25

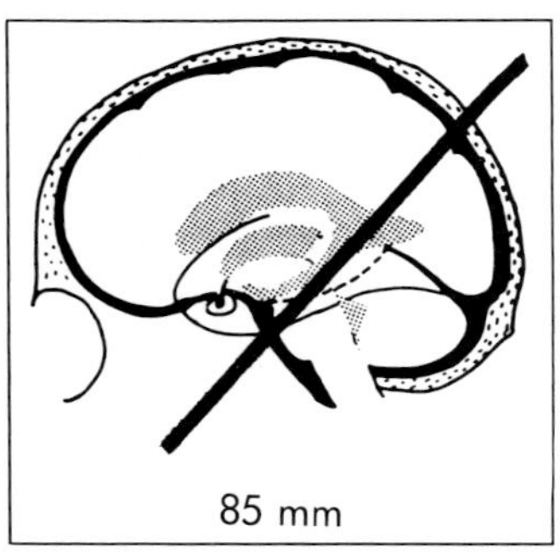

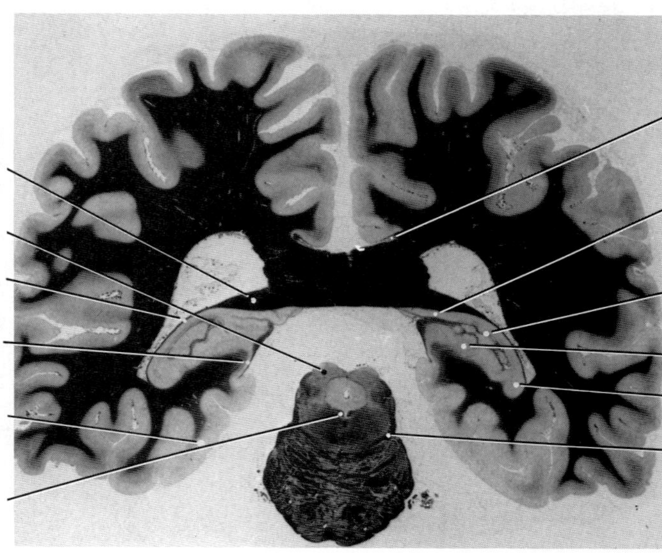

Figure 3-26

CORONAL IMAGES

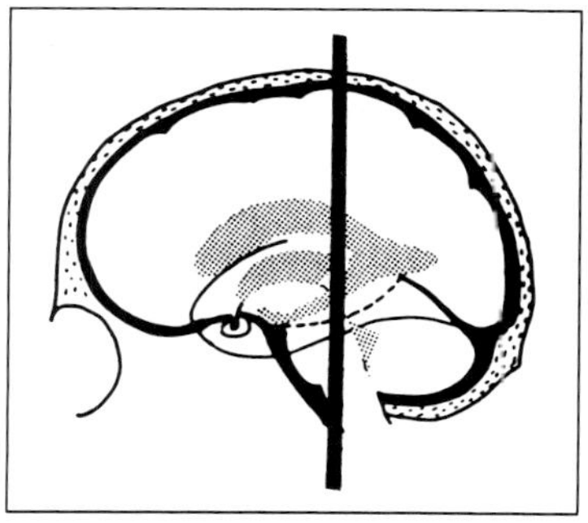

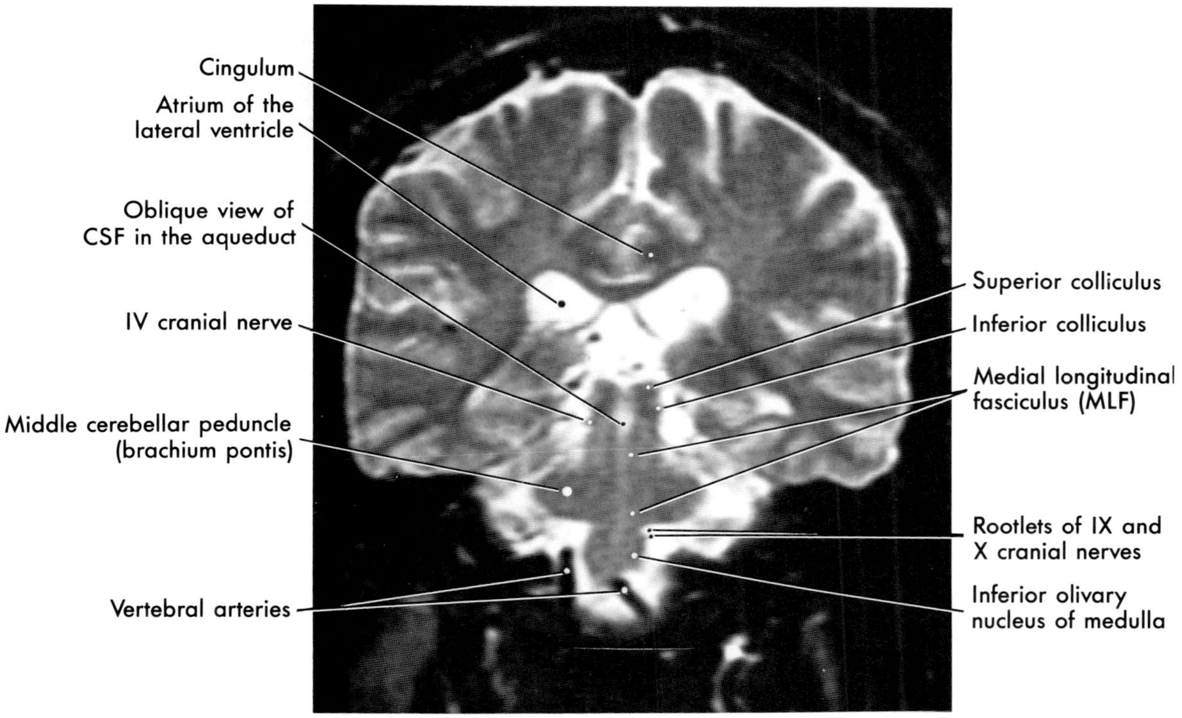

Figure 3-27

CORONAL IMAGES

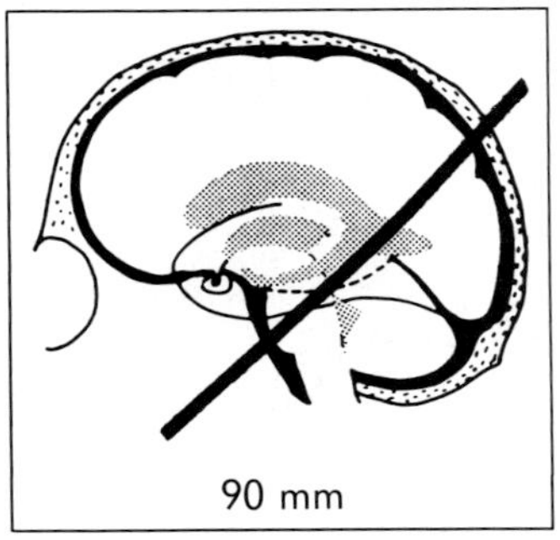

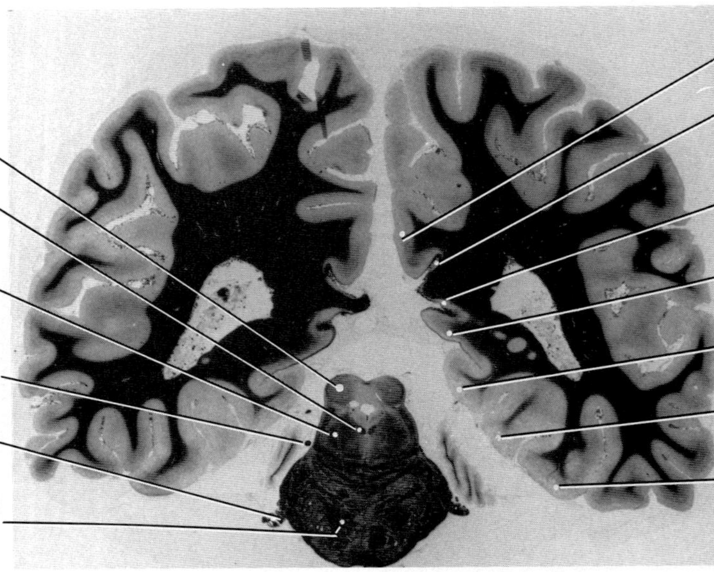

Figure 3-28

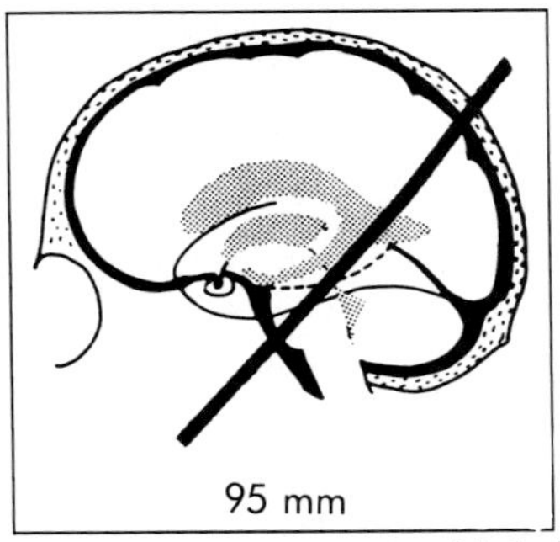

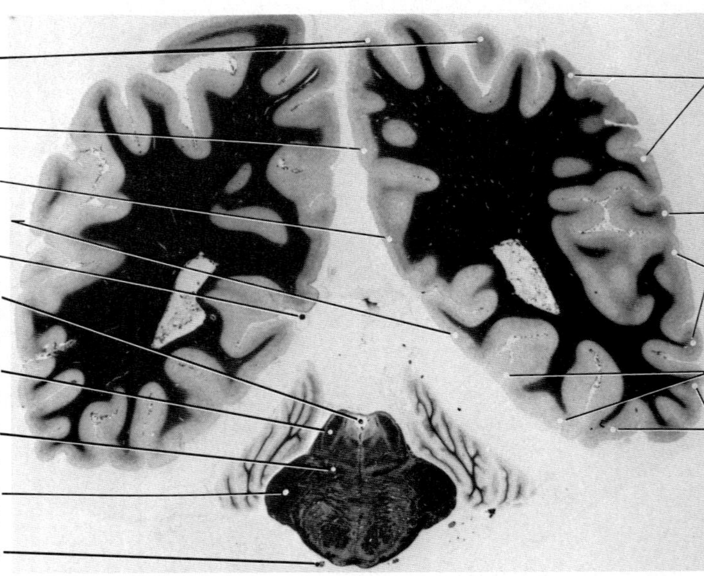

Figure 3-29

CORONAL IMAGES

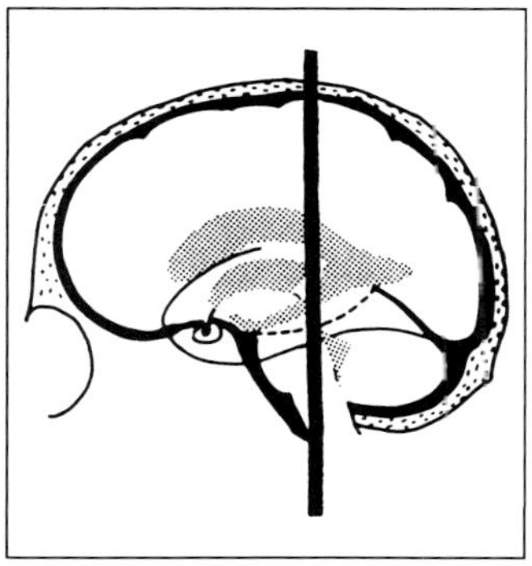

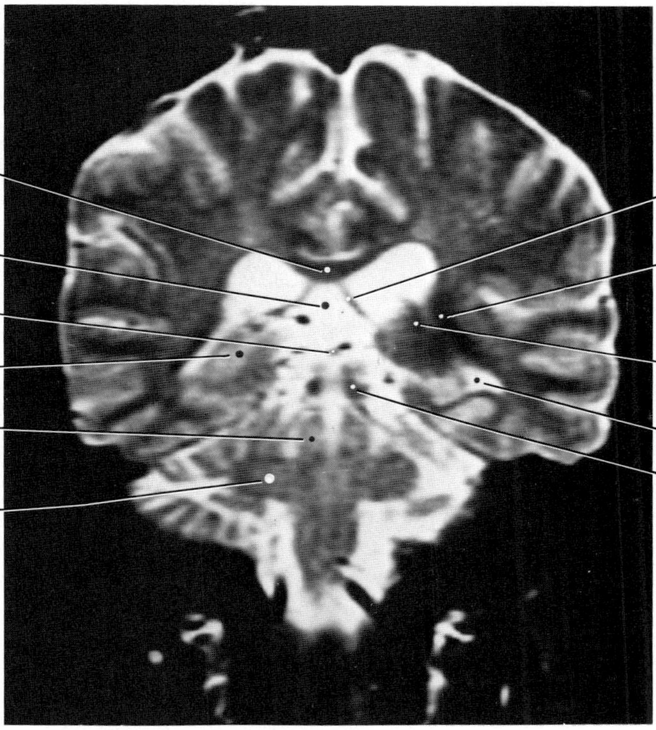

Figure 3-30

CORONAL IMAGES

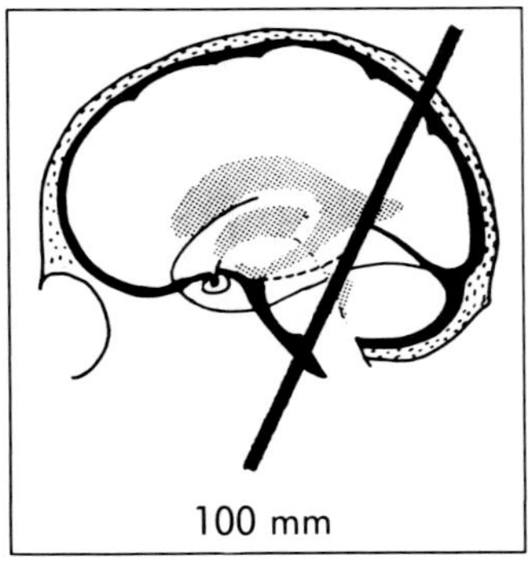

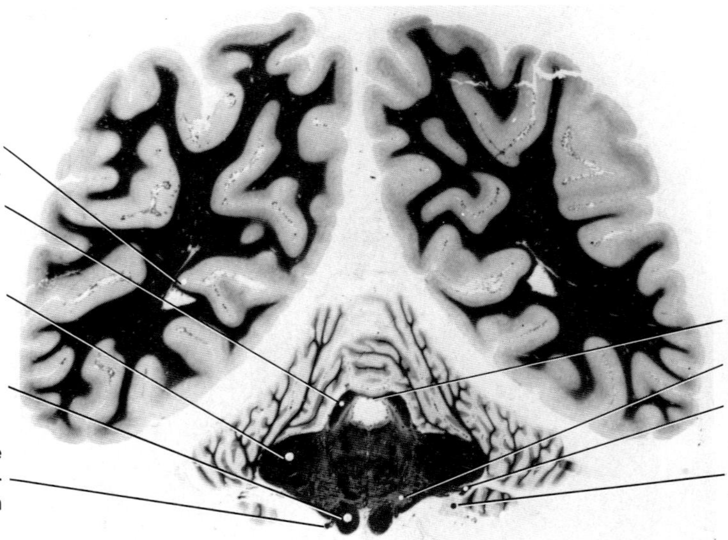

Figure 3-31

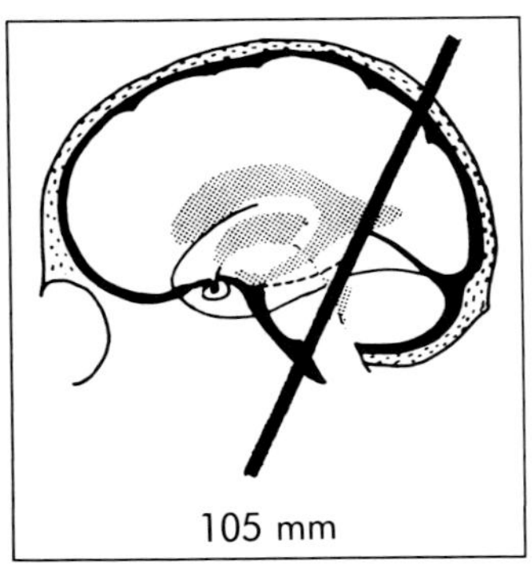

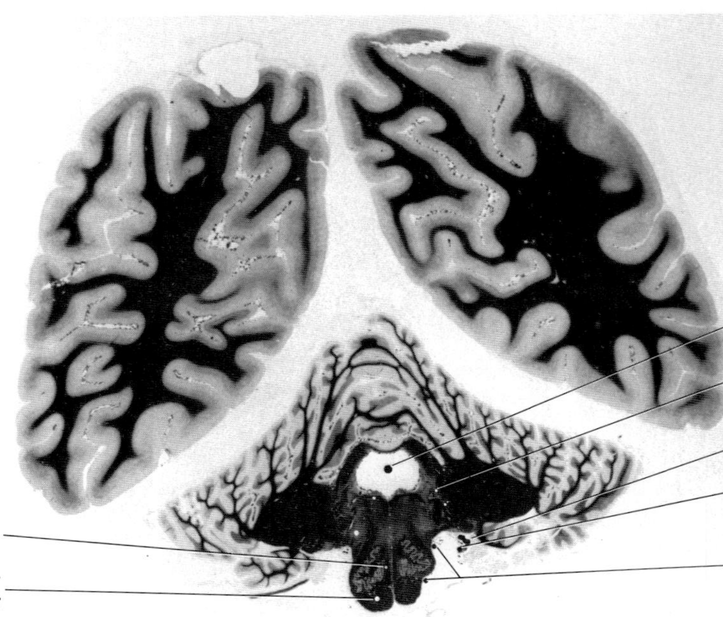

Figure 3-32

CORONAL IMAGES

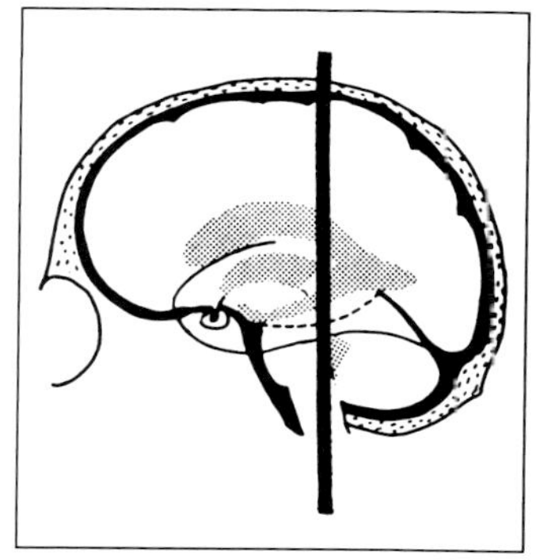

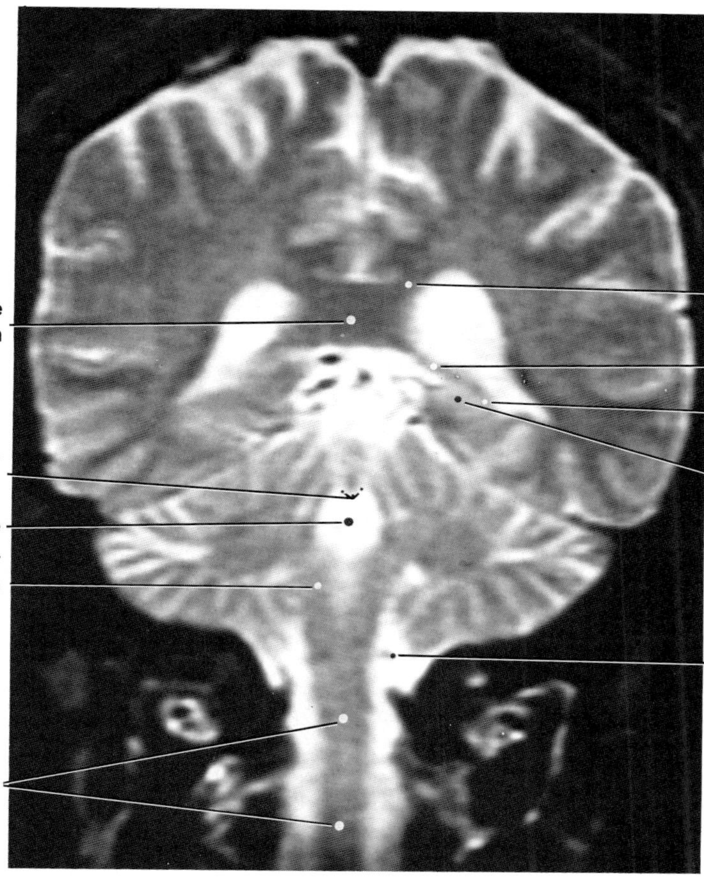

Figure 3-33

CORONAL IMAGES

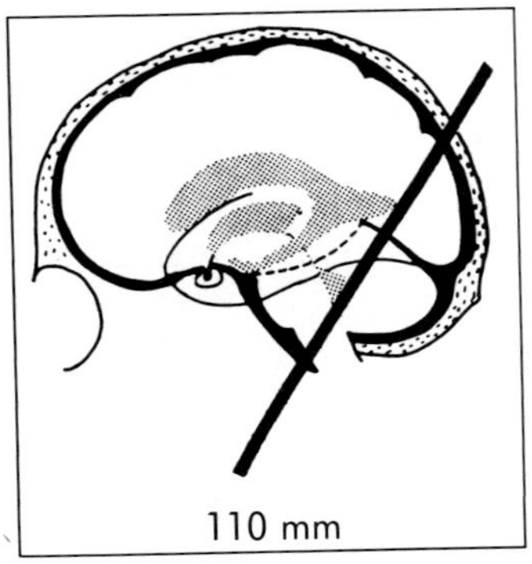

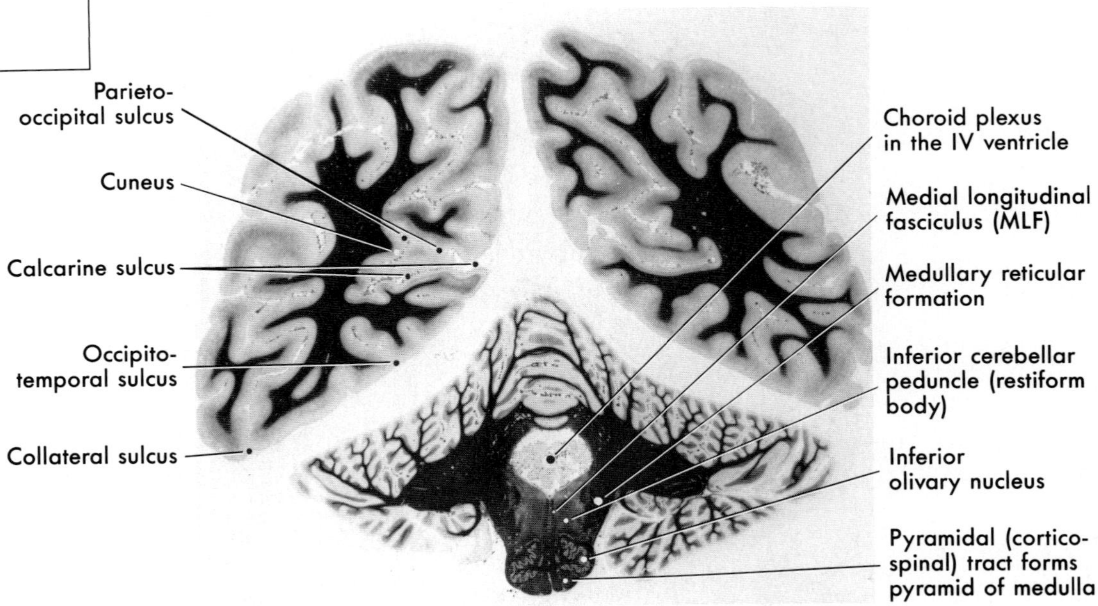

Figure 3-34

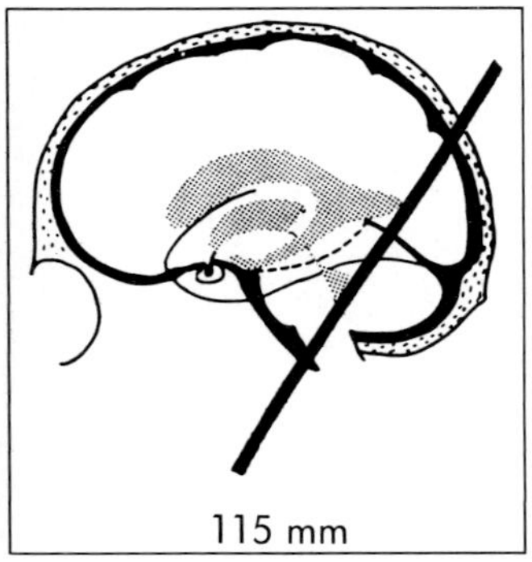

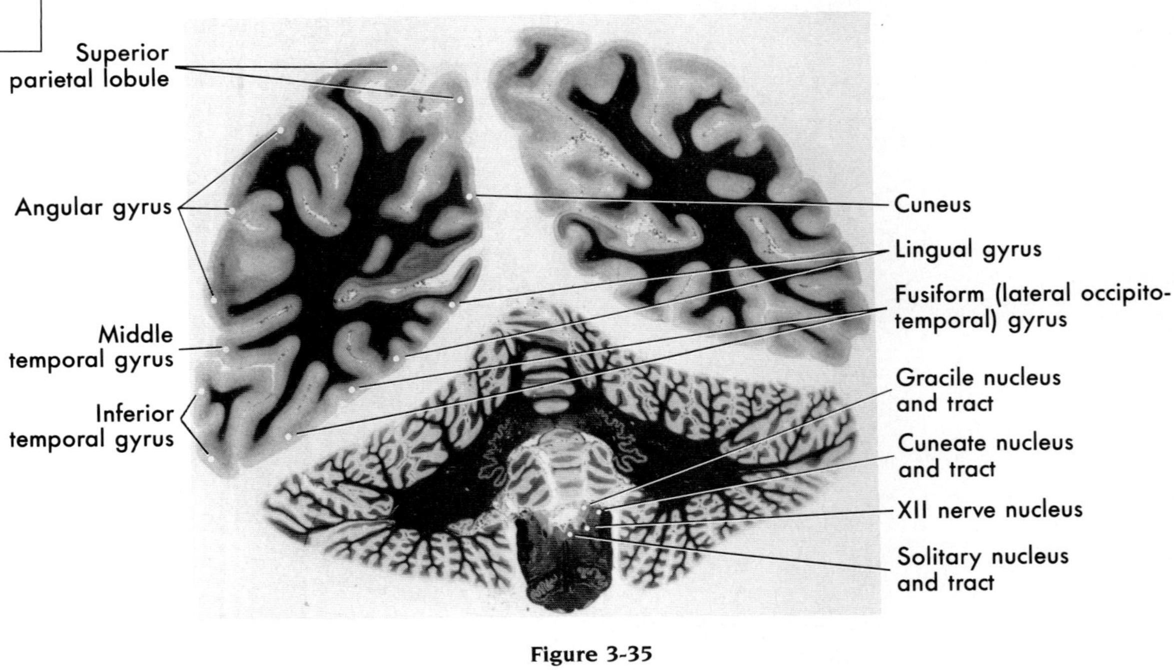

Figure 3-35

CORONAL IMAGES

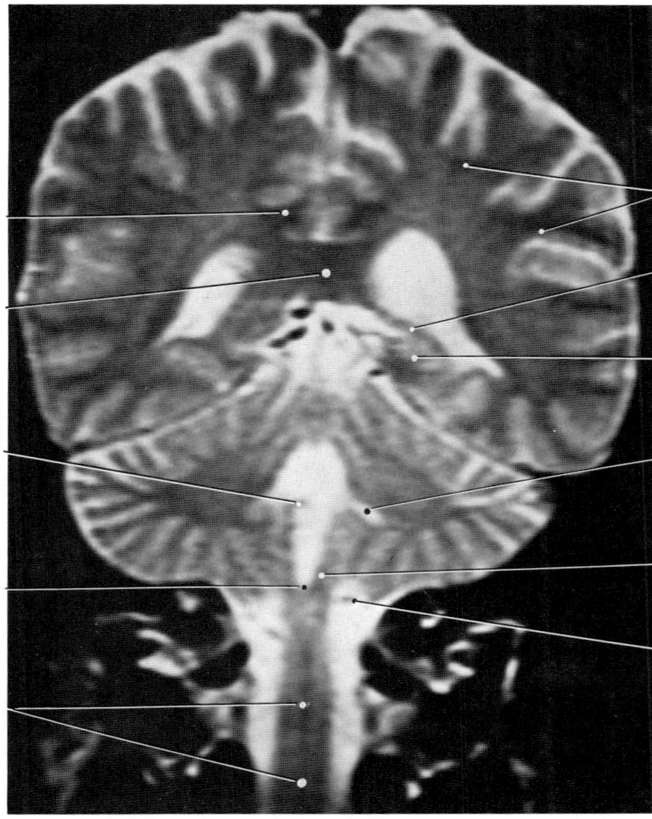

Figure 3-36

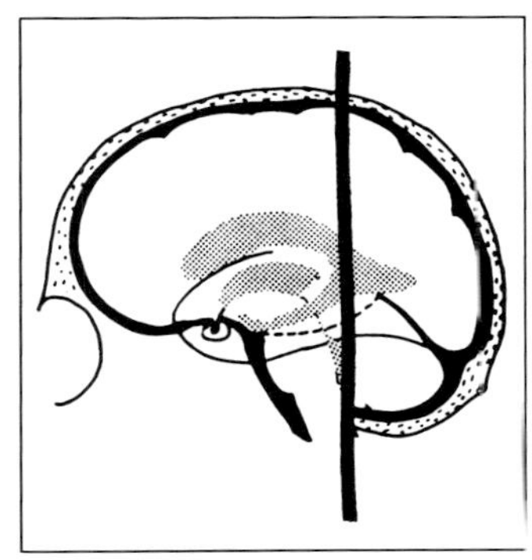

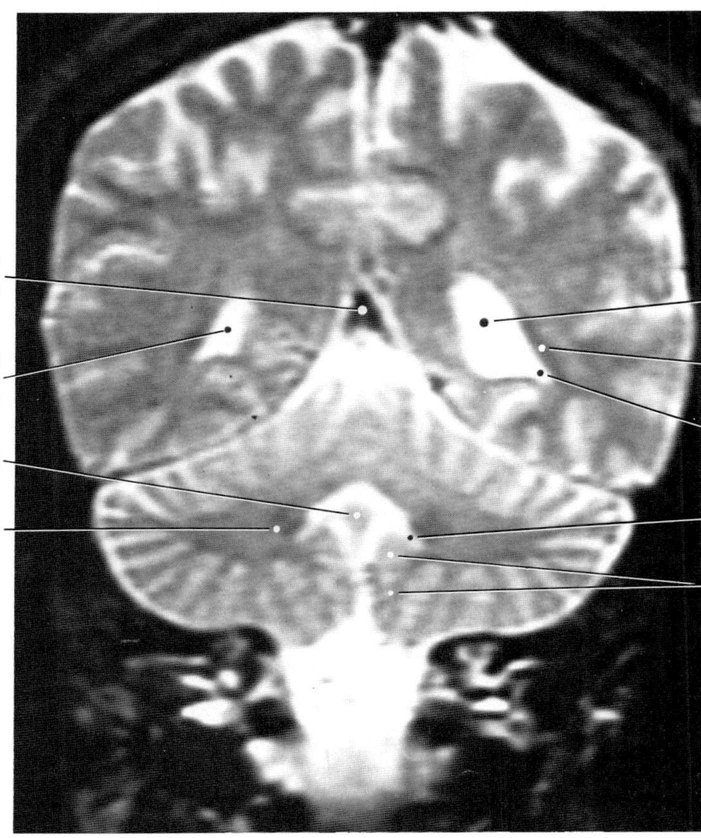

Figure 3-37

CORONAL IMAGES

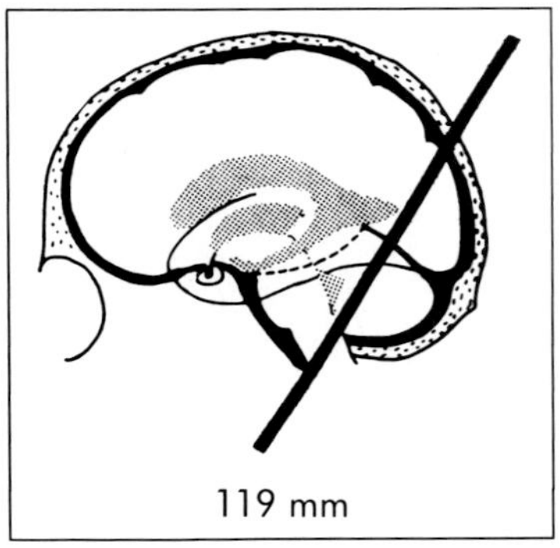

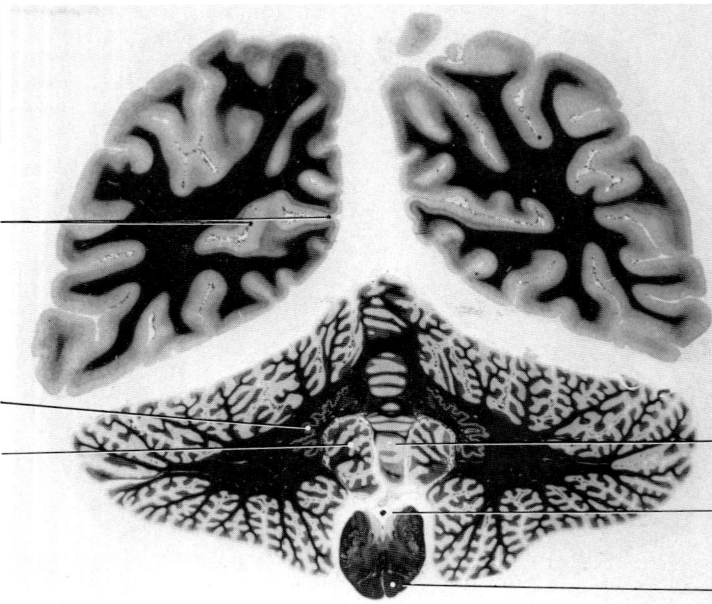

Figure 3-38

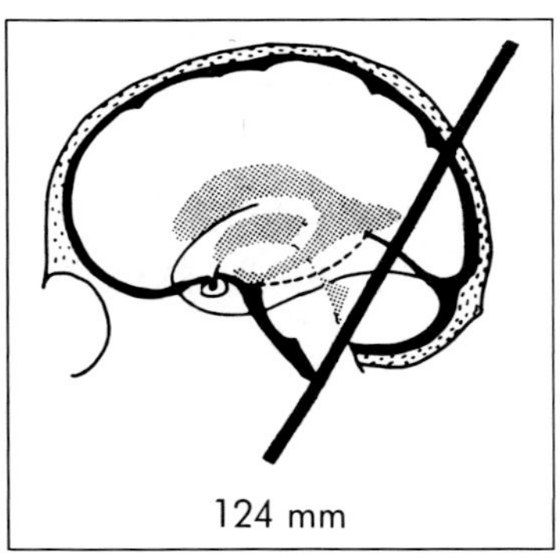

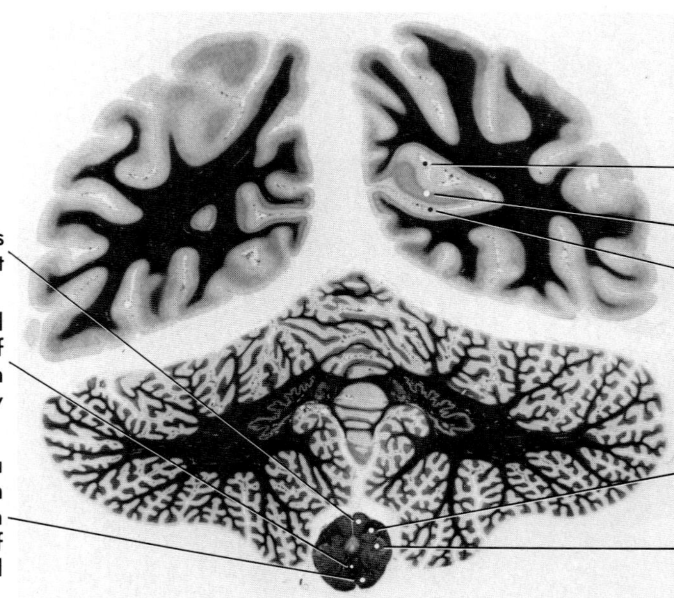

Figure 3-39

CORONAL IMAGES

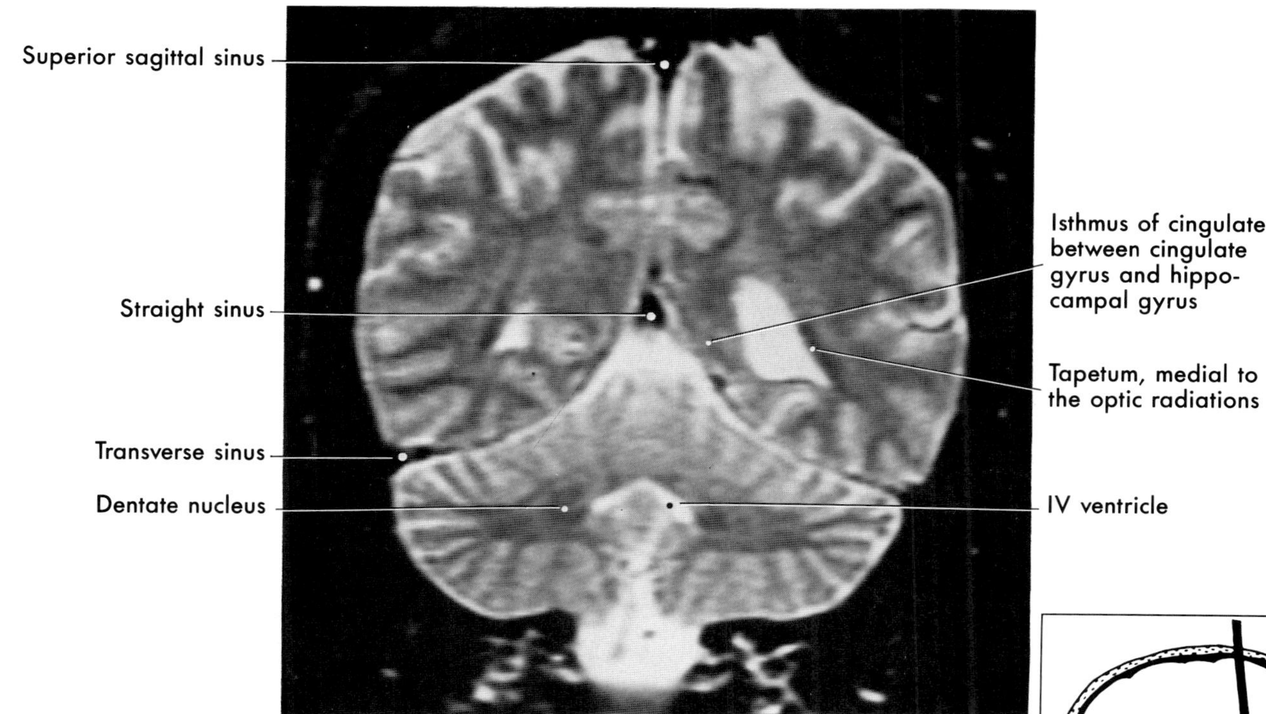

Figure 3-40

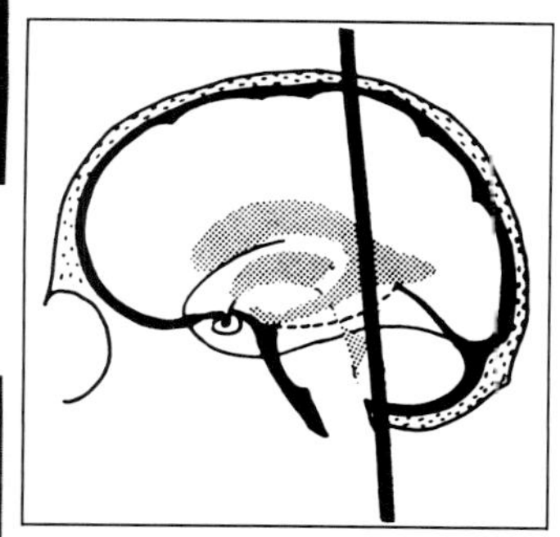

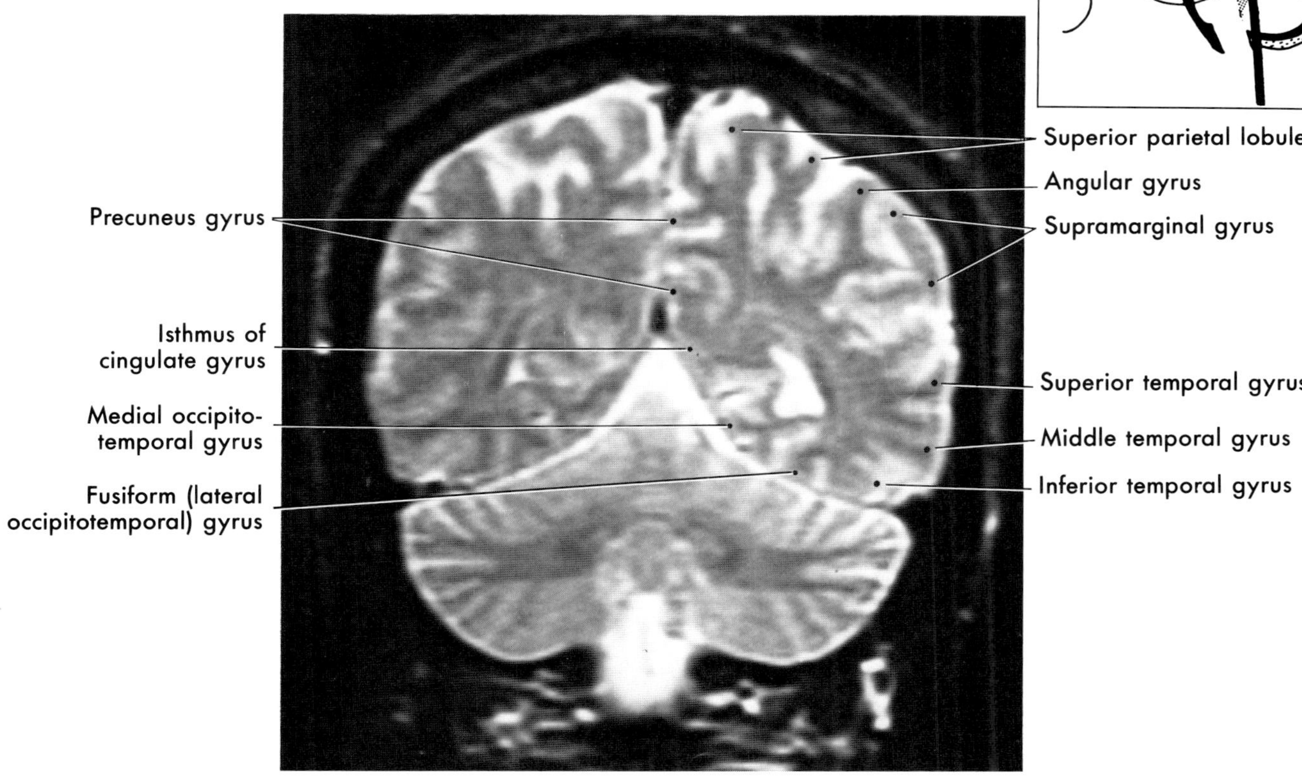

Figure 3-41

CORONAL IMAGES

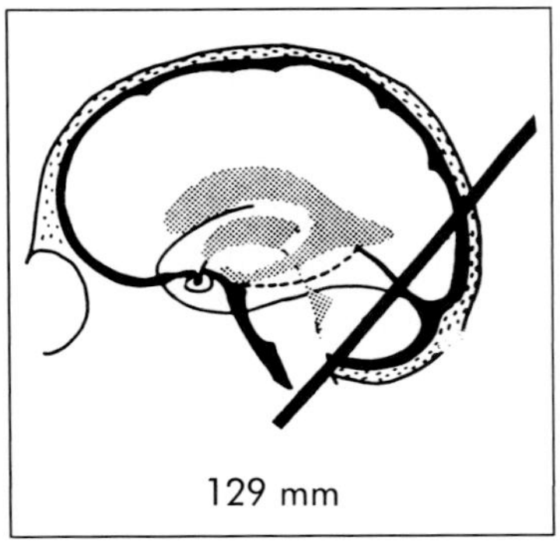

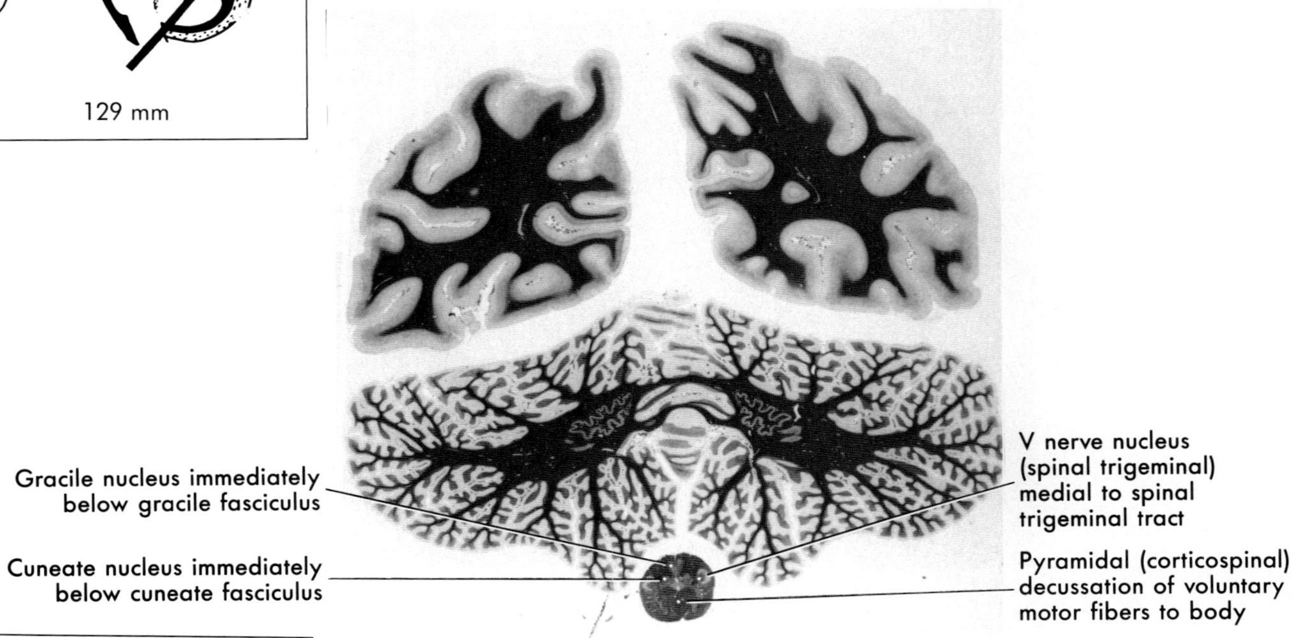

Figure 3-42

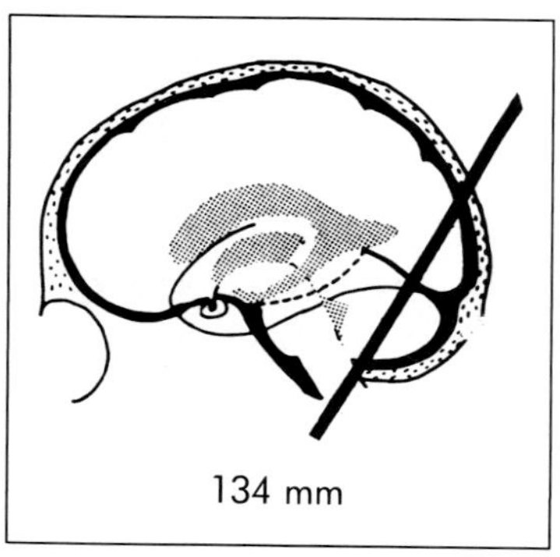

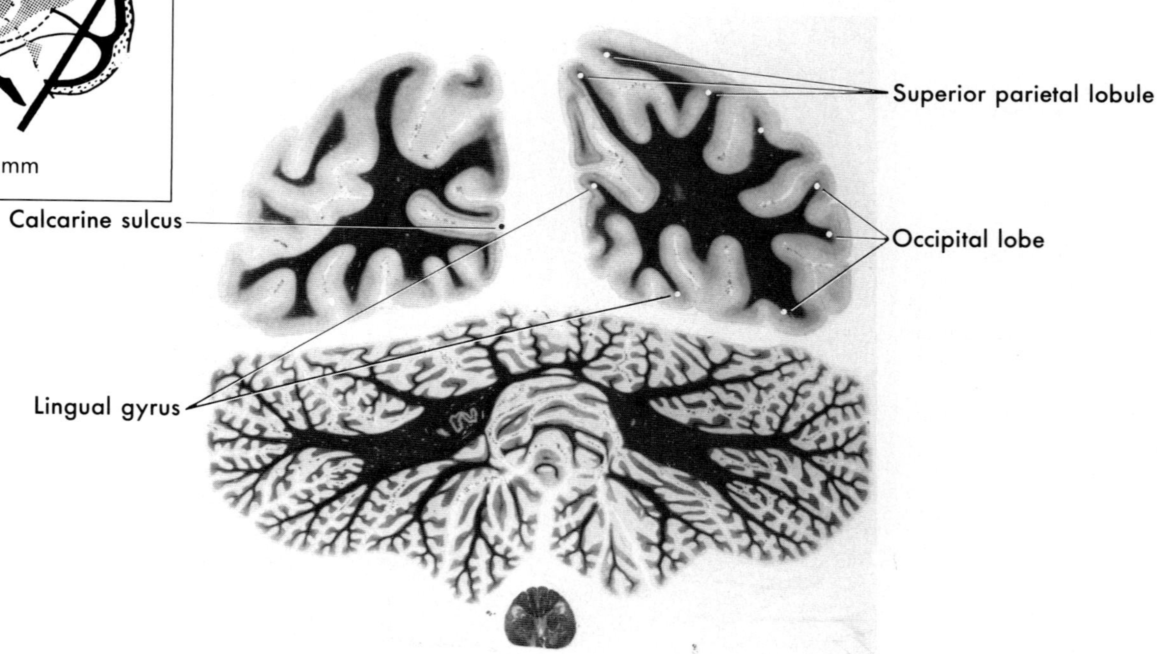

Figure 3-43

AXIAL IMAGES

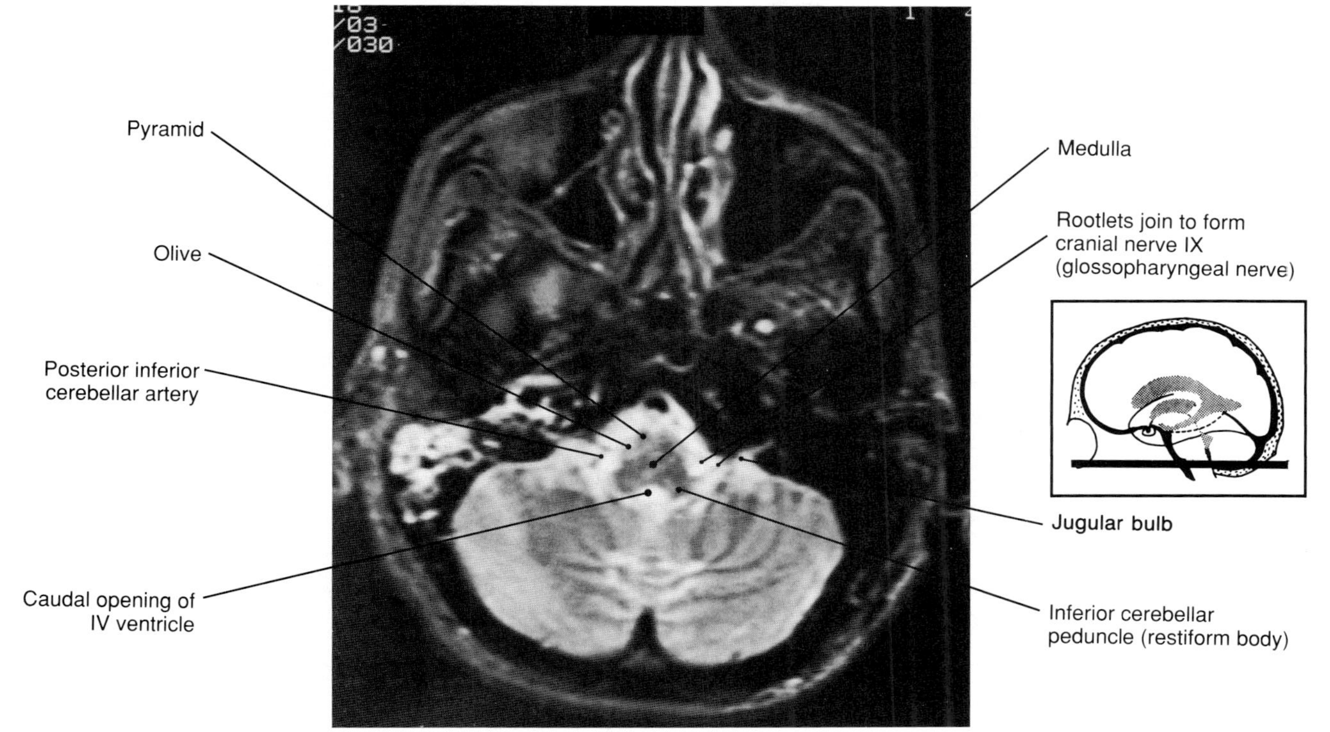

Figure 3-44

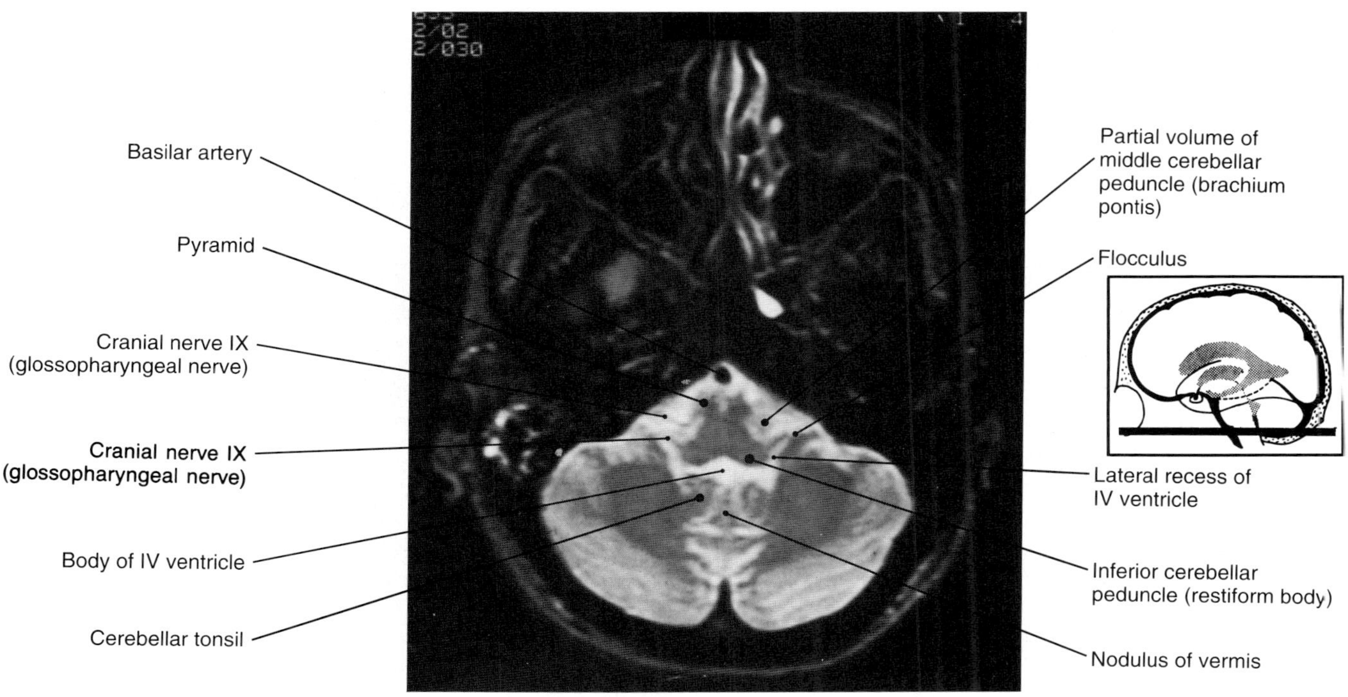

Figure 3-45

AXIAL IMAGES

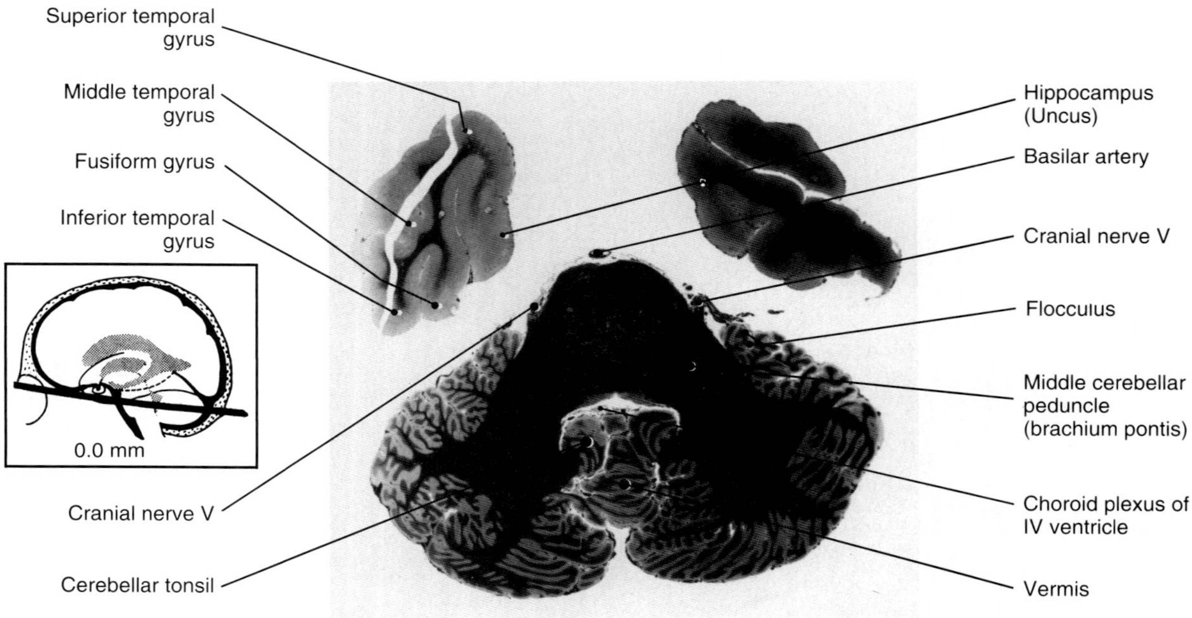

Figure 3-46

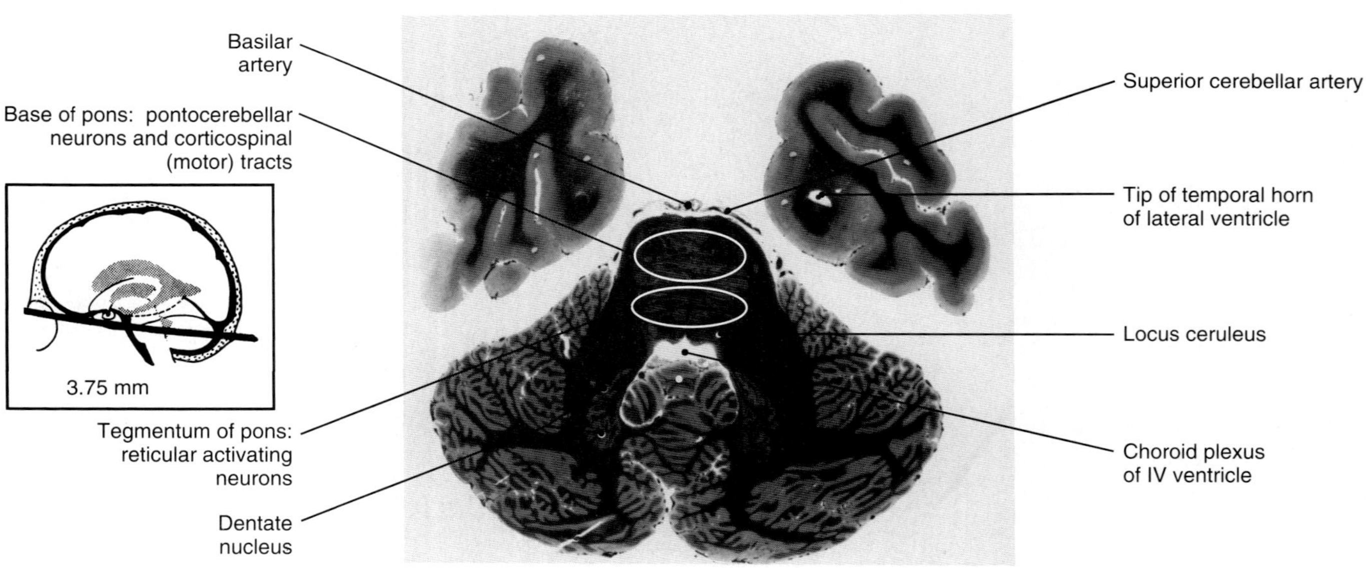

Figure 3-47

AXIAL IMAGES

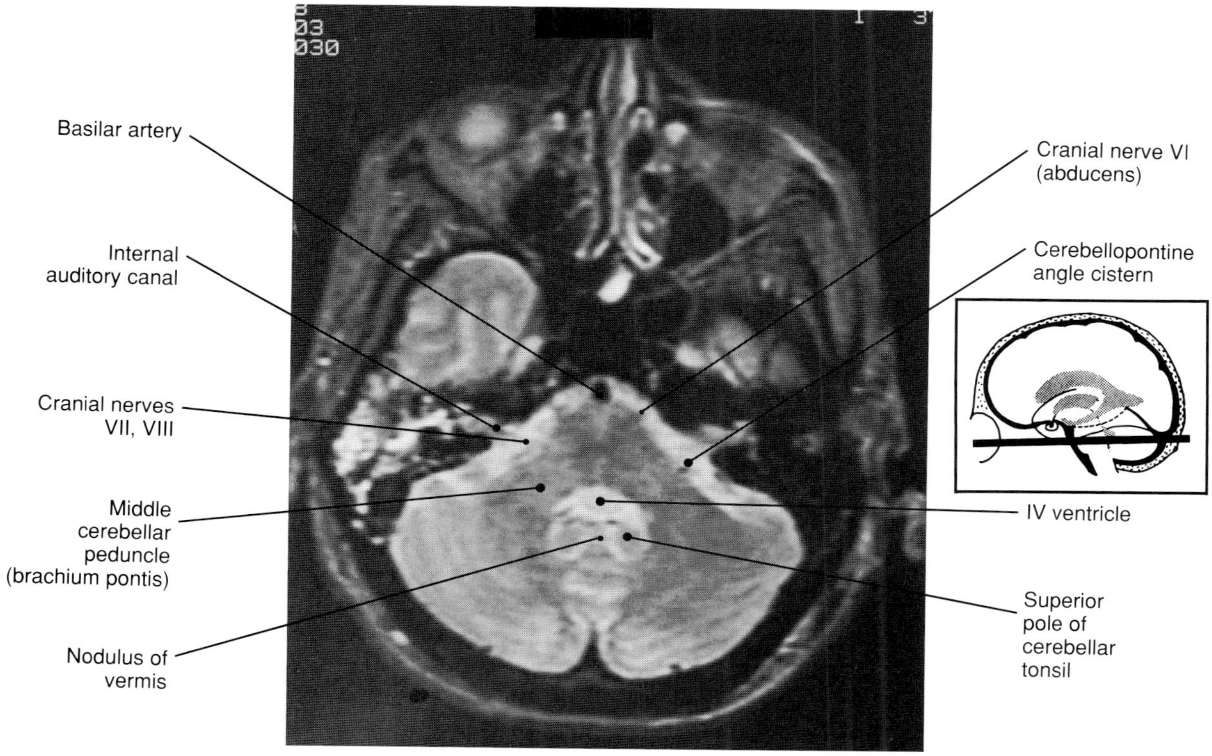

Figure 3-48

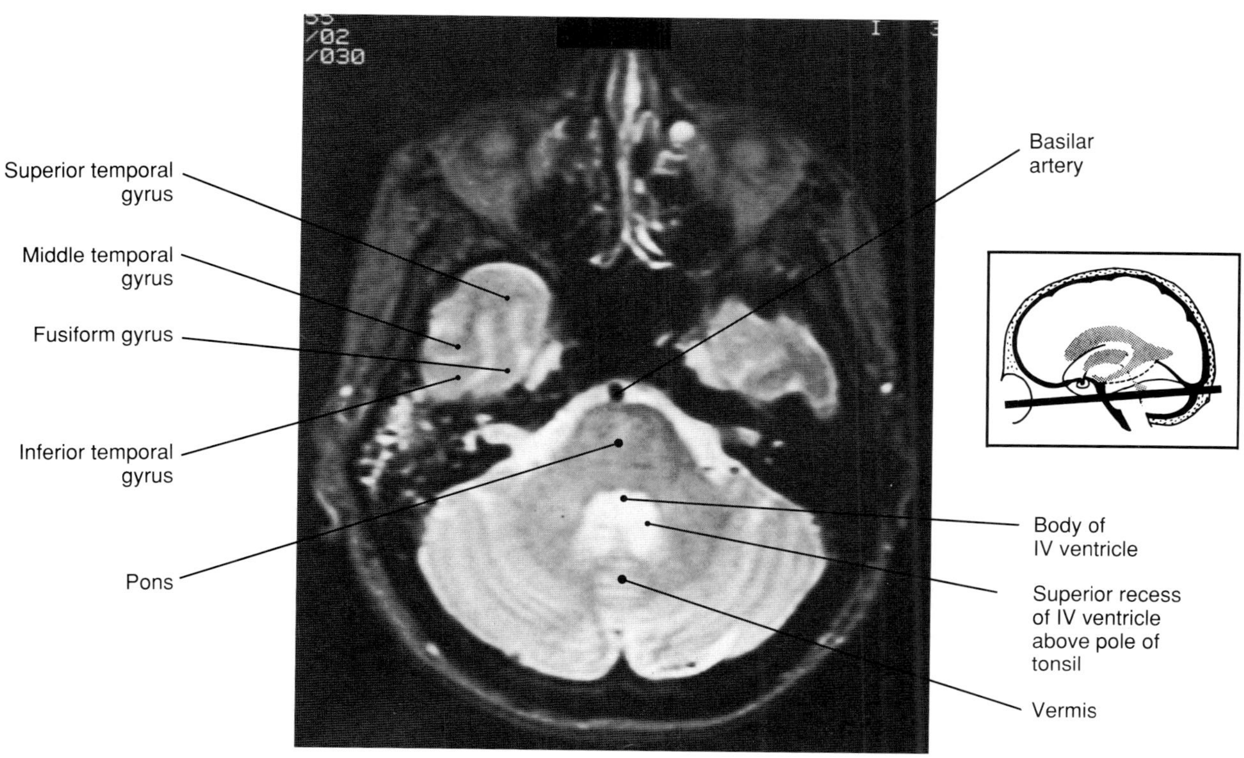

Figure 3-49

AXIAL IMAGES

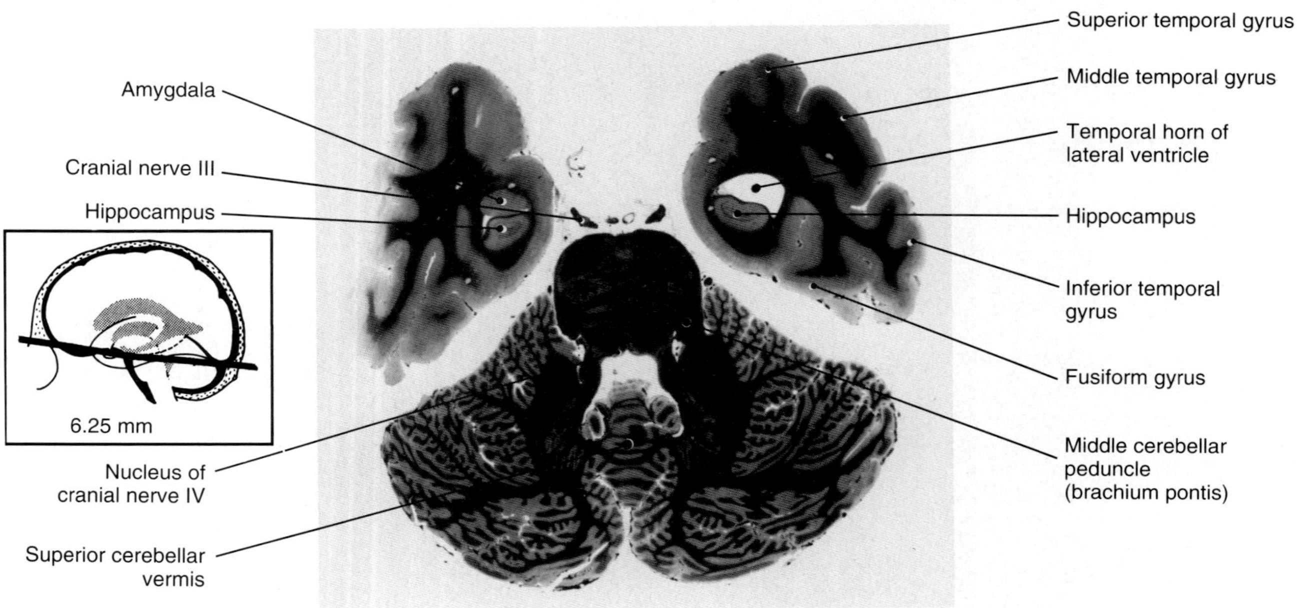

Figure 3-50

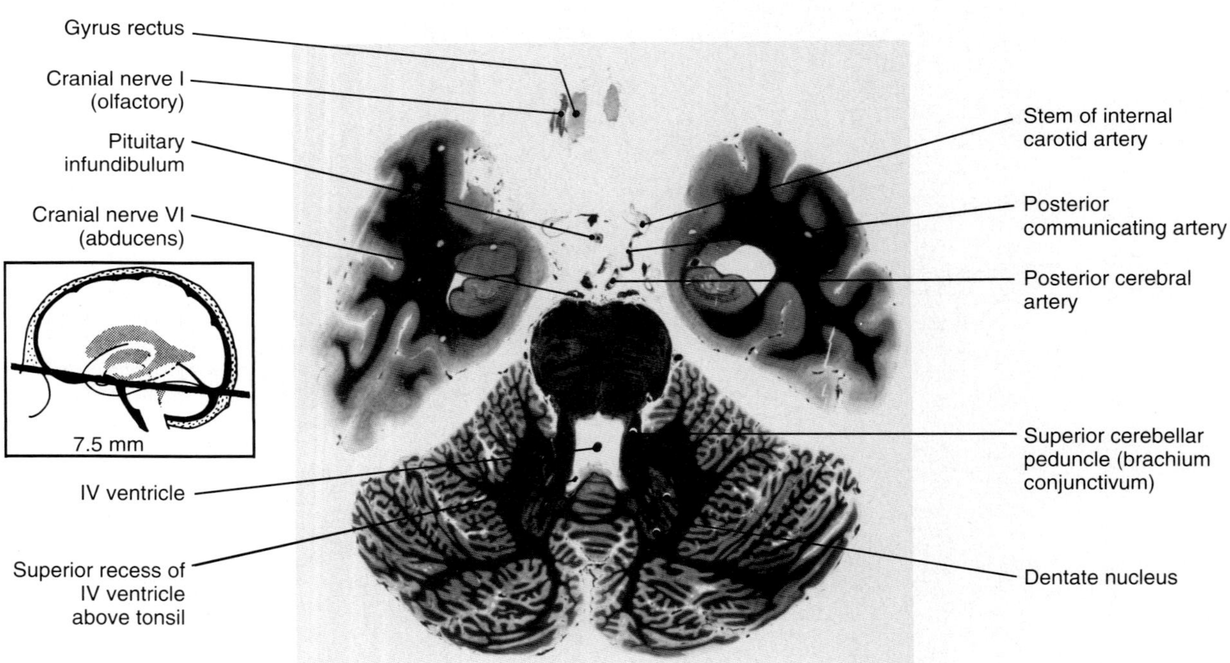

Figure 3-51

AXIAL IMAGES

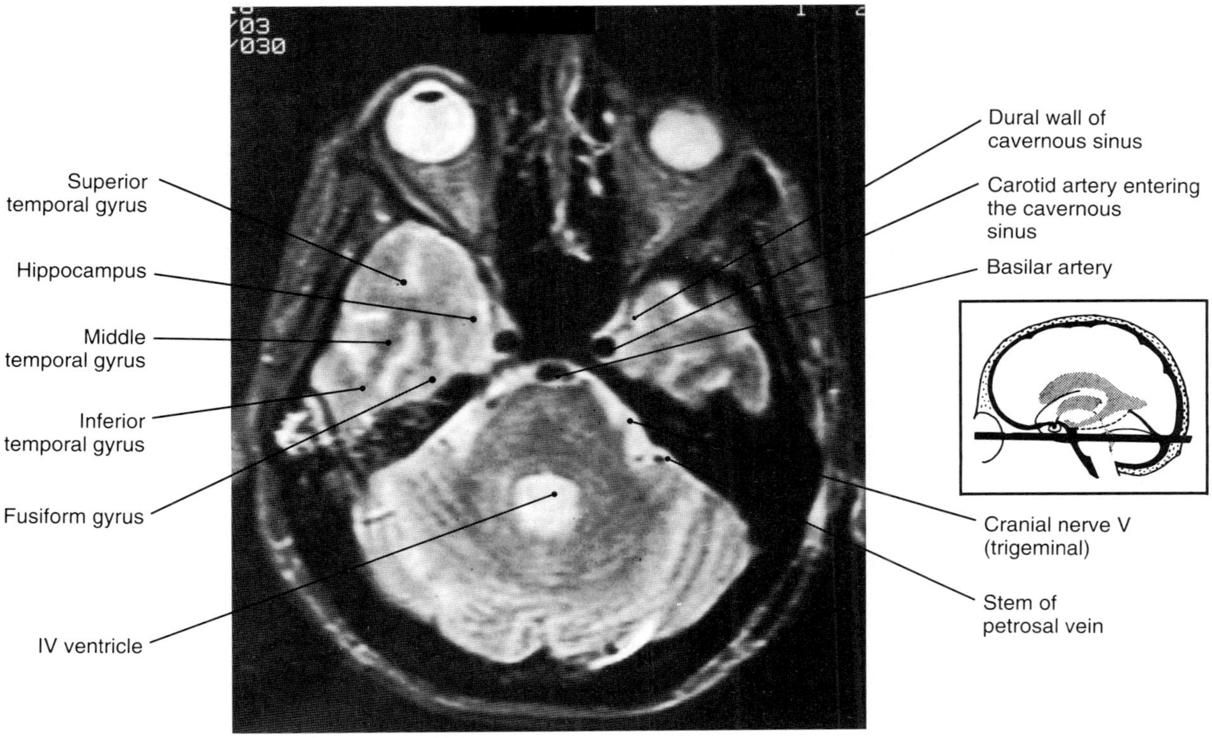

Figure 3-52

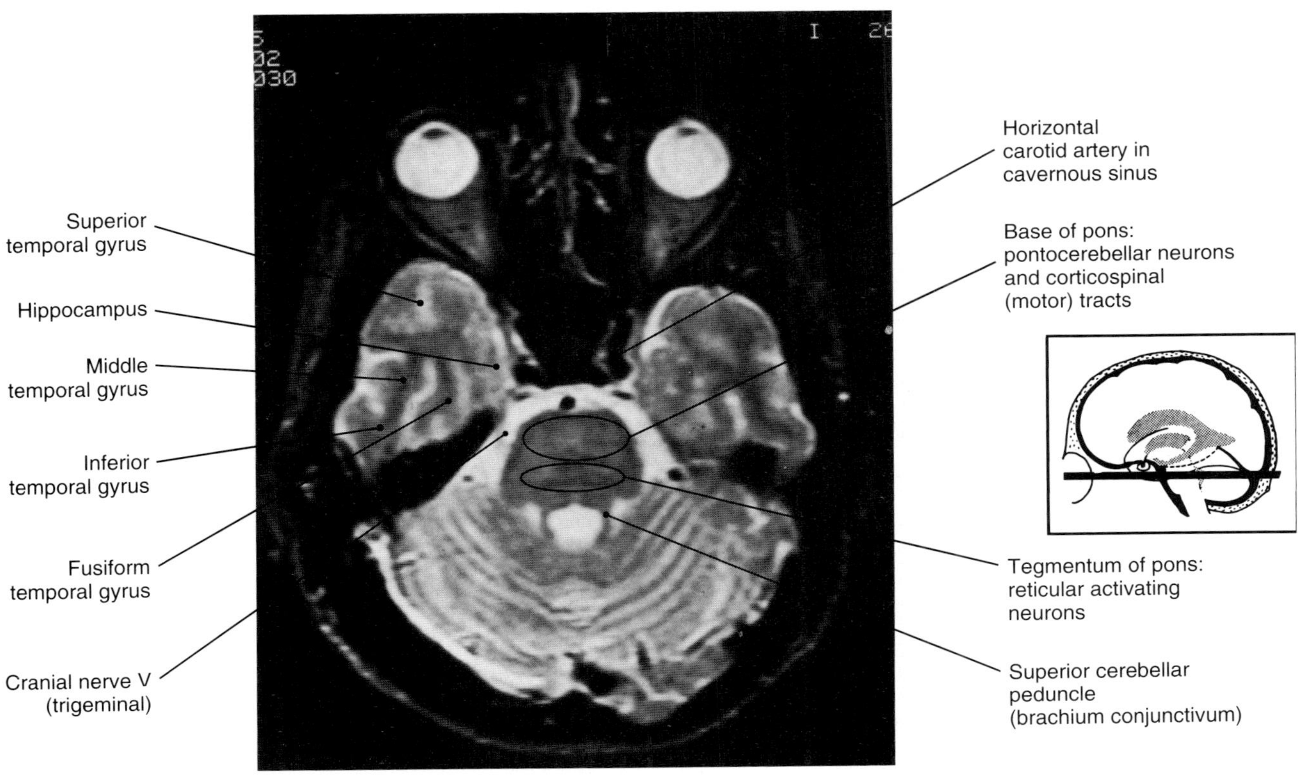

Figure 3-53

AXIAL IMAGES

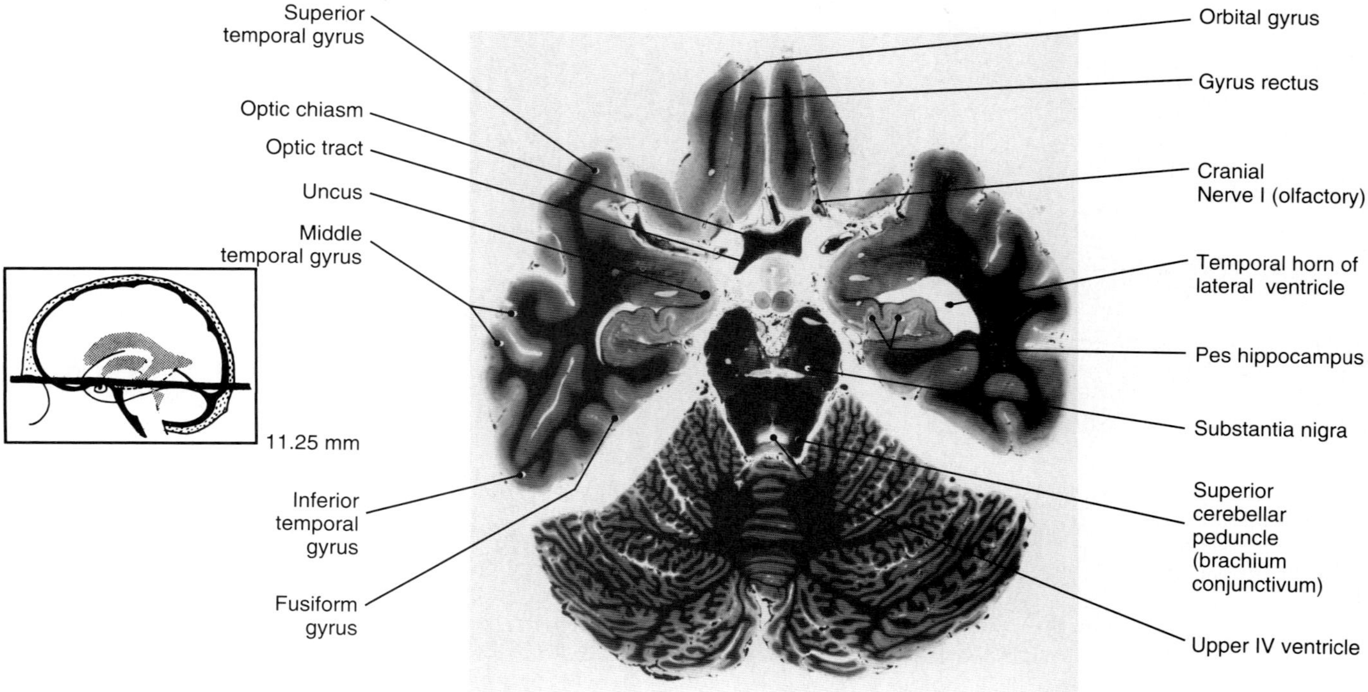

Figure 3-54

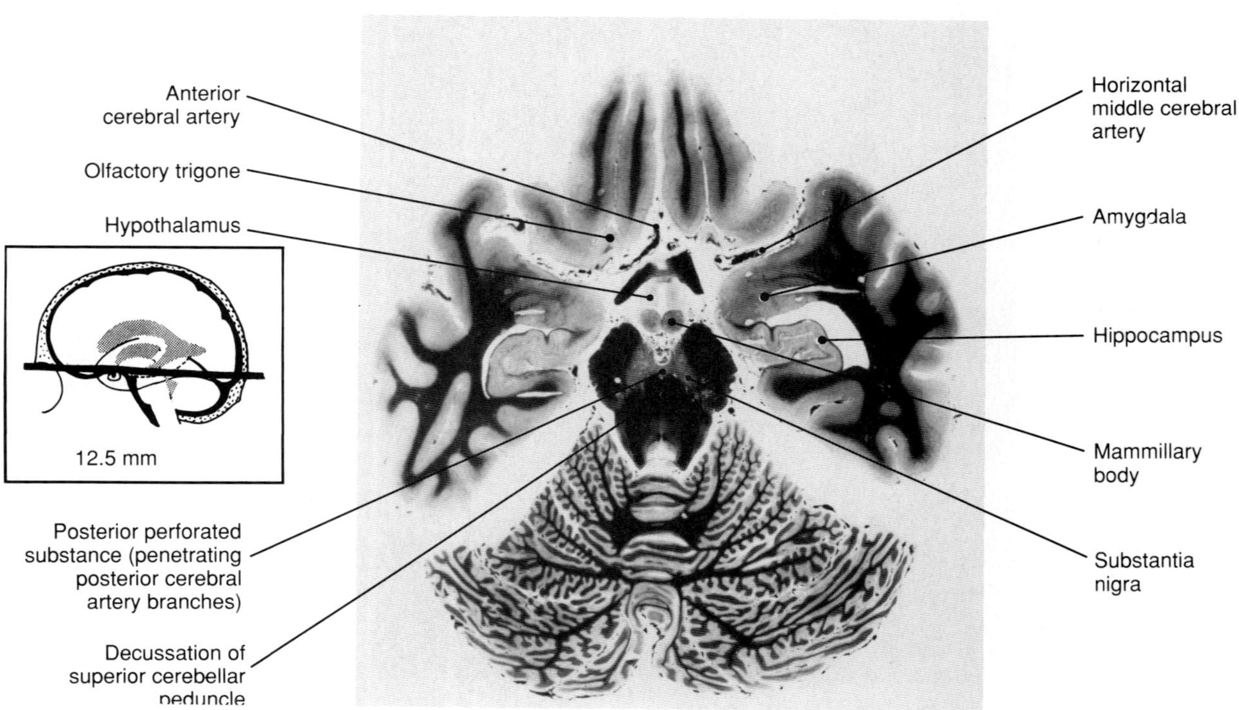

Figure 3-55

AXIAL IMAGES

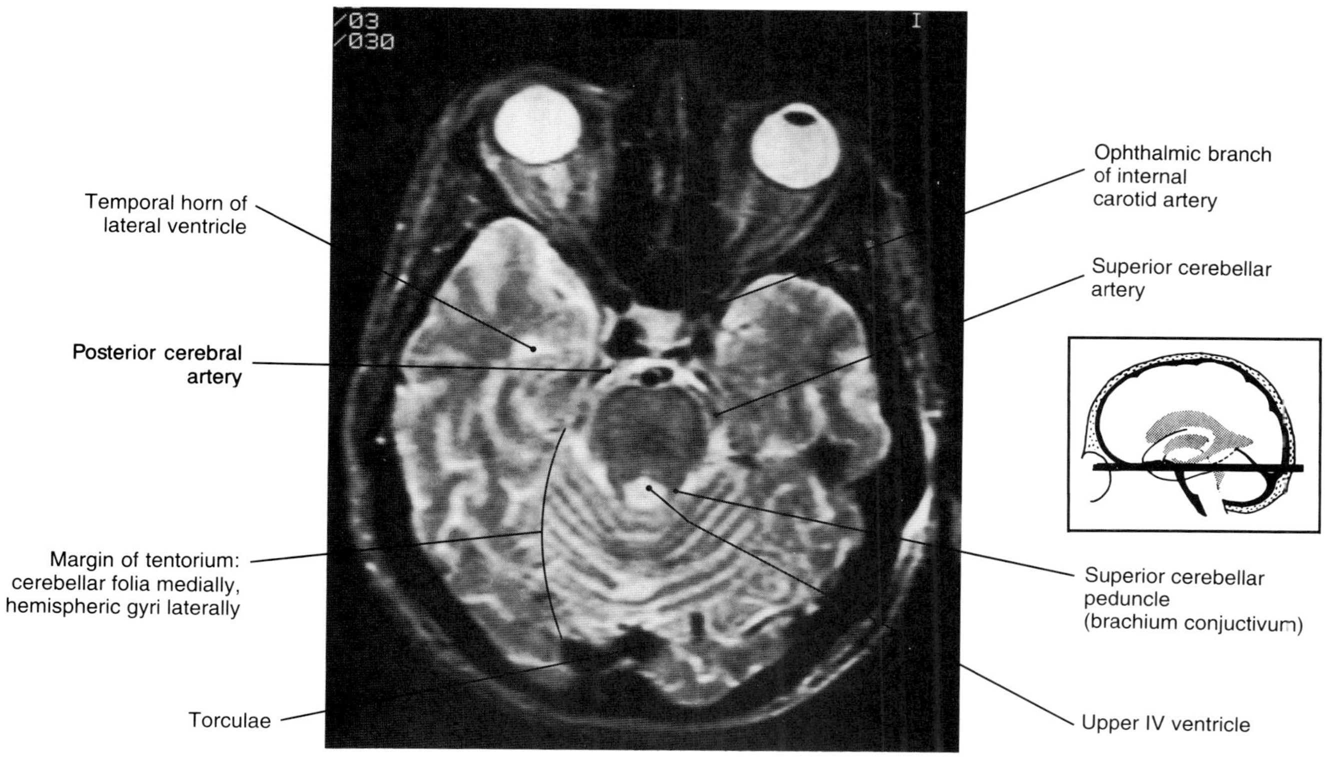

Figure 3-56

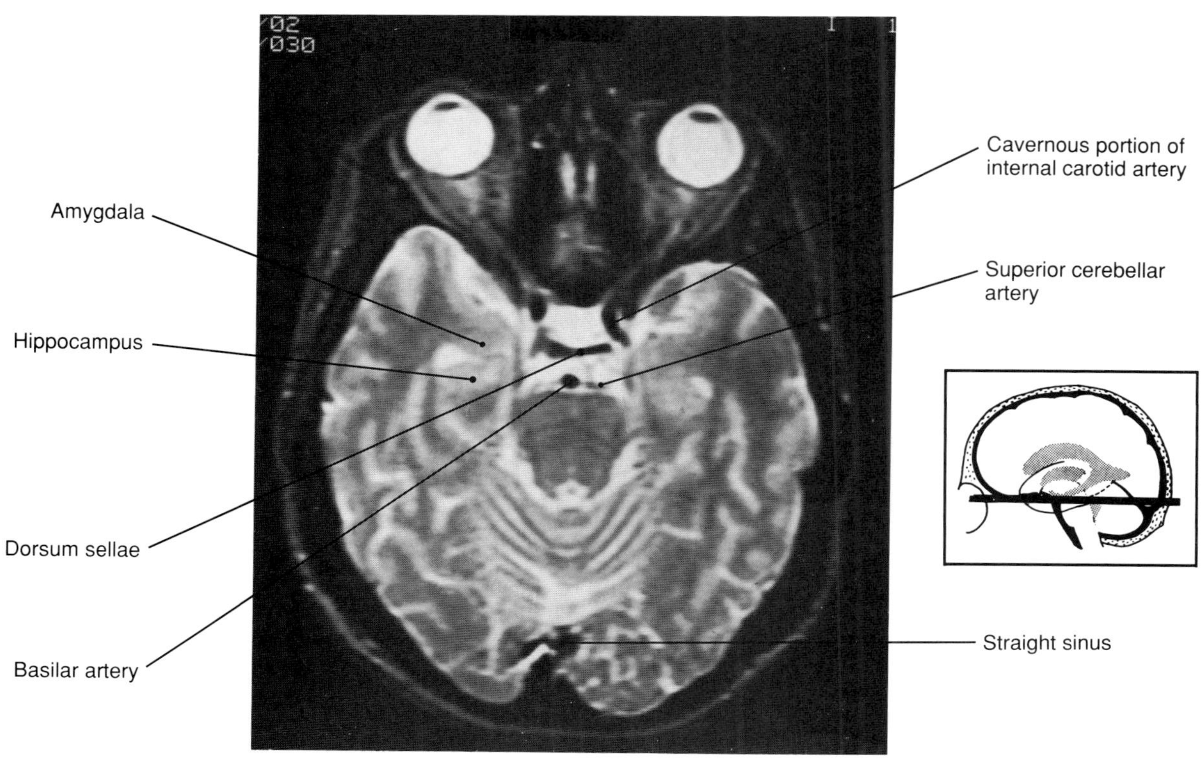

Figure 3-57

AXIAL IMAGES

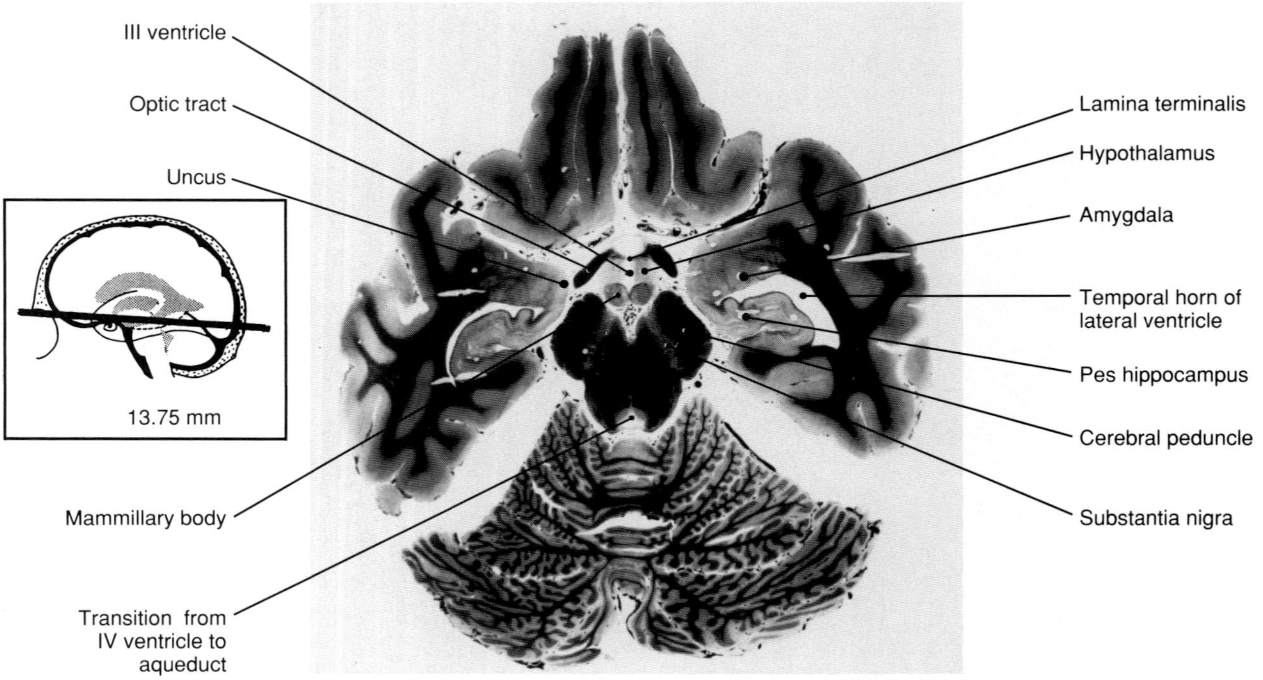

Figure 3-58

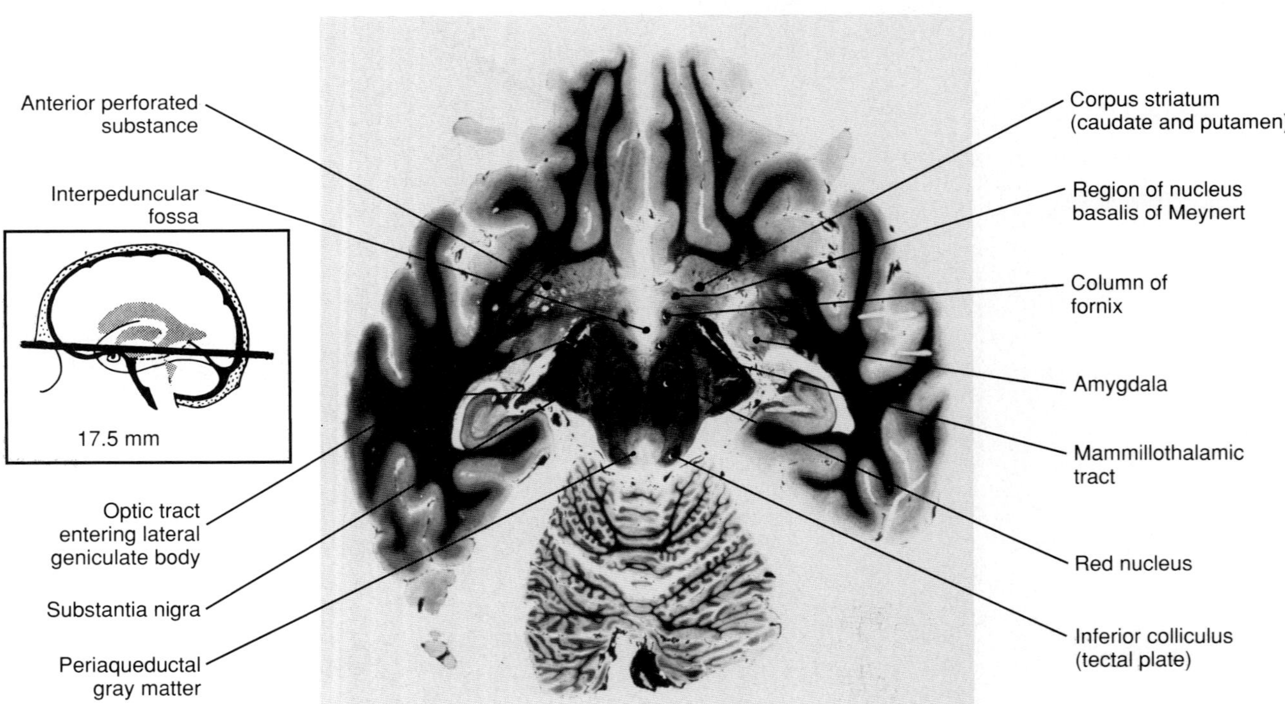

Figure 3-59

AXIAL IMAGES

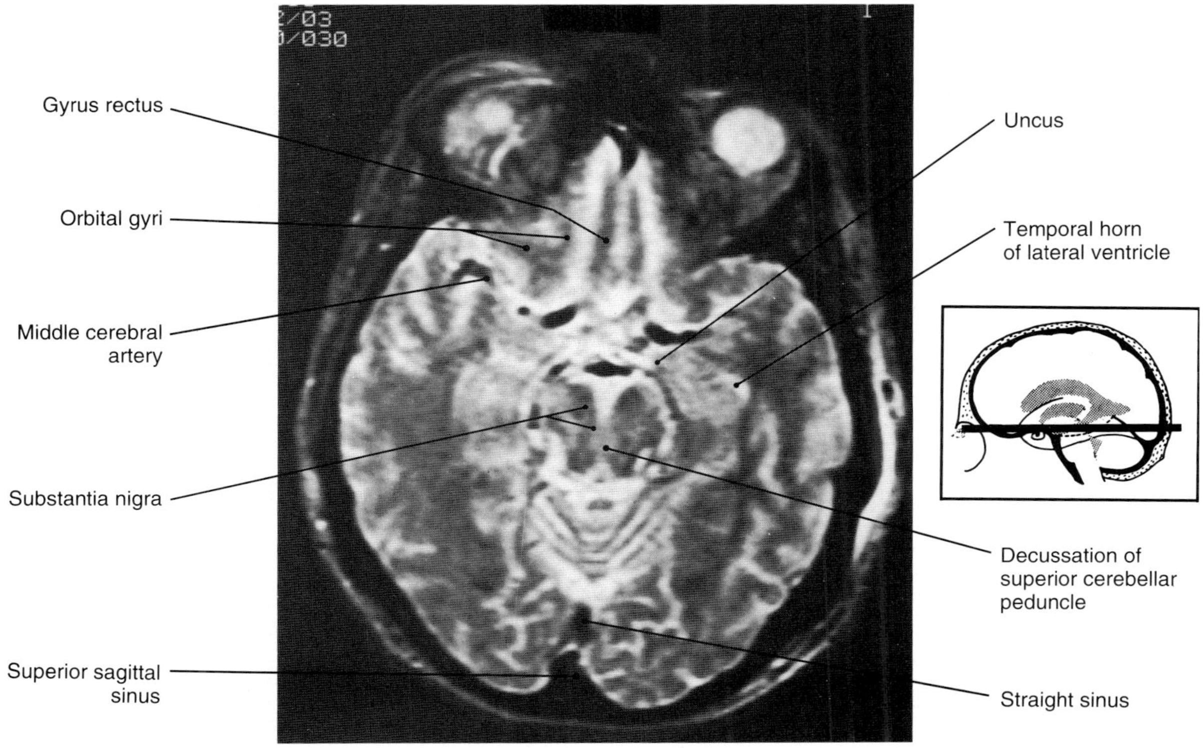

Figure 3-60

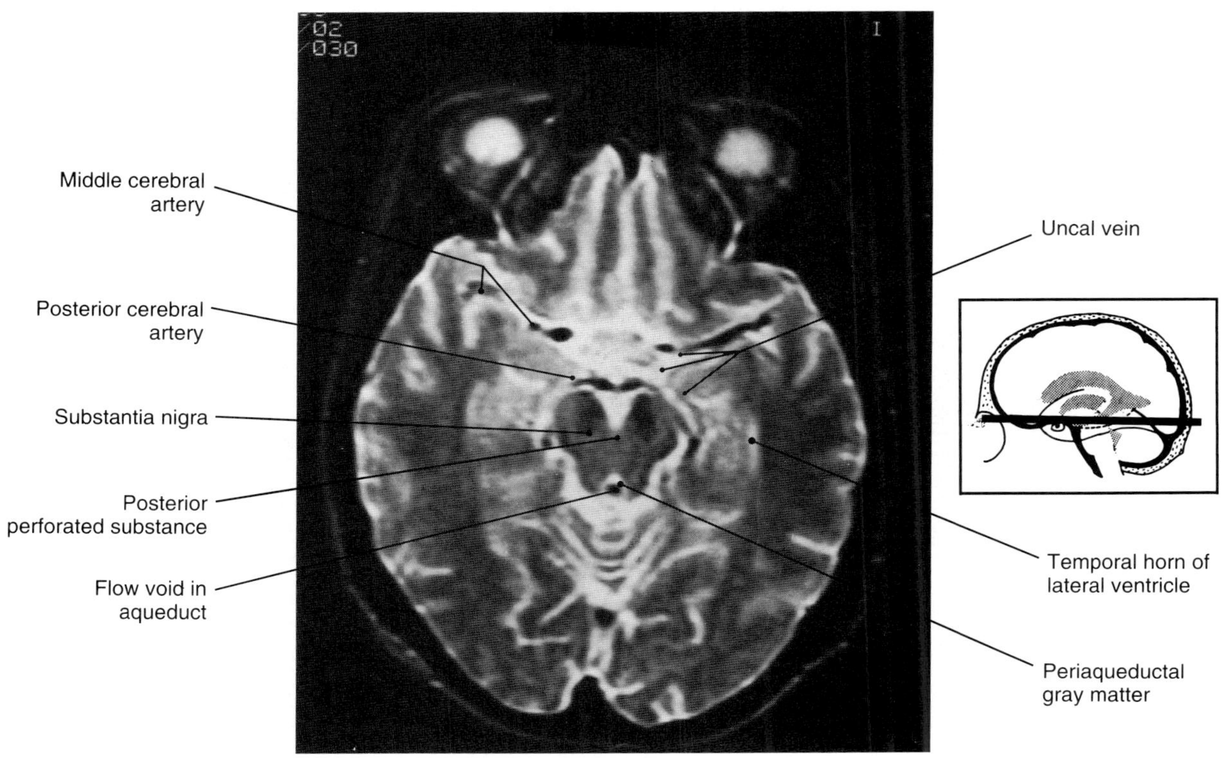

Figure 3-61

AXIAL IMAGES

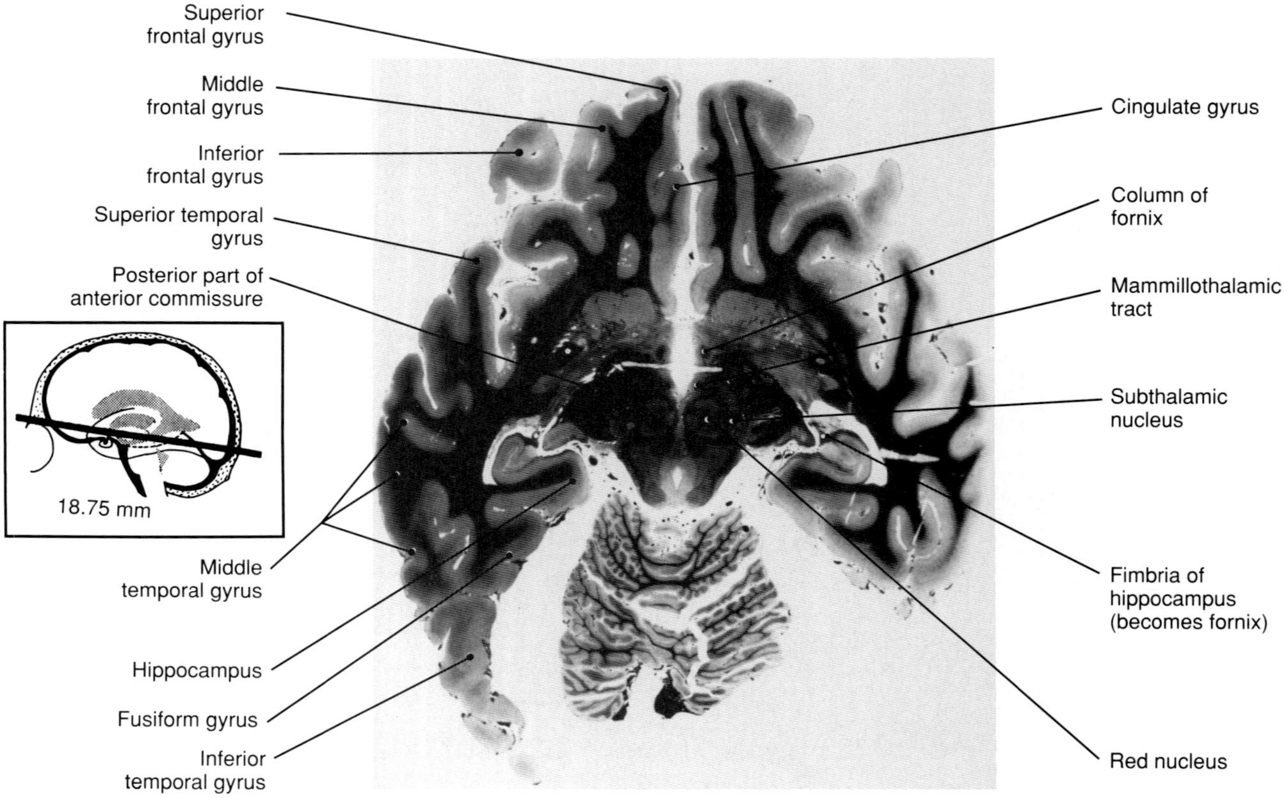

Figure 3-62

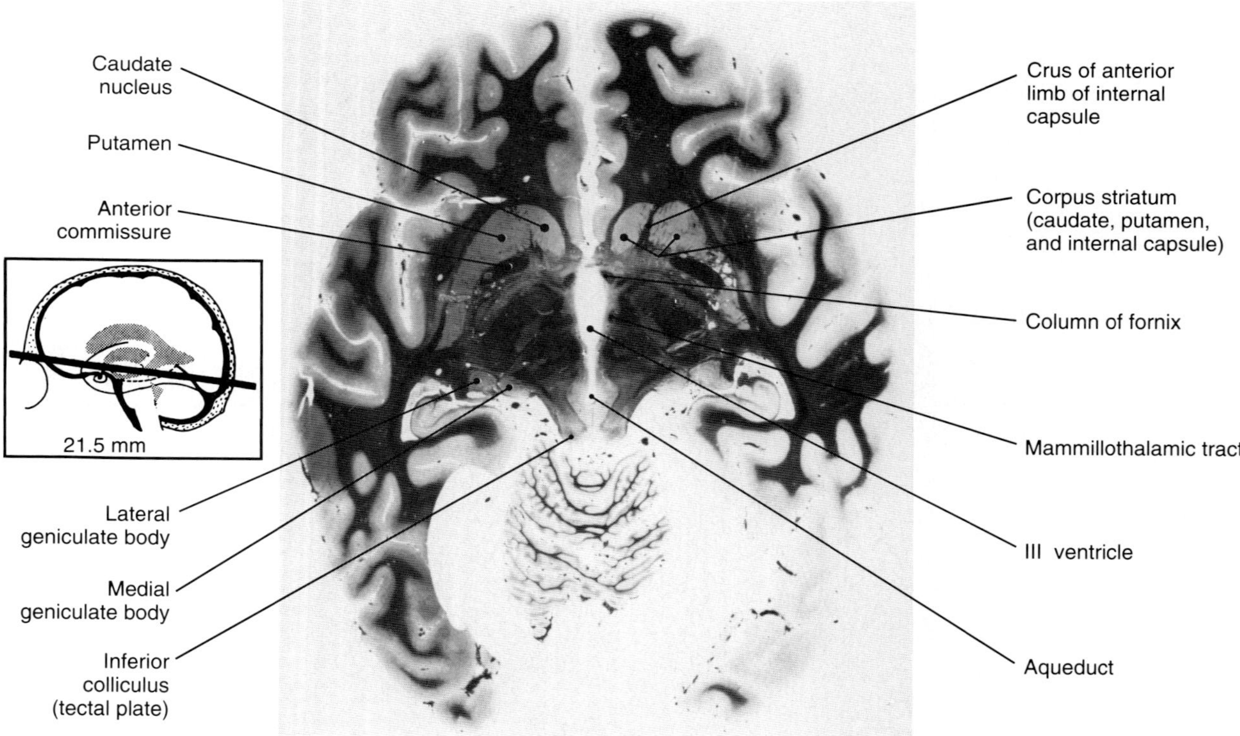

Figure 3-63

AXIAL IMAGES

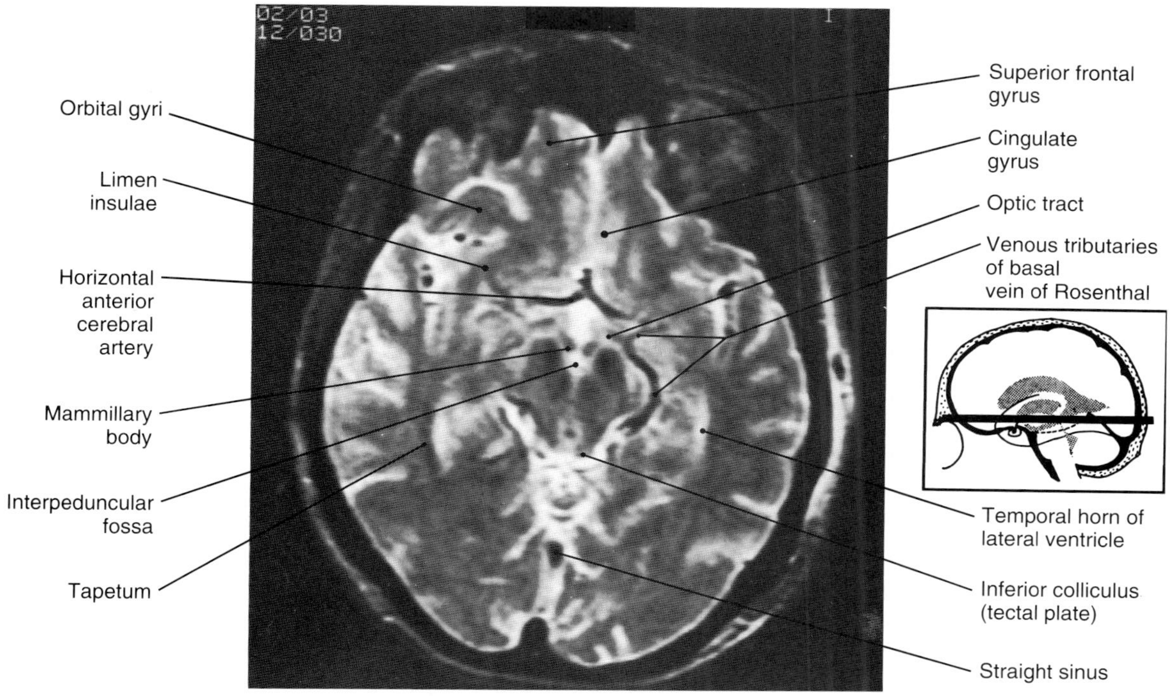

Figure 3-64

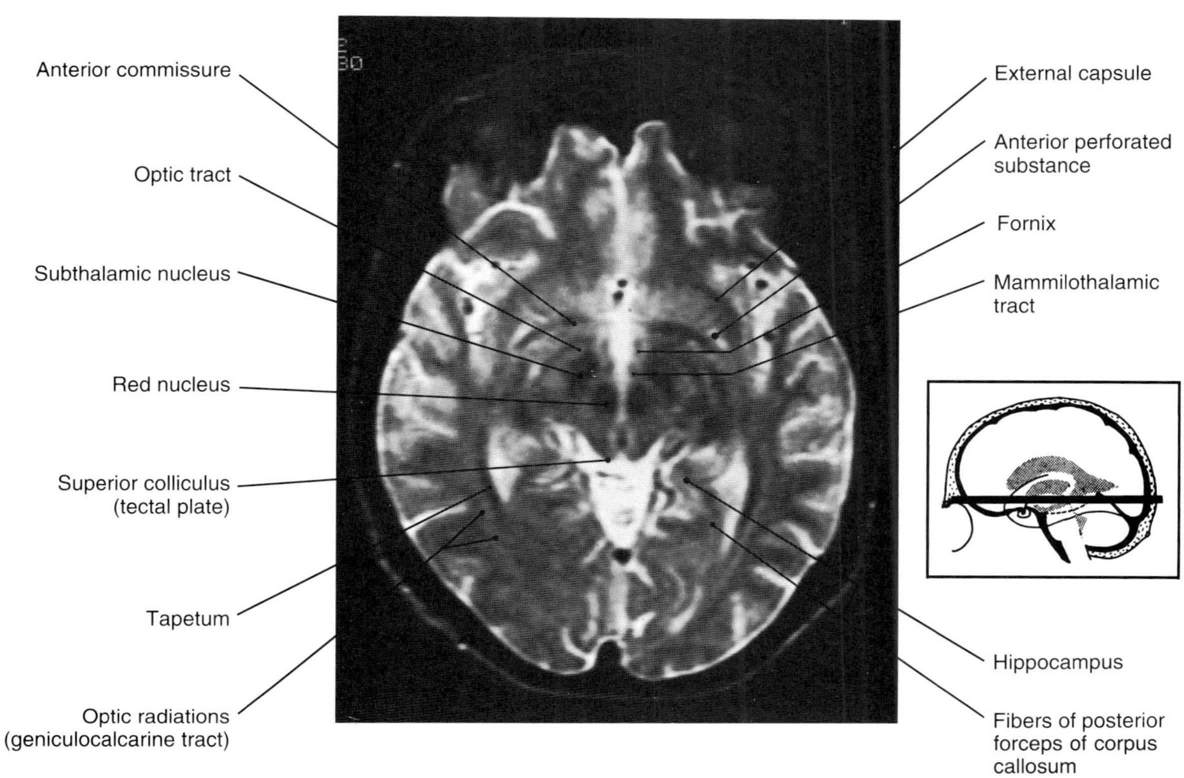

Figure 3-65

AXIAL IMAGES

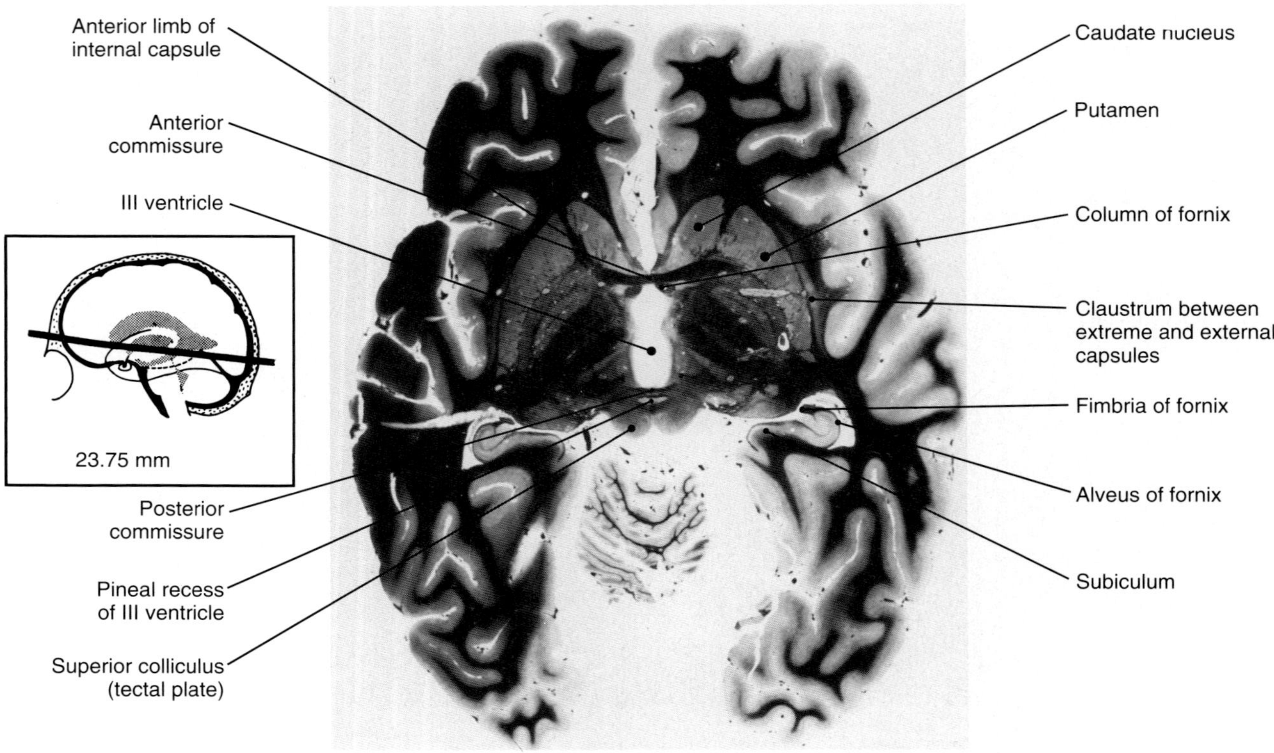

Figure 3-66

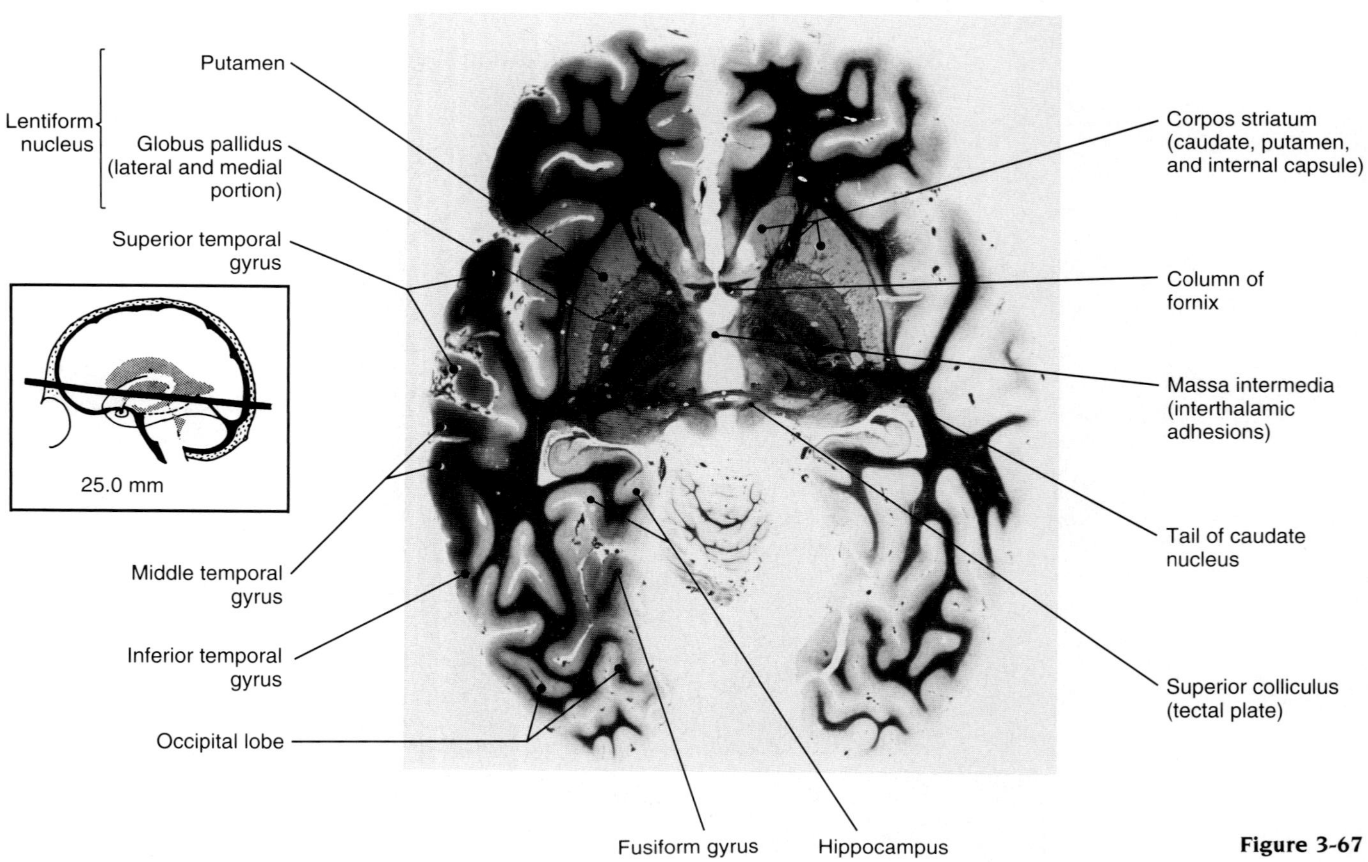

Figure 3-67

AXIAL IMAGES

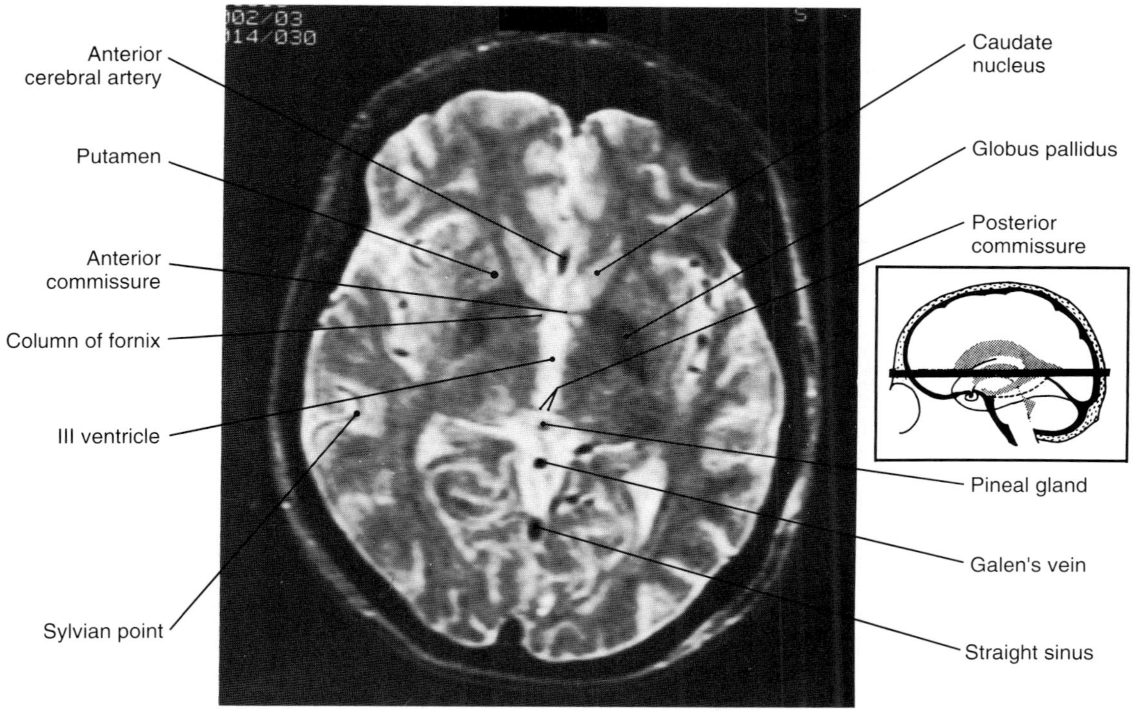

Figure 3-68

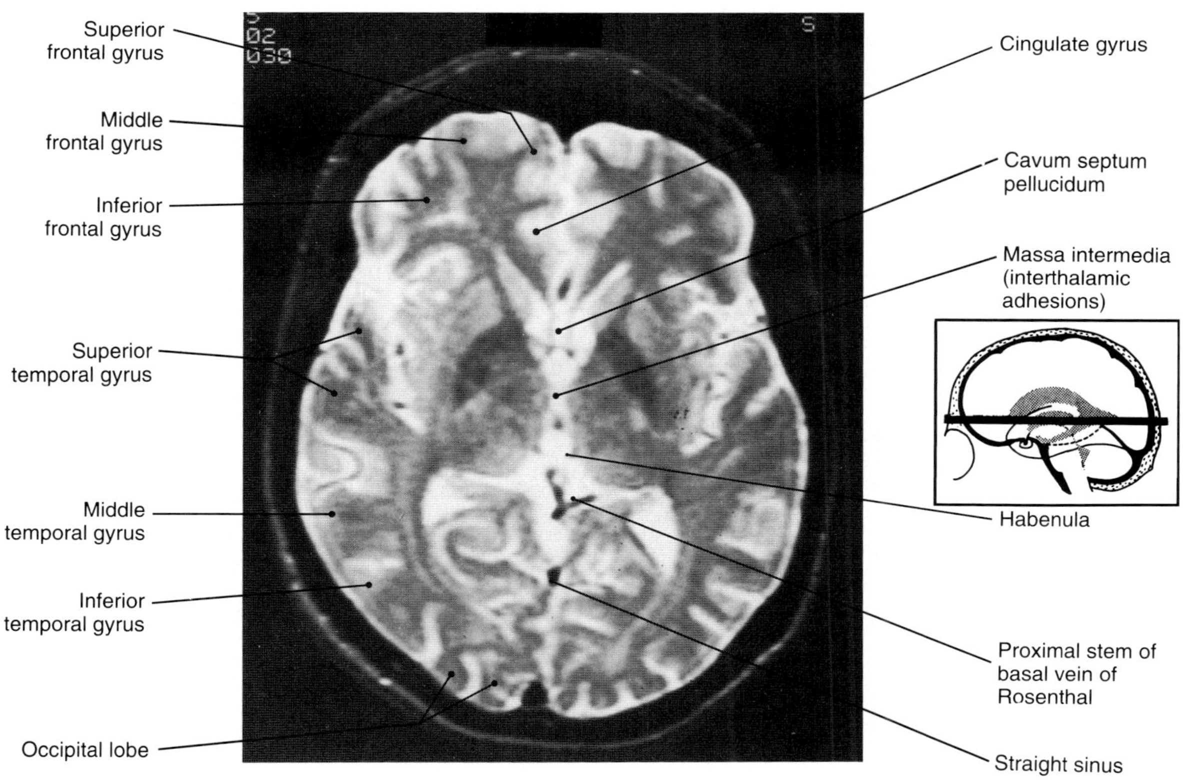

Figure 3-69

AXIAL IMAGES

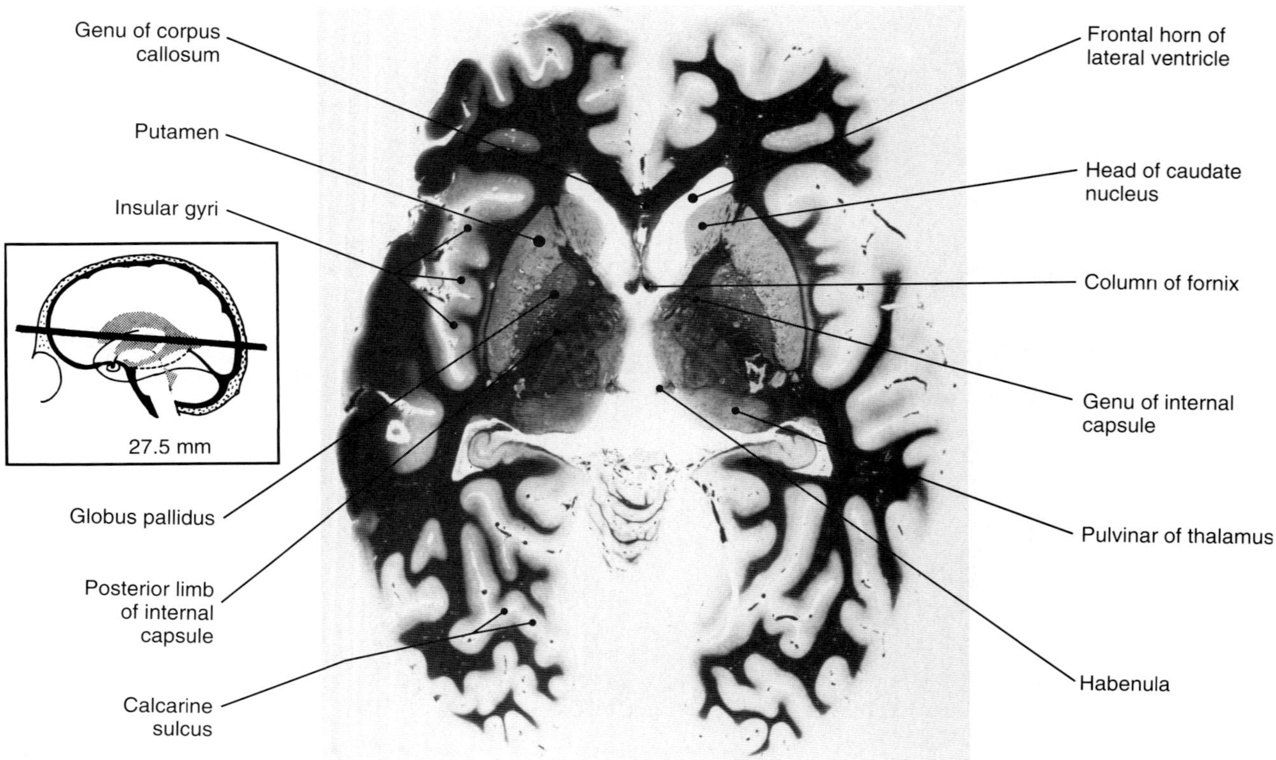

Figure 3-70

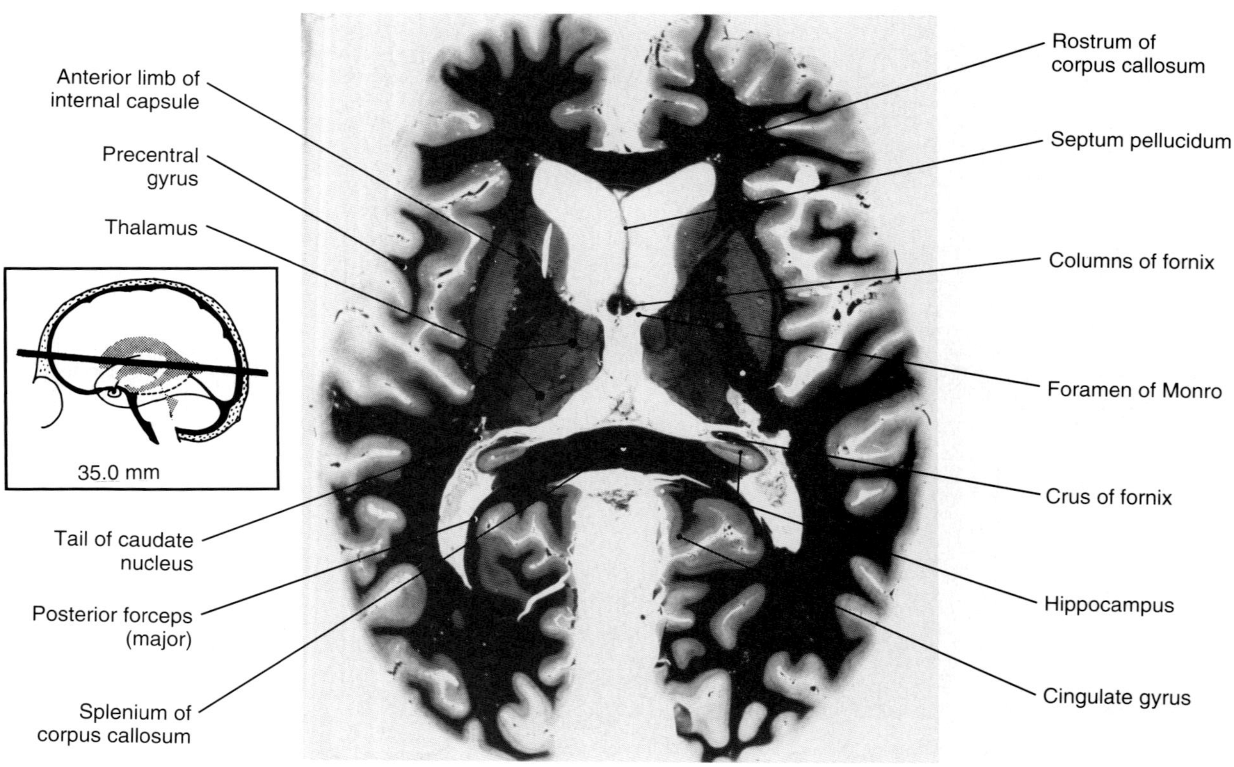

Figure 3-71

AXIAL IMAGES

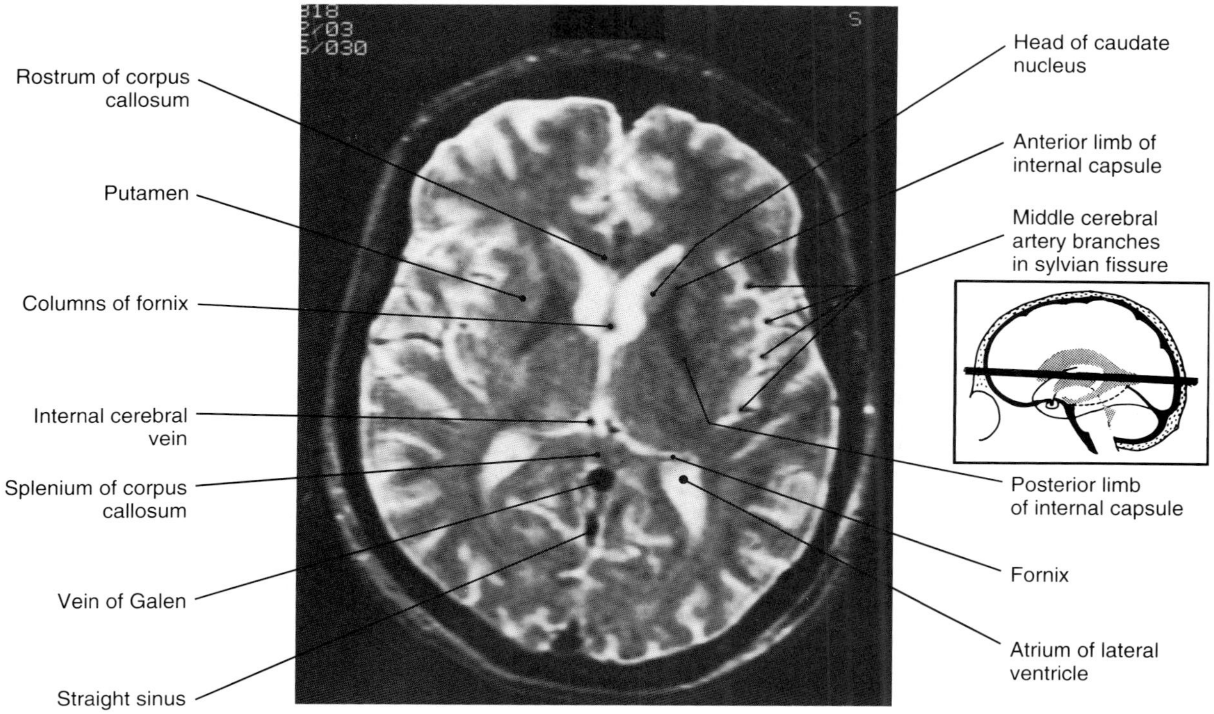

Figure 3-72

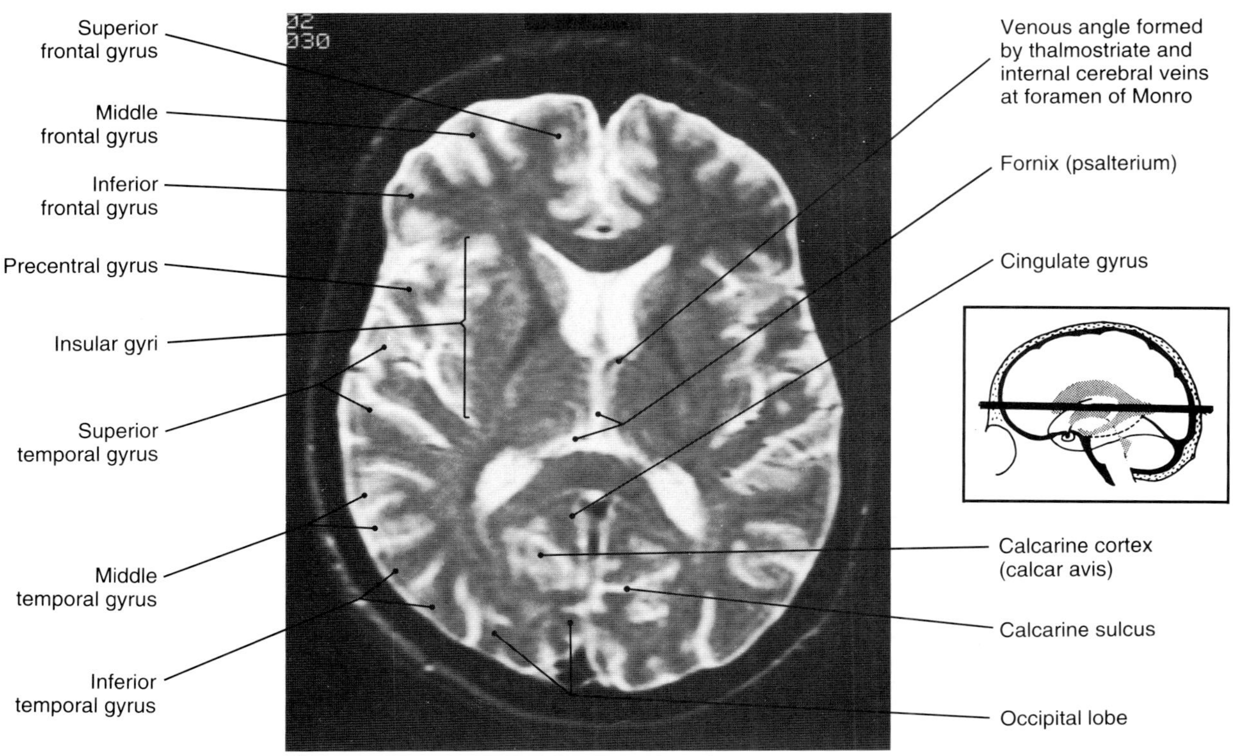

Figure 3-73

AXIAL IMAGES

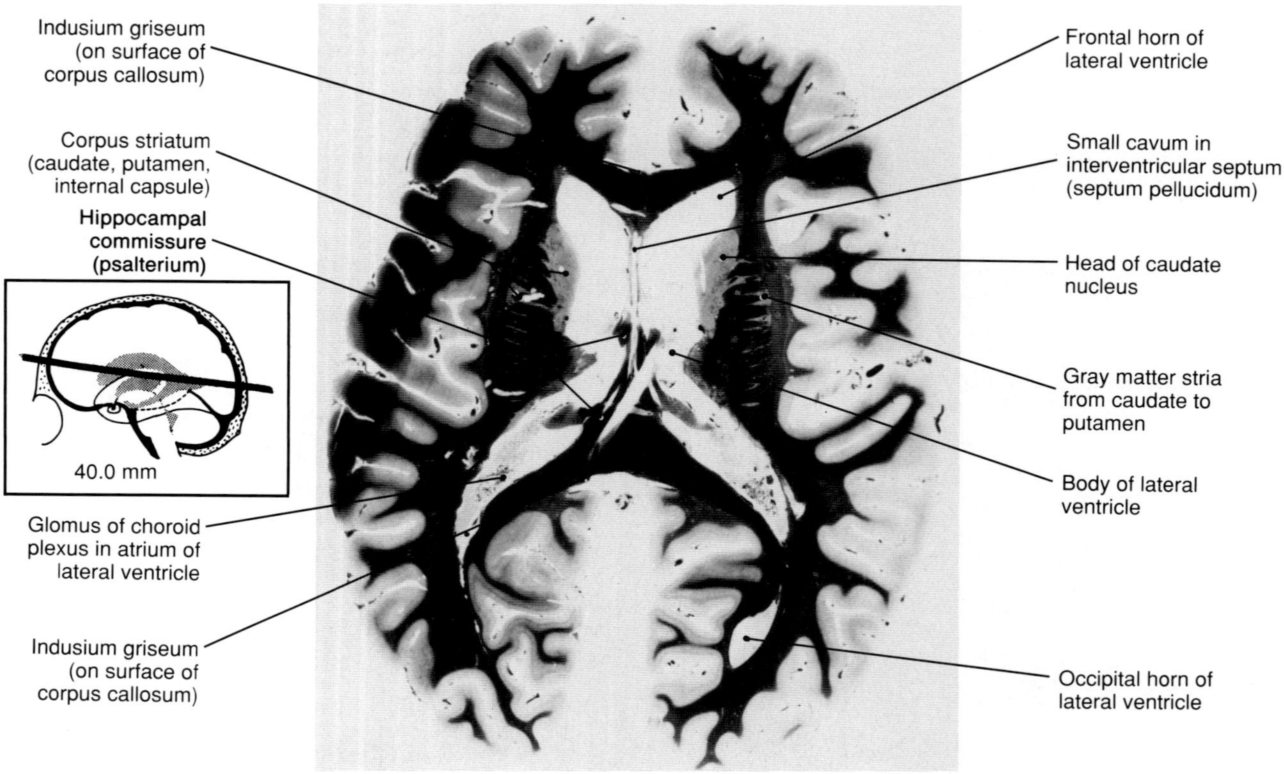

Figure 3-74

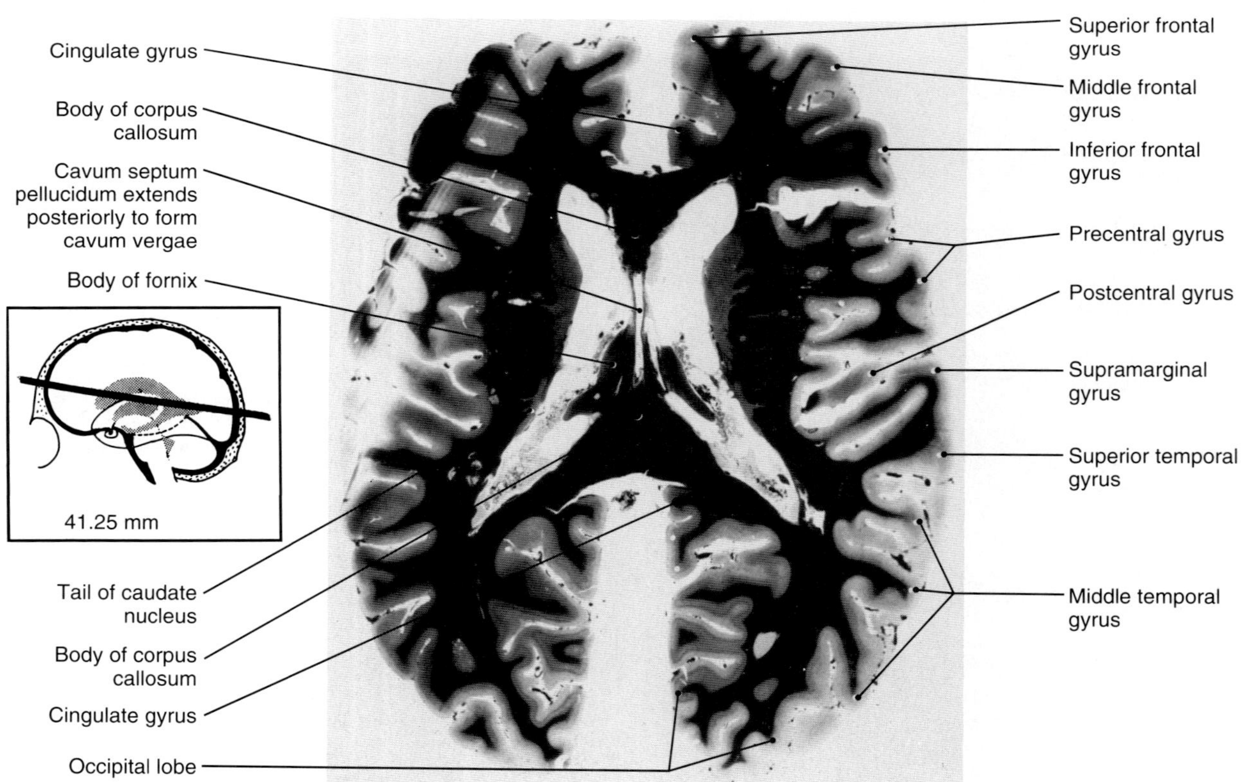

Figure 3-75

AXIAL IMAGES

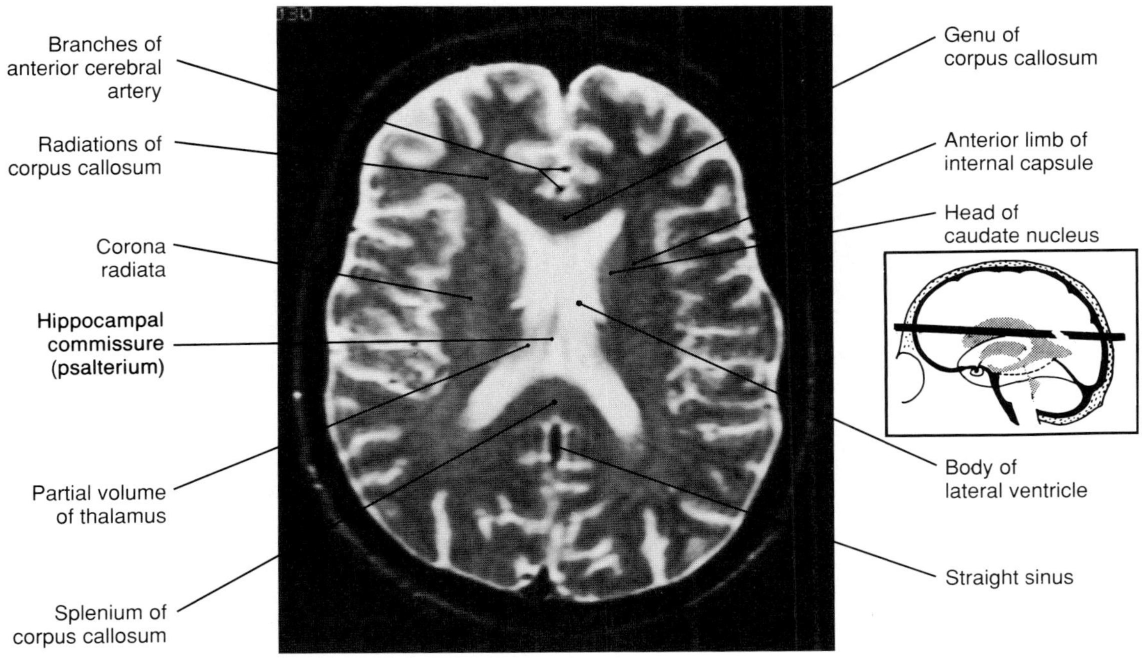

Figure 3-76

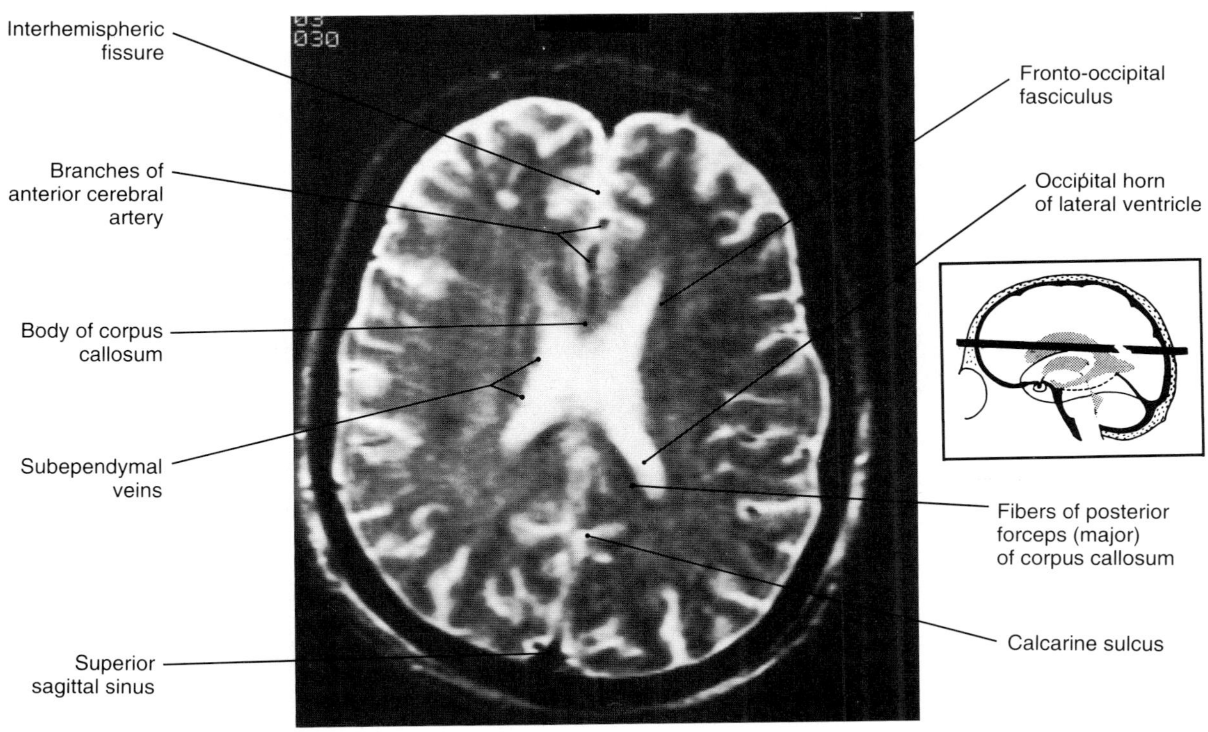

Figure 3-77

AXIAL IMAGES

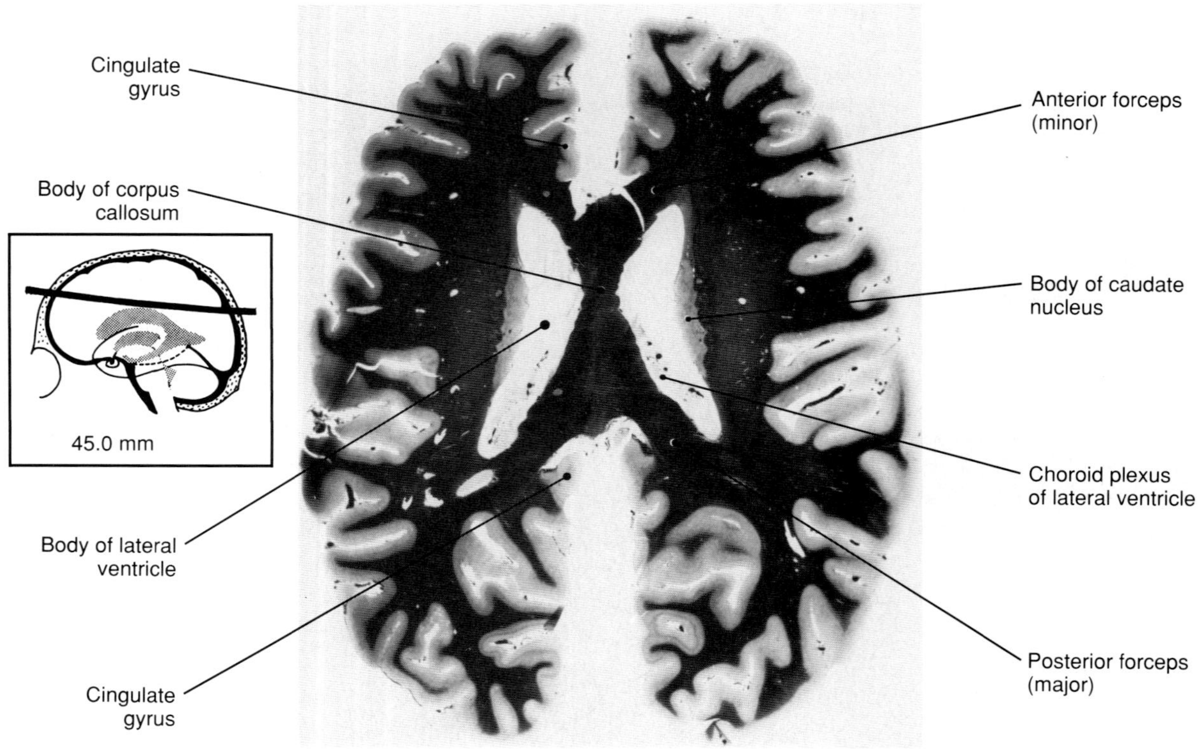

Figure 3-78

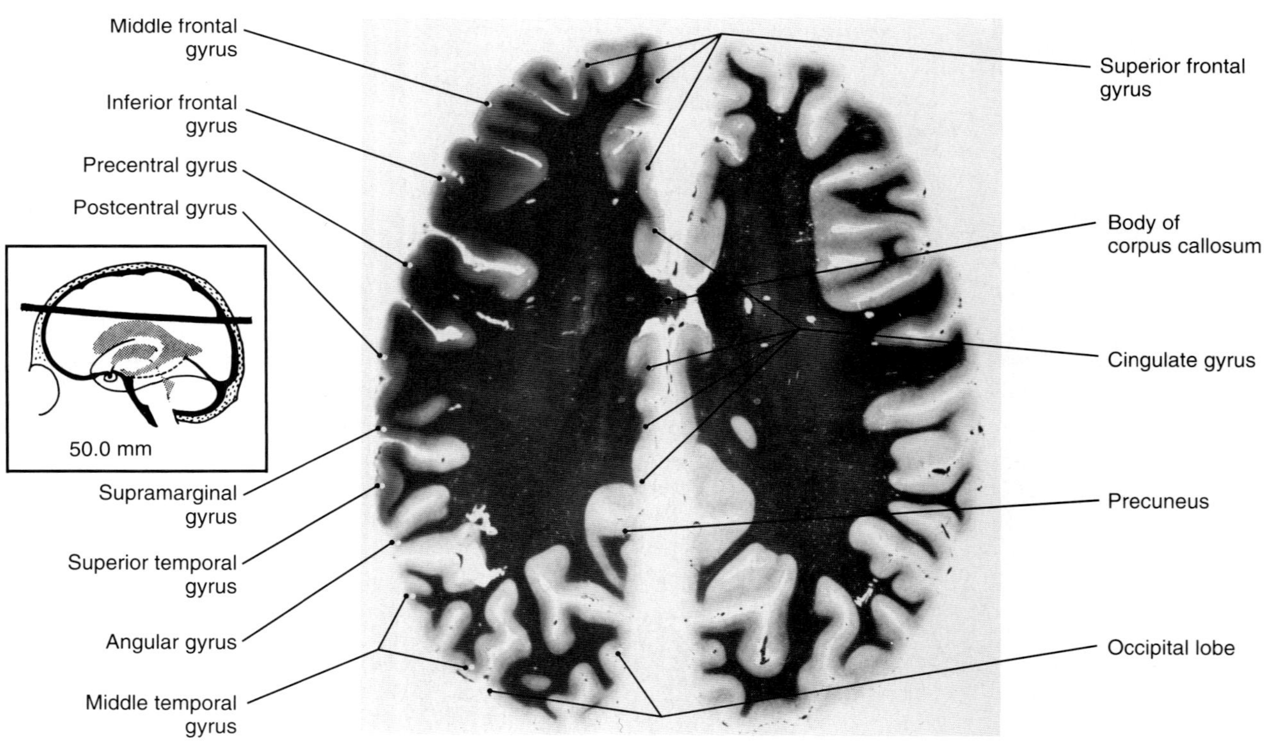

Figure 3-79

AXIAL IMAGES

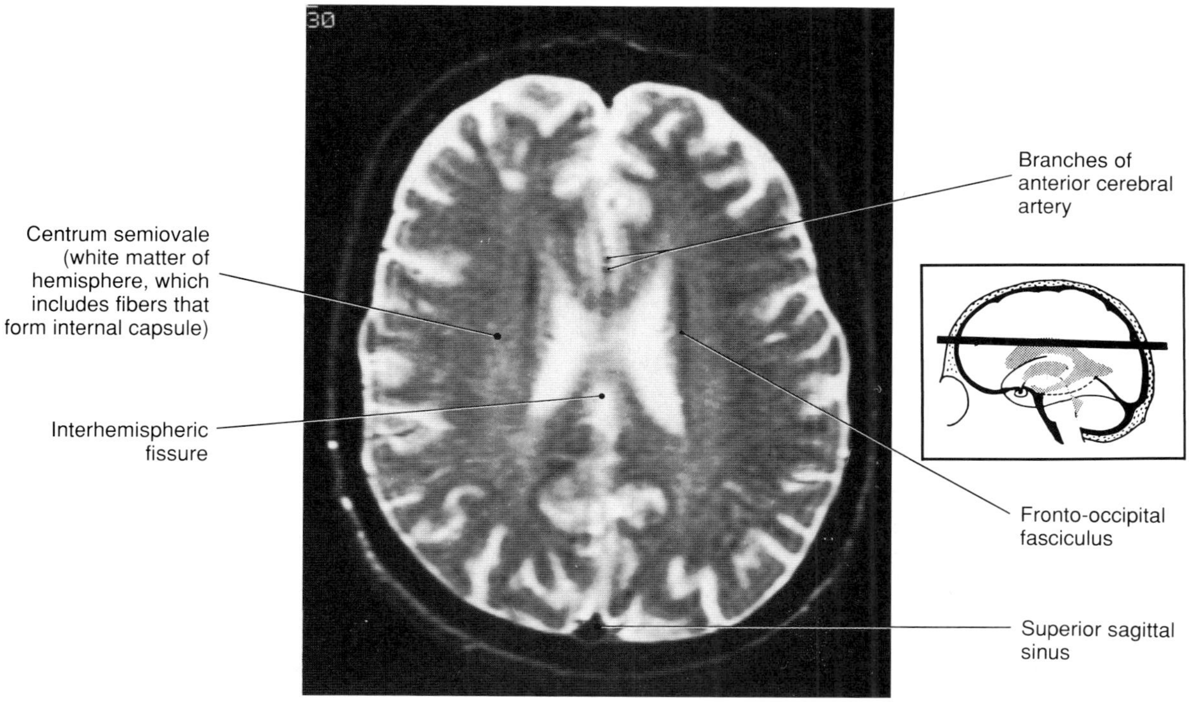

Figure 3-80

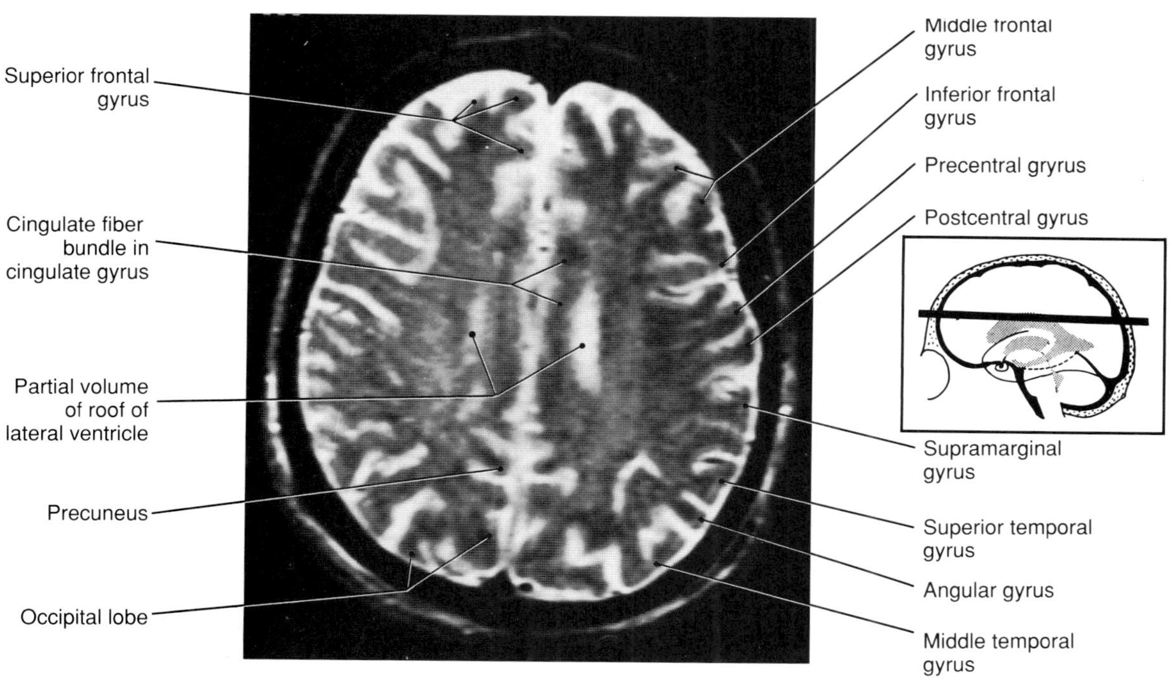

Figure 3-81

SAGITTAL IMAGES

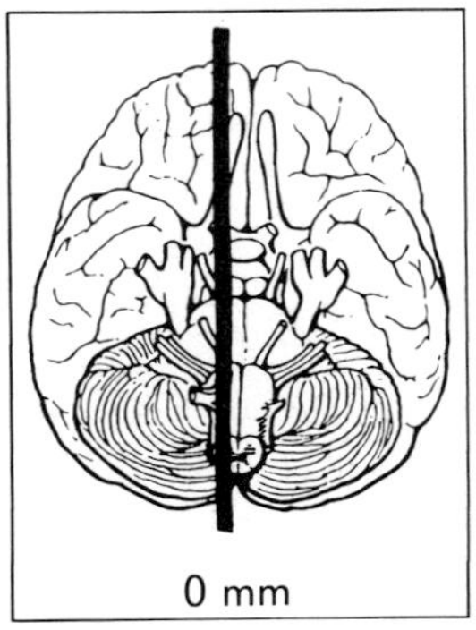

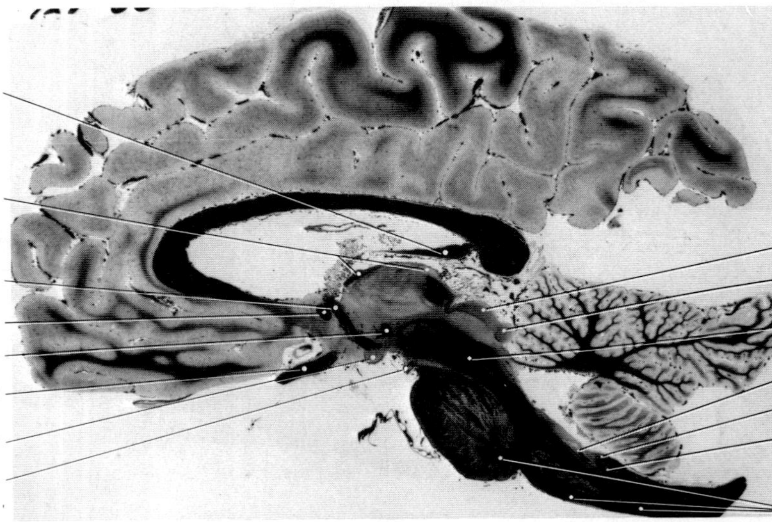

Figure 3-82

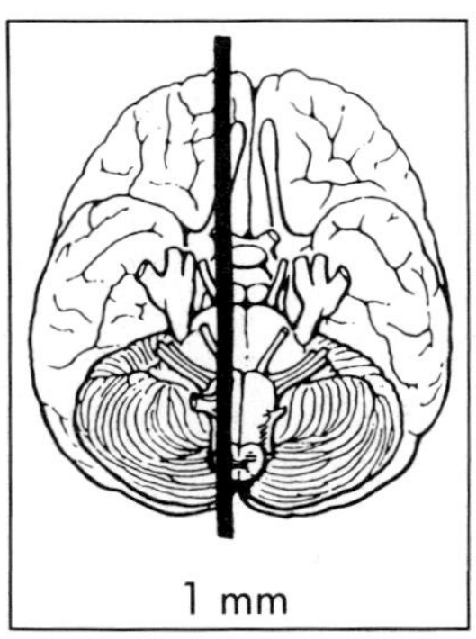

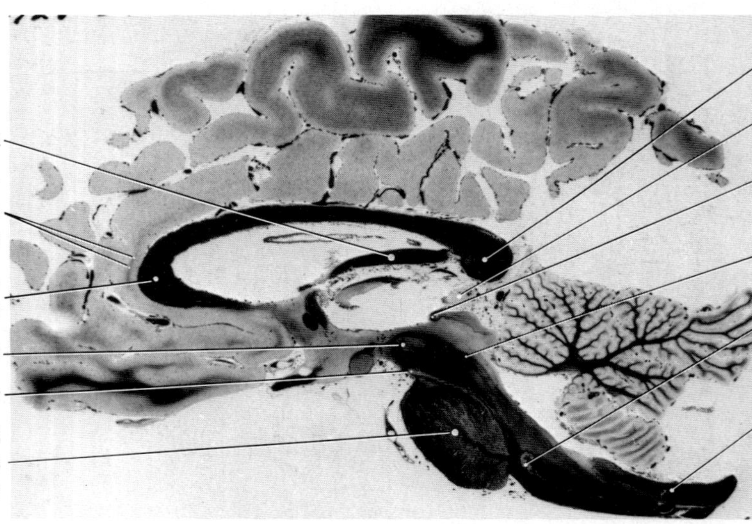

Figure 3-83

SAGITTAL IMAGES

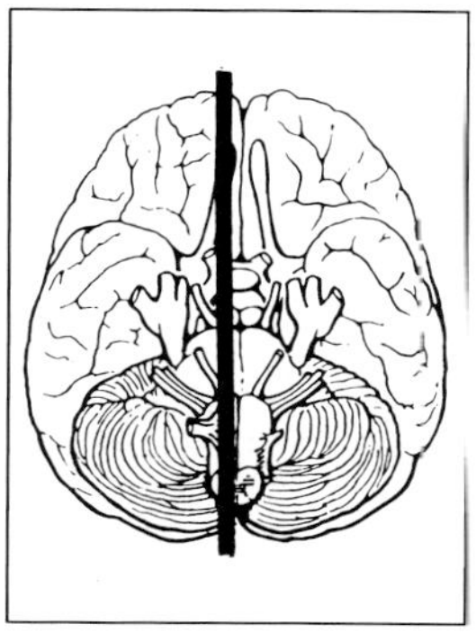

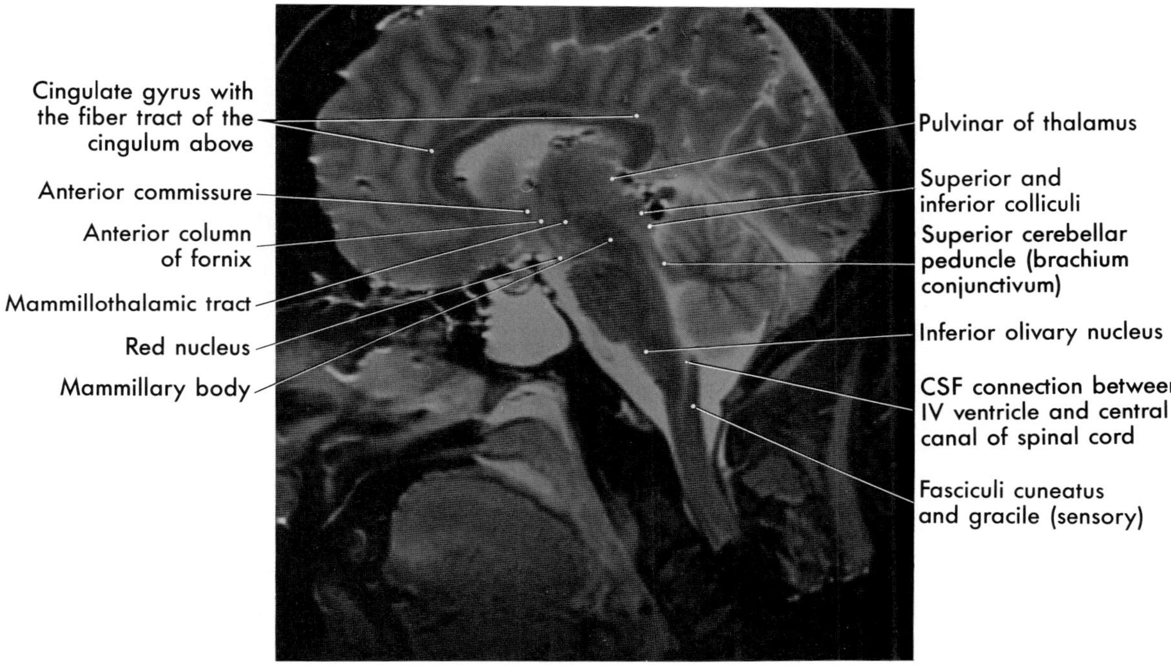

Figure 3-84

SAGITTAL IMAGES

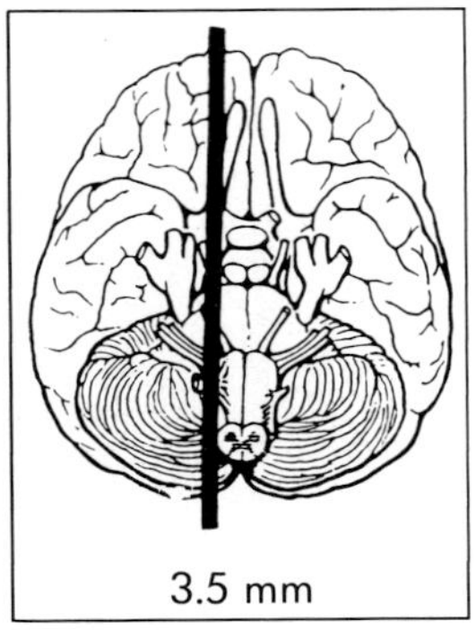

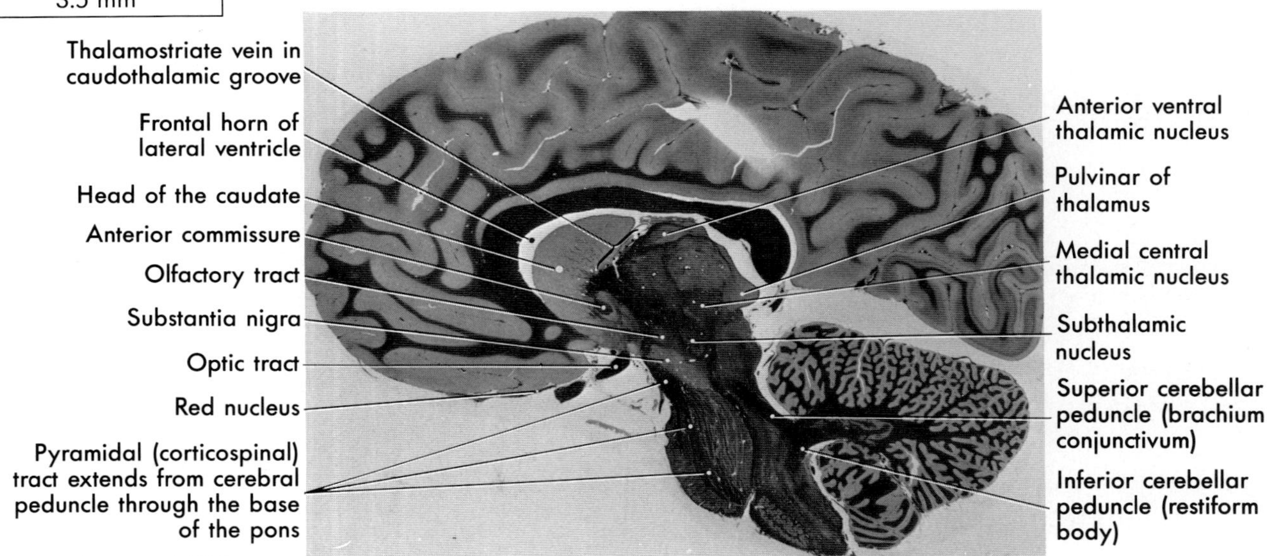

Figure 3-85

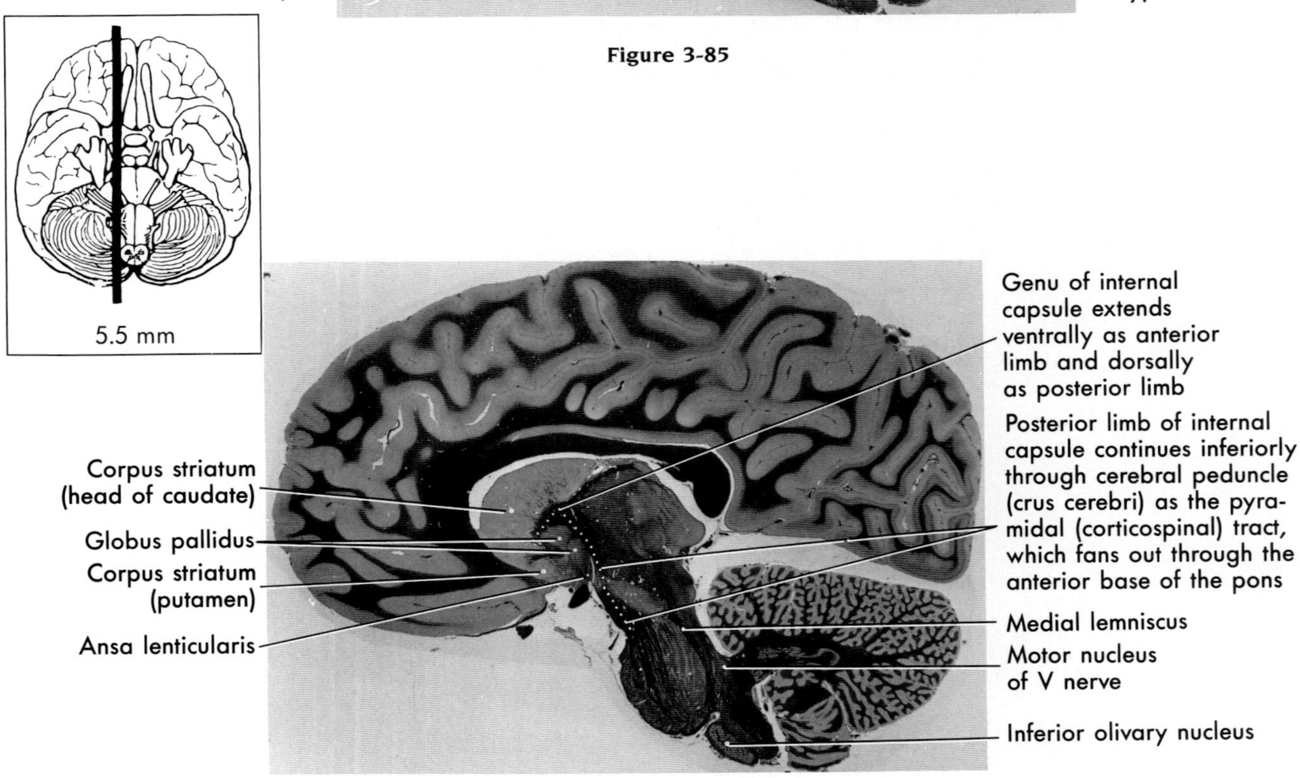

Figure 3-86

SAGITTAL IMAGES

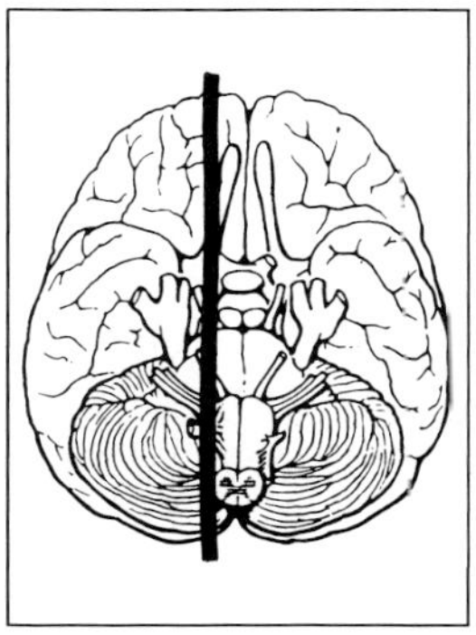

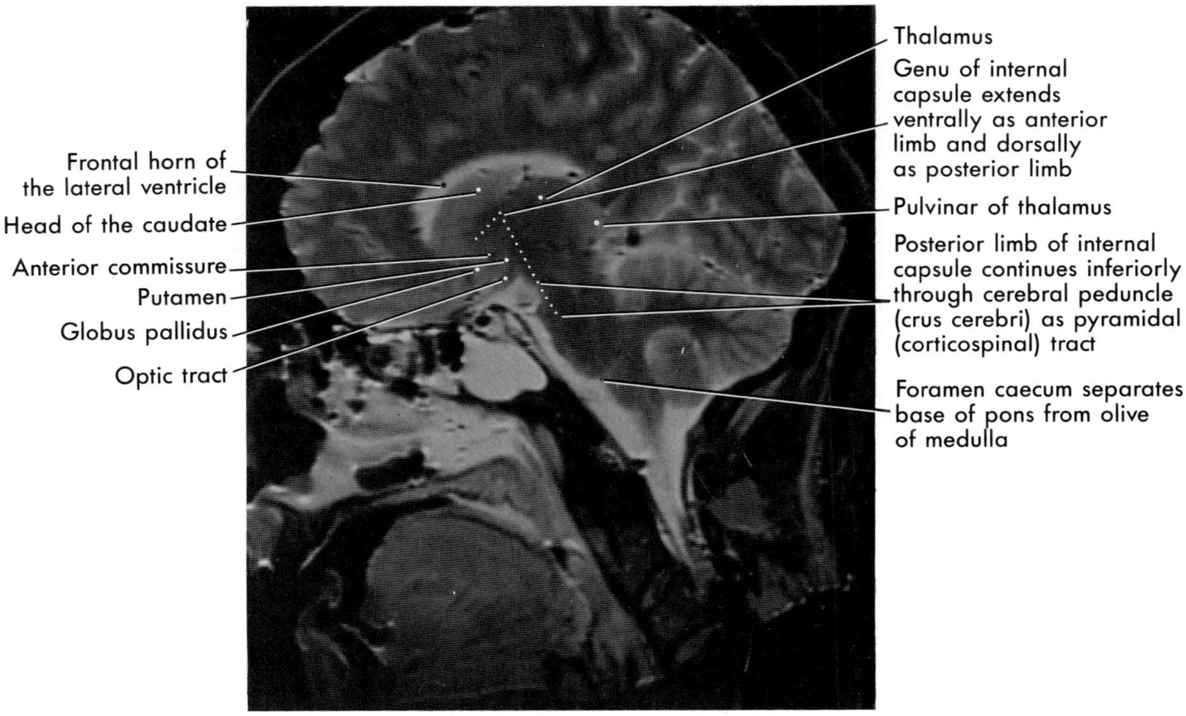

Figure 3-87

SAGITTAL IMAGES

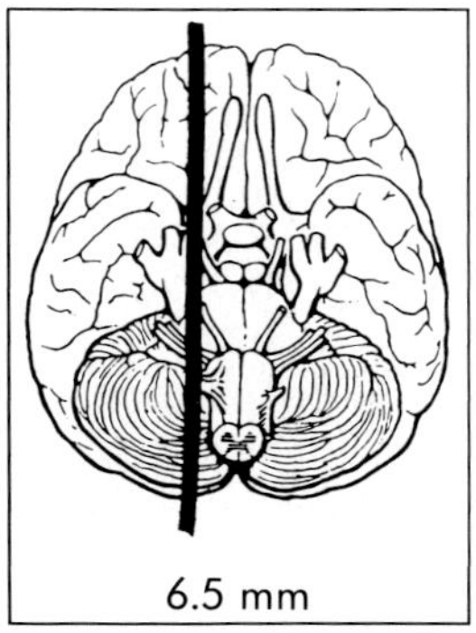

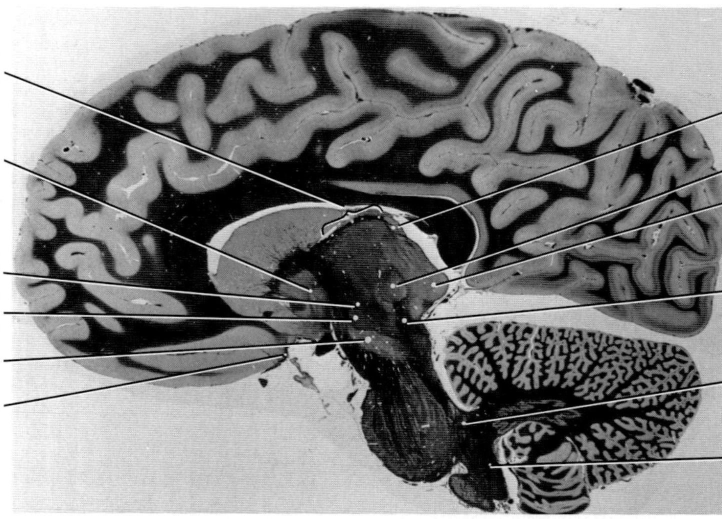

Figure 3-88

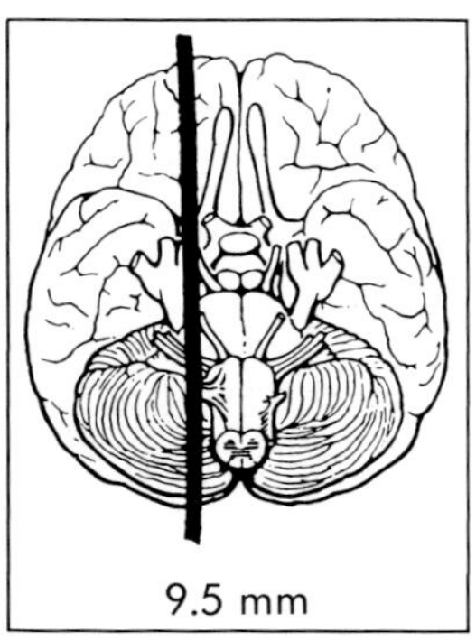

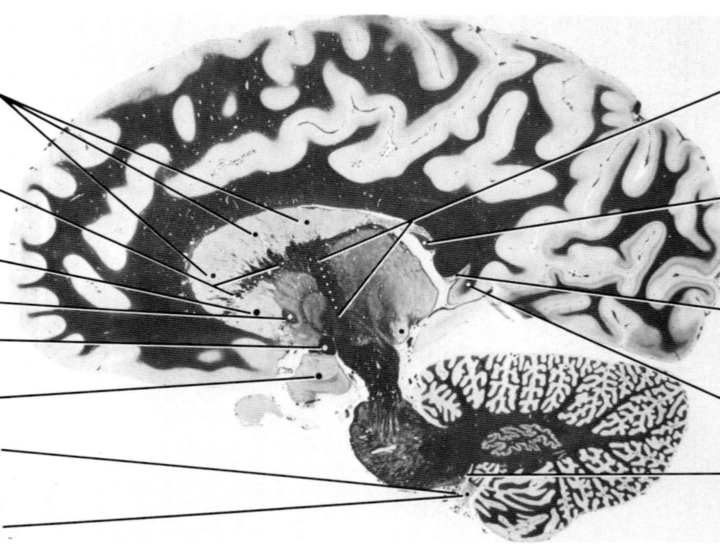

Figure 3-89

SAGITTAL IMAGES

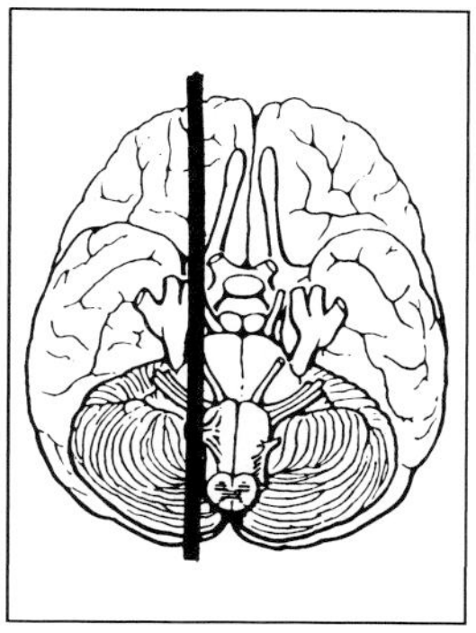

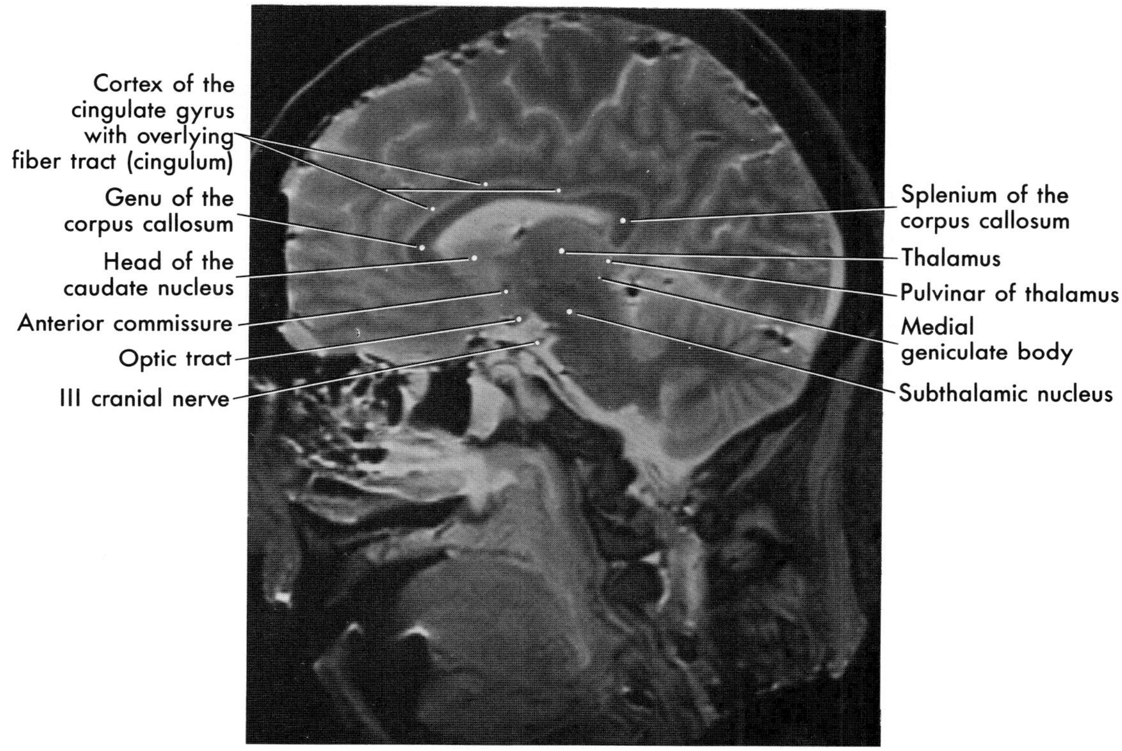

Figure 3-90

SAGITTAL IMAGES

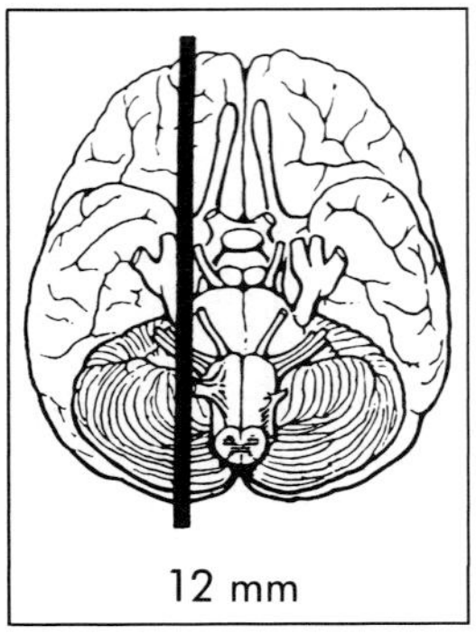

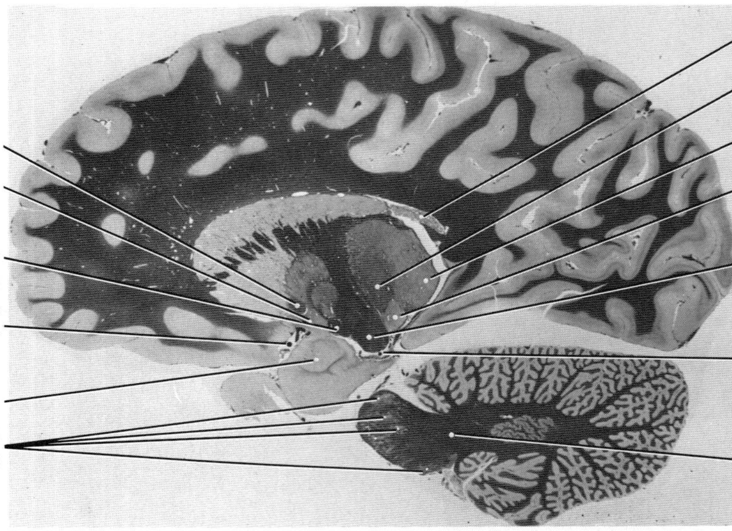

Figure 3-91

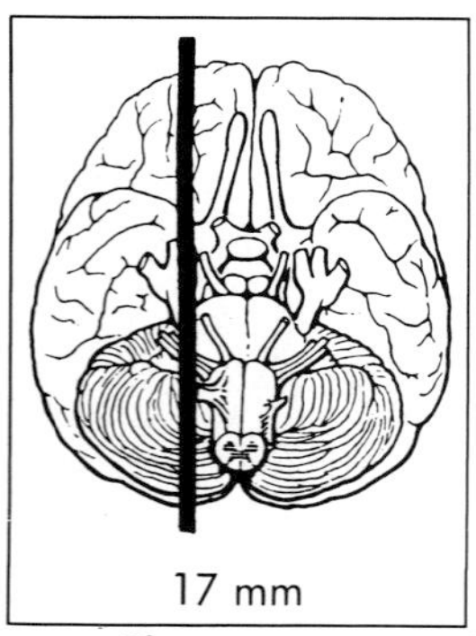

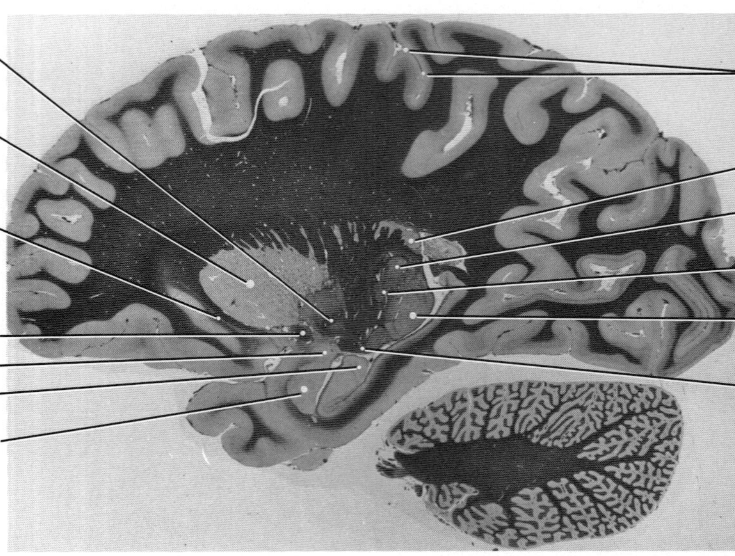

Figure 3-92

SAGITTAL IMAGES

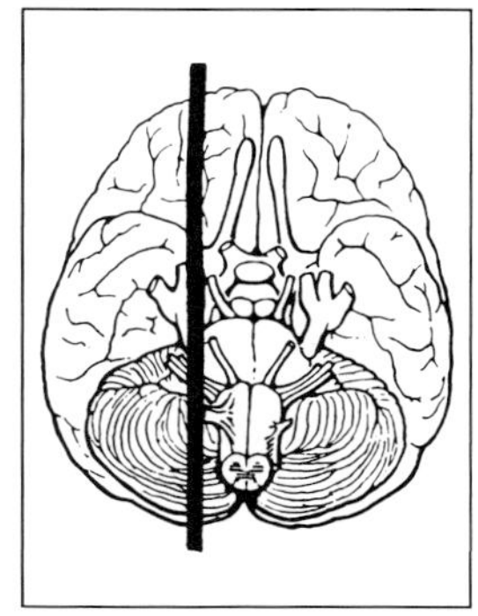

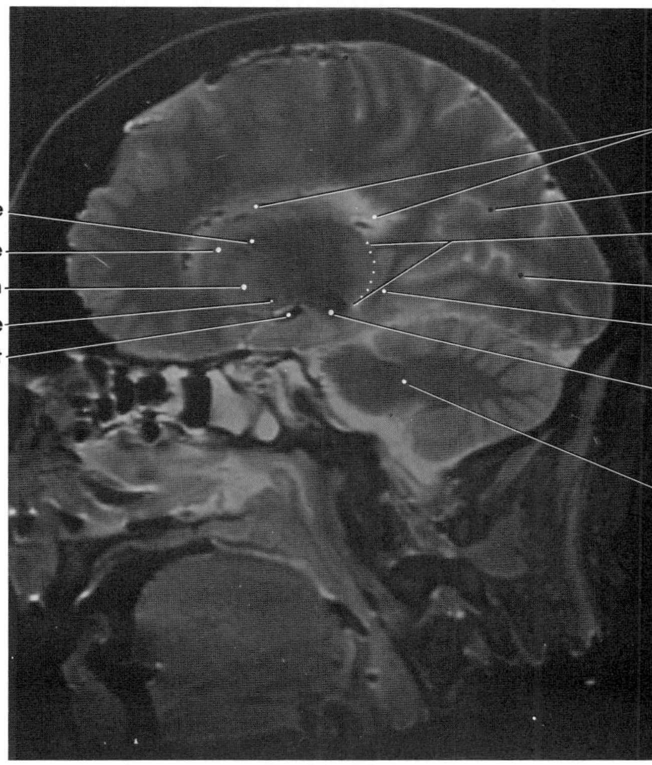

Figure 3-93

SAGITTAL IMAGES

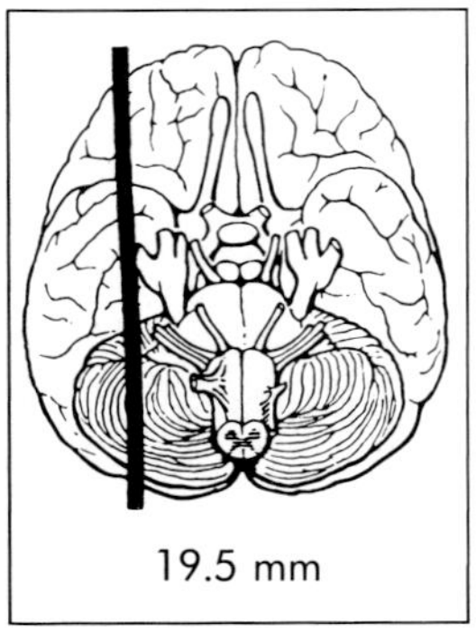

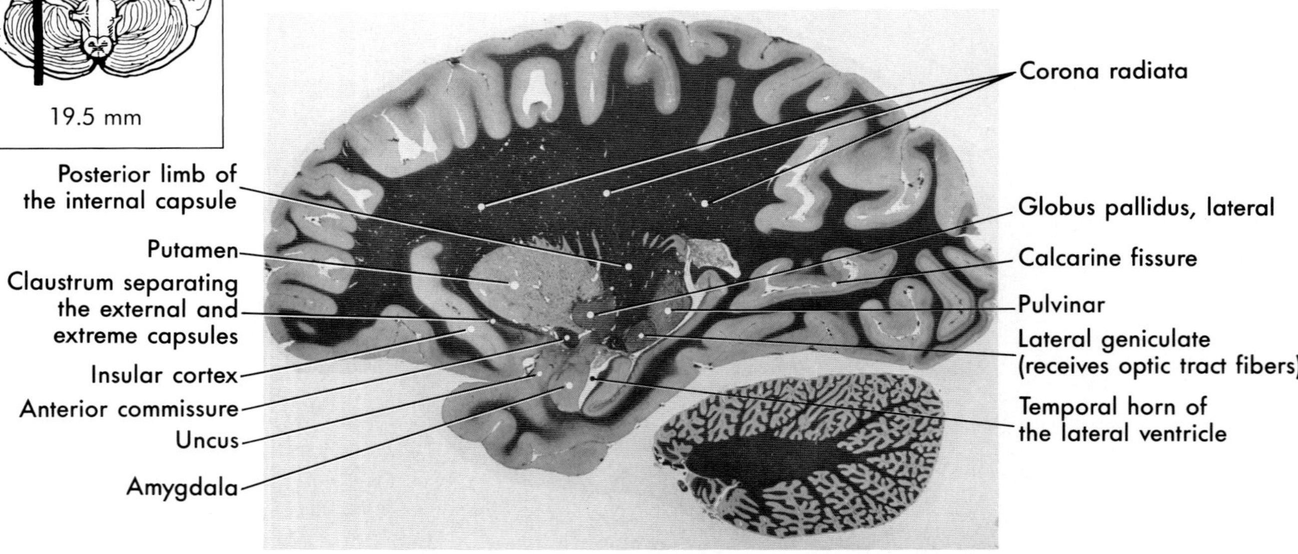

Figure 3-94

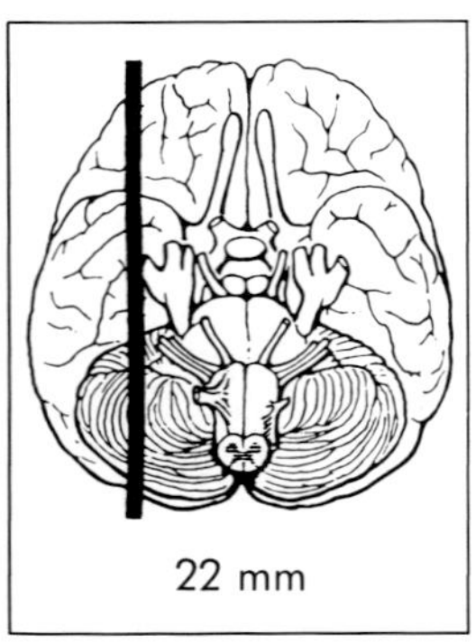

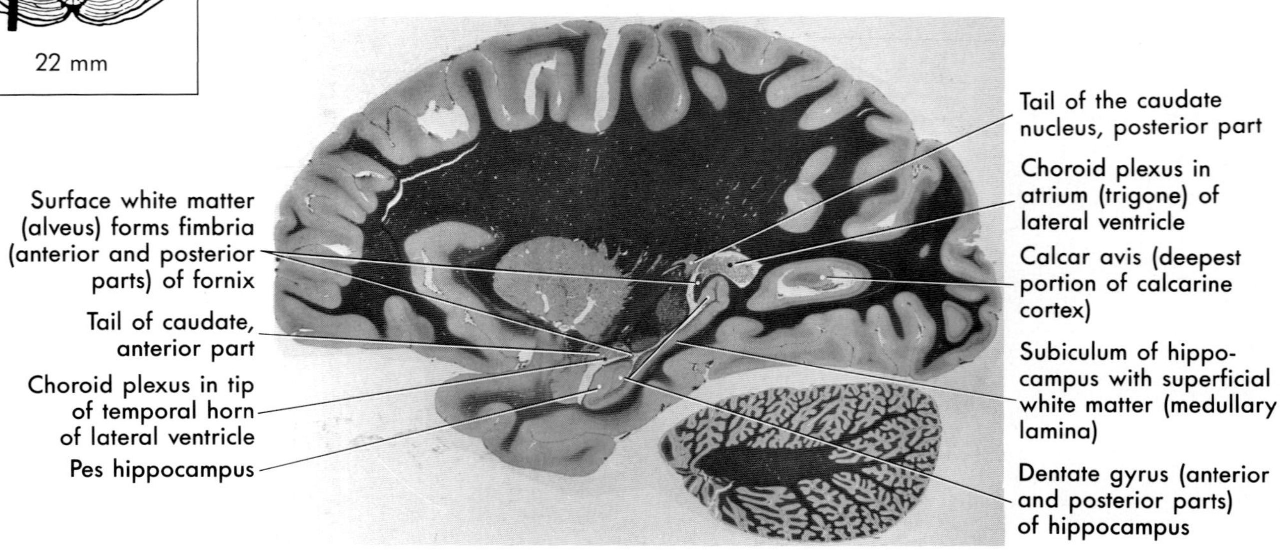

Figure 3-95

SAGITTAL IMAGES

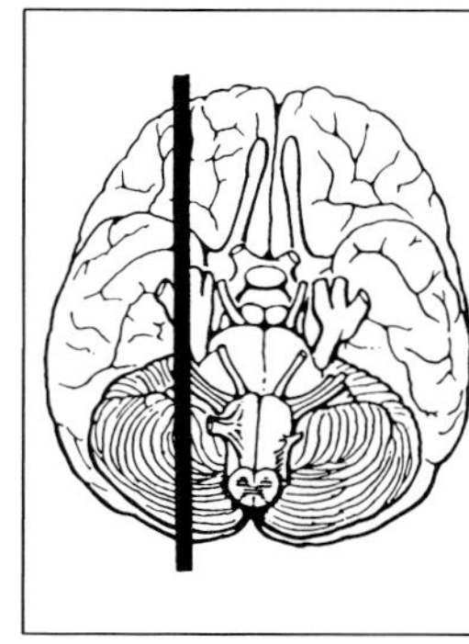

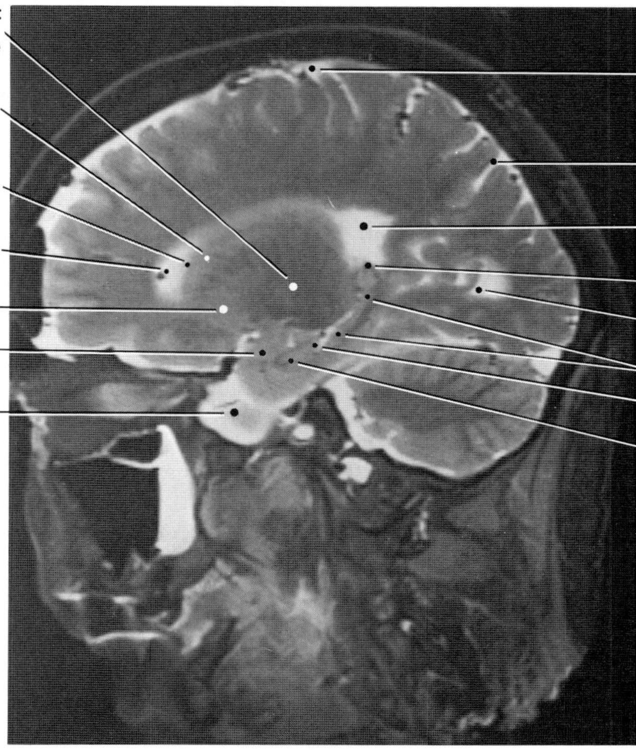

Figure 3-96

SAGITTAL IMAGES

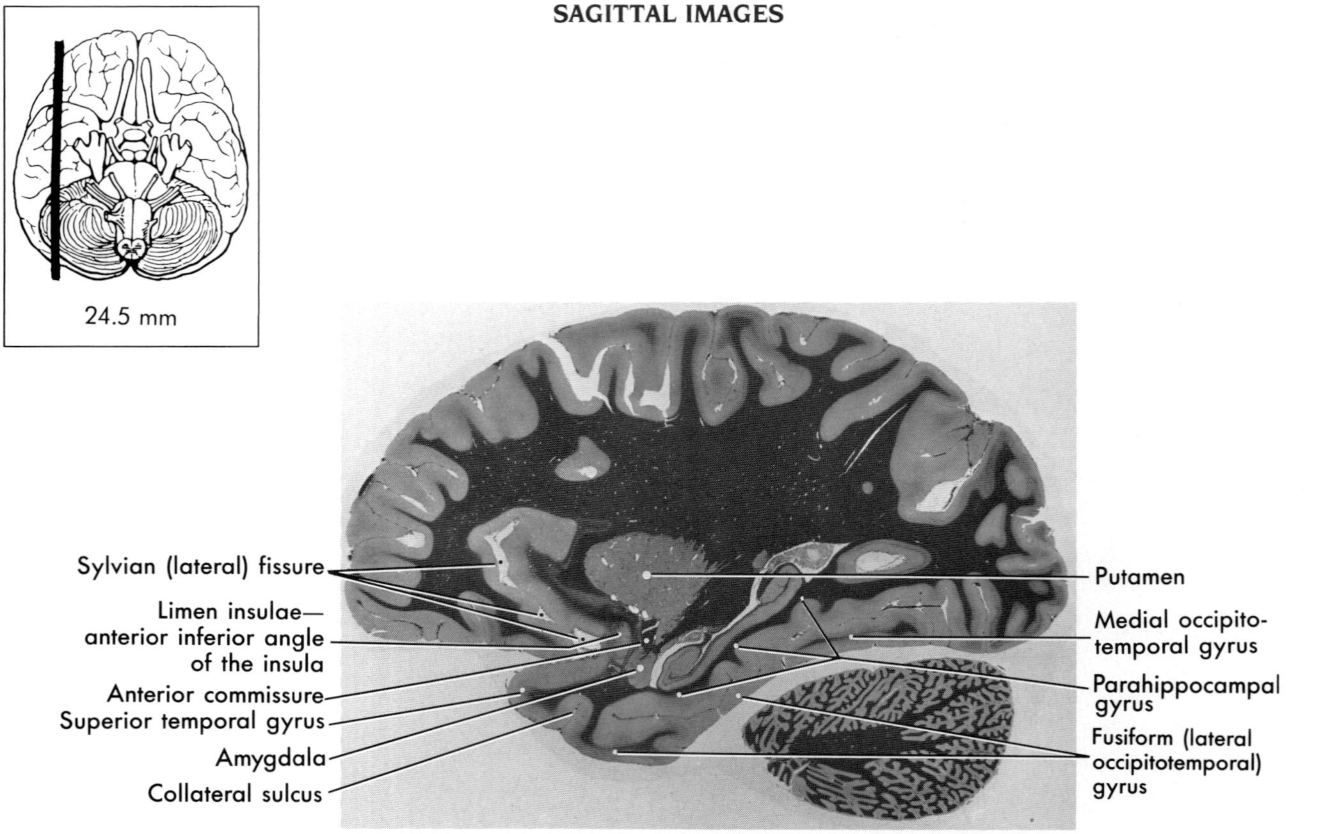

Figure 3-97

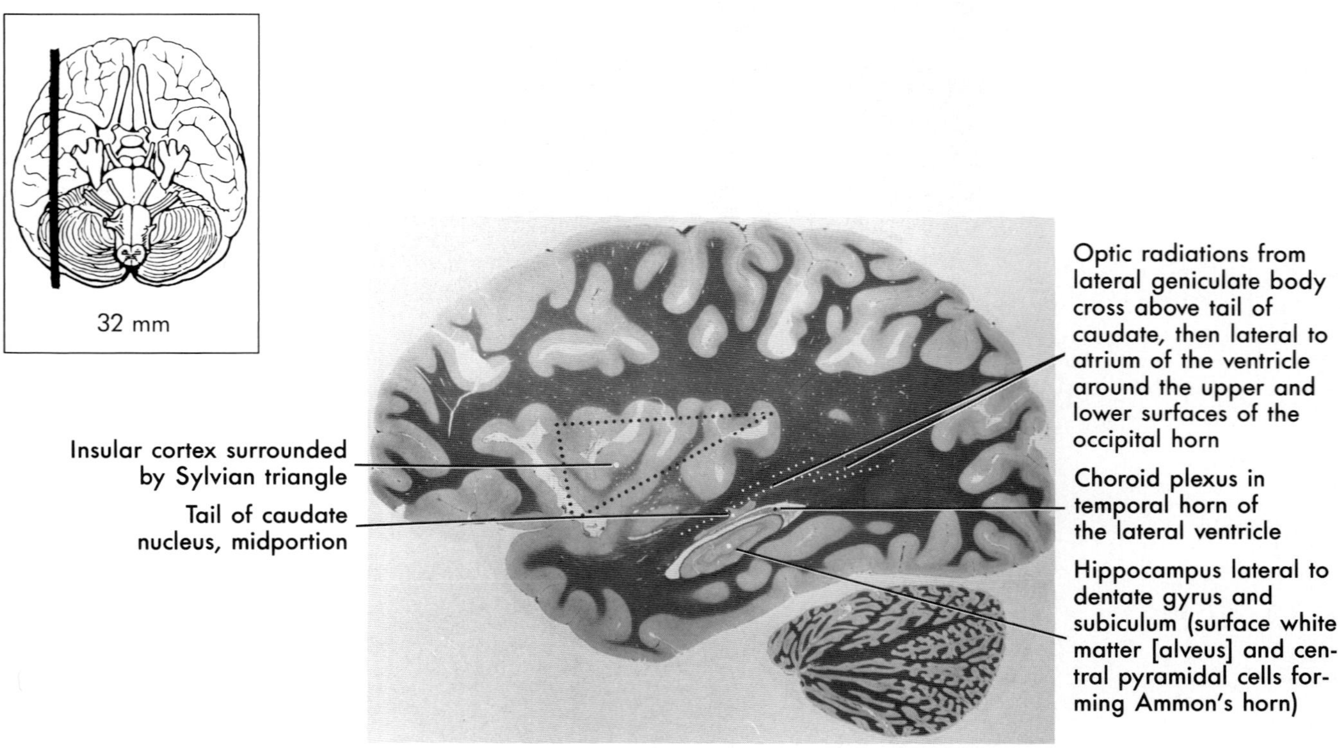

Figure 3-98

SAGITTAL IMAGES

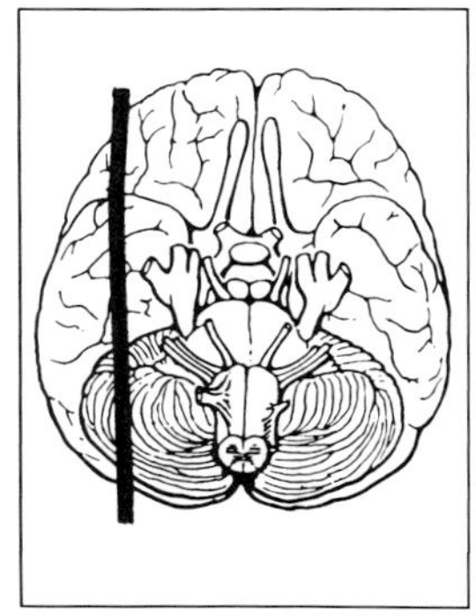

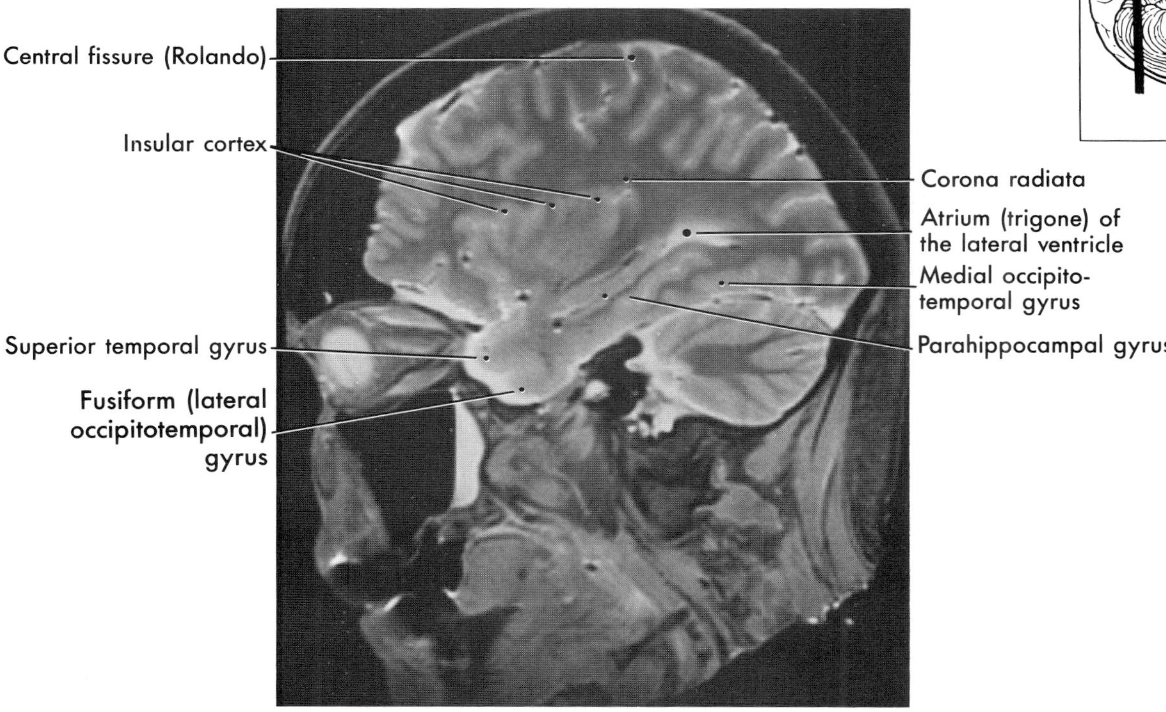

Figure 3-99

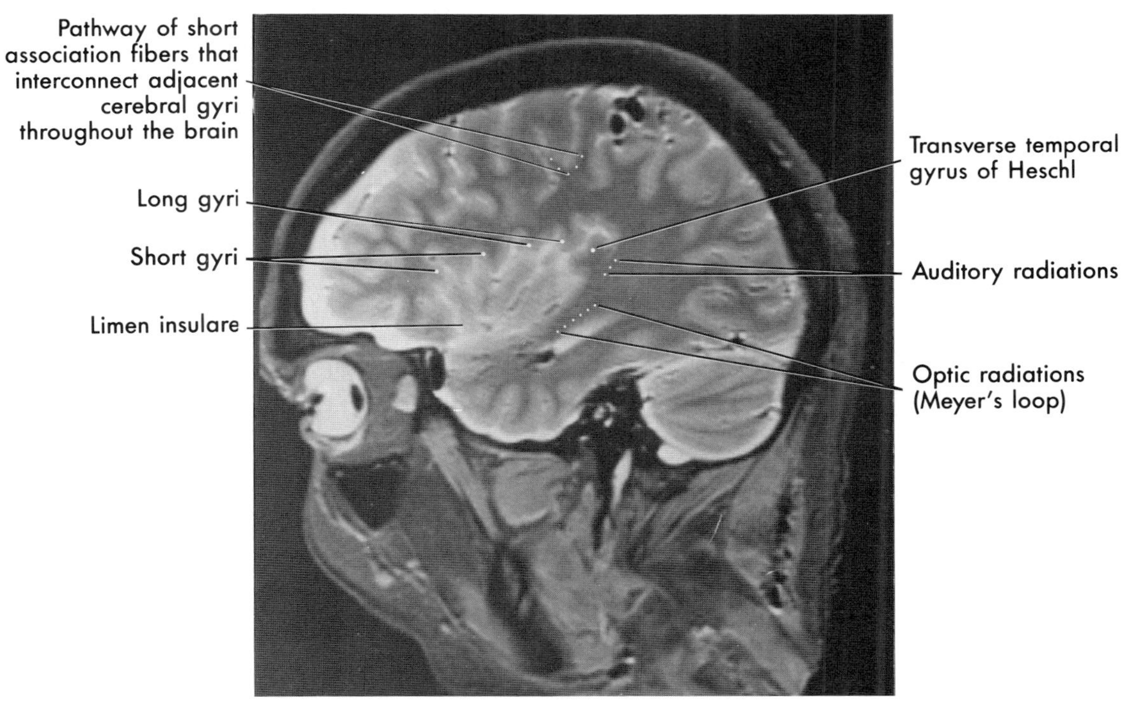

Figure 3-100

SAGITTAL IMAGES

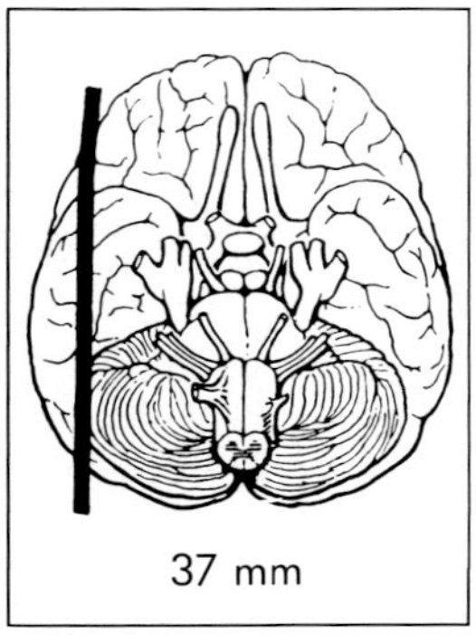

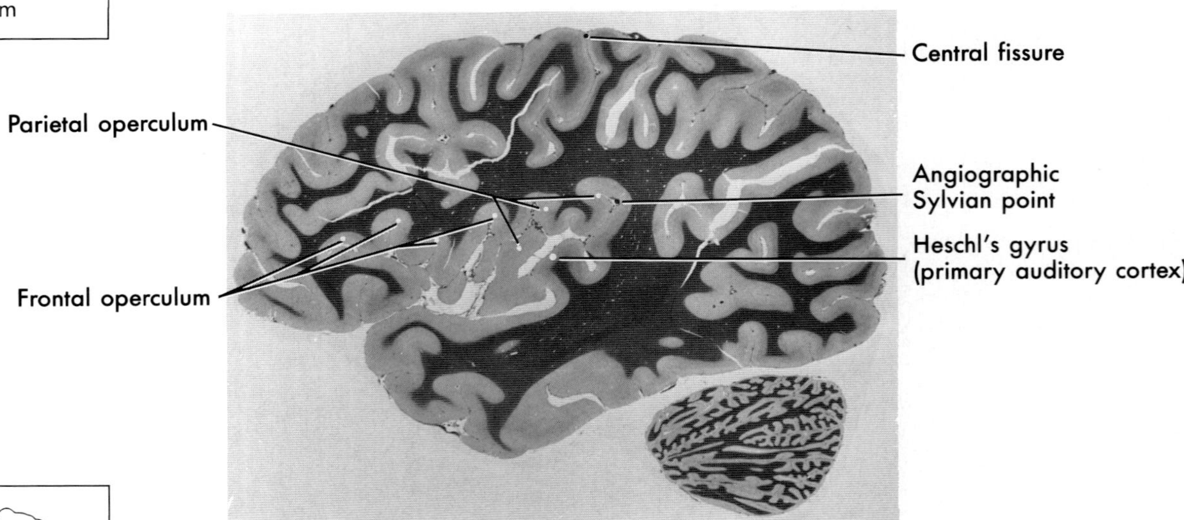

Figure 3-101

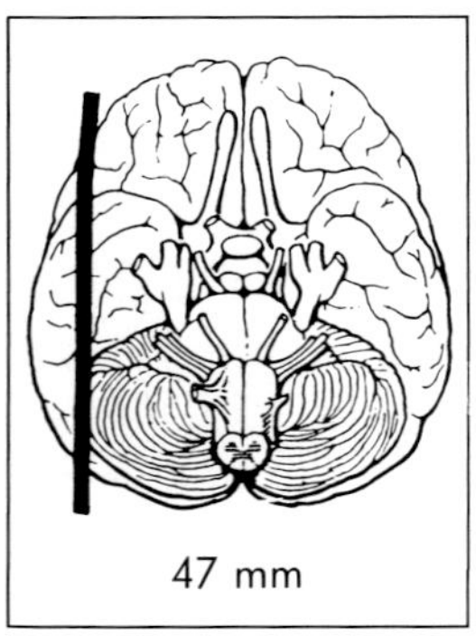

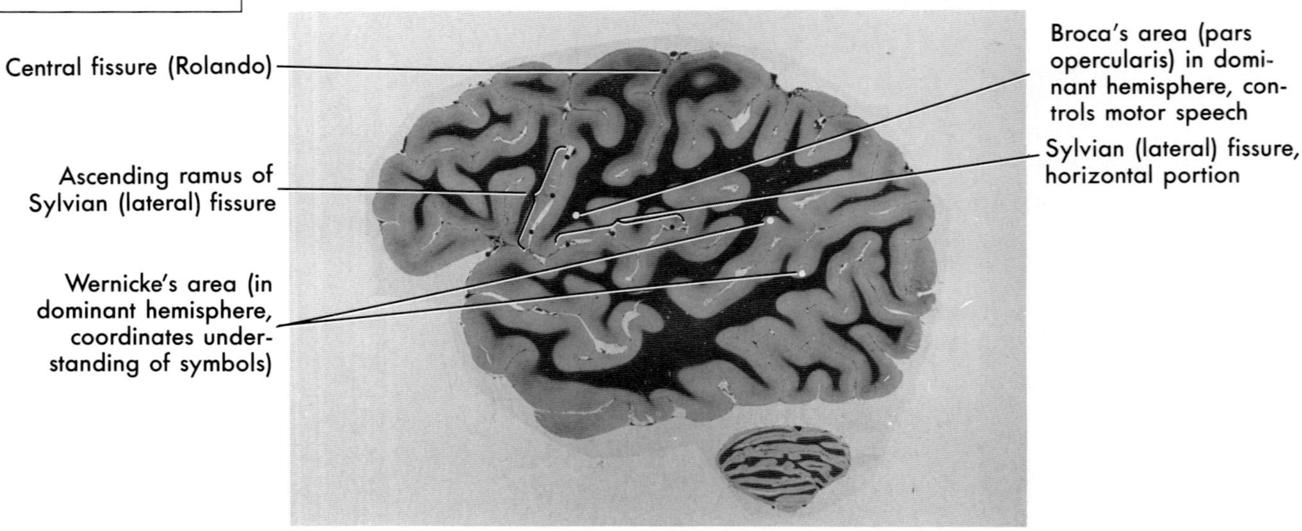

Figure 3-102

SAGITTAL IMAGES

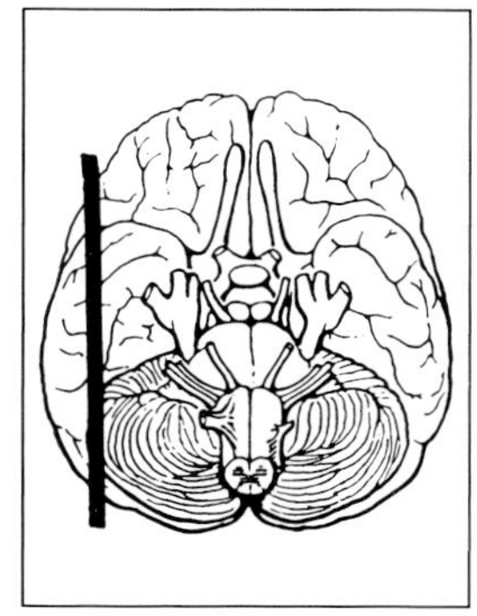

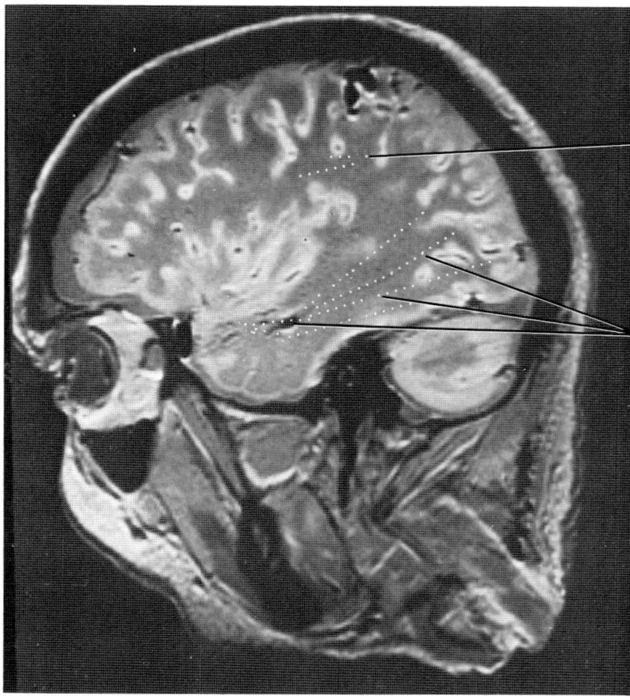

Figure 3-103

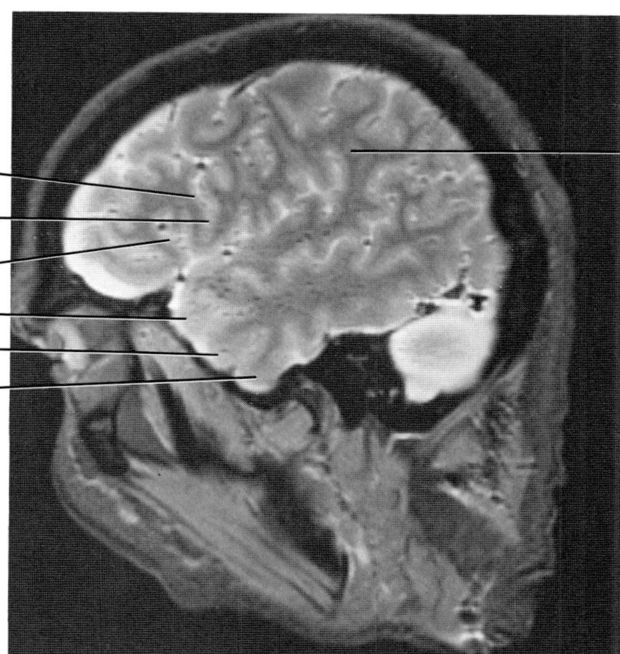

Figure 3-104

INDEX TO THE ILLUSTRATIONS

Entries refer to figures in which the specific structures are labeled.

CHAPTER 4

L. Anne Hayman
Richard A. Bronen
Dale A. Charletta

Adult Cerebrum

IMAGING TECHNIQUES

The adult cerebrum can be imaged directly with either computed tomography (CT) or magnetic resonance imaging (MRI). The decision concerning when each examination is appropriate depends on many factors. MR scans are usually obtained from cooperative patients with medical conditions that require the extreme sensitivity of long TR/long TE (T2-weighted) sequences (TR, repetition time; TE, echo delay time; T2, transverse relaxation time). MRI is also particularly useful when sagittal and coronal images are needed to clarify the anatomic features of a lesion. In general, MR images obtained with long TR/TE sequences, cardiac gating, and motion suppression techniques supplemented by short TR/TE sequences provide more anatomic information concerning brain structure than conventional CT scans.[1] High field strength (1.5 T) scanners afford greater resolution of anatomic detail than the current generation of lower field strength MR scanners.

The adult cerebrum can be adequately examined with the standard clinical MR axial, coronal, and sagittal images. This protocol should be varied when images of the *central sulcus* or the *limbic lobe* are needed. The positioning of axial and sagittal scan levels that best demonstrate the central sulcus (between the motor and sensory cortex) is illustrated and described in Chapters 11 and 12. These projections should be obtained if surgical removal of lesions near this area is planned.[2,3]

A specialized MR protocol is also needed in patients with partial complex seizures. MRI may be used to lateralize the temporal seizure focus and augment the complex and time-consuming electrophysiologic testing now used to determine which temporal lobe should be removed in patients who are refractory to medical management.[4] T1-weighted (T1, longitudinal relaxation time) coronal MR slices angled so that they are perpendicular to the long axis of the hippocampus have proved to be the most accurate way in which to evaluate the size of the hippocampus in these patients.[5] Thin slices (3 mm or less) with a small field of view (16 cm) are best for accurately quantitating the volume of the hippocampus (see the later section on the limbic lobe). Spoiled gradient-echo pulse sequences provide better anatomic resolution than angled spin-echo images, but gradient-echo sequences cannot be oriented obliquely with the current software.[6] Coronal T2-weighted MR images are helpful for detecting signal abnormalities within the hippocampus.

CT has been shown to be a useful examination for determining the degree of focal limbic lobe atrophy in the patients with symptoms of Alzheimer's disease.[7] The standard CT protocol should be altered in such patients to optimize visualization of these particular structures on axial images. Thin sections (5 mm or less) of the limbic and temporal lobes should be obtained, and the scan angle should be oriented 20 degrees negative (caudal) to the plane of the canthomeatal line (Figure 4-1). Using this protocol, one study showed that focal enlargement of the choroid and/or hippocampal fissures created a hypodense focus in the hippocampus in 82% of patients with Alzheimer's disease.[7] The superior anatomic resolution and multiplanar capability of MRI make it the preferred modality for evaluating findings in Alzheimer's disease in patients who can cooperate for this imaging study.

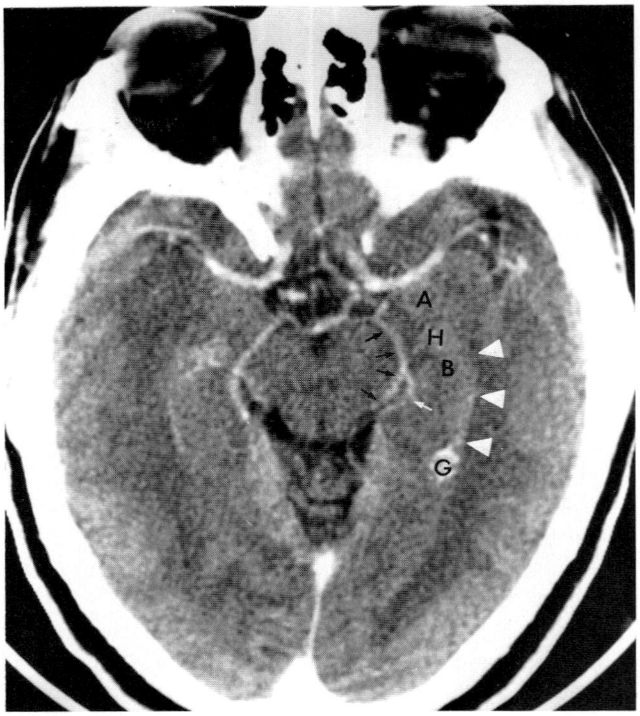

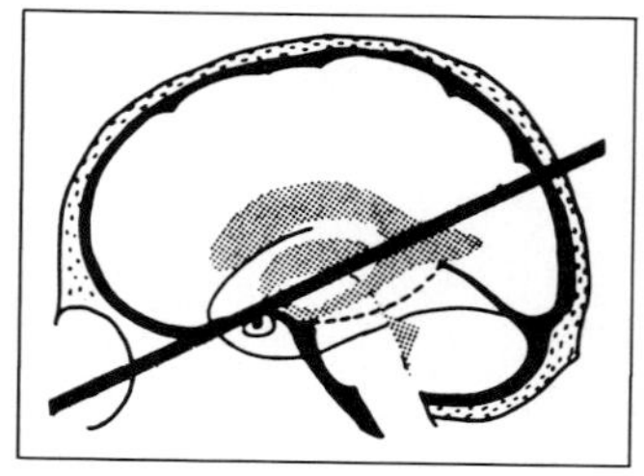

Figure 4-1 Axial intravenous iodine contrast–enhanced CT scan angled 20 degrees negative to the canthomeatal line (see *inset*). Arrowheads mark the enhancement of the choroid plexus and hippocampus (H = head; B = body) in the floor of the temporal horn. Lucencies in the body are noted in many subjects with Alzheimer's disease when this scan angle is used.[7] The posterolateral choroidal artery marks the choroidal fissure (*white arrow*). *Black arrows* mark posterior cerebral artery in ambient cistern. A, Amygdala; G, glomus of choroid plexus.

NORMAL ANATOMY

Cerebral Cortex

In the adult brain, a superficial layer of neurons 3 to 5 mm thick forms the cortex of the cerebral hemispheres. This cortex can be divided into six individual lobes that are partially separated from each other by sulci. These are the limbic, temporal, frontal, parietal, occipital, and insular lobes. Although this classification separates the cortex into somewhat arbitrary regions, it is widely used by neurologists, neurosurgeons, and neuroradiologists to locate a hemispheric lesion. The following discussion describes the borders of each of these lobes, as well as the functions of the cortical regions they encompass.

Limbic Lobe

The limbic lobe is found on the medial surface of each cerebral hemisphere. A simplified overview of the cortical functions mediated by this lobe is labeled in Figure 4-2, *A*. In most subjects the left limbic lobe mediates verbal memory and language functions, whereas the right mediates nonverbal and spatial functions. The location of this lobe on axial images is shown in Figure 4-2, *B*. The extensive connections between subcortical nuclei and the limbic lobe form the limbic system, which is discussed later in the section on major functional pathways.

The limbic lobe is a difficult region for several reasons. The anatomy is complex, the terminology is redundant and confusing, and the two gyri have been subdivided and renamed many times. To assist the reader, Tables 4-1 and 4-2 list the common nomenclature for hippocampal and limbic structures.[8-26] For clarity, most of the terms used in this chapter are based on work by Duvernoy.[10]

The limbic lobe consists of two concentric gyri surrounding the corpus callosum and extending anteriorly, medial to the temporal lobe. Broca named the larger, outer one the *limbic gyrus* and the smaller, inner one the *intralimbic gyrus*.* Each gyrus can be divided in the sagittal plane into three segments based on their relationship to the corpus callosum: (1) a rostral (anterior) segment, (2) a superior segment, and (3) a temporal (inferior) segment (Figure 4-3).

The larger, outer limbic gyrus (Figure 4-3, *A*) contains a bundle of fibers known as the *cingulum*. The anterior segment, known as the *subcallosal area,* is found beneath the rostrum and genu of the corpus callosum. The second segment, above the corpus callosum, is known as the *cingulate gyrus*. The inferior component curves under the splenium of the corpus callosum. At this point, it is referred to as the *isthmus* of the cingulate gyrus. The isthmus of the cingulate gyrus continues anteriorly along the medial surface of the temporal lobe and is renamed the *parahippocampal gyrus*. The parahippocampal gyrus hooks medially at its anterior end to form the uncus.

*Unfortunately, the term *intralimbic gyrus* is currently used to refer to a portion of the uncus. For clarity, this chapter refers to the smaller, inner limbic ring as *Broca's intralimbic gyrus*.

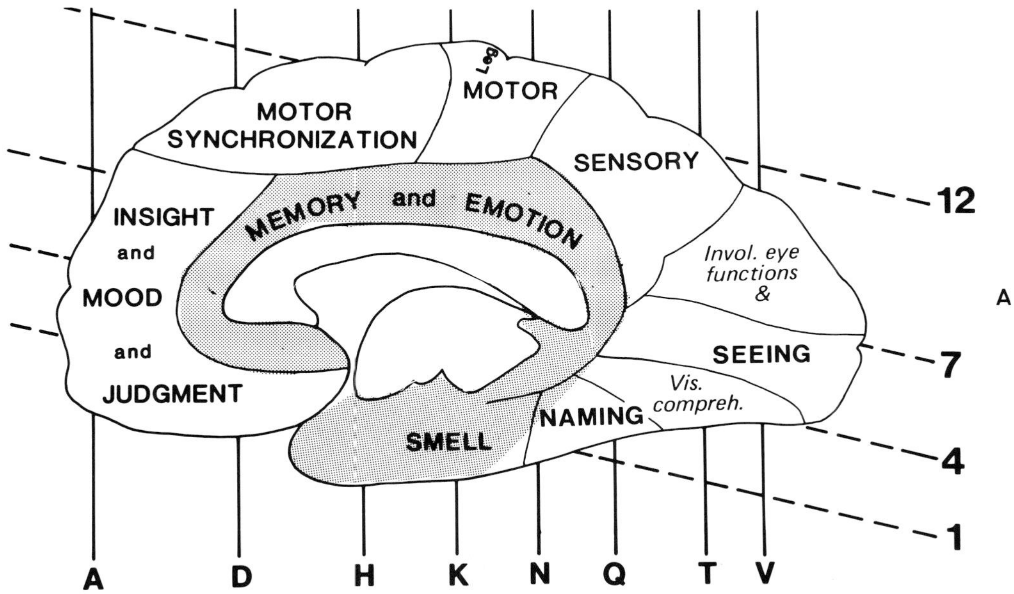

Figure 4-2 Limbic cortex is shaded on the medial surface of the right cerebral hemisphere **(A)** and on axial and coronal brain slices **(B)**.

Continued.

The division of the *anterior* parahippocampal gyrus into upper and lower parts is best visualized in the coronal plane (Figure 4-4). The upper part is called the *subiculum*. The lower portion is known as the *entorhinal area*. The entorhinal area is not present in the posterior sections of the parahippocampal gyrus. This anatomic distinction has clinical significance because the entorhinal area invariably reveals abnormality in autopsy studies of patients with Alzheimer's disease. The onset of confusion, which is an early finding in Alzheimer's disease, is undoubtedly caused by changes in this cortical area.[27,28]

The smaller, inner limbic gyrus (i.e., Broca's intralimbic gyrus) is also divided into three segments (Figure 4-3, *B*). The paraterminal gyrus (anterior segment) and supracallosal gyrus (superior segment) are vestigial in man, whereas the hippocampus (inferior segment) is well formed. The *paraterminal gyrus* is situated between the subcallosal area and the lamina terminalis. Above the corpus callosum, but below the cingulate gyrus, Broca's intralimbic gyrus is renamed the *supracallosal gyrus* or *indusium griseum*. (This gray matter is flanked by white matter fibers of the lateral and medial longitudinal stria.) The inferior segment is referred to as the *hippocampus*.* It is bordered superiorly by the choroidal fissure, medially by the ambient cistern, and inferiorly by the upper segment of the parahippocampal gyrus, the subiculum. Laterally, the hippocampus protrudes into the temporal horn of the lateral ventricle. Macroscopically, the hippocampus is divided into three segments as it curves around the lateral margin of the brainstem: (1) the bulbous anterior head, (2) the body, and (3) the slender posterior tail. These are best demonstrated in the axial plane (Figure 4-5).

The *internal* macroscopic architecture of the hippocampus is complex. When viewed in the coronal plane, it consists of two interlocking laminae of gray matter. These have been named the *cornu ammonis* and the *dentate gyrus*. Both are primitive cortical areas that have three, rather than the usual six, layers of neurons. The peculiar arrangement of the cornu ammonis (Ammon's horn) and dentate gyrus is caused by the folding of cortex that occurs during fetal development (Figure 4-6). This fold becomes the hippocampal fissure, or sulcus. It separates the dentate gyrus (above) from the cornu ammonis and subiculum (below). The deepest (lateral) portion of this fissure is usually obliterated in utero, but a residual cavity of this fissure can be seen on MR images in 10% of the normal population.[24] The hippocampal fissure is present in the head, body, and tail of the hippocampus. Anteriorly, this fissure merges with the uncal sulcus. The MR appearance of the medial hippocampal fissure is that of a slitlike cerebrospinal fluid (CSF) space in most normal subjects[24] but has been noted to be dilated in those with Alzheimer's disease.[7]

The *microscopic* anatomy of the hippocampus is also complex. The principal neuronal layer of the cornu ammo-

*The term *hippocampal formation* refers to the functional unit that includes the hippocampus, the subiculum, and the entorhinal cortex. However, many authors use this interchangeably with the term *hippocampus*.

B

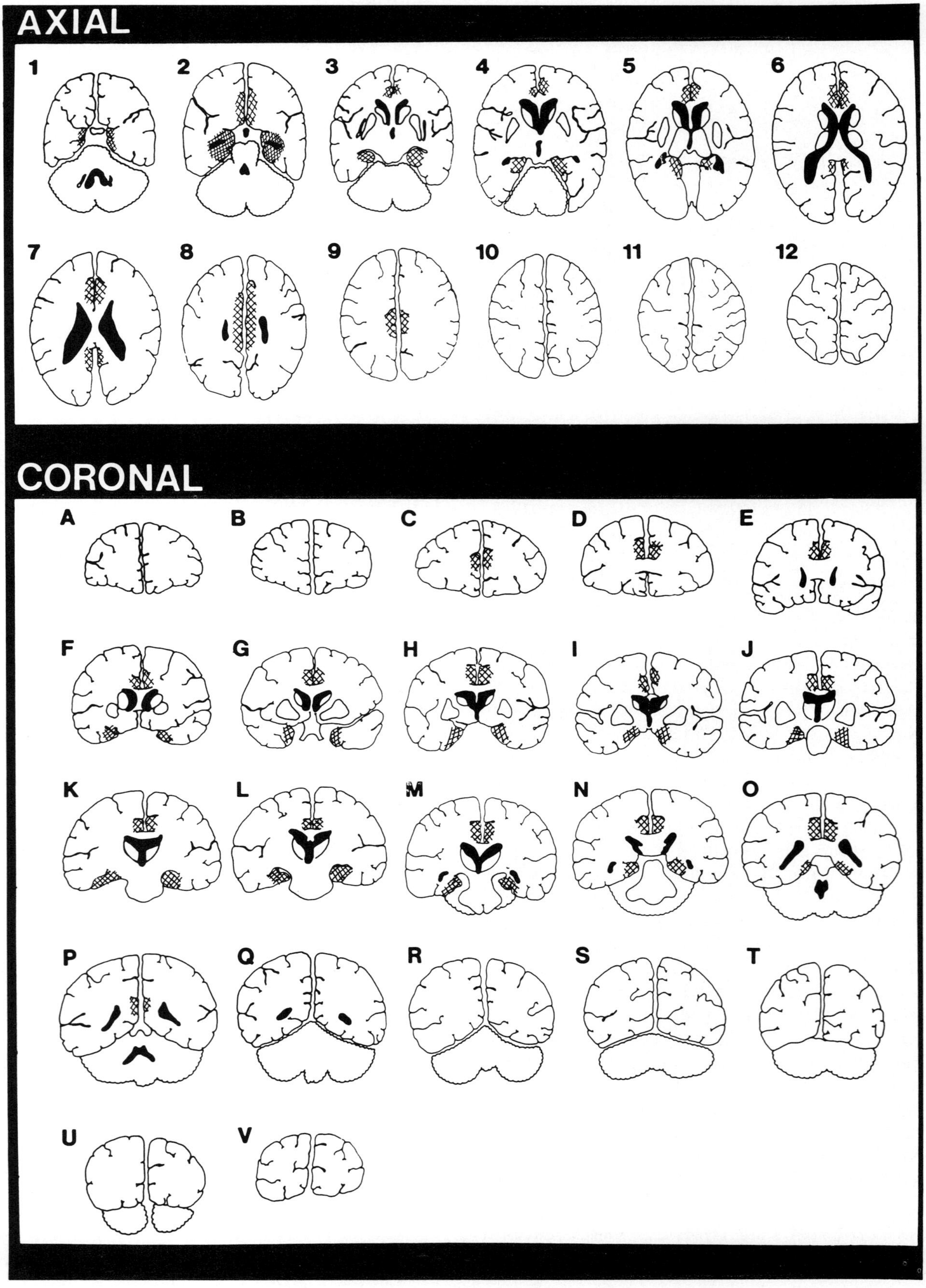

Figure 4-2, cont'd. **B,**For legend see p. 119.

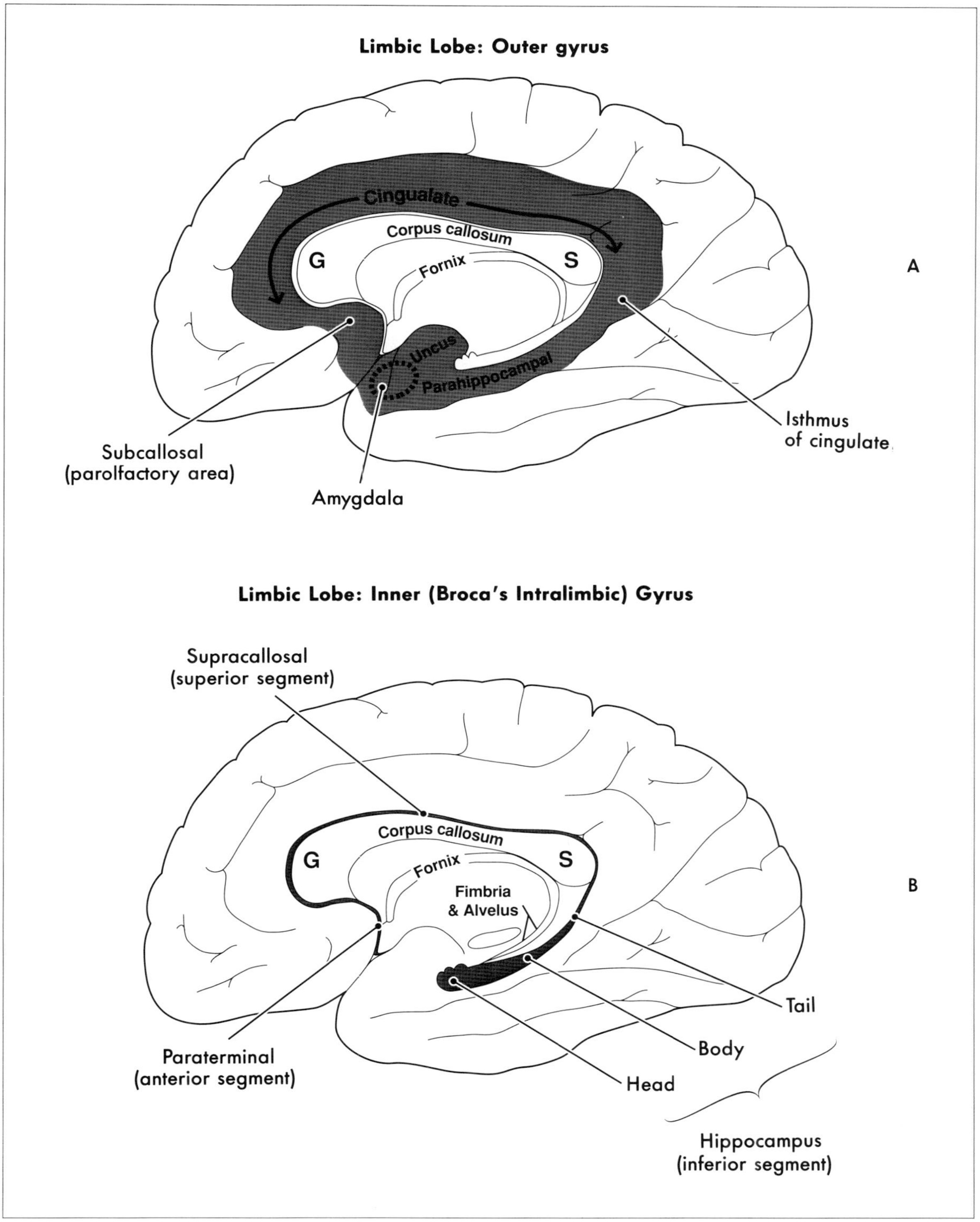

Figure 4-3 Schematic diagrams of the medial surface of the right cerebral hemisphere illustrate nomenclature for the (shaded) outer **(A)** and inner **(B)** cortical gyri that form the limbic lobe. Tables 4-1 and 4-2 should be consulted for synonyms. The amygdala is labeled to orient the reader.

◆ **TABLE 4-1** Hippocampal Terminology

Described entity	Best term	Synonyms	Other terms
HIPPOCAMPUS*	Hippocampus	Hippocampal formation	Ram's horn, Ammon's horn, cornu ammonis, pes hippocampus, pes hippocampus major
CORNU AMMONIS	Cornu ammonis (CA)	Ammon's horn, hippocampus proper	Hippocampus
Lorente de No's CA1	CA1	Sommer sector, vulnerable sector	Rose's H1, Vogt's H1, Retzius' gyri,† retrosplenial gyrus,† subcallosal eminence†
Lorente de No's CA2	CA2		Rose's H2, Vogt's H2
Lorente de No's CA3	CA3	Resistant sector, Spielmeyer sector	Rose's H3, Vogt's H2
Lorente de No's CA4	CA4	Hilus of fascia dentata, endfolium	Rose's H4, H5; Vogt's H4; endblade; Bratz sector
DENTATE GYRUS	Dentate gyrus	Gyrus dentatus, fascia dentata	
Visible dentate gyrus			
In uncus	Band of Giacomini		
In head and body	Margo denticulatus		
In tail	Fasciola cinerea		
Area dentata			
CA4			
Dentate gyrus			
FORNIX			
Hippocampal segment			
Fimbria			
Alveus			
Crus of fornix			
Commissure of fornix		Hippocampal commissure, psalterium	Lyre of David
Body of fornix			
Column of fornix			
Precommissural fornix			
Retrocommissural fornix		Postcommissural fornix	
SULCI			
Hippocampal fissure		Hippocampal sulcus	
Dentatofimbrial fissure		Fimbriodentate sulcus	
HIPPOCAMPAL TAIL			
Retrosplenial gyrus	Retzius' gyri†	Subcallosal eminence,† bulge of CA1 in tail	
Subsplenial gyrus§	Terminal segment of tail, inferior to splenium; bridge of cornu ammonis to indusium griseum‡		
Fasciolar gyrus‖	As fimbria separates and forms fornix crus, fimbriodentate sulcus widens to form this structure, which is CA3 covered by alveus		
Fasciola cinerea	Visible portion of dentate gyrus		

*Originally based on its intraventricular appearance.
†Names in hippocampal tail only.
‡It is controversial as to whether indusium griseum is continuation of cornu ammonis (as thought by Duvernoy) or dentate gyrus.
§Some use subsplenial gyrus to refer to entire tail.
‖Some use fasciolar gyrus interchangeably with fasciola cinerea/dentate gyrus.

◆ **TABLE 4-2** Limbic Terminology

Described entity	Best term	Synonym	Other terms
LIMBIC SYSTEM	Limbic system		
I. Limbic lobe	Limbic lobe		Rhinencephalon
A. Limbic gyrus			
1. Subcallosal area	Subcallosal area	Paraolfactory area	
2. Cingulate gyrus	Cingulate gyrus		
3. Isthmus of cingulate gyrus	Isthmus of the cingulate gyrus		
4. Parahippocampal gyrus (PHG)	Parahippocampal gyrus		Hippocampal gyrus
a. Anterior portion including uncus	Entorhinal cortex or area	Brodmann's area 28	
(anterior folded PHG)	Uncus		
b. Subiculum*	Subiculum		
B. Intralimbic gyrus†			
1. Anterior segment	Paraterminal gyrus	Prehippocampal rudiment, precommissural hippocampus‡	
2. Superior segment	Supracallosal gyrus	Indusium griseum, supracommissural hippocampus‡	
a. Indusium griseum gray matter			
b. Lateral longitudinal stria white matter			
c. Medial longitudinal stria white matter			
3. Inferior segment	Hippocampus	Hippocampal formation, retrocommissural hippocampus‡	
a. Anterior hippocampal digitations	Hippocampal head	Pes hippocampi, digitationes hippocampi	
b. Middle segment	Hippocampal body		
c. Posterior segment	Hippocampal tail	Subsplenial gyrus	
II. Subcortical structures: amygdala, septal nuclei, thalamus, habenula, hypothalamus, midbrain, mamillary body			
SEPTAL AREA	Septal area	Paraterminal body	
I. Subcallosal area	Subcallosal area	Paraolfactory area	
II. Paraterminal gyrus	Paraterminal gyrus	Subcallosal gyrus	

*Some include subiculum as part of hippocampal formation.
†Coined by Broca, note that this is also term for portion of posterior uncus (this term is more widely used to denote that portion of uncus).
‡In relationship to corpus callosum.

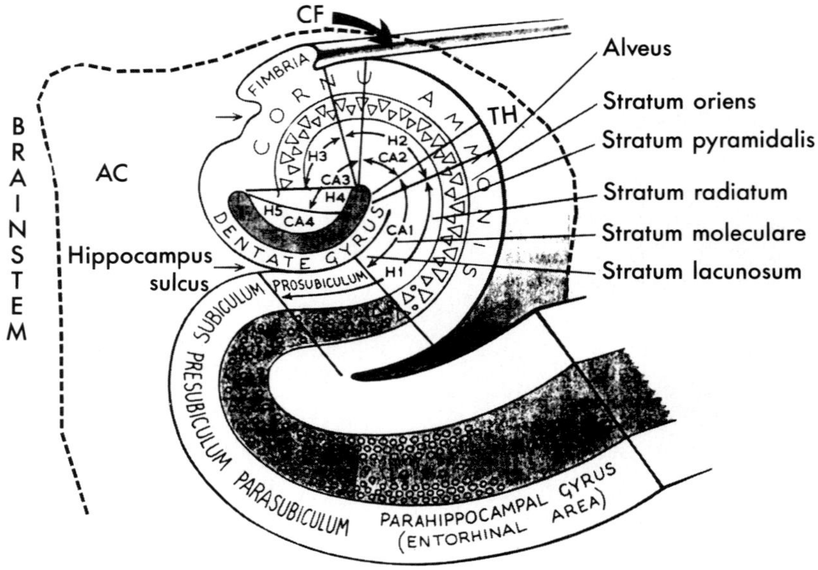

Figure 4-4 Labeled coronal schematic through the body of the adult left hippocampal formation. The brainstem, perimesencephalic or ambient cistern (AC), choroidal fissure (CF), and upper part of the temporal horn of the lateral ventricle (TH) are labeled to orient the reader. The microscopic fields of the cornu ammonis are labeled with the terminology of Lorente de No (CA1 to CA-4) and Rose (H1 to H5) (see Table 4-1). The alveus is a subependymal layer of white matter that contains fibers entering and leaving the hippocampus. The exiting (efferent) fibers of the alveus converge to form the fimbria of the fornix. The striatum oriens, pyramidalis, radiatum, moleculare, and lacunosum refer to microscopically distinct layers of the hippocampus. (Modified from Williams PL, Warwick R: *Gray's anatomy*, ed 36 (British), Edinburgh, 1973, Churchill Livingstone.)

nis (Ammon's horn) is composed of pyramidal cells, whereas in the dentate gyrus, this layer is formed of the granule cells. The axons of these granule cells form the mossy system that projects to the cornu ammonis. The cornu ammonis (CA) can be divided into four microscopic zones of the granule cells: CA1, CA2, CA3, and CA4. The zone of CA4 forms the hilus of the U-shaped dentate gyrus that surrounds it. The zone of CA1 is the most vulnerable to hypoxia. Neuronal loss associated with gliosis often occurs in CA1, CA4, and the dentate gyrus in patients with temporal lobe epilepsy caused by hippocampal sclerosis. The CA3 is sometimes referred to as the *fasciolar gyrus*. This anatomy is best demonstrated on a coronal slice at the level of the hippocampal body (see Figure 4-4).

The principal pathway into the hippocampus is a perforating pathway. Fibers from the entorhinal cortex "perforate" the subiculum to synapse with neurons located in either the dentate gyrus or the cornu ammonis. The major pathway exiting the hippocampus is the *alveus,* a thick layer of white matter on the surface of the cornu ammonis. These fibers converge medially to form the *fimbria,* which travels *beneath* the splenium of the corpus callosum to become the *fornix* (see Figure 4-3, *B*). The fibers of the fimbria are separated from the dentate gyrus by the fimbriodentate sulcus (see Figure 4-4).

A system has been developed to help the imaging clinician identify the complex anatomy of the hippocampus in the coronal plane. Easily identified coronal MR landmarks are used to identify each hippocampal level (Figure 4-7). The hippocampal *head* can be seen on coronal MR slices that include the basilar artery or interpeduncular fossa (Figure 4-7, *C*). The cornu ammonis, dentate gyrus, and subiculum cannot be resolved separately on coronal MR studies. At the level of the hippocampal body, these structures appear as a confluent oval or almond-shaped region of gray above the parahippocampal gyrus. The hippocampal *body* is located on sections that extend from the red nucleus to the superior colliculus (Figure 4-7, *E, F,* and *G*). The body is the most uniform segment of the hippocampus and the easiest and most reliable section to quantify by histology and MRI. Although the right hippocampus is normally quantitatively slightly larger than the left (regardless of age, sex, or handedness), this slight difference cannot be perceived visually on MR studies.[11,24] On coronal MR studies, the alveus and fimbria are easily visualized as a sliver of white matter capping the superior aspect of the hippocampal gray matter and separating the hippocampus from the choroidal fissure and temporal horn[8,9,24] (see Figures 4-4 and 4-7, *E, F,* and *G*).

The hippocampal *tail* ascends from the hippocampal

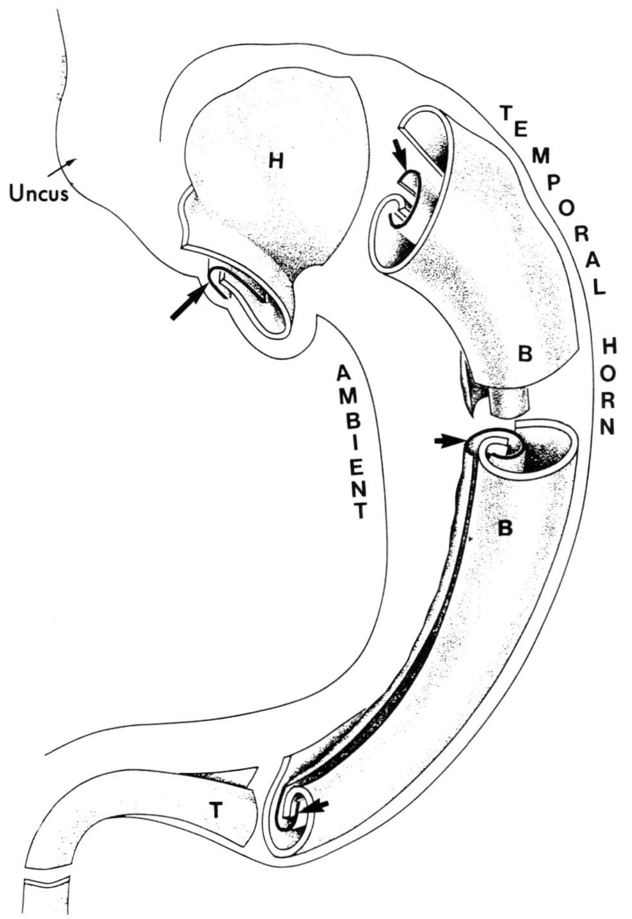

Figure 4-5 Axial schematic diagram of the left hippocampus seen from above. The head (H), body (B), and tail (T) indent the inferomedial surface of the temporal horn. Cross sections of the hippocampus along its length allow the reader to observe that the cells of the dentate gyrus (dark zones indicated by *arrows*) always form a C-shaped cap around cells of the cornu ammonis (Ammon's horn) as this structure rotates in space. The ambient cistern is labeled to orient the reader. (Modified from Duvernoy HM: *The human hippocampus: an atlas of applied anatomy*, München, 1988, JF Bergmann, Verlag.)

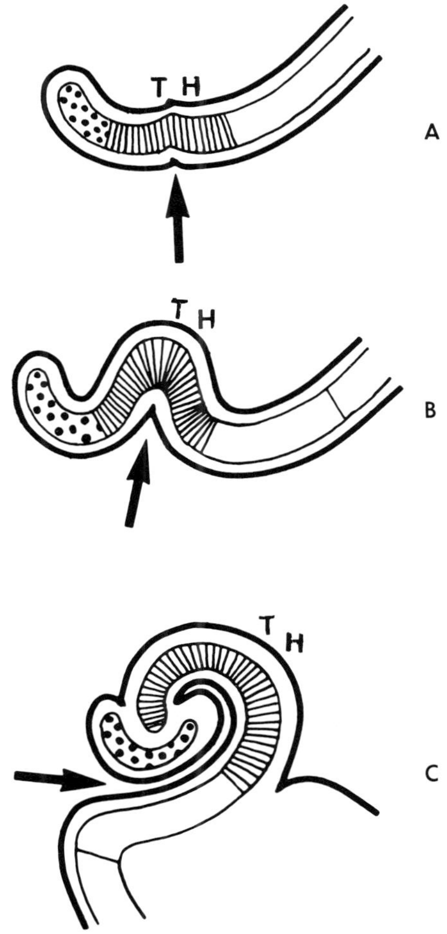

Figure 4-6 Simplified schematic coronal sections through the body of the developing left hippocampus. The dotted portion represents the dentate gyrus; the hatched portion represents the cornu ammonis (Ammon's horn). The unmarked zone represents the subiculum and entorhinal area. **A,** Initially, the tissues that will become the medial floor of the left temporal horn (TH) fold to form the hippocampal sulcus (*arrow*). **B** and **C,** Further growth and infolding create the hippocampal bulge in the inferomedial floor of the temporal horn (TH). Note that migration of the cells that form the dentate gyrus creates a C-shaped cap on the reverse S shape formed by the cornu ammonis and the subiculum. Compare with adult configuration in Figure 4-4. (Modified from Duvernoy HM: *The human hippocampus: an atlas of applied anatomy*, München, 1988, JF Bergmann, Verlag.)

body (at the back of the brainstem) to the supracallosal gyrus (posterior to the splenium) (Figures 4-3, *B*, and 4-7, *H* and *I*). The tail is much thinner than the hippocampal body. The anatomic terms applied to this region are particularly complex and confusing. Terms for all or part of the tail include the *subsplenial gyrus, retrosplenial gyrus, fasciolar gyrus,* and *fasciola cinerea* (see Table 4-1).

Some authors consider the limbic lobe part of the temporal lobe. Thus MR studies are often requested in patients with medically refractory temporal lobe epilepsy caused by hippocampal sclerosis (also called mesial temporal sclerosis). Several MR findings have been reported in the limbic lobe ipsilateral to the seizure focus.[5,12-22,25] The "temporal" lobe is often small (or atrophic). The hippocampal gray matter is usually atrophic and often increased in signal intensity on long TR scans. The adjacent temporal horn may be secondarily enlarged, but this is a less reliable finding, since some variation of temporal horn size occurs in normal subjects, especially adjacent to the hippocampal head.[26] MR evidence of bilaterally small or atrophic hippocampi has also been reported in patients with Alzheimer's disease, schizophrenia, and amnesia.[27-32]

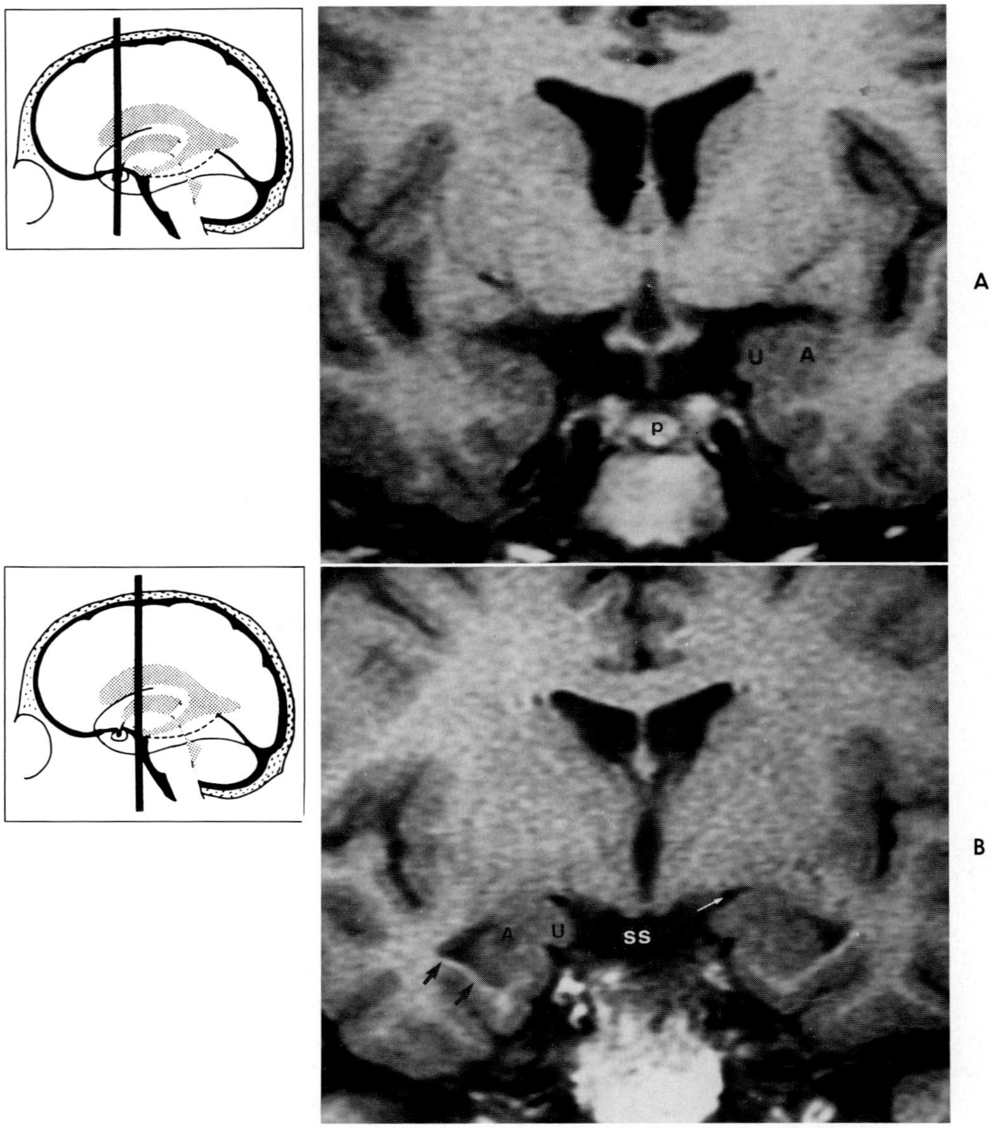

Figure 4-7 Coronal MR scans of the hippocampus at eight levels, which begin anteriorly and proceed posteriorly in 5 mm sections. All images were obtained with T1-weighted sequences (TR/TE, 400/20 msec), except for the companion T2-weighted (1700/75) image shown in **F** for Level V. The hippocampal structures are labeled, and surrounding anatomic landmarks are included to orient the reader. **A,** *Level* I. The boundaries of the amygdala (A) and uncus (U) are indistinguishable from one another. Note the pituitary stalk and posterior pituitary gland (P) are seen at this level. **B,** *Level* II. Amygdala is superior to temporal horn tip (*small black arrows*). Amygdala (A) and uncus (U) form a gray matter complex. Note the suprasellar (SS) cistern contains neither the pituitary nor the basilar artery bifurcation at this level. The entorhinal sulcus is marked by a *small white arrow*.[10]

C

D

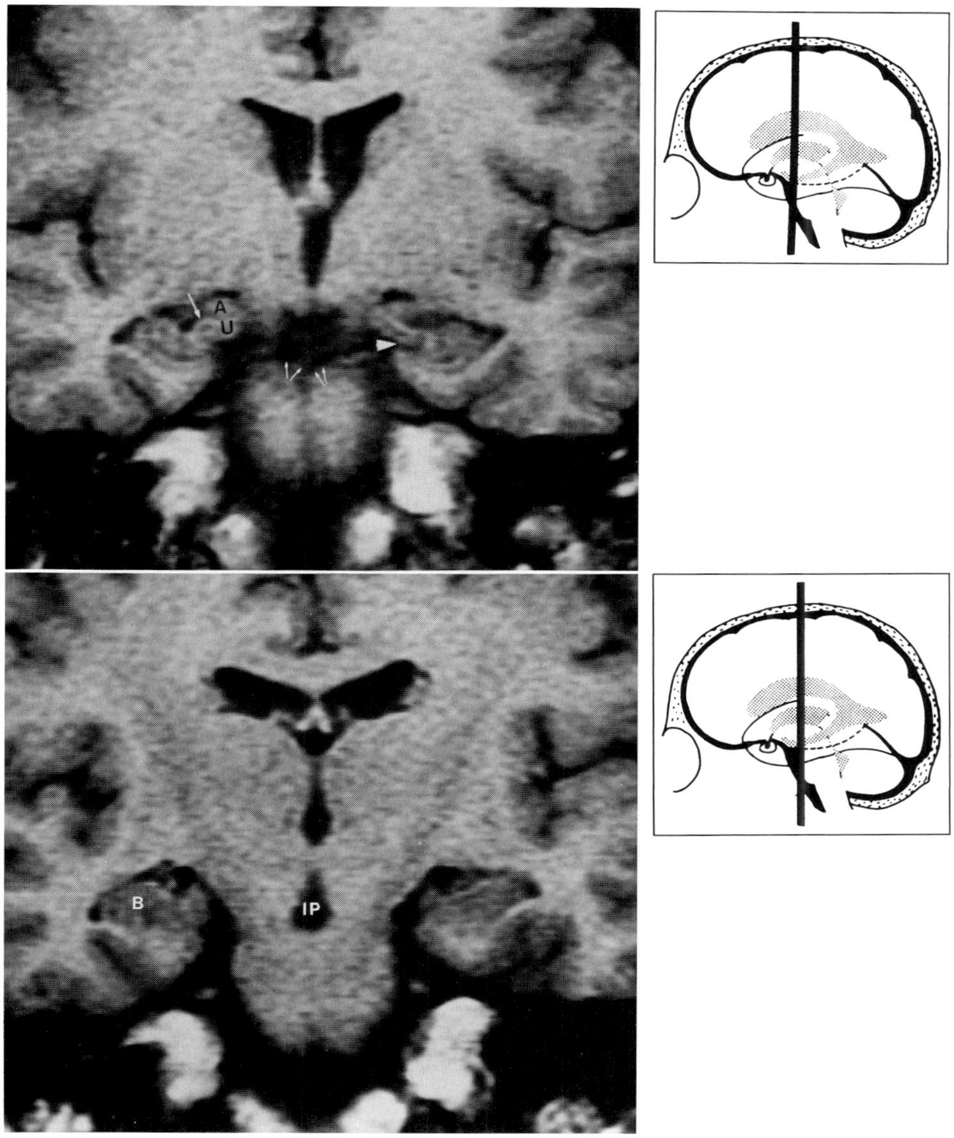

Figure 4-7, cont'd. **C,** *Level* III. The digitations (*white arrow*) identify the hippocampal head. The amygdala (A) and uncus (U) are also seen in this transitional section (between the head and body of the hippocampus). Note the basilar artery as it bifurcates into the posterior cerebral arteries (*small white arrows*) in the prepontine cistern at this level. An *arrowhead* marks the uncal sulcus,[10] that has been unfortunately misnamed the hippocampal sulcus in some texts. **D,** *Level* IV. The bulbous head becomes the hippocampal body (B) at this level. Note the interpeduncular (IP) cistern between cerebral peduncles is also visualized at this level.

Continued.

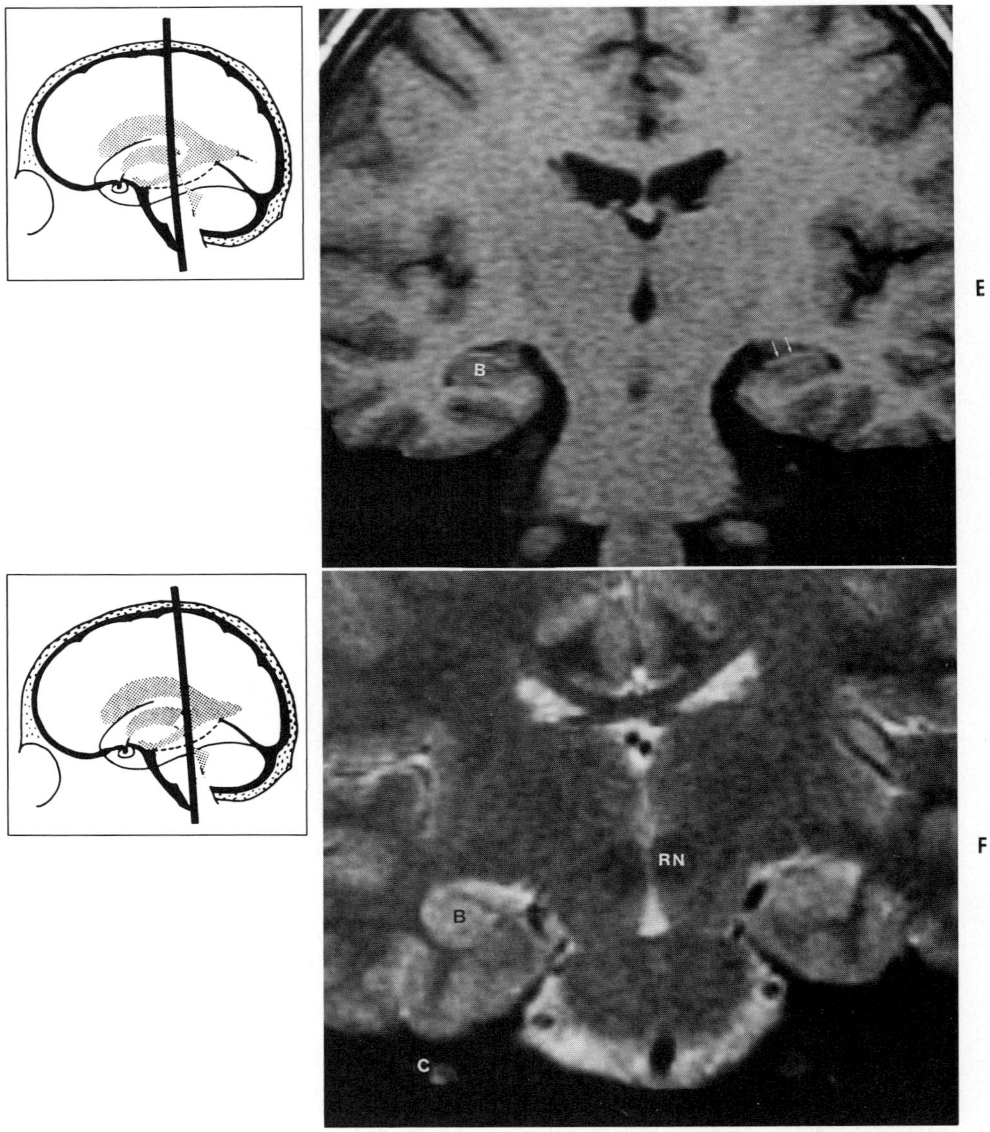

Figure 4-7, cont'd. **E,** *Level* V. The hippocampal body (B) has an oval shape, capped superiorly by the alveus and fimbria (*small white arrows*) below the wing of the ambient cistern. Note the uniform appearance of the hippocampal body on Levels IV to VI. **F,** *Level* V. The hippocampal body (B) is present at this level. Note that the red nucleus (RN) and cochlea (C) are found at this level. Because these structures are difficult to discern on T1-weighted images **(E)**, the companion T2-weighted sequence (TR/TE 1700/75) is shown in this illustration. **G,** *Level* VI. The hippocampal body (B) and the overlying alveus and fimbria (*small arrows*) are again seen at this level. Note the adjacent brainstem does not include either the red nucleus or the colliculi. **H,** *Level* VII. The body of the hippocampus becomes the tail (T) in this section. The pineal gland (*arrow*) is seen at this level just above the superior colliculus. **I,** *Level* VIII. The hippocampal tail (T) ascends vertically behind the brainstem in this section. The inferior colliculi (IC) and superior colliculi (SC) are seen at this level. (Reproduced with permission from Brown, Cheung J, Bronen RA: *Magn Reson Imaging* 9(3):449-457, 1991.)

G

H

I

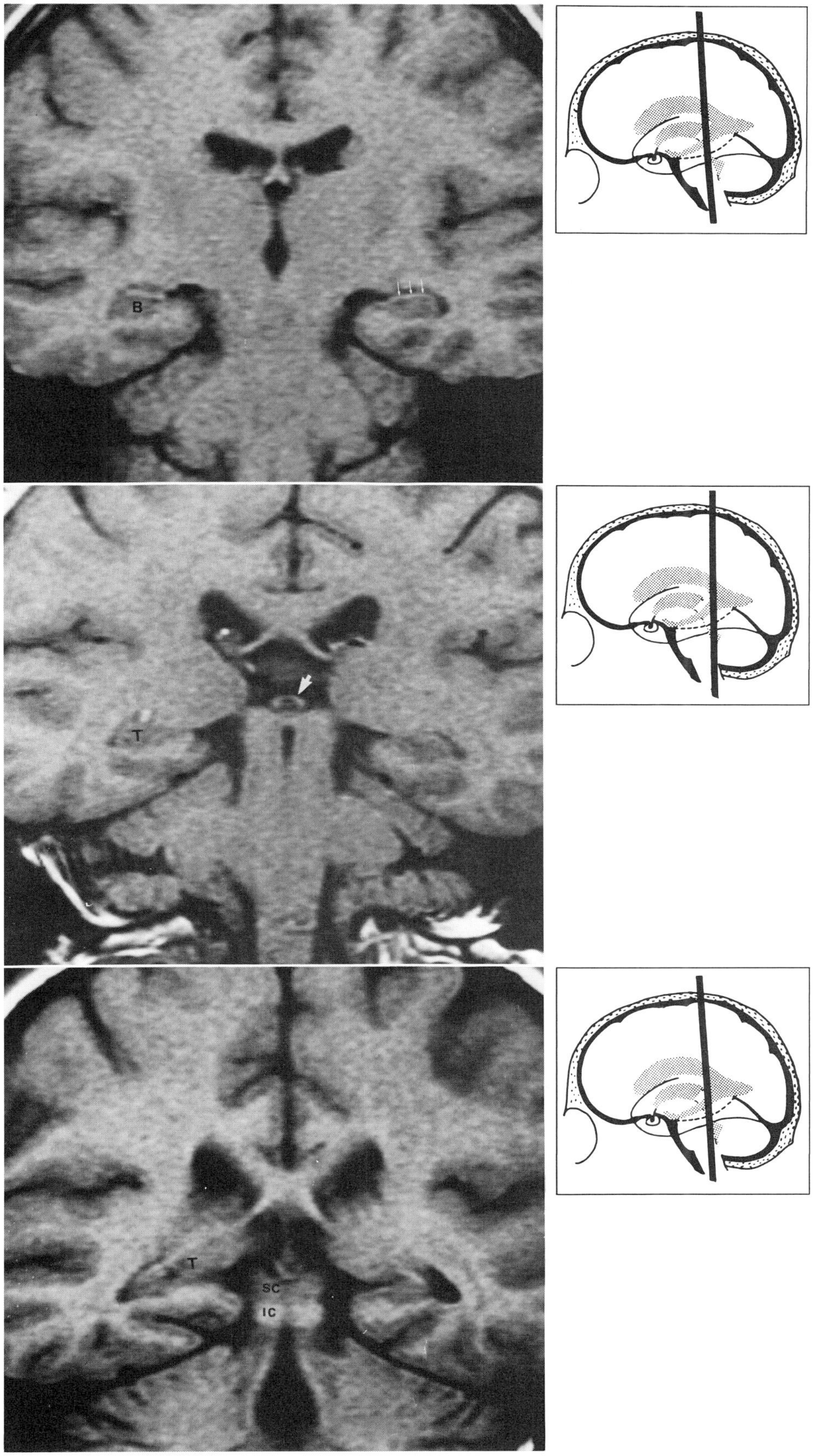

Figure 4-7, cont'd. **G** to **I**, For legend see opposite page.

Temporal Lobe

The temporal lobe lies below the sylvian fissure. It consists of parallel gyri that extend forward from the occipital region toward the temporal pole. The location and the cortical functions mediated by the temporal lobe are labeled on the lateral surface of the brain in Figure 4-8, *A*. The location of the temporal lobe on axial and coronal brain slices[33] is shown in Figure 4-8, *B*. The individual gyri are categorized and labeled on serial sagittal MR scans in Chapter 11. A detailed discussion of the functions of this cortical region can be found in the description of the hemispheric branches of the middle and posterior cerebral arteries in Chapter 16.

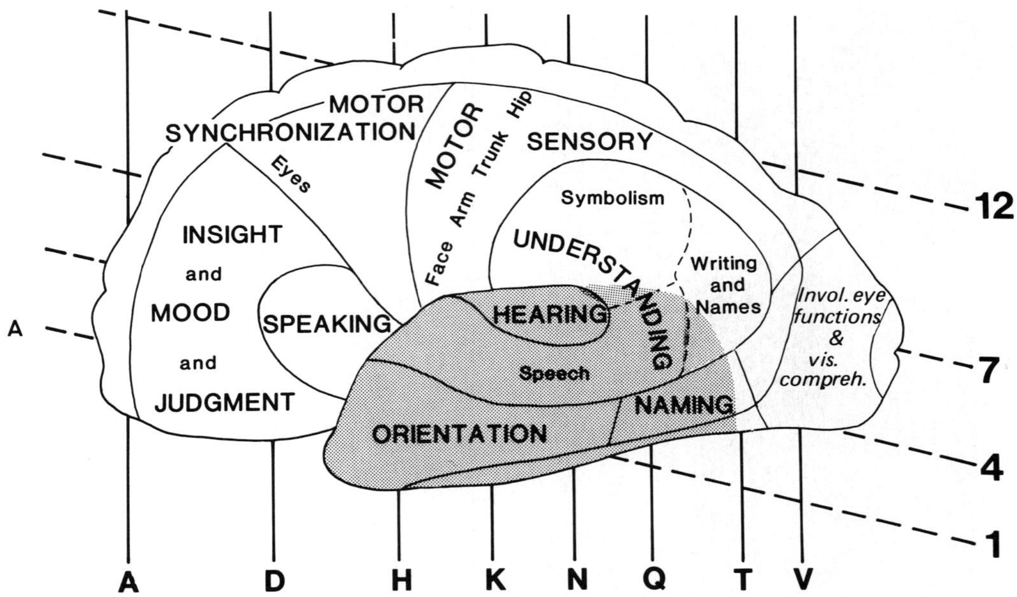

Insular cortex – autonomic function and taste

Figure 4-8 Temporal cortex is shaded on the lateral surface of the left cerebral hemisphere **(A)** and on axial and coronal brain slices **(B)**. The numbers correspond to the axial schematics, and the letters indicate coronal levels of the brain slices.

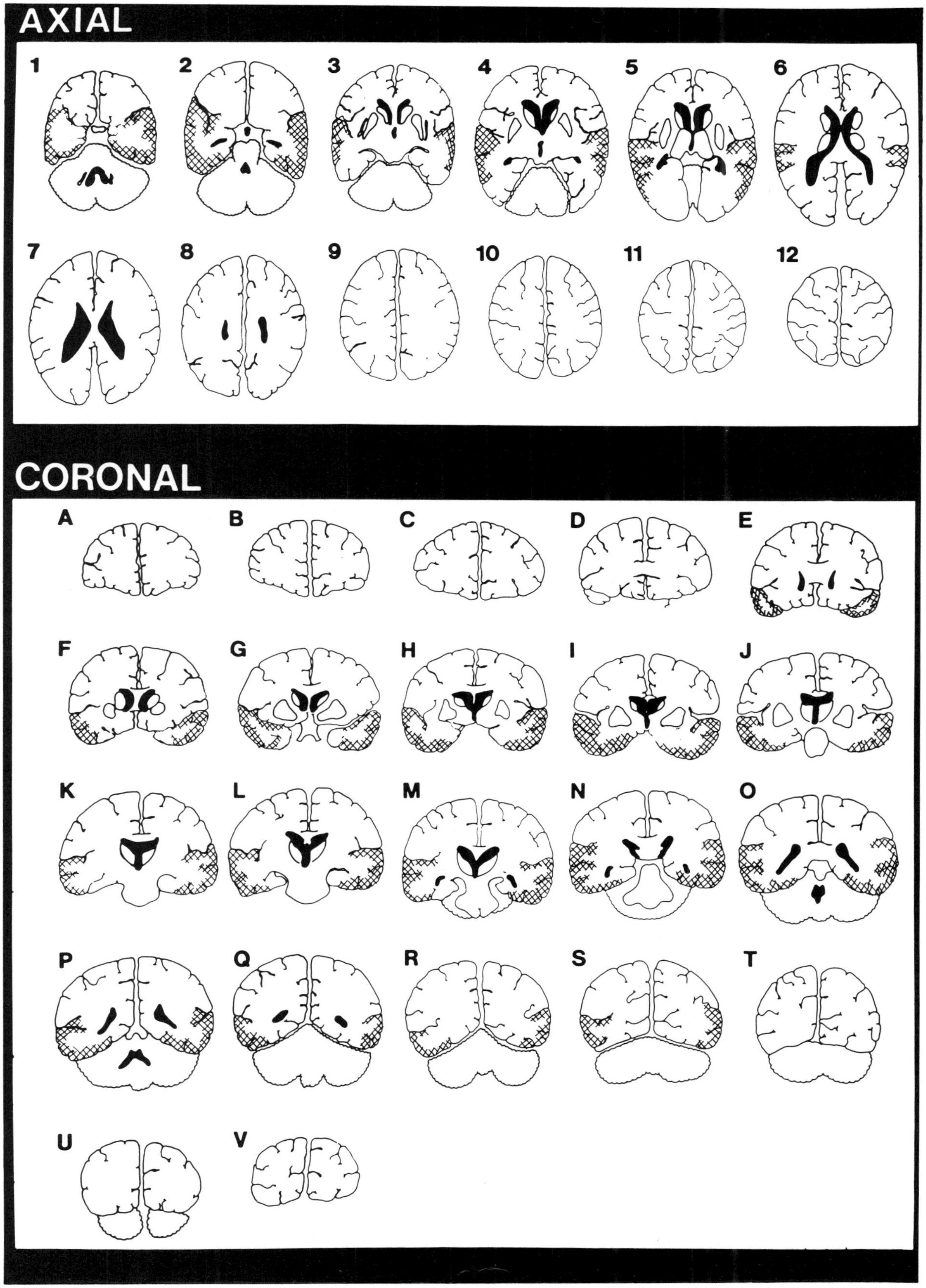

B

Figure 4-8, cont'd. **B,** For legend see opposite page.

Frontal Lobe

The frontal lobe comprises the anterior one third of the hemisphere. It is bounded below by the sylvian fissure and behind by the central sulcus. The location and the cortical functions mediated by this lobe are labeled on the medial and lateral surfaces of the brain[33] in Figure 4-9, *A* and *B*. The location of the frontal lobe on axial and coronal brain slices is shown in Figure 4-9, *C*. The individual gyri are identified and labeled on serial sagittal MR scans in Chapter 11. A detailed discussion of the functions of this cortical region can be found in the description of the hemispheric branches of the anterior and middle cerebral arteries in Chapter 16.

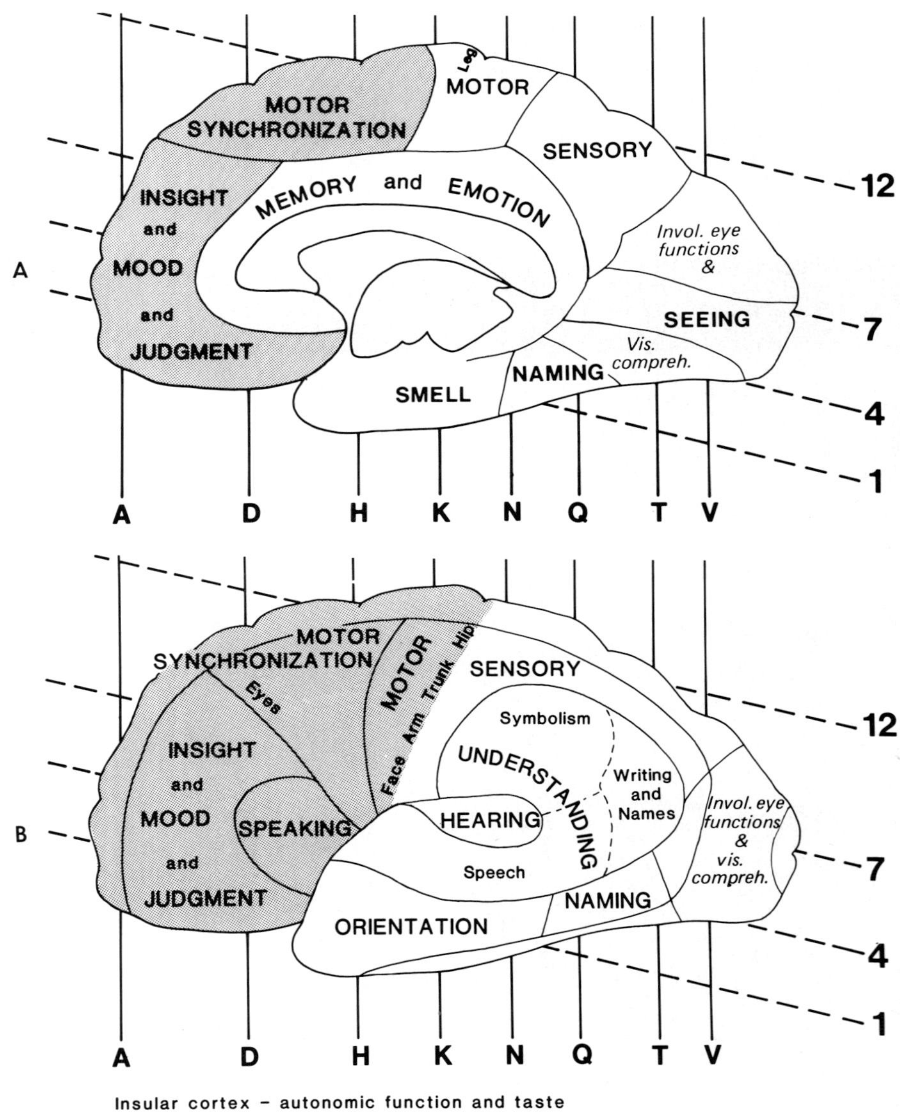

Figure 4-9 Frontal cortex is shaded on the medial surface of the right cerebral hemisphere **(A)**, on the lateral surface of the left cerebral hemisphere **(B)**, and on axial and coronal brain slices **(C)**. The numbers indicate the level of the axial schematics, and the letters correspond to the levels of the coronal brain slices. The general cortical regions that contain motor neurons for the leg, hip, trunk, arm, and face are indicated.

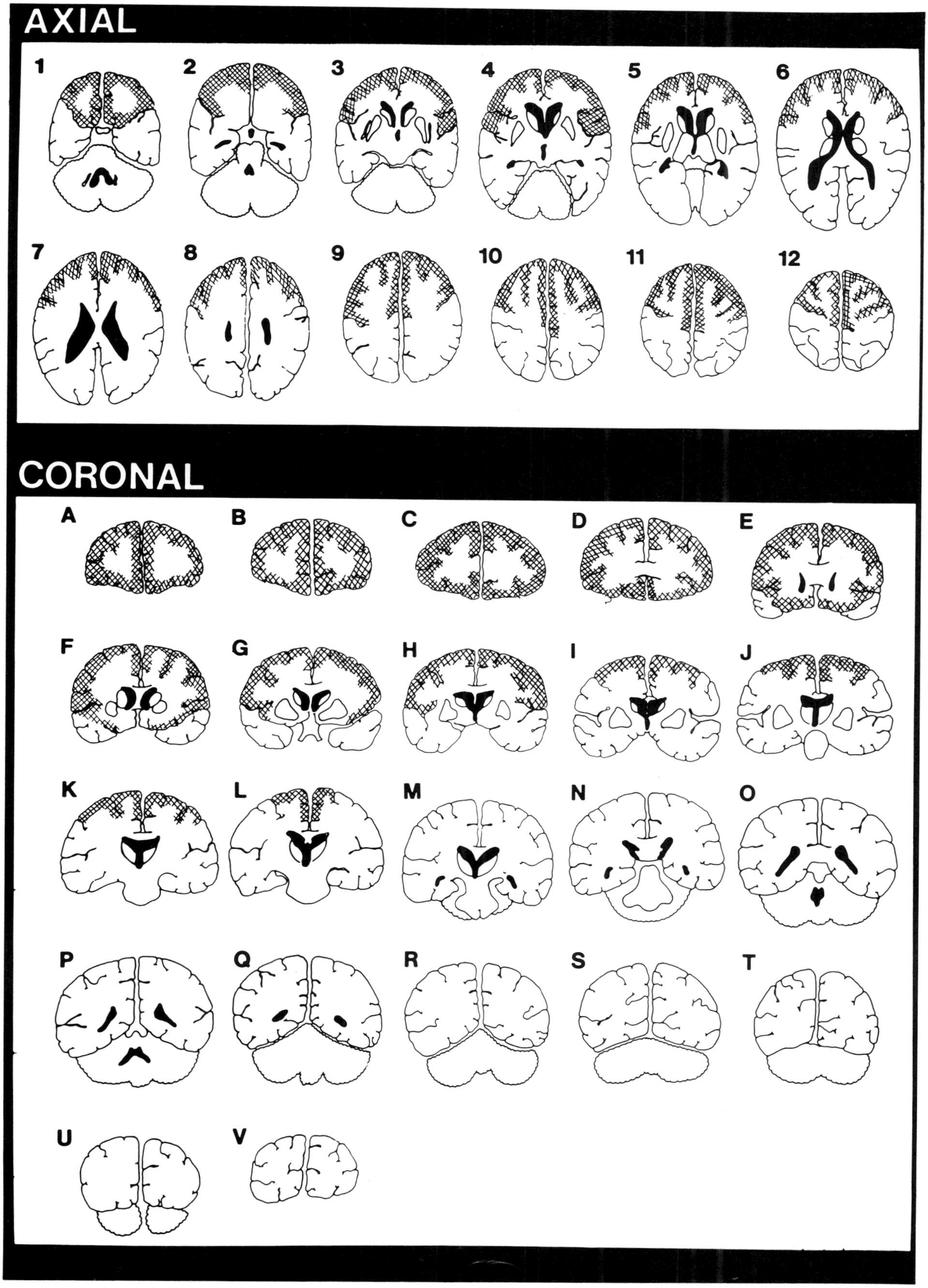

C

Figure 4-9, cont'd C, For legend see opposite page.

Parietal Lobe

From the central sulcus, the parietal lobe extends dorsal on the *medial* surface of the hemisphere to the parieto-occipital fissure. On the *lateral* surface, no gross anatomic landmarks separate the parietal lobe from the occipital and temporal lobes. The parietal lobe's inferior border is a backward continuation of the lateral fissure. The location and the cortical functions mediated by this lobe are labeled on medial and lateral surfaces of the brain[33] in Figure 4-10, *A* and *B*. The location of the parietal lobe on axial and coronal brain slices is shown in Figure 4-10, *C*. The individual gyri are categorized and labeled on serial sagittal MR scans in Chapter 11. A detailed discussion of the functions of this cortical region can be found in the description of the hemispheric branches of the anterior and middle cerebral arteries in Chapter 16.

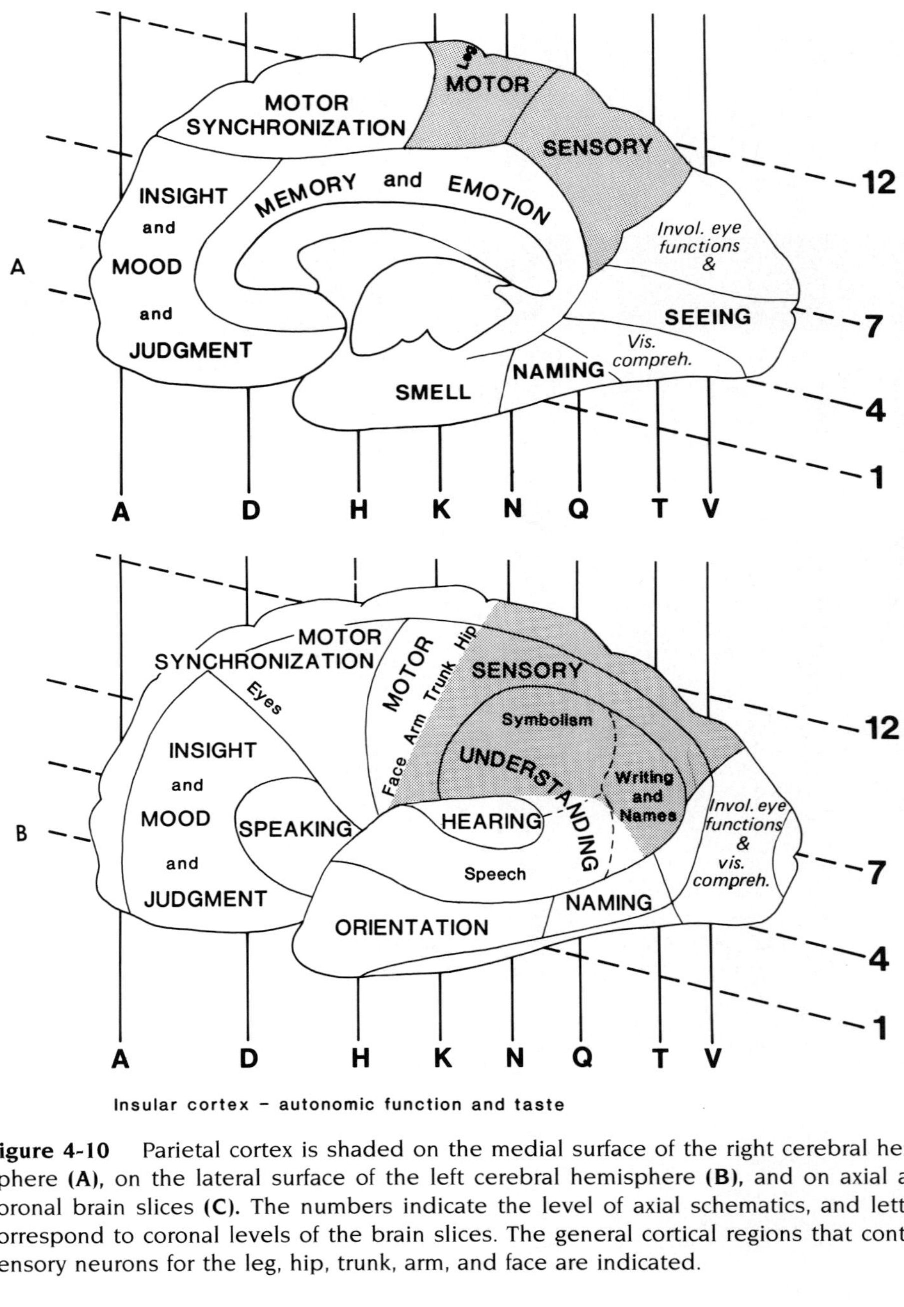

Figure 4-10 Parietal cortex is shaded on the medial surface of the right cerebral hemisphere **(A)**, on the lateral surface of the left cerebral hemisphere **(B)**, and on axial and coronal brain slices **(C)**. The numbers indicate the level of axial schematics, and letters correspond to coronal levels of the brain slices. The general cortical regions that contain sensory neurons for the leg, hip, trunk, arm, and face are indicated.

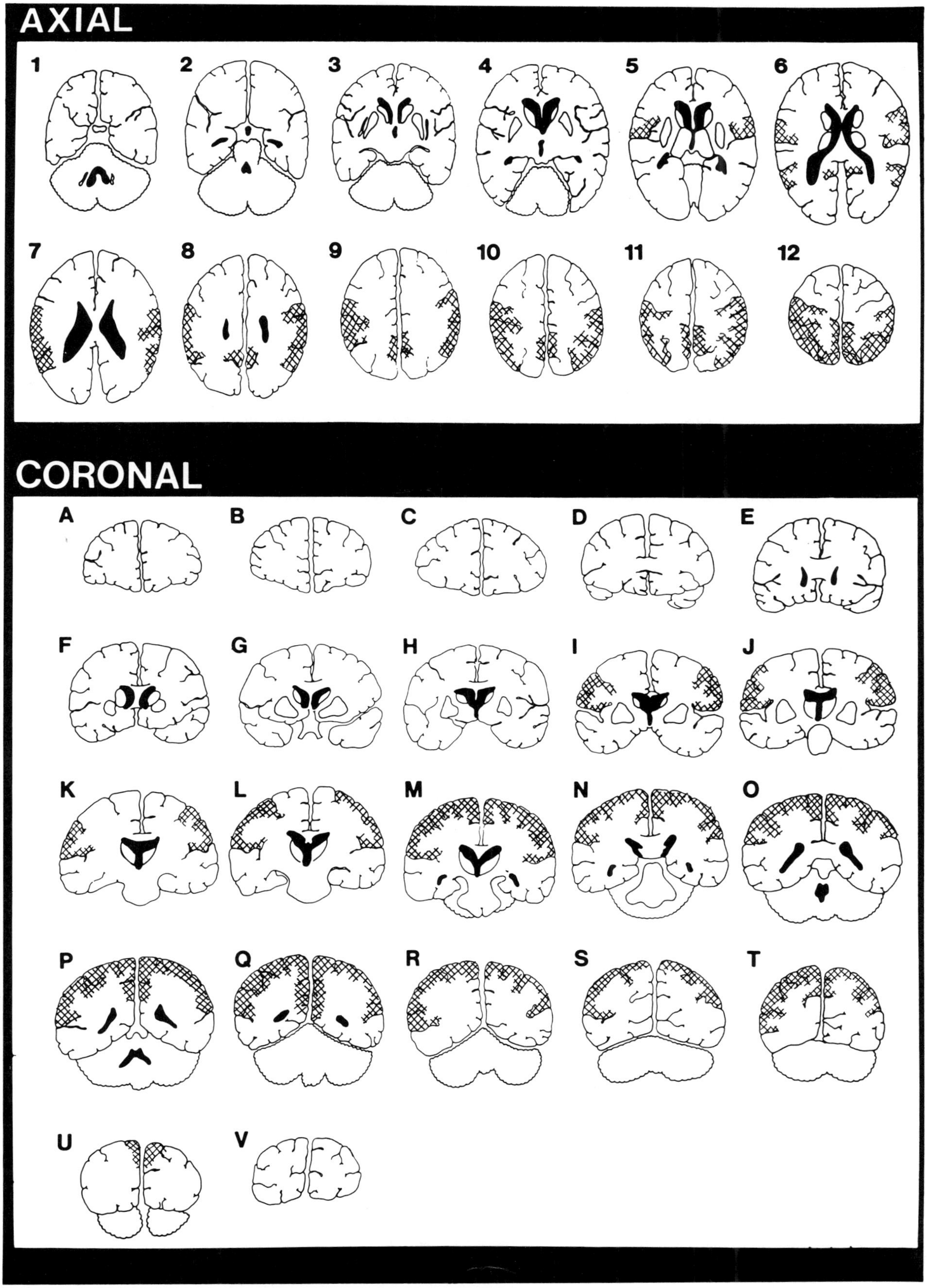

C

Figure 4-10, cont'd. C, For legend see opposite page.

Occipital Lobe

The occipital lobe is the portion of cortex that is behind an arbitrary line drawn from the parieto-occipital fissure to the preoccipital notch. The occipital lobe is primarily located on the medial aspect of the hemisphere. The location and the cortical functions mediated by this lobe are labeled on the medial and lateral surfaces of the brain[33] in Figure 4-11, *A* and *B*. The location of the occipital lobe is shown on axial and coronal brain slices in Figure 4-11, *C*. The individual gyri of this lobe are categorized and labeled on serial sagittal MR scans in Chapter 11. A detailed discussion of the functions of this cortical region can be found in the description of the hemispheric branches of the posterior cerebral artery in Chapter 16.

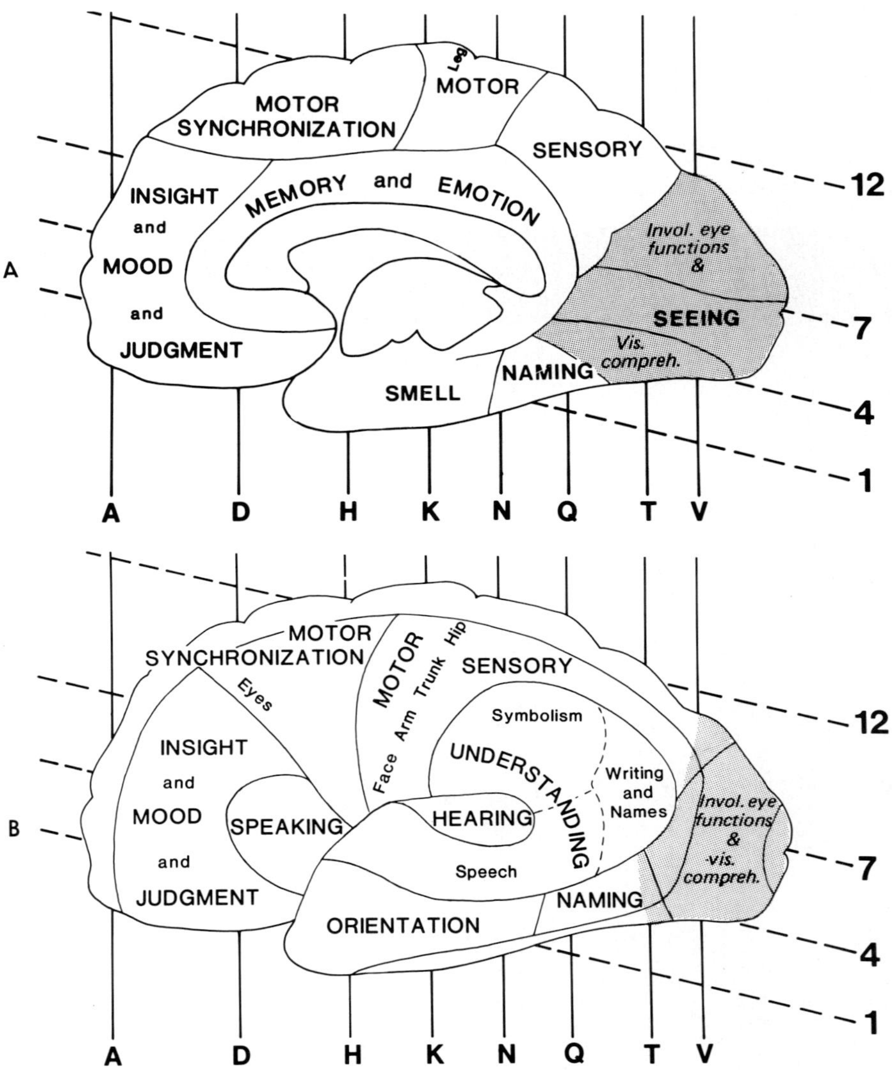

Insular cortex – autonomic function and taste

Figure 4-11 Occipital cortex is shaded on the medial surface of the right cerebral hemisphere **(A)**, on the lateral surface of the left cerebral hemisphere **(B)**, and on axial and coronal brain slices **(C)**. The numbers indicate the level of the axial schematics, and letters correspond to the levels of the coronal brain slices.

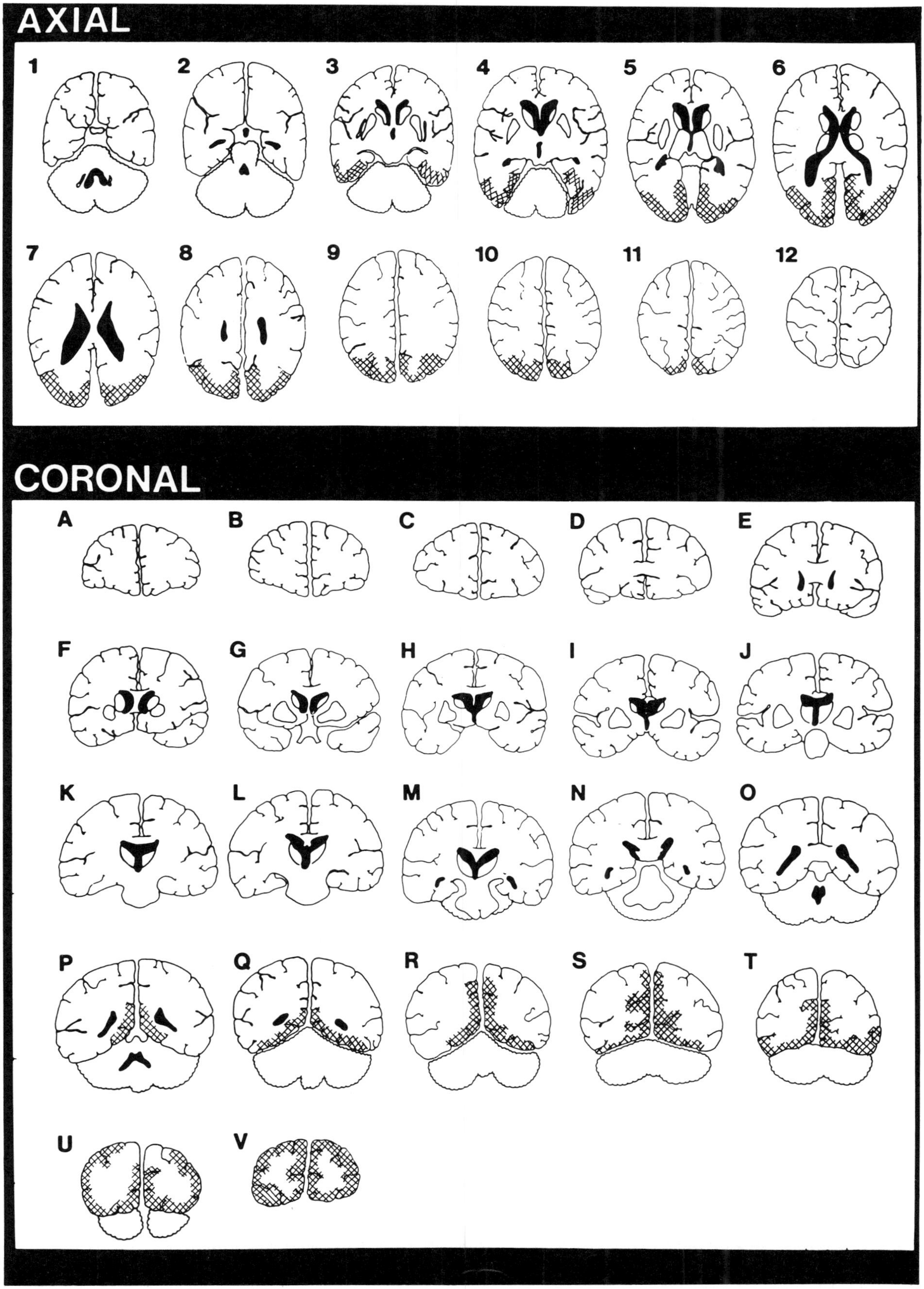

C

Figure 4-11, cont'd. **C,** For legend see opposite page.

Insular Lobe

The insular lobe is located on the lateral surface of the hemisphere. It can be exposed by spreading the lips of the sylvian fissure. The location of this lobe is shown on axial and coronal brain slices[33] in Figure 4-12. The insular cortex appears to mediate the motor and sensory functions of the viscera. (Electrical stimulation of the region at surgery has been observed to cause increased peristaltic activity.) The common epigastric sensation premonitory to many epileptic seizures may result from involvement of insular cortex in the seizure discharge.[34] The gyri of this lobe are identified and labeled in Chapter 9.

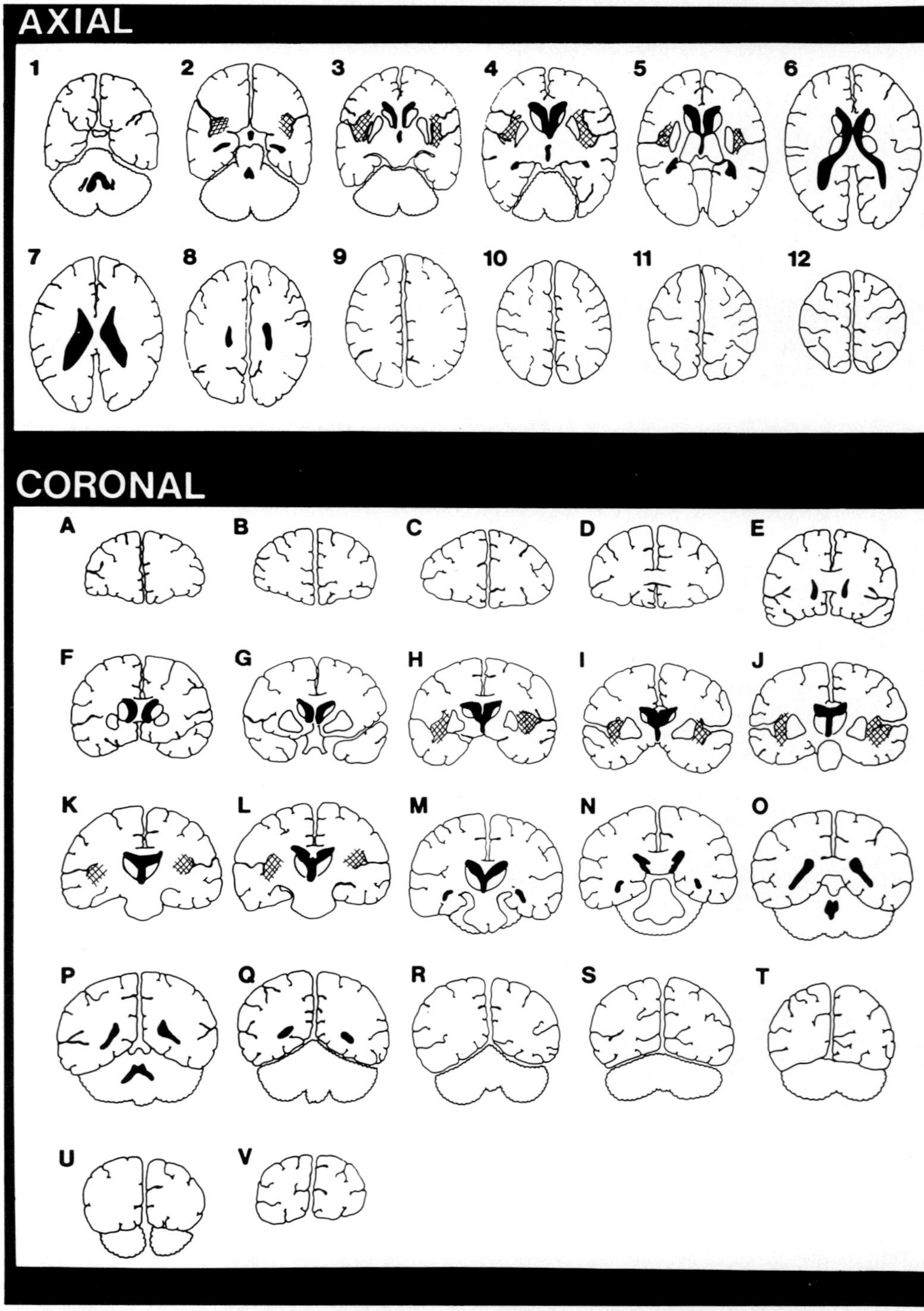

Figure 4-12 Insular cortex is shaded on axial and coronal brain slices.

Subcortical Nuclei

Several important neuronal clusters (nuclei) lie beneath the cerebral cortex. The major groups of hemispheric nuclei are the basal ganglia (primarily the putamen, globus pallidus, caudate, claustrum, subthalamus, and substantia nigra), basal forebrain nuclei, thalamus, hypothalamus, and amygdala. They are all closely associated with the ventricular system. These nuclei are identified in axial, coronal, and sagittal planes on MR scans and brain slices in Chapter 3. They are shown schematically[35] in Figure 4-13, *A* to *E*.

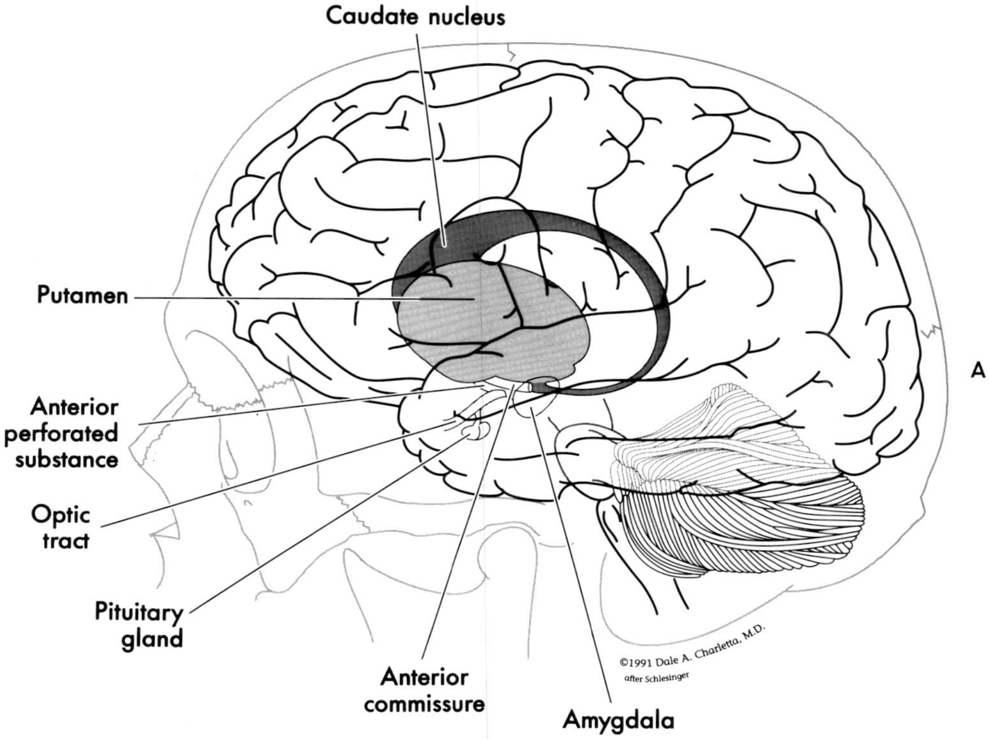

Figure 4-13 Sagittal schematics of the brain from lateral **(A)** to medial **(E)** show the positions of the major subcortical nuclei. The anterior perforated substance shown in **A** marks the *lateral* boundary of the substantia innominata, which contains the basal forebrain nuclei. (Modified from Schlesinger B: *The upper brainstem in the human: its nuclear configuration and vascular supply*, New York, 1976, Springer-Verlag.)

Continued.

B

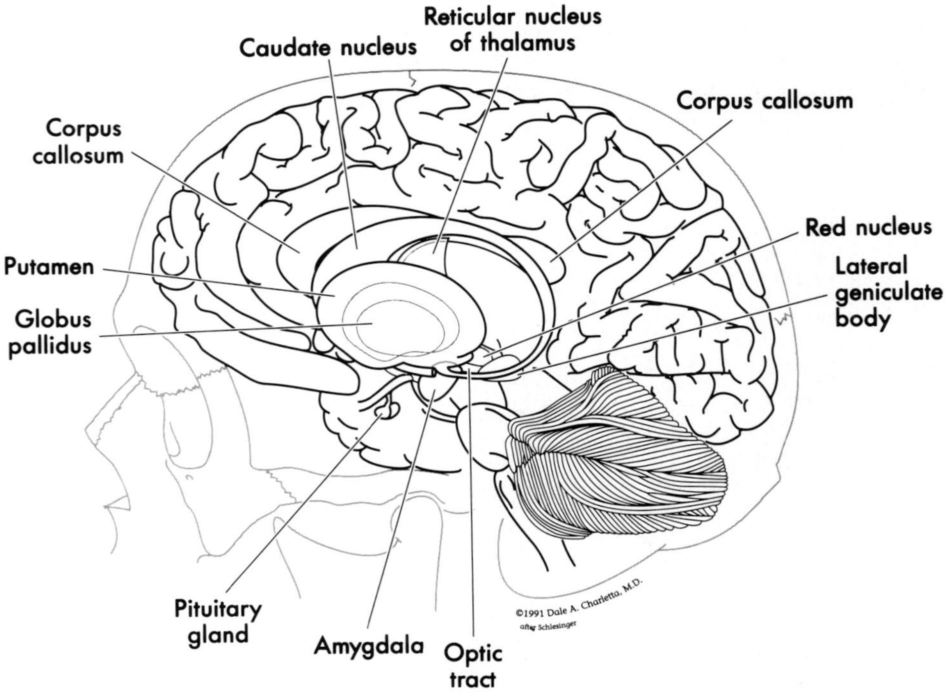

C

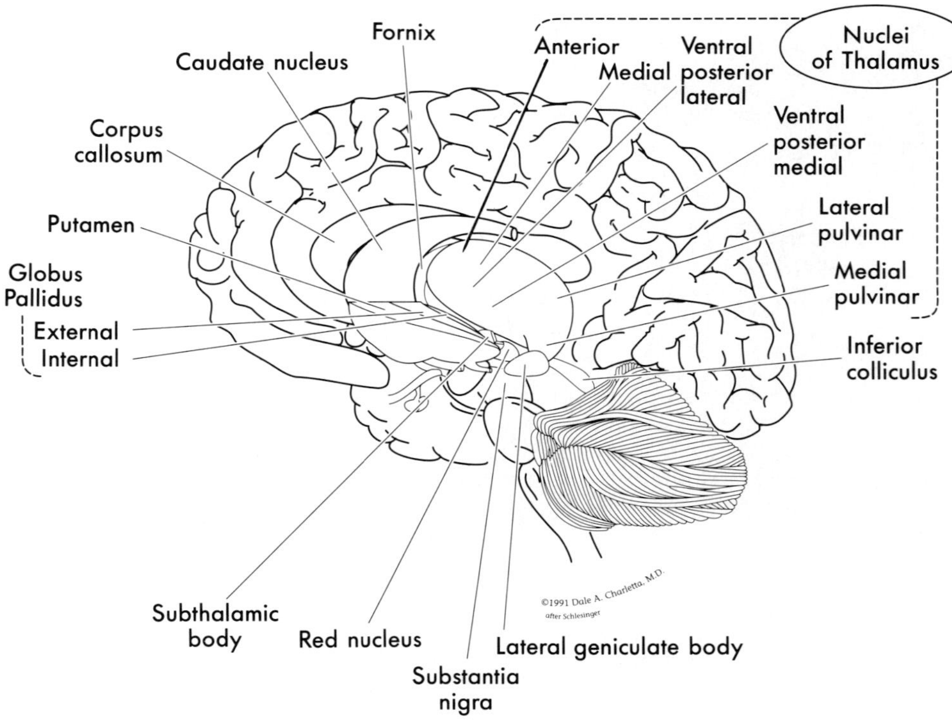

Figure 4-13, cont'd. For legend see p. 139.

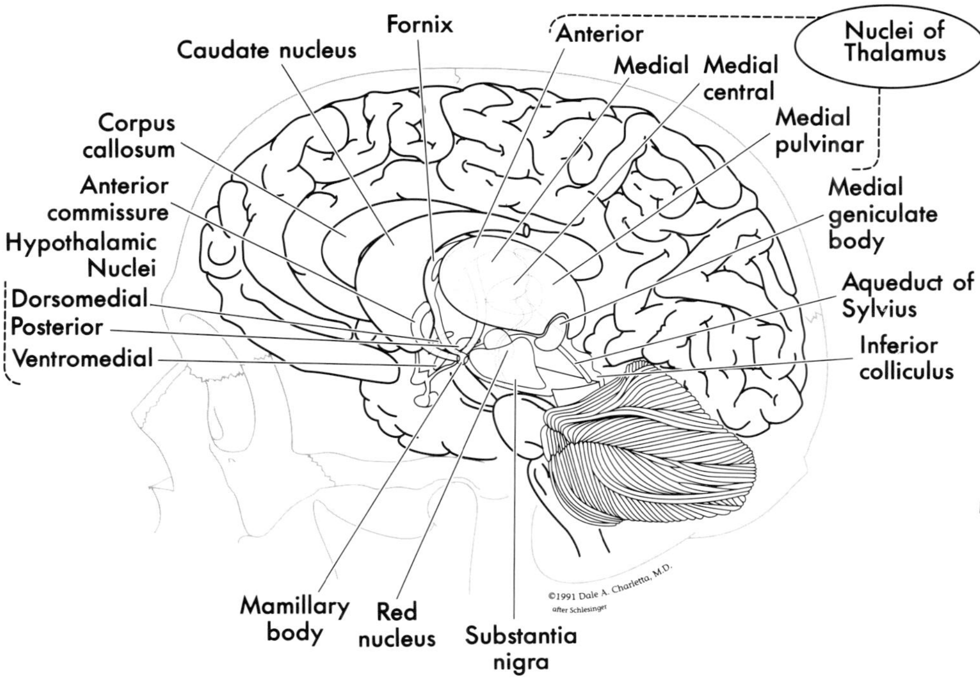

D

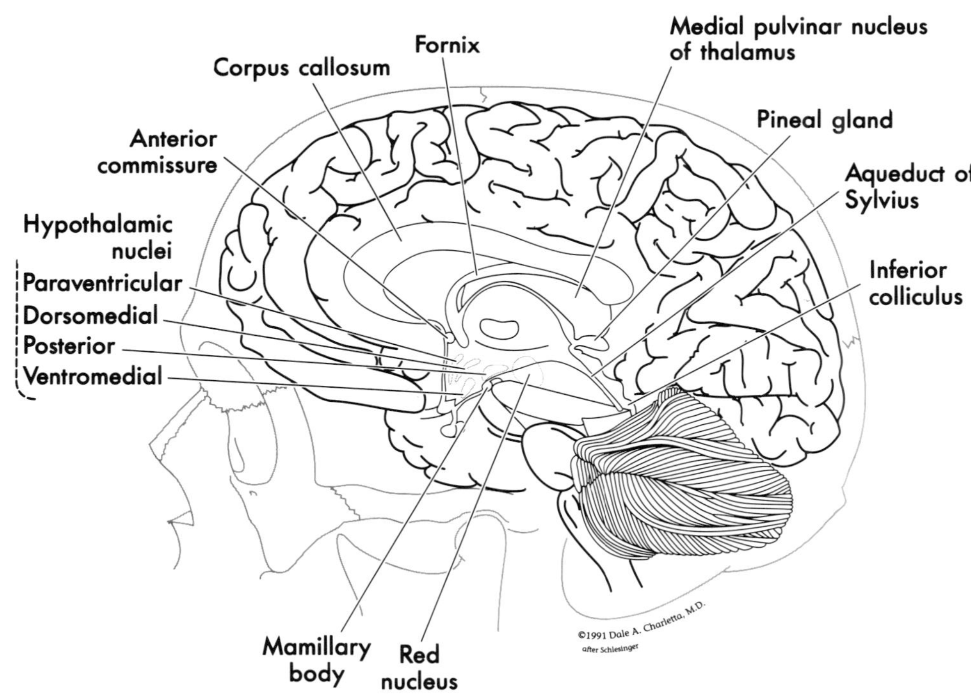

E

Figure 4-13, cont'd. For legend see p. 139.

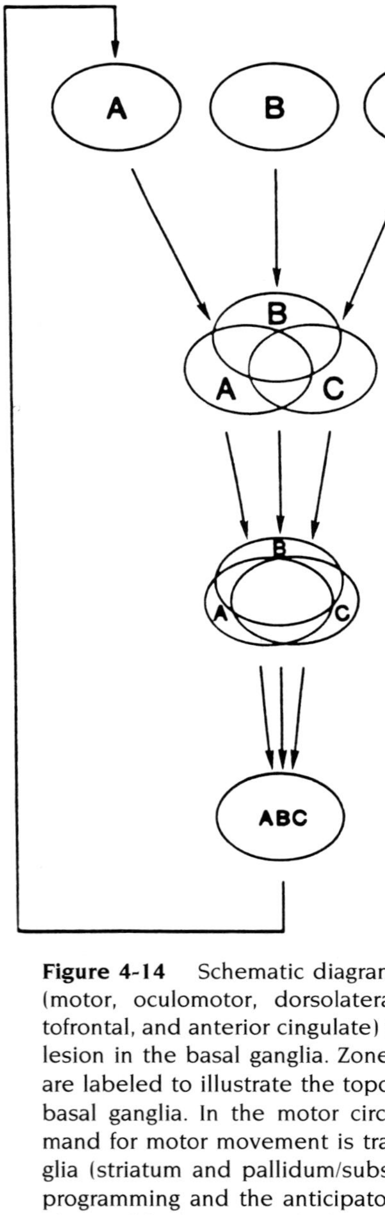

Figure 4-14 Schematic diagram of one of the five circuits (motor, oculomotor, dorsolateral prefrontal, lateral orbitofrontal, and anterior cingulate) that may be disrupted by a lesion in the basal ganglia. Zones A, B, and C in the cortex are labeled to illustrate the topographic organization of the basal ganglia. In the motor circuit, for example, the command for motor movement is transmitted to the basal ganglia (striatum and pallidum/substantia nigra), which inserts programming and the anticipatory aspects of a movement. The modified "command" then travels via the thalamus and returns to the cortex of origin. Disruption of this basal ganglia circuit disturbs the sequencing of movement. The specific anatomic interconnections for each of the five circuits can be found in reference 37. (Reproduced with permission from DeLong HR, Alexander GE, Miller WC, et al: In Franks AJ, Ironside JW, Mindham RHS, et al, editors: *Function and dysfunction in basal ganglia,* Manchester, England, 1990, Manchester University.)

Basal Ganglia

The basal ganglia are a collection of subcortical neuronal cell clusters that cannot be strictly grouped by their location, embryology, or interconnections. These nuclei are considered together principally because when they are damaged, characteristic abnormal movements or motor deficits occur. These are referred to as *extrapyramidal* symptoms because they are clearly distinct from the paralysis produced by lesions in the motor cortex or pathways of the pyramidal (corticospinal) system. The basal ganglia contribute to the planning and programming of movement.

Models of basal ganglia function in humans have been constructed using the clues provided by patients with the two forms of dyskinesia, parkinsonism and Huntington's disease. Initially, the basal ganglia were thought to synthesize input from the *whole* cortex.[36] Newer evidence shows that fibers from five separate cortical areas form five separate discrete circuits that enter specific sites in the basal ganglia, travel to specific locations in the thalamus, and from there return to the same cortex from which the signals originated. The details of these circuits can be found elsewhere[37] (Figure 4-14). Some of these pathways are discussed in the later section on the extrapyramidal system.

Preliminary data suggest that the basal ganglia may have neural functions beyond those modulating motor functions.[38] In fact, the basal ganglia may be the point at which the medical subspecialties of neurology and psychiatry interface. Evidence for cognitive and affective basal ganglia functions comes from clinicians who have noted dementia and a peculiar form of depression that leads to suicide in patients with dyskinesia caused by Huntington's disease. Several clinical studies have noted cognitive impairments and a form of dementia without aphasia and apraxia.[38] This has been termed *subcortical dementia* and has been reported in patients with hydrocephalus. A high frequency of depression has also been seen in patients with movement disorders resulting from Parkinson's disease.[38] Speculation concerning these functions was strengthened by the recently discovered limbic pathways through the basal ganglia.[37]

The six *principal* subcortical nuclear areas are collectively known as the basal ganglia of the cerebral hemisphere. These are the caudate, putamen, globus pallidus, claustrum, subthalamus, and substantia nigra. The nomenclature of the basal ganglia can be confusing because occasionally these large nuclei are subgrouped and renamed. For example, the *corpus striatum* refers to the head of the caudate nucleus, the anterior limb of the internal capsule, and the putamen. The *neostriatum* is formed from the caudate and putamen. The *lentiform nucleus* is formed by both portions of the globus pallidus and the putamen.

The three largest basal ganglia nuclei are the caudate nucleus, putamen, and globus pallidus (medial and lateral segments). Each of them serves as a relay station between the ipsilateral cerebral cortex and thalamus (Figure 4-14).

The MR appearance on long TR scans of the basal ganglia is discussed in the later section on normal aging.

MR scans may show areas of symmetric increased signal intensity on T1-weighted scans in the globus pallidus in cirrhotic patients who have no neuropsychiatric abnormalities. These areas demonstrate no mass effect or enhancement after intravenous contrast administration. It is postulated that they are caused by blood-borne gut-derived toxins that create ultrastructural changes in the astrocytes of the globus pallidus.[39] These toxins are thought to arrive via the large portal-systemic collateral vessels that have been found originating from the superior mesenthalamic vein in all patients with these MR findings.

The three remaining nuclear groups of the basal ganglia are so small that they are located primarily by identifying surrounding structures. For example, the *claustrum* is a small, linear, nuclear area immediately beneath the insular cortex. Unlike other basal ganglia nuclei, which connect with the thalamus, the claustrum only has connections to and from the ipsilateral cortex. The *subthalamic nucleus* surrounds the inferolateral aspect of the third ventricle. This nucleus is grouped with the other basal ganglia nuclei because of its functional interconnections. The *substantia nigra* is found below the subthalamic nucleus immediately dorsal to the red nucleus in the midbrain. The substantia nigra is also considered a functional component of the basal ganglia.

Recently, a seventh, small, *pedunculopontine nucleus*, which is located lateral to the medial longitudinal fasciculus in the midbrain, has been included in the basal ganglia group. This nucleus appears to interrelate basal ganglia nuclei that have no cortical input or reciprocal connections with one another.[40]

Basal Forebrain Nuclei

Large, prominent cellular groups can be found in the forebrain. The zone that contains these cells can be identified on MRI because it is surrounded by structures that are clearly shown on coronal images. The optic tract, anterior commissure, and fornix are inferior to the forebrain nuclei, and the anterior column of the fornix is immediately medial to these nuclei (Figures 4-13, *A*, and 4-15).

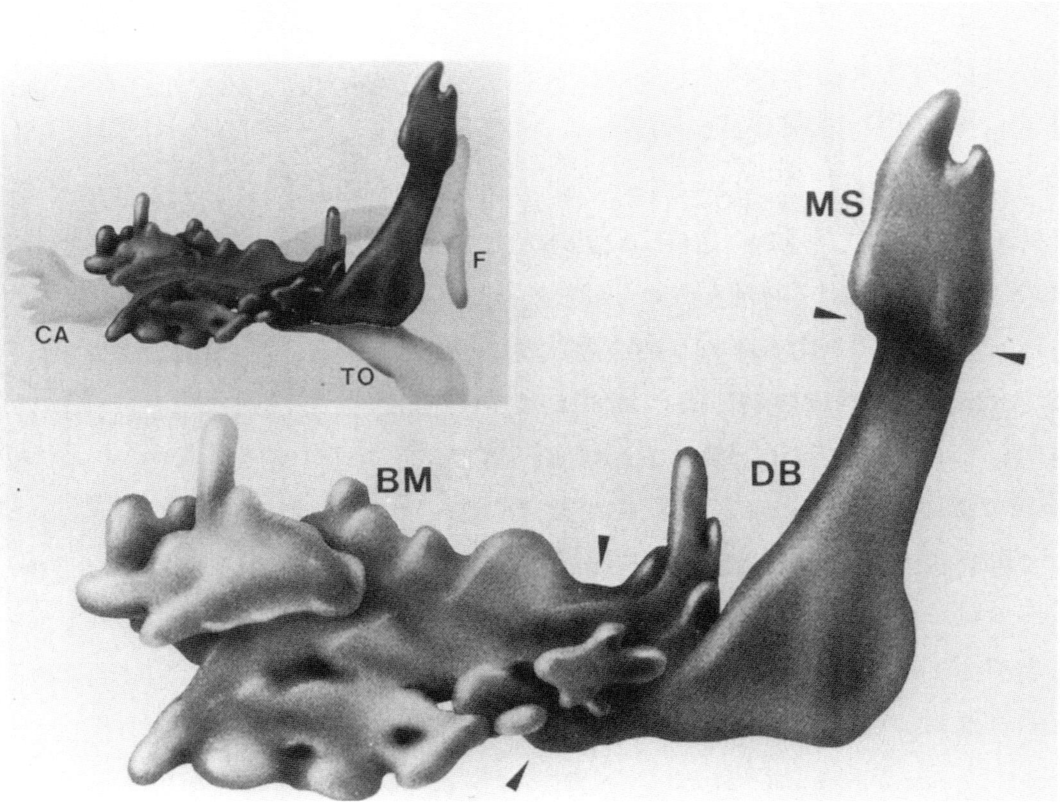

Figure 4-15 Three-dimensional coronal view of the cells of the *right* forebrain nuclei. The landmarks of the anterior column of the fornix (F), the optic tract (TO), and the anterior commissure (CA) are provided to orient the reader. *Arrowheads* separate these cells into three subgroups: the medial septal nucleus (MS), the nucleus of the diagonal band (DB), and the basal nucleus of Meynert (BM). (Reproduced with permission from Ulfig N: *Acta Anat (Basel)* 134:100-105, 1989.)

All the cells of the forebrain nuclei contain acetyl transferase and acetyl cholinesterase. They have traditionally been divided into three groups based on their cortical projection(s). The most important group is the *basal nucleus of Meynert*. A reduction in the cholinergic input to the cortex from this region appears to be a constant feature in patients with Alzheimer's disease.[41-45]

Thalamus

The nine major nuclear groups in the thalamus are schematically illustrated in Figures 4-13 and 4-16.[46] The anatomic location of the thalamus is shown in axial, coronal, and sagittal projections in Chapter 3. It is interconnected with most other regions of the central nervous system (CNS) by a vast array of fiber tracts. Myelinated fiber tracts course through the thalamus and divide it into three parts. These have been termed the *anterior, medial,* and *lateral nuclear groups*. The anterior and lateral groups contain many myelinated fibers. Demyelination of these fibers can mimic abnormalities in the neurons of the thalamus itself on MR scans.[46]

The complex function(s) of the thalamus can generally be divided into four categories: (1) memory and emotion, (2) motor stabilization, (3) sensation, and (4) interconnections between the visual and auditory system (Figure

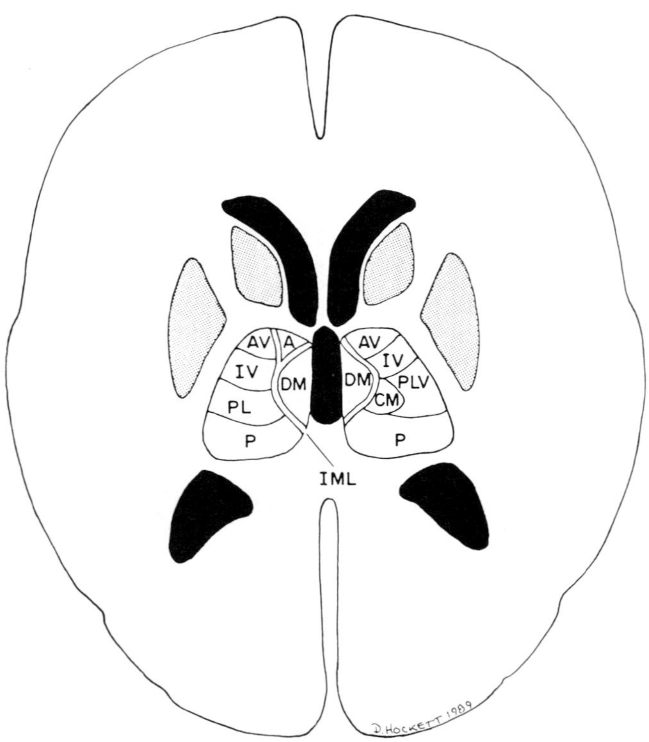

Figure 4-16 Diagrammatic representation of major thalamic nuclei at middorsal thalamic level (portion of diagram to reader's left) and midventral thalamic level (reader's right). A, Anterior nucleus; AV, anteroventral nucleus; IV, intermediate ventral nucleus; PL, posterolateral nucleus; P, pulvinar; DM, dorsomedial nucleus; PLV, posterolateral ventral nucleus; CM, centromedian nucleus; IML, internal medullary lamina. (Reproduced with permission from Koci TM, Chiang F, Chow P, et al: AJNR 11:1229-1233, 1990.)

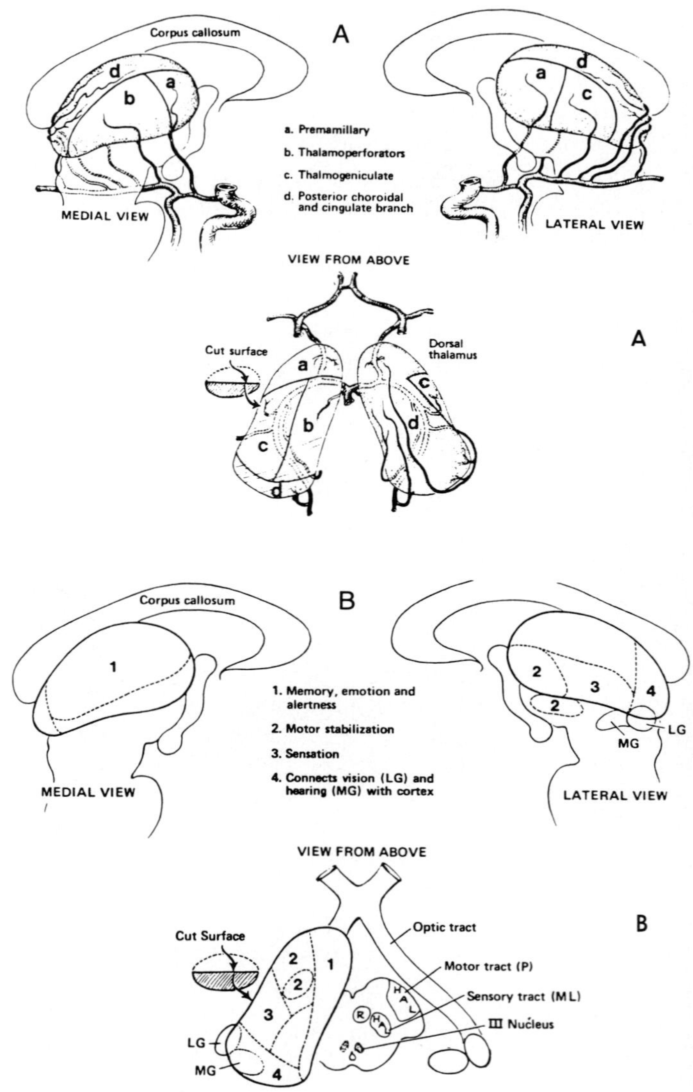

Figure 4-17 Schematic diagram of thalamic functions shows the four functional relay areas of the thalamus: (1) memory and emotion (anteromedial and dorsomedial nuclei), (2) motor stabilization (ventroanterior, ventrolateral, and subthalamic nuclei), (3) sensation (ventroposteromedial and ventroposterolateral nuclei), and (4) connections of visual (LG, lateral geniculate) and auditory (MG, medial geniculate) areas with the parietal cortex via the pulvinar. Unmarked areas are nonspecific association areas that require further investigation. (Reproduced with permission from Hayman LA, Berman SA, Hinck VC: ASNR 2:219-225, 1981.)

4-17). Lesions in area 1 result in neuropsychologic symptoms; in area 2, they result in hemiballismus (or curb Parkinson's disease contralaterally); in area 3, lesions result in Déjérine-Roussy (thalamic) syndrome; and in area 4, they cause aphasia if the left thalamus is affected. The vessels that supply the thalamus are described in the section on the posterior cerebral artery in Chapter 16.

Hypothalamus

The poorly defined clusters of neurons found in the floor and lateral walls of the third ventricle have been called the hypothalamus. Numerous "nuclei" and countless interconnections have been described in the region. These can be classified into three principal groups (regions): the supraoptic (anterior), tuberal (central), and mamillary (posterior). The specific function of the mamillary group is unknown. Efforts to relate this area to memory because of its association with the fornix have not been successful. The neuroendocrine functions of the hypothalamus are described in Chapter 17. The limbic system, brainstem reticular formation, and cortex are all connected with the hypothalamic nuclei.[47]

Amygdala

The amygdala (amygdaloid body, amygdaloid nuclear complex) is an almond-shaped structure located anterior to the hippocampus. It consists of multiple groups of nuclei. The two major collections of cells are the corticomedial and basolateral groups. The amygdala forms the anterior and superior walls of the tip of the lateral ventricle's temporal horn. The temporal horn separates the amygdala from the head of the hippocampus. The uncal portion of the parahippocampal gyrus lies medial to the amygdala. The claustrum and lentiform nucleus are situated above it. The tail of the caudate nucleus is connected to the amygdala.[6] The amygdala itself is connected to the other regions of brain via three major fiber tracts: (1) the lateral olfactory stria (to the olfactory bulb), (2) the stria terminalis (to the septal area and hypothalamus), and (3) the ventral amygdala–fugal pathway (to the hypothalamus and entorhinal cortex).

The amygdala is a pivotal structure in the limbic system. It has been studied intensely in the hope of elucidating the basic mechanisms of some forms of epilepsy. Twenty years ago, the amygdala was considered to be an intermediary link between the olfactory system and the hypothalamus. Recent studies have significantly advanced our understanding of this structure. Five monoamine neurotransmitters, five amino acids, and more than 13 peptides have been isolated in the amygdala.[48,49] Evaluation of epileptic patients with stereotactic electrical stimulation of the amygdala often elicits fear. Less frequently, these patients have complex perceptions and recollections of past events after such stimulation.[48] Amygdalectomy in monkeys produces behavioral changes that have been termed the *Klüver-Bucy syndrome* (primarily tameness and hyperorality).

The most recent data suggest the amygdala is the site in the brain that attaches emotional significance to the sensory information the brain receives from the temporal cortex. Connections between the amygdala, hypothalamus, and brainstem autonomic motor nuclei appear to integrate an emotional response. Thus animals with lesions in the amygdala show a reduction in fear response. As a consequence, these animals show deficits in learning tasks that are reinforced by painful stimuli.[48,50]

Major Functional Pathways

The internal interconnections of the cerebral hemisphere are very complex and at present are not fully understood. The largest fiber tracts are labeled in Chapter 3. The connections *between* each of the cerebral hemispheres are discussed in detail in Chapter 5. Interconnections *among* the various subcortical nuclei and between these nuclei and the cortex create the four major functional systems of the brain: the limbic, voluntary motor (pyramidal), involuntary motor (extrapyramidal), and sensory systems. Each is briefly described in this section. The extensions of the sensory and pyramidal (motor) systems to the brainstem are diagrammed in Chapter 7.

Limbic System

The cortex of each limbic lobe connects with six ipsilateral structures: the hypothalamic nuclei, including the mamillary body, the thalamus, amygdala, frontal association cortex, and reticular activating system. These connections form the limbic system, which is shown schematically[51] in Figure 4-18. Interhemispheric connections also exist among many of these structures. This system is critical for memory, attention, regulation of emotion and affect, and processing of olfactory information. The following discussion briefly summarizes what is presently known about the clinical aspects of the limbic system.[10,52]

The connection between the cortex of the limbic lobe and the hypothalamus (via the fornix) appears to be important in modulating visceral activities. The cortex of the limbic lobe is also connected with the septal nuclei found above the hypothalamus. These connections are important in social and sexual behavior. Connections between the hypothalamus and the amygdala are important in fight-or-flight responses. The connections between the thalamus (i.e., the dorsal medial nucleus) and the mamillary bodies play a role in memory. The hippocampal formation is part of the brain involved in storing declarative memory (i.e., the ability to recall specific facts). The fibers that interconnect the right and left hippocampi are described in Chapter 5.

Lesions in the limbic system are generally microscopic and/or biochemical. The anatomic abnormalities seen in patients with temporal lobe seizures and dementia have been discussed in the section on the limbic lobe.

Motor System

In classic literature the motor system of the brain was divided into separate pathways: the pyramidal (voluntary)

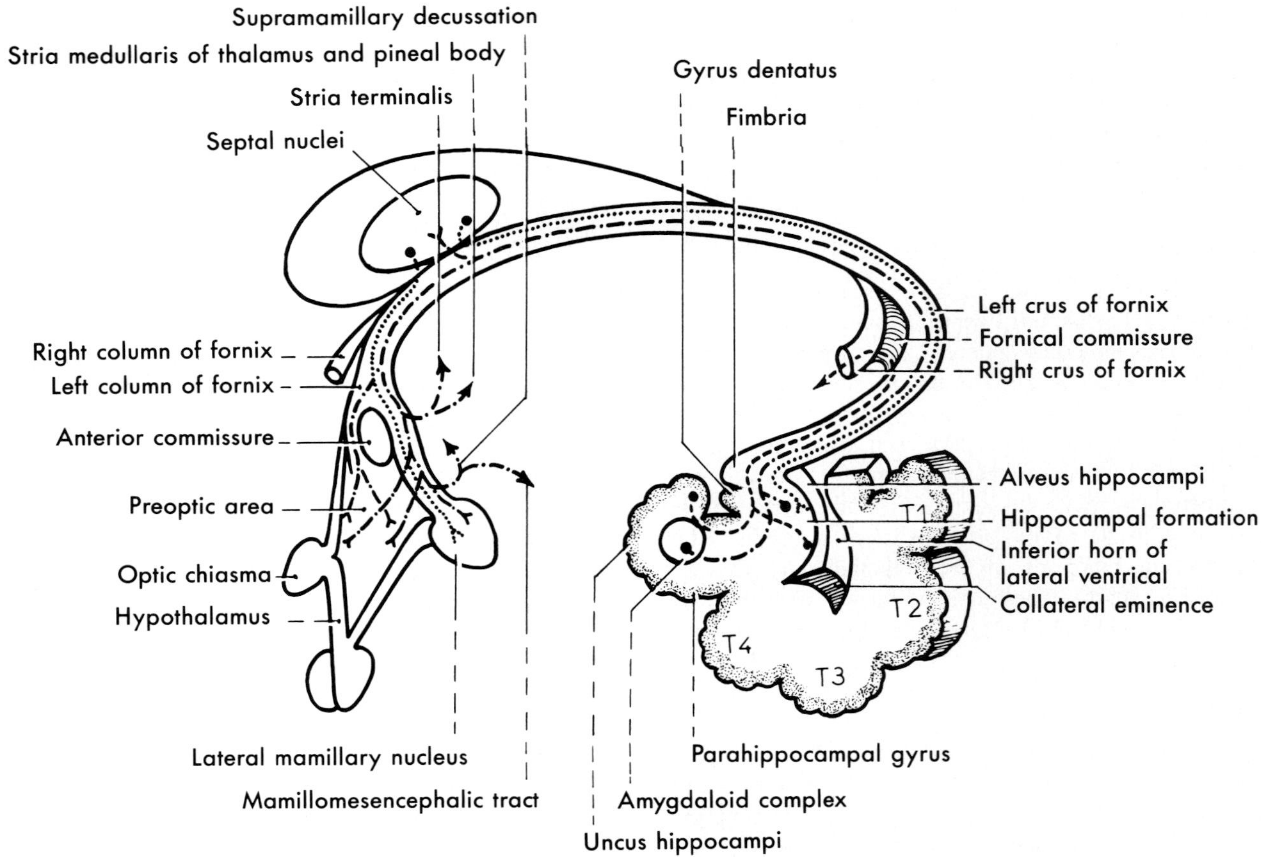

Figure 4-18 Schematic diagram of the interconnections of the limbic system. T1 to T4 refer to the gyri of the temporal lobe: T1, superior temporal gyrus; T2, middle temporal gyrus; T3, inferior temporal gyrus; T4, lateral occipitotemporal gyrus. (Reproduced with permission from Bossy J: *Atlas of neuroanatomy and special sense organs*, Philadelphia, 1970, WB Saunders.)

and the extrapyramidal (involuntary). Relatively recent studies of this system indicate that the pyramidal and extrapyramidal pathways interconnect via feedback loops between the cortical and subcortical neurons. These connections can be illustrated by observing a simple voluntary motor activity, such as walking or running, in which the subject involuntarily swings the arms. Although this mixture of voluntary and involuntary pathways does occur, it is still *clinically* useful to divide the motor system into pyramidal and extrapyramidal components.

PYRAMIDAL (VOLUNTARY). The cortex of the frontal lobe contains most of the neurons that control voluntary movements, but some motor cells are found in the sensory cortex located immediately behind the motor cortex. The pyramidal system is shown on axial brain slices in Figure 4-19. The general anatomic areas (leg, hip, trunk, arm, face) controlled by various zones of this cortex are indicated in Figure 4-19, *B*. Lesions involving these cells, or their axons, cause neurologic findings referred to as *upper motor neuron deficits*. These are characterized by paralysis, loss of polysynaptic reflexes, and the appearance of pathologic reflexes. Eventually, an increase in muscle tone (spasticity) develops in the affected area. Irritative lesions of the motor cortex may produce epileptic seizures.

Some of the motor nuclei in the facial region of the face are connected with the motor nuclei of the cranial nerves (V, VII, IX, X, XII, and part of XI) that are located in the brainstem. These *corticonuclear* connections are discussed individually for each of the motor cranial nerves in Chapter 8.

Most of the cortical motor neurons connect with contralateral spinal neurons. These *corticospinal* connections are shown in Chapter 7. Their motor axons extend through the internal capsule, cerebral peduncles, and basal pons to form the pyramids of the medulla oblongata. For this reason, these connections have also been named the *pyramidal* pathways. Approximately 75% of these fibers cross to the opposite side of the lower medulla at the pyramidal de-

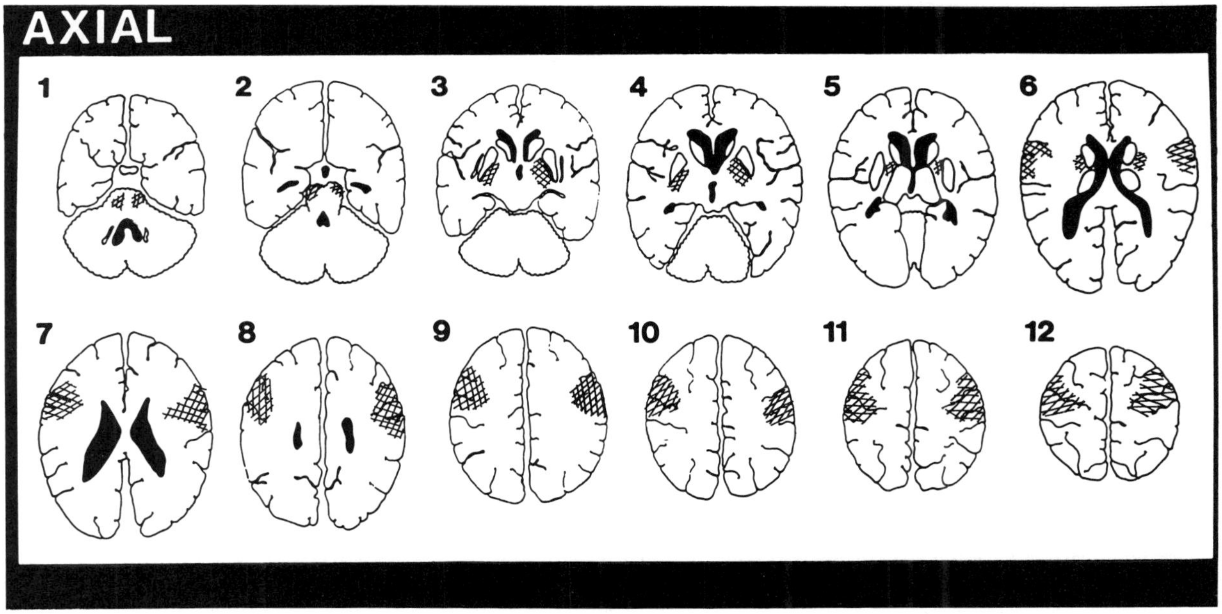

Figure 4-19 Pyramidal (motor) system shaded on axial brain slices. (Adapted from Kretschmann HJ, Weinrich W: *Neuroanatomy and cranial computed tomography*, New York, 1986, Thieme.)

cussation. The crossing fibers form the *lateral* corticospinal tract, and the uncrossed fibers form the *anterior* corticospinal tract. Motor cells called *interneurons* connect groups of the descending axons to the spinal motor neurons. Other connections form feedback loops. These complex interconnections account for the frequency of *incomplete* paralysis in patients with lesions involving the motor cortex.

EXTRAPYRAMIDAL (INVOLUNTARY). The fine control of motor movement is regulated by the subcortical nuclei that form the claustrum, putamen, caudate nucleus, globus pallidus, subthalamic nucleus, substantia nigra, and the lateral thalamic nuclei (i.e., ventroanterior and ventrolateral). These have been discussed in the previous sections on the basal ganglia and thalamus. The extrapyramidal system is shown on axial brain slices in Figure 4-20. These nuclei have extensive interconnections, as well as connections with the motor cortex (just described), reticular formation of the brainstem and cerebellum (i.e., dentate nucleus), and the limbic system (via the thalamic nuclei).[53,54]

Lesions of this system cause characteristic deficits of motor function: spontaneous hyperkinesia, hypokinesia, changes of muscle tone (especially rigidity), tremor, and characteristic postural disorders (Figure 4-21 and Table 4-3). Atrophy of some neurons of the caudate nuclei causes enlargement of the frontal horns of the lateral ventricles in hereditary Huntington's chorea. Usually, extrapyramidal symptoms are not associated with gross anatomic lesions; rather, they are caused by abnormalities in the neurotransmitters, gamma aminobutyric acid (GABA) and dopamine. For example, Parkinson's disease is caused by a deficiency of dopamine synthesis in the substantia nigra. In this disease, gradient-echo, high field strength MR scans reliably show only a decrease in the width of the pars compacta of the substantia nigra.[55] This finding may be the result of abnormally increased iron deposition in this area or cellular loss[55-57] (see following section on deposition of calcium and iron).

◆ **TABLE 4-3** Definitions of Terms Descriptive of Movement Disorders

Term	Definition
Tremor	Involuntary, rhythmic, oscillatory movements of opposing muscles
Myoclonus	Abrupt, shocklike contraction of a single muscle or group of muscles
Hemiballismus	Sudden, violent, swinging movements of arm and/or leg
Dystonia	Usually slow, sustained, continual, repetitive, and twisting contractions that can result in postural abnormality
Athetosis	Slow, sinuous, writhing, purposeless movements flowing into one another
Chorea	Rapid, arrhythmic, nonrepetitive, nontwisting, flowing movements affecting proximal and distal muscles

Reproduced with permission from Rutledge JN, Hilal SK, Silver AJ, et al: AJNR 8:397-411, 1987.

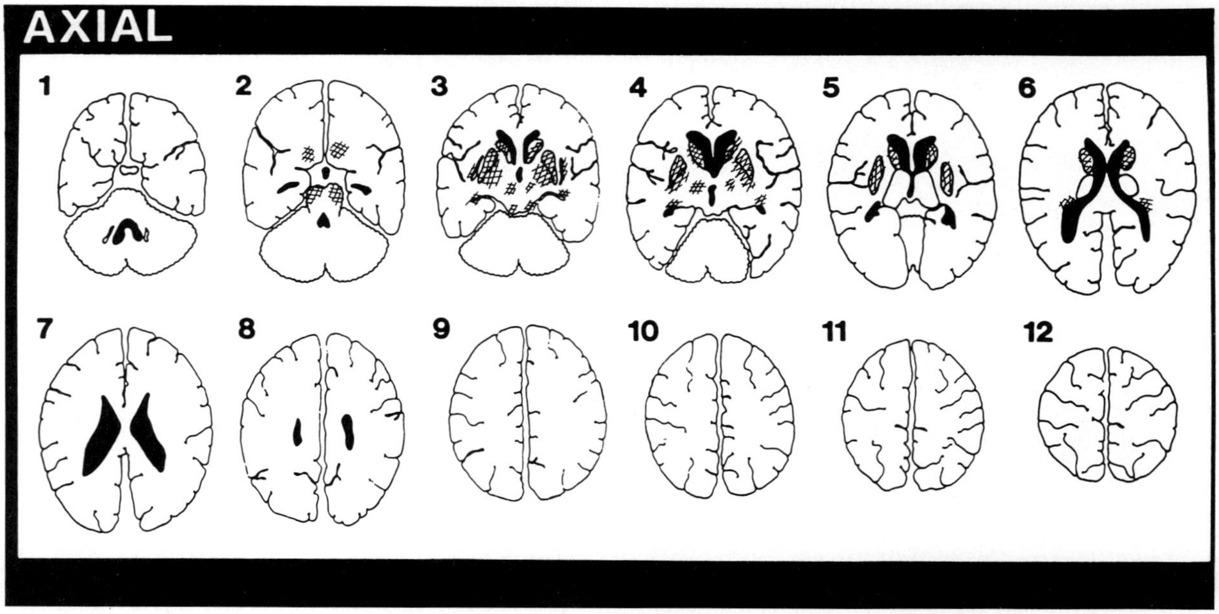

Figure 4-20 Extrapyramidal motor system shaded on axial brain slices. (Adapted from Kretschmann HJ, Weinrich W: *Neuroanatomy and cranial computed tomography*, New York, 1986, Thieme.)

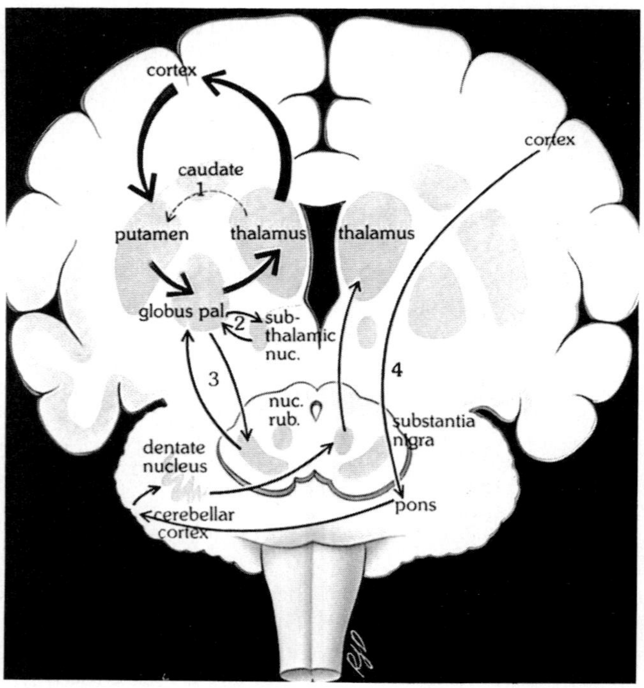

Figure 4-21 Coronal schematic of simplified extrapyramidal pathways. The circuit marked 1 is involved in disorders that result in dystonias and choreas. The circuit marked 2 is involved in disorders that result in hemiballismus. Circuits 3 and 4 are involved in parkinsonism. (Reproduced with permission from Rutledge JN, Hilal SK, Silver AJ, et al: AJNR 8:397-411, 1987.)

Sensory System

The subcortical neurons of the thalamus receive sensory information from the face via the *trigeminothalamic tract* (see Chapter 8). In addition, the thalamus receives *two* sets of sensory information from the legs, trunk, arms, and neck. Sensations of pain, temperature, and simple or crude touch are carried by the *anterolateral system* to the thalamus. Vibratory sensations, proprioception, two-point discrimination, and the ability to identify objects and contours are carried by the *lemniscal system* to the same thalamic area. From the thalamus, fibers of both systems extend through the posterior limb of the internal capsule to the sensory cortex of the postcentral gyrus (see Figures 4-10, *B*, and 4-17). The pathway of these thalamocortical fibers is shaded in Figure 4-22. The pathways of the anterolateral and lemniscal sensory systems in the brainstem are described in Chapter 7.

NORMAL AGING

The radiographic, CT, or MR evaluations of elderly patients are challenging because various changes normally occur as the brain ages. Familiarity with these alterations will be increasingly important, since more than 30% of the population will soon be over 50 years of age.[58]

Loss of Brain Volume

One of the major changes that can be observed in MR or CT images of neurologically normal, elderly patients is the loss of brain volume and the concomitant enlargement of the cortical sulci, ventricles, and paravermian subarach-

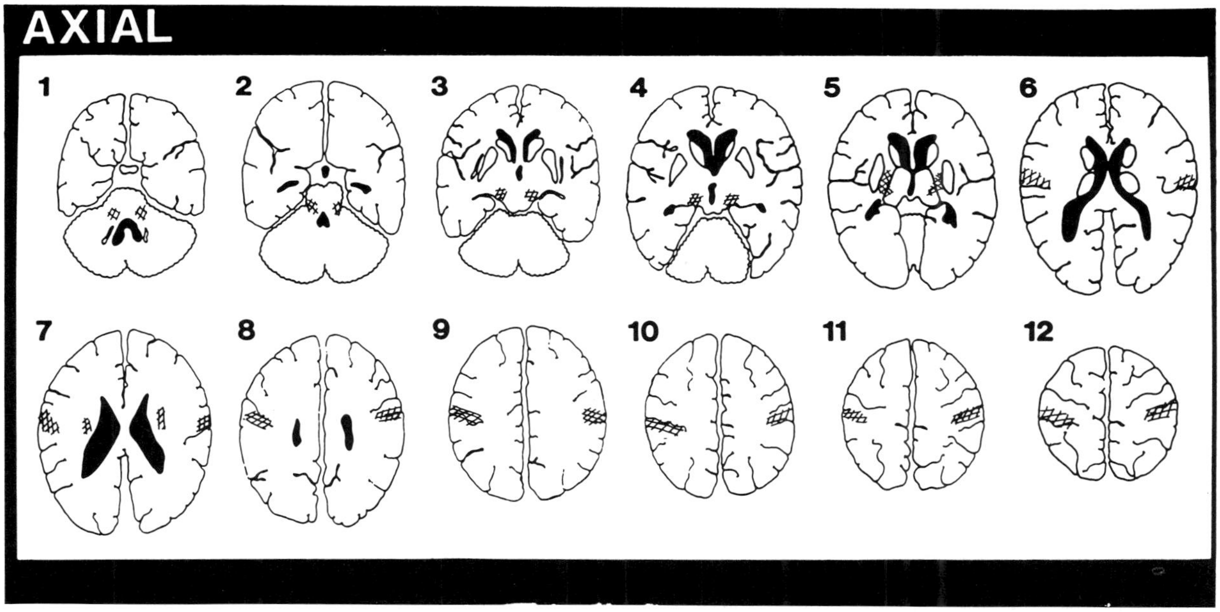

Figure 4-22 Sensory system shaded on axial brain slices. (Adapted from Kretschmann HJ, Weirich W: *Neuroanatomy and cranial computed tomography*, New York, 1986, Thieme.)

noid space. These changes are discussed in detail in Chapter 12.

Focal Cerebral White Matter "Lesions"

Thirty to eighty percent of elderly individuals without neurologic deficits demonstrate focal cerebral white matter "lesions" on neuropathologic slices and imaging studies.[59-73] On MRI, these are seen as small, focal, usually multiple and occasionally confluent areas of increased signal intensity on long TR images. These areas are typically located in the deep frontoparietal cerebral white matter, in the basal ganglia, and bordering the lateral ventricular margins (Figure 4-23). They have been called *subcortical hyperintensities* or "unidentified bright objects" (UBOs).[58-60]

Various neuropathologic findings have been reported in the periarteriolar regions in brains with subcortical hyperintensity on long TR images. Neuronal atrophy, demyelination, gliosis, vascular hyalinosis and ectasia, and enlargement of water-filled perivascular spaces are the most common findings. Each of these would be associated with increased periarteriolar water, which might produce localized areas of MR signal hyperintensity.[71-73] These areas, however, are not always associated with pathologic changes on MRI.[70,73] A careful MRI-histopathologic comparative study by Grafton et al.[70] found that *neither* myelin-stained nor axon-stained brains showed histologic abnormalities that corresponded to high signal intensity, white matter foci on T2-weighted MR scans. Thus it is likely that as yet undiscovered factors account for at least some of these subcortical hyperintensities.

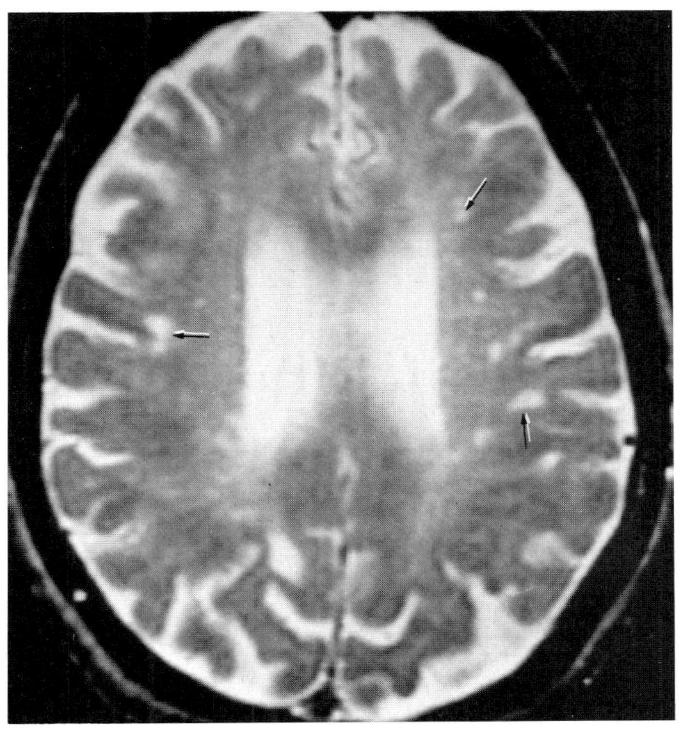

Figure 4-23 MR image (TR/TE, 2000/80) shows multiple, small, focal areas of increased signal intensity in the centrum ovale of a 40-year-old male with no cerebrovascular risk factors. These regions were unchanged on a follow-up scan 1 year later.

Many studies have attempted to correlate these nonspecific white matter and basal ganglia hyperintensities with underlying clinical conditions or predisposing factors. The most frequently associated processes include ischemic cerebrovascular disease, hypertension, and aging itself. Interestingly, these hyperintense regions may also be found in healthy adults without such underlying risk factors.

Deposition of Calcium and Iron

Autopsy series indicate that calcium and iron are normally deposited in the basal ganglia as the brain ages. Gross physiologic calcifications can be found in 3.4% of autopsy specimens. Histologically, these deposits may be arterial or capillary in location. Fine, punctate parenchymal or large, laminated concretions may also be present. On older-generation CT scans, patients greater than 40 years of age often have calcifications in the globus pallidus (Figure 4-24).[74] Several theories exist to explain the susceptibility of the globus pallidus to anoxic injury and consequent dystrophic calcification. These theories are (1) the peculiar arterial supply via the lenticulostriate branches, (2) the abundance of oxidative enzymes, and (3) disturbances in vasomotor regulation.[74] When calcification occurs, it is located in and around the fine blood vessels. The initial deposition of a colloid substrate in these areas changes to a gel that accepts the calcium salts. This entire process can occur over a period as short as 31 days.[74] Calcification in other brain regions or in patients under age 40 years may indicate the presence of endocrine, familial, inflammatory, or toxic/anoxic pathology.[75,76]

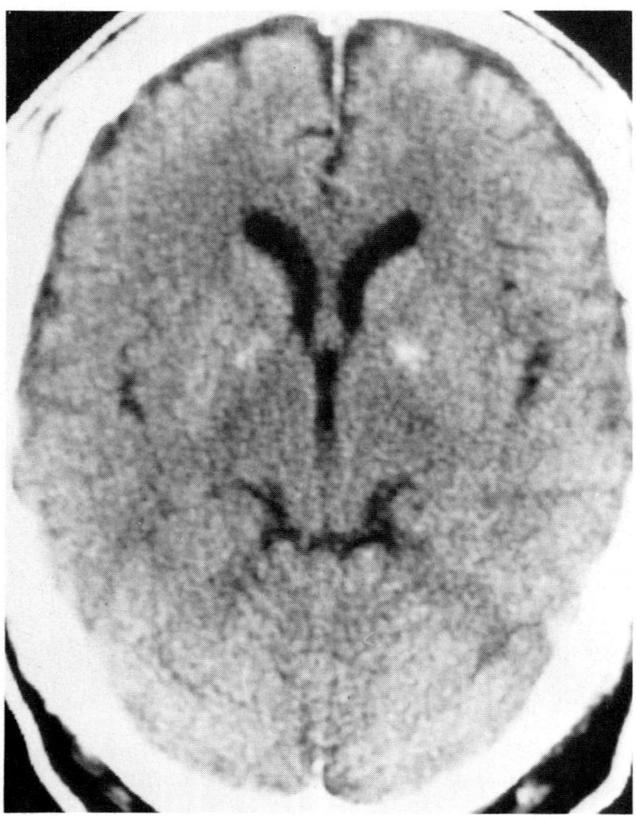

Figure 4-24 Axial CT image shows typical symmetric appearance of physiologic calcifications in the medial globus pallidus (*arrowheads*) of the lentiform nucleus.

By 25 years of age, a hypointense signal on T2-weighted MR scans can *normally* be detected in the same region of the lentiform nucleus (i.e., the globus pallidus) that shows calcification on CT scans. *In vivo* MRI virtually never demonstrates this finding in *normal* children under 10 years of age.[77] This finding was initially attributed (on the basis of circumstantial evidence) to iron deposition, which occurs first in the globus pallidus and later in the pars reticulata of the substantia nigra and red nucleus, and even later in the dentate nuclei[78-82] (Figure 4-25). The temporal accumulation of iron in these regions is thought to cause them to lose their initial hyperintense MR appearance and appear isointense and then hypointense relative to the surrounding normal white matter of the brain on long TR/TE spin-echo or gradient-echo sequences.[77] The etiology for these changes is controversial,[80-83] but probably represents a gradual loading of iron atoms within ferritin molecules with resulting antiferromagnetic and superparamagnetic effects.[84]

Abnormal levels of brain iron have been reported in parkinsonisms, which are characterized by degeneration of dopaminergic nigrostriatal neurons. There are conflicting reports, however of both increased and decreased iron.[80,85] Dopamine manipulation and axon sparing lesions of intrinsic striatal neurons in animal models have shown fluctuating, increased, and decreased signals, suggesting that changes seen clinically may represent progression in the complex metabolic processes associated with parkinsonisms and neuronal degeneration.[85,86]

Cerebral infarction in children can cause axonal disruption, which results in a nonspecific *abnormal* accumulation of iron in the basal ganglia.[84] This accumulation probably results because axonal damage prevents the iron, which is normally accumulated by the capillaries in the basal ganglia and thalamic nuclei, from being transported to distal sites that require iron for normal brain metabolism.[87] Other pathologic conditions (i.e., multiple sclerosis, cerebral infarctions in children, and other movement disorders)[84] have also been associated with an increase of iron in the basal ganglia. Although tissue studies are limited, Hallevorden-Spatz disease has been clearly associated with increased iron in the globus pallidus. Huntington's chorea and Striato-nigral degeneration has been associated with increase iron in the neostriatum (caudate and putamen).[88,89]

Some authors have suggested that abnormalities of iron deposition in the basal ganglia may be useful in diagnosing patients with Parkinson's disease. Braffman et al. have recently shown that the finding of hypointense signal on T2-weighted MR scans in these patients is not statistically significant. However, patients with Parkinson's disease reliably demonstrate a reduction in the width of the pars compacta of the substantia nigra.[55] Axial MR scans oriented 0 to 20 degrees positive to the inferior orbitomeatal line show a normal width of the pars compacta of 2.67 ± 0.5 mm. In age-matched and gender-matched control subjects, this value falls to 2.12 ± 0.82 mm in patients with Parkinson's disease.[55]

Loss of Gray-White Matter Discriminability

CT density measurements of gray and white matter in the region of the basal ganglia of normal elderly subjects have been conducted.[90] These measurements confirmed prior subjective assessment[90] by reporting loss of gray-

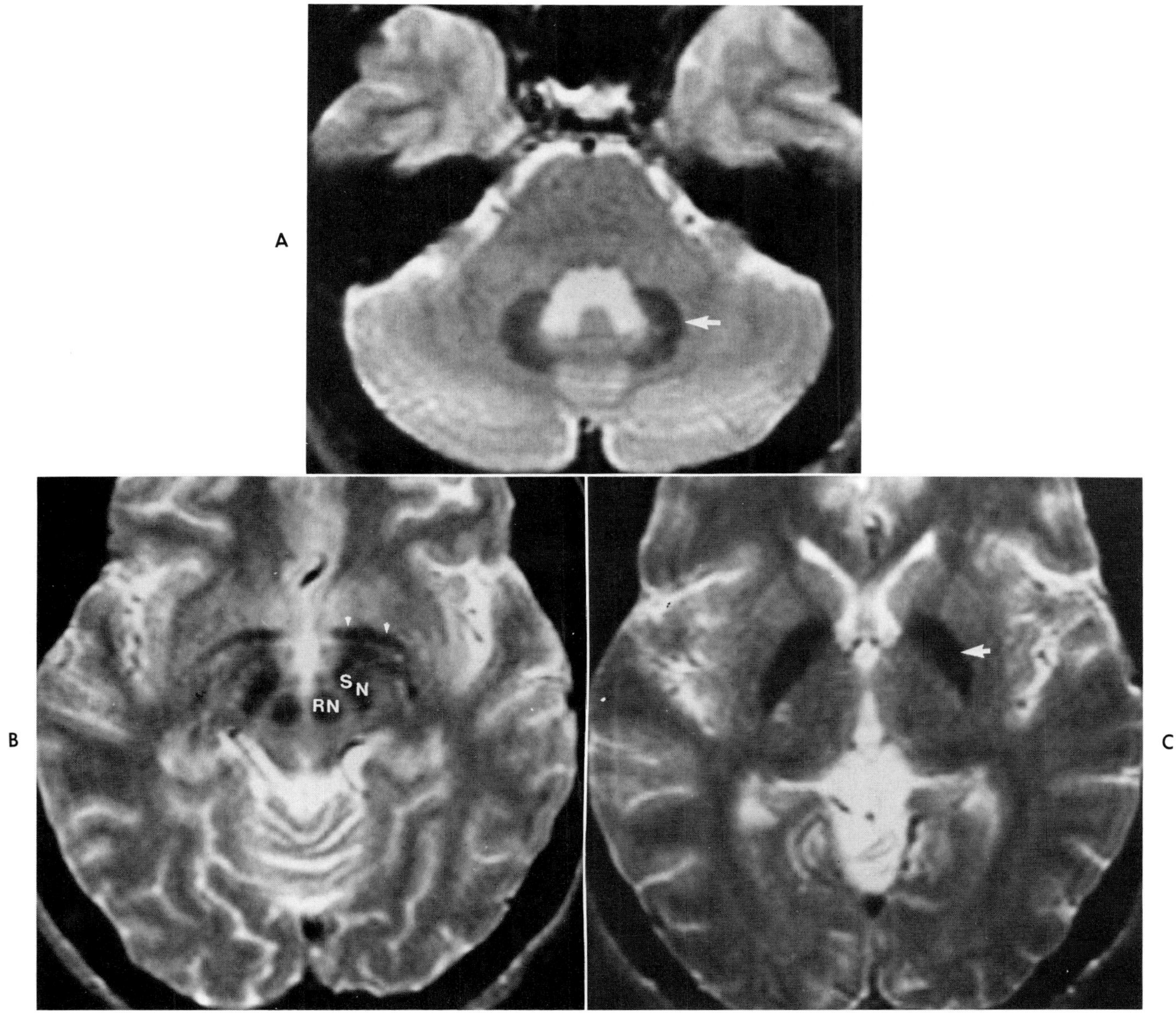

Figure 4-25 Axial MR images (TR/TE, 2000/80) demonstrate an age-related decrease in signal in selected regions of a normal brain. **A,** In the posterior fossa, hypointense signal can be seen in the dentate nuclei (*arrow*). **B,** At the brainstem level, a partial volume of subthalamic nucleus/substantia nigra (SN) and red nucleus (RN) are symmetrically hypointense. The pars compacta of the substantia nigra is the relatively hyperintense band of tissue between the red nucleus and the reticular substantia nigra (SN). The width of this region is reduced in patients with Parkinson's disease. The anterior commissure (*arrowheads*) is identified because of the presence of tightly compacted, heavily myelinated fibers.[89] Iron is not deposited in this structure.[90] The lateral nucleus of the globus pallidus is particularly well seen on the left in **B** as a prominent hypointense band immediately beneath the anterior commissure. At level **C,** the frontal horns of the lateral ventricle and the symmetric hypointensity in the globus pallidus are seen (*arrow*).

white matter discriminabilities in elderly patients with large ventricles. A diminished ability to separate the signal intensity of the gray and white matter zones has been subjectively noted clinically in the elderly population.[91-93]

REFERENCES

1. Enzmann DR, Rubin JB, O'Donohue J, et al: Use of cerebrospinal fluid gating to improve T2-weighted images. Part II. Temporal lobes, basal ganglia, and brain stem, *Radiology* 162:768-773, 1987.
2. Ebeling U, Steinmetz H, Huang Y, et al: Topography and identification of the inferior precentral sulcus in MR imaging, *AJNR* 10:937-942, 1989.
3. Kido DK, LeMay M, Levinson AW, et al: Computed tomographic localization of the precentral gyrus, *Radiology* 135:373-377, 1980.
4. Duncan R, Patterson J, Hadley DM, et al: CT, MR and SPECT imaging in temporal lobe epilepsy, *J Neurol Neurosurg Psychiatry* 53:11-15, 1990.
5. Jack CR, Sharbough FW, Twomey CK, et al: Temporal lobe seizures: lateralization with MR volume measurements of the hippocampal formation, *Radiology* 175:423-429, 1990.
6. Brown, Cheung G, Bronen RA: Relationship of hippocampus and amygdala to coronal MRI landmarks, *Magn Reson Imaging* 9(3):449-457, 1991.
7. George AE, de Leon MJ, Stylopoulos LA, et al: CT diagnostic features of Alzheimer disease: importance of the choroidal/hippocampal fissure complex, *AJNR* 11:101-107, 1990.
8. Naidich TP, Daniels D, Haughton VM, et al: Hippocampal formation and related structures of the limbic lobe: anatomic-MR correlation. Part I. Surface features and coronal sections, *Radiology* 162:747-754, 1987.
9. Naidich TP, Daniels DL, Haughton VM, et al: Hippocampal formation and related structures of the limbic lobe: anatomic-MR correlation. Part II. Sagittal sections, *Radiology* 162:755-761, 1987.
10. Duvernoy HM: *The human hippocampus: an atlas of applied anatomy,* München, 1988, JF Bergmann, Verlag.
11. Jack CR, Twomey CK, Zinsmeister AR, et al: Anterior temporal lobes and hippocampal formations: normative volumetric measurements from MR images in young adults, *Radiology* 172:549-554, 1989.
12. Sperling MR et al: Magnetic resonance imaging in intractable partial epilepsy: correlative studies, *Ann Neurol* 20:57-62, 1986.
13. Kuzniecky R et al: Magnetic resonance imaging in temporal lobe epilepsy: pathological correlations, *Ann Neurol* 22:341-347, 1987.
14. Schorner W et al: Temporal lobe epilepsy: comparison of CT and MR imaging, *AJNR* 8:773-781, 1987.
15. McLaughlan RS et al: Nuclear magnetic resonance imaging, a new approach to the investigation of refractory temporal lobe epilepsy, *Epilepsia* 26:555-562, 1985.
16. Chronister RB, White LE: Fiber architecture of the hippocampal formation: anatomy, projections and structural significance. In Isaacson RL, Pribram KH, editors: *The hippocampus, vol 1, Structure and development,* New York, 1975, Plenum.
17. Convers P, Bierme T, Ryvlin P, et al: Contribution of magnetic resonance imaging in 100 cases of refractory partial epilepsy with normal CT scans, *Rev Neurol (Paris)* 146:330-337, 1990.
18. Franceschi M, Triulzi F, Ferini SL, et al: Focal cerebral lesions found by magnetic resonance imaging in cryptogenic nonrefractory temporal lobe epilepsy patients, *Epilepsia* 30:540-546, 1989.
19. Furune S, Negoro T, Maehara M, et al: Magnetic resonance imaging in complex partial seizures, *Jpn J Psychiatry Neurol* 43:361-367, 1989.
20. Jackson GD, Berkovic SF, Tress BM, et al: Hippocampal sclerosis can be reliably detected by magnetic resonance imaging, *Neurology* 40:1869-1875, 1990.
21. Matsuda K, Yagi K, Mihara T, et al: MRI lesion and epileptogenic focus in temporal lobe epilepsy, *Jpn J Psychiatry Neurol* 43:393-400, 1989.
22. Stefan H, Schneider S, Abraham FK, et al: Magnetic source localization in focal epilepsy: multichannel magnetoencephalography correlated with magnetic resonance brain imaging, *Brain* 113:1347-1359, 1990.
23. Bronen RA: Anatomy of the temporal lobe. In Spencer SS, Spencer DD, editors: *Surgery for epilepsy,* Boston, 1991, Blackwell.
24. Bronen RA, Cheung G: MRI of the normal hippocampus, *Magn Reson Imaging* 9:497-500, 1991.
25. Bronen RA, Cheung G, Charles JT, et al: Imaging of hippocampal sclerosis: correlation with pathology, *AJNR,* September/October 1991.
26. Bronen RA, Cheung G: MRI of the temporal lobe: normal variations, with special reference toward epilepsy, *Magn Reson Imaging* 9(5):501-507, 1991.
27. Van Hoesen GW, Hyman BT, Damasio AR: Entorhinal cortex pathology in Alzheimer's disease, *Hippocampus* 1(1):1-8, 1991.
28. Ball MJ, Hachinski V, Fox A, et al: A new definition of Alzheimer's disease: a hippocampal dementia, *Lancet* 14-16, 1985.
29. Roberts GW: Schizophrenia: a neuropathological perspective, *Br J Psychiatry* 158:8-17, 1991.
30. Suddath RL, Christison GW, Torrey EF, et al: Anatomic abnormalities in the brains of monozygotic twins discordant for schizophrenia, *N Engl J Med* 322:789-794, 1990.
31. Press GA, Amaral DG, Squire LR: Hippocampal abnormalities in amnesic patients revealed by high-resolution magnetic resonance imaging, *Nature* 341:54-57, 1989.
32. Seab JP, Jagust WJ, Wong STS, et al: Quantitative NMR measurements of hippocampal atrophy in Alzheimer's disease, *Magn Reson Med* 8:200-208, 1988.
33. Kretschmann HJ, Weinrich W: *Neuroanatomy and cranial computed tomography,* New York, 1986, Thieme.
34. Garoutte B: *Survey of functional neuroanatomy,* ed 2, Greenbrae, Calif, 1987, Jones.
35. Schlesinger B: *The upper brainstem in the human: its nuclear configuration and vascular supply,* New York, 1976, Springer-Verlag.
36. McKenzie JS, Kemm RE, Wilcock LN, editors: *The basal ganglia: structure and function,* New York, 1984, Plenum.
37. DeLong HR, Alexander GE, Miller WC, et al: Anatomical and functional aspects of basal ganglia–thalamocortical circuits. In Franks AJ, Ironside JW, Mindham RHS, et al, editors: *Function and dysfunction in the basal ganglia,* Manchester, England, 1990, Manchester University.
38. McHugh PR: The basal ganglia: the region, the integration of its systems and implications for psychiatry and neurology. In Franks AJ, Ironside JW, Mindham RHS, et al, editors: *Function and dysfunction in the basal ganglia,* Manchester, England, 1990, Manchester University.
39. Inoue E, Hori S, Narumi Y, et al: Portal-systemic encephalopathy: presence of basal ganglia lesions with high signal intensity on MR images, *Radiology* 179:551-555, 1991.
40. Carpenter MB: Interconnections between the corpus striatum and brainstem nuclei. In McKenzie JS, Kemm RE, Wilcock LN, editors: *The basal ganglia: structure and function,* New York, 1984, Plenum.
41. Arendt T, Bigl V, Arendt A, Tennstedt KA: Loss of neurons in the nucleus basalis of Meynert in Alzheimer's disease, paralysis agitans and Korsakoff's disease, *Acta Neuropathol* 61:101-108, 1983.
42. Averbeck P: Lesions of the nucleus ansae peduncularis in neuropsychiatric disease, *Arch Neurol* 38:230-235, 1981.
43. Coyle JT, Price DL, DeLong MR: Alzheimer's disease: a disorder of cortical cholinergic innervation, *Science* 219:1184-1190, 1983.
44. Etienne P, Robitaille Y, Wood P, et al: Nucleus basalis: neuronal loss, neuritic plaques and choline acetyltransferase activity in advanced Alzheimer's disease, *Neuroscience* 19:1279-1291, 1986.

45. Ulfig N: Configuration of the magnocellular nuclei in the basal forebrain of the human adult, *Acta Anat (Basel)* 134:100-105, 1989.
46. Koci TM, Chiang F, Chow P, et al: Thalamic extrapontine lesions in central pontine myelinolysis, *AJNR* 11:1229-1233, 1990.
47. Netter FH: Nervous system, vol 1. Part I. Anatomy and physiology. In Brass A, Dingle RV, editors: *The CIBA collection of medical illustration,* West Caldwell, NJ, 1983, CIBA Pharmaceutical.
48. Ben-Ari Y, editor: *The amygdaloid complex: INSERM Symposium 20,* Amsterdam, 1981, Elsevier/North Holland.
49. Fallon JH, Ben-Ari Y: Transmitters and modulators—chairman's comments. In Ben-Ari Y, editor: *The amygdaloid complex: INSERM Symposium 20,* Amsterdam, 1981, Elsevier/North Holland.
50. Kapp BS, Kesner RP: Behavioral functions—chairman's comments. In Ben-Ari Y, editor: *The amygdaloid complex: INSERM Symposium 20.* Amsterdam, 1981, Elsevier/North Holland.
51. Bossy J: *Atlas of neuroanatomy and special sense organs,* Philadelphia, 1970, WB Saunders.
52. Baulac M, Vitte E, Dormont D, et al: The limbic system: identification of its structures on brain slices. In Gouaze A, Salamon G, editors: *Brain anatomy and magnetic resonance imaging,* New York, 1988, Springer-Verlag.
53. Albin RL, Reiner A, Anderson KD, et al: Striatal and nigral neuron subpopulations in rigid Huntington's disease: implications for the functional anatomy of chorea and rigidity-akinesia, *Ann Neurol* 27:357-365, 1990.
54. Albin RL, Young AB, Penney JB: The functional anatomy of basal ganglia disorders, *Trends Neurol Sci* 12:366-375, 1989.
55. Braffman BH, Grossman RI, Goldberg HI, et al: MR imaging of Parkinson disease with spin-echo and gradient-echo sequences, *AJNR* 9:1093-1099, 1988.
56. Duguid JR, DeLaPaz R, DeGroot J: Magnetic resonance imaging of the midbrain in Parkinson's disease, *Ann Neurol* 20(6):744-747, 1986.
57. Stern MB, Braffman BH, Skolnick BE, et al: Magnetic resonance imaging in Parkinson's disease and parkinsonian syndromes, *Neurology* 39:1524-1525, 1989.
58. Drayer BP: Imaging of the aging brain. Part I. Normal findings, *Radiology* 166:785-796, 1988.
59. Tomlinson BE, Blessed G, Roth M: Observations on the brains of nondemented old people, *J Neurol Sci* 7:331-356, 1968.
60. Bradley WG, Waluch V, Brant-Zawadzki M, et al: Patchy, periventricular white matter lesions in the elderly: a common observation during NMR imaging, *Noninvasive Med Imaging* 1(1):35-41, 1984.
61. Brant-Zawadzki M, Fein G, Van Dyke C, et al: MR imaging of the aging brain: patchy white-matter lesions and dementia, *AJNR* 6:675-682, 1985.
62. Fazekas F, Chawluk JB, Alavi A, et al: MR signal abnormalities at 1.5 T in Alzheimer's dementia and normal aging, *AJNR* 8:421-426, 1987.
63. George AE, de Leon MJ, Gentes CI, et al: Leukoencephalopathy in normal and pathologic aging. I. CT of brain lucencies, *AJNR* 7:561-566, 1986.
64. George AE, de Leon MJ, Kalnin A, et al: Leukoencephalopathy in normal and pathologic aging. II. MRI of brain lucencies, *AJNR* 7:567-570, 1986.
65. Goto K, Ishii N, Fukasawa H: Diffuse white-matter disease in the geriatric population, *Radiology* 141:687-695, 1981.
66. Tomlinson BE, Blessed G, Roth M: Observations on the brains of demented old people, *J Neurol Sci* 11:205-242, 1970.
67. Zatz LM, Jernigan TL, Ahumada AJ Jr: White matter changes in cerebral computed tomography related to aging, *J Comput Assist Tomogr* 6:19-23, 1982.
68. Gerard G, Weisberg L: MRI periventricular lesions in adults, *Neurology* 36:998-1001, 1986.
69. Blessed G, Tomlinson BE, Roth M: The association between quantitative measures of dementia and of senile change in the cerebral grey matter of elderly subjects, *Br J Psychiatry* 114:797-811, 1968.
70. Grafton ST, Sumi SM, Stimac GK, et al: Comparison of postmortem magnetic resonance imaging and neuropathologic findings in the cerebral white matter, *Arch Neurol* 48:293-298, 1991.
71. Awad IA, Johnson PC, Spetzler RF, et al: Incidental subcortical lesions identified on magnetic resonance imaging in the elderly. II. Postmortem pathological correlations, *Stroke* 17(6):1090-1097, 1986.
72. Awad IA, Spetzler RF, Hodak JA, et al: Incidental subcortical lesions identified on magnetic resonance imaging in the elderly. I. Correlation with age and cerebrovascular risk factors, *Stroke* 17(6):1084-1089, 1986.
73. Kirkpatrick JB, Hayman LA: White-matter lesions in MR imaging of clinically healthy brains of elderly subjects: possible pathologic basis, *Radiology* 162:509-511, 1987.
74. Sarwar M, Ford K: Rapid development of basal ganglia calcification, *AJNR* 2:103-104, 1981.
75. Cohen CR, Duchesneau PM, Weinstein MA: Calcification of the basal ganglia as visualized by computed tomography, *Radiology* 134:97-99, 1980.
76. Reyes PF, Gonzalez CF, Zalewska MK, et al: Intracranial calcification in adults with chronic lead exposure, *AJR* 146:267-270, 1986.
77. Aoki S, Okada Y, Nishimua K, et al: Normal deposition of brain iron in childhood and adolescence: MR imaging at 1.5 T, *Radiology* 172:381-385, 1989.
78. Hallgren B, Sourander P: The effect of age on the nonhaemin iron in the human brain, *J Neurochem* 3:41-51, 1958.
79. Cumings JN: The copper and "inorganic" iron content of human tissues, *Biochem J* 29:480-486, 1935.
80. Drayer B, Burger P, Darwin R, et al: Magnetic resonance imaging of brain iron, *AJNR* 7:373-380, 1986.
81. Koenig SH, Brown RD III: Relaxometry of ferritin solutions and the influence of the Fe^{3+} core ions, *Magn Reson Med* 3:755-767, 1986.
82. Chen JC, Hardy PA, Clauberg M, et al: T2 values in the human brain: comparison with quantitative assays of iron and ferritin, *Radiology* 173:521-526, 1989.
83. Drayer BP: Basal ganglia: significance of signal hypointensity on T2 weighted MR images, *Radiology* 173:311-312, 1989.
84. Bizzi A, Brooks R, Brunetti A, et al: Role of iron and ferritin in MR imaging of the brain: A study in primates at different field strengths, *Radiology* 177:59-65, 1990.
85. Rutledge JN: MR of movement disorders. In *Parkinson's disease and movement disorders,* 1988, Urban & Schwarzenberg.
86. Hall S, Rutledge JN, Schallert T: Neurological disorders and brain iron visualized by MRI, *J Clin Exp Neuropsychol* 2(1):92-93, 1989.
87. Cross PA, Atlas SW, Grossman RI: MR evaluation of brain iron in children with cerebral infarction, *AJNR* 11:341-348, 1990.
88. Schaffert D, Johnson S, Johnson P, et al: Magnetic resonance imaging in pathologically proven Hallervorden-Spatz disease, *Neurology* 39:440-442, 1989.
89. O'Brien C, Sung JH, McGeachie R, et al: Striatonigral degeneration: Clinical MRI and pathologic correlation, *Neurology* 40:710-711, 1990.
90. Gado M, Danziger WL, Chi D, et al: Brain parenchymal density measurements by CT in demented subjects and normal controls, *Radiology* 147:703-710, 1983.
91. George AE, de Leon MJ, Ferris SH, et al: Parenchymal CT correlates of senile dementia (Alzheimer disease): loss of gray-white matter discriminability, *AJNR* 2:205-213, 1981.
92. George AE, de Leon MJ, Ferris SH, et al: Authors' response to invited commentary, *AJNR* 2:212-213, 1981.
93. Heier LA, Orenstein A, Schwartz L, et al: Decreasing gray/white contrast: an aging phenomenon, *Neuroradiology* 33(S):607-608, 1991.

CHAPTER 5

L. Anne Hayman
J. Randy Jinkins
Joel B. Kirkpatrick

Cerebral Commissures

IMAGING TECHNIQUES

Groups of neural association fibers that cross the midline to interconnect the cerebral hemispheres are termed *commissures*. Functionally similar, and occasionally dissimilar, cortical regions are interconnected by these fiber tracts, which are closely associated with the third ventricle. Four commissural groups develop in the anterior wall of the third ventricle: the *corpus callosum, commissure of the fornix, anterior commissure,* and *supraoptic commissures*. The *habenular* and *posterior commissures* are found in the posterior wall of the third ventricle. The floor of the third ventricle contains very small commissural bundles termed the *subthalamic* and *hypothalamic commissures*. These tracts have clinical importance because they are the pathways by which some tumors (e.g., gliomas) cross from one hemisphere to another. In addition, commissural tracts can serve as discrete landmarks on sagittal magnetic resonance (MR) scans. Absence of the largest commissural tract, the corpus callosum, can sometimes have a confusing appearance on imaging studies when it occurs as an incidental finding in clinically normal patients.

Although axial computed tomographic (CT) projections can visualize these cerebral commissures, they are best examined by sagittal MR scans, which can be supplemented by coronal and axial views. Magnetic resonance imaging (MRI) is superior to ultrasonography, even in the newborn, because MRI avoids distortions caused by angling the sonographic transducer through the anterior fontanelle.[1] MRI also provides information on the rate and pattern of myelination and maturation of the fiber tracts in the neonatal brain. Despite these advantages, the high cost and limited availability of MRI have restricted its use. Therefore the cerebral commissures in the neonate are usually evaluated initially by ultrasound (see Chapters 1 and 2).

NORMAL ANATOMY

Commissures of Anterior Wall of Third Ventricle

Corpus Callosum

The corpus callosum has traditionally been divided from anterior to posterior into four parts: the rostrum, genu, body, and splenium (Figure 5-1). Isolated agenesis or postsurgical section of the corpus callosum is usually not associated with overt neurologic symptoms or gross changes in intellect, behavior, or emotion. Only the use of specific, sophisticated neuropsychologic tests will detect subtle signs of absence of callosal fibers.[2-4]

The following discussion outlines the development of the corpus callosum in utero and in the postnatal period. The information on fetal development is intended to help the reader understand the normal adult appearance of this region. Anomalies of the corpus callosum that originate during embryogenesis of the forebrain are briefly discussed, since anomalies in this commissural tract can be seen in otherwise normal subjects.

DEVELOPMENT IN UTERO: ASYMPTOMATIC INITIATIVE AGENESIS. Uncomplicated or isolated callosal agenesis is found in only 0.7% of patients.[5] This condition is caused by events that occur very early in fetal development. Between 6 and 8 weeks of gestation, shortly after closure of the neural tube, the thin tissue precursor of the corpus callosum begins to thicken and migrate into the adjacent mesenchyme. This region in the anterior aspect of the third ventricle develops into the commissural plate, which provides a bridge through which callosal fibers may cross the midline from one hemisphere to the other. This decussational process begins anteriorly in the 12th week of gestation. By the 20th week, the corpus callosum has reached its adult configuration, but not its adult size.

If an insult occurs in the very earliest stage of development, this commissural plate may not form. Consequently, the commissural fibers from the cerebral hemispheres cannot cross the midline, and accordingly, the callosal decussation has no guidance. Some of the decussating fibers may join the anterior commissure, causing enlargement, or *hypertrophy,* of this tract. Other fibers deflect posteriorly to form bundles and extend parallel to the interhemispheric fissure. In such circumstances, these fibers terminate randomly without forming neurologically meaningful connections. Each bundle contains fewer fibers than one would expect to find in a normal corpus callosum[6,7] (Figure 5-2). These anomalous bundles of fibers create characteristic indentations in the medial aspect of each lateral ventricle that have been named the *callosal bundles of Probst.*[8] These bundles can be seen on MR scans as hypointense bands lying medial to the lateral ventricles on both long TR/TE and short TR/TE scans (TR, repetition time; TE, echo delay time). The characteristic concavity of the medial border of the lateral ventricles is caused by these fibers, by hypertrophy of the cingulate gyrus,[6] and by a splaying of the components of the septum pellucidum.

Absence of the corpus callosum also causes an unusually wide separation and mild dilation of the lateral ventricles, as well as a midline extension of the dilated third ventricle dorsad. This occurs because formation of the corpus callosum normally pushes the fetal third ventricle ventrad. In the absence of a corpus callosum, the third ventricle remains in its higher fetal position. Absence of the corpus callosum alters the mechanical stresses in the developing brain, which in turn causes a characteristic, abnormal, radial arrangement of the gyri and sulci on the medial surface of the brain.[6] The features of callosal agenesis can be demonstrated best on coronal MR images.[7-9] In this projection, one can identify the distinctive anatomic distortions that occur at and behind the level of the foramen of Monro. These are illustrated in Figures 5-3 and 5-4.

DEVELOPMENT IN UTERO: ASYMPTOMATIC INTERRUPTIVE HYPOGENESIS. This anomaly results from an insult that occurs after the anterior decussational bed, which forms the rostrum of the corpus callosum, has developed. In this anomaly's mild form, only the most dorsal aspect of the corpus callosum, the splenium, is absent. In the more severe forms, one finds progressively more loss of the corpus callosum and, in the most severe cases, only a remnant of the callosal rostrum. The appearance of interruptive hypogenesis on coronal MR images is identical to that

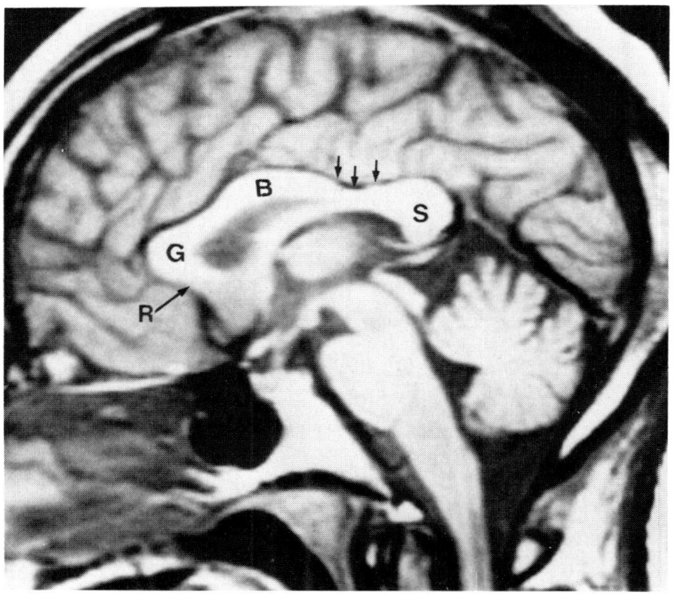

Figure 5-1 Midsagittal MR image (TR/TE, 600/20 msec) of the normal adult corpus callosum. R, Rostrum; G, genu; B, body; S, splenium. Although the thinning between the body and splenium (*arrows*) is within the normal range, this is a somewhat exaggerated example of this highly variable region. NOTE: The sulci on the medial surface of the hemisphere do not extend past the cingulate gyrus, which encircles the corpus callosum.

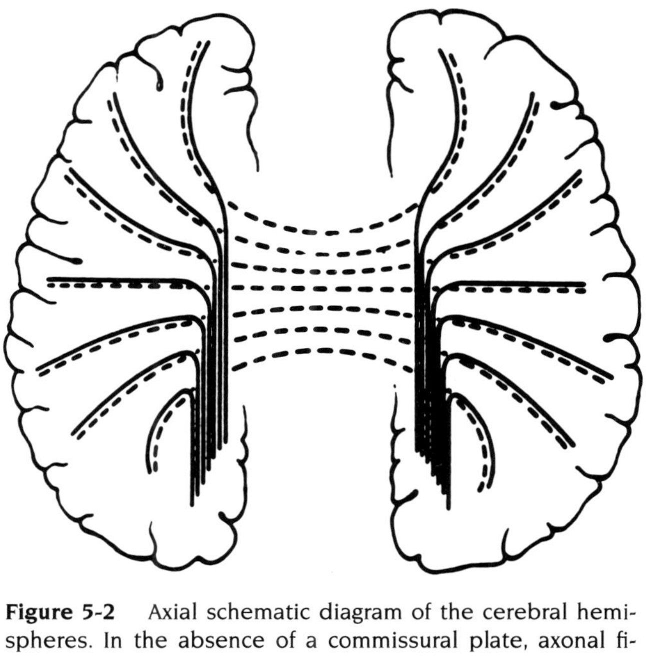

Figure 5-2 Axial schematic diagram of the cerebral hemispheres. In the absence of a commissural plate, axonal fibers from the cerebral hemispheres fail to cross the midline. Instead, these fibers reach the medial hemispheric wall and turn to course parallel to the interhemispheric fissure, indenting the medial wall of each lateral ventricle (*solid lines*). These fibers have been termed the lateral *callosal bundles of Probst.* Broken lines represent the normal course of the corpus callosal fibers.

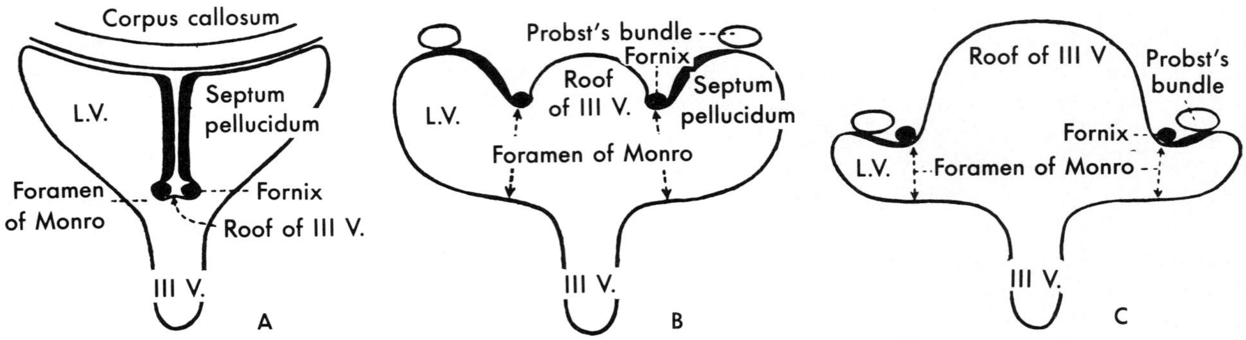

Figure 5-3 Schematic coronal brain sections. **A**, Normal brain at the level of the foramen of Monro. Callosal agenesis creates moderate **(B)** and severe **(C)** derangements of the normal anatomy at this level. LV, Frontal horn of lateral ventricle; III V, third ventricle. (Reproduced with permission from Hernandez-Schulman MM, Dohan FC, Jones T, et al: AJNR 6:361-368, 1985.)

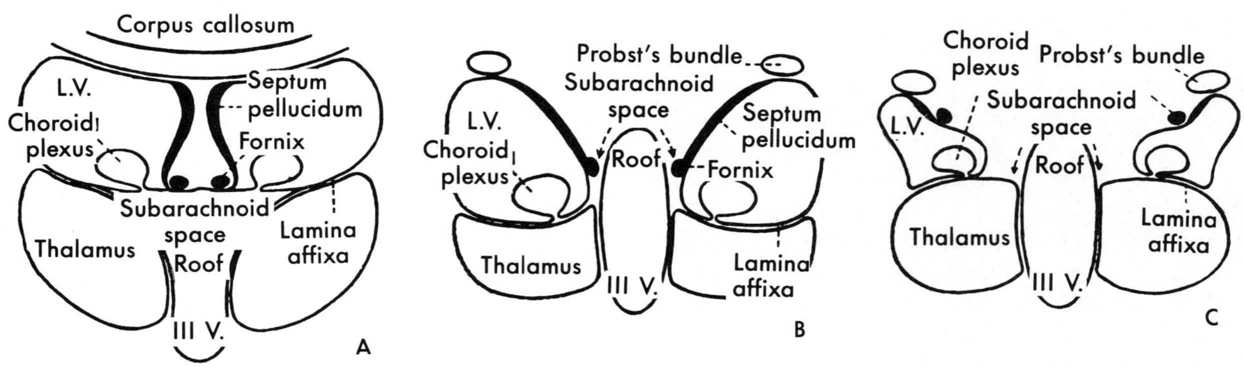

Figure 5-4 Schematic coronal brain sections. **A**, Normal brain posterior to the level of the foramen of Monro. Callosal agenesis creates moderate **(B)** and severe **(C)** derangements of normal anatomy at this level. LV, Frontal horn of lateral ventricle; III V, third ventricle. (Reproduced with permission from Hernandez-Schulman MM, Dohan FC, Jones T, et al: AJNR 6:361-368, 1985.)

of initiative agenesis, except that anteriorly, part of the corpus callosum persists (Figures 5-4, *A* and *B*, 5-5, and 5-6).

A subsection of interruptive hypogenesis includes an anomaly that has been called an *embryonic collision* or *obstructive hypogenesis*. This occurs if an ectopic collection of cellular material develops in the path of the caudally growing corpus callosum. In such cases the posteriorly developing corpus callosum collides with and indents the ectopic mass. Ultimately, the mass may cloak the posterior, superior, and inferior surfaces of the developing corpus callosum[10,11] (Figure 5-7).

So-called lipomas of the corpus callosum are formed by such a collision of the developing corpus callosum with ectopic fat cells. When this occurs, additional ectopic fat cells can be found in the ventricles and cisterns in 20% to 25% of patients.[11] This condition causes no consistently identifiable clinical deficits, although seizures have been reported. On MR images the pericallosal lipoma of the corpus callosum appears as a strikingly hyperintense zone cloaking the superior and posterior aspects of the corpus callosum on long TR/long TE and short TR/short TE acquisitions (Figure 5-8). Vessels can sometimes be identified within the lipoma by their flow void characteristics.[10] The pathogenesis and MR appearance of this congenital malformation have recently been reviewed in 42 patients.[12] Current theories postulate several etiologies for this condition: embryonic inclusion, lipoma formation caused by an abnor-

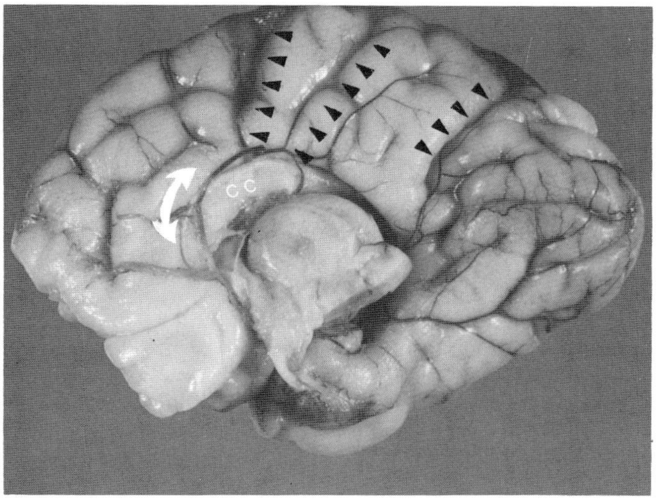

Figure 5-5 Midsagittal section of the lateral aspect of the right hemisphere in a neonate. The normal anterior corpus callosum (*cc*) and cingulate gyrus (*white double-headed arrow*) terminate abruptly in this patient, who has interruptive hypogenesis of the corpus callosum. Note the abnormal, radiating gyral pattern on the posterior aspect of the hemisphere (*arrowheads*) and the absence of the posterior cingulate gyrus. This occurs because the structural support from the corpus callosum is absent. (Compare with Figure 5-1, B). (Reproduced with permission from Hernandez-Schulman MM, Dohan FC, Jones T et al: AJNR 6:361-368, 1985.)

A

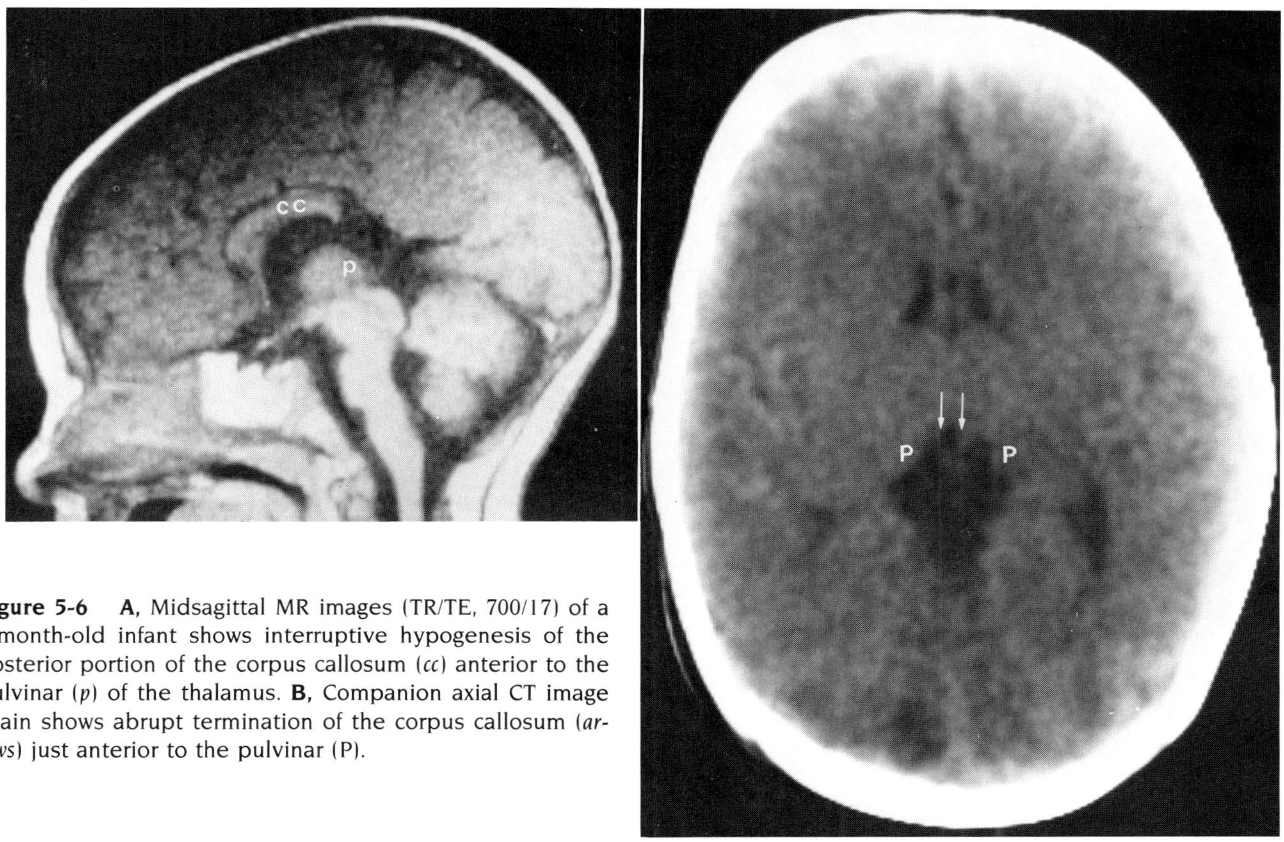

B

Figure 5-6 **A,** Midsagittal MR images (TR/TE, 700/17) of a 5-month-old infant shows interruptive hypogenesis of the posterior portion of the corpus callosum (*cc*) anterior to the pulvinar (*p*) of the thalamus. **B,** Companion axial CT image again shows abrupt termination of the corpus callosum (*arrows*) just anterior to the pulvinar (P).

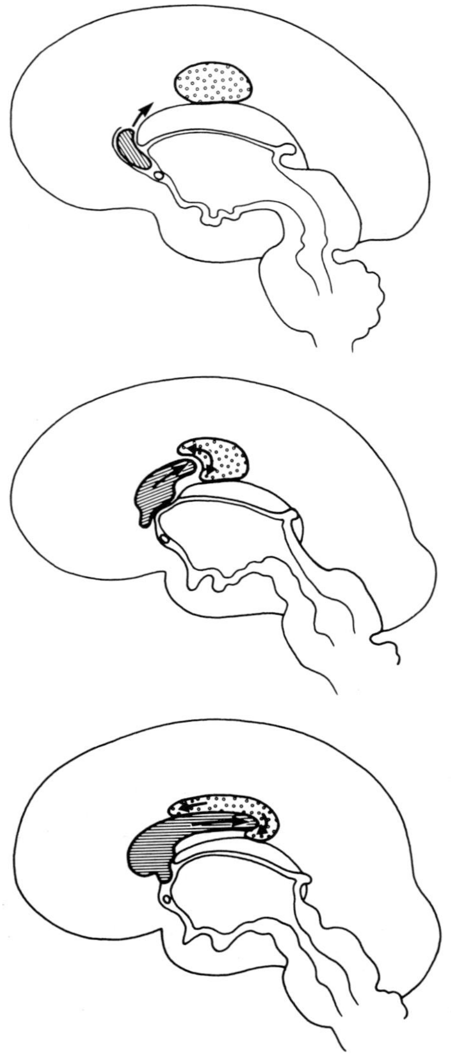

Figure 5-7 Serial sagittal illustrations depicting embryonic callosal collision. **A,** As callosal induction begins at 12 weeks of gestation, a deep midline neural tube mass (i.e., lipoma) is seen blocking the path of future callosal growth (*arrow*). **B,** With further advance (*arrow*), the corpus callosum collides with the mass, indenting it (*curved double arrow*). **C,** The mass, if sufficiently pliable (e.g., lipomatous tissue), becomes invaginated by corpus callosum. As a result, varying degrees of obstructive callosal hypogenesis and "commalike" cloaking of the corpus callosum occur. (Reproduced with permission from Jinkins JR, Whittemore AR, Bradley WG: AJNR 10:339-344, 1989.)

mal fetal persistence, and/or a maldifferentiation of the tissues that form the meninges.[10,12]

CT images of patients with "lipomas of the corpus callosum" have a striking, hypodense area caused by the fatty tissue (Figure 5-9, *A*). On ultrasound, these "lipomas" appear as hyperechoic zones in the same characteristic location (Figure 5-9, *B*). Associated dysgenesis of the corpus callosum (e.g., hypogenesis) is found with 30% to 50% of these lipomas.[11]

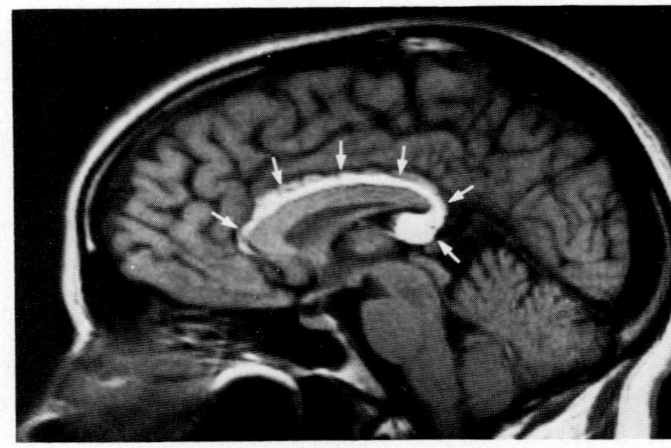

Figure 5-8 Midsagittal MR scan (TR/TE, 500/40) demonstrates "commalike" lipomatous cloaking (*arrows*) of the corpus callosum with minimum obstructive hypogenesis of the splenium. (Reproduced with permission from Davidson HD, Abraham R, Steiner RE: *Radiology* 155:371-373, 1985.)

DEVELOPMENT IN UTERO: SYMPTOMATIC HYPOPLASIA. Autopsy results indicate that 88% of brains with callosal anomalies also have various other cerebral malformations.[6] In many of these cases, hypoplasia of the corpus callosum occurs because the cerebral cortex, which supplies the commissural axons, is dysgenetic.[10] In these brains, abnormal migration, lamination, and destruction of the cortical elements result in *polymicrogyria*. Polymicrogyria can only be reliably detected microscopically, and thus it is a histologic diagnosis. On imaging studies, polymicrogyria grossly appears as a thick cortical band of gray matter without discernible sulci. This abnormal fetal cortex projects a subnormal complement of axons to the midline,[13] which in turn results in hypoplasia of the corresponding portion of the corpus callosum.[10] Such cortical and callosal abnormalities may be multifocal.

Associated hypoplasia of the hemispheric white matter caused by reduced numbers of commissural, associational, and projectional fibers (i.e., hypoplasia of the posterior forceps) may also result in enlargement of the adjacent ventricles *(colpocephaly)*.[1,10] Cortical dysgenesis may be superimposed on either initiative or interruptive callosal anomalies[14] and, when present, typically causes severe clinical deficits.[10,15] Accordingly, 2.3% of mentally retarded persons have agenesis of the corpus callosum.

Associated anomalies of other, nonneural systems are also frequently encountered.[6] The causes of these congenital malformations are unknown, but multiple intrauterine factors have been suggested.[16,17]

POSTNATAL DEVELOPMENT. At birth and throughout the first month of life, the corpus callosum is visualized on MR images as a thin band that has the same signal

A 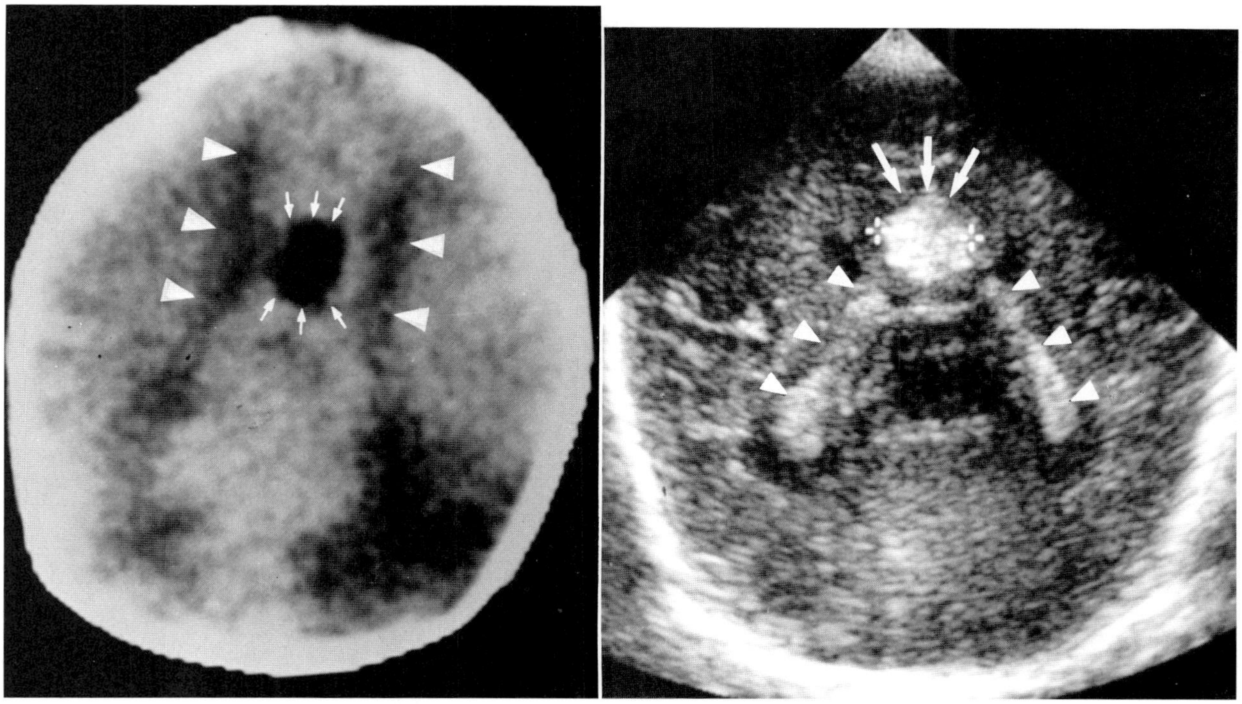 B

Figure 5-9 **A,** Axial CT image showing the characteristic hypointense appearance of the "lipoma" (*arrows*) between the widely separated lateral ventricles (*arrowheads*). Unrelated cortical and white matter damage is present in the left hemisphere. **B,** The companion axial ultrasound image shows the characteristic, highly echogenic appearance and location of the lipoma (*arrows*) and lateral ventricles (*arrowheads*). Two cursor markers to determine lipoma size are incidentally seen.

intensity as the other nonmyelinated white matter fibers of the cerebral hemispheres. Shape and signal intensity of the corpus callosum gradually change until a child's brain achieves normal adult configuration at age 8 to 13 months.[1]

The first noticeable change in *size* of the corpus callosum can be seen in some infants as early as the second or third month of life. The first noticeable change in *shape* is a substantial thickening of the anterior part of the corpus callosum (i.e., the rostrum). This parallels development of the precentral (motor) and postcentral (sensory) cortices in early life.[1] In the fifth and sixth months after birth, a rapid increase occurs in size of the splenium of the corpus callosum because of arrival of commissural fibers from the primary visual and visual association areas of the occipital lobe.

The successive changes in *signal intensity* of the corpus callosum on short TR/TE MR scans also occur during the first year after birth. These are thought to reflect progressive myelination.[1] Unlike the formation of the corpus callosum (which progresses from anterior to posterior), myelination progresses from the splenium rostrad. At 4 months of age, an increase in MR signal intensity is seen in the splenium, which progresses rostrally over the next 2 months. High signal intensity (relative to gray matter) on short TR/TE MR images is uniform throughout the corpus callosum by the eighth month after birth. A concomitant decrease in signal intensity is seen on long TR/TE MR images in the splenium at approximately 6 months and in the genu at 8 months of age. These changes in signal intensity of the corpus callosum appropriately reflect the relatively short T1 (longitudinal relaxation time) and T2 (transverse relaxation time) MR values (relative to gray matter) of myelinated axons of the adult brain and may be useful for gauging normal progress of brain development and maturation.[18,19] Myelination of the corpus callosum is complete early in the second decade of life.[20]

ADULT FEATURES. A thinning is seen at the junction between the body and the splenium of the corpus callosum in 22% of patients and is thought to be a normal variant of no clinical significance[21] (see Figure 5-1). Other normal variations in configuration of the corpus callosum have been described in a small series of patients examined at autopsy or by imaging studies. These variations appeared to be related to the sex or handedness of the subject. The volume (cm^3) of the corpus callosum can be measured and has been described as being larger in left-handed than in right-handed subjects,[22] but this was not substantiated in an MR study of 80 normal subjects.[23] The splenium may be found to be wider and more bulbous in female than in male subjects,[23] but these normal variations in shape of the corpus callosum appear to be clinically irrelevant. The thickness of the genu and the splenium of the corpus callosum also has been measured. In one study the distance from the callosal sulcus to the innermost margin was 7.98 mm for the genu and 8.37 mm for the splenium in the average adult.[24] Measurements greater than 10 mm should be considered abnormal.

The corpus callosum is a white matter tract with two unique characteristics that have only been observed in vivo by modern imaging techniques. First, the corpus callosum seldom, if ever, displays the commonly identified foci of hyperintense signal seen on long TR/TE MR images in many elderly patients. Second, the corpus callosum does not allow transmission of edema fluid.[25] These findings have been attributed to certain microscopic features of normal callosal vessels, which are described below.[26]

The corpus callosum is supplied by arterioles 80 to 100 μm in length that enter its upper surface to descend vertically and obliquely backward for a short distance. In contrast, the centrum semiovale and the outer one quarter of the lateral ventricular roof are supplied by longer (20 to 50 mm) arterioles that are, with rare exception, end arteries. Unlike the callosal arteries, these vessels appear to be susceptible to atherosclerotic disease and occlusion. Accordingly, the shorter callosal vessels appear to protect the corpus callosum and may thereby account for the absence of hyperintense foci in this fiber tract. A full discussion of these hyperintense areas can be found in Chapter 4.

The presence and orientation of unusual perivascular fibrous alae (which extend laterally from the callosal vessels) may form the microscopic barrier that prevents edema from spreading across or within the corpus callosum.[23]

Commissure of Fornix (Hippocampal)

The fornix is an intrahemispheric tract that primarily connects each hippocampus to the ipsilateral septal region and mamillary body of the hypothalamus. Some fibers of the fornix cross the midline to provide access to the contralateral hippocampus. These fibers are called the *fornical* or *hippocampal commissure*. The fornix functions as part of the limbic system, which is described in detail in Chapter 4. In utero, the decussational bed of this tract lies directly beneath that of the corpus callosum in the anterior wall of the third ventricle. The unusual path of the fornix is caused by the growth and subsequent rotation of the cerebral hemispheres around the brainstem during development (see Chapter 12). The fibers of the fornix form the base of the septum pellucidum, which has the corpus callosum as its roof. The location of these fibers can be seen schematically in Figure 5-10.[27]

Even though the fornical commissure begins anteriorly in the wall of the third ventricle, it is found in the adult brain at the posterior aspect of the fornix below the splenium of the corpus callosum (Figure 5-11). When the overlying corpus callosum is completely absent, the com-

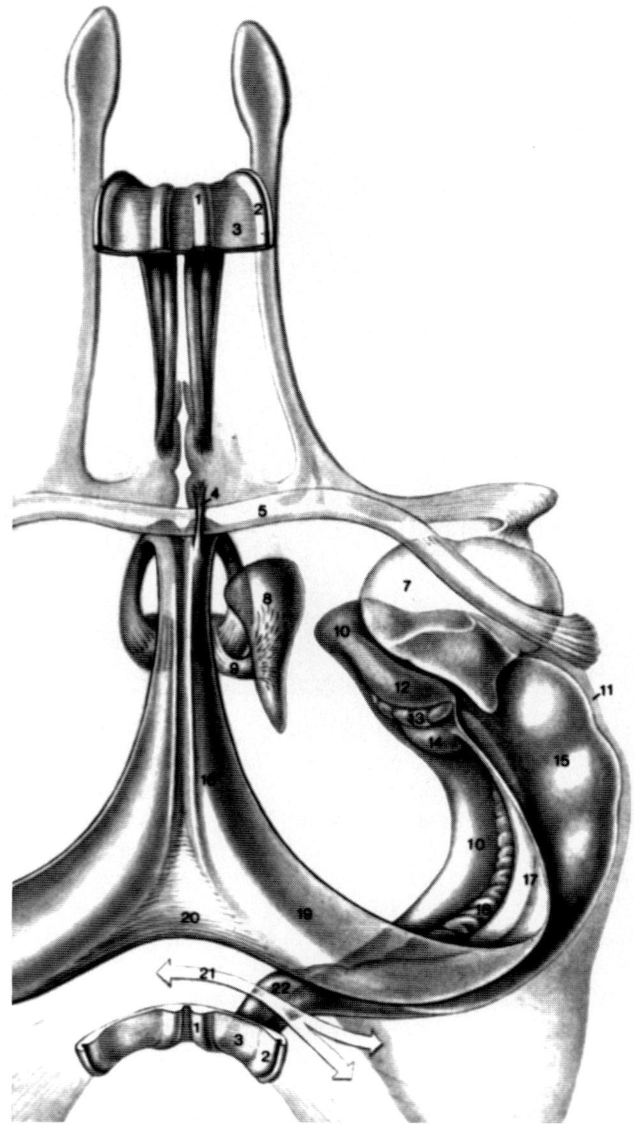

Figure 5-10 Axial schematic drawing of the limbic system from above. Most of the surrounding brain structures have been removed. The fimbria of the hippocampus (17) forms the crus of the fornix (19). Some fibers of the crus cross the midline below the corpus callosum (which has been removed) to form the fornical commissure (20). A portion of the body of the fornix continues anteriorly to form the column of the fornix (6), which is located below the anterior commissure (5). Incidentally identified structures shown in this schematic are medial longitudinal striae (1), lateral longitudinal striae (2), indusium griseum (3), precommissural fibers of fornix to septal area (4), amygdala (7), anterior thalamic nucleus (8), mamillothalamic tract (9), subiculum (10), temporal horn of lateral ventricle (11), uncinate gyrus (12), band of Giacomini (fibers from uncinate gyrus to dentate gyrus) (13), caudal portion of uncinate gyrus (14), pes hippocampus (15), body of the fornix (16), dentate (18), site of resected splenium of corpus callosum (21), fasciolar gyrus (22). (Reproduced with permission from Nieuwenhuys R, Voogd J, van Huijzen C: *The human central nervous system: a synopsis and atlas*, ed 3, New York, 1981, Springer-Verlag.)

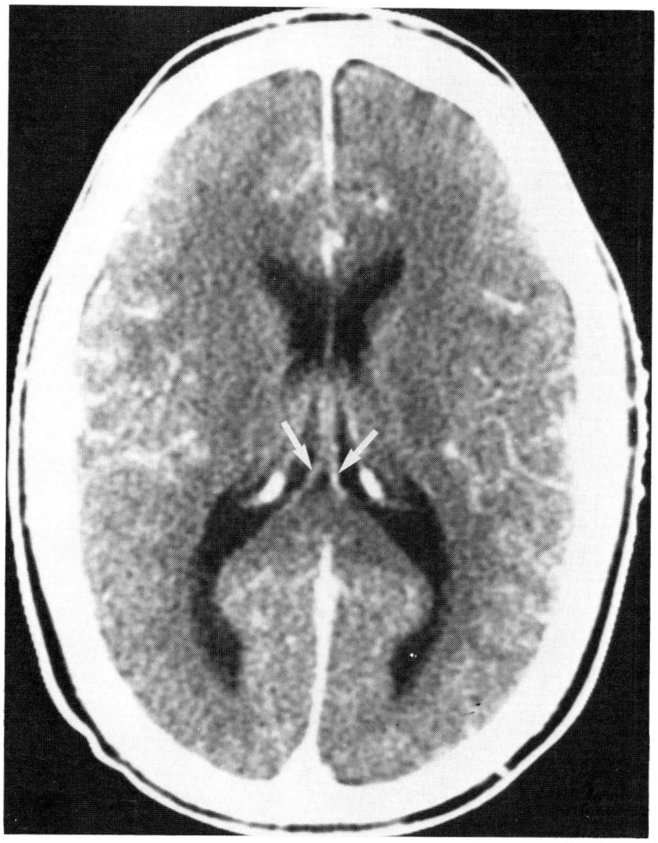

missure of the fornix may become enlarged and thus may be mistaken for the absent splenium.[28]

Anterior Commissure (Olfactory Chiasm)

In utero, the anterior commissure, as with the corpus callosum and the fornical commissure, forms within the anterior wall of the third ventricle (i.e., the lamina terminalis). However, the anterior commissure does not migrate with hemispheric growth.

Initially, the anterior commissure connects the paired olfactory bulbs. For this reason, it is sometimes referred to as the *olfactory chiasm*. Later in development, other fibers also pass through the anterior commissure to connect those portions of the temporal lobes that physically cannot interconnect through the corpus callosum.[29,30] A more complete picture of the areas interconnected by the fibers of the anterior commissure in the adult is schematically illustrated in Figure 5-12.[31] Little is known of the functions of this fiber tract.

The anterior commissure is an important landmark on MR images. It is well defined on MRI because it is sur-

Figure 5-11 Contrast-enhanced axial CT image shows the enhanced septum pellucidum as it attaches to the fornix (*arrows*). The cerebrospinal fluid space between the diverging septal leaves is the cavum velum interpositum. The fornical (hippocampal) commissure blends with the corpus callosum as it crosses the midline between the cura of the fornix to form the roof of the cavum velum interpositum. (Compare with Figure 5-10.)

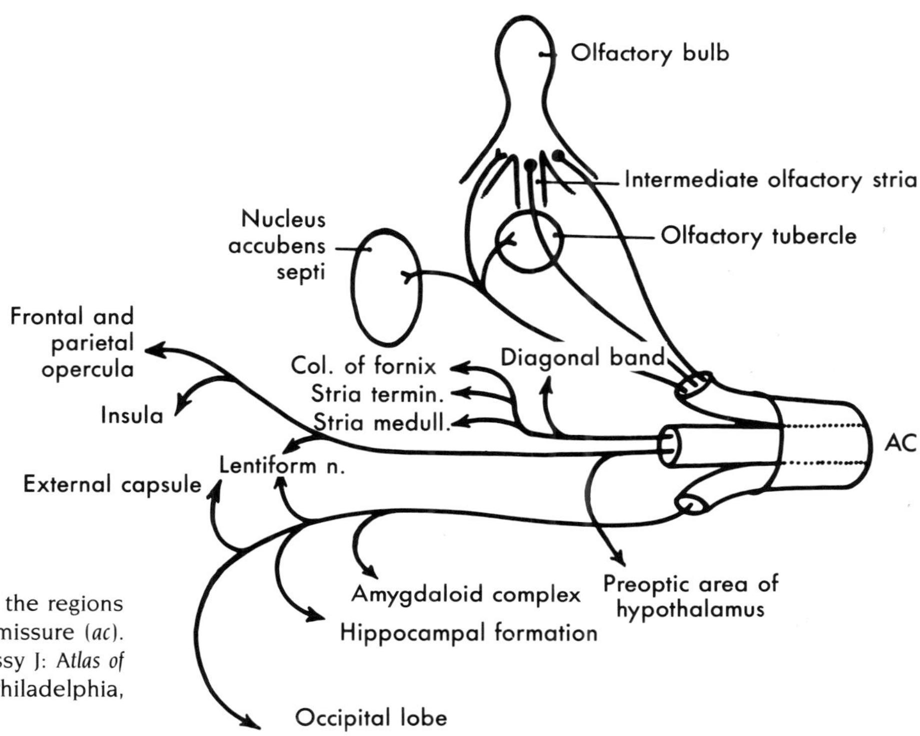

Figure 5-12 Schematic illustration of the regions that supply fibers to the anterior commissure (*ac*). (Reproduced with permission from Bossy J: *Atlas of neuroanatomy and special sense organs*, Philadelphia, 1970, WB Saunders.)

rounded by gray matter structures throughout most of its path. Correct identification of this structure localizes the less well-defined basal ganglia, the nuclear boundaries of which are often obscured on MR images by iron deposition.[29] Figures 5-13 and 5-14 define the location of the anterior commissure on axial and sagittal MR images, respectively.

Figure 5-15 reviews the interrelated anatomy of the corpus callosum, fornix, and the anterior commissure in the adult brain.

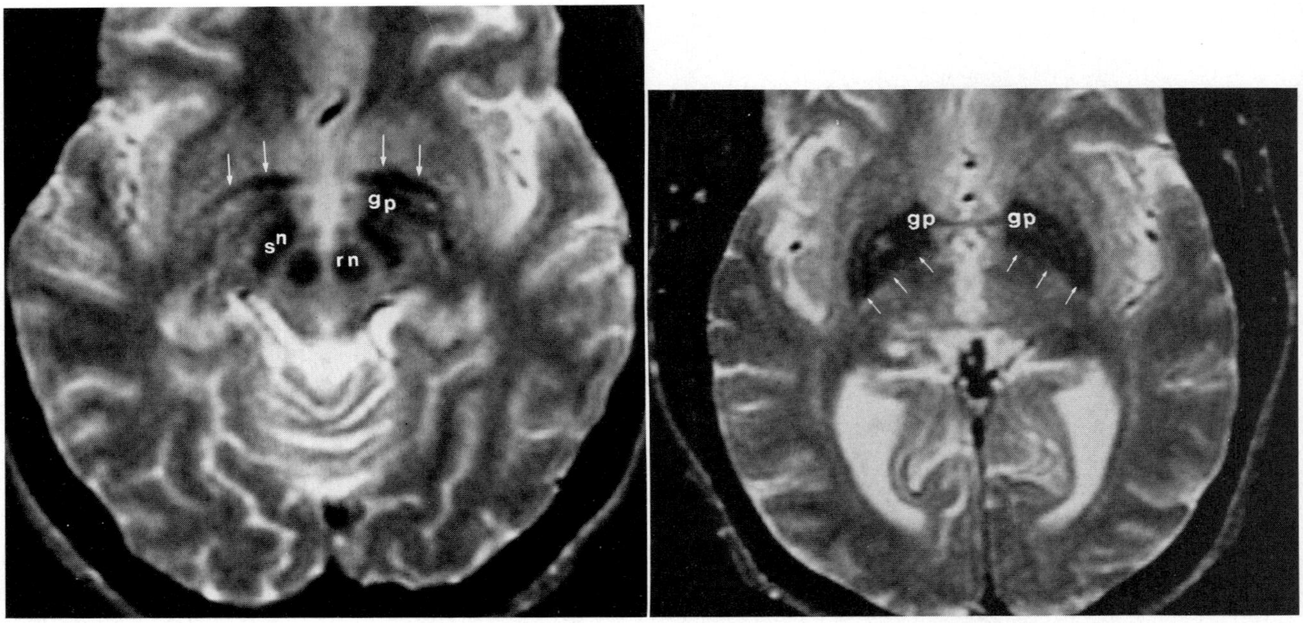

Figure 5-13 **A,** Axial MR images (TR/TE, 2000/80) at the midbrain level show the hypointense signal in the anterior commissure (*arrows*). Iron deposition causes hypointense signal in the globus pallidus (*gp*), substantia nigra (*sn*), and red nucleus (*rn*) in this elderly subject. **B,** MR image slightly above the midbrain in another patient shows the anterior commissure crossing the midline beneath the hypointense lateral globus pallidus (*gp*), which is part of the lentiform nucleus (*arrows*).

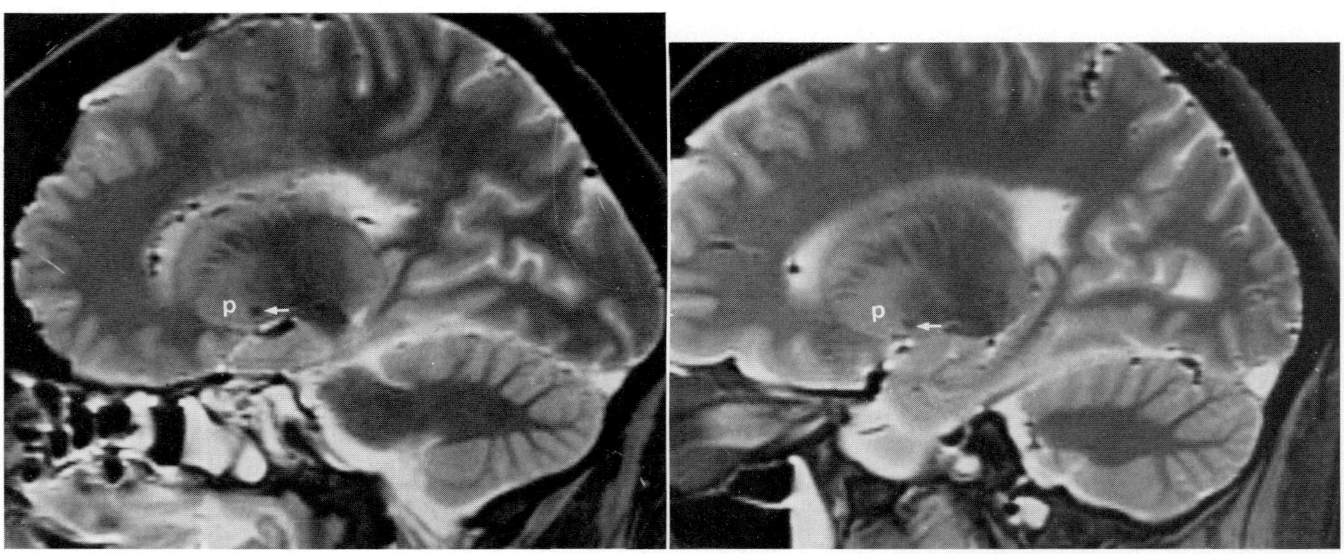

Figure 5-14 **A** and **B,** Serial sagittal MR images of a cadaver brain show the anterior commissure (*arrow*) immediately below the lateral globus pallidus and posterior to the putamen (*p*).

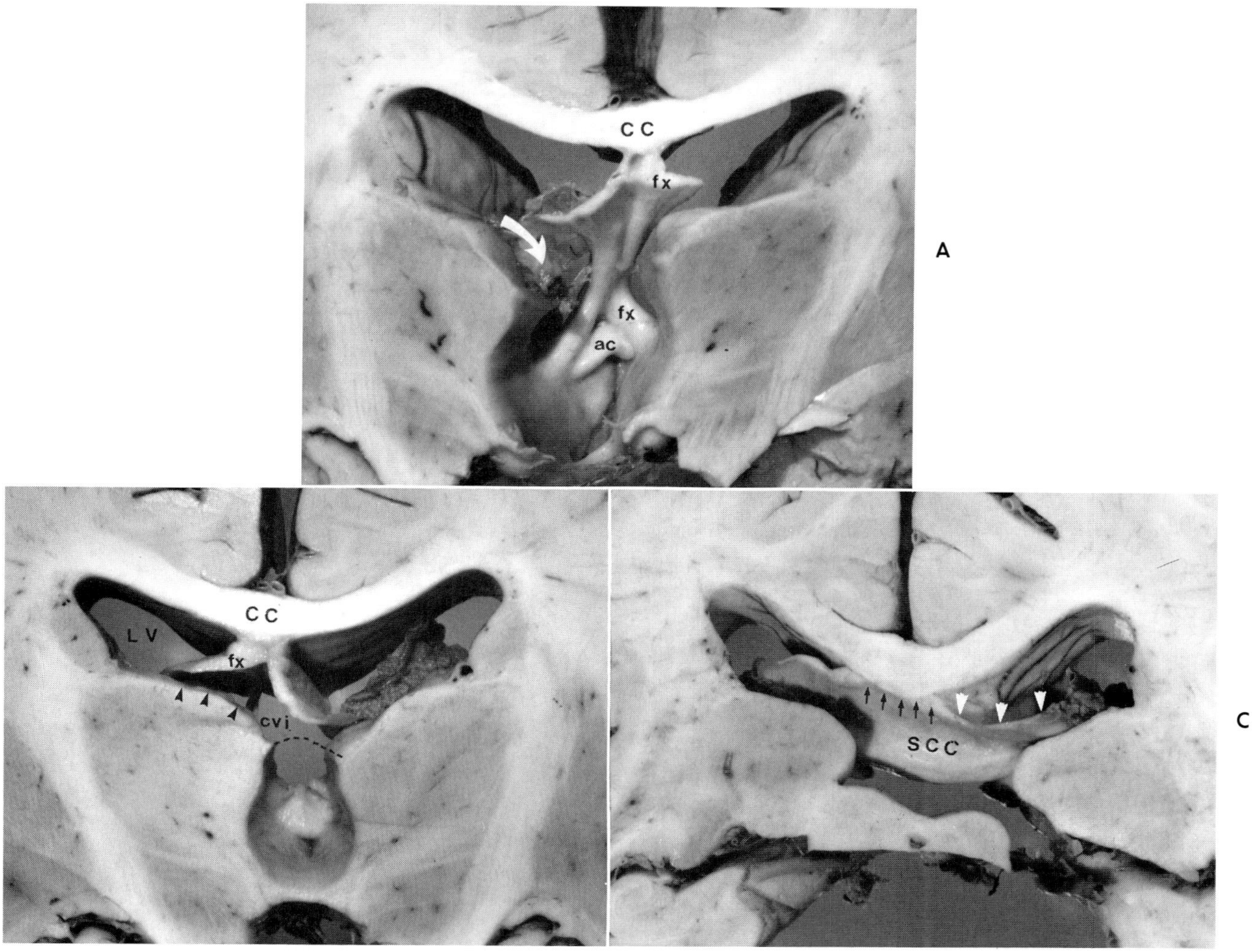

Figure 5-15 Serial coronal sections of formalin-fixed brain. **A,** At the foramen of Monro (*arrow*), the commissural anatomy is best seen if the dorsal (posterior) surfaces are shown. In this projection the columns of the fornix (*fx*) descend to the mamillary bodies. The fibers of the anterior commissure (*ac*) cross the midline in this region. The roofs of the lateral ventricles are formed by the corpus callosum (CC). **B,** At the middle of the third ventricle, the fibers of the fornix (*fx*) can be seen below the corpus callosum (CC). Centrally, these fibers form the roof of the cavum velum interpositum (*cvi*) and laterally the choroidal fissure (*arrowheads*). A dotted line marks the position of the roof of the third ventricle between the stria medullaris on the thalamic surfaces. The fornix forms the medial aspect of the floor of the lateral ventricles (LV) and the inferior attachment of the septum pellucidum, which has almost terminated at this level. (The unmarked fornix on the reader's right is artifactually depressed.) **C,** At the splenium of the corpus callosum (SCC), the commissural anatomy is best seen if the ventral (anterior) surface is shown. In this projection the fornical fibers form the floor of the lateral ventricles (*arrowheads*). As these fibers join in the midline, they form the fornical commissure (*arrows*), which is the roof of the cavum velum interpositum.

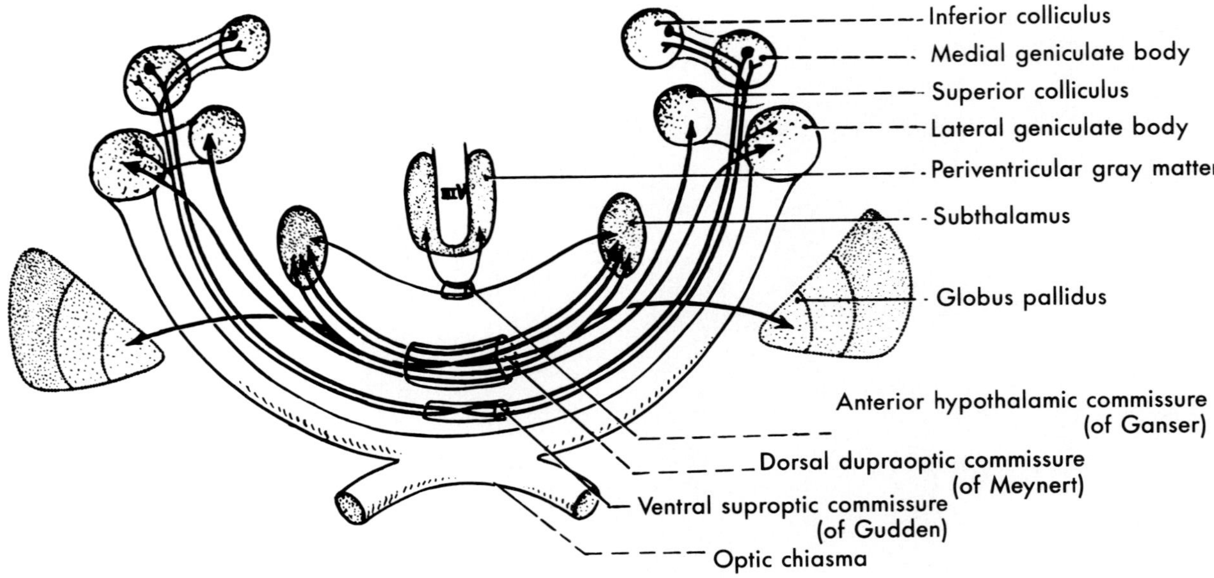

Figure 5-16 Schematic illustration of the brain regions that supply fibers to the supraoptic commissures. (Reproduced with permission from Bossy J: *Atlas of neuroanatomy and special sense organs*, Philadelphia, 1970, WB Saunders.)

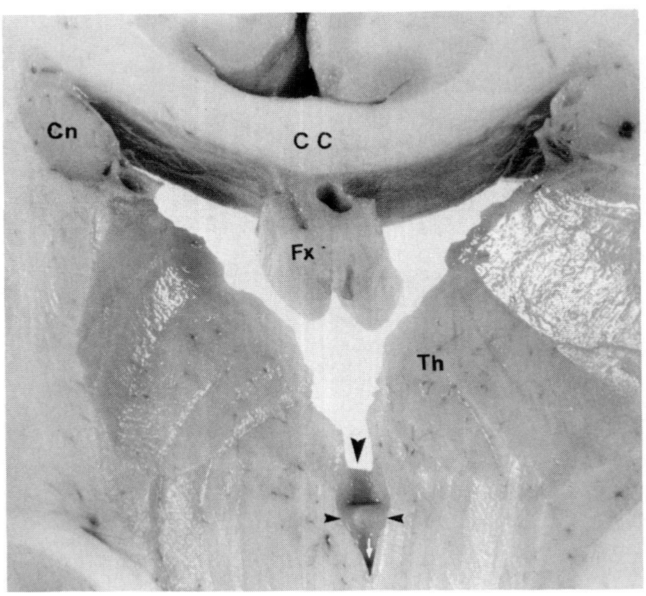

Figure 5-17 Coronal brain section. Removal of the medial thalamus (T*h*) exposes the habenular commissure (*vertical arrowhead*) and the posterior commissure (*horizontal arrowheads*) above the aqueduct (*small white arrow*). The pineal recess is the dark depression (not labeled) between the habenular and posterior commissures. CC, Corpus callosum; *fx*, fornix; *cn*, body of caudate nucleus.

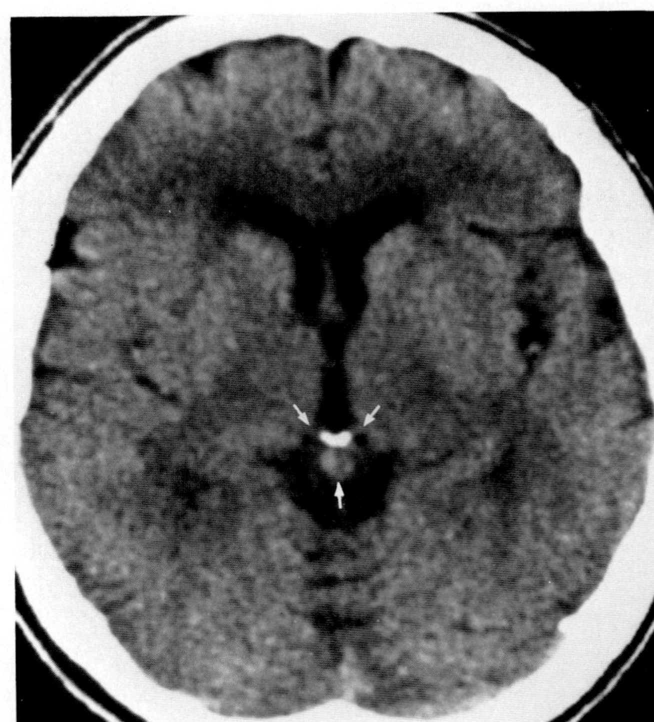

Figure 5-18 Axial nonenhanced CT image shows characteristic shape of the calcified habenular commissure extending between the habenular nuclei (*arrows*) anterior to the pineal gland (*arrowhead*).

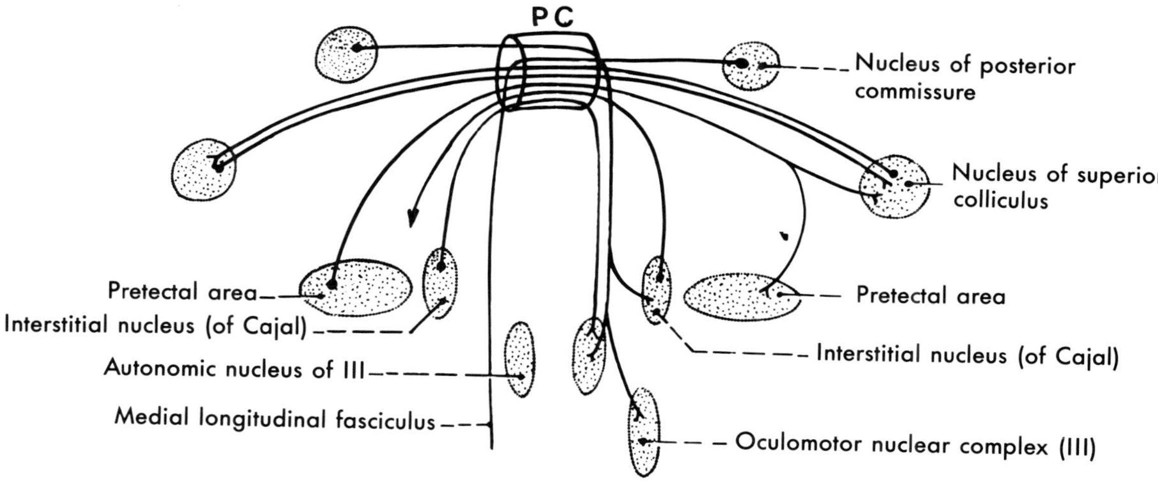

Figure 5-19 Schematic illustration of the regions that supply fibers to posterior commissure (PC). (Reproduced with permission from Bossy J: *Atlas of neuroanatomy and special sense organs*, Philadelphia, 1970, WB Saunders.)

Supraoptic Commissures

Three extremely small commissural bundles are found immediately dorsal to the optic chiasm in the anterior wall of the third ventricle. These commissures interconnect important regions of the cerebral hemispheres, which are schematically illustrated in Figure 5-16.[31] Tumors that arise in these regions can spread across the midline in these commissural tracts. The anterior hypothalamic *commissure of Ganser* interconnects the gray matter around the third ventricle and subthalamic region. The dorsal supraoptic *commissure of Meynert* also interconnects the subthalamic nuclei, the lateral geniculate bodies, the superior colliculus, and the globus pallidus. The ventral supraoptic *commissure of Gudden* connects the medial geniculate bodies.

Commissures of Posterior Wall of Third Ventricle

Habenular Commissure

The habenular commissure interconnects the habenular nuclei. It forms part of the posterosuperior wall of the third ventricle (Figure 5-17). Calcification is sometimes seen on lateral skull radiographs and CT images in the habenular nuclei and/or the commissural tract (Figure 5-18). The clinical significance of this thalamic interconnection is unknown. The principal fiber tracts associated with the habenular nuclei are the stria medullaris thalami, which connects the habenular commissure with the hypothalamus, and the fasciculus retroflexus, which terminates in the midbrain.

Posterior Commissure

This bundle of association fibers crosses the midline at the junction of the mesencephalon and diencephalon, immediately below the stalk of the pineal gland. The posterior commissure forms the roof of the aqueduct (Figure 5-17). The brain regions that are interconnected by the fibers of this commissure are outlined in Figure 5-19.[31] The function of this fiber tract is poorly understood.

Commissures of Floor of Third Ventricle

Two very small fiber tracts cross the midline in the floor of the third ventricle: the *posterior subthalamic commissure of Forel* and the *posterior hypothalamic (supramamillary) commissure*. These tracts are seldom mentioned in anatomic texts, and their function has not yet been clarified.[2,32] They are mentioned in this chapter because they can serve as unusual pathways for interhemispheric spread of tumor (e.g., glioma).

REFERENCES

1. Barkovich AJ, Kjos BO: Normal postnatal development of the corpus callosum as demonstrated by MR imaging, *AJNR* 9:487-491, 1988.
2. Brodal A: *Neurological anatomy in relation to clinical medicine,* ed 2, New York, 1969, Oxford University.
3. Ettlinger G, Blakemore CB, Milner AD, et al: Agenesis of the corpus callosum: a further behavioral investigation, *Brain* 97:225-234, 1974.
4. Sperry RW: Cerebral organization and behavior, *Science* 133:1749-1757, 1961.
5. Jellinger K, Gross H, Kaltenback E, et al: Holoprosencephaly and agenesis of the corpus callosum: frequency of associated malformations, *Acta Neuropathol (Berl)* 55:1-10, 1981.
6. Hernandez-Schulman MM, Dohan FC, Jones T, et al: Sonographic appearance of callosal agenesis: correlation with radiologic and pathologic findings, *AJNR* 6:361-368, 1985.
7. Rakic P, Yakovlev PI: Development of the corpus callosum and cavum septi in man, *J Comp Neurol* 132:45-72, 1968.
8. Barkovich AJ, Norman D: Anomalies of the corpus callosum: correlation with further anomalies of the brain, *AJNR* 9:493-501, 1988.
9. Davidson HD, Abraham R, Steiner RE: Agenesis of the corpus callosum: magnetic resonance imaging, *Radiology* 155:371-373, 1985.
10. Jinkins JR, Whittemore AR, Bradley WG: MR imaging of callosal and corticocallosal dysgenesis, *AJNR* 10:339-344, 1989.
11. Truwitt CL, Williams RG, Armstrong EA, et al: MR imaging of choroid plexus lipomas, *AJNR* 11:202-204, 1990.
12. Truwitt CL, Barkovich AJ: Pathogenesis of intracranial lipoma: an MR study in 42 patients, *AJNR* 11:665-674, 1990.
13. Larroche J: Malformations of the nervous system. In Adams HJ, Corsellis J, Duchen LW, editors: *Greenfield's neuropathology,* New York, 1984, John Wiley & Sons.
14. Brun A, Probst F: The influence of associated cerebral lesions on the morphology of the acallosal brain: a pathological and encephalographic study, *Neuroradiology* 6:121-131, 1973.
15. Parrish ML, Roessmann U, Levinsohn MW: Agenesis of the corpus callosum: a study of the frequency of associated malformations, *Ann Neurol* 6:349-354, 1979.
16. Langman J: Congenital malformations and their causes. In *Medical embryology,* Baltimore, 1975, Williams & Wilkins.
17. Ludwin SK, Norman MG: Congenital malformations of the nervous system. In Davis RI, Robertson DM, editors: *Textbook of neuropathology,* Baltimore, 1985, Williams & Wilkins.
18. Johnson MA, Bydder GM: NMR imaging of the brain in children, *Br Med Bull* 40:175-178, 1983.
19. Rorke LB, Riggs HE: *Myelination of the brain in the newborn,* Philadelphia, 1969, JB Lippincott.
20. Yakolev PI, Lecours AR: The myelogenetic cycles of regional maturation in the brain. In Minkowski A, editor: *Regional development of the brain in early life,* Oxford, 1967, Blackwell Scientific.
21. McLeod NA, Williams JP, Machen B, et al: Normal and abnormal morphology of the corpus callosum, *Neurology* 37:1240-1242, 1987.
22. Witelson SF: The brain connection: the corpus callosum is larger in left-handers, *Science* 229:665-668, 1985.
23. Reinarz SJ, Coffman CE, Smoker WRK, et al: MR imaging of the corpus callosum: normal and pathologic findings and correlation with CT, *AJNR* 9:649-656, 1988.
24. Rakic P, Yakovlev PI: Development of the corpus callosum and cavum septi in man, *J Comp Neurol* 132:45-72, 1968.
25. Cowley AR: Influence of fiber tracts on the CT appearance of cerebral edema: anatomic-pathologic correlation, *AJNR* 4:915-925, 1983.
26. Moody DM, Bell MA, Challa VR: The corpus callosum, a unique white-matter tract: anatomic features that may explain sparing in Binswanger disease and resistance to flow of fluid masses, *AJNR* 9:1051-1059, 1988.
27. Nieuwenhuys R, Voogd J, van Huijzen C: *The human central nervous system: a synopsis and atlas,* ed 2, New York, 1981, Springer-Verlag.
28. Barkovich AJ: Apparent atypical callosal dysgenesis: analysis of MR findings in six cases and their relationship to holoprosencephaly, *AJNR* 11:333-339, 1990.
29. Nadich TP, Daniels DL, Pech P, et al: Anterior commissure: anatomic-MR correlation and use as a landmark in three orthogonal planes, *Radiology* 158:421-429, 1986.
30. FitzGerald MJT: *Human embryology: a regional approach,* New York, 1978, Harper & Row.
31. Bossy J: *Atlas of neuroanatomy and special sense organs,* Philadelphia, 1970, WB Saunders.
32. Truex RC, Carpenter MB: *Strong and Elwyn's human neuroanatomy,* ed 5, Baltimore, 1964, Williams & Wilkins.

CHAPTER 6

Michel E. Mawad
L. Anne Hayman
Joel B. Kirkpatrick
Robert B. Lufkin

Atlas of Brainstem and Cranial Nerves

◆

Cranial Nerves—Relationships
Anatomy of Brainstem — Serial Axial Sections

This chapter is designed to provide the reader with the detailed *anatomy* of the brainstem and its associated cranial nerves III to XII. The *function* of these structures can be found in Chapters 7 and 8. Before examining the axial sections that constitute the bulk of this chapter, the reader may find it useful to review the relationships of the cranial nerves. The points at which these nerves enter or exit the skull base are illustrated in Figure 6-1. The relationship between these nerves and the complex surface anatomy of the brainstem is best summarized on a sagittal whole-brain schematic (Figure 6-2). Unfortunately, magnetic resonance imaging (MRI) in the sagittal plane is less satisfactory because only the largest cranial nerves, III and V, are usually visible (Figure 6-3).

The remainder of this chapter is devoted to labeling brainstem structures in serial axial sections. The axial scan plane is best suited to examining cranial nerves III to XII and internal brainstem anatomy because it reveals site-specific shapes that can be used to localize small structures accurately. The internal anatomy of the brainstem in sagittal and coronal planes has been carefully illustrated and labeled in Chapter 3.

To assist the reader, the axial anatomy in this chapter is not presented in traditional anatomic format (viewed from **above** with the subject's nose toward the **bottom** of the page). The anatomy is shown instead in an *imaging* format (viewed from **below** with the patient's nose toward the **top** of the page). In addition, the brain is sectioned along the conventional *imaging* plane rather than the standard anatomic plane, which is perpendicular to the long axis of the brainstem.

To assist the reader further, the brainstem has been divided into nine site-specific axial levels, each having an easily recognized, distinctive external contour. These levels are indicated on labeled dorsal and ventral schematic illustrations of the brainstem (Figure 6-4). Each level is then described separately in Figures 6-5 to 6-13. The surface anatomy and surrounding imaging landmarks are shown on schematic drawings taken directly from in vivo axial images. Many of these drawings are accompanied by anatomic sections. Supplemental companion MR images also are included at many levels to provide further clarification of the most difficult regions. These T2-weighted images (T2, transverse relaxation time) were obtained from a thawed cadaver head using the technical factors described in Chapter 3. An index is provided so that the reader can more easily locate unfamiliar structures on the images provided in this chapter and locate unfamiliar terms in other chapters. Several anatomic references were consulted in the preparation of these figures.[1-8]

REFERENCES

1. Mawad ME, Silver AJ, Hilal SK, et al: Computed tomography of the brain stem with intrathecal metrizamide. Part I. The normal brain stem, *AJNR* 4:1-11, 1983.
2. DeArmond SJ, Fusco MM, Dewey MM: *Structure of the human brain: a photographic atlas,* ed 3, Oxford, 1989, Oxford University.
3. Riley HA: *An atlas of the basal ganglia, brainstem and spinal cord,* Baltimore, 1943, Williams & Wilkins.
4. Solsberg MD, Fournier D, Potts DG: MR imaging of the excised human brainstem: a correlative neuroanatomic study, *AJNR* 11:1003-1013, 1990.
5. Hirsch WL, Kemp SS, Martinez AJ, et al: Anatomy of the brainstem: correlation of *in vitro* MR images with histologic sections, *AJNR* 10:923-928, 1989.
6. Ho PSP, Shiwei Y, Czervionke LF, et al: MR appearance of grey and white matter at the cervicomedullary region, *AJNR* 10:1051-1055, 1989.
7. Flannigan B, Bradley W, Mazziotta J, et al: Magnetic resonance imaging of the brainstem: normal structure and basic functional anatomy, *Radiology* 154:375-383, 1985.
8. Wilson-Paules L, Akesson EJ, Stewart PA: *Cranial nerves: anatomy and clinical comments,* Toronto, 1988, BC Decker.

CRANIAL NERVES—RELATIONSHIPS

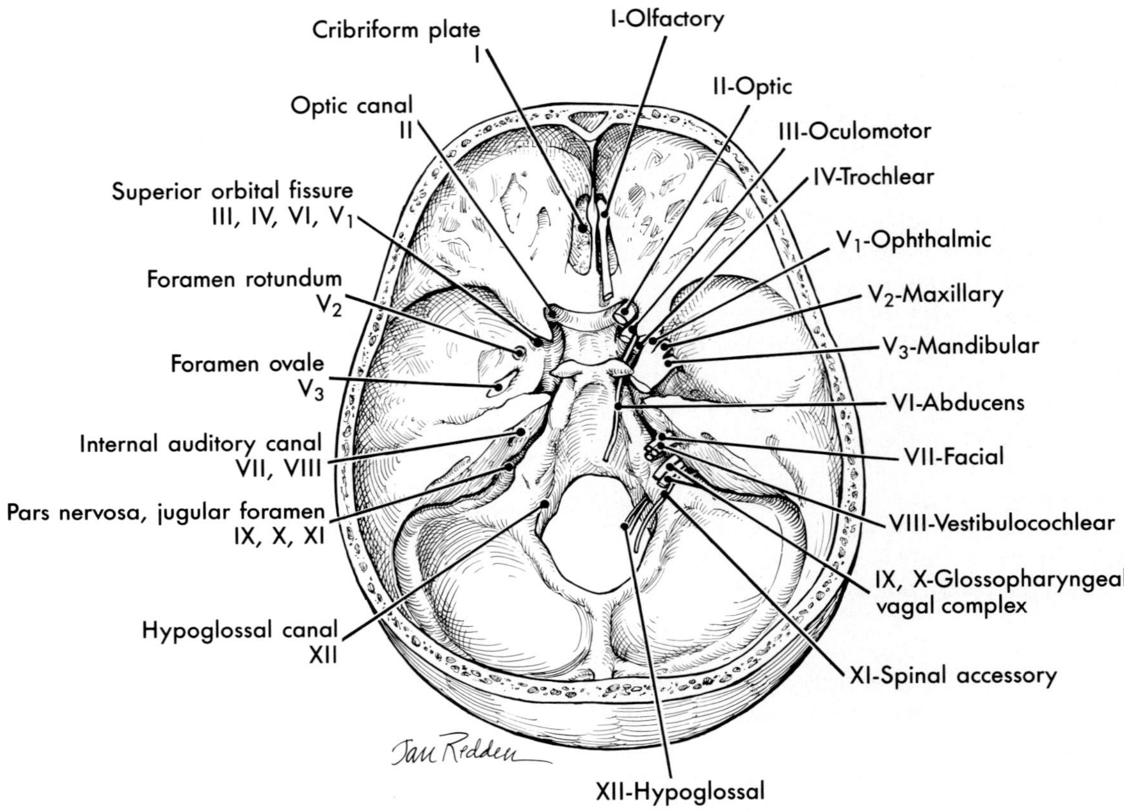

Figure 6-1 Schematic illustration of the skull base from above showing the cranial nerves and the foramina through which they leave the skull.

CRANIAL NERVES—RELATIONSHIPS

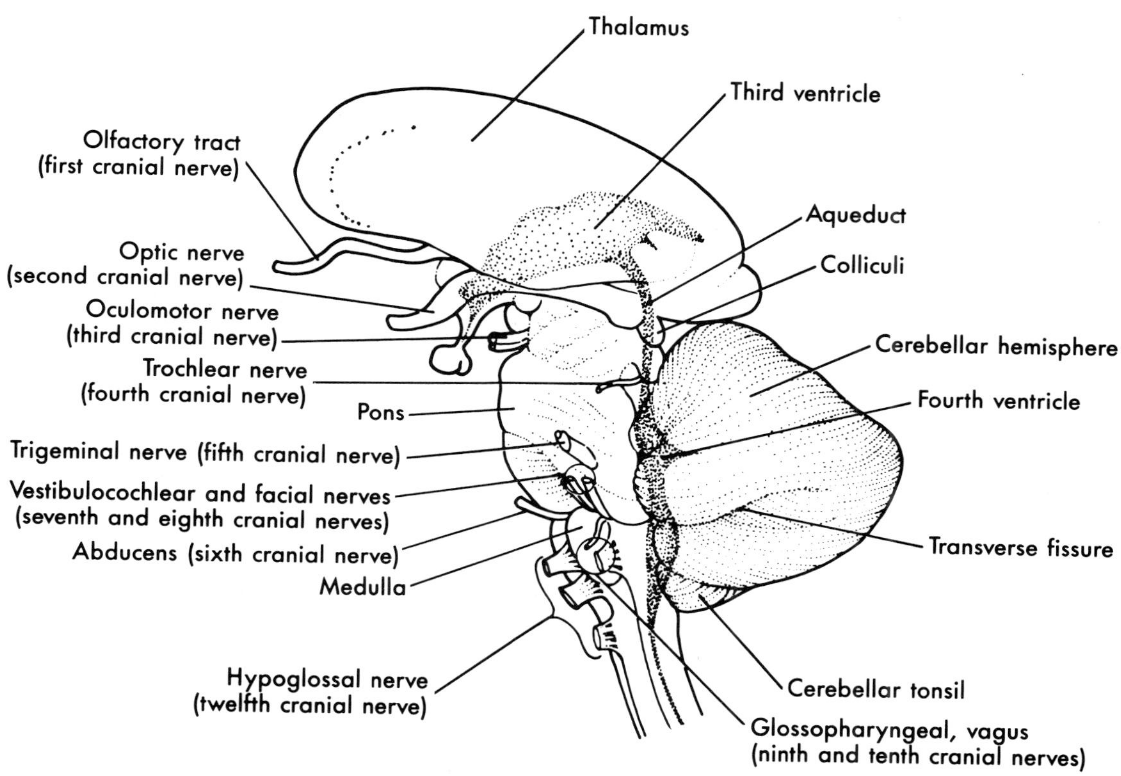

Figure 6-2 Sagittal schematic illustration of the brainstem showing the origin of the cranial nerves. The spinal accessory nerve (eleventh cranial nerve) is not included in this diagram. (Reproduced with permission from Chakeres DW, DW, Kapild A: *Radiology* 149(3): 709-715, 1983.)

CRANIAL NERVES—RELATIONSHIPS

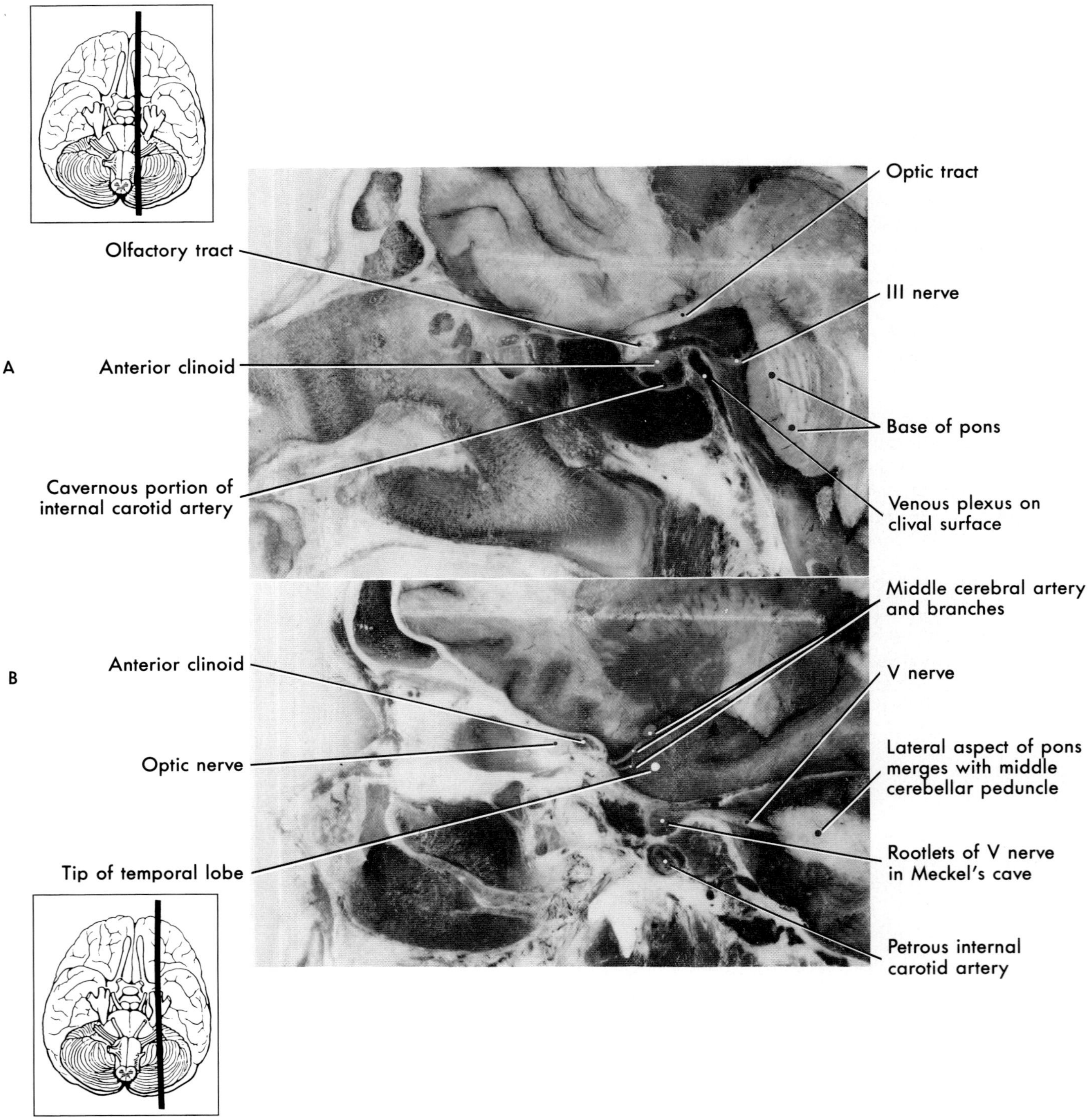

Figure 6-3 **A** and **B**, Labeled parasagittal sections of the sellar region in an anatomic specimen.

ANATOMY OF BRAINSTEM—SERIAL AXIAL SECTIONS

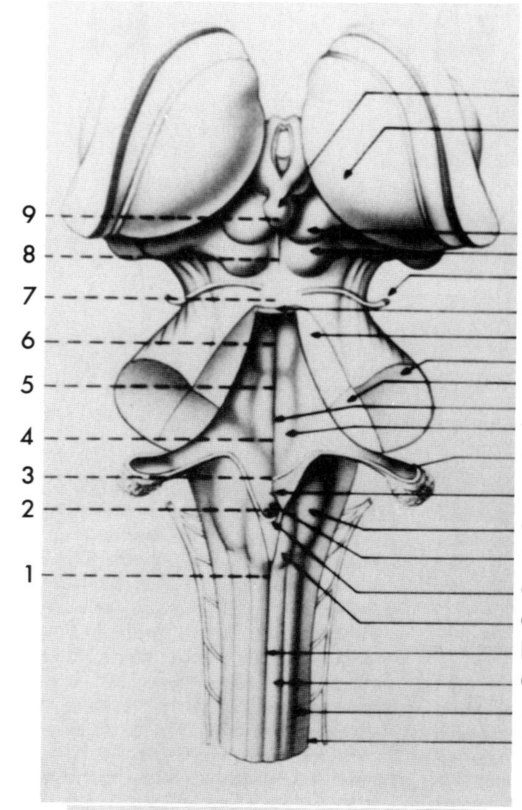

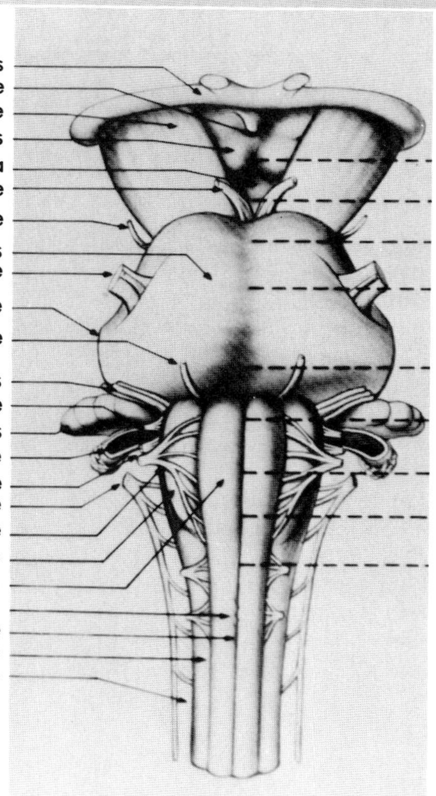

Figure 6-4 Labeled dorsal **(A)** and ventral **(B)** schematics of the brainstem showing the plane of section for the nine axial brainstem sections in Figures 6-5 to 6-13.

ANATOMY OF BRAINSTEM—SERIAL AXIAL SECTIONS

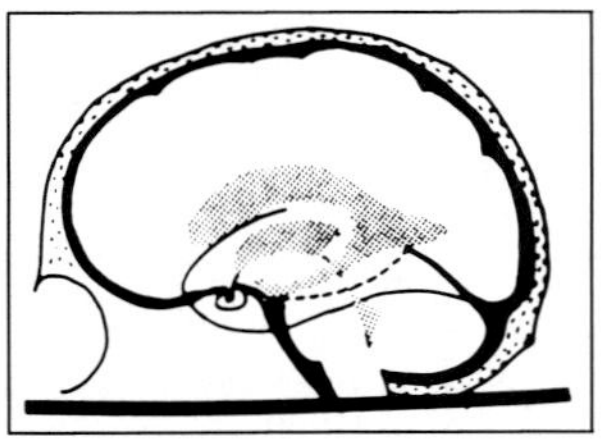

A

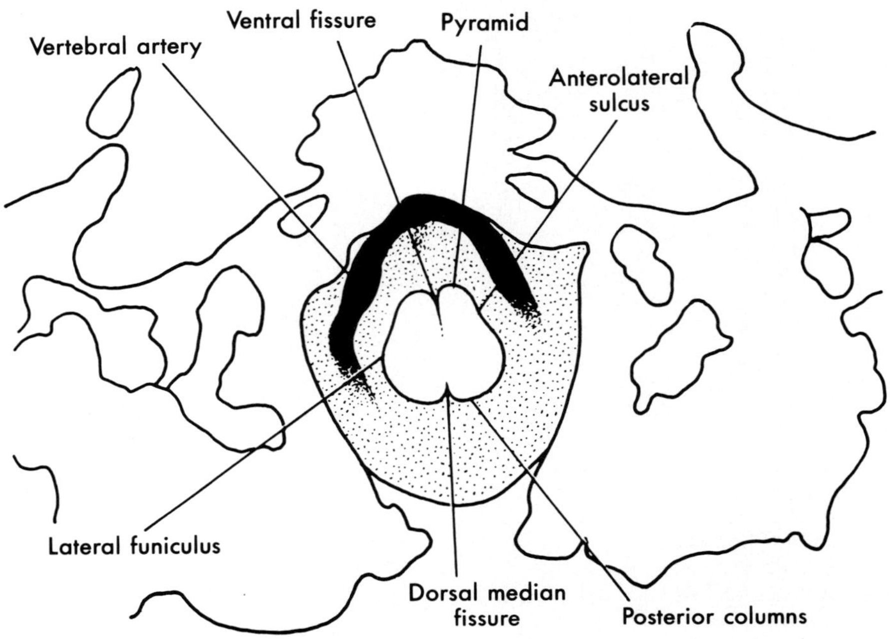

Figure 6-5 ***Level 1: closed medulla at foramen magnum***

This region extends from just above the first roots of the cervical spinal cord, which are usually slightly below the foramen magnum, to the obex of the fourth ventricle. **A,** In the schematic cross section, the upper portion of the closed medulla has a pear-shaped appearance, with a narrow ventral surface featuring a short, often oblique, ventral fissure and a broader, dorsal surface with a less pronounced dorsal median fissure. Axial rotation of the medulla at this level is a normal variant. The vertebral arteries usually lie close to the anterolateral sulcus, which is a very shallow groove posterior and lateral to the pyramidal eminence.

Anteriorly, on either side of the ventral fissure are two eminences, the *voluntary motor tracts,* which form the *pyramids* of the medulla. These pyramids become progressively smaller as most of the fibers cross the midline to the lateral column of the spinal cord. Thus the diminishing size of the pyramids indicates a progressively lower level in the medulla. This region is referred to as the *pyramidal decussation.* Lesions of motor fibers *above the decussation* cause loss of motor function on the opposite side of the body. Lesions in the motor tracts *below the decussation* cause motor loss on the same side of the body.

ANATOMY OF BRAINSTEM—SERIAL AXIAL SECTIONS

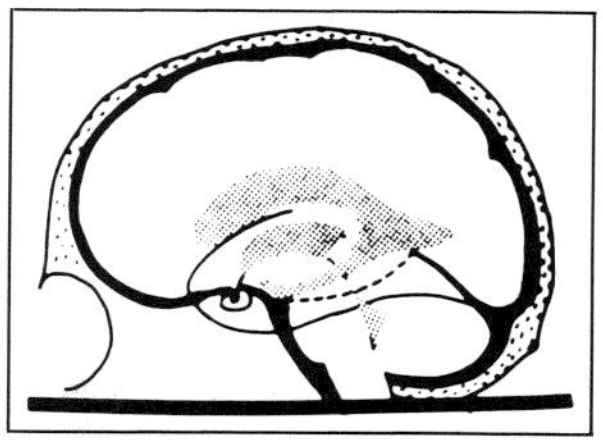

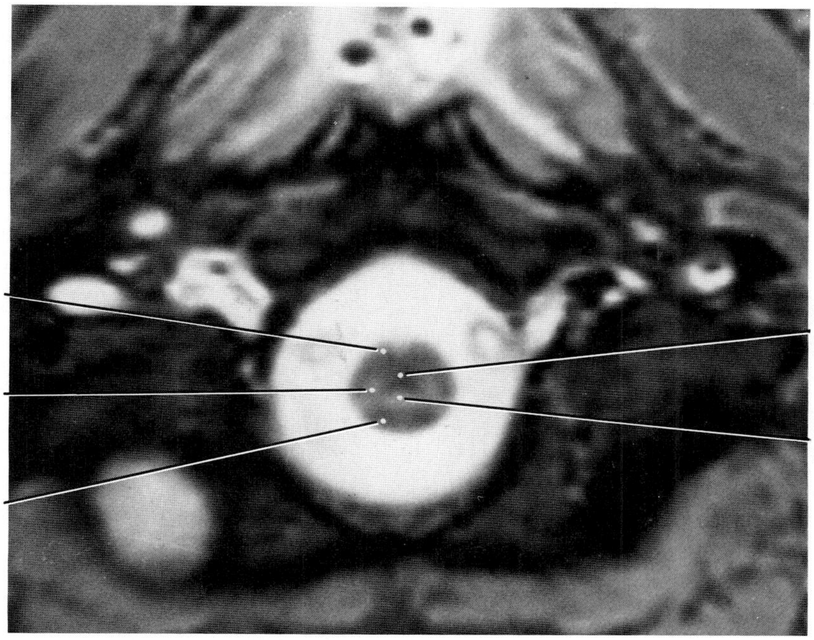

B

Figure 6-5, cont'd. ***Level 1: closed medulla at foramen magnum***

B, The labeled MR image (TR/TE, 2000/80 msec) of a cadaver shows some of the nuclei and fiber tracts of the closed medulla at the motor (pyramidal) decussation. Note that the pyramids are smaller than those shown in schematic **A** because the MR image is at a slightly lower medullary level.

The small rootlets of cranial nerve XI are rarely visualized at Level 1 as they exit the lateral aspect of the medulla.

ANATOMY OF BRAINSTEM—SERIAL AXIAL SECTIONS

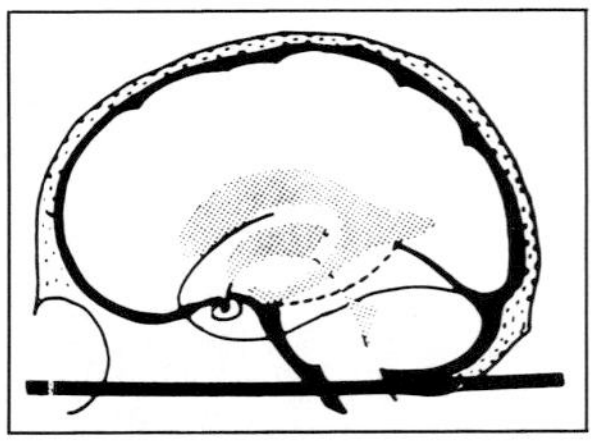

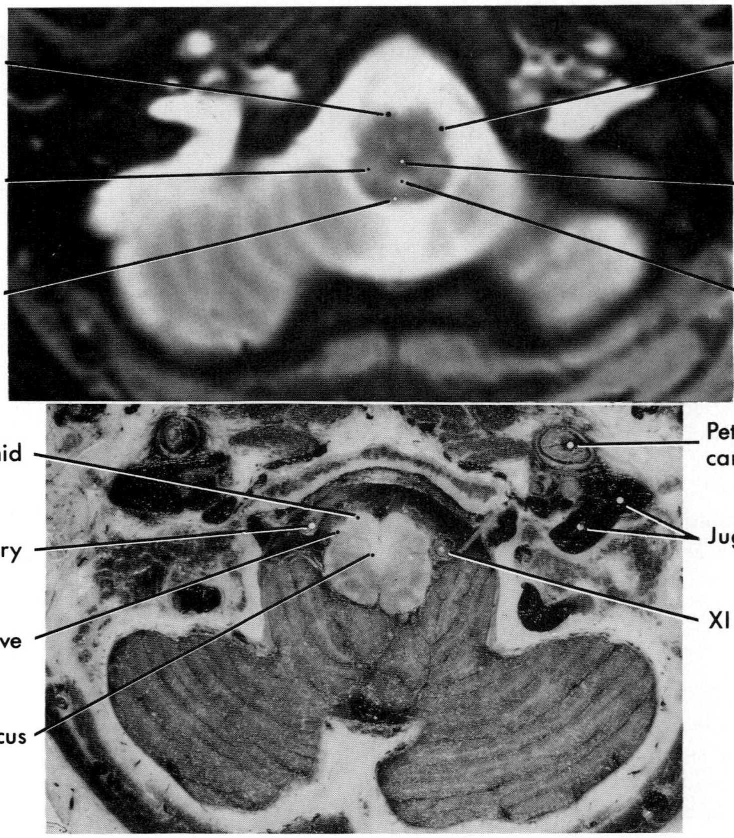

Figure 6-6 ***Level 2: transitional medulla***

This extremely short segment of the medulla can be distinguished from Level 1 (Figure 6-5) because it contains the lowest portion of the *olive*, which is located lateral to the pyramid. Two distinct segments make up this level. The *lower segment* begins at the obex of the fourth ventricle. **A,** The MR image (TR/TE, 4000/80) of a cadaver shows this segment. The sensory fibers from the cuneate and gracile nuclei and tracts are smaller than they are in Level 1, since these fibers are moving medially to cross and then form the midline medial lemniscus. **B,** The anatomic section at this level shows one of the many rootlets of cranial nerve XI as it exits the lateral medulla to enter the pars nervosa of the jugular bulb. The very small rootlets of cranial nerve XII that exit between the olive and pyramid at this level are not seen.

ANATOMY OF BRAINSTEM—SERIAL AXIAL SECTIONS

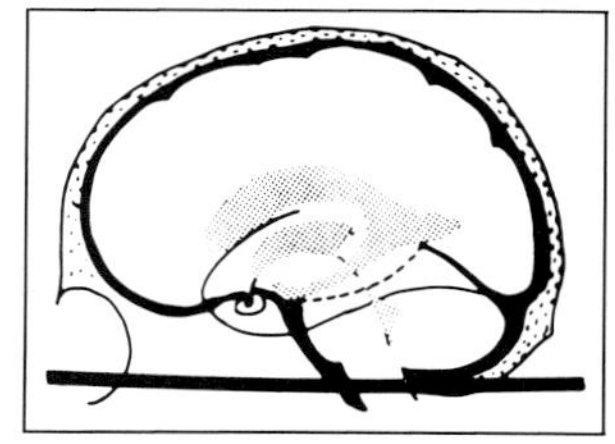

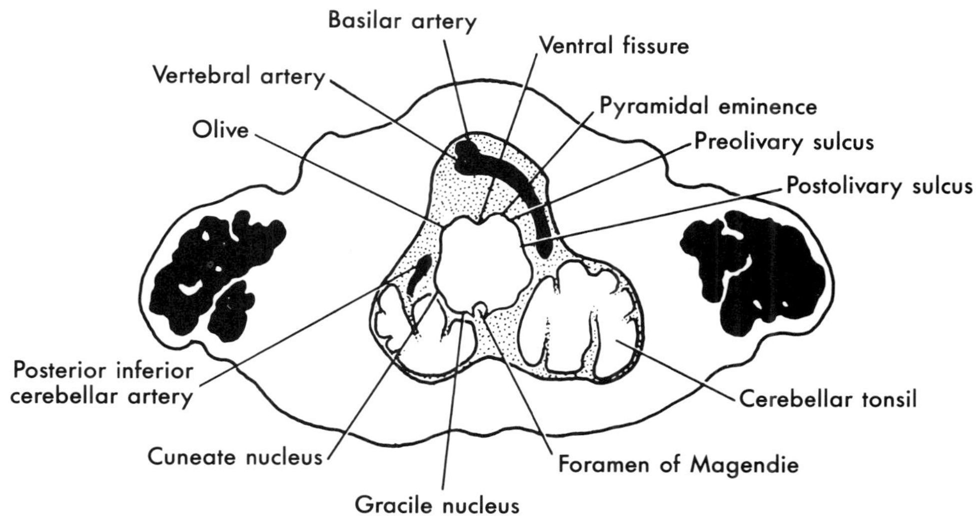

C

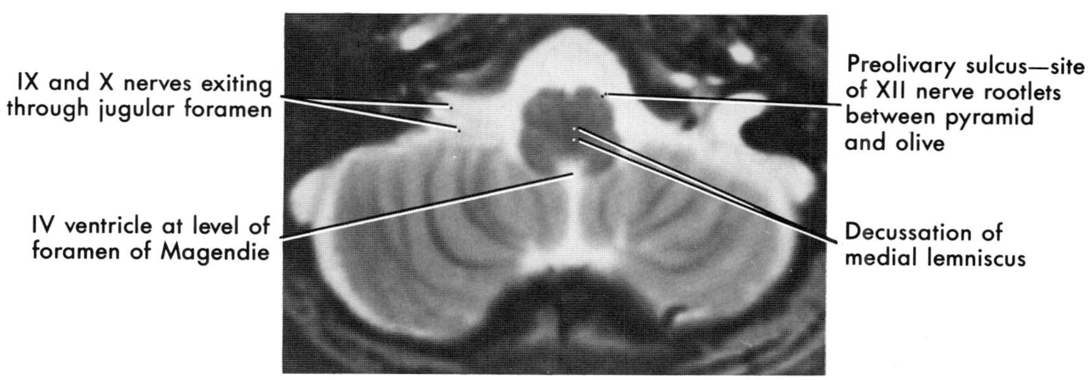

D

Figure 6-6, cont'd. ***Level 2: transitional medulla***

The second segment is the *uppermost transitional medulla* at the foramen of Magendie (i.e., the caudal midline opening of the fourth ventricle). This segment is shown in the schematic diagram **(C)** and the MR image (4000/80) of a cadaver **(D)**. Note that the gracile and cuneate nuclei and tracts make only a small contribution to the dorsal boundary of the medulla, since most of the fibers are in the medial lemniscus.

ANATOMY OF BRAINSTEM—SERIAL AXIAL SECTIONS

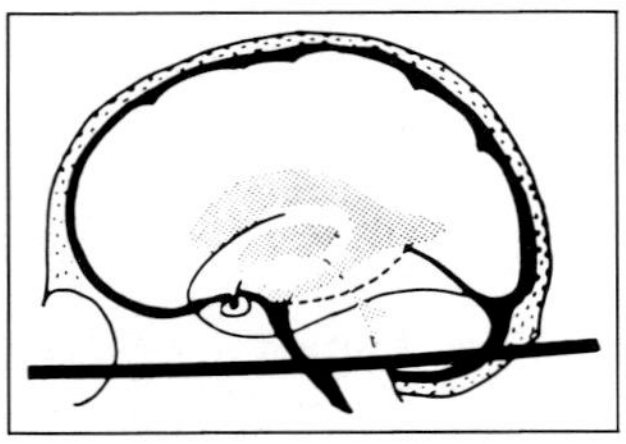

A

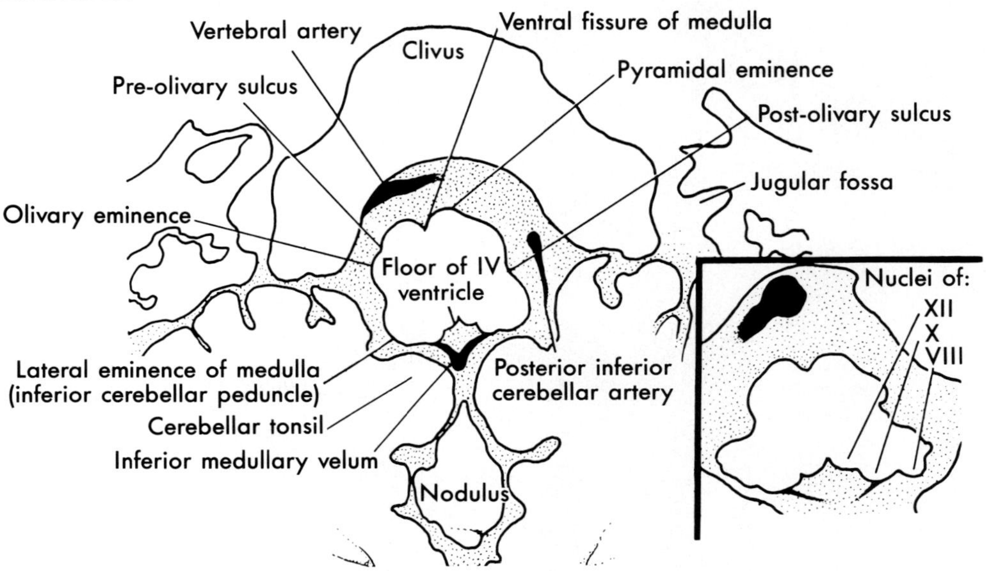

Figure 6-7 ***Level 3: open (upper) medulla***

Above the foramen of Magendie, the medulla (now open posteriorly) has a characteristic shape on cross section because of the appearance of the *inferior cerebellar peduncle* (*restiform body*). This peduncle is separated from the olive by the shallow postolivary sulcus. **A,** The axial schematic shows the preolivary sulcus separating the olive from the pyramid. Asymmetric flattening of the medullary pyramid and olivary protuberance is often observed as a result of impression by an adjacent, tortuous, vertebral or basilar artery. Mild asymmetry is seen often and may even be the rule. The lateral and posterior medullary segments of the posteroinferior cerebellar artery may be seen lateral and posterior to the medulla within the medullary cistern at this level.

At Level 3 the dorsal aspect of the medulla is the "floor" of the fourth ventricle. Here one can sometimes recognize the eminences of the *nuclei* of cranial nerves XII (hypoglossal), X (vagus), and VIII (vestibulocochlear). These nuclei are located on either side of the midline median sulcus.

ANATOMY OF BRAINSTEM—SERIAL AXIAL SECTIONS

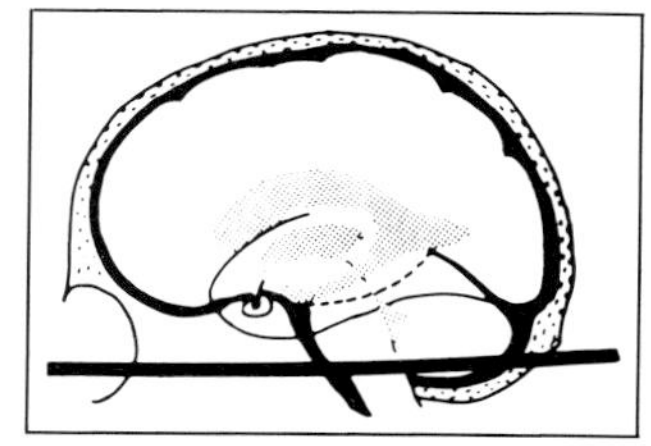

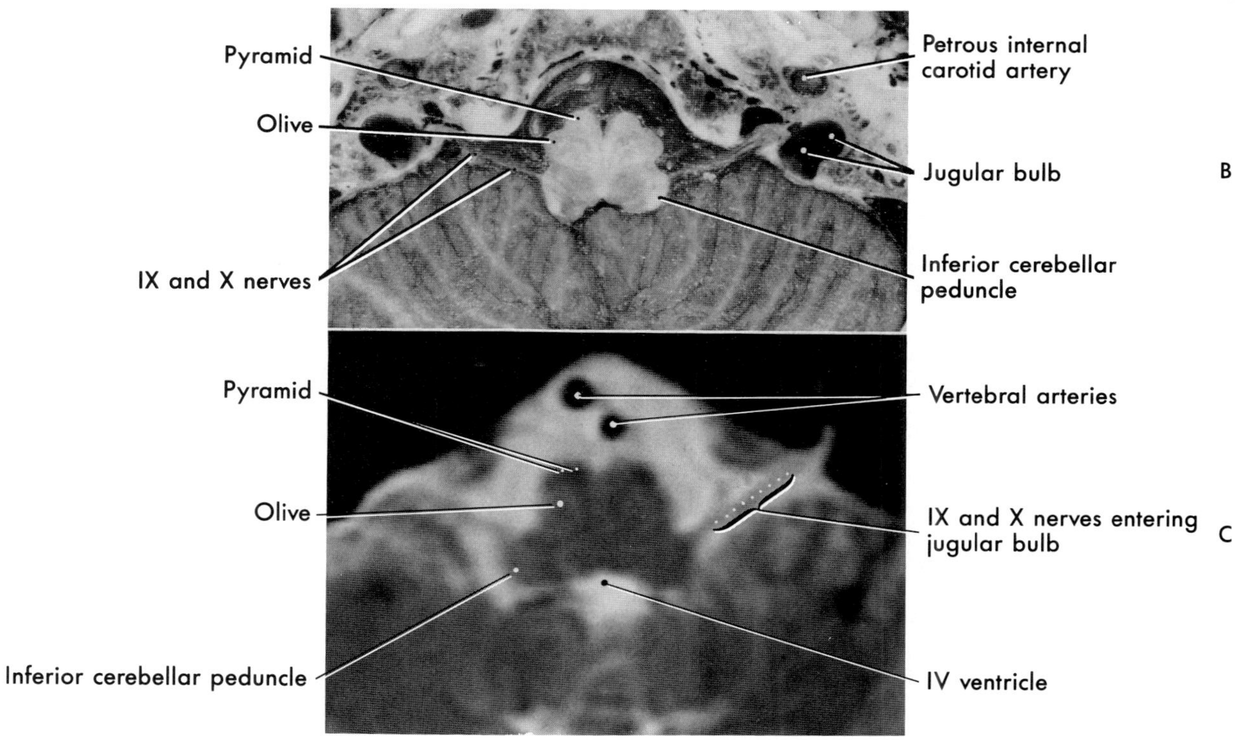

Figure 6-7, cont'd. ***Level 3: open (upper) medulla***

The anatomic section **(B)** and the MR image (TR/TE, 4000/80) of a cadaver **(C)** show cranial nerves IX and X, which exit the lateral medulla and travel to the pars nervosa of the jugular bulb.

ANATOMY OF BRAINSTEM—SERIAL AXIAL SECTIONS

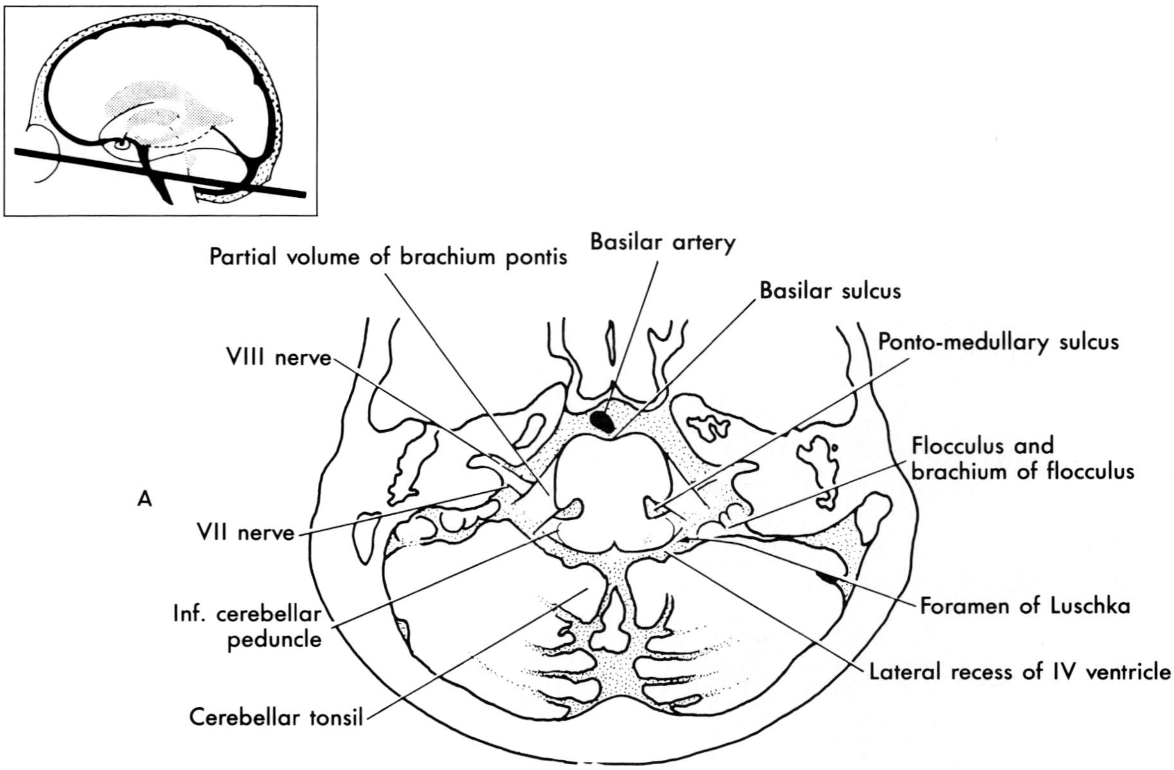

Figure 6-8 ***Level 4: medullary pontine junction***

The cross section of the brainstem at this level has a characteristic "mushroomlike" appearance on radiographic images because the angle of the scan often includes a portion of the inferior pons and the *middle cerebellar peduncle* (*brachium pontis*). **A,** The axial schematic shows the *pontine midline groove* (*basilar sulcus*), which often contains the basilar artery. This groove is not as deep as the ventral fissure of the medulla. The *inferior cerebellar peduncles* (*restiform bodies*), which were first identified in Level 3 (Figure 6-7), can be seen as they move posteriorly to connect the medulla to the cerebellum. These peduncles appear as a posteriorly diverging, biped structure in continuity with the floor of the fourth ventricle.

At Level 4 the lateral recess of the fourth ventricle extends anterolaterally and opens into the cerebellopontine angle cistern through the foramen of Luschka, which is posterior and lateral to the inferior cerebellar peduncle.

Although three cranial nerves (VI, VII, VIII) exit the brainstem at the medullopontine junction, they are not seen at Level 4. They are seen on the pontine levels as they travel superiorly.

ANATOMY OF BRAINSTEM—SERIAL AXIAL SECTIONS

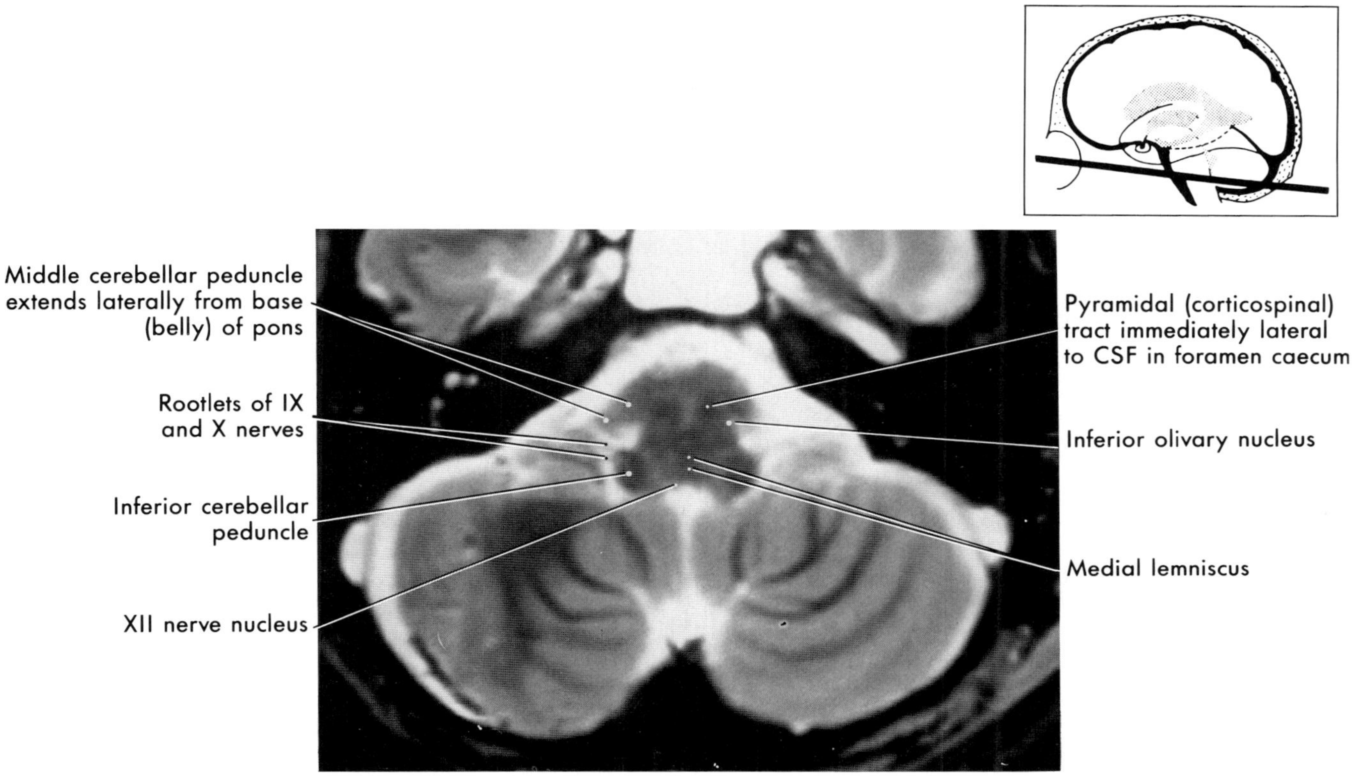

B

Figure 6-8, cont'd. ***Level 4: medullary pontine junction***
B, The labeled MR image (TR/TE, 4000/80) of a cadaver shows the rootlets of cranial nerves IX and X and the nuclei and fiber tracts of the medullopontine junction.

ANATOMY OF BRAINSTEM—SERIAL AXIAL SECTIONS

A

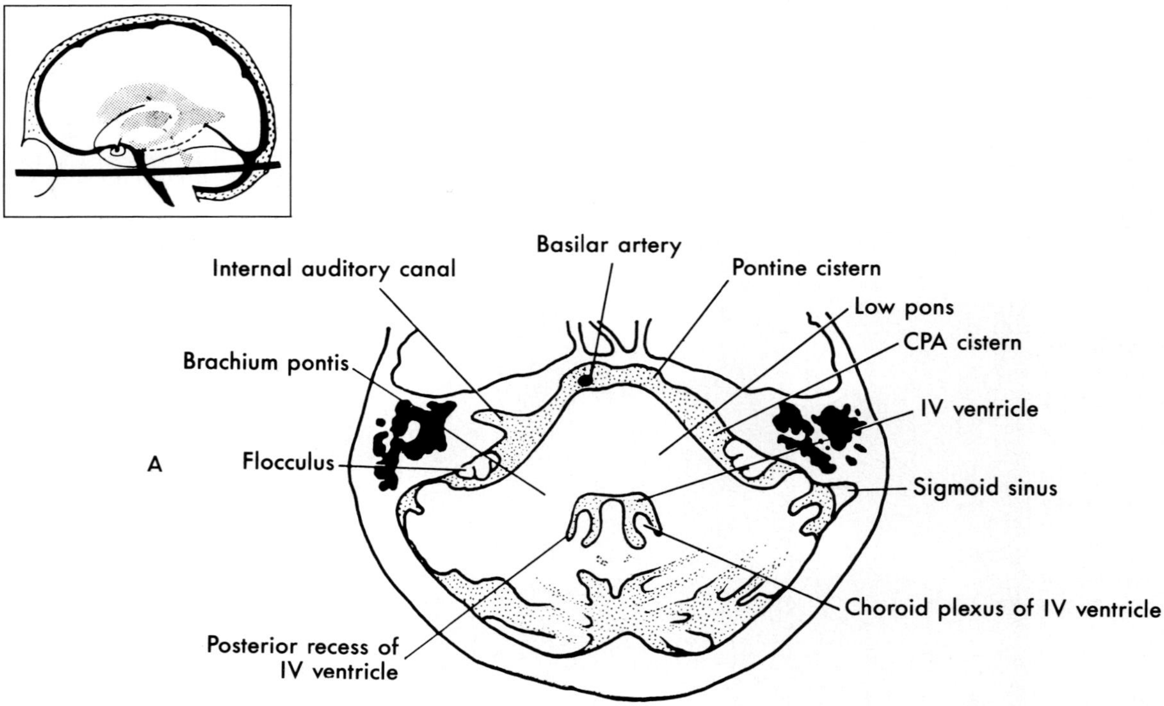

Figure 6-9 ***Level 5: lower pons***
The lower pons extends from the medullopontine junction upward to a level *below* the origin of cranial nerve V. This part of the pons, largely formed by the pyramidal tracts and the pontine nuclei, is connected to the cerebellum by the *middle cerebellar peduncle* (*brachium pontis*), which was partially seen in Level 4 (Figure 6-8). **A,** The schematic diagram of the pons shows a shallow, anterior midline groove. The basilar artery, which is anterior to the pons in the pontine cistern, may be tortuous and often lies off the midline.

At Level 5 the posterior recesses of the fourth ventricle and the choroid plexus of the fourth ventricle can be demonstrated. The space between the brachium pontis and the petrous bone constitutes the *cerebellopontine angle cistern*, which extends posteriorly and laterally from the pontine cistern. This angle cistern is limited posterolaterally by the *flocculus*, which projects into the cistern.

ANATOMY OF BRAINSTEM—SERIAL AXIAL SECTIONS

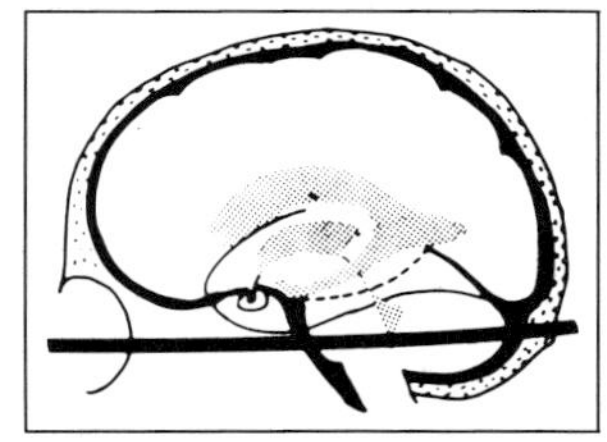

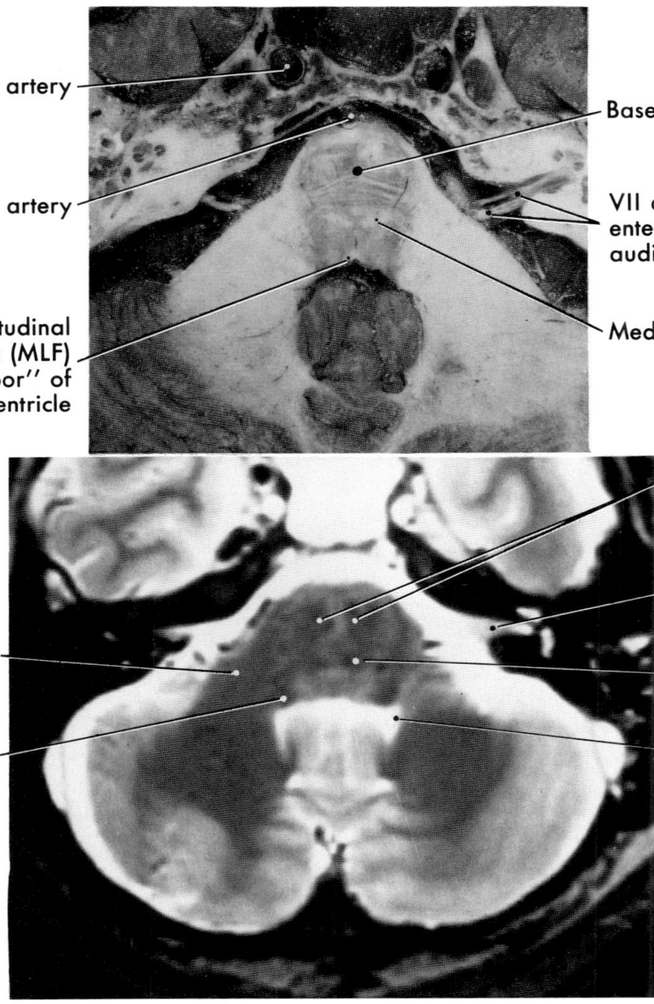

Figure 6-9 cont'd. ***Level 5: lower pons***
B, The axial brain section shows cranial nerves VII and VIII in the angle cistern. Very small cranial nerve IV is not seen as it travels superiorly. **C**, The MR image (TR/TE, 2000/80) of a cadaver shows the nuclei and fiber tracts of the lower pons.

ANATOMY OF BRAINSTEM—SERIAL AXIAL SECTIONS

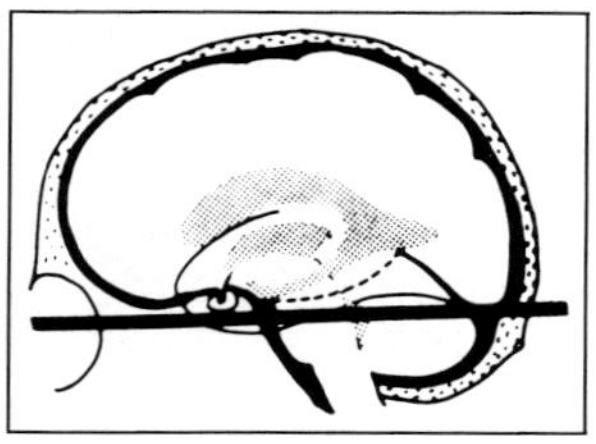

A

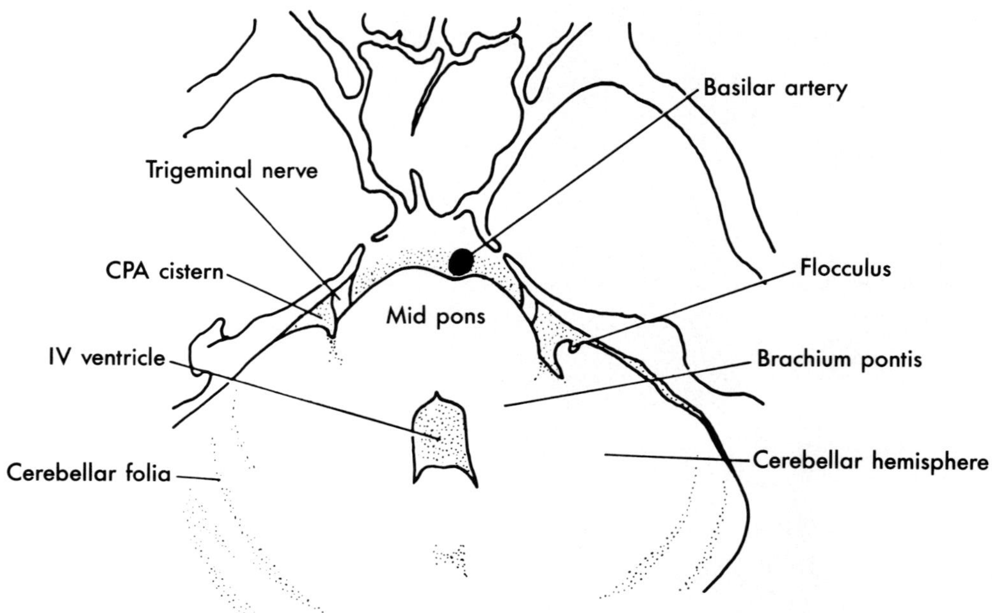

Figure 6-10 ***Level 6: midpons***

The middle third of the pons is distinguished primarily by the easily recognizable origin of the *trigeminal nerves,* which travel in an anterosuperior direction from the lateral aspect of the pons to Meckel's cave. **A,** The axial schematic shows the pontine and cerebellopontine angle cisterns surrounding the midpons. They contain a large number of vascular structures, such as the basilar artery and its branches, which can be identified because they are usually tortuous and wavy compared with the rectilinear course of cranial nerve V.

At Level 6 the fourth ventricle is a fairly symmetric structure in the midline of the posterior fossa, but some asymmetry in the sizes of its two halves can often be seen. The dorsal aspect of the fourth ventricle is usually indented by the nodulus of the vermis and the fastigial nucleus. The floor of the fourth ventricle may show the *median sulcus* with the *medial eminences* on either side. Both features are important aspects of the anatomy of the floor of the fourth ventricle. The obliteration of these features is often the earliest indication of a swelling or mass in the pons.

ANATOMY OF BRAINSTEM—SERIAL AXIAL SECTIONS

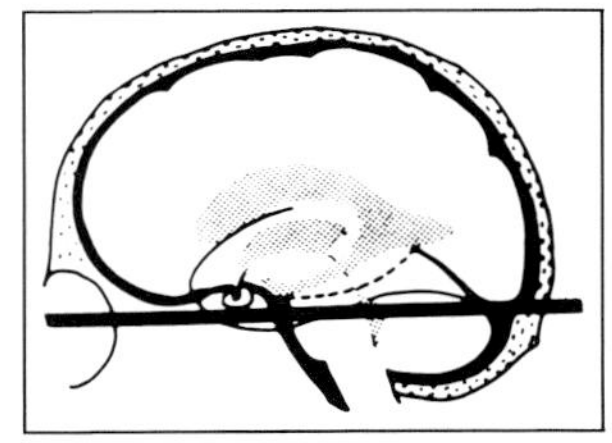

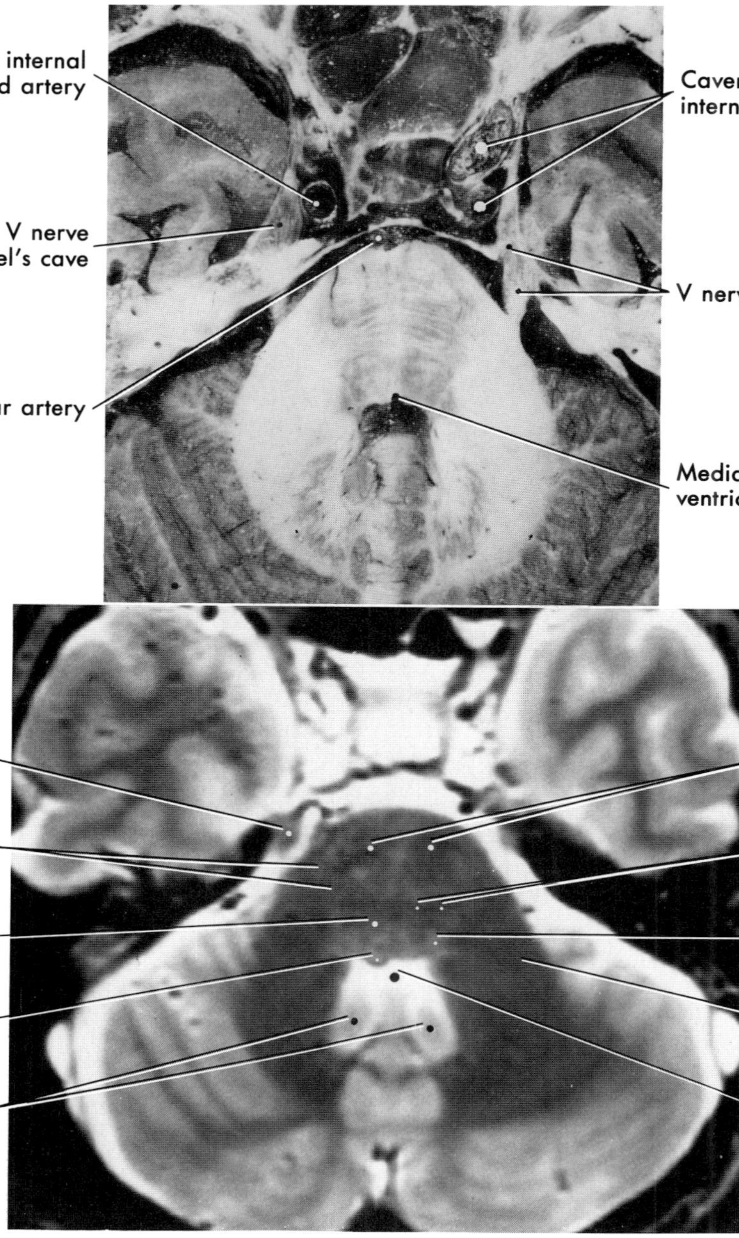

Figure 6-10, cont'd. ***Level 6: midpons***

B, The axial brain slice shows cranial nerve V. **C,** The MR image (TR/TE, 2000/80) of a cadaver shows the nuclei and fiber tracts of the midpons.

ANATOMY OF BRAINSTEM—SERIAL AXIAL SECTIONS

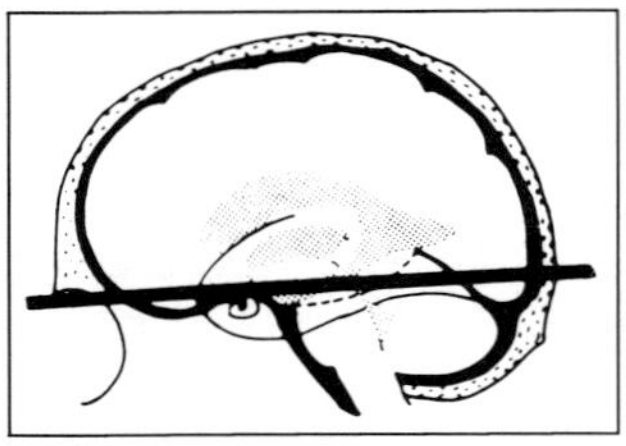

A

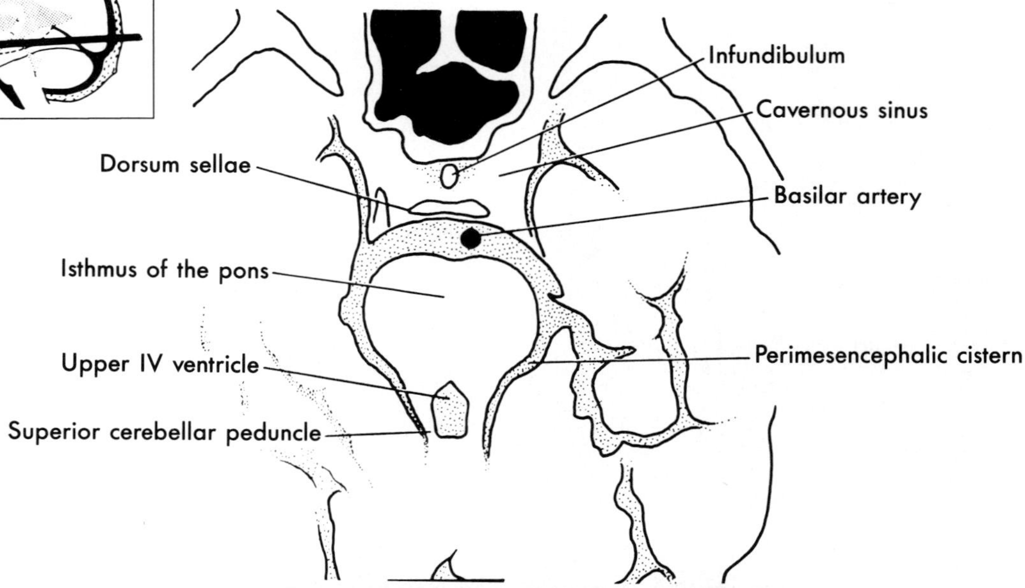

B

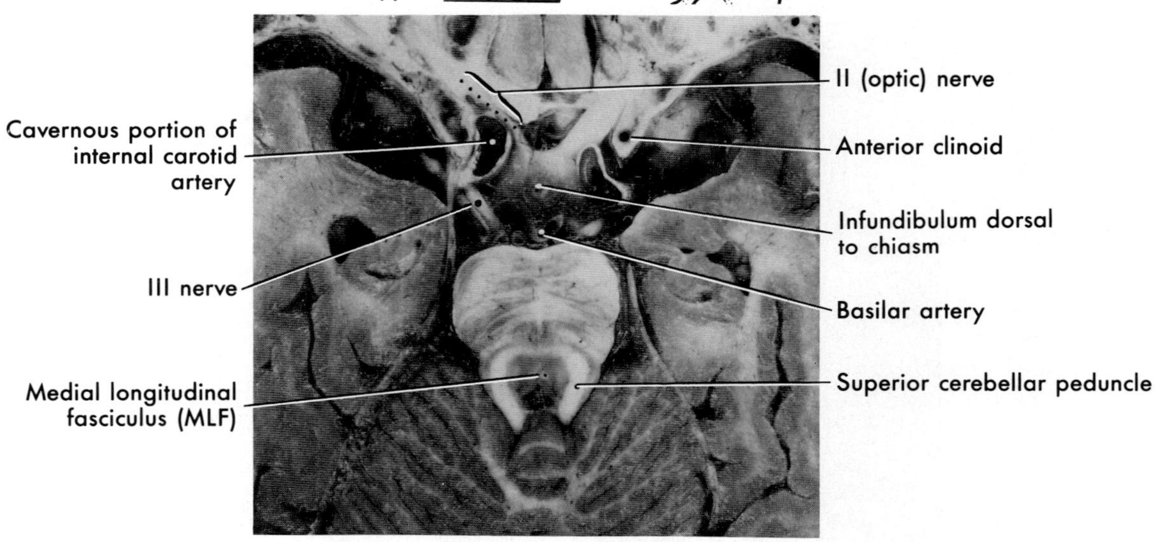

Figure 6-11 ***Level 7: isthmus of pons***

The isthmus of the pons is the transition between the pons and the midbrain. It is only a few millimeters thick and almost entirely surrounded by cerebrospinal fluid. **A,** The axial schematic shows that the continuity of the *perimesencephalic cistern* at this level is interrupted by the *superior cerebellar peduncles* (*brachium conjunctivum*) and the upper end of the fourth ventricle. Ventrally, the isthmus has the same shallow basilar groove seen in the lowest two levels of the pons. This section typically passes above the origin of the rootlets of cranial nerve V, which have already entered Meckel's cave. The upper end of the fourth ventricle is bounded on both sides by the superior cerebellar peduncles and posteriorly by the superior medullary velum. The "roof" of the fourth ventricle is usually flat at this level, but its "floor" is indented by the *median sulcus.* Obliteration of this median sulcus is an early sign of a mass in the brainstem.

The petrous bone is usually not visualized in this section, and only the central portion of the cerebellum is represented at Level 7. Anterior to the pons, the upper end of the basilar artery is usually recognizable, and some of its branches (e.g., the superior cerebellar artery) may be seen. The dorsum sellae is anterior to the basilar artery.

B, The axial brain section shows distal cranial nerve III as it travels inferiorly to the lateral wall of the cavernous sinus.

ANATOMY OF BRAINSTEM—SERIAL AXIAL SECTIONS

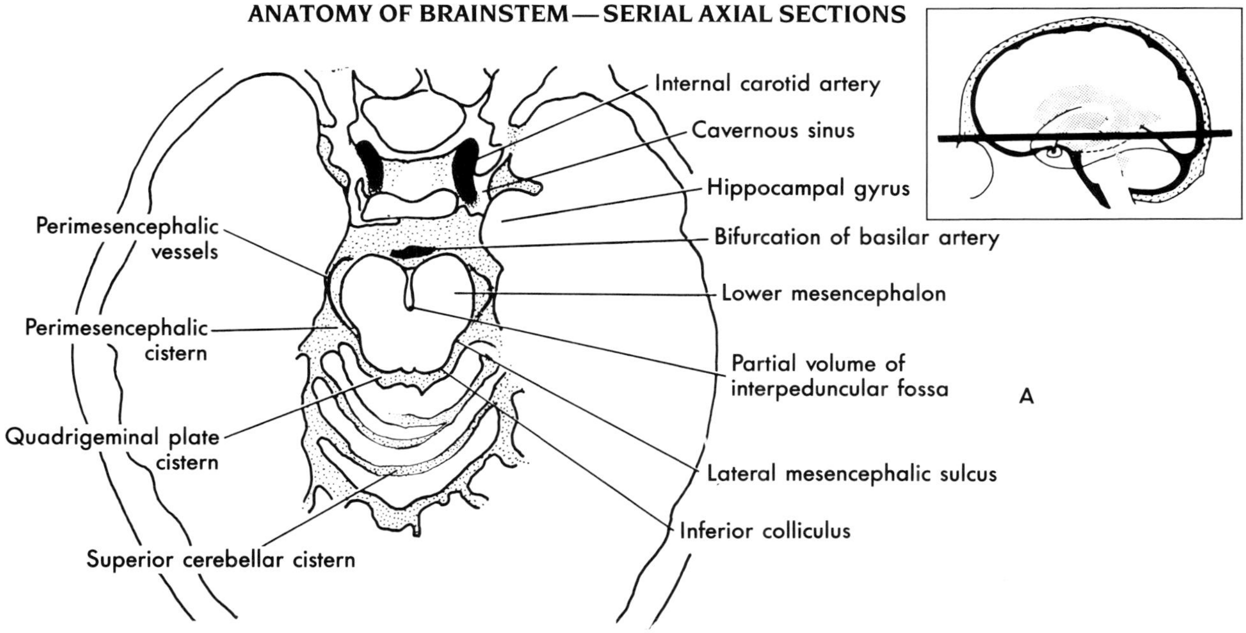

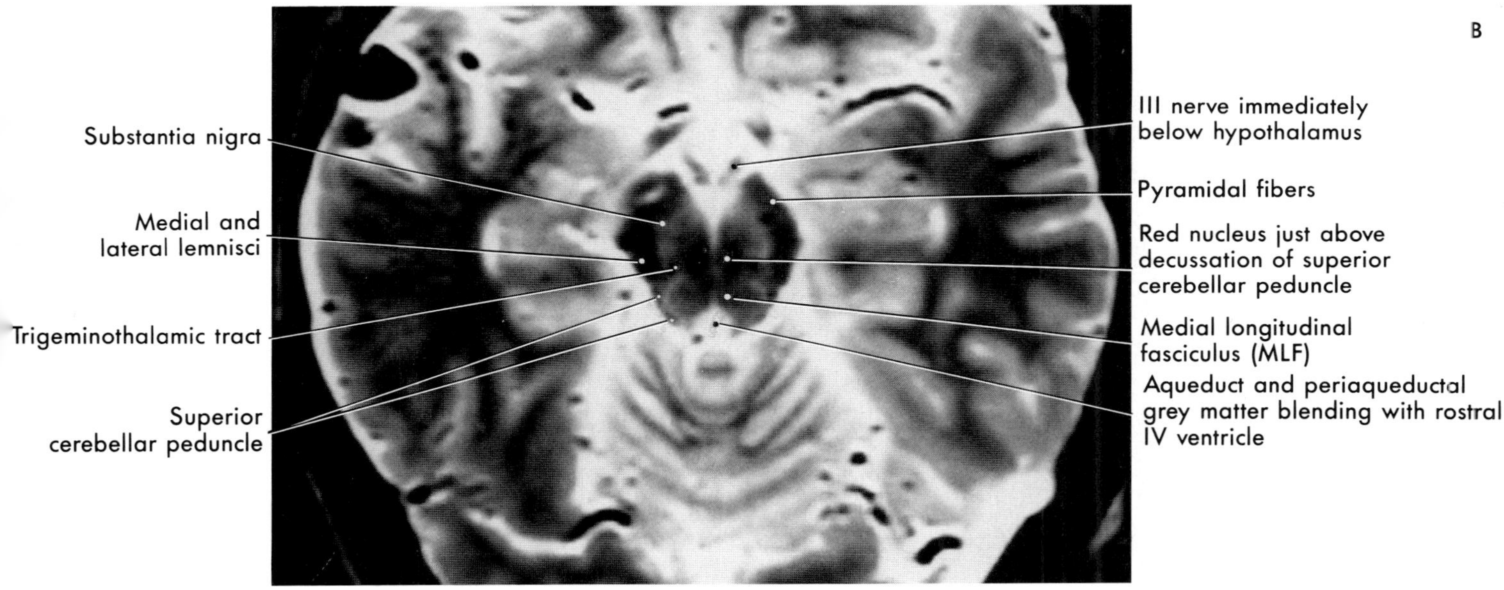

Figure 6-12 ***Level 8: lower midbrain, inferior colliculus***

At this level, the brainstem has the characteristic heart shape of the midbrain created by the shallow *lateral mesencephalic sulcus*. **A,** The axial schematic shows that the lower midbrain is formed posteriorly by the inferior colliculus and anteriorly by the cerebral peduncles.

Occasionally, a partial-volume display of the lowest part of the *interpeduncular fossa* may be seen at this level. Very small cranial nerve IV arises from the posterior aspect of the midbrain at this level (not shown). The *pontine* and *perimesencephalic cisterns* contain the basilar artery ventrally and branches of the superior cerebellar artery and veins on both sides of the midbrain. These vessels are readily recognized by their characteristic wavy appearance. Posterior to the collicular plate is the *quadrigeminal plate cistern*, which is bounded posteriorly by the central lobule of the *vermis*. The *cerebellar folia* can be identified in the central region of this section. The change from parallel cerebellar folia to the cerebral sulci on the inferior surfaces of the temporal lobes marks the boundary of the *tentorial incisura*.

B, The MR image (TR/TE, 2000/80) of a cadaver shows the distal oculomotor nerves (cranial nerve III), which have originated from the upper midbrain, Level 9 (Figure 6-13).

ANATOMY OF BRAINSTEM—SERIAL AXIAL SECTIONS

A

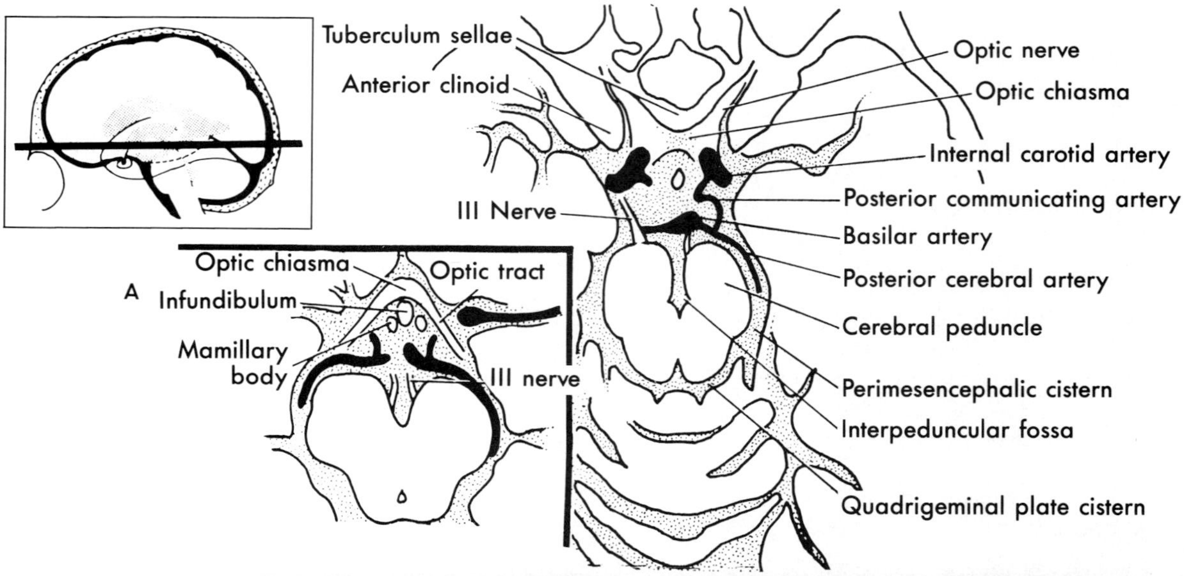

B

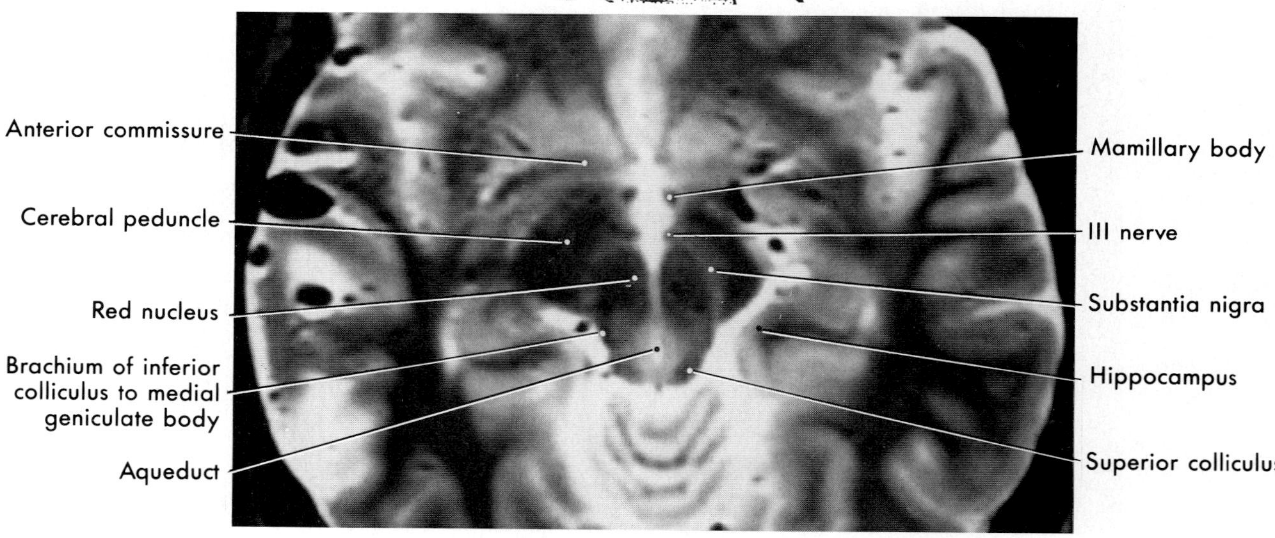

Figure 6-13 ***Level 9: upper midbrain, superior colliculus***

The brainstem has a characteristic heart shape at this midbrain level, which is created by the waistlike indentation of the shallow *lateral mesencephalic sulcus* located immediately behind the cerebral peduncle. The origin of cranial nerve III from the medial aspect of the cerebral peduncle distinguishes this level from Level 8 (Figure 6-12). **A,** The axial schematic shows the pathway of cranial nerve III as it passes between the posterior cerebral artery (above) and the superior cerebellar artery (below), crossing the interpeduncular fossa parallel and lateral to the posterior communicating artery.

At Level 9, the *suprasellar cistern* may show the two mamillary bodies and the base of the pituitary infundibulum. Anterior to the stalk, the optic chiasm and tract are usually seen. In the *perimesencephalic cistern,* branches of the posterior cerebral artery and the basal vein of Rosenthal may be detected. The upper end of the *vermis* and the *cerebellar folia* can still be demonstrated at this level, posterior to the *quadrigeminal plate cistern,* in a small triangular cistern.

B, The MR image (TR/TE, 2000/80) of a cadaver shows the nuclei and fiber tracts of the lower midbrain and the origin of cranial nerve III.

INDEX TO THE ILLUSTRATIONS

Entries refer to figures in which the specific structures are labeled.

CHAPTER 7

Stephen Alan Berman
John Gundzik
L. Anne Hayman

Brainstem

IMAGING TECHNIQUES

The complex anatomy of the brainstem is best imaged by magnetic resonance imaging (MRI) that employs techniques to minimize cerebrospinal fluid (CSF) motion artifacts.[1] This MR technique provides the first in vivo definition of some internal structures in the brainstem. Despite this advance, the imaging clinician must continue to rely on the distinctive surface anatomic features of the brainstem to deduce the positions of the important tracts and nuclei that are below the resolution limit of even the best clinical MR images. This surface anatomy was first elegantly described on *axial* computed tomographic (CT) images that used water-soluble contrast or air to define the boundaries of the brainstem.[2] The axial imaging plane remains the most reliable for accurately localizing brainstem anatomy. Coronal and sagittal MR planes are currently used to help the clinician locate a lesion in the brainstem. The anatomy of the brainstem in these planes is labeled in Chapter 4.

The sensitivity of MR images presents a problem for the imaging clinician because it can demonstrate clinically *insignificant* bright regions in the brainstem on long TR/TE sequences (TR, repetition time; TE, echo delay time). Some of these regions have a characteristic location near the substantia nigra of the midbrain and have been attributed to enlarged perivascular spaces[3] (see Chapter 12). Other bright regions have no obvious cause, and only with a detailed knowledge of the nuclei and tracts in the brainstem can one hope to distinguish these clinically irrelevant zones from actual lesions responsible for clinical symptoms.

Currently, changes in brainstem size can be determined on midline sagittal MR images.[4] Figure 7-1 illustrates the sites at which the anteroposterior diameter of the brainstem is normally measured. Table 7-1 lists the normal dimensions for each level. Table 7-2 provides ratios at each level. To obtain these normal measurements, Koehler et al.[4] used partial-saturation images with 250 to 400 msec TRs, a 9 to 10 mm slice thickness, and clinical window settings. The authors noted several potential difficulties with this technique. Variations in placement of the "midline" sagittal plane occasionally prevented identification of the interpeduncular fissure and thus precluded precise measurement of the anteroposterior diameter of the midbrain. Errors from cursor placement were reported to result in variations of about 1 mm in the values listed in Table 7-1. Despite these problems, this MR technique is preferable to measurements derived from axial CT images. Small variations in axial CT scan angle cause *wide* variations in anteroposterior diameter measurements. These are reflected in the variations of normal measurements reported in the literature using this technique.[5,6]

FUNCTIONAL-ANATOMIC CORRELATIONS

In this section, information concerning the functional anatomy of the brainstem is organized into two parts. The first allows the reader to find the function of an area on selected axial schematic brainstem maps (Figures 7-2 to 7-9 and Boxes 7-1 to 7-7). An index for these terms has been compiled to assist the reader. The second part presents an overview of the motor, sensory, and cerebellar pathways in the brainstem. These pathways are illustrated on axial brainstem sections that are viewed from *behind* (rather than in the standard anatomic presentation). A general discussion of the reticular and autonomic systems is also presented in the second part of this section. Tables 7-3 to 7-5 summarize the features that can be used to distinguish hemispheric from brainstem lesions in comatose patients. The details concerning the cranial nerves that arise from the brainstem (III to XII) are given in Chapter 8, which provides a summary table of the clinically important brainstem syndromes.

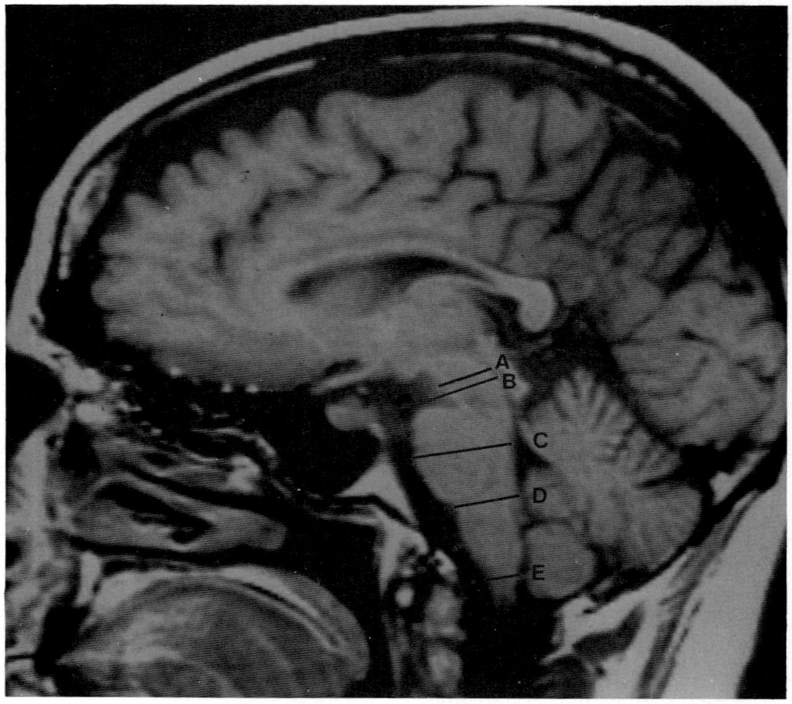

Figure 7-1 Midsagittal MR image showing anatomic placement for brainstem diameters listed in Table 7-1. Five measurements were made: the distance between the interpeduncular fissure and the aqueduct (A), the distance from the anterior surface of the cerebral peduncles to the aqueduct (B), the distance between the anterior surface of the pons (midway between the mesencephalon and medulla) and the fourth ventricular floor (C), the shortest anteroposterior diameter of the medulla at the pontomedullary junction (D), and the shortest anteroposterior diameter of the medulla at the medullospinal junction (E).

◆ **TABLE 7-1** Brainstem Diameters (in Millimeters) for 28 Normal Subjects

Regions measured*	Minimum	Mean	Maximum
A. Interpeduncular fissure to aqueduct	11.1	13.2	15.3
B. Cerebral peduncle to aqueduct	15.0	18.1	21.2
C. Midpons to floor of fourth ventricle	24.5	26.6	28.7
D. Pontomedullary junction	14.0	15.3	16.6
E. Medullospinal junction	8.1	9.4	10.7

Adapted with permission from Koehler PR, Haughton VM, Daniels DL, et al: AJNR 6:425-427, 1985.
*See Figure 7-1.

◆ **TABLE 7-2** Ratio of Midpons (C) to Other Brainstem Measurements

Ratios*	Minimum	Mean	Maximum
Interpeduncular fissure to aqueduct (C/A)	2.2	2.0	1.9
Cerebral peduncle to aqueduct (C/B)	1.6	1.5	1.4
Pontomedullary junction (C/D)	1.8	1.7	1.7
Medullospinal junction (C/E)	3.0	2.8	2.6

Adapted with permission from Koehler PR, Haughton VM, Daniels DL, et al: AJNR 6:425-427, 1985.
*Letters correspond to regions as listed in Table 7-1.

Axial Schematic Maps

This section divides the brainstem into seven axial slices (Figure 7-2). These are presented as schematic illustrations in the conventional axial imaging format (i.e., the patient's nose toward the top of the page). To assist the reader, only structures with a clearly defined function are included in these schematic maps. Each level (Figures 7-3 to 7-9) is accompanied by a box that briefly describes the functions of the structures labeled in the accompanying axial section (Boxes 7-1 to 7-7). The parallel lines, stippling, and unmarked rectangles in the boxes identify the reticular, sensory, and motor areas, respectively, on the corresponding figures. Various anatomic and neurologic sources were consulted to construct these figures.[7-27] Axial MR images (TR/TE, 4000/80) of a cadaver that correspond to these seven brainstem levels can be found in Chapter 6.

Text continued on p. 207.

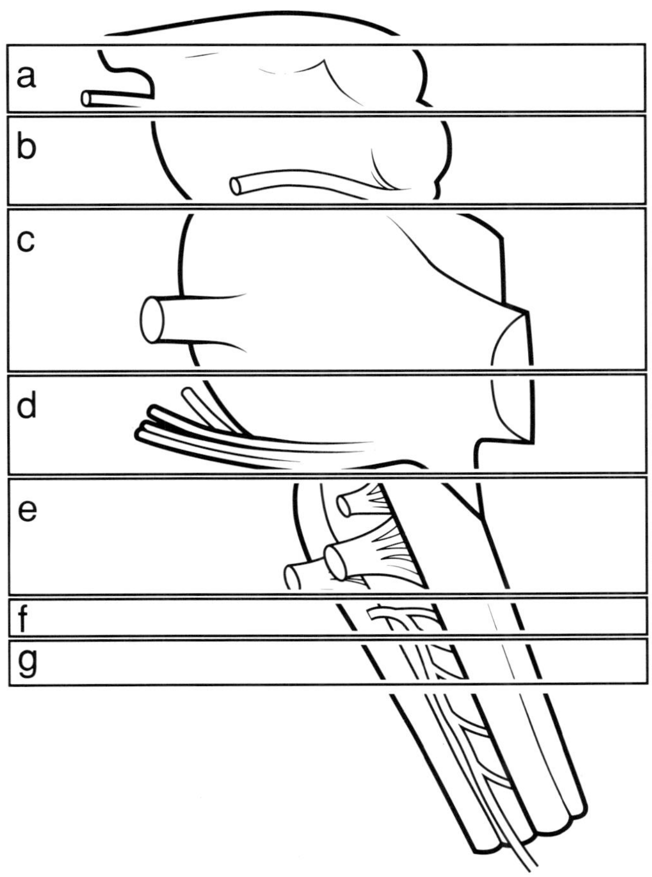

Figure 7-2 Midsagittal schematic illustration of the brainstem demonstrates the seven axial sections illustrated in Figures 7-3 to 7-9. Note that section thickness varies from one level to the next. This was done to assist the reader in understanding important vertical interconnections between nuclei and tracts that would have to be presented at several axial levels if thinner sections were used.

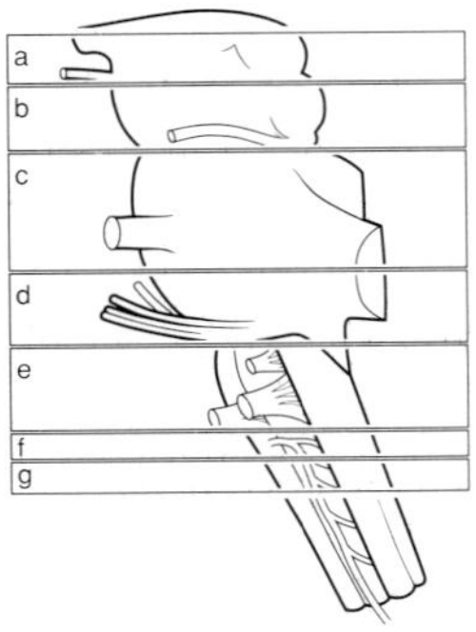

MIDBRAIN—SUPERIOR COLLICULUS

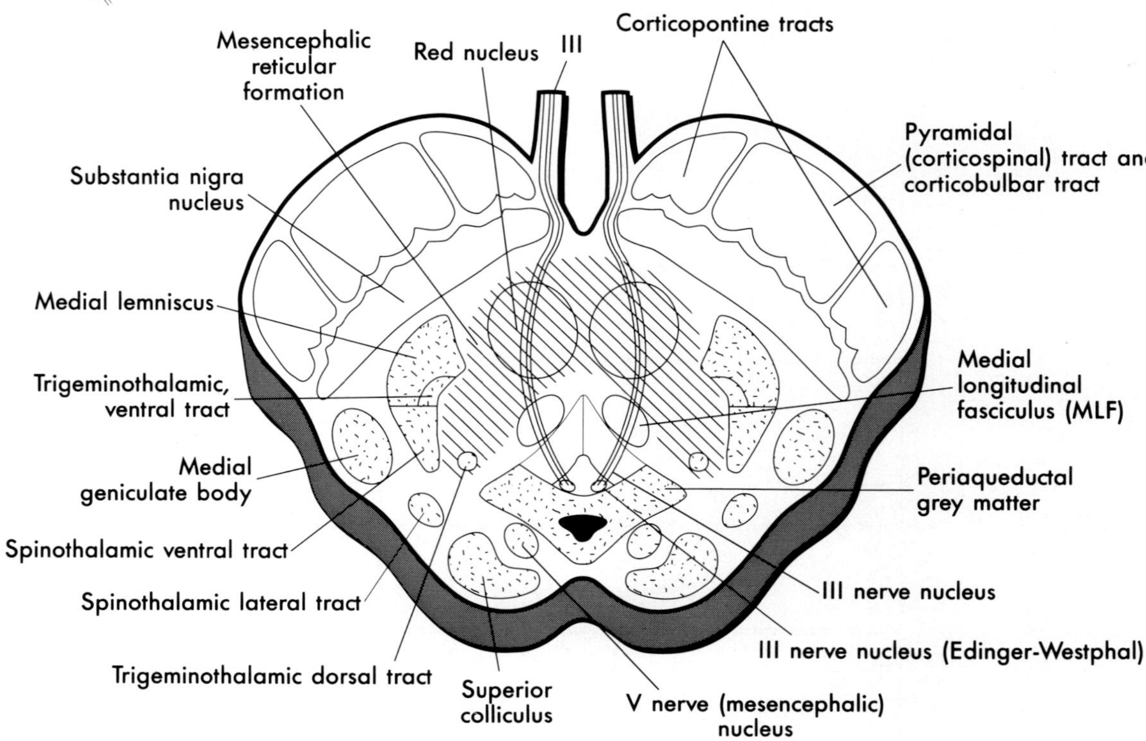

Figure 7-3 *Level a: upper midbrain (superior colliculus)*

This axial brainstem section has the characteristic heart shape of the midbrain. It can be distinguished from the level of the inferior colliculus by the origin of cranial nerve III from the interpeduncular fossa. The fibers of this motor nerve can be traced back to their origin in the cranial nerve III nuclei. (See Chapter 8 for further details on this cranial nerve.)

The region of the reticular system is marked by *parallel lines*, the sensory tracts and nuclei are *stippled*, and the motor structures are *unmarked*. (See Box 7-1.) The aqueduct is shown but not labeled. It is the dark region surrounded by the periaqueductal gray matter.

The anatomic nomenclature of the brainstem is reversed when the brainstem is viewed (as presented here) in an imaging format. The *crus cerebri*, which is formed by the corticospinal and corticopontine fibers, represents the anatomic "base" of the midbrain. The aqueduct divides the remainder of the midbrain into an anatomic *tegmentum* ("attic") and *tectum* ("roof"). The tectum is also referred to as the *quadrigeminal plate*.

BOX 7-1

Midbrain—Superior Colliculus (see Figure 7-3)

Reticular Formation

Mesencephalic reticular formation: lesion causes an inability to stay fully awake

Red nucleus: lesion causes contralateral tremors, ataxia, choreiform activity, and ipsilateral eye movement disorders

Sensory Systems

Medial geniculate body: transmits auditory input from both cochleae

Medial lemniscus: transmits contralateral discriminative touch, proprioception (vibration, stereognosis) from body

Cranial nerve V (mesencephalic) nucleus: transmits ipsilateral proprioception for mandible

Periaqueductal gray matter: reduces the sensation of pain; stimulation causes anesthesia

Spinothalamic, lateral tract: transmits contralateral pain and temperature from body

Spinothalamic, ventral tract: transmits contralateral light touch from body

Superior colliculus: coordinates reflex eye responses to visual, auditory, and somatic stimuli and visual tracking; lesion causes loss of pupillary reflexes, ocular convergence, and Parinaud's syndrome (inability to look up)

Trigeminothalamic, dorsal tract: transmits mainly ipsilateral touch and pressure from face

Trigeminothalamic, ventral tract: transmits contralateral pain and temperature from face

Motor Systems

Corticobulbar tract: controls motor cranial nerves V, VII (contralateral); IX, X (bilateral); XI (mainly ipsilateral); to XII (contralateral)

Corticopontine tracts: connect frontal, temporal, occipital, and parietal cortex with cerebellum; lesion causes transient ataxia and hypotonia

Medial longitudinal fasciculus (MLF): coordinates eye movements; lesion causes internuclear ophthalmoplegia

Nerve III nucleus: controls ipsilateral voluntary eye and upper lid movement

Nerve III (Edinger-Westphal) nucleus: lesion dilates the ipsilateral pupil

Pyramidal (corticospinal) tract: controls contralateral voluntary motor function of body

Substantia nigra nucleus: controls contralateral involuntary motor movements of body and face (abnormal in Parkinson's disease)

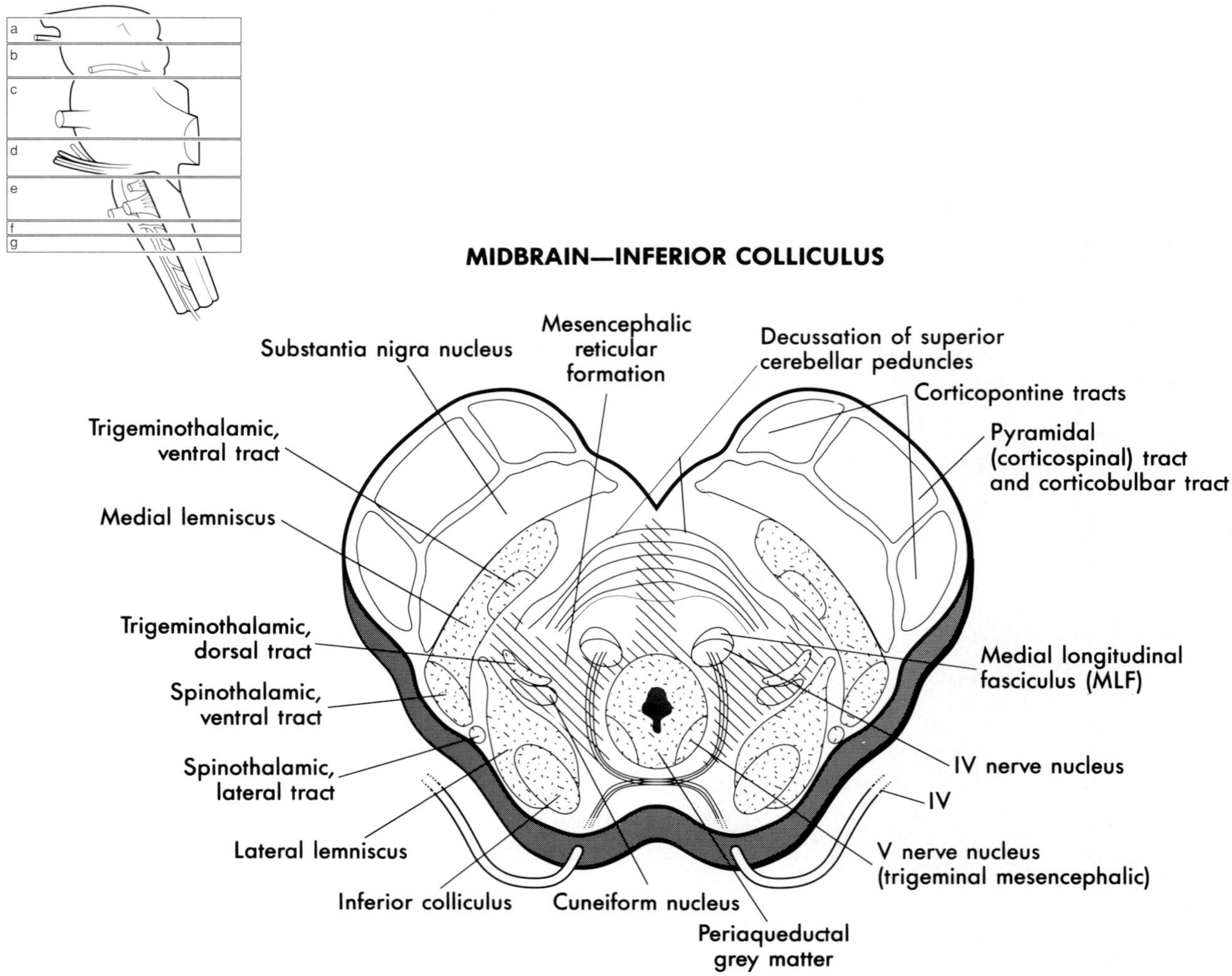

Figure 7-4 *Level b: lower midbrain (inferior colliculus)*

This axial brainstem section has the characteristic heart shape of the midbrain. The inferior colliculus can be distinguished from the level of the superior colliculus because it is *below* the origin of cranial nerve III in the interpeduncular fossa. The origin of cranial nerve IV from the dorsal aspect of the brainstem is below the resolution limit of modern imaging. The fibers of cranial nerve IV are shown as they cross and enter this nerve's nucleus. (See Chapter 8 for further details on this cranial nerve.)

The region of the reticular system is marked by *parallel lines*, the sensory tracts and nuclei are *stippled*, and the motor structures are *unmarked*. (See Box 7-2.) The aqueduct is shown but not labeled. It is the dark region surrounded by the periaqueductal gray matter.

The anatomic nomenclature of the brainstem is reversed when the brainstem is viewed (as presented here) in an imaging format. The crus cerebri, which is formed by the corticospinal and corticopontine fibers, represents the anatomic "base" of the midbrain. The aqueduct divides the remainder of the midbrain into an anatomic tegmentum ("attic") and tectum ("roof"). The tectum is also referred to as the quadrigeminal plate. The tegmentum at this level contains the decussation of the *superior cerebellar peduncles*.

BOX 7-2

Midbrain—Inferior Colliculus (see Figure 7-4)

Reticular Formation

Cuneiform nucleus: site where conscious motor commands from above (e.g., cortex) activate complex motor patterns (e.g., walking)

Mesencephalic reticular formation: lesion causes inability to stay fully awake

Sensory Systems

Inferior colliculus: acts as an auditory relay station that helps to localize the source of sound

Lateral lemniscus: transmits auditory input from both cochlea; lesion causes bilateral partial deafness

Medial lemniscus: transmits contralateral discriminative touch, proprioception (vibration, stereognosis) from body

Nerve V nucleus (trigeminal mesencephalic): transmits ipsilateral proprioception from face, mainly the mandible

Periaqueductal gray matter: stimulation of this area reduces pain perception

Spinothalamic, lateral tract: transmits contralateral pain and temperature from body

Spinothalamic, ventral tract: transmits contralateral light touch from body

Trigeminothalamic, dorsal tract: transmits mainly ipsilateral touch and pressure from face

Trigeminothalamic, ventral tract: transmits contralateral pain and temperature from face

Motor Systems

Corticobulbar tract: controls motor cranial nerves V, VII (contralateral); IX, X (bilateral); XI (mainly ipsilateral); to XII (contralateral)

Corticopontine tracts: connect frontal, temporal, occipital, and parietal lobes with the cerebellum; lesion causes transient ataxia and hypotonia

Decussation of superior cerebellar peduncles: controls motor coordination; lesion causes intention tremor

Medial longitudinal fasciculus (MLF): coordinates eye movements; lesion causes internuclear ophthalmoplegia

Nerve IV nucleus: lesion causes contralateral weakness of downward and lateral gaze

Pyramidal (corticospinal) tract: controls contralateral voluntary motor function of body

Substantia nigra nucleus: controls contralateral involuntary motor movements of body (abnormal in Parkinson's disease)

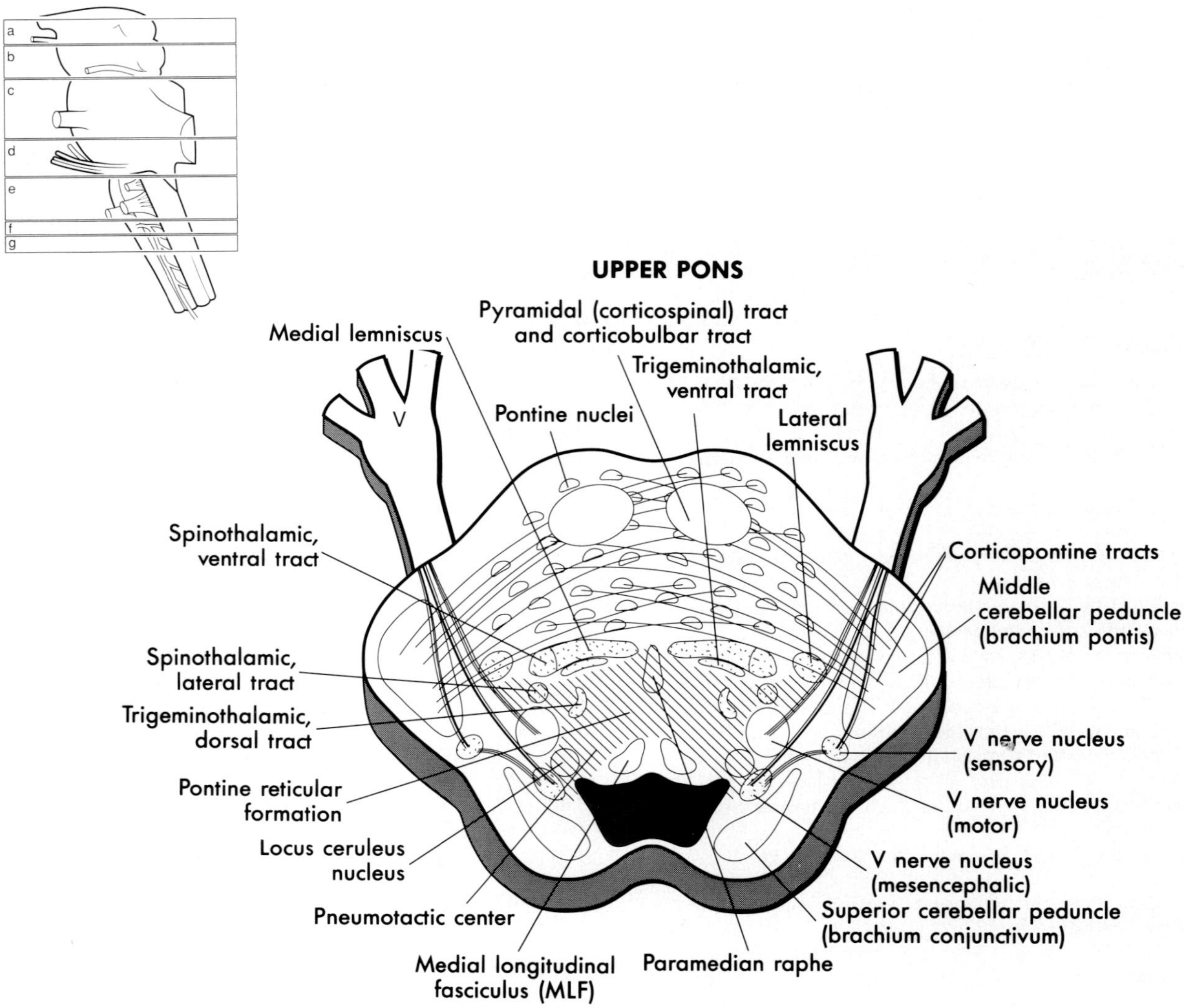

Figure 7-5 *Level c: upper pons*

This axial brainstem section is easily distinguished from the lower pontine level because the cranial nerve V exits at this level. The fibers of cranial nerve V are shown as they enter this nerve's motor, sensory, and mesencephalic nuclei. (See Chapter 8 for further details on this cranial nerve.)

The region of the reticular system is marked by *parallel lines*, the sensory tracts and nuclei are *stippled*, and the motor structures are *unmarked*. (See Box 7-4.) The fourth ventricle and a small portion of the medullary velum, that forms its "roof," are shown as an unlabeled, dark area which merges posteriorly with the cut surfaces of the brainstem.

The "base" of the pons contains numerous individual fascicles of the descending *pyramidal* (*corticospinal*) and *corticobulbar tracts*. The *corticopontine tracts* arise from the frontal, parietal, temporal, and occipital lobes and descend to synapse in the pontine nuclei. These fibers create horizontal bands in the base of the pons. The tegmentum ("attic") of the pons is the region between the base and the fourth ventricle.

BOX 7-3

Upper Pons—Components and Their Functions (Figure 7-5)

Reticular Formation

Locus ceruleus nucleus: inhibits painful stimuli; regulates circadian rhythms

Paramedian raphe: part of pathway for coordinated movements (e.g., of eye)

Pneumotactic center: controls the rate of breathing; lesion causes deep respirations

Pontine reticular formation: lesion causes inability to go to sleep

Sensory Systems

Lateral lemniscus: transmits auditory input from both cochlea; lesion causes bilateral deafness

Medial lemniscus: transmits contralateral discriminative touch and proprioception (vibration, stereognosis) from body

Nerve V nucleus (mesencephalic): transmits ipsilateral proprioception for face, mainly the mandible

Nerve V nucleus (sensory): transmits ipsilateral proprioception and vibration from face and scalp

Spinothalamic, lateral tract: transmits contralateral pain and temperature from body

Spinothalamic, ventral tract: transmits contralateral light touch from body

Trigeminothalamic, dorsal tract: transmits mainly ipsilateral touch and pressure from face

Trigeminothalamic, ventral tract: transmits contralateral pain and temperature from face

Motor Systems

Corticobulbar tract: controls motor cranial nerves V, VII (contralateral); IX, X (bilateral); XI (mainly ipsilateral); to XII (contralateral)

Corticopontine tracts: connect frontal, temporal, occipital, and parietal lobes with cerebellum; lesion causes transient ataxia and hypotonia

Medial longitudinal fasciculus (MLF): coordinates eye movements; lesion causes internuclear ophthalmoplegia

Middle cerebellar peduncle (brachium pontis): controls motor coordination; lesion causes incoordination and ataxia

Nerve V nucleus (motor): controls ipsilateral chewing and palatal muscles

Pontine nuclei: relay motor cortex information to cerebellum via corticopontine tract

Pyramidal (corticospinal) tract: controls contralateral voluntary motor function of body

Superior cerebellar peduncle (brachium conjunctivum): controls motor coordination; lesion causes tremors

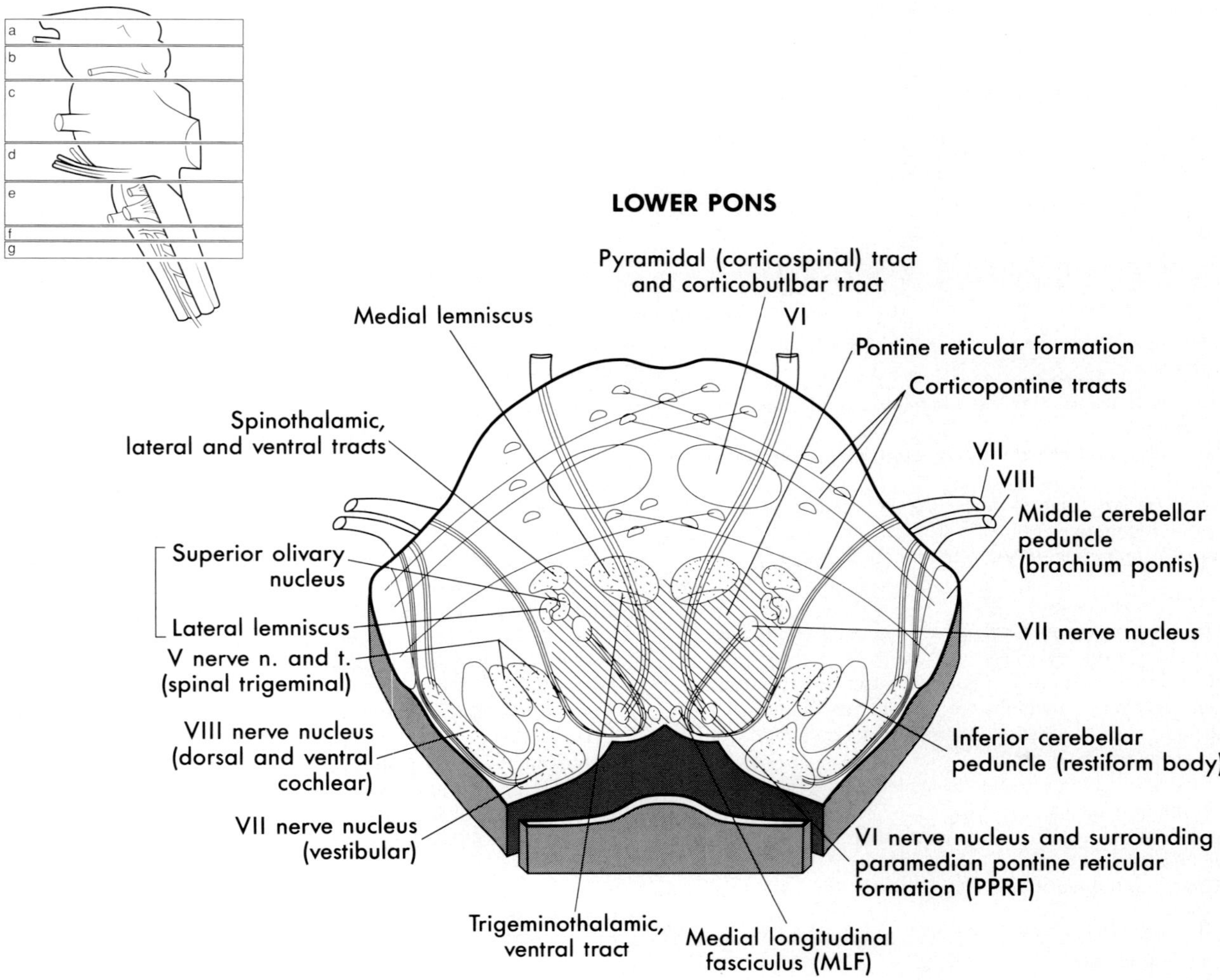

Figure 7-6 *Level d: lower pons*

This axial brainstem section is found immediately below the origin of cranial nerve V. This nerve passes through the middle cerebellar peduncles (shown as cut surfaces) as they attach to the cerebellar hemisphere. Three cranial nerves (VI, VII, VIII) exit the brainstem at the pontomedullary junction. The fibers, nuclei, and points at which these nerves leave the brainstem are all shown on this thick schematic slice of the lower pons. The fibers of cranial nerve VII loop around the cranial nerve VI nucleus to form a "facial colliculus" that protrudes into the floor of the fourth ventricle. (See Chapter 8 for further details on these cranial nerves.)

The region of the reticular system is marked by *parallel lines*, the sensory tracts and nuclei are *stippled*, and the motor structures are *unmarked*. (See Box 7-4.) The fourth ventricle and a small portion of the medullary velum, that forms its "roof," are shown as an unlabeled, dark area which merges posteriorly with the cut surfaces of the brainstem.

The "base" of the pons contains numerous individual fascicles of the descending pyramidal (corticospinal) and corticobulbar tracts. The corticopontine tracts arise from the frontal, parietal, temporal, and occipital lobes. They descend to synapse in the pontine nuclei. These fibers create horizontal bands in the base of the pons. The tegmentum ("attic") of the pons is the region between the base and the fourth ventricle.

BOX 7-4

Lower Pons—Components and Their Functions (Figure 7-6)

Reticular Formation

Pontine reticular formation: lesion causes loss of the ability to go to sleep

Paramedian pontine reticular formation (PPRF): helps coordinate conjugate eye movements

Sensory Systems

Lateral lemniscus and superior olivary nuclei: transmit auditory input from both cochleae; lesion causes bilateral partial deafness

Medial lemniscus: transmits contralateral discriminative touch and proprioception (vibration, stereognosis) from body

Nerve VIII nucleus (dorsal and ventral cochlear): lesion causes ipsilateral deafness

Nerve VIII nucleus (vestibular): transmits equilibrium information; lesion causes dizziness, falling, and abnormal eye movements with nausea and vomiting

Nerve V nucleus and tract (spinal trigeminal): transmit ipsilateral pain and temperature from face

Spinothalamic, lateral tract: transmits contralateral pain and temperature from body

Spinothalamic, ventral tract: transmits contralateral light touch from body

Spinotrigeminal tract: transmits ipsilateral pain and temperature from face

Trigeminothalamic, ventral tract: transmits contralateral pain and temperature from face

Motor Systems

Corticobulbar tract: controls motor nuclei of cranial nerves VII (contralateral); IX, X (bilateral); XI (mainly ipsilateral); to XII (contralateral)

Corticopontine tracts: connect frontal, temporal, occipital, and parietal lobes with cerebellum; lesion causes transient ataxia and hypotonia

Inferior cerebellar peduncle (restiform body): controls coordination of motor movements; lesion causes ipsilateral ataxia

Middle cerebellar peduncle (brachium pontis): coordinates motor movements; lesion causes incoordination and ataxia

Nerve VII nucleus: lesion causes ipsilateral paralysis of entire face

Nerve VI nucleus: lesion causes ipsilateral paralysis of lateral gaze

Medial longitudinal fasciculus (MLF): coordinates eye movements; lesion causes internuclear ophthalmoplegia

Pyramidal (corticospinal) tract: controls contralateral voluntary motor function of body

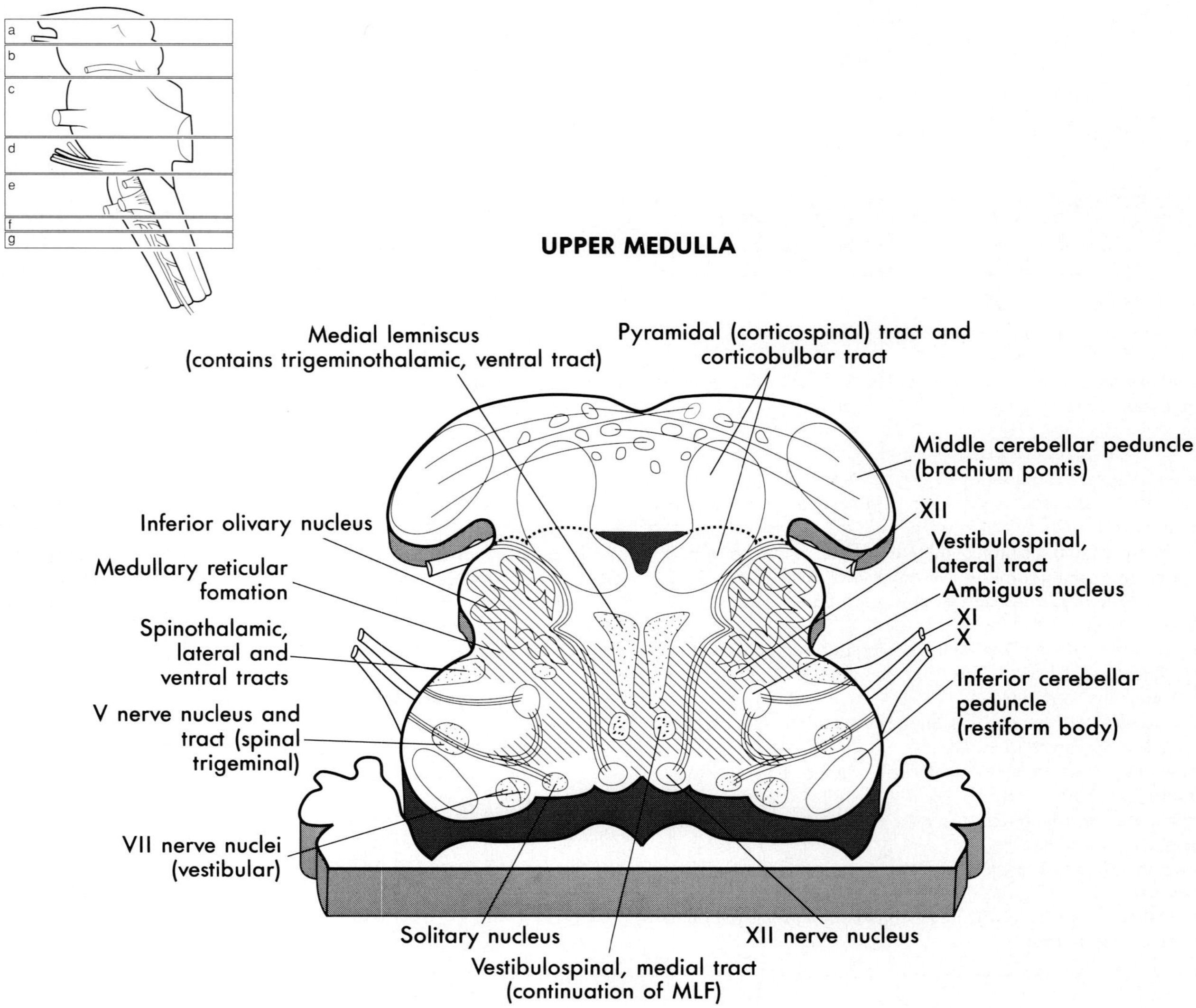

Figure 7-7 *Level e: upper (open) medulla*

This distinctive axial brainstem level usually contains a partial-volume image of the base of the inferior pons. Often, the CSF-filled *foramen cecum*, which is formed between the inferior pons and the pyramidal tracts, is visualized in this section. This foramen is shown in here as a triangular, unlabeled, dark area. This medullary level can be distinguished from the lower medulla because it contains the *inferior olivary nucleus*, which produces a characteristic shape anterolaterally. (The fibers from this nucleus, which cross the midline to enter the opposite inferior cerebellar peduncle, are not shown.) The small rootlets of cranial nerves X, XI, and XII are often not visible. The fibers and nuclei of these nerves are shown on this schematic illustration. (See Chapter 8 for further details on these nerves.)

The region of the reticular system is marked by *parallel lines*, the sensory tracts and nuclei are *stippled*, and the motor structures are *unmarked*. (See Box 7-5.) The fourth ventricle and its lateral recesses are shown as an unlabeled, dark area covering the entire posterior surface of the medulla. A small section of vermis and cerebellum has been included to create the posterior silhouette of the fourth ventricle.

BOX 7-5

Upper Medulla—Components and Their Functions (Figure 7-7)

Reticular Formation

Inferior olivary nucleus: relays sensory information to cerebellum to help with motor coordination; may promote motor learning

Medullary reticular formation: the central region mediates pain suppression; vomiting center adjacent to the solitary nucleus; chemoreceptor trigger zone centrally located between the cranial nerve XII nuclei

Sensory Systems

Medial lemniscus: transmits contralateral discriminative touch and proprioception (vibration, stereognosis) from body

Nerve V nucleus and tract (spinotrigeminal): transmit ipsilateral pain and temperature from face

Nerve VIII nuclei (vestibular): transmit equilibrium information; lesion causes dizziness, falling, and abnormal eye movements with nausea and vomiting

Solitary nucleus: transmits taste and visceral sensation

Spinothalamic, lateral tract: transmits contralateral pain and temperature from body

Spinothalamic, ventral tract: transmits contralateral light touch from body

Trigeminothalamic, ventral tract: transmits contralateral pain and temperature from face

Vestibulospinal, lateral, and medial tracts: transmit balance information to muscles of head and body

Motor Systems

Ambiguus nucleus: controls motor fibers for speech and swallowing from nerves IX, X, and XI

Corticobulbar tract: controls activity of motor cranial nerves IX, X (bilateral); XI (mainly ipsilateral); XII (contralateral)

Inferior cerebellar peduncle (restiform body): coordinates motor movements; lesion causes ipsilateral ataxia

Middle cerebellar peduncle (brachium pontis): coordinates motor movements; lesion causes incoordination and ataxia

Nerve XII nucleus: controls ipsilateral motor function of tongue

Pyramidal (corticospinal) tract: controls contralateral voluntary motor function of body

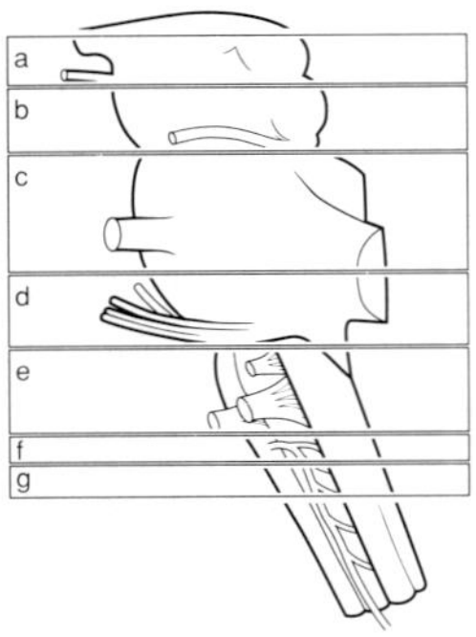

LOWER MEDULLA—SENSORY [MEDIAL LEMNISCAL] DECUSSATION

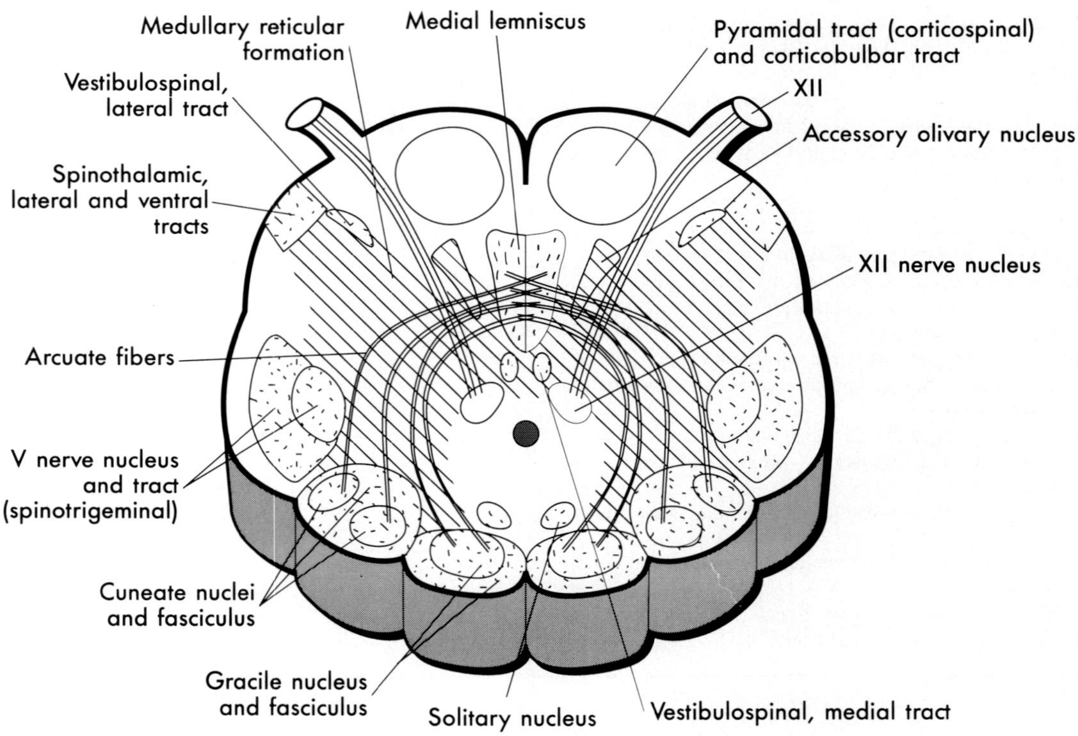

Figure 7-8 *Level f: lower (closed) medulla—sensory decussation*

This axial brainstem section can be distinguished from the next lower medullary section by the comparatively prominent eminences of the *pyramidal (motor) tracts* and the comparatively smaller eminences of the *cuneate* and *gracile (sensory) tracts*. The relative smallness of these sensory tracts occurs because fibers exit these ascending tracts and cross the midline at the lemniscal decussation to form the medial lemniscus. The small rootlets of cranial nerve XII may be seen at this level. Their path from the motor nucleus of cranial nerve XII is shown. (See Chapter 8 for further details on this nerve.)

The region of the reticular system is marked by *parallel lines*, the sensory tracts and nuclei are *stippled*, and the motor structures are *unmarked*. (See Box 7-6.) The central canal is shown as an unlabeled, dark circle between the cranial nerve XII nuclei.

BOX 7-6

Lower Medulla: Sensory (Medial Lemniscal) Decussation—Components and Their Functions (Figure 7-8)

Reticular Formation

Accessory olivary nucleus: relays sensory information to cerebellum to help with motor coordination; may facilitate motor learning

Medullary reticular formation: central areas suppress pain; cardiovascular pressor and depressor areas; inspiratory and expiratory centers

Sensory Systems

Arcuate fibers: connect gracile and cuneate nuclei to contralateral medial lemnisci

Cuneate nucleus and fasciculus: transmit ipsilateral discriminative touch and proprioception (vibration, stereognosis) from upper extremities

Gracile nuclei and fasciculus: transmit ipsilateral discriminative touch and proprioception (vibration, stereognosis) from lower extremities

Medial lemniscus: transmits contralateral discriminative touch and proprioception (vibration, stereognosis) from body

Nerve V nucleus and tract (spinotrigeminal): transmit ipsilateral pain, temperature, and crude touch in face

Solitary nucleus: transmits taste and visceral sensation

Spinothalamic, lateral tract: transmits contralateral pain and temperature from body

Spinothalamic, ventral tract: transmits contralateral light touch from body

Vestibulospinal, lateral, and medial tracts: relay balance information to muscles of head and body

Motor Systems

Corticobulbar tract: controls activity of motor cranial nerves XI (mainly ipsilateral) and XII (mainly contralateral)

Nerve XII nucleus (hypoglossal): controls ipsilateral tongue movement

Pyramidal (corticospinal) tract: controls contralateral voluntary motor function of body

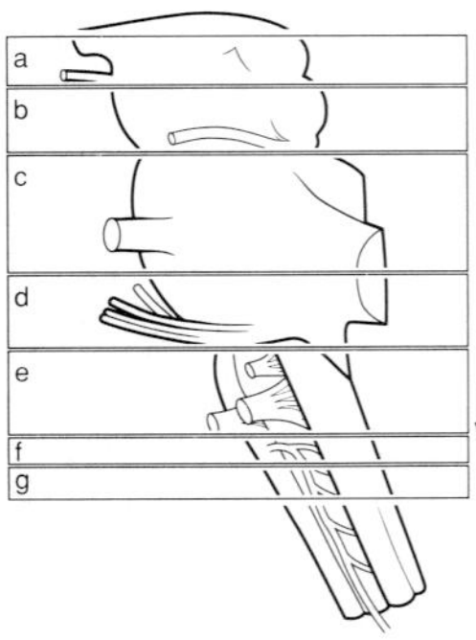

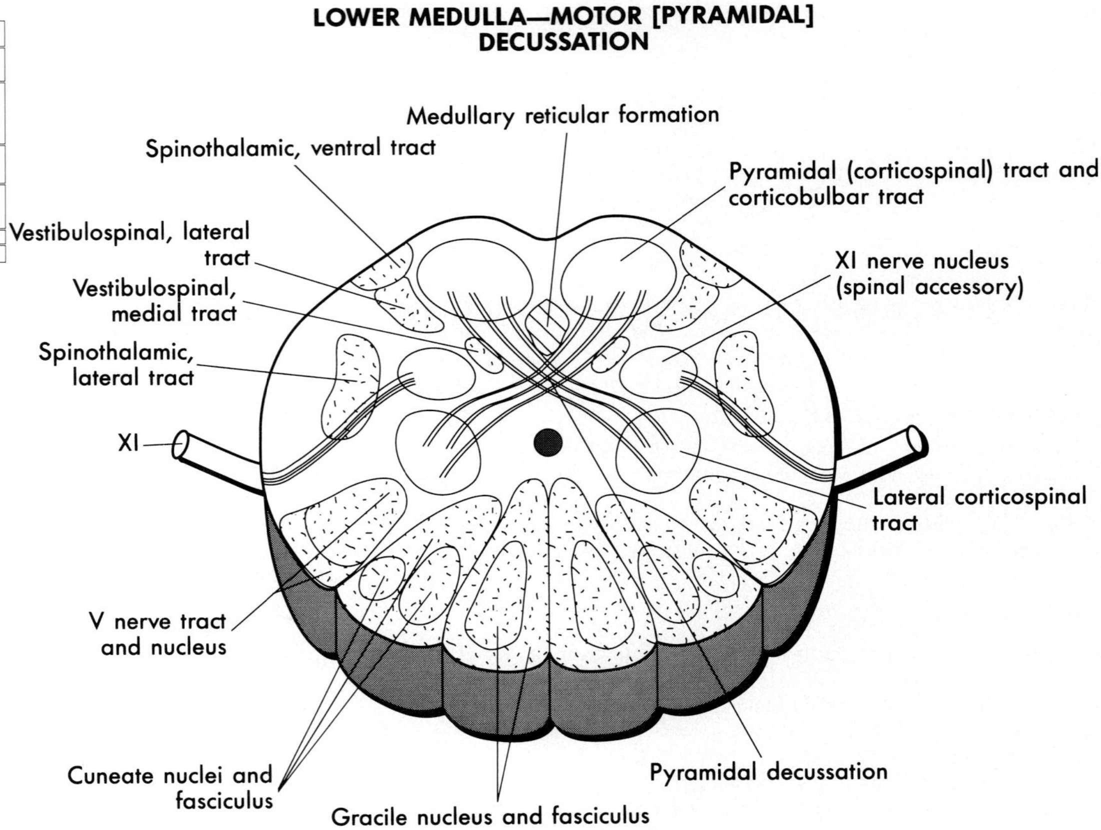

Figure 7-9 *Level g: lower (closed) medulla—motor decussation*

This axial brainstem section can be distinguished from the previous medullary level by the presence of the relatively smaller eminences of the pyramidal tracts and the relatively larger eminences of the cuneate and gracile (sensory) tracts. The reduction in size of the descending motor tracts occurs because almost all these fibers cross the midline at the pyramidal decussation to form the lateral corticospinal tracts. The small rootlets of cranial nerve XI may be seen at this level. Their path from the motor nucleus of this nerve is shown. (See Chapter 8 for further details on this nerve.)

The region of the reticular system is marked by *parallel lines*, the sensory tracts and nuclei are *stippled*, and the motor structures are *unmarked*. (See Box 7-7.) The central canal at this level is shown as an unlabeled, dark circle between the lateral corticospinal tracts.

BOX 7-7

Lower Medulla: Motor (Pyramidal) Decussation—Components and Their Functions (Figure 7-9)

Reticular Formation

Medullary reticular formation: suppresses pain; stimulation causes anesthesia and sleep

Sensory Systems

Cuneate nuclei and fasciculus: transmit ipsilateral discriminative touch and proprioception (vibration, stereognosis) from upper extremities

Gracile nuclei and fasciculus: transmit ipsilateral discriminative touch and proprioception (vibration, stereognosis) from lower extremities

Nerve V nucleus and tract (spinotrigeminal): transmit ipsilateral pain, temperature, and crude touch from face

Spinothalamic, lateral tract: transmits contralateral pain and temperature from body

Spinothalamic, ventral tract: transmits contralateral light touch from body

Vestibulospinal, lateral and medial tracts: relay balance information to muscles of head and body

Motor Systems

Corticobulbar tract: controls predominantly contralateral motor function of cranial nerve XI

Lateral corticospinal tract: controls ipsilateral voluntary motor function of body

Cranial nerve XI nucleus (spinal accessory): controls ipsilateral shrugging of shoulder and turning of head to opposite side

Pyramidal decussation: connects corticospinal fibers of pyramidal tract to contralateral corticospinal tracts

Pyramidal (corticospinal) tract: controls contralateral voluntary motor function of body

◆ **TABLE 7-3** Localizing Features of Response Patterns In Comatose Patients

Clinical findings	Cerebral hemispheres	Midbrain/pons/medulla
CLASSIC SYNDROMES		
1. Decerebrate rigidity: arms extended, adducted, hyperpronated; legs extended with plantar flexion; occasional arching of back and clenching of teeth	Bilateral (sometimes in combination with a midbrain lesion; often metabolic)	*Midbrain*: in animals, between superior and inferior colliculi, sparing vestibular nuclei and pontine reticular formation. *This is not a reliable localization in the human patient.*
2. Decorticate rigidity: upper extremity flexed (at elbows, wrist, fingers) and adducted; legs extended as in decerebrate rigidity	Bilateral (diffuse, widespread hemispheric dysfunction, usually not as severe as in decerebrate rigidity)	
ALTERNATIVE CLASSIFICATION		
1. Arms abnormally flexed; legs flexed, extended, or flaccid	Bilateral (usually diffuse, supratentorial; less likely to involve deep structures than syndromes described in following 2, 3, and 4)	
2. Arm and legs extended	Bilateral (likely to be severe problem involving deeper structures; often metabolic)	*Midbrain*: usually in combination with hemispheric lesion
3. Arms extended, legs flaccid or weakly flexed		*Pons*: tegmentum at about vestibular level
4. Flaccidity*		*Pons*: destruction of vestibular nuclei and pontine reticular formation *Medulla*: destruction of motor tracts in medulla

Summarized from Plum F, Posner JB: *The diagnosis of stupor and coma*, Philadelphia, 1980, FA Davis.

*By itself, flaccidity in coma is not highly localizing. Spinal shock and peripheral denervation can produce flaccidity. Also in coma, because of bilateral hemispheric dysfunction, decreased tone can be seen, which might be difficult to distinguish from the flaccidity. The development of flaccidity, however, can indicate the progression of rostral-caudal herniation. In this context, the key point might be to recognize that loss of an extended posture can often mean deterioration rather than improvement.

◆ **TABLE 7-4** Localizing Features of Respiratory Patterns In Comatose Patients

Clinical findings	Midbrain/pons/medulla
HYPERPNEA	
Rapid, deep breathing "central neurogenic hyperventilation"*	Rostral brainstem tegmentum, between low *midbrain* and middle third of *pons*
APNEUSTIC BREATHING	
Long (2 to 3 seconds or more) pause after a full inspiration	Mid-to-lower *pons* (often, a large lesion in dorsal tegmentum also extending to dorsolateral pontine nuclei)
ATAXIC BREATHING	
Completely irregular breathing	*Medulla*: dorsomedial, approximately down to obex
Cluster of breaths followed by pauses	Low *pons* High *medulla*
ONDINE'S CURSE	
Loss of automatic breathing while asleep	*Medulla*: dorsomedial respiratory centers

Summarized from Plum F, Posner JB: *The diagnosis of stupor and coma*, Philadelphia, 1980, FA Davis.

*True "central neurogenic hyperventilation" is very rare. For deep rapid breathing to be hyperventilation, blood gas evidence of hyperventilation must be present (i.e., low carbon dioxide tension, high oxygen tension). One rarely finds such evidence. However, at least some correlation exists between rapid deep breathing and midbrain/pons tegmental damage, even though the oxygen tension is often depressed rather than elevated.

◆ **TABLE 7-5** Localizing Features of Eye Movement (Including Eyelids) In Comatose Patients

Clinical findings	Cerebral hemispheres/midbrain/pons
ABSENT BLINKING ON ONE SIDE	
Corneal reflex test	*Pons*: ipsilateral cranial nerve VII
1. Absent Bell's phenomenon (i.e., eyes do not go up)	*Pons*: pontine tegmental damage (above cranial nerve V)
2. Bell's phenomenon present; no blink on one side	*Pons*: damage of ipsilateral cranial nerve VII or its nucleus
Oculocephalic (doll's head) and oculovestibular (ice water caloric) responses	
1. Internuclear ophthalmoplegia (eye on side irrigated with cold water moves laterally, but other eye moves only to midline)	*Pons*: medial longitudinal fasciculus (MLF; on side of eye that moves only to midline)
2. No response	*Pons*: damage between vestibular nucleus and cranial nerve VI nucleus
SPONTANEOUS EYE MOVEMENTS	
1. Roving	*Cerebral hemispheres*: bilateral (may be metabolic)
2. Retractory nystagmus (eyes jerk back into orbit at irregular intervals because of simultaneous contraction of extraocular muscles)	*Midbrain*: tegmentum
3. Convergence nystagmus (eyes slowly drift apart, then jerk back into convergence)	*Midbrain*
4. Ocular bobbing (quick downward motion of both eyes, then slow movement upward)	Caudal *pons*
5. Nystagmoid jerking of single eye	Mid-to-lower *pons*
6. Lateral gaze problems	
a. Eyes deviate away from paralyzed side	*Cerebral hemispheres*: unilateral* (side to which eyes look)
b. Eyes deviate toward side of body exhibiting unilateral seizure	*Cerebral hemispheres*: unilateral* (side opposite to which eyes look)
c. Eyes deviate toward paralyzed side	*Pons*: often near cranial nerve VI nucleus
d. Eye(s) deviate(s) outward (often increased diameter of pupil[s])	*Midbrain*: cranial nerve III
e. Eye(s) deviate(s) inward	*Pons*: cranial nerve VI
7. Vertical gaze problems	
a. Conjugate downward gaze at rest (i.e., without specific stimulation by examiner)	*Midbrain*: tectum (may be metabolic)
b. Paralysis of upward gaze (i.e., no response to corneal touch or oculocaloric or oculovestibular maneuvers)	*Midbrain*: pretectum, posterior commissure
c. Skew deviation (one eye up, one eye down)	*Pons*: usually brachium pontis or dorsolateral medulla on side of up eye or MLF on side of down eye
Oculocephalic-oculovestibular responses	
1. Internuclear ophthalmoplegia	*Pons*: MLF (on side of eye that does not fully adduct)
2. No response	*Pons*: damage between vestibular nucleus and cranial nerve VI nucleus
3. Able to overcome conjugate lateral eye deviation	*Cerebral hemispheres*: lesion on side of eye deviation
4. Unable to overcome conjugate lateral eye deviation	*Pons*: usually at cranial nerve VI nucleus
5. Unable to produce upward gaze	*Pons*: pretectum
6. One eye lacks all movement except abduction	*Pons*: cranial nerve III nucleus on side of affected eye
7. Doll's head maneuver normal, but ice water caloric tests cause no movement	*Pons*: bilateral destruction of vestibular nucleus (or labyrinth)

Summarized from Plum F, Posner JB: *The diagnosis of stupor and coma*, Philadelphia, 1980, FA Davis.

*For a person to be in coma, significant bilateral cerebral dysfunction or significant dysfunction of the brainstem reticular activating system is required. *Unilateral* refers to the side of the brain most likely to have a specific structural lesion.

Functional Systems

Sensory Pathways

The pathway for sensory impulses *from the body* that travel through the brainstem consists of fibers that convey (1) pain and temperature, (2) light touch (Figure 7-10), and (3) proprioception and vibration (Figure 7-11). The transmission of these sensations from the face via cranial nerve V is discussed in Chapter 8.

Motor Pathways

The pathway for motor impulses *to the body* that travel through the brainstem is summarized in Figure 7-12. Motor impulses to the eyes, face, and neck are discussed in Chapter 8.

Cerebellar Pathways

The pathways to and from the cerebellum that travel in the brainstem are summarized in Figures 7-13 and 7-14. Considerable disagreement exists among neurology texts concerning these pathways and their functions.[28-31] In addition, clinical neurologists frequently disagree about whether tremors or other findings in a specific patient are really "cerebellar." Given these disagreements, it is possible to provide the reader with only a broad discussion of the cerebellar pathways.

In general, three overlapping cerebellar systems exist and are designated somewhat arbitrarily: the vestibular, spinal, and cerebral systems. The *vestibular system* regulates equilibrium and also influences muscle tone and affects posture. The *spinal system* regulates gross and automatic types of motor output. The *cerebral system* facilitates the more complex motor patterns.

Incoming information arrives at the cerebellum via one of the three cerebellar peduncles. These tracts are outlined in Figure 7-13. Information leaves the cerebellum via either the superior or the inferior cerebellar peduncles (Figure 7-14). Despite (or perhaps because of) the myriad of complicated cerebellar connections that pass through the brainstem, it is usually not possible to discern specific syndromes corresponding to these tracts in the brainstem. Thus specific cerebellar problems are rarely the *sole* localizing factors in a given brainstem lesion, since most lesions encompass more than just the cerebellar tracts. A few notable brainstem syndromes combine cerebellar dysfunction with other types of problems (see Chapter 8).

Reticular System

The reticular areas of the brainstem are marked by diagonal lines in Figures 7-3 to 7-9. The neuron groups in this system regulate vital functions such as blood pressure, respiration, levels of brain activity, and sleep/wake cycles. For example, it is known that lesions of the midbrain reticular formation may lead to a loss of the ability to stay awake and that lesions of the pontine reticular formation, conversely, may result in the loss of the ability to sleep. Abnormalities in these functions are frequently caused by conditions other than brainstem lesions. These include infections, emotional states, and medically induced changes in vital functions.[32] Thus the protean signs and symptoms that can arise from reticular lesions are usually not specific in localizing a brainstem lesion. Nevertheless, information about the reticular formation and the reticular system may help rationalize the connection between structural pathology and clinical signs and symptoms. Such information could give valuable clues about which levels of the brainstem require special attention.

The reticular formation is divided into three main nuclear zones: *paramedian* (which contains the raphe nuclei), *medial*, and *lateral*. The central tegmental tract travels vertically through the brainstem to interconnect these reticular nuclei. The reticular formation is part of an extensive *reticular system* that extends above the midbrain into the midline nuclei, interlaminar nuclei, reticular nucleus, and the ventroanterior nucleus of the thalamus. This system extends into part of the hypothalamus, as well as into the zona incerta of the ventral thalamus. The reticular system is also considered to extend into the septal nuclei and the substantia innominata. Even the subthalamic nucleus and the globus pallidus are sometimes included in the reticular system, although they are definitely part of the basal ganglia. The reticular system sends output to the spinal cord via the reticular spinal tracts that influence the motor neurons of the spinal cord. This system also sends information to the cerebellum.

The reticular system also includes all the fibers that enter the reticular formation. The spinal cord inputs arrive via the spinoreticular tracts, spinotemporal tracts, and spinothalamic tracts. Interestingly, the medial lemniscus, which carries proprioceptive information, does *not* contribute to the reticular formation. All the sensory cranial nerves, however, do contribute. Cerebral influences are transmitted by corticobulbar and corticoreticular tracts, as well as by collaterals from the corticospinal tract, basal ganglia projections, and projections from the limbic lobe and the hypothalamus. Fibers also come from the cerebellum.

Autonomic System

The parasympathetic preganglionic neurons in the brainstem form the bulk of the autonomic system in the brain. These neurons are part of cranial nerves III, VII, IX, and X. The specific autonomic functions of these fibers are summarized in the following text.

Fibers of the *Edinger-Westphal nucleus* (cranial nerve III) innervate the ciliary ganglion. They are generally responsible for pupillary constriction, as well as light and accommodation reflexes. The fibers of the *superior salivatory nucleus* (cranial nerve VII) form the greater superficial petrosal nerve, which innervates the pterygopalatine ganglion. These fibers in turn innervate the lacrimal glands and the mucosa of the nose and palate. The chorda tympani and lingual nerves that arise from this ganglion

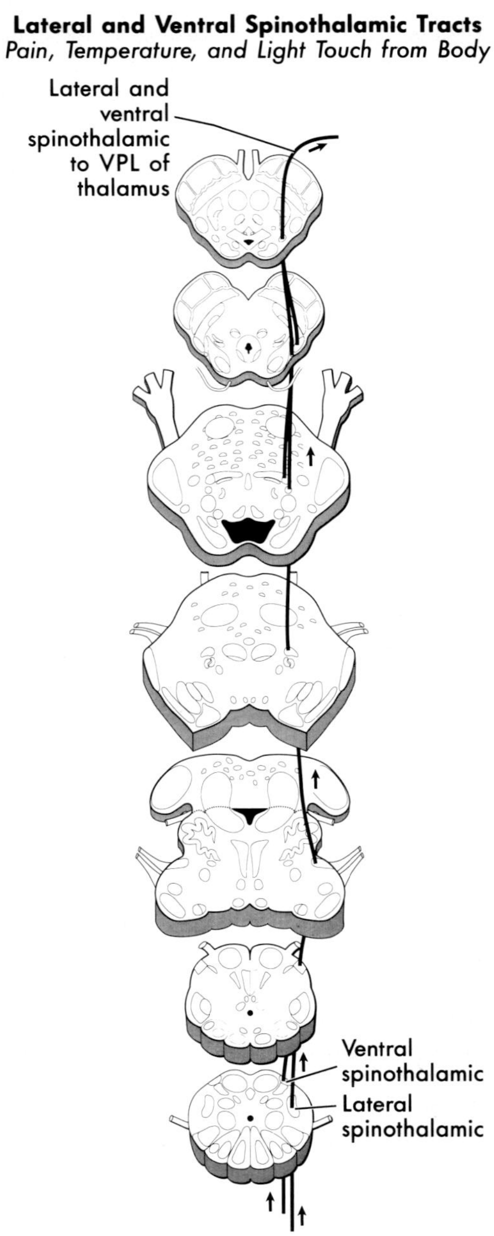

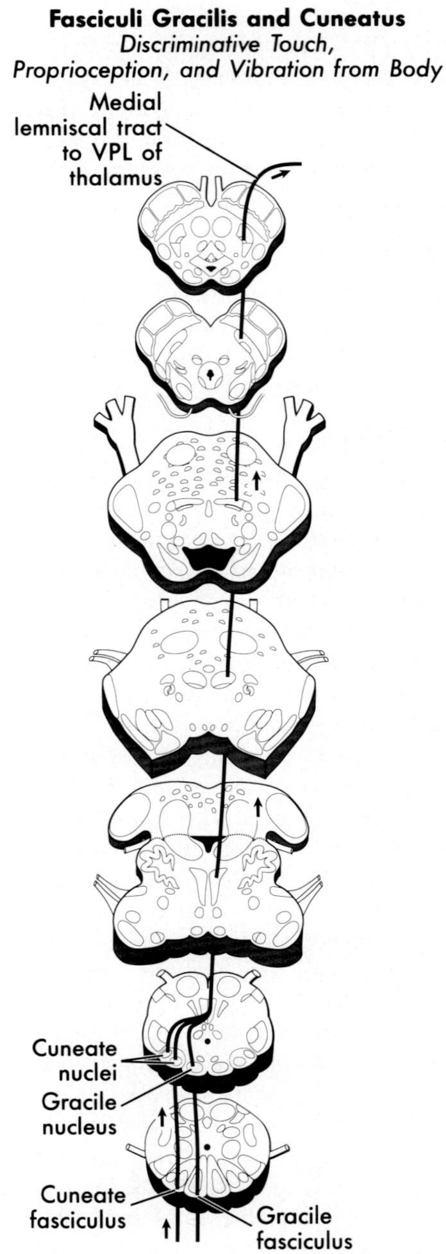

Figure 7-10 The lateral and ventral spinothalamic tracts convey sensations of pain and temperature, as well as aspects of light touch (including pressure) from the body. Both tracts begin in the dorsal horn (on the same side as the original sensory input). There they receive the sensory input either directly from a primary sensory neuron or sometimes from an interneuron. These tracts cross almost immediately to the other side of the spinal cord and ascend as shown. With regard to the different types of sensation, the pain and temperature sense primarily ascends in the lateral spinothalamic tract, and touch mainly ascends in the anterior spinothalamic tract.

Figure 7-11 Sensation that underlies discriminative touch, proprioception, and vibration begins in the periphery at the skin and joint receptors and ascends the spinal cord without crossing until it reaches the cervical spinal cord levels. Classically, this sensory information has been thought to travel through the posterior columns and synapse at the cuneate (upper extremity) and gracile (lower extremity) nuclei. Now it is known that other pathways exist as well, but for purposes of this discussion, only the classic spinal pathways are shown because the others are relatively unimportant. After synapsing, the information crosses and becomes part of the medial lemniscus, which rises through the whole brainstem and eventually synapses in the thalamus.

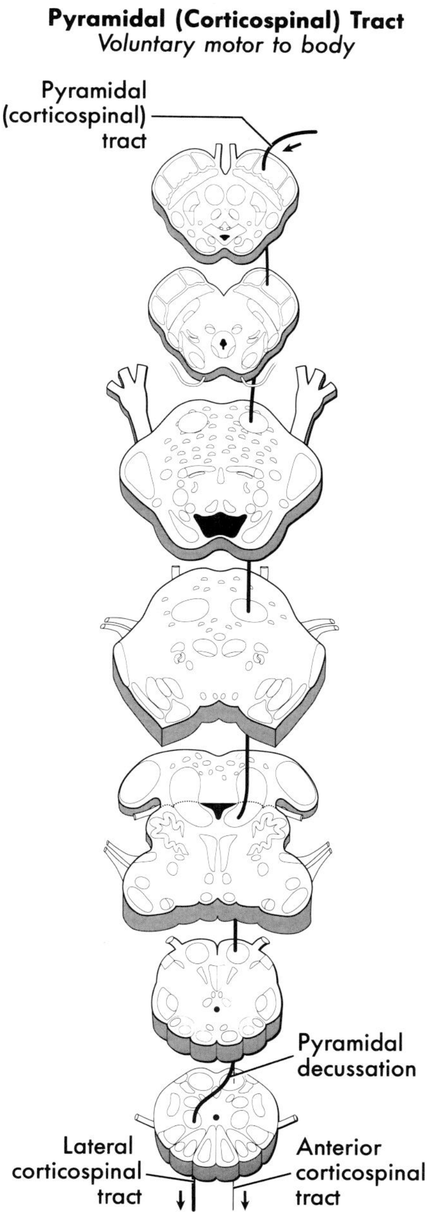

Figure 7-12 The major voluntary motor output travels through the corticospinal pathway. This pathway descends ipsilaterally, as shown, until it reaches the pyramidal decussation in the medulla, where most of it crosses to the opposite side, becoming the lateral corticospinal tract of the spinal cord. Some fibers do not cross (5% to 20%). These, which are more concerned with proximal (e.g., trunk) muscles than with those of the extremities, become the anterior corticospinal tract.

synapse at the submandibular ganglion and innervate the submandibular and sublingual salivary glands. Fibers of the *inferior salivatory nucleus* (cranial nerve IX) form the glossopharyngeal nerve and the otic ganglion, which innervates the parotid gland and the mucosa of the mouth. Fibers of the *dorsal motor nucleus of the vagus nerve* (cranial nerve X) form various vagal branches and ganglia in the walls of the abdominal and thoracic viscera (e.g., heart muscle, smooth muscle, glandular tissue).

The remainder of the descending preautonomic outflow that travels through the brainstem comes from the hypothalamus to the preganglionic autonomic neurons. Such descending pathways not only supply the previously mentioned cranial parasympathetic preganglionic neurons, but also extend to the spinal cord levels to supply the sympathetic nerves (first thoracic to second lumbar) and the sacral parasympathetic nerves. These are complicated, multisynaptic pathways that do not take a clearly defined route through the brainstem.

The descending influences on the autonomic system can be summarized as follows.

1. The *median forebrain bundle* projects to the midbrain ventral tegmental region, including the ventral (deep) tegmental nucleus, portions of the central gray matter, and other nearby regions. These then further project downward through largely multisynaptic pathways.
2. The *dorsolongitudinal fasciculus* conveys information from the medial and periventricular parts of the hypothalamus to the central gray matter and tectum of the midbrain. Some fibers may also extend to the dorsotegmental nucleus. Information then descends further through poorly understood pathways, often through parts of the reticular system.

One clinically interesting component of the autonomic downflow is the pupillodilator pathway and other sympathetic components that travel through the lateral part of the medulla. Damage to this region produces the *lateral medullary syndrome* (Wallenberg's syndrome), which is discussed in Chapter 8 (see also Table 7-6).

VASCULAR TERRITORIES

The vascular supply to the brainstem is variable. Therefore the patients with syndromes produced by occlusion of these branches show a wide range of symptomatology. This is manifested by some inconsistency in the definition of these syndromes among various neurology texts. For purposes of this chapter, the neurologic syndromes produced by occlusion of these branches are taken from Heilman et al.[26] (Table 7-6). The axial brainstem sections in the figures for this chapter are marked and indicate the general areas supplied by the major brainstem arteries.

◆ **TABLE 7-6** Syndromes Involving Vascular Territories of Brainstem

Vessel	Syndrome	Major symptoms	Major structures involved	
Medial penetrating midbrain arteries from basilar artery	Medial midbrain syndrome (Weber's syndrome)	Ipsilateral complete cranial nerve III palsy	CN III rootlets	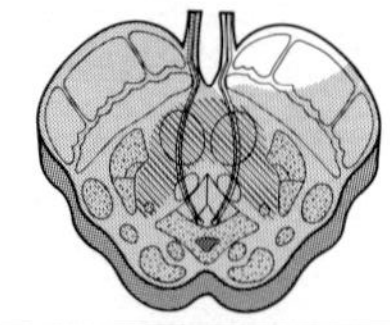
		Contralateral hemiplegia	Corticospinal and corticobulbar tracts	
Penetrating midbrain arteries from the basilar artery	Paramedial midbrain syndrome	Ipsilateral complete CN III palsy, so that eye looks down and laterally, lid has ptosis, and pupil is dilated and not responsive to light	Roots of CN III	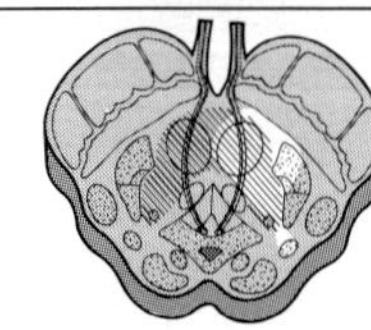
		Contralateral ataxia and intention tremor of arm	Red nucleus and decussation of superior cerebellar peduncle after its crossover (not shown)	
		Sometimes contralateral loss of position and vibration sensation	Medial lemniscus	
		Sometimes contralateral loss of pain and temperature sensation	Lateral spinothalamic tract and ventral secondary ascending tract of CN V	
Superior cerebellar artery	Superolateral pontine syndrome	Ipsilateral ataxia and intention tremor of arm and leg	Superior and/or middle cerebellar peduncle	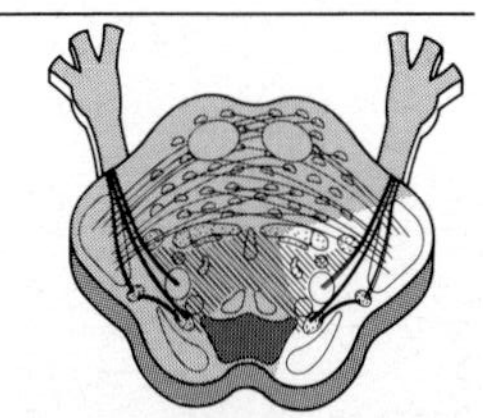
		Ipsilateral Horner's syndrome	Descending sympathetic fibers (not labeled)	
		Contralateral loss of pain and temperature sensation on face and body	Lateral spinothalamic and ventral ascending CN V fibers	
Medial penetrating pontine arteries from basilar artery	Medial pontine syndrome (Millard-Gubler syndrome, Gubler's syndrome)	Ipsilateral lateral rectus muscle palsy	CN VI	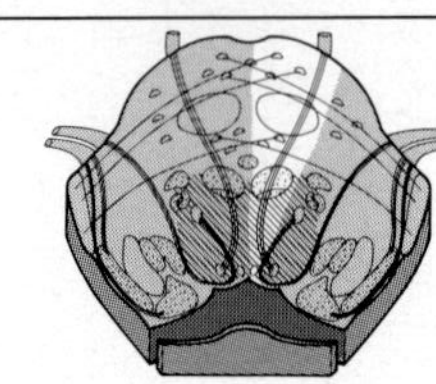
		Contralateral hemiplegia, with face usually involved	Corticospinal and corticobulbar tracts	
		Sometimes contralateral loss of position and vibration sensation	Medial lemniscus	
		Sometimes loss of adduction of ipsilateral eye during conjugate gaze	Medial longitudinal fasciculus	

Anteroinferior cerebellar artery (AICA)	Inferolateral pontine syndrome (Foville's syndrome)	Ipsilateral lower motor neuron facial weakness and loss of taste sensation on anterior two thirds of tongue	CN VII	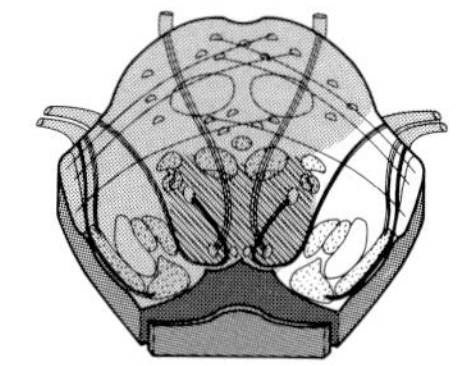
		Ipsilateral deafness	CN VIII	
		Ipsilateral loss of pain and temperature sensation on face	Descending CN V	
		Ipsilateral loss of horizontal conjugate gaze	Pontine paramedial reticular formation	
		Ipsilateral Horner's syndrome	Descending sympathetic tract (not labeled)	
		Contralateral loss of pain and temperature sensation of body	Lateral spinothalamic tract	
Anterior spinal artery	Medial medullary syndrome (Déjérine's syndrome)	Ipsilateral flaccid tongue weakness	CN XII	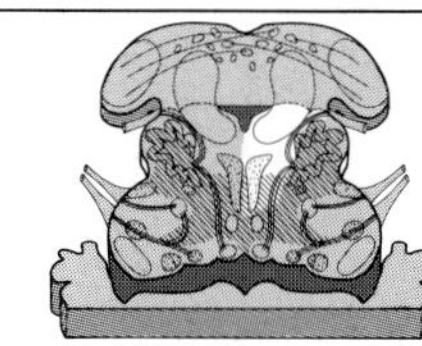
		Contralateral hemiplegia	Pyramidal tract	
		Sometimes contralateral loss of position and vibration sensation	Medial lemniscus	
Posteroinferior cerebellar artery (PICA) or vertebral artery	Lateral medullary syndrome (Wallenberg's syndrome)	Voice change from ipsilateral vocal cord paralysis	Nucleus ambiguus	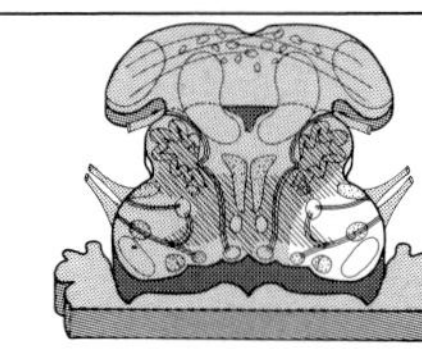
		Ipsilateral decreased gag response	Nucleus solitarius or roots of CN IX	
		Ipsilateral loss of pain and temperature sensation on face	Descending tract and nucleus of CN V	
		Ipsilateral Horner's syndrome	Descending sympathetic tract (not labeled)	
		Ipsilateral cerebellar findings	Inferior cerebellar peduncle	
		Contralateral loss of pain and temperature sensation of body	Lateral spinothalamic tract	
		Vertigo, nystagmus, vomiting	Vestibular nuclei	

Adapted with permission from Heilman KM, Watson RT, Green M: *Handbook for differential diagnosis of neurological signs and symptoms*, New York, 1977, Appleton-Century-Crofts.

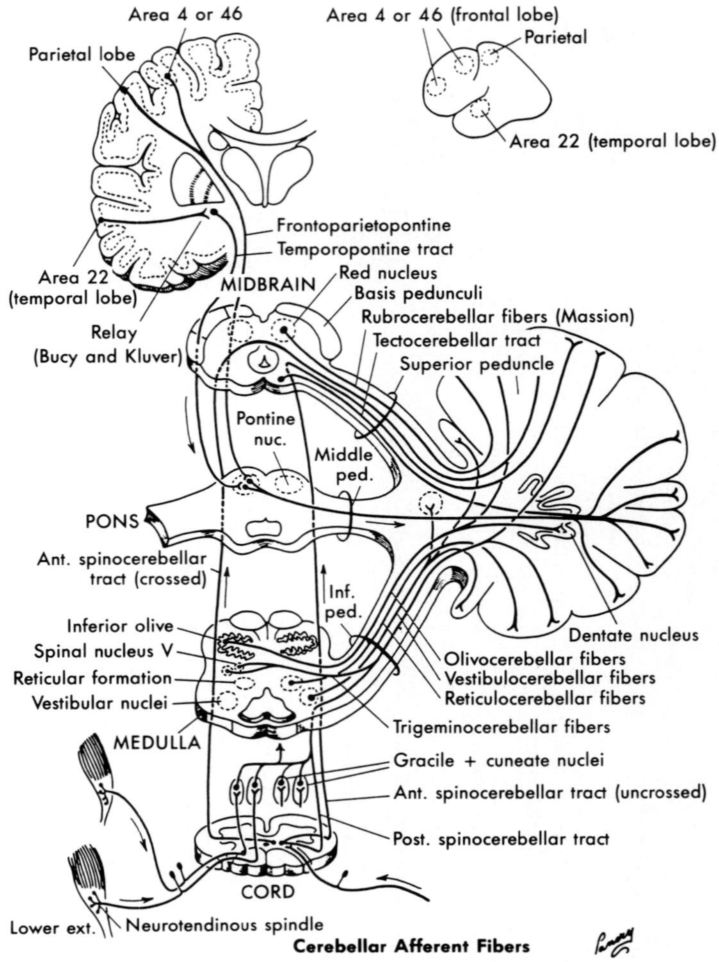

Figure 7-13 Afferent (incoming) cerebellar pathways. The cerebellum receives information from all three brainstem levels (midbrain, pons, medulla) via the superior, middle, and inferior cerebellar peduncles, respectively. The *inferior cerebellar peduncles* carry sensory information from the body (posterior spinocerebellar tracts) and head (trigeminocerebellar and vestibulocerebellar tracts), as well as more complex information from the reticular formation and the inferior olives. The *superior cerebellar peduncles* also carry sensation from the body (anterior spinocerebellar tracts) and contain fibers that transmit visual information, as well as data from the red nucleus and other areas. The *middle cerebellar peduncles* carry output from the cerebral cortex (pontocerebellar fibers, which mediate motor movement). (Reproduced with permission from Pansky B, Allen DJ: In *Review of neuroscience*, New York, 1980, Macmillan.)

REFERENCES

1. Enzmann DR, Rubin JB, O'Donohue J, et al: Use of cerebrospinal fluid gating to improve T2-weighted images, *Radiology* 162:768-773, 1987.
2. Mawad ME, Silver AJ, Hilal SK, et al: Computed tomography of the brain stem with intrathecal metrizamide. Part I. The normal brain stem, *AJNR* 4:1-11, 1983.
3. Elster AD, Richardson DN: Focal high signal on MR scans of the midbrain caused by enlarged perivascular spaces: MR-pathologic correlation, *AJNR* 11:1119-1122, 1990.
4. Koehler PR, Haughton VM, Daniels DL, et al: MR measurement of normal and pathologic brainstem diameters, *AJNR* 6:425-427, 1985.
5. Steele JR, Hoffman JC: Brainstem evaluation with CT cisternography, *AJNR* 1:521-526, 1980.
6. Abe S, Miyasaka K, Tashiro K, et al: Evaluation of the brainstem with high-resolution CT in cerebellar atrophic processes, *AJNR* 4:446-449, 1983.
7. Flannigan B, Bradley W, Mazziotta J, et al: Magnetic resonance imaging of the brainstem: normal structure and basic functional anatomy, *Radiology* 154:375-383, 1985.
8. Hirsch WL, Kemp SS, Martinez AJ, et al: Anatomy of the brainstem: correlation of *in vitro* MR images with histologic sections, *AJNR* 10:923-928, 1989.
9. Chakeres DW, Kapila A: Brainstem and related structures: normal CT anatomy using direct longitudinal scanning with metrizamide cisternography, *Radiology* 149:709-715, 1983.
10. Berns TF, Daniels DL, Williams AL, et al: Mesencephalic anatomy: demonstration by computed tomography, *AJNR* 2:65-67, 1981.

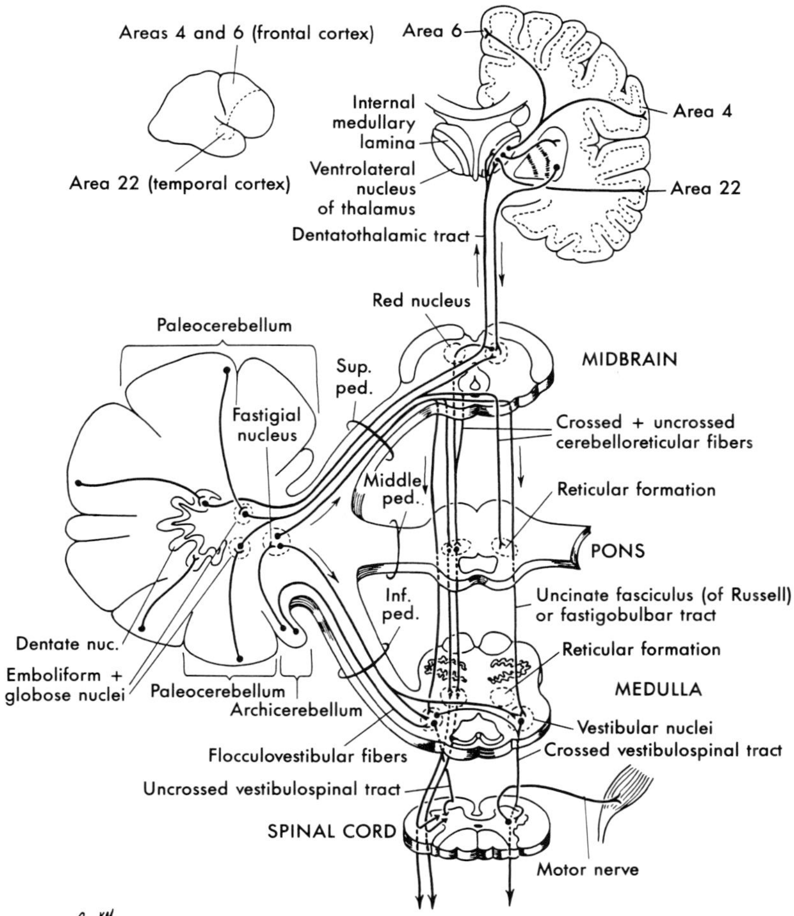

Figure 7-14 Efferent (outgoing) cerebellar pathways. The cerebellum sends information to only two brainstem levels: the midbrain (via the *superior cerebellar peduncle*) and the medulla (via the *inferior cerebellar peduncle*). Both these peduncules carry output to the vestibular system that influences balance and muscle tone. The superior cerebellar peduncle also sends considerable information to the basal ganglia, then to the cerebral cortex. These pathways travel near, but do not necessarily synapse in, the red nucleus of the midbrain. Some superior cerebellar output does synapse in (or near) the red nucleus, and much of it projects downward through the reticular formation to reach spinal levels. The basal ganglia, under the influence of the cerebral cortex as well as the cerebellum, feeds back into the downward-projecting midbrain levels (see Figure 7-13). (Reproduced with permission from Pansky B, Allen DJ: In *Review of neuroscience*, New York, 1980, Macmillan.)

11. Daniels DL, Williams AL, Haughton VM: Computed tomography of the medulla, *Radiology* 145:63-69, 1982.
12. Patten J: *Neurological differential diagnosis*. New York, 1977, Springer-Verlag.
13. Watson C: *Basic human neuroanatomy: an introductory atlas*, ed 3, Boston, 1985, Little, Brown.
14. Carpenter MB: *Human neuroanatomy*, ed 7, Baltimore, 1976, Williams & Wilkins.
15. Noback CR, Demarest RJ: *The human nervous system: basic principles of neurobiology*, ed 2, New York, 1975, McGraw-Hill.
16. Ingram WR: *A review of anatomical neurology*, Baltimore, 1976, University Park.
17. Brazis PW, Masdeu JC, Biller J: *Localization in clinical neurology*, Boston, 1985, Little, Brown.
18. Daube JR, Sandok BA, Reagan TJ, Westmoreland BF: *Medical neurosciences: an approach to anatomy, pathology, and physiology by systems and levels*, Boston, 1978, Little, Brown.
19. Lockhart RD, Hamilton GF, Fyfe FW: *Anatomy of the human body*, London, 1974, JB Lippincott.
20. DeArmond SJ, Fusco MM, Dewey MM: *Structure of the human brain: a photographic atlas*, ed 3, Oxford, 1989, Oxford University.
21. Haines DE: *Neuroanatomy: an atlas of structures, sections, and systems*, ed 2, Baltimore-Munich, 1987, Urban & Schwarzenberg.
22. Riley HA: *An atlas of the basal ganglia, brainstem and spinal cord*, Baltimore, 1943, Williams & Wilkins.
23. Stratton DB: *Neurophysiology*, New York, 1981, McGraw-Hill.
24. Han JS, Bonstelle CT, Kaufman B, et al: Magnetic resonance imaging in the evaluation of the brainstem, *Radiology* 150:705-712, 1984.

25. Solsberg MD, Fournier D, Potts DG: MR imaging of the excised human brainstem: a correlative neuroanatomic study, *AJNR* 11:1003-1013, 1990.
26. Heilman KM, Watson RT, Green M: *Handbook for differential diagnosis of neurological signs and symptoms,* New York, 1977, Appleton-Century-Crofts.
27. Wall M: Brainstem syndromes. In Bradley WG, editor: *Neurology in clinical practice,* Boston, 1991, Butterworth-Heinemann.
28. Pansky B, Allen DJ: The cerebellum. In *Review of neuroscience,* New York, 1980, Macmillan.
29. Gilman S, Newman SW: The cerebellum. In *Manter and Gatz's essentials of clinical neuroanatomy and neurophysiology,* Philadelphia, 1987, FA Davis.
30. Carpenter MB, Sutin J: The cerebellum. In *Human neuroanatomy,* ed 8, Baltimore, 1983, Williams & Wilkins.
31. Brodal A: The cerebellum. In: *Neurological anatomy in relation to clinical medicine,* ed 3, New York, 1981, Oxford University.
32. Wilson JD, Braunwald E, Isselbecher KJ: *Harrison's principles of internal medicine,* New York, 1991, McGraw-Hill.

INDEX TO THE ILLUSTRATIONS

Entries refer to figures in which the specific structures are labeled.

CHAPTER 8

L. Anne Hayman
Loren A. Rolak
John M. Gundzik
Robert B. Lufkin

Cranial Nerves

IMAGING TECHNIQUES

Relatively few imaging techniques can trace the complex anatomy of the cranial nerves. Intrathecal metrizamide-enhanced computed tomography (CT) and pneumoencephalography can outline the cranial nerves and adjacent brainstem, but these invasive procedures have been virtually replaced by magnetic resonance imaging (MRI). The MRI is noninvasive and affords excellent soft tissue contrast resolution in an unlimited variety of scanning planes. When specialized high-performance radiofrequency (RF) receiver coils and thin sections are used, the spatial resolution of MRI is superior to that of CT. Additionally, MR images are not degraded by the beam-hardening artifacts from the petrous bones that are often seen on CT scans.

Several technical factors must be carefully controlled to perform MR evaluation of the cranial nerves properly. They are usually best demonstrated on short TR/short TE images, but the largest cranial nerves may also be seen on long TR/long TE images (TR, repetition time; TE, echo delay time). Confusing cisternal artifacts caused by cerebrospinal fluid (CSF) pulsation may be minimized by the use of gradient moment nulling strategies, presaturation pulses, cardiac gating, or similar techniques. Imaging techniques with high in-plane spatial resolution and thin sections should be used to minimize partial-volume errors.

Table 8-1 describes the cisternal pathway of each cranial nerve and the imaging plane in which it can best be visualized. Specialized techniques have been proposed to evaluate better the cranial nerves in the region of the skull base, face, and neck. These techniques are beyond the scope of this text, which focuses on the brain. However, to assist the reader, these references are also listed in Table 8-1. The brainstem nuclei and their associated fiber tracts are generally not visible even on the long TR/TE images that optimize tissue contrast. MRI can be used to evaluate these areas adequately only if the imaging clinician accurately locates them by using some of the adjacent internal anatomic landmarks and surface configuration of the brainstem as a guide (see Chapters 6 and 7).

CT air cisternography is occasionally useful for evaluation of masses in the cerebellopontine angle cisterns and internal auditory canals when an MR scan is not definitive. Otherwise, the superior contrast resolution, multiplanar imaging capabilities, and lack of beam-hardening artifact make MRI the modality of choice for evaluation of cranial nerve pathology. Occasionally, MRI with intravenous contrast enhancement may be useful in identifying lesions involving cranial nerve nuclei or in the nerve. This is particularly true if the patient has a multiple sclerosis or viral inflammation of the nerve. MR procedures have thus far not been successful in selecting patients who might benefit from microvascular decompression of cranial nerve V.

◆ **TABLE 8-1** Imaging Cisternal Portions of the Cranial Nerves

Cranial nerve	Cisternal pathway	Optimum imaging plane	Optimum techniques (sources)
I (olfactory)	Olfactory groove below gyrus rectus of frontal lobe	Coronal	Reference 8
II (optic)	Enters optic canal and travels through suprasellar (chiasmatic) cistern to lateral geniculate body	Axial, coronal, sagittal	Chapter 18
III (oculomotor)	Exits interpeduncular fossa of midbrain and travels through prepontine cistern to lateral wall of cavernous sinus	Sagittal, coronal, axial	Chapter 18
IV (trochlear)*	Exits above lateral inferior colliculus, travels around midbrain in perimesencephalic cistern, through prepontine cistern to lateral wall of cavernous sinus	Sagittal, coronal	Chapter 18
V (trigeminal)	Exits lateral aspect of pons, travels through prepontine cistern and Meckel's cave to trigeminal ganglion	Axial, coronal, sagittal	References 9 and 10
VI (abducens)*	Exits at junction of pons and medulla (just above pyramid) and travels superiorly in prepontine cistern to enter cavernous sinus	Sagittal, axial	Chapter 18
VII and VIII (facial and vestibulocochlear)	Exits just lateral to cranial nerve VI (see above) and travels through cerebellopontine angle cistern to internal auditory canal	Axial, coronal, sagittal	References 11 to 22
IX, X, and XI (glossopharyngeal, vagus, and spinal accessory)	Exits medulla between olive and inferior cerebellar peduncle and travels to pars nervosa of jugular bulb	Axial, coronal	References 23 to 26
XII (hypoglossal)	Exits medulla between olive and pyramid (posterior olivary sulcus) and travels to hypoglossal canal	Axial, coronal	References 27 and 28

*These nerves are very small, and their cisternal portions are seldom visualized.

DEVELOPMENTAL ANATOMY

The brainstem contains various sensory and motor nuclei. Most of the cell groups are related to the cranial nerves and appear to have a random orientation. Understanding the development of these cell groups offers some insight into their general position in the brainstem.

Before the growth of the cerebral hemispheres, the cranial portion of the neural tube is the brainstem. This portion has the same basic structure as the spinal cord (i.e., a ventral plate that contains motor neurons and a dorsal plate that contains sensory neurons). However, continued asymmetric growth of the brainstem results in a bending of the cranial neural tube, which changes the location of the motor and sensory nuclei in the upper medulla and pons.

Figure 8-1 illustrates the location of motor and sensory cells as one proceeds rostrally along the brainstem. At the level of the closed medulla, the structural plan of the spinal cord is preserved. At the open medullary level, the brainstem is flattened by the pontine flexure. This displaces the dorsal sensory nuclei laterally. In addition, some of these sensory neurons migrate ventrally to form the olivary nuclei dorsal to the motor nuclei, thereby further disrupting the simple spinal pattern. As one progresses rostrally into the pons, the disruption caused by the pontine flexure completely reverses the spinal pattern (i.e., the sensory nuclei are now ventral to the motor nuclei). The spinal pattern is reinstated at the midbrain level, and the motor nuclei are *again* found ventral to the sensory nuclei.

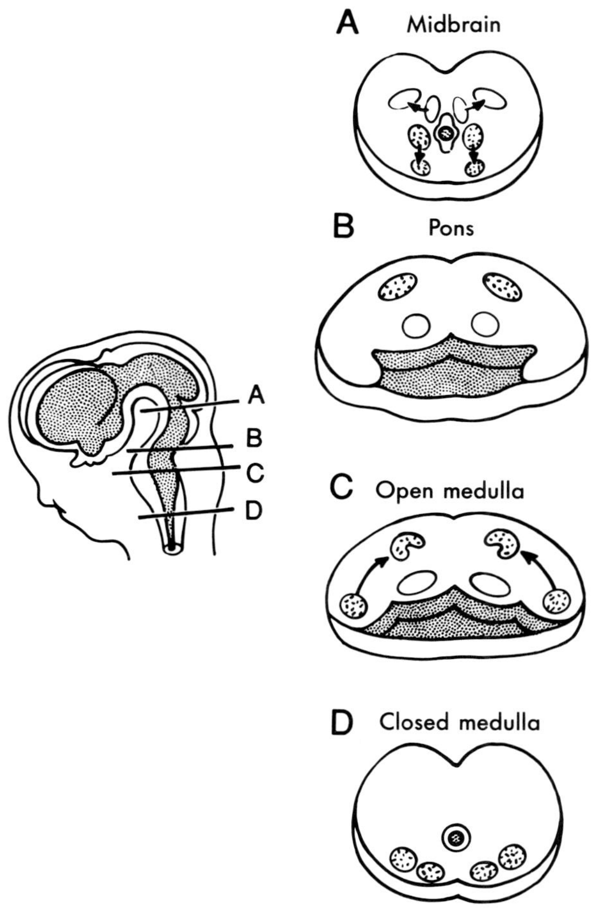

Figure 8-1 Axial brainstem schematics of the fetal development of cranial nerve nuclei III to XII illustrate the disruption of the spinal pattern of ventral motor nuclei (*open circle*) and dorsal sensory nuclei (*lightly stippled areas*) at the pontine flexure (**B** and **C**). Note that the spinal pattern of dorsal sensory nuclei is preserved in the midbrain and closed medulla (**A** and **D**). The cerebrospinal fluid (CSF) spaces are also shown (*heavily stippled areas*).

FUNCTIONAL-ANATOMIC CORRELATIONS

This section is designed to provide the reader a compact assessment of only the clinically most significant functions of each cranial nerve. The diagrams of the anatomic pathways for each nerve have been tailored to illustrate only these clinically relevant features. The following section was compiled after consulting various anatomic texts and reviews.[1-7] For completeness, Table 8-2 lists each cranial nerve and all its functions. To assist in tailoring the imaging study for patients in whom the only clinical information provided is a neurologic syndrome (rather than a specific cranial nerve deficit), Table 8-3 indicates the appropriate anatomic areas to be examined, as well as clinical features of each syndrome.

In the ensuing discussion, those nerves that are closely related anatomically, functionally, and/or clinically are discussed as a group. This causes cranial nerve (CN) VI to appear before CN V nerve in the following text. The analysis of each cranial nerve describes the anatomic location of clinically relevant nuclei and their connections with other brain regions. These connections are often complex and cross the midline. Therefore the accompanying illustrations diagram only *one* of each of the paired cranial nerves. The text also describes the neurologic symptoms caused by a lesion at various points along the pathway of the nerve.

◆ **TABLE 8-2** Summary of Cranial Nerve Functions

Nerve	Component	Function
Olfactory (I)	Special sensory (special afferent)	To provide sensation of olfaction, or smell
Optic (II)	Special sensory (special afferent)	To convey visual information from retina
Oculomotor (III)	Somatic motor (general somatic efferent)	To supply superior levator palpebrae, superior rectus, medial rectus, inferior rectus, and inferior oblique muscles of eye
	Visceral motor (general visceral efferent)	To provide parasympathetic supply to constrictor pupillae and ciliary muscles via ciliary ganglion
Trochlear (IV)	Somatic motor (general somatic efferent)	To supply superior oblique muscle of eye
Trigeminal (V)	Branchial motor (special visceral efferent)	To innervate muscles of mastication: tensor tympani, tensor veli palatini, mylohyoid, and anterior belly of digastric
	General sensory (general somatic afferent)	To provide general sensation from face and scalp as far as top of head, conjunctiva, eyeball, mucous membranes of paranasal sinuses, nasal and oral cavities including tongue and teeth, part of external aspect of tympanic membrane, and from meninges of anterior and middle cranial fossae
Abducens (VI)	Somatic motor (general somatic efferent)	To supply lateral rectus muscle of eye
Facial (VII)	Branchial motor (special visceral efferent)	To supply stapedius, stylohyoid, posterior belly of digastric muscles; and muscles of facial expression: buccinator, platysma, and occipitalis
	Visceral motor (general visceral efferent)	To stimulate lacrimal, submandibular, and sublingual glands, as well as mucous membranes of nose and hard and soft palates
	General sensory (general somatic afferent)	To supply skin of concha of auricle, a small area of skin behind ear, and possibly to supplement cranial nerve V_3, which supplies wall of acoustic meatus and external tympanic membrane
	Special sensory (special afferent)	To provide taste from anterior two thirds of tongue and hard and soft palates
Vestibulocochlear (VIII)	Special sensory (special afferent)	To convey auditory information from cochlea To convey balance information from semicircular canals
Glossopharyngeal (IX)	Branchial motor (special visceral efferent)	To supply striated muscle, the stylopharyngeus
	Visceral motor (general visceral efferent)	To supply otic ganglion, which sends fibers to stimulate parotid gland
	Visceral sensory (general visceral afferent)	To carry sensation (subconscious) from carotid body and from carotid sinus
	General sensory (general somatic afferent)	To provide general sensation from posterior one third of tongue, skin of external ear, and internal surface of tympanic membrane
	Special sensory (special afferent)	To provide sensation from taste receptors in posterior one third of tongue
Vagus (X)	Branchial motor (special visceral efferent)	To supply striated muscles of pharynx, tongue (palatoglossus), and larynx (except stylopharyngeus [IX] and tensor veli palatini [V_3])
	Visceral motor (general viscerent efferent)	To stimulate smooth muscle and glands of pharynx, larynx, and thoracic and abdominal viscera
	Visceral sensory (visceral afferent)	To carry sensation from larynx, trachea, esophagus, thoracic and abdominal viscera, stretch receptors in walls of aortic arch, and chemoreceptors in aortic bodies adjacent to arch
	General sensory (general somatic afferent)	To provide sensation from skin at back of ear and in external acoustic meatus, part of external surface of tympanic membrane, and pharynx
Spinal accessory (XI)	Branchial motor (special visceral efferent)	To supply sternocleidomastoid and trapezius muscles
Hypoglossal (XII)	Somatic motor (general somatic efferent)	To supply all intrinsic and extrinsic muscles of tongue except palatoglossus

Adapted with permission from Wilson-Paules L, Akesson EJ, Stewart PA: *Cranial nerves: anatomy and clinical comments*, Toronto, 1988, BC Decker.

◆ **TABLE 8-3** Cranial Nerve, Brainstem, and Related Syndromes

Syndrome	Anatomy and pathology of lesion	Clinical features	Comments
Avellis' syndrome	Vascular infarction of tegmentum of medulla from vertebral artery thrombosis	Ipsilateral paralysis of soft palate, pharynx, and vocal cord from involvement of nucleus ambiguus; contralateral loss of pain and temperature sense from involvement of lateral spinothalamic tract; occasionally, contralateral hemianesthesia from involvement of medial lemniscus. Horner's syndrome may be present from involvement of descending sympathetic pathways.	
Benedikt's syndrome	Lesion in tegmentum of midbrain involving red nucleus, brachium conjunctivum, fascicles of CN III, and corticospinal tract	Oculomotor palsy with contralateral hyperkinesia, ataxia, and intention tremor involving arm only; contralateral hemiparesis	
Central pontine myelinolysis syndrome	Selective, noninflammatory demyelination with relative sparing of axons and neurons in variable area in base of pons	Rapid onset of flaccid quadriplegia, with paralysis of bulbar muscles and inability to talk, chew, or swallow. Pupillary reflexes, movements of eyes and lids, and corneal reflexes may be normal. Patients generally are critically ill. Clinical picture may simulate locked-in syndrome. CT may show hypodense lesion in pons.	Etiologic factors are diverse. Nutritional deficiency in alcoholism is most frequent cause. Severe hyponatremia has been shown to induce syndrome clinically and experimentally.
Claude's syndrome	Lesion in tegmentum of midbrain involving red nucleus, brachium conjunctivum, and fascicles of CN III	Ipsilateral oculomotor palsy and contralateral cerebellar ataxia and tremor	Minor variant of Benedikt's syndrome
Collet-Sicard syndrome	Lesions in retropharyngeal and retroparotid space in high neck, such as tumors of parotid gland or metastatic tumor in lymph nodes; invasive tumors at base of skull near jugular foramen and anterior condylar canal	Paralysis of CN IX, X, XI, and XII	
Duane's syndrome (retraction syndrome)	Etiology obscure. Aplasia of CN VI with anomalous innervation of lateral rectus muscle by CN III or fibrosis of lateral rectus and levator muscles are postulated as possibilities.	Limitation of lateral gaze, widening of palpebral fissure on abduction, and narrowing of fissure during adduction	Despite apparent limitation of lateral gaze in affected eye, patient does not complain of diplopia.

Reproduced and modified with permission from Rengachary SS: In Wilkins RH, Rengachary SS, editors: *Neurosurgery*, New York, 1988. McGraw-Hill.

Continued.

◆ **TABLE 8-3** Cranial Nerve, Brainstem, and Related Syndromes—cont'd

Syndrome	Anatomy and pathology of lesion	Clinical features	Comments
Foster Kennedy's syndrome	Large olfactory groove or medial third sphenoidal wing tumor, usually a meningioma	Ipsilateral anosmia resulting from pressure on olfactory tract; ipsilateral central scotoma and optic atrophy from pressure on cranial nerve (CN) II; contralateral papilledema from increased intracranial pressure; occasionally ipsilateral proptosis from invasion of orbit by tumor	Very rare syndrome, especially in view of early detection of intracranial masses with CT
Foville's syndrome (anteroinferior cerebellar artery syndrome)	Lesion in dorsolateral pontine tegmentum	Ipsilateral paralysis of lateral gaze resulting from involvement of para-abducens area, ipsilateral lower-motor-neuron type facial palsy from involvement of CN VII nucleus, ipsilateral Horner's syndrome from involvement of descending sympathetic pathways in reticular formation, ipsilateral analgesia of face from involvement of descending tract of CN V, and ipsilateral deafness from involvement of auditory pathways	Incomplete expression of this clinical syndrome frequently occurs.
Gradenigo's syndrome	Initial lesion is usually an acute mastoiditis. If uncontrolled, infection spreads to involve petrous temporal bone up to its apex (apical petrositis); epidural abscess may form at this location. Infection may then extend into intradural space.	In patients with known acute mastoiditis, onset of pain around eye and forehead suggests irritation of gasserian ganglion. Corneal anesthesia may be present. Diplopia results from CN VI palsy. CN VIII may be involved infrequently.	Rarely, tumors at petrous apex (meningioma, trigeminal neurinoma) may give rise to this syndrome.
Jackson's syndrome	Vascular infarction of tegmentum of medulla	Involvement of nuclei of CN X, XI (nucleus ambiguus), and XII, resulting in ipsilateral paralysis of palate, pharynx, larynx, tongue, and sternocleidomastoid and trapezius muscles.	
Locked-in syndrome (pseudocoma)	Lesion in base of pons from basilar artery thrombosis, trauma, or neoplasm. Such a lesion spares pathways for somatic sensation and reticular activating system responsible for consciousness but disrupts corticobulbar and corticospinal pathways.	All motor functions are absent except for ocular and eyelid movements. Patient is speechless and motionless but yet may respond to simple questions requiring "yes" and "no" answers by blinking once or twice when instructed to do so.	Terms *coma vigil* and *akinetic mutism* have been used synonymously with locked-in syndrome. Unfortunately, however, the former terms have also been used to describe patients with large bifrontal lesions (butterfly glioblastoma) or bilateral cingulate lesions who remain speechless and immobile although motor and sensory pathways are intact.
Millard-Gubler syndrome (Gubler's syndrome)	Lesion in ventral paramedian pons, usually an ischemic infarct, affecting CN VI and VII nuclei and corticospinal tract	Ipsilateral lateral rectus weakness and facial paralysis of lower-motor-neuron type with contralateral hemiplegia	

Reproduced and modified with permission from Rengachary SS: In Wilkins RH, Rengachary SS, editors: *Neurosurgery*, New York, 1988. McGraw-Hill.

◆ **TABLE 8-3** Cranial Nerve, Brainstem, and Related Syndromes—cont'd

Syndrome	Anatomy and pathology of lesion	Clinical features	Comments
Nothnagel's syndrome	Lesion in tectum of midbrain	Unilateral oculomotor palsy combined with ipsilateral cerebellar ataxia resulting from involvement of CN III and brachium conjunctivum	
Parinaud's syndrome (sylvian aqueduct syndrome)	Lesion around tectum (superior colliculus) of midbrain, such as pineal or posterior third ventricular tumor; may also result from vascular lesion or demyelinating disease	Paralysis of conjugate movements of eyes in vertical plane. Patient unable to elevate eyes voluntarily or elevate and depress eyes. Pupils may be dilated and fail to react to light. Papilledema may be present from obstructive hydrocephalus.	Often associated with convergence spasm and reaction nystagmus. Skew deviation may represent a unilateral variant of Parinaud's syndrome. Passive head movements may include vertical eye movements in patient who may be unable to look upward voluntarily. This confirms clinical notion that Parinaud's syndrome results from supranuclear vertical gaze palsy.
Raymond-Cestan syndrome	Same as for Raymond's syndrome, plus ipsilateral CN VII palsy		Varient of Raymond's syndrome
Raymond's syndrome	Lesion in ventral paramedian pons, usually an ischemic infarct, affecting CN VI nucleus and corticospinal tract	Ipsilateral lateral rectus weakness and contralateral hemiplegia	Minor variant of the Millard-Gubler syndrome
Steele-Richardson-Olszewski syndrome (progressive supranuclear palsy)	Degenerative changes in basal ganglia, brainstem, and cerebellum	Supranuclear ophthalmoplegia, especially for downward gaze. With progression of disease, there is supranuclear paresis of other eye movements and muscles of facial expression, speech, and deglutition. There may be dystonia of neck muscles, masklike facies, and rigidity in muscles. Progressive dementia may occur.	Thought to be related to Parkinson's disease
Tapia's syndrome	Parotid or other tumors or penetrating injuries to high cervical region	Vagal and hypoglossal paralysis with or without involvement of CN XI	Tapia's syndrome or vagohypoglossal palsy may also result from intrinsic lesion in medulla.
Tolosa-Hunt syndrome (painful ophthalmoplegia)	Indolent granuloma of unknown etiology around anterior cavernous sinus, superior orbital fissure, and orbital apex	Presents with steady "gnawing" or "boring" pain behind eye and in forehead. Pain usually precedes ophthalmoplegia by several days or may not appear until sometime later. Neurologic involvement may begin in any of the cranial nerves passing through cavernous sinus: III, IV, VI, or first division of CN V. Periarterial sympathetic fibers and CN II may be involved. Spontaneous remission occurs, sometimes with residual neurologic deficit. Attacks may occur at intervals of months or years.	Differential diagnosis includes collagen diseases (temporal arteritis, periarteritis nodosa), cavernous carotid aneurysm, diabetes, lymphoma, carcinoma, meningioma, specific granulomata such as syphilitic periostitis, and ophthalmoplegic migraine. Diagnosis of Tolosa-Hunt syndrome is established through process of exclusion and rapid response to administration of steroids. Carotid angiography may show irregular narrowing of carotid siphon. Orbital venography may show venous occlusions.

Continued.

◆ **TABLE 8-3** Cranial Nerve, Brainstem, and Related Syndromes—cont'd

Syndrome	Anatomy and pathology of lesion	Clinical features	Comments
Vernet's syndrome (jugular foramen syndrome)	Tumors (glomus jugulare tumor, metastatic tumor, meningioma); basilar skull fracture across jugular foramen	Paralysis of CN IX, X, and XI; possible occlusion of jugular bulb	
Villaret's syndrome	Same as for Collet-Sicard syndrome	In addition to cranial nerve paralyses described in Collet-Sicard syndrome, cervical sympathetic paralysis results in Horner's syndrome	
Wallenberg's syndrome (lateral medullary syndrome, posteroinferior cerebellar artery syndrome)	Infarction of dorsolateral medulla from atheromatous occlusion of vertebral artery or posteroinferior cerebellar artery, more often the former; rarely, results from aneurysms, intramedullary hematomas, or metastatic neoplasms	Onset is acute with ipsilateral facial pain and paresthesias resulting from involvement of descending tract and nucleus of CN V. Intense vertigo and vomiting may occur from involvement of the inferior vestibular nucleus and its central connections. Impairment of swallowing and hoarseness of voice result from involvement of nucleus ambiguus and motor paralysis of CN IX, X, and XI. Involvement of spinocerebellar tract, inferior cerebellar peduncle, and inferior vestibular nuclei may result in nystagmus, ipsilateral dysmetria, intention tremor, and ataxia with tendency to fall toward side of lesion. Ipsilateral Horner's syndrome results from destruction of descending sympathetic pathways in medullary reticular formation. Loss of pain and temperature sensation in ipsilateral half of face and contralateral half of body results from destruction of descending trigeminal pathways and spinothalamic tract.	Syndrome has also been reported from vertebral artery occlusion following chiropractic manipulation, yoga exercises, and trauma to head and neck.
Weber's syndrome (superior alternating hemiplegia)	Lesion in cerebral peduncle of midbrain affecting pyramidal tract and exiting fascicles of CN III.	Ipsilateral oculomotor palsy and contralateral hemiplegia	

Cranial Nerve I (Olfactory)

The pathway of CN I is best illustrated by a schematic basal view of the brain (Figure 8-2). Impulses from the olfactory epithelium of the nasal cavity are carried by special sensory nerves that join into 20 or fewer bundles and perforate the cribriform plate of the skull and attach to the olfactory bulb. The secondary sensory neurons for smell are in the olfactory bulb, and their projections are actually a central nervous system tract, even though they are sometimes referred to as the olfactory "nerve." This olfactory tract subdivides into three olfactory striae: the medial, intermediate, and lateral. The thin gray matter covering the medial and lateral striae has been termed the *olfactory gyri*. The *medial striae* enter the anterior commissure and communicate with nuclear cells in the opposite olfactory bulb. The *intermediate striae* (not shown in Figure 8-2) enter the olfactory trigone in the region of the anterior perforated substance. The *lateral striae* primarily enter the amygdala.

The inability to detect an odor *(anosmia)* indicates a peripheral lesion in the olfactory pathway (mucosa, olfactory nerves, bulb or tract). Clinically significant lesions are usually bilateral and are caused by trauma damaging the olfactory fibers. Such patients generally have anosmia but may complain of *parosmia* (a perverted sense of smell) instead. The gradual onset of unilateral anosmia is often caused by a subfrontal tumor that may also produce other symptoms (see Foster Kennedy's syndrome in Table 8-3). Cortical lesions per se cannot produce anosmia. However, since the olfactory fibers project to the uncus, a seizure focus in this region may produce "uncinate fits," in which the patient describes a powerful, usually unpleasant smell or taste. This may be followed by other seizure manifestations, such as loss of consciousness, chewing, or smacking of the lips.

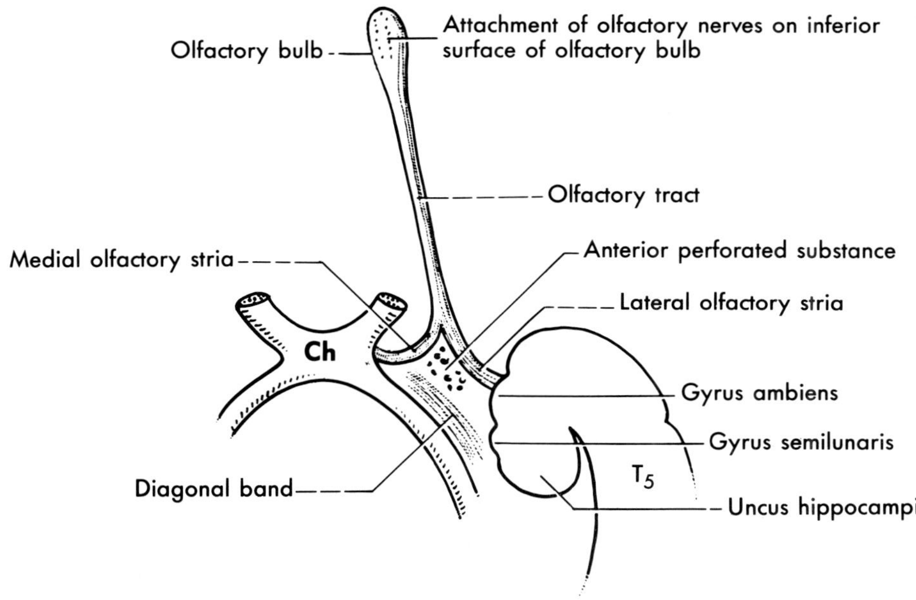

Figure 8-2 Schematic of the olfactory pathways (CN I) on the basal surface of the brain. The medial olfactory striae enter the anterior commissure. They interconnect the anterior olfactory nuclei present at the base of the olfactory bulb. The lateral olfactory striae enter the ipsilateral amygdala. The minor contribution of the intermediate olfactory striae to the ipsilateral anterior perforated substance has been omitted in this diagram. For orientation, the fibers of the optic chiasm (*Ch*) and the diagonal band (a continuation of the paraterminal gyrus) are shown. (Reproduced with permission from Bossy J: *Atlas of neuroanatomy and special sense organs*, Philadelphia, 1970, WB Saunders.)

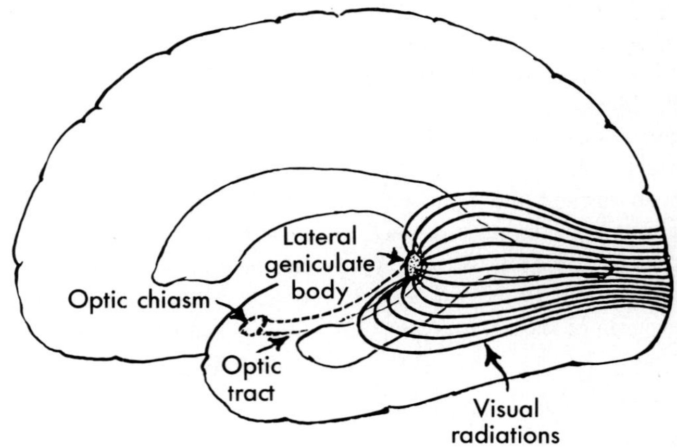

Figure 8-3 Schematic lateral view of the brain shows the pathway of the optic tract (CN II) from the chiasm to the calcarine cortex of the occipital lobe. Note that the optic radiations are closely related to the walls of the lateral ventricle. Those that encircle the anterior aspect of the temporal horn of the lateral ventricle are referred to as Meyer's loop.

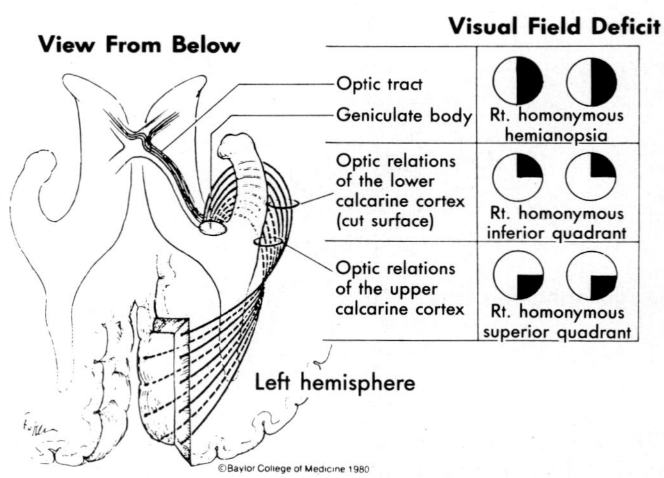

Figure 8-4 Schematic of the brain from below shows the pathway of the optic tract (CN II) from the chiasm to the calcarine cortex. The visual field deficits that occur from disruptions of various portions of the tract are shown. (Reproduced with permission from Hayman LA, Berman SA, Hinck VC: AJNR 2:219-225, 1981.)

Cranial Nerve II (Optic)

The optic nerves are technically not nerves. They are actually evaginated fiber tracts and, unlike true cranial nerves, the optic nerves can be involved in central nervous system diseases such as multiple sclerosis and glial neoplasia. Figure 8-3 is a schematic lateral diagram of the brain that illustrates the path of the optic fibers as they continue beyond the chiasm as bilateral optic tracts to terminate in the lateral geniculate bodies. The optic radiations then course over the tail of the caudate nucleus and the temporal horn of the lateral ventricle. The anterior portion of these fibers is referred to as *Meyer's loop* (Meyer-Archambault loop). The optic fibers reach the calcarine portion of the occipital cortex by closely following the lateral walls of the temporal horn and atrium of the lateral ventricle. They travel superiorly, laterally, and inferiorly, encircling all but the medial surface of the occipital horn of the ventricle.

Damage to these fibers causes visual loss, the precise nature of which is determined by the specific location of the lesion, as shown in Figure 8-4. The anatomy of these "nerves," as depicted on the planar scans within the suprasellar cistern, is reviewed in detail in Chapter 18.

Ocular Nerve Group: Cranial Nerves III, IV, and VI (Oculomotor, Trochlear, Abducens)

These cranial nerves are considered as a group because each controls muscles that move the eyes and because each travels in the lateral wall of the cavernous sinus to reach the orbital apex. Clinically, a patient may have either an isolated nerve deficit or a deficit caused by a lesion that affects more than one of these cranial nerves. The imaging implications of each of these presentations are discussed in this section.

Many lesions that affect eye movements occur in one of three regions: the cavernous sinus or superior orbital fissure, the frontal lobe, and the periaqueductal gray matter. The distinguishing clinical features present in each instance are discussed separately. A lesion in the cavernous sinus or the superior orbital fissure can damage all three nerves that move the eye. These lesions can be localized by the clinician because they usually also involve the first and/or second divisions of CN V, which mediates facial sensation. The anatomy of this region is discussed in detail in Chapter 17.

The frontal lobe (via the corticomesencephalic portion of the pyramidal system) helps regulate the motor nuclei of CN III, IV, and VI. The frontal cortex (and its connecting tract) allows the patient to turn the eyes voluntarily to the opposite side. The left frontal lobe turns the eyes to the right, and vice versa. After sustaining a lesion in one frontal lobe, the patient may not be able to look in the direction opposite the lesion. If this occurs, both eyes may be deviated to the side of the lesion by the unopposed action of the normal frontal lobe so that the patient "looks at his or her (frontal lobe or pyramidal tract) lesion." Thus a patient with a left frontal lobe stroke may have a right hemiparesis, and the eyes will look to the left.

In addition to the frontal lobe connections that control voluntary eye movement (see previous discussion), CN III, IV, and VI are interconnected via brainstem pathways. The gray matter around the aqueduct coordinates vertical gaze by way of its connections to the nuclei of CN III and IV. Quadrigeminal plate lesions that compress this region may affect the patient's ability to direct the eyes upward (see Parinaud's syndrome in Table 8-3). The coordination of lateral gaze can be affected if the connections between the CN III and VI nuclei are interrupted. Lesions in the (paired) medial longitudinal fasciculus or in the pontine reticular formation will disrupt these connections.

In addition to these regions, lesions in either the cisterns or the brainstem nuclei of the CN III, IV, and VI may cause an isolated, complete deficit in the function of that cranial nerve. Identical symptoms can also be produced by lesions distal to the skull base, although peripheral lesions are more likely to cause a partial loss of function.

Cranial Nerve III (Oculomotor)

The pathway of the motor components of CN III is illustrated on the schematic axial and coronal drawings (Figure 8-5, *A* and *B*). Impulses from the motor cortex of both hemispheres travel via the internal capsule to the ipsilateral superior colliculus. These fibers cross between the red nuclei in what is termed the *dorsal tegmental decussation*. They travel down the brainstem in the paramedian raphe to synapse in the paramedian pontine reticular formation (PPRF). Both ipsilateral and contralateral fibers then ascend in the medial longitudinal fasciculus (MLF) to reach the motor nucleus of CN III. Fibers from the nucleus exit anteriorly at the pontomidbrain junction between the superior cerebellar artery and the posterior cerebral artery. They traverse the interpeduncular cistern to reach the lateral wall of the cavernous sinus. The oculomotor nerves pass anterior and superolateral to the cavernous carotid arteries.

Damage to CN III causes predictable neurologic symptoms. An isolated CN III palsy usually causes outward deviation of the eye (external strabismus), inability to turn the eye inward, drooping of the upper eyelid (ptosis), and inability to raise the lid. Pupillary changes help to localize the lesion further. For example, dilation of the pupil (mydriasis) results from compression of the parasympathetic fibers that surround the nerve.

Patients with symptoms of a CN III palsy in which no lesion is identified by imaging studies may have a peripheral lesion caused by infarction of the nerve from occlusion of the vasonervorum. In these cases the parasympathetic fibers that supply the pupillary constrictor muscles are spared, and the pupil is not dilated. This sparing is virtually never seen in CN III lesions caused by extrinsic compression. The most common cause of a CN III palsy is compression of the nerve in the cisternal or cavernous sinus region, often by an aneurysm of the circle of Willis.

Nuclear lesions of CN III may have the same clinical presentation as peripheral lesions, but they are rarer. A lesion that completely destroys the CN III nucleus results in ophthalmoplegia on the side of the lesion, but nuclear lesions also produce deficits in the opposite eye. With this type of lesion, bilateral ptosis occurs because only a single levator nucleus is present in the brainstem. Brainstem lesions that cause CN III dysfunction are often observed in syndromes that produce wider areas of deficit (see Benedikt's and Weber's syndromes in Table 8-3).

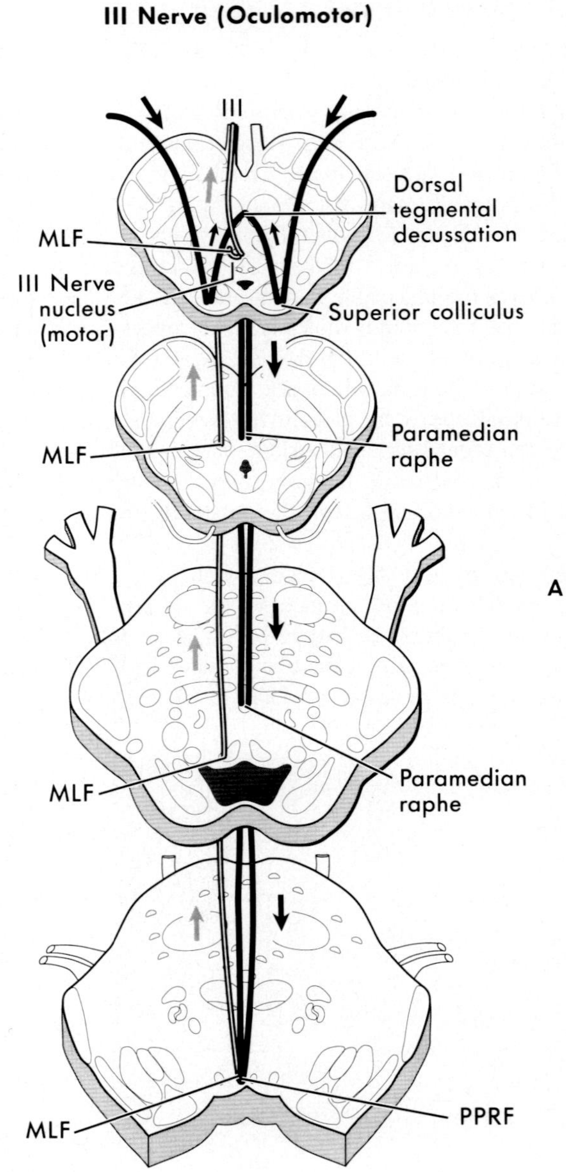

Figure 8-5 For legend see opposite page.

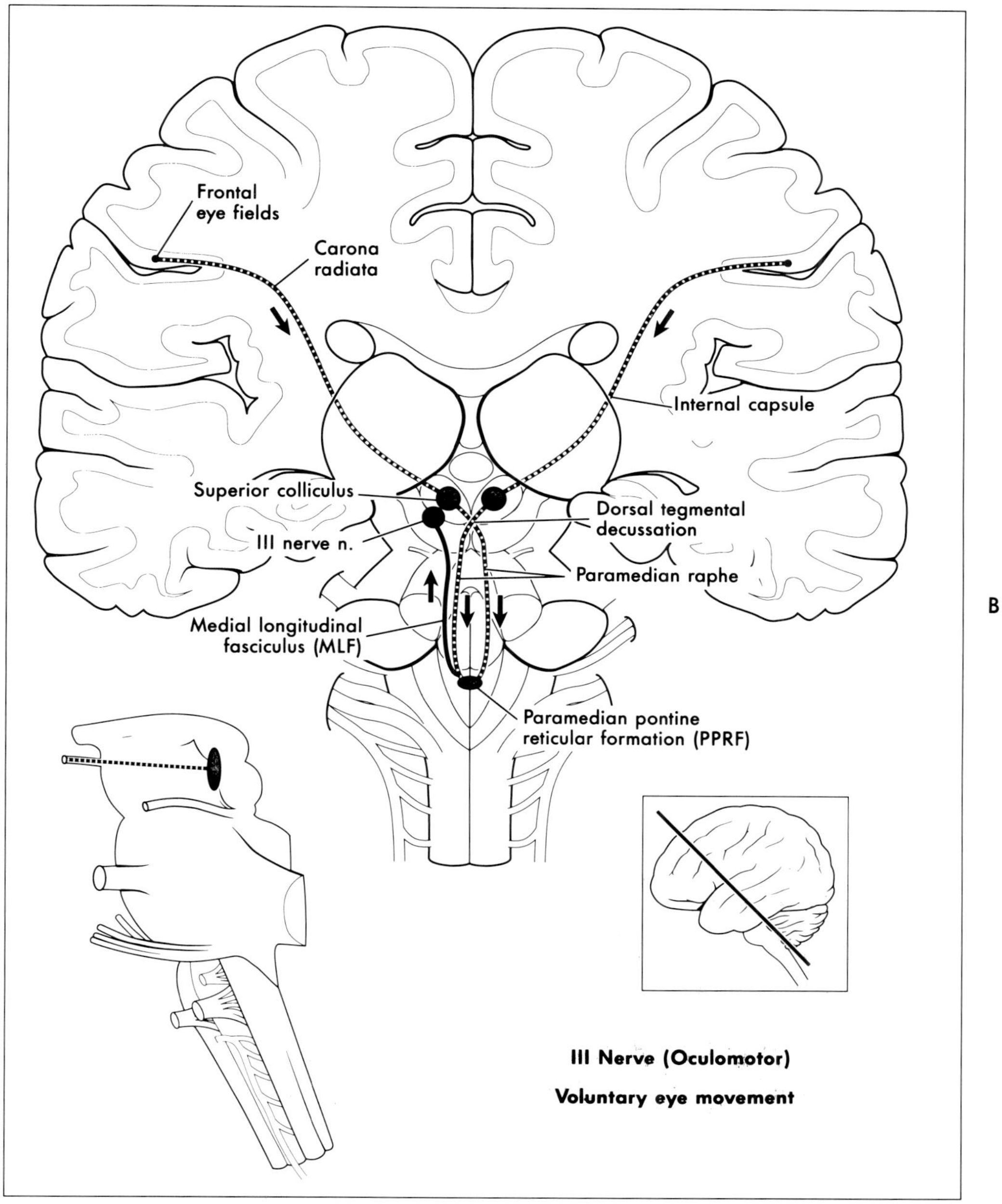

Figure 8-5 **A,** Brainstem pathway of CN III (oculomotor). Individual structures in each brainstem slice are labeled in Chapter 7. **B,** Coronal schematic shows pathway of CN III. Sagittal schematic shows only the location of CN III and its brainstem nucleus.

Cranial Nerve IV (Trochlear)

The pathway of CN IV is illustrated on the schematic axial and coronal drawings (Figure 8-6, *A* and *B*). Impulses from the motor cortex in both hemispheres travel via the internal capsule to the ipsilateral superior colliculus. These fibers cross between the red nuclei in the dorsal tegmental decussation. They travel down the brainstem in the paramedian raphe to synapse in the parapontine reticular formation (PPRF). Both ipsilateral and contralateral fibers then ascend in the medial longitudinal fasciculus (MLF) to reach the motor nucleus of CN IV. Fibers from the nucleus cross the midline and exit from the posterior surface of the midbrain tectum below the inferior colliculus. These fibers travel around the brainstem and enter the cavernous sinus. They can be found lateral to the carotid artery and inferior to the oculomotor nerve (CN III).

An isolated lesion of CN IV (which supplies the superior oblique muscle) occurs infrequently. When it does occur, ability to turn the eye downward and inward is compromised. In severe cases the patient may tilt the head to the unaffected side to align the eyes and achieve binocular vision.

IV Nerve (Trochlear)

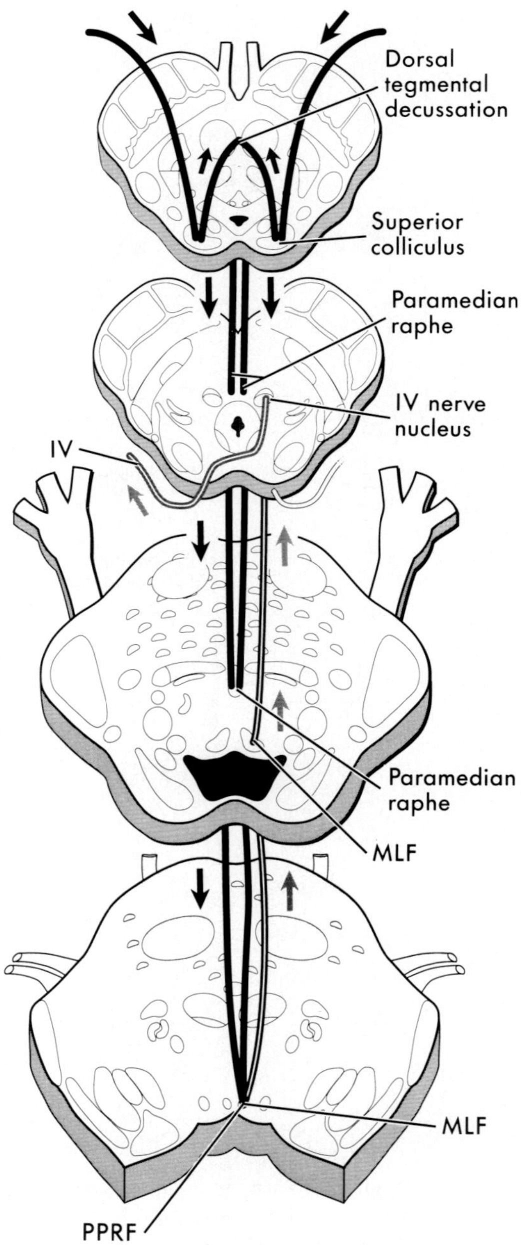

A

Figure 8-6 For legend see opposite page.

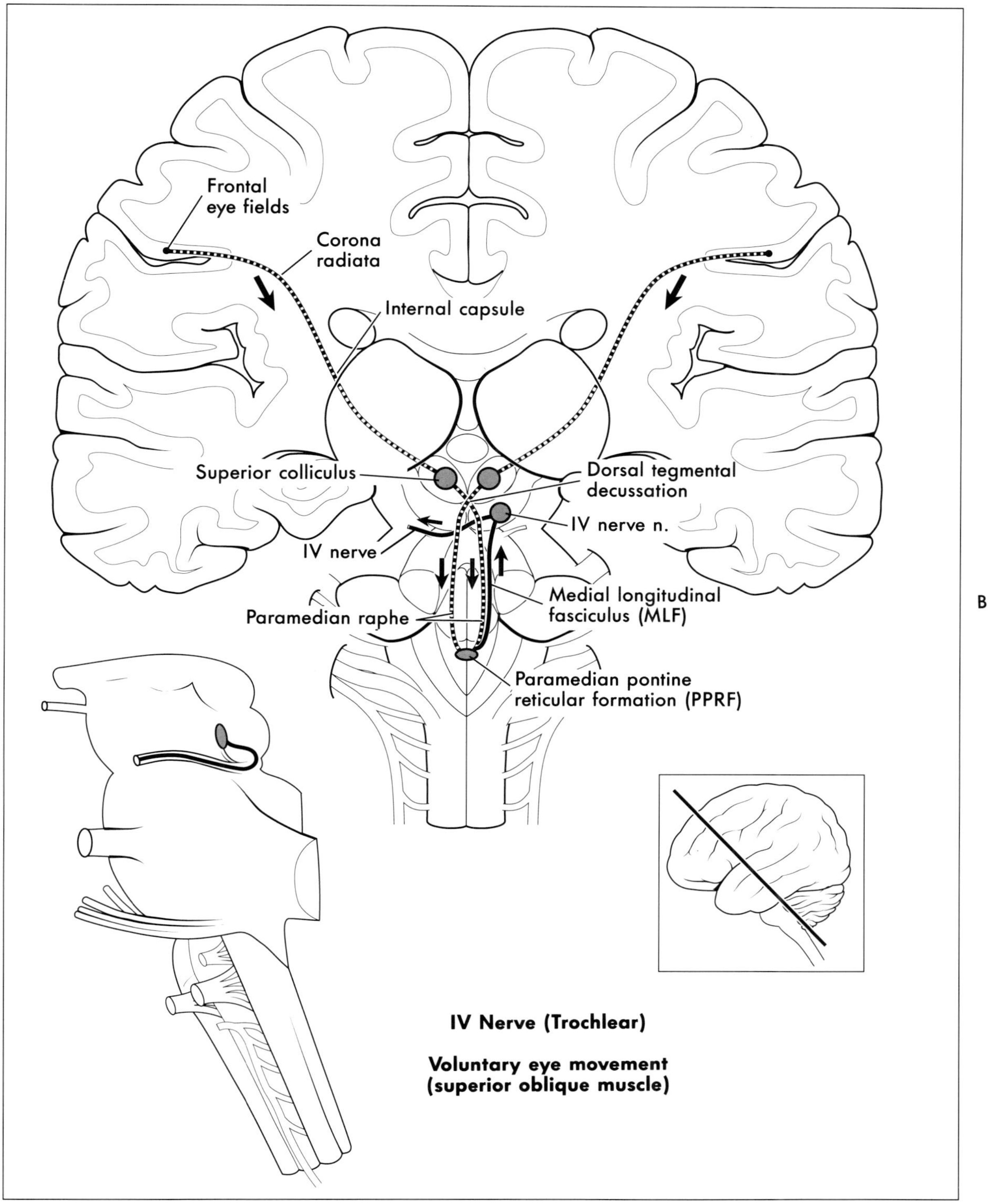

Figure 8-6 **A,** Brainstem pathway of CN IV (trochlear). Individual structures in each brainstem slice are labeled in Chapter 7. **B,** Coronal schematic shows pathway of CN IV. Sagittal schematic shows only the location of CN IV and its brainstem nucleus.

Cranial Nerve VI (Abducens)

The pathway of CN VI is illustrated on the schematic axial and coronal drawings (Figure 8-7, *A* and *B*). Impulses from the motor cortex in both hemispheres travel via the internal capsule to the ipsilateral superior colliculus. These fibers cross between the red nuclei in the dorsal tegmental decussation. They travel down the brainstem in the paramedian raphe to synapse in the parapontine reticular formation (PPRF). Both ipsilateral and contralateral fibers then ascend in the medial longitudinal fasciculus (MLF) to reach the nucleus of CN VI. Fibers from the nucleus exit from the anterior aspect of the brainstem at the junction of the medulla and pons. CN VI travels superiorly and enters the cavernous sinus. CN VI courses anteriorly just below CN III and IV.

An isolated CN VI deficit is usually caused by a lesion in the cisternal portion of the nerve. The lesion may be focal or a prolonged increase in intracranial pressure may cause the nerve to be stretched. Abducens nerve damage produces paralysis of the lateral rectus muscle of the eye on the side of the lesion. This causes an inward deviation of the eye (internal strabismus), which will in turn cause double vision (diplopia) unless the head position is adjusted so as to bring the affected eye into line with the object.

A lesion involving the CN VI nucleus can produce symptoms identical to those described for the cisternal lesions, but with nuclear lesions these symptoms are usually part of a more extensive neurologic syndrome (see Foville's, Millard-Gubler, Raymond's, and Raymond-Cestan syndromes in Table 8-3).

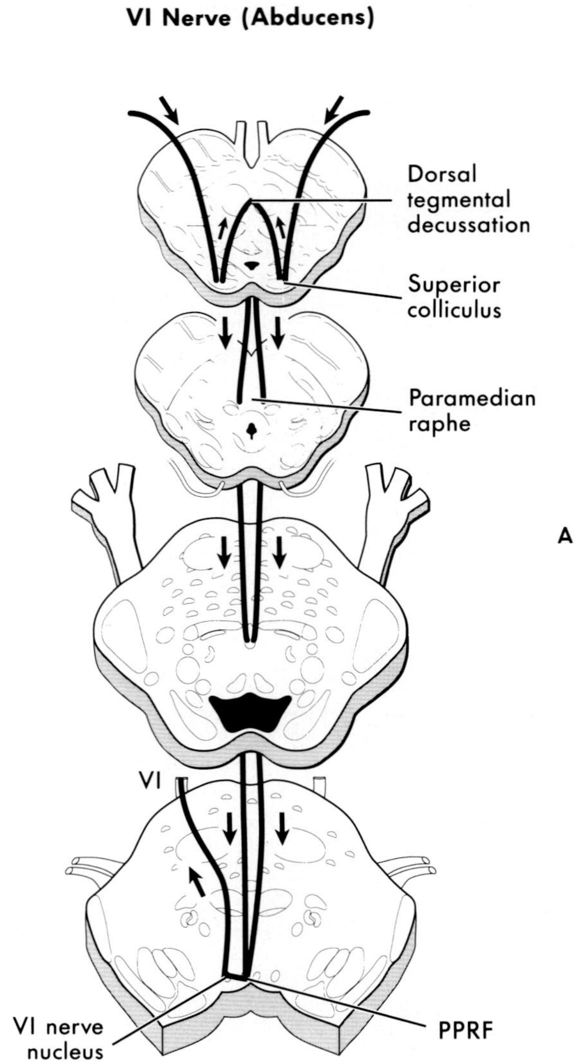

Figure 8-7 For legend see opposite page.

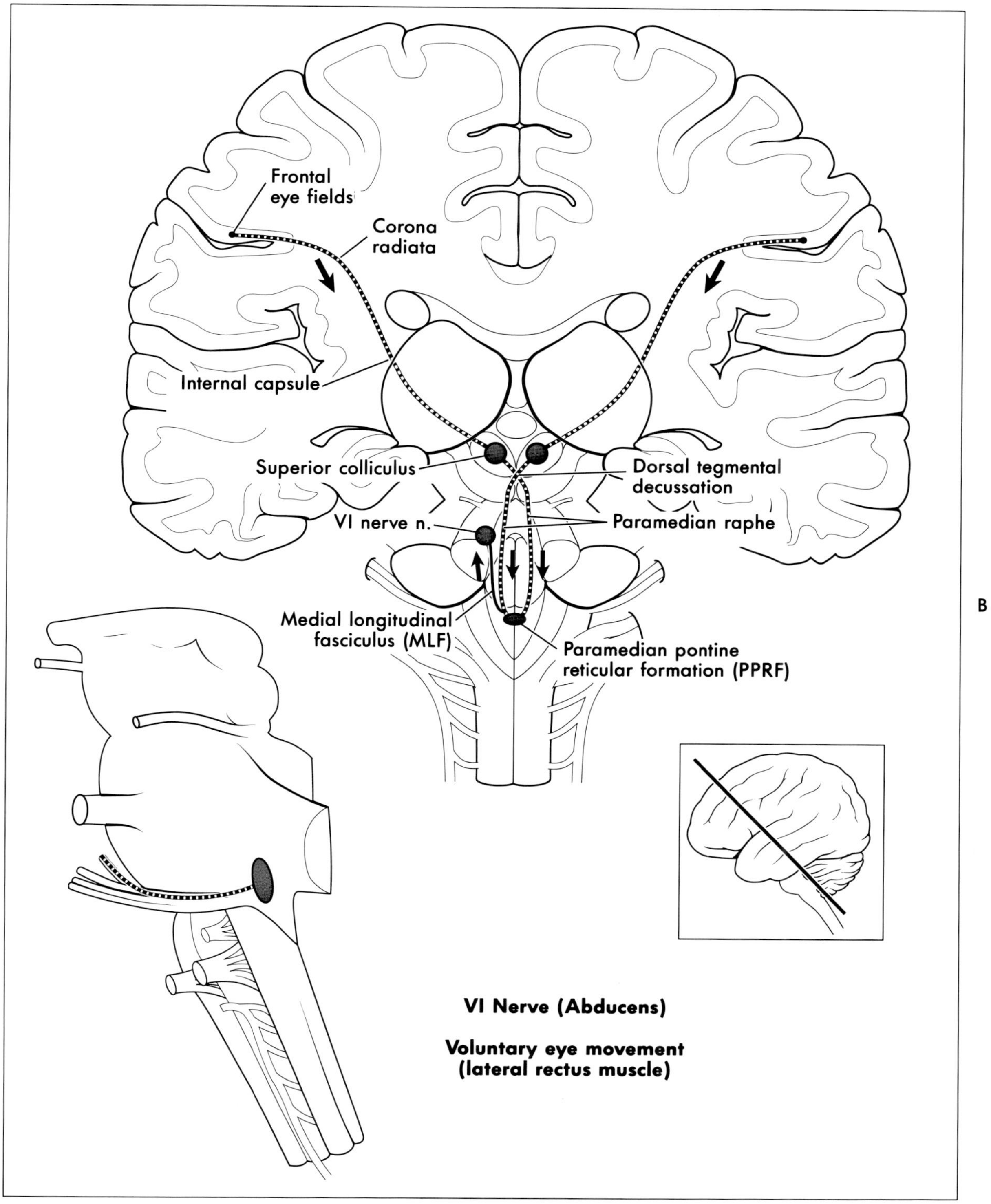

Figure 8-7 **A,** Brainstem pathway of CN VI (abducens). Individual structures in each brainstem slice are labeled in Chapter 7. **B,** Coronal schematic shows pathway of CN VI. Sagittal schematic shows only the location of CN VI and its brainstem nucleus.

Cranial Nerve V (Sensory Trigeminal—Pain and Temperature)

The sensory impulses from the face travel through CN V to the midlateral pons. As the axons enter the brainstem, many of them separate and send branches to the three sensory nuclei of CN V: the *principal* sensory nuclei, mesencephalic nucleus, and spinal nucleus. The *principal* sensory nucleus is involved with touch, whereas the mesencephalic nucleus handles proprioceptive information from facial muscles. These are discussed in detail in the section entitled Cranial Nerve V (Sensory Trigeminal—Proprioception and Touch).

The fibers that mediate pain and temperature are the clinically most important group. They descend and synapse in the spinal nucleus of CN V. Neurons from this nucleus cross the midline and reach the contralateral ventral posteromedial (VPM) nucleus of the thalamus via the ventral trigeminothalamic tract (Figure 8-8, *A* and *B*). The thalamocortical tract then travels in the internal capsule to the lower third of the postcentral gyrus (sensory cortex).

Lesions in the ganglion of CN V and/or the cavernous and cisternal portions of CN V produce a loss of all sensation in the entire ipsilateral face. A loss of sensation in the upper, middle, or lower part of the face indicates a lesion of a peripheral branch of CN V. These branches, which originate in the gasserian ganglion, are named for the sensory regions they supply: the *ophthalmic* (V_1), *maxillary* (V_2), and *mandibular* (V_3) *divisions*. Detecting lesions involving these peripheral nerves requires imaging of the face, neck, and skull base. The ophthalmic branch enters the skull via the superior orbital fissure. The maxillary and mandibular divisions enter the skull via the foramen rotundum and ovale, respectively.

Lesions in the spinal nucleus of CN V can sometimes be distinguished from peripheral lesions because they produce characteristic sensory deficits. A lesion in the medulla or upper cervical cord, such as syringobulbia, or a cervical disk above C4 can compromise the descending spinal nucleus of CN V and produce a loss of pain and temperature sensation with the preservation of touch (i.e., dissociated anesthesia), since touch is processed in the principal sensory nucleus. This may also be seen with an infarction of the medulla (see Wallenberg's syndrome in Table 8-3). Peripheral lesions, on the other hand, abolish all sensation, including touch.

The sensory divisions of the trigeminal nerve must also be evaluated in several facial pain syndromes, such as trigeminal neuralgia (tic douloureux), atypical facial pain, and Raeder's paratrigeminal syndrome. These syndromes all produce sharp pain in the face and are frequently confused with dental problems or paranasal sinus disease.

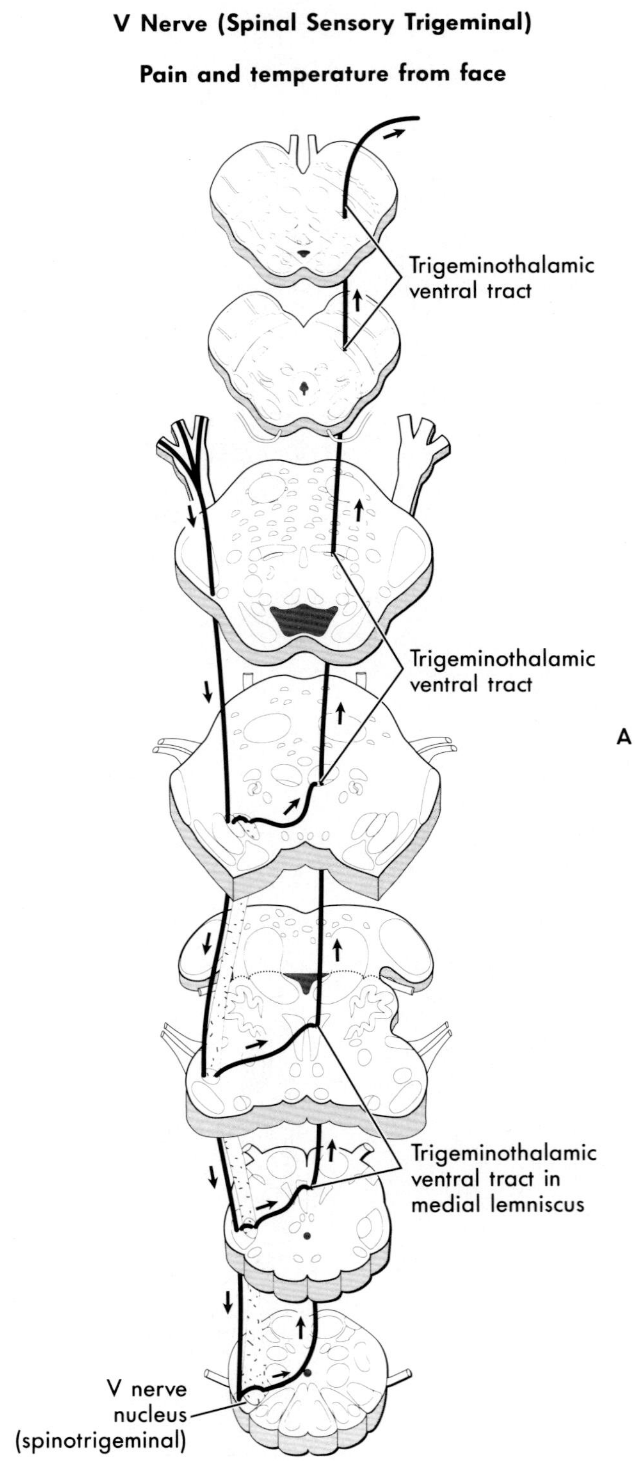

Figure 8-8 For legend see opposite page.

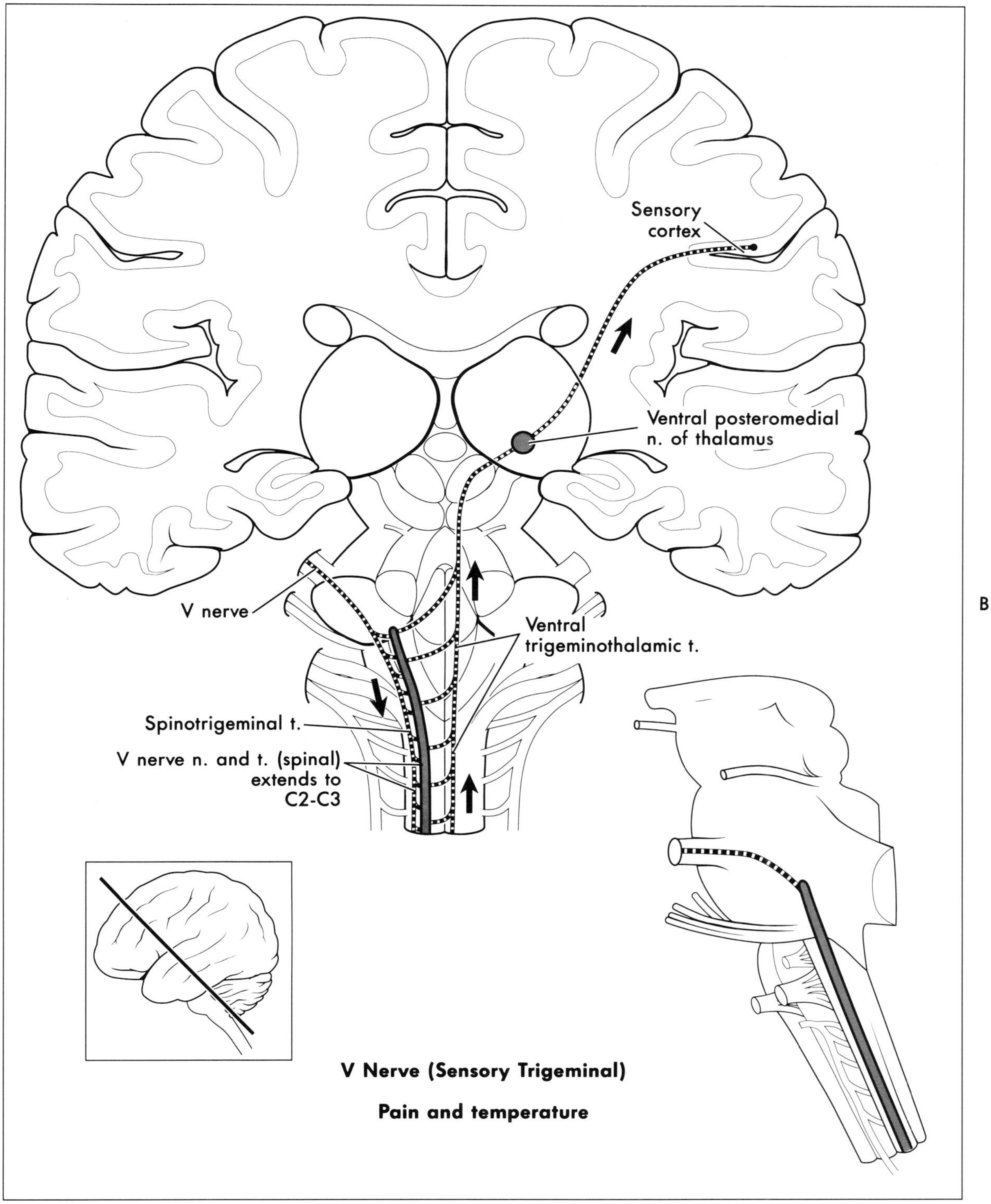

Figure 8-8 **A,** Brainstem pathway of CN V (sensory trigeminal—pain and temperature). Individual structures in each brainstem slice are labeled in Chapter 7. **B,** Coronal schematic shows pathway of the fibers of CN V (sensory trigeminal—pain and temperature). Sagittal schematic shows only the location of CN V and the brainstem nucleus, which mediates pain and temperature. (See Figure 8-9 for a description of the V nerve pathways for proprioception and touch.)

Cranial Nerve V (Sensory Trigeminal—Proprioception and Touch)

Sensory impulses that mediate proprioception from the face (mainly from the mandible) synapse in the mesencephalic nucleus of CN V (Figure 8-9, *A*). The nucleus extends through the mesencephalon (midbrain) and sends fibers that join the principal sensory nucleus of CN V. The exact pathway of these fibers beyond this point is unknown.

Sensory fibers of CN V that mediate touch and pressure from the face synapse in the principal sensory nucleus of CN V (Figure 8-9, *B*) and ascend to the ventral posteromedial nucleus of the thalamus via the ipsilateral and contralateral dorsal trigeminothalamic tract. From there, the thalamocortical tract travels in the internal capsule to the lower third of the postcentral gyrus (sensory cortex).

Lesions in the ganglion of the CN V and/or the cavernous and cisternal portions of CN V produce a loss of *all* sensation in the entire ipsilateral face. A loss of sensation in the upper, middle, or lower part of the face indicates a lesion of the peripheral branch of CN V. These branches, which originate in the gasserian ganglion, are named for the sensory regions they supply: the ophthalmic (V_1), maxillary (V_2), and mandibular (V_3) divisions. Detecting lesions involving these peripheral nerves requires imaging of the face, neck, and skull base. The ophthalmic branch enters the skull via the superior orbital fissure. The maxillary and mandibular divisions enter the skull via the foramen rotundum and ovale, respectively.

Lesions in the principal sensory and mesencephalic nuclei of CN V can sometimes be distinguished from peripheral lesions because peripheral lesions usually cause a loss of all sensation. Damage to the mesencephalic nucleus causes almost no clinical deficit, whereas damage to the principal sensory nucleus should cause only a loss of touch (with preservation of pain and temperature).

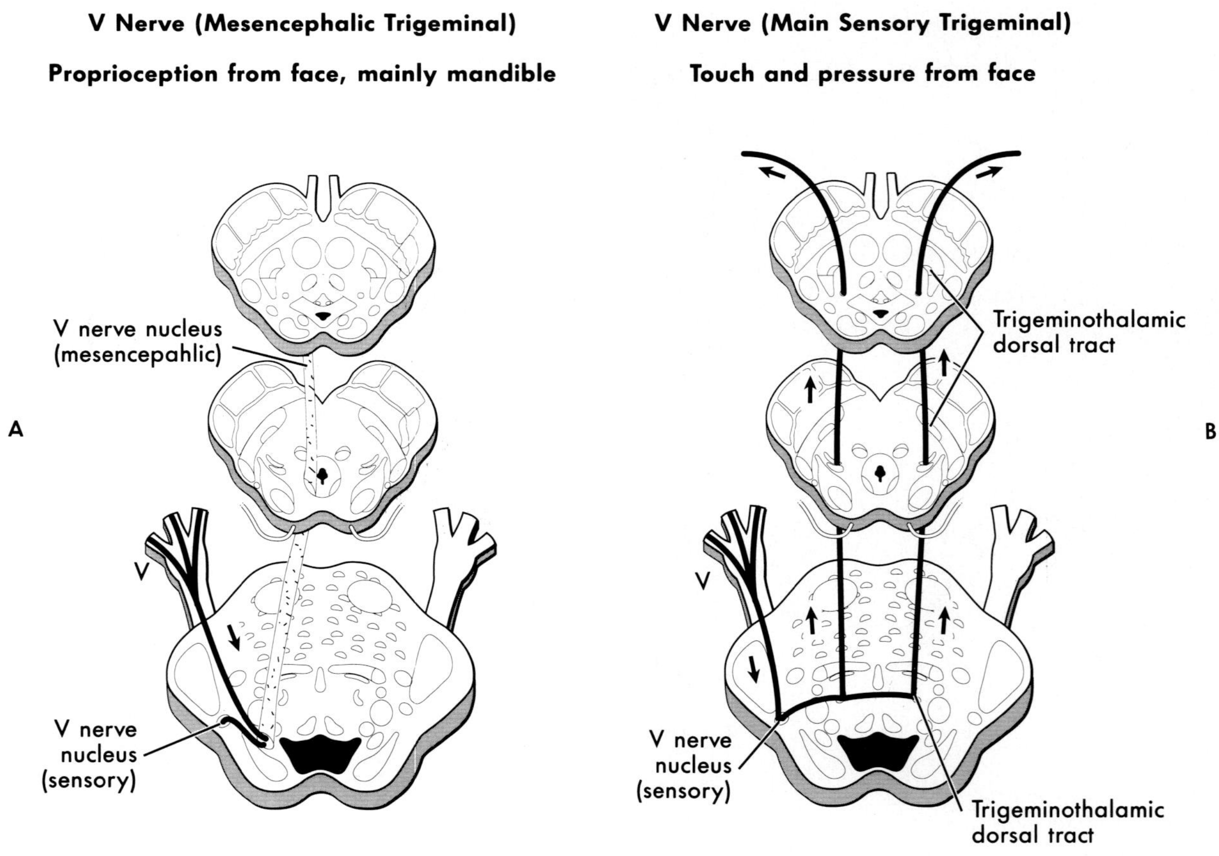

FIGURE 8-9 **A,** Brainstem pathway of CN V (sensory trigeminal—proprioception). Individual structures in each brainstem slice are labeled in Chapter 7. **B,** Brainstem pathway of CN V nerve (sensory trigeminal—touch and pressure). Individual structures in each brainstem slice are labeled in Chapter 7. **C,** Coronal schematic shows pathway of the fibers of CN V (mesencephalic and sensory trigeminal—proprioception and touch). Sagittal schematic shows only the location of the CN V, the rostral brainstem nucleus, which mediates proprioception, and the caudal nucleus, which mediates touch and pressure from the face. (See Figure 8-8 for a description of the V nerve pathways for pain and temperature.)

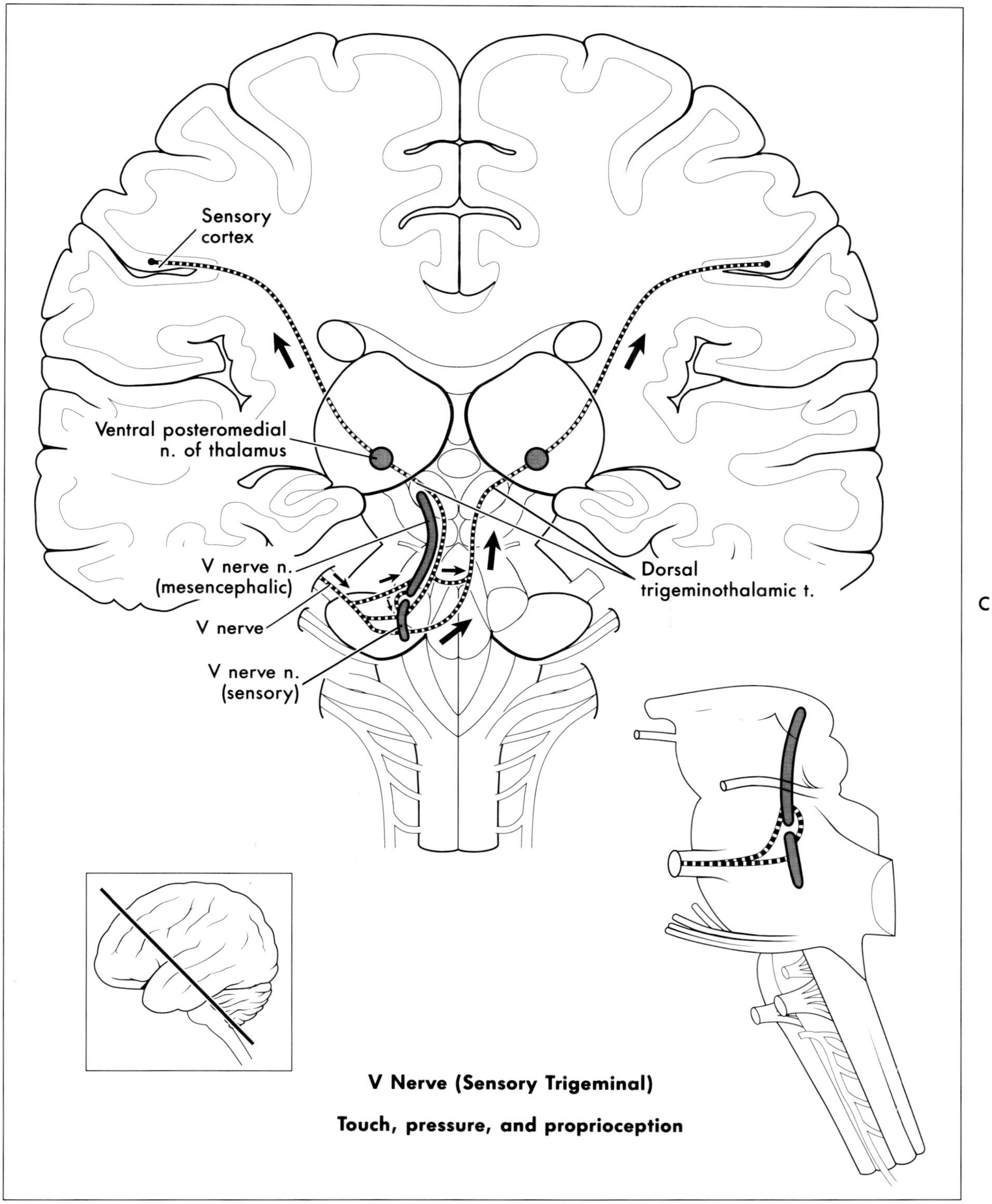

Figure 8-9, cont'd. For legend see opposite page.

Cranial Nerve V (Motor Trigeminal)

The pathway of the motor components of the CN V is illustrated on the schematic axial and coronal drawings (Figure 8-10, *A* and *B*). Impulses from the motor cortex of both hemispheres travel via the genu of the internal capsule and through the cerebral peduncles to the motor nucleus of CN V. Fibers from the nucleus join to form a separate nerve that joins the mandibular branch after it exits through the foramen ovale.

A lesion involving the motor fibers of CN V in the cisternal and/or ganglionic region causes atrophy and weakness of the ipsilateral muscles of mastication. This can be assessed in the masseter by feeling the tautness and size of this muscle with the jaws clenched. Because the muscle is denervated, fasciculations may be noted. When the jaw is opened, the chin may deviate toward the paralyzed side because of the action of the unaffected pterygoid muscles.

A unilateral, cortical, hemispheric lesion does not produce marked clinical symptoms if the connections from the opposite hemisphere are intact, since the motor cortex of both hemispheres innervates both motor nuclei of CN V. The normal minimal jaw jerk, which can be elicited by tapping the middle of the chin while the mouth is slightly open, also becomes exaggerated by bilateral lesions located in the cortex or the corticobulbar tracts that project to the motor nucleus of CN V.

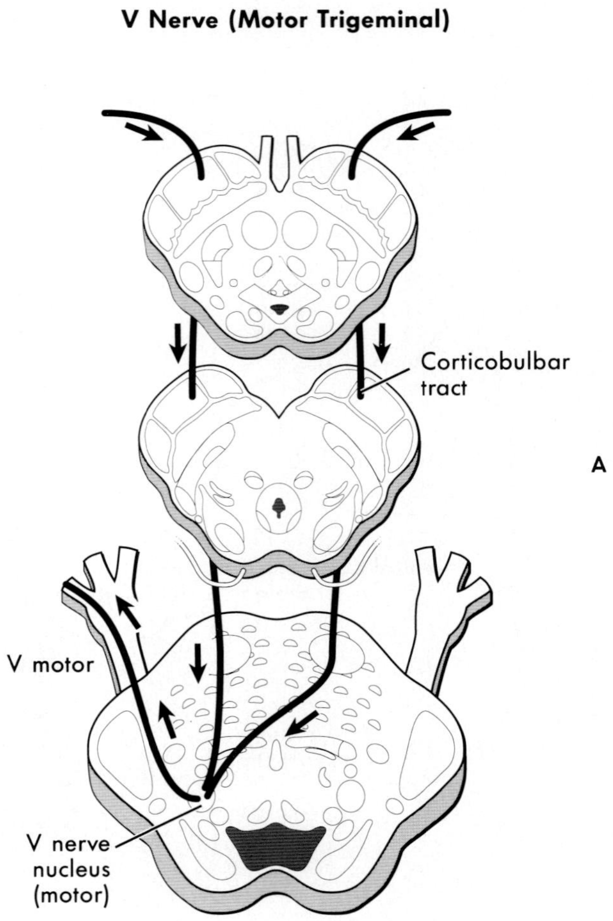

Figure 8-10 For legend see opposite page.

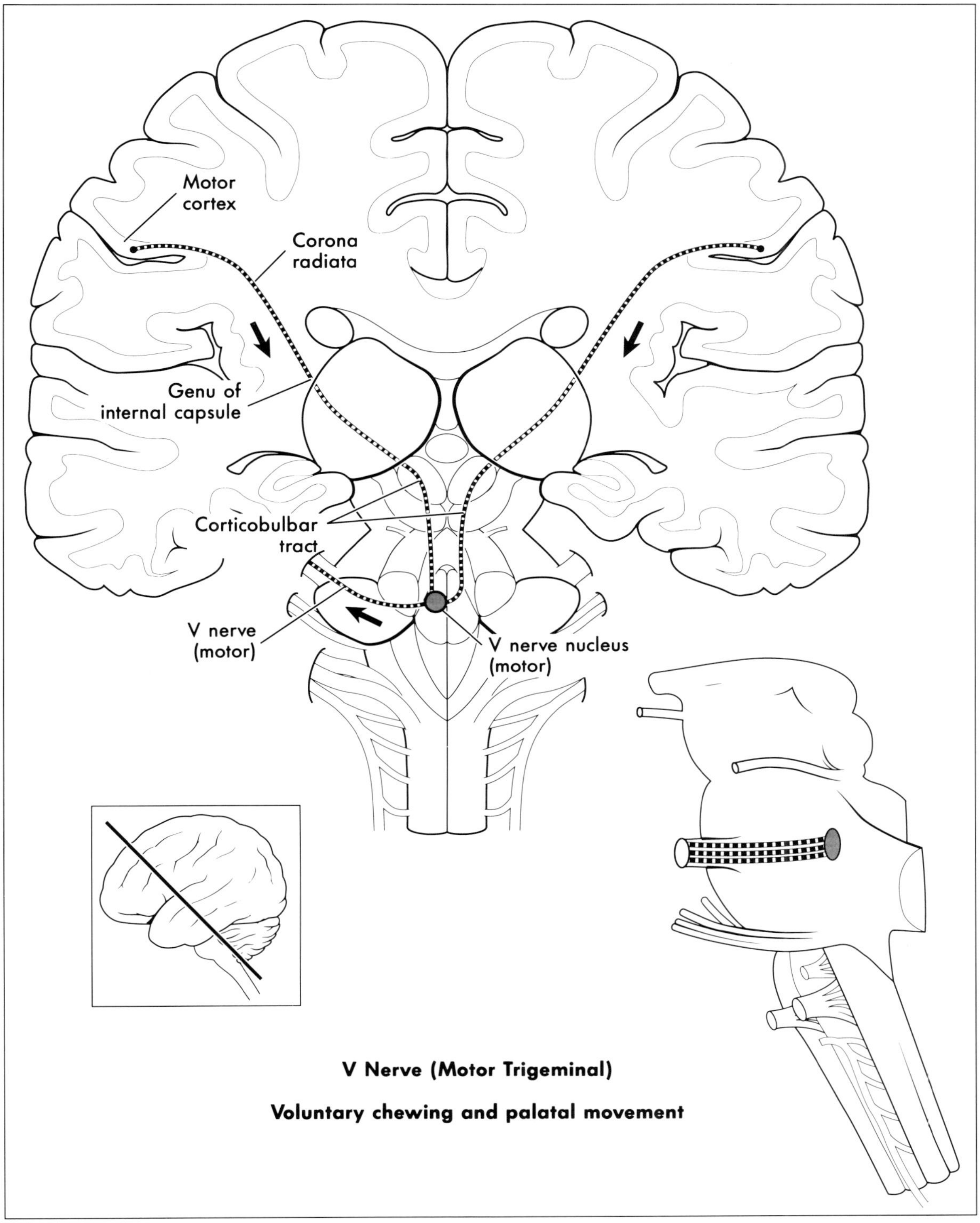

B

Figure 8-10 **A,** Brainstem pathway of CN V (motor trigeminal). Individual structures in each brainstem slice are labeled in Chapter 7. **B,** Coronal schematic shows pathway of CN V (motor trigeminal). Sagittal schematic shows only the location of the motor fibers of CN V and its brainstem nucleus.

Cranial Nerve VII (Facial)

The pathway of CN VII nerve is illustrated on the schematic axial and coronal drawings (Figure 8-11, *A* and *B*). Impulses from the motor cortex of both cerebral hemispheres travel via the genu of the internal capsule and through the cerebral peduncles to the nucleus of CN VII. Fibers from the nucleus travel dorsally around the nucleus of CN VI to form the genu of CN VII. These fibers then course ventrally to exit the brainstem at the pontomedullary junction. They course laterally in the cerebellopontine angle cistern until they enter the anterosuperior quadrant of the internal auditory canal. From there, the facial nerve passes through the temporal bone superior to the cochlea to reach the anterior genu. CN VII then turns posteriorly to travel beneath the lateral semicircular canal to the posterior genu. From there, CN VII descends to exit the skull base through the stylomastoid foramen. Then the facial nerve passes anterolaterally through the substance of the parotid gland, where it divides into smaller branches.

Damage to the facial nerve, whether extracranial or intracranial (cisternal portion or brainstem nucleus), produces weakness in all the muscles of facial expression on the side of the lesion. The most frequent cause of such damage is an idiopathic inflammation of the extracranial segment of the nerve known as *Bell's palsy*. Usually in these patients, facial strength slowly recovers over a period of weeks.

Sometimes, damage may occur in either the motor cortex or the descending pyramidal tracts that project to the motor nucleus of CN VII. A loss of innervation from such an upper motor neuron lesion causes volitional facial palsy, in which complete paralysis of only the lower one half of the face occurs, on the side opposite the lesion. The upper one half of the face remains functional, possibly because it receives fibers from both corticobulbar tracts and the motor cortex of the opposite hemisphere.

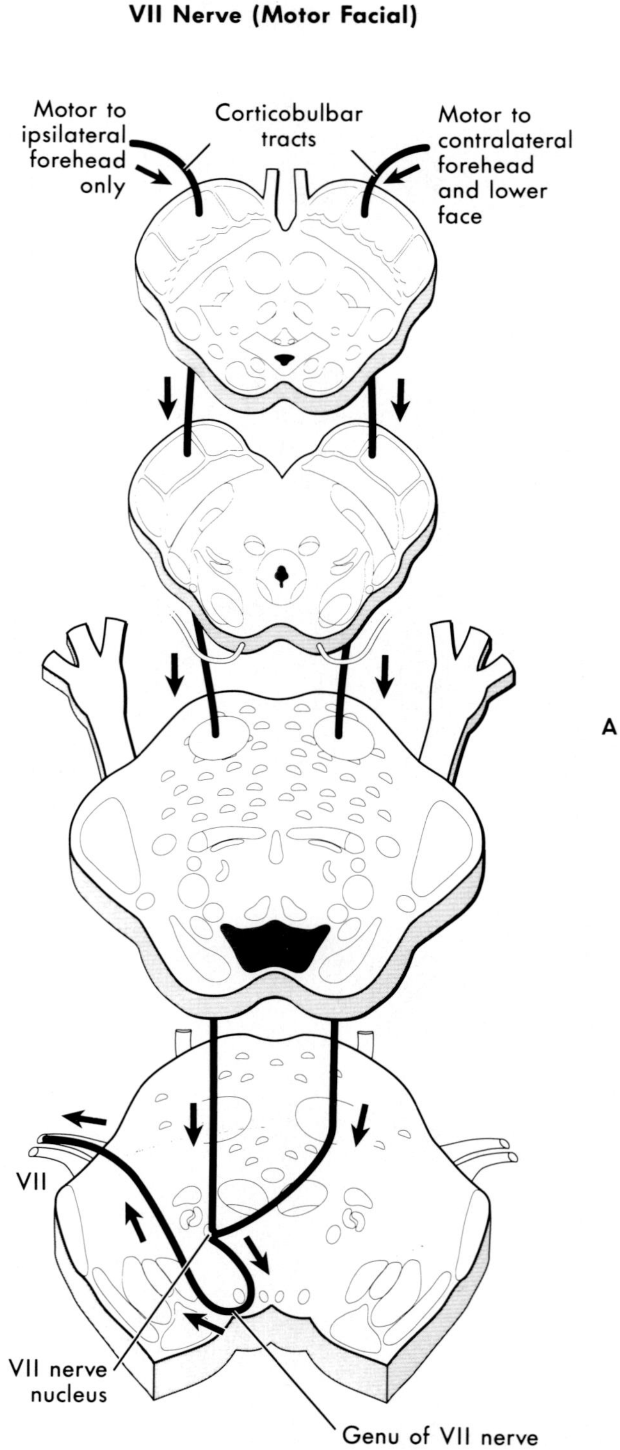

Figure 8-11 For legend see opposite page.

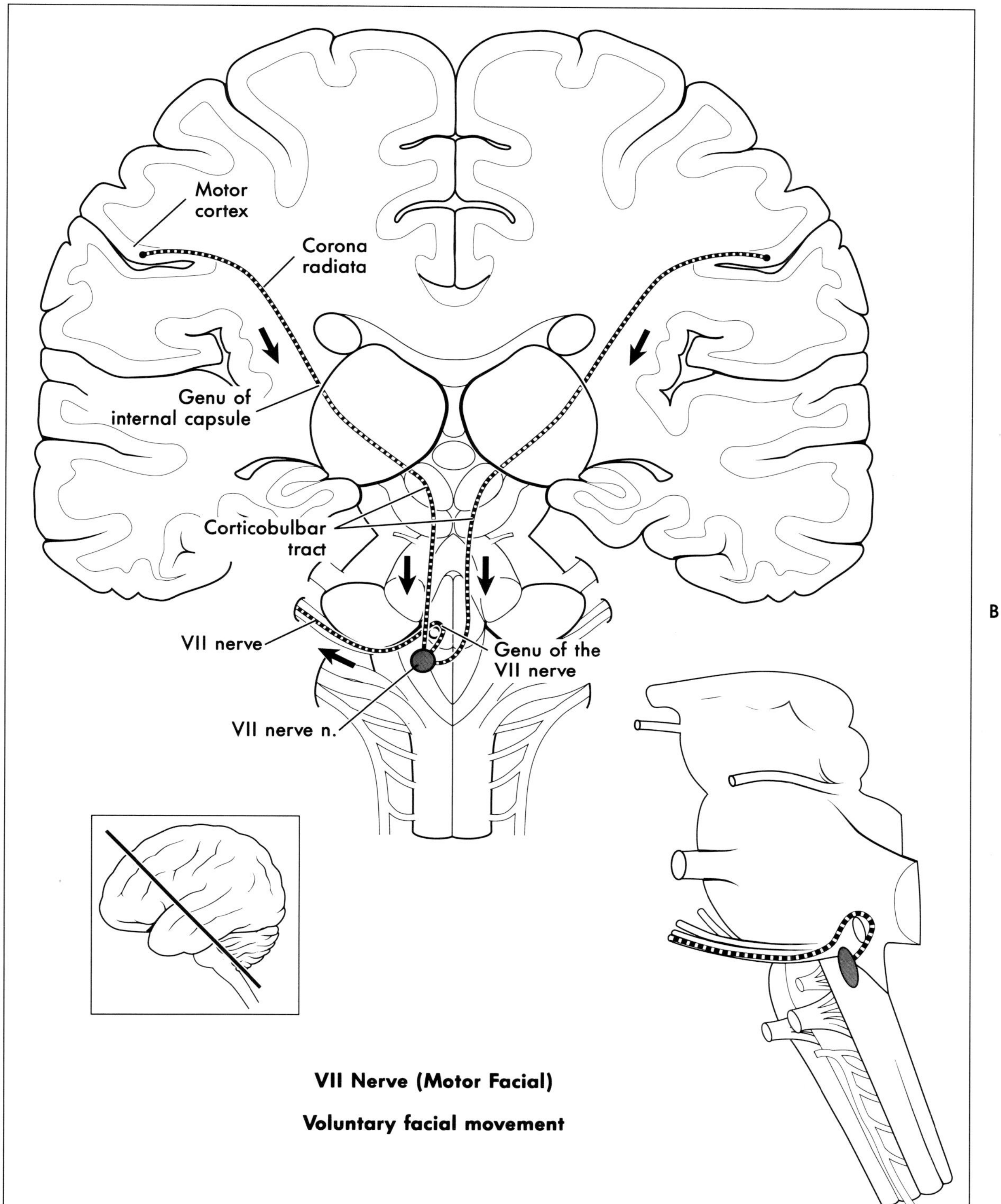

FIGURE 8-11 **A,** Brainstem pathway CN V nerve (facial). Individual structures in each brainstem slice are labeled in Chapter 7. **B,** Coronal schematic shows pathway of CN VII. Sagittal schematic shows only the location of CN VII and its brainstem nucleus.

Cranial Nerve VIII (Vestibular)

Impulses from the cristae in the ampullae of the three semicircular canals and the hair cells of the maculae of the utricle and saccule are transmitted through the superior and inferior vestibular nerves. These nerves pass through the posterior portion of the internal auditory canal and enter the anterior aspect of the brainstem at the pontomedullary junction after crossing the cerebellopontine angle cistern. The pathway of CN VIII is illustrated on the schematic axial and coronal drawings in Figure 8-12, *A* and *B*. Fibers enter the vestibular nuclei and information concerning equilibrium is transmitted via the medial longitudinal fasciculus (MLF) bilaterally to the paired CN III, IV, and VI nuclei that coordinate eye movements. Fibers are also sent to the cerebellum via the juxtarestiform body and to the muscles of the head and body via the medial and lateral vestibulospinal tracts. These pathways connect the vestibular apparatus (saccule, utricle, three semicircular canals) with the cerebellum and motor nuclei that control the eyes and the muscles of balance. When this system is properly functioning, it detects the effects of gravity and adjusts the body and eyes in space via its motor and cerebellar connections.

Lesions of this component of CN VIII result in dizziness, falling, and nystagmus. Clinically, lesions in the portion of the nerve within the temporal bone (i.e., the spiral and vestibular ganglia and their sensory projections) may mimic lesions in the cistern or the brainstem nuclei. However, cisternal lesions are often accompanied by deficits in the adjacent cochlear division of CN VIII and by damage to CN VII. Brainstem lesions rarely cause isolated dizziness because they usually involve adjacent nuclei and/or fiber tracts.

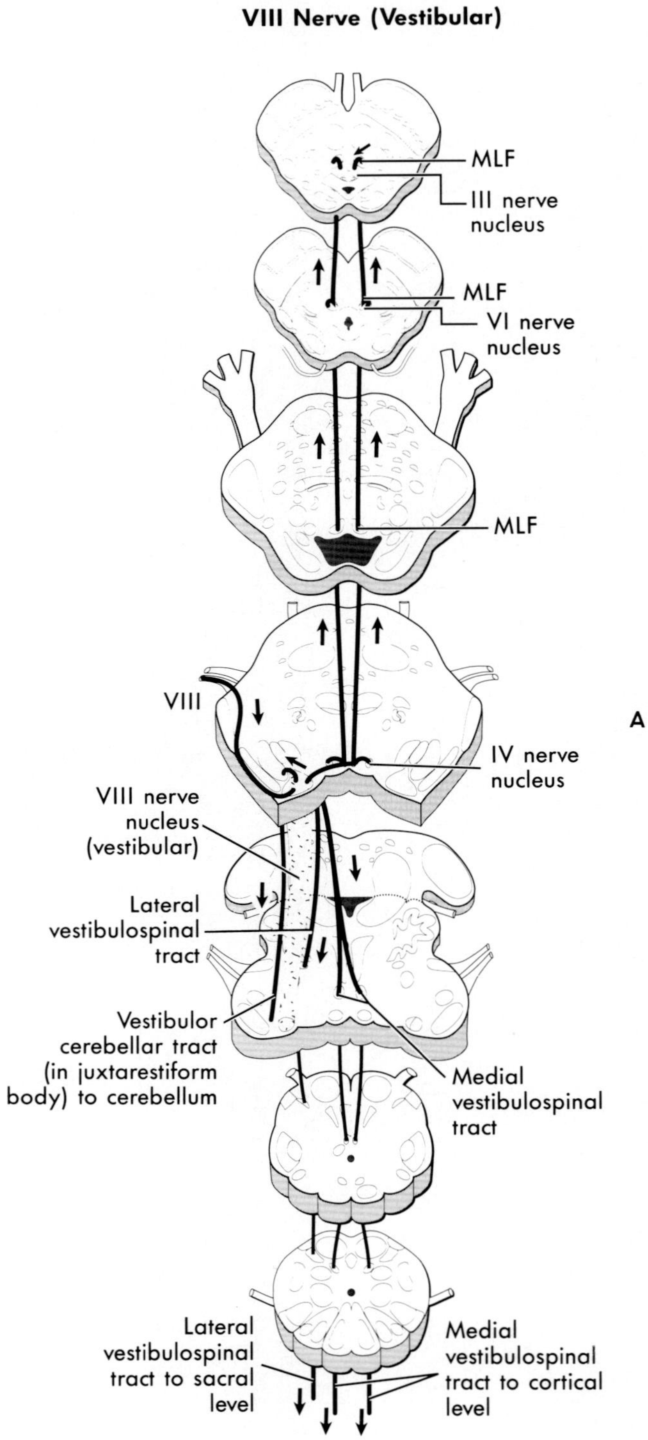

Figure 8-12 For legend see opposite page.

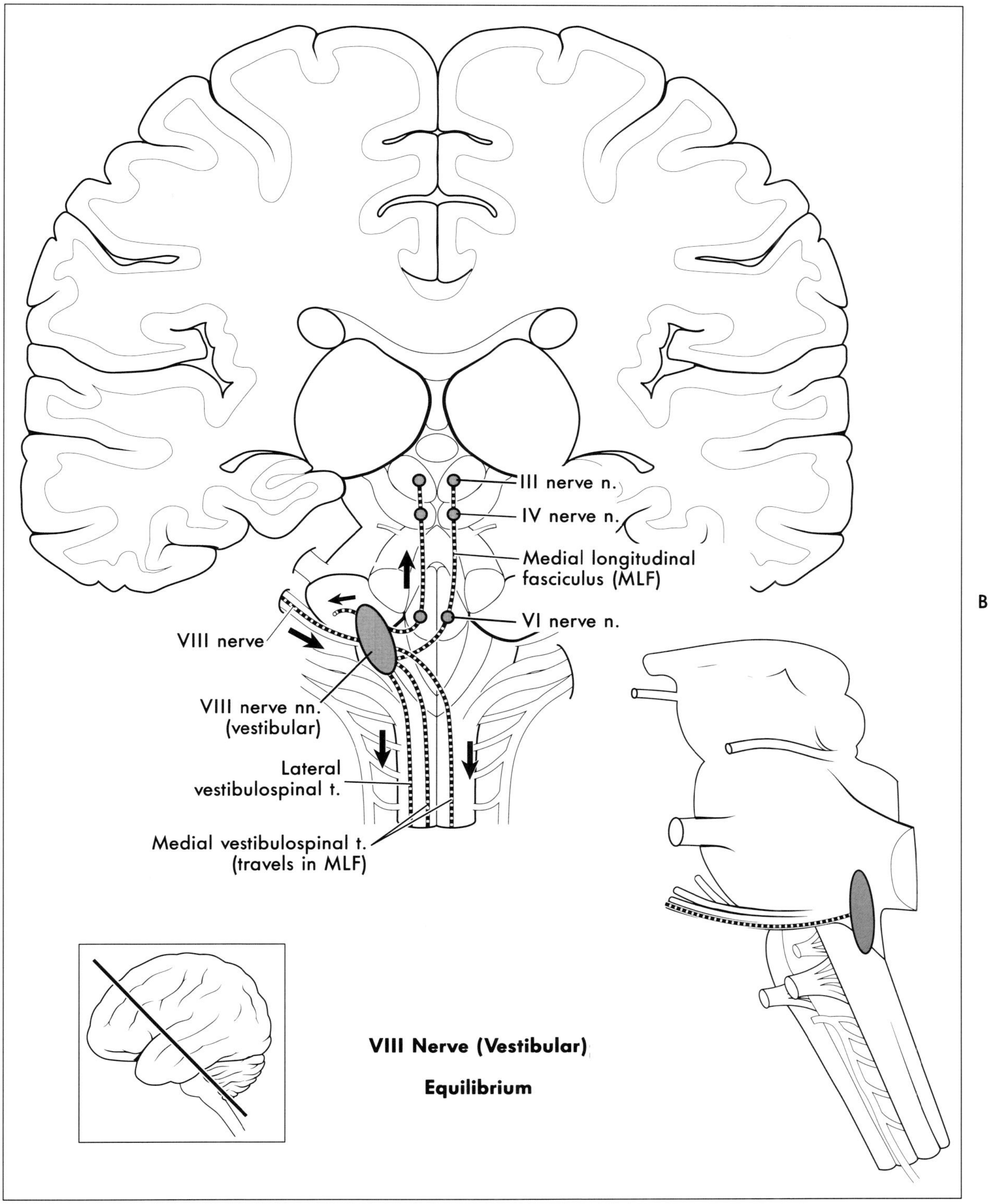

Figure 8-12 **A,** Brainstem pathway of CN VIII (vestibular). Individual structures in each brainstem slice are labeled in Chapter 7. **B,** Coronal schematic shows pathway of CN VIII (vestibular). Sagittal schematic shows only the location of CN VIII and its vestibular brainstem nucleus. (See Figure 8-13 for a description of the cochlear pathways.)

Cranial Nerve VIII (Cochlear)

Impulses from the cochlea travel through CN VIII. This nerve passes through the internal auditory canal and enters the anterior aspect of the brainstem at the pontomedullary junction after crossing the cerebellopontine angle cistern (Figure 8-13, *A* and *B*). Fibers then enter the superior olivary nucleus and trapezoid body on both sides of the pons and ascend in the lateral lemniscus to the inferior colliculus. From each of the inferior colliculi, these fibers travel to the medial geniculate bodies and terminate in the auditory cortex (transverse temporal gyri) of both cerebral hemispheres.

Lesions of this component of peripheral CN VIII or its nuclei may cause tinnitus (ringing in the ear) or deafness on the side of the lesion. A lesion in the cisternal portion of the nerve is often accompanied by symptoms related to the adjacent vestibular component of CN VIII and to CN VII. Because the auditory cortex, superior olivary nucleus, and trapezoid body receive input from both ears, lesions involving these regions (or their connecting fiber tracts) produce no clinical symptoms. Cortical lesions seldom affect hearing.

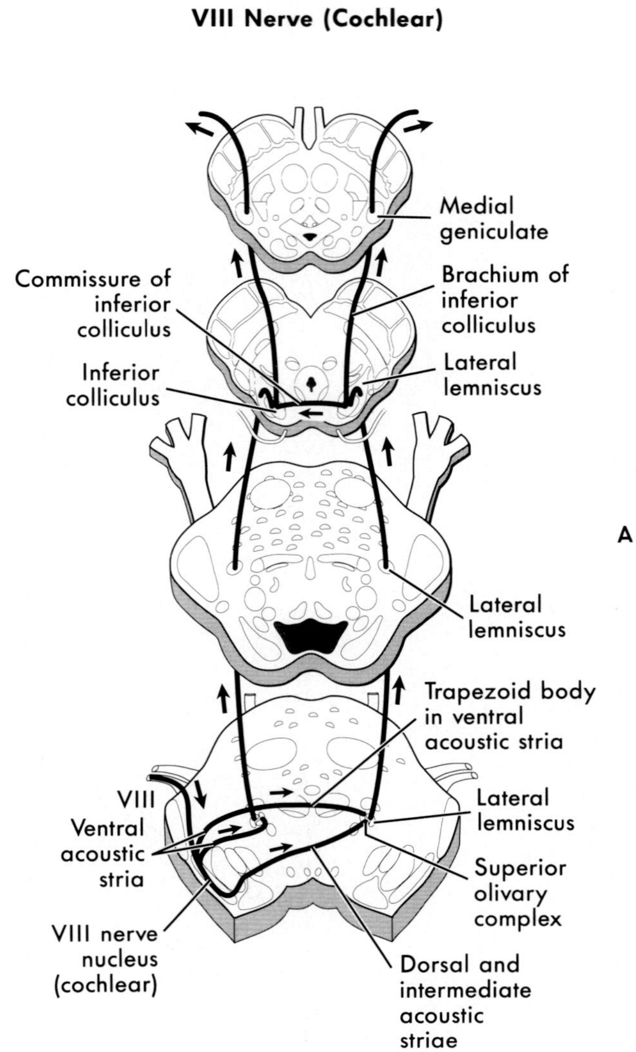

Figure 8-13 For legend see opposite page.

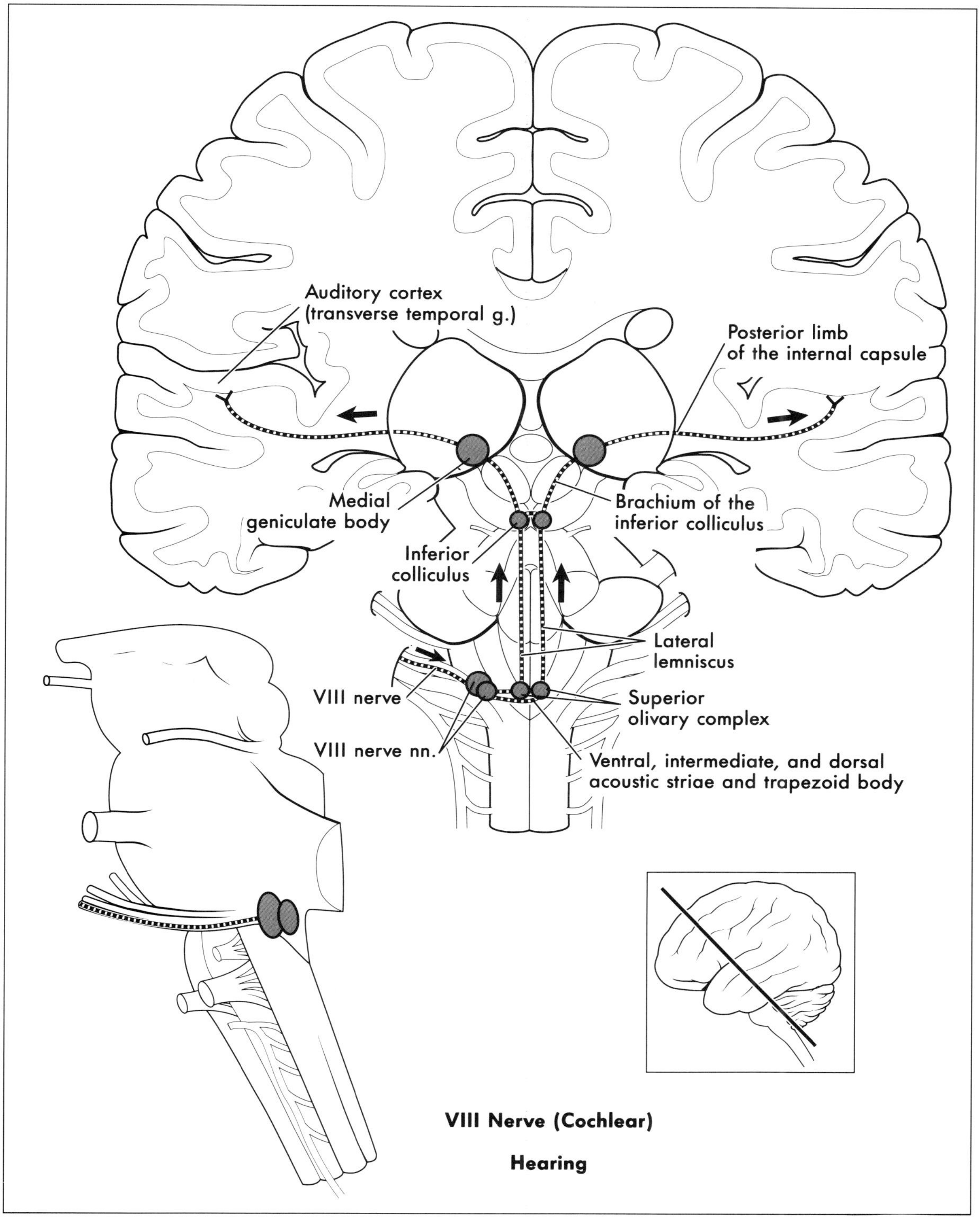

B

FIGURE 8-13 **A,** Brainstem pathway of CN VIII (cochlear). Individual structures in each brainstem slice are labeled in Chapter 7. **B,** Coronal schematic shows pathway of CN VIII (cochlear). Sagittal schematic shows only the location of CN VIII and its cochlear brainstem nucleus. (See Figure 8-12 for a description of the vestibular pathways.)

Cranial Nerves IX and X (Glossopharyngeal-Vagal Motor Complex)

The pathway of CN IX and X is illustrated on the schematic axial and coronal drawings (Figure 8-14, *A* and *B*). Impulses from the motor cortex of both hemispheres travel via the genu of the internal capsule through the cerebral peduncles to the nucleus ambiguus. Fibers from this nucleus leave the medulla at the postolivary sulcus and pass anterolaterally to enter the jugular foramen. The fibers of CN IX travel inferiorly to the surface of the stylopharyngeus and constrictor muscles of the pharynx, to the mucosa of the palatine tonsils, and to the posterior one third of the tongue. The fibers of CN X pass vertically through the jugular foramen, down the neck along the carotid sheath to the thorax.

Lesions of the cisternal and nuclear components of CN IX (glossopharyngeal) result in paralysis of the stylopharyngeus muscle on the side of the lesion. Lesions of the cisternal and nuclear components of CN X (vagus) cause paralysis of the striated muscles of the pharynx and larynx on the side of the lesion. Symptoms are minimal, given a unilateral lesion, although a decreased gag reflex may be found on examination. Rarely, the patient may suffer from hoarseness, dysphagia, or choking. Cisternal lesions can sometimes be distinguished from nuclear lesions because the cisternal lesions often involve the adjacent CN XI.

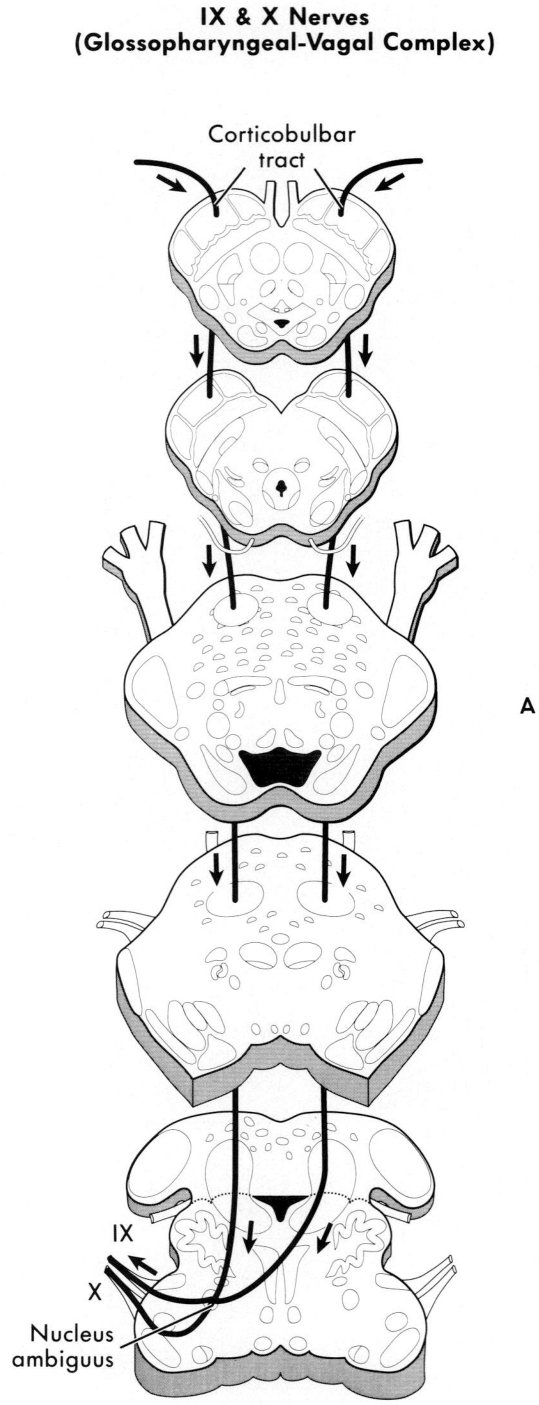

Figure 8-14 For legend see opposite page.

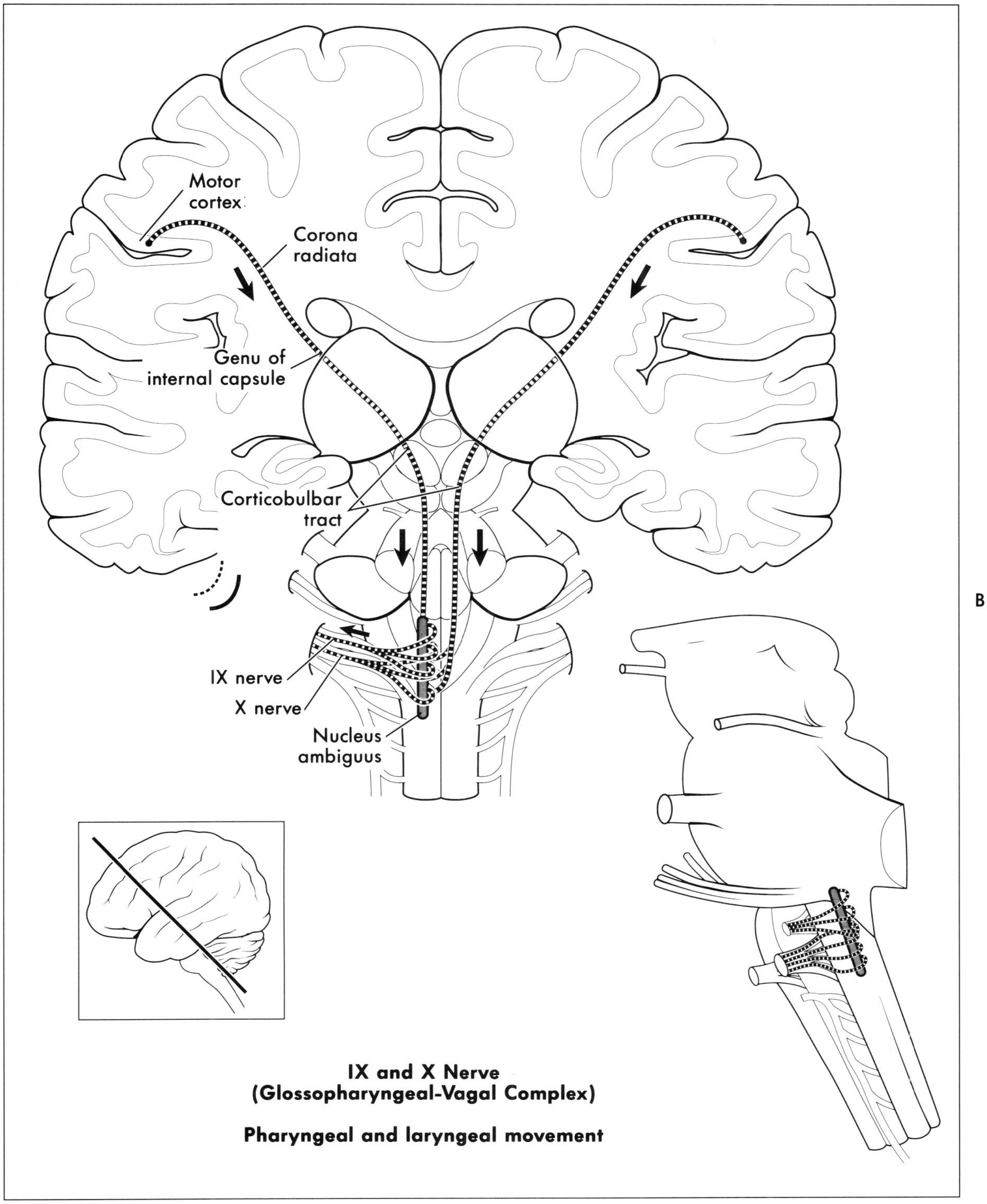

FIGURE 8-14 **A,** Brainstem pathway of CN IX-X (glossopharyngeal-vagal) complex. Individual structures in each brainstem slice are labeled in Chapter 7. **B,** Coronal schematic shows pathway of CN IX-X complex. Sagittal schematic shows only the location of CN IX-X and its brainstem nucleus.

Cranial Nerve XI (Spinal Accessory)

The pathway of CN XI is illustrated on the schematic axial and coronal drawings (Figure 8-15, *A* and *B*). Impulses from the motor cortex of primarily the opposite cerebral hemisphere travel via the genu of the internal capsule, through the cerebral peduncle to the nuclei of CN XI. Fibers from the bulbar nucleus (accessory component) exit the medulla at the postolivary sulcus and follow CN X into the neck (see Figure 8-14). These fibers are not shown in Figure 8-15.

Additional fibers from the spinal nucleus (C1-C5) ascend through the foramen magnum to join the bulbar root and pass anteriorly through the pars nervosa of the jugular bulb. These fibers then descend in the neck to innervate the sternocleidomastoid and trapezius muscles.

Lesions of the spinal component of CN XI cause inability to shrug the ipsilateral shoulder and weakness against resistance to turning the head contralaterally. At rest, the ipsilateral scapula may be rotated downward and laterally because of muscle paralysis. Cisternal lesions are usually associated with deficits in adjacent CN IX and X. Although nuclear lesions are extremely rare, the nucleus for CN XI is located in the cervical spinal cord (perhaps as low as C4), making it important to include this region in the radiographic examination. Lesions in the motor cortex or the fiber tracts that connect with the CN XI nucleus sometimes produce an ipsilateral deficit. In other words, destruction of the right nucleus impairs the right sternocleidomastoid muscle, which weakens head turning toward the left.

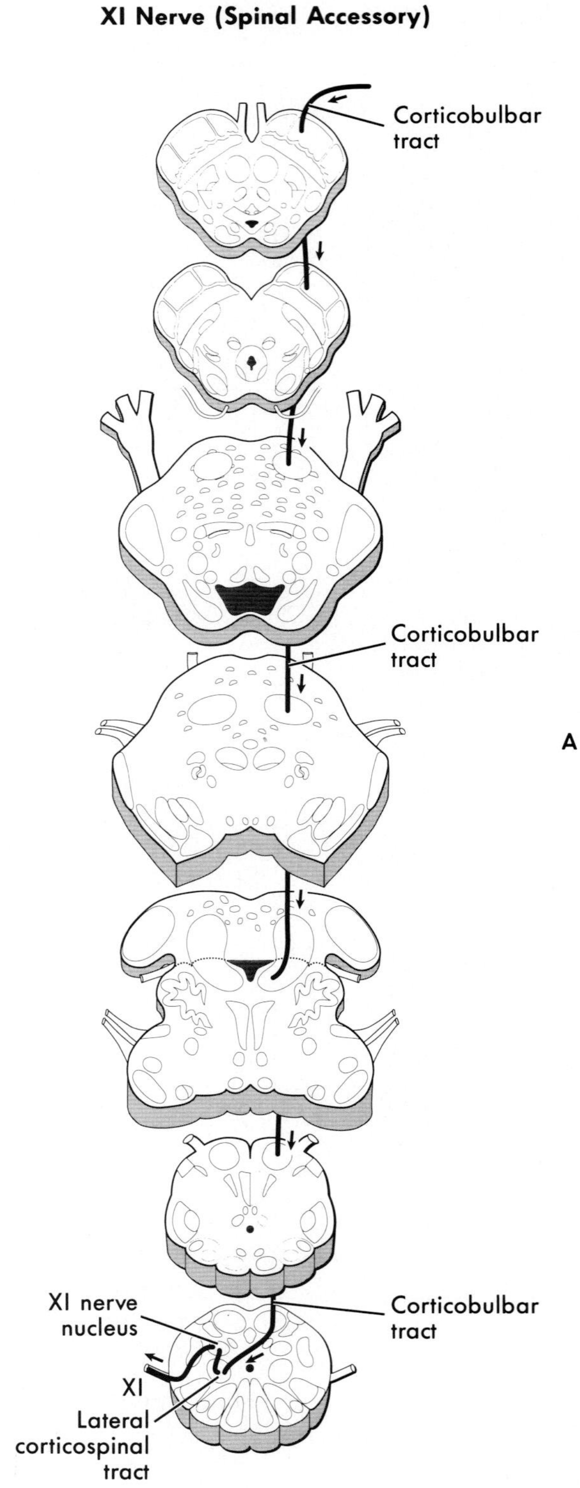

Figure 8-15 For legend see opposite page.

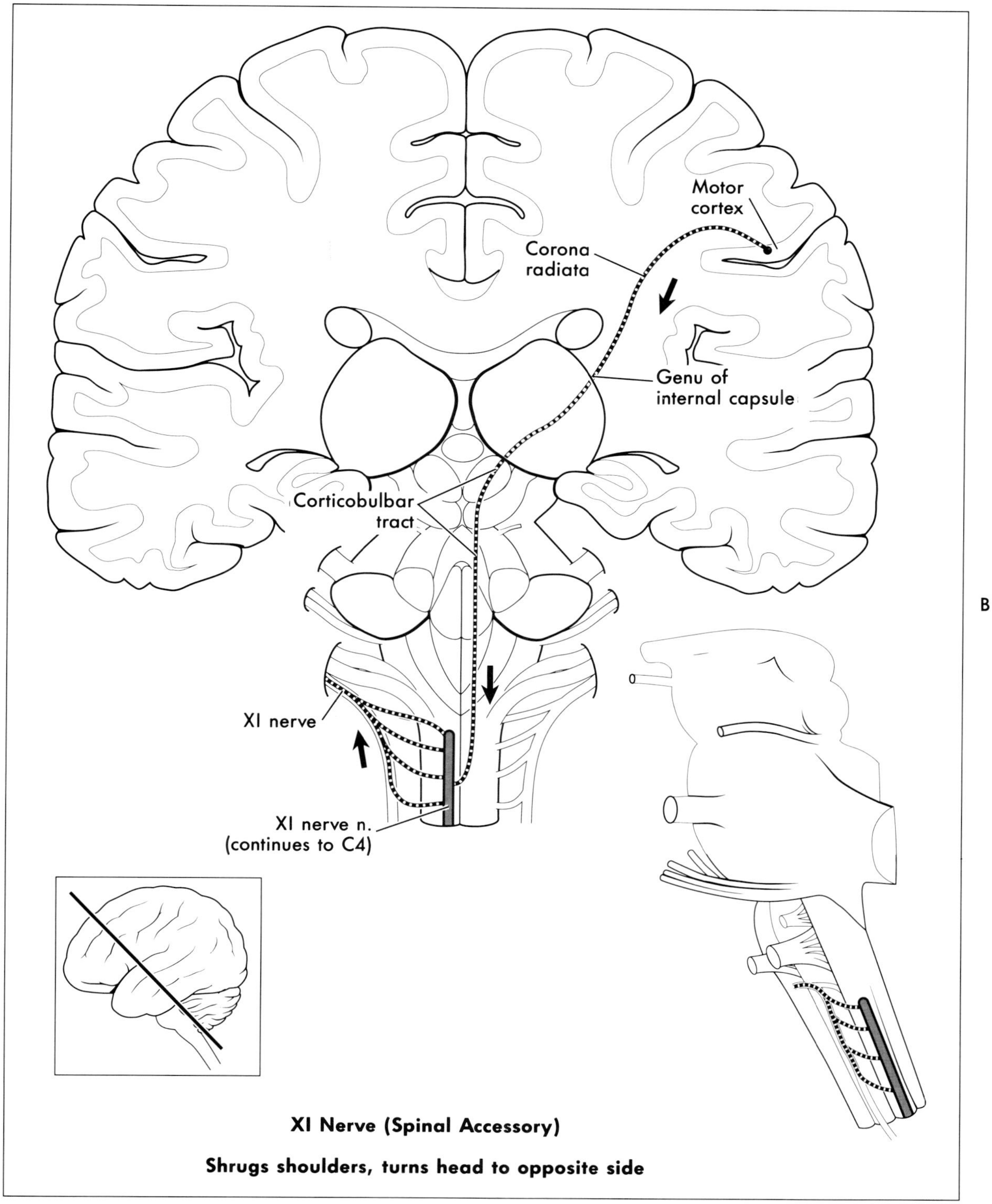

FIGURE 8-15 **A,** Brainstem pathway CN XI (spinal accessory). Individual structures in each brainstem slice are labeled in Chapter 7. **B,** Coronal schematic shows pathway of the fibers of spinal CN XI. Sagittal schematic shows only the location of CN XI and its spinal nucleus. (The bulbar accessory fibers, which arise from the nucleus ambiguus, follow the pathway of CN X shown in Figure 8-14, B. They are not shown in this diagram.)

Cranial Nerve XII (Hypoglossal)

The pathway of CN XII is illustrated on the adjacent axial and coronal drawings (Figure 8-16, *A* and *B*). Impulses from the motor cortex of the opposite cerebral hemisphere travel via the genu of the internal capsule through the cerebral peduncle to the CN XII nucleus. Fibers from the nucleus exit the medulla at the preolivary sulcus and pass anterolaterally through the hypoglossal canal. From here the fibers travel inferiorly to supply the tongue muscles and infrahyoid strap muscles.

Lesions of CN XII result in flaccid paralysis, atrophy, and/or fatty replacement of the tongue on the side of the cisternal or nuclear lesion. The tongue deviates to the side of the lesion. Damage in the cortex or the motor fiber tracts before they cross the midline may result in weakness but no atrophy of the contralateral tongue muscles.

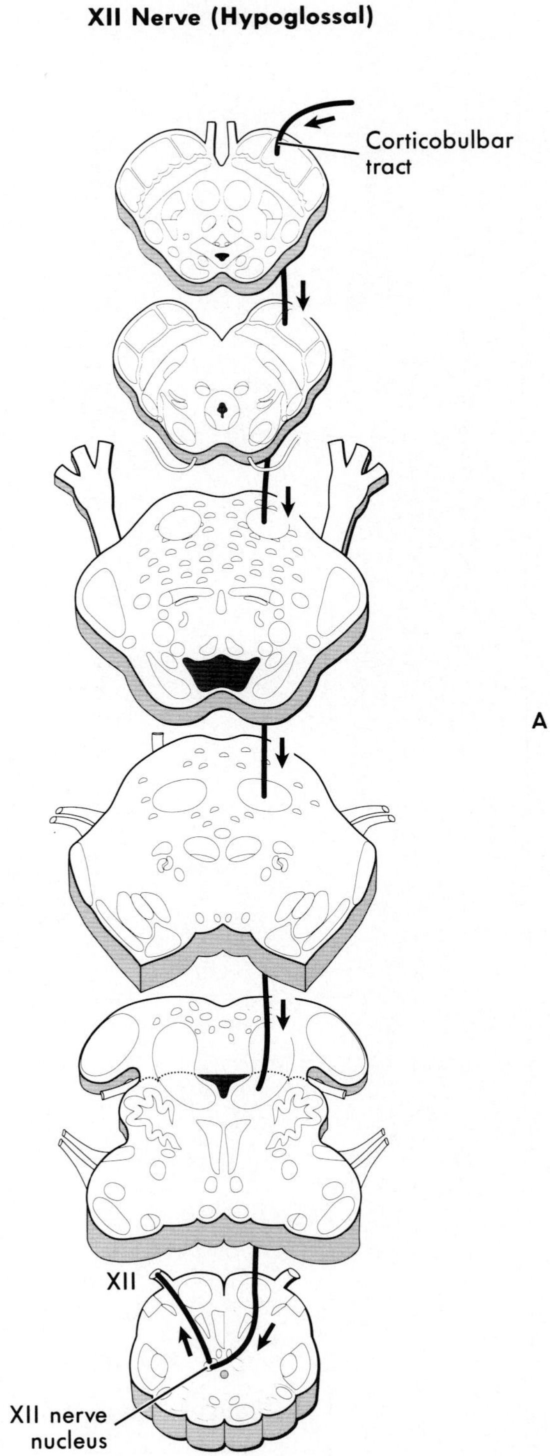

Figure 8-16 For legend see opposite page.

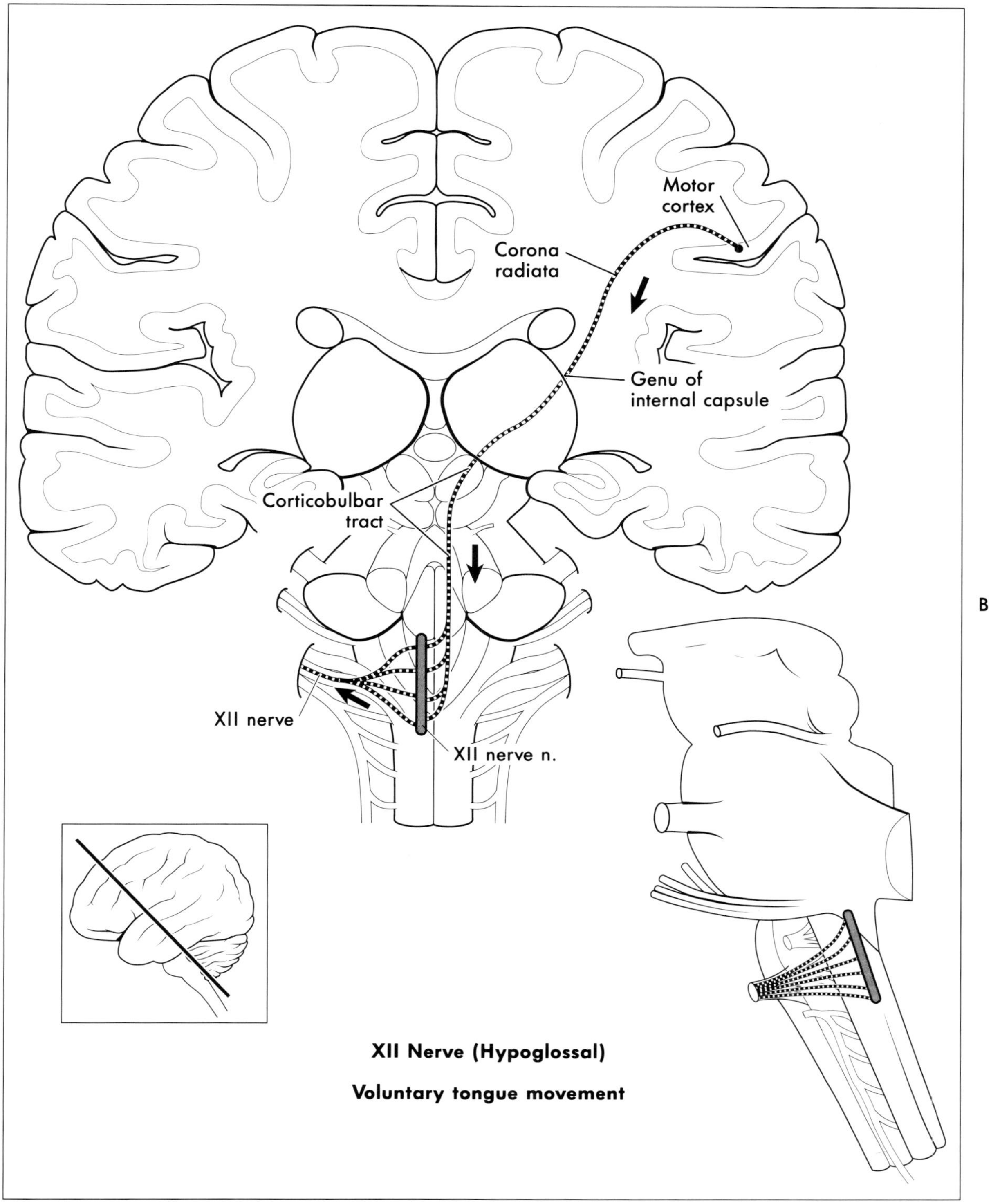

FIGURE 8-16 **A,** Brainstem pathway of CN XII (hypoglossal). Individual structures in each brainstem slice are labeled in Chapter 7. **B,** Coronal schematic shows pathway of CN XII. Sagittal schematic shows only the location of CN XII and its brainstem nucleus.

REFERENCES

1. Wilson-Paules L, Akesson EJ, Stewart PA: *Cranial nerves: anatomy and clinical comments,* Toronto, 1988, BC Decker.
2. Gatz AJ: *Manter's essentials of clinical neuroanatomy and neurophysiology,* ed 4, Philadelphia, 1989, FA Davis.
3. Rosenbery M: Neuro-ophthalmology. In Wilkins RH, Rengachary SS, editors: *Neurosurgery,* New York, 1988, McGraw-Hill.
4. Rengachary SS: Cranial nerve examination. In Wilkins RH, Rengachary SS, editors: *Neurosurgery,* New York, 1988, McGraw-Hill.
5. Flannigan B, Bradley W, Mazziotta J, et al: Magnetic resonance imaging of the brainstem: normal structure and basic functional anatomy, *Radiology* 154:375-383, 1985.
6. Lufkin R, Bentson J, Wilson G, et al: MRI of the brainstem and cranial nerves, *Surg Radiol Anat* 8:49-66, 1986.
7. Daniels DL, Williams AL, Haughton VM: Computed tomography of the medulla, *Radiology* 145:63-69, 1982.
8. Suzuki M, Takashima T, Kadoya M, et al: MR imaging of olfactory bulbs and tracts, *AJNR* 10:955-957, 1989.
9. Laine FJ, Braun IF, Jensen ME, et al: Peritumoral tumor extension through the foramen ovale: evaluation with MR imaging, *Radiology* 174:65-71, 1990.
10. Hutchins LG, Harnsberger HR, Jacobs JM, et al: Trigeminal neuralgia (tic douloureux): MR imaging assessment, *Radiology* 175:837-841, 1990.
11. Gentry LR, Jacoby CG, Turski PA, et al: Cerebellopontine angle–petromastoid mass lesions: comparative study of diagnosis with MR imaging and CT, *Radiology* 162:513-520, 1987.
12. Press GA, Hesselink JR: MR imaging of cerebellopontine angle and internal auditory canal lesions at 1.5 T, *AJR* 150:1371-1381, 1988.
13. Bird CR, Hasso AN, Drayer BP, et al: The cerebellopontine angle and internal auditory canal: neurovascular anatomy on gas CT cisternograms, *Radiology* 154:667-670, 1985.
14. Lee SH, Lewis E, Montoya JH, Seelaus JF: Bilateral cerebellopontine angle air-CT cisternography, *AJNR* 2:105-106, 1981.
15. Enzmann DR, O'Donohue J: Optimizing MR imaging for detecting small tumors in the cerebellopontine angle and internal auditory canal, *AJNR* 8:99-106, 1987.
16. Daniels DL, Czervionke LF, Millen SJ, et al: MR imaging of facial nerve enhancement in Bell's palsy or after temporal bone surgery, *Radiology* 171:807-809, 1989.
17. Disbro MA, Harnsberger HR, Osborn AG: Peripheral facial nerve dysfunction: CT evaluation, *Radiology* 155:659-663, 1985.
18. Mafee MF, Kumar A, Valvassori GE, et al: CT in the evaluation of the vestibulocochlear nerves and their central pathways: evaluation of neurotologic disorders, *Radiol Clin North Am* 22(1):45-66, 1984.
19. Harnsberger HR, Davis RK, Parkin JL, et al: The tailored CT evaluation of persistent facial nerve paralysis, *Laryngoscope* 96:347-352, 1986.
20. Braun JP, Tournade A, Adynowski J: A comparative anatomical CT study of the vascular and nervous structures of the cerebello-pontine angle, *Neuroradiology* 26:3-7, 1984.
21. Teresi L, Lufkin R, Nitta K, et al: MRI of the facial nerve: normal anatomy and pathology, *Semin Ultrasound, CT, MR* 8:240-255, 1987.
22. Mafee MF: Acoustic neuroma and other acoustic nerve disorders: role of MRI and CT: an analysis of 238 cases, *Semin Ultrasound, CT, MR* 8:256-283, 1987.
23. Remley K, Harnsberger HR, Smoker WRK, Osborn AG: CT and MRI in the evaluation of glossopharyngeal, vagal and spinal accessory neuropathy, *Semin Ultrasound, CT, MR* 8:284-300, 1987.
24. Jacobs SJM, Harnsberger HR, Lufkin RB, et al: Vagal neuropathy: evaluation with CT and MRI, *Radiology* 164:97-102, 1987.
25. Daniels DL, Czervionke LF, Pech P, et al: Gradient recalled echo MR imaging of the jugular foramen, *AJNR* 9:675-678, 1988.
26. Daniels DL, Schenck JF, Foster T, et al: Magnetic resonance imaging of the jugular foramen, *AJNR* 6:699-703, 1985.
27. Larsson SG: Hemiatrophy of the tongue and floor of the mouth demonstrated by computed tomography, *J Comput Assist Tomogr* 9(5):914-918, 1985.
28. Smoker WRK, Harnsberger HR, Osborn AG: The hypoglossal nerve, *Semin Ultrasound, CT, MR* 8:301-312, 1987.

CHAPTER 9

Atlas of Cerebellar Hemispheres and Vermis

Gary A. Press
Eric Courchesne

This chapter is designed to serve as a quick reference for identifying the complex anatomy of the cerebellar hemispheres and vermis. It is a summary of previous work done by the authors on this subject.[1-3] An index of anatomic terms is included. This allows the reader to find unfamiliar regions on these illustrations. The images used were obtained with a 1.5 T superconducting magnetic resonance (MR) scanner (Signa, General Electric).

Figures 9-1 to 9-7 describe serial sagittal sections of the cerebellum and vermis. Figures 9-8 to 9-13 describe coronal sections of this area. For all of these figures, image *A* is either a sagittal or coronal microtome section through a formalin-fixed normal brain specimen. Each section was stained for myelin using Luxol fast blue–cresyl violet. Image *B* is the corresponding proton-density-weighted image of the same brain specimen before sectioning. Images *C* and *D* are T1-weighted and cardiac-gated T2-weighted MR images, respectively, from a normal young volunteer (T1, longitudinal relaxation time; T2, transverse relaxation time). A key to the abbreviations used in Figures 9-1 to 9-13 precedes the illustrations. The anatomic text of Angevine et al. was consulted for assistance in labeling these figures.[4]

Optimum visualization of detailed cerebellar anatomy was provided by the following protocol. In all instances a 28-second T1-weighted scout sequence (TR/TE/TI, 200/20/1; 24 cm FOV; and 256 × 128 matrix) in the axial and sagittal plane was performed initially to verify precise positioning of the subject or brain specimen (TR, relaxation time; TE, echo delay time; TI, inversion recovery time; FOV, field of view). Subsequent high-resolution, short TR/TE/TI sequences had the parameters, 600/20/4 to 6 with a 12 to 18 cm FOV. Living subjects underwent long TR (T2-weighted) examinations that were cardiac gated to every other or every third heartbeat. The pulse sequence parameters were 2400 to 3800/20, 70/2 to 4. A presaturation radiofrequency (RF) pulse was also used for eliminating blood flow artifacts along the z axis (flow void = 1). Nongated long TR sequences performed on cadaver brains had the parameters, 1800 to 3000/20,70/4. The 5 mm thick slices obtained in all sequences were separated by a 2.5 mm gap.

REFERENCES

1. Courchesne E, Press GA, Murakami J, et al: The cerebellum in sagittal plane: anatomic-MR correlation. 1. The vermis, *AJNR* 10:659-665, 1989.
2. Press GA, Murakami J, Courchesne E, et al: The cerebellum in sagittal plane: anatomic-MR correlation. 2. The cerebellar hemispheres, *AJNR* 10:667-676, 1989.
3. Press GA, Murakami JW, Courchesne E, et al: The cerebellum. 3. Anatomic-MR correlation in the coronal plane, *AJNR* 11:41-50, 1990.
4. Angevine JB Jr, Mancall EL, Yakovlev PI: *The human cerebellum: an atlas of gross topography in serial sections,* Boston, 1961, Little, Brown.

KEY TO ABBREVIATIONS USED IN FIGURES 9-1 TO 9-13

A	artifact of sectioning
An	anterior aspect of section
Ant Lobe	anterior lobe of cerebellar hemisphere
ao	atlantooccipital joint
A Ve	lobules of anterior lobe of vermis
Bi	biventer
C	central lobule
Ce	centralis
Ci	cisterna magna
cl	clivus
Cm	corpus medullare
cpa	cerebellopontine angle cistern
Cu	culmen
C1	posterior arch of C1 vertebra
D	dentate nucleus
De	declive
dm	digastric muscle
F	flocculus
fm	foramen magnum
Fo	folium vermis
Gr	gracile lobule
iac	internal auditory canal
ibf	intrabiventral fissure
icp	inferior cerebellar peduncle
jb	jugular bulb
jt	jugular tubercle
jv	jugular vein
Li	lingula
M	medulla
ma	rectus capitis posterior major muscle
mcp	middle cerebellar peduncle
Mi	midbrain
mi	rectus capitis posterior minor muscle
mv	medullary velum
No	nodulus
P	pons
pb	petrous bone
pl	posterior cortical lip of foramen magnum
pt	primary white-matter tract
P Ve	lobules of posterior lobe of vermis
Py	pyramis
Qu A	quadrangular lobule, anterior posterior
Qu P	quadrangular lobule, posterior portion
sc	semicircular canal
scp	superior cerebellar peduncle
Se I	semilunar lobule, inferior portion
Se S	semilunar lobule, superior portion
so	superior oblique muscle
tf	transverse fossa
tmj	temporomandibular joint
To	tonsil
Tu	tuber vermis
Uv	uvula
V	fourth ventricle
1	precentral fissure
2	preculminate fissure
3	primary fissure
4	superior posterior fissure
5	horizontal fissure
6	prepyramidal fissure (vermis only)
6′	inferior posterior fissure (hemisphere only)
6″	inferior anterior fissure (hemisphere only)
7	secondary fissure
8	posterolateral fissure
9	vallecula
10	paramedian sulcus

Figure 9-1 *Midline sagittal scan plane.*
A, Myelin-stained brain specimen. **B,** Proton-density-weighted MR image of brain specimen. **C,** T1-weighted MR image of normal volunteer. **D,** T2-weighted MR image of normal volunteer. White matter branching within vermis is seen with remarkable fidelity on MR images. Anterior division of white matter of corpus medullare (C*m*) innervates lingula (L*i*), centralis (C*e*), and culmen (C*u*) of anterior lobe of vermis. Posterior division innervates declive (D*e*), folium vermis (F*o*), tuber vermis (T*u*), pyramis (P*y*), and uvula (U*v*) of posterior lobe, as well as the nodulus (N*o*) of flocculonodular lobe of cerebellum. Fine secondary and tertiary white matter branches to some regions (U*v*) are shown well. Images **C** and **D** best show surface landmarks of vermis by accentuating signal intensity difference between cerebellar parenchyma and cerebrospinal fluid (CSF). Precentral (1), preculminate (2), primary (3), superoposterior (4), horizontal (5), prepyramidal (6), secondary (7), and posterolateral (8) fissures around periphery of vermis are readily identified. Vallecula (9) separates vermis from inferior medulla (M), whereas cisterna magna (C*i*) separates vermis from meninges of the overlying occipital bone. Curvilinear CSF flow artifact (A) may be identified within fourth ventricle (V) anterior to lingula on T2-weighted image. T2-weighted image also shows well the pattern of white matter branching within vermis (compare with **A** and **B**). Flow void within posteroinferior cerebellar arteries (*arrowheads*) is seen posterior to medulla.

SAGITTAL SECTIONS

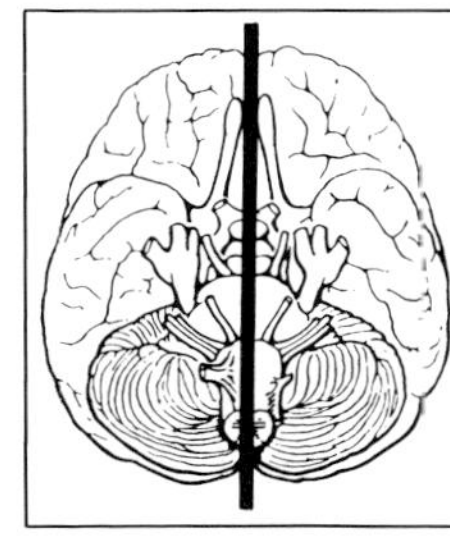

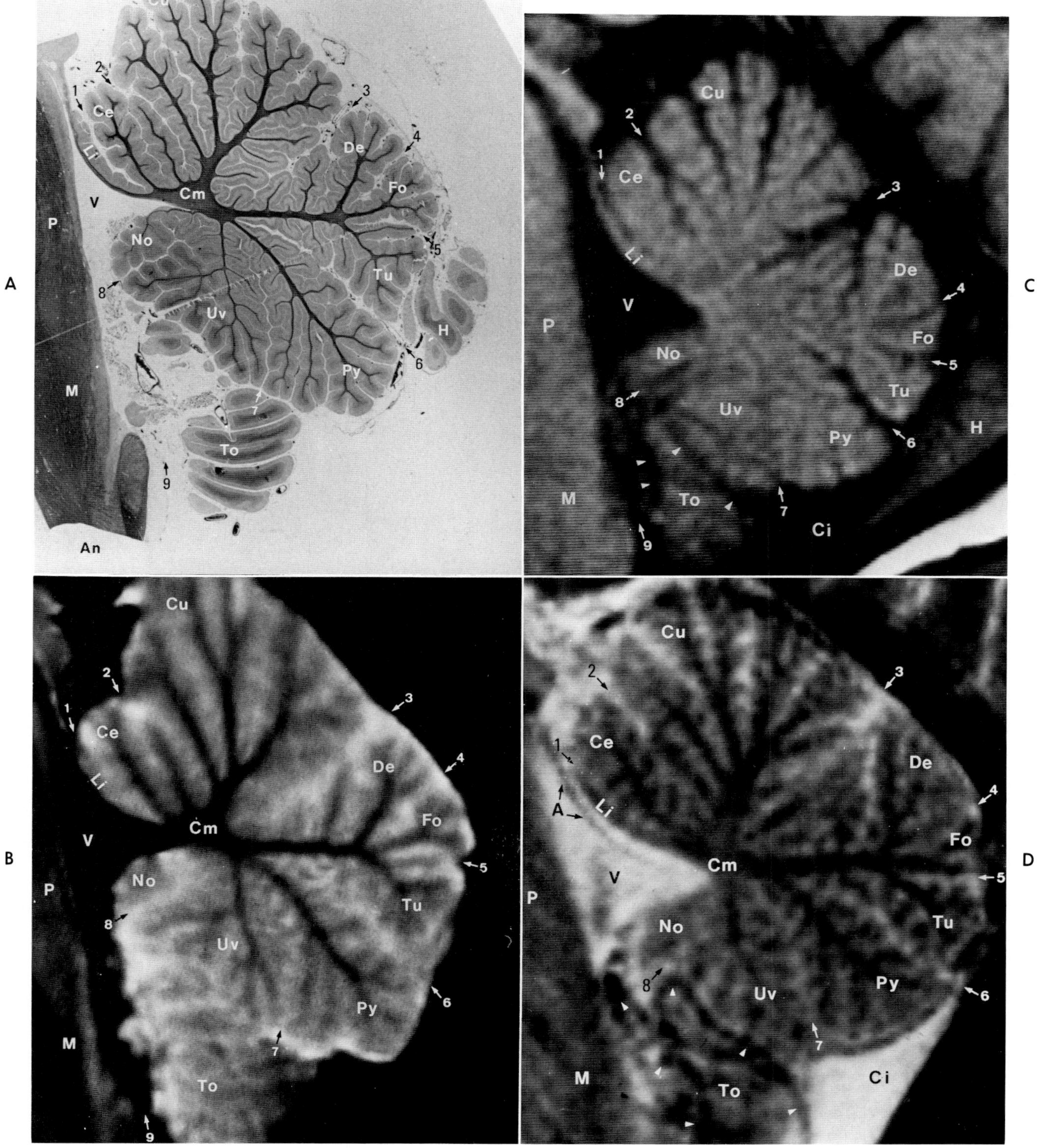

SAGITTAL SECTIONS

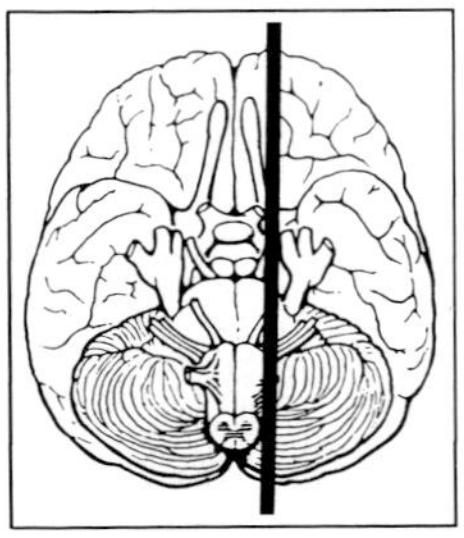

A

B

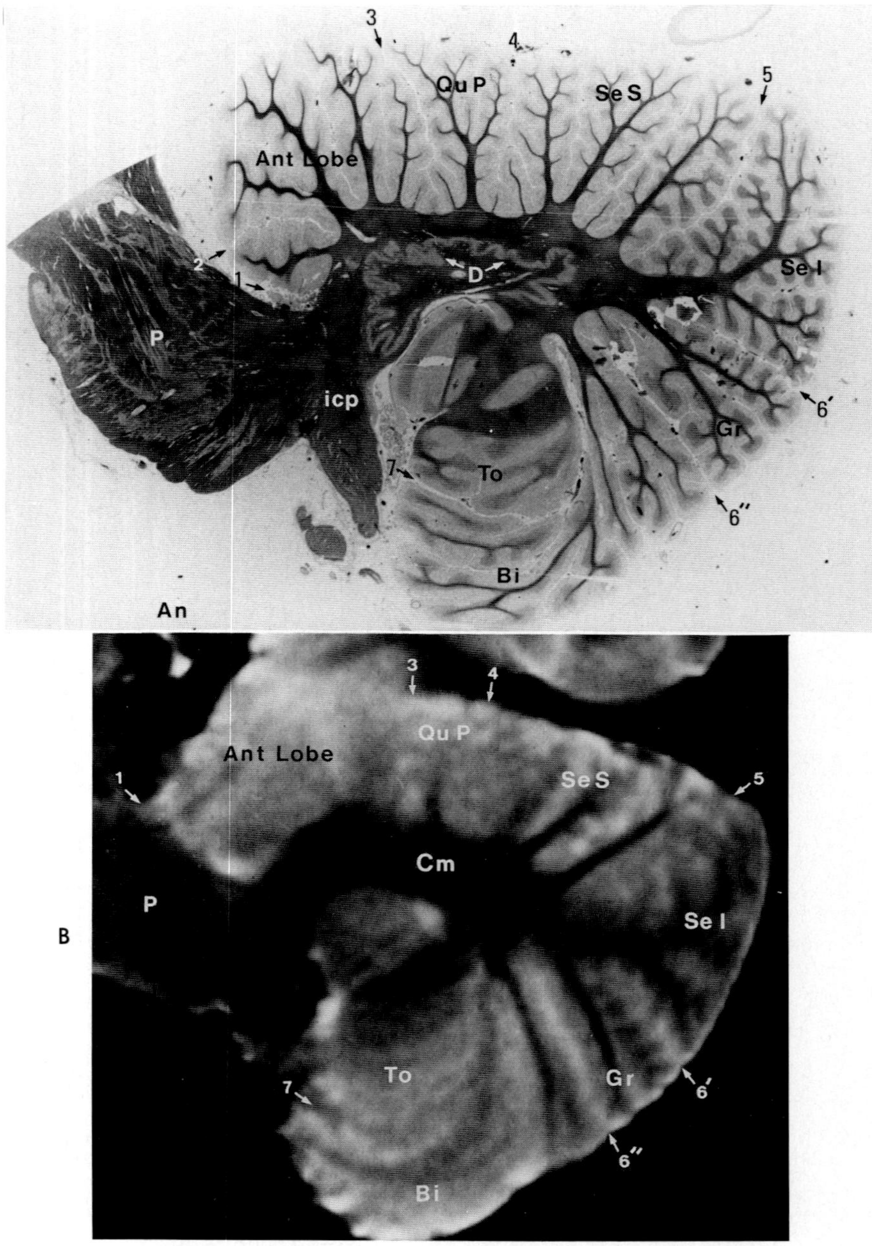

Figure 9-2 *Parasagittal scan plane through tonsil.*
A, Myelin-stained brain specimen. **B**, Proton-density-weighted MR image of brain specimen. **C**, T1-weighted MR image of normal volunteer. **D**, T2-weighted MR image of normal volunteer. Pons (P) and cerebellar hemisphere are continuous. Corpus medullare (C*m*) arches over tonsil (T*o*). Primary white matter tracts innervating posterior quadrangular (Q*u* P), inferior and superior semilunar (S*e* I, S*e* S), and gracile (G*r*) lobules and posterior portion of the biventer (B*i*) are well delineated on images **A** and **B.** Note hatchmarklike horizontal arrangement of gray and white matter within tonsil **(A, B, and D).**

SAGITTAL SECTIONS

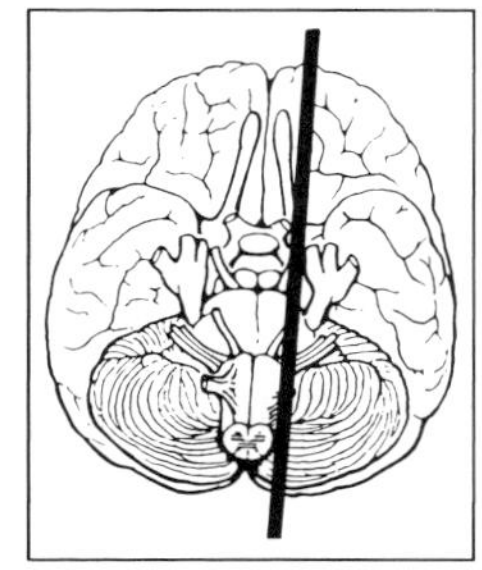

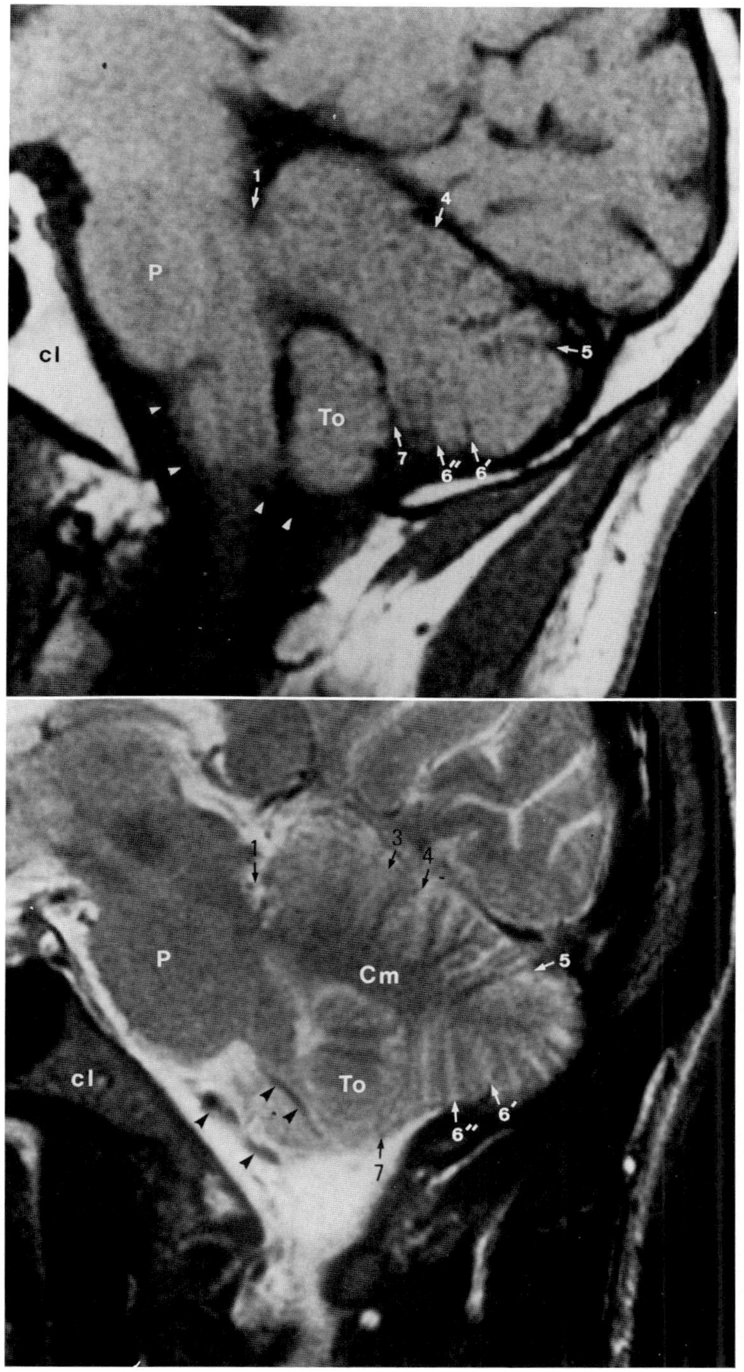

C

D

Figure 9-2, cont'd. *Parasagittal scan plane through tonsil.*
Several primary white matter tracts to anterior lobe of hemisphere are obscured because of volume averaging on **B** and **D.** For the same reason, characteristic undulating contour of dentate nucleus (D) is identifiable only on thin (15 μm) section used for the anatomic image **(A).** Gray and white matter have similar signal intensity on **C;** however, margins of hemisphere and fissures are well defined on this image. Extraparenchymal landmarks in this plane include a paramidline section through the clivus (*cl*), intraarachnoid course of vertebral artery (*ventral arrowheads*), and lateral medullary segment of postero-inferior cerebellar artery (*dorsal arrowheads*).

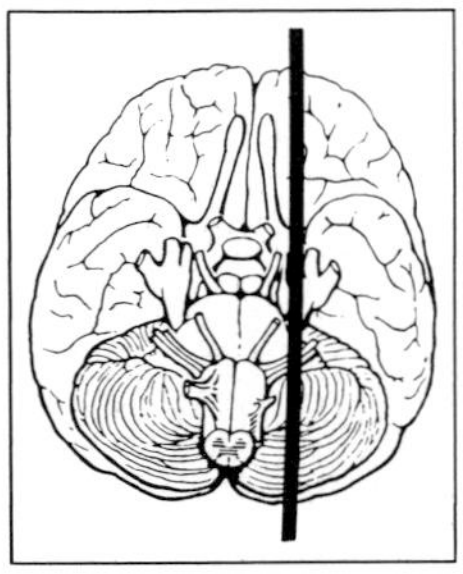

SAGITTAL SECTIONS

A

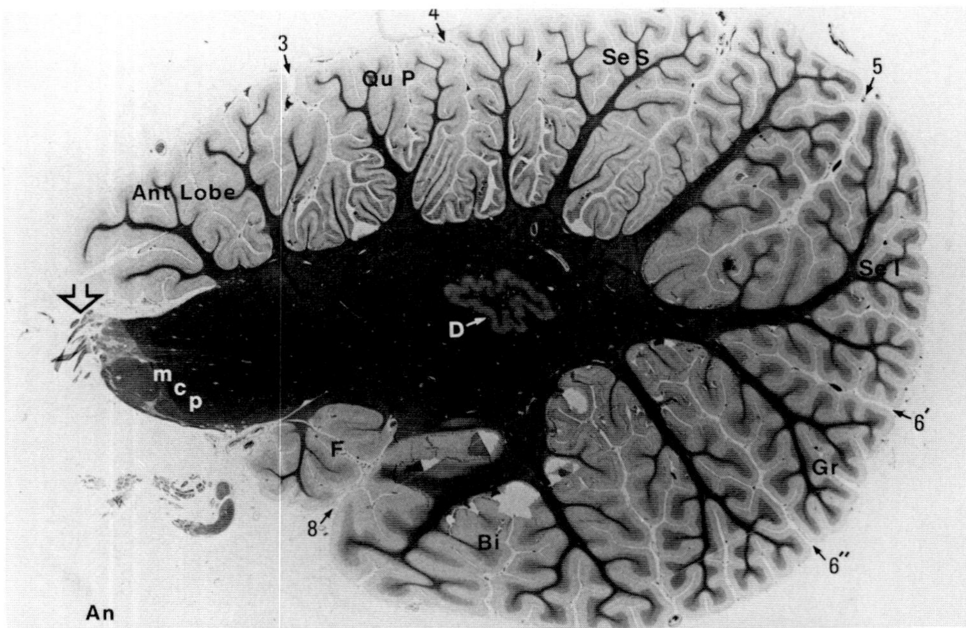

B

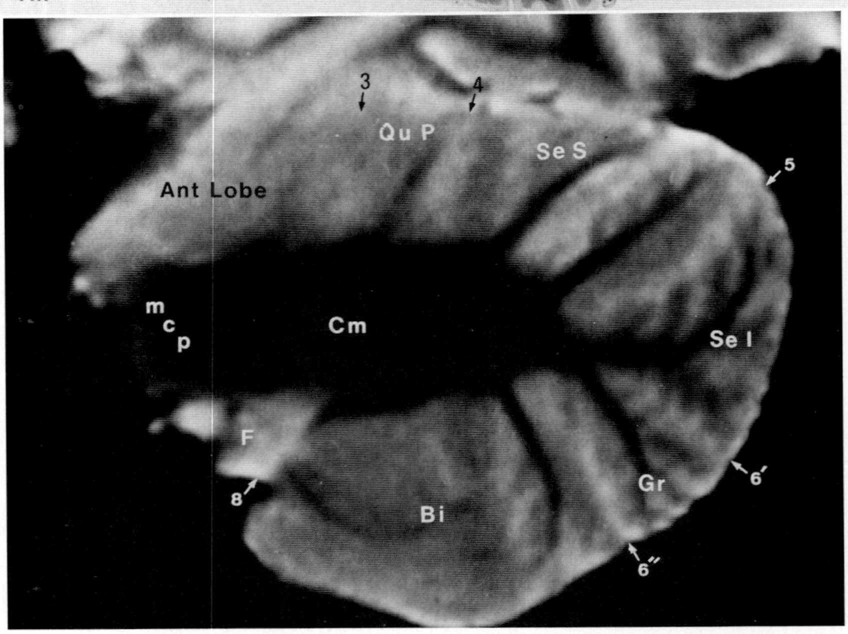

Figure 9-3 *Parasagittal scan plane through middle cerebellar peduncle.*
A, Myelin-stained brain specimen. **B,** Proton-density-weighted MR image of brain specimen. **C,** T1-weighted MR image of normal volunteer. **D,** T2-weighted MR image of normal volunteer. In this plane, lateral to brainstem and tonsil, corpus medullare (C*m*) becomes oval in shape. Middle cerebellar peduncle (*mcp*) extends from corpus medullare to anterior aspect of hemisphere. Biventer (B*i*) alone is sectioned at anteroinferior aspect of cerebellar hemisphere. Anterior lobe of hemisphere (A*nt* L*obe*) is smaller than in Figure 9-2. Flocculus (F) may appear as a small, globular lobule at anteroinferior aspect of corpus medullare **(A** and **B).**

SAGITTAL SECTIONS

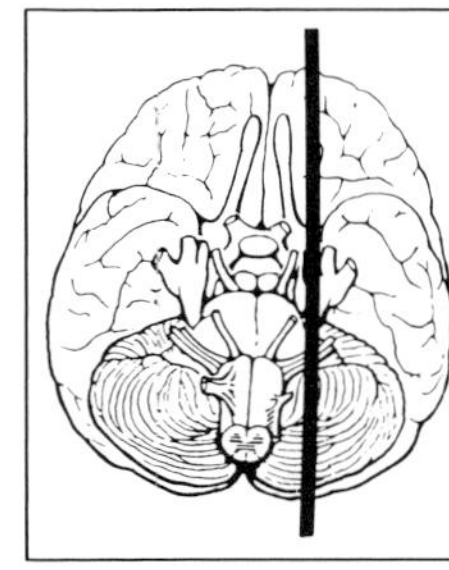

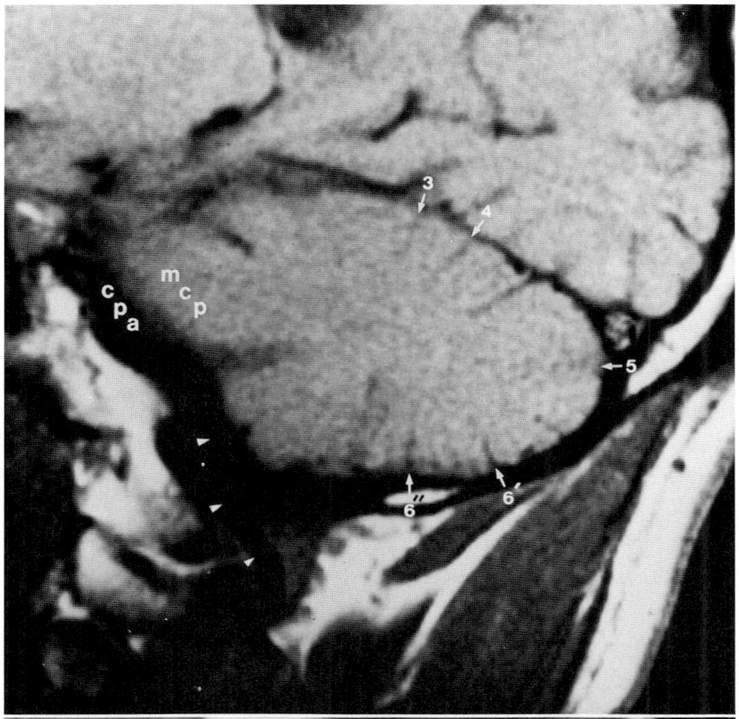

C

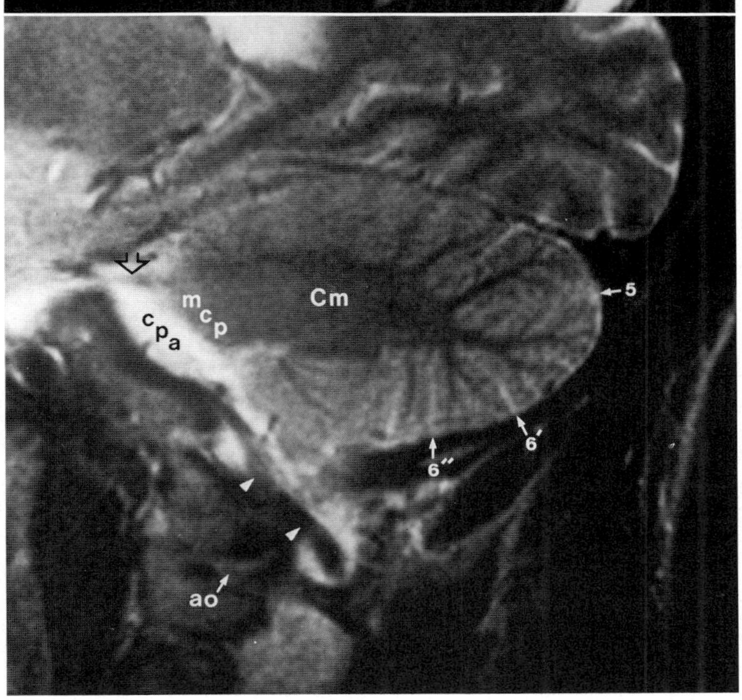

D

Figure 9-3, cont'd. *Parasagittal scan plane through middle cerebellar peduncle.*
Posterolateral aspect of dentate nucleus (D) appears as a complete ring within corpus medullare and is best seen on anatomic image **(A)**. Within superior aspect of cerebellopontine angle cistern (*cpa*) is trigeminal nerve root (*open arrow*, **A** and **D**), which courses over petrous bone to end in Meckel's cave **(D)**. Extraparenchymal landmarks identified in vivo include atlanto-occipital joint and vertebral artery (*arrowheads*) passing over posterior arch of the first cervical vertebra (C1) to enter cranial cavity.

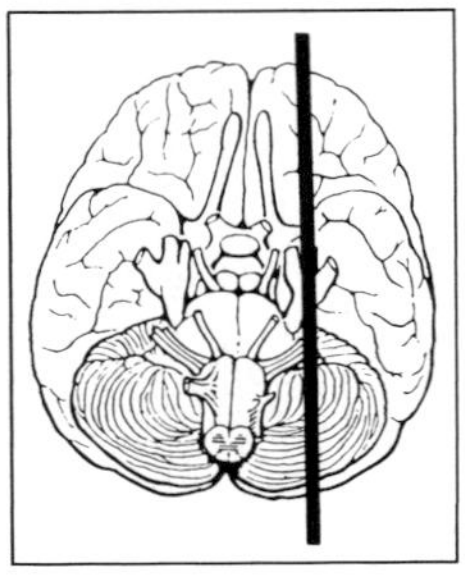

SAGITTAL SECTIONS

A

B

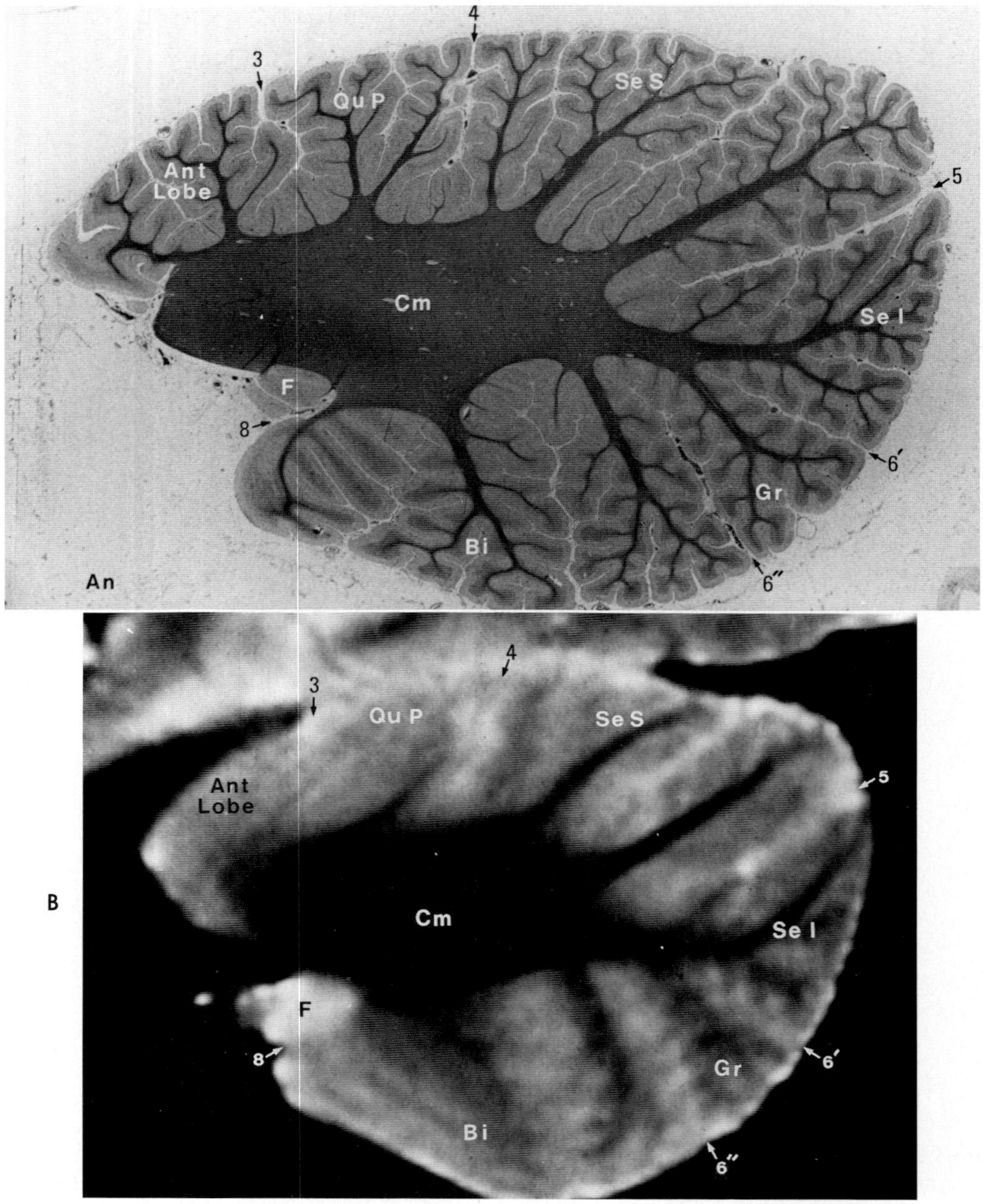

Figure 9-4 *Parasagittal scan plane lateral to middle cerebellar peduncle.*
A, Myelin-stained brain specimen. **B,** Proton-density-weighted MR image of brain specimen. **C,** T1-weighted MR image of normal volunteer. **D,** T2-weighted MR image of normal volunteer. This is the final section to include a portion of the anterior lobe of the cerebellar hemisphere. Dentate nucleus is not present in image **A.**

SAGITTAL SECTIONS

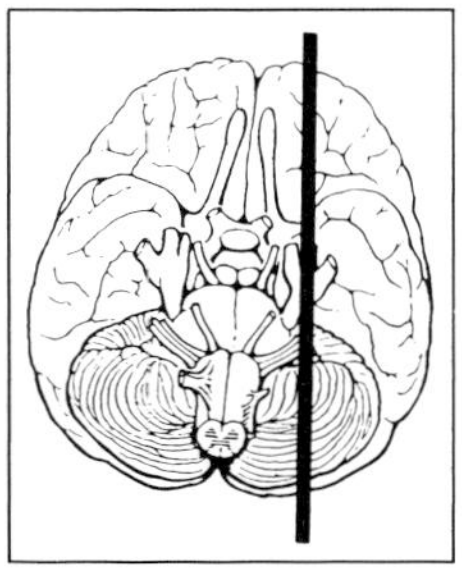

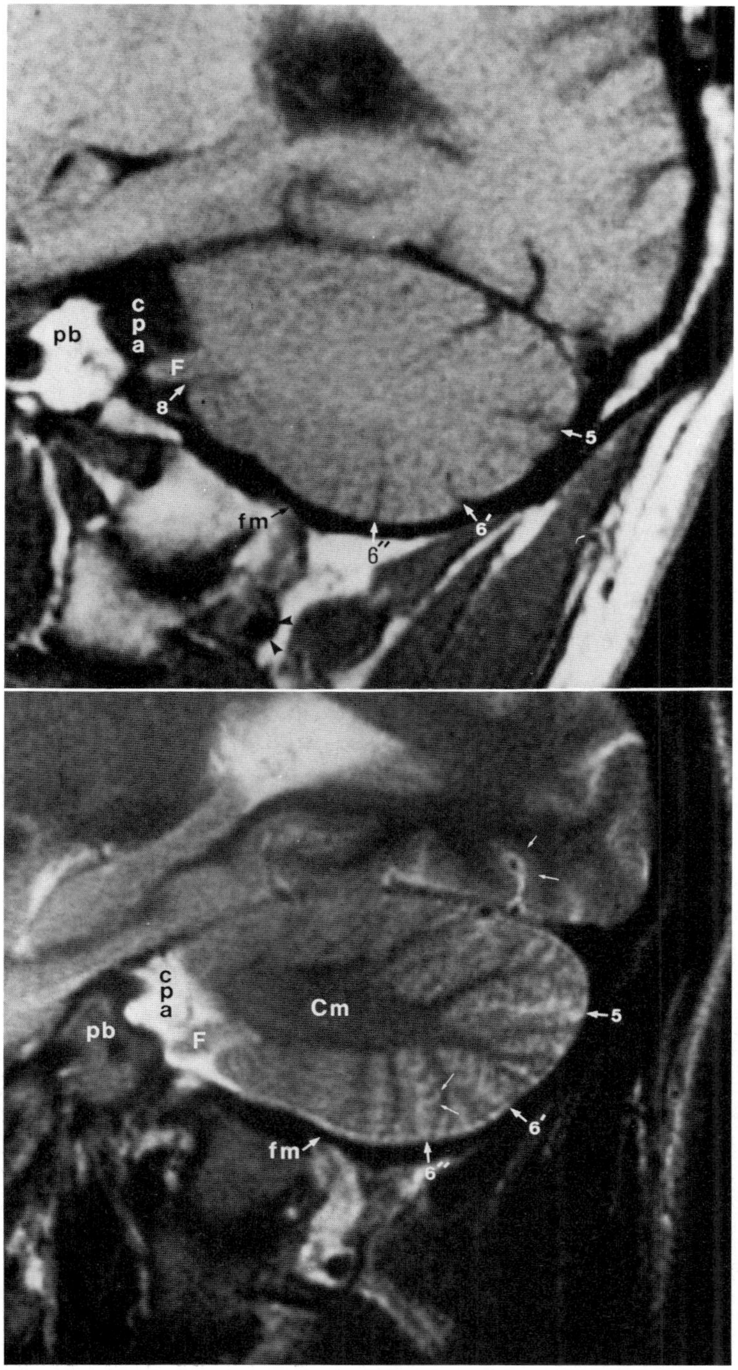

C

D

Figure 9-4, cont'd. *Parasagittal scan plane lateral to middle cerebellar peduncle.*
Flocculus (F) protrudes tonguelike into inferior aspect of cerebellopontine angle cistern **(C** and **D)**. Three-layered cortex of cerebellum is thinner than six-layered cortex of inferior occipital lobe (*smallest arrows*, **D**). Extraparenchymal landmarks identified in this plane in vivo include apex of petrous bone (*pb*) anterior to porus acusticus, lateral edge of foramen magnum (*fm*), and vertebral artery (*arrowheads*).

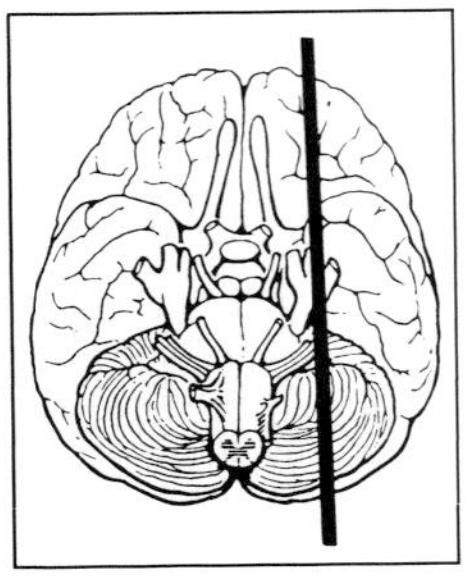

SAGITTAL SECTIONS

A

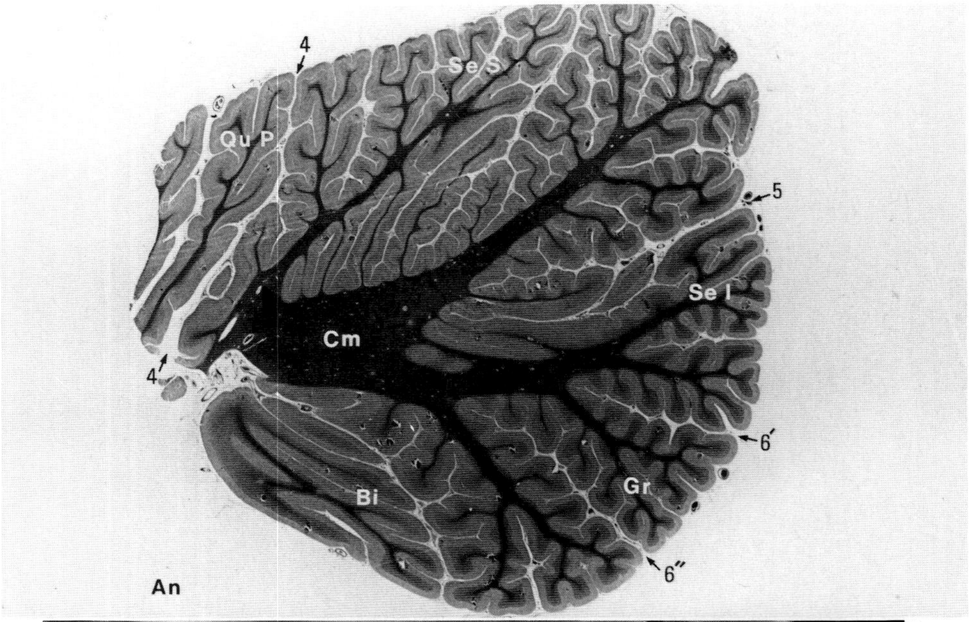

B

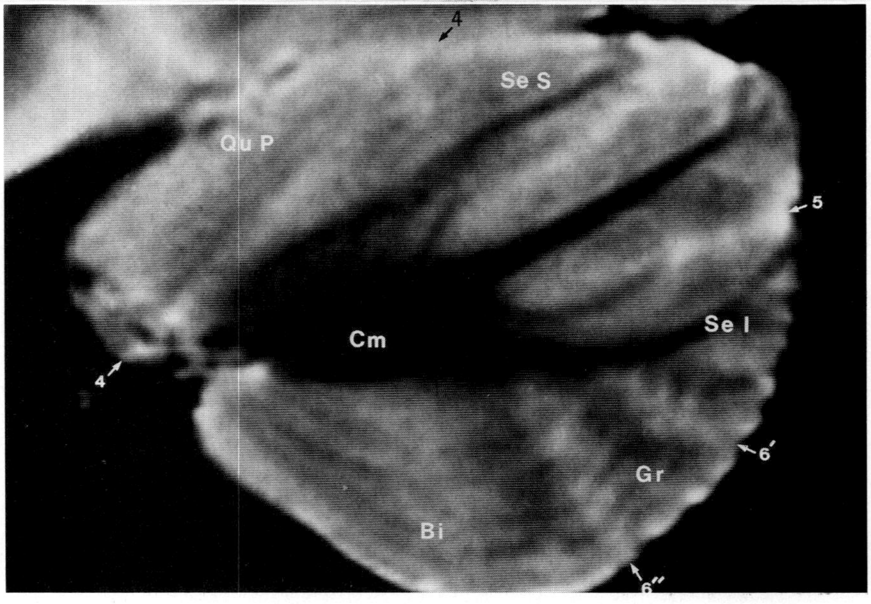

Figure 9-5 *Parasagittal scan plane lateral to flocculus.*
A, Myelin-stained brain specimen. **B**, Proton-density-weighted MR image of brain specimen. **C**, T1-weighted MR image of normal volunteer. **D**, T2-weighted MR image of normal volunteer. Lateral to anterior lobe of hemisphere, corpus medullare (C*m*) becomes smaller, with linear upper and lower margins. Profile of hemisphere as a whole is more rounded.

SAGITTAL SECTIONS

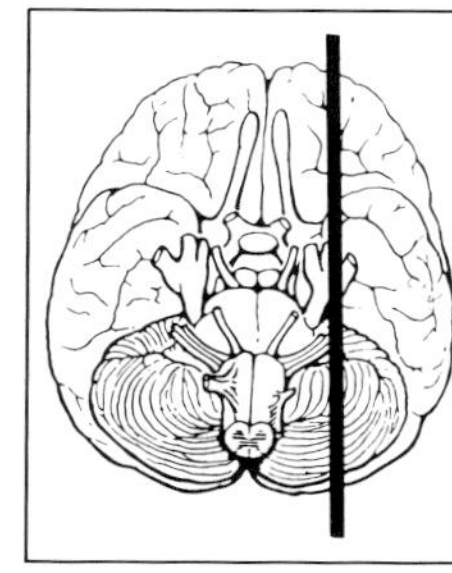

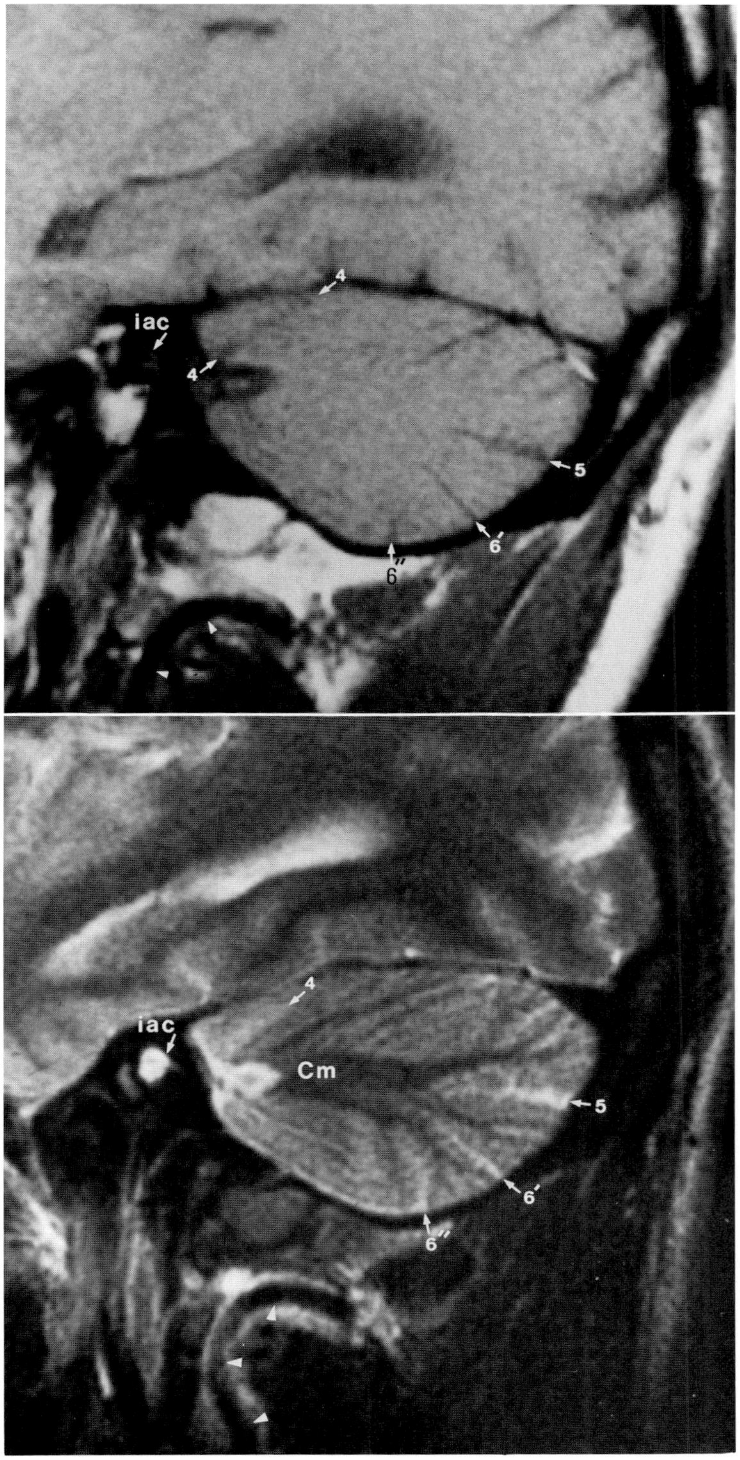

C

D

Figure 9-5, cont'd. *Parasagittal scan plane lateral to flocculus.*
Flocculus is no longer present. Extraparenchymal landmarks identified in this plane in vivo include cranial nerves VII and VIII within internal auditory canal (*iac*) and vertebral artery (*arrowheads*) coursing posteromedially from transverse foramen to posterior arch of atlas.

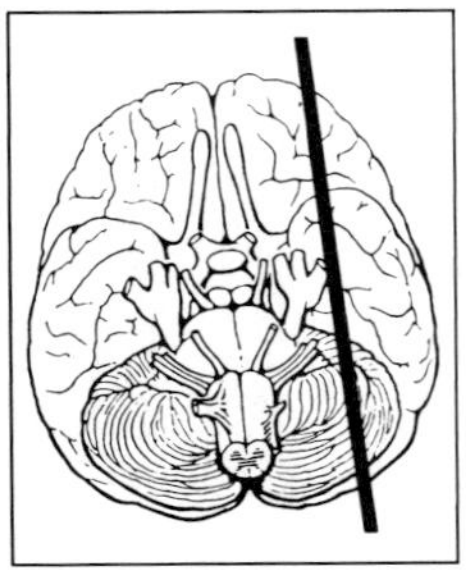

SAGITTAL SECTIONS

A

B

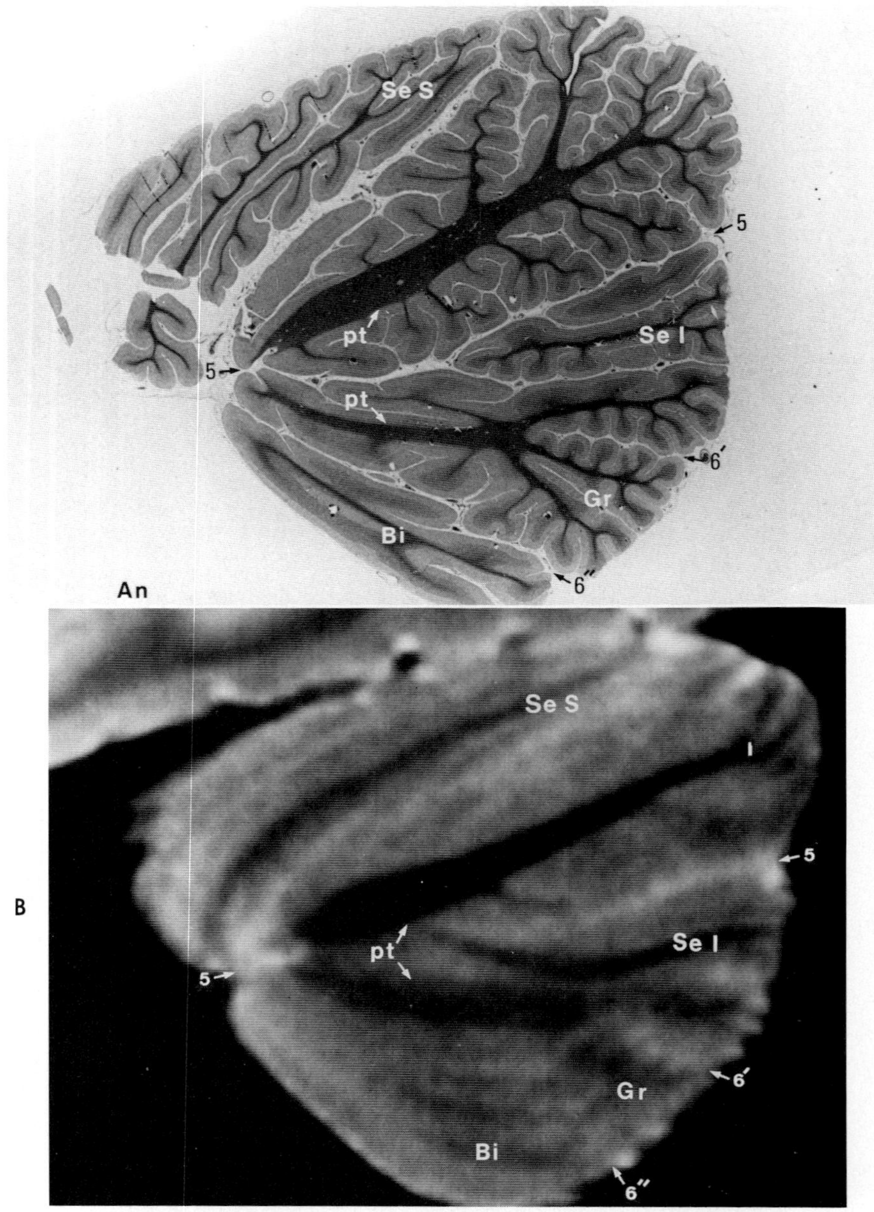

Figure 9-6 *Parasagittal scan plane lateral to corpus medullare.*

A, Myelin-stained brain specimen. **B,** Proton-density-weighted MR image of brain specimen. **C,** T1-weighted MR image of normal volunteer. **D,** T2-weighted MR image of normal volunteer. Primary white matter tracts (*pt*) innervating superior and inferior portions of semilunar lobule (*Se* S, *Se* I) diverge posteriorly. This is the final section to include a portion of the biventer (B*i*) and gracile lobules (G*r*). Extraparenchymal landmarks identified in this plane include semicircular canals (*sc*) and vestibule within petrous bone and internal jugular vein (*jv*).

SAGITTAL SECTIONS

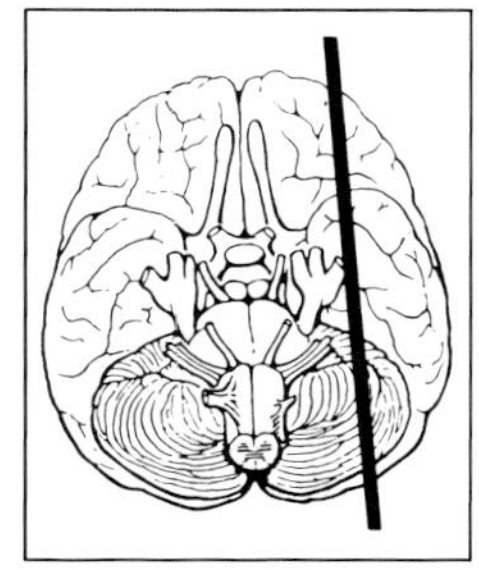

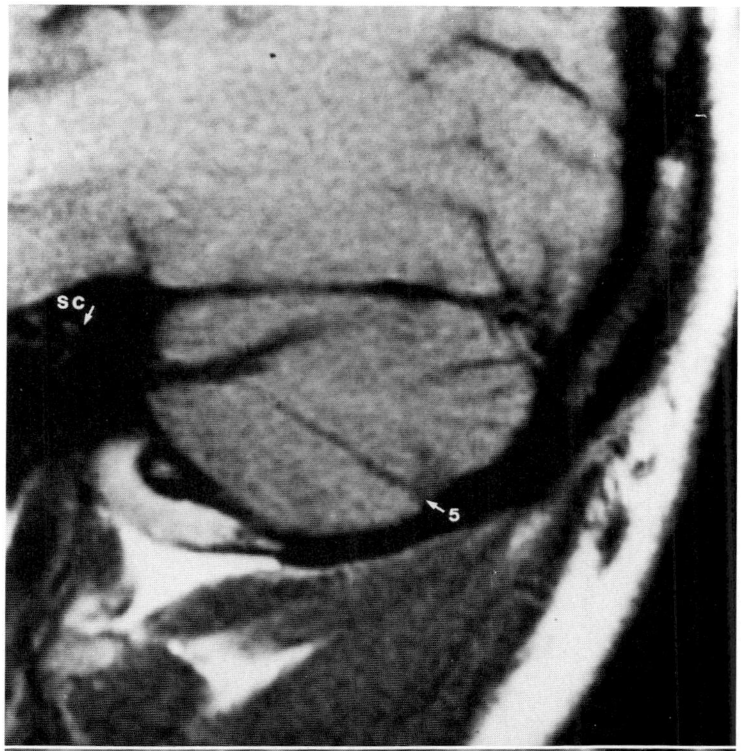

C

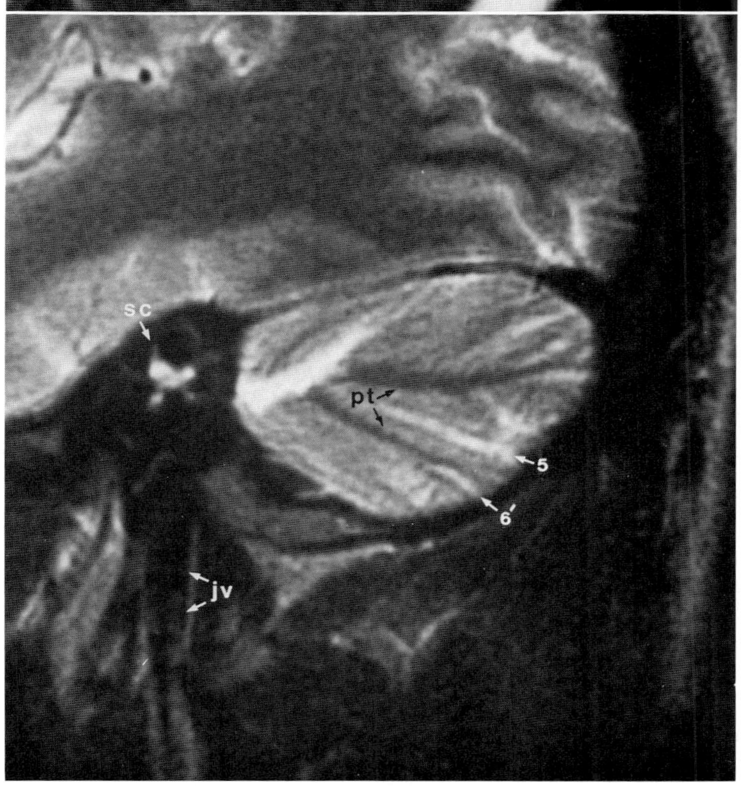

D

Figure 9-6, cont'd. *Parasagittal scan plane lateral to corpus medullare.* For legend see opposite page.

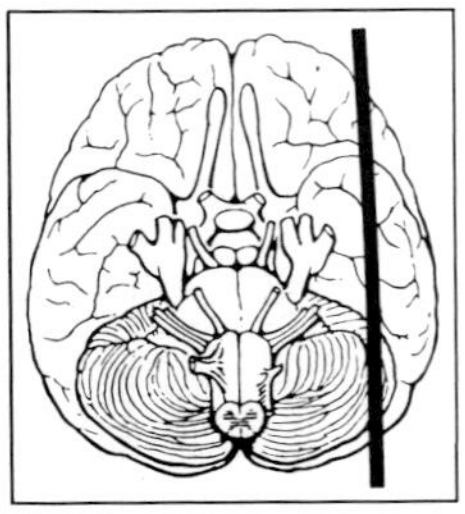

SAGITTAL SECTIONS

A

B

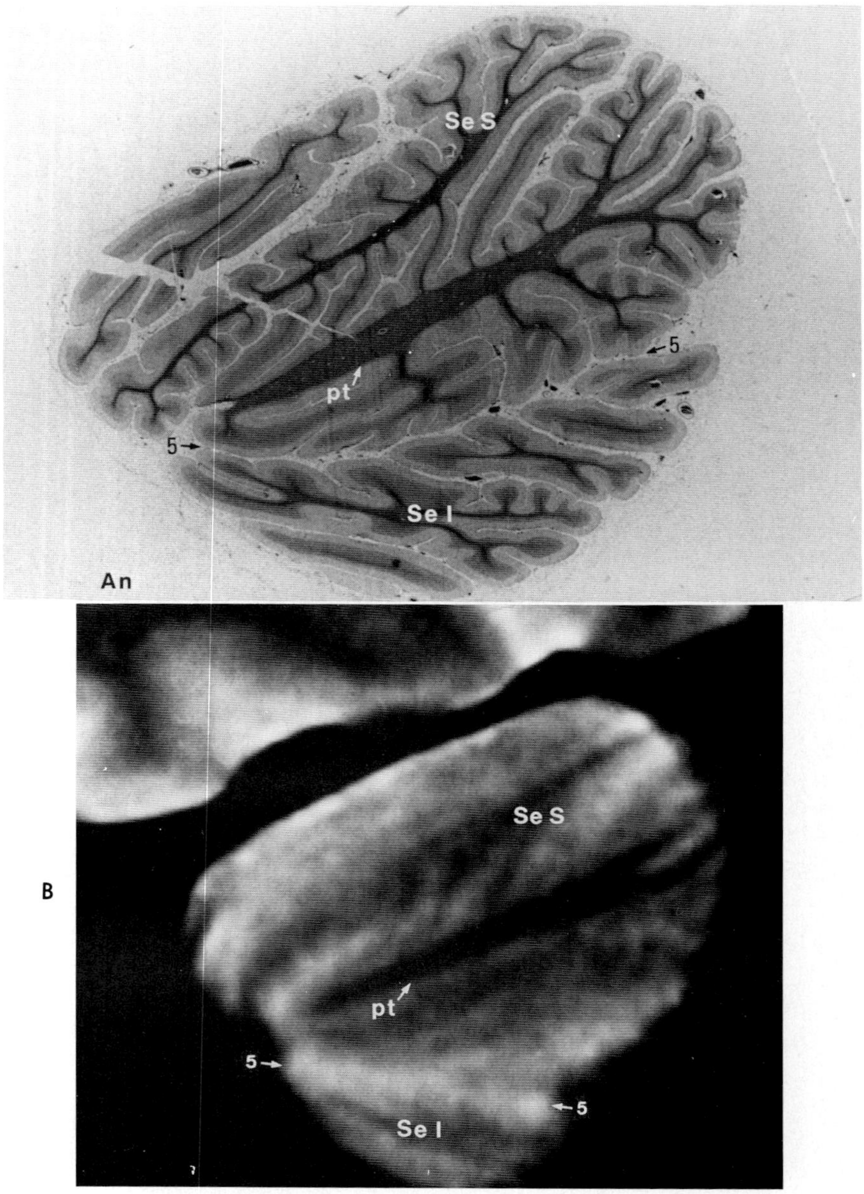

Figure 9-7 *Parasagittal scan plane through lateralmost part of cerebellum.*
A, Myelin-stained brain specimen. **B,** Proton-density-weighted MR image of brain specimen. **C,** T1-weighted MR image of normal volunteer. **D,** T2-weighted MR image of normal volunteer. Horizontal fissure (5) divides completely the remainder of the hemisphere into upper and lower portions containing lateralmost aspects of superior and inferior semilunar lobules (*Se* S, *Se* I), respectively. Temporomandibular joint (*tmj*) is extraparenchymal landmark consistently identified in this plane in vivo.

SAGITTAL SECTIONS

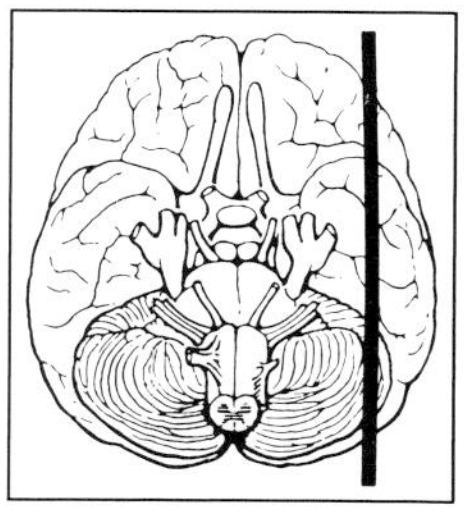

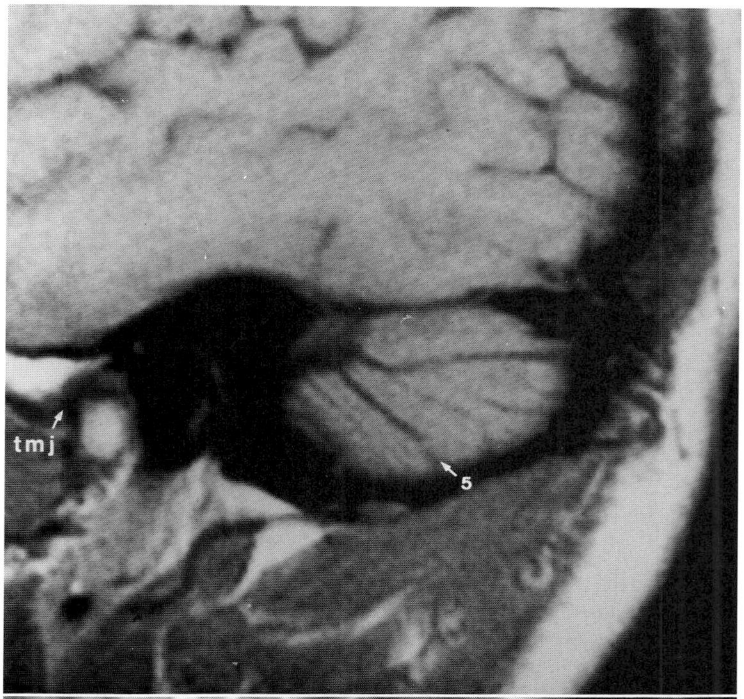

C

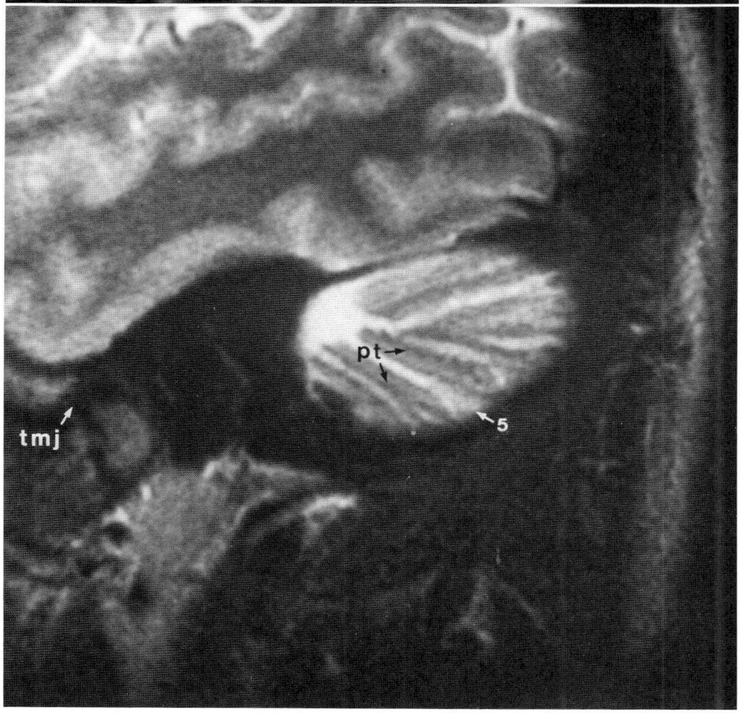

D

Figure 9-7, cont'd. *Parasagittal scan plane through lateralmost part of cerebellum.* For legend see opposite page.

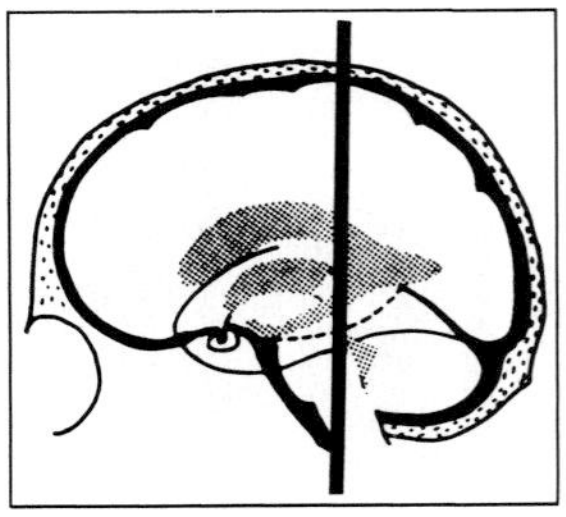

CORONAL SECTIONS

A

B

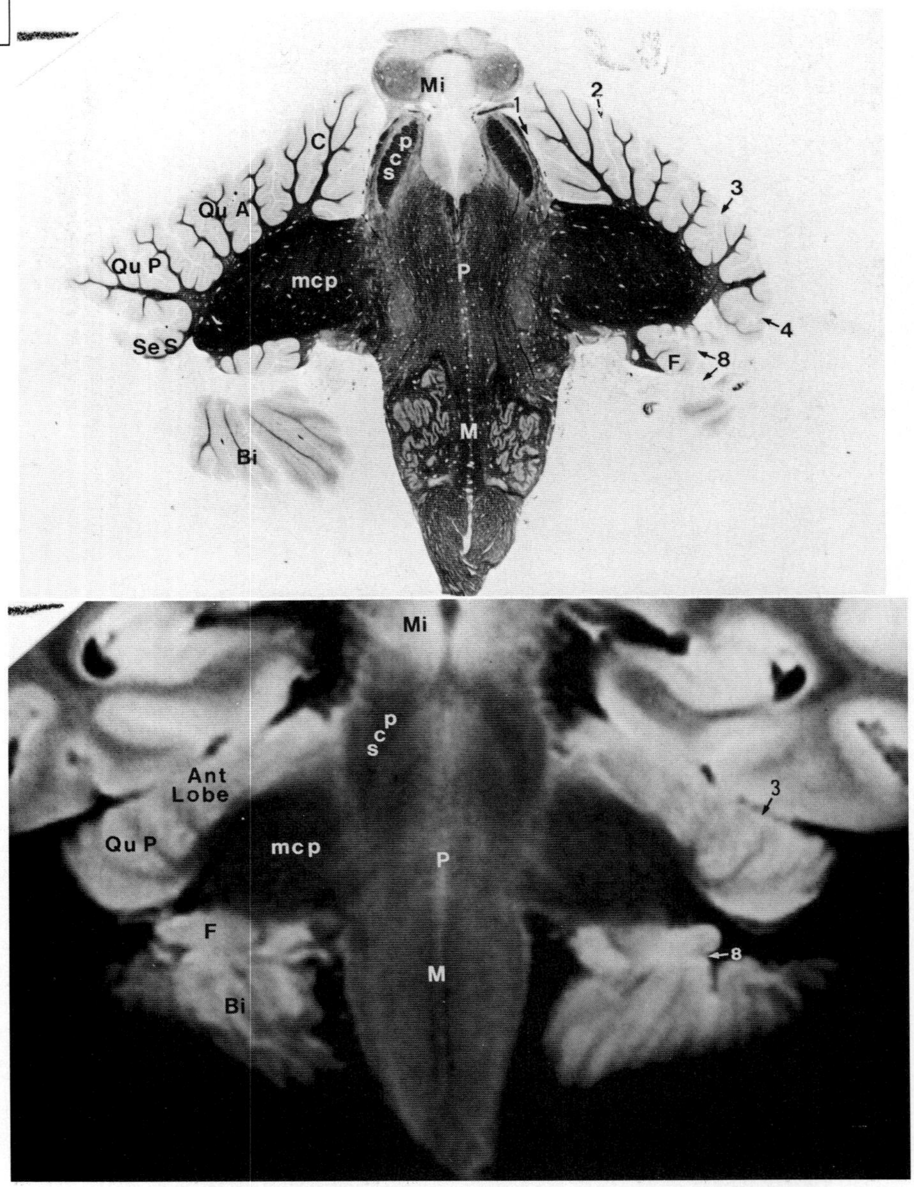

Figure 9-8 *Coronal scan plane through the brainstem.*
A, Myelin-stained brain specimen. **B,** Proton-density-weighted MR image of brain specimen. **C,** T1-weighted MR image of normal volunteer. **D,** T2-weighted MR image of normal volunteer. The midbrain (Mi), pons (P), and medulla (M) are continuous; the middle cerebellar peduncles (*mcp*) join the pons to the cerebellar hemispheres. The superior cerebellar peduncles (*scp*) diverge within the midbrain just beneath their decussation. Three distinct symmetric bands of cerebellar parenchyma arranged above and below the middle cerebellar peduncles appear to converge laterally in this plane. The single band above the peduncle represents the anterior aspect of the anterior quadrangular lobules (Q*u*A).

CORONAL SECTIONS

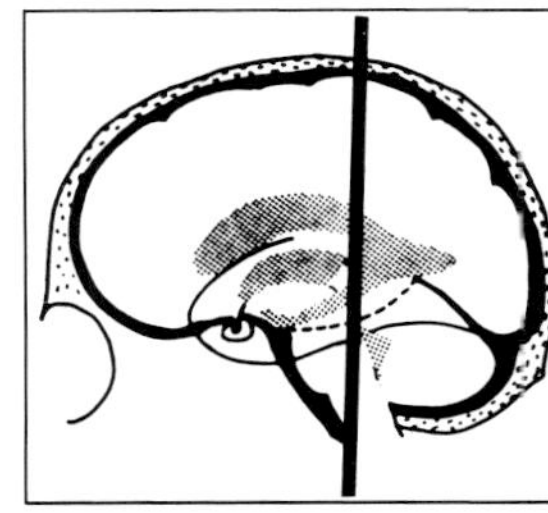

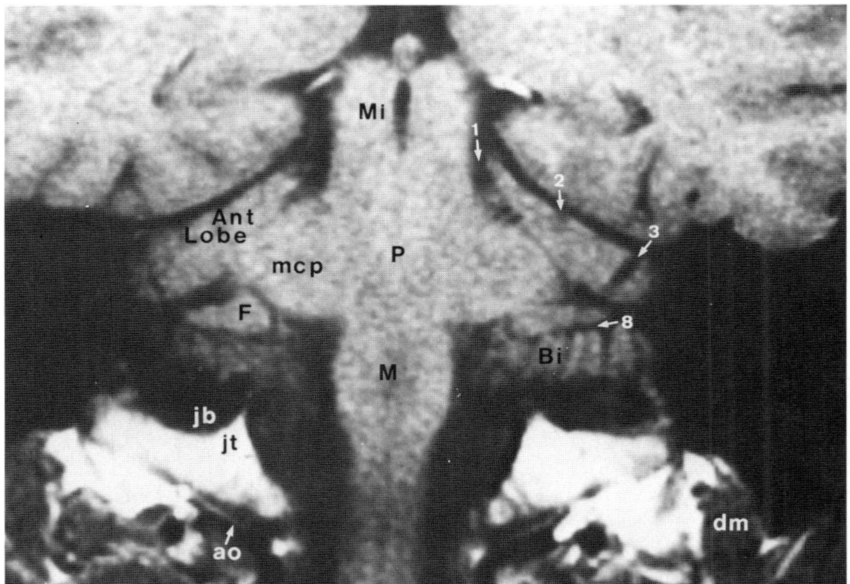

C

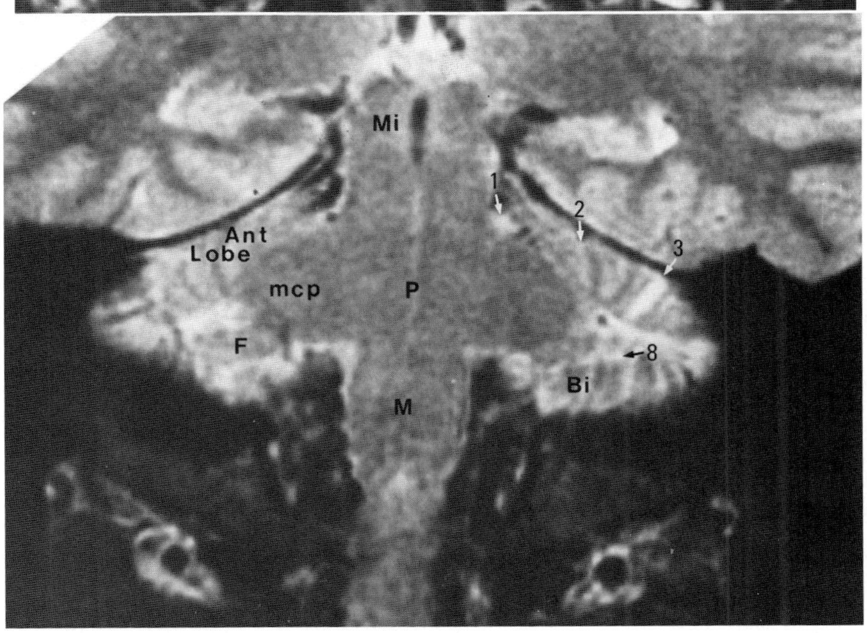

D

Figure 9-8, cont'd. *Coronal scan plane through the brainstem.*
Depending on the precise angle of section and the size of the lobules, small portions of the posterior quadrangular lobule (Q*u*P) and superior semilunar lobule (S*e* S) may be sectioned at the lateralmost aspect of this band. The middle band of tissue situated immediately beneath the middle cerebellar peduncle represents the flocculus (F) of the cerebellar hemisphere. The posterolateral fissure (8) separates the flocculus (F) from the third band of hemispheric tissue situated most inferiorly. This third band is the anterior aspect of the biventer (B*i*) (image **B**). Extraparenchymal landmarks in this plane are best demonstrated on **C** and include the posterior aspect of the jugular tubercle (*jt*), jugular bulb (*jb*), atlanto-occipital joint (*ao*), and insertion of posterior belly of digastric muscle (*dm*) medial to mastoid tip **(C)**.

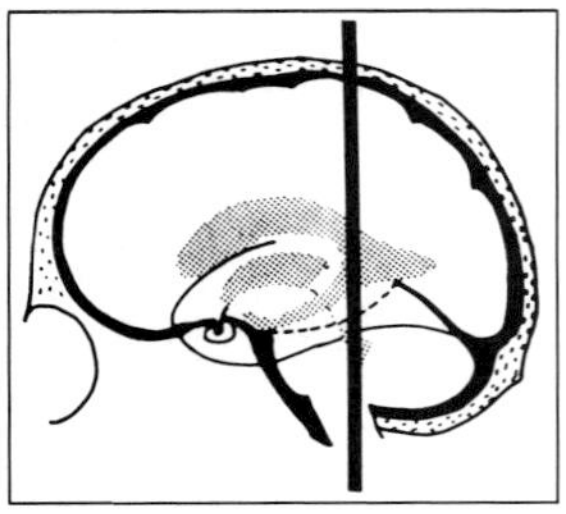

CORONAL SECTIONS

A

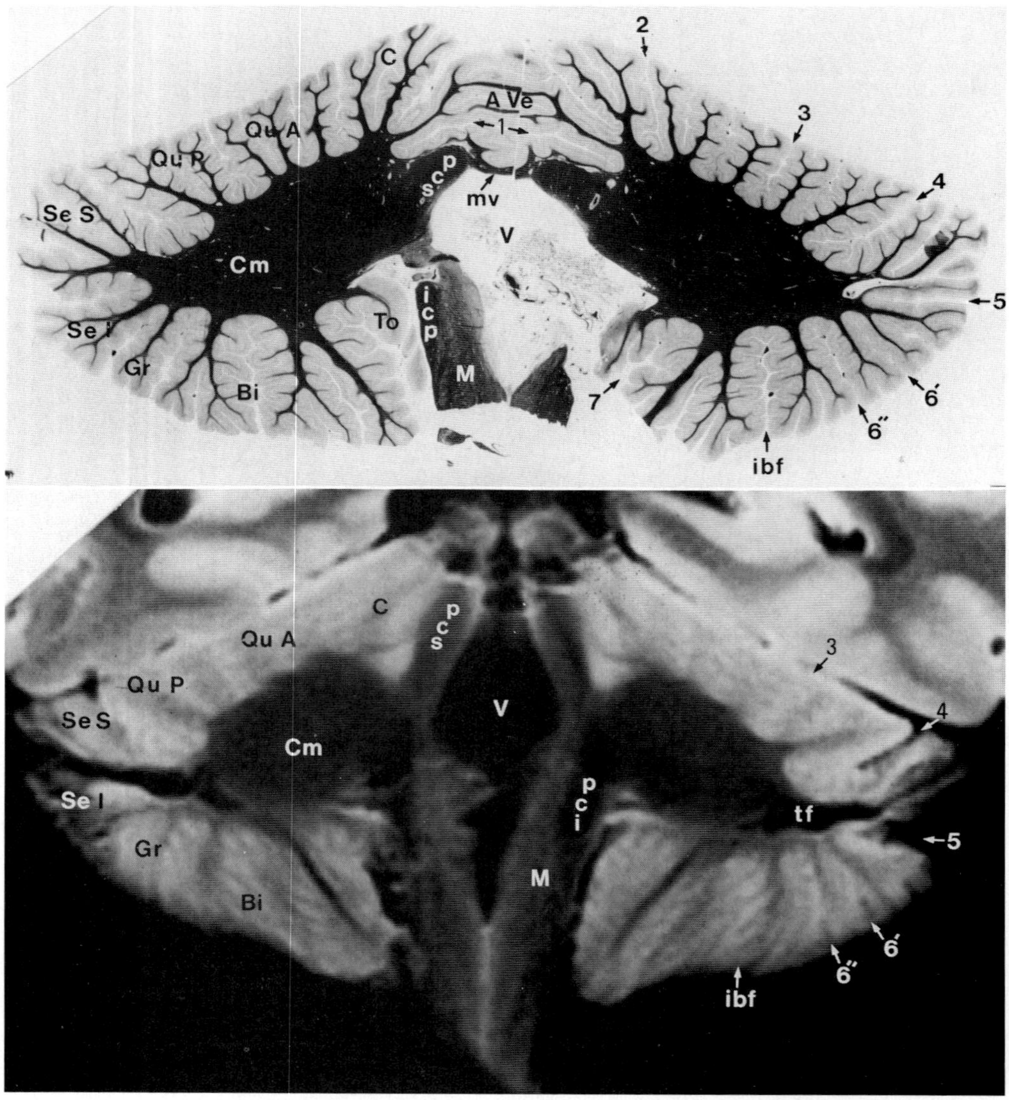

B

Figure 9-9 *Coronal scan plane through fourth ventricle.*
A, Myelin-stained brain specimen. **B,** Proton-density-weighted MR image of brain specimen. **C,** T1-weighted MR image of normal volunteer. **D,** T2-weighted MR image of normal volunteer. The superolateral margins of the fourth ventricle are formed by the superior cerebellar peduncles (*scp*); the inferior cerebellar peduncles (*icp*) are separated from the inferolateral margins of the fourth ventricle by the vestibular nuclei. A laterally directed cerebrospinal fluid (CSF) space, the transverse fossa (*tf,* images **B** to **D**), is formed by the converging folia of the superior, lateral, and inferior hemispheric surfaces. It is not a true cerebellar fissure **(C** and **D)**. Depending on the plane of section, the quadrigeminal plate or the anterior extreme of the anterior lobe of the vermis (A *Ve*) may be sectioned above the fourth ventricle.

CORONAL SECTIONS

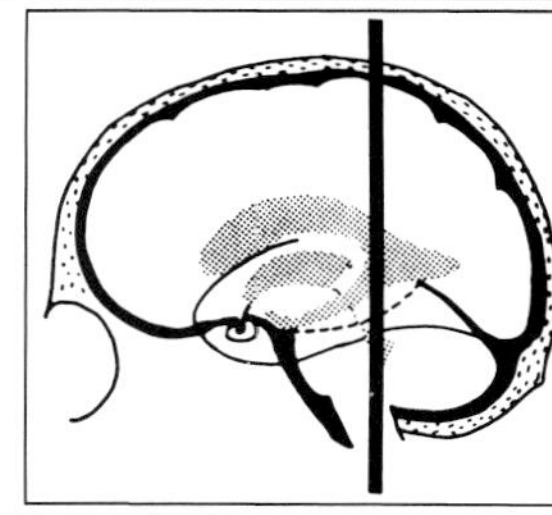

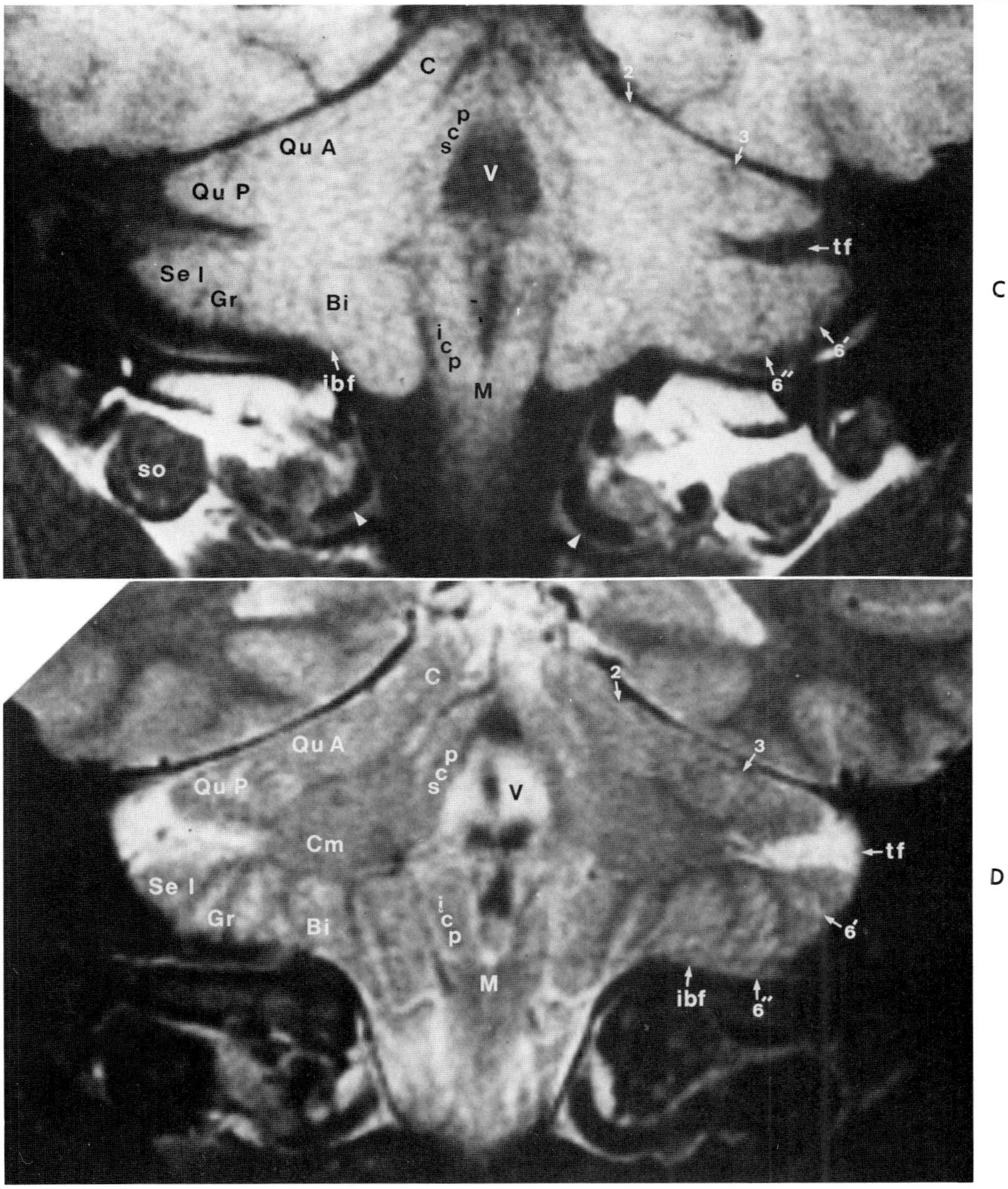

Figure 9-9, cont'd. *Coronal scan plane through fourth ventricle.*
In **C**, gray and white matter have similar signal intensity. Nevertheless, the borders of the parenchyma with surrounding CSF are better defined in **C** than **D** because of persistent CSF flow artifacts adjacent to the medulla that resemble parenchyma in **D.** In **B** and **C**, note that the biventer (*Bi*) forms the inferomedial border of each hemisphere where it abuts the medulla. Extraparenchymal landmarks identified in this image in vivo include the vertebral arteries (*arrowheads*) entering the subarachnoid space above the sulcus arteriosus, and the superior oblique muscles (*so*) sectioned transversely beneath the occipital bone in **C.**

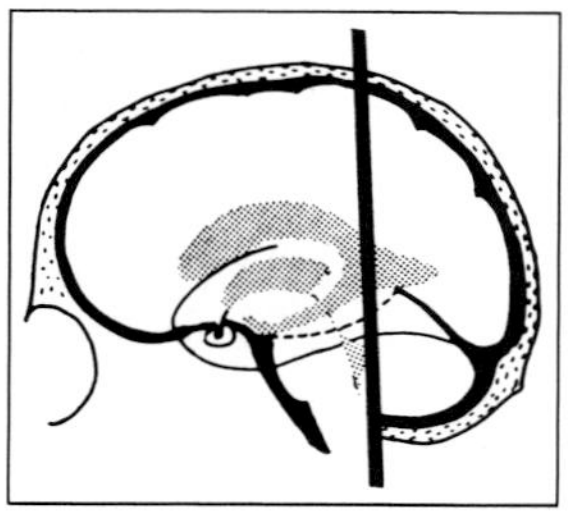

CORONAL SECTIONS

A

B

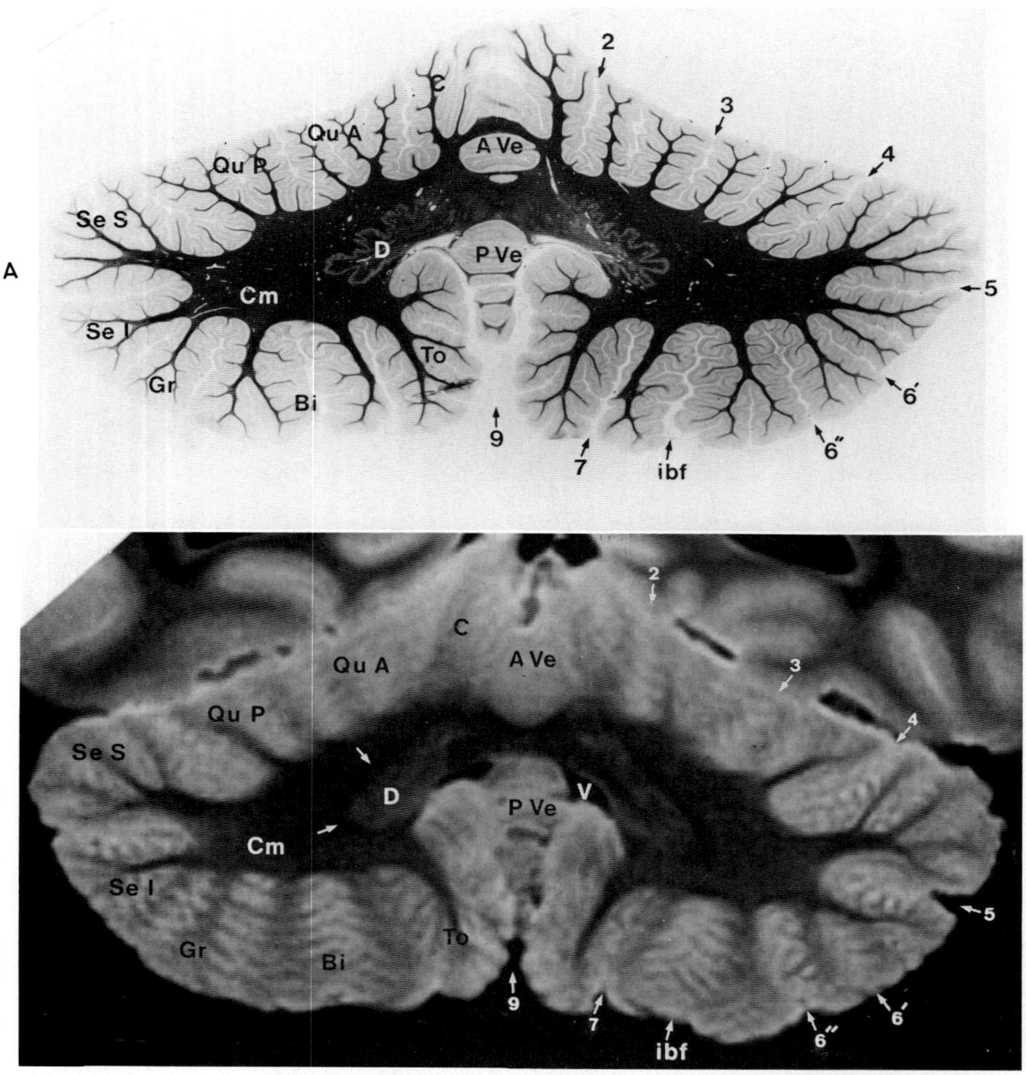

Figure 9-10 *Coronal scan plane through the tonsils.*

A, Myelin-stained brain specimen. **B,** Proton-density-weighted MR image of brain specimen. **C,** T1-weighted MR image of normal volunteer. **D,** T2-weighted MR image of normal volunteer. This is the initial section posterior to the medulla; only the posterolateral recesses of the fourth ventricle (V) are included. The inferomedial aspect of each hemisphere is now formed by the tonsils, which abut the inferior aspect of the vermis (P V*e*) medially and may abut each other inferiorly in the midline. This is the final section to include a small portion of the central lobule (C). The corpus medullare (C*m*) attains its greatest size on this image. The dentate nucleus (D) is seen clearly within the medial aspect of each corpus medullare (C*m*) in image **B.** The white matter immediately peripheral to the nucleus (*arrows* in **B**) has lower signal intensity than the remainder of the white matter, most likely because of iron deposition.

CORONAL SECTIONS

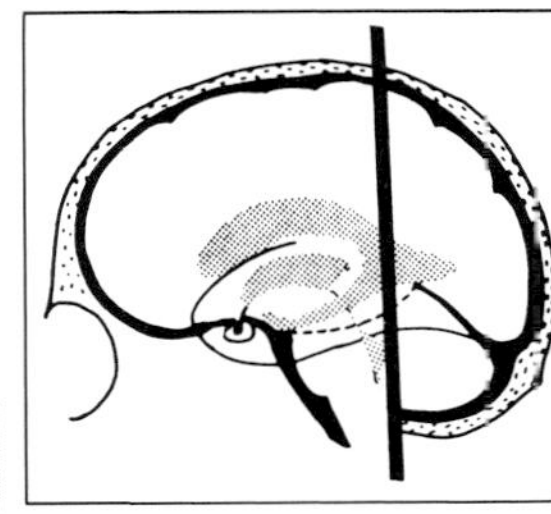

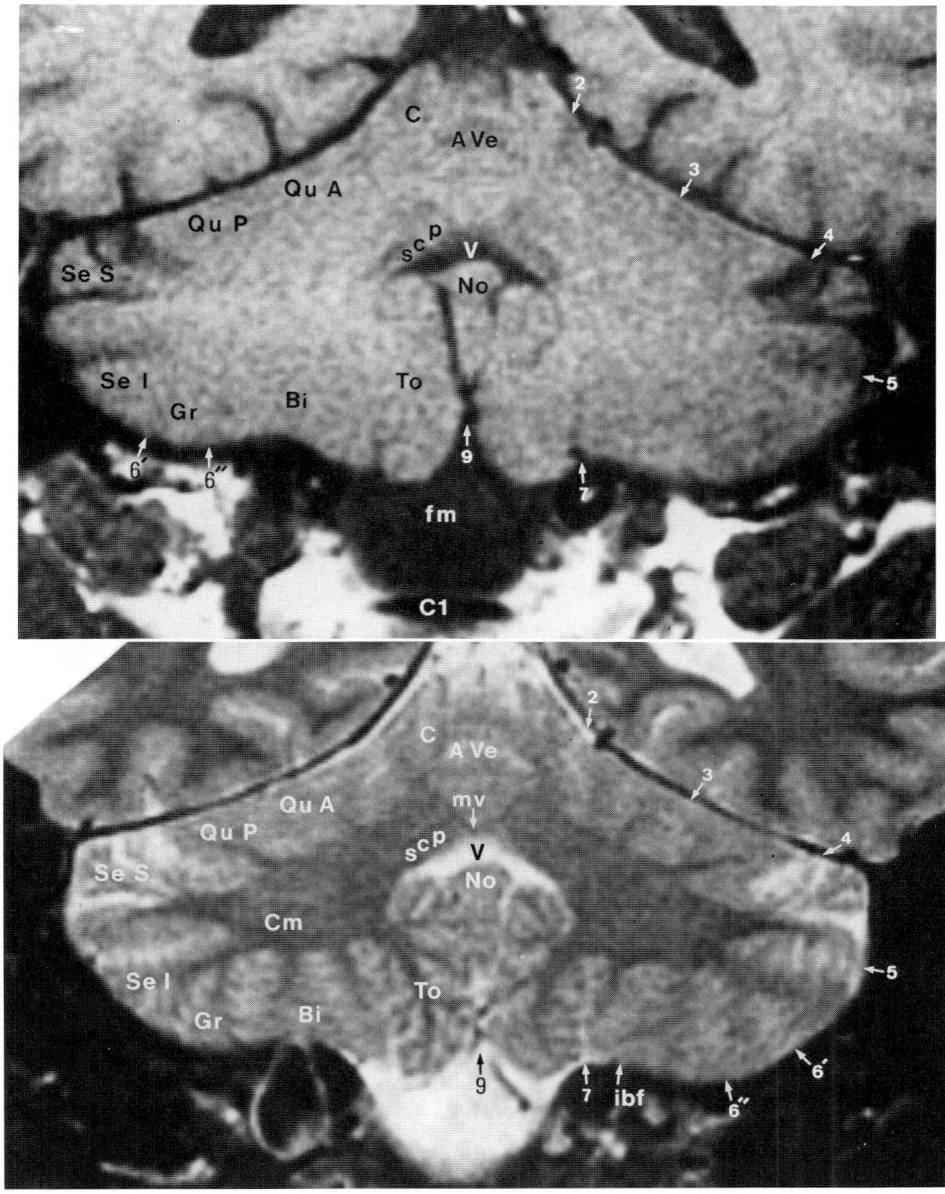

C

D

Figure 9-10, cont'd. *Coronal scan plane through the tonsils.*
The transverse fossa is no longer present. The horizontal fissure (5) separates the superior and inferior semilunar lobules (*Se* S, *Se* I) in **C**. Note the intracrural sulcus (unlabeled) divides the superior semilunar lobule into an upper and lower portion. (In all the images, only the upper portion of the superior semilunar lobule is labeled *Se* S.) The detailed anatomy of the vermis is not well defined in this coronal plane. Nevertheless, the fourth ventricle, overlying medullary velum (*mv*), and central confluence of vermian white matter provide the landmark for dividing the lobules of the anterior lobe of the vermis (A *Ve*) from those of the posterior lobe (P *Ve*) and the nodulus (N*o*). Extraparenchymal landmarks in this plane include the cerebrospinal fluid (CSF) within the foramen magnum (*fm*), vallecula (9), and the posterior arch of the first cervical vertebra (C1) in **C** and **D**.

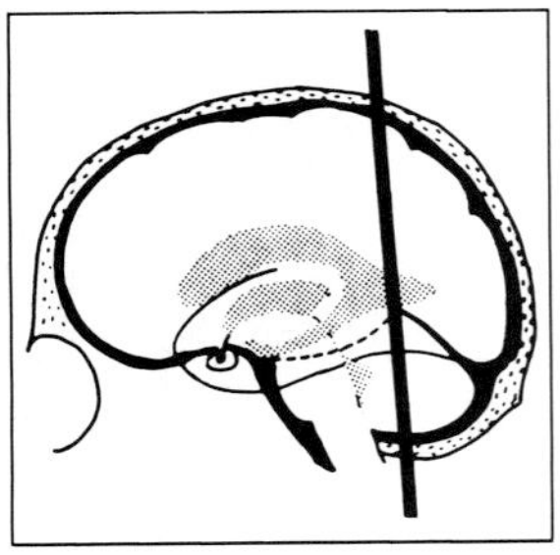

CORONAL SECTIONS

A

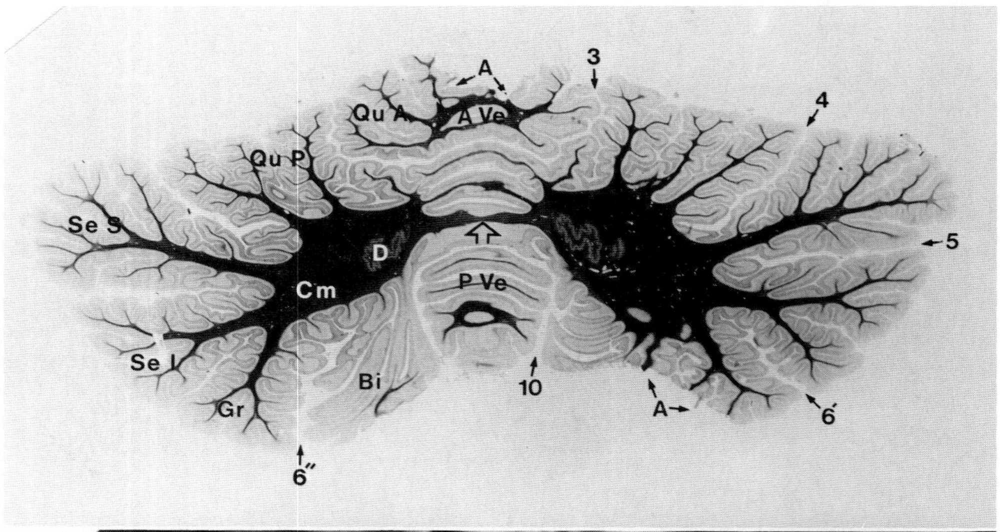

B

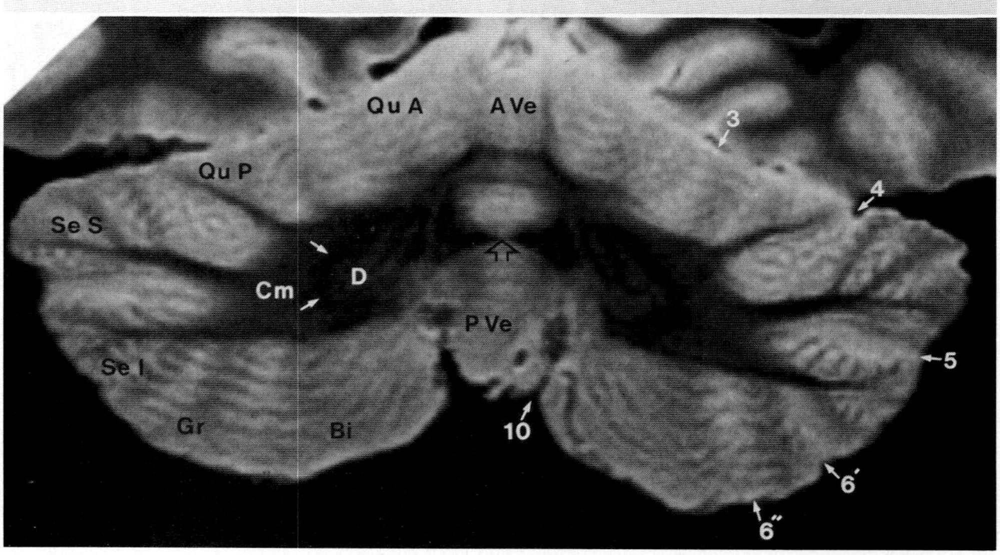

Figure 9-11 *Coronal scan plane through posterior tonsils.*
A, Myelin-stained brain specimen. **B,** Proton-density-weighted MR image of brain specimen. **C,** T1-weighted MR image of normal volunteer. **D,** T2-weighted MR image of normal volunteer. The corpora medullare (C*m*) begin to decrease in size in this section. This is the last section to include a small portion of the tonsils (T*o*) (images **C** and **D**). Two major bands of white matter crossing the vermis are resolved on MR images **(B** and **D).** They connect regions not visualized in this section. The superior band (unlabeled) is a portion of the primary tract to the culmen that ascends in a nearly vertical course; the inferior band (*open arrow,* **A, B,** and **D**) is the horizontally oriented, primary tract connecting to the declive, folium, and tuber.

CORONAL SECTIONS

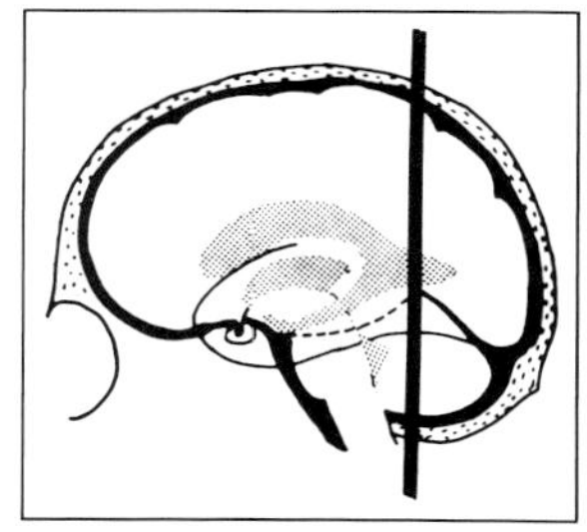

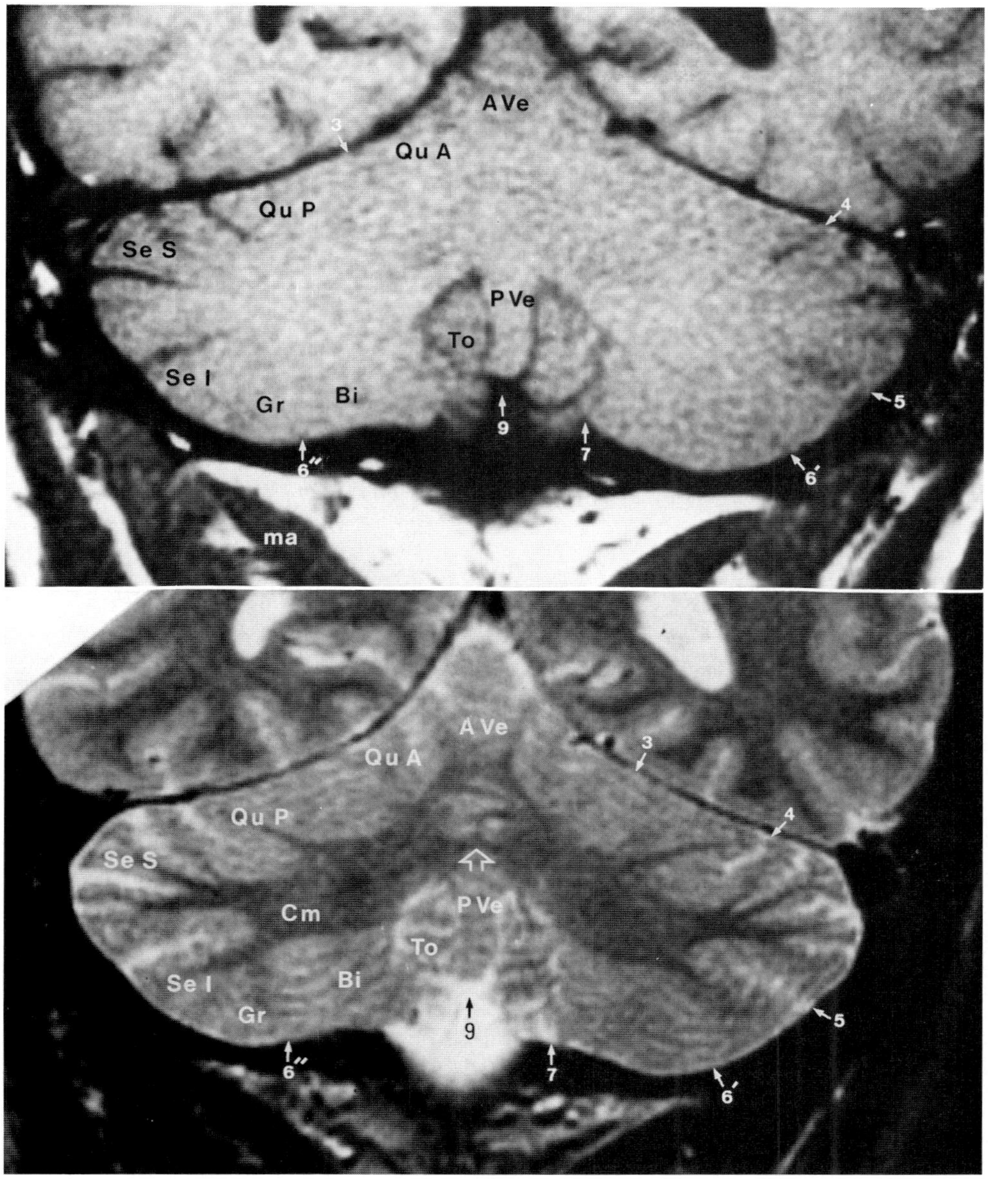

C

D

Figure 9-11 cont'd. *Coronal scan plane through posterior tonsils.*
These white matter bands help distinguish the anterior lobe of the vermis (A *Ve*), which is above the upper band, from the posterior lobe of the vermis (P *Ve*), which is below the lower band **(B** and **D)**. The portion of the vermis *between* the two bands represents a region of overlap between the anterior and posterior lobes of the vermis. Small solid arrows indicate iron deposition in the region of the dentate **(B)**. The distinctive V-shaped configuration of the rectus capitis posterior major (*ma*) muscles is an extraparenchymal landmark identified in **C**.

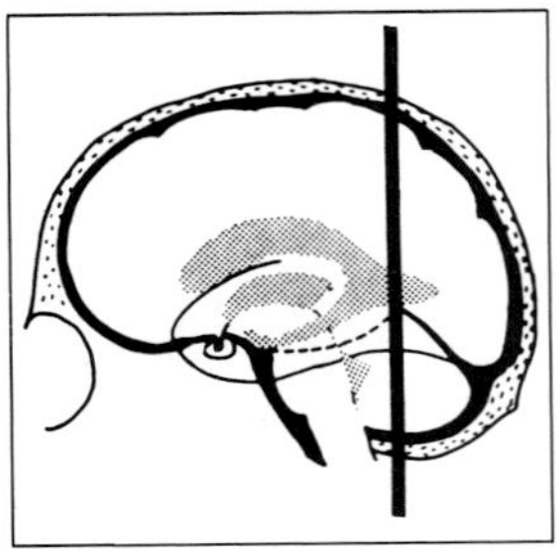

CORONAL SECTIONS

A

B

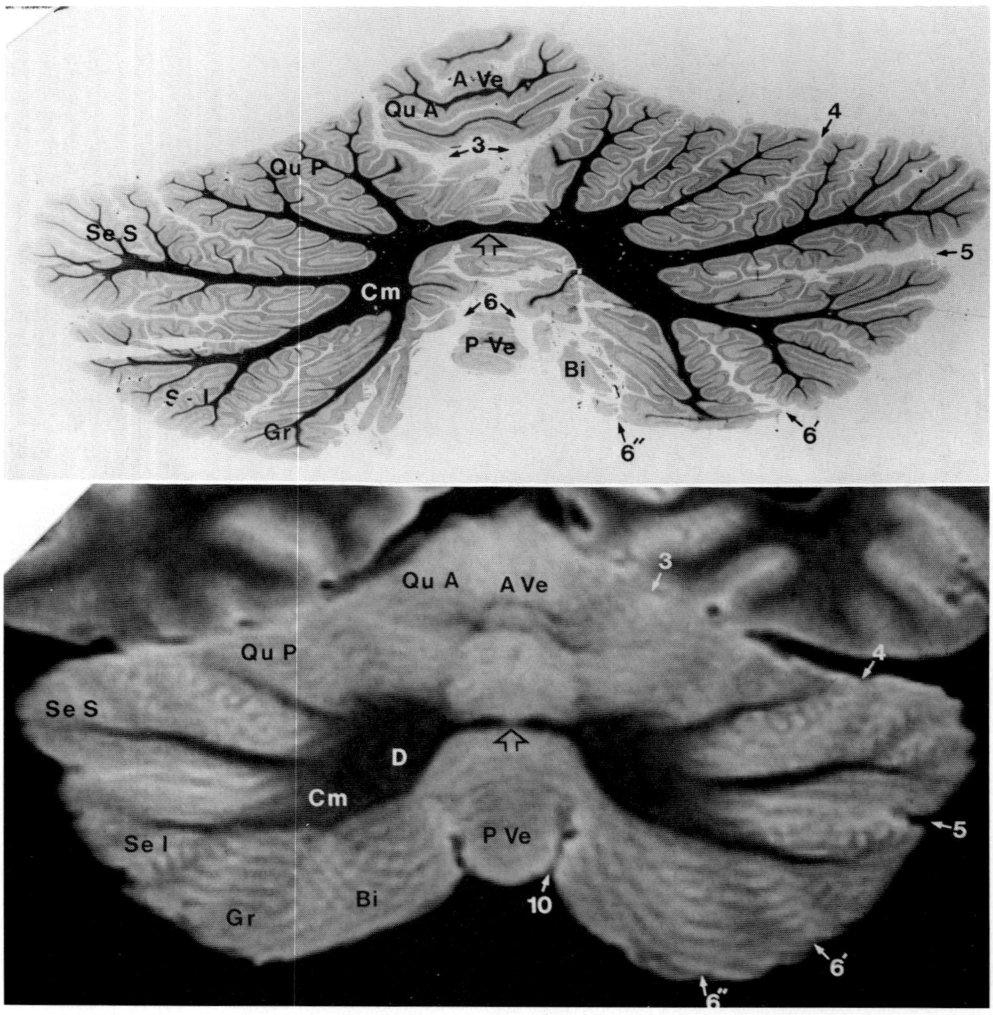

Figure 9-12 *Coronal scan plane posterior to the tonsils.*
A, Myelin-stained brain specimen. **B**, Proton-density-weighted MR image of brain specimen. **C**, T1-weighted MR image of normal volunteer. **D**, T2-weighted MR image of normal volunteer. This section usually includes mainly the lobules of the posterior lobe of the hemispheres. Only a small portion of the anterior quadrangular lobule (*Qu* A) may be seen (images **A** and **B**). The primary fissure (3) in **A**, **C**, and **D** traverses the vermis above the white matter tract (*open arrow*) that connects the declive, folium, and tuber regions, which are not seen on this section. The prepyramidal fissure of the vermis (6) is identified beneath this tract and is especially well seen in **A**.

CORONAL SECTIONS

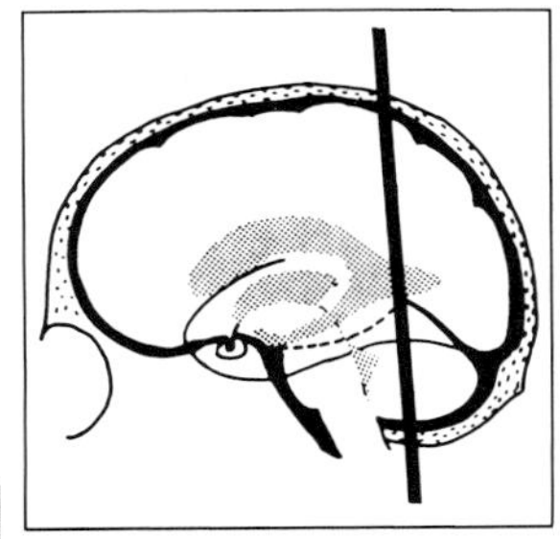

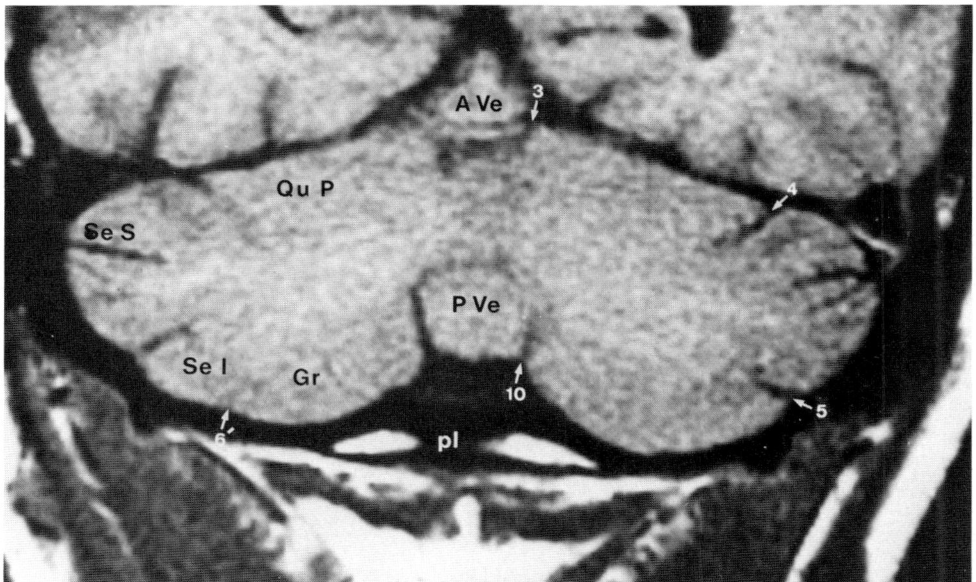

C

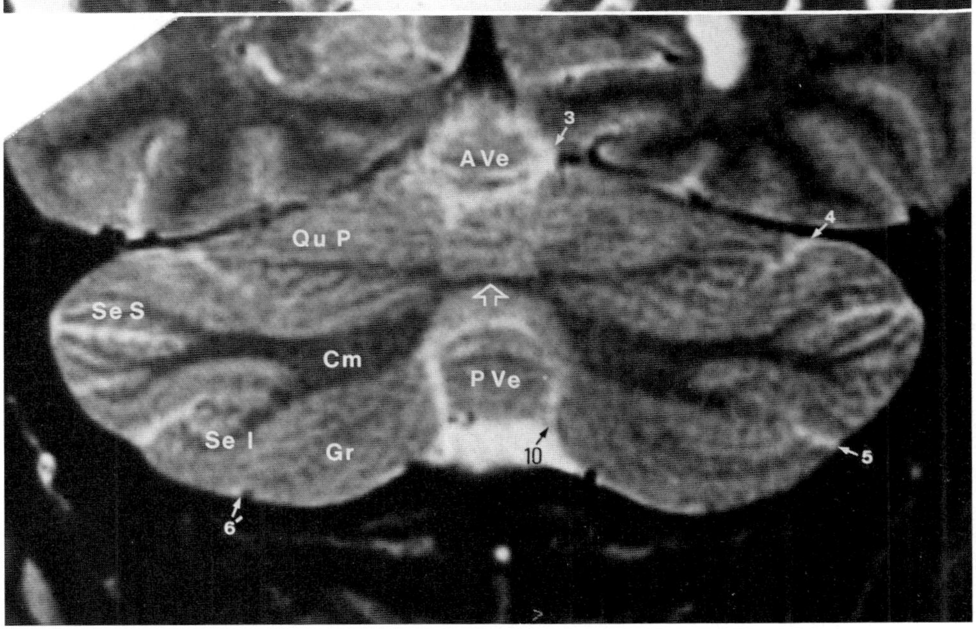

D

Figure 9-12, cont'd. *Coronal scan plane posterior to the tonsils.*
Since this plane lies posterior to the tonsils, it is the biventer (B*i*) or gracile lobule (G*r*) that forms the inferomedial margin of the cerebellar hemispheres. This is the final section to include a portion of the corpora medullare (C*m*). An extra-parenchymal landmark identified in this plane *in vivo* is the posterior lip (*pl*) of the foramen magnum **C.**

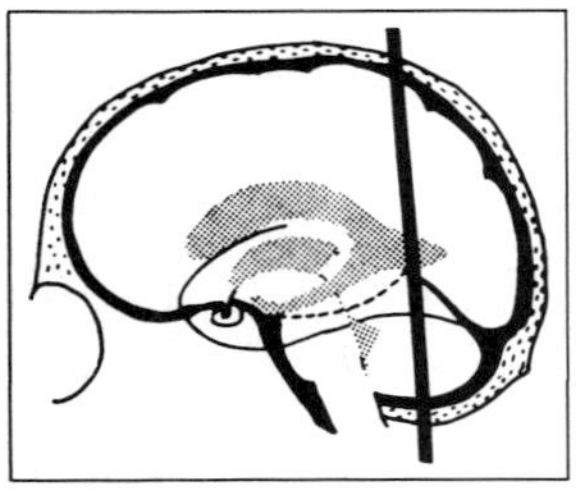

CORONAL SECTIONS

A

B

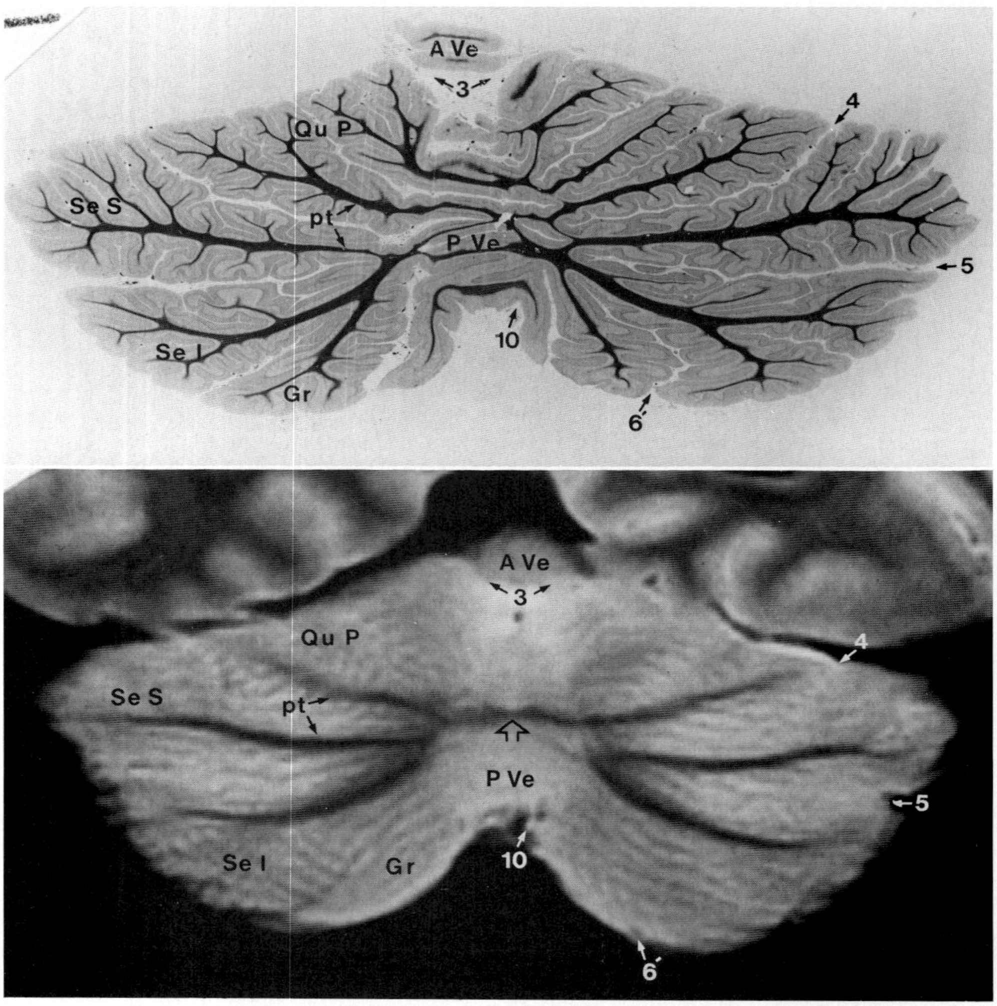

Figure 9-13 *Coronal scan plane posterior to the corpora medullare.*
A, Myelin-stained brain specimen. **B**, Proton-density-weighted MR image of brain specimen. **C**, T1-weighted MR image of normal volunteer. **D**, T2-weighted MR image of normal volunteer. The primary white matter tracts innervating the posterior quadrangular (*Qu* P) and the superior and inferior semilunar (*Se* S, *Se* I) lobules on either side diverge laterally (images **B** and **D**).

CORONAL SECTIONS

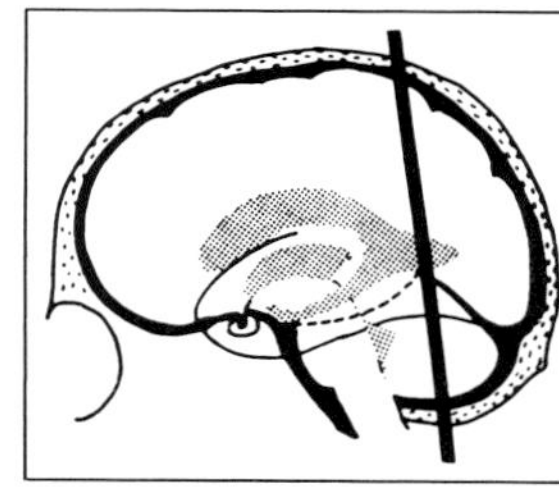

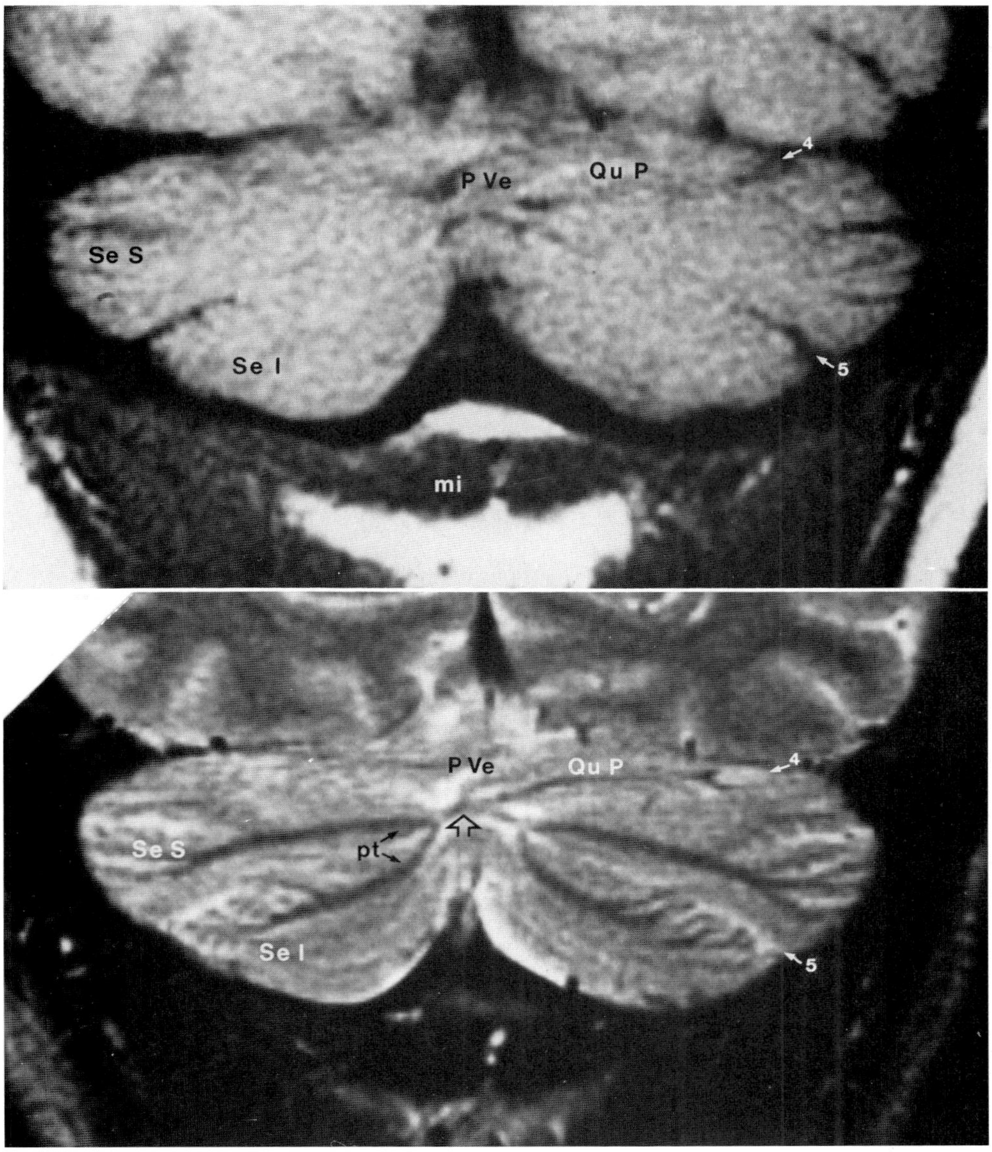

C

D

Figure 9-13, cont'd. *Coronal scan plane posterior to the corpora medullare.*
The posterior extreme of the vermis is sectioned in the vicinity of the termination of the primary tract (*open arrow*) to the declive, folium, and tuber, which are not seen on this section **(B** and **D)**. An extra-parenchymal landmark consistently identified in this plane in vivo is the horizontally oriented junction of the rectus capitis posterior minor (*mi*) muscles in the midline immediately beneath the occipital bone **(C)**.

INDEX TO THE ILLUSTRATIONS

Entries refer to figures in which the specific structures are labeled.

CHAPTER 10

Cerebellar Hemispheres and Vermis

Gary A. Press
Eric Courchesne

IMAGING TECHNIQUES

Before the advent of magnetic resonance imaging (MRI), very little cerebellar and vermian anatomy could be visualized *in vivo*. Computed tomography (CT), limited by streak artifacts because of x-ray beam hardening at the base of the skull and by relatively poor soft tissue contrast, was suboptimal for demonstrating the contents of the posterior fossa. MR spin-echo images are not plagued by significant bone-induced artifacts and therefore have superior soft tissue contrast. Moreover, definition of the transverse-oriented, boundary-forming fissures and white matter tracts of the cerebellum is best understood when sagittal and coronal planes of section (perpendicular to these landmarks) are used. For the first time, the multiplanar capability of MRI has afforded this luxury *without* requiring patient repositioning. Thin (3 to 5 mm) sections, special flow-compensating spin-echo pulse sequences, and cardiac gating facilitate display of anatomic features of the cerebellum not shown previously.[1-3]

Surface features of the cerebellum (e.g., precentral, primary, horizontal, secondary, posterolateral fissures) are best delineated on long TR/TE or short TR/TE images (TR, relaxation time; TE, echo delay time) that provide the greatest contrast between cerebrospinal fluid (CSF) and parenchyma. Long TR and intermediate or long TE images provide the best gray-white matter contrast and optimally display the nearly constant branching pattern of the hemispheric and vermian white matter tracts.[1-3]

Using a combination of these surface and deep features, one can confidently identify all lobules of the vermis (e.g., culmen, declive, folium, tuber) and hemispheres (e.g., central, semilunar, biventer) that appear on any coronal or sagittal MR image. The relative size and morphology of the major lobules appear to be constant when imaged in the coronal or sagittal planes. The dentate nucleus is visualized reliably within the medial aspect of each corpus medullare; it appears as an oval-shaped, curvilinear structure with an undulating margin, best seen on coronal long TR/intermediate TE images. The opportunity for side-to-side comparison is a distinct advantage provided by the coronal view.[3]

DEVELOPMENTAL ANATOMY

A brief review of key stages in the development of the cerebellum contributes greatly to understanding its adult appearance. Figure 10-1 provides a visual key that identifies the important anatomic features of the adult cerebellar hemispheres. Table 10-1 organizes the various nomenclatures used to describe the cerebellar and vermian anatomy. Figure 10-2 illustrates the sequence of changes that occur to produce the adult cerebellar hemispheres and vermis.

Neuroblasts that form the cerebellum derive ultimately from symmetric "alar plates" on both sides of the rhombencephalon beneath the level of the roof of the fourth ventricle, sites of intense neuroblastic activity.[4,5] At the beginning of the second month of life, the proliferating neuroblasts form paired rhombic lips (cerebellar rudiments) that thicken, project further into the fourth ventricle, and extend progressively toward the midline (Figure 10-2, *A* and *B*). At the end of the second month of gestation, the rhombic lips of the two sides fuse in the midline beginning rostrally, and the anterior lobe of the vermis is thereby formed before the posterior lobe. During the third month, the cerebellum acquires additional cells at such a rate that it begins to bulge extraventricularly (Figure 10-2, *C* and *D*). The middle regions of the vermis and hemispheres proliferate more extensively than the rostral or caudal extremes, and the simple linear structure of the developing cerebellum becomes mushroom shaped.[4,5]

The growth of the cerebellum posterior to the roof of the fourth ventricle creates the posterolateral fissure early in

◆ **TABLE 10-1** Components of the Human Cerebellum

	Vermian lobule nomenclature		Hemispheric lobule nomenclature	
Cerebellar lobe	**Name**	**Roman numeral**	**Name**	**Roman numeral**
Anterior	Lingula	I		(HI*)
	Centralis	II, III	Central lobule	HII, HIII
	Culmen	IV, V	Quadrangular lobule, anterior portion	HIV, HV
Posterior	Declive	VI	Quadrangular lobule, posterior portion	HVI
	Folium vermis	Superior VIIA	Semilunar lobule, superior portion	HVIIA
	Tuber vermis	Inferior VIIA	Semilunar lobule, inferior portion	HVIIA
		VIIB	Gracile lobule	HVIIB
	Pyramis	VIIIA, VIIIB	Biventer	HVIII
	Uvula	IX	Tonsil	HIX
Flocculonodular	Nodulus	X	Flocculus	HX

Reproduced with permission from Courchesne E, Press GA, Murakami J, et al: AJNR 10:659-665, 1989.
*Hemispheric counterpart of vermian lobule I is usually absent in humans.

the third month.[4,5] All the remaining horizontally oriented fissures, which divide the cerebellar vermis and hemispheres into transverse lobules, are visible by the end of the fourth month (Figure 10-2, *E* and *F*). Eventually, continued hemispheric growth outstrips growth of the vermis, creating the sagittally directed paravermian sulci between the hemispheres and the vermis (Figure 10-2, *F*). Moreover, to accommodate the expansion of lobules HVIIA and HVIIB (see Table 10-1), a shift in the hemispheric lobules occurs. The biventral lobules (HVIII), tonsils (HIX), and flocculi (HX) are pushed anteriorly, inferiorly, and medially from their initially lateral position, attaining their final position along the anteroinferior aspect of the hemispheres (Figure 10-2, *E* to *G*). This shifting process, together with growth of the tonsils themselves, results in a sagittally oriented furrow between them and the vermis.[4-6] The maturation of the fiber tracts in the neonatal cerebellum is reviewed in detail in Chapter 2.

FUNCTIONAL ANATOMY AND CONNECTIONS

Motor Functions

A major responsibility of the cerebellum is the coordination of motor responses. The fiber tracts that pass to and from the cerebellum are summarized in Chapter 7. These interconnections allow the cerebellum and vermis to interact in a synergistic fashion, which coordinates reflex and voluntary motor acts.[6] In broad general terms, distinct clinical abnormalities can be referred to two major sagittal zones of function (midline and lateral) within the cerebellum that correspond closely to its anatomic organization. These zones have distinct but overlapping functions.[7]

Vermis

The *midline zone,* containing the vermis and fastigial nuclei, regulates and coordinates somatic motor (midline musculature) and vestibulo-ocular activities.[7,8] Cortical (Purkinje) neurons project to the fastigial nuclei, which project in turn to reticular and vestibular neurons of the brainstem. Subsequent ascending pathways controlled by Purkinje cells within the declive, folium, and tuber influence brainstem nuclei governing ocular movements (e.g., oculomotor nucleus); descending (reticulospinal and vestibulospinal) pathways controlled by other regions of the vermian cortex reach anterior horn cells of the spinal cord. The cortex of the vermis also influences neural pathways involved with the level of attention,[7,9] sensory function,[10] corticoneostriatal interactions,[11] autonomic activities,[12] motivation,[13,14] memory,[15,16] and behavior.[13,14,17]

Such functional diversity is reflected in regional specialization of the vermis.[7] For instance, the anterior lobe receives mainly spinal input (from spinocerebellar and cuneocerebellar fibers) and relatively little cerebral cortical input. Efferent fibers from the anterior lobe are sent primarily to lower brainstem systems. The posterior lobe receives major input from the cerebral cortex (motor, somatosensory, visual, auditory, and association areas), tectum, and hippocampus but receives sparse spinal input. Efferents from the posterior lobe connect with the midbrain, thalamus, and hypothalamus, as well as with lower brainstem systems.[7] Specialization is epitomized by the declive, folium, and tuber—the auditory and visual areas of the vermis—which are critical for establishing certain types of long-term memory traces.[16]

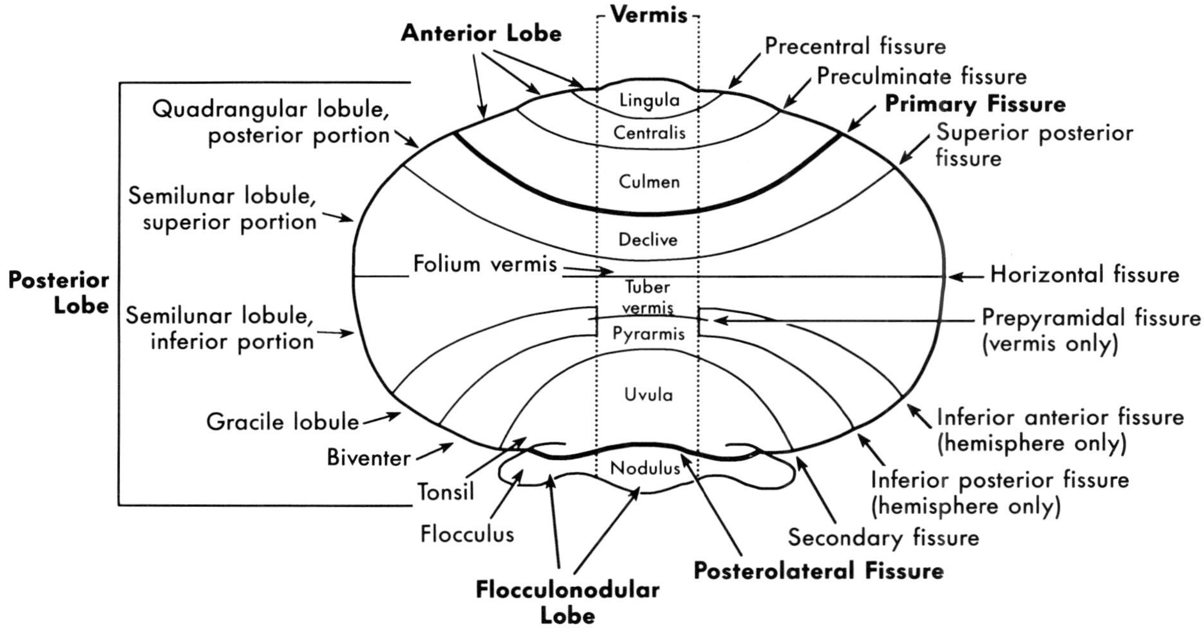

Figure 10-1 Schematic diagram of the *flattened* surface anatomy of the globe formed by the two cerebellar hemispheres and the central vermis. The surface anatomy is distorted by the artist to help the reader appreciate the relative positions of the labeled anatomic structures. In this schematic representation, the lingulae of the vermis and the nodulus, which anatomically face each other across the fourth ventricle, are shown at the top and bottom of the illustration, respectively.

On the *left* side of the diagram, the major divisions of the hemisphere are labeled. The posterior lobe is further divided into six lobules. The *right* side of the diagram locates the fissures subdividing the cerebellar hemispheres and vermis (the thickest lines indicating the primary fissure and the posterolateral fissure, which separate the anterior from the posterior lobes and the posterior lobes from the flocculonodular lobes, respectively). The lobules of the vermis are labeled.

Lesions of the vermis generally result in disorders of eye movements (e.g., horizontal nystagmus), abnormal posture of the head, disturbances of stance and gait, dysmetria, succession deficits, and kinetic tremor.[7] Impairments in memory and consciousness, dysarthria, and past pointing occur less often.[7]

Cerebellar Hemispheres

The *lateral (hemispheric) zone* of the cerebellum consists of the hemisphere and the dentate, globose, and emboliform nuclei of each side. The cerebellar hemispheres are phylogenetically younger than the midline structures and are involved with movements of the proximal and distal extremities. Neurons of the lateral hemispheric cortex (including the most lateral region of the anterior lobe and the lateral portions of the superior and inferior semilunar lobules, HVIIA) project to the dentate nuclei, which then project to the ventrolateral thalamic nucleus.[7] Nerve fibers from this portion of the thalamus ascend to the precentral gyrus and influence finely coordinated movements of the distal extremities. Cortical neurons of the medial portions of the cerebellar hemispheres project to the globose and emboliform nuclei. These nuclei project subsequently to the red nucleus and ventrolateral thalamic nucleus. The rubrospinal tract (originating from cells of the red nucleus) synapses with both medial and lateral groups of anterior horn cells of the spinal cord, thereby influencing the activity of proximal and distal limb musculature, respectively. This pathway is involved in several motor functions, including phasic limb movements, maintained positions of an extremity, stance, gait, and posture.[7]

Motor signs accompanying lesions involving mainly the cerebellar hemispheres include ipsilateral static and kinetic tremors of the extremities, dysmetria, dysdiadochokinesia (abnormal rapid alternating movements), excessive rebound, impaired check reflex, decomposition of movements, past pointing, and hypotonia.[7]

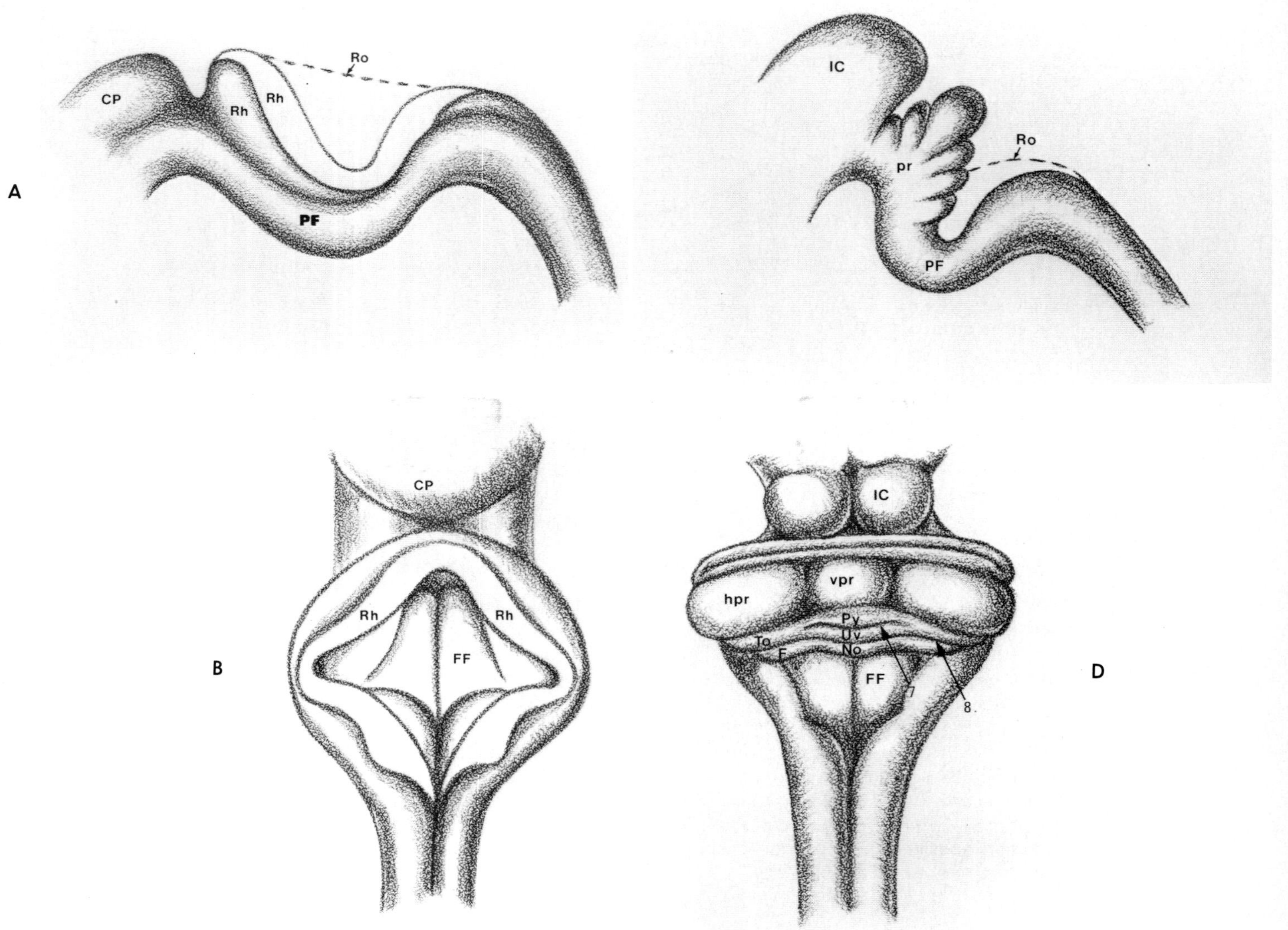

Figure 10-2 Schematic diagrams of normal cerebellar development. **A** and **B,** At 5 weeks, the fourth ventricle forms at the pontine flexure (PF) below the collicular plate (CP). Symmetric alar plates (cerebellar rudiments) are noted beneath membranous roof of fourth ventricle (R*o*) on both sides of rhombencephalon (R*h*). These sites of proliferating neuroblasts grow toward the midline and fuse to form the vermis. This begins rostrally; therefore the anterior lobe of vermis is formed before the posterior lobe. **C,** At 3 months, the lateral view shows the continuing cellular proliferation, which causes the enlarging cerebellar primordium (*pr*) to bulge extraventricularly. **D,** On the posteroinferior view, the vermis primordium has fused in midline. Note the pyramis (P*y*), uvula (U*v*), and nodulus (N*o*) above the floor of the fourth ventricle (FF). The tonsil (T*o*) and flocculus (F) are located laterally below the hemispheric primordium (*hpr*). The posterolateral fissure (8), secondary fissure (7), and inferior colliculus (IC) can all be identified at 3 months. **E,** By 4 months, several additional horizontally oriented vermian fissures are visible on the posteroinferior view. These are the horizontal (5), prepyramidal of the vermis (6), and the superoposterior fissure (4). **F,** By 5 months, the posteroinferior view shows that these fissures extend across entire cerebellum and that the inferoposterior (6') and inferoanterior (6") fissures of the hemispheres appear. Sagittally oriented paravermian sulci (unmarked indentations between vermis and hemisphere) form because of hemispheric overgrowth. **G,** At birth, the posteroinferior view shows that the inferior vermis is covered nearly entirely by expanded hemispheres. Flocculus (F), tonsil (T*o*), and biventer (B*i*) become wedged anteromedially because of growth of superior and inferior semilunar (S*e* I) and gracile (G*r*) lobules. Similarly, overgrowth of anterior and posterior lobules of vermis causes apparent "tucking in" of nodulus, which comes to indent the inferior aspect of the fourth ventricle. (For orientation, the resected brainstem is lightly indicated by a *broken line*.)

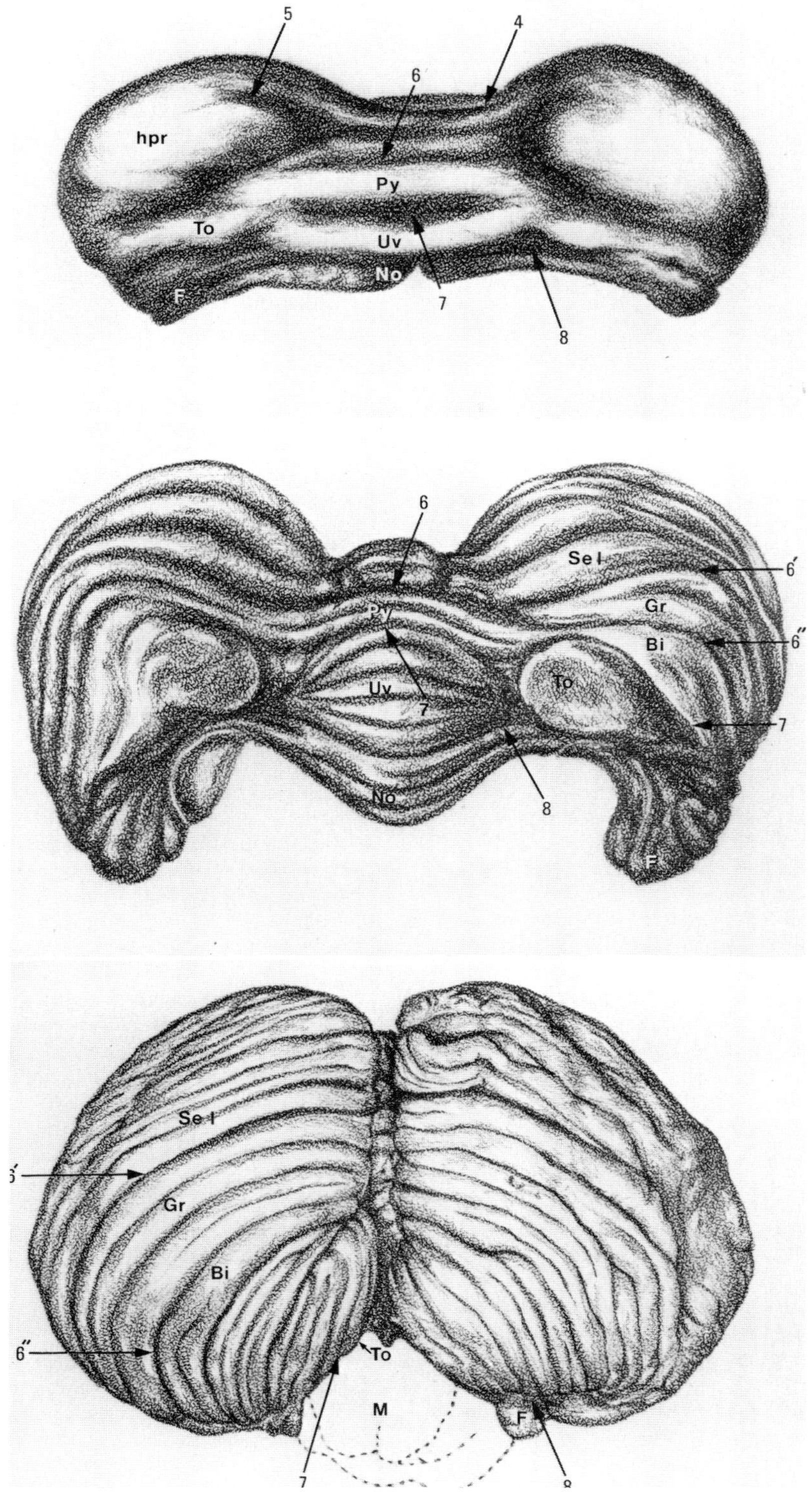

Figure 10-2, cont'd. For legend see opposite page.

Nonmotor Functions

Clinical and basic research indicates that the cerebellum (particularly the posterior lobes of the hemispheres and vermis) regulates, integrates, and coordinates a wide variety of additional, nonmotor concerns, including level of consciousness, learning, memory, and motivated behavior. For example, early investigators recognized that cerebellar damage occurring in adulthood may be associated with lethargy and coma[7] or psychosis.[7,18] Others observed that retarded intellectual functioning is typically associated with developmental disorders of the cerebellum ranging from hypoplasia[19-21] to near total agenesis.[22,23] In many such instances, lesions found in the central nervous system (CNS) outside the cerebellum were insufficient to explain the severity of the mental retardation.[19] More recently, in a test of word meaning and association, the cerebellum was one of three sites of significant neural activity defined by positron emission tomography.[24] In addition, the posterior lobe of the cerebellum has been shown to be an "obligatory part" of the discrete adaptive response circuit for associative learning; the cerebellum may be the locus of the memory trace for learned responses of this type.[25,26]

Such clinical data and experimental observations require a reassessment of the role of the cerebellum in normal CNS function. Indeed, one investigator has proposed that the role of the cerebellum may extend far beyond regulation of simple motor activities to encompass global coordination of many additional types of behavior for the purpose of optimizing information acquisition (sensory reception) during active exploration of the environment.[27] MRI will likely facilitate redefining the bounds of the "expanding" role of the cerebellum by providing improved in vivo identification, localization, and quantification of cerebellar disease in patients whose clinical deficits can be thoroughly tested.[28]

REFERENCES

1. Courchesne E, Press GA, Murakami J, et al: The cerebellum in sagittal plane: anatomic-MR correlation. 1. The vermis, *AJNR* 10:659-665, 1989.
2. Press GA, Murakami J, Courchesne E, et al: The cerebellum in sagittal plane: anatomic-MR correlation. 2. The cerebellar hemispheres, *AJNR* 10:667-676, 1989.
3. Press GA, Murakami JW, Courchesne E, et al: The cerebellum. 3. Anatomic-MR correlation in the coronal plane, *AJNR* 11:41-50, 1990.
4. Larsell O: The development of the cerebellum in man in relation to its comparative anatomy, *J Comp Neurol* 87:85-129, 1947.
5. Lemire RJ, Loeser JD, Leech RW, Alvord EC Jr: *Normal and abnormal development of the human nervous system,* Hagerstown, Md, 1975, Harper & Row.
6. Crosby EC, Humphrey T, Lauer EW: *Correlative anatomy of the nervous system,* New York, 1962, Macmillan.
7. Gilman S, Bloedel J, Lechtenberg R: *Disorders of the cerebellum,* Philadelphia, 1981, FA Davis.
8. Ito M: *The cerebellum and neural control,* New York, 1984, Raven.
9. Nieuwenhuys R, Voogd J, Huijzen C: *The human central nervous system: a synopsis and atlas,* ed 2, New York, 1981, Springer-Verlag.
10. Crispino L, Bullock TH: Cerebellum mediates modality-specific modulation of sensory responses of midbrain and forebrain in rat, *Proc Natl Acad Sci USA* 81:2917-2920, 1984.
11. Ryan LI: Personal communication.
12. Haines DE, Dietrichs E: On the organization of interconnections between the cerebellum and hypothalamus. In King JS, editor: *New concepts in cerebellar neurobiology,* vol 12, New York, 1987, Alan R Liss.
13. Supple WF, Leaton AN, Fanselow MS: Effects of cerebellar vermal lesions on species-specific fear responses, neophobia, and taste-aversion learning in rats, *Physiol Behav* 39:579-586, 1987.
14. Ball G, Micco DJ Jr, Berntson G: Cerebellar stimulation in the rat: complex stimulation-bound oral behaviors and self-stimulation, *Physiol Behav* 13:123-127, 1974.
15. Newman PP, Reza H: Functional relationships between the hippocampus and the cerebellum: an electrophysiological study of the cat, *J Physiol (Lond)* 287:405-426, 1979.
16. Leaton RN, Supple WF: Cerebellar vermis: essential for long-term habituation of the acoustic startle response, *Science* 232:513-515, 1986.
17. Reis DJ, Doba N, Nathan MA: Predatory attack, grooming, and consummatory behaviors evoked by electrical stimulation of cat cerebellar nuclei, *Science* 182:845-847, 1973.
18. Keddie KMG: Hereditary ataxia, presumed to be of the Menzel type, complicated by paranoid psychosis in a mother and two sons, *J Neurol Neurosurg Psychiatry* 32:82-87, 1969.
19. Jervis GA: Early familial cerebellar degeneration (report of three cases in one family), *J Nerv Ment Dis* 111:398-407, 1950.
20. Joubert M, Eisenring JJ, Robb JP, Andermann F: Familial agenesis of the cerebellar vermis, *Neurology* 19:813-825, 1969.
21. Sarnet HB, Alcala H: Human cerebellar hypoplasia, *Arch Neurol* 37:300-305, 1980.
22. Rubinstein HS, Freeman W: Cerebellar agenesis, *J Nerv Ment Dis* 92:489-502, 1943.
23. Mercuri S, Curatolo P, Giuffre R, DiLorenzo N: Agenesis of the vermis cerebelli and malformations of the posterior fossa in childhood and adolescence, *Neurochirurgia (Stuttg)* 22:180-188, 1979.
24. Petersen SE, Fox PT, Posner MI, et al: Positron emission tomographic studies of the processing of single words, *J Cognitive Neuropsychol,* (in press).
25. McCormick DA, Thompson RF: Cerebellum: essential involvement in the classically conditioned eyelid response, *Science* 223:296-299, 1984.
26. Thompson RF: Neuronal substrates of simple associative learning: classical conditioning, *Trends Neurosci* 6:270-275, 1983.
27. Brower J: Personal communication.
28. Press GA, Courchesne E, Yeung-Courchesne R, Hesselink JR: Cerebellar hypoplasia and autism, *N Engl J Med* 319:1154, 1988 (letter).

CHAPTER 11

Mark J. Pfleger
L. Anne Hayman
John J. Pagani

Atlas of Cerebrospinal Fluid Spaces

This chapter provides a review of the cerebrospinal fluid (CSF) spaces. The ventricles and cisternal spaces that surround the brain are labeled on axial and sagittal short TR/short TE (T1-weighted) magnetic resonance (MR) images in Figure 11-1 (TR, relaxation time; TE, echo delay time; Tl, longitudinal relaxation time). The ventricular spaces are labeled in the frontal and lateral schematics shown in Figure 11-2.

The cerebral sulci and fissures are comprehensively listed in Table 11-1. The nomenclature of the temporal lobe sulci is a source of confusion in the literature. In this chapter the newest terminology is used, and the *inferior temporal sulcus* replaces the previous term, middle temporal sulcus. In addition, the *occipitotemporal sulcus* is now used to designate what was once known as the inferior temporal sulcus. Table 11-2 comprehensively lists the gyri of the cerebral hemispheres. Figures 11-3, *A* and *B,* and 11-4, *A* and *B,* schematically summarize these tables by displaying the gyri and sulci of the lateral surface of the left cerebral hemisphere and the medial surface of the right cerebral hemisphere. The functions mediated by the cerebral cortex are shown in Figures 11-3, *C,* and 11-4, *C.*

The complicated anatomy of the sulcal CSF spaces is shown on consecutive sagittal MR images in Figures 11-5 to 11-20. These spaces and the gyri that form their boundaries are indexed so that unfamiliar terms mentioned in other chapters can be quickly located. It should be noted that significant variations exist in the sulcal pattern of the cerebral hemispheres. Therefore these images can only provide a general guide for the reader. Variability in the macroanatomy of the sulci and gyri necessitates individual mapping when precise localization of anatomic regions must be performed for positron emission tomography (PET) or cerebral blood flow studies; sagittal MR images are ideally suited for this purpose.[1]

The short TR/TE (600/20 msec) MR images used for figures in this chapter were obtained on a 1.5 T Signa (General Electric) scanner with a 256 × 256 matrix, two averages, and a 24 cm field of view. Two separate acquisition series of 5 mm sections were obtained. These were interleaved to obtain the closely spaced sagittal slices. Several anatomic references were consulted to label these images.[2-7] In general, the sulci are labeled on one image and gyri on the adjacent scan.

REFERENCES

1. Steinmetz H, Furst G, Freund H-J: Variation of perisylvian and calcarine anatomic landmarks within stereotaxic proportional coordinates, *AJNR* 11:1123-1130, 1990.
2. Kreig WJS: *Functional neuroanatomy,* ed 3, Evanston, Ill, 1966, Brain Books.
3. Riley HA: *An atlas of the basal ganglia, brainstem and spinal cord,* Baltimore, 1943, Williams & Wilkins.
4. Elliott HC: *Textbook of neuroanatomy,* Philadelphia, 1963, JB Lippincott.
5. Clemente CD, editor: *Gray's anatomy of the human body,* ed 30 (American), Philadelphia, 1985, Lea & Febiger.
6. Di Chiro G: *An atlas of detailed normal pneumoencephalographic anatomy,* Springfield, Ill, 1961, Charles C Thomas.
7. Newton TH, Potts DG: *Radiology of the skull and brain,* vol IV, *Ventricles and cisterns,* St Louis, 1978, Mosby–Year Book.

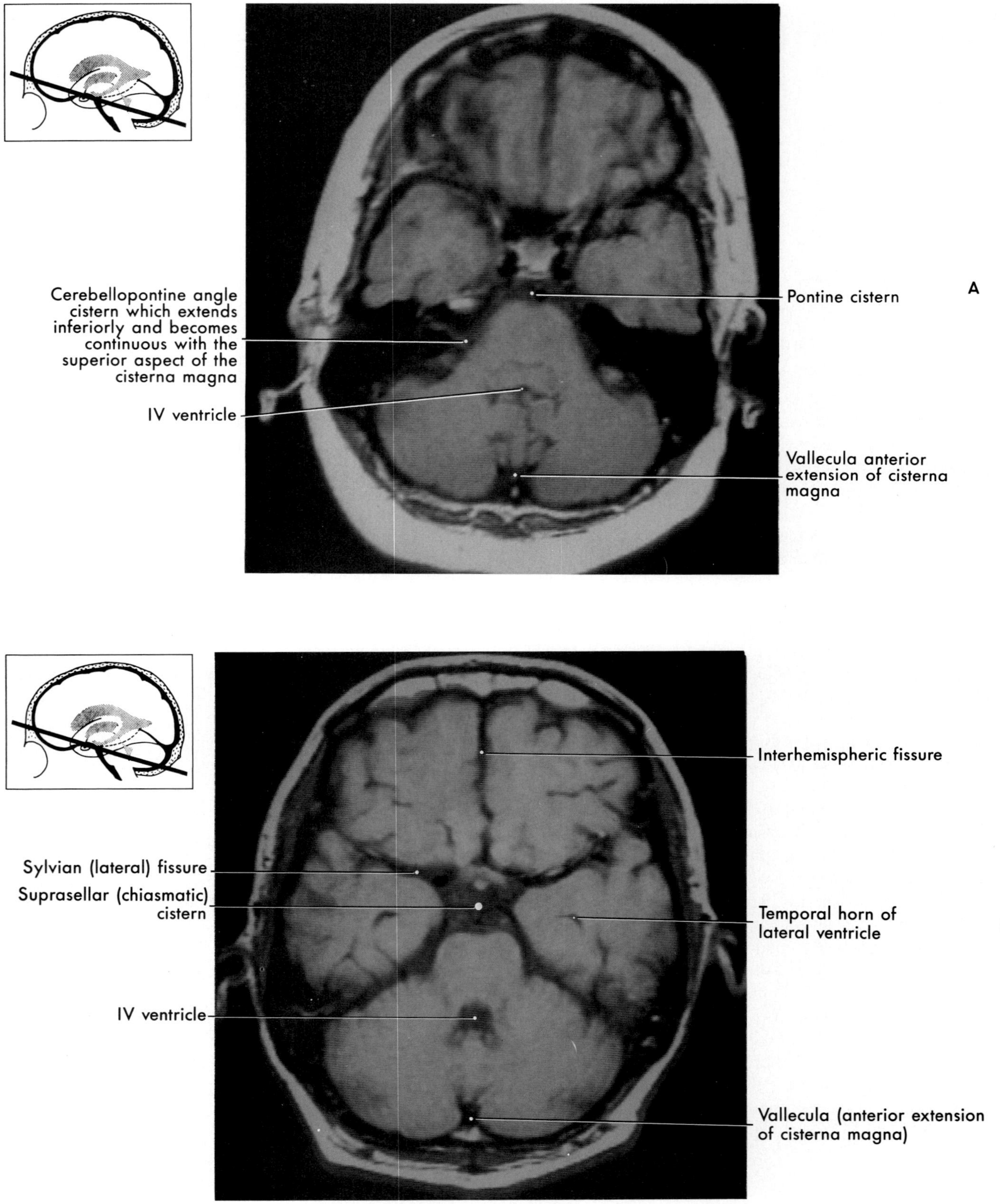

Figure 11-1 MR images (TR/TE, 800/20) in axial **(A** to **F)** and sagittal **(G)** scan planes illustrate the ventricles and cisternal spaces of the brain.

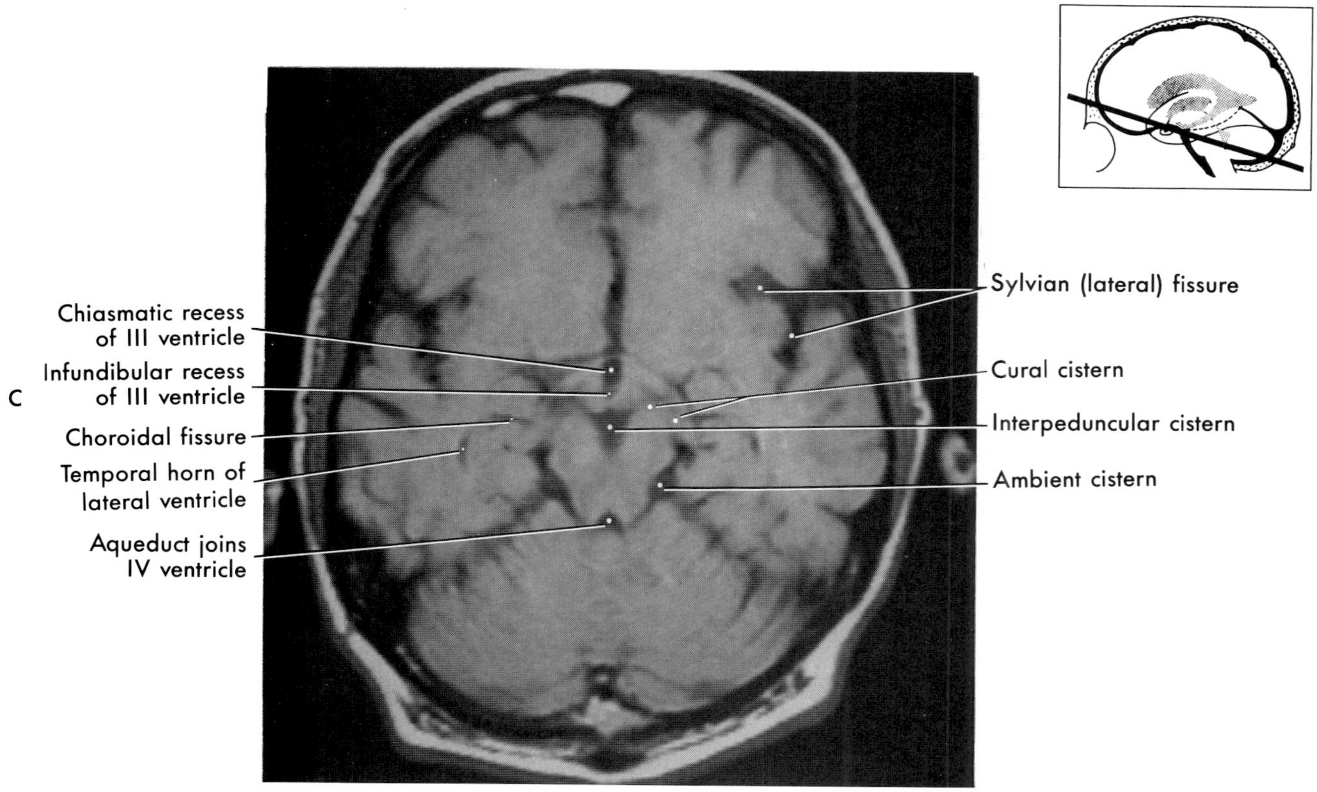

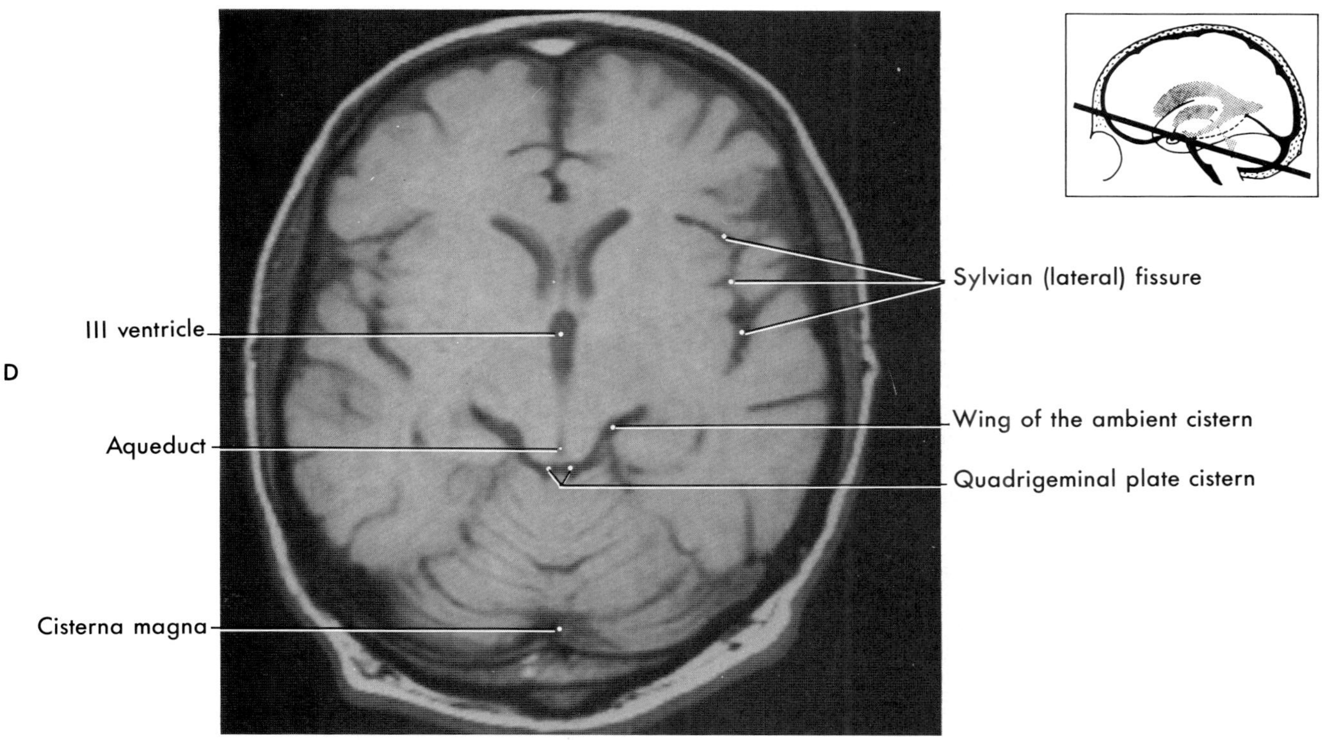

Figure 11-1, cont'd. MR images (TR/TE, 800/20) in axial (**A** to **F**) and sagittal (**G**) scan planes illustrate the ventricles and cisternal spaces of the brain.

E

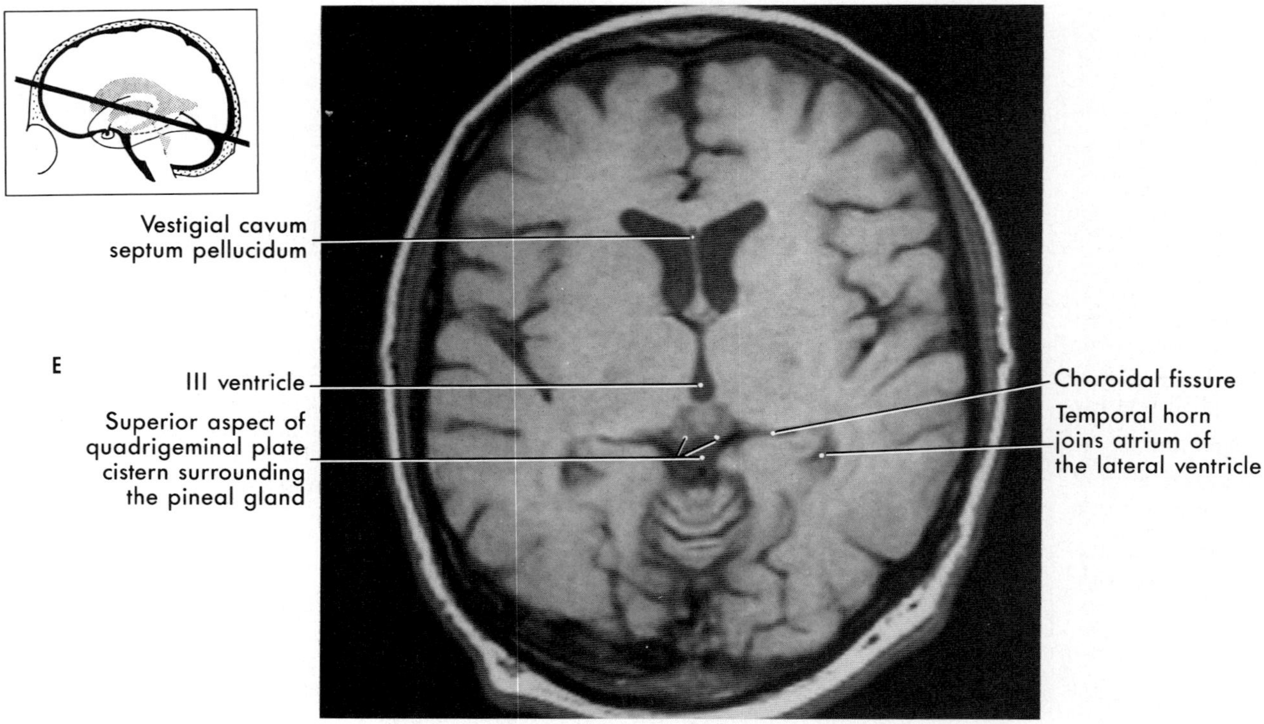

F

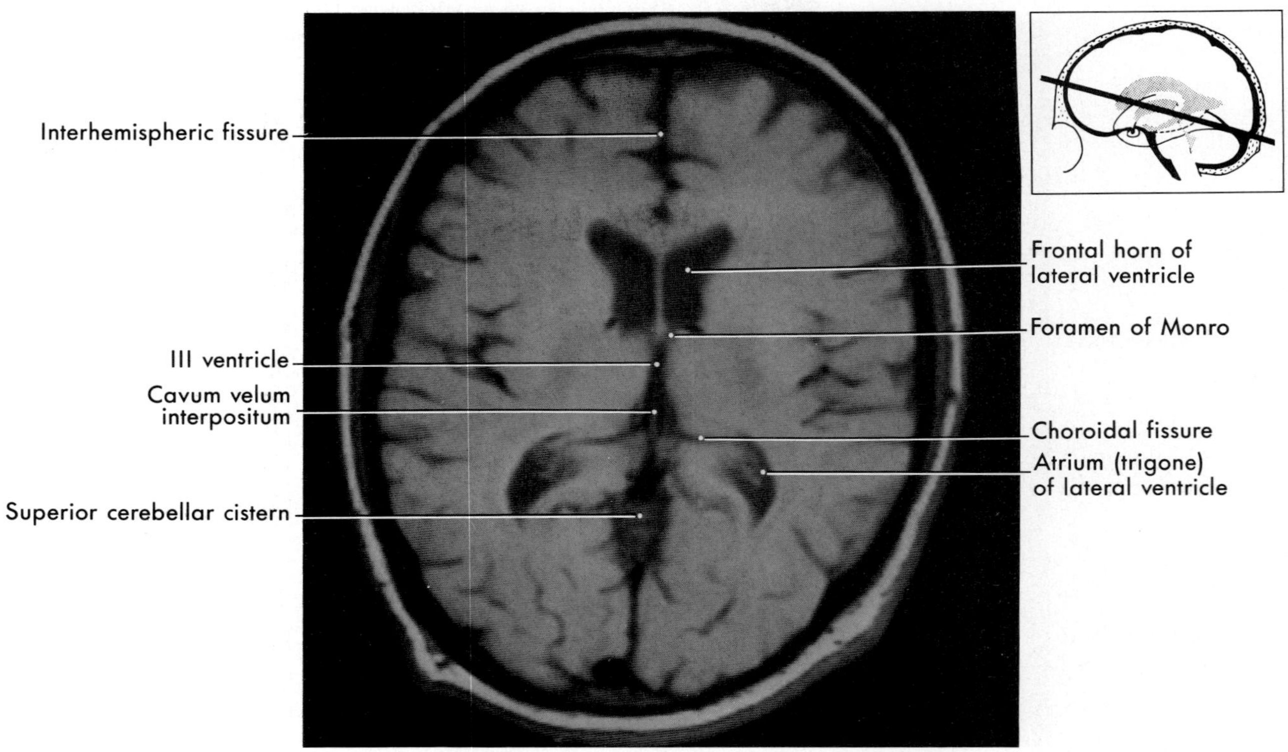

Figure 11-1, cont'd. MR images (TR/TE, 800/20) in axial (**A** to **F**) and sagittal (**G**) scan planes illustrate the ventricles and cisternal spaces of the brain.

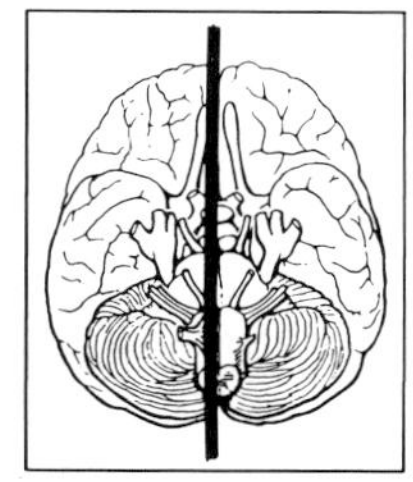

G

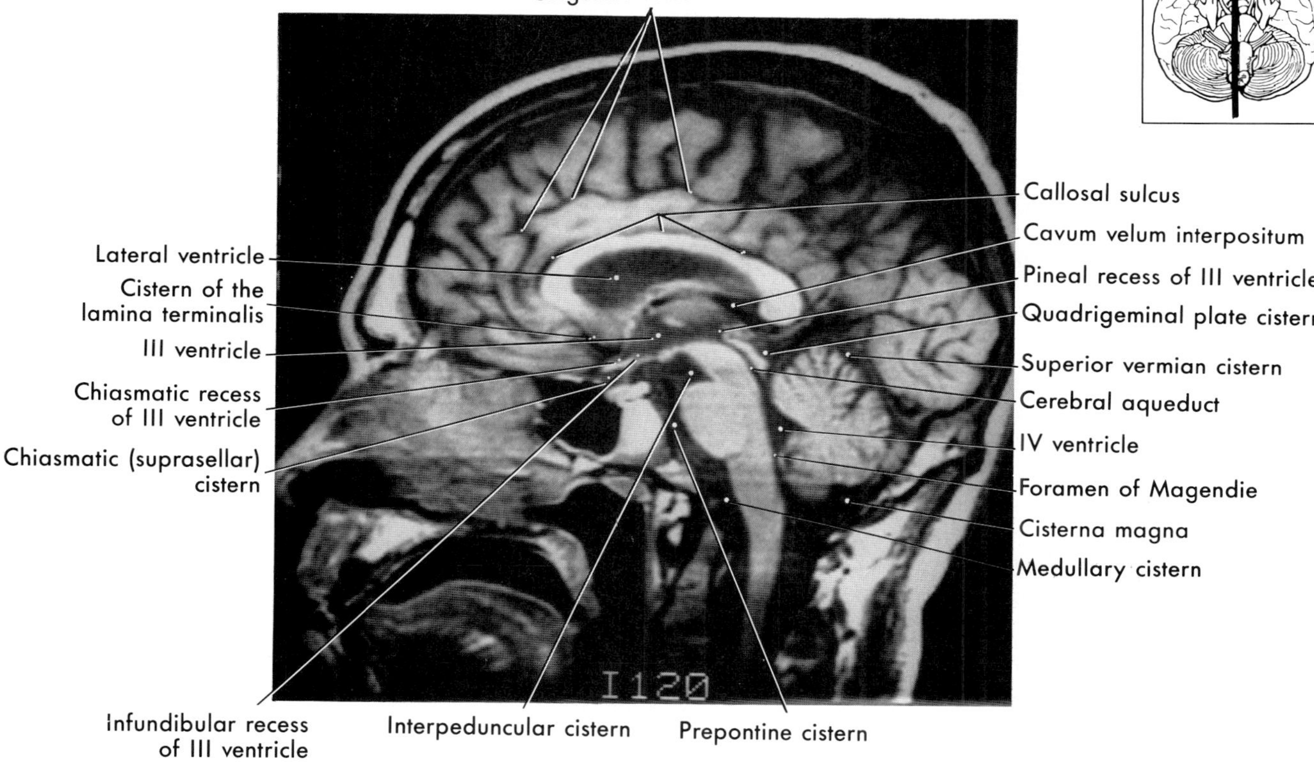

Figure 11-1, cont'd. MR images (TR/TE, 800/20) in axial (**A** to **F**) and sagittal (**G**) scan planes illustrate the ventricles and cisternal spaces of the brain.

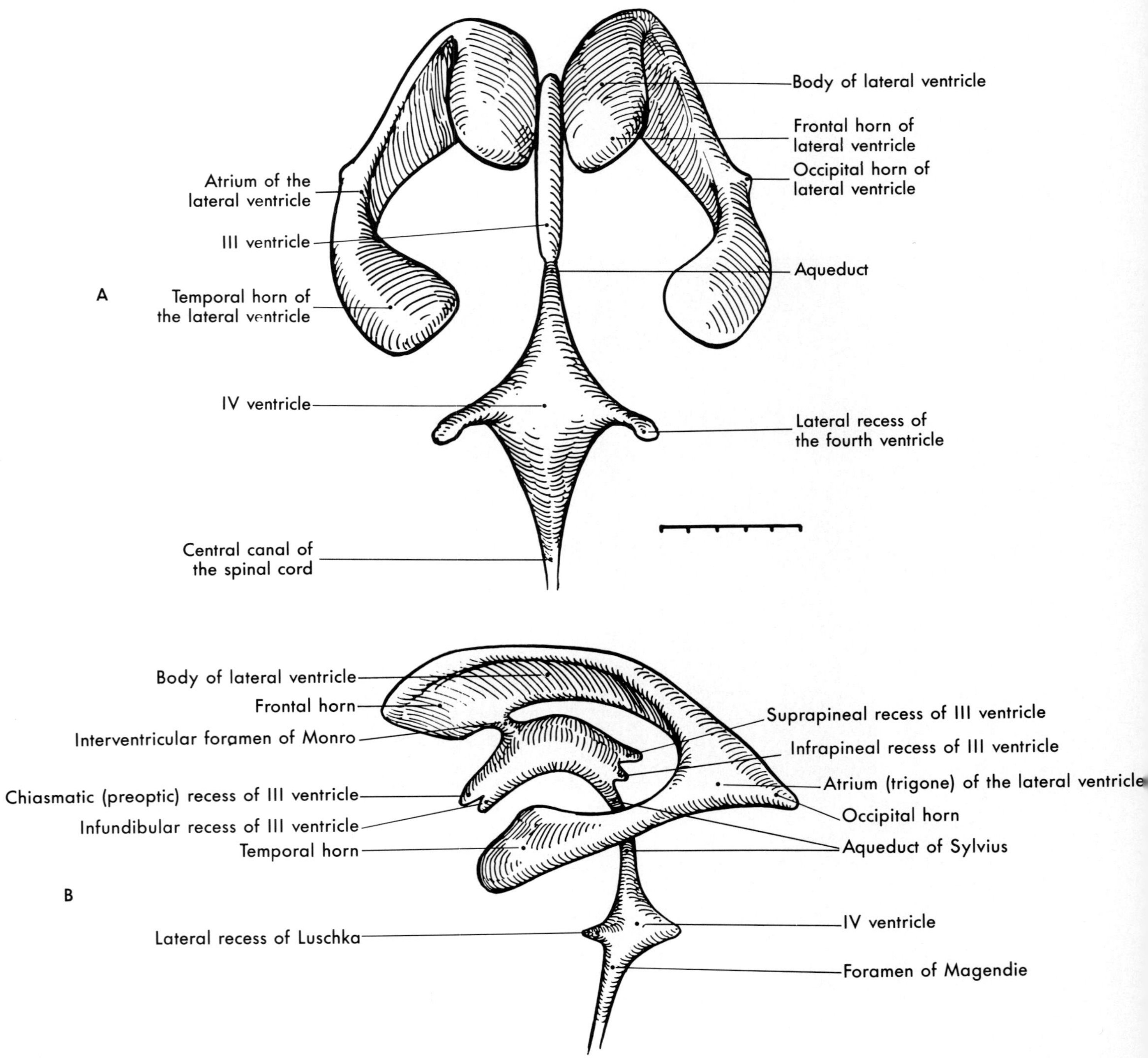

Figure 11-2 Labeled schematics of the ventricular system in frontal **(A)** and lateral **(B)** projections were traced from pneumoencephalograms. (Adapted from Kreig WJS. Functional neuroanatomy, Evanston, Ill, 1966, Brain Books.)

◆ **TABLE 11-1** Sulci (s) and Fissures (f) of the Cerebral Hemispheres*

Frontal lobe	Parietal lobe	Occipital lobe	Temporal lobe	Limbic lobe	Insula
Central s.	**Postcentral s.**	**Calcarine f.**	**Sylvian (lateral) f., posterior ramus**	**Hippocampal f.**	Circular s.
Precentral s.	Intraparietal s.	**Parietooccipital f.**	Superior temporal s.	Rhinal s.	Central s. of insula
Superior frontal s.	Marginal s. (ramus)	Lunate s.	Inferior temporal s.	Callosal s.	
Inferior frontal s.			Occipitotemporal s.	Cingulate s.	
Sylvian (lateral) f., anterior ramus			Collateral f.	Subparietal s.	
Sylvian (lateral) f., ascending ramus				Choroidal f.	
Paraolfactory s.					
Orbital s.					

Adapted from Elliott HC: *Textbook of neuroanatomy*, Philadelphia, 1963, JB Lippincott; and Clemente CD, editor: *Gray's anatomy of the human body*, ed 30 (American), Philadelphia, 1985, Lea & Febiger.
*Clinically significant sulci and fissures are noted in bold type.

◆ **TABLE 11-2** Gyri (g) and Other Ridges of the Cerebral Hemispheres*

Frontal lobe	Parietal lobe	Occipital lobe	Temporal lobe	Limbic lobe	Insula
Precentral g.	**Postcentral g.**	Lingual g.	Superior temporal g.	**Hippocampal g.**	Short g.
Superior frontal g. (marginal g.)	Supramarginal g.	Cuneus	Middle temporal g.	Cingulate g.	Long g.
Middle frontal g.	Angular g.		Inferior temporal g.	Subcallosal gg.	
Inferior frontal g.	**Paracentral lobule (partly frontal)**		Fusiform (lateral occipito-temporal) g.	Isthmus of cingulate	
Pars orbitalis	Precuneus		Medial occipitotemporal g.	Parahippocampal	
Pars triangularis (Broca's area)			**Transverse temporal g. (Heschl's)**		
Pars opercularis					
G. rectus					
Orbital gg.					

Adapted from Elliott HC: *Textbook of neuroanatomy*, Philadelphia, 1963, JB Lippincott.
*Clinically significant gyri are noted in bold type.

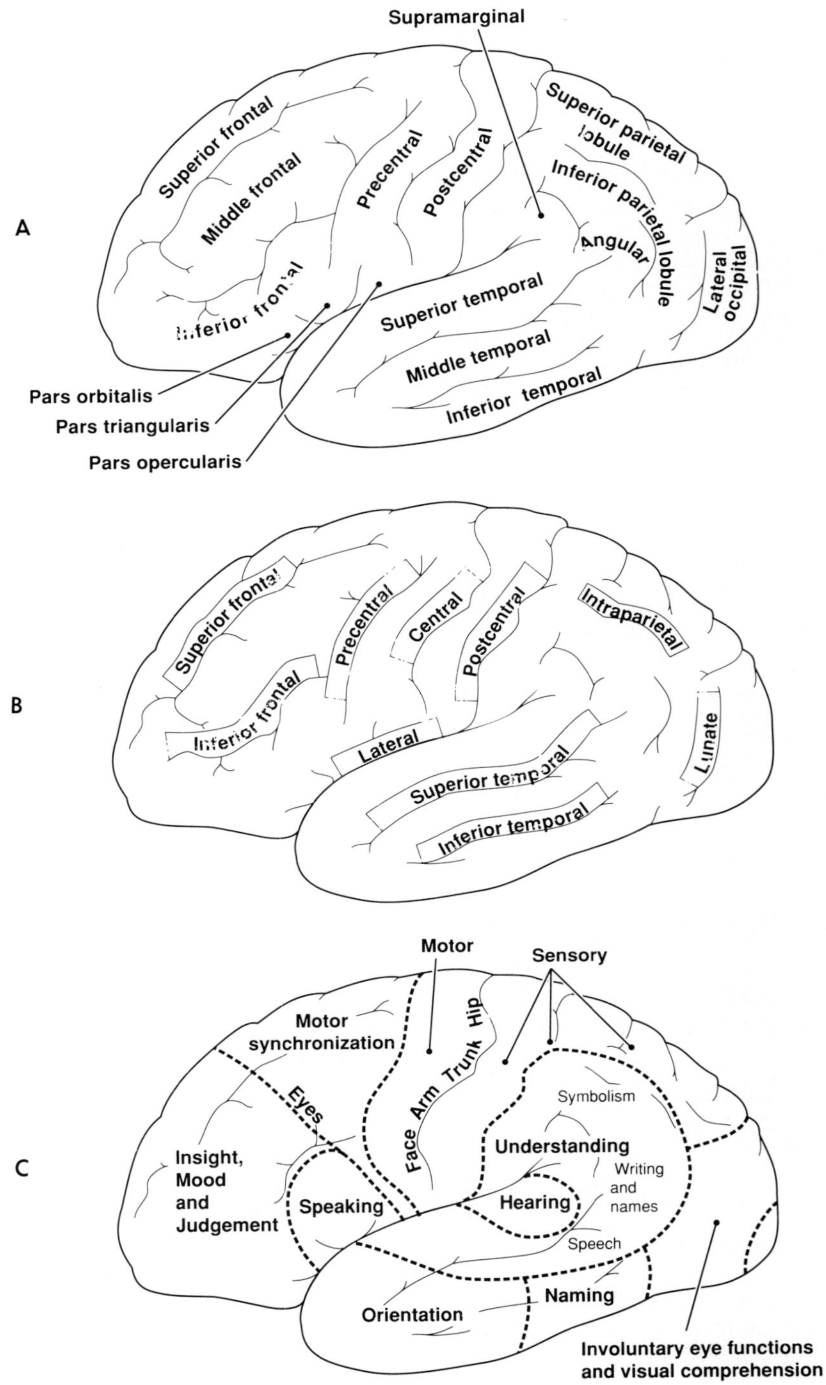

Figure 11-3 Schematics of the lateral aspect of the left cerebral hemisphere. **A,** With gyri labeled; **B,** with sulci labeled; **C,** with cortical functions labeled. Note the cortices for speaking (Broca's area) and understanding (Wernicke's area) are usually found in the dominant left hemisphere. Only in some left-handed individuals will these areas be present in the right hemisphere.

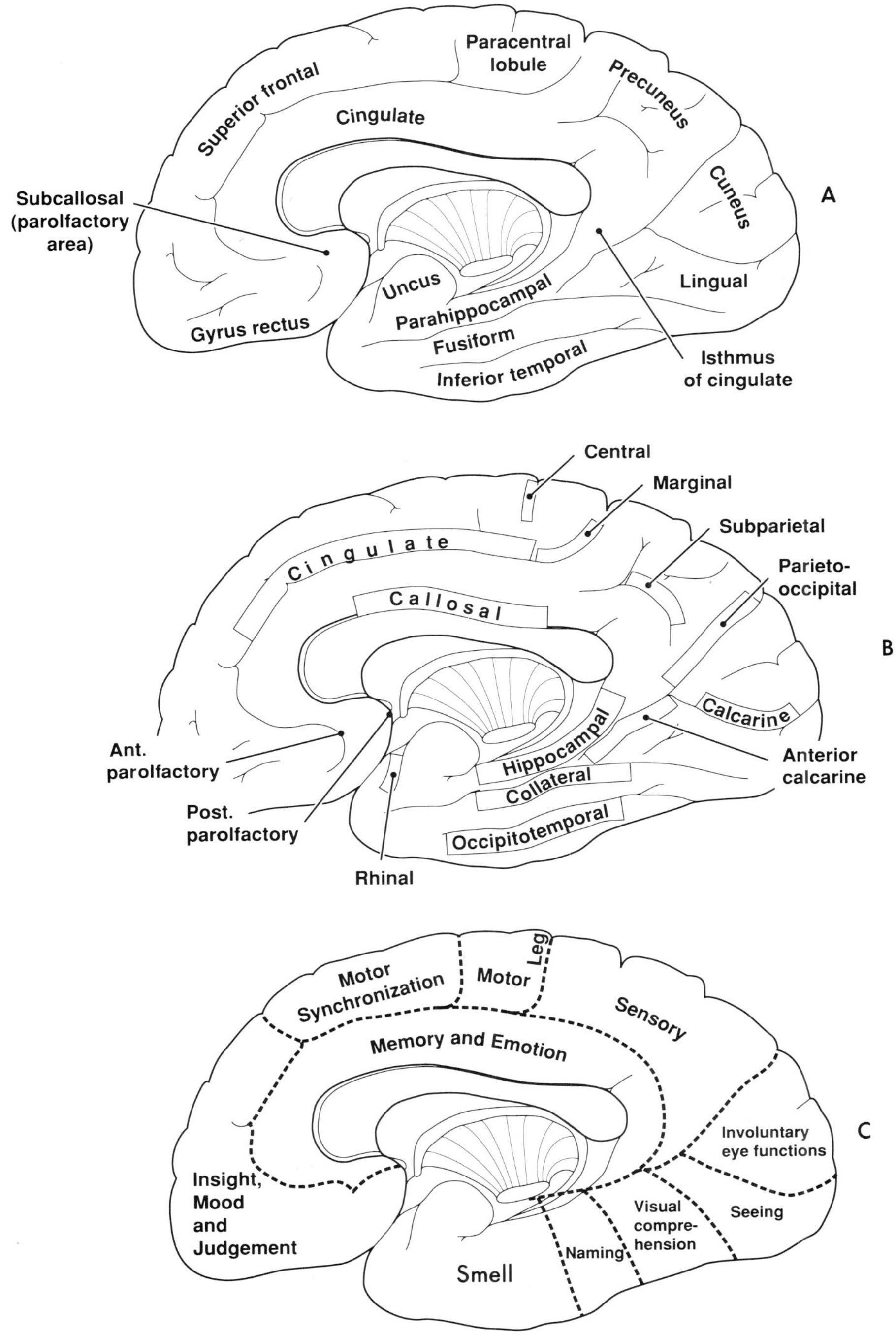

Figure 11-4 Schematics of the medial aspect of the right cerebral hemisphere. **A,** With gyri labeled; **B,** with sulci labeled; **C,** with cortical functions labeled.

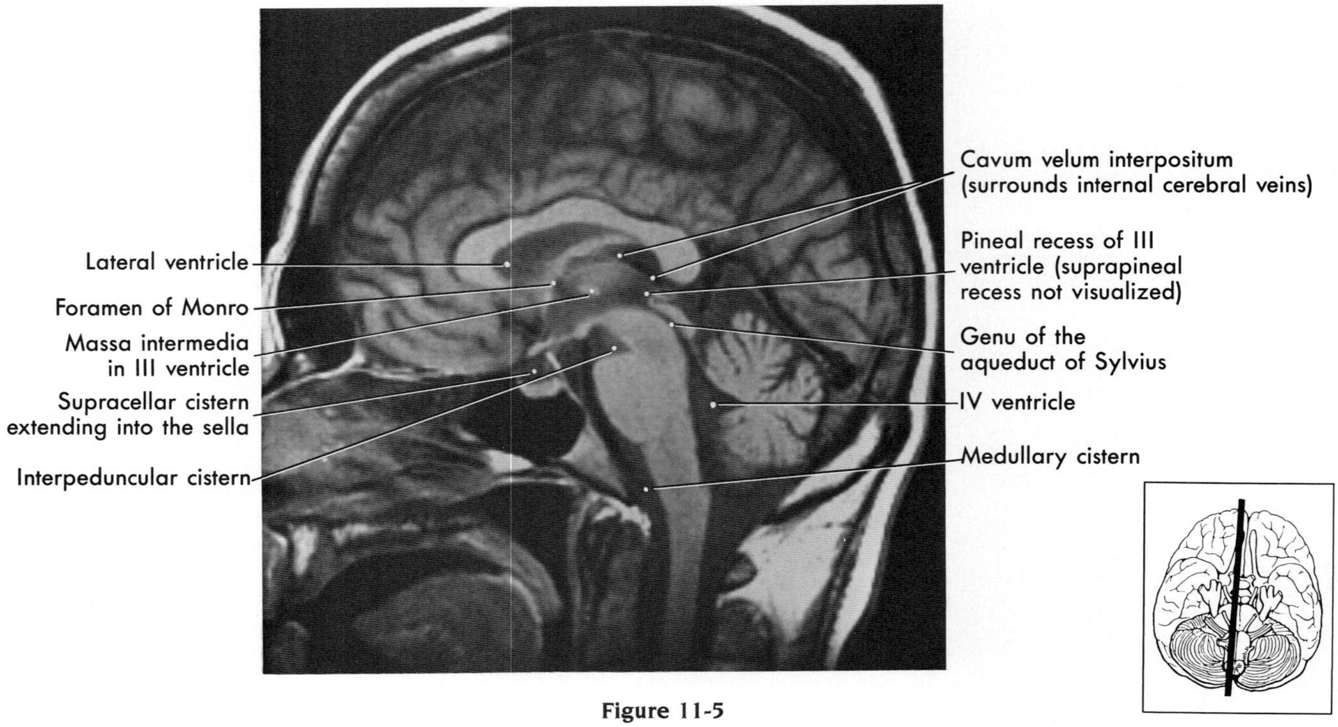

Figure 11-5

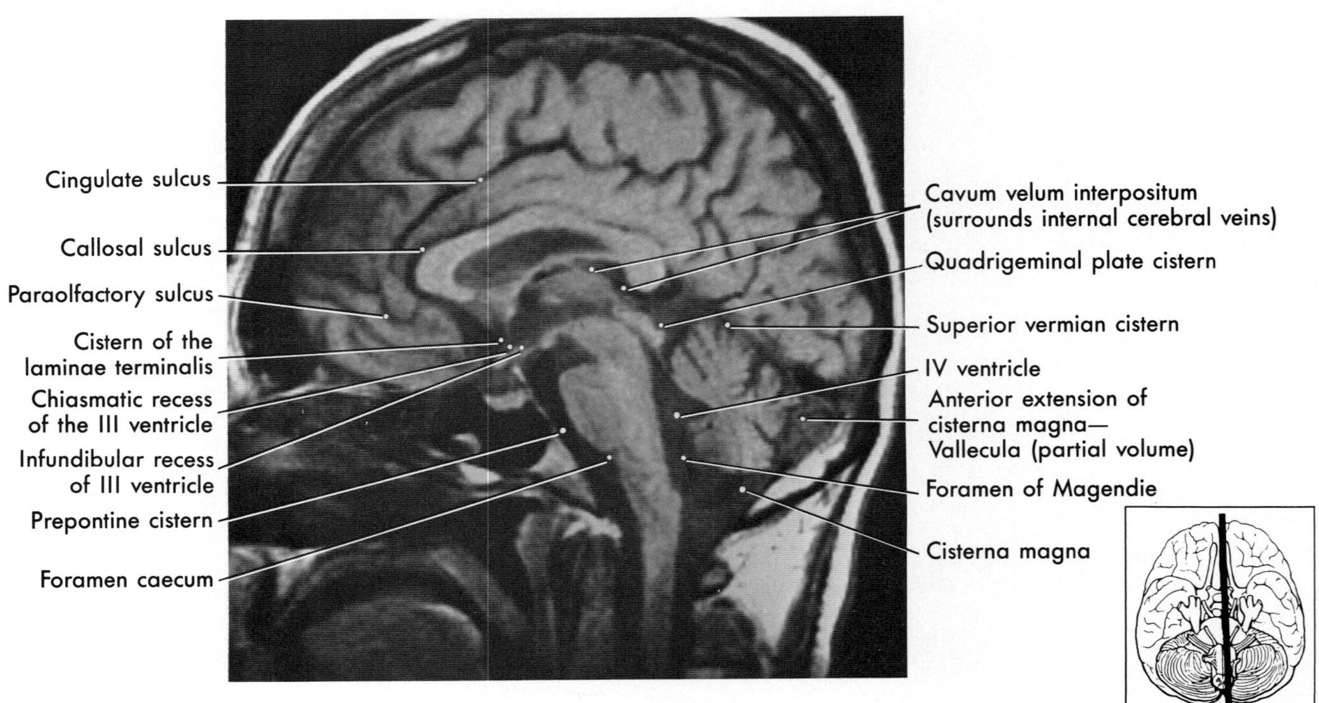

Figure 11-6

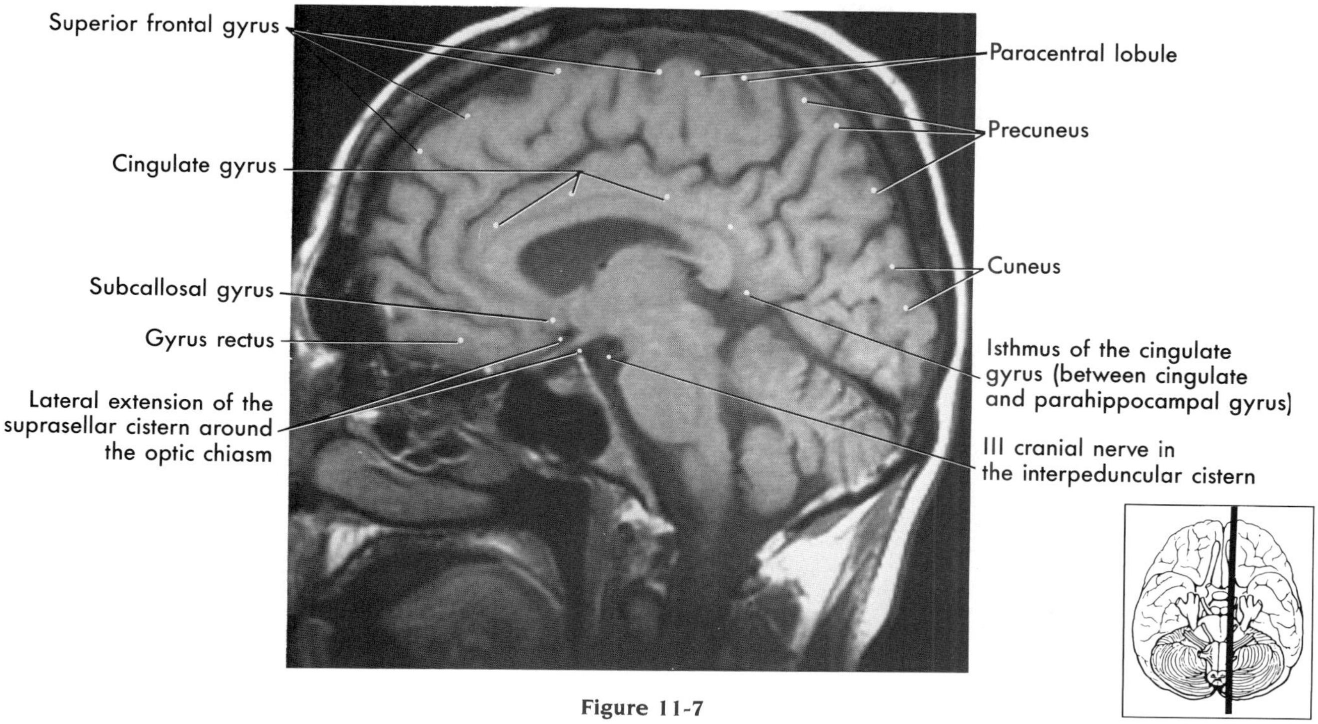

Figure 11-7

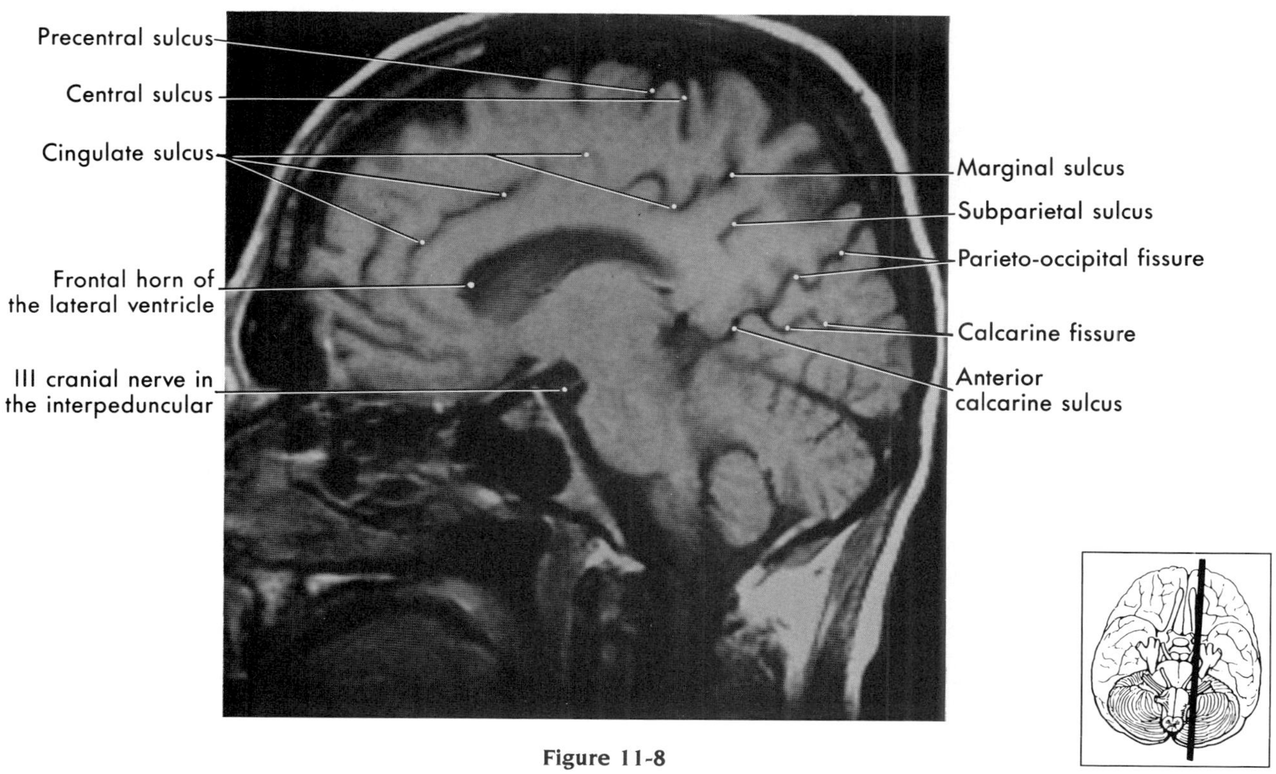

Figure 11-8

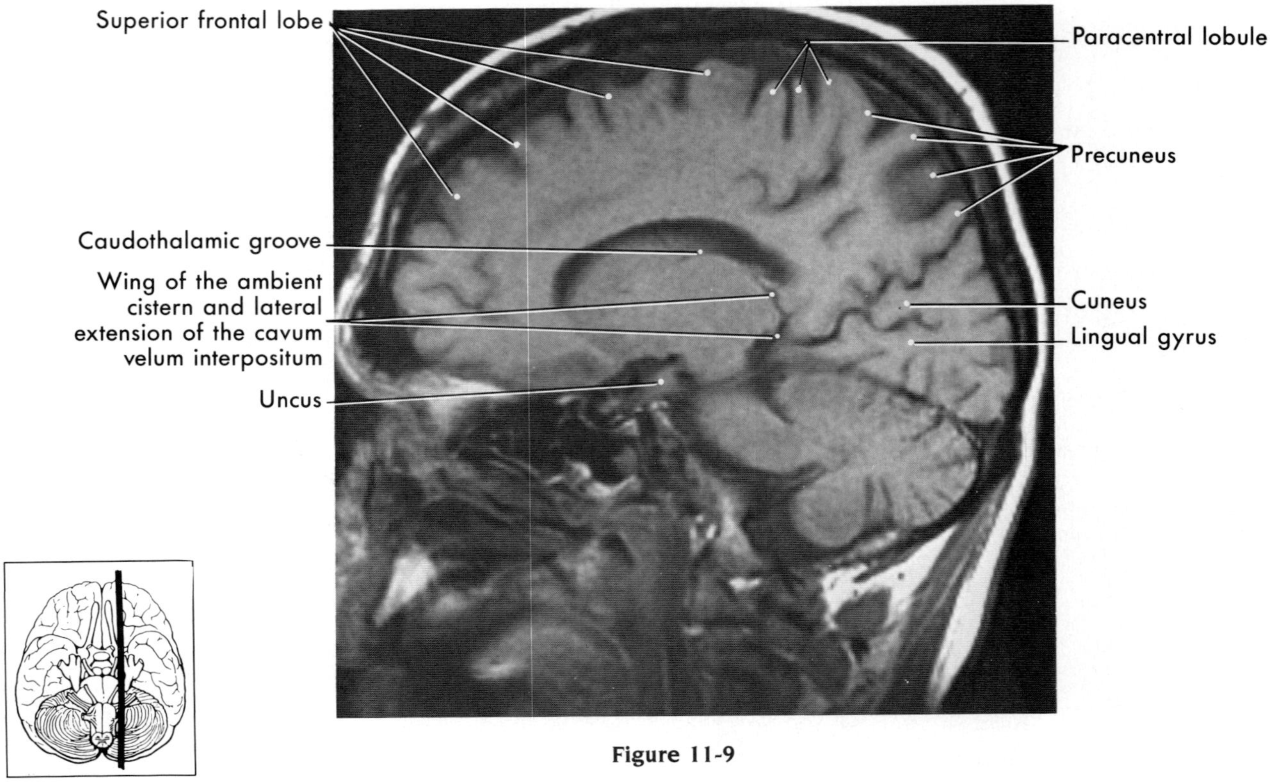

Figure 11-9

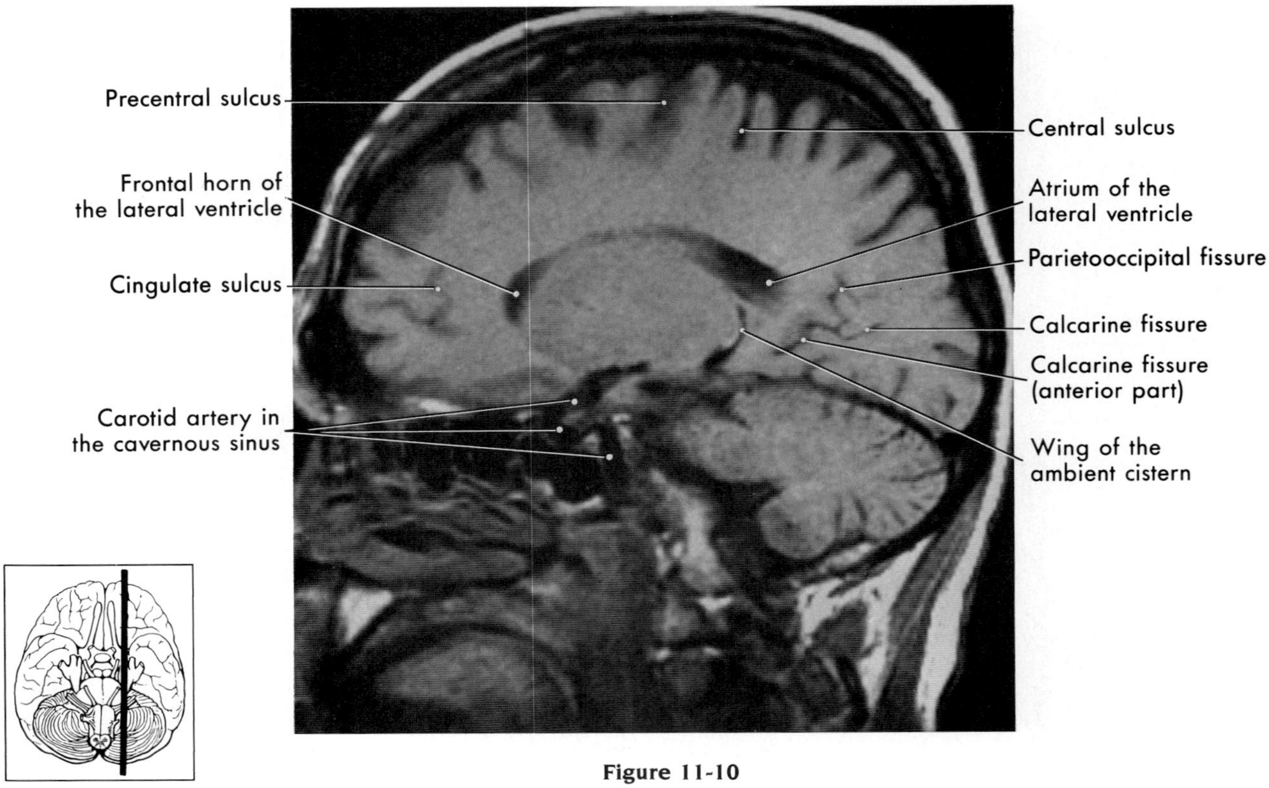

Figure 11-10

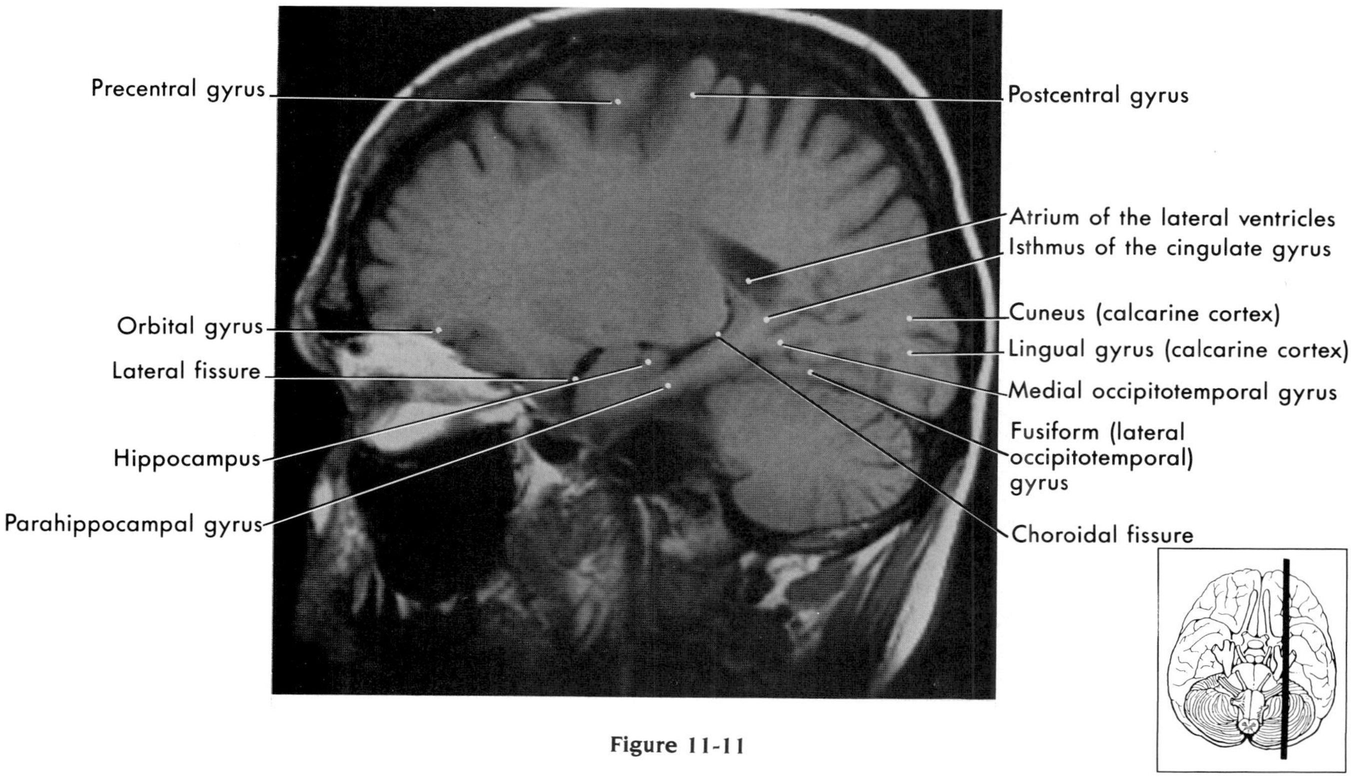

Figure 11-11

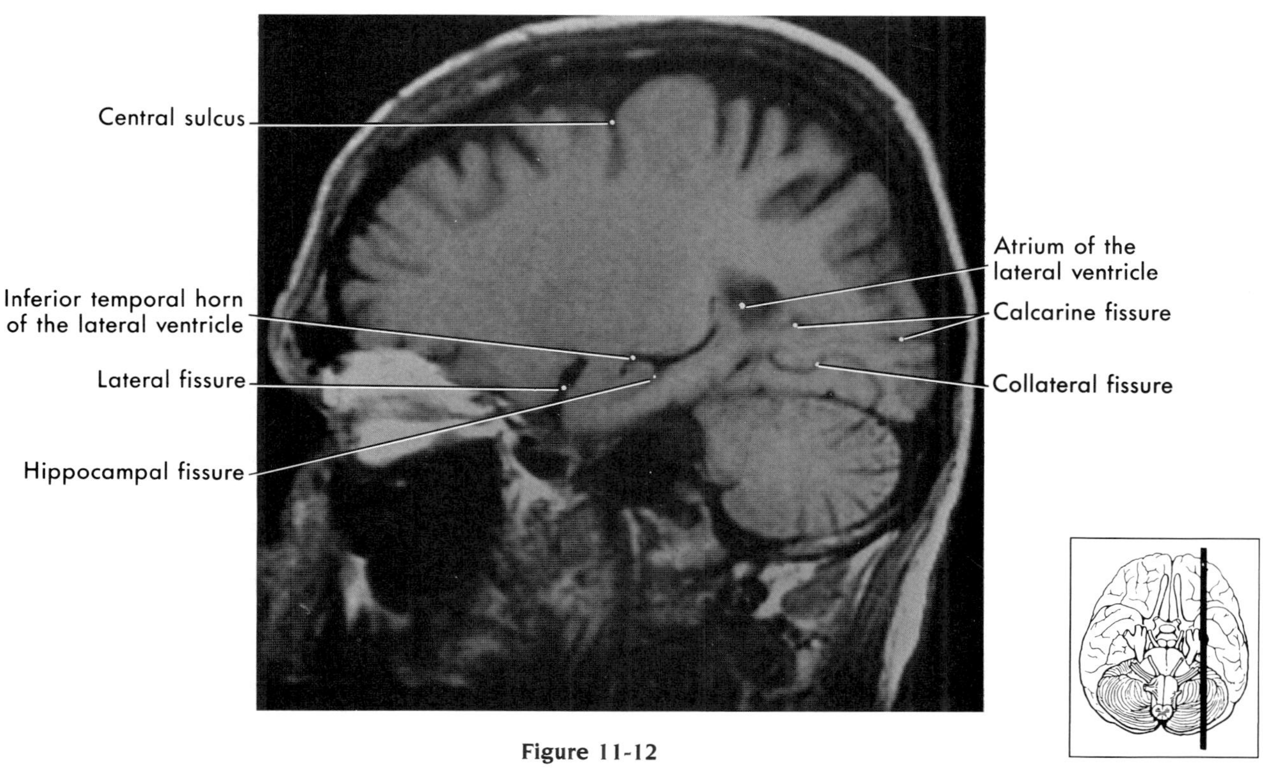

Figure 11-12

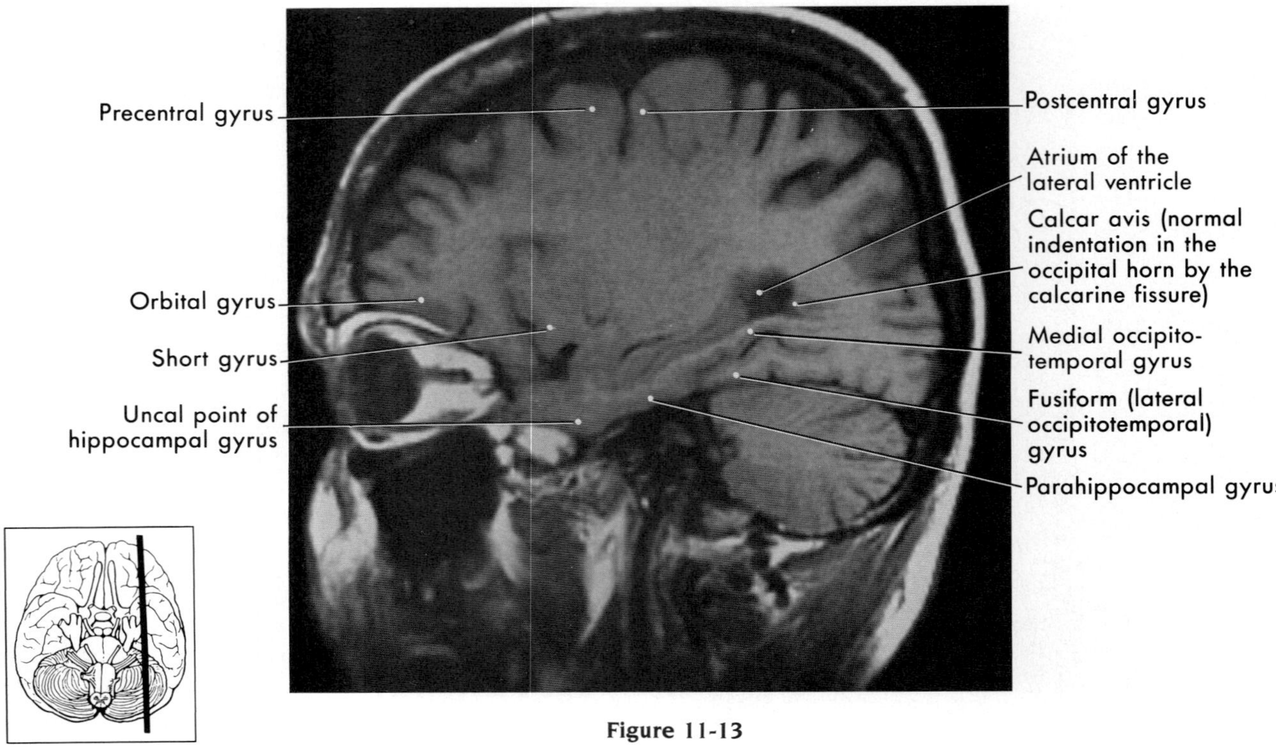

Figure 11-13

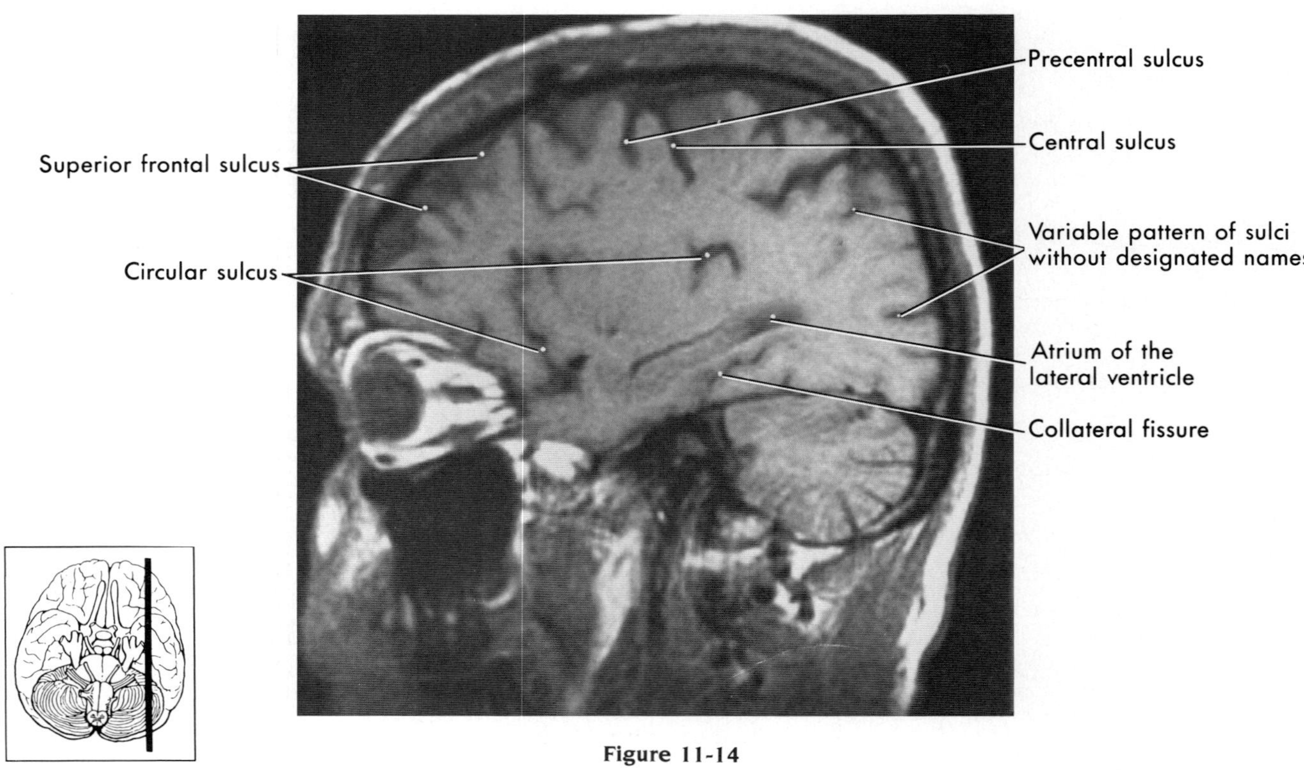

Figure 11-14

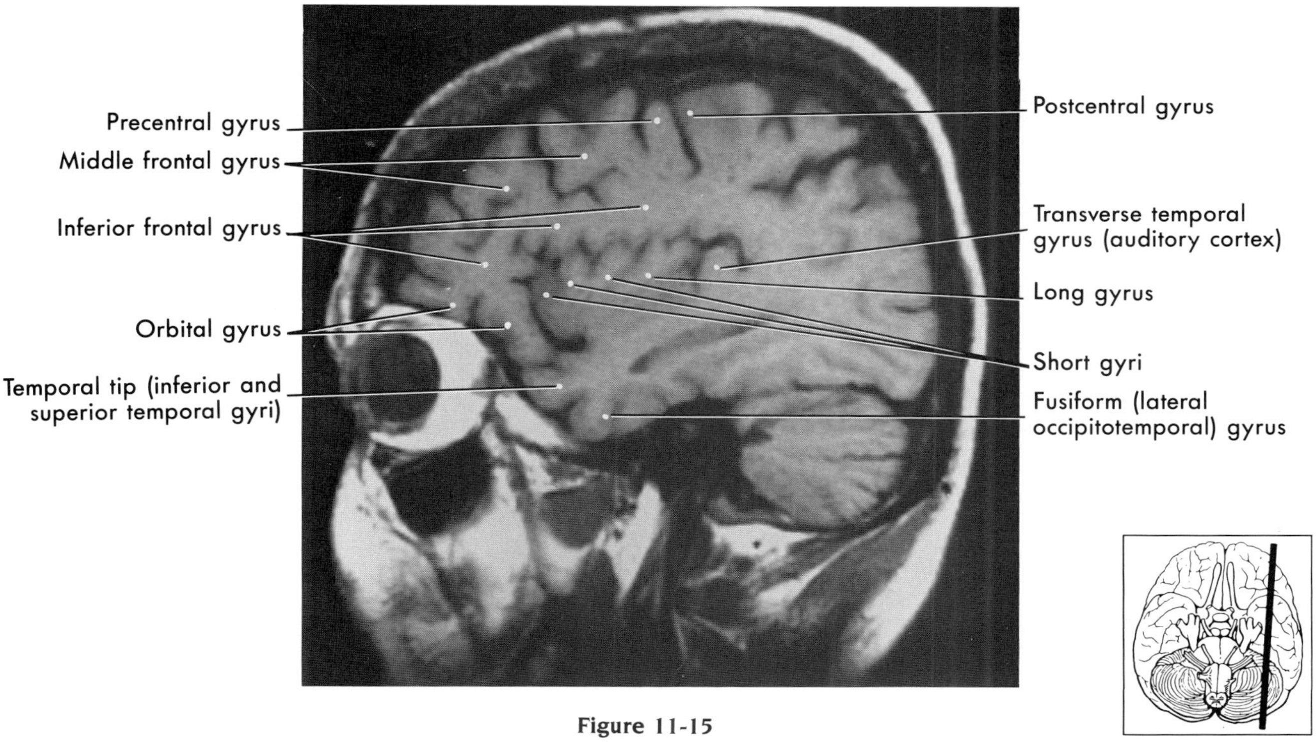

Figure 11-15

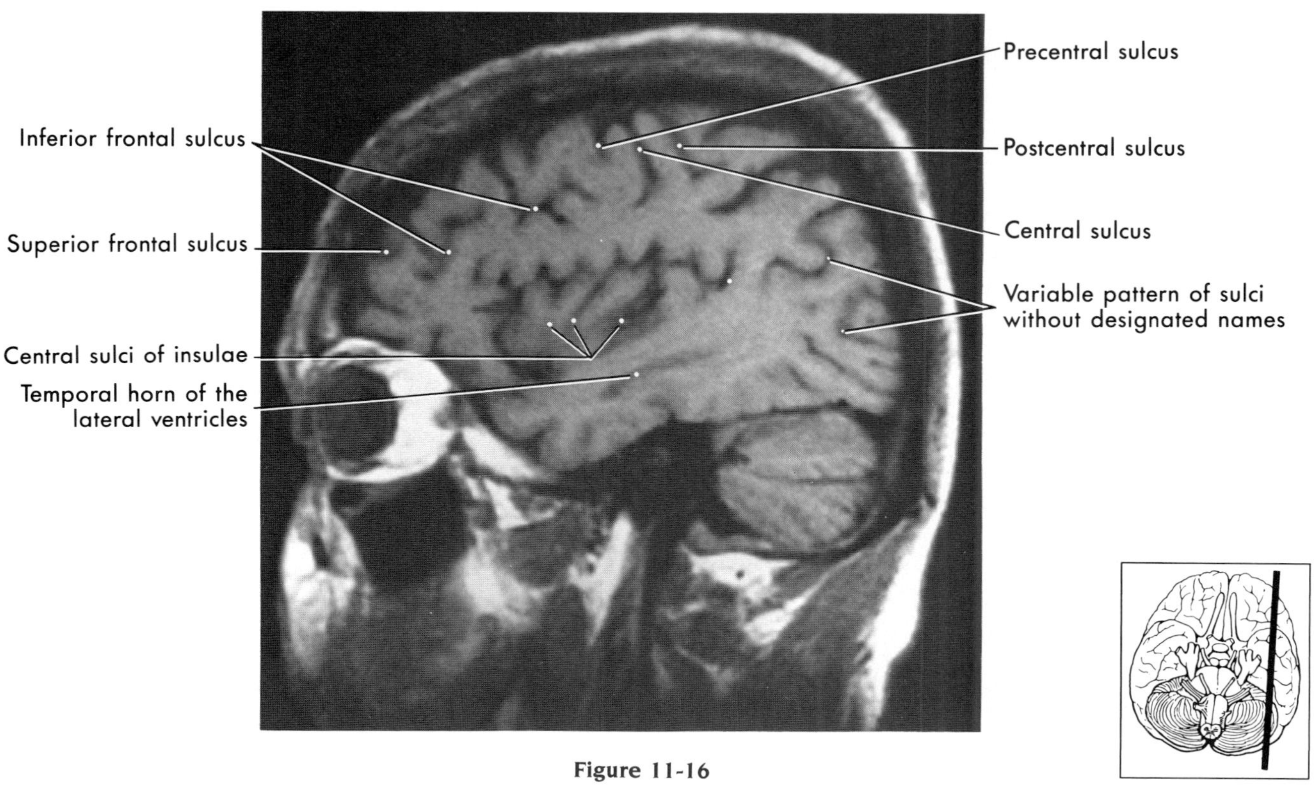

Figure 11-16

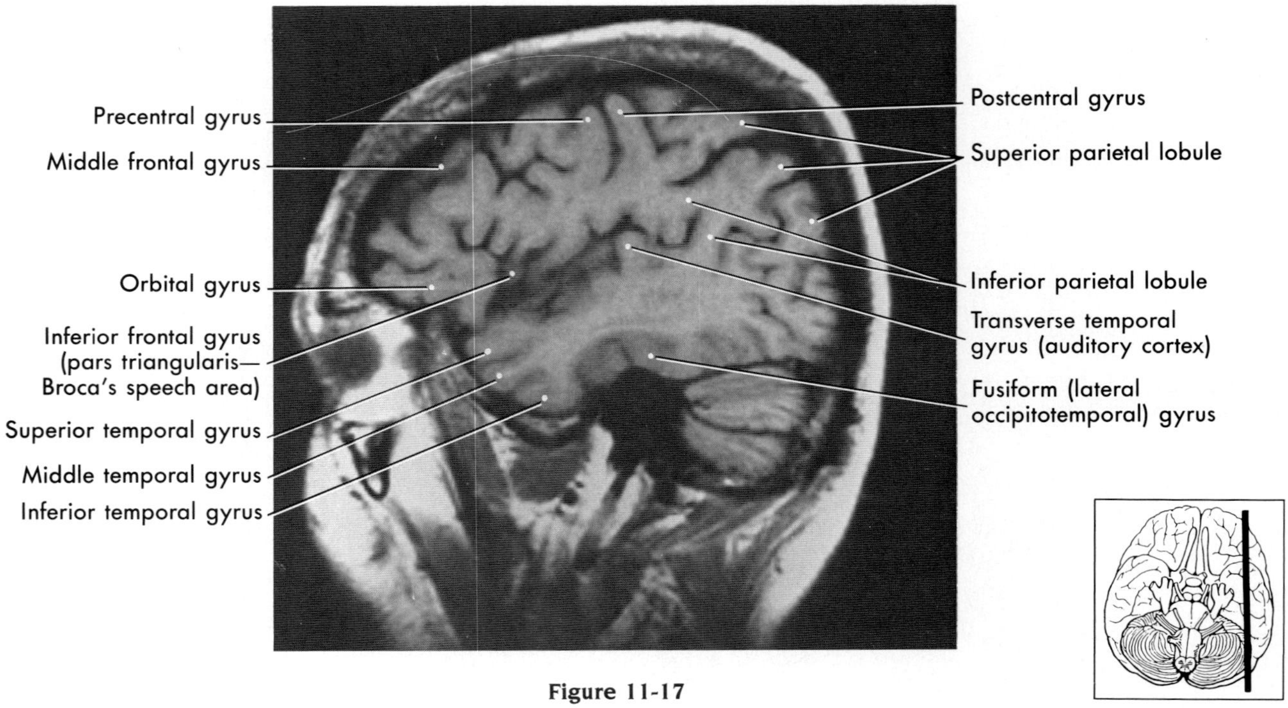

Figure 11-17

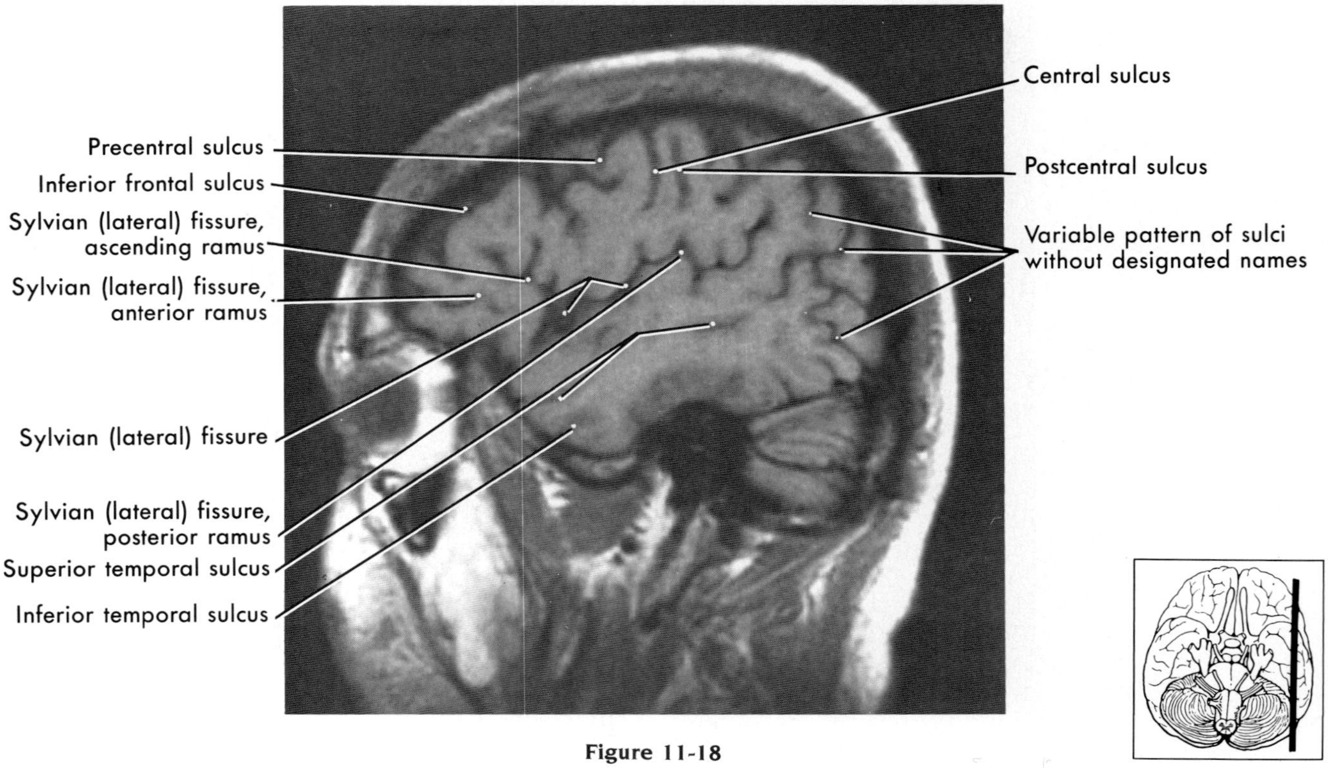

Figure 11-18

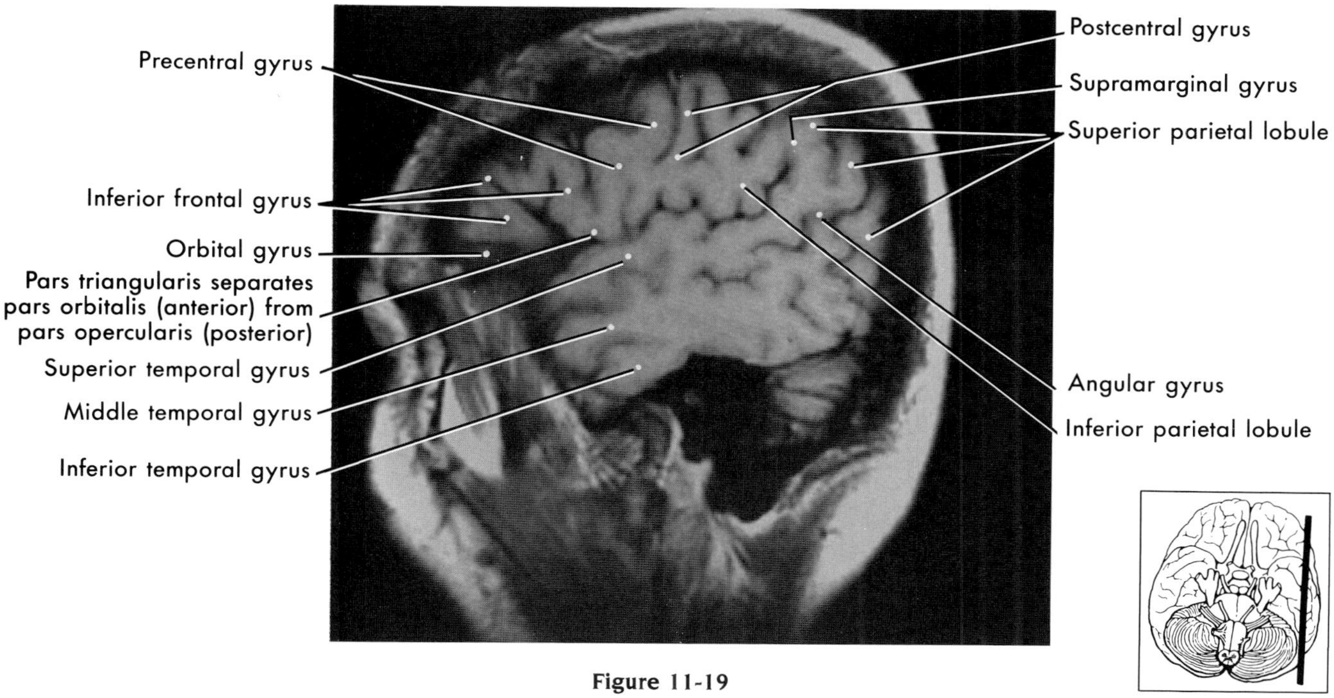

Figure 11-19

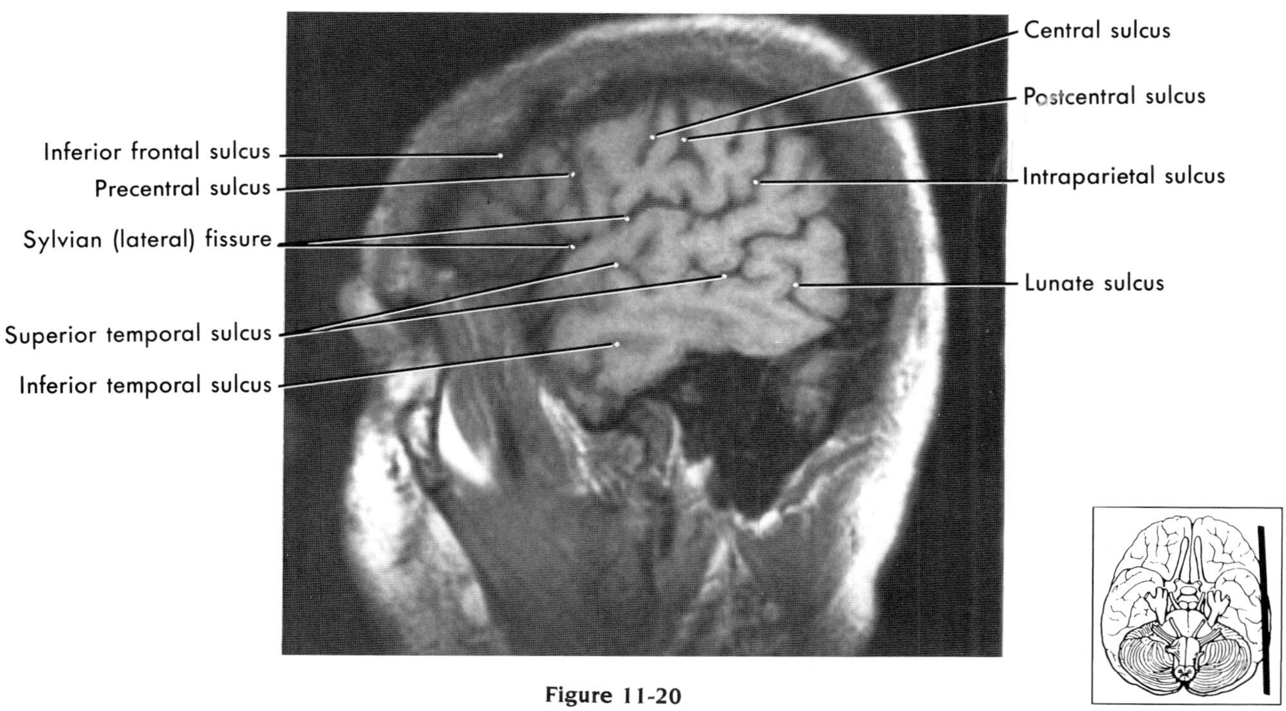

Figure 11-20

INDEX TO THE ILLUSTRATIONS

Entries refer to figures in which the specific structures are labeled.

CHAPTER 12

L. Anne Hayman
Susan Wheeler Weathers
Joel B. Kirkpatrick

Cerebrospinal Fluid Spaces and Choroid Plexuses

IMAGING TECHNIQUES

Ventricles

Within a few years of its introduction, computed tomography (CT) completely replaced pneumoencephalography as a method of visualizing cerebrospinal fluid (CSF) spaces.[1] Non-contrast-enhanced scans usually suffice for study of CSF spaces, but intraventricular injection of nonionic contrast agents is sometimes required to demonstrate masses or obstructions. Direct CT scanning is feasible only in axial and coronal planes, the latter sometimes suffering some image degradation because of dental and bone artifacts. Magnetic resonance imaging (MRI) offers advantages, particularly for imaging the fourth ventricle, aqueduct, and temporal horns because of the flexibility of scan plane selection. Sagittal magnetic resonance (MR) scans are particularly important for evaluating brainstem gliomas in which displacement of the fourth ventricle may be difficult to assess on axial CT scans.[2] The MR pulse sequences should be chosen to maximize CSF/brain contrast. Short TR/TE sequences are optimal for this purpose, although sequences that are heavily weighted for either spin density (TR greater than 6 seconds) or long TR/TE sequences may be adequate (TR, relaxation time; TE, echo delay time).

Although CT and MRI are the primary modalities for imaging adult ventricles, ultrasonography is the technique of choice for infants. The portability of ultrasound equipment permits bedside imaging of the critically ill patient and does not involve ionizing radiation. Using the anterior and posterior fontanelles as acoustic windows, one can image all four ventricles (see Chapter 1).

Except in cases of vascular malformation and intraventricular neoplasm, angiography seldom yields more information than CT or MRI. Nevertheless, the radiologist should be familiar with those vessels that relate closely to the ventricles and are typically seen on angiograms.

Subarachnoid Spaces (Cisterns)

The subarachnoid spaces (SAS) are best demonstrated with either CT or MRI. If MRI is unavailable, a CT scan that uses thin sections (less than 5 mm) and intrathecal iodinated contrast material can identify many small neural and vascular structures that traverse the SAS. In the posterior fossa, the presence of contrast material in the SAS mitigates the problem of beam-hardening artifacts on CT, since these result from the abrupt transition from dense petrous bone to adjacent, lucent CSF.

With either CT or MRI, the posterior fossa spaces are best seen in the axial plane. The coronal projection is often useful for evaluating the suprasellar and pericallosal areas. Coronal scans of the brainstem are possible with CT, but they are more easily obtained with MRI. MRI also offers the option of direct sagittal scanning, which provides an ideal way to visualize the midline cisterns. Cardiac gating with MRI improves resolution of finer details, particularly in the posterior fossa, by "stopping" brainstem motion and thereby reducing artifacts. Short TR/TE spin-echo pulse sequences offer maximum contrast of CSF with brain and fine neural structures and permit multiple repetitions to be performed, thus improving signal-to-noise ratio (SNR) and thereby spatial resolution. Long TR/TE images may also be used for SAS visualization.

Angiography provides little information about the conformation of the cisterns. Although large extraaxial masses may alter the course of vessels, most pathology is seen better with CT or MRI. Nevertheless, angiography can be helpful when the exact location of a lesion (intraaxial vs. extraaxial) is unclear on CT or MRI (see Chapter 15).

FUNCTION AND MOVEMENT OF CEREBROSPINAL FLUID

The CSF that surrounds the brain has several important functions. CSF provides physical support for the brain, regulates chemical environment, and provides a moving pathway for transporting both nutrients and substances that must be excreted.[3] The most easily documented of these functions is the role of the CSF in physically supporting the brain. A 1500 g brain afloat in CSF weighs only 50 g.[3] This support also protects the brain from acute changes in venous, arterial, and pulse pressure because CSF volume fluctuates reciprocally with changes in intracranial blood volume, if the skull is intact. CSF may also serve to dampen the effects of arterial pulsations that may damage the cisternal portions of adjacent cranial nerves (see Chapter 14).

The role of CSF in regulating the chemical environment by distributing biologically active substances is the subject of intensive investigation.[3] Nuclear medicine and MR studies have demonstrated the movements of CSF around the brain and spinal cord.[4-8] This motion cannot be explained by the rate of CSF formation, which is only 0.35 ml/minute.[3] A portion of the CSF movement can be attributed to the surges in blood pressure during the cardiac cycle that cause brain pulsations. In vivo, quantitative MR techniques have been developed to show the effects of vascular-driven brain motion on CSF.[9] Ejection of CSF from the cerebral ventricles and reversal of CSF flow in the foramen of Monro and cerebral aqueduct during systole have all been observed. These observations have changed the traditional views concerning movement of CSF.[9]

DEVELOPMENTAL ANATOMY

In the adult brain the close relationship between the ventricular system, SAS, and meninges may not be readily apparent, but a study of their embryogenesis reveals their close interdependence both developmentally and anatomically. A review of this development helps one to form a better three-dimensional concept of the relationships among some of the more complex brain structures[10-12] (Figure 12-1).

In early development the central nervous system (CNS) exists as a hollow tube covered by the mesenchyme, which will eventually become the meninges. The hollow tube develops a central ependymal lining that is not completely continuous even in the adult. This tube develops three expansions (forebrain, midbrain, hindbrain). Figure 12-1 illustrates the growth and rotation in each of these regions, and the following text describes how the lumen of the neural tube develops into the adult ventricular system.

The roof of the *hindbrain* thins and the neural cavity expands from side to side to form the fourth ventricle. Folds of tela invaginate into this cavity. Accompanied by blood vessels, the tela form the choroid plexus of the fourth ventricle. The lateral aspects of the hindbrain at this level expand symmetrically to form the cerebellar hemispheres, which protrude medially into the fourth ventricle. The medial surfaces of the cerebellar hemispheres join and induce the formation of the cerebellar vermis, which indents the posterior aspect of the fourth ventricle (see Chapter 10). The tela that lines the fourth ventricle eventually ruptures in three locations. The opening in the caudal midline area becomes the foramen of Magendie, and the symmetric lateral openings form the foramina of Luschka.

The neural cavity of the *midbrain* persists as the sylvian aqueduct in the mature brain. The marked relative reduction in size of this channel can be ascribed to enlargement of the collicular plate and an increase in the number of fiber tracts ventral to the aqueduct.

The rostralmost *forebrain* contains a central cavity that persists as the third ventricle. Its roof becomes greatly thinned so that ependyma and pia abut to form the tela choroidea of the third ventricle, which protrudes from above into the ventricle, forming the choroid plexus of the third ventricle. Vesicles bud off anterolaterally from the anterosuperior aspect of the third ventricle. These eventually become the lateral ventricles, which communicate with the third ventricle by way of the widely patent interventricular foramina of Monro. Forward and upward extension of these cerebral buds (also referred to as the telencephalon) occurs as the cerebral hemispheres begin to approach each other above the diencephalon (Figure 12-2). Further growth of the primitive cerebral hemispheres proceeds posteriorly and then inferolaterally, eventually covering the midbrain and diencephalon. This folding of the cerebral hemispheres into the available intracranial space produces the ram's horn shape of the cerebral hemispheres and lateral ventricles.

The thick basal plates of the cerebral hemispheres that lie inferolateral to the lateral ventricles give rise to the *caudate nuclei*. This relationship between caudate nuclei and ventricles is maintained during the growth and rotation of the cerebral hemispheres already described. Thus, the tail of each caudate nucleus lies superolateral to its temporal horn.

The primitive cerebral hemisphere becomes very thin near its attachment to the roof of the forebrain (i.e., the third ventricle). At this pial-ependymal interface, the tela invaginates into the lateral ventricle to form the choroid plexus. This process begins at the interventricular foramen of Monro and follows the posterior and inferolateral move-

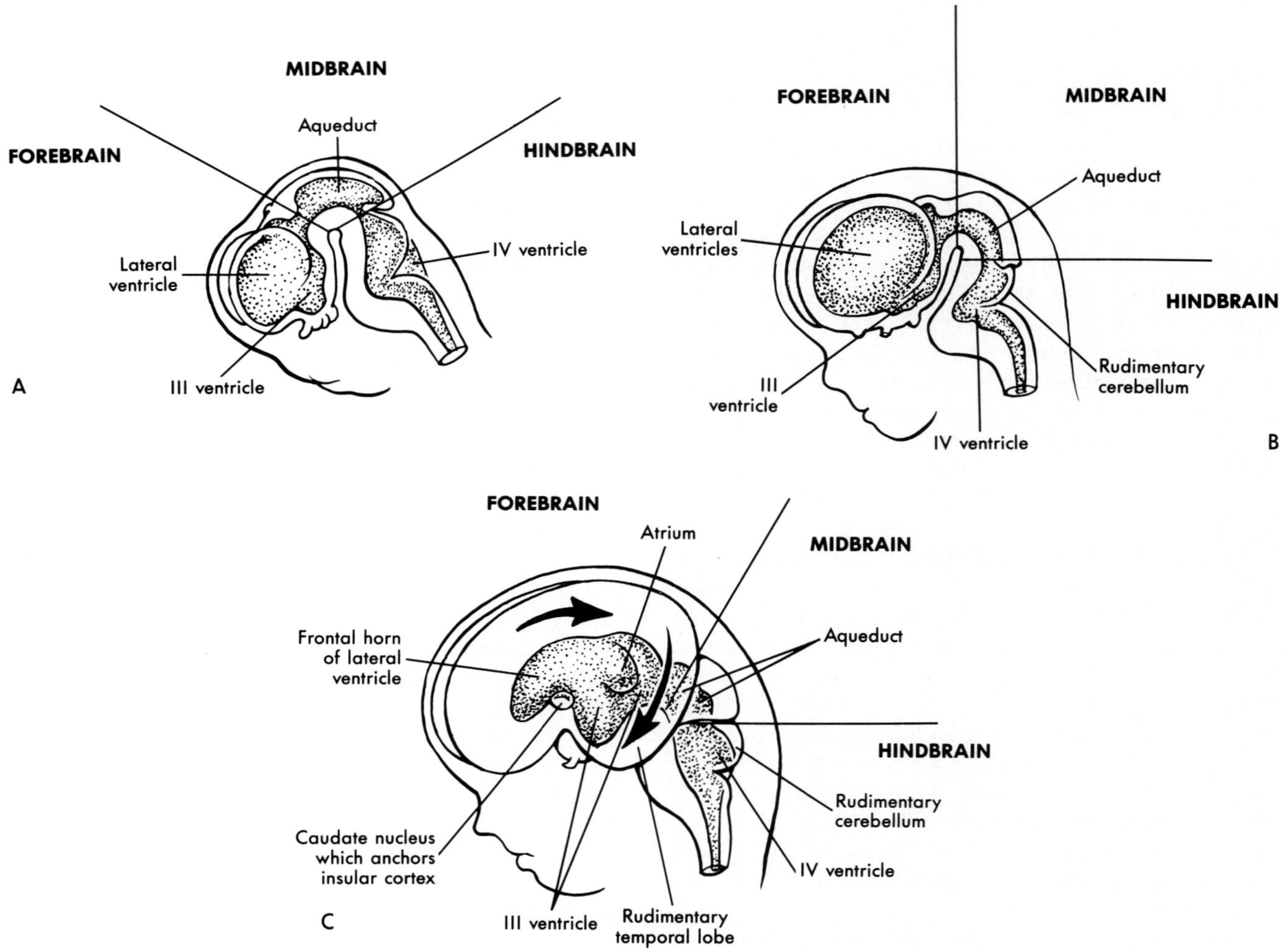

Figure 12-1 Lateral schematic illustrations showing the growth of the brain. **A,** At approximately 6 weeks of gestation, the third ventricle buds laterally into the rudimentary cerebral hemispheres to form the lateral ventricles. **B,** At approximately 8 weeks of gestation, the forebrain and the lateral ventricle have grown and shifted the midbrain and hindbrain caudally. **C,** At approximately 10 weeks of gestation, the forebrain has almost covered the midbrain, and the temporal lobes of the hemispheres have begun to form. The choroidal fissure is formed by this growth of the cerebral hemispheres. The rudimentary cerebellum has enlarged and, with additional growth, will cover the posterior and lateral aspects of the fourth ventricle. (Reproduced with permission from Smith CP, Williams PL, Treadgold S: *Basic human embryology*, London, 1984, Pitman.)

ment of the lateral ventricle previously described. This rotation of the primitive cerebral hemisphere over the midbrain creates a narrow cleft in the mature brain between the medial aspect of the cerebral hemisphere and the thalamus. This cleft has been termed the *choroidal fissure* (see Figure 12-1). Throughout the length of the choroidal fissure, ventricle and SAS are separated only by a very thin membrane.

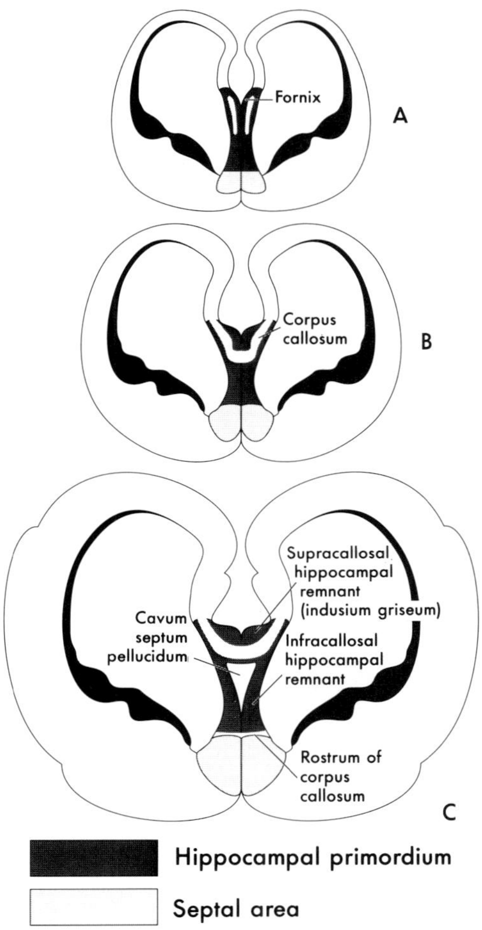

Figure 12-2 Coronal schematics anterior to the foramen of Monro show progressive stages of brain development. **A,** Lateral expansions of the neural foramina have become the fetal lateral ventricles. The dark periventricular rim, also seen in **B** and **C,** represents the germinal matrix. **B,** Development of the corpus callosum between the cerebral hemispheres. Note that the cortex is extremely thin at this stage of development. **C,** The triangular, CSF-filled cavum septum pellucidum between the body (above) and the rostrum (below) of the corpus callosum. The smallest and innermost of the concentric gyri of the limbic lobe (i.e., the indusium griseum) is also identified. (Reproduced with permission from Sarwar M: AJNR 10:989-1005, 1989.)

Above the choroidal fissure, the cortex develops a thickening, the *hippocampus;* as with the caudate nucleus, the hippocampus elongates and rotates with the cerebral hemisphere. However, most of the hippocampus subsequently degenerates, leaving only a small portion medial to the temporal horn. The fiber tract that connects the hippocampus to the diencephalon betrays its circuitous migration. This fiber tract has been named the *fornix*. It forms part of the medial wall of the adult lateral ventricle and curves around the thalamus, from which the fornix is separated by the choroidal fissure. The bodies of the paired fornices exchange fibers above the thalamus, whereas the anterior columns descend, medial to the interventricular foramen, to reach the hypothalamus.

Closure of the rostral end of the neural tube results in the formation of the anterior wall of the third ventricle (i.e., the *lamina terminalis*). Development of the cerebral hemispheres is accompanied by thickening of the upper portion of the lamina terminalis. This thickened area becomes a commissural plate from which several interhemispheric commissural tracts develop, including the anterior and hippocampal commissures (see Chapter 5).

Development of the cerebral hemisphere also creates another interhemispheric tract, the *corpus callosum,* which forms the roof of the lateral ventricle. According to one theory, the rapid growth of the corpus callosum from anterior to posterior causes stretching of the commissural plate between the corpus callosum and the fornices, thus forming the septum pellucidum.

As the hemispheres and corpus callosum grow posteriorly over the diencephalon, the meningeal layers between them are apposed, forming a two-layer membrane, the *velum interpositum,* which overlies the roof of the third ventricle. Incomplete apposition or fusion of these layers results in the formation of a *cavum velum interpositum* (Figure 12-3). In the process of folding over, the primitive internal cerebral veins and choroidal vessels, which were formerly on the dorsal surface of the neural tube, become entrapped in the velum interpositum between the cerebral hemispheres and the thalamus. Although these vessels appear centrally situated, they do not course through brain tissue.

Although the ventricular system may seem to be deep within the brain, it is only separated from the SAS by a thin membrane in several places, specifically at the choroidal fissures of the lateral ventricles, at the lamina terminalis and roof of the third ventricle, and at the superior and inferior medullary vela of the fourth ventricle. Except for the superior medullary velum and lamina terminalis, which have no associated choroid plexus, these membranes provide easy access for vessels supplying the choroid plexuses. Despite the proximity of ventricular cavity to SAS, the only direct communications between the intraventricular and subarachnoid CSF are the foramina of the fourth ventricle.

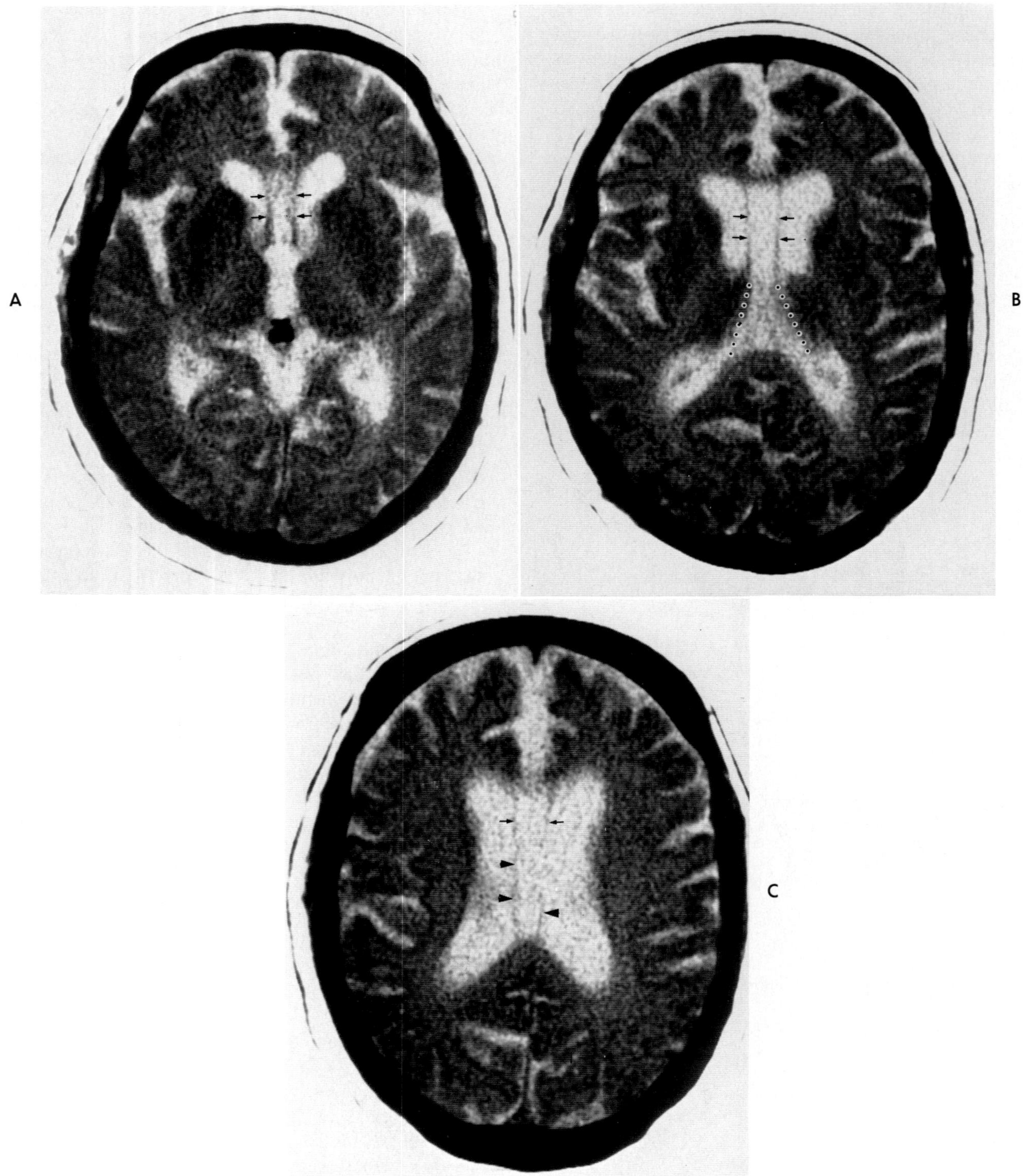

Figure 12-3 **A** to **C**, Serial axial CT scans, photographed with video reversal of the contrast settings. The triangular-shaped cavum velum interpositum, which is located below the velum interpositum, is outlined by dotted lines in **B.** The cavum septum pellucidum persists between the walls of the septum pellucidum (*arrows*). Note that this CSF-filled space extends posteriorly only to the level of the foramen of Monro. This space continues posterosuperiorly as the cavum vergae between the medial walls of the lateral ventricles (*arrowheads*).

In the formation of the SAS, the patency of the fourth ventricular outlet foramina is crucial. Initially, a sheet of *mesenchyme* covers the brain surface. This sheet has an outer layer, which develops into the *dura mater* and *cranium,* and an inner layer, which forms the *arachnoid* and *pia mater.* At 3 months' gestational age, the two lateral and single midline outlet foramina of the fourth ventricle become patent, allowing the CSF to escape and seep into the endomeninx, dissecting this inner membrane into two layers, which become the arachnoid and the pia mater. The dissection is incomplete, leaving strands, the trabeculae, which bridge between the two layers. Formation of the SAS begins around the fourth ventricle, but the process of dissection eventually extends to cover the entire CNS.

In most areas, only a thin collection of CSF exists between the pial and arachnoid layers. In some areas, however, a large CSF space is present between the surface pia and the bridging arachnoid membrane. These spaces are the cisterns and fissures, which are categorized in Box 12-1.

BOX 12-1

*Subarachnoid Cisterns and Fissures**

A. Ventral spaces
   1. Median (unpaired)
      a. Medullary cistern (caudally)
      b. Pontine cistern
      c. Interpeduncular cistern
      d. Suprasellar (chiasmatic) cistern (rostrally)
   2. Paramedian (paired)
      a. Cerebellopontine angle cisterns
      b. Crural cisterns
      c. Sylvian fissures
B. Dorsal spaces
   1. Median (unpaired)
      a. Superior cerebellar cistern
      b. Quadrigeminal cistern (cistern of great vein of Galen)
      c. Callosal sulcus
   2. Paramedian (paired)
      a. Wings of ambient cisterns (retropulvinar cisterns)
      b. Interhemispheric fissures
C. Vertical spaces
   1. Median (unpaired)
      a. Cistern of lamina terminalis (rostrally)
      b. Cisterna magna (caudally)
   2. Paramedian (paired)
      a. Ambient cisterns (around midbrain)
      b. Choroidal fissures (medial wall: midbrain and thalamus; lateral wall: temporal and atrial portions of lateral ventricles)

Adapted from Wilson ME: *The anatomic foundation of neuroradiology of the brain,* Boston, 1972, Little, Brown.

*Excludes calcarine, collateral, hippocampal, and parietooccipital fissures (see Chapter 11).

NORMAL ANATOMY

Dural Compartments

The outermost fibrous covering of the brain is the *dura.* This layer forms the periosteum of the bone and the walls of the venous sinuses. Folds of dura extend into the cranial cavity to provide support for the brain. These folds divide the CSF spaces into compartments and create pockets of CSF.

The largest dural fold is the *falx,* which divides the interhemispheric fissure into a right and a left half. This CSF space is extremely narrow in normal subjects less than 30 years of age. However, the anterior aspect of the interhemispheric fissure dilates with advancing age. This aspect can be clearly demonstrated by axial scans after age 30.[13] The posterior interhemispheric space is unique because it rarely becomes enlarged with advancing age. These features have clinical significance because acute collections of subarachnoid blood in the interhemispheric fissure of adults result in a linear hyperdense region on CT that is confined to the *anterior* portion of this SAS. Acute collections of blood in the subdural space (between the dura of the falx and the arachnoid membrane) widen the normally narrow *posterior* aspect of the interhemispheric fissure.[14]

The second largest dural fold, the *tentorium,* forms the roof of the posterior fossa and creates the infratentorial and supratentorial compartments. The infolding of a pocket of dura around the rootlets of cranial nerve V creates a CSF-filled space within the cavernous sinus that has been termed *Meckel's cave* (see Chapter 18) (Figure 12-4).

Cavum Septum Pellucidum and Cavum Vergae

In most adults the *septum pellucidum* is identified as a thin, straight membrane that separates the frontal horns of the lateral ventricles. In patients with minimum asymmetry of the frontal horns, the septum pellucidum may be tilted 1 to 2 mm to the side opposite the larger frontal horn.[15] If the tilt is curved instead of rectilinear, an intraventricular lesion should be sought.

In some normal subjects, a vertical CSF-filled cleft is found between the two leaves of the septum pellucidum (see Figure 12-3). This has been named the *cavum septum pellucidum.* It is always present in the neonatal brain (see Chapter 1) and is bounded posteroinferiorly by the fornix and anteroinferiorly by the genu and rostrum of the corpus callosum and the anterior commissure. The cavum septum pellucidum does not extend beyond the interventricular foramina. It communicates only with the lateral ventricles.[16] In almost 98% of brains imaged in vivo, this cavum is obliterated during the first few months after birth by the rapid growth of the hippocampus and the corpus callosum. (The cavum septum pellucidum can be seen in 15% to 20% of brains at autopsy when in vivo pressure from the adjacent lateral ventricles is no longer present.) This CSF collection is considered abnormal if it has a width greater than 1 cm and if the lateral walls are convex rather than parallel.[16]

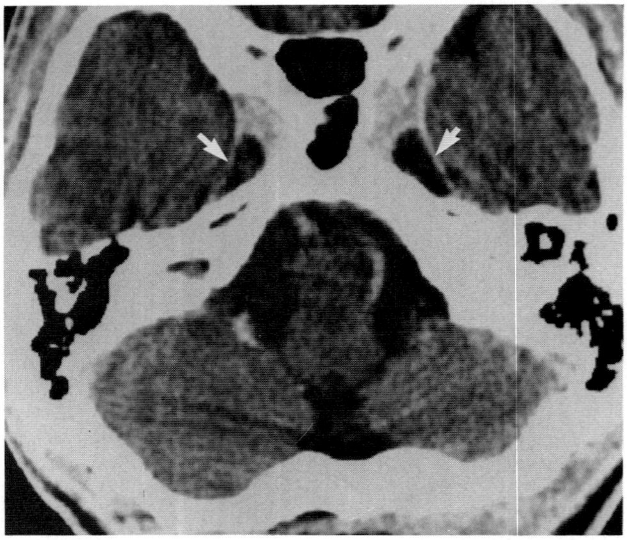

Figure 12-4 Axial CT scan after the intravenous administration of contrast material. Arrows mark the large CSF spaces (Meckel's caves) within the enhanced cavernous sinuses. This dural compartment contains the rootlets of cranial nerve V.

Only recently has the importance of the septum pellucidum been understood. It serves as an important relay station for fibers that connect the hippocampus and the hypothalamus. The septum pellucidum is linked with the hippocampus by precommissural fornix fibers. It is also connected to the preoptic and hypothalamic nuclei by the median forebrain bundle of Broca, which also connects the limbic system with the olfactory system and the amygdaloid nuclei by way of the striae terminalis. In addition, the septum pellucidum connects the habenular nucleus of the thalamus and colliculi by way of the striae medullaris and the midbrain by its connection with the anterior fornix. This septum has a connection with the infracallosal, precommissural, primordial hippocampi through the paraterminal body[16] (Figure 12-5).

In the fetus the cavum septum pellucidum is continuous caudally with a CSF-filled space found *above* the fornical or hippocampal commissure between the diverging medial walls of the lateral ventricles. This posterior space has been named the *cavum vergae*. It is obliterated in 70% of newborn infant brains studied in an autopsy series. The persistence of a CSF-filled cavum septum pellucidum and a cavum vergae was found in 3% of children aged 1 to 14 years old who had CT scans for convulsive, developmental, or neurologic syndromes[16] (see Figure 12-3). Since this space closes in a caudal to rostral direction, an *isolated* cavum vergae is extremely rare and probably represents an abnormal pattern of development of the fornix and splenium of the corpus callosum.[16]

The cavum vergae should not be confused with the cavum velum interpositum, which is a triangular CSF-filled cisternal space present *below* the fornical or hippocampal commissures in all brains (Figures 12-3; 12-5, *A;* and 12-6). Although both these CSF spaces are found above the third ventricle, the cavum velum interpositum merges with the CSF space of the quadrigeminal plate cistern and does *not* extend into the septum pellucidum.

Ventricular System

The following discussion provides an overview of the cerebral structures adjacent to the CSF spaces. It is designed to help the reader to select quickly the anatomic terms with which to describe a periventricular lesion(s) and to identify correctly the vessels that supply the choroid plexuses. The location of the largest of the choroidal vessels is shown in Chapter 13 on axial CT sections.

Lateral Ventricles and Choroidal Fissure

PERIVENTRICULAR ANATOMY. The boundaries of the lateral ventricles are formed by the thalami, caudate nuclei, fornices, and corpus callosum. As described in the section on developmental anatomy, the growth of the cerebral hemispheres folds these structures around the paired thalami. This accounts for the curved shape of the lateral ventricles, which are flanked inferomedially by the fornices and laterally by the caudate nuclei. The corpus callosum sits on top of the bodies of the lateral ventricles but dips down between their anterior and posterior horns.

The superior surface of the *thalamus* provides a floor for the body of the lateral ventricle. The anterior margin of the thalamus is marked by the foramen of Monro, which connects the floor of the lateral ventricle with the anterosuperior aspect of the third ventricle. The frontal horn of the lateral ventricle extends anteriorly beyond the thalamus.

Unlike other structures, the caudate nucleus and ventricle always remain in contact. The *caudate nucleus* lies adjacent to the inner curve of the lateral ventricle. Thus this nucleus occupies a position inferolateral to the body of the ventricle, anterolateral to the atrium, and superolateral to the temporal horn as they both curve around the thalamus.

The *corpus callosum* is often thought of in terms of its appearance on the medial surface of a bisected brain. However, one must remember that its fiber tracts course transverse to, not parallel with, the long axis of the lateral ventricle. Therefore the corpus callosum provides the roof over the entire suprathalamic portions of both lateral ventricles. In addition, its genu and rostrum, curving around the rostral end of each ventricle, provide the anterior and inferior walls of the most anterior portions of the frontal horns.

Extending down from the corpus callosum is the *septum pellucidum,* which forms the medial walls of the contiguous lateral ventricles, extending from the anterior horns almost as far posteriorly as the atria. Anterior to the thala-

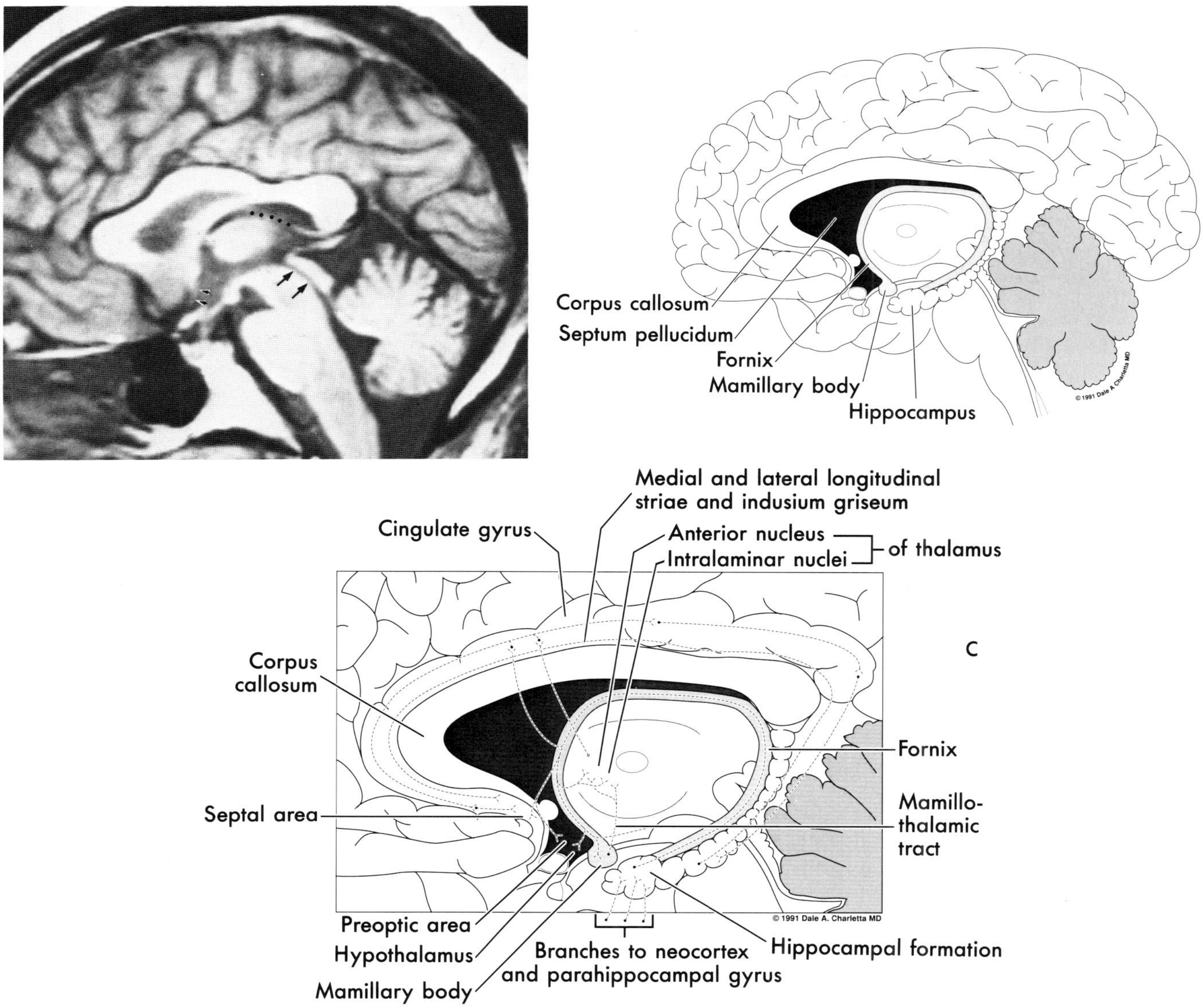

Figure 12-5 **A,** Sagittal MR image (TR/TE, 700/20) shows the anterior wall of the third ventricle (the lamina terminalis, *arrowheads*), the cavum velum interpositum (located above the roof of the third ventricle, *black dotted line*), and the aqueduct (*black arrows*). **B,** Schematic diagram of sagittal brain section shows these anatomic relationships. **C,** Fiber tracts within the septum pellucidum. (**B** and **C** reproduced with permission from Sarwar M: AJNR 10:989-1005, 1989.)

mus, this membranous sheet extends between the body and rostrum of the corpus callosum. At the level of the foramen of Monro, the rostrum ends and the fornix takes over as the inferior boundary of the septum pellucidum (Figure 12-5, *A*).

Each anterior pillar of the *fornix* passes superiorly and medially from the hypothalamus to form the anteromedial boundary of the foramen of Monro. Each fornix continues superiorly and then posteriorly and laterally above its thalamus, from which it is separated by the choroidal fissure. As the height of the septum pellucidum decreases, each fornix approaches the corpus callosum and eventually blends into the medial aspect of the cerebrum as it curves around the thalamus. As with the caudate nuclei, the fornices abut the inner curves of the lateral ventricles so that, above the thalami, they run along the inferomedial aspects of the ventricles. However, each fornix continues (as the fimbria of the hippocampus) along the superomedial aspect of the temporal horn.

Along the entire course of the choroidal fissure, the SAS is separated from the temporal horn of the lateral ventricle by only a very thin membrane. The invaginated portion of this membrane is the choroid plexus.

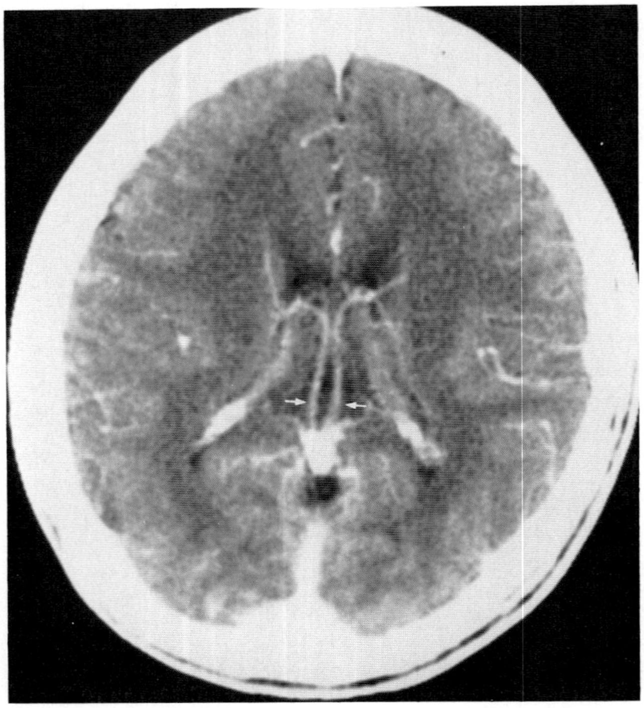

Figure 12-6 Axial, contrast-enhanced CT image of brain shows cavum velum interpositum containing the paired internal cerebral veins (*arrows*).

VASCULATURE AND CHOROID PLEXUS. Vessels frequently seen at angiography that provide information about the lateral ventricles include the anterior choroidal and posterior choroidal arteries and the septal, thalamostriate, and other subependymal veins. All the choroidal vessels travel in a narrow CSF cleft that is formed when the cerebral hemispheres grow over and around the thalami and midbrain (see Figure 12-1). The superior portion of this space is the *cavum velum interpositum*. It contains the internal cerebral veins and their tributaries, as well as the medial branch of the posterior choroidal artery (see Figures 12-3, 12-5, and 12-6). The anterolateral extension of this cleft has been named the *choroidal fissure*. It is lined laterally by the pia mater on the surface of the limbic lobe and medially by the pial lining of the thalamus and midbrain. These layers unite laterally to form the *choroid plexus,* which extends anteriorly into the medial tip of the temporal horn. The CSF in the choroidal fissure communicates with the ambient (circummesencephalic) cistern posteriorly. The choroidal fissure contains the anterior and posterior lateral choroidal arteries and tributaries of the basal vein of Galen.

The *anterior choroidal artery* arises from the internal carotid artery just distal to the origin of the posterior communicating artery. The anterior choroidal artery dips into the choroidal fissure of the temporal horn and atrium; accordingly, it reflects the position of the inner curve of the temporal horn of the lateral ventricle (Figure 12-7). The *lateral posterior choroidal artery* has anterior and posterior branches that supplement the anterior choroidal artery's blood supply to the choroid plexus of the temporal horn, atrium, and posterior portion of the body of the lateral ventricle. The lateral posterior choroidal artery, which is usually identifiable at angiography, arises from the posterior cerebral artery in the ambient cistern, enters the choroidal fissure, and ascends in the ventricle around the pulvinar of the thalamus in a smooth arc (Figure 12-7).

The *subependymal veins,* which receive blood from the caudate nucleus and central white matter, consist of two major groups: those that outline the *lateral* wall and floor of the body and atrium and those that outline the *medial* wall and roof (i.e., septum and corpus callosum). These vessels, which are relatively numerous and much more intimately related to the walls of the lateral ventricles than are the arterial markers, are the most sensitive angiographic indicators of ventricular size and configuration (Figure 12-8).

The principal vein of the lateral group is the *thalamostriate,* which originates in the atrium. The thalamostriate runs anteriorly along the inferolateral wall of the ventricle between the caudate nucleus and the thalamus, then passes inferiorly and medially across the ventricular floor to go through the foramen of Monro deep to the choroid plexus. Its course reverses at this point (the venous angle) as the thalamostriate converges with the septal vein to become the internal cerebral vein (Figure 12-8).

Other veins in the lateral group include the *anterior caudate* and the *long caudate,* which drain the caudate nucleus and more rostral white matter before joining the thalamostriate vein (Figure 12-8). Veins that run along the lateral wall of the atrium include the *lateral atrial vein* (which drains into the basal vein of Rosenthal), the thalamostriate vein (which usually drains into the internal cerebral vein), and the *inferior ventricular vein* (which continues along the superior wall of the temporal horn and eventually drains into the basal vein). Drainage of this area may also occur via the hippocampal venous complex (Figure 12-8).

The medial group of subependymal veins includes the *posterior septal veins,* which run along the inferior surface of the corpus callosum before passing down the septum to join the internal cerebral vein (Figure 12-8). The septal vein itself originates in the anteromedial wall of the anterior horn, where it drains the genu of the corpus callosum and frontal polar white matter (Figure 12-8). The septal vein runs first posteromedially to enter the inferior portion of the septum pellucidum and then directly posteriorly in the septum to the fornix. The septal vein passes lateral to the fornix at the foramen of Monro to the internal cerebral vein, usually anteriorly.

The *medial atrial veins* course along the roof and medial wall of the atrium and occipital horn and then penetrate the

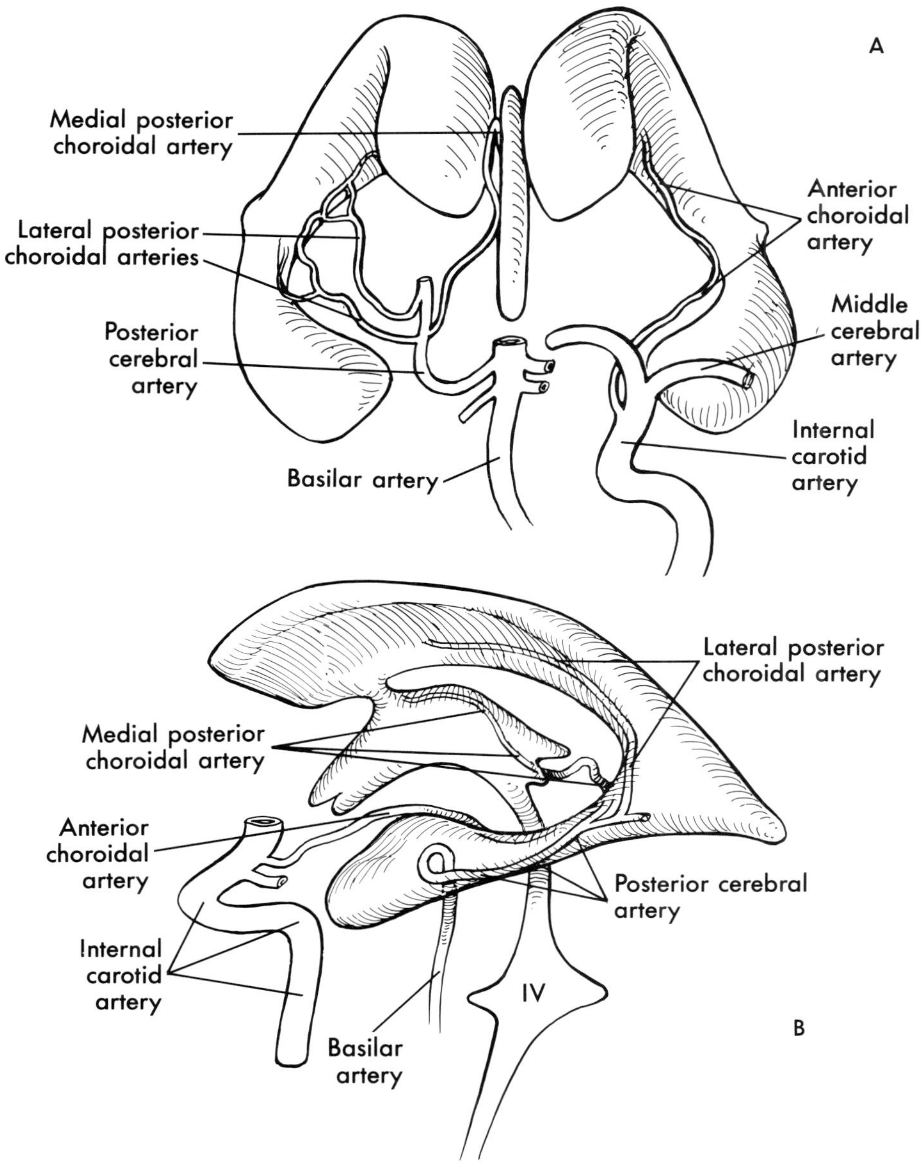

Figure 12-7 Schematic illustration of ventricles and choroidal arteries in anteroposterior **(A)** and lateral **(B)** projections.

posterior crus of the fornix as they leave the ventricle to join the internal cerebral vein or great vein of Galen (Figure 12-8). Veins draining the medial aspect of the temporal horn are seldom seen.

Third Ventricle

PERIVENTRICULAR ANATOMY. The third ventricle is a single midline cavity. It communicates with each lateral ventricle through one of the paired foramina of Monro, which are located in the anterior roof of the third ventricle. Rostrally, the third ventricle is bounded by the anterior commissure and lamina terminalis, these being the attenuated continuation of the corpus callosum inferior to the rostrum. Continuing inferiorly, one encounters the *optic recess,* which is a beaklike projection of the third ventricle anterosuperior to the optic chiasm. The *infundibular recess* is located immediately posteroinferior to the optic chiasm and extends down into the hypophyseal infundibulum. The remainder of the floor of the third ventricle is formed by the hypothalamus anteriorly and the subthalamus posteriorly.

The roof of the third ventricle consists only of the very thin tela choroidea, tela caverna, and velum interpositum, the folded-over layer of primitive mesenchyme that formed as a result of the posterior growth of the cerebral hemispheres over and above the diencephalon. At the roof of the third ventricle posteriorly, a projection, the *suprapi-*

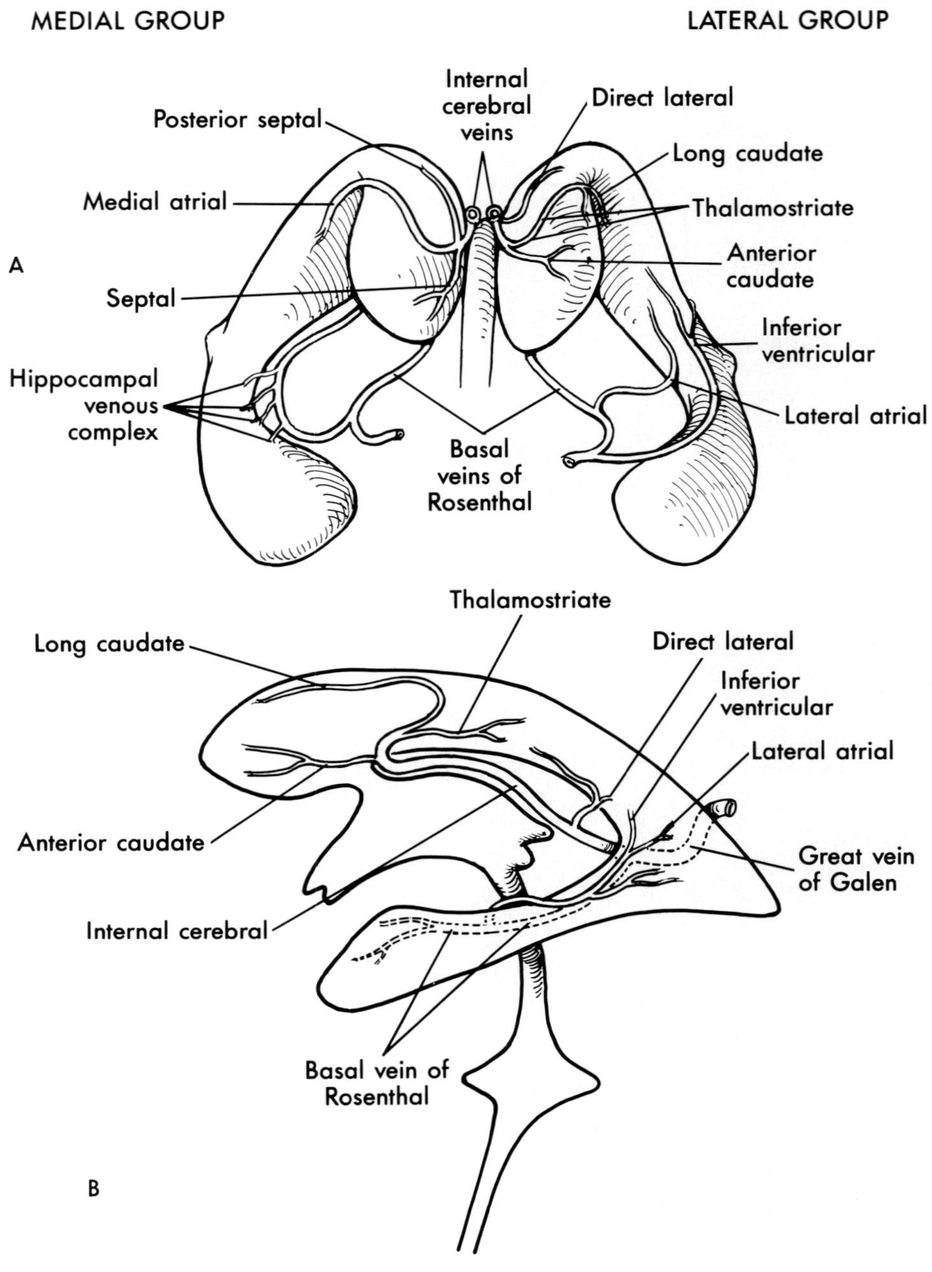

Figure 12-8 Schematic illustration of ventricles and choroidal veins in anteroposterior **(A)** and lateral **(B** and **C)** projections. Note that the veins are divided into lateral (**B**) and medial (**C**) groups.

neal recess, lies below the splenium of the corpus callosum and above the pineal gland. Inferior to this recess is the habenular commissure. The next more inferior structure is the pineal recess of the third ventricle, followed by the posterior commissure and finally the cerebral aqueduct. The lateral boundaries of the third ventricle are the hypothalamus anteriorly and inferiorly and the thalamus posteriorly and superiorly.

Because the lamina terminalis and velum interpositum are such delicate structures, the anterior, superior, and posterior limits of the third ventricle are seldom identifiable on CT but can be seen on sagittal MRI (see Figure 12-5).

VASCULATURE AND CHOROID PLEXUS. Angiography is another method for assessing (although indirectly) the position of the roof of the third ventricle. Vascular structures that can serve as reference markers of the third ventricular roof include the medial posterior choroidal artery and the

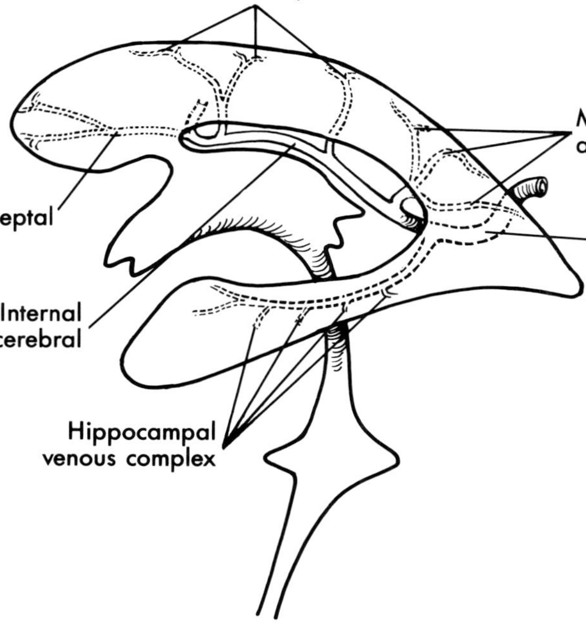

Figure 12-8, cont'd. For legend see opposite page.

internal cerebral vein. The *medial posterior choroidal artery* (see Figure 12-7) arises from the posterior cerebral artery and courses posterosuperiorly around the midbrain to the quadrigeminal cistern. On a lateral arteriogram, this choroidal artery resembles a "3," the center point reflecting proximity to the pineal gland as the artery passes lateral to that structure. This artery continues between the layers of the velum interpositum in the roof of the third ventricle to supply the choroid plexus.

The paired *internal cerebral veins* also lie in the roof of the third ventricle near midline. Each is formed from the confluence of the ipsilateral thalamostriate and septal veins. The internal cerebral veins pass posteriorly through the quadrigeminal cistern, where they empty into the great vein of Galen.

Invaginated into the roof of the third ventricle from the tela is the *choroid plexus* of the third ventricle. This plexus is continuous anteriorly through the foramen of Monro with the choroid plexuses along the floors of the lateral ventricles (see Figure 12-8). The choroid plexus extends posteriorly to terminate in the suprapineal recess of the third ventricle.

Cerebral Aqueduct

The aqueduct arises from the posteroinferior region of the third ventricle and courses inferiorly through the midbrain to the superior recess of the fourth ventricle. In the midbrain the aqueduct is located between the tegmentum ventrally and the tectum or roof (which includes the colliculi) posteriorly. Although not consistently seen on CT scans, the aqueduct is invariably visible on both axial and midline sagittal MRI (Figure 12-9). The MR signal intensity of the aqueduct on short TR/TE images is identical to that of the CSF. On long TR/TE images the signal intensity becomes hypointense compared with the ventricular CSF. This may be the result of CSF pulsations in the aqueduct. This phenomenon can be seen at other points of narrowing in the CSF pathways where flow velocity is greatest. It has been termed the *flow-void sign*.[4-8] It has recently been demonstrated that this sign is unreliable if the patient has a fresh, intraventricular hemorrhage. Fresh blood can mimic the hypointense signal in the aqueduct.[17]

Absence of the flow-void sign may indicate obstructive hydrocephalus, but the flow void in the aqueduct is absent on MR scan sequences that employ techniques that eliminate flow artifacts. These methods are called *flow compensation* or *gradient motion rephasing* (GMR).

A zone of increased signal intensity can sometimes be seen around the aqueduct on these long TR/TE images in normal patients. This does not represent periaqueductal CSF absorption, although the actual cause of the increased signal is unknown (Figure 12-9).[18]

Fourth Ventricle

PERIVENTRICULAR ANATOMY. The floor of the fourth ventricle has a diamond shape, the most rostral point of which narrows to the cerebral aqueduct. The two lateral recesses curve anteriorly around the upper medulla and communicate via the foramina of Luschka with the ventral subarachnoid space. The midline foramen of Magendie repre-

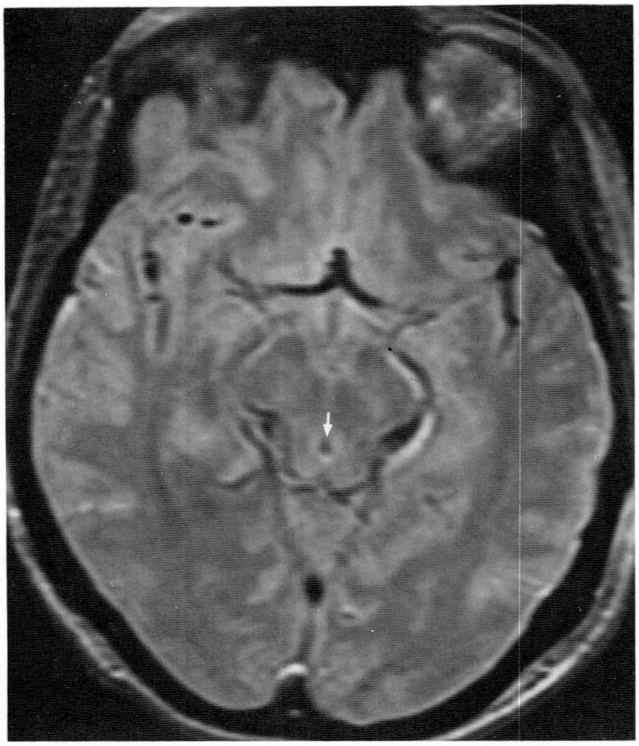

Figure 12-9 Axial MR image (TR/TE, 4000/80) shows flow void in the aqueduct (*arrow*). Note the normally increased signal in the zone surrounding the aqueduct.

sents the most caudal point of the diamond. CSF exiting from this foramen passes between the cerebellar tonsils in a space known as the *vallecula* to flow into the cisterna magna. Ventral to the fourth ventricle is the tegmentum of the pons and medulla. The roof of the ventricle has a pyramidal configuration because of the convergence of its superior, inferior, and lateral walls. The superior and inferior walls are the superior and inferior medullary vela, respectively. The very apex of the pyramid, however, is indented by the vermis of the cerebellum. This divides the pyramid into two apices, resembling little ears, side by side. The superior, middle, and inferior cerebellar peduncles form the lateral walls.

VASCULATURE AND CHOROID PLEXUS. The choroid plexus of the fourth ventricle is not continuous with that of the third ventricle. The plexus is actually a paired structure with two basic components. A paramedian *medial limb* parallels the long axis of the brainstem and lies against the lateral surface of the vermis. This limb joins a horizontal *lateral limb* that lies in the lateral recess of the ventricle. The two parts were found to be symmetric in 96.5% of 57 brain dissections.[19]

The plexus can be demonstrated by an anatomic dissection in which the ventricular chamber is viewed from below to show the exit of the medial limbs through the foramen of Magendie and of the lateral limbs through the foramina of Luschka (Figure 12-10). The bulbous terminal expansions of the lateral limbs (i.e., the *cornucopiae*) at the foramina of Luschka are particularly well demonstrated in this view. The cornucopiae mark the anterior surface of each cerebellar hemisphere at the level of the seventh and eighth cranial nerve roots. In this dissection the superior aspects of the medial limbs are hidden within the depths of the superior recesses of the fourth ventricle. The appearance of the choroid plexus on axial scans is shown in Figure 12-11.

The vessels that supply the plexus are small and difficult to visualize on angiograms. The medial portion of the plexus is supplied by the posterior inferior cerebellar artery. The lateral component has a variable contribution from the basilar, the anterior inferior cerebellar, and/or the posterior inferior cerebellar arteries.[20] The veins of the plexus enter the vein of the lateral recess of the fourth ventricle. This vein is found in the posterolateral fissure, which is parallel to, below, and behind the lateral recess of the fourth ventricle.

MR scans routinely demonstrate the fourth ventricle. If MRI is unavailable, CT scans after intravenous contrast injection can be used for visualizing the choroid plexus to identify significant small distortions or displacements of the fourth ventricle by adjacent masses (see Chapter 15).[21]

Cisterns, Fissures, and Sulci

The SAS is continuous around the brain and spinal cord and is filled with CSF. Irregular pockets and focal enlargements reflect that the pia on one side of the SAS adheres closely to the brain surface, whereas the arachnoid and dura on the other side adhere to the skull. For convenience, the cisterns are named according to the brain structures on which they abut, but they all communicate with each other across arbitrary boundaries. The cisterns and the cerebral gyri that form the boundaries of the hemispheric sulci are labeled in Chapter 11. Box 12-1 categorizes these cisterns by their location (i.e., ventral, dorsal, or vertical).

The major cerebral fissures are formed during the midtrimester of fetal life. These have relatively constant positions on the surface of the hemisphere and extend deeply into the brain. Only a few of the secondary fissures and sulci are even approximately constant in form and position in all brains.[22] However, a working knowledge of these landmarks is needed clinically, since they can be used to locate the cortical regions that usually mediate speech, motor, sensory, and visual function. Sparing of these regions is critical when planning radiation therapy or surgery. The fissures and gyri that form these cortical boundaries are illustrated schematically in Chapter 11.

The surface anatomy of the hemisphere, as seen on axial CT scans, is difficult to interpret because the relative anterior or posterior position of a given sulcus depends on de-

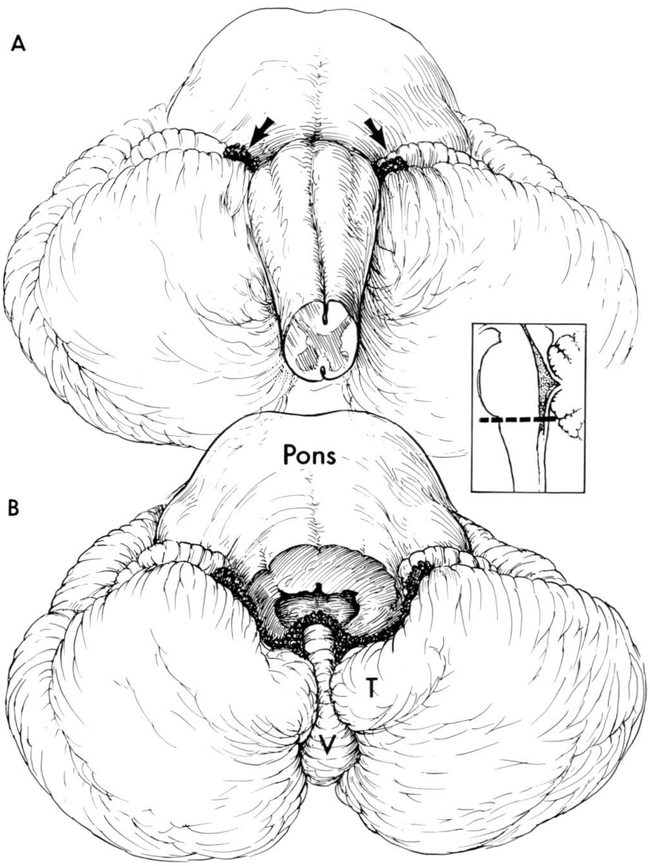

Figure 12-10 **A,** Ventral aspect of brainstem and cerebellum seen from below. Seventh and eighth cranial nerves removed bilaterally to uncover bulbous cornucopiae of choroid plexuses (*arrows*), which protrude from foramina of Luschka to cerebellopontine angle cisterns. **B,** Same specimen after removal of medulla oblongata. Inferior aspects of medial components of choroid plexuses on either side of vermis (V). Horizontal limbs of plexuses in lateral recesses terminate at cornucopiae. Superior extensions of medial limbs disappear in upper end of transected fourth ventricular lumen. T, Tonsil. (Reproduced with permission from Hayman LA, Evans RA, Hinck VC: AJR 133:285-288, 1979.)

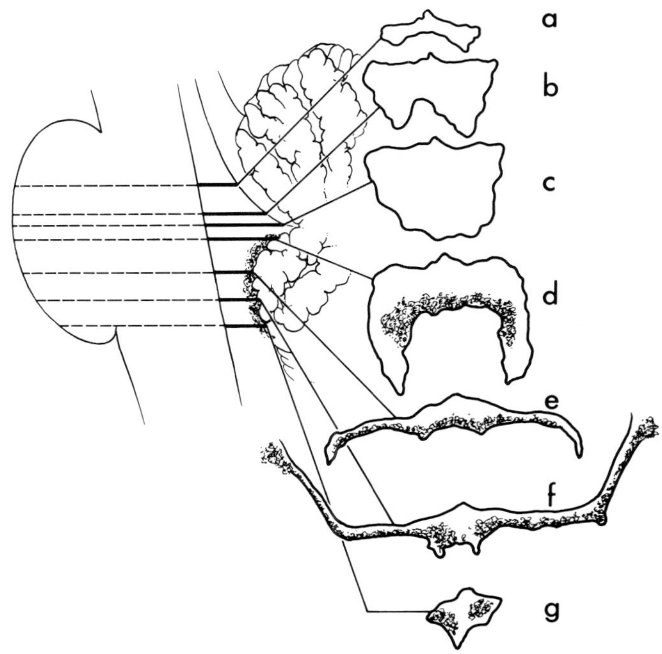

Figure 12-11 Serial axial sections of the fourth ventricle illustrate the extremely different configurations present at each level. The choroid plexus is shown in the posteroinferior wall of the ventricle in levels *d* to *g*. (Reproduced with permission from Hayman LA, Evans RA, Hinck VC: AJR 133:285-288, 1979.)

gree of head flexion or extension. To a lesser extent, this difficulty is also noted on axial MR scans. One can identify reliably the *superior precentral* and *superior postcentral gyri,* which control the motor and sensory functions of the lower half of the body, respectively. This is possible because in 92% of hemispheres examined with axial scans, the superior frontal sulcus joins the superior precentral sulcus to form a *wedge*. The superior precentral gyrus can be located behind this wedge, and the superior postcentral gyrus can be identified immediately behind the precentral gyrus (Figure 12-12).[23] When masses that distort and compress the cerebral sulci are present at the convexity, the pattern of the white matter between the gyri can serve as a useful guide.[24]

Localizing the inferior extent of these important gyri requires the use of sagittal MR scans.[25] A consistent anatomic pattern (described as Type I) was found in 81% of a series of 102 hemispheres.[26] Using this pattern, one can localize the motor and sensory cortices that mediate function in the face and arm (i.e., the *inferior precentral* and *inferior postcentral gyri,* respectively). One can also locate Broca's area, which governs speech (see Chapter 11). Perhaps the most reliable method of defining the motor cortex is to note that it is almost twice the thickness of the sensory cortex, a fact long known to neuroanatomists but unreported in the radiologic literature (Figure 12-12).

MRI in the sagittal plane is particularly helpful to the neurosurgeon, since it can provide a view of the hemispheric surface that corresponds to the operative field. This allows variations and distortions of gyral pattern to be studied preoperatively and functional regions tentatively to be identified in advance. One must remember, however, that the boundaries of functional areas do not *always* fall within the anatomic zones prescribed. Intraoperative electrical cortical stimulation may be needed to ensure the accuracy of preoperative topographic MR assessment.

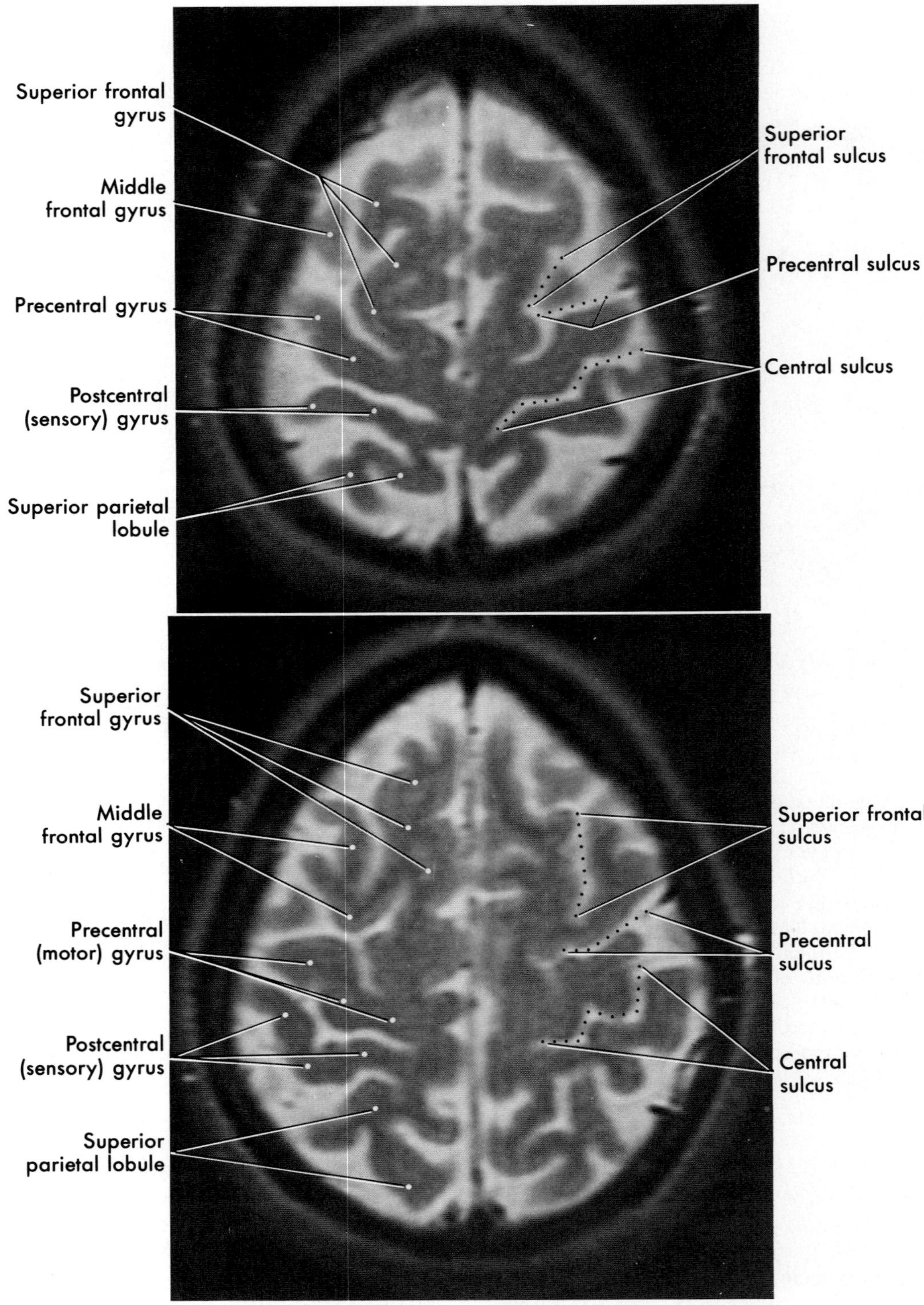

Figure 12-12 Serial axial MR images (2000/80) at the vertex show the middle frontal gyrus within the wedge formed by the frontal sulcus anteriorly and the precentral sulcus posteriorly. The precentral gyrus controls the motor functions of the opposite side of the body. The gyrus immediately posterior is the postcentral gyrus, which controls the sensory functions of the opposite side of the body. Note that the motor cortex of the precentral gyrus is almost twice the thickness of the sensory (postcentral) cortex. The central sulcus separates the precentral and postcentral gyri.

Perivascular Spaces

The CSF in the SAS is in contact with the extracellular fluid spaces within the brain.[27] These spaces communicate with each other via innumerable tiny channels that form around the cerebral arterial branches that penetrate into the brain substance (Figure 12-13) (see Chapter 11). These channels are the *Virchow-Robin perivascular spaces*. They can inadvertently be displayed on CT scans of the brain if high concentrations of intrathecal, nonionic, myelographic contrast medium reach the cerebral SAS. The diffusion of contrast agent into these channels causes uniform enhancement of the cortical brain surfaces on CT images.[28-30] However, exposure of the brain to these levels of intrathecal contrast media must be avoided, since it may cause neurotoxic side effects. Although the Virchow-Robin channels communicate with the SAS, the flow of CSF through them is relatively slow. This in turn may enhance the toxicity of contrast agents by prolonging neuronal exposure to the chemical agent. It should be noted that brain penetration of contrast media will not be identified in regions of cerebral edema, presumably because of counterpressure caused by the edema.

NORMAL AGING

Enlargement of Perivascular Spaces

Patulous (patent) perivascular spaces of Virchow-Robin (5 mm and occasionally larger) are frequently found at autopsy in otherwise normal elderly brains. These spaces typically occur in the lower one third of the basal ganglia region (i.e., the anterior perforated substance below the anterior commissure), especially in the area of the putamen and medial temporal lobes (Figure 12-14). Their appearance has variously been reported in 23% to 61% of MR scans. The incidence with which perivascular spaces are visualized appears to be age related.[31] On MR images, their signal intensity resembles that of CSF in every pulse sequence, and these spaces do not produce a mass effect on surrounding tissues. They can best be visualized in relation to the perforating arteries of the basal ganglia on coronal or sagittal images. These same perivascular spaces may also be seen in the cortical region on axial MR images (Figure 12-15). Dilated perivascular spaces can be seen in the lower midbrain along the penetrating branches of the collicular and accessory arteries. These small foci can be seen near the substantia nigra and cerebral peduncle in 20% of normal subjects if 4 mm sections are obtained (Figures 12-16 and 12-17).[32]

Occasionally, differentiation of perivascular spaces from small lacunar infarcts may be difficult. However, infarcts are most often seen in the upper or more distal reaches of the lenticulostriate vessels, where these vessels supply the basal ganglia. Also, perivascular spaces may not resemble CSF on every pulse sequence.[31,33,34]

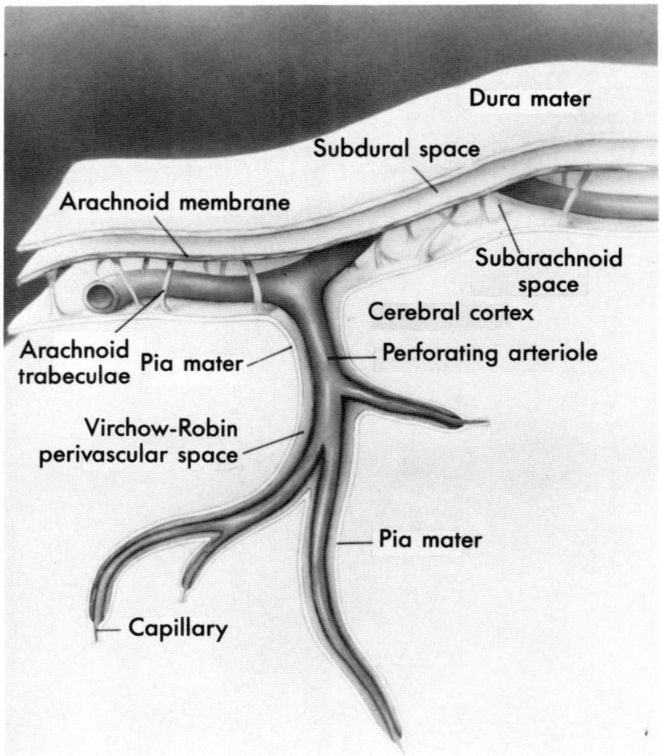

Figure 12-13 Schematic representation of one of the innumerable perivascular CSF spaces surrounding penetrating arterial branches.

Enlargement of Ventricular and Cisternal Spaces

Mild to moderate enlargement of the ventricles, cortical sulci, and pericerebellar SAS occurs as a normal aging process.[35-41] The pericerebellar (especially superior vermian) SAS also dilates in the elderly, perhaps because of gray matter atrophy or subjacent white matter loss. It has been shown that, white matter atrophies faster than gray.[42]

Neuronal loss occurs with aging in certain regions,[43-50] including the superior frontal and temporal gyri, precentral gyrus, corpus striatum, hippocampus, thalamus (especially the median nuclei), amygdaloid body, inferior olive, Purkinje cells, and dentate nucleus. Because of age-related involutionary changes in the temporal lobes, the anterior end of the circular sulcus (sylvian fissure) may become prominent in the fifth decade of life.[42] At all times of life, the left circular (sylvian) sulcus is larger than the right; this should not be taken to indicate adjacent ischemic changes.

Some investigators have shown a decrease in dendritic branching and a possible diminution in number of synapses in the temporal, frontal, and limbic lobes.[51] For further study of the histochemical and neuropathologic changes in the normally aging brain, the reader is referred to selected references.[35,45]

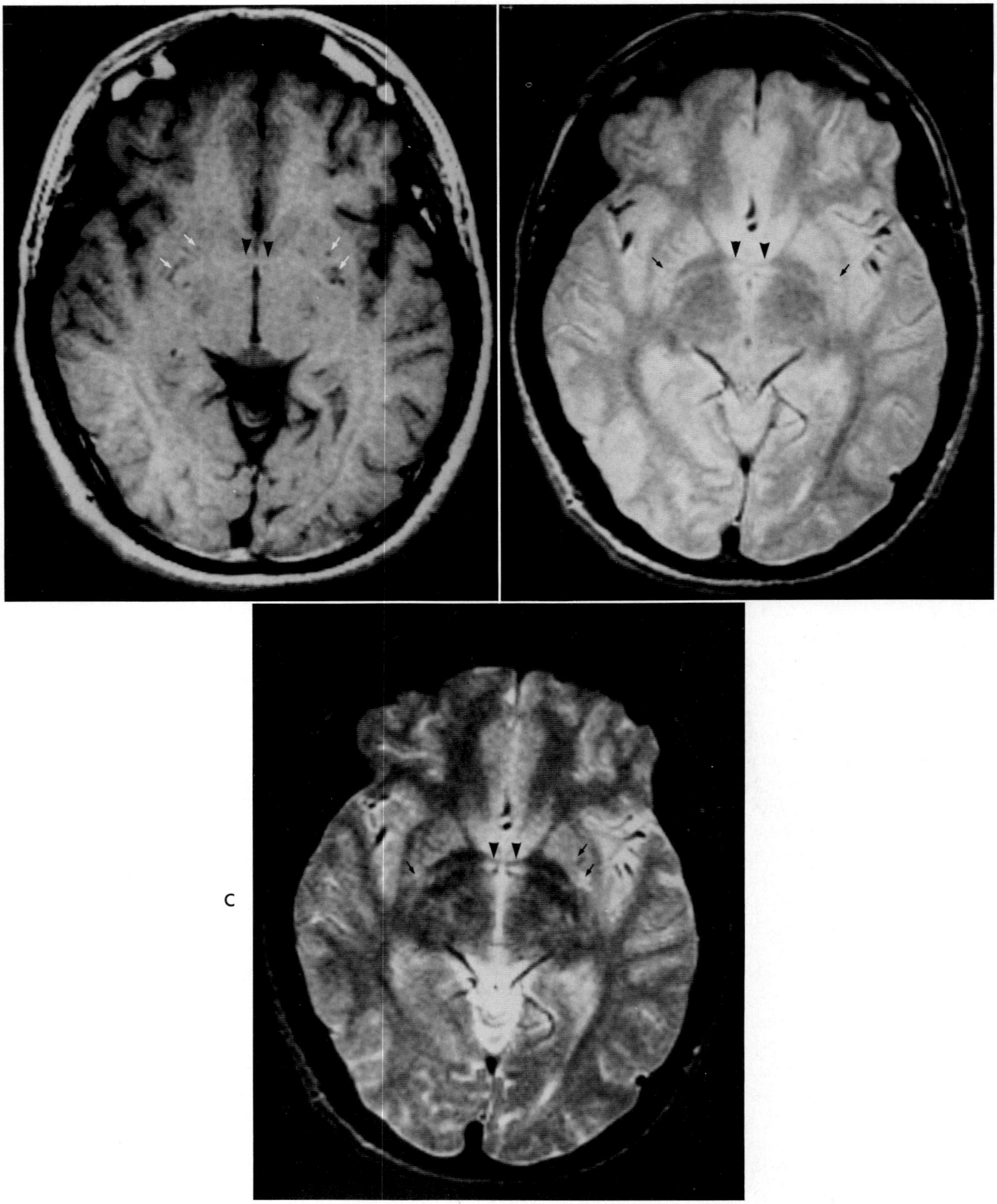

Figure 12-14 Axial MR images in a 40-year-old patient complaining of headache. **A,** TR/TE, 800/20; **B,** 2000/40; **C,** 2000/80. Arrows indicate dilated perivascular spaces in the putamen at the level of the anterior commissure (*arrowheads*). These spaces can be distinguished from lacunar infarcts and other pathologic processes because of (1) their characteristic location, (2) the absence of mass effect on surrounding tissue, and (3) the presence of a signal intensity matching that of CSF on all pulse sequences. (Courtesy Linda A. Heir, New York Hospital, Cornell Medical Center, New York.)

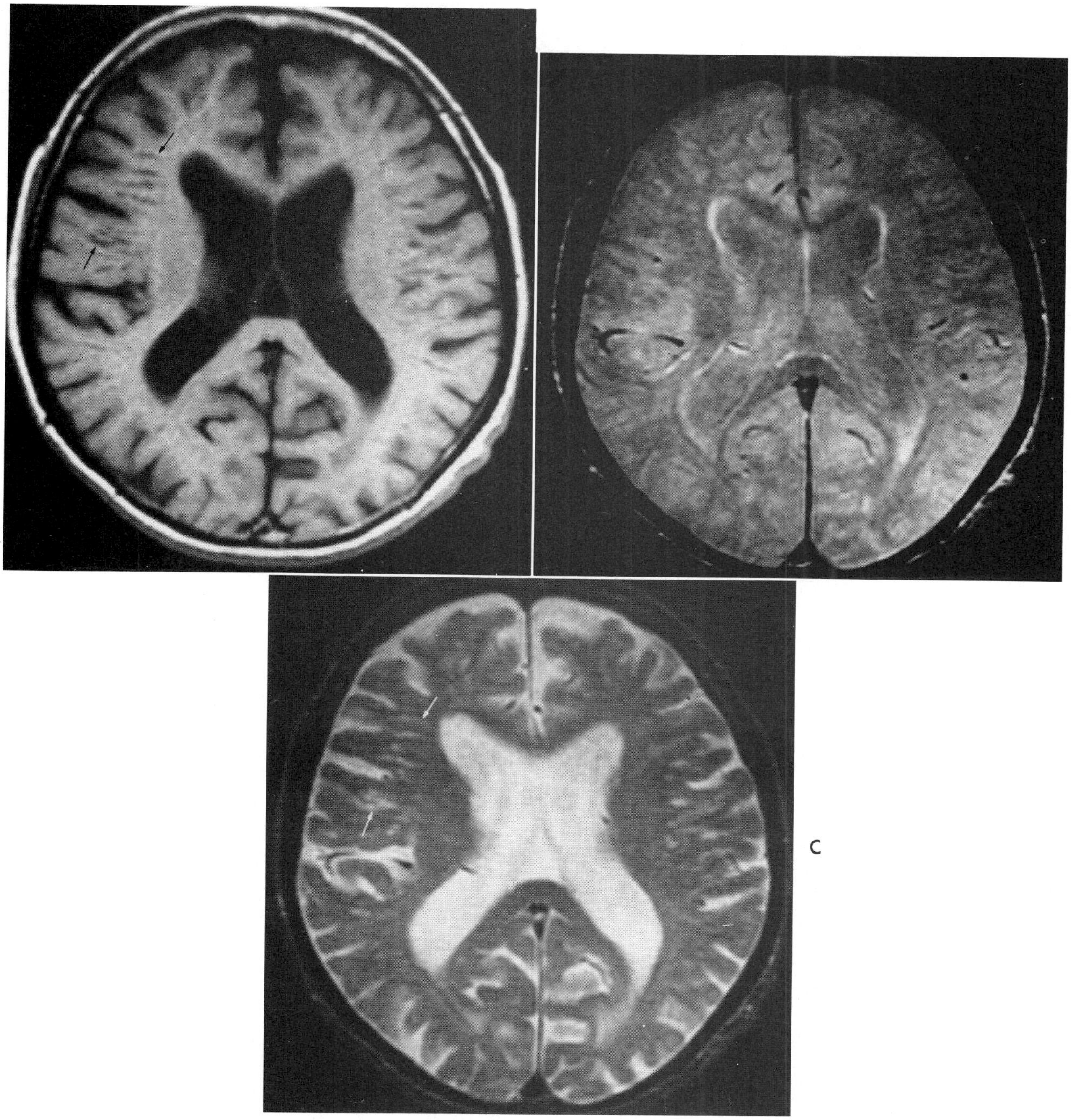

A

B

C

Figure 12-15 Axial MR images in an 83-year-old subject with vertebrobasilar ischemia. **A,** TR/TE, 800/20; **B,** 2000/40; **C,** 2000/80. Arrows indicate dilated perivascular spaces radiating medially from the cortex. Note the absence of mass effect on surrounding tissues and the presence of a signal intensity matching that of CSF on all pulse sequences. (Courtesy Linda A. Heir, New York Hospital, Cornell Medical Center, New York.)

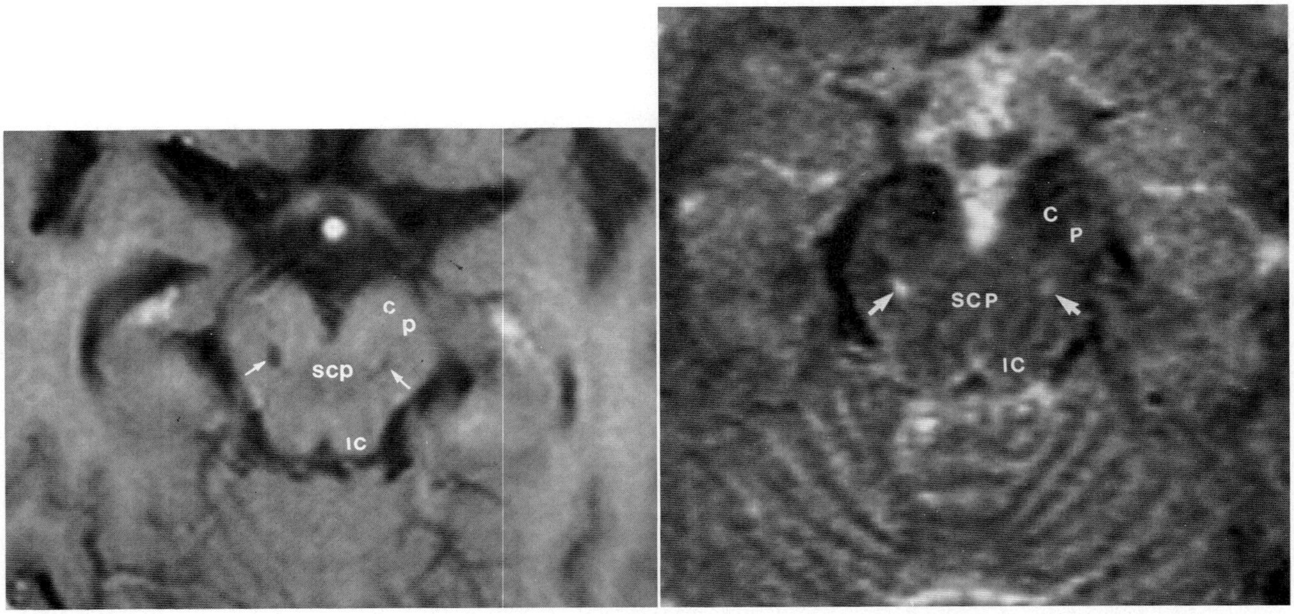

Figure 12-16 Axial MR images (**A**, 600/20, **B**, 2000/120) of the lower midbrain show the enlarged perivascular CSF spaces that surround the branches of the collicular and accessory collicular arteries (*arrows*). *cp*, Cerebral peduncle; *ic*, inferior colliculus; *scp*, superior cerebellar peduncle decussation. (Reproduced with permission from Elster AD, Richardson DN: AJNR 11:1119-1122, 1991.)

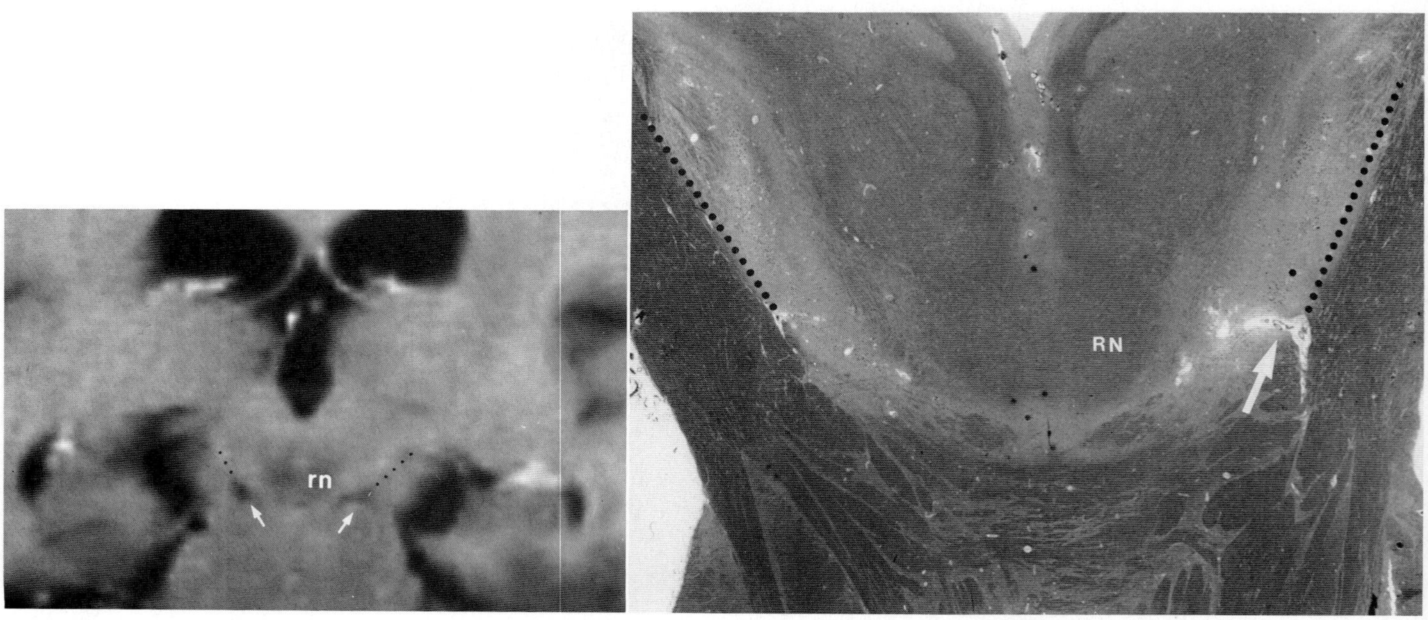

Figure 12-17 Coronal MR image (600/20) **(A)** and enlarged companion anatomic section **(B)** shows the Virchow-Robin perivascular spaces (*arrows*) between the cerebral peduncle (*immediately below dotted lines*) and the substantia nigra (*immediately above dotted lines*). RN, Red nucleus (on the reader's right). (Reproduced with permission from Elster AD, Richardson DN: AJNR 11:1119-1122, 1991.)

Numerous imaging investigations to delineate normal aging have centered around CT and MRI measurement techniques.[52] These studies have shown that the CSF/brain volume ratio is relatively constant from ages 10 to 50 years, but that variable (although progressive) CSF space enlargement occurs thereafter.[53-60] These studies have correlated well with autopsy findings of normal brain atrophy with aging.

Degeneration of Choroid Plexus and Arachnoid Granulations

Choroid Plexus

The ependymal lining of the ventricles is invaginated at specific sites by the vessels of the pia mater. These vessels and the ependymal and interstitial connective tissue form the choroid plexus. Extensive sympathetic innervation surrounds the choroidal vessels and may provide a mechanism by which the secretion of CSF can be inhibited.[3] With increasing age, microscopic *psammoma bodies* (i.e., calcification) occur in the interstitial tissue of the choroid plexus, and microcystic degeneration can be seen. Occasionally, bone is formed. The imaging features of each of these changes is described separately in the following text.

The frequency and extent of *physiologic calcification* in the choroid plexus depends on the imaging modality chosen. CT is 15 times more sensitive than skull radiographs for detecting these calcifications.[61] The incidence of choroid calcifications on CT in a series of 1000 consecutive examinations was 0.5% in the first decade and 86% in the eighth decade of life.[62] However, children with neurofibromatosis (with or without intraventricular meningioma), toxoplasmosis, tuberous sclerosis, or choroid plexus papilloma may have calcifications that can mimic these physiologic calcifications.

Physiologic calcification of the choroid plexus (except for the glomus in the lateral ventricle or in the roof of the fourth ventricle) is rarely visualized on CT (Figure 12-18).[62] Calcification of the choroid plexus in the roof of the third ventricle and in the temporal horns of the lateral ventricles has been reported. Rarely, the choroid plexus of one lateral ventricle will calcify anterior to, and sometimes instead of, the glomus of the lateral ventricle. Marked asymmetry of choroid calcification is occasionally observed, and the position of the glomera can change significantly with postural changes. Calcifications of the choroid usually appear as zones of absent signal on MR scans.

On short TR/TE MR pulse sequences, the entire choroid plexus shows a low signal intensity comparable to CSF. At 0.5 Tesla (T), the glomera in the atria of the lateral ventricles have a highly variable appearance on long TR/TE MR images. As many as 40% may show areas of hyperintense signal relative to CSF. These zones may measure from 3 to 22 mm in size (Figure 12-19). Microscopically, they appear to represent early, age-related, xanthogranulomatous degeneration (i.e., minimum lipid deposits, neuroepithelial microcysts, peripheral psammoma calcifications). Contrast-enhanced CT scans show an absence of the normal choroid enhancement in these areas, but *peripheral* flecks or clumps of calcification can be seen. Occasionally, small zones of fat density can be visualized by CT in the choroid plexus. At present, these zones are considered to have no clinical significance.[63] Serial MR scans of enlarged glomera have not shown a change in size over a 6-month follow-up period, but some authors have suggested that they may progress and coalesce to form intraventricular, neuroepithelial cysts.[64] At field strengths of 1 to 1.5 T, the glomera are isointense with the CSF and are not visualized.[65]

Arachnoid Granulations

Certain regions of the arachnoid membrane project through the dura. These projections are microscopic villi in the newborn, but they become macroscopic by 6 months of age. By age 4 years, more than 50 large granulations are present on the surface of the brain.[3] These arachnoid granulations, or *pacchionian bodies,* usually project into the main venous sinus channels of the brain and the venous lakes that parallel these sinuses. However, they may also be found projecting into extradural, intradiploic, or cerebral veins. These granulations generally occur in the parasagittal area. In adults, they can be seen as calcifications on the parasagittal surfaces of the brain (Figure 12-20). Occasionally, they can erode the inner and middle tables of the skull and cause a thinning, and rarely even an outward bulging, of the outer table of the skull.

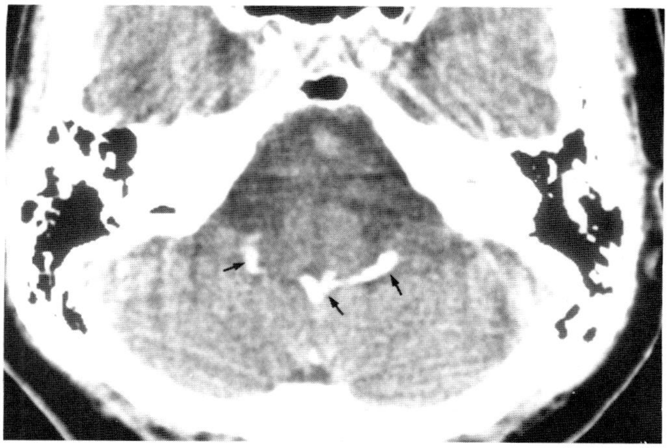

Figure 12-18 Axial CT scan shows physiologic calcification in portions of the choroid plexus of the fourth ventricle (*arrows*).

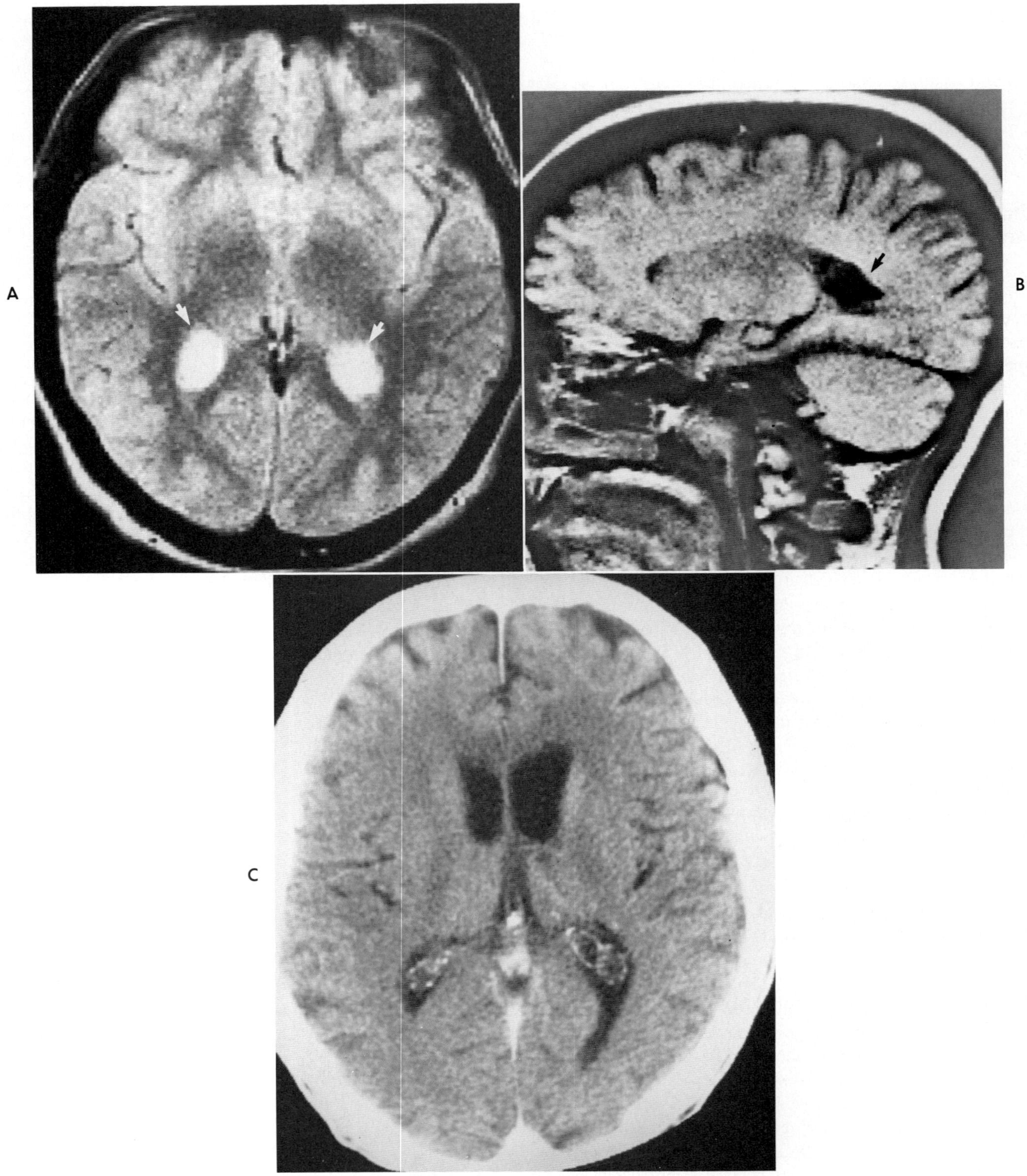

Figure 12-19 **A**, Axial MR image (1800/70) shows bilaterally bright, choroid plexus glomera (*arrows*) in the atria of the lateral ventricles that measure approximately 15 × 12 mm. **B**, Sagittal MR image (500/30) shows the expected hypointense signal in this region (*arrow*). **C**, CT scan after intravenous iodinated contrast injection shows only small peripheral zones of calcification in the choroid glomerula and subependymal veins. Note the absence of enhancement in the choroid plexus glomera. (**A** and **B** reproduced with permission from Hinshaw DB, Fahmy JL, Peckham N, et al: AJNR 9:483-486, 1988.)

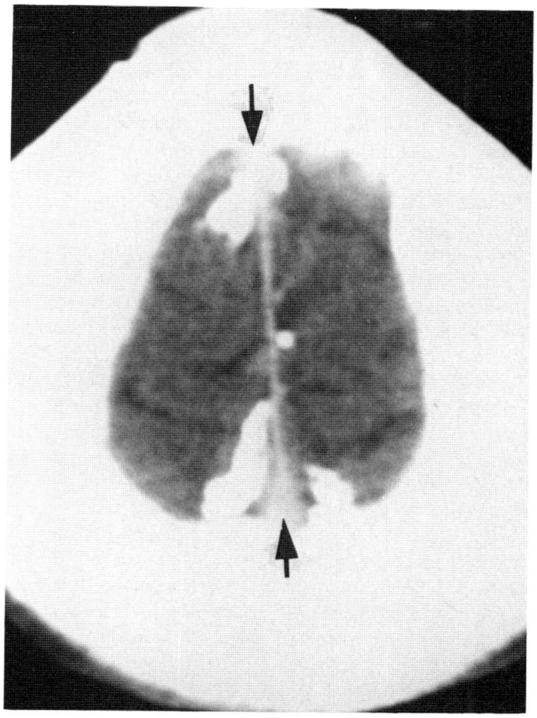

Figure 12-20 Axial contrast-enhanced CT scan at the cerebral convexity shows the characteristic calcification of the arachnoid granulations typically seen in adults adjacent to the superior sagittal sinus. Arrowheads mark the anterior and posterior portions of the contrast-enhanced superior sagittal sinus.

REFERENCES

1. Tondreau RL: Ventriculography and pneumoencephalography: contributions of Dr. Walter E. Dandy, *Radiographics* 5(4):553-555, 1985.
2. Zimmerman RD, Russel EJ, Leeds NE: Axial CT recognition of anteroposterior displacement of fourth ventricle, *AJNR* 1:65-70, 1980.
3. Fishman RA: *Cerebrospinal fluid in diseases of the nervous system,* Philadelphia, 1980, WB Saunders.
4. Sherman JL, Citrin CM: Magnetic resonance demonstration of normal CSF flow, *AJNR* 7:3-6, 1986.
5. Bradley WG, Kortman KE, Burgoyne B: Flowing cerebrospinal fluid in normal and hydrocephalic states: appearance on MR images, *Radiology* 159:611-616, 1986.
6. Bergstrand G, Bergstrom M, Nordell B, et al: Cardiac gated MR imaging of cerebrospinal fluid flow, *J Comput Assist Tomogr* 9(6):1003-1006, 1985.
7. Sherman JL, Citrin CM, Gangarosa RE, Bowen BJ: The MR appearance of CSF pulsations in the spinal canal, *AJNR* 7:879-884, 1986.
8. Sherman JL, Citrin CM, Bowen BJ, Gangarosa RE: MR demonstration of altered cerebrospinal fluid flow by obstructive lesions, *AJNR* 7:571-579, 1986.
9. Feinberg DA, Mark AS: Human brain motion and cerebrospinal fluid circulation demonstrated with MR velocity imaging, *Radiology* 163:793-799, 1987.
10. Moore KL: *The developing human: clinically oriented embryology,* ed 4, Philadelphia, 1988, WB Saunders.
11. Fitzgerald MJT: *Human embryology: a regional approach,* New York, 1978, Harper & Row.
12. Netter FH: Vol 1, *Nervous system.* Part 1, Anatomy and physiology. In Brawss A, Dingle RV, editors: *The CIBA collection of medical illustrations,* West Caldwell, NJ, 1986, CIBA.
13. Zimmerman RD, Yurberg E, Russell EJ, Leeds NE: Falx and interhemispheric fissure on axial CT. I. Normal anatomy, *AJNR* 3:175-180, 1982.
14. Zimmerman RD, Russell EJ, Yurberg E, Leeds NE: Falx and interhemispheric fissure on axial CT. II. Recognition and differentiation of interhemispheric subarachnoid and subdural hemorrhage, *AJNR* 3:635-642, 1982.
15. Shapiro R, Galloway SJ, Shapiro MC: Minimal asymmetry of the brain: a normal variant, *AJR* 147:753-756, 1986.
16. Sarwar M: The septum pellucidum: normal and abnormal, *AJNR* 10:989-1005, 1989.
17. Augustyn GT, D'Amour PG, Scott JA, Worth RM: Thrombus simulating flow void: a pitfall in diagnosing aqueductal patency by high field MR imaging, *AJNR* 8:1139-1141, 1987.
18. Lee BCP: Magnetic resonance imaging of peri-aqueductal lesions, *Clin Radiol* 38:527-533, 1987.
19. Bradac GB, Simon RS, Fiegler W, Schneider H: A radioanatomical study of the choroid plexus of the fourth ventricle, *Neuroradiology* 11:87-91, 1976.
20. Kumar AJ, Naidich TP, George AE, et al: The choroidal artery to the fourth ventricle and its radiological significance, *Radiology* 126:431-439, 1978.

21. Hayman LA, Evans RA, Hinck VC: Choroid plexus of the fourth ventricle: a useful CT landmark, *AJR* 133:285-288, 1979.
22. Elliott HC: *Textbook of neuroanatomy*, Philadelphia, 1969, JB Lippincott.
23. Kido DK, LeMay M, Levinson AW, Benson WE: Computed tomographic localization of the precentral gyrus, *Radiology* 135:373-377, 1980.
24. Iwasaki S, Nakagawa H, Fukusami A, et al: Identification of pre- and postcentral gyri on CT and MR images on the basis of the medullary pattern of cerebral white matter, *Radiology* 179:207-213, 1991.
25. Steinmetz H, Furst G, Freund HJ: Variation of perisylvian and calcarine anatomic landmarks within stereotaxic proportional coordinates, *AJNR* 11:1123-1130, 1990.
26. Ebeling U, Steinmetz H, Huang Y, Kahn T: Topography and identification of the inferior precentral sulcus in MR imaging, *AJNR* 10:937-942, 1989.
27. Cserr HF: Relationship between cerebrospinal fluid and interstitial fluid of brain, *Fed Proc* 33:2075-2078, 1974.
28. Drayer BP, Rosenbaum AE: Metrizamide brain penetrance, *Acta Radiol* 355:280-293, 1977.
29. Winkler SS, Sackett JF: Explanation of metrizamide brain penetrance: a review, *J Comput Assist Tomogr* 4:191-193, 1980.
30. Sage MR, Wilcox J, Evill CA, Benness GT: Brain parenchyma penetration by intrathecal ionic and nonionic contrast media, *AJNR* 3:481-483, 1982.
31. Heir LA, Bauer CJ, Schwartz L, et al: Large Virchow-Robin spaces: MR-clinical correlation, *AJNR* 10:929-936, 1989.
32. Elster AD, Richardson DN: Foci of high-T2 signal in the midbrain: anatomic correlates, *AJNR* 11:1119-1122, 1991.
33. Jungreis CA, Kanal E, Hirsh WL, et al: Normal perivascular spaces mimicking lacunar infarction: MR imaging, *Radiology* 169:101-104, 1988.
34. Braffman BH, Zimmerman RA, Trojanowski JQ, et al: Brain MR: pathologic correlation with gross and histopathology. I. Lacunar infarction and Virchow-Robin spaces, *AJNR* 9:621-628, 1988.
35. Creasey H, Rapoport SI: The aging human brain, *Ann Neurol* 17:2-10, 1985.
36. Dekaban AS, Sadowsky D: Changes in brain weights during the span of human life: relation of brain weights to body heights and body weights, *Ann Neurol* 4:334-356, 1978.
37. David PJM, Wright EA: A new method for measuring cranial cavity volume and its application to the assessment of cerebral atrophy at autopsy, *Neuropathol Appl Neurobiol* 3:341-358, 1977.
38. Roessmann U, Ho KC, Straumfjord JV, et al: The weight of the infratentorial portion of the adult brain and analysis of the infratentorial/whole brain weight ratio, *J Neuropathol Exp Neurol* 41:536-547, 1982.
39. LeMay M: Radiologic changes of the aging brain and skull, *AJR* 143:383-389, 1984.
40. Gomori JM, Steiner I, Melamed E, et al: The assessment of changes in brain volume using combined linear measurements: a CT-scan study, *Neuroradiology* 26:21-24, 1984.
41. Tomlinson BE, Blessed G, Roth M: Observations on the brains of nondemented old people, *J Neurol Sci* 7:331-356, 1968.
42. Miller AKH, Alston RL, Corsellis JAN: Variation with age in the volumes of grey and white matter in the cerebral hemispheres of man: measurements with an image analyser, *Neuropathol Appl Neurobiol* 6:119-132, 1980.
43. Brody H: Organization of the cerebral cortex. III. A study of aging in the human cerebral cortex, *J Comp Neurol* 102:511-556, 1955.
44. Anderson JM, Hubbard BM, Coghill GR, et al: The effect of advanced old age on the neurone content of the cerebral cortex: observations with an automatic image analyser point counting method, *J Neurol Sci* 58:235-246, 1983.
45. Brody H, Vijayashankar N: Anatomical changes in the nervous system. In Fince CE, Hayflick L, editors: *Handbook of the biology of aging*, New York, 1977, Van Nostrand.
46. Yakovlev PL: Morphological criteria of growth and maturation of the nervous system in man, *Ment Retard* 39:3-46, 1961.
47. Terry RD: Some biological aspects of the aging brain, *Mech Ageing Dev* 14:191-201, 1980.
48. Peress NS, Kane WC, Aronson SM: Central nervous system findings in a tenth decade autopsy population, *Prog Brain Res* 40:473-483, 1973.
49. Miquel J, Johnson JE Jr, Cervos-Navarro J: Comparison of CNS aging in humans and experimental animals. In Cervos-Navarro J, Sarkander HI, editors: *Brain aging: neuropathology and neuropharmacology*, New York, 1983, Raven.
50. Huag H: Quantitative investigation of the human cerebral cortex, *Gerontology* 27:105-111, 1981.
51. Huttenlocher PR: Synaptic density in human frontal cortex: developmental changes and effects of aging, *Brain Res* 163:195-205, 1979.
52. Drayer BP: Imaging of the aging brain. Part I. Normal findings, *Radiology* 166:785-796, 1988.
53. Jacoby RJ, Levy R, Dawson JM: Computed tomography in the elderly. I. The normal population, *Br J Psychiatry* 136:249-255, 1980.
54. Nagata K, Basugi N, Fukushima T, et al: A quantitative study of physiological cerebral atrophy with aging: a statistical analysis of the normal range, *Neuroradiology* 29:327-332, 1987.
55. Gyldensted C: Measurements of the normal ventricular system and hemispheric sulci of 100 adults with computed tomography, *Neuroradiology* 14:183-192, 1977.
56. Damasio H, Eslinger P, Damasio AR, et al: Quantitative computed tomographic analysis in the diagnosis of dementia, *Arch Neurol* 40:715-719, 1983.
57. Yamaura H, Ito M, Kubota K, et al: Brain atrophy during aging: a quantitative study with computed tomography, *J Gerontol Aging* 35:492-498, 1980.
58. Schwartz M, Creasey H, Grady CL, et al: Computed tomographic analysis of brain morphometrics in 30 healthy men, aged 21 to 81 years, *Ann Neurol* 17(2):146-157, 1985.
59. Malko JA, Hoffman JC, Green RC: MR measurement of intracranial CSF volume in 41 elderly normal volunteers, *AJNR* 12:371-374, 1991.
60. Wahlund LO, Agartz I, Almqvist O, et al: The brain in healthy aged individuals: MR imaging, *Radiology* 174:675-679, 1990.
61. Norman D, Diamond C, Boyd D: Relative detectability of intracranial calcifications on computed tomography and skull radiography, *J Comput Assist Tomogr* 2:61-64, 1978.
62. Modic MT, Weinstein MA, Rothner AD, et al: Calcification of the choroid plexus visualized by computed tomography, *Radiology* 135:369-372, 1980.
63. Hinshaw DB, Fahmy JL, Peckham N, et al: The bright choroid plexus on MR: CT and pathologic correlation, *AJNR* 9:483-486, 1988.
64. Czervionke LF, Daniels DL, Meyer GA, et al: Neuroepithelial cysts of the lateral ventricles: MR appearance, *AJNR* 8:609-613, 1987.
65. Hinshaw DB: Personal communication.

CHAPTER 13

L. Anne Hayman
Todd Ellison Lanier
Vincent C. Hinck
John W. Wright

Atlas of Cerebral Vessels

This chapter is designed to provide the reader with information concerning the relationship of cerebral vessels to the surfaces of the brain. The location of cerebral vessels on axial images and in standard angiographic projections is presented in atlas form. An index allows the reader to locate unfamiliar vessels on all the images provided. Chapter 12 provides additional figures that illustrate the relationship between the ventricular surfaces and the choroidal arteries and subependymal veins. Chapter 15 uses axial and angiographic schematics to illustrate how intracranial mass lesions displace both the superficial and the ventricular surfaces of the brain.

In the angiographic section, the carotid arteries and veins are labeled in Figures 13-1 to 13-3. The vertebral vessels are shown in Figures 13-4 to 13-6. The schematic illustrations of the cerebrovascular anatomy that accompany these angiograms have been drawn to scale, allowing the reader mentally to superimpose the arterial and venous phases of the angiogram on the anatomic drawings.

In this chapter, serial axial, contrast-enhanced computed tomographic (CT) images are used to identify the intracranial vessels, as well as their relationship to the brain surfaces (Figures 13-7 to 13-25). This imaging modality was chosen because, unlike their appearance on magnetic resonance imaging (MRI), the cerebral vessels are consistently hyperdense and highly visible on contrast-enhanced CT scans. Several anatomic references were consulted to label all the enhanced structures that appear on these images.[1-8] A General Electric 9800 Quick Scanner was used to obtain the 10 mm thick scans shown in this atlas. A bolus infusion of 42.3 g iodine was given in the form of diatrizoate meglumine. The examinations of several normal patients were used to illustrate the variations in vascular patterns that may be encountered at each level.

REFERENCES

1. Hayman LA, Evans RA, Hinck VC: Rapid high dose (RHD) contrast cranial computed tomography: a concise review of normal anatomy, *J Comput Assist Tomogr* 3(2):147-154, 1979.
2. Naidich TP, Pudlowski RM, Leeds NE, et al: The normal contrast-enhanced computed axial tomogram of the brain, *J Comput Assist Tomogr* 1:16-29, 1977.
3. Stephens RB, Stilwell DL: *Arteries and veins of the human brain,* Springfield, Ill, 1969, Charles C Thomas.
4. Newton TH, Potts DG, editors: *Radiology of the skull and brain: angiography,* vol 2, book 2, St Louis, 1974, Mosby–Year Book.
5. Newton TH, Potts DG, editors: *Radiology of the skull and brain: angiography,* vol 2, book 3, St Louis, 1974, Mosby–Year Book.
6. DeArmond SJ, Fusco MM, Dewey MM: *Structure of the human brain: a photographic atlas,* ed 3, New York, 1989, Oxford University.
7. Osborn AG, Maack JG: *Introduction to cerebral angiography,* Hagerstown, Md, 1980, Harper & Row.
8. Zimmerman RD, Yurberg E, Russel EJ, et al: Falx and interhemispheric fissure on axial CT. I. Normal anatomy, *AJNR* 3:175-180, 1982.

KEY: ICA — Internal carotid artery
PCA — Posterior cerebral artery
ACA — Anterior cerebral artery
MCA — Middle cerebral artery

CAROTID VESSELS

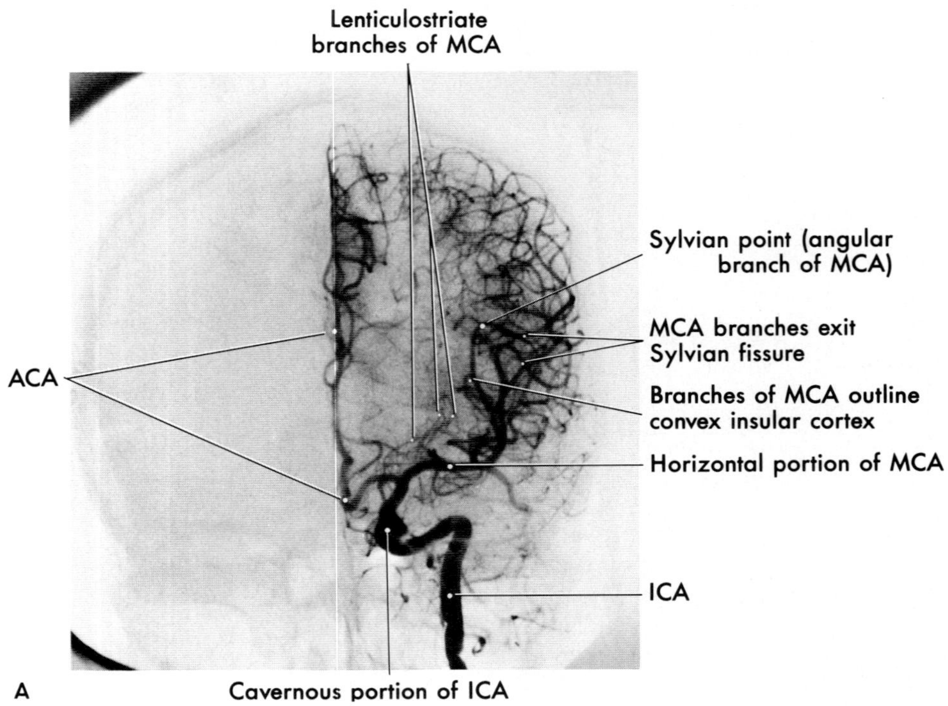

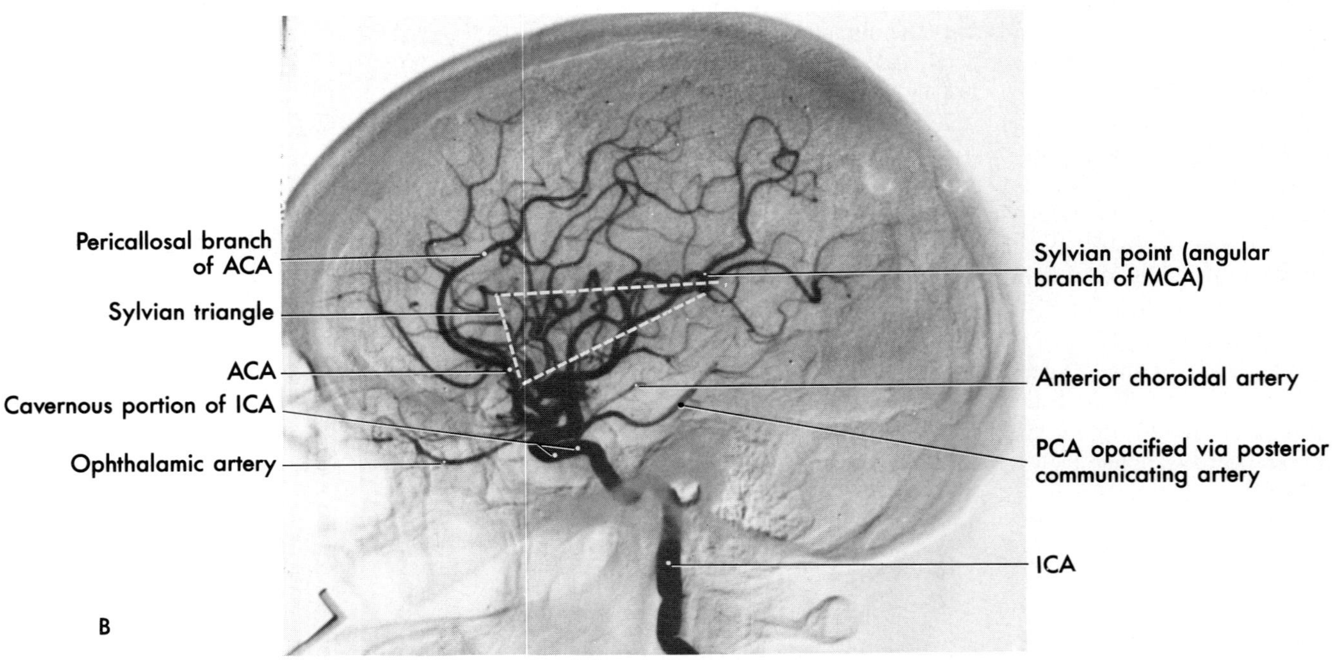

Figure 13-1 *Carotid arteriogram: arterial phase.*
A, Anteroposterior projection.
B, Lateral projection.

CAROTID VESSELS

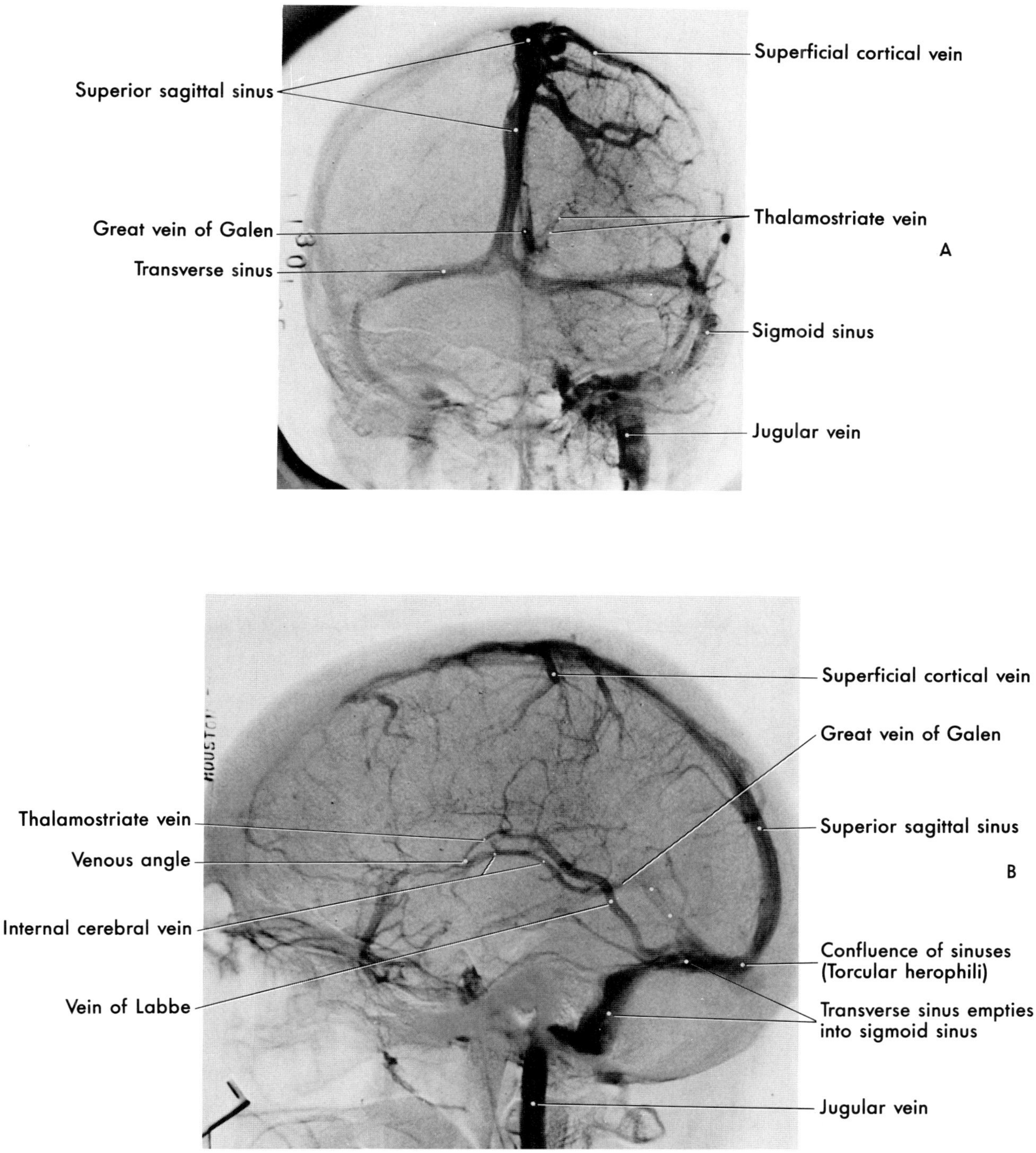

Figure 13-2 *Carotid arteriogram: venous phase.*
A, Anteroposterior projection.
B, Lateral projection.

CAROTID VESSELS

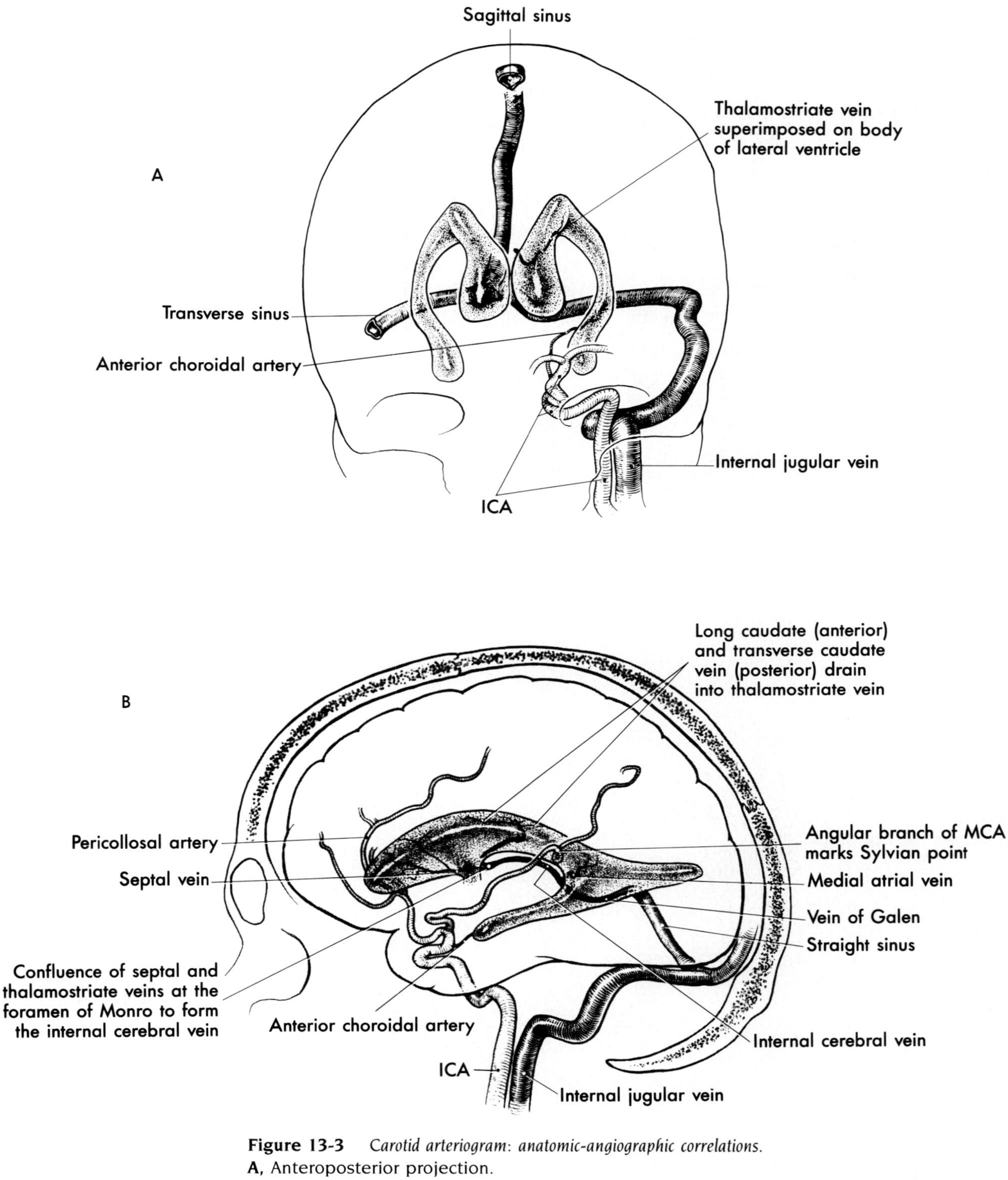

Figure 13-3 *Carotid arteriogram: anatomic-angiographic correlations.*
A, Anteroposterior projection.
B, Lateral projection.

CAROTID VESSELS

C

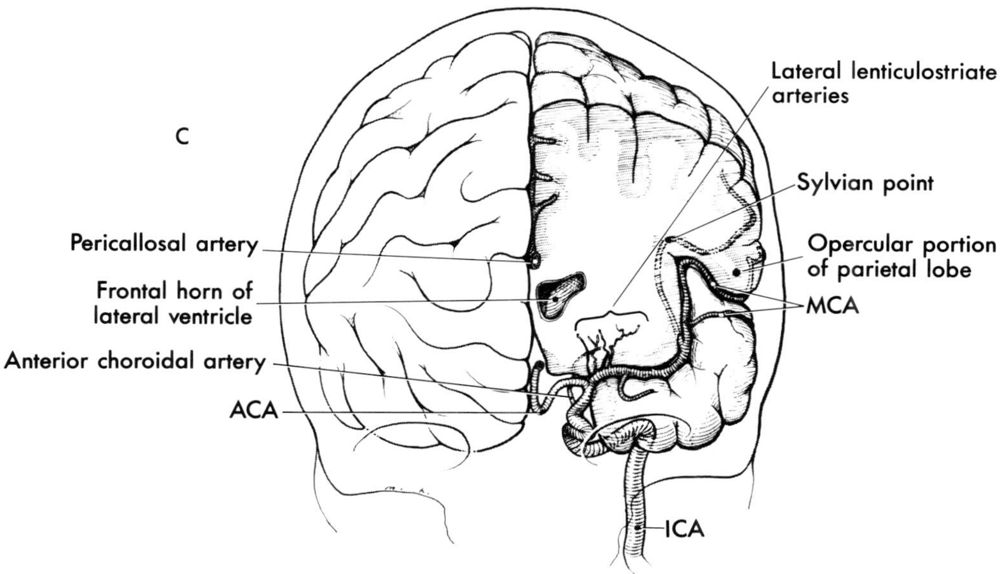

D

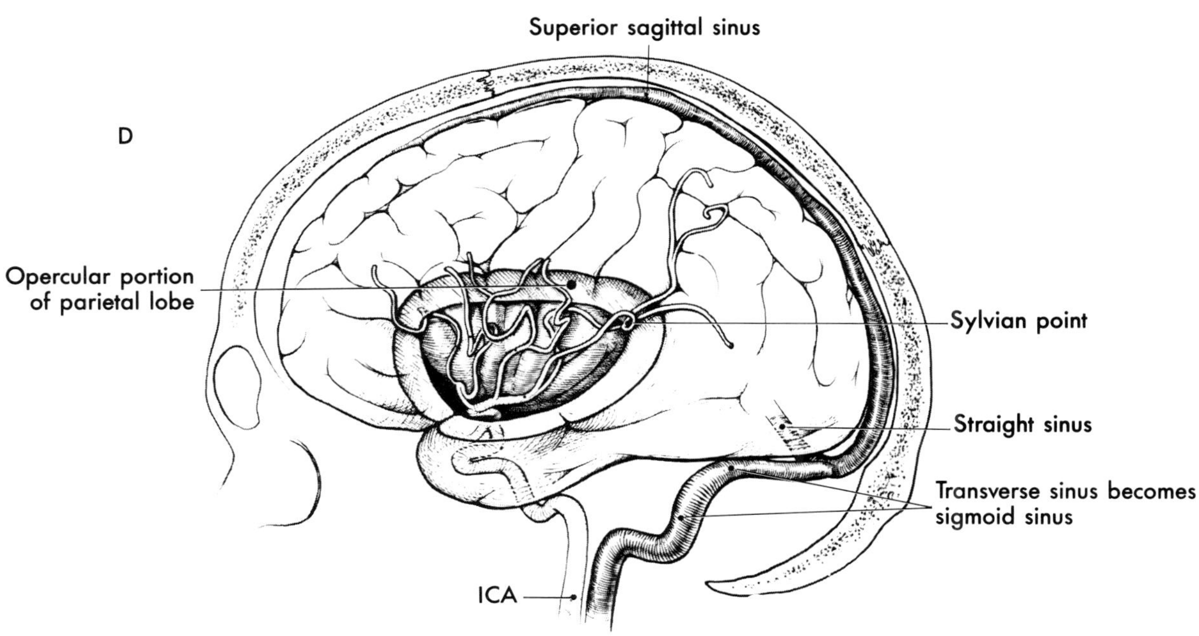

Figure 13-3, cont'd *Carotid arteriogram: anatomic-angiographic correlations.*
C, Anteroposterior projection.
D, Lateral projection.

VERTEBRAL VESSELS

A

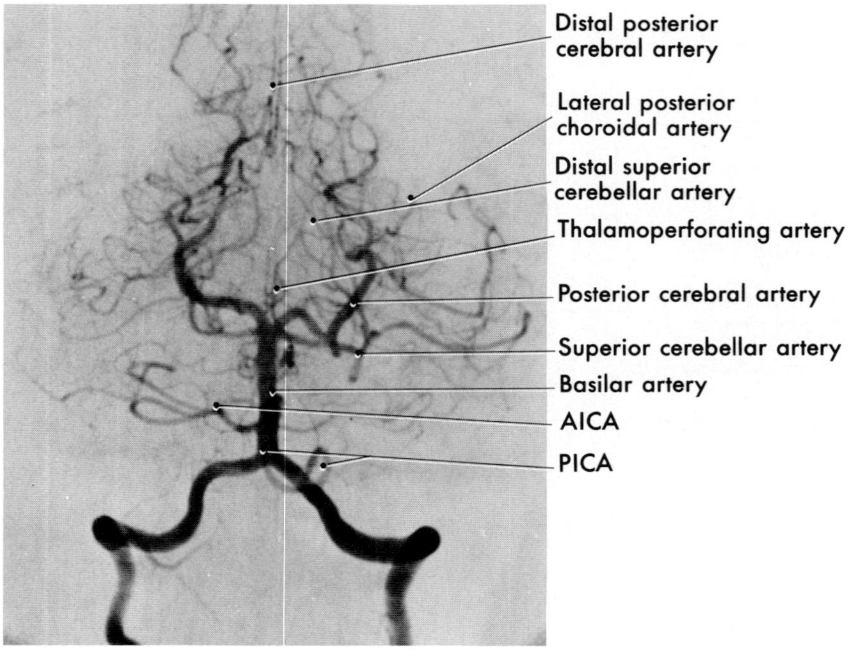

B

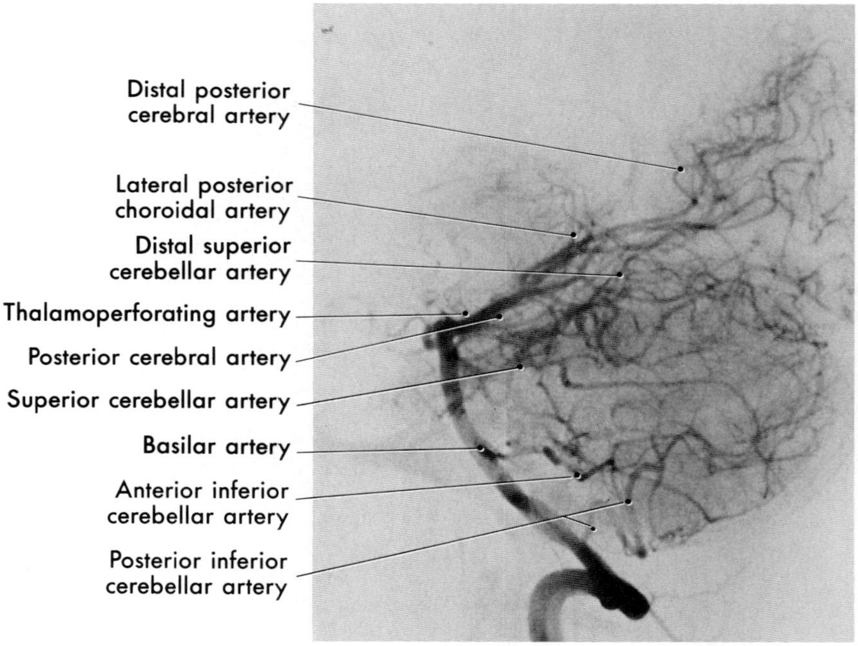

Figure 13-4 *Vertebral arteriogram: arterial phase.*
A, Anteroposterior projection.
B, Lateral projection.

VERTEBRAL VESSELS

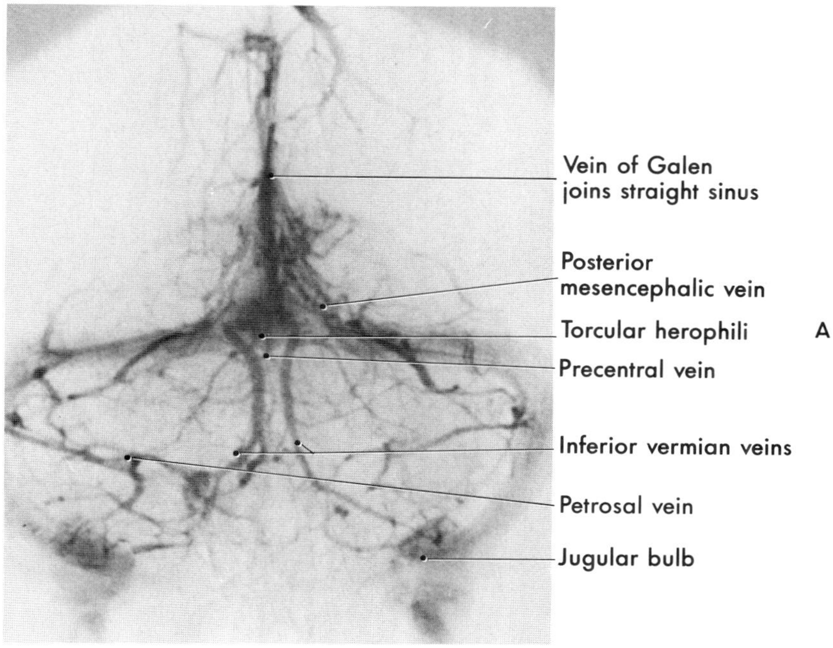

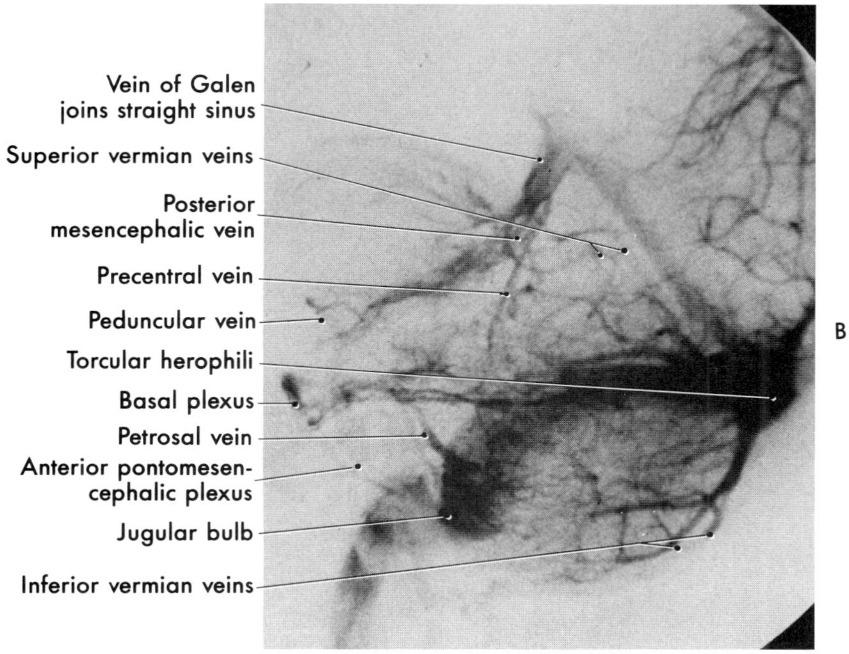

Figure 13-5 *Vertebral arteriogram: venous phase.*
A, Anteroposterior projection.
B, Lateral projection.

VERTEBRAL VESSELS

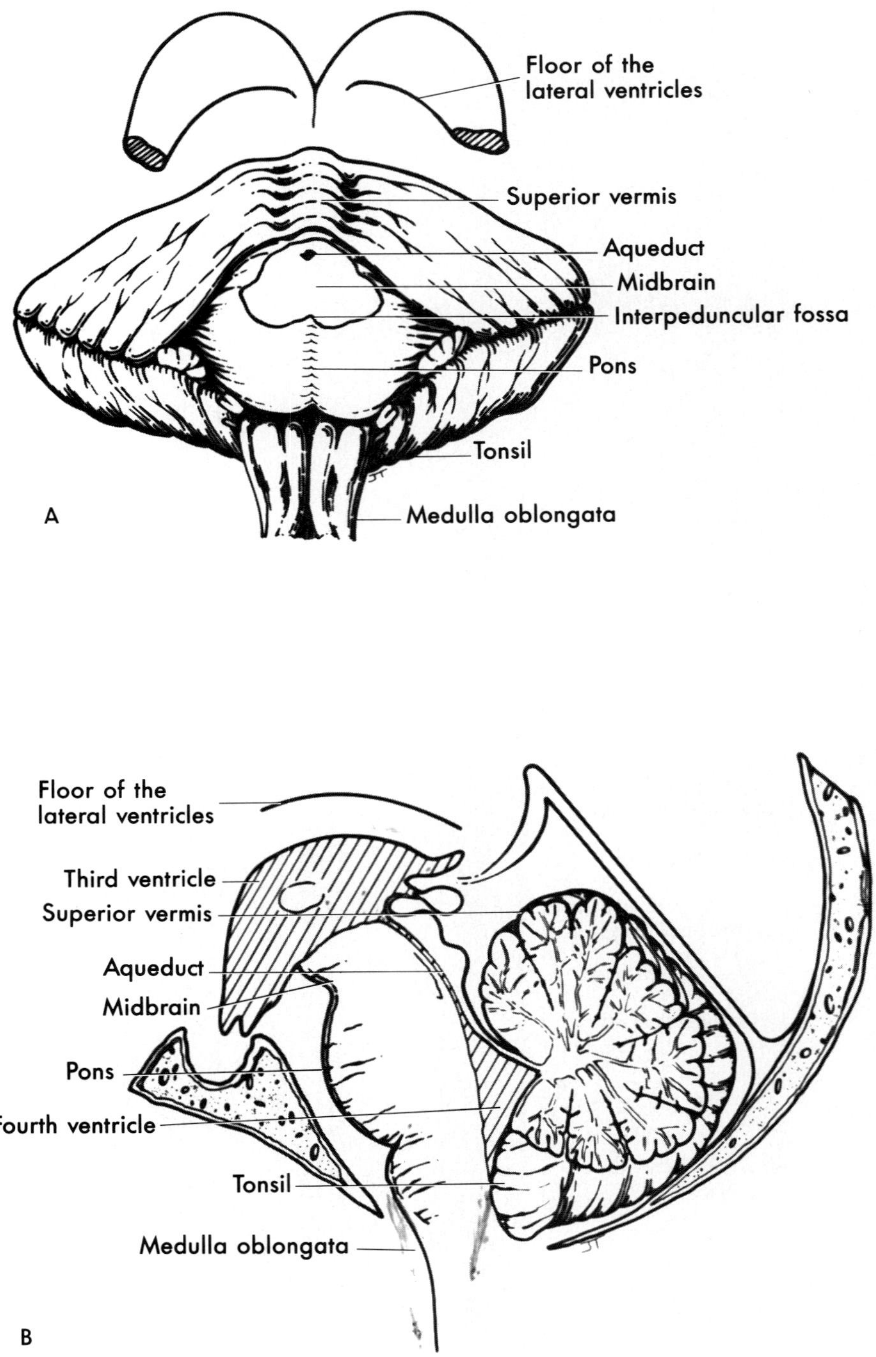

Figure 13-6 *Vertebral arteriogram: anatomic-angiographic correlations.*
A, Anteroposterior projection.
B, Lateral projection.

AXIAL CT SCANS OF CEREBRAL VESSELS

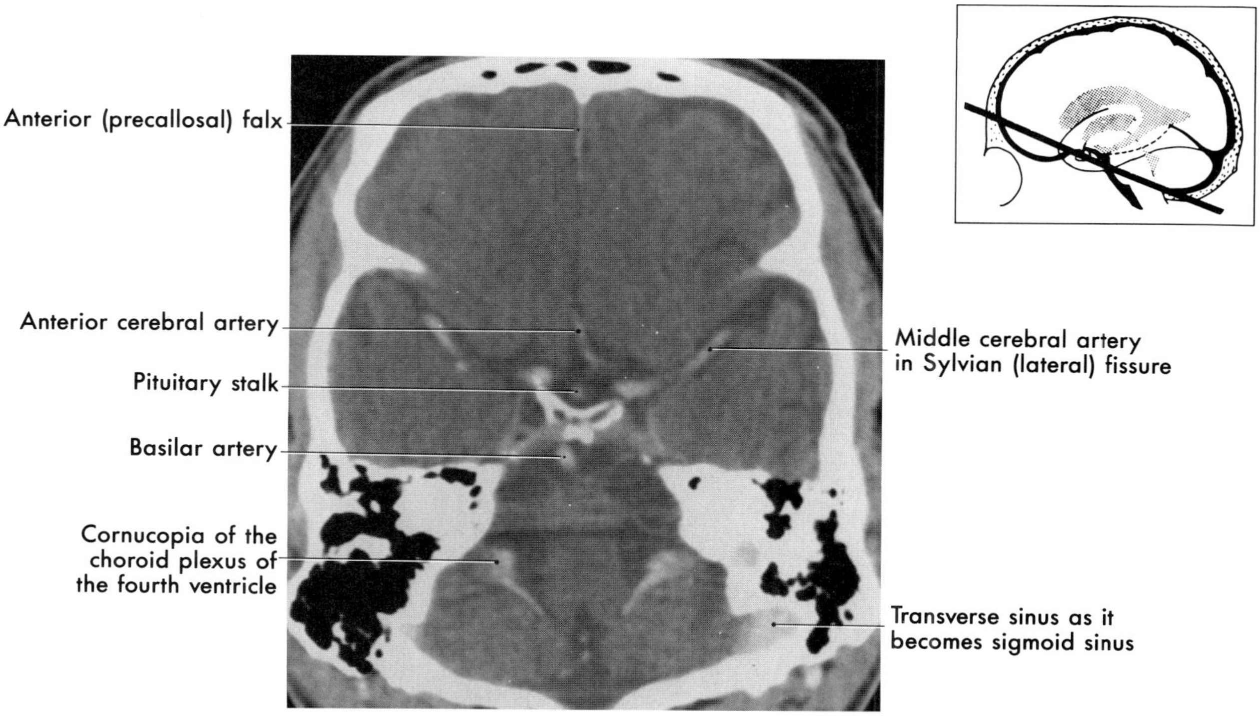

Figure 13-7

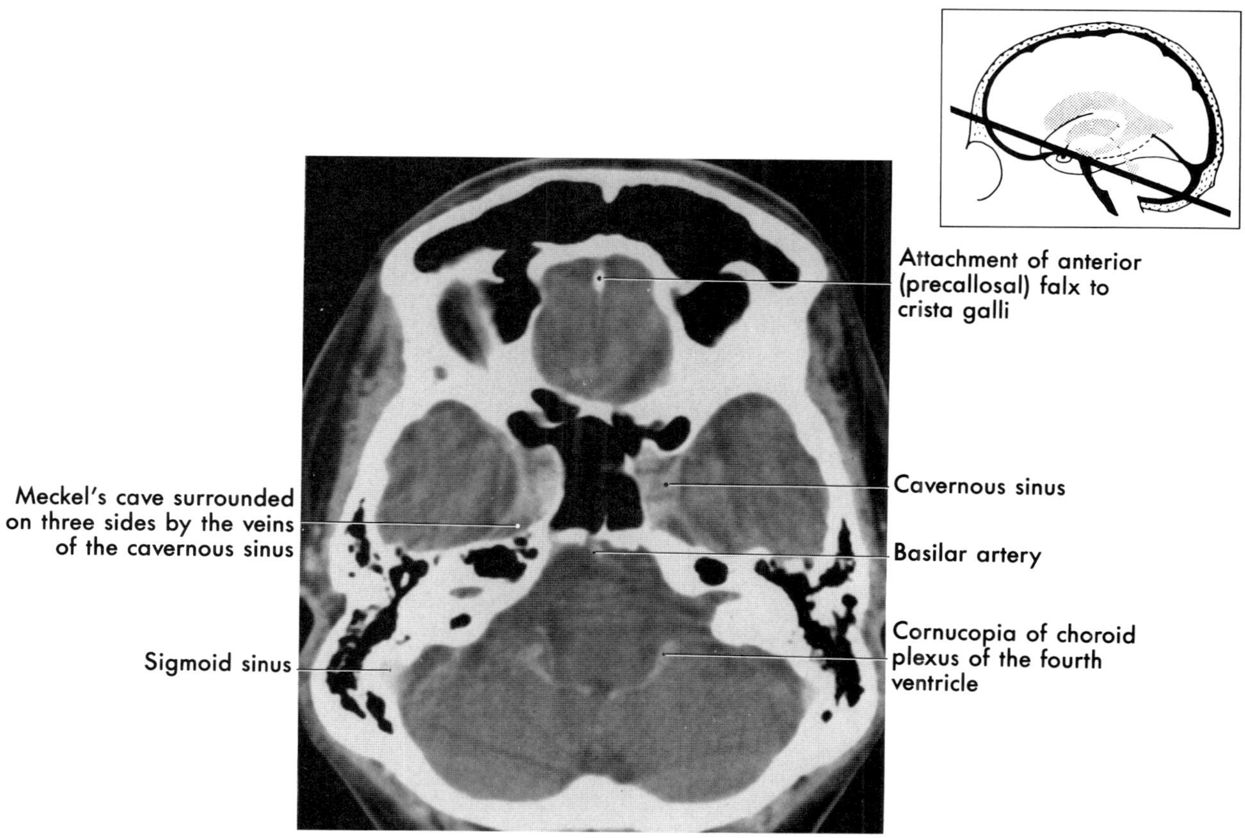

Figure 13-8

AXIAL CT SCANS OF CEREBRAL VESSELS

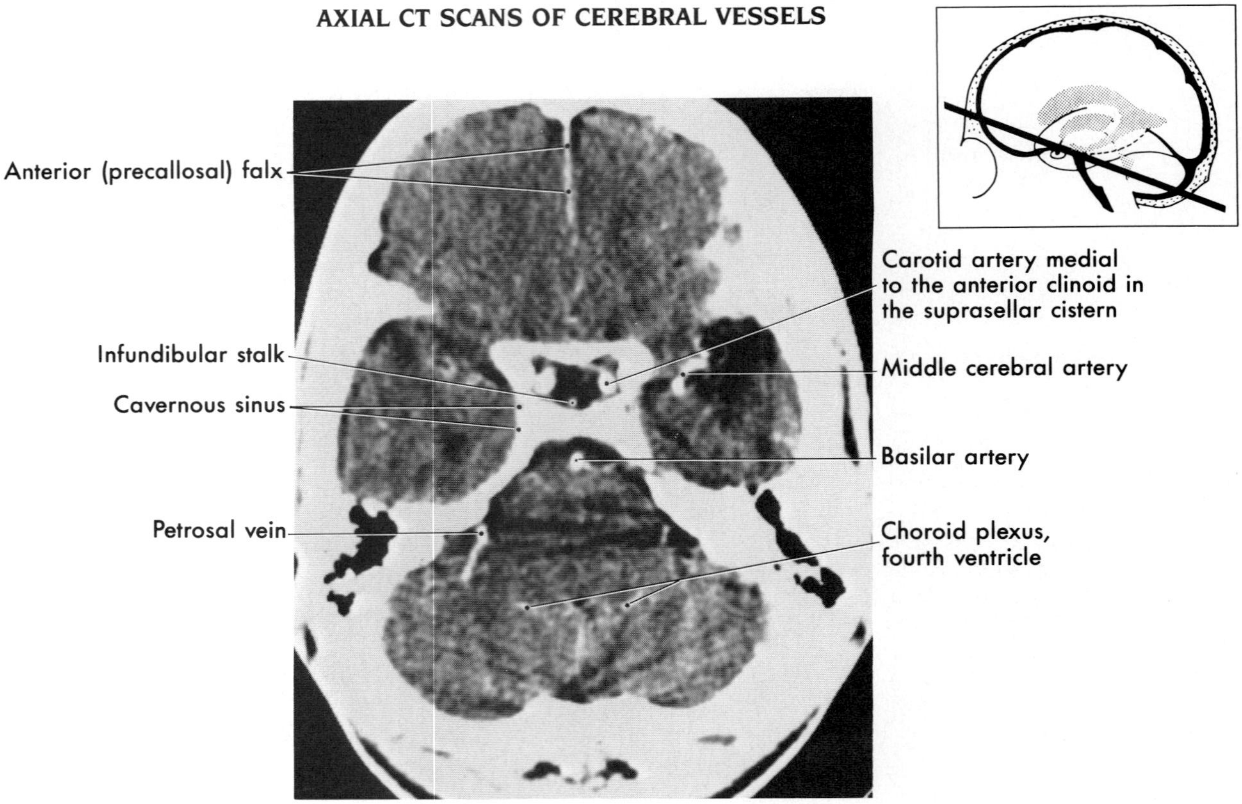

Figure 13-9

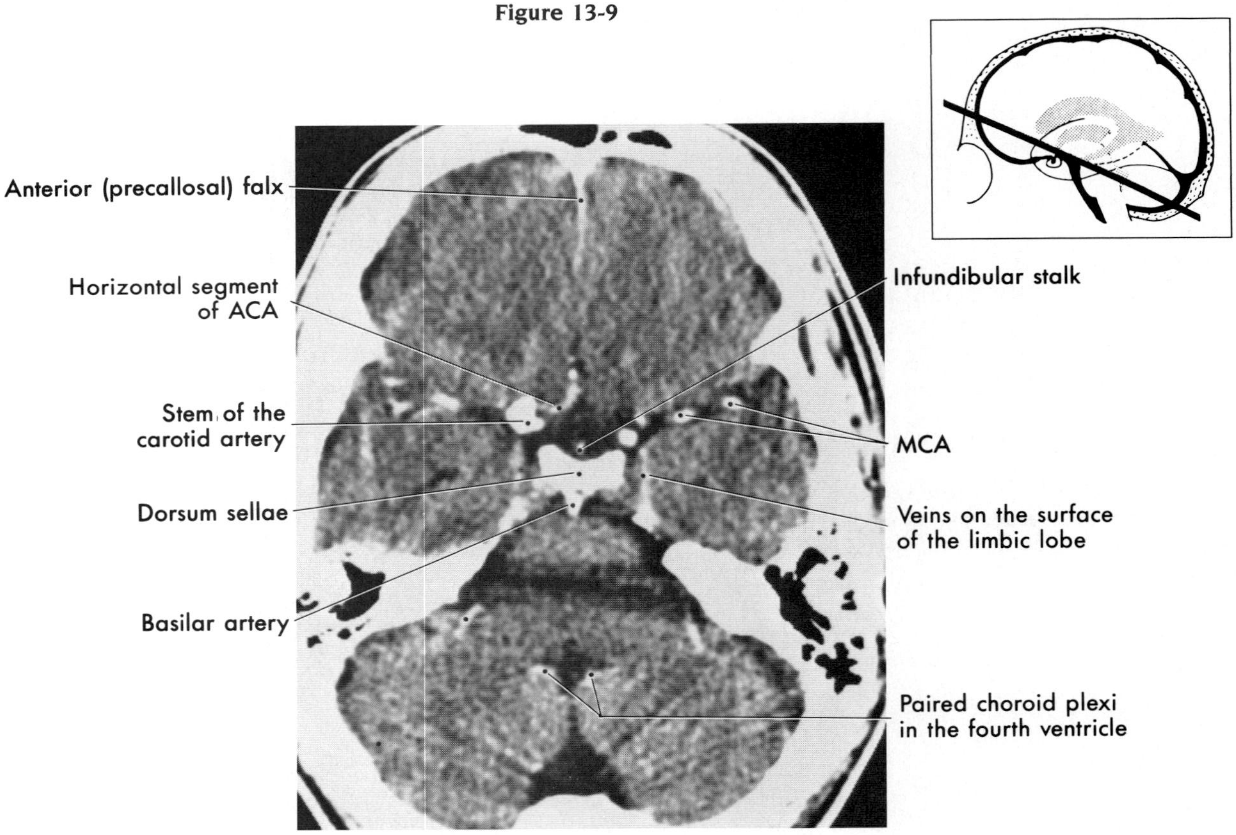

Figure 13-10

AXIAL CT SCANS OF CEREBRAL VESSELS

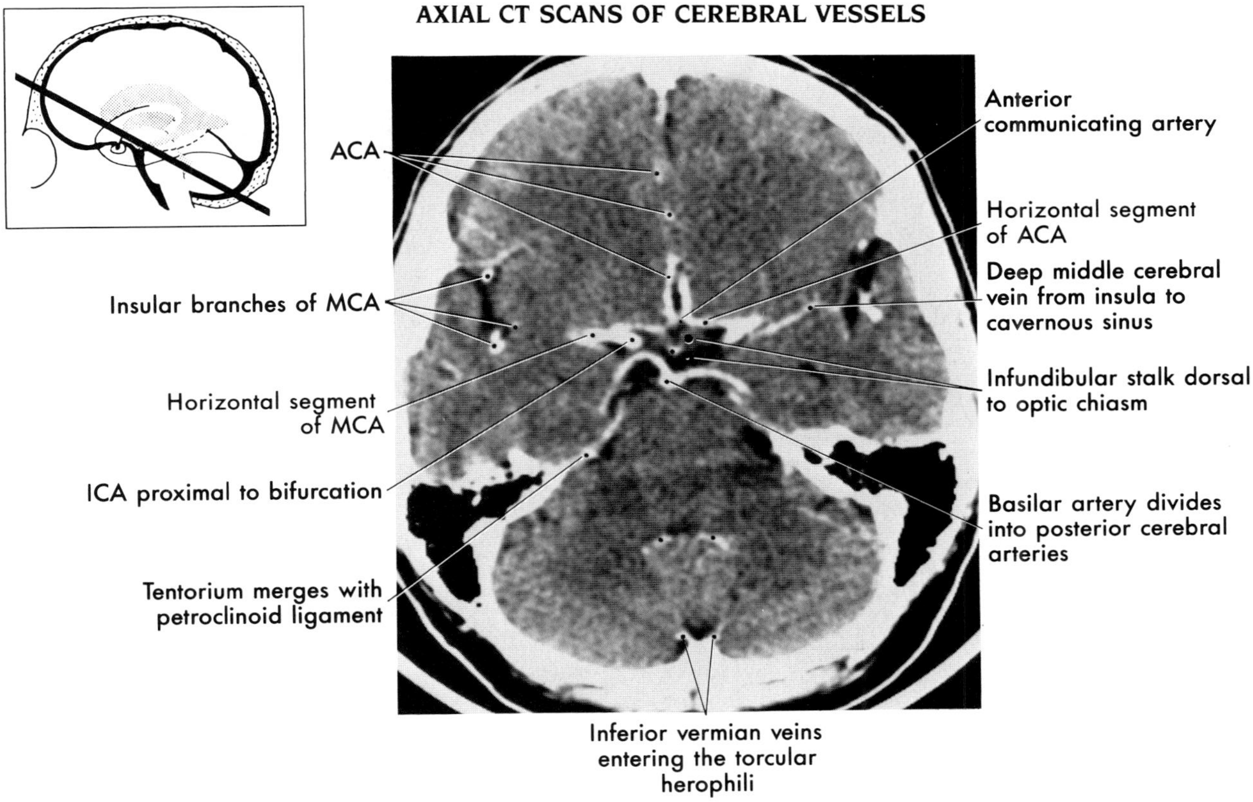

Figure 13-11

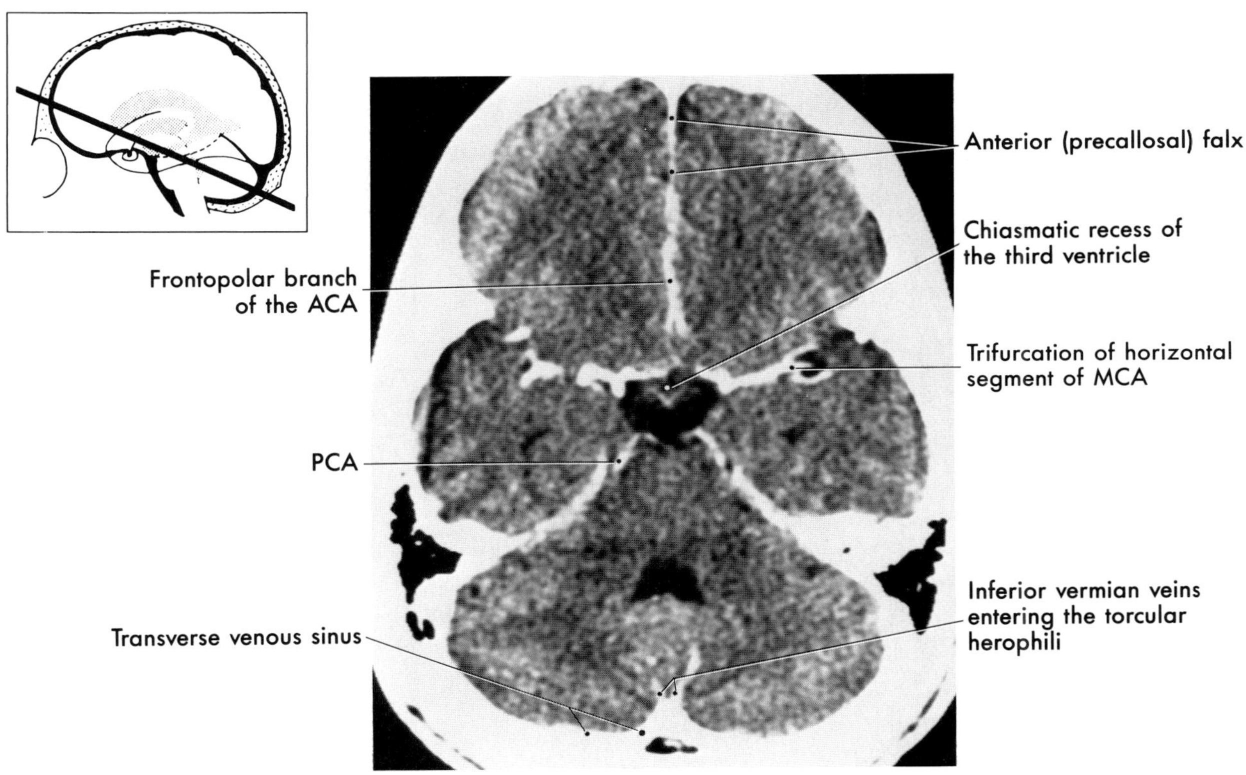

Figure 13-12

AXIAL CT SCANS OF CEREBRAL VESSELS

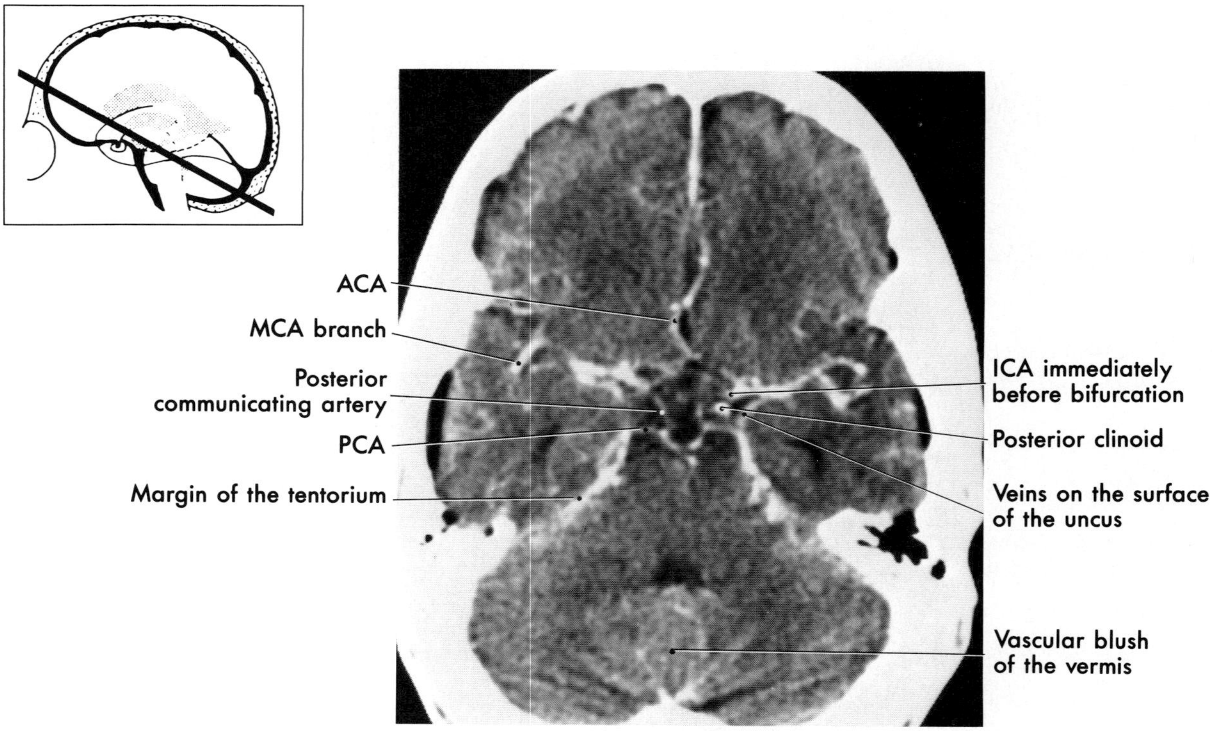

Figure 13-13

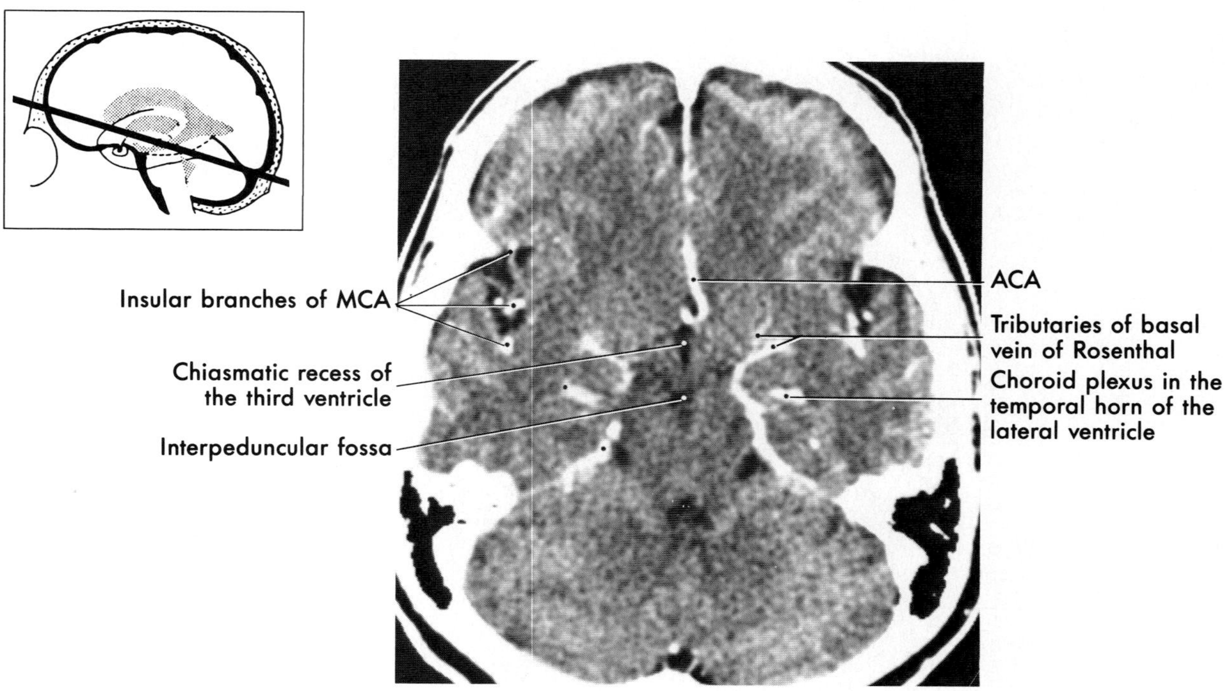

Figure 13-14

AXIAL CT SCANS OF CEREBRAL VESSELS

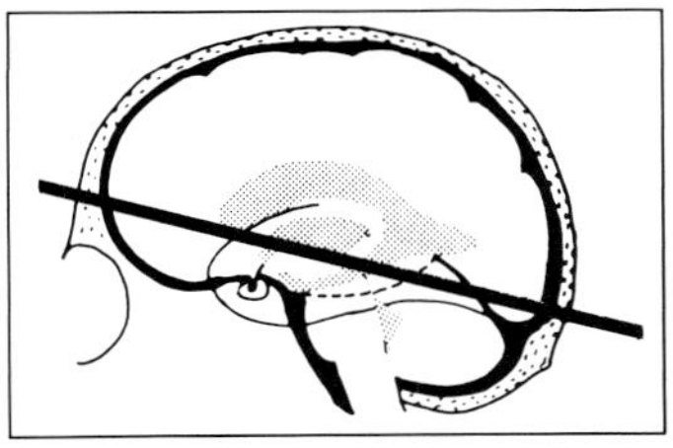

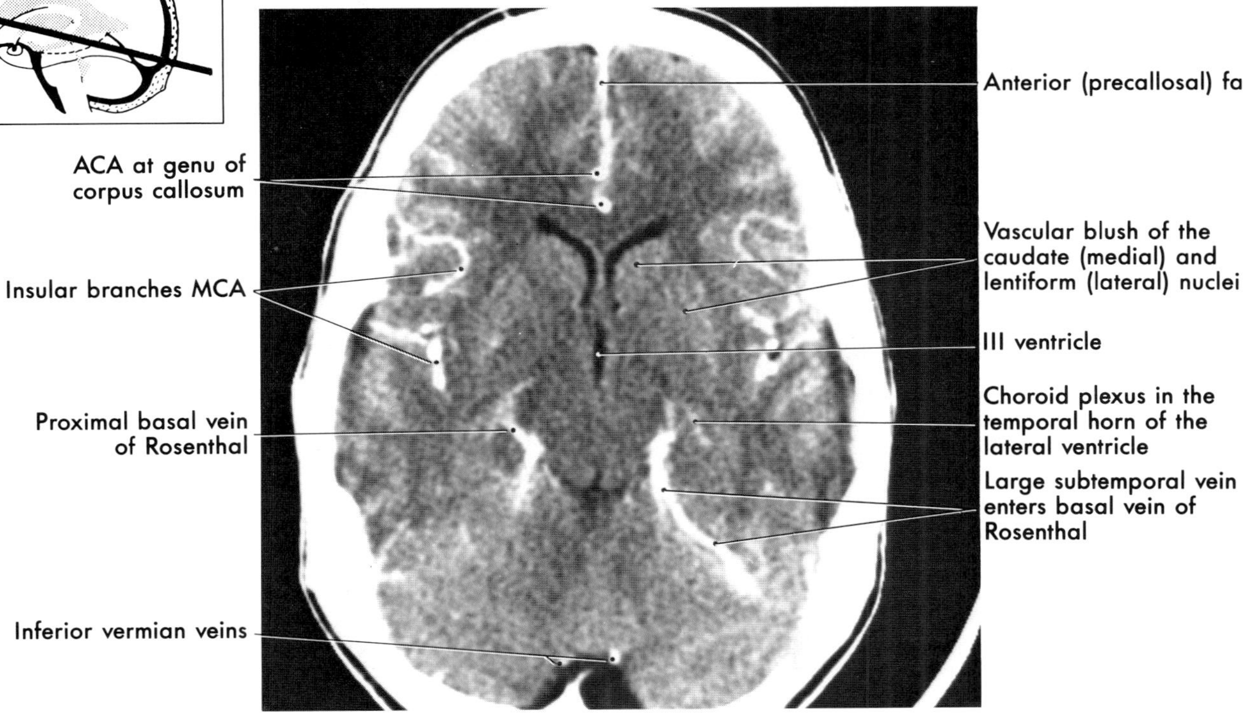

Figure 13-15

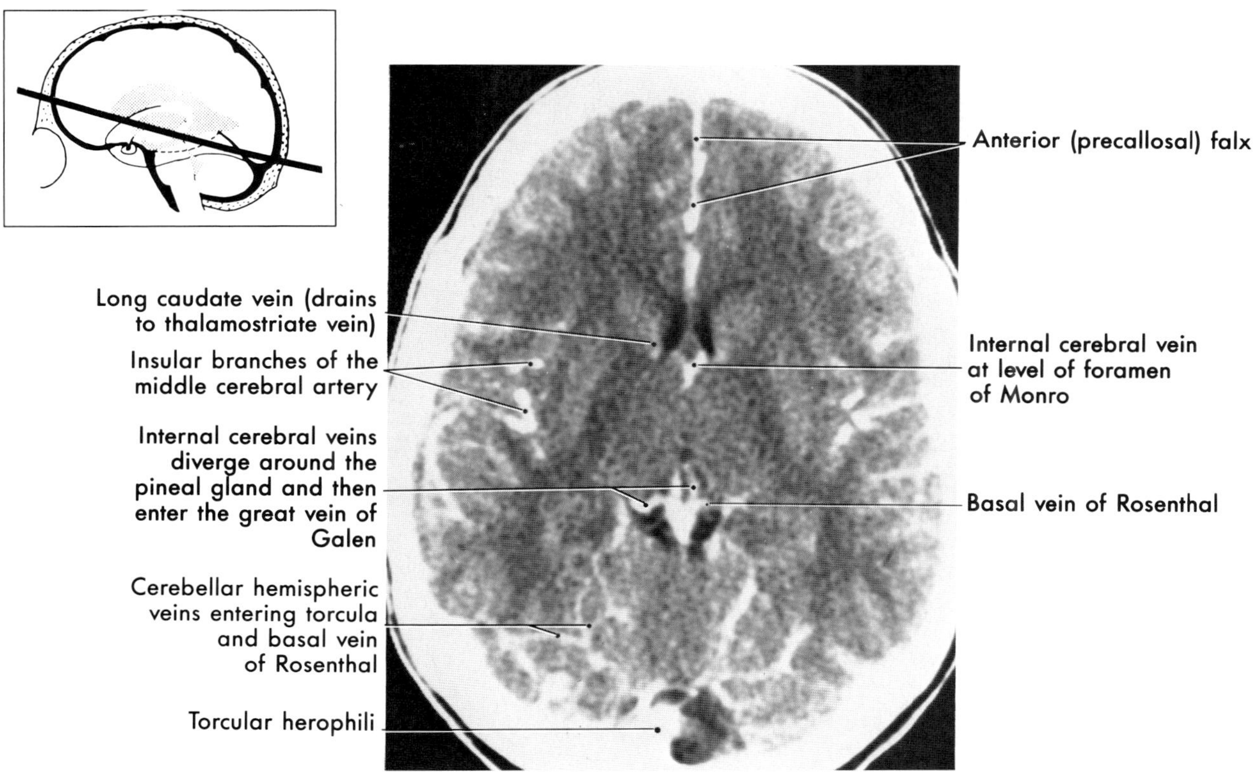

Figure 13-16

AXIAL CT SCANS OF CEREBRAL VESSELS

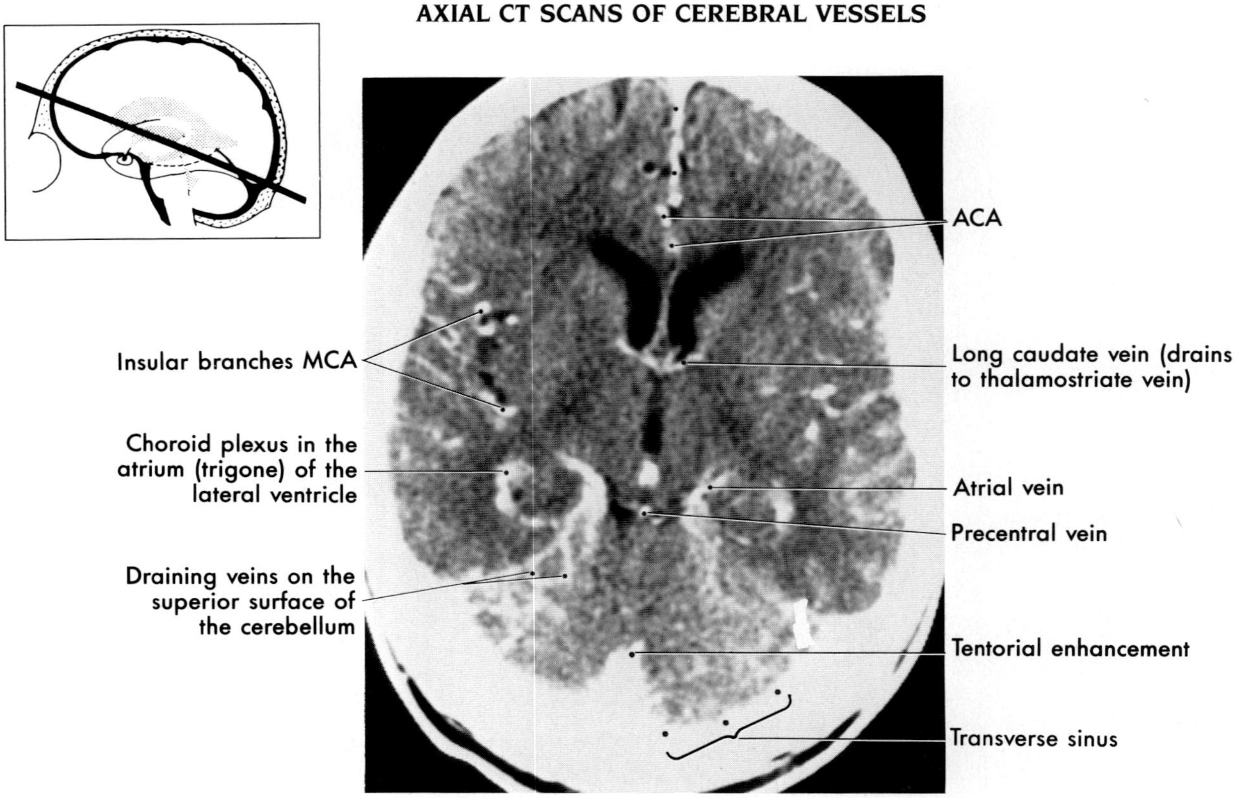

Figure 13-17

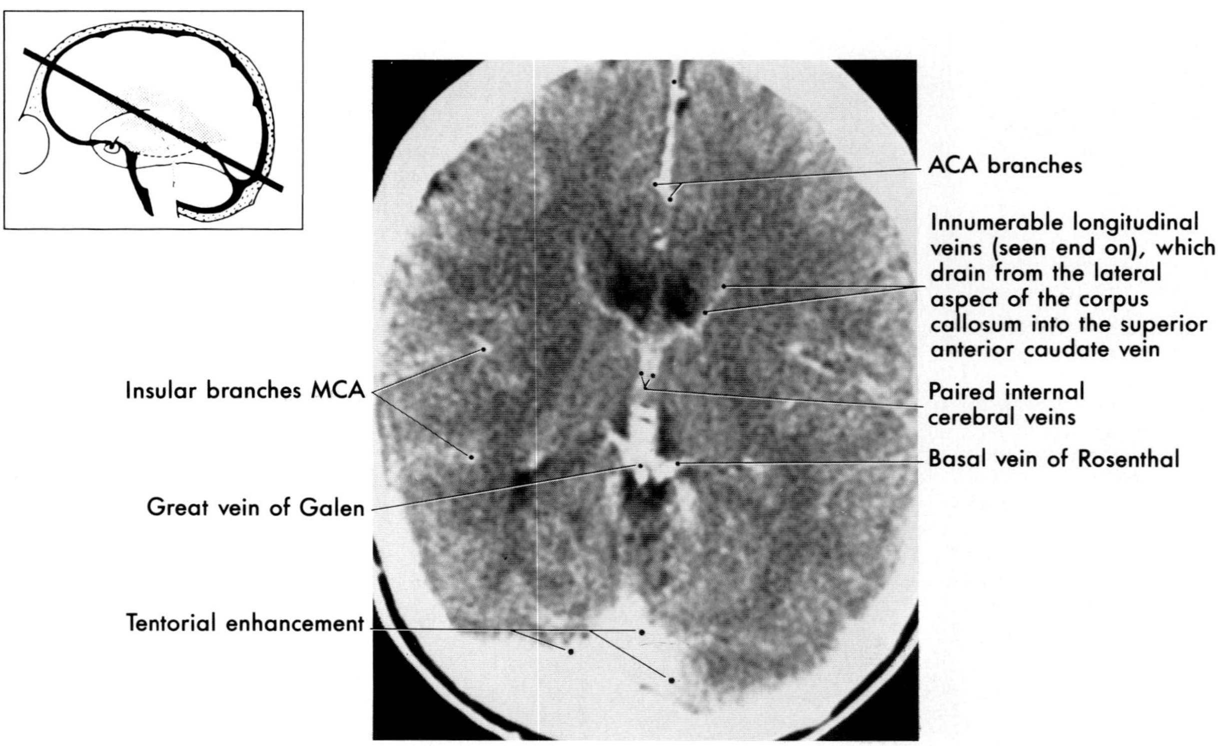

Figure 13-18

AXIAL CT SCANS OF CEREBRAL VESSELS

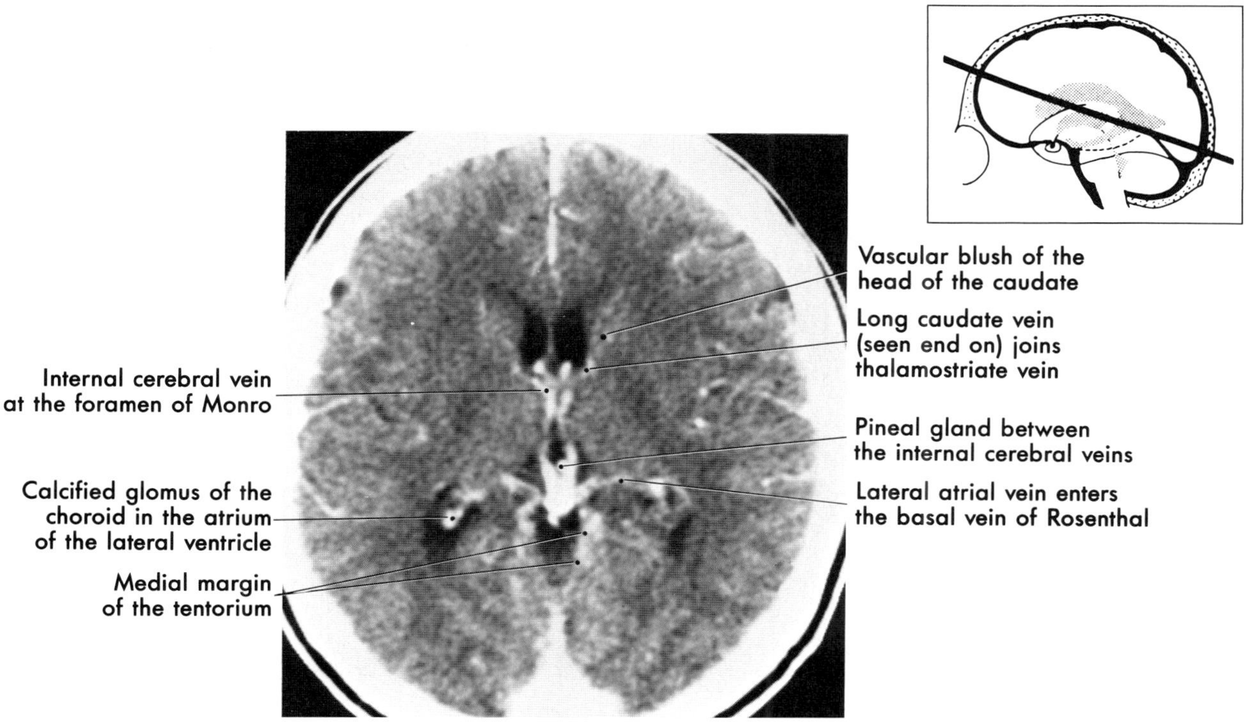

Figure 13-19

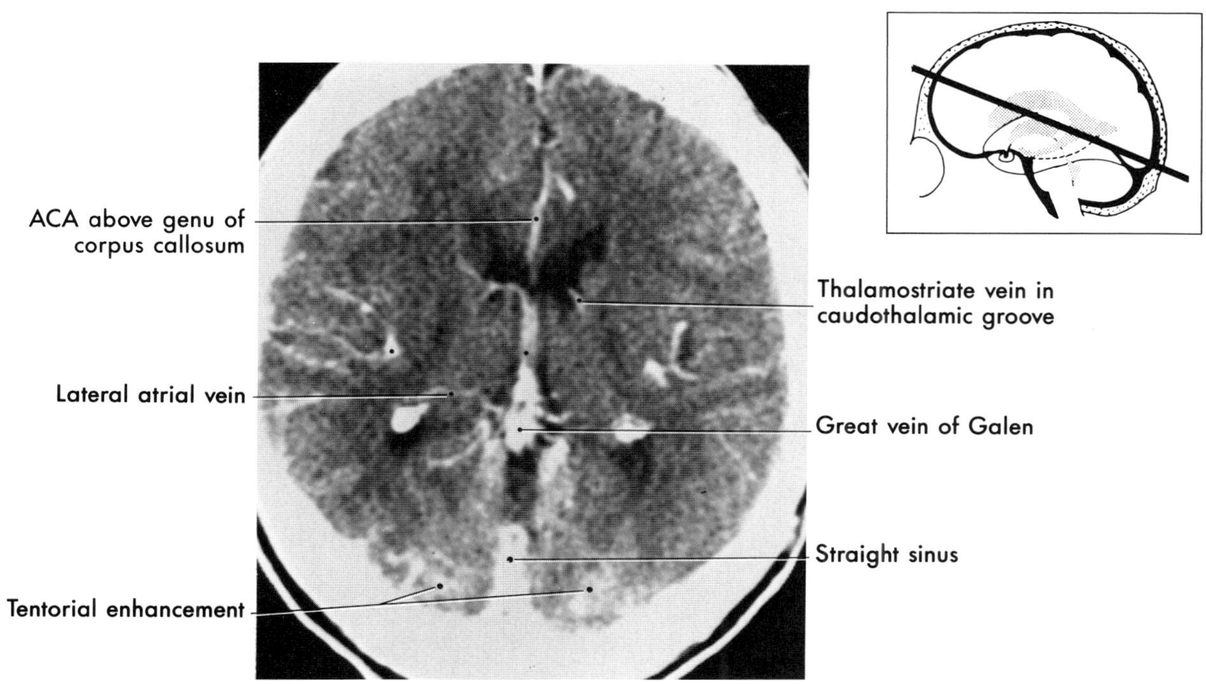

Figure 13-20

AXIAL CT SCANS OF CEREBRAL VESSELS

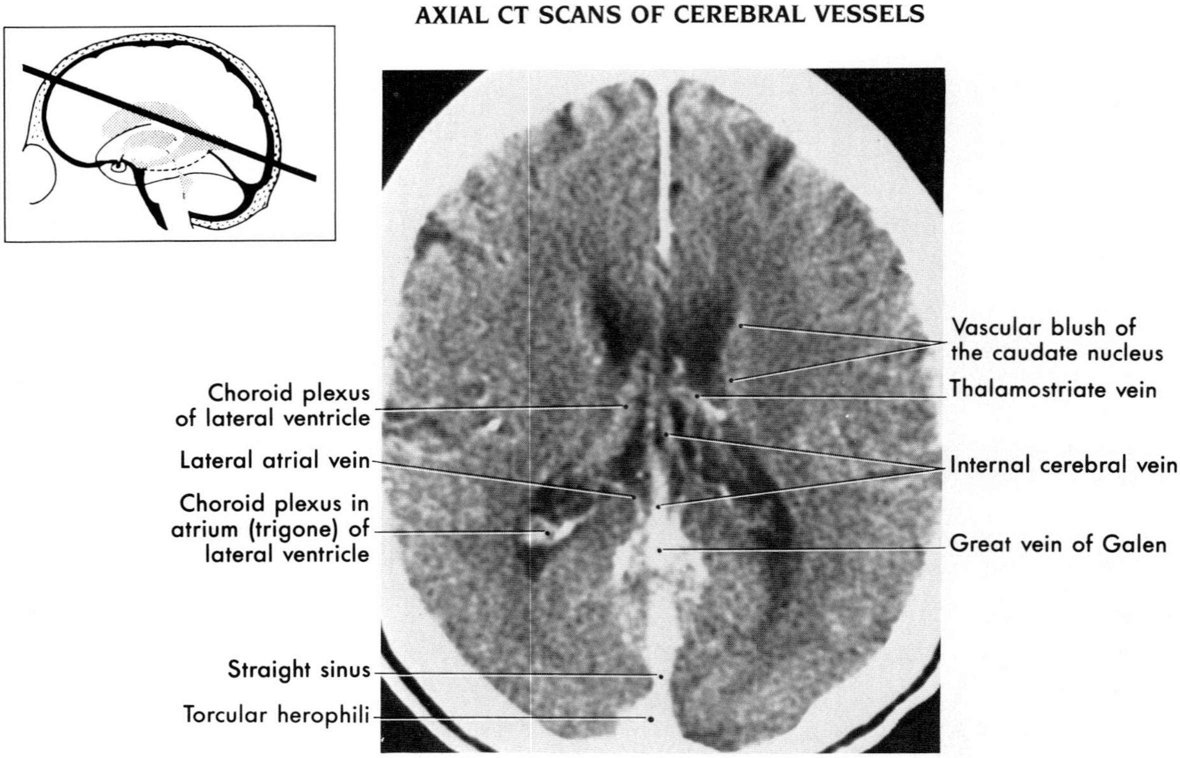

Figure 13-21

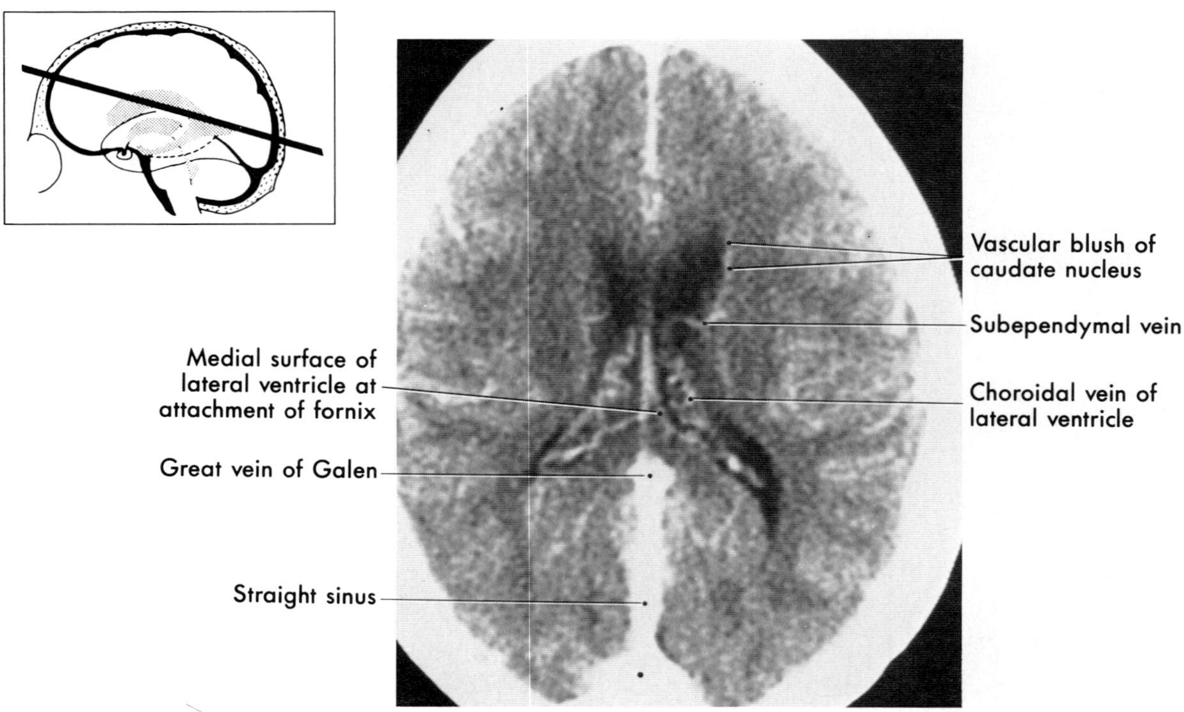

Figure 13-22

AXIAL CT SCANS OF CEREBRAL VESSELS

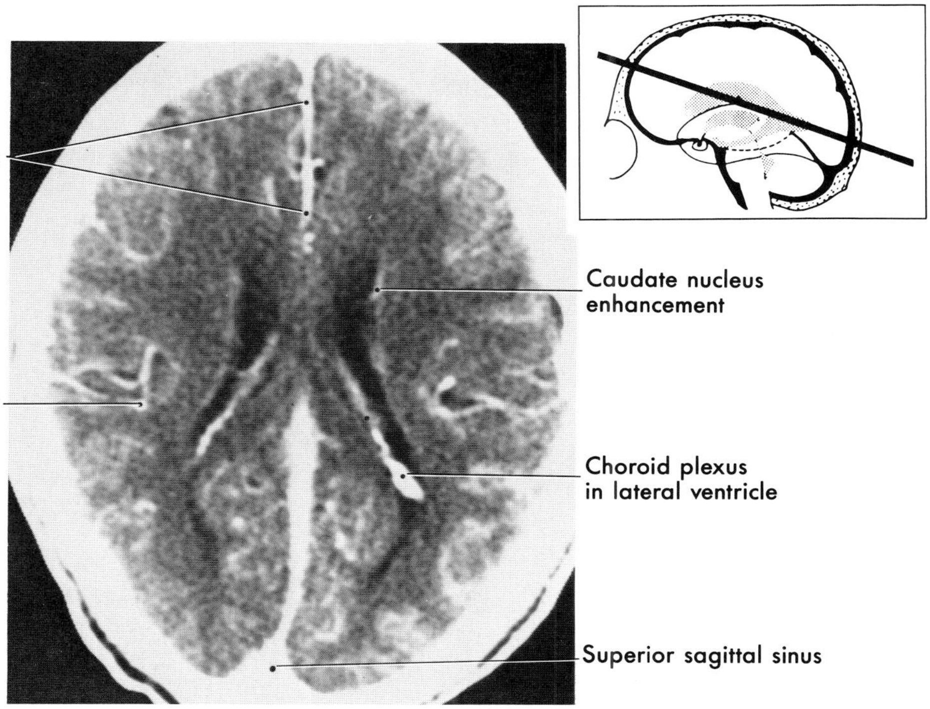

Figure 13-23

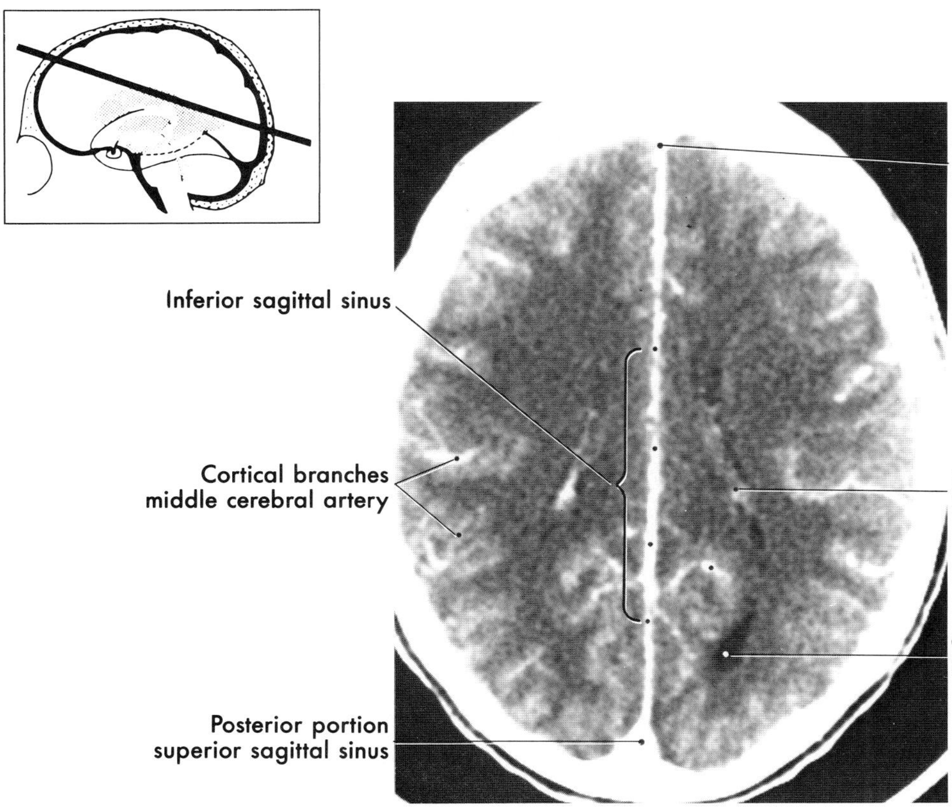

Figure 13-24

AXIAL CT SCANS OF CEREBRAL VESSELS

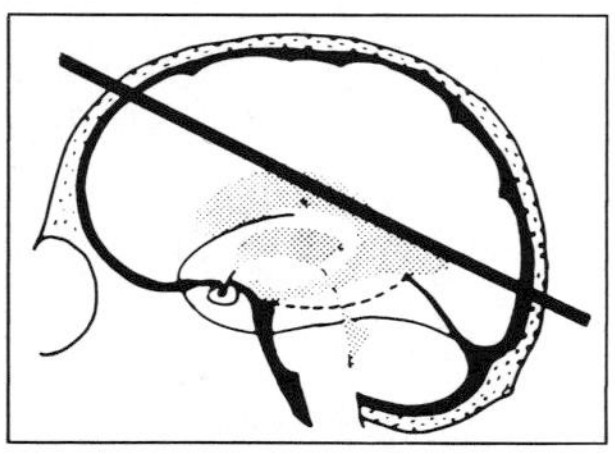

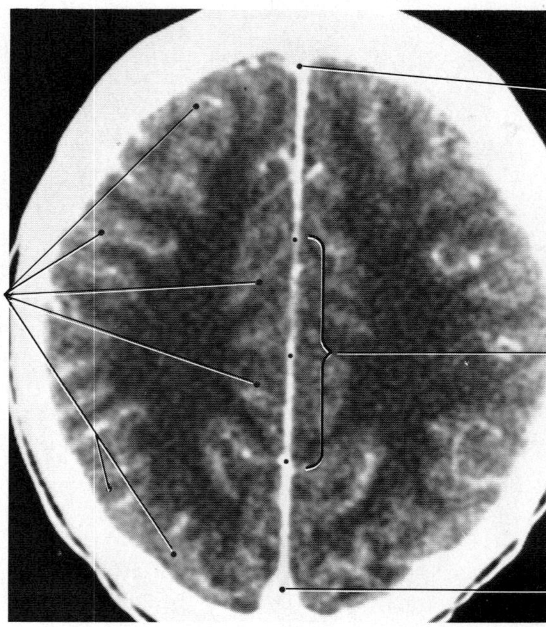

Figure 13-25

INDEX TO THE ILLUSTRATIONS

Entries refer to figures in which the specific structures are labeled.

CHAPTER 14

David A. Feinberg
Richard Ernest Wendt, III
Julie Wendt
L. Anne Hayman
Joel B. Kirkpatrick

Cerebral Vessels

IMAGING TECHNIQUES

Large Cerebral Vessels

Angiography

Conventional angiography remains the "gold standard" for many neuroradiologic diagnoses. This modality is particularly useful in determining the origin and degree of neovascularity in intracranial tumors and for mapping cerebral vessels for operative planning. Occasionally, angiography is needed to determine if a mass is within or outside the brain. Angiography continues to be useful when evaluating patients with vasospasm, intracerebral atherosclerotic disease, and vascular malformations.

The principal disadvantage of angiography is its invasiveness and potential morbidity. The incidence of complications has been reduced by the introduction of nonionic contrast media, advances in catheter and guide wire technology, and digital imaging.[1-4] Because of these innovations, modern neuroangiography is no longer a lengthy, painful procedure. In fact, it can now be performed in outpatients, thereby dramatically reducing cost.

Despite enhanced safety, the number of patients who require this examination has fallen each year because of improvements in vessel recognition with computed tomography (CT) and magnetic resonance imaging (MRI). *Doppler ultrasound* with color flow imaging for screening the cervical carotid artery at the bifurcation has reduced the number of normal carotid arteriograms performed.[5-8] This technique has replaced angiography in some medical centers. However, the inability of ultrasound to assess intracranial diseases limits its usefulness. The diagnostic criteria for carotid artery ultrasound are well established in the literature.[8] One should remember that this is a technically demanding technique that is machine and operator dependent.

The use of conventional neuroangiography may decline still further if technical advances in MR technology produce clinically useful, noninvasive angiograms. MR angiographic images would be able to depict moving blood and, theoretically, would not be limited to demonstrating only blood that contains a contrast agent.

Computed Tomography

Modern, thin-section CT images can detect focal mural calcifications in cerebral vessels. These have been associated with hemodynamically significant vascular stenosis in the vertebral arteries. Diffuse thickening and associated microscopic calcifications in the vascular wall of the horizontal portion of the middle cerebral artery can mimic the hyperdense appearance of intraluminal clot.[9,10] Intravascular clot within cortical veins and the dural sinuses can be reliably detected as an abnormally increased density on nonenhanced CT scans.[11] The cerebral arteries and veins may also be abnormally dense in patients who have increased blood viscosity (hematocrit greater than 60%).[12]

For most purposes, CT evaluation of cranial vasculature requires intravenous (IV) infusion of iodinated contrast material. The dose of contrast medium, the speed with which it is given, and the time elapsed between injection and scan all influence CT's ability to image vessels. In general, an iodinated contrast agent given rapidly, immediately before imaging, shows the vascular detail per se to best advantage. If the CT images cannot be obtained rapidly and vascular anatomy is clinically important, the initial contrast bolus (approximately 40 g iodine) can be supplemented by a drip infusion of contrast agent to replace the amount continually lost through renal excretion. Most modern CT scanners can now attain speeds that render a supplemental contrast injection unnecessary.

Absence of the normal IV contrast medium–induced hyperdensity in a large cerebral artery or the superior sagittal sinus indicates focal clot within the vascular lumen. This has been called the *delta sign* when it is seen in the sagittal sinus.[13] Arteries that contain clot do not always exhibit this absence of contrast medium–induced enhancement.

Magnetic Resonance Imaging

Clinical MRI routinely visualizes flowing blood in the larger cranial vessels (greater than 1 mm diameter) without IV contrast enhancement. The signal intensity of vessels on routine clinical MR images is variable because (1) each pulse sequence has different technical factors that can influence the appearance of flowing blood; (2) the blood flow in a given individual may vary during the time span of an MR examination; and (3) the technique is prone to a variety of artifacts that are specific for the imaging sequence chosen. Several simple physical concepts and terms help to explain why intracranial vessels appear as they do on MR images. The appearance of large vessels on spin-echo images and gradient-echo clinical images is discussed next. A separate third section describes the developing MR angiographic sequences.

SPIN ECHO SEQUENCES. The spin-echo (SE) technique is used to create the brain images used in routine clinical practice. Before the reader can understand why cerebral vessels have a variable appearance on SE images, it is necessary to review how this MR image is obtained. All typical SE pulse sequences consist of four basic steps: excitation, spatial encoding, measurement, and recovery. These are repeated over and over until all the information needed for an image has been acquired. The duration of these four basic steps is called the *repetition time* (TR). The SE sequence first uses a 90-degree radiofrequency (RF) pulse to excite the spins within the imaging plane. This rotates their axis of rotation 90 degrees with respect to their equilibrium orientation (which is parallel to the static magnetic field). To refocus the spins, another RF pulse, the 180-degree pulse, is used (Figure 14-1). In the presence of intravascular flow, the 180-degree RF pulse in effect encodes the spatial location of the spins.[14] A spin must be affected by *both* of the RF pulses to contribute a signal to the MR image. The time interval from the 90-degree RF pulse to the center of the SE signal is called the *time of echo,* or *echo delay time* (TE). The SE signal is measured, digitized, and stored by the imager during the readout (measurement) period. The fourth step, the recovery time, allows the spins in the slice to relax (to a greater or lesser extent depending on their T1 parameters) in the longitudinal axis, which is the direction of the static magnetic field. A number (typically 128, 192, or 256) of such signals are used to encode the *phase axis* of the image, produced by a *two-dimensional Fourier transform* (2DFT).

The clinician can manipulate both TR and TE to create T1 (longitudinal relaxation time), T2 (transverse relaxation time), or proton density contrast between normal and abnormal tissues. In clinical practice, three SE images are desirable. A short TR/short TE gives a T1-weighted image. A long TR/short TE gives a proton-density-weighted image. A long TR/long TE gives a T2-weighted image. The proton-density-weighted and T2-weighted images, both of which use a long TR, are usually acquired together in a *double-echo* sequence.

On SE images, the vascular lumen almost always appears darker than surrounding brain ("black blood") because no signal is detected from flowing blood (Figure 14-2). This happens because, in most patients, the flow in the vessel is fast enough (10 cm/second or longer) to remove physically the excited spins of the blood from the imaging slice before the refocusing (180-degree) pulse occurs (see Figure 14-1). This escape of blood from the imaging slice has been termed a *time-of-flight effect*. It causes what has been termed *high-velocity signal loss*. These terms do not apply to blood that travels within (but does not leave) the imaging slice during SE imaging.[1]

Flowing blood that travels within the imaging plane has a diminished signal because of *dephasing* or defocusing of its net signal. Also, the flow velocities vary between systole and diastole during the cardiac cycle, and in the absence of cardiac gating (see following discussion), further destructive phase interference results with the combining of signals in the image construction process. A loss of intensity from the lumen results when signals from different spin velocities within a voxel destructively interfere or cancel each other.

Occasionally, cerebral vessels will appear brighter than brain on SE images. This has been called the *in-flow phenomenon, flow-related vascular enhancement,*[1] or *paradoxic enhancement*.[3] It can be caused by two mechanisms. First, this enhancement occurs when the flow in a vessel that is perpendicular to the image slice is slower than a few centimeters per second. In these circumstances, little motion of the fully magnetized spins exists between the two pulses of the SE sequence (i.e., TE), but the time between pulses (i.e., TR) is sufficient to allow significant replacement of saturated blood by fresh blood. This gives the appearance of a shorter T1 interval for flowing blood than for stationary blood.

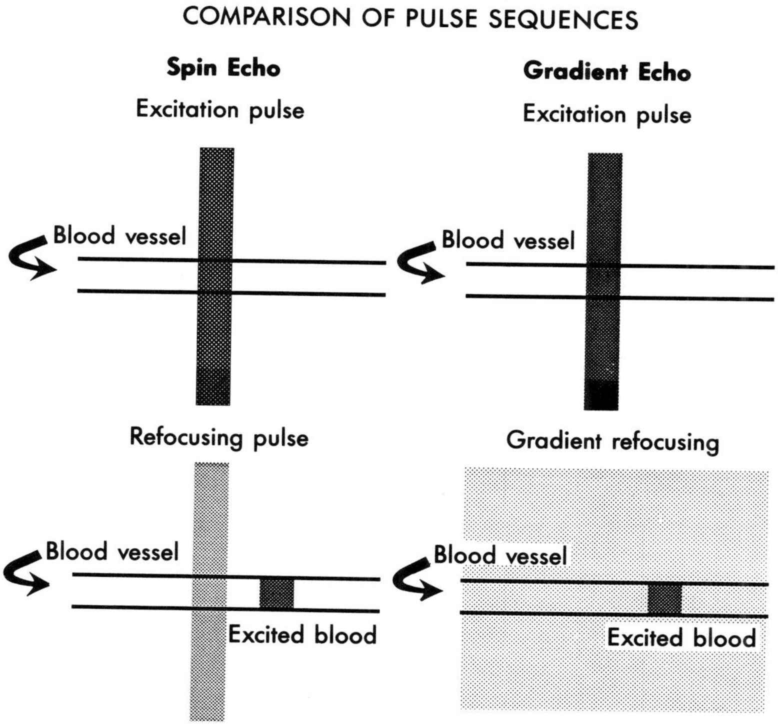

Figure 14-1 Comparison of effects of spin-echo (SE) and gradient-echo (GE) MR sequences on a bolus of flowing blood. The excitation of the bolus is the same for both sequences, as shown in the top row. The SE sequence employs a spatially selective pulse (*reader's lower left*) and thus misses the bolus that has flowed out of the slice. Therefore the vessel will appear dark. The GE sequence (*lower right*) refocuses all the spins in or out of the slice. (Only those that were excited contribute to the SE.) Thus, even though the bolus has flowed out of the slice, it can still contribute to the signal, and the vessel may appear bright on GE images.

Second, cerebral vessels also appear brighter than brain on SE images when blood *outside* the image volume that flows into the imaged slice during the pulse sequence appears brighter than brain. In clinical practice, many slices of the entire brain are obtained simultaneously so that this can only occur at the entry and exit margins of the stack of slices. This inflow of unsaturated blood can be avoided or manipulated to determine directionality of flow by using what have been termed *presaturation pulses*. These reduce the net magnetizations of the tissues above and below the area of interest so that inflowing spins do not produce high-magnitude signals.

Thus far we have discussed (1) diminution of signal intensity caused by high-velocity flow through the image slice, (2) destructive interference of signal caused by flow variables within (or through) the slice, and (3) flow-related or paradoxic vascular enhancement. It is also possible, however, for signal from an artery to be affected by cardiac variations. The pulse sequence randomly samples flow in the cardiac cycle when there is slow flow (diastole) or fast flow (midsystole). The final image is a summation or average of these signals. The vessel, therefore, has an unpredictable signal intensity. This can be overcome by use of *cardiac gating* (synchronization to one point in the cardiac cycle), which forces the TR of the pulse sequence to be equal to an integral number of heartbeats. In cardiac-gated images, diastolic-phase blood and systolic-phase blood may appear bright and dark, respectively, rather than an average, gray, intermediate intensity.

Other techniques used in clinical practice to reduce the effects of flow in vessels have been termed *motion compensating gradients*,[15] *motion artifact suppression technique* (MAST),[16] and *gradient moment nulling*.[17] These techniques use additional gradients to prevent dephasing of the signal from the blood. They are complementary to cardiac gating and are best used for short TR/TE sequences. They cannot completely prevent signal loss in areas of turbulent flow.

GRADIENT ECHO SEQUENCES. Gradient echo (GE), or gradient-refocused echo (GRE), is another type of pulse sequence that can be used clinically to generate images of the brain and its vessels. This sequence uses only one RF pulse (which typically rotates the vector of magnetization less than 90 degrees from the field induced by the magnet). An image is generated without the use of the 180-degree pulse that is used for SE images. As with SE sequences, the time between pulse (TR) and the data acquisition from the echo (TE) can be varied by the imaging clinician. The capabilities of the MR scanner limit how much the TR can be shortened.

Several versions of these GE scans produce images much more quickly than SE sequences. These have been named by the acronyms FLASH, FISP, FFE, FAST and CE-FAST, and GRASS, and all are considered fast T1-weighted MR techniques. Images generated using these techniques usually show vessels with flowing blood to be brighter than brain (Figure 14-3).

Blood inside vessels that course perpendicularly through a slice often appears more intense on GE images than on SE images. The mechanism that accounts for the effect of flow on image intensity in SE images is both inflow phenomena and nonselective gradient refocusing. The signal of flowing blood is increased because of the inflow of fully magnetized blood into the slice of interest. In contrast, tissues that remain in the slice have diminished signal because of their short TR recovery time.

The GE sequence also refocuses high-velocity blood that leaves the image plane because the gradient is experienced over the entire body. This "global" refocusing is dissimilar to SE images, where any blood that leaves the slice after the 90-degree excitation does not experience the slice-selective 180-degree pulse. Thus the blood that has flowed out of the slice is not refocused to form an echo (Figure 14-1).

Additional mechanisms contribute to the high intensity of flowing blood in GE images. First, an even larger contrast is possible between the inflow of unsaturated blood into a slice and the greatly saturated stationary tissue because of the short TR. As discussed, a GE sequence cannot discriminate between blood that remains within a particular slice and blood that has left that slice. All the blood inside the slice at the time of the RF pulse contributes to the measured signal, even if it has flowed into another slice at the time of measurement.

GE imaging substantially reduces the streaking artifact caused by blood flow in SE images, especially in the arteries. The streaking arises from differences in the speed of blood flow during each of the sequential TR intervals. Even when it is used, cardiac synchronization does not remove all the variabilities in speed. These variations in speed produce variations in signal phase from cycle to cycle, just as phase encoding of spatial position is also accomplished by inducing phase shifts that vary from cycle to cycle. Thus motion can introduce erroneous phase shifts that mislead the reconstruction algorithm. Consequently, flow-related artifacts are visualized on the image axis that is phase encoded (Figure 14-4).

The phase shifts arising from motion greatly increase with the length of TE (those from constant velocity increase as the square of TE, those from constant accelera-

A

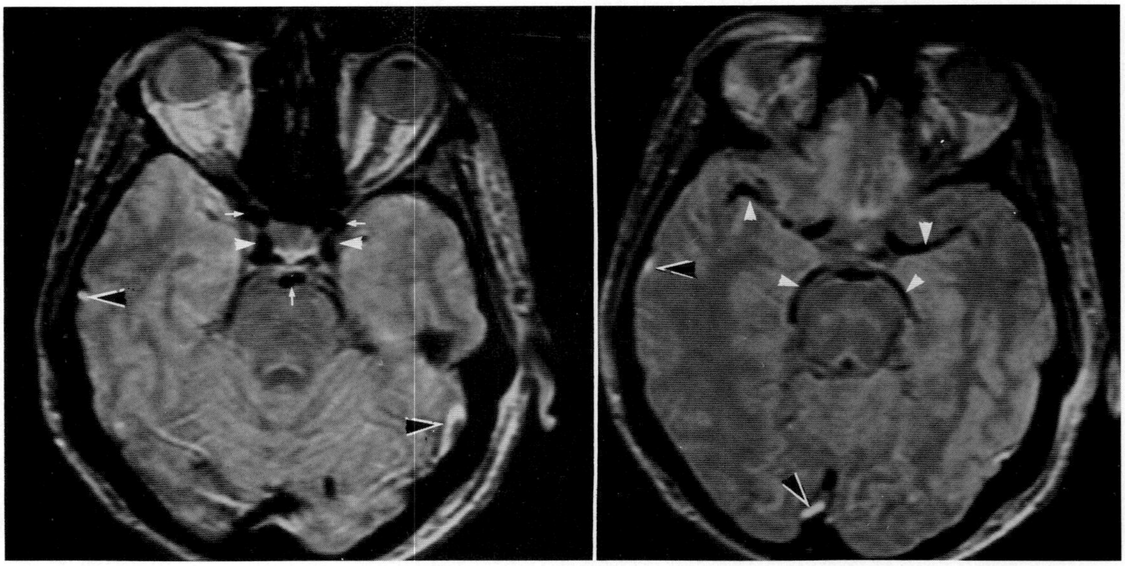

B

Figure 14-2 Spin-echo MR images (TR/TE, 800/20 msec) show absence of signal in some cranial vessels. This is caused by MR signal loss in presence of high-velocity blood flow. Such signal void occurs from *time-of-flight effects* in vessels that are *perpendicular to the scan plane* (*white arrows*). A second flow effect, the variable velocities within the lumina of vessels *within the scan plane*, produces the signal loss seen in the lumen of these vessels (*white arrowheads*). Slow flow in surface veins has a hyperintense signal (*black arrowheads*).

tion increase as the cube of TE, etc.). Thus it is highly desirable to use a short TE to reduce flow-related artifacts. The GE pulse sequences can achieve echo times as short as 3 to 7 msec (compared with 12 to 22 msec for the minimum TEs of SE sequences) and thus can significantly reduce the smearing and ghosting artifacts resulting from phase-encoding errors in the data.

ANGIOGRAPHIC SEQUENCES. MR angiography is a rapidly developing technique that has recently become available commercially. It seems most likely that MR angiography will be used in conjunction with routine SE imaging.[4,18] However, investigators are developing pulse sequences that give a T1-weighted three-dimensional (3D) data set with bright vessels and thus reduce the need for a complete SE study.

3D data sets for angiographic reconstructions can be produced either by 3D Fourier transform (3DFT) methods or by contiguous 2DFT multislice techniques. Given the interrelationships among blood velocity, slice thickness, and time between excitation and refocusing pulses, the most successful approaches to date have been 3D acquisitions for faster flow and sequential 2D acquisitions for slower flow. One must be aware that vessels with slow flow running in the plane of the image may not be seen well with either technique.

The future holds the prospect of smaller voxel sizes and thus improved resolution and detection of smaller vessels. Quantitative techniques that combine an angiographic de-

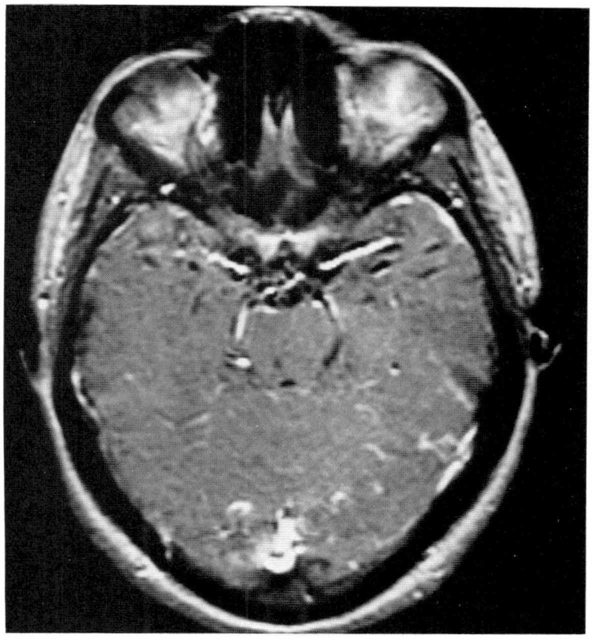

Figure 14-3 Gradient-echo MR images with bright blood. The signal from blood is high because of constant inflow of nonmagnetized spins that have not experienced the previous in-plane RF pulses. The GE technique refocuses spins that have moved downstream, out of the excitation plane. The stationary brain tissue produces low signal intensity because of the experienced short TR interval.

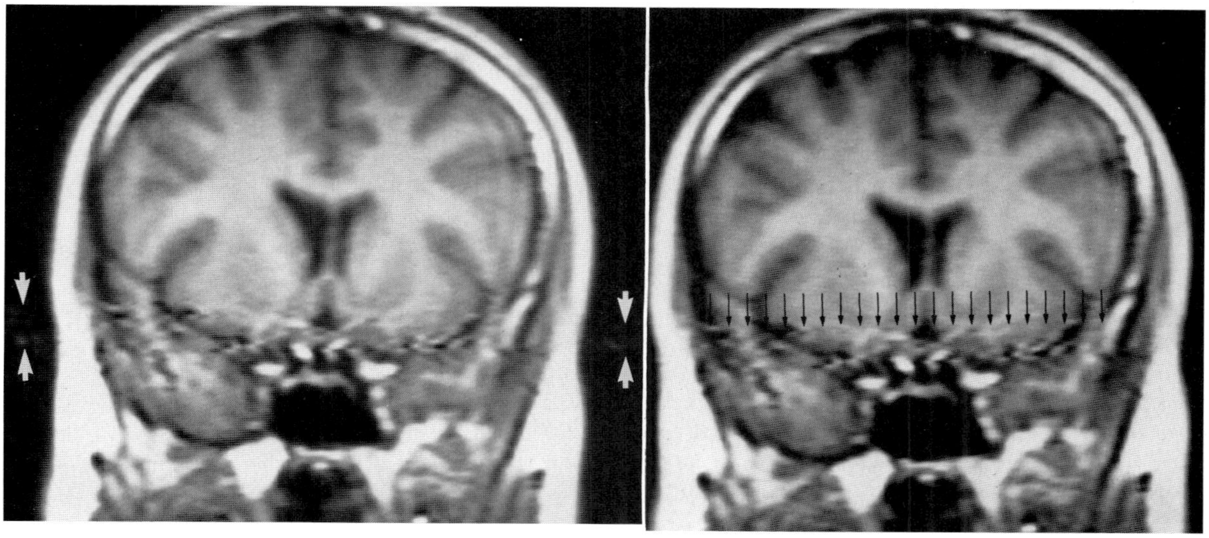

Figure 14-4 Spin-echo coronal MR images (TR/TE, 200/15). **A,** Window settings are adjusted to show streak artifact, which extends beyond the head (*arrows*). This artifact is created by flow in the carotid arteries. **B,** Clinical window settings are used to minimize the extracranial portion of the artifact. Note that the distortion in the adjacent brain is still present (*below the row of arrows*).

piction with accurate velocity or volumetric flow information are under development. To be useful, any new techniques must accurately detect vessel patency and cross-sectional area of the lumen (i.e., the size of stenoses).

The first step in producing MR angiograms is to enhance the contrast between the vessels and their surrounding tissue, either by making blood "bright" (using inflow phenomena) or "dark" (using outflow and/or dephasing phenomena). This is done by creating a 3D MR data set of the brain and vessels, which is then manipulated to separate the vessels (which contain moving blood) from the brain (which is relatively stationary). The contrast between vessels and brain may already be adequate in a "bright blood" acquisition; if necessary, however, contrast may be enhanced by subtracting a "dark blood" data set to reduce the intensity of the stationary tissue. Another way to identify the vessels in the 3D MR data set is to allow the motion of blood flow to alter the phase of the signal, known as *phase-contrast* angiography.

Once the vessels are identified in the MR data set, they can be displayed in the standard angiographic views (i.e., anteroposterior, lateral, and base positions) and in others if necessary (Figures 14-5 and 14-6).

These MR angiograms are easier to interpret than the raw data, which can only be displayed as multiple, sequential, orthogonal images. In the MR angiogram, tortuous vessels can be traced more easily, and the vascular anatomy is projected in a format familiar to imaging clinicians (i.e., similar to conventional angiograms). One should remember, however, that information is lost when MR angiograms are formed. Therefore clinical interpretation of these studies will probably require a careful scrutiny of differing projection images, since MR angiograms often underestimate the caliber of arteries with "unusual" flow, and since the images currently available do not depict small vessels well.[19]

GADOLINIUM ENHANCEMENT. The first contrast agent approved by the Food and Drug Administration for MRI was gadolinium diethylenetriaminepentaacetic acid (Gd-DTPA).[20] The incidence of serious side effects from this agent has thus far been low,[21] perhaps because only small doses of Gd^{+3} (0.5 to 2.9 g) have been administered intravenously. However, patients with renal failure may not be able to excrete the compound, so particular caution has been advised with this group.

The molecular weight and biodistribution of present MR contrast agents are similar to those of the iodinated contrast materials used for conventional angiography. Other paramagnetic metal ion chelates (Gd-DOTA, Gd-DOBA) are under development.[22] These are more stable, have better MR relaxation characteristics, and may become the preferred agents.

All these paramagnetic contrast agents act indirectly to cause contrast enhancement by altering the local magnetic environment, thereby facilitating proton T1 and T2 relaxation. Zones that accumulate contrast agent become brighter on short TR/short TE images. The normal appearance of vessels on a Gd-enhanced MR study is illustrated in Figure 14-7, *A*. Unfortunately, the increase in vessel signal on these enhanced scans can be associated with exaggerated motion artifacts, which are caused by pulsation of the cerebral vessels (Figure 14-7, *B*). It has been suggested that MAST be used to reduce these artifacts.

The IV administration of gadolinium produces enhancement (i.e., hyperintense signal) on T1-weighted images *only* in vessels that have slow flow. Thus the arterial flow appears as a hypointense flow void (see preceding sections). MR angiography techniques that use 3D reconstructions of the venous structures can be augmented by the administration of Gd. The separation of slow from fast flow on Gd-enhanced MR images is clinically useful in predicting regions of acute (less than 26 hours old) cortical cerebral infarction, since this separation demonstrates abnormal enhancement in *cortical* arteries that have greatly slowed collateral circulation. This technique cannot, however, detect basal ganglia infarctions.[23]

Cerebral Perfusion (Microcirculation)

Various techniques have been developed to measure cerebral blood flow (CBF); some are less useful than others. They have been used clinically to identify seizure foci, manage cerebrovascular occlusive disease, and predict the neurologic sequelae after transient or permanent carotid artery occlusions.

The advantages and disadvantages of each technique have been recently reviewed.[24] The following sections briefly discuss several of these techniques: xenon-enhanced CT, single-photon emission CT (SPECT), and MR perfusion imaging. Absolute quantitative measurement of CBF is currently performed using probe measurements with xenon-133 or *positron emission tomography* (PET). These procedures have restricted clinical use because they require specialized equipment.

The clinical role of PET continues to evolve and is likely to increase in the future. At present, PET plays an important role in research and as a standard with which other clinical imaging modalities can be compared. PET imaging allows for absolute quantification of CBF using various radionuclides. These are incorporated into physiologically important substances, such as oxygen-15 incorporated into carbon dioxide and fluorine-18 incorporated into fluorodeoxyglucose (FDG). Versatile PET scanners achieve spatial resolution in the range of 3 mm (full-width at half-maximum), but high resolution is achieved at the expense of other characteristics, such as temporal and contrast resolution.[25] PET scanners achieve spatial resolution in the range of 1.0 to 1.7 cm, depending on the mode (high resolution vs. dynamic) of image acquisition used.[26] At present, PET is only available in specialized medical institutions, since the production of positron-emitting radionuclides is complex and often requires on-site production with a cyclotron.[27]

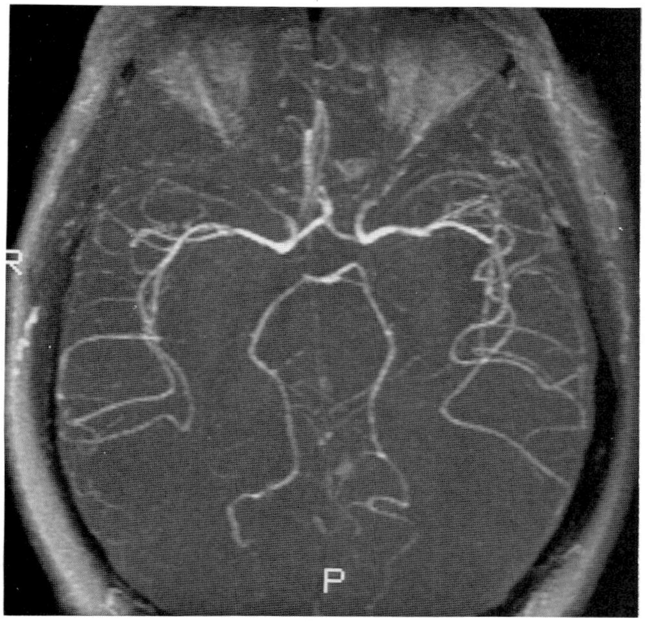

Figure 14-5 3D time-of-flight, axial MR arteriographic base view (bright blood using maximum intensity projection [MIP] algorithm) of the cerebral arteries at the circle of Willis.

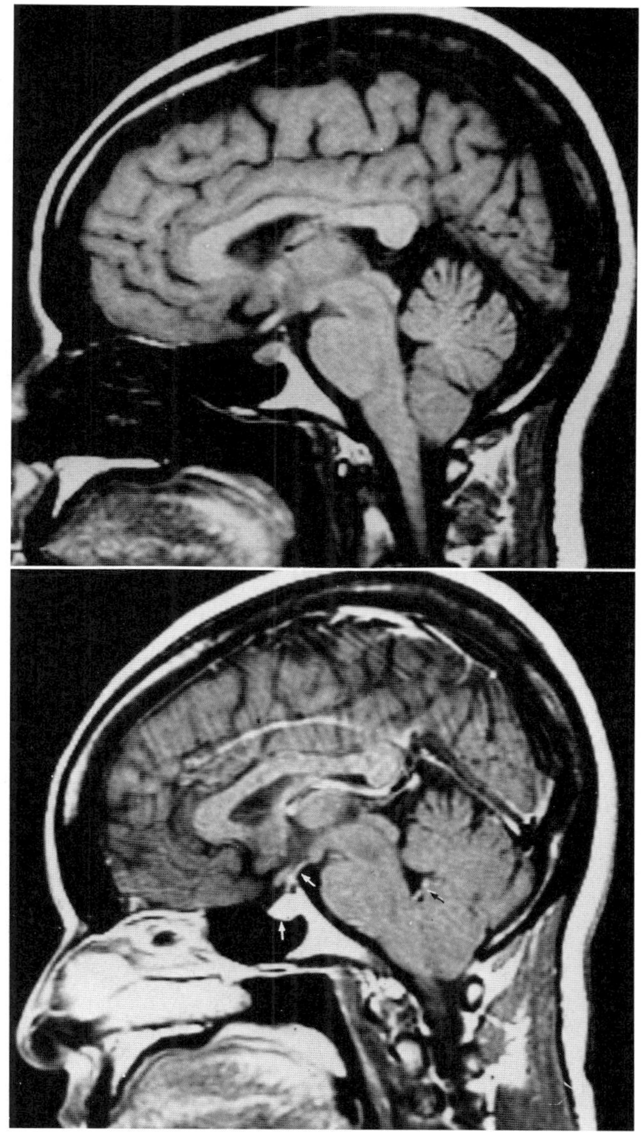
A

B

Figure 14-7 Sagittal MR images (800/20) before **(A)** and after **(B)** intravenous gadolinium (Gd) injection. Gd enhancement increases the signal intensity of the blood within vessels with slow flow (i.e., superior and inferior sagittal sinuses and internal cerebral veins). This intensifies the motion artifacts produced by pulsation of these vessels (note linear artifacts in **B** compared with **A**). Contrast enhancement is also seen in the choroid plexus of the fourth ventricle (*black arrow*), pituitary stalk and gland (*white arrows*), and the nasal mucosa.

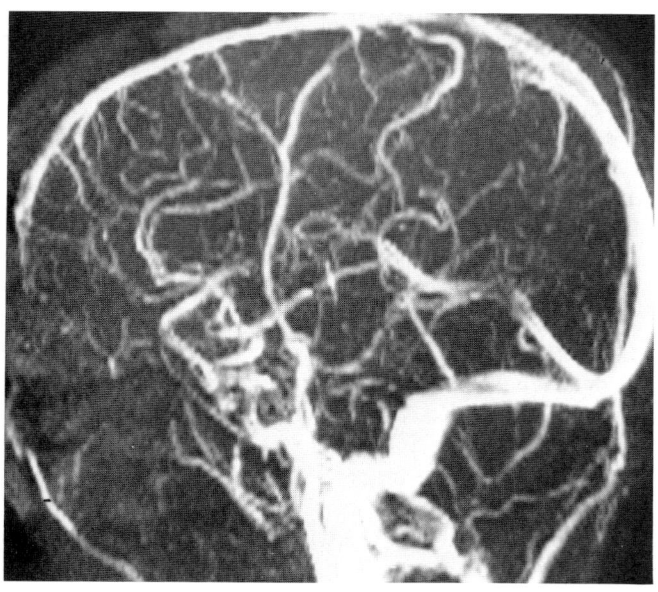

Figure 14-6 2D time-of-flight, MR angiogram of normal cerebral veins in lateral projection. Axial gradient-recalled-echo scans (50/9, 60-degree flip angle, slice thickness of 1.5 mm, without presaturation pulse). A 3D reprojection was obtained using a maximum intensity projection (MIP) postprocessing algorithm. (Courtesy Orest B. Boyko, Duke University Medical Center, Durham, NC.)

Computed Tomography

IODINATED CONTRAST MEDIA. Several authors have proposed using rapid-sequence CT scans to evaluate CBF following the IV injection of iodinated contrast material.[28,29] Their calculations assumed that the contrast medium was a *nondiffusible* indicator (i.e., it remained within the vessel lumen). However, serial temporal measurements of the CT attenuation coefficient in brain indicate that a small portion of the contrast medium normally leaks out of the cerebral vessels. This occurs independent of the osmolarity of the medium and probably results from the liposolubility of the agent.[30] This leakage prevents the use of iodinated IV contrast medium for reliably measuring cerebral blood volume or CBF.

Iodine contrast–enhanced CT can, however, provide a rough estimate of *cerebral perfusion,* which may be useful in detecting large infarctions in zones of gray matter (i.e., these areas will not show a normal increase in density) (see Chapter 13). This technique is usually not needed, since the current generation of CT scanners can detect cortical infarctions by imaging subtle density changes in the cortex caused by edema formation. Recent reports indicate that the insular cortex becomes isodense compared with white matter as early as 6 hours after middle cerebral artery infarction.[31]

NONRADIOACTIVE XENON. Various investigators have used CT scans after patient inhalation of xenon in an attempt to measure CBF. This technique requires patients to place a gas mask over their mouth and nose. The mask must fit tightly enough to prevent air leaks, which would dilute the inhalation of a gas containing 25% to 30% xenon and/or contaminate the measurement of exhaled xenon. In addition, the patient must remain absolutely motionless while a minimum of five CT scans are performed at a single axial level over 5 to 7 minutes.[32] Given these requirements, it is not surprising that 20% of patients cannot tolerate this procedure.[24]

Several other problems interfere with use of xenon CT to quantify CBF.[24,32,33] The most serious is that the xenon itself significantly increases the velocity of blood flow. The effects of this change cannot be corrected mathematically because it varies unpredictably between individuals. In addition, the size of the region of interest (ROI) sampled must be large enough to overcome sampling error. Thus blood flow is calculated for regions that contain both gray and white matter, each of which has physiologically different CBFs. This causes the CBF numbers to reflect the mixture of tissues, with varying CBFs in the ROI, rather than the correct CBF for white and gray matter.[24]

Single-Photon Emission Computed Tomography (SPECT)

Planar imaging of cerebral perfusion using radionuclides was largely replaced by x-ray CT in the 1970s. Currently, the most frequent indication for planar radionuclide brain imaging is the evaluation of cerebral death. With a mobile gamma camera, planar cerebral scintiangiography is easily performed in the intensive care unit. Technetium-99m-labeled agents such as pertechnetate, DTPA, and glucoheptanate are most often used. Quantitative measurements of CBF are *not* obtained with these methods. They provide a qualitative measure of cerebral *perfusion*.

Absolute quantification of CBF can be obtained with xenon-133 (^{133}Xe) probe measurements without arterial sampling, but the patient must be able to cooperate for the ^{133}Xe inhalation procedure. Probe measurements do not provide cerebral images. SPECT imaging with this agent is possible but requires a dedicated gamma camera capable of rapid, dynamic image acquisition. ^{133}Xe SPECT images have poor spatial resolution compared with images obtained with newer radiopharmaceuticals developed for SPECT imaging.

Radiopharmaceuticals for SPECT imaging with high blood-brain barrier permeability and uptake in the *normal* brain that is proportional to regional CBF became available in the 1980s. The two frequently used clinical agents are *iodine-123* (^{123}I) *isopropyl iodoamphetamine* (IMP) and *technetium-99m* (^{99m}Tc) *hexamethyl-propyleneamine oxime* (HM-PAO). An additional agent, *^{99m}Tc ethyl cysteinate dimer* (ECD), is likely to be approved for clinical use in the near future. Each of these agents has certain advantages based on characteristics of uptake and redistribution in the brain and other tissues, as well as on characteristics of the radionuclide label itself.[27,34] None of them provides the absolute quantification of CBF as is obtained with PET and ^{133}Xe probe measurements. With these agents, comparison of regional count densities between the symmetric areas of the brain allows for semiquantitative analysis of regional CBF. Because the uptake of these agents depends on metabolic processes, SPECT images of brain lesions often show a greater extent of derangement than do CT studies, which depend on structural derangement. Spatial resolution is comparable among these radiopharmaceuticals and depends, in part, on the type of imaging system used. Resolution varies from approximately 0.7 to 1.6 cm full-width at half-maximum.[34,35] Adequate brain SPECT images are obtained with the standard, single-head rotating gamma cameras typically used in nuclear medicine facilities. These images require 30 to 40 minutes of acquisition time. Dedicated multidetector systems have much shorter image acquisition times and better spatial resolution, and the chance of error being introduced in the process of image reconstruction is reduced (Figure 14-8).

Qualitative imaging of *cerebral perfusion* can be obtained by administering an IV injection of radionuclide.[36] A recent review of regional CBF measurements compared ^{123}I-IMP–enhanced, ^{133}Xe-enhanced, and ^{99m}Tc-HM-PAO–enhanced SPECT images in a group of 24 patients. The results of this comparison are summarized in the following discussion.[24]

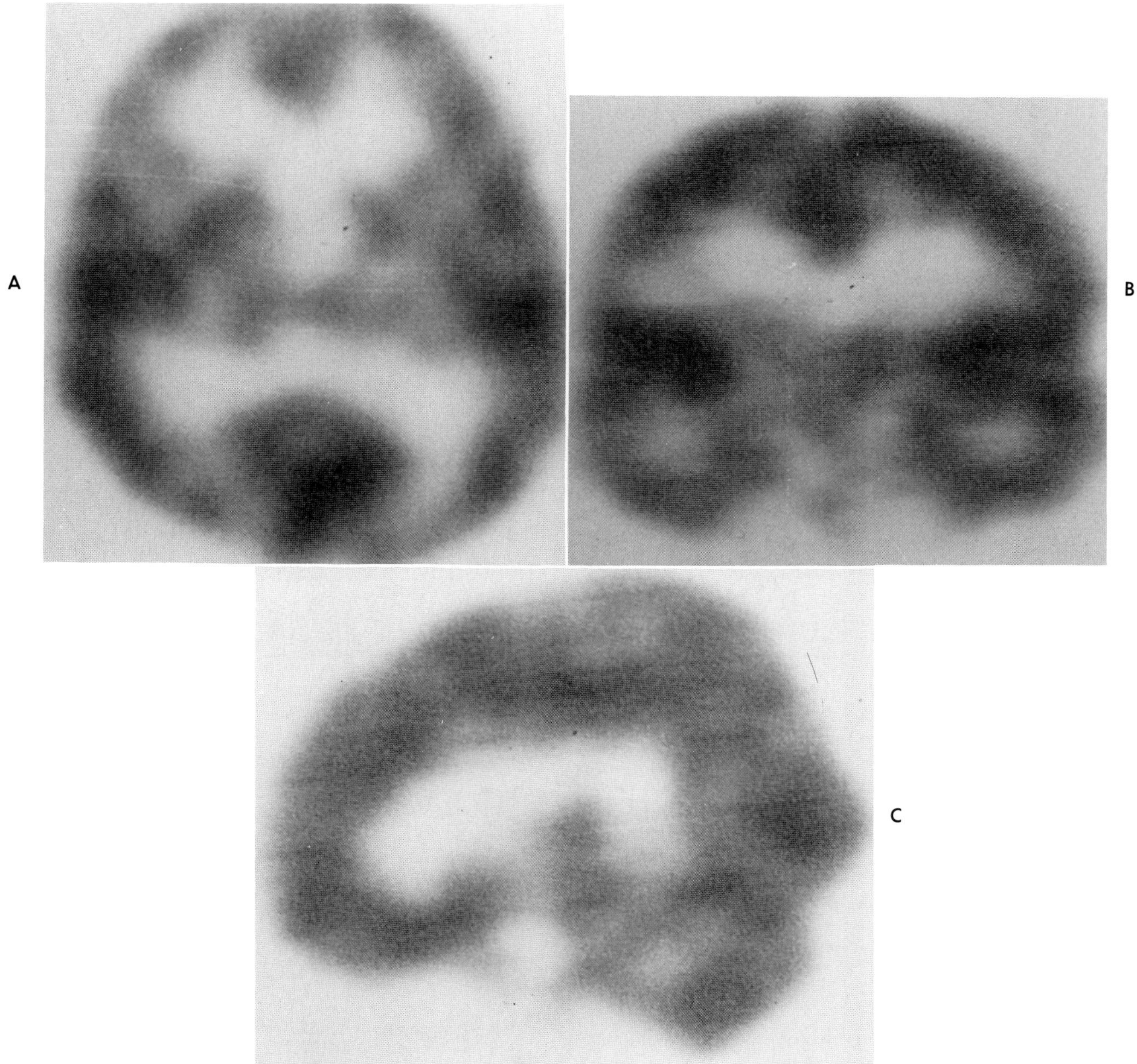

Figure 14-8 Technetium-99m HM-PAO SPECT images of *normal* cerebral blood flow in axial **(A)**, coronal **(B)**, and sagittal **(C)** projections. Note the symmetric hemispheric signal. If regional decreases or absence of signal were present, they would indicate *relative* perfusion deficits. (Courtesy Lamk M. Lamki, University of Texas Health Science Center, Houston.).

IODINE-123 IMP SPECT. This agent was considered superior to SPECT studies that use ^{99m}Tc-HM-PAO and ^{133}Xe to detect cortical perfusion deficits. Although this technique is only qualitative, it has a high degree of patient acceptance and is easily obtained in the clinical setting. Tomograms of the brain after IV injection of ^{123}I-IMP should be taken within 10 minutes to maximize the distinction between gray and white matter areas in the brain. However, since only minimum redistribution occurs in the first hour after administration, clinically useful images may be obtained during this time frame. Images obtained 4 hours after injection are not clinically acceptable.[24]

XENON-133 SPECT. ^{133}Xe SPECT scans have poor spatial resolution and are therefore inferior to scans using other

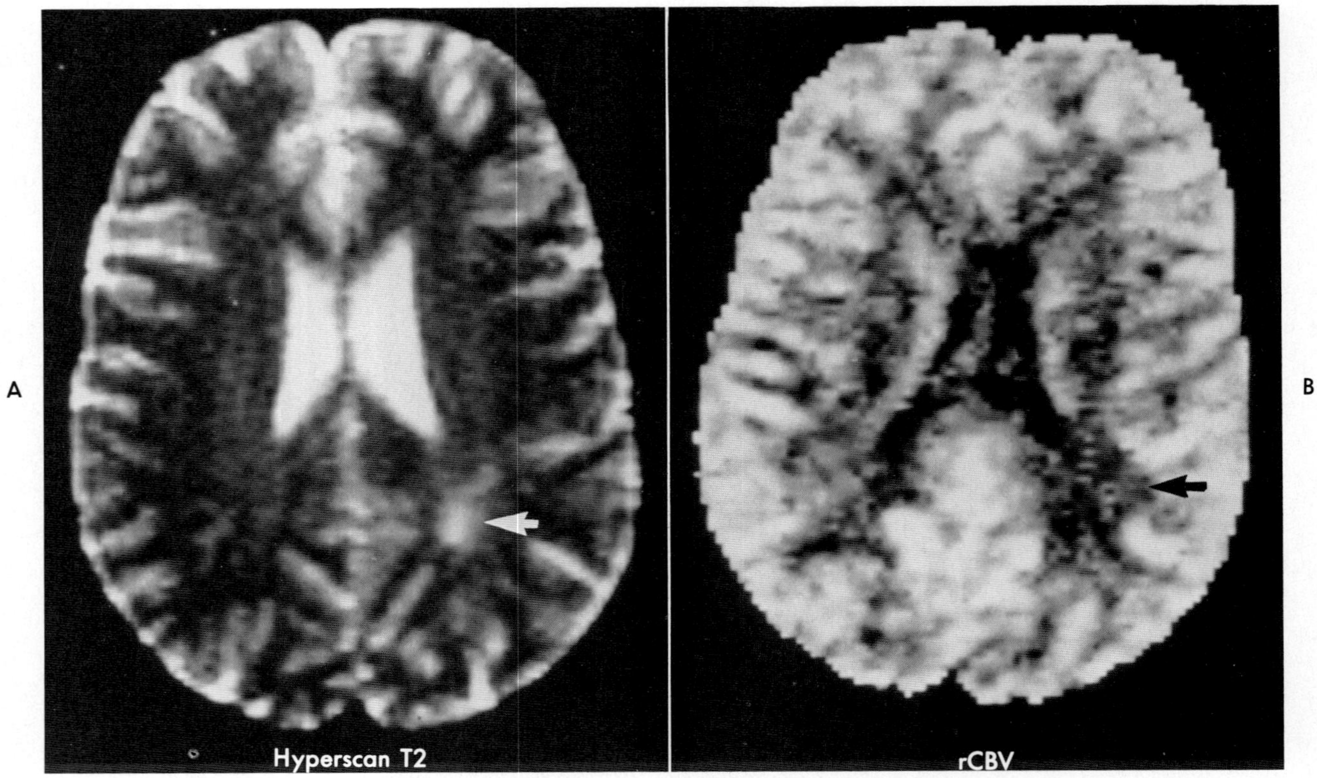

Figure 14-9 **A,** Axial echo-planar T2-weighted MR image shows a hyperintense signal in the posterior right centrum ovale (*arrow*). This area was unchanged on a 1-year follow-up image. **B,** Perfusion MR image (map of regional cerebral blood volume [rCBV]). Note the slightly decreased blood flow (*arrow*) in the same area noted in **A.** This is consistent with a metabolically inactive process. **B** was obtained after an IV bolus injection of 0.1 mmol/kg Gd-DTPA. A series of 60 images (one per second) was acquired over 1 minute using an echo-planar imaging technique. Magnetic susceptibility signal loss from the paramagnetic contrast agent's passage through the capillary bed was converted into a concentration-time curve. The area under this curve is calculated pixel by pixel and shown as an rCBV image. (Courtesy Bruce Rosen, Massachusetts General Hospital, Boston.)

agents for assessing cerebral perfusion. The accumulation of ^{133}Xe gas in the paranasal sinuses can obscure skull base lesions. In addition, the administration of this agent requires the patient to understand and comply with instructions. This limits its usefulness in many patients with cerebrovascular accident (CVA, stroke), despite the lower radiation dose delivered by this agent and the ability to perform serial ^{133}Xe SPECT examinations.[24]

TECHNETIUM-99m HM-PAO SPECT. This agent should only be used as a screening examination in emergency cases, since the presence of a significant amount of intravascular radioactivity can mask hypoperfused cortical areas. Tomograms of the brain after IV injection of ^{99m}Tc-HM-PAO demonstrate stable gray-white matter enhancement ratios within 10 minutes.[24] These persist for several hours (Figure 14-8).

Magnetic Resonance Perfusion Imaging

Recently, MR techniques have been proposed that may measure the fraction of MR signal arising within the lumina of brain capillaries containing actively flowing blood.[37-39] Preliminary multisection work has been done yielding images of brain with good spatial resolution by using cardiac gating. Noninvasive measurement of the microcirculation of the brain, once achieved clinically, could open new realms to research that can be expected directly to influence patient care. The techniques described make the basic assumption that no fluid is exchanged across the capillary walls during TE. Further research will be needed to determine if this is true. If not, the technique could still have clinical potential for measuring capillary permeability.[40]

The fundamental key to measuring diffusion with MRI is the reduction of signal intensity caused by signal cancellation within a voxel. When strong magnetic field gradients are applied and spins move in random directions (as might be the case in diffusive motion or some models of the microcirculation), there will be an incoherent addition (dispersion) of phase shifts within the pixel and a reduction of signal intensity, just as occurs in the vessels mentioned previously that contain a range of velocities (Figure 14-9). Very strong gradient pulses (0.5 to 1.0 gauss/cm or greater) with rather long durations (30 msec or more) are needed to achieve adequate sensitivity to very slow motion. These gradient-pulse methods of detecting slow blood movement are greatly hampered by the relatively small fraction of blood volume in the voxel, in which signal changes are often dominated by diffusion effects and noise.

Another promising class of pulse sequences that is sensitive to diffusion or slow motion is based on *steady-state free precession.* These sequences establish a steady-state magnetization of the spins by using a very short TR. The maintenance of the steady state requires identical conditions in each TR interval. Random motion violates this requirement, causing the pulse sequence to give a weaker signal in regions experiencing random motion.

NORMAL ANATOMY

Large Cerebral Vessels

Information concerning many of the features of the large cerebral vessels can be found in other chapters. Chapter 12 describes the arterial supply and venous drainage of the choroid plexuses. Chapter 13 describes the anatomic location of the cerebral and cerebellar vessels that can be seen by angiography. Chapter 15 summarizes the vascular displacements caused by cerebral masses. Chapter 16 describes the cerebral arteries as well as the structure and function of the regions they supply. This section describes the *arrangement* and *composition* of the major cerebral vessels.

The arteries that supply oxygenated blood to the brain are divided into a carotid and a vertebrobasilar system. The development of this arrangement in the fetus is illustrated in the frontal and lateral projections in Figure 14-10. This figure correctly illustrates that at this stage of development, all the intracranial arteries are on the surface of the brain. The later growth of the cerebral hemispheres over the brainstem and thalamus folds the proximal components of these arteries to the basal surface of the hemispheres to overlie the surface arteries of the thalamus (i.e., posterior choroidal). This causes some of these vessels to appear to be within the brain.

Since the growth of the vascular system only occurs in response to the presence of neural tissue, the mere presence of angiographically demonstrable cerebral vessels reliably testifies to the presence of neural tissue. This is clinically useful in the radiologic evaluation of children with midline neural tube defects. Angiography can be used in these patients to differentiate encephalocele, which contains brain and therefore is supplied by cerebral vessels, from meningocele, which does not.

The large arteries that supply the brain are structurally different from arteries in other parts of the body in many important ways.[41] The walls of cerebral vessels are considerably thinner because their media (smooth muscle) and adventitia are thinner. The vasa vasorum that supply other arteries are notably absent in nonatherosclerotic cerebral arteries. In addition, cerebral arteries are not supported by perivascular tissue; rather, they lie within the cerebrospinal fluid (CSF), which dampens the potentially damaging effects of their systolic pulsations.

A further difference in the cranial arteries can be found in the distribution of their elastic fibers. They are concentrated in the internal lamina rather than throughout the wall. This may help further to reduce pulsatile movements in the intracranial vessels.[41] The thickness of this internal elastic lining varies in thickness. It is thinnest at sites that receive the full force of the arterial pulsations (i.e., the outermost surface along a curve). Calcifications in the internal elastic lamina of the carotid siphon can be seen in normal children as young as 1 year of age if special staining techniques are used.[42] These intimal calcifications are thought to be caused by hemodynamic stresses along the outer surface of the vessel's curve. They are considered *primary calcifications,* which can be distinguished histologically from the secondary calcifications that occur in atherosclerotic intima.[42]

The caliber of a cerebral artery is governed by the volume of blood flowing through it. Thus reductions in blood flow caused by a distal vascular occlusion or a loss of metabolically active tissue will lead to a reduction in caliber of the cerebral artery supplying that region.

The cerebral veins are less rigid than arteries, and their walls are always much thinner. Most cerebral veins empty into the large venous sinuses found between the dural layers. The negative pressure that develops in these sinuses when the patient is erect or seated will enable development of a potentially fatal air embolus if they are inadvertently opened during neurologic surgery or by cranial trauma. The anatomy of the veins and sinuses at the skull base is of particular interest to those obtaining venous blood samples from the petrosal sinus, as may be obtained in patients with Cushing's syndrome.[43] The relevant anatomy is schematically illustrated in Figure 14-11.

Cerebral Microvessels

The microvasculature of the brain consists of the capillary bed, which is supplied by the terminal arterial branches (i.e., the arterioles) and the progressively larger series of venules that unite to form small veins. These vessels are too small to be seen individually by angiography. Rather, they appear as a *capillary blush* following the arterial phase of the arteriogram. An arteritic process con-

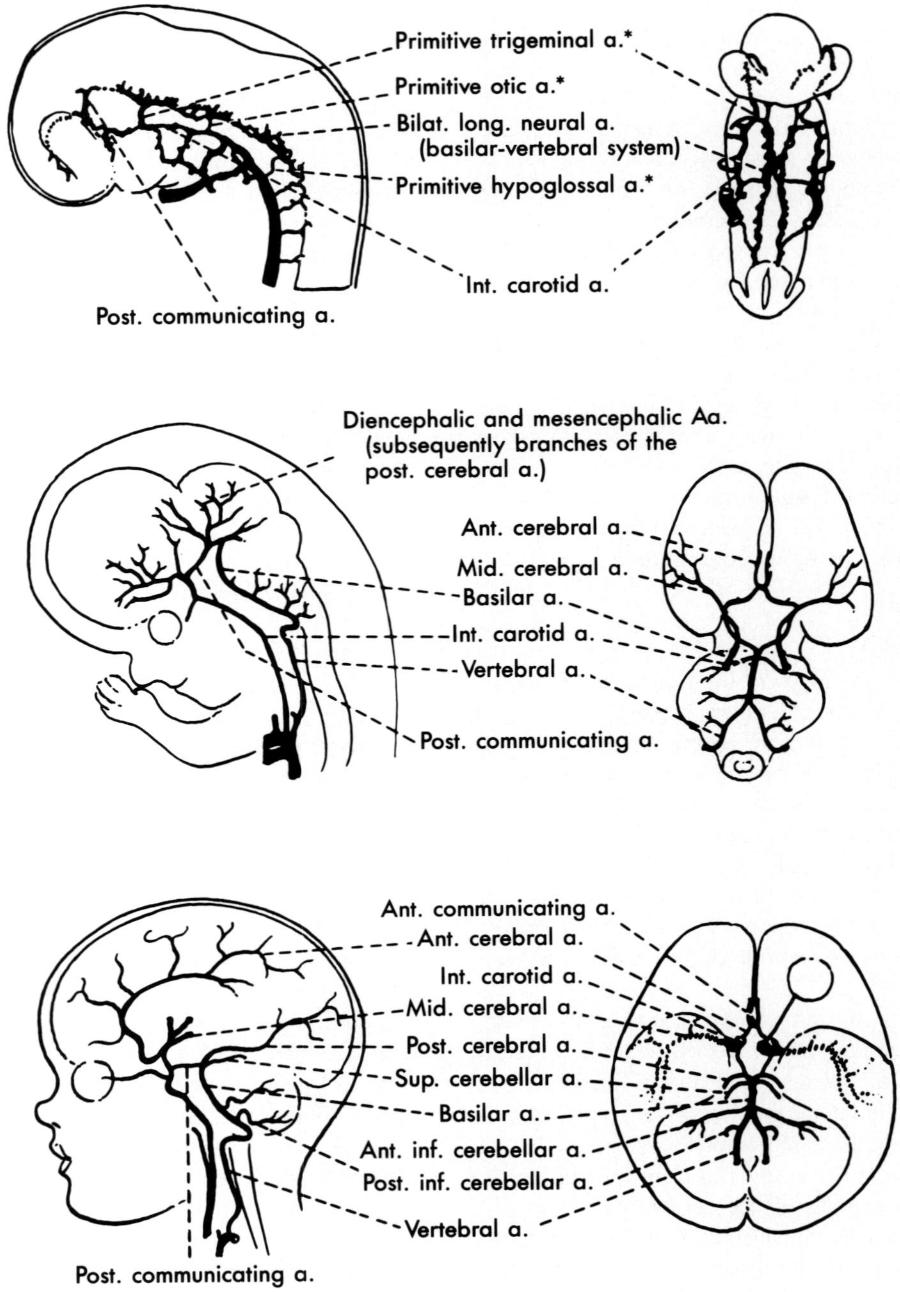

Figure 14-10 Companion schematic illustrations in frontal and lateral projections show the development of the carotid and vertebral systems. See text for details. (Reproduced with permission from Burger PC, Vogel LFS: Cerebrovascular disease: teaching monograph, *The American Association of Pathologists*, 1978.)

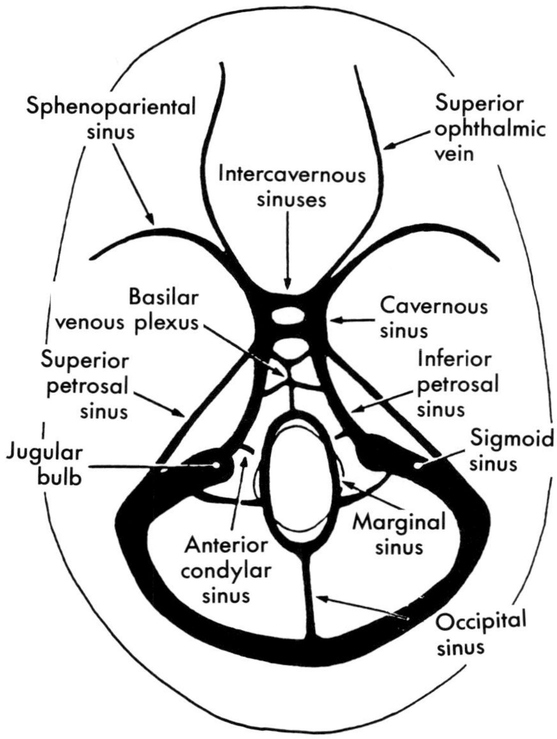

Figure 14-11 Schematic drawing of the skull base seen from above shows the venous sinuses in the skull base. Variations in this venous drainage pattern have been described. (Reproduced with permission from Miller DM, Doppman JL: *Radiology* 178:37-47, 1991.)

fined to these small vessels will, of course, not be detected by arteriography.

The brain tissue *immediately* surrounding these arterioles appears to derive its nutrients and oxygen from the arterioles rather than from the capillary network. A disturbance of the nurturing artery (which may be a normal consequence of aging) is thought to cause loss of brain substance with consequent enlargement of the perivascular space.[44] Generally, the normal artery and its perivascular space are invisible on CT and MR images; however, with current technology, one can visualize focally dilated perivascular spaces.[45,46] (These perivascular Virchow-Robin spaces are discussed in Chapter 11.) The points at which these arteries enter the brain are thought by some investigators to function as canaliculi joining the extracellular fluid space surrounding the neurons and glia with the CSF surrounding the brain itself. Other investigators note that the pia mater of the brain appears to join the basement membrane of the penetrating artery and thereby prevent communication between the CSF and the extracellular spaces of the brain.

The arrangement of cerebral arterioles and their lengths, sizes, and potential for collateral flow vary throughout the brain. These differences in microvascular construction are important because they probably explain why some regions are relatively resistant to ischemia and/or hypotension and others are vulnerable (Table 14-1).[47]

The centrum ovale and basal ganglia may be especially prone to lacunar infarctions because they are supplied by *long* arteries and arterioles which do *not* interdigitate. The increased length of the vessel theoretically exaggerates the intravascular pressure drop that occurs during episodes of hypotension. In addition, these arteries are selectively subject to narrowing from atherosclerosis (especially in patients with diabetes mellitus and hypertension) and other degenerative vascular conditions.[47]

Some researchers have postulated that the vascular supply to the centrum ovale is responsible for the "border zone" infarctions that surround the lateral ventricles. These areas have been referred to as *periventricular leukomalacia*. Recent work in the adult brain[47] and in fetal and childhood brains[48] has not verified the existence of a "border zone" of arterial supply in the centrum ovale.

Areas of the brain supplied by different parent arteries and with interdigitating arteriolar territories presumably provide collateral supply to each other and mutually protect the brain they supply from the potential complications of hypotension. Thus lacunar infarcts are not found in the white matter immediately beneath the cortex (i.e., the subcortical U fibers) or the external capsule–claustrum–extreme capsule area. These infarcts also occur infrequently in the corpus callosum or cortex, except at the border zones between major cerebral vessels. These areas are presumably spared because they are supplied directly from the overlying surface arterial and arteriolar pial plexus by *short* penetrating arterioles, which are usually not subject to atherosclerosis.

The peculiar microvascular architecture of the hippocampal region does not appear to be the cause of the selective neuronal loss that occurs in this region of the brain.[47,49] Instead, excessive stimulation by excitatory neurotransmitters is thought to trigger calcium entry, which kills the neurons in this brain region.[50]

Regardless of their microvascular patterns, almost all cerebral arteries and arterioles eventually enter the capillary bed, which also supplies nutrients and oxygen to the brain substance. Most investigators believe that the capillary network of the brain allows weak collateral flow from one arteriolar territory to the next.[47] Only the choroidal arteries appear to have direct connections to cerebral veins.[47] These connections may explain why large microspheres may be found in the venous sinuses following their injection into a carotid artery.

The capillaries of the brain are unlike those supplying nonneural tissues in that their endothelial cells restrict

◆ **TABLE 14-1** Six Patterns of Cerebral Hemispheric Microvascular Arteries and Arterioles

Microvascular pattern	Location	Risk
Short arterioles from a single source	Cortex	Anoxia (hypoperfusion at watershed)
Short-to-intermediate-length arteriole from a single source	Anterior two thirds of corpus callosum	—
Short-to-intermediate-length arterioles and arteries, dual source, with interdigitation of arterioles from different parent vessels	Subcortical U fibers	—
Intermediate-length arterioles and arteries, triple source, with interdigitation of arterioles from different parent vessels	Extreme/external capsule and claustrum	—
Long arteries and arterioles from a single source	Centrum ovale	Hypoperfusion
Large, long, muscular arteries from a single source	Thalamus, basal ganglia	Anoxia, hypoperfusion, rupture

Data from Moody DM, Bell MA, Challa VR: AJNR 11:431-439, 1990.

movement of many molecules from the lumen to the brain. This unique quality of capillary impermeability has been called the *blood-brain barrier* (bbb) and results from complex physiologic processes that have been summarized by Sage.[51] These features may be highlighted as follows. The microscopically observed association between astrocytes and cerebral capillaries appears to result in a unique, continuous basement membrane and "tightly" connected vascular endothelial cells.[52] The astrocytes appear virtually to eliminate the capacity of the cerebral capillary to carry material by vesicular transport or pinocytosis.[53] Others have noted a lack of enzymes in cerebral capillaries that alters the uptake of substances from blood.[54,55] Transport through the brain capillary endothelium (i.e., the bbb) is also regulated by dynamic inputs from pericytes and neurons.[56]

The bbb can be summarized by outlining the permeability of cerebral capillaries to various substances. The bbb prevents most protein-bound substances from entering the extracellular spaces of the brain. Lipid-soluble compounds pass easily and quickly through the bbb. It only allows small, water-soluble molecules to pass through the vessel wall if specific active or passive "transporter" mechanisms are in place. (Glucose enters the brain via passive transport across the bbb.)

The presence of a normal bbb prevents large amounts of iodinated contrast medium or Gd-DTPA from entering the brain. However, when a pathologic lesion is present, the bbb may be damaged, allowing extravascular accumulation of either contrast agent. The growth of new capillaries, which have not yet formed a bbb, occurs in regions of cerebral damage. These areas consequently will also show interstitial accumulation of contrast medium. Thus the orthogonal contrast-enhanced MR or CT image is "positive" only when the bbb is deficient.

There are small regions in the brain in which the capillary bbb is normally absent. Obviously, contrast enhancement in these areas should not be considered pathologic. These areas include the choroid plexus, hypophysis, tuber cinereum, area postrema, subcommissural body, subfornical organ, paraphysis, pineal gland, and preoptic recess (see Chapter 17). On a Gd-enhanced MR image, the choroid plexus and the stalk of the pituitary gland consistently enhance, possibly because of both the relatively larger volume of blood per voxel and the slow flow in the venous plexus that contains contrast agent.

The cerebral capillary bed drains into numerous venules. The gross architecture of these vessels is difficult to envision because it has not been possible to display them in brain specimens injected with barium sulfate. These venules join to form larger venous channels, which drain either to the brain surfaces or inwardly to the walls of the ventricles. Eventually, all venules drain into larger veins that are angiographically identifiable (see Chapter 13).

NORMAL AGING

The aging of cerebral vessels is presumably the natural result of the hemodynamic stress inflicted over the course of the person's lifetime. With age, the elastic tissue in the cerebral vessel degenerates, and the pulsatile flow causes dilation and elongation of the vessel. The increase in length occurring between sites that are fixed at points of branching creates tortuosity. In severe cases, coiling and even kinking of a vessel may occur. This is frequently seen in the cervical internal carotid artery, but loops in the vertebral artery have been reported to cause erosion of cervical vertebrae.

These changes also occur in intracranial vessels (Figure 14-12). Pulsation in elongated arteries can mechanically

A

B

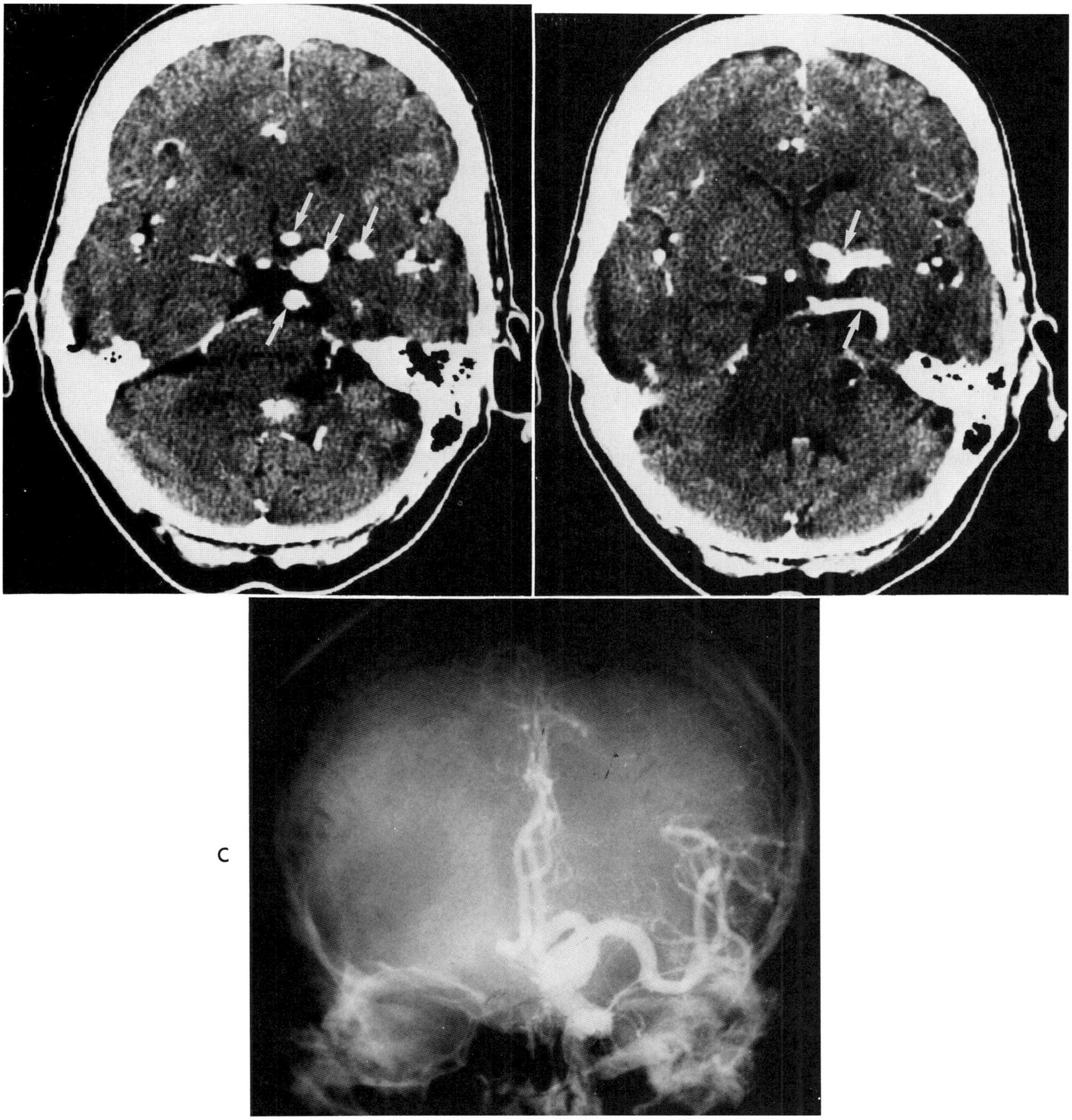

C

Figure 14-12 **A** and **B**, Axial CT images after administration of IV iodinated contrast material demonstrate extremely tortuous and dilated left internal carotid and basilar arteries (*arrows*). **C**, Companion anteroposterior arteriogram confirms the atherosclerotic dilation and tortuosity in the intracranial left carotid artery.

compress the brainstem and/or root entry zones of a cranial nerve. This phenomenon has been associated with trigeminal neuralgia, hemifacial spasm, tinnitus and vertigo, glossopharyngeal neuralgia, and even essential hypertension.[57] Microsurgical decompression of these vessels for patients with these findings is a controversial mode of treatment.[58]

Age-related changes in the caliber and length of cerebral vessels occur without atherosclerotic vascular involvement.[41] However, since artherosclerotic changes inevitably increase in severity with advancing age, some authors consider them part of the aging process. The vascular changes caused by atherosclerosis occur at sites of greatest hemodynamic stress. Initially, lipid is deposited in and beneath the intima. Later, the lesion involves the internal elastic membrane and muscular wall. These deposits frequently calcify. Vasa vasora, which are not normally present in cerebral vessels, form in atherosclerotic vessels. Changes associated with aging are also seen in cerebral veins at sites of hemodynamic stress.

Only a few studies have been done to assess the age-dependent changes that occur in the cerebral microcirculation. No agreement exists on whether capillaries, arterioles, or arteries are primarily involved.[59-61] The little information available on the state of the vessel wall varies. All authors agree that aging produces convoluted microvessels in the cerebral hemisphere with relative cerebellar sparing. Blood flow at these sites of microvascular elongation and convolution is focally reduced.[61] The significance of these reductions as a cause for neurologic aging awaits further study. It is known, however, that the mean cerebral arterial blood pressure and cerebrovascular resistance are significantly elevated in normal elderly men (mean age, 71 years) compared with young men (mean age, 21 years). This change does not translate into a significant difference in *mean* cerebral blood flow.[62]

Cerebral capillary density is only weakly correlated with age.[63] However, this density is strongly related to the number of metabolically active synapses in a region. Thus the relatively inactive newborn brain has a capillary density that is only one-third that of the adult brain.[54] Decreased capillary density in dementia is generally considered to result from the primary loss of functioning neural tissue and is not considered the *cause* of neuron loss. The hippocampal regions of the cornu ammonis most severely affected by tangles and granulovacuoles[63] have been found to have the best vascular capacity when capillary and arteriolar measurements are made.[64]

Preliminary indirect evidence suggests that other changes may occur in aging intracranial vessels. The density of the nerves that innervate the cerebral vessels and produce vascoconstriction and vasodilation is altered in aging animals. Preliminary studies have shown that these changes are minor and that the motor activity of the cerebrovascular bed is therefore unaffected.[65] Other investigators have reported preliminary data suggesting that certain aspects of capillary bbb function are altered in the elderly.[56]

REFERENCES

1. Von Schulthess GK, Higgins CB: Blood flow imaging with MR: spin-phase phenomena, *Radiology* 157:687-695, 1985.
2. Kido DK, Paulin S, Alenghat JA, et al: Thrombogenicity of heparin- and non-heparin-coated catheters: clinical trial, *AJNR* 3:535-539, 1982.
3. Manelfe C, Mark AS, Berry I: Magnetic resonance imaging of the cerebral vessels. In Gouaze A, Salmon G, editors: *Brain anatomy and magnetic resonance imaging,* New York, 1988, Springer-Verlag.
4. Haacke EM, Masaryk TJ: The salient features of MR angiography, *Radiology* 173:611-612, 1989.
5. Steinke W, Kloetzsch C, Hennerici M: Carotid artery disease assessed by color Doppler flow imaging: correlation with standard Doppler sonography and angiography, *AJNR* 11:259-266, 1990; *AJR* 154:1061-1068, 1990.
6. Beckett WW Jr, Davis PC, Hoffman JC: Duplex Doppler sonography of the carotid artery: false-positive results in an artery contralateral to an artery with marked stenosis, *AJNR* 11:1049-1053, 1990; *AJR* 155:1091-1095, 1990.
7. Erickson SJ, Mewissen MW, Foley WD, et al: Stenosis of the internal carotid artery: assessment using color Doppler imaging compared with angiography, *AJR* 152:1299-1305, 1989.
8. Foley WD, Erickson SJ: Color Doppler flow imaging, *AJR* 156:3-13, 1991.
9. Schuierer F, Huk W: The unilateral hyperdense middle cerebral artery: an early CT sign of embolism or thrombosis, *Neuroradiology* 30:120-122, 1988.
10. Pressman BD, Tourje EJ, Thompson JR: An early sign of ischemic infarction: increased density in a cerebral artery, *AJNR* 8:645-658, 1987.
11. Eick JJ, Miller KD, Bell KA, et al: Computed tomography of deep cerebral venous thrombosis in children, *Radiology* 140:399-402, 1981.
12. Nelson MD, Thompson JR, Hinshaw DB, et al: Radiodense dural sinuses: new CT sign in patients at risk for hypoxemic insult, *AJNR* 2:545-548, 1981.
13. Buonanno FS, Moody DM, Ball MR, et al: Computed cranial tomographic findings in cerebral sinovenous occlusion, *J Comput Assist Tomogr* 2:281-290, 1978.
14. Feinberg DA, Crooks LE, Hoenninger J, et al: Pulsatile blood velocity in human arteries displayed by magnetic resonance imaging, *Radiology* 153:177-180, 1984.
15. Constantinesco A, Mallet JJ, Bomartin A, et al: Spatial or flow velocity phase encoding gradients in NMR imaging, *Magn Reson Imaging* 2:335-340, 1984.
16. Pradip M, Pattany PM, Phillips JJ, et al: Motion artifact suppression technique (MAST) for MR imaging, *J Comput Assist Tomogr* 11(3):369-377, 1987.

17. Haacke EM, Lenz GW: Improving MR image quality in the presence of motion using rephasing gradients, *Am J Roentgenol* 148:1251-1258, 1987.
18. Rippe DJ, Boyko OB, Spritzer CE, et al: Demonstration of dural sinus occlusion by the use of MR angiography, *AJNR* 11:199-201, 1990.
19. Anderson C, Saloner D, Tsuruda J, et al: Artifacts encountered in maximum intensity projection display of MR angiography. Paper presented at Society of Magnetic Resonance in Medicine, Amsterdam, The Netherlands, Aug 12-18, 1989.
20. Weinmann H-J, Gries H, Speck U: Gd DTPA and low osmolar Gd chelates. In Runge VM, editor: *Enhanced magnetic resonance imaging,* St Louis, 1989, Mosby–Year Book.
21. Brasch RC, Bennett HF: Considerations in the choice of contrast media for MR imaging, *Radiology* 166:897, 1987.
22. Doucet D, Meyer D, Bonnemain B, et al: Gd DPTA. In Runge VM, editor: *Enhanced magnetic resonance imaging,* St Louis, 1989, Mosby–Year Book.
23. Sato A, Takahashi S, Soma Y, et al: Cerebral infarction: early detection by means of contrast-enhanced cerebral arteries at MR imaging, *Radiology* 178:433-439, 1991.
24. Purdy PD: Imaging cerebral blood flow in interventional neuroradiology: choice of technique and indications, *AJNR* 12:424-427, 1991.
25. Tilyou SM: The evolution of positron emission tomography, *J Nucl Med* 32(4):15N-26N, 1991.
26. Yamamoto YL, Meyer E, Menon D, et al: Dynamic positron emission tomography for measurement of regional cerebral blood flow using Kr-77 and 0-15 labeled tracers. In Magistretti PL, editor: *Functional radionuclide imaging of the brain,* New York, 1983, Raven.
27. Kung HF, Ohmomo Y, Kung M-P: Current and future radiopharmaceuticals for brain imaging with single photon emission computed tomography, *Semin Nucl Med* 20(4):290-302, 1990.
28. Axel L: Cerebral blood flow determination by rapid-sequence computed tomography, *Radiology* 137:679-686, 1980.
29. Ladurner G, Zilkha E, Iliff LD, et al: Measurement of regional cerebral blood volume by computerized axial tomography, *J Neurol Neurosurg Psychiatry* 39:152-158, 1976.
30. Calle JM, Guibert-Tranier F, Orgogozo JM, et al: Vascular phenomenon and computerized (CAT) tomography. In Bes A, Geraud G, editors: *Excerpta Medica International Congress,* series 507.
31. Truwit CL, Barkovich AJ, Gean-Marton A, et al: Loss of the insular ribbon: another early CT sign of acute middle cerebral artery infarction, *Radiology* 176:801-806, 1990.
32. Gur D, Yonas H, Good WF: Local cerebral blood flow by xenon-enhanced CT: current status, potential improvements, and future directions, *Cerebrovasc Brain Metab Rev* 1:68-86, 1989.
33. Good WF, Gur D: Xenon-enhanced CT of the brain: effect of flow activation on derived cerebral blood flow measurements, *AJNR* 12:83-85, 1991.
34. Holman BL, Hellman RS, Goldsmith JJ, et al: Biodistribution, dosimetry and clinical evaluation of the technetium-99m ethyl cysteinate dimer in normal subjects and in patients with chronic cerebral infarction, *J Nucl Med* 30(6):1018-1024, 1989.
35. Hellman RS, Tikovsky RS: An overview of the contribution of regional cerebral blood flow studies in cerebrovascular disease: is there a role for single photon emission computed tomography? *Semin Nucl Med* 20(4):303-304, 1990.
36. Van Heertum RL, Tikofsky RS: *Advances in cerebral SPECT imaging: an atlas and guidelines for practitioners,* New York, 1989, Trivirum.
37. LeBihan DL, Breton E, Lallemand D, et al: MR imaging of intravoxel incoherent motions: application to diffusion and perfusion in neurologic disorders, *Radiology* 161:401-407, 1986.
38. LeBihan DL, Breton E, Lallemand D, et al: Separation of diffusion and perfusion in intravoxel incoherent motion MR imaging, *Radiology* 168:497-505, 1988.
39. Feinberg DA, Jacob P: Tissue perfusion in humans studied by Fourier velocity distribution, line scan, and echo-planar imaging, *Magn Reson Med* 16:280-293, 1990.
40. Dixon WT: Separation of diffusion and perfusion in intravoxel incoherent motion MR imaging: a modest proposal with tremendous potential, *Radiology* 168:566-567, 1988.
41. Stehbens WE: *Hemodynamics and the blood vessel wall,* Springfield, Ill, 1979, Charles C Thomas.
42. Meyer WW, Lind J: Calcifications of the carotid siphon—a common finding in infancy and childhood, *Arch Dis Child* 47:355, 1972.
43. Miller DL, Doppman JL: Petrosal sinus sampling: technique and rationale, *Radiology* 178:37-47, 1991.
44. Kirkpatrick J, Hayman LA: Brain lesions in neurologically normal elderly autopsy subjects: a possible explanation of MR cerebral white matter findings, *Radiology* 162:509-511, 1987.
45. Heir LA, Bauer CJ, Schwartz L, et al: Large Virchow-Robin spaces: MR-clinical correlation, *AJNR* 10:929-936, 1989.
46. Elster AD, Richardson DN: Foci of high-T2 signal in the midbrain: anatomic correlates, *AJNR* 11:1119-1122, 1991.
47. Moody DM, Bell MA, Challa VR: Features of the cerebral vascular pattern that predict vulnerability to perfusion or oxygenation deficiency: an anatomic study, *AJNR* 11:431-439, 1990.
48. Nelson MD Jr, Gonzales-Gomez I, Gilles FH: The search for human telencephalic ventriculofugal arteries, *AJNR* 12:215-222, 1991.
49. Duvernoy HM: *The human hippocampus: an atlas of applied anatomy,* Bergmann JF, Munchen, 1988, Verlag.
50. Meldrum BS, Evans MC, Swan JH, et al: Protection against hypoxic/ischemic brain damage with excitatory amino acid antagonists, *Med Biol* 65(2-3):153-157, 1987.
51. Sage MR: Blood-brain barrier: phenomenon of increasing importance to the imaging clinician, *AJNR* 3:127-138, 1982.
52. Reese TS, Karnovsky MJ: Fine structural localization of a blood-brain barrier to exogenous peroxidase, *J Cell Biol* 34:207-217, 1967.
53. Bradbury MWB: Why a blood-brain barrier? *Trends Neurosci* 2:36-38, 1979.
54. Bradbury M, editor: *The concept of a blood-brain barrier,* New York, 1979, John Wiley & Sons.
55. Katzman R, Pappius HM: Brain electrolytes and fluid metabolism. In Bradbury M, editor: *The concept of a blood-brain barrier,* New York, 1979, John Wiley & Sons.
56. Pardridge WM: Does the brain's gatekeeper falter in aging? *Neurobiol Aging* 9:44-46, 1988.
57. Jannetta PJ: Neurovascular compression in cranial nerve and systemic disease, *Ann Surg* 192:518-528, 1980.
58. Sweet WH: The treatment of trigeminal neuralgia (tic douloureux), *N Engl J Med* 315(3):174-177, 1986.
59. Cervos-Navarro J, Gertz HJ, Frydl V: Cerebral blood vessel changes in old people, *Mech Ageing Dev* 39:223-231, 1987.
60. Hassler O: Vascular changes in senile brains: a micro-angiographic study, *Acta Neuropathol* 5:40-53, 1965.
61. Hassler O: Arterial deformities in senile brains: the occurrence of the deformities in a large autopsy series and some aspects of their functional significance, *Acta Neuropathol* 8:219-229, 1967.
62. Dastur DK: Cerebral blood flow and metabolism in normal human aging, pathological aging, and senile dementia, *J Cereb Blood Flow Metab* 5(1):1-9, 1985.
63. Mann DM, Eaves NR, Marcyniuk B, et al: Quantitative changes in cerebral cortical microvasculature in aging and dementia, *Neurobiol Aging* 7(5):321-330, 1986.
64. Bell MA, Ball MJ: The correlation of vascular capacity with parenchymal lesions of Alzheimer's disease, *Can J Neurol Sci* 13(4):456-461, 1986.
65. Hamel E, MacKenzie ET: Influence of age on cerebrovascular function. In Bes A, Geraud G, editors: *Circulation cerebrale et vieillissement,* London, 1990, John Libbey Eurotext.

CHAPTER **15**

L. Anne Hayman
Ronald Quisling
Edward Callaway
R. Nick Bryan

Displacement of Cerebral Vessels by Mass Lesions

Recent advances in magnetic resonance (MR) technology have made it possible to obtain ever-improving images of cerebral vessels. Noninvasive MR arteriography (MRA) may soon be a routine part of the radiographic analysis of the brain, since the displacement of important vessels contributes to the diagnostic interpretation of masses located on computer-generated images. For example, the displacement of the superficial cerebral vessels can be used to differentiate extraaxial from intraaxial masses in the subtemporal and tentorial regions. In other instances, the origin of a mass can best be determined by studying cerebrovascular displacements.

This chapter summarizes the vascular displacements caused by various cerebral masses. Only masses that cause a distinctive array of diagnostic vascular displacements have been illustrated, since these patterns of displacement have clinical significance in preoperative planning. Masses in areas with few identifiable vascular landmarks have been omitted, since they are best localized on appropriate cross-sectional images. This chapter uses schematic diagrams of the adult cerebral vasculature as depicted on anteroposterior (AP) and lateral cerebral MR or conventional arteriograms. These images are matched with related schematic axial brain slices that show the epicenter of a given mass and its effect on adjacent structures. The anatomic landmarks used in these schematics have been identified in Chapter 14 on normal vascular anatomy.

Detailed charts accompany each mass. They are organized vertically and horizontally. The three vertical columns list the various anatomic changes that can be confidently detected in the accompanying illustrations. Horizontally, the charts are cross-referenced to allow correlation of the anatomic changes seen on brain sections with either the AP or the lateral arteriogram projection. This allows the reader to delete arteriographic findings that may not occur if the mass discovered clinically is smaller than the mass illustrated.

In this chapter, cerebral masses have been classified according to location as *supratentorial* or *infratentorial*. Within each of these major regions, these masses are further subdivided by location. For example, Figure 15-1 demonstrates seven supratentorial loci close to the sylvian triangle. Each could be even further subdivided as medial, lateral, or central; however, in most cases this is not necessary because the relevant angiographic signs will be minimally affected. Therefore masses central to each location are depicted, and companion footnotes indicate any additional vascular displacements that would be expected from a mass located more medially or laterally. Footnotes also indicate whether the mass is *above* or *below* important vascular landmarks. For example, a mass in the central part of the anteroinferior sylvian area could be above or below the anterior choroidal artery. Masses below would elevate the artery, and vice versa.

Axial schematics and the accompanying vascular chart for masses located in 17 separate areas in the cerebral hemispheres are shown in Figures 15-2 to 15-18. The same format is used to locate masses in five separate regions of the posterior fossa in Figures 15-19 to 15-23. Box 15-1 lists the abbreviations used in these figures. Three major texts were consulted to compile these illustrations.[1-3]

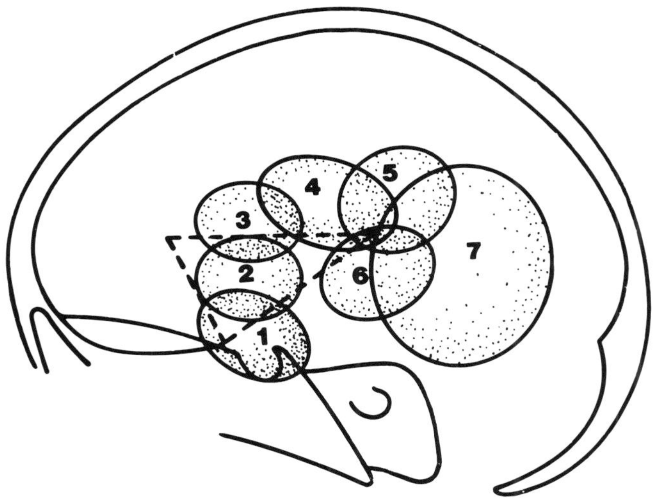

Figure 15-1 Seven masses related to the periphery of the Sylvian triangle: (1) Anterior Infra-Sylvian, (2) Centro-Sylvian, (3) Anterior Supra-Sylvian mass, (4) Posterior Supra-Sylvian, (5) Superior Retro-Sylvian, (6) Posterior and Medial Infra-Sylvian, and (7) Inferior Retro-Sylvian.

BOX 15-1

Key to Abbreviations for Figures 15-2 to 15-23

ACA	Anterior cerebral artery
AICA	Anterior inferior cerebellar
BVR	Basilar vein of Rosenthal
ICV	Internal cerebral vein
ICA	Internal carotid artery
MCA	Middle cerebral artery
PCA	Posterior cerebral artery
PICA	Posterior inferior cerebellar artery
SCA	Superior cerebellar artery

REFERENCES

1. Newton TH, Potts DG: Radiology of the skull and brain, vol II, *Angiography*, St Louis, 1974, Mosby–Year Book.
2. Taveras JM, Wood EH: *Diagnostic neuroradiology*, vol II, Baltimore, 1976, Williams & Wilkins.
3. Quisling RG: *Correlative neuroradiology: intracranial radiographic analysis with computed tomography, angiography, and magnetic resonance imaging*, New York, 1985, John Wiley & Sons.

FRONTOPOLAR MASS

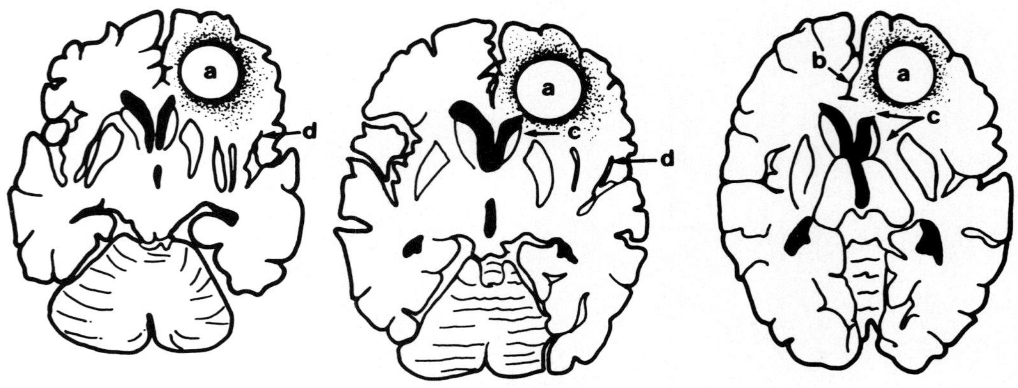

Figure 15-2 Frontopolar Mass

Axial brain sections	AP carotid arteriogram	Lateral carotid arteriogram
a. Mass within the frontal pole.	a. Frontal ACA branches stretch around the mass.	a. (−)
b. Herniation of pericallosal portion of frontal lobe.	b. Pericallosal segment of ACA displaced across the midline (round shift).	b. Pericallosal and/or callosomarginal ACA branches displaced posteriorly.
c. Compression of frontal horn and basal ganglia.	c. Stretched lenticulostriate arteries, basal ganglia region.	c. Posterior displacement of (1) anterior septal and (2) anterior caudate veins* (not shown).
d. Posterolateral displacement of the anterior Sylvian fissure.	d. Lateral displacement of the anterior Sylvian branches of MCA.	d. Posterior displacement of anterior Sylvian point.

*A larger frontopolar mass will also posteriorly displace the venous angle formed by the thalamostriate as it joins the internal cerebral vein at the foramen of Monro.

AP CAROTID ARTERIOGRAM

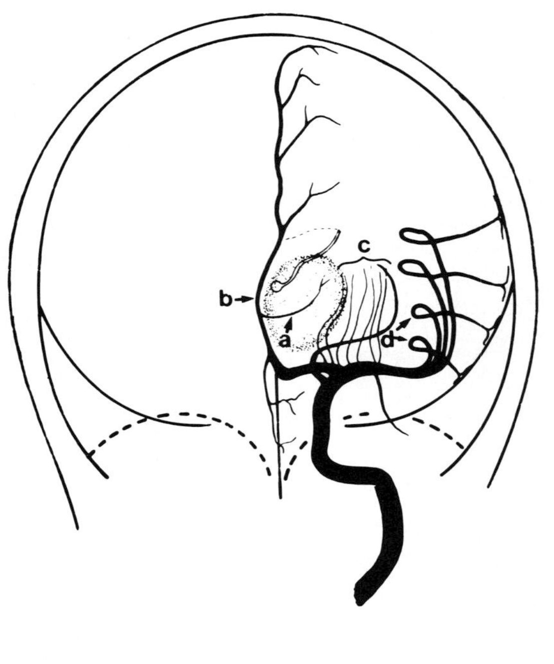

LATERAL CAROTID ARTERIOGRAM

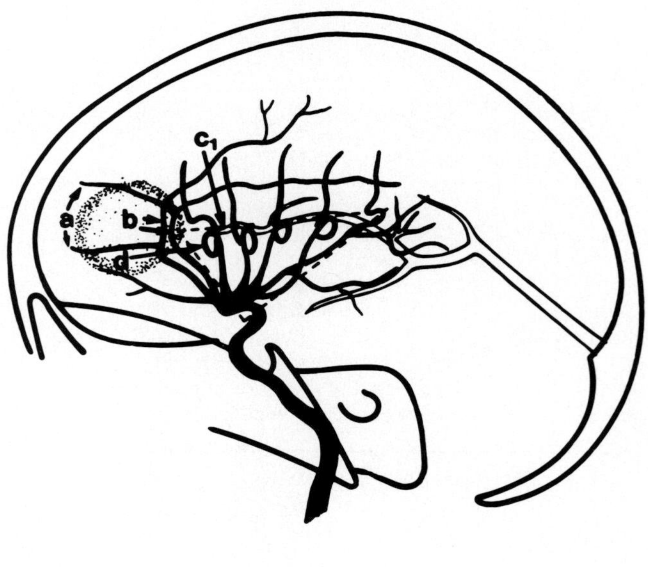

BASIFRONTAL MASS

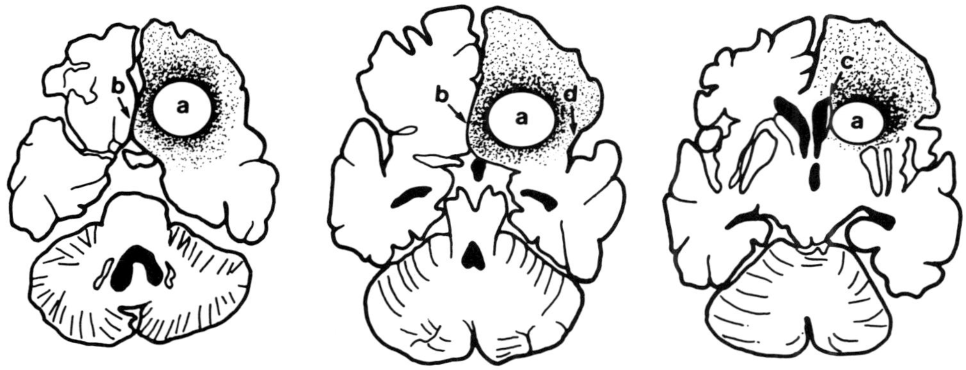

Figure 15-3 Basifrontal Mass

Axial brain sections	AP carotid anteriogram	Lateral carotid anteriogram
a. Mass within the inferior frontal lobe.	a. Inferior frontal arteries stretched and displaced around the mass.	a. Inferior frontal arteries stretched and displaced around the mass.
b. Herniation of inferior frontal lobe.	b. Infracallosal segment of ACA displaced across the midline (proximal shift).	b. Infracallosal segment of ACA and bifurcation of ICA displaced posteriorly.
c. Compression of the frontal horn and anterior caudate nucleus.	c. Lenticulostriate vessels are stretched; distortion of the anterior septal and caudate veins (not shown).	c. Elevation of: (1) anterior septal and (2) anterior caudate veins† (not shown).
d. Mild compression of the inferior aspect of the anterior Sylvian fissure.	d. lateral displacement of anterior Sylvian branches of MCA.*	d. (−)

*A laterally situated frontal mass will cause posterior displacement and greater medial displacement of the anterior MCA vessels.

†A large mass will also elevate the venous angle formed by the thalamostriate vein as it joins the internal cerebral vein.

AP CAROTID ARTERIOGRAM

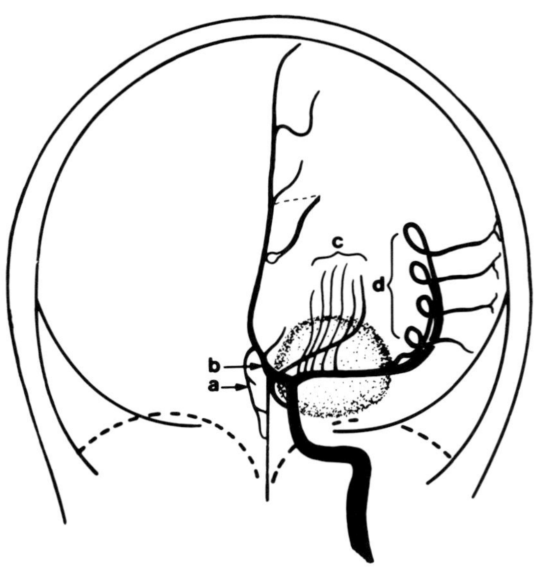

LATERAL CAROTID ARTERIOGRAM

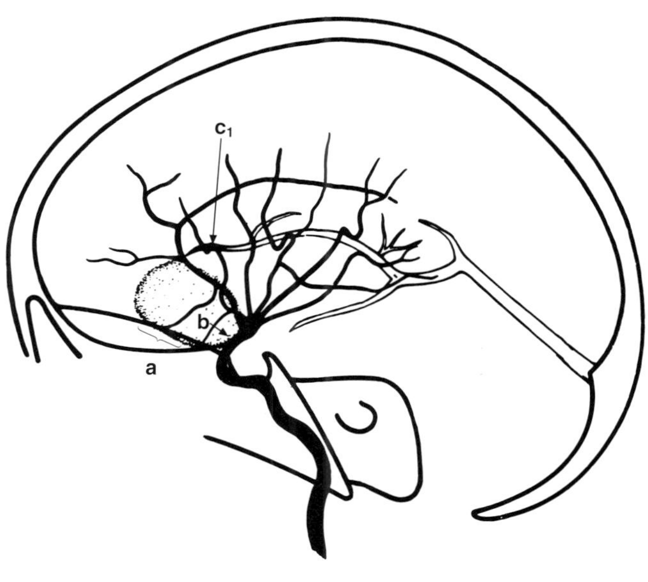

SYMMETRICAL ANTERIOR SUPRASELLAR MASS

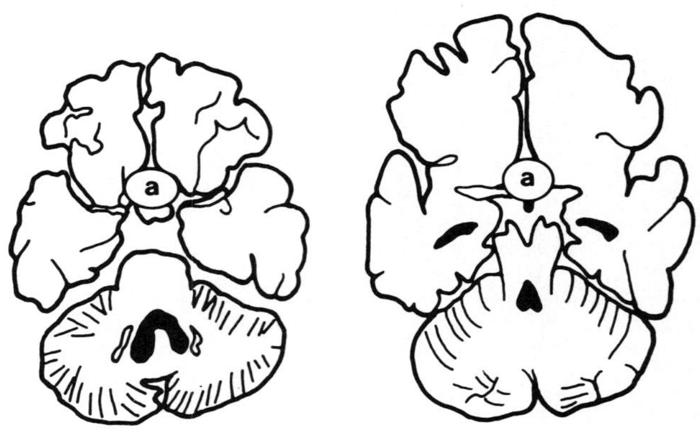

Figure 15-4 Symmetrical Anterior Suprasellar Mass

Axial brain sections	AP carotid arteriogram	Lateral carotid arteriogram
a. Mass within the anterior suprasellar cistern. b. Elevation of the inferior surface of the frontal lobes (not visible on axial sections).	a. Lateral displacement of the supraclinoid segment of ICA. b. Elevation of the proximal segment of ACA.	a. Posterior displacement of the supraclinoid segment of ICA. b. Elevation of the proximal segment of ACA.

AP CAROTID ARTERIOGRAM

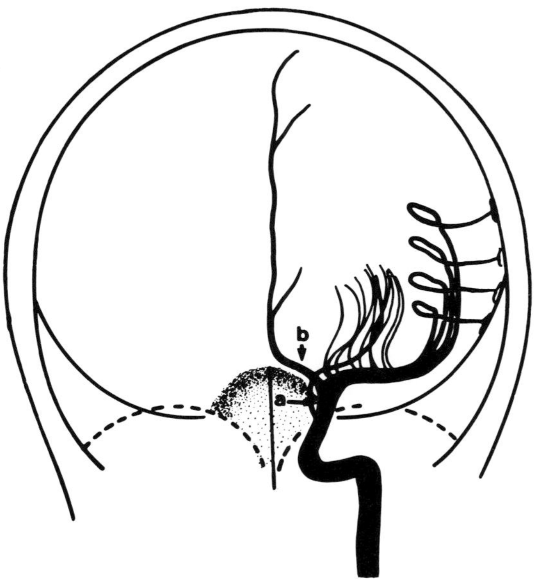

LATERAL CAROTID ARTERIOGRAM

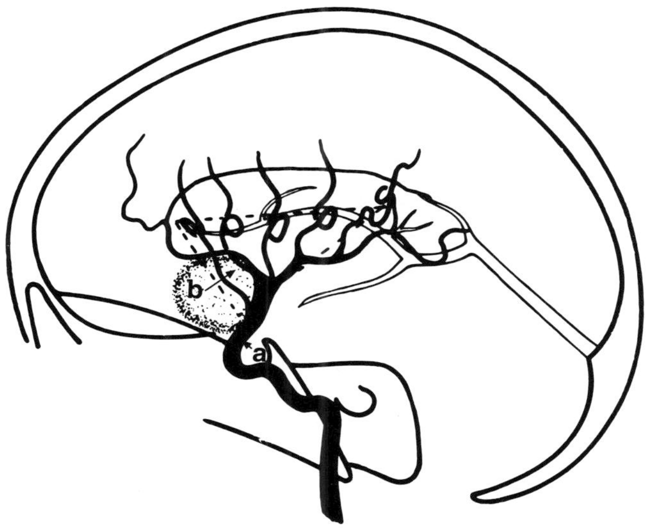

SYMMETRICAL POSTERIOR SUPRASELLAR MASS (ORIGIN ABOVE CHIASM)

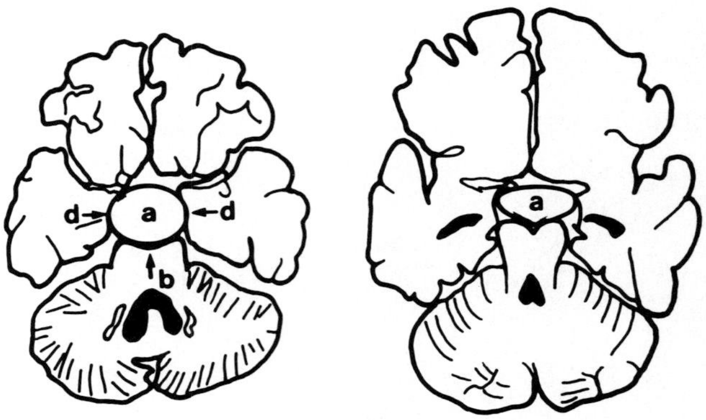

Figure 15-5 Symmetrical Posterior Suprasellar Mass (origin above chiasm)

Axial brain sections	AP vertebral and carotid arteriograms	Lateral vertebral and carotid arteriograms
a. Mass within the posterior suprasellar cistern; elevation and posterior displacement of the hypothalamus, floor of the third ventricle, and optic chiasm.	a. (−)	a. (−)
b. Posterior displacement of the upper brainstem.	b. (−)	b. Focal posterior displacement of the upper basilar artery; veins on the anterior surface of the pons and mesencephalon reflect the posterior displacement of the brainstem (not shown).
c. Focal elevation of the inferior thalamic surfaces (not visible on axial brain sections).	c. Stretching of the thalamoperforating vessels* (not shown).	c. Stretching and posterior displacement of the thalamoperforating branches of the PCA and posterior communicating arteries.
d. Lateral displacement of the uncus.	d. Lateral displacement of the cisternal part of the anterior choroidal artery.	d. Depression of the cisternal part of the anterior choroidal artery.

*An asymmetric mass will displace these vessels in the appropriate direction on the AP vertebral arteriogram.

AP CAROTID ARTERIOGRAM

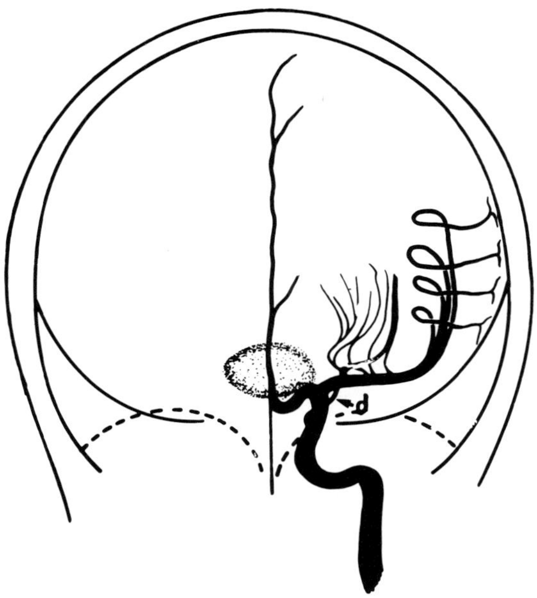

LATERAL CAROTID ARTERIOGRAM

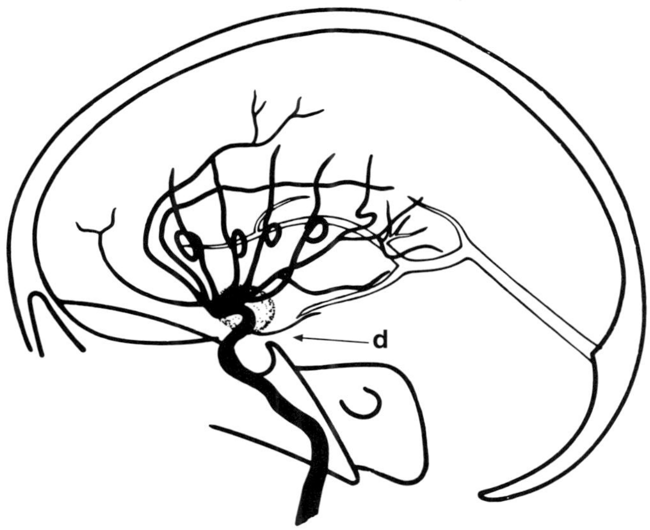

AP VERTEBRAL ARTERIOGRAM

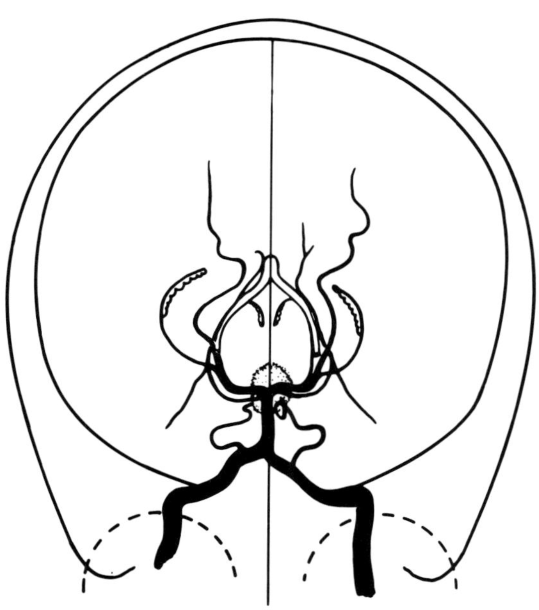

LATERAL VERTEBRAL ARTERIOGRAM

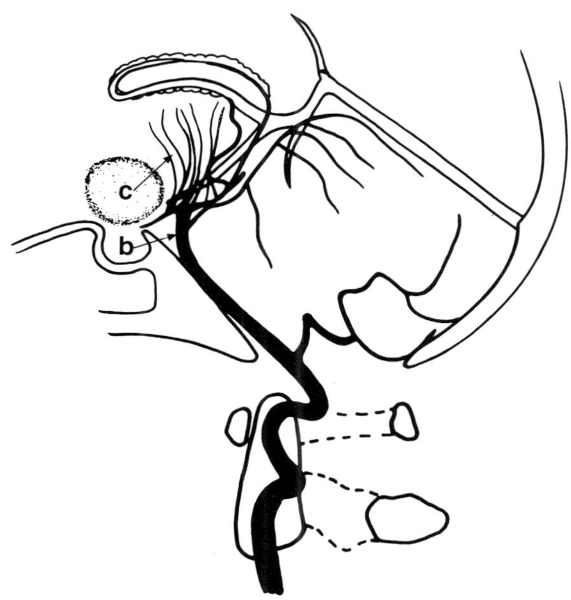

SYMMETRICAL POSTERIOR SUPRASELLAR MASS (ORIGIN BELOW CHIASM)

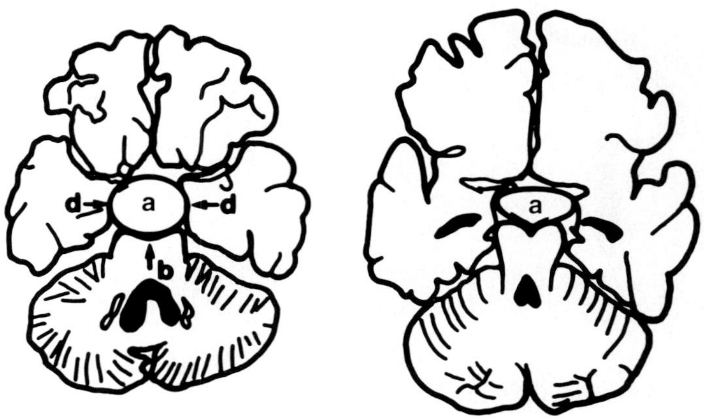

Figure 15-6 Symmetrical Posterior Suprasellar Mass (origin below chiasm)

Axial brain sections	AP vertebral and carotid arteriograms	Lateral vertebral and carotid arteriograms
a. Mass within the posterior suprasellar cistern; elevation of the hypothalamus, floor of the third ventricle and optic chiasm.	a. (−)	a. (−)
b. Posterior displacement of the upper brainstem.	b. (−)	b. Focal posterior displacement of the upper basilar artery; veins on the anterior surface of the pons and mesencephalon reflect the posterior displacement of the brainstem (not shown).
c. Focal elevation of the inferior thalamic surfaces (not visible on axial brain sections).	c. Stretching of the thalamoperforating vessels* (not shown).	c. Stretching and posterior displacement of the thalamoperforating branches of the PCA and posterior communicating arteries.
d. Lateral displacement of the uncus.	d. Lateral displacement of the cisternal part of the anterior choroidal artery.	d. Elevation of the cisternal part of the anterior choroidal artery.†

*An asymmetric mass will displace these vessels in the appropriate direction on the AP vertebral arteriogram.

†The normal variations in the course of the distal Basal Vein of Rosenthal prevent confident identification of elevation of this vessel.

AP CAROTID ARTERIOGRAM

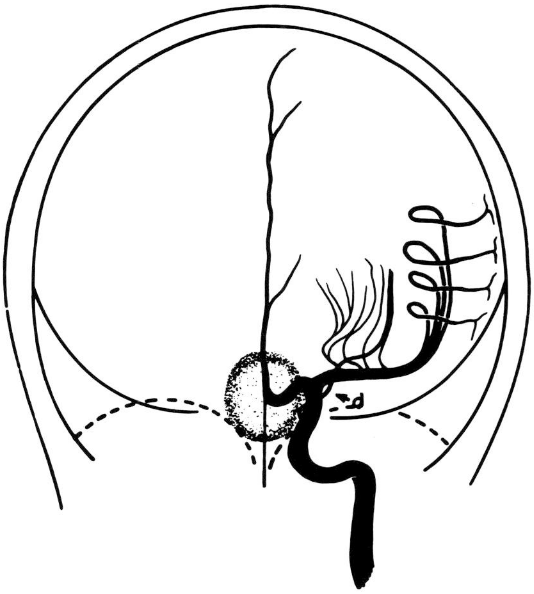

LATERAL CAROTID ARTERIOGRAM

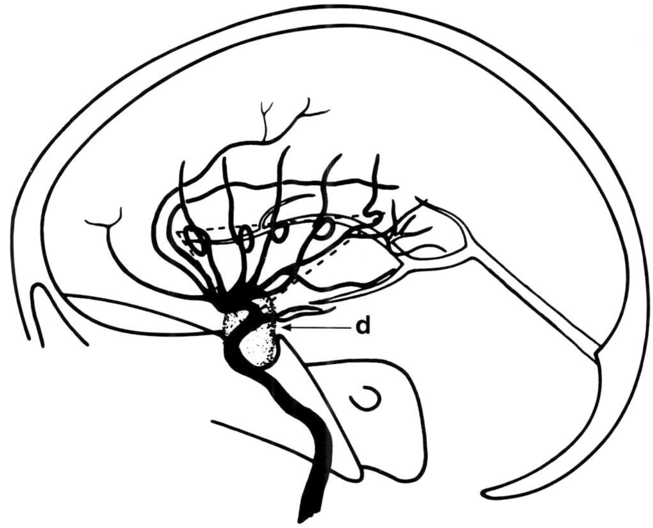

AP VERTEBRAL ARTERIOGRAM

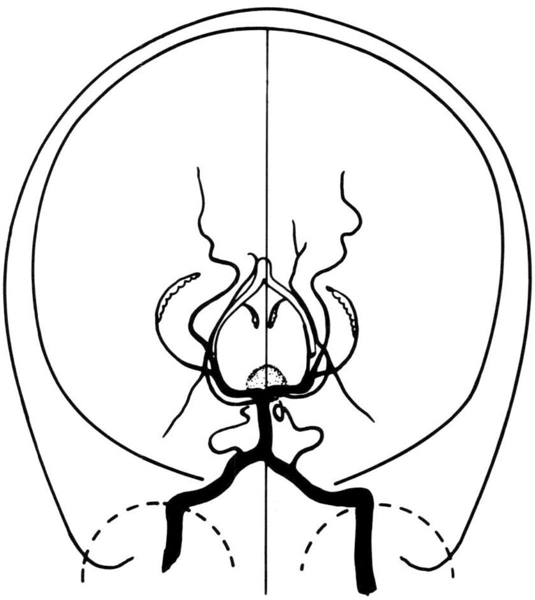

LATERAL VERTEBRAL ARTERIOGRAM

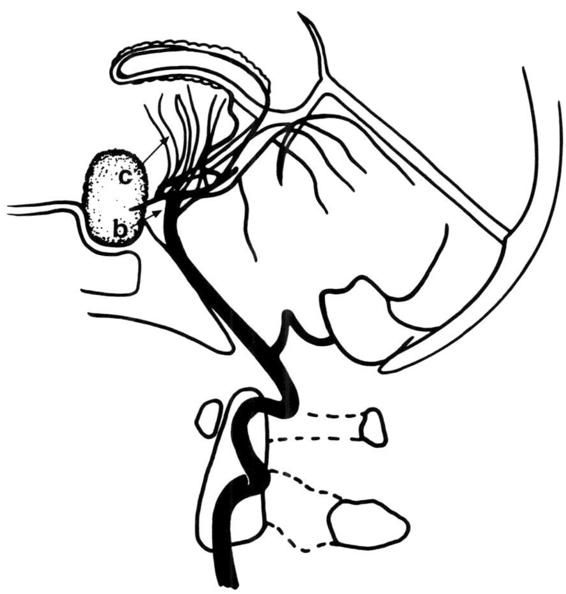

ANTERIOR INFRASYLVIAN MASS: INTRAAXIAL

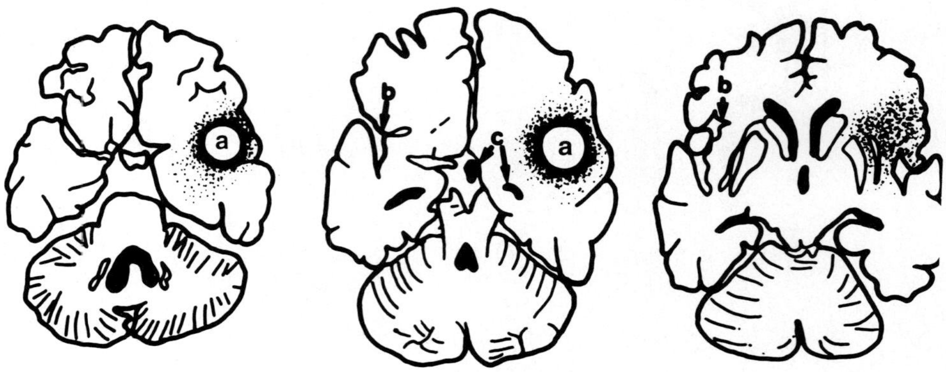

Figure 15-7 Anterior Infrasylvian Mass: Intraaxial
(below the anterior Sylvian point at the plane of the anterior choroidal artery)

Axial brain section	AP carotid	Lateral carotid
a. Mass within the anterior temporal lobe below the anterior aspect of the Sylvian fissure.	a. (1) Distal superficial temporal MCA branches stretched over intra-axial mass ("draping sign"); (2) elevation of proximal MCA trunk.	a. (1) Distal portion of temporal MCA stretched by mass; (2) elevation of proximal MCA; and (3) elevation of supraclinoid ICA.
b. Obliteration of anterior aspect of Sylvian triangle (normal side marked for comparison).	b. (−)*	b. Elevation of anterior Sylvian point.
c. Uncal herniation evidenced by asymmetry of suprasellar cistern and medial displacement of temporal horn of lateral ventricle.	c. Medial displacement of anterior choroidal artery.†	c. Straightening of the normal undulations of the anterior choroidal artery.†
d. Compression of the adjacent basal ganglia.	d. Medial displacement of lenticulostriate vessels.	d. (−)

*Masses medial or lateral to the anterior Sylvian point will displace it in the appropriate direction on the AP carotid arteriogram.
†The normally variable course of the Basal Vein of Rosenthal obscures mild medial deflection of this vessel on the AP and focal distal elevation on the lateral.

AP CAROTID ARTERIOGRAM

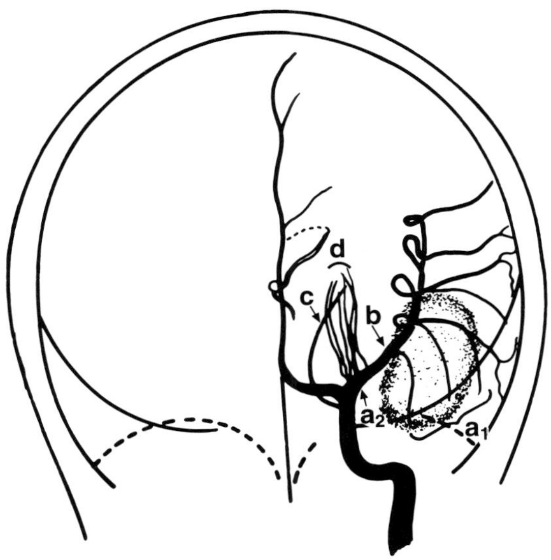

LATERAL CAROTID ARTERIOGRAM

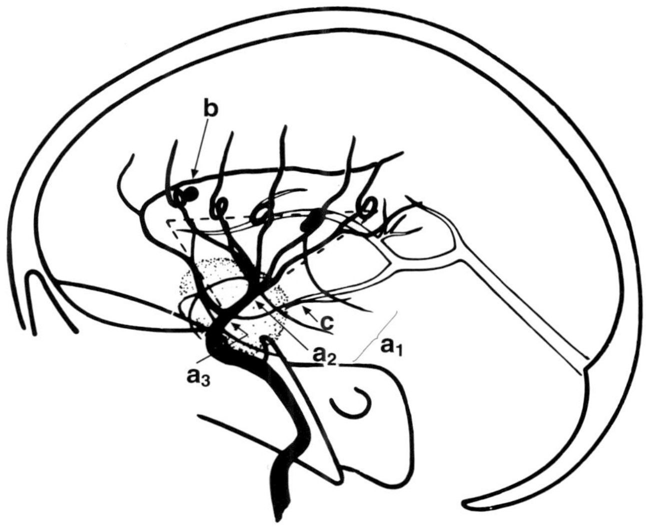

ANTERIOR INFRASYLVIAN MASS: EXTRAAXIAL

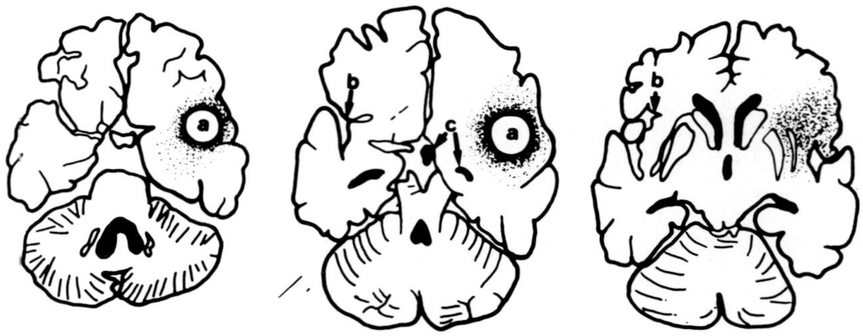

Figure 15-8 Anterior Infrasylvian Mass: Extraaxial
(below anterior Sylvian point and below the plane of the anterior choroidal artery)

Axial brain section	AP carotid	Lateral carotid
a. Mass beneath the anterior temporal lobe.	a. (1) Elevation of the temporal branches by the extraaxial mass and (2) the proximal MCA trunk.	a. (1) Distal portion of temporal MCA elevated and stretched apart by mass; (2) elevation of the proximal MCA; (3) elevation of supraclinoid ICA.
b. Obliteration of anterior aspect of Sylvian triangle (normal side marked for comparison).	b. (−)*	b. Elevation of anterior Sylvian point.
c. Uncal herniation evidenced by asymmetry of suprasellar cistern and medial displacement of temporal horn of lateral ventricle.	c. Medial displacement and elevation of anterior choroidal artery.†	c. Elevation of (1) anterior choroidal artery and (2) anterior segment of the Basal Vein of Rosenthal.†
d. Compression of the adjacent basal ganglia.	d. Medial displacement of lenticulostriate vessels.	d. (−)

*Masses medial or lateral to the anterior Sylvian point will displace it in the appropriate direction on the AP carotid arteriogram.
†The normally variable course of the Basal Vein of Rosenthal obscures mild medial deflection of this vessel.

AP CAROTID ARTERIOGRAM

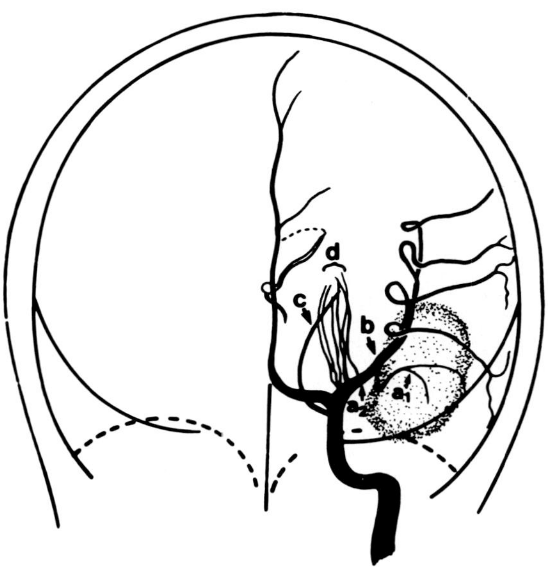

LATERAL CAROTID ARTERIOGRAM

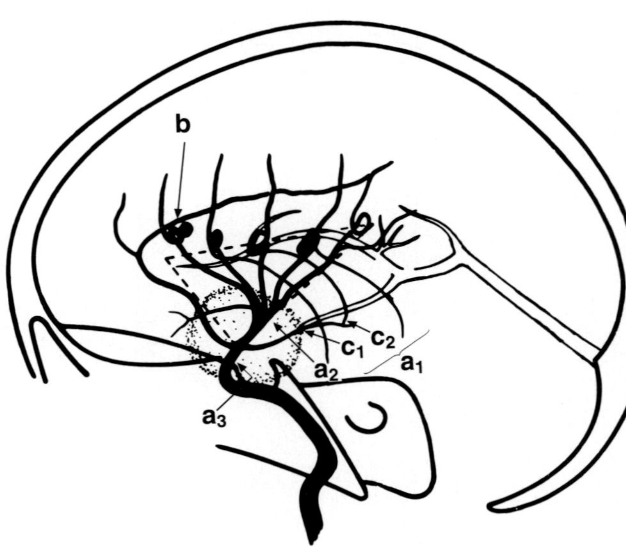

LATERAL CENTROSYLVIAN MASS

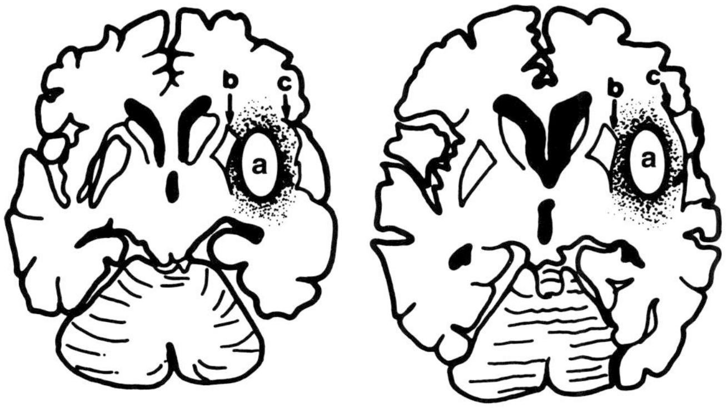

Figure 15-9 Lateral Centrosylvian Mass

Axial brain section	AP carotid arteriogram	Lateral carotid
a. Mass in the region of the insula, putamen, and external capsule.	a. Opening of the knee of the MCA.	a. (−)
b. Medial displacement of the basal ganglia.	b. Lenticulostriate arteries are stretched and bowed medially.	b. Mild straightening of lenticulostriate arteries (not shown).
c. Compression of the insula and lateral displacement of the Sylvian fissure.	c. Lateral displacement of the insular portions of (1) the MCA branches and (2) the posterior Sylvian point.	c. (−)

AP CAROTID ARTERIOGRAM

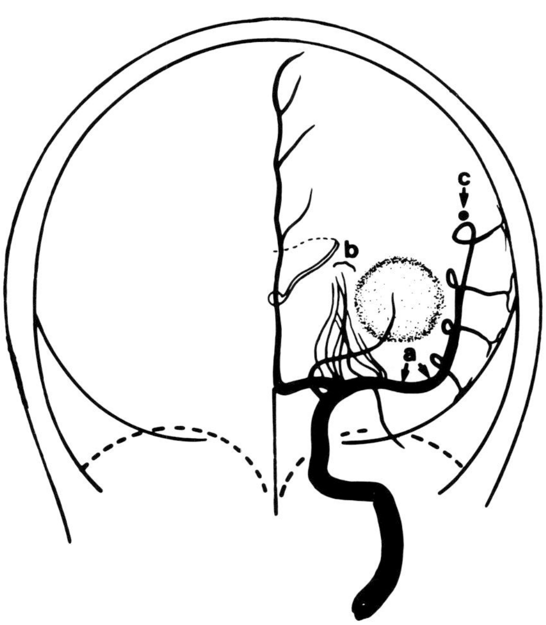

LATERAL CAROTID ARTERIOGRAM

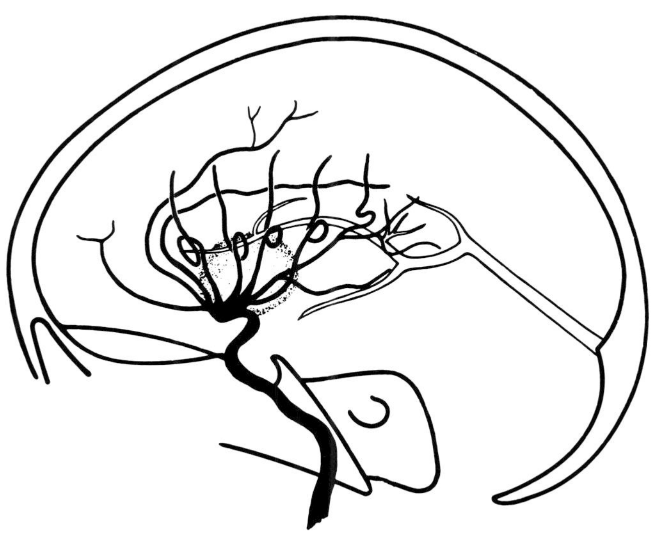

MEDIAL CENTROSYLVIAN MASS: INTRAXIAL

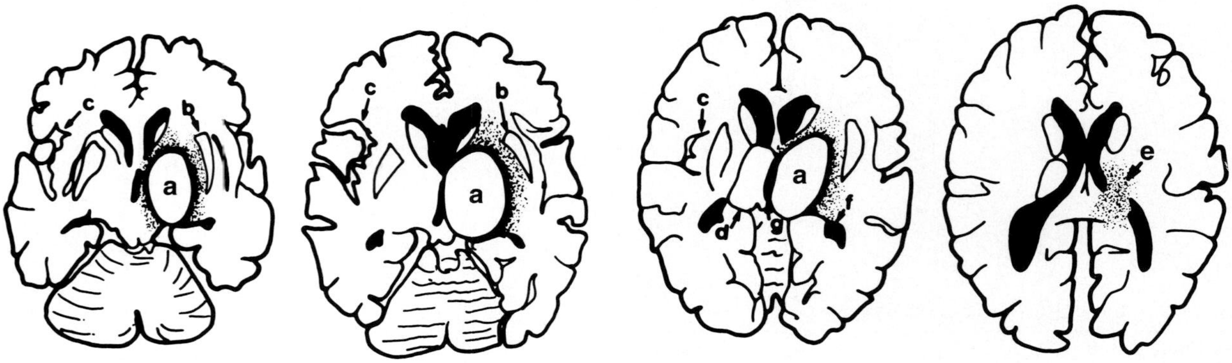

Figure 15-10 Medial Centrosylvian Mass: Intra-axial (thalamus and posterior deep frontal region)

Axial brain sections	AP carotid and vertebral arteriogram	Lateral carotid and vertebral arteriogram
a. Thalamic and posterior deep frontal region mass.	a. (−)(Thalamoperforating arteries superimposed on the ambient part of PCA.)	a. Straightened and stretched thalamoperforating arteries from PCA and posterior communicating artery.
b. Downward and lateral displacement of the basal ganglia.	b. Lenticulostriate arteries are stretched and bowed around the intraaxial mass.*	b. Straightening of lenticulostriate arteries (not shown).
c. Compression of the insula and obliteration of the Sylvian fissure (normal side marked for comparison).	c. Straightening and lateral displacement of the insular portions of the MCA branches and lateral displacement of the posterior Sylvian point.	c. (−)
d. Obliteration of the retrothalamic cistern (normal side marked for comparison).	d. Medial and lateral choroidal PCA branches outline the superior and lateral surfaces of the thalamic mass and are stretched and displaced laterally and superiorly.	d. Medial and lateral choroidal PCA branches outline the posterior and superior surfaces of the thalamic mass and are stretched and displaced posteriorly and superiorly.
e. Elevation of the floor of the lateral ventricle.	e. Elevation and medial displacement of the choroid plexus within the floor of the lateral ventricle and the thalamostriate vein.	e. Elevation of: (1) chorid plexus and ICV and (2) thalamostriate vein in the floor of the lateral ventricle.
f. Posterior and lateral displacement of the atrium of the lateral ventricle.	f. Lateral displacement of the atrial choroidal plexus which is supplied by the anterior choroidal artery.	f. Posterior displacement of the atrial choroid which is supplied by the anterior choroidal artery.
g. Elevation and medial displacement of the roof of the third ventricle.	g. Elevation and medial displacement across the midline of the choroid plexus in the roof of the third ventricle and the ICV.	g. Elevation of: (1) the choroidal plexus of the roof of the third ventricle (not shown) and (2) the ICV.

*Thalamic masses without a deep posterior frontal component will displace the lenticulostriate vessels forward.

AP CAROTID ARTERIOGRAM

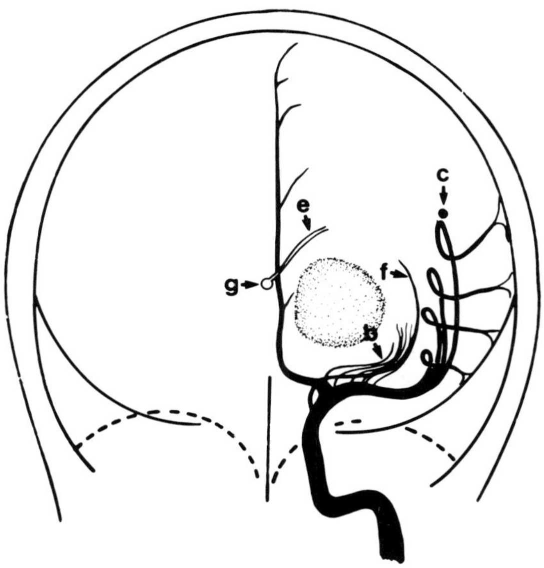

LATERAL CAROTID ARTERIOGRAM

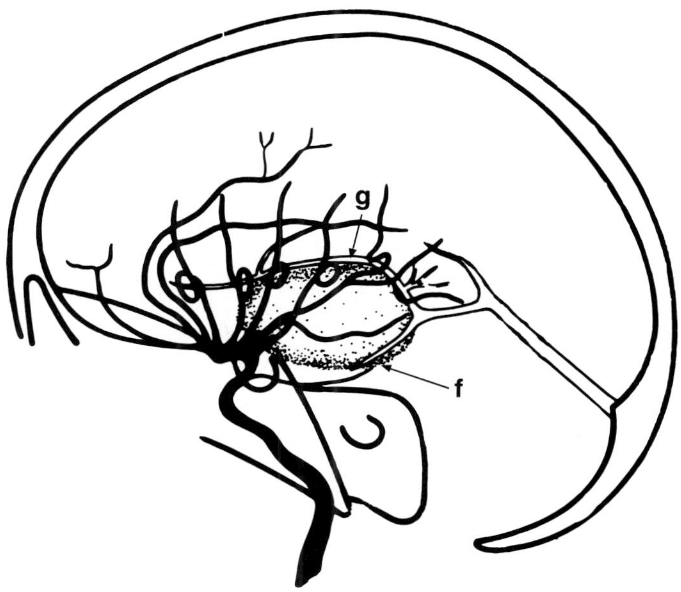

AP VERTEBRAL ARTERIOGRAM

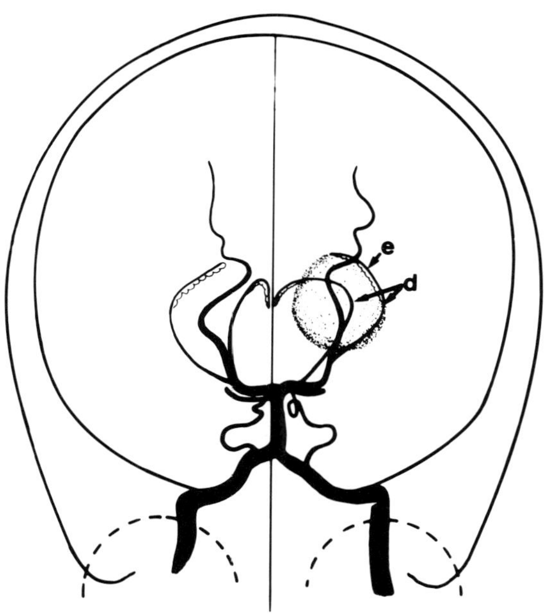

LATERAL VERTEBRAL ARTERIOGRAM

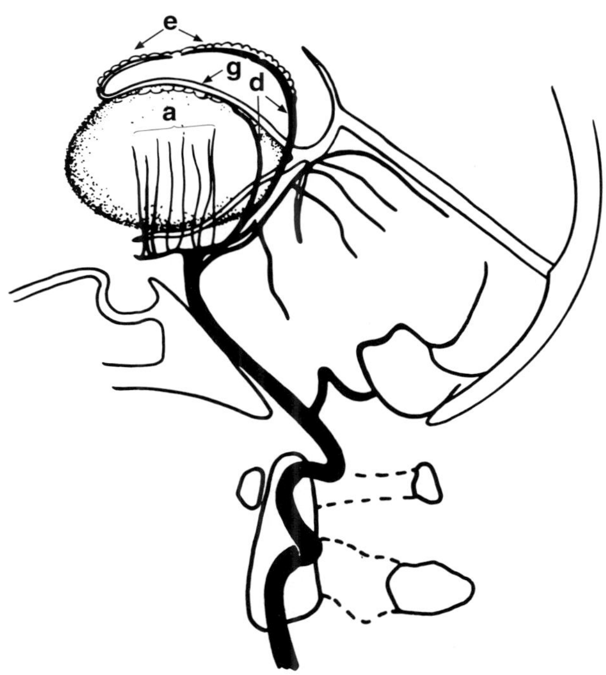

MODERATE "SYMMETRICAL" NON-ATROPHIC HYDROCEPHALUS (THIRD-LATERAL VENTRICLES)

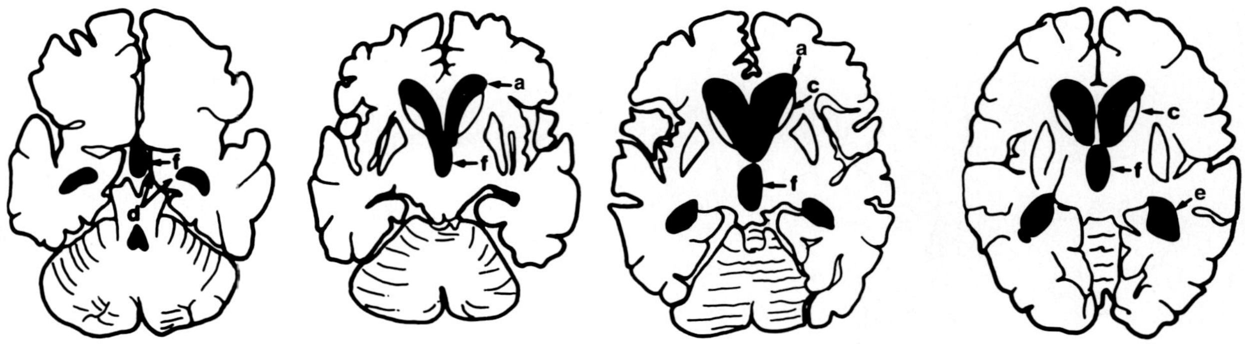

Figure 15-11 Moderate "Symmetrical" Non-Atrophic Hydrocephalus (third and lateral ventricles)

Axial brain sections	AP carotid and vertebral arteriogram	Lateral carotid and vertebral arteriogram
a. Enlargement of frontal horns and bodies of the lateral ventricles.	a. (1) Depression of the ICV; (2) lateral displacement and outward bowing of the thalamostriate vein; (3) normal septal vein.	a. Flattened (1) ICV and (2) thalamostriate veins; (3) elongated septal veins.
b. Elevation of the corpus callosum (not visible on axial sections).	b. Straightening of the pericallosal branch of the ACA.	b. Upward displacement and rounding of the curve of the (1) pericallosal branch of the ACA; (2) posterior pericallosal branch of the PCA (not shown); and (3) the splenial vein.
c. Lateral displacement of the caudate nucleus.	c. Lateral and downward displacement of lenticulostriate branches.	c. Straightening of lenticulostriate branches (not shown).
d. Enlargement of temporal horn causes uncal herniation (concomitant dilation of the third ventricle opposes medial displacement of the temporal horn).	d. Cisternal anterior choroidal artery stretched around the medially displaced uncus (plexal portion of anterior choroid artery is not medially displaced).	d. Stretching of cisternal portion of anterior choroidal artery.
e. Enlargement of the atria of the lateral ventricle.	e. Straightened medial atrial veins (visualized medial to the thalamostriate vein).	e. Elongated (1) medial and lateral atrial subependymal veins; (2) depression of the choroid in the floor of the atrium of the lateral ventricle. (NOTE: Increased distance between the elevated pericallosal PCA and the depressed choroid plexus.)
f. Enlargement of the third ventricle.	f. (−)	f. Elevation of the medial posterior choroidal artery and ICV is prevented by the hydrocephalic lateral ventricles above the third ventricle, which depress these vessels.

In massive nonatrophic hydrocephalus the enlarged frontal horn will displace the horizontal part of the ACA posteriorly, medially, and inferiorly. The temporal horn enlargement will elevate the Sylvian triangle and the horizontal portion of the MCA. Occipital and atrial enlargement will stretch the PCA and separate the posterior temporal and parietal occipital branches. Third ventricle enlargement will depress the posterior communicating arteries, elevate the horizontal ACA, displace the ICA and ascending ACA forward, depress the top of the basilar artery, and if unopposed by hydrocephalus of the lateral ventricle, elevate the medial posterior choroidal artery and ICV.

AP CAROTID ARTERIOGRAM

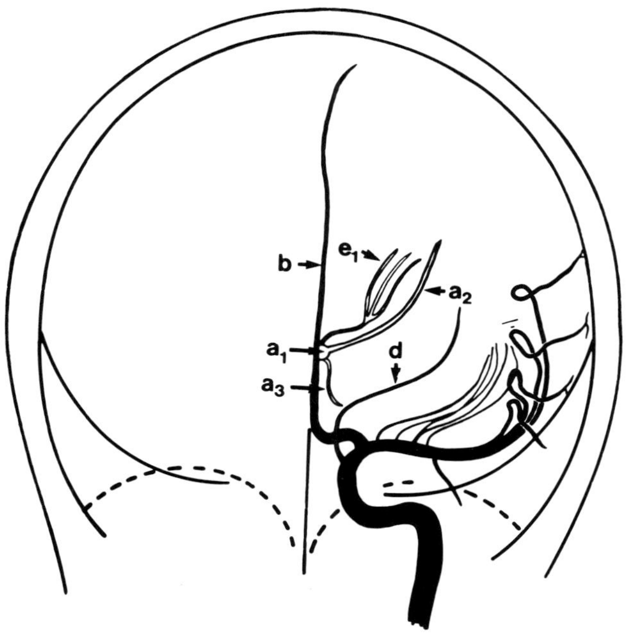

LATERAL CAROTID ARTERIOGRAM

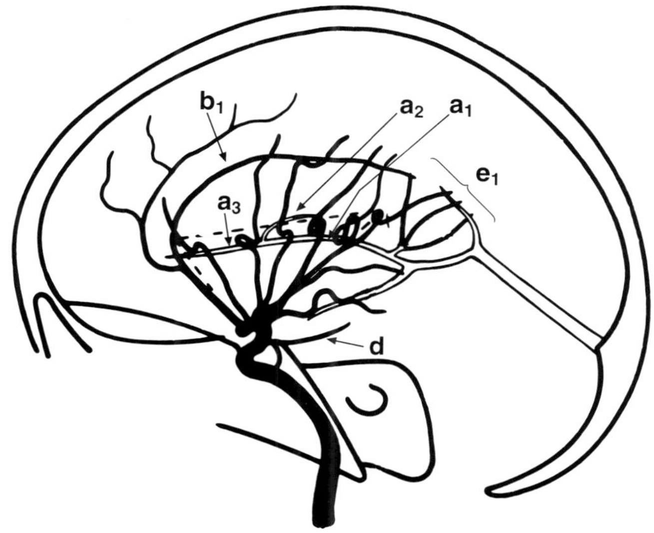

AP VERTEBRAL ARTERIOGRAM

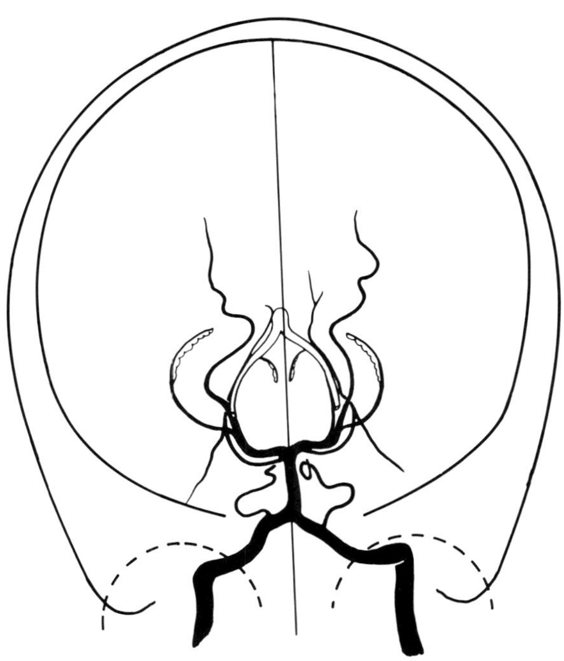

LATERAL VERTEBRAL ARTERIOGRAM

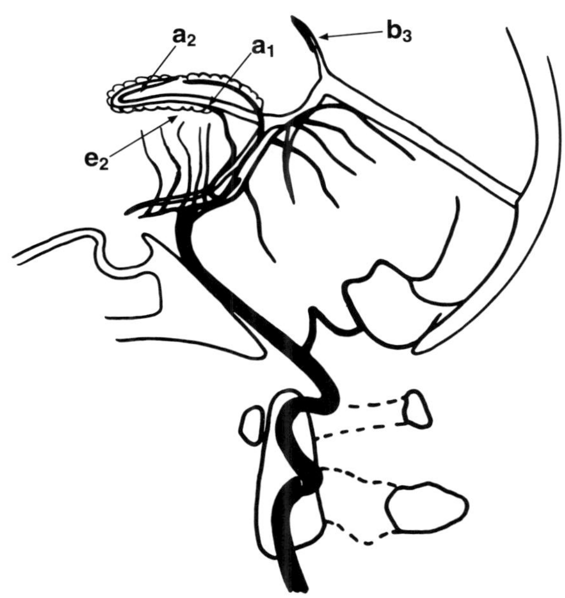

ANTERIOR SUPRASYLVIAN MASSES: INTRAAXIAL

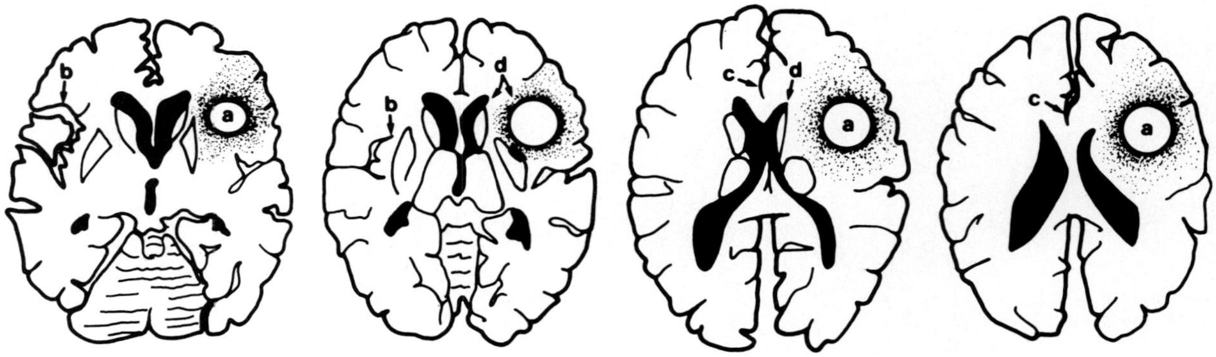

Figure 15-12 Anterior Suprasylvian Masses: Intraaxial (above the anterior Sylvian point*)

Axial brain sections	AP cartoid anteriogram	Lateral cartoid anteriogram
a. Frontal mass above the anterior part of the Sylvian fissure.	a. (−)	a. Distal portions of Sylvian MCA stretched and spread apart by mass.
b. Obliteration of anterior aspect of Sylvian fissure (normal side marked for comparison).	b. (−)*	b. Depression of (1) the anterior Sylvian point and (2) Sylvian branches below the mass.
c. Transtentorial herniation of proximal supracallosal segment of frontal lobe.	c. Proximal supracallosal segment of ACA displaced across midline.	c. (−)
d. Compression of the anterior part of the lateral ventricle and adjacent basal ganglia.	d. Medial deflection of distal lenticulostriate vessels.	d. (−)†

*Intraaxial masses medial and lateral to the Sylvian point will displace it in the approximate direction on the AP arteriogram.
†Minimal medial displacement cf the distal septal vein is difficult to confidently recognize.

AP CAROTID ANTERIOGRAM

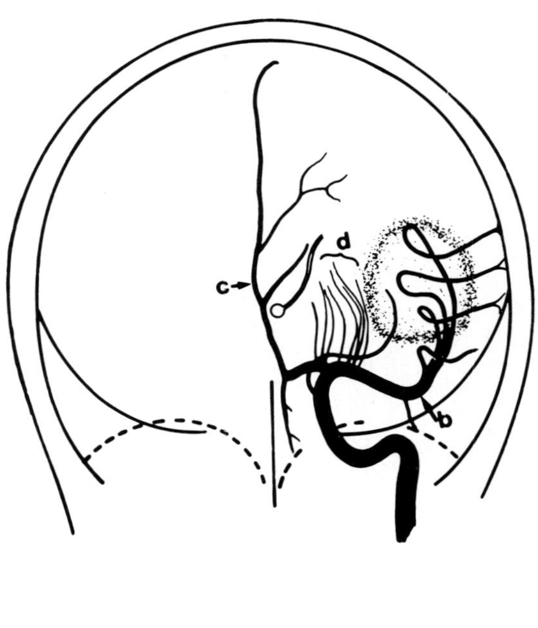

LATERAL CAROTID ARTERIOGRAM

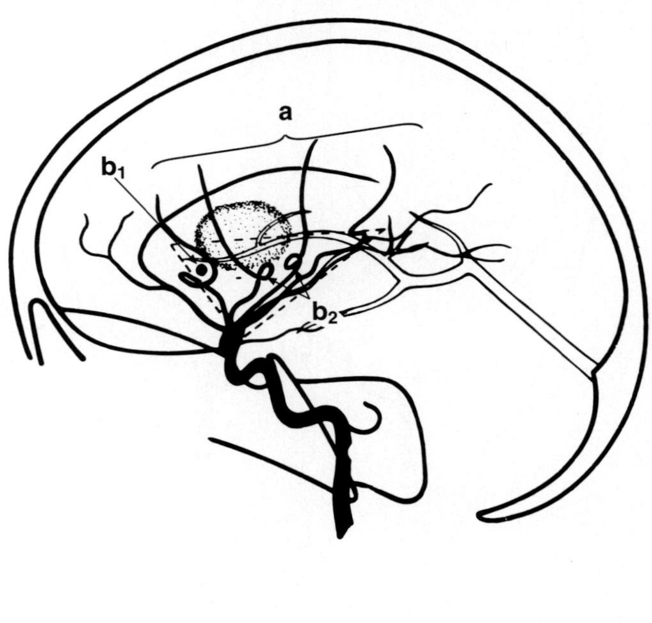

POSTERIOR SUPRASYLVIAN MASS (INTRAAXIAL)

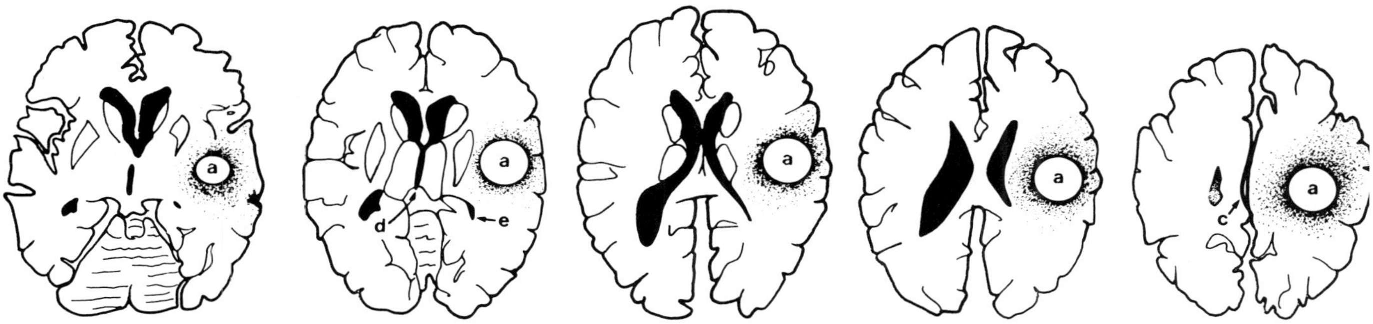

Figure 15-13 Posterior Suprasylvian Mass: Intraaxial

Axial brain sections	AP carotid arteriogram	Lateral carotid arteriogram
a. Mass within the parietal lobe directly above the posterior part of the Sylvian fissure.	a. Distal branches of the posterior Sylvian MCA stretched around intraaxial mass.	a. Distal branches of posterior Sylvian MCA stretched and spread apart by mass.
b. Obliteration of the posterior aspect of the Sylvian triangle (normal side marked for comparison).	b. Depression of the posterior Sylvian point.*	b. Depression of: (1) the posterior Sylvian point and (2) Sylvian branches beneath the mass.
c. Transfalcine herniation of the anterior parietal lobe.	c. Distal (supracallosal) segment of ACA displaced across the midline.	c. (−)
d. Transfalcine herniation of the posterior third ventricle.	d. Transfalcine herniation of the ICV. (NOTE: IVC shift is greater than ACA shift.)	d. Mild depression of the proximal ICV.
e. Compression of the trigone of the lateral ventricle.	e. Subtle distortion of medial atrial subependymal vein (not shown).	e. Subtle distortion of medial atrial subependymal vein.

*Intraaxial masses medial or lateral to the posterior Sylvian point will displace it in the appropriate direction on the AP carotid arteriogram.

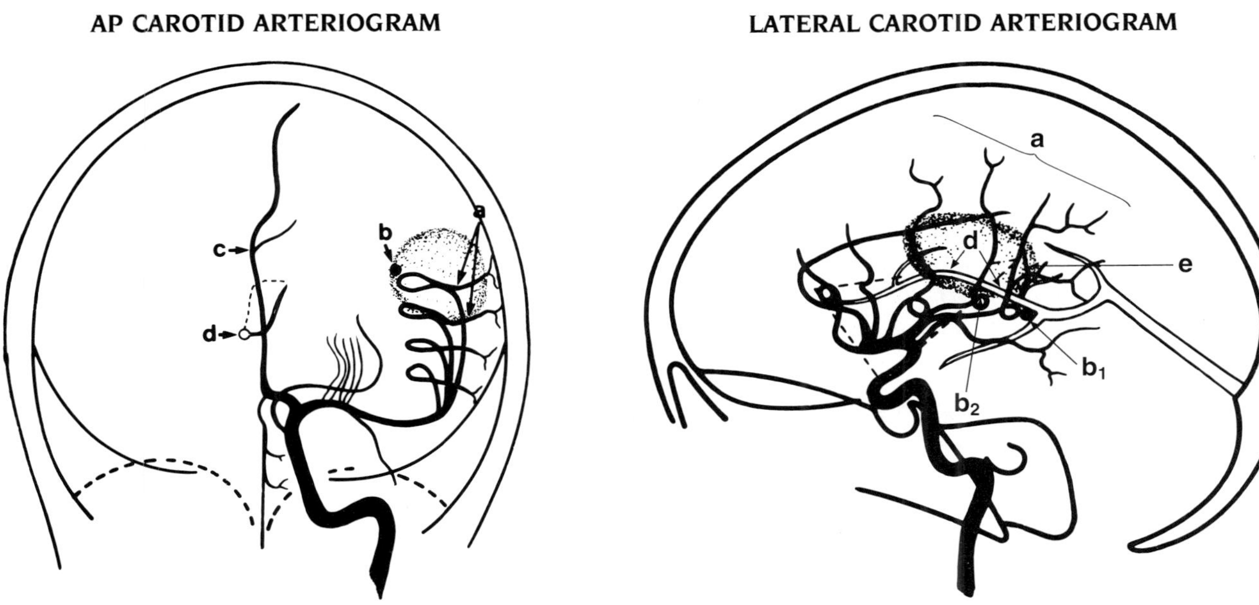

SUPERIOR RETROSYLVIAN MASS: INTRAAXIAL

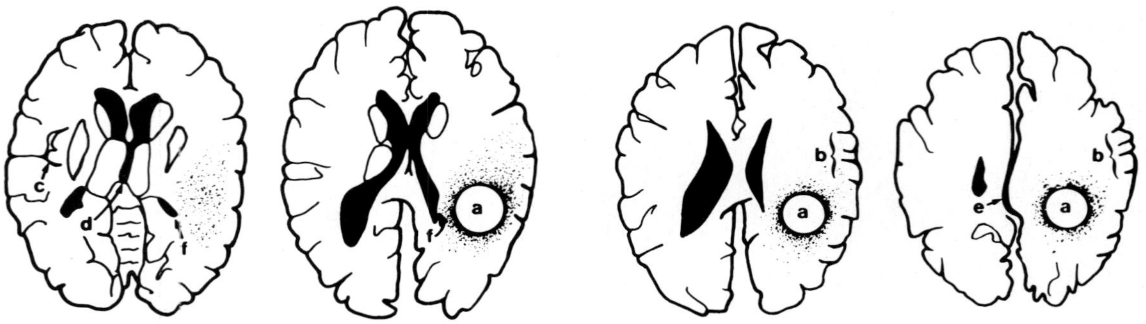

Figure 15-14 Superior Retrosylvian Mass: Intraaxial (mass above and behind the posterior Sylvian point)

Axial brain sections	AP carotid arteriogram	Lateral carotid arteriogram
a. Mass within the posterior superior parietal lobe.	a. (−)	a. Distal branches of posterior MCA spread apart by mass.
b. Cortical gyri anterior to the mass are compressed due to the forward displacement of brain.	b. (−)	b. Anterior Sylvian MCA branches are stretched and have a forward convexity.
c. Compression of the posterior aspect of Sylvian fissure (see normal side for comparison).	c. Posterior Sylvian point is moved forward which causes it to "appear" depressed on a Towne's view.*	c. Forward displacement of posterior Sylvian point results in telescopic or closed accordian appearance of Sylvian branches. NOTE: There is no actual depression of the posterior Sylvian point.
d. Depression of the posterior aspect of the third ventricle roof and shift across the midline.	d. ICV depressed and shifted across the midline.	d. Flattened posterior slope of internal cerebral vein.
e. Focal transtentorial herniation of the parietal cortex adjacent to the mass.	e. Shift across the midline of the distal ACA.	e. (−)
f. Compression of the trigone and occipital horn of the lateral ventricle.†	f. Distortion of the medial atrial vein (not shown).	f. (−)

*Intraaxial masses medial or lateral to the posterior Sylvian point will displace it in the appropriate direction on the AP arteriogram.
†In some normal cases, this appearance is due to congenital coaptation of the occipital horn and has no clinical significance.

AP CAROTID ARTERIOGRAM

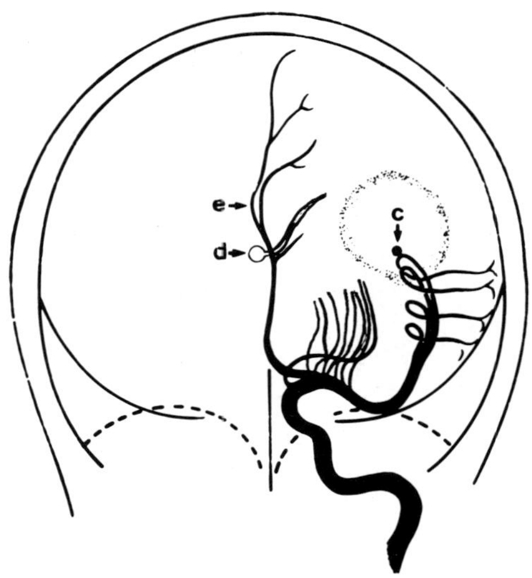

LATERAL CAROTID ARTERIOGRAM

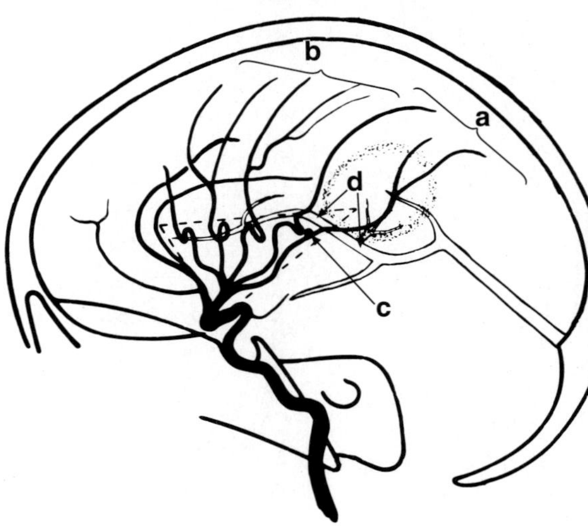

POSTEROMEDIAL INFRASYLVIAN MASS: INTRAAXIAL

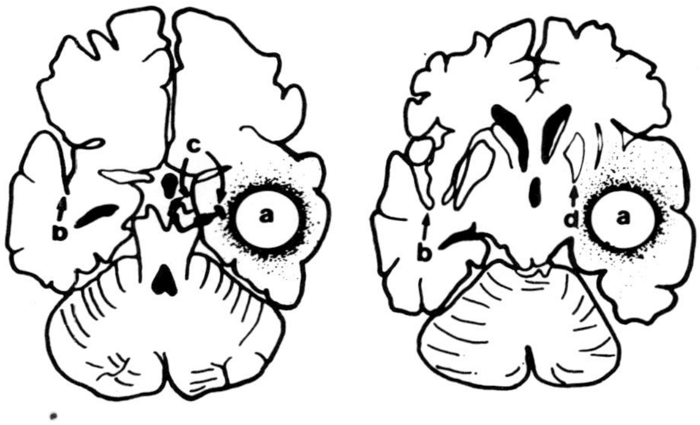

Figure 15-15 Posteromedial Infrasylvian Mass: Intraaxial
(below the posterior Sylvian point and above the plane of the anterior choroidial artery)

Axial brain sections	AP carotid arteriogram	Lateral carotid arteriogram
a. Mass within the inferior temporal lobe below the posterior and middle aspects of the Sylvian triangle.	a. Distal superficial temporal MCA branches stretched over the intraaxial mass.	a. Distal superficial temporal MCA branches stretched and spread apart by mass.
b. Obliteration of posterior and middle aspects of Sylvian fissure (normal side marked for comparison).	b. Elevation of the posterior Sylvian point*.	b. Elevation of (1) posterior Sylvian point and (2) adjacent Sylvian branches.
c. Uncal herniation evidenced by asymmetry of suprasellar cistern and medial displacement of temporal horn of lateral ventricle.	c. Medial displacement of anterior choroidial artery.†	c. Elevation of the anterior choroidal artery.†
d. Compression and slight anterior displacement of the adjacent basal ganglia region.	d. Medial displacement of lenticulostriate vessels.	d. (−)

*Masses medial or lateral to the posterior Sylvian point will displace it in the appropriate direction on the AP arteriogram.
†The normal variation in the course of the Basal Vein of Rosenthal prevents confident detection of medial elevation on the AP or elevation on the lateral views.

AP CAROTID ARTERIOGRAM

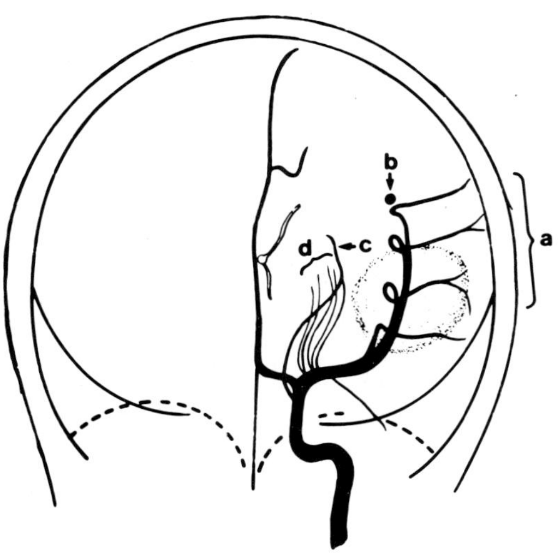

LATERAL CAROTID ARTERIOGRAM

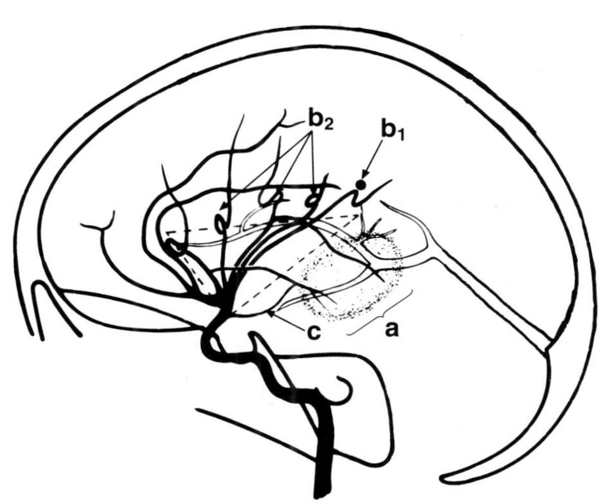

INFERIOR RETROSYLVIAN MASS: INTRAAXIAL

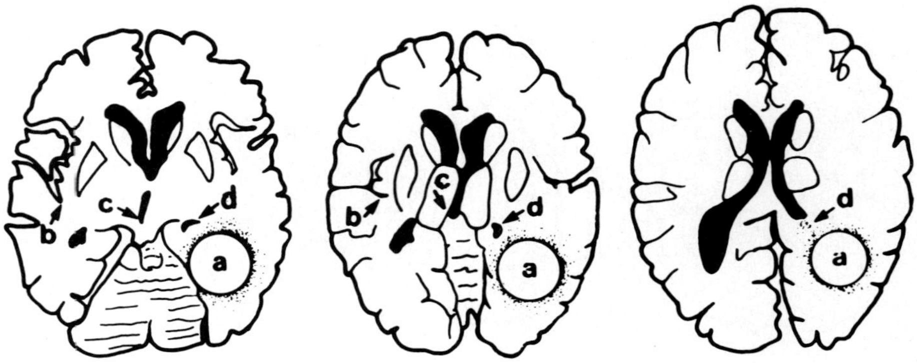

Figure 15-16 Inferior Retrosylvian Mass: Intraaxial (mass below and behind the posterior Sylvian point)

Axial brain sections	AP carotid arteriogram	Lateral carotid arteriogram
a. Mass within the temporooccipital region.	a. (−)	a. Distal branches of posterior Sylvian MCA and PCA are stretched around the mass.
b. Compression of posterior aspect of the Sylvian fissure (see normal side for comparison).	b. Posterior Sylvian point is moved forward* which causes it to "appear" depressed on a Towne's view.	b. Forward displacement of posterior Sylvian point results in telescoped or closed accordian appearance of Sylvian branches. NOTE: There is no actual depression of the posterior Sylvian point despite appearance on AP.
c. Compression of the posterior aspect of the third ventricle with shift across the midline.	c. ICV displaced across midline.	c. (−)
d. Medial and forward displacement of the atrium of the lateral ventricle; compression of the occipital horn.†	d. Distortion of the atrial subependymal veins (not shown).	d. Distortion of the atrial subependymal veins (not shown).

*Intraaxial masses medial or lateral to the posterior Sylvian point will also displace it in the opposite direction on the AP arteriogram.
†In some normal cases this appearance of the occipital horn is due to congenital coaptation and has no clinical significance.

AP CAROTID ARTERIOGRAM

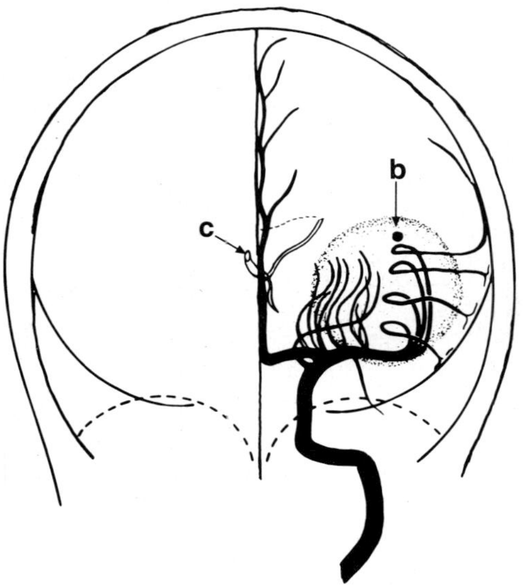

LATERAL CAROTID ARTERIOGRAM

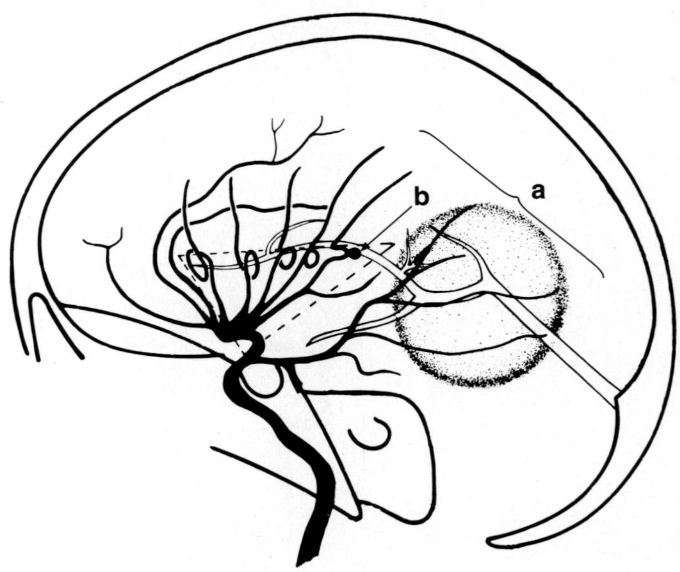

INFERIOR RETROSYLVIAN MASS: EXTRAAXIAL

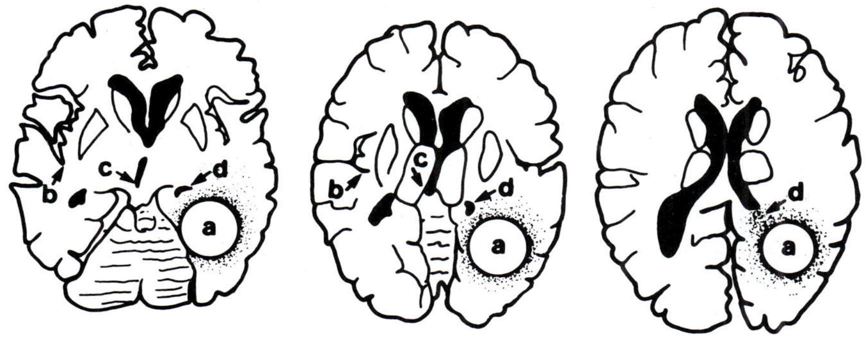

Figure 15-17 Inferior Retrosylvian Mass: Extraaxial
(centrally positioned between the tentorium and the inferior surface of the cerebral hemisphere)*

Axial brain sections	AP carotid arteriogram	Lateral carotid arteriogram
a. Mass between the temporooccipital region and the tentorium.	a. (−)	a. Distal branches of (1) the posterior MCA and (2) PCA are stretched, spread apart, and elevated by the mass.
b. Compression of posterior aspect of the Sylvian fissure (see normal side for comparison).	b. Posterior Sylvian point is moved forward which causes it to "appear" depressed on a Towne's view.	b. Forward displacement of posterior Sylvian point results in telescopic or closed accordian appearance of Sylvian branches. NOTE: There is no actual depression of the posterior Sylvian point.
c. Compression of the posterior aspect of the third ventricle with shift across the midline.	c. ICV displaced across the midline.	c. (−)
d. Medial and forward displacement of the atrium of the lateral ventricle; compression of the occipital horn.†	d. Distortion of the atrial subependymal veins (not shown).	d. Distortion of the atrial subependymal veins (not shown).

*A medial extraaxial mass will elevate the PCA branches but have minimal effect on the posterior Sylvian MCA branches; a lateral extrasylvian mass will displace the PCA branches medially and elevate the posterior Sylvian branches of the MCA.

†In some normal cases this appearance of the occipital horn is due to congenital coaptation and has no clinical significance.

AP CAROTID ARTERIOGRAM

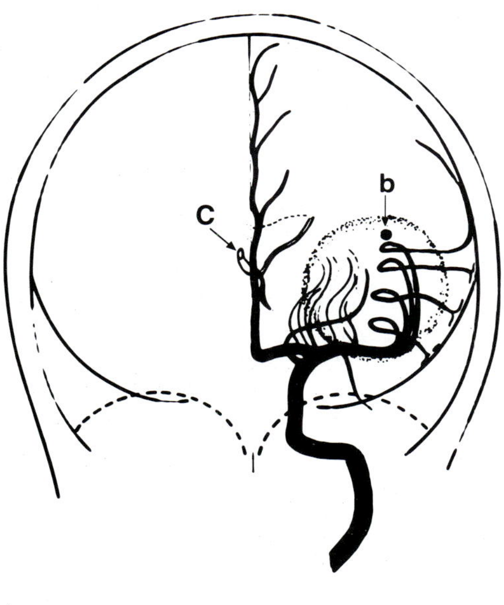

LATERAL CAROTID ARTERIOGRAM

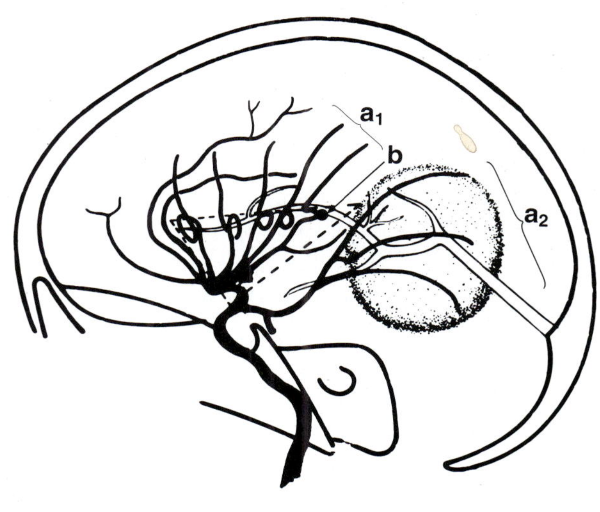

SYMMETRICAL PINEAL REGION MASS

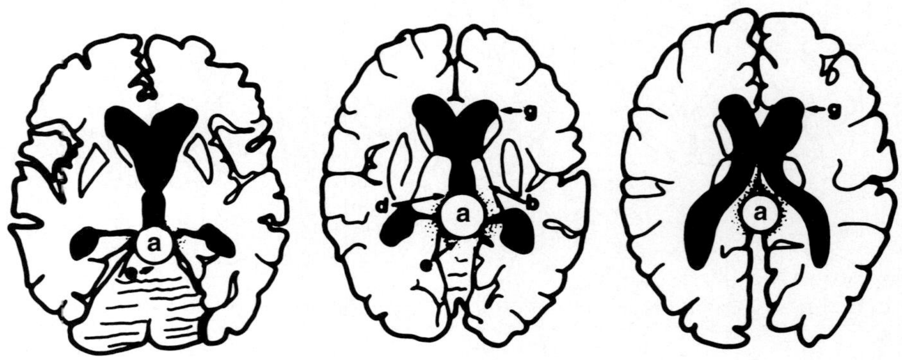

Figure 15-18 Symmetrical Pineal Region Mass Causing Aqueduct Stenosis*

Axial brain slice	AP vertebral arteriogram	Lateral vertebral arteriogram
a. Pineal cistern mass (exclude stippled area).	a. Separation and superolateral bowing of the posterior segment of the Basal Vein or Rosenthal (BVR) around the mass.†	a. Elevation of (1) the distal ICV, (2) posterior segment of Basal Vein of Rosenthal (BVR), (3) the Great Vein of Galen (GVG) by the mass.‡
b. Forward displacement of the thalamus and separation of the medial thalamic walls.	b. (−)	b. Stretching and posterior displacement of the thalamoperforating branches of PCA.
c. Elevation of the splenium of the corpus callosum (not visible on axial sections).	c. (−)	c. Elevation of (1) the posterior pericallosal arteries of PCA (not shown) and (2) the vein of the splenium of the corpus callosum.
d. Compression of the posterior third ventricle.	d. Lateral displacement of the posteromedial choroidal arteries.§	d. (1) Anterior (or posterior) bowing of the distal posterior medial choroidial arteries around the mass§ and (2) focal elevation and forward displacement of the choroid in the roof of the third ventricle.
e. Extension below the tentorium into (1) the superior cerebellar and vermian cisterns and (2) indentation of the superior vermis and cerebellar hemispheres.	e. (−)	e. (1) Posterior bowing of the SCA branches on the anterior surface of the vermis and superior cerebellar hemisphere and (2) posterior displacement of the precentral vein (reversal of colliculocentral angle).
f. (1) Extension into the quadrigeminal cistern and (2) compression of the midbrain which results in obstruction of the aqueduct (not shown).	f. (−)	f. (−)
g. Symmetrical obstructive hydrocephalus of the third and lateral ventricles.	g. Consult Hydrocephalus in this section (Figure 15–11).	g. Consult Hydrocelphalus in this section (Figure 15–11).

*The pattern of vascular displacements caused by a pineal region mass cannot be used to distinguish intraaxial (pineal) tumors from extraaxial masses (cyst, aneurysm of the Vein of Galen, tentorial tumor, etc.). The clinical history, presence, and character of neovascularity as well as the appearance of the mass on CT and MR must be evaluated.

†The ambient segment of PCA does not reliably define the brainstem surface; therefore lateral displacement of this vessel can be confidently detected only when the mass is huge.

‡The positions of the inferior and superior thalamic veins cannot be reliably identified.

§This is seldom recognized on AP or lateral arteriogram because it is concealed by overlapping vascular images.

AP VERTEBRAL ARTERIOGRAM

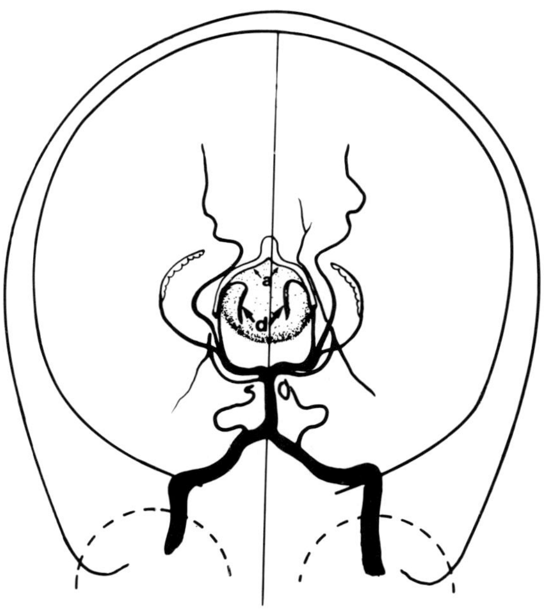

LATERAL VERTEBRAL ARTERIOGRAM

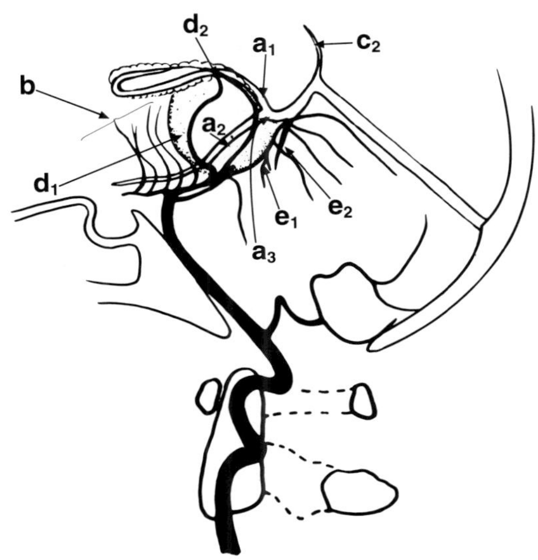

FOURTH VENTRICLE MASS

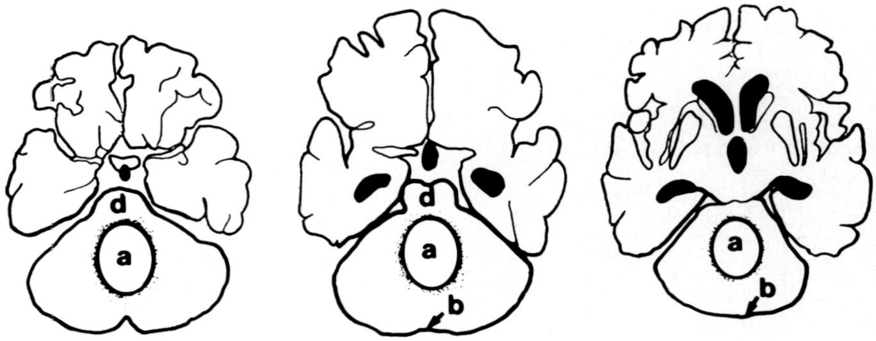

Figure 15-19 Fourth Ventricle Mass

Axial brain sections	AP vertebral arteriogram	Lateral vertebral arteriogram
a. Mass within the fourth ventricle. b. Posterior and superior displacement of the vermis.	a. (−) b. (−)	a. (−) b. Superior displacement of the colliculocentral point; fissural and parenchymal segments of precentral cerebellar vein are displaced upward and somewhat backward (colliculocentral angle becomes acute).
c. Mass between the tonsils separates, flattens, and elongates them (not shown).	c. (1) Separation of the choroidal points of PICA and the copular points of the retrotonsillar vein and (2) lateral displacement of the medial tonsillar tributary of the vein of the lateral recess of the fourth ventricle.	c. (1) Posterior displacement of the choroidal points of the PICA and (2) the copular point of both retrotonsillar veins; (3) elongation of the medial tonsillar vein and the supratonsillar vein.
d. Anterior displacement and minimal widening of the brainstem.	d. (−)	d. Anterior displacement of the pontomesencephalic veins and the basilar artery (when it is midline).
e. Absence of the fourth ventricle lumen causes obstruction of CSF passage. (Consult hydrocephalus in supratentorial section.)	e. Consult Hydrocephalus in supratentorial section (see Figure 15–11).	e. Consult Hydrocephalus in supratentorial section (see Figure 15–11).

AP VERTEBRAL ARTERIOGRAM—ARTERIAL PHASE

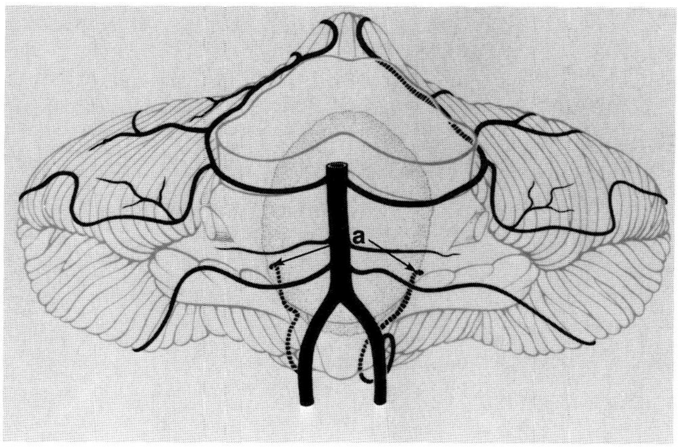

AP VERTEBRAL ARTERIOGRAM—VENOUS PHASE

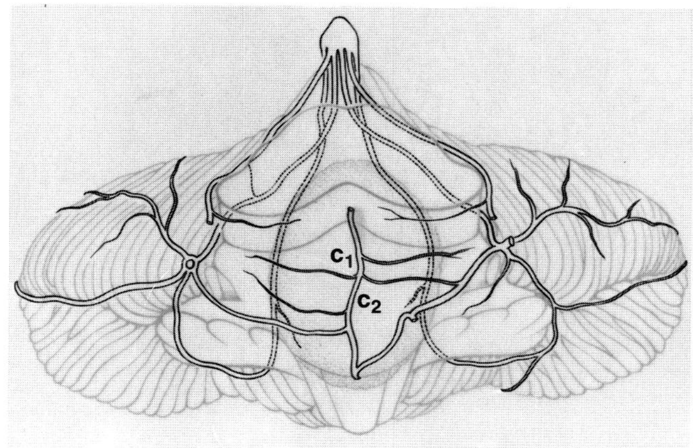

LATERAL VERTEBRAL ARTERIOGRAM

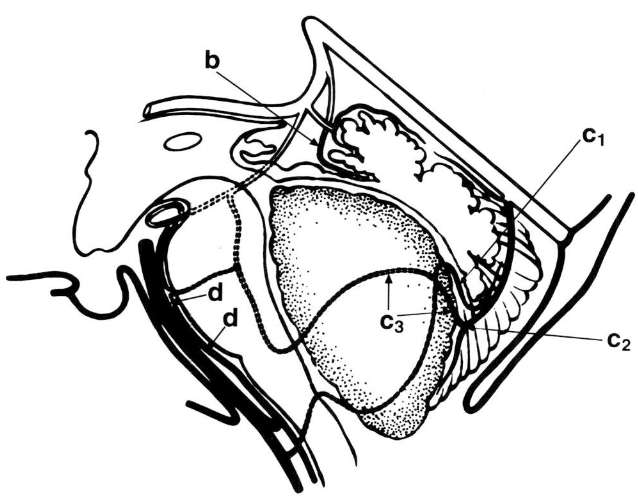

INTRAVERMIAN MASS

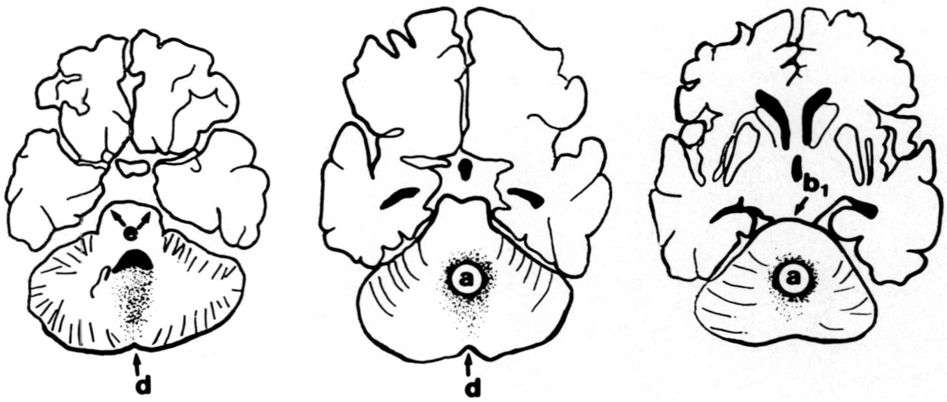

Figure 15-20 Intravermian Mass*

Axial brain sections	AP vertebral arteriogram	Lateral vertebral arteriogram
a. Mass within the central vermis.	a. (−)	a. (−)
b. Superior expansion of the vermis compresses the (1) quadrigeminal plate and (2) superior vermian cisterns (not visible on axial sections).	b. Separation of vermian branches of SCA.	b. Focal forward and superior displacement and stretching of the precentral vein† (effaced and widened colliculo-central angle).
c. Inferior expansion of the vermis causes symmetrical tonsillar herniation, which obliterates the cisterna magna (not shown).	c. (1) Depression of the superior tonsillar pole veins (tonsillar tributary of the lateral recess of the fourth ventricle and the superior retrotonsillar vein); (2) depression of the inferior retrotonsillar vein; (3) depression of the choroid point of both PICAs	c. (1) Depression of the superior tonsillar pole veins (tonsillar tributary of the vein of the lateral recess of the fourth ventricle and the superior retrotonsillar vein); (2) depression of the inferior retrotonsillar vein‡; (3) depression of the choroid point of PICA.
d. Posterior expansion of the vermis causes AP compression of the vallecula.	d. (−)	d. Posterior displacement of the inferior vermian veins.§
e. Anterior expansion of the vermis compresses and broadens the pons.	e. Stretching of (1) AICA and (2) transverse pontine veins around the broadened pons.	e. Anterior displacement of (1) the anterior pontomesencephalic vein and (2) the basilar artery (when it is midline).
f. Lateral expansion of the vermis causes widening of the vallecula, which separates the medial tonsillar surfaces (not shown).	f. Lateral displacement of (1) inferior vermian veins and (2) PICA.	f. (−)

(*) A mass of the inferiormost aspect of the vermis will cause anterior displacement of the tonsils in addition to the inferolateral displacement described for a central vermian mass. Also, relatively greater displacement and separation of the inferior vermian vein will occur with an inferior vermian mass.

†Elevation of the superior vermian branch of SCA is usually unrecognizable due to overlapping vessels in the routine lateral.

‡Normal variations in the tonsillar branch of PICA preclude its use as a reliable marker.

§Posterior displacement of the vermian branch of PICA is usually unrecognized due to overlapping vessels.

AP VERTEBRAL ARTERIOGRAM—ARTERIAL PHASE

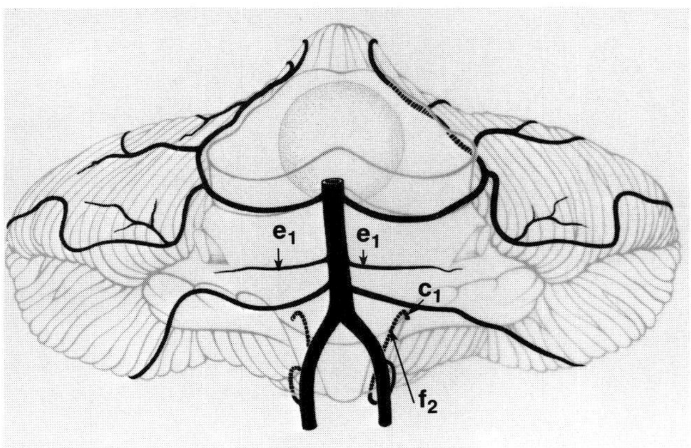

AP VERTEBRAL ARTERIOGRAM—VENOUS PHASE

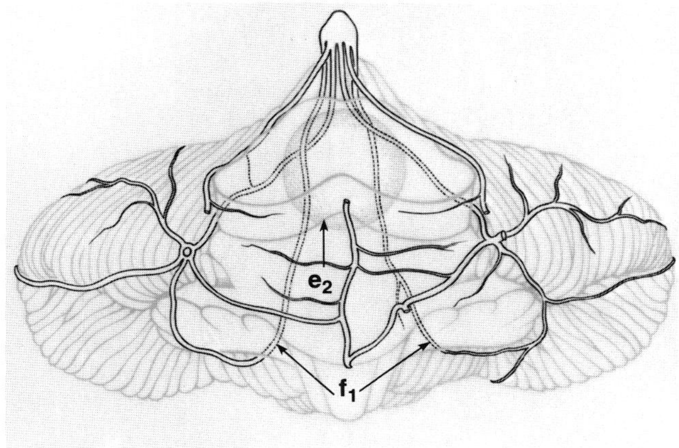

LATERAL VERTEBRAL ARTERIOGRAM

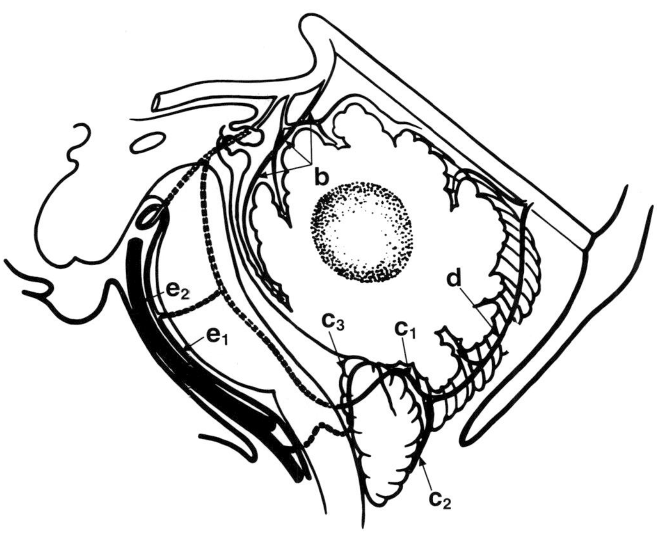

SUPERIOR CEREBELLAR HEMISPHERE MASS

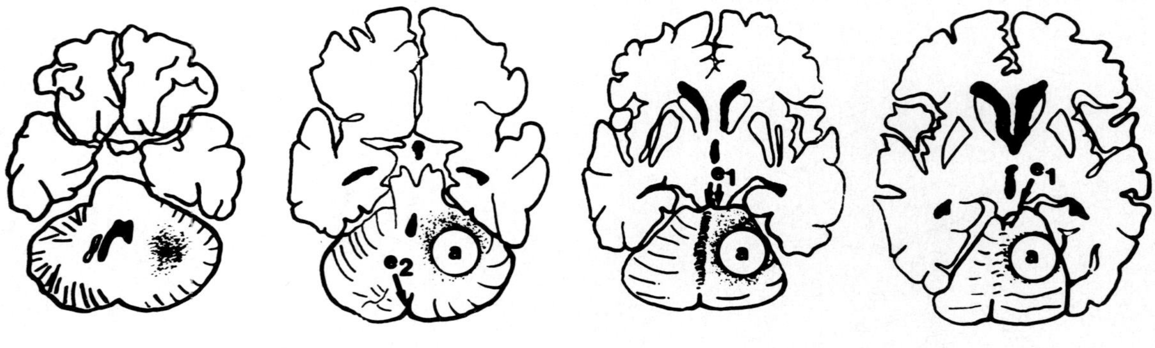

Figure 15-21 Superior Cerebellar Hemisphere Mass*

Axial brain images	AP vertebral arteriogram	Lateral vertebral arteriogram
a. Mass within or above the superior aspect of the cerebellar hemisphere.	a. Stretching of the superior cerebellar arteries and the surface veins.†	a. (−)
b. Expansion of superior cerebellum causes compression of the superior cerebellar cistern and the posterior aspect of the ambient cistern (not visible on axial sections).	b. Mild flattening of the distal ambient segment of SCA.	b. (−)
c. Obliteration of the superior recess of the fourth ventricle and depression and medial displacement of the posterior surface of the fourth ventricle (which is the superior pole of the tonsil).	c. (1) Depression and medial displacement of the superior tonsillar pole veins (tonsillar tributary of the vein of the lateral recess of the fourth ventricle and the superior retrotonsillar vein); (2) depression and medial displacement of the choroidal point of PICA (not shown).	c. (1) Depression of the superior tonsillar pole veins (supratonsillar branch of inferior vermian vein); (2) downward displacement of the choroid point of the PICA.§
d. Depression of the Great Horizontal fissure (not visible on axial sections).	d. Depression of the marginal branch of SCA and the petrosal tributary vein within the Great Horizontal fissure.	d. (−)
e. Compression of the medial aspect of the vermis causes: (1) superior and forward movement of its upper surface which obliterates the quadrigeminal plate cistern and (2) backward and downward movement of its inferior surface which compresses the vallecula.	e. Medial displacement of the inferior vermian vein.‖	e. (1) Forward and superior displacement of the precentral vein. NOTE: There is no focal deformity of the vein to indicate intravermian pathology (consult vermian mass). (2) Backward and downward displacement of the inferior vermian vein.

(*) A mass in the inferior cerebellum creates a relatively greater focal effect on the adjacent tonsil than described for a cerebellar mass.

†Axial images and routine angiography of intraaxial and extraaxial masses appear the same. Stereoscopic angiography or oblique orbital AP films (which places the tentorial surface of the appropriate side in profile) are needed to detect the superior or inferior displacement of the superior hemispheric veins and arteries caused by intraaxial or extraaxial superior cerebellar masses.

‡Increased pressure in the posterior fossa may result in delayed or absent opacification of these veins.

§The wide range of normal in the configuration of PICA precludes its use in evaluating the tonsil.

‖The wide range of normal in the position of the vermian and hemispheric branches of PICA preclude their use.

AP VERTEBRAL ARTERIOGRAM—ARTERIAL PHASE

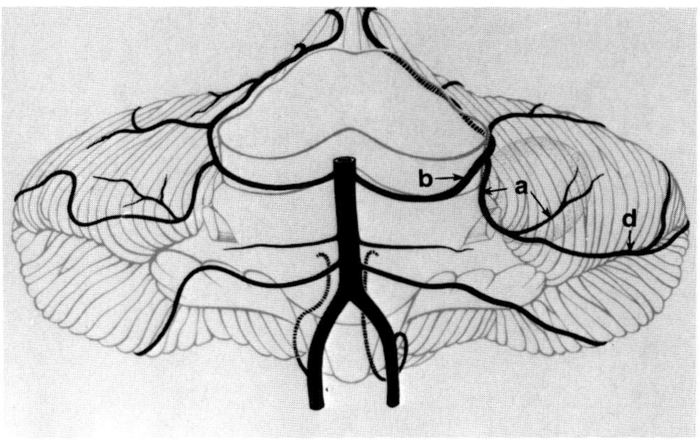

AP VERTEBRAL ARTERIOGRAM—VENOUS PHASE

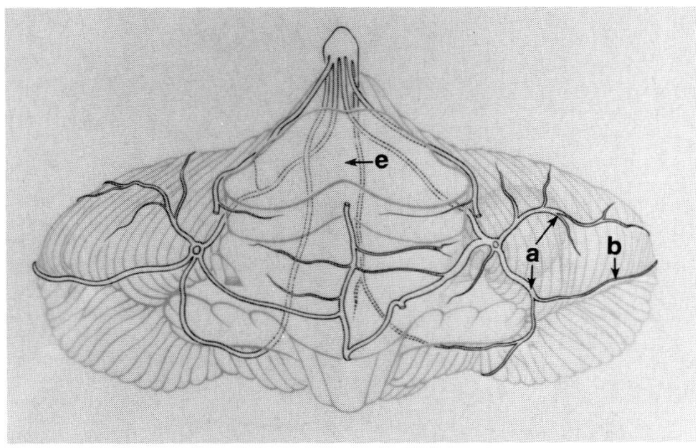

LATERAL VERTEBRAL ARTERIOGRAM

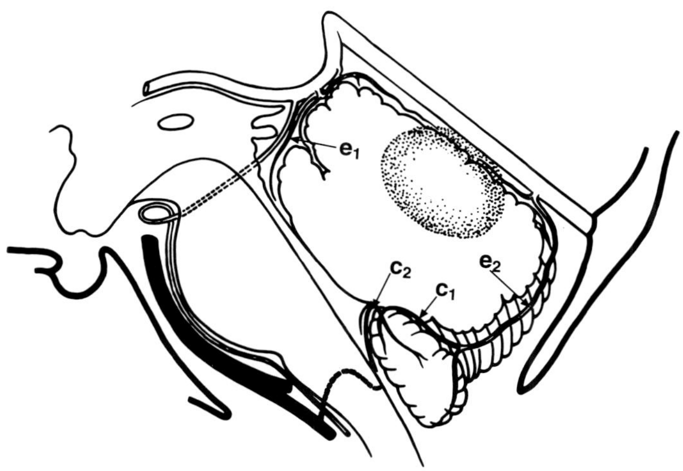

BRAINSTEM MASS

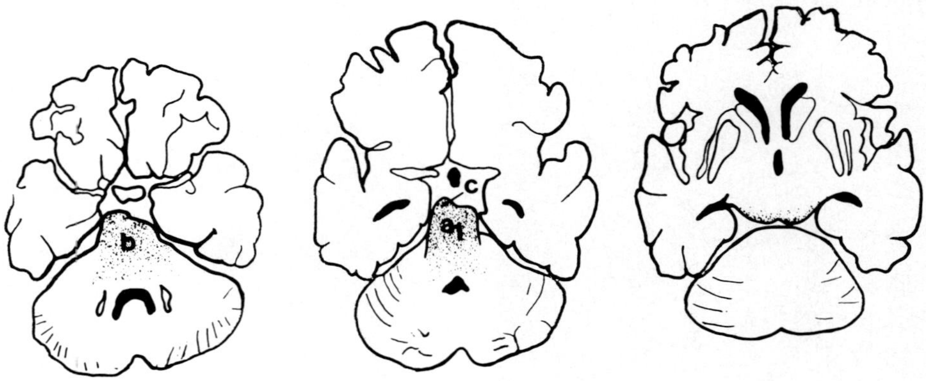

Figure 15-22 Brainstem Mass

Axial brain sections	AP vertebral arteriogram	Lateral vertebral arteriogram
a. (1) Circumferential enlargement and (2) elongation of the midbrain (mesencephalon) which deforms the posterior aspect of the suprasellar cistern.	a. (1) Stretching and lateral displacement of both the ambient segments of: (1) SCA and (2) PCA (not shown) which encircle the enlarged midbrain.	a. Upward displacement of the ambient portions of (1) SCA; PCA (not shown); and (2) BVR.‡
b. Generalized circumferential enlargement of the pons compresses the prepontine cistern.	b. Generalized stretching of the proximal AICAs and all of the transverse pontine veins.	b. (1) Posterior displacement of the precentral vein (causes flattening of the colliculocentral angle); (2) anterior displacement of the pontomesencephalic veins and basilar artery (when it is midline).
c. Eccentric exophilic pontine mass in the prepontine cistern.*	c. Focal stretching and lateral displacement of the proximal AICAs and the transverse veins around the mass (not shown).	c. Relatively greater focal outward bowing of the transverse pontine veins and AICA around the mass compared to midline vessels on the pontine surface.
d. Generalized circumferential enlargement of the medulla oblongata (not shown).	d. (−)†	d. Posterior displacement of: (1) the medullary segments of PICA and (2) the veins on the posterior surface of the brainstem (restiform vein, medial posterior spinal vein).
e. Posterior displacement and AP compression of the tonsils (not shown).	e. Retrotonsillar veins are displaced laterally (not shown).	e. Posterior displacement of the choroidal point of PICAs; (2) posterior displacement of the copular point of the retrotonsillar veins; (3) decreased AP diameter of the tonsil decreases the distance between the retrotonsillar and retromedullary veins (tonsillar compression).

*Compression of the anterior brainstem surface by the exophytic component of the intrinsic brainstem mass may mimic a prepontine lesion.
†Lateral displacement and stretching of the lateral medullary segment of PICA cannot be reliably differentiated from normal variations in the course of this artery.
‡The posterior mesencephalic vein(s) duplicate the course of the Basal Vein of Rosenthal (BVR) around the midbrain. If the BVR is absent, it can be used as the primary venous landmark for this region.

AP VERTEBRAL ARTERIOGRAM—ARTERIAL PHASE

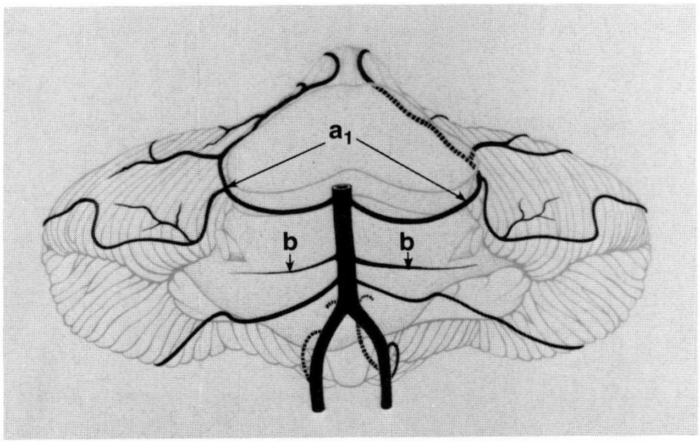

AP VERTEBRAL ARTERIOGRAM—VENOUS PHASE

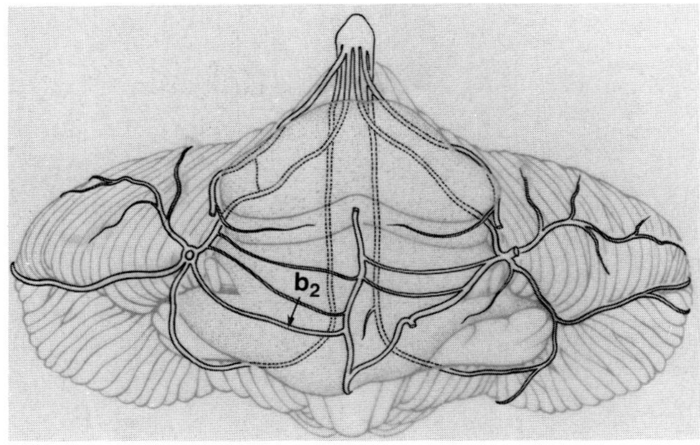

LATERAL VERTEBRAL ARTERIOGRAM

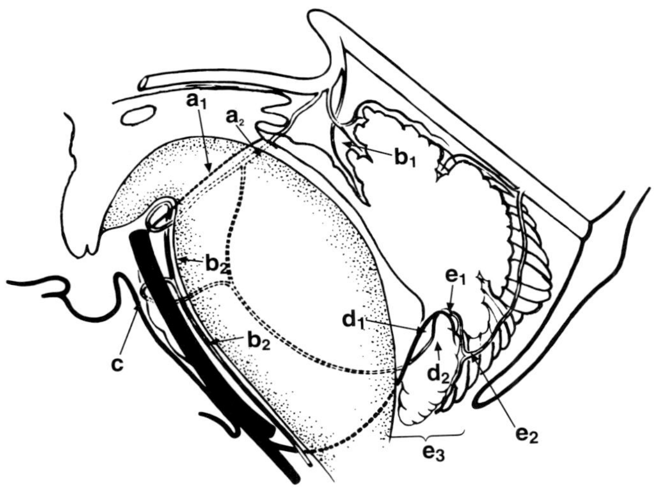

CEREBELLOPONTINE ANGLE MASS

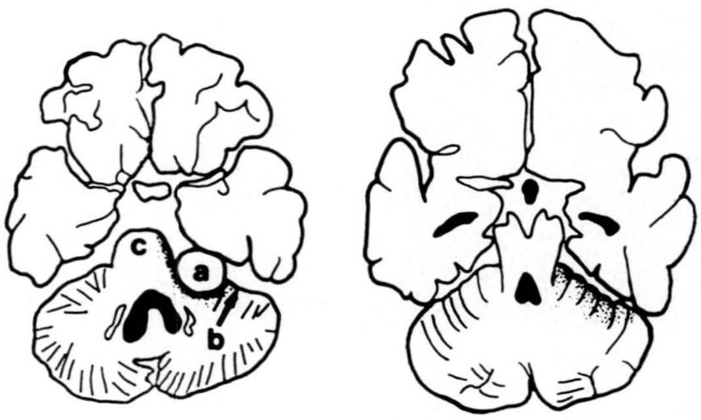

Figure 15-23 Cerebellopontine Angle Mass (greater than 2 cm)

Axial brain sections	AP vertebral arteriogram	Lateral vertebral arteriogram
a. Mass within the cerebellopontine (CP) angle cistern.	a. (−)	a. (−)
b. Posterior displacement of the anterior cerebellar surface causing AP widening of the CP angle cistern.	b. (1) Stretching of the petrosal vein* around the mass; (2) stretching of the AICA and marginal branch of SCA with superior or inferior displacement.	b. Posterior displacement of (1) the petrosal vein (not shown) and (2) AICA by the mass.†
c. Compression of the lateral pontine surface.	c. (1) Medial displacement of the transverse pontine veins; (2) deflection of the trigeminal artery.	c. (−)

*Pressure from the mass may cause absence, delayed and/or diminished filling of this vessel at angiography.

†Stereoscopic filming or a base projection may be needed to demonstrate the posterior displacement of these vessels which may not be visualized confidently on the lateral vertebral arteriogram.

AP VERTEBRAL ARTERIOGRAM—ARTERIAL PHASE

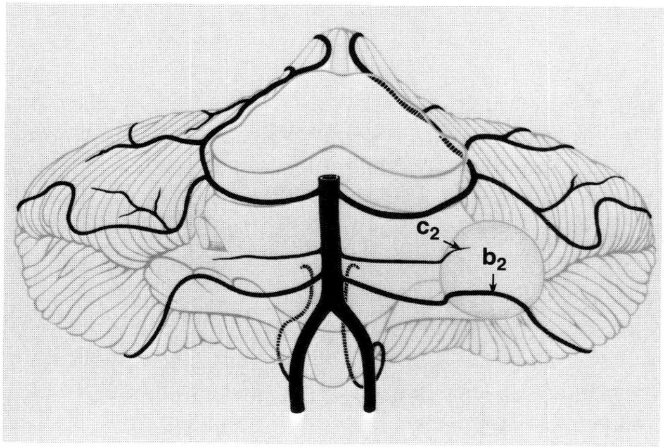

AP VERTEBRAL ARTERIOGRAM—VENOUS PHASE

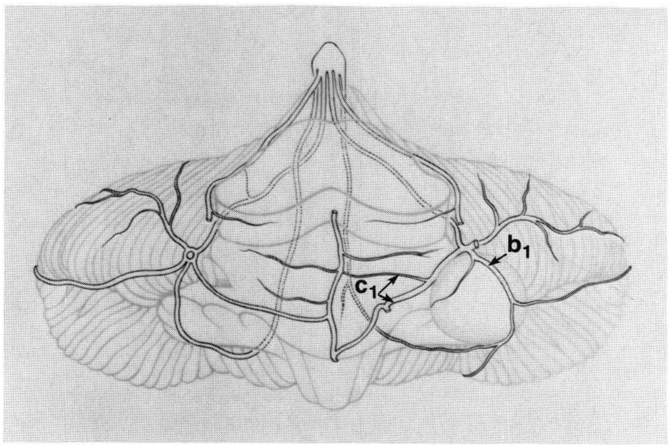

LATERAL VERTEBRAL ARTERIOGRAM

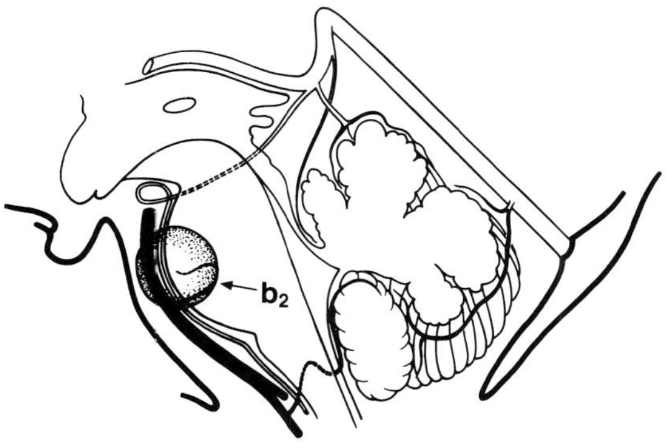

CHAPTER 16

Stephen Alan Berman
L. Anne Hayman
Vincent C. Hinck

Cerebrovascular Territories

This chapter summarizes the functional neuroanatomy and the three vascular territories of the cerebrum in a format directly applicable to axial and coronal images. This simplifies correlation of these images, clinical signs and symptoms, and vascular territories in everyday practice. When using this material, after finding a lesion by computed tomography (CT) or magnetic resonance imaging (MRI), one may choose the axial or coronal images that correspond to the abnormal level(s) and determine whether the lesion is confined to a single vascular territory. If it is, the schematic diagrams can be used to determine which branches supply the area. If arteriography is indicated, the whole-brain schematic of the affected vascular territory can be used to interpret the lateral, arterial phase of the angiogram. Broad functional correlation is then provided by the companion whole-brain schematic that maps the function of the cortex. Further information outlining the fiber tracts encompassed within a territory can be found from accompanying text and diagrams provided in the detailed description of each arterial territory.

Knowledge of vascular territories provided in this chapter can help in differentiating infarction from other pathologic processes. If, for example, the position and extent of a lesion and the usual position and extent of a vascular territory are incongruous, the diagnosis of infarction should receive a relatively low priority, and vice versa. Knowledge of vascular territories can also facilitate correct interpretation of cerebral angiograms by pinpointing specific vessels for particularly close attention. For example, analysis of a patient's clinical findings in terms of functional neuroanatomy can improve detection of subtle lesions by pinpointing specific territories for special attention on CT and specific vessels for attention on angiograms.

Before examining the following sections, the reader should be aware that an occlusion of *all* the branches of a cerebral territory will rarely produce a lesion on CT that is larger than that defined on the coronal or axial images. In fact, collateral supply, which often interfaces at the periphery of an infarction, may cause the area of involvement to be smaller than that depicted. Furthermore, the area of involvement may have a patchy appearance, since only selected branches within the territory are occluded by emboli or affected by failure of collateral circulation. Very rarely, occlusion results in infarction of an area that is larger than the territory ascribed to it. In these cases the territory supplied by the infarcted vessel has "extended" via collateral vessels into adjacent territory(ies), the natural supply of which has previously been compromised. Thus, when the rescuing vessel is compromised, territory outside the usual vascular limit is also compromised. MRI of completed infarctions may demonstrate the wallerian degeneration in fiber tracts that originated in the now absent or damaged neurons. Therefore the reader should pay particular attention to descriptions of these tracts.

ANTERIOR CEREBRAL ARTERY TERRITORY

In Figures 16-1 and 16-2, the branches of the anterior cerebral artery have been divided into three groups: (1) the medial lenticulostriate arteries, (2) the pericallosal branches to the corpus callosum, and (3) the branches to the cerebral hemisphere.[1] Figure 16-3 is a companion dia-

This chapter is adapted with permission from Latchaw RE: *MR and CT imaging of the head, neck, and spine,* ed 2, St Louis, 1991, Mosby–Year Book.

gram of the medial aspect of the right cerebral hemisphere. It is provided to localize the axial and coronal images of Figures 16-1 and 16-2. The regions supplied by the hemispheric branches and the cortical function of each region are shown.

Medial Lenticulostriate Arteries

The medial lenticulostriate arteries include the artery of Heubner (long central artery) and basal branches of the anterior cerebral artery. The artery of Heubner supplies the anterior aspects of the putamen and caudate nucleus, as well as the anteroinferior part of the internal capsule. Infarction causes weakness of the contralateral face and arm without sensory loss. A transient aphasia is often seen in which spontaneous speech is lost, whereas repetition and comprehension are preserved.[2] Occasionally, the patient has dysarthria. Although the lower extremity is unaffected, the patient has a halting gait because of difficulty in initiating movements.[2,3]

The basal branches supply the dorsal aspect of the chiasm and the hypothalamus. The anterior portion of the hypothalamus is supplied by small, perforating branches from the anterior cerebral artery. Infarctions in this area can cause abnormalities in temperature regulation, fluid electrolyte balance, synchronization of sleep and wakefulness, and perhaps some aspects of cardiac rhythm. Infarction of the hypothalamus may cause transient memory disorders or more protean psychological manifestations of anxiety, agitation, or a feeling of weakness.[3]

If a bilateral occlusion of the lenticulostriate arteries occurs, a profound alteration of mental activity develops, at times resulting in a state of *akinetic mutism,* a comalike condition in which the patient's eyes remain open and cause him or her to appear awake to superficial inspection. More often, a classic picture of coma evolves.[4,5]

Infarction of the medial lenticulostriate arteries occurs much less frequently than hypertensive hemorrhage from these vessels. Unlike infarction, hemorrhage that arises medial to the putamen crosses vascular boundaries, destroys the hypothalamus, and ruptures into the ventricle. Therefore the radiologist can differentiate a hemorrhagic infarct, in which hemorrhage occurs secondarily, from a primary hemorrhage *(intracerebral hematoma).*

Callosal Branches

The callosal arteries arise from the pericallosal branch of the anterior cerebral artery, penetrate the upper surface of the corpus callosum, and from there extend inferiorly into the septum pellucidum. Usually, 7 to 20 short callosal branches exist, although these are sometimes replaced by a single artery. Infarction can result in isolation of the language-dominant left hemisphere from the right hemisphere, which mediates function of the left side of the body. As a result, the patient experiences difficulty in moving the left side of the body in response to verbal commands *(ideomotor apraxia),* even though no paralysis may exist. Furthermore, the patient cannot recognize words written on the left side of the body, although sensation may be unimpaired *(tactile agnosia),* and the patient has difficulty writing with the left hand *(left-sided agraphia).*[6,7]

Hemispheric Branches

Usually, nine hemispheric branches are present (Figure 16-3, *A*), each supplying a segment of the medial surface of the hemisphere. The medial surface of the hemisphere can be supplied in whole or in part by either anterior cerebral artery. Sometimes both hemispheres are supplied by a single pericallosal artery, the so-called azygous artery. Occlusion of the azygous results in infarction of the medial surfaces of both hemispheres.

In view of the large number of branches and numerous variations of cross-perfusion that can occur, one might expect that the compromise of hemispheric branches could lead to a wide variety of possible clinical sequelae. However, the patterns of infarction can be simplified by comparing the whole-brain schematics of the vascular territories of Figure 16-3, *A,* with the functional areas in Figure 16-3, *B*.

For example, Figure 16-3, *A* and *B,* reveals that the frontal association areas that mediate judgment, insight, and mood receive arterial supply from the orbitofrontal, frontopolar, and anterior internal frontal arteries and, to a lesser extent, from the middle internal frontal arteries.[8] (The posterior internal frontal and paracentral territories may sometimes include a small part of the frontal association area that mediates judgment, insight, and mood [Figure 16-3, *B*].) These functions would be impaired by occlusion of those branches. Some degree of *aphasia* (disturbance of language function) may develop because the arterial supply of subjacent white matter, related to the frontal speech area of Broca, is also disturbed (see the later discussion of aphasia, especially under the hemispheric branches of the middle cerebral artery territory). A release of grasping, groping, and sucking reflex patterns may be seen in addition to impairment of those functions indicated in Figure 16-3, *B*.[2]

Figure 16-3, *A* and *B,* also shows that the motor synchronization area is supplied by the middle and posterior internal frontal branches and, to a small extent, by the anterior internal frontal and paracentral branches. Infarction of the anterior part of the motor synchronization areas affects contralateral conjugate eye deviation, whereas involvement of the posterior part affects coordination of contralateral eye, head, and trunk movement.[9]

Note that the motor function area is supplied by the paracentral branch. Unilateral damage of this branch causes weakness of the contralateral lower extremity (see Figure 16-3). Bilateral damage causes incontinence as well.[8] Note further that the sensory area is supplied by the paracentral and superior and inferior parietal branches. Rarely, a parieto-occipital branch (not shown in Figure

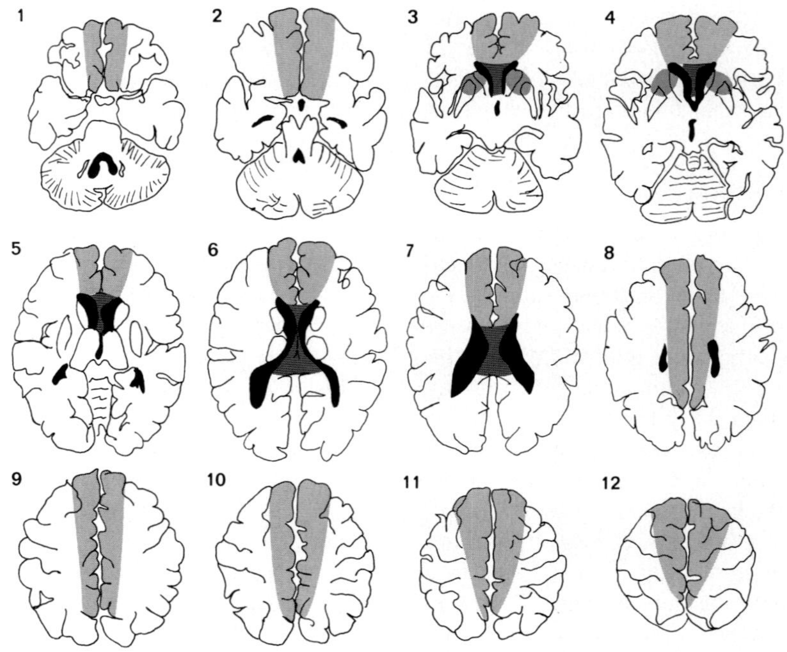

Figure 16-1 Axial diagrams arranged in sequence from base to vertex. Angle and levels of scan planes are shown in Figure 16-3. Territory of the anterior cerebral artery is divided into three regions: medial lenticulostriate (*medium shading*), callosal (*dark shading*), and hemispheric (*light areas*). (Adapted from Matsui T, Hirano A: *An atlas of the human brain for computerized tomography*, Tokyo, 1978, Igaku-Shoin.)

16-3, *A*) may supply the posterior part of this area. Damage to the anterior part of the sensory region impairs but does not abolish appreciation of primary sensory modalities such as touch and pain. Damage to the posterior part impairs more complex sensory appreciation, such as recognition of objects by touch *(stereognosis),* recognition of shapes written on skin *(graphesthesia),* and two-point discrimination.[10]

The supply of the cingulate gyrus, which "controls" memory and emotion, comes from the pericallosal, orbitofrontal, frontopolar, posterior internal frontal, paracentral, and superior and inferior parietal arteries. The cingulum fiber tract within this area is part of the limbic system that is supplied by the posterior cerebral and anterior cerebral arteries. Therefore memory and emotional disturbance may occur as a result of damage to either vascular territory.[2,8]

Finally, infarction in the region of the parieto-occipital fissure, which is sometimes supplied by the parieto-occipital branch of the anterior cerebral artery, has been reported in one patient with anterior cerebral artery compromise. The patient experienced disturbance of recognition in the contralateral visual field *(visual agnosia).* The rarity of such cases can be ascribed to the same area usually being well supplied by the posterior circulation.[2]

MIDDLE CEREBRAL ARTERY TERRITORY

In Figures 16-4 and 16-5, branches of the middle cerebral artery have been divided into two groups: (1) the lateral lenticulostriate branches to the basal ganglia and adjacent fiber tracts and (2) the hemispheric branches to the cerebral convexity.[11] Figure 16-6 is a companion diagram of the lateral aspect of the *left* cerebral hemisphere. It is provided to localize the axial and coronal images of Figures 16-4 and 16-5. The regions supplied by the hemispheric branches and the cortical function of each region are shown.

Lateral Lenticulostriate Arteries

In 20% of brains, the lateral lenticulostriate branches arise from one of the hemispheric branches of the middle cerebral artery. In the other 80%, these branches arise from the trunk of the middle cerebral artery. They supply the substantia innominata, the lateral part of the anterior commissure, most of the putamen and the lateral segment of the globus pallidus, the superior half of the internal capsule and adjacent corona radiata, and the body and head (except the anteroinferior portion) of the caudate nucleus. Portions of the optic radiation, which originate from the lateral geniculate body, and the arcuate fasciculus are supplied by the striate branches.[12]

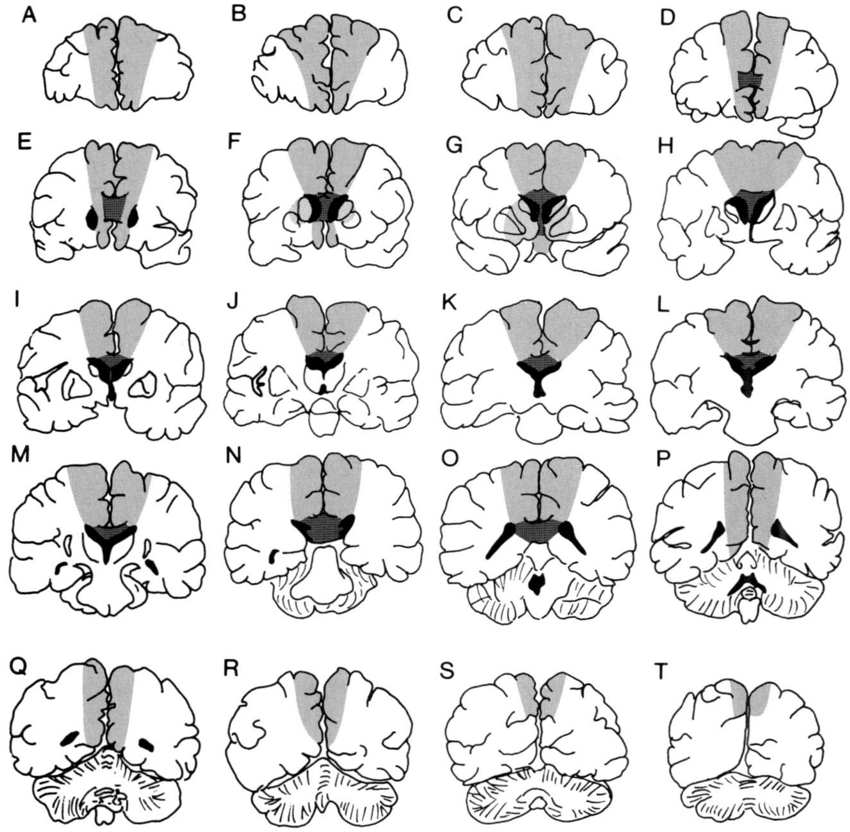

Figure 16-2 Coronal diagrams arranged in sequence from front to back. Angle and levels of scan planes are shown in Figure 16-3. Territory of the anterior cerebral artery is divided into three regions: medial lenticulostriate (*medium shading*), callosal (*dark shading*), and hemispheric (*light areas*). (Adapted from Matsui T, Hirano A: *An atlas of the human brain for computerized tomography*, Tokyo, 1978, Igaku-Shoin.)

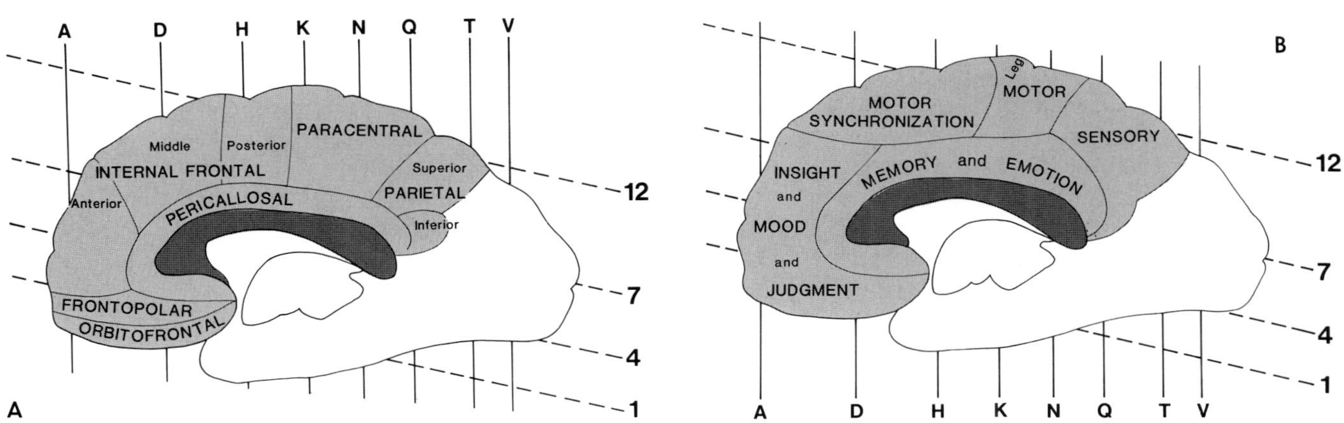

Figure 16-3 **A,** Regions supplied by the nine hemispheric branches of the anterior cerebral artery localized on a medial view of the cerebral hemisphere. **B,** Functional regions supplied by the anterior cerebral artery localized on a medial view of the cerebral hemisphere. See axial and coronal diagrams in Figures 16-1 and 16-2 for correlation.

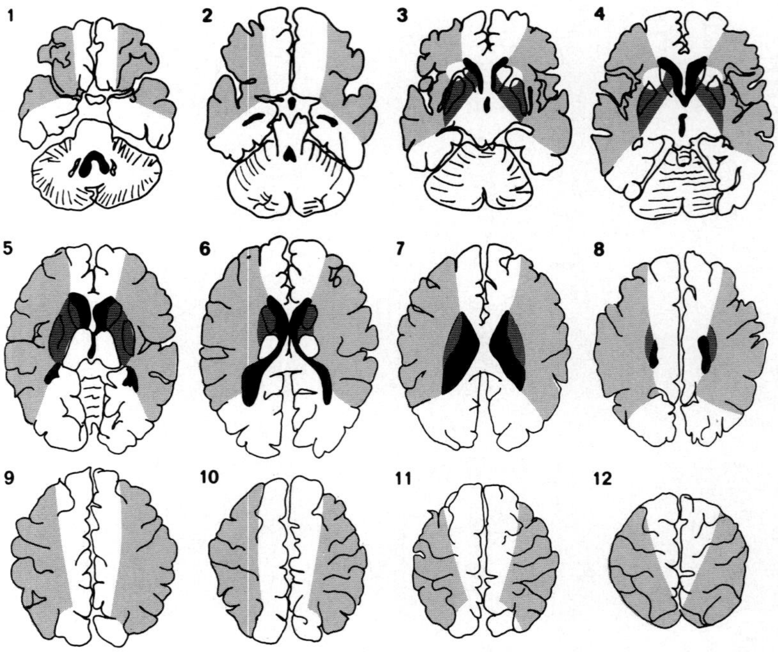

Figure 16-4 Axial diagrams arranged in sequence from base to vertex. Angle and levels of scan planes are shown in Figure 16-6. Territory of the middle cerebral artery is divided into two regions: lateral lenticulostriate (*medium shading*) and hemispheric (*light areas*).

The largest area of the brain normally supplied by the striate vessels is shown in Figures 16-4 and 16-5. This area will be smaller if a large recurrent artery of Heubner or the anterior choroidal artery (or both) is present, since these vessels may nourish the anterior inferomedial part of the striate territory (Figures 16-4 and 16-5).

The striate branches of the middle cerebral artery are "end branches" in that they have few, if any, major anastomotic connections other than those of the capillary bed. The striate branches do not supply the claustrum and extreme capsule, which are nourished by the hemispheric branches that supply the insular cortex.[13]

Vascular lesions in the striate distribution can disturb four functions: (1) movement, (2) tactile sensation, (3) speech, and (4) vision. The deficiency of movement is that of contralateral hemiparesis of the face, arm,* and leg,* which is caused by damage to the motor fibers in the internal capsule. Weakness, slowness, and changes in passive tone accompany the hemiparesis because the basal ganglia and extrapyramidal pathways are affected. A true parkinsonian syndrome is not a recognized feature of basal ganglia infarction. However, the slowness, increased tone, and spasticity associated with capsular infarction may sometimes be mistaken for early parkinsonism. The basal ganglia component of the hemiplegia in striate lesions may partly account for the greater degree of spasticity sometimes seen when these lesions are contrasted with hemispheric lesions that produce hemiplegia.[14]

The sensory tracts lie close to the motor tracts in the region of the internal capsule. Thus both functions are often affected in lesions of the striate territory. *Pure* motor cerebrovascular accidents (CVAs, strokes), involving face, arm, and leg, sometimes occur in patients with striate lesions.[15,16] However, this is not diagnostic of a lesion in the striate area. Pure motor CVA may be seen with infarctions at (1) the base of the pons (from occlusion of the paramedian branches of the basilar artery), (2) the medullary pyramids (vertebral branches), or (3) rarely, at the cerebral peduncle (basilar or posterior cerebral artery).[15-19] Since the striate branches of the middle cerebral artery may not supply the entire posterior limb of the internal capsule, occlusion of the anterior choroidal artery may be the cause of identical deficits.[15,17,20] Occlusion of any of these vessels can cause a very small infarction that may be difficult to detect.

Striate lesions that damage the sensory fibers in the posterior limb of the internal capsule can cause elevation of the threshold for primary modalities of touch, pain, temperature, and vibration in the contralateral face, arm, and leg. Lesions in the posterior cerebral territory in subcortical or thalamic nuclei may mimic these findings. Finally, infarctions of the other vessels that supply the posterior internal capsule can mimic striate artery lesions, as previously discussed.

*In this chapter, the terms *arm* and *leg* are used to represent the upper and lower extremity, respectively.

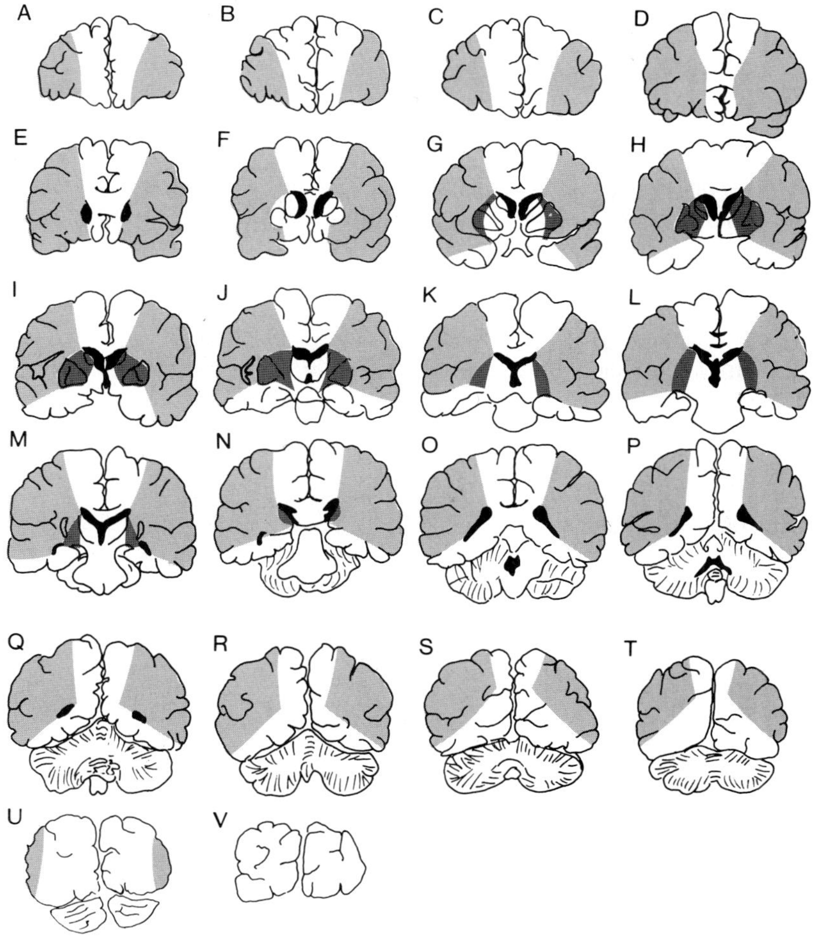

Figure 16-5 Coronal diagrams arranged in sequence from front to back. Angle and levels of scan planes are illustrated in Figure 16-6. Territories of the middle cerebral artery are identified as in Figure 16-4.

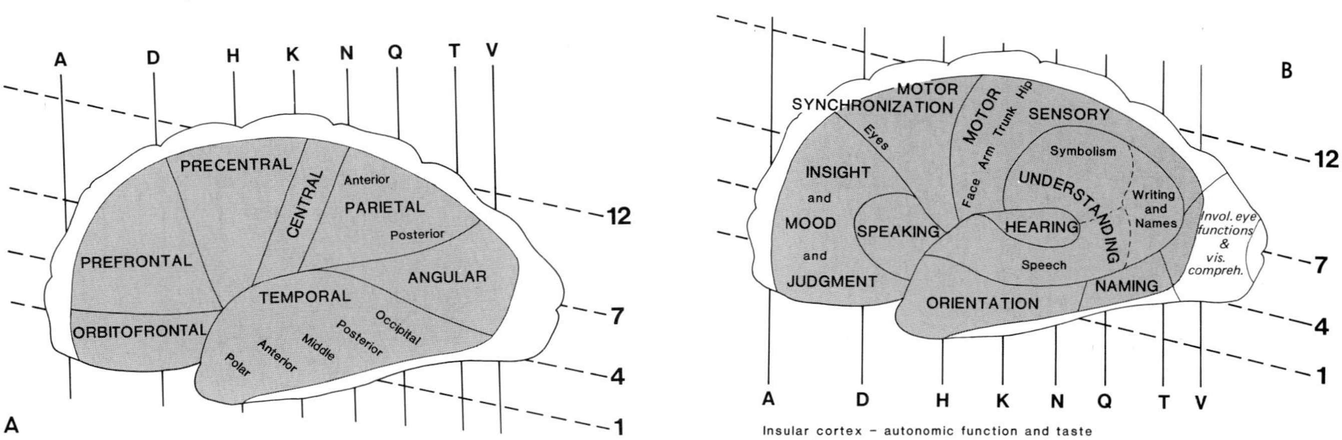

Figure 16-6 Arterial territories and function correlated. **A,** Regions supplied by the hemispheric branches of a middle cerebral artery on a lateral view of the left cerebral hemisphere. Axial and coronal scan levels marked in Figures 16-4 and 16-5 are indicated for cross-referencing. **B,** Functional cortical regions supplied by the middle cerebral artery localized on a lateral view of the left cerebral hemisphere. Areas labeled "speaking" and "understanding" are found only in the dominant hemisphere (usually the left). These zones have poorly understood functions in the nondominant hemisphere. Axial and coronal scan levels marked in Figures 16-4 and 16-5 are indicated for correlation.

Lesions in the lateral striate territory may produce speech and language impairment. Damage to the nearby Broca's area (roughly the posterior portion of the third frontal gyrus) causes *Broca's syndrome,* which consists of reduced language output, impaired repetition and naming, along with (largely) preserved comprehension.[21,22] Although Broca's area is supplied by the hemispheric branches (see next section), lateral striate infarction sometimes causes similar impairments, at least transiently.

Striate lesions may also involve the arcuate fasciculus. This subcortical fiber tract connects the area of the brain labeled "understanding" in Figure 16-6, *B* (Wernicke's area) with the area labeled "speaking" (Broca's area). Damage to this tract causes *conduction aphasia* (an impaired ability to repeat words or phrases).[22,23]

The visual deficit produced by lesions in the striate territory is that of a contralateral homonymous hemianopsia and may be complete or subtle and difficult to detect clinically.[24,25] This deficit is caused when damage occurs to the optic radiations that traverse the striate territory as they originate from the geniculate body.

Hemispheric Branches

Twelve major cortical branches are illustrated in Figure 16-6, *A*. Given the large number of branches, one might expect a great variety of clinical sequelae. The overall picture can be simplified by comparing the vascular territories of Figure 16-6, *A,* with the functional areas of Figure 16-6, *B*. The areas marked "speaking" and "understanding" are present only in the dominant hemisphere, which is the left hemisphere in almost all right-handed patients and in about half of the left-handed patients. In the nondominant hemisphere, these areas have no well-accepted, clinically demonstrable function.

The term *speaking* in this context refers to the complex language function associated with verbal output, including speaking, writing, and even sign language. This definition excludes the purely motor aspects of these functions, such as movements of facial muscles or hands, which relate to the motor region for face or arm, respectively. Similarly, *understanding* means understanding of language, whether written, spoken, sign, or Braille, and is conceptually separate from a loss of the sensory modalities of sight, hearing, or touch, which can mediate language. More detail on this complex subject can be found in relevant references.[21,22,26,27]

The cortical area marked "hearing" receives impulses from both ears. Therefore deficits in this area must be bilateral to cause clinical symptoms. The insular cortex is not shown in Figure 16-6, *A* or *B,* since it lies buried within the sylvian fissure. This infolded cortex is supplied by the major hemispheric branches that course over its surface. Small branches arise from these surface vessels and penetrate the insular cortex, extreme capsule, and claustrum.

Damage to the insular cortex can produce the opercular syndrome of Foix-Chavany-Marie, which is characterized by impairments of speech, articulation (dysarthria) and clarity (dysphonia), swallowing (dysphagia), and chewing (dysmasesia).[28,29] These problems are caused by the interruption of signals to cranial nerves V, VII, and IX to XII. This syndrome is a type of pseudobulbar palsy.[28,29]

The lateral surface of the frontal lobe mediates judgment, insight, and mood. This surface receives arterial supply from the orbitofrontal and prefrontal branches of the middle cerebral artery. The medial surface of the frontal lobe contains the remainder of the judgment, insight, and mood areas, which are supplied by the anterior cerebral artery.[12,20,24,25]

The prefrontal and precentral arteries supply that area of the dominant hemisphere that is essential for "speaking" (Figure 16-6, *B*). Damage here causes *Broca's (motor) aphasia,* which, as previously noted, causes greatly reduced verbal output (agrammatic and telegraphic) and impaired ability to repeat sentences and phrases or name objects.[22,23] The patient's ability to understand speech remains largely intact.[22,23]

A much less common type of aphasia, *transcortical motor aphasia,* results from lesions rostral or superior to Broca's area.[22,30] Infarctions of the territories of the orbitofrontal, prefrontal, and precentral middle cerebral arterial branches (Figure 16-6, *A*) or a watershed infarction of the zone between the anterior and middle cerebral arteries may produce this syndrome. The patient has an aphasia identical to Broca's, except that repetition of sentences and phrases is not impaired.[23,30]

As shown in Figure 16-6, *A,* the precentral artery also supplies those parts of the frontal lobe that facilitate "motor synchronization." One area in this region controls coordination of eye and head movement. Damage here deprives the patient of the ability to look in the direction opposite the side of the lesion.[31]

The cortex marked "motor" in Figure 16-6, *B,* is supplied by the central branch of the middle cerebral artery. Damage in this territory causes contralateral weakness of the face, arm, trunk, and hip. The motor cortex of the medial surface of the frontal lobe that controls the leg is supplied by the anterior cerebral artery.[20] The leg, however, may be weakened after occlusion of the central branch of the middle cerebral artery. This occurs if the lesion also damages the motor fiber tracts to the leg as they travel downward beneath the cortical areas (marked "face" and "arm" in Figure 16-6, *B*). Leg weakness may also occur when the cortical, middle cerebral lesion causes edema in the medial frontal lobe and this edema compresses the motor fiber tracts of the leg. The leg weakness associated with middle cerebral cortical lesions is usually less severe and more transient than that seen with cortical infarcts of the anterior cerebral artery, which controls motor function of the leg.[14,24,25,31]

The cortex marked "sensory" in Figure 16-6, *B*, is supplied by central and anterior parietal branches.[25] Damage to this region causes loss of high-order sensory functions in the face, arm, trunk, and hip. Occasionally, the leg is involved, presumably by the mechanisms described previously. These lesions cause loss of (1) position sense; (2) tactile localization; (3) stereognosis (recognizing the object one is feeling); (4) ascertainment of shape, size, and texture; (5) two-point discrimination; and (6) recognition of letters or numbers written on the skin (graphesthesia).[14,31,32] This cortical sensory loss contrasts with the loss of primary sensory perception (pain, temperature, vibration, touch) that is found with lesions in the lateral striate territory of the middle cerebral artery.

The posterior parietal, angular, occipital, and posterior temporal arteries (Figure 16-6, *A*) vascularize a part of the cortex that, in the dominant hemisphere, mediates understanding.[12,25] Damage to this region, which is known as Wernicke's area, causes striking neuropsychological symptoms.[14,22,25,31] Involvement of the lower part of the area impairs perception and understanding of speech. Damage to the rest of it impairs written, visual, and auditory language integration.[22,23] Lesions tend to involve the entire Wernicke's area and produce an aphasia in which language comprehension, repetition, and naming are all severely affected, although the spontaneity and fluency of speech remain intact. As a result, the patient with *Wernicke's aphasia* speaks meaningless gibberish that has normal intonation and fluency, and he or she cannot understand written or spoken language.[22,23]

Lesions in part of the dominant hemisphere supplied by the angular artery may produce a neuropsychological deficit known as *Gerstsmann's syndrome,* in which the patient exhibits a variety of problems in understanding. Acalculia (loss of arithmetic ability), alexia (inability to read), finger agnosia (inability to identify one's fingers), and right-left confusion may be present.[33] Aphasia is sometimes also encountered.

Infarction of the parietal lobe occurs when there is occlusion of the central, anterior, and/or posterior parietal arteries. In the *nondominant* hemisphere, occlusion produces disturbances in the ability to use or synthesize geometric and spatial information *(amorphosynthesis)*.[34] These disturbances can take many forms. Some are syndromes of unilateral neglect. For example, the patient may ignore the existence of the half of the world contralateral to the lesion. Only part of such neglect that produces a contralateral hemianopsia may result from concomitant lesions of the sensory cortex or involvement of the optic radiations.[10] Other neglect syndromes are the denial of illness, hemiplegia, or pain in the contralateral body *(anosognosia)*. The patient may also have difficulty with clothing himself, which is often worse contralateral to the lesion *(dressing apraxia)*. These syndromes cannot be explained by concomitant paralysis, sensory loss, or dementia. Another difficulty that may be encountered with nondominant parietal lesions is loss of orientation or spatial memory. In these instances, the subject has difficulty finding his or her way around a town, house, or room.

All the syndromes described for the nondominant parietal lobe may also be seen with lesions of the *dominant* parietal lobe, but they are difficult to detect because of concomitant aphasia.[10]

The anterior temporal and temporal polar arteries supply the inferior temporal areas and a portion of the insular cortex. Occlusion of these branches does not produce readily discernible clinical signs and symptoms. However, autonomic disturbances such as contralateral *mydriasis* (enlargement of the pupil) and *hyperhydrosis* (increased perspiration) may be associated with damage in this area.[10]

POSTERIOR CEREBRAL ARTERY TERRITORY

In Figures 16-7 and 16-8, the branches of the posterior cerebral artery have been divided into three groups: (1) the penetrating arteries to the brainstem, thalamus, and other deep structures; (2) the splenial branch to the corpus callosum; and (3) the branches to the cerebral hemisphere.[1,35] Figure 16-9 is a companion diagram of the medial aspect of the right cerebral hemisphere. It is provided to localize the axial and coronal images in Figures 16-7 and 16-8. The regions supplied by the hemispheric branches and the cortical function of each region are shown.

Penetrating Branches

Numerous very small branches arise from the proximal part of the posterior cerebral artery as it encircles the midbrain. These have arbitrarily been divided into one group that supplies the thalamus and hypothalamus and another that supplies the midbrain.[36]

Thalamus and Hypothalamus

The approximate origin and termination of the vessels that supply the thalamus are indicated in Figure 16-10, *A*. Each vessel in the drawing represents numerous very small branches. The pattern of arterial supply to the thalamus is variable. That shown in Figure 16-10, *A*, is the most common and represents 30% of the brains studied.[36] In general, four groups of perforating vessels supply the thalamus: (1) premamillary, (2) thalamoperforating, (3) thalamogeniculate, and (4) posterior choroidal and cingulate.

As illustrated in Figure 16-10, *A*, the *premamillary arterial group* supplies the anterior thalamus (anterior, medial, ventral anterior, and ventral lateral nuclei). The anterior nucleus connects with the mamillary bodies and the hippocampus and is part of the memory and emotion circuit of Papez.[37,38] The dorsomedial nucleus connects with the frontal lobe, the amygdala, and possibly the hypothalamus. Damage to either of these nuclei can cause profound memory loss and personality change (Figure 16-10, *B*). Usually, the recent memory is most severely affected

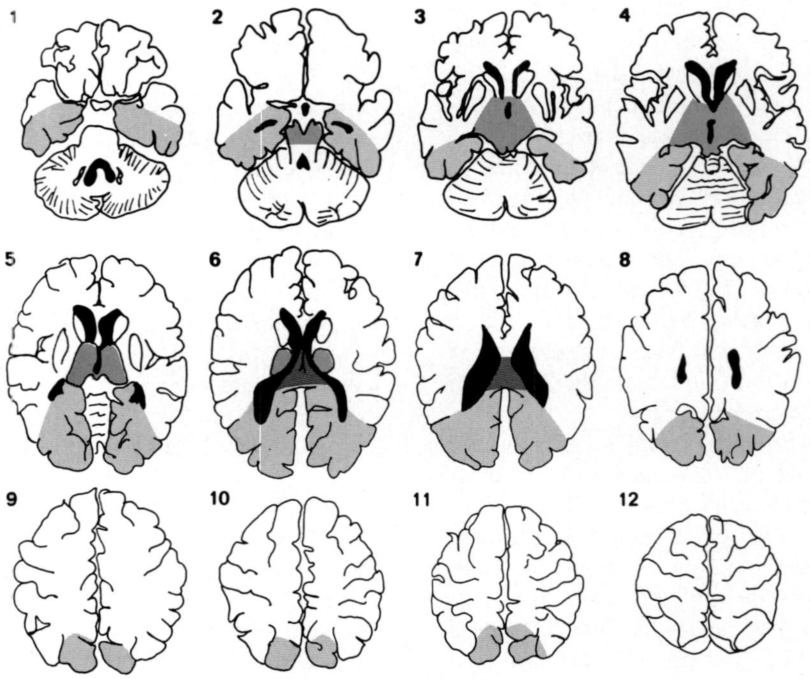

Figure 16-7 Axial diagrams arranged in sequence from base to vertex. Angle and levels of scan planes are shown in Figure 16-9. Territory of the posterior cerebral artery is divided into three regions: thalamic and midbrain perforators (*medium shading*), callosal (*dark shading*), and hemispheric (*light areas*).

(Wernicke-Korsakoff syndrome).[39] The specific anatomic pathophysiology underlying these effects is a subject of controversy.[40,41] The ventroanterior and ventrolateral nuclei influence the motor system, particularly the extrapyramidal and cerebellar systems; their ablation may relieve some symptoms of Parkinson's disease.[42] The lateral nucleus helps coordinate motor and sensory impulses but has no clinically defined function (Figure 16-10, *B*).

In addition to the thalamus, the premamillary arteries supply the intermediate part of the hypothalamus, an area that forms the central one third of the walls of the third ventricle and the mamillary bodies. There is collateral supply to this area from internal carotid branches.[43] This part of the hypothalamus is the source of somatostatin[44] (which blocks the release of growth hormone and thyroid-stimulating hormone) and thyroid-releasing hormone.[45] Neuropathways carrying vasopressin and oxytocin to the posterior pituitary gland, as well as pathways for luteinizing hormone–releasing hormone, corticotropic-releasing factor, and prolactin-inhibiting factor, travel through this region.[45] Therefore lesions in this area can cause a complete loss of endocrine function that simulates total section of the pituitary stalk, as well as hyperphasia, anorexia, and rage attacks.[44]

The premamillary artery, together with branches from the thalamoperforating arteries, supplies the posterior part of the hypothalamus.[43] Tumors in this area produce precocious puberty,[44] disturbances of temperature regulation,[46] and disturbances of consciousness with somnolence.[44] The anterior hypothalamus is supplied by the anterior cerebral artery (see earlier section on medial lenticulostriate arteries).

As illustrated in Figure 16-10, *A*, the *thalamoperforating arterial group* supplies the medioventral part of the thalamus (centromedian and parafascicular nuclei). This territory mediates many aspects of arousal, attention, and alertness.[37] Thalamoperforating branches derived from one posterior cerebral artery usually supply all or part of the contralateral territory, as well as the ipsilateral territory.[47]

As illustrated in Figure 16-10, *A*, the *thalamogeniculate group* supplies the lateroventral part of the thalamus (pulvinar, ventroposterior lateral, and ventroposterior medial nuclei). The pulvinar may coordinate visual and auditory information by receiving input from the lateral and medial geniculate bodies and projecting to the occipital and temporal lobes.[37] Lesions of the left pulvinar area can produce language dysfunction (aphasia or dysphasia).[48] The ventro-

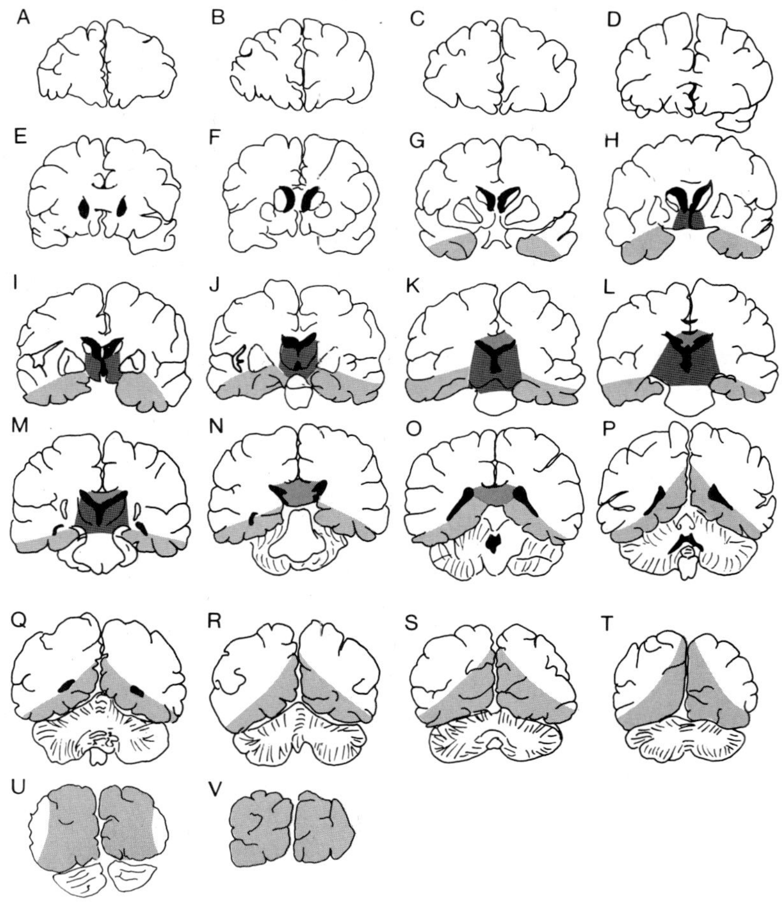

Figure 16-8 Coronal CT scan diagrams arranged in sequence from front to back. Angle and levels of scan planes are shown in Figure 16-9. Territories of the posterior cerebral artery are identified as in Figure 16-7.

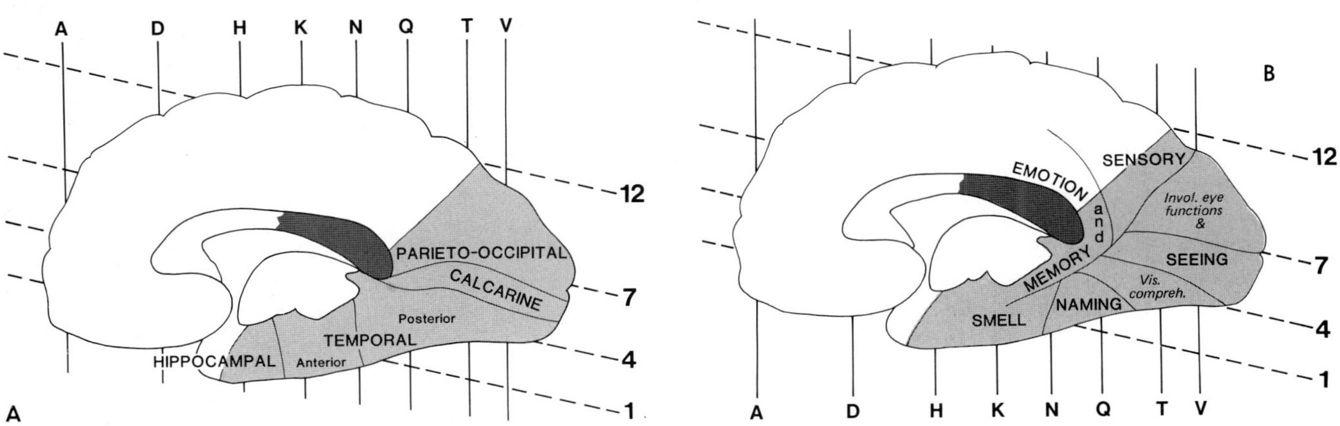

Figure 16-9 **A,** Regions supplied by the five hemispheric branches of the posterior cerebral artery localized on a medial view of the right cerebral hemisphere. **B,** Functional cortical regions supplied by the posterior cerebral artery localized on a medial view of the right cerebral hemisphere. See axial and coronal scan levels in Figures 16-7 and 16-8 for correlation.

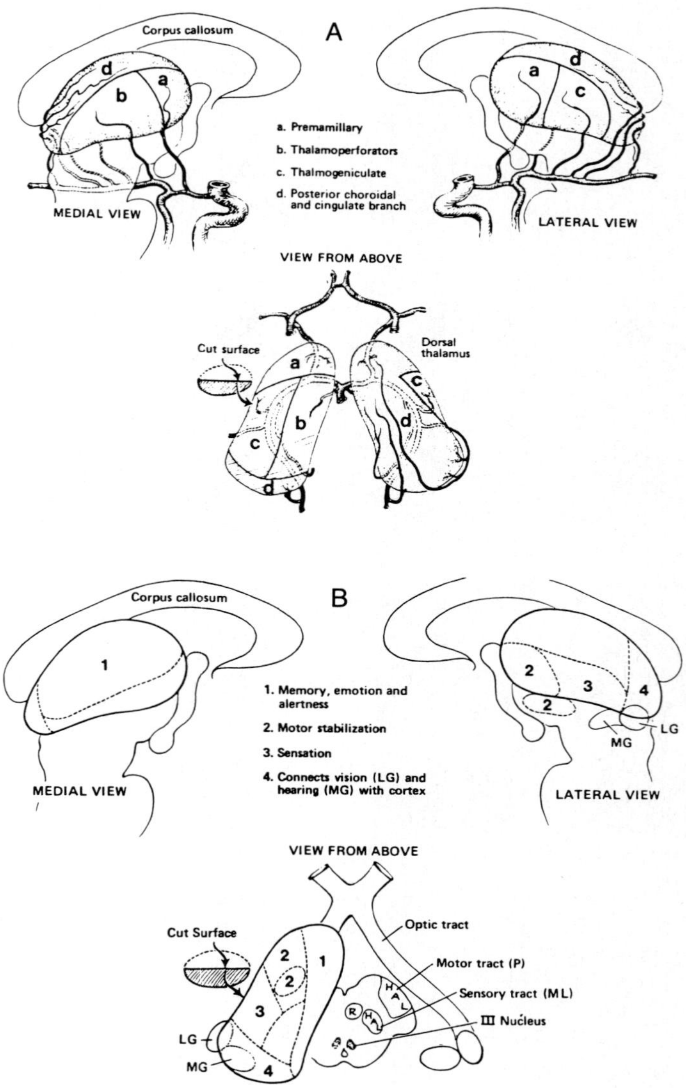

Figure 16-10 **A,** Schematic view of four vascular territories on the thalamus. Each is represented by a single arterial branch at the approximate origin and termination of numerous small perforating branches: (*a*) premamillary, (*b*) thalamoperforator, (*c*) thalamogeniculate, and (*d*) posterior choroidal and cingulate branches. This pattern represents 30% of brains. Midbrain perforators (the largest of which is the quadrigeminal plate artery) are not illustrated. **B,** Four functional relay areas of thalamus: (1) memory and emotion (anteromedial and dorsomedial nuclei); (2) motor stabilization (ventroanterior, ventrolateral, and subthalamic nuclei); (3) sensation (ventroposteromedial and ventroposterolateral nuclei); and (4) connections of visual (LG, lateral geniculate) and hearing (MG, medial geniculate) areas with the parietal cortex via the pulvinar. Unmarked areas are nonspecific association areas that are poorly understood. Lesions in area 1 result in neuropsychological symptoms; in area 2, they result in hemiballismus (or curb Parkinson's disease contralaterally); in area 3 they result in Déjérine-Roussy syndrome; and in area 4 they cause aphasia, if the left thalamus is affected. Midbrain sectioned at level below inferior colliculi shows major midbrain motor tract (P, pyramidal) and sensory tract (ML, medial lemniscus) divided into areas for head (H), arm (A), and leg (L) fibers. These tracts control side of body opposite lesion. Red nucleus (R) is pathway for fibers from cerebellum to thalamus. Lesions here affect coordination contralaterally.

posterior lateral and ventroposterior medial nuclei relay sensory information from body and face, respectively.[37] Lesions produce an initial insensitivity to pain that evolves over months into spontaneous or inappropriately elicited pain in the affected body part. This has been named *anesthesia dolorosa* and is found in the Déjérine-Roussy (thalamic) syndrome[49] (see Figure 16-10).

The thalamogeniculate branches also supply the lateral geniculate body, the medial geniculate body, and structures below the anterior and medial part of the thalamus (e.g., the Forel fields in the subthalamic area). Lesions of the lateral geniculate body cause loss of sight in the half of the visual field opposite the lesion.[37] The medial geniculate body is part of the hearing pathway, but unilateral lesions of the medial geniculate body do not cause clinical hearing problems, since bilateral representation of hearing exists at this level because of previous decussation. Lesions in the vicinity of the subthalamic area and Forel fields can cause violent flinging movements of the opposite extremities *(hemiballismus)* as well as uncontrollable jerking and writhing movements *(choreoathetosis)*.[50,51] However, only hemiballismus has good localizing value and suggests a lesion in the subthalamic nucleus. Since the subthalamic region receives collateral supply from the anterior choroidal artery, these manifestations are rare in infarction but common in hemorrhage.[51]

As shown in Figure 16-10, *A*, the *choroidal and cingulate branches* supply the posterior and superior thalamus (anterior, medial, pulvinar, and habenular nuclei). There are extensive anastomoses in these areas, and infarction is rare.[47,52] Symptoms resulting from lesions in the first three of these thalamic nuclei have been described in the previous discussion. No known specific clinical deficit is produced by habenular lesions per se. In addition to the thalamus, the posterior choroidal branches supply the pineal gland, choroid plexus, crus, commissure and body of the fornix, part of the anterior columns of the fornix, and part of the lateral geniculate body.[47]

Midbrain

The second group of small penetrating branches supplies the midbrain.[52] They enter the midbrain substance perpendicularly, either directly at their point of origin from the posterior cerebral artery or after accompanying the parent artery around the midbrain for some distance.[52,53] Others term these "thalamoperforators" and the syndromes produced by their occlusion "thalamoperforate syndromes."[54] Since this group of vessels does not supply the thalamus, it would be better to call them *midbrain perforators* and the associated syndromes *midbrain perforate syndromes*.*

Damage to parts of the midbrain can lead to (1) cranial nerve (CN) III paralysis, which causes symptoms in both eyes but most marked in the eye on the same side as the lesion; (2) disturbed sensation, strength, and/or coordination on the side opposite the lesion; (3) depression of consciousness; and (4) decerebrate rigidity. A detailed description of these deficits follows. The reader will find it helpful to refer to Figure 16-10, *B*, to localize the CN III nucleus, red nucleus, and motor and sensory tracts in the midbrain because these structures are discussed.

A total *CN III paralysis* results in ptosis, a dilated unreactive pupil, and downward and outward deviation of the eye ipsilaterally. Injury to peripheral CN III fibers (after they leave the brainstem or as they travel through the cisterns to reach the eye) causes some or all of these symptoms ipsilaterally. Brainstem lesions may cause CN III symptoms bilaterally because the nuclei are close together. Isolated brainstem lesions involving a single CN III nucleus are therefore very rare (see Figure 16-10, *B*). Brainstem lesions may simulate peripheral CN III lesions by compromising nerve fibers in the brainstem before they exit. Some authors state that CN III paralysis without pupillary abnormality indicates infarction rather than compression by a mass, but this distinction is unreliable.[4,56-58]

Fibers of CN III at the collicular level of the midbrain can be damaged by tumor compression (e.g., pinealoma) so as to produce *Parinaud's syndrome*.[58,59] This consists of a loss of upward gaze, impaired pupillary reactivity, and *convergence nystagmus,* which is not true nystagmus but rather a simultaneous contraction of all the extraocular muscles. Convergence results because the medial rectus muscles are the strongest in the group.[58]

Disturbances of sensation or movement are caused by damage to the major sensory tract (medial lemniscus) or motor tract (pyramidal) (Figure 16-10, *B*). Lesions here cause contralateral hemianesthesia and/or hemiparesis and may affect the head, arm, or leg in varying degrees.[60]

Damage to the red nucleus, which coordinates cerebellar-thalamic fiber tracts (Figure 16-10, *B*), results in impaired coordination and control of movement contralaterally.[61] Tremor occurs during movement (perpendicular to the direction of motion), which worsens as the target is approached. One also finds *dysmetria,* difficulty with rapidly alternating movements, and inability to check or stop a previously initiated movement.[59,62,63] Another related type

*The midbrain contains many vital pathways and nuclei. Lesions here have a variety of clinical manifestations. Many midbrain syndromes have eponyms (e.g., Claude's, Nothnagel's, Weber's, and Benedikt's syndromes), but we think that it is simpler and more fruitful to emphasize the functional anatomy. Familiarity with *combinations* of the deficits described in this chapter is the key to localizing lesions to the midbrain. Any isolated deficit can always be caused by a lesion outside the midbrain, but if one looks for the combinations of deficits described, one can frequently make an accurate localization of a lesion to the midbrain and/or find satisfying correlations between the CT anatomy and the clinical presentation. This is usually better than trying to fit the signs and symptoms to the eponymic syndromes, which are specific examples of combinations of deficits and worthy of attention after one is familiar with the basic functional anatomy.[52,54,55] of tremor, *rubral tremor,* may also be seen. This tremor is present at rest (although it increases during movement) and involves the limb more proximately than does the usual cerebellar tremor. A third type of tremor, seen only at rest, and similar to that of Parkinson's disease, may also be encountered.[59,62,63] In addition to the tremor, there may be contralateral hemiballismus and choreoathetosis (as described previously) if associated damage occurs to the adjacent substantia nigra and/or subthalamic region.[54,61,62,64]

Depression of consciousness is presumably caused by damage to the central or paramedian reticular midbrain activating system. It can also be caused by destruction or depression of the reticular system in the pons or medulla or by bilateral hemispheric dysfunction. Thus impairment of consciousness by itself is of little localizing value.[59]

Decerebrate rigidity can be produced in animals by lesions in the regulating structures between the quadrigeminal plate and the lateral vestibular nucleus in the pons.[59,65] The subject assumes a position in which the legs are rigidly extended and the arms are extended, abducted, and hyperpronated.[57] This posture is not as reliable a localizing indicator in humans as it is in other animals.[4]

Callosal Branches

The callosal arteries are a plexus of small vessels that arise from the parieto-occipital or lateral choroidal branches and penetrate the upper surface of the posterior half of the corpus callosum. The plexus may be replaced by a single branch.[47] Infarction can result in separation of the language-dominant left hemisphere from the right hemisphere, which mediates function of the left side of the body. If the patient's left occipital lobe and splenium are infarcted, he or she can speak, write, and understand speech. However, the patient becomes unable to read with the remaining left visual field despite being able to see the letters. (The patient cannot transfer the visual images received by the right occipital lobe for interpretation in the left hemisphere.) This is called *alexia without agraphia*. It is rare and may be partial.[66]

Hemispheric Branches

The posterior cerebral artery has five cortical branches. The patterns of infarction can be simplified by comparing the vascular territories (Figure 16-9, *A*) with corresponding functional areas (Figure 16-9, *B*). Infarction of cortical branches of the posterior cerebral artery is responsible for several interesting clinical syndromes. The calcarine artery (sometimes together with the parieto-occipital artery) supplies the calcarine cortex ipsilaterally. Infarction of this artery causes homonymous hemianopsia of the contralateral visual fields. It is often stated that with lesions of the calcarine cortex, the central macular part of the visual field is spared because of collateral circulation.[67] A recent study reported macular sparing in 5 of 25 patients with cortical blindness.[68]

Infarction of the calcarine cortex bilaterally may result in complete blindness. However, an unusual constellation of symptoms known as *Anton's syndrome* also may occur, in which the patient, although blind, is unaware of the blindness and denies it.[69] Sometimes the patient will construct elaborate descriptions of surroundings. If allowed, the patient may walk into walls or trip over objects.

Apraxia of ocular movements (inability to shift the direction of gaze on command) may also be encountered. This may be accompanied by *optic ataxia* (poor control of movements, e.g., hand movements, performed under visual guidance) and decreased attention to the visual periphery. This combination of optic apraxia, optic ataxia, and peripheral visual inattention is called *Balint's syndrome*. Many cases actually result from bilateral tumors rather than vascular lesions.[70] It is in bilateral occipital infarction that macular sparing is most frequently reported. Macular sparing in these patients may actually represent partial recovery from total blindness.[66] Damage to the calcarine cortex can also produce unformed visual hallucinations, *metamorphopsia* (distortion of shape), *teleopsia* (an illusion in which near objects appear to be at a great distance), distortion of visual outlines, and other aberrations of visual perception.[69]

Damage to the nondominant calcarine cortex and to the nondominant lingual gyrus, which are supplied by the calcarine and temporal branches (Figure 16-9, *A*), may produce topographic disorientation and prosopagnosia. *Prosopagnosia* is the inability to recognize familiar faces even though they can be clearly seen.[69]

Damage to the cortex above and below the calcarine fissure, particularly in the dominant hemisphere, destroys the visual association areas that control involuntary eye function and visual comprehension. These areas are supplied by the parieto-occipital and posterior temporal branches of the posterior cerebral artery. Patients with lesions in these areas may continue for several seconds to see the image of an object that is quickly removed from view. They may also not perceive an object in the damaged visual field if another identical object is simultaneously presented in the normal visual field. This phenomenon is called *extinction*.[69]

The anterior temporal branch supplies only the inferior aspect of the anterior temporal lobe; the tip of the temporal lobe is supplied by the middle cerebral artery. The cortex in this area is involved in naming objects.

The hippocampal branches of the posterior cerebral artery supply the hippocampal formation, including its projections, the fornices, and the psalterium (fornical commissure) (Figure 16-9, *B*). The most frequently observed clinical finding in patients with bilateral hippocampal infarcts is *memory deficit*. This may also be seen in unilateral deficits on the dominant side. Lesions in this area may also impair the sense of smell.[69] CT studies have suggested that damage to the anterior temporal lobe may cause both taste and smell dysfunctions.[71]

REFERENCES

1. Matsui T, Hirano A: *An atlas of the human brain for computerized tomography,* Tokyo, 1978, Igaku-Shoin.
2. Critchley M: Anterior cerebral artery and its syndromes, *Brain* 53:120-165, 1930.
3. Denny-Brown D: The nature of apraxia, *J Nerv Ment Dis* 126:9-32, 1958.
4. Plum F, Posner JB: *The diagnosis of stupor and coma,* Philadelphia, 1980, FA Davis.
5. Fisher CM: Clinical syndromes in cerebral arterial occlusion. In Fields WS, editor: *Pathogenesis and treatment of cerebrovascular disease,* Springfield, Ill, 1961, Charles C Thomas.
6. Geschwind N, Kaplan E: A human cerebral disconnection syndrome: a preliminary report, *Neurology* 12:675-685, 1962.
7. Strub RL, Black FW: *The mental status examination in neurology,* Philadelphia, 1977, FA Davis.
8. Chusid JG: *Correlative neuroanatomy and functional neurology,* ed 16, Los Altos, Calif, 1976, Lange.
9. Cogan DG: *Neurology of the ocular muscles,* ed 2, Springfield, Ill, 1956, Charles C Thomas.
10. Critchley M: *The parietal lobes,* London, 1953, Edward Arnold.
11. Berman SA, Hayman LA, Hinck VC: Correlation of CT cerebral vascular territories with function. III. Middle cerebral artery, *AJR* 142:1035-1040, 1984.
12. Stephens RB, Stillwell DL: *Arteries and veins of the human brain,* Springfield, Ill, 1969, Charles C Thomas.
13. Gibo H, Carver CC, Rhoton AL, et al: Microsurgical anatomy of the middle cerebral artery, *J Neurosurg* 54:151-169, 1981.
14. Vick N: *Grinker's neurology,* ed 7, Springfield, Ill, 1976, Charles C Thomas.
15. Fisher CM: Capsular infarcts, the underlying vascular lesions, *Arch Neurol* 36:65-73, 1979.
16. Fisher CM, Curry HB: Pure motor hemiplegia of vascular origin, *Arch Neurol* 13:130-140, 1965.
17. Mohr JP: Lacunes, *Stroke* 13:3-11, 1982.
18. Ho K: Pure motor hemiplegia due to infarction of the cerebral peduncle, *Arch Neurol* 39:524-526, 1982.
19. Fisher CM: Lacunar strokes and infarcts: a review, *Neurology* 32:871-876, 1982.
20. Berman SA, Hayman LA, Hinck VC: Correlation of cerebral vascular territories with cerebral function by computed tomography. I. Anterior cerebral artery, *AJNR* 1:259-263, 1980; *AJR* 135:352-357, 1980.
21. Naeser MA, Hayward RW: Lesion localization in aphasia with cranial computed tomography and the Boston diagnostic aphasia exam, *Neurology* 28:545-555, 1978.
22. Benson DF, Geschwind N: The aphasias and related disturbances. In Baker AB, Baker LH, editors: *Clinical neurology,* vol 1, Hagerstown, Md, 1971, Harper & Row.
23. Goldstein K: *Language and language disturbances,* New York, 1948, Grune & Stratton.
24. Foix C, Levy M: Les ramollissement Sylviens, syndromes des lesions en foyer du territories de l'artere Sylviens en de ses branches, *Rev Neurol (Paris)* 48:1-51, 1927.
25. Waddington MM, Ring BA: Syndromes of occlusion of middle cerebral artery branches: angiographic and clinical correlation, *Brain* 91:685-696, 1968.
26. Geschwind N: Current concepts in aphasia, *N Engl J Med* 284:654, 1971.
27. Benson SF: *Aphasia, alexia, and agraphia,* New York, 1979, Churchill Livingstone.
28. Foix C, Chavany A, Marie P: Deplegie facio-linguomasticatrice cortico-sous-corticale sans paralysie des membres, *Rev Neurol (Paris)* 33:214-219, 1926.
29. Bruyn GW, Gathier JC: The operculum syndrome. In Vinken PJ, Bruyn GW, editors: *Handbook for clinical neurology,* vol 2, Amsterdam, 1969, Elsevier.
30. Rubens AB: Transcortical motor aphasia. In Whitaker H, Whitaker HA, editors: *Studies in neurolinguistics,* vol 1, New York, 1976, Academic.
31. Adams RD, Victor M: *Principles of neurology,* ed 2, New York, 1981, McGraw-Hill.
32. Déjérine J, Mouzon J: Un nouveau type de syndrome sensit corticale observe dans un cas de monoplegie corticale dissocies, *Rev Neurol (Paris)* 28:1265-1273, 1914.
33. Gerstmann J: Zur symptomatologie der hirnlasionen im ubergangsgebiet der unteren parietal und mittleren occipitalwindung, *Nervenarzt* 3:691-695, 1930.
34. Denny-Brown D, Banker B: Amorphosynthesis from left parietal lesions, *Arch Neurol Psychiatry* 1:302-312, 1954.
35. Hayman LA, Berman SA, Hinck VC: Correlation of CT cerebral vascular territories with function. II. Posterior cerebral artery, *AJR* 137:13-19, 1981.
36. Schlesinger B: *The upper brainstem in the human,* Berlin, 1976, Springer.
37. Ingram WR: *A review of anatomical neurology,* Baltimore, 1976, University Park.
38. Papez JW: A proposed mechanism of emotion, *Arch Neurol* 38:725-743, 1937.
39. Victor M: The amnestic syndrome and its anatomical basis, *Can Med Assoc J* 100:1115-1125, 1969.
40. Horel JA: The neuroanatomy of amnesia: a critique of the hippocampal memory hypothesis, *Brain* 101:403-445, 1978.
41. Scoville WB, Milner B: Loss of recent memory after bilateral hippocampal lesions, *J Neurol Neurosurg Psychiatry* 20:11-21, 1957.
42. Cooper IS: An investigation of neurosurgical alleviation of Parkinsonism, chorea, athetosis and dystonia, *Ann Intern Med* 45:381-392, 1956.
43. Haymaker W: Blood supplies of the human hypothalamus. In Haymaker W, Anderson E, Nauta WJH, editors: *The hypothalamus,* Springfield, Ill, 1969, Charles C Thomas.
44. Zimmerman EA: Neuroendocrine disorder. In Rosenberg RN, editor: *Neurology,* New York, 1980, Grune & Stratton.
45. Rudelli R, Deck JHN: Selective traumatic infarction of the human anterior hypothalamus, *J Neurosurg* 50:645-654, 1979.
46. Pelletier G, Leclerc R, Dube D: Morphologic basis of neuroendocrine function in the hypothalamus. In Tolis G, Labrie F, Martin J, et al, editors: *Clinical neuroendocrinology: a pathophysiological approach,* New York, 1979, Raven.
47. Percheron G: The anatomy of the arterial supply of the human thalamus and its use for the interpretation of the thalamic vascular pathology, *J Neurol* 205:1-13, 1973.
48. Brown JW: Language, cognition and the thalamus, *Appl Neurophysiol* 36:33-60, 1974.
49. Scherbel ME, Scherbel A: The basis of thalamic pain: a structurofunctional hypothesis, *Trans Am Neurol Assoc* 94:149-152, 1969.
50. Carpenter MB: *Human neuroanatomy,* Baltimore, 1976, Williams & Wilkins.
51. Whittier JR: Ballism and the subthalamic nucleus (nucleus hypothalamicus; corpus Luysi), *Arch Neurol* 58:672-692, 1947.
52. Zeal AA, Rhoton AL: Microsurgical anatomy of the posterior cerebral artery, *J Neurosurg* 48:534-559, 1978.
53. Stephens RB, Stillwell DL: *Arteries and veins of the human brain.* Springfield, Ill, 1969, Charles C Thomas.
54. Merritt HH: *A textbook of neurology,* Philadelphia, 1967, Lea & Febiger.
55. Walton JN: *Brain diseases of the nervous system,* New York, 1977, Oxford University.
56. Sears ES, Franklin G: Diseases of the cranial nerves. In Rosenberg RN, editor: *Neurology,* New York, 1980, Grune & Stratton.
57. Warwick R: Representation of the extra-ocular muscles in the oculomotor nuclei of the monkey, *J Comp Neurol* 98:449-495, 1953.
58. Gay AJ, Newman NM, Keltner JL, et al: *Eye movement disorders,* St Louis, 1974, Mosby–Year Book.

59. Fog M, Hein-Sorensen O: Mesencephalic syndromes. In Vinken PJ, Bruyn GW, editors: *Handbook of clinical neurology,* vol 2, *Localization in clinical neurology,* Amsterdam, 1969, Elsevier.
60. Walton C: *Basic human neuroanatomy,* Boston, 1977, Little, Brown.
61. Aronson AE, Bastron JA, Brown JR, et al: *Mayo Clinic, clinical examinations in neurology,* Philadelphia, 1971, WB Saunders.
62. Foix C, Masson A: Le syndrome de l'artere cerebrale posteriere, *Presse Med* 32:361-365, 1923.
63. Holmes G: The cerebellum of man, *Brain* 62:1-30, 1939.
64. De Jong R: *The neurologic examination,* Hagerstown, Md, 1979, Harper & Row.
65. Daube JR, Sandok BA: *Medical neurosciences,* Boston, 1978, Little, Brown.
66. Benson DF, Geschwind N: The alexias. In Vinken PJ, Bruyn GW, editors: *Handbook of clinical neurology,* vol 4, Amsterdam, 1969, Elsevier.
67. Ross Russell RW: The posterior cerebral circulation, *J R Coll Physicians Lond* 7:331-346, 1973.
68. Aldrich MS, Alessi AG, Beck RW, et al: Cortical blindness: etiology, diagnosis, and prognosis. *Ann Neurol* 21:149-158, 1987.
69. Walsh KW: *Neuropsychology: a clinical approach,* Edinburgh, 1978, Churchill Livingstone.
70. Hecaen H, DeAjuriaguerra J: Balint's syndrome (psychic paralysis of visual fixation and its minor forms), *Brain* 77:373-400, 1984.
71. Schellinger D, Henkin RT, Smirniotopoulos JG: CT of the brain in taste and smell dysfunctions, *AJNR* 4:752-754, 1983.

CHAPTER 17

Neurosecretory Regions

Eric M. Spickler
William L. Hirsch, Jr.
L. Anne Hayman

IMAGING TECHNIQUES

Adjacent to the third and fourth ventricles lie specialized circumventricular organs that produce secretory substances. These substances may be true hormones that are released into the circulating blood or factors that eventually cause the elaboration of hormones at other sites. By definition, *hormones* alter the function and sometimes the structure of one or more organs. Nine regions have the histologic configuration necessary for a neurohumoral control center: (1) pineal gland, (2) hypothalamus, (3) anterior and (4) posterior lobes of the pituitary gland, (5) median eminence, (6) subcommissural organ, (7) subfornical organ, (8) organ vasculosum, and (9) area postrema (Figure 17-1).

Only three of these regions—the anterior lobe of the pituitary gland, the hypothalamus, and the subcommissural organ—have a blood-brain barrier (bbb). The remainder of these specialized areas are structurally similar in that they contain a large capillary surface and no bbb. This allows them to be identified on enhanced magnetic resonance (MR) images (Figure 17-2). Lack of a barrier also allows easy flow of substances between vascular lumina, cerebrospinal fluid (CSF) spaces, and unmyelinated neurons, thereby enabling feedback to the neurons from the extraneuronal environment. The absence of a bbb in these areas may also allow retroviruses to enter brain substance. Accordingly, viruses associated with multiple sclerosis, leukemia, and acquired immunodeficiency syndrome (AIDS) might conceivably be taken up in these neurosecretory areas and even transported from them to other regions of the brain.

These circumventricular organs govern the hormones that control behavioral, physiologic, and endocrine responses to a variety of peripheral stimuli. Regulation of homeostatic functions, such as lactation, parturition, gestation, reproduction, metabolism, temporal rhythms, arousal, and cardiovascular dynamics, requires such communication between the neurosecretory regions of the brain and the rest of the body. Further research into the functions of these areas will undoubtedly increase our understanding of these complex mechanisms.

NORMAL ANATOMY

Pineal Gland

The pineal gland (or *epiphysis*) is one of the neurosecretory organs that does not have a bbb. The pineal gland secretes serotonin, norepinephrine, melatonin, thyroid-releasing hormone (TRH), luteinizing hormone–releasing hormone (LRH), and somatostatin. This gland is thought also to regulate the circadian rhythms because light deprivation decreases melatonin production. Retinal input reaches the pineal gland by a complicated pathway through the suprachiasmatic nucleus and medial forebrain bundle to the superior cervical ganglion. The latter directly innervates the pineal gland.[1]

Experimental evidence suggests that the pineal gland may also play a major role in regulating the onset of puberty.[2] In theory, pineal production of melatonin affects the hypothalamus, midbrain, and pituitary gland by depressing production of the luteinizing hormone (LH) and follicle-stimulating hormone (FSH). A relationship appears to exist between melatonin production and the progressive aggregation of particulate hydroxyapatite and calcium carbonate that occurs during the first 2 decades of life. This process has radiographic significance, since these calcified areas (which are most frequently located in the connective tissue at the base of the gland) are visible on computed tomographic (CT) scans and radiographs.

The incidence of pineal calcification varies with the genetic makeup of the population. In Americans, calcification in children under age 6 years should prompt follow-up

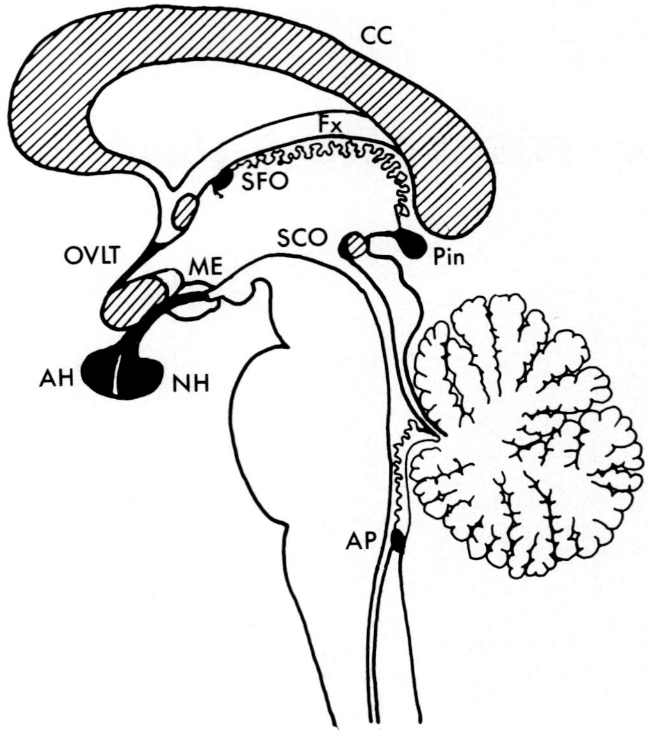

Figure 17-1 Midline sagittal diagram of the brain showing eight of the nine neurosecretory regions as black areas. AH, Adenohypophysis of the pituitary gland; NH, neurohypophysis of the pituitary gland; ME, termination of the pituitary stalk in the median eminence; OVLT, organum vasculosum of the lamina terminalis; SFO, subfornical organ below the fornix (*Fx*); SCO, subcommissural organ above the aqueduct; *Pin*, pineal gland; AP, area postrema in the medulla. The hypothalamus on either side of the third ventricle is not visualized in this midline section. The midline fiber tracts are indicated by diagonal lines. The anterior column of the fornix is shown between the OVLT and SFO. The anterior commissure is located between the OVLT and the pituitary stalk. The posterior commissure is shown above and behind the SCO.

studies and clinical examinations to exclude pathologic conditions.[2] CT scans show calcification in the pineal gland in 8% to 11% of children 8 to 14 years of age, 30% at 15 years, and 40% at 20 years.[2] Calcified foci gradually become more numerous, and by old age, almost all pineal glands are so involved. These calcifications do not correlate with loss of function or degree of fibrosis in the gland. A calcified deposit greater than 1 cm in diameter found at any age must be considered abnormal because the pineal gland itself measures only 5 to 9 mm in length, 3 to 6 mm in width, and 3 to 5 mm in height.[2]

Pineal capillaries do not have the bbb characteristic of arteries in most other regions of the brain.[3] Thus the gland enhances normally on CT scans after administration of iodinated contrast material and on MR scans after administration of gadolinium.

The pineal gland is formed from parenchymal cells that arise from the neuroectoderm of the roof of the third ventricle and the pia of the tela choroidea. Proliferation of these cells creates a diverticulum that eventually forms the pineal recess of the third ventricle. Sequestration of portions of this diverticulum within the pineal gland or degeneration of those cells that differentiate into ependyma or neuroglia may cause formation of *cysts* within the gland.[4,5] These cysts can be found in 30% to 40% of pineal glands at autopsy.[5-7] The cysts may become large enough to be visualized on either CT or MR images (Figure 17-3). On CT scans, the fluid within the cyst generally resembles the surrounding cerebrospinal fluid (CSF). On MR images, the cyst may have a slightly greater signal intensity than CSF on long TR/TE spin-echo sequences (TR, relaxation time; TE, echo delay time). Some have suggested that this signal intensity results from absence of fluid motion within the cyst.[6] Others have attributed this appearance to elevated protein content and describe one case in which a fluid-fluid level (presumably representing cellular debris or

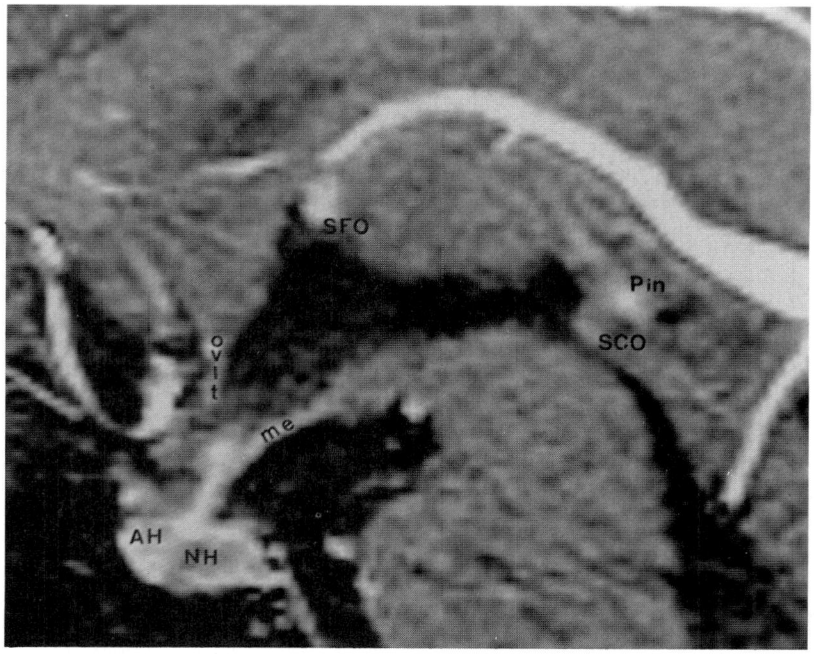

Figure 17-2 Gadolinium-enhanced MR image (0.7 mm slice, three-dimensional gradient-recalled echo, T1 weighted) shows enhancement resulting from absence of the blood-brain barrier in the pineal gland (*Pin*), posterior lobe of the pituitary gland (neurohypophysis, NH), median eminence (*me*), organum vasculosum of the lamina terminalis (*ovlt*), and the subfornical organ (SFO). Enhancement of the anterior pituitary gland (adenohypophysis, AH) and the subcommissural organ (SCO) is caused by the high capillary density in these areas.

A

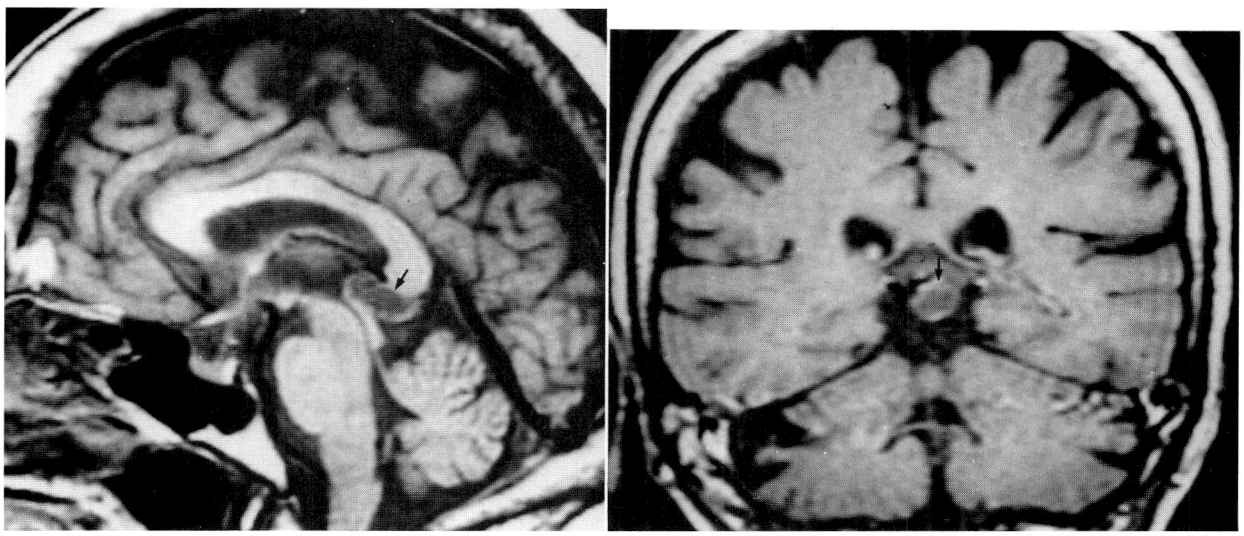

B

Figure 17-3 T1-weighted MR images demonstrate a large pineal cyst (*arrow*) in sagittal **(A)** and coronal **(B)** scan planes in a patient with cerebral and cerebellar atrophy. Follow-up scans at 1 year showed no change.

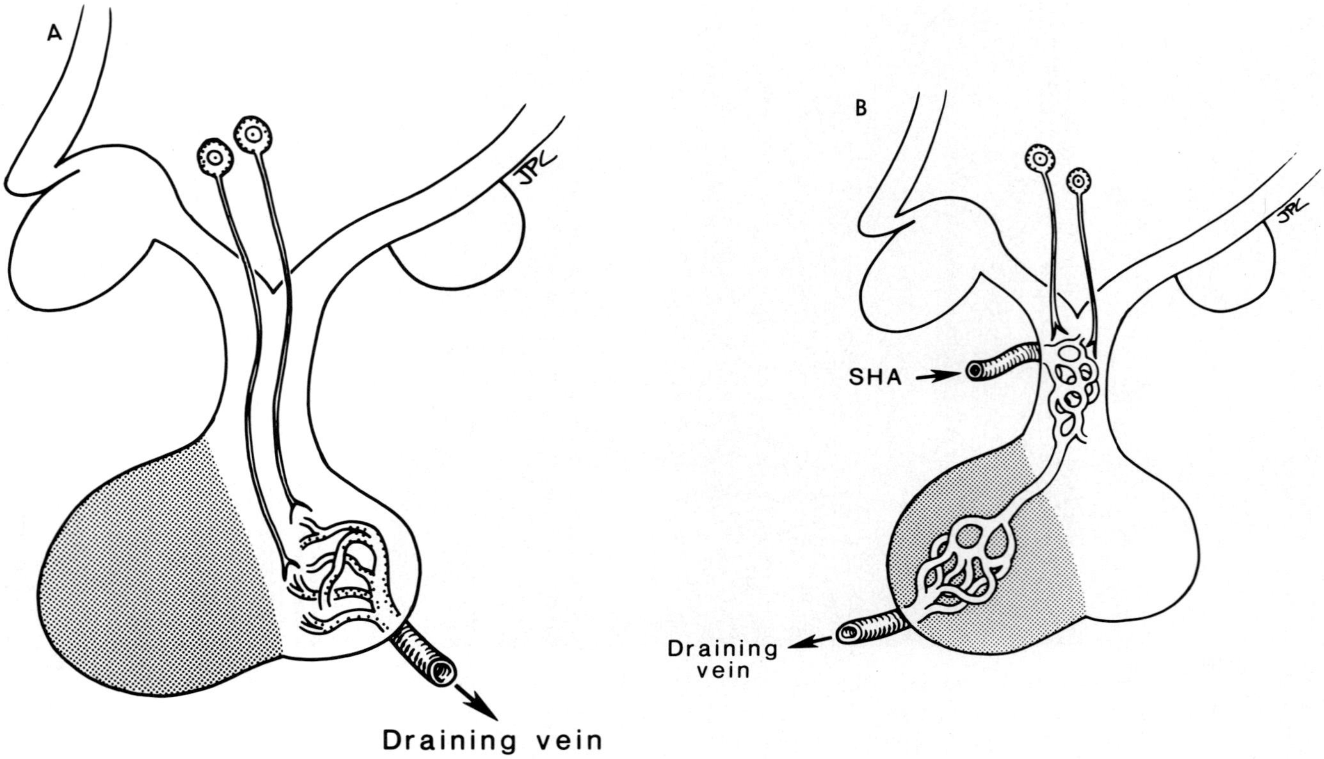

Figure 17-4 **A,** *Neurohypophysis.* Antidiuretic hormone (ADH) and oxytocin are synthesized in the neurons of the supraoptic and paraventricular nuclei. These octapeptides are bound to *neurophysines* (carrier proteins) and transported down the nerve axons in the infundibulum to bulbous axon terminals in the posterior lobe. From here, ADH or oxytocin is released directly into systemic veins. *Pituicytes,* modified glial cells supporting the axon terminals, accumulate intracytoplasmic fat in proportion to their neurosecretory activity. **B,** *Adenohypophysis.* Releasing factors are synthesized by hypothalamic neurons. From axon terminals in the median eminence, these factors are released into the superior part of the hypothalamic portal system. They are carried by blood flow inferiorly to the vascular sinusoids of the anterior pituitary gland, where they stimulate (in the case of GH, ACTH, TSH) or inhibit (in the case of prolactin) the release of systemically active anterior pituitary hormones. (Diagrams based on Kelly WM, Kucharczyk W, Kucharczyk J, et al: AJNR 9:453-460, 1988.)

coagulated fluid) was evident.[5] In both reports, these cysts generally had a signal intensity on short TR/TE MR images that was hypointense relative to brain.

Pineal cysts can share MR signal intensity characteristics with other cystic lesions (e.g., dermoid, epidermoid, arachnoid cyst, cysticercosis), so care must be taken in interpreting these MR scans. Absence of symptoms or hydrocephalus referable to a pineal mass is generally enough to suggest that a given pineal cyst is simply a normal variant. However, MR images have been described that met all these signal intensity criteria for pineal cysts in a 45-year-old patient with no neurologic evidence of abnormality other than dizziness. Histologic examination of a surgical specimen in this case revealed the presence of a *pinocytoma* with astrocytomatous differentiation. Therefore, in effect, the appearance of this rare tumor cannot be reliably distinguished from that of normal cysts known to occur in this region.[8]

Hypothalamus

The hypothalamus is a small but important structure responsible for such varied functions as temperature regulation, water balance, feeding and drinking behavior, and sexual activity.[9] This thin layer of tissue forms the floor and lower lateral walls of the third ventricle, thereby separating the ventricular cavity from the suprasellar cistern. The inferior surface of the hypothalamus is therefore exposed to the CSF of the suprasellar (chiasmatic) cistern and appears as a ridge of gray matter extending from the lamina terminalis and optic chiasm anteriorly to include the mammillary bodies posteriorly. This ridge of tissue (excluding the mammillary bodies) is called the *tuber ci-*

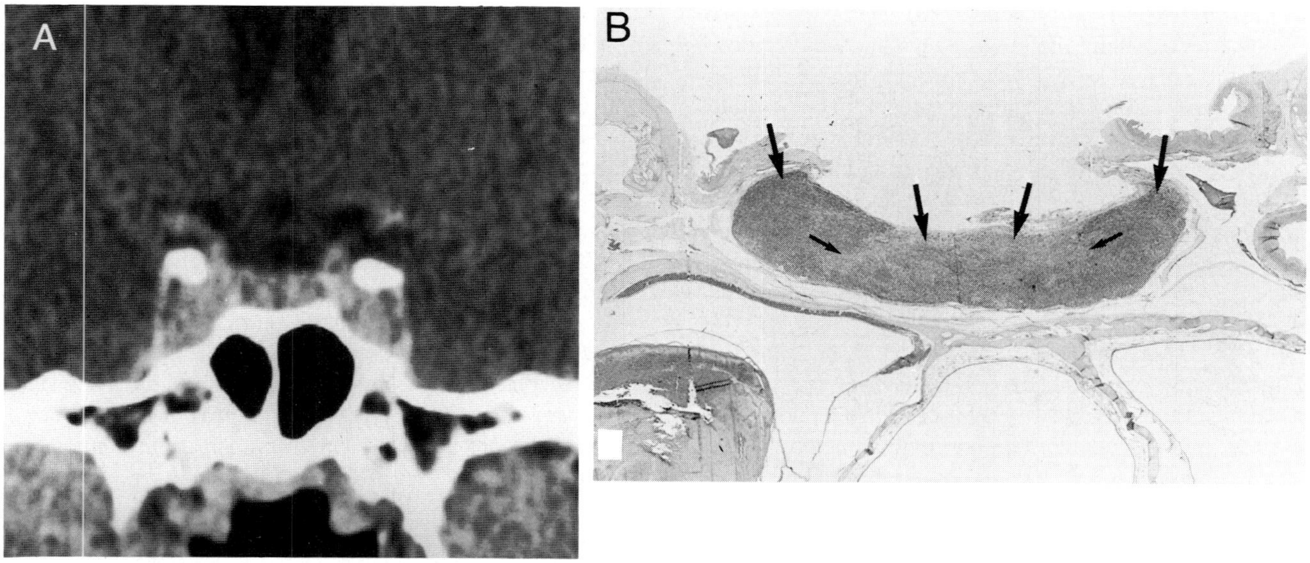

Figure 17-5 Normal inhomogeneity of the pituitary gland's anterior lobe. **A,** Contrast-enhanced coronal CT image through the anterior lobe shows vertical bands of hypointense signal. **B,** Coronal histologic section (hematoxylin-eosin stain) shows the inhomogeneity of the anterior lobe. Strongly staining areas (*large arrows*) consist of tightly compacted, heavily granulated cells. Weakly stained areas (*small arrows*) consist of loosely compacted, mildly granulated cells. (From Latchaw RE: MR *and* CT *imaging of the head, neck, and spine,* St Louis, 1991, Mosby–Year Book.)

nereum. A swelling on its surface, the *median eminence,* is continuous with the infundibulum and posterior lobe of the pituitary gland. These structures are discussed in the following sections on the pituitary gland and median eminence. Collectively, they constitute the neurohypophysis. At each lateral margin of the hypothalamus are the ipsilateral optic tract and the sulci of the adjacent temporal lobe.[9]

The hypothalamus controls pituitary function through direct neuronal links with the *posterior lobe (neurohypophysis)* and a vascular link with the *anterior lobe (adenohypophysis).*[10] The supraoptic and paraventricular nuclei of the hypothalamus consist of neurosecretory cells where *antidiuretic hormone* (ADH, vasopressin) is produced (Figure 17-4, *A*). This octapeptide (with a carrier protein) is transported via the unmyelinated axons. The modified axon terminals are located either along the infundibulum or, more often, in the posterior lobe of the pituitary gland. When stimulated, these terminals release ADH into the systemic circulation via a plexus of veins in the posterior lobe. *Oxytocin* is a similar octapeptide that is produced and transported in an analogous fashion. This hormone causes uterine contractions during parturition and mammary smooth muscle contraction during milk ejection.

Control of the anterior lobe is different (Figure 17-4, *B*), since no direct neuronal links exist from the hypothalamus. Instead, releasing factors are produced by hypothalamic cells and delivered to the anterior lobe by the hypophyseal portal system, which runs from hypothalamic veins to the vascular sinusoids of the anterior pituitary gland. These hypothalamic factors may inhibit tonic hormone release, as in the case of prolactin, or may stimulate hormone production and release, as with growth hormone (GH), thyroid-stimulating hormone (TSH), and adrenocorticotrophic hormone (ACTH).[11]

The details of production and transport of these hormones are described in the next section, since they may be important in understanding the MR signal characteristics of the pituitary gland's posterior lobe.

Pituitary Gland and Stalk

The pituitary gland is connected to the hypothalamus by a stalk referred to as the *pituitary infundibulum.* In an MR study of 20 normal subjects, the upper limit of width on nonenhanced short TR/short TE (T1-weighted) images was 3.5 mm near the median eminence and 2.8 mm at the midpoint.[12] The uniform intense enhancement of the stalk on MR and CT studies can in part be attributed to the numerous veins present within this structure.

In one study, coronal views of the pituitary stalk showed a tilt from a vertical midline position in 46% of patients without pituitary pathology. This tilt occurred because the pituitary gland itself was off midline or the stalk inserted eccentrically into a midline gland.[13]

The pituitary gland consists of two embryologically distinct structures, the *adenohypophysis (anterior lobe)* and the *neurohypophysis (posterior lobe)*. They have close functional and anatomic relationships. The adenohypophysis arises from Rathke's pouch, an upgrowth of rudimentary ectoderm from the primitive mouth. The neurohypophysis arises as a downgrowth of neuroectoderm from the diencephalon. The adenohypophysis and neurohypophysis are separated by the *pars intermedia,* a thin layer of tissue that has numerous, usually small, colloid-containing cysts.[14] Each of these components is discussed separately next.

Anterior Lobe

The adenohypophysis occupies the anterior two thirds of the sella and is composed of glandular cells responsible for the production of numerous hormones, including GH, TSH, FSH, LH, ACTH, and prolactin. On enhanced CT images, the anterior lobe is normally inhomogeneously dense. Histologic correlations demonstrate that areas dense on CT images consist of tightly packed cells, often containing numerous intracellular secretory granules. Areas lucent on CT images consist of less tightly packed cells with fewer intracellular granules (Figure 17-5).[15] On enhanced CT images, differences in vascularity also produce variations of density. For instance, a collection of venous sinusoids is seen on the superior aspect of the mid–anterior lobe. On dynamic bolus-contrasted CT images, this vascular bed enhances more than the adjacent pituitary tissue. Displacement of this vascular tuft may be a secondary indicator of a pituitary mass *(tuft sign).*[16] Areas lucent on CT images are also frequently seen separating the anterior

Figure 17-6 Normal pituitary gland in 15-year-old woman examined after minor head trauma. Extensive endocrinologic testing revealed no abnormality. **A,** Contrast-enhanced coronal CT image shows symmetrically convex superior surface of the gland *(arrow)*. Variations in anterior lobe density are normal. MR images (TR/TE, 600/20 msec) of same patient in coronal **(B)** and sagittal **(C)** planes. Note the superior surface of the gland almost touches the optic chiasm *(arrow* in **B**). (From Latchaw RE: MR *and* CT *imaging of the head, neck, and spine,* St Louis, 1991, Mosby–Year Book.)

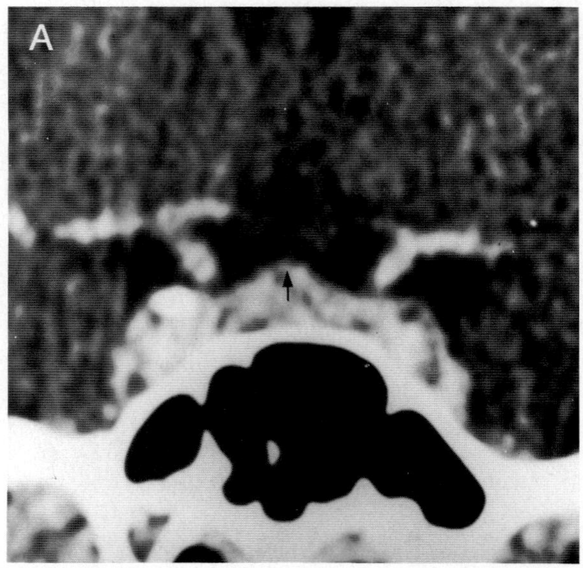

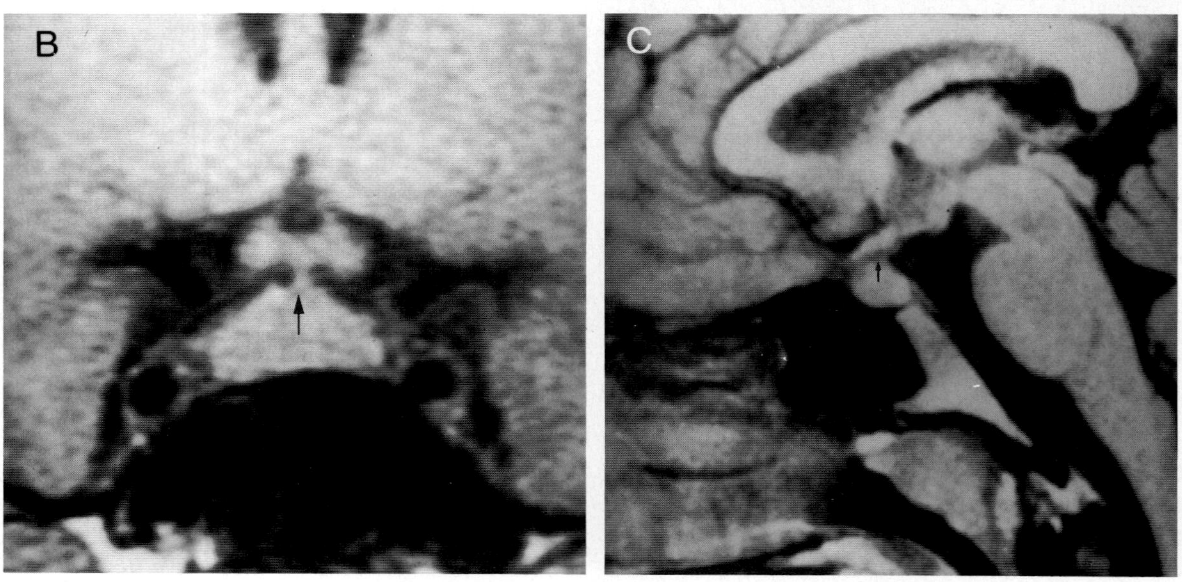

lobe from the adjacent cavernous sinus. Histologically, these hypodense areas are found to be composed of adipose or connective tissue.

Tissue variations within the anterior lobe are probably less noticeable on MR images because the thicker cuts (3 mm as opposed to 1.5 mm) result in obscurement from partial-volume averaging. The anterior lobe typically is isointense with brain on both short and long TR, spin-echo MR images. The appearance of the anterior lobe on contrast enhanced MR scans is complex (see Figure 18-1 in Chapter 18).

The size and shape of the anterior lobe vary with age, sex, and stage of the menstrual cycle. A large series of MR scans indicates that the normal pituitary gland undergoes a period of physiologic hypertrophy in all teenagers. In girls, the gland frequently has a convex upper margin and may reach a vertical diameter of 10 mm. In boys, no change is seen in shape, but the gland could enlarge to a maximum of 7 mm.[17] Young adult women also have large pituitary glands, which normally may be up to 9 mm in height. The average adult values for the pituitary gland are 4.2 mm in women and 3.5 mm in men. The upper margin of the gland may be concave, flat, or symmetrically convex (Figure 17-6). Asymmetric upward convexities in the gland may indicate an underlying pituitary mass.[18,19]

Pars Intermedia

The pars intermedia is an inconspicuous tissue layer separating the adenohypophysis from the neurohypophysis. It is nonfunctional but important from an imaging standpoint, since the pars normally contains small vesicles that represent the embryologic remnants of the posterior wall of Rathke's pouch.[14] Histologically, these vesicles are true cysts, with an epithelial lining, and contain variable numbers of goblet cells. In aggregate, these tiny cysts can appear as lucent areas on CT images (Figure 17-7).[15] Usually, they are not evident on MR images. Occasionally, these cysts enlarge and compress adjacent structures.

Posterior Lobe

The neurohypophysis occupies the posterior one third of the sella. It consists of the bulbous terminal axons of hypothalamic neurons and pituicytes. The latter are modified glial cells. On axial, enhanced CT images, the posterior lobe is visualized in one third of normal subjects, presumably because this region has no bbb. The posterior lobe is less dense than the anterior lobe, probably a result of reduced cellular density.

The posterior lobe is distinctive in that it usually has a very high signal intensity on short TR/TE MR images. This high signal has been attributed to the neurosecretory granules that contain arginine, vasopressin, and neurophysin, which are substances formed by the hypothalamus.[20] Others ascribe this signal intensity to lipid found within modified astrocytes (pituicytes), which are associated with the terminal axons.[11] This theory is supported by histologic and MR phantom studies.[11,21] These theories are not mutually exclusive, since pituicytes contain vari-

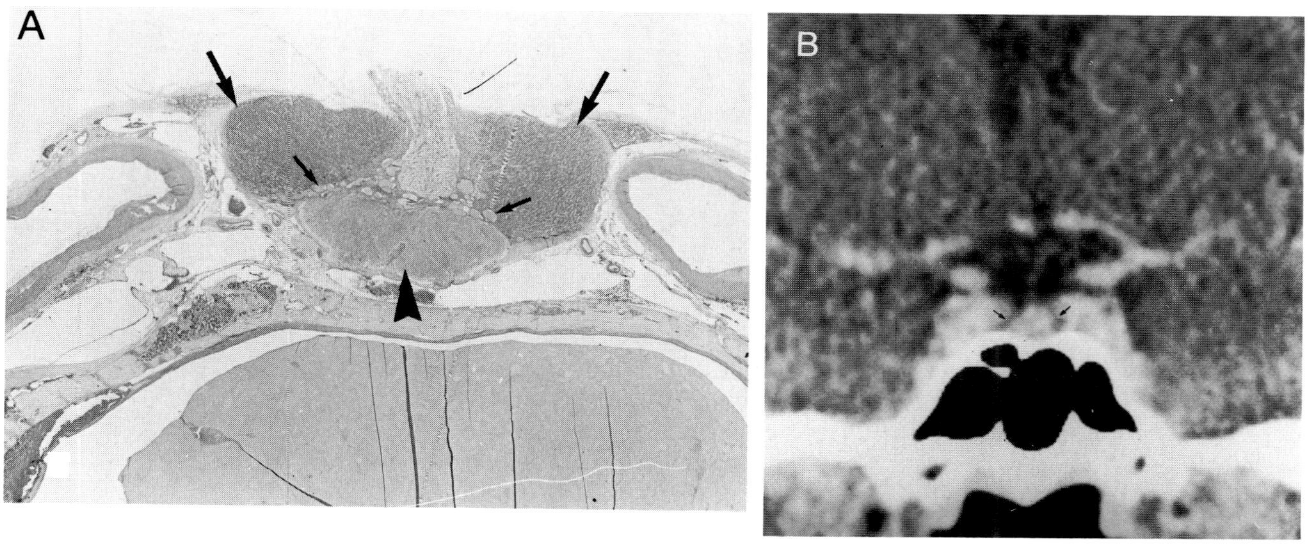

Figure 17-7 Pars intermedia. **A**, Coronal histologic section (hematoxylin-eosin stain) at the level of the pituitary infundibulum. The posterior lobe of the pituitary gland (*arrowhead*) is separated from the posterolateral extensions of the anterior lobe (*large arrows*) by the pars intermedia (*small arrows*), which contains numerous tiny colloid cysts. **B**, Corresponding enhanced CT image. The pars intermedia (*arrows*) is less dense than the surrounding tissue. This lucent band may be unilateral if the pars intermedia is asymmetric. (From Latchaw RE: MR *and* CT *imaging of the head, neck, and spine*, St Louis, 1991, Mosby–Year Book.)

able amounts of both lipid and neurosecretory granules, which vary with the level of ADH release and synthesis. In either case, the posterior lobe has high signal intensity in most infants and adults on short TR images.[22,23] This high signal is absent in 10% to 50% of the healthy population.[10,24] In a study of the size and signal intensity of the posterior lobe in 36 patients who had at least two MR scans, it was concluded that variations in size and signal intensity of the posterior lobe over time were typical.[24]

The high signal intensity in the posterior lobe on short TR/TE MR images may also be absent in patients with conditions that disturb hypothalamic secretion or axonal transport to the neurohypophysis. Such conditions include physical compression of the infundibulum by a suprasellar mass or infiltration of the hypothalamus or infundibulum, as by a hypothalamic glioma, optic glioma, germinoma, or histiocytosis X.[12] In one study, loss of bright signal intensity in the posterior lobe was found in all 13 children with diabetes insipidus.[23]

Physical disruption of axonal transport may lead to high signal intensity in the infundibulum itself, as has been observed after hypophysectomy or when a large macroadenoma compresses the infundibulum.[26] These findings support the hypothesis that the bright signal may result from accumulation of neurosecretory material proximal to a block in the axonal transport system.[10,26] Recent research has indicated that phospholipid vesicles present in the cell membranes of the neurohypophyseal cells have a hydrophilic pole that acts as a relaxation enhancer, thereby shortening T1 (longitudinal relaxation time) on MR images without a chemical shift.[21]

Rarely, the posterior lobe is located within a small fossa in the posterior wall of the bony sella. Very rarely, high signal intensity, attributable to the posterior pituitary gland, is seen in the suprasellar cistern. This has been described as a normal variant,[24,25] but it is also seen in patients with pituitary dwarfism.[27]

The MR appearance of the posterior lobe after gadolineum enhancement is complex. The reader is referred to Chapter 18 for a review of the temporal pattern of signal change in this region. On delayed MR images, after gadolinium enhancement, the posterior lobe blends with the anterior lobe or may even have less intense signal on MR images. This reflects the relatively greater enhancement of the anterior lobe and is analogous to the density pattern seen on enhanced CT scans.[28] The border between the posterior lobe and the pars intermedia may be convex, flat, or concave. The posterior lobe is occasionally off midline, in which case the infundibulum may be deviated as well.

Median Eminence

The median eminence is a neurosecretory region of the brain that does not possess a bbb.[29] It forms the floor of the third ventricle where the infundibular stem attaches to the base of the brain (see Figure 17-4, *B*). The ependymal cells of this area differ from those in the hypothalamus because they have surface specializations, as well as basal processes that extend to the perivascular spaces around the portal capillaries of the infundibular stalk. Accordingly, substances from the CSF and releasing and inhibitory factors secreted by adjacent unmyelinated nerve fibers of the hypothalamus can enter the capillary plexus of the median eminence.[30] These substances are carried through the portal vascular plexus to the anterior lobe of the pituitary.

Subcommissural Organ

In the adult the subcommissural organ consists of isolated remnants of secretory parenchymal ependyma under the posterior commissure at the junction of the third ventricle and the cerebral aqueduct.[31] This area is unusual because it is a neurosecretory region that has a bbb. Enhancement on MR images appears to result from the high capillary density in this region (see Figure 17-2). One surface of the subcommissural organ contacts the third ventricle, and the other is in contact with the vascular system. The processes of these neurons penetrate the posterior commissure. This area produces an aldosteronotropic factor and therefore may be important in water and electrolyte metabolism.[32]

Subfornical Organ

The subfornical organ is a highly vascularized zone 1 mm in diameter that is located on the inferior surface of

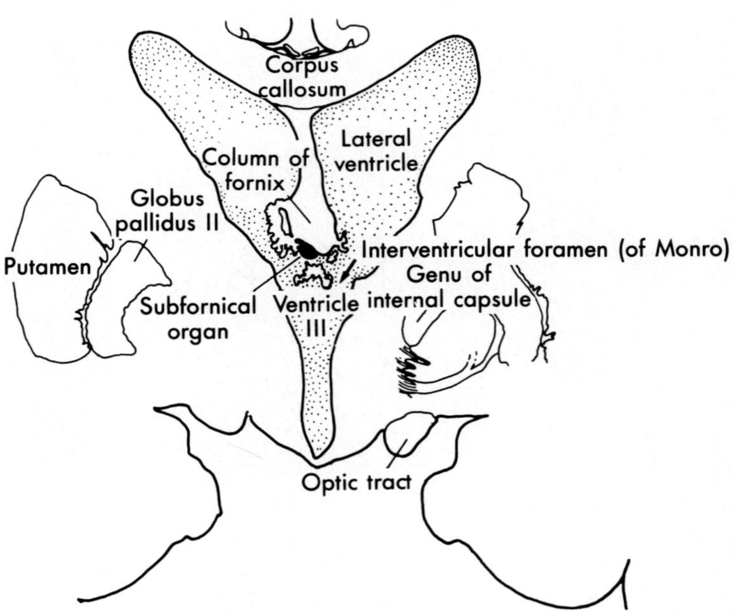

Figure 17-8 Coronal diagram at the level of the foramen of Monro showing the location of the subfornical organ immediately below the column of the fornix.

the columns of the fornix (Figure 17-8).[33] The vessels in this area lack a bbb. They connect with those of the adjacent choroid plexus and drain into the medial septal veins. The ependymal channels in this area are in contact with the adjacent CSF. This area appears to contribute to the regulation of ADH and water homeostasis.[32,34]

Organum Vasculosum

The organum vasculosum is located at the lamina terminalis immediately in front of the optic chiasm (see Figures 17-1 and 17-2). This zone lacks a bbb, and the cells in this region appear to be in communication with the CSF in the anterior part of the third ventricle.[35] The organum vasculosum may function to some extent as an accessory anterior lobe of the pituitary gland. Certain peptides, proteins, and amines present in blood are detected by neurons in the organum vasculosum.[36] These neurons may send feedback to the supraoptic nucleus of the hypothalamus, where ADH is produced, and thus may contribute to the regulation of body water. Oxytocin, which is produced in the paraventricular nucleus of the hypothalamus, may also be regulated in a similar manner.[37]

Area Postrema

The area postrema is a paired midline structure located on the dorsal surface of the medulla oblongata just dorsal to the obex of the fourth ventricle (Figure 17-9).[38,39] No specialized neurosecretory factor has yet been ascribed to this area. However, it has the same structure as is found in other neurosecretory regions. The area postrema is surrounded by capillaries that form sinusoids, and it is continuous with the subarachnoid CSF via these perivascular spaces. Large molecules and protein-bound dyes in the bloodstream easily permeate the extravascular spaces of the area postrema and filter through the ependymal cell junctions into the fourth ventricular CSF. This area is the chemoreceptor trigger zone for vomiting. It has been shown that selective destruction of this area results in permanent immunity to certain emetic agents. Thus the enhancement seen in this area may be responsible for the vomiting sometimes encountered in patients after iodinated contrast administration. Enhancement in the area postrema can also be seen on gadolinium-enhanced MR images.[39] This enhancement in the medulla should not be confused with enhancement of the choroid plexus of the fourth ventricle, which is found ventral to the inferior medullary velum of this ventricle.

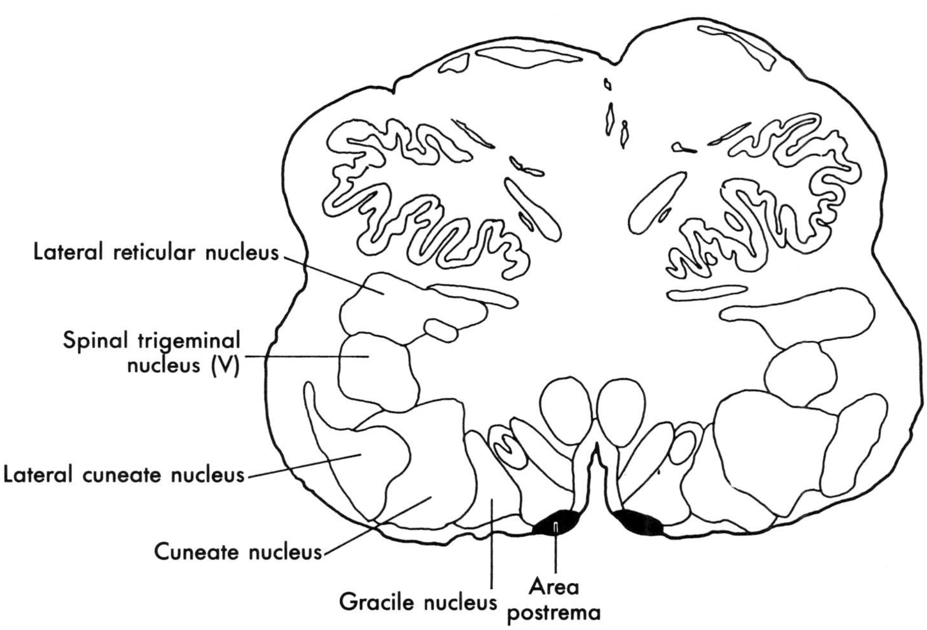

Figure 17-9 Axial schematic diagram of the medulla at the level of the caudal fourth ventricle demonstrating the paired area postrema organs.

REFERENCES

1. Reiter RJ: The pineal and its hormones in the control of reproduction in mammals, *Endocr Rev* 1:109, 1980.
2. Zimmerman RA, Bilaniuk L: Age-related incidence of pineal calcification detected by computed tomography, *Radiology* 142:659-662, 1982.
3. Sage MR: Blood-brain barrier: phenomenon of increasing importance to the imaging clinician, *AJNR* 3:127-138, 1982.
4. Reyes PF: Age related histologic changes in the human pineal gland, *Prog Clin Biol Res* 92:253-261, 1982.
5. Mamourian AC, Towfighi J: Pineal cysts: MR imaging, *AJNR* 7:1081-1086, 1986.
6. Lee DH, Norman D, Newton TH: MR imaging of pineal cysts, *J Comput Assist Tomogr* 11(4):586-590, 1987.
7. Lum GB, Williams JP, Machen BC, et al: Benign cystic pineal lesions by magnetic resonance imaging, *J Comput Tomogr* 11:228-235, 1987.
8. Nakagawa H, Iwasaki S, Kichikawa K, et al: MR imaging of pineocytoma: report of two cases, *AJNR* 11:195-198, 1990.
9. Nolte J: *The human brain: introduction to its functional anatomy,* St Louis, 1981, Mosby–Year Book.
10. Columbo N, Berry I, Kucharczyk J, et al: Posterior pituitary gland: appearance on MR images in normal and pathologic states, *Radiology* 165:481-485, 1987.
11. Kucharczyk J, et al: Histochemical characterization and functional significance of the hyperintense signal on MR images of the posterior pituitary, *AJNR* 9:1079-1083, 1988.
12. Tien RD, Newton TH, McDermot MW, et al: Thickened pituitary stalk on MR images in patients with diabetes insipidus and Langerhans cell histiocytosis, *AJNR* 11:703-708, 1990.
13. Ahmadi H, Larsson EM, Jinkins JR: Normal pituitary gland: coronal MR imaging of infundibular tilt, *Radiology* 177:389-392, 1990.
14. Tinall GT, Barrow DL: *Disorders of the pituitary,* St Louis, 1986, Mosby–Year Book.
15. Roppolo HMN, Latchaw RE: The normal pituitary gland. Part II. Microscopic anatomy–CT correlation, *AJNR* 4:937, 1983.
16. Bonneville JF, Cattin F, Moussa-Bacha K, et al: Dynamic computed tomography of the pituitary gland: the tuft sign, *Radiology* 149:145-148, 1983.
17. Elster AD, Chen MYM, Williams DW III, Key LL: Pituitary gland: MR imaging of physiologic hypertrophy in adolescence, *Radiology* 174:681-685, 1990.
18. Peyster RG, Hoover ED, Viscarello RR, et al: CT appearance of the adolescent and preadolescent pituitary gland, *AJNR* 4:411-414, 1983.
19. Wolpert SM, Molitich ME, Goldman JA, et al: Size, shape and appearance of the normal female pituitary gland, *AJR* 143:37-38, 1984.
20. Fujisawa I, Asato R, Nishimura K, et al: Anterior and posterior lobes of the pituitary gland: assessment by 1.5 T MR imaging, *J Comput Assist Tomogr* 11:214-220, 1987.
21. Kucharczyk W, Lenkinski RE, Kucharczyk J, Henkelman RM: The effect of phospholipid vesicles on the NMR relaxation of water: an explanation for the MR appearance of the neurohypophysis? *AJNR* 11:693-700, 1990.
22. Wolpert SM, Osborne M, Anderson M, et al: The bright pituitary gland—a normal MR appearance in infancy, *AJNR* 9:1-3, 1988.
23. Gudinchet F, Brunelle F, Barth MO, et al: MR imaging of the posterior hypophysis in children, *AJNR* 10:511-514, 1989.
24. Brooks BS, El Gammal T, Allison JD, et al: Frequency and variation of the posterior pituitary bright signal on MR images, *AJNR* 10:943-948, 1989; *AJR* 153, 1989.
25. Benshoff ER, Katz BH: Ectopia of the posterior pituitary gland as a normal variant: assessment with MR imaging, *AJNR* 11:709-712, 1990.
26. El Gammal T, Brooks BS, Hoffman WH: MR imaging of the ectopic bright signal of posterior pituitary regeneration, *AJNR* 10:323-328, 1989.
27. Kelly WM, Kucharczyk W, Kucharczyk J, et al: Posterior pituitary ectopia: an MR feature of pituitary dwarfism, *AJNR* 9:453-460, 1988.
28. Bonneville JF, Cattin F, Portha C, et al: Computed tomographic demonstration of the posterior pituitary, *AJNR* 6:889-892, 1985.
29. Knisgek SD, Weindl A: *Brain endocrine interaction—median eminence: structure and function,* Basel, 1972, Karger.
30. Kelly D: Circumventricular organs. In *Histology and histopathology of the nervous system,* Springfield, Ill, 1982, Charles C Thomas.
31. Rodriguez E, Oksche A, Rodriguez S, et al: The subcommissural organ and Reissner's fiber: fine structure and cytochemistry. In *Circumventricular organs and body fluids,* vol 22, Boca Raton, Fla, 1987, CRC.
32. Weindl A: Neuroendocrine aspects of circumventricular organs. In Ganong W, Martini L, editors: *Frontiers in neuroendocrinology,* London, 1973, Oxford University.
33. Dellman H, Simpson J: The subfornical organ, *Int Rev Cytol* 58:333-421, 1979.
34. Bouchard C, Bosler O: The circumventricular organs of the mammalian brain with special reference to monoaminergic innervation, *Int Rev Cytol* 105:283-327, 1986.
35. Gross P, Weindl A: Peering through the windows of the brain, *J Cereb Blood Flow Metab* 7:663-672, 1987.
36. Davison H, Welch SM: The physiology and pathophysiology of the cerebrospinal fluid, Edinburgh, 1987, Churchill Livingstone.
37. Cross B, Leng G: The neurohypophysis: structure, function and control, *Prog Brain Res* 60, 1983.
38. Borison H: Area postrema, *Fed Proc* 43:2937-2971, 1984.
39. Williams KD, Dean B, Drayer BP: Demonstration of the area postrema with contrast-enhanced MR, *AJNR* 11:733-734, 1990.

CHAPTER 18

William L. Hirsch, Jr.
Reed Shankwiler
L. Anne Hayman

Sella and Parasellar Structures

IMAGING TECHNIQUES

Computed Tomography

Sellar Contents

The pituitary gland and sella are optimally imaged using direct coronal computed tomography (CT) with the following scan parameters: contiguous cuts 1.5 mm thick, 256 × 256 matrix, 12.8 cm field of view (FOV), head calibration, soft tissue resolution with a technique of 120 kV, 170 milliamperes (mA), and 3-second scan time. Bone windows are usually adequate for evaluation of the sella, but bone algorithms provide superior detail and require little additional reconstruction time using modern scanners. Coronal scanning requires hyperextension of the neck and may be performed either in the prone or the supine position, whichever is better tolerated by the patient. If the patient is unable to hyperextend the neck, 1.5 mm axial cuts through the sella and suprasellar cistern are used to generate reformatted sagittal and coronal images.

All patients are scanned after intravenous (IV) contrast infusion and receive a total of 40 to 45 g of iodine unless contraindicated. Half the contrast is given as a bolus, and the other half is administered as a rapid-drip infusion during scanning.

Portions of this chapter are adapted from Latchaw RE: *MR and CT imaging of the head, neck, and spine,* ed 2, vol 2, St Louis, 1991, Mosby–Year Book.

Parasellar Region

Optimum imaging of parasellar lesions requires examination in two planes using both soft tissue and bone algorithms. The following scanning parameters are recommended: contiguous sections 3 mm thick, 3 mm spacing, 120 kV, 170 mA, 3-second scan time, and soft tissue as well as bone algorithms. Coronal sections are made perpendicular to the sellar floor and extend from the orbital apex to the prepontine cistern using a 17 cm FOV. Axial images are made parallel to the hard palate, extending from hard palate up to the top of the orbit using a 19 cm FOV. Wide scan margins are needed around the parasellar region to evaluate for spread of lesions into surrounding structures, particularly in evaluation of perineural extension.

Magnetic Resonance Imaging

Sellar Contents

To identify small pituitary lesions with magnetic resonance imaging (MRI), contrast resolution must be maximized and voxel volume minimized to eliminate partial-volume averaging. The specific pulsing sequences used continue to change as MR technology evolves. Gradient-echo (GE) techniques (fast low-angle shot, or FLASH) produce susceptibility artifacts at the border of the pituitary gland and air in the sphenoid sinus. At present, the following spin-echo (SE) sequences are obtained using a 1.5 Tesla (T) magnet and the following parameters: coronal and sagittal planes; repetition time (TR), 400 msec; echo delay time (TE), 15 msec; 256 × 200 acquisition matrix; four excitations; 20 cm FOV; sections 3 mm thick; 0.5 mm interslice gap; and a total of seven cuts through the sella. A "square" pulse wave is used to reduce interslice "cross talk."

The MR scans are performed before and after IV injection of gadolinium (Gd) contrast agent. Information concerning the optimum dose and timing of this injection is evolving. The use of only half the maximum recommended dose reduces the problematic marked sellar hyper-

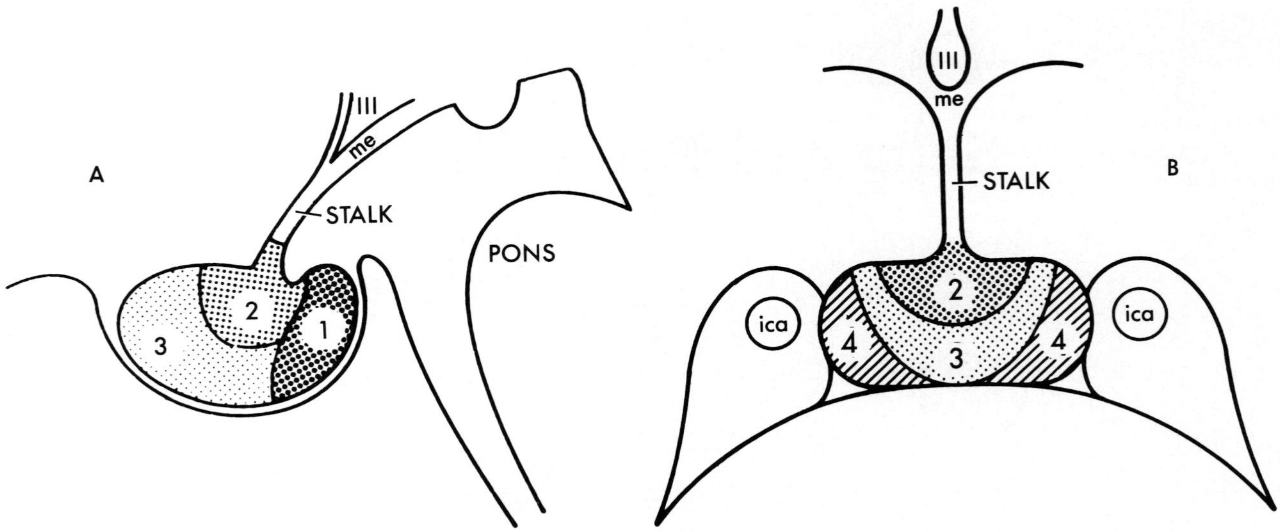

Figure 18-1 Temporal sequence of enhancement in the normal pituitary gland is shown on sagittal **(A)** and coronal **(B)** schematics. Within 20 seconds after bolus injection of gadolinium, contrast accumulates in the pituitary's posterior lobe (*zone* 1). This occurs because the posterior lobe is supplied by the inferior hypophyseal branch of the meningohypophyseal artery, or as a direct branch from the cavernous portion of the internal carotid artery (*ica*). Simultaneous enhancement is also seen in the infundibular stalk, since it is also supplied directly by the internal carotid and posterior communicating arteries. The pituitary's anterior lobe, which is adjacent to the stalk (*zone* 2), enhances 50 seconds after injection of contrast. This is followed by a gradual increase in contrast in the periphery of the gland (*zones* 3 *and* 4), which reaches a peak 60 to 90 seconds after injection. This relatively delayed enhancement occurs because the pituitary's anterior lobe is supplied by an *indirect* route. The superior hypophyseal arteries that arise from the supraclinoid portion of the internal carotid and the posterior communicating arteries supply the median eminence (*me*) and the infundibular stalk. The blood is then shunted into the portal venous system, which carries it to the sinusoids of the anterior pituitary gland. (Modified with permission from Sakamoto Y, Takahashi M, Korogi Y, et al: *Radiology* 178:441-445, 1991.)

intensity, which occurs at full-dose techniques. Immediate imaging (i.e., 3 minutes after Gd injection) seems preferable to delayed scans.[1,2]

Recently, dynamic coronal MRI has been advocated to visualize serially the anatomy of this region.[3] This technique requires the rapid injection of a bolus of Gd followed by serial coronal SE scans on a 1.5 T magnet using the following parameters: TR/TE 600/15; 128 × 256 acquisition matrix; one excitation; 25 cm FOV; sections 5 mm thick; and a total of five cuts through the sella. A total of 7 to 10 images is obtained every 20 to 30 seconds to assess the serial enhancement of normal structures in the region (Figure 18-1). This technique produces better visualization of the cranial nerves in the cavernous sinus and the dura between the pituitary and cavernous sinus. The coronal scans are most important for detection of small pituitary microadenomas, which enhance later than the normal gland and thus are hypointense when this dynamic technique is used. Pituitary adenomas have a variable appearance several minutes after contrast administration. They may be isointense or hypointense to the gland, since contrast appears to leave some adenomas more slowly than it clears from the normal gland. Additional MR views in the sagittal plane may be used to evaluate the size of the sella and the relationship of large sellar masses to the sphenoid sinus, clivus, and suprasellar structures.

Parasellar Region

When confronted with a parasellar lesion, MRI is performed to evaluate the lesion's relationship to the parasellar segment of the carotid artery, the cavernous sinus, and cranial nerves II, III, IV, V, and VI. To examine for possible extracranial extension through nearby skull base foramina, the scan margin must extend sufficiently below the skull base.

Currently the following routine SE sequences are used: axial; TR/TE, 800/20; 256 × 256 acquisition matrix; 16 cm FOV; four excitations; cuts 3 mm thick; 1 mm interslice gap; and a total of 16 cuts. Scans are made from the hard palate through the suprasellar cistern. Coronal scans

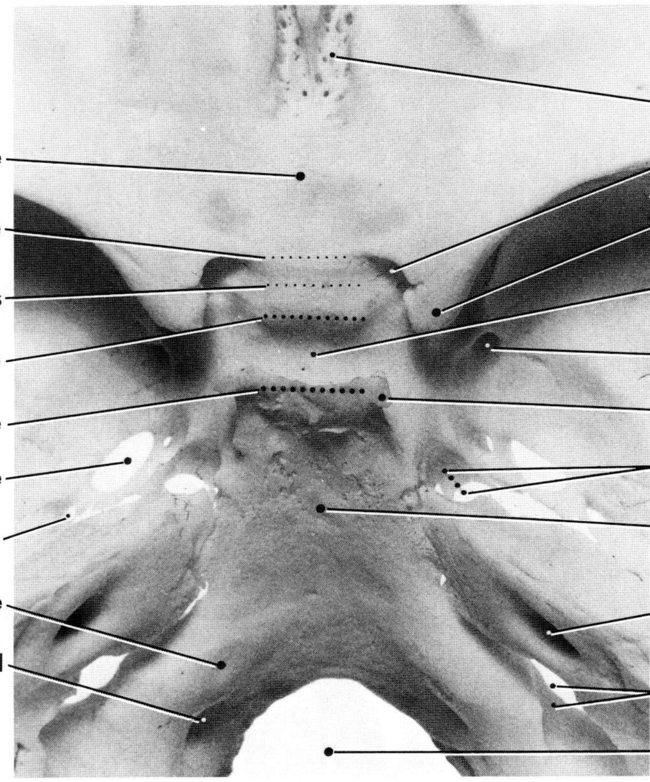

Figure 18-2 View of skull base from above shows the bony anatomy of the sella.

are made from the orbital apex to the prepontine cistern using the same parameters. Scans are performed before and after contrast infusion. The preinfusion scans exploit the inherent contrast between fat planes adjacent to the skull base and neoplastic tissue. If only contrast studies were performed, these boundaries might be obscured. This is particularly true for densely enhancing tumors (e.g., meningioma), which may become isointense with surrounding fat on postcontrast MR studies. In addition, an axial T2-weighted series (T2, transverse relaxation time) is performed using the following parameters: TR/TE, 2500/30,80; 256 × 128 acquisition matrix; 20 cm FOV; two excitations; 5 mm slice thickness; and 1 mm interslice gap.

NORMAL ANATOMY

Bony Sella

The bony landmarks of the sellar area are labeled in Figure 18-2. The anterior wall and floor of the sella consist of cortical bone, which varies from several millimeters to only a few microns in thickness depending on degree of *pneumatization* of the underlying sphenoid sinus.[4] Pneumatization of the body of the sphenoid bone begins at age 3 years, but the extent of pneumatization is variable and is sometimes even absent in adult life (Figure 18-3, *A* to *C*).[5]

If the sphenoid sinus is well pneumatized, the parasellar carotid artery can be expected to impress a groove in its posterosuperior wall. The bone between artery and sinus is very thin or even incomplete in one third of individuals. In these individuals, the carotid artery is covered only by sinus mucosa and is therefore vulnerable to injury during transsphenoidal surgery.[5] The carotid arteries are particularly vulnerable to intraoperative injury when they course within 4 mm of the midline.[6] If the sphenoid sinus is incompletely pneumatized, transsphenoidal surgery is more difficult. Infection of the sphenoid sinus is another relative contraindication to transsphenoidal surgery.[7]

The configuration of the sellar floor is quite variable. Localized defects or depressions are sometimes encountered normally (Figure 18-3, *A*). Attempts have been made to correlate dips in the sellar floor with location of microadenomas, but correlation has proved to be very poor. Carin et al.[8] reviewed 205 autopsies and found only four abnormal pituitary glands, none of which had sellar abnormalities. It is best to disregard the shape of the floor when evaluating for pituitary adenomas.[4,9]

Coronal CT images with bone algorithms are ideal for evaluation of the bony sella and skull base. Hyperostosis, erosion, and remodeling are better demonstrated by CT than by MRI,[10] but MRI is useful for demonstrating replacement of normal bone marrow. This may occur in neoplastic infiltration of marrow cavities.

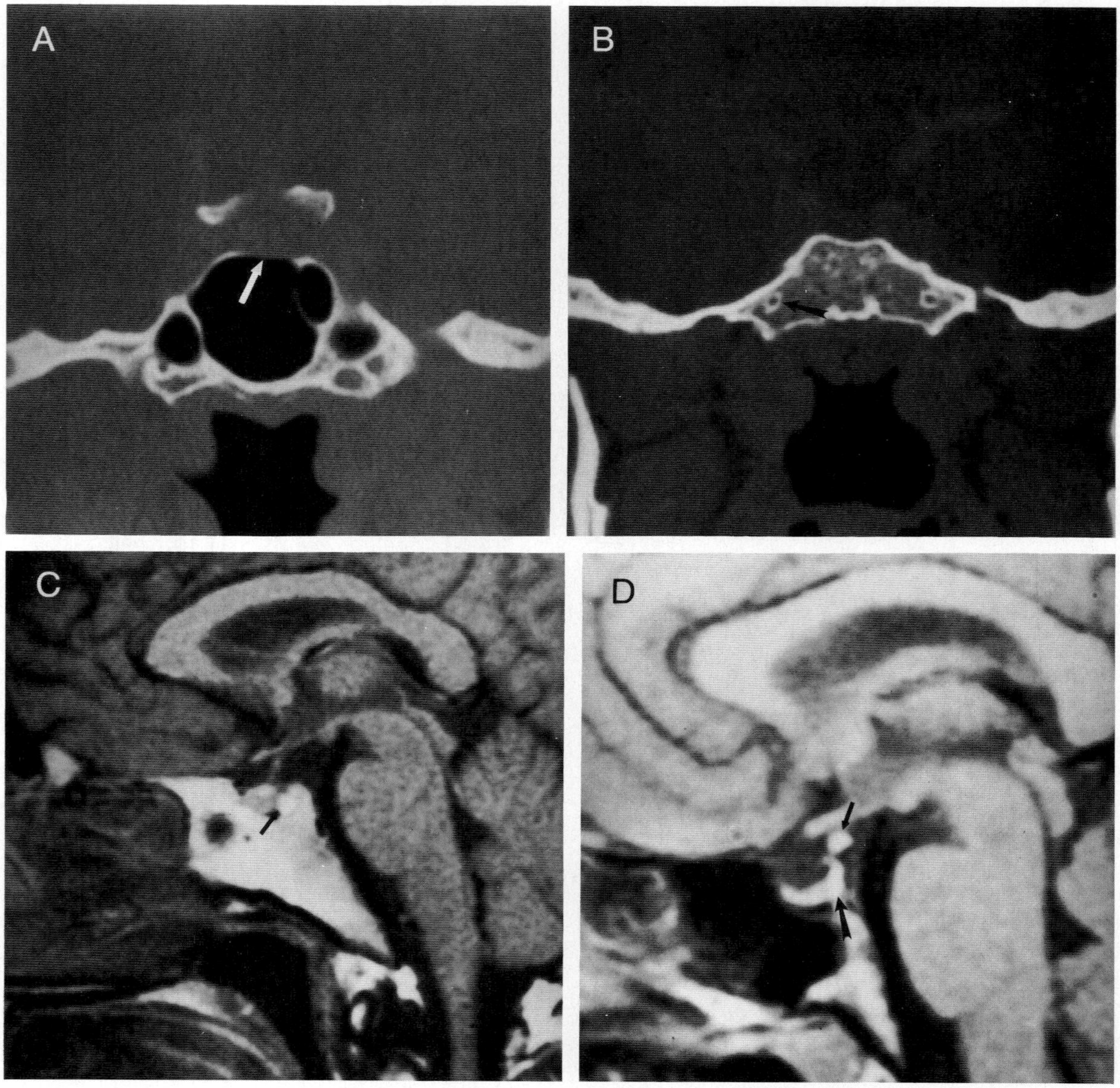

Figure 18-3 Normal imaging variants of the bony sella. **A,** CT image (bone windows) shows a well-pneumatized sphenoid sinus. Focal thinning of the floor (*arrow*) is normal. **B,** Coronal CT image (bone algorithm) of a nonpneumatized sphenoid bone. Transsphenoidal surgery is difficult in this situation. Incidentally, the vidian (pterygoid) canal is well seen (*arrow*). **C,** Sagittal MR images (TR/TE, 500/20) of nonpneumatized sphenoid sinus. The sphenoid bone marrow has high signal intensity on short TR images. Normal high signal intensity is seen in the posterior pituitary lobe (*arrow*). **D,** Sagittal MR images (TR/TE, 500/20). Prominent fat in the dorsum sellae (*small arrow*) mimics ectopic posterior pituitary tissue. Note the normal posterior pituitary lobe (*large arrow*). (From Latchaw RE: MR *and* CT *imaging of the head, neck, and spine,* ed 2, vol 2, St Louis, 1991, Mosby–Year Book.)

Dural Relationships

During life the bony sella is invested with dura. As the dura passes anteriorly from the dorsum, it divides into an outer layer, which lines the floor, and an inner layer, which forms the roof of the pituitary fossa. The latter is the *diaphragma sellae,* which is perforated, usually in the center, by a foramen for passage of the pituitary infundibulum. This foramen varies in size from small (just large enough to allow passage of the infundibulum) to large, with only a narrow rim of surrounding dura (Figure 18-4, *A* and *B*).[4,11]

On MRI, the diaphragma sellae is sometimes seen as a thin band between the pituitary fossa and the suprasellar cistern on proton-density-weighted (long TR/short TE SE) images. When visible, this structure helps to differentiate suprasellar from intrasellar pathology (Figure 18-5, *B*).[12,13]

Lateral to the sella, the dura splits into two layers, one forming the medial wall and the other the lateral wall and roof of the cavernous sinus. Between these dural reflections lie numerous venous channels (Figures 18-4, *D,* and 18-5, *A*).[11] Winslow coined the term *cavernous sinus* in 1732 because he thought it was a trabeculated venous space that resembled the corpus cavernosum of the penis.[14,15] Other investigators claim that the cavernous sinus is really a plexus of small veins.[11,16] The paired cavernous sinuses connect with each other through variable intrasellar channels, which may be anterior or posterior to the pituitary gland, as well as through extrasellar communications. These anastomotic channels are usually small but occasionally bleed severely during transsphenoidal surgery.

The cavernous sinus drains the superior and inferior ophthalmic veins, middle and inferior cerebral veins, and the sphenoparietal sinus. These vessels, in turn, drain into the basilar plexus, the transverse sinus (via the superior petrosal sinus), the jugular bulb (via the inferior petrosal sinus), and the pterygoid plexus (via a vein passing through the foramen ovale) (Figure 18-4, *D*).[17]

On contrast-enhanced CT images, the veins of the cavernous sinus blend together. A similar effect is seen on Gd-enhanced MR images. On nonenhanced MR images, the cavernous sinus has a speckled appearance, probably related to flow rate differentials within the venous plexus. Small globules of fat are also found normally within the cavernous sinuses and are visible on both CT and MR images (Figure 18-6).[18,19]

The internal carotid artery passes between the dural leaves of the cavernous sinus, giving off small branches to supply the tentorium, pituitary capsule, and gasserian ganglion. These intracavernous branches are not seen on CT or MR images and are only rarely demonstrated by angiography. The ophthalmic artery usually arises from the carotid artery after it has pierced the dura and entered the cranial cavity, but it originates from the intracavernous portion of the carotid artery in 8% of anatomic dissections.[4,16] This variation, difficult to recognize angiographically or by other imaging modalities, is nonetheless important when aneurysms are discovered arising at the origin of the ophthalmic artery. This variation makes it difficult to determine preoperatively whether or not the cavernous sinus will have to be entered to clip the aneurysm's neck. The carotid artery is fixed at its exit from the cavernous sinus by a tight dural band, but its intracavernous course is variable. Usually, the carotid artery is separated from the pituitary gland by a distance of about 1 mm. However, in one third of autopsy specimens, the artery is more medial and actually indents the pituitary gland (Figure 18-7).[20,21] Occasionally, both carotid arteries bow medially and may be separated from each other by as little as 4 mm (Figure 18-8). Transsphenoidal surgery in such patients may be contraindicated. MRI is ideal for noninvasively demonstrating intercarotid distance.

In addition to the venous plexus and the carotid artery, two other structures course within the dural envelope of the cavernous sinus: (1) the plexus of sympathetic nerves that accompanies the cavernous carotid artery and (2) cranial nerve VI, which penetrates the posterior wall of the cavernous sinus at Dorello's canal, courses superiorly and laterally through the sinus, and exits through the superior orbital fissure (Figure 18-4, *C* and *D*).[4,22,23]

The lateral wall of the cavernous sinus consists of a tough, outer layer and a thin, inner reticular layer. The inner layer is formed by the sheaths of cranial nerves III, IV, and V_1 (Figure 18-5, *A*).[24] These nerves converge anteriorly, pass through the superior orbital fissure, and supply motor fibers to the extraocular muscles and sensory fibers to the cornea, upper face, and scalp. The superior ophthalmic vein also courses through the superior orbital fissure to drain into the cavernous sinus.

Just lateral to the posterior part of the cavernous sinus is an almost vertical pocket of dura, *Meckel's cave* (Figure 18-9, *C*). After exiting from the ventral surface of the pons, the axons of cranial nerve V traverse this oval- or triangular-shaped dural pocket. These axons exit anteriorly and synapse in the gasserian (semilunar) ganglion. Cranial nerve V_3 does not enter the cavernous sinus but instead courses laterally to exit through the foramen ovale. Cranial nerve V_2 travels through only a small portion of the inferior aspect of the cavernous sinus before exiting through the foramen rotundum. Cranial nerve V_1 traverses the entire length of the cavernous sinus to exit through the superior orbital fissure (Figure 18-4, *C*).[4,22,24]

On careful inspection of nonenhanced coronal MR images, cranial nerves III, V_1, V_2, and VI are difficult to recognize as they run in the lateral wall of the cavernous sinus (Figure 18-6). They are sometimes more readily seen on CT or MR images following contrast enhancement.[18,22]

The cavernous sinuses should be symmetric in size. The lateral walls may be flat or slightly convex laterally. On

Text continued on page 438.

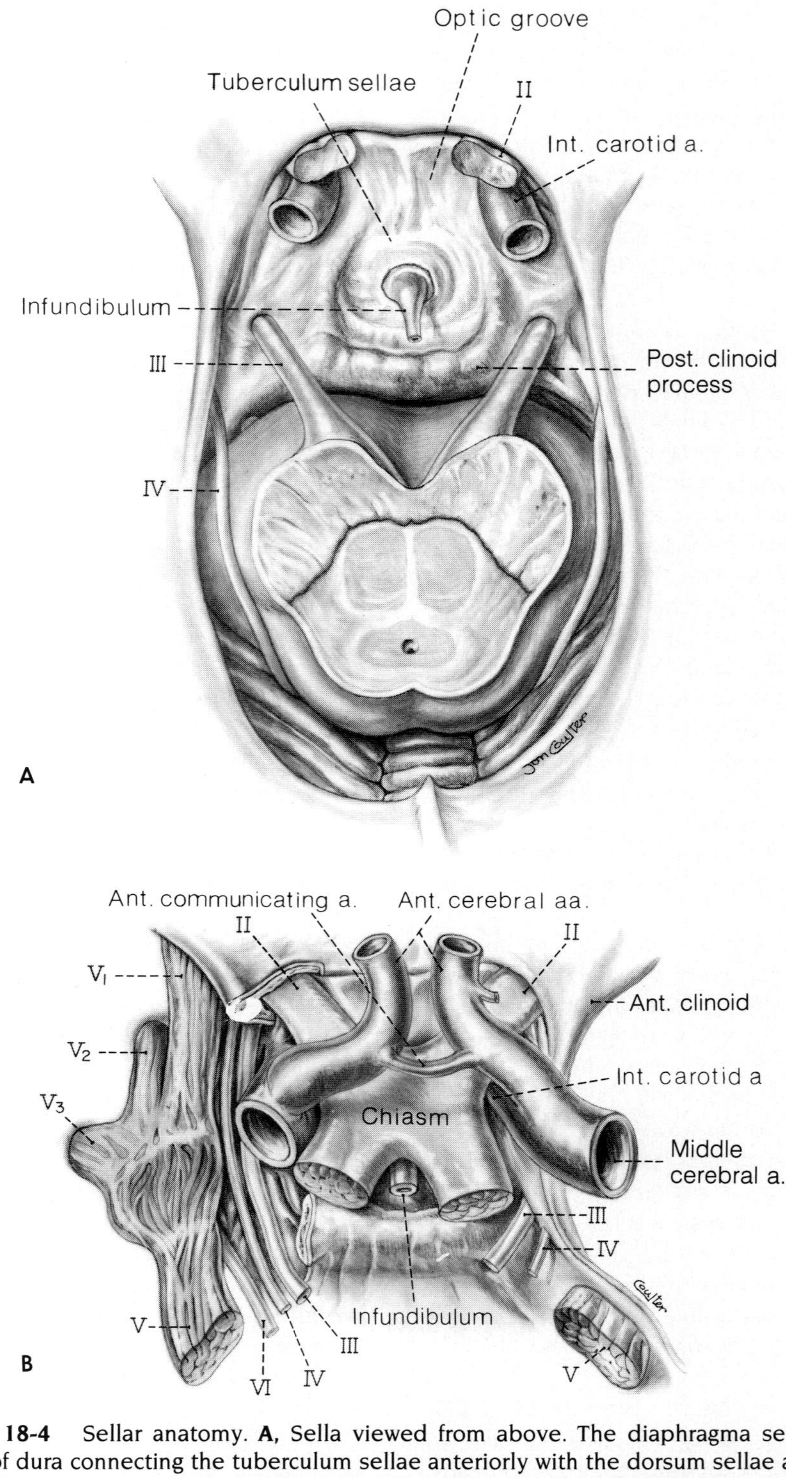

Figure 18-4 Sellar anatomy. **A,** Sella viewed from above. The diaphragma sellae is a sheet of dura connecting the tuberculum sellae anteriorly with the dorsum sellae and posterior clinoid processes. The diaphragma sellae is perforated by a foramen for passage of the infundibulum. The tentorium blends into the superolateral border of the cavernous sinus bilaterally. **B,** Sella and suprasellar cistern from above. The dura of the left cavernous sinus has been removed. The A1 segments and the anterior communicating artery course just superior to the optic chiasm. The origin of the recurrent artery of Heubner (long central artery) from the right anterior cerebral artery is shown.

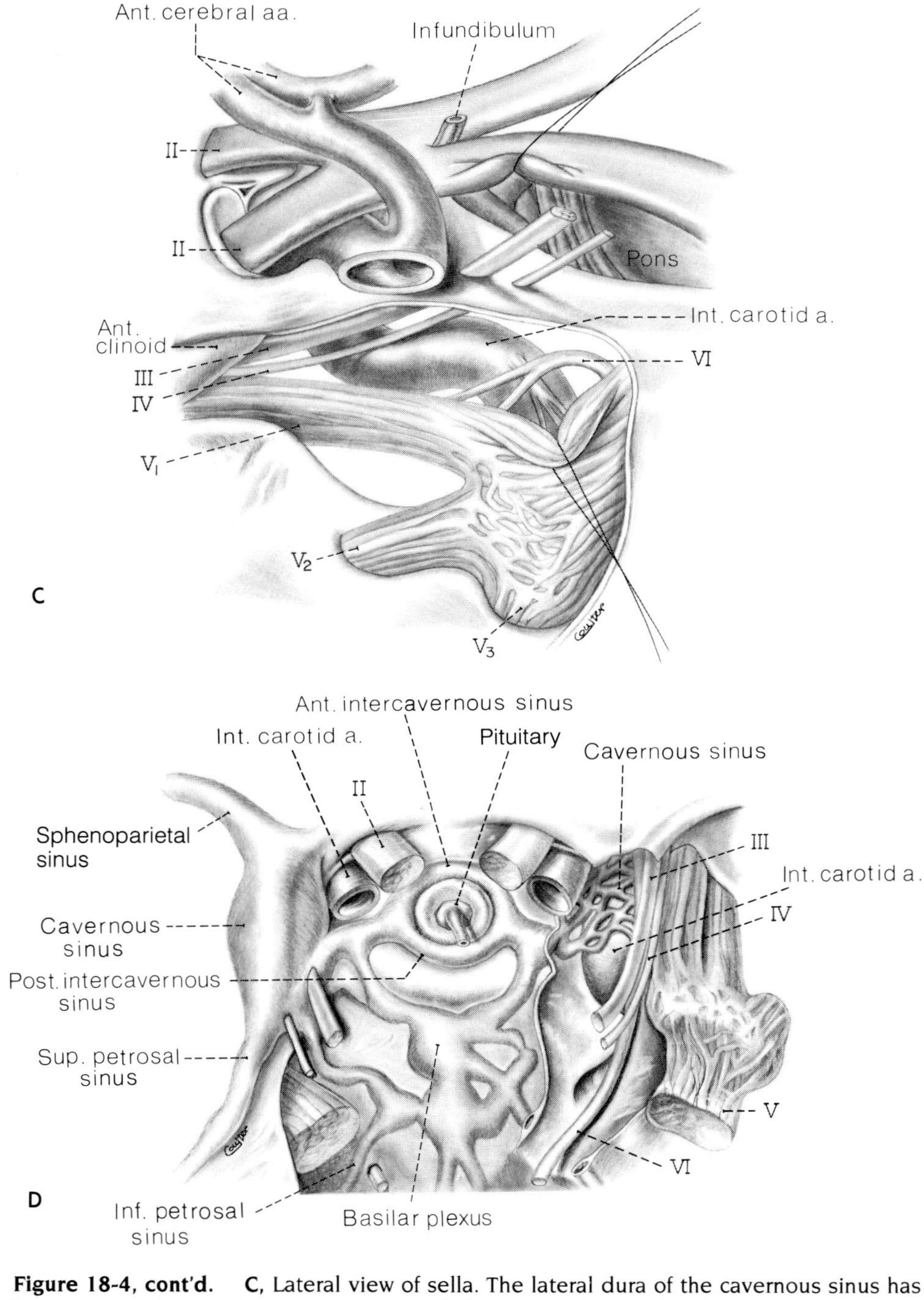

Figure 18-4, cont'd. **C,** Lateral view of sella. The lateral dura of the cavernous sinus has been removed. Cranial nerve V_3 exits Meckel's cave and immediately passes through the foramen ovale to the masticator space; V_3 never enters the cavernous sinus. Cranial nerve V_2 courses through the most inferior aspect of the cavernous sinus, then exits through foramen rotundum into the pterygopalatine fossa. Cranial nerves V_1, VI, IV, and III all run in the cavernous sinus and exit through the superior orbital fissure to enter the orbit. **D,** Venous anatomy viewed from above. The dural covering of the right cavernous sinus has been removed to expose the venous anatomy. (From Latchaw RE: MR *and* CT *imaging of the head, neck, and spine,* ed 2, vol 2, St Louis, 1991, Mosby–Year Book.)

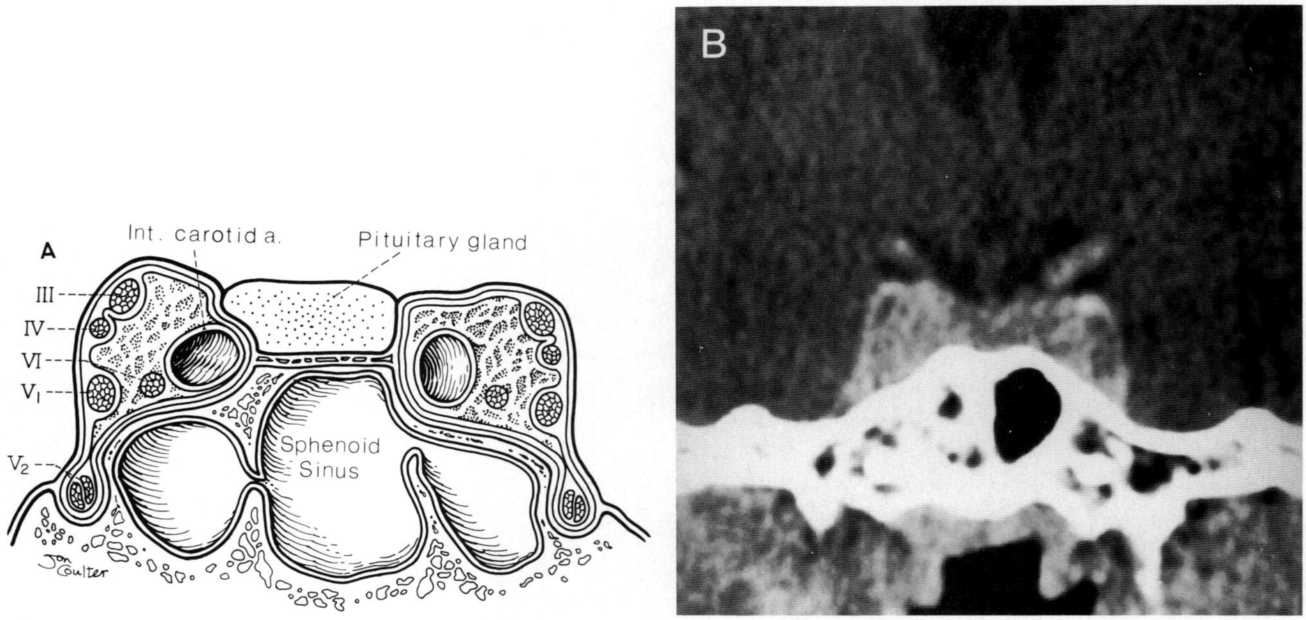

Figure 18-5 Normal sella and cavernous sinus. **A,** Coronal section of the pituitary gland and cavernous sinus. Note that cranial nerves III, IV, and V_1 run adjacent to the lateral wall of the cavernous sinus; VI runs more medially within the venous plexus. **B,** Enhanced coronal CT image. Intravascular contrast causes enhancement of the cavernous venous plexus. Extravasated contrast enhances the pituitary gland because its vessels lack an effective blood-brain barrier. The thin pituitary capsule (medial wall of cavernous sinus) is not visualized. (From Latchaw RE: MR *and* CT *imaging of the head, neck, and spine,* ed 2, vol 2, St Louis, 1991, Mosby–Year Book.)

Figure 18-6 Pairs of coronal MR images (TR/TE, 401/15) before and several minutes after gadolinium (Gd) contrast injection in a normal subject. **Section A,** MR image before Gd enhancement shows the supraclinoid internal carotid artery (sICA) and cavernous internal carotid artery (*c*ICA), cranial nerve III (III), and the anterior pituitary gland (AP). Note that enhancement defines the lateral margin of the cavernous sinus on the right (*small dots*), the mucosa of the septum of the sphenoid sinus (*s*), and the dura around the anterior clinoid process (*ac*). Enhancement of the central part of the anterior pituitary gland is marked by three vertical dots.

Section B, MR image before Gd enhancement shows the supraclinoid internal carotid artery (sICA) and the vertical portion of the internal carotid artery (*c*ICA). Note that the boundary between the pituitary gland and the cavernous sinus is well seen (*small dots*). Enhancement shows the veins at the sellar floor that interconnect the cavernous sinuses (*small dots*). The most anterior extension of Meckel's cave (*mc*), which contains the rootlets of the cranial nerve V, is seen in the left cavernous sinus.

Section C, MR image before Gd enhancement shows the optic chiasm (*ch*) above the infundibular stalk (*s*). The posterior lobe of the pituitary (*pp*) is the hyperintense area in the floor of the sella. The foramen ovale (*fo*) is also seen. Minor patient movement before the Gd-enhanced scan allows visualization of the symmetric peripheral enhancement in the anterior pituitary gland (AP) and the infundibular stalk (*s*). Meckel's cave (*mc*) is seen just lateral to the vertical part of the cavernous carotid artery (*c*ICA).

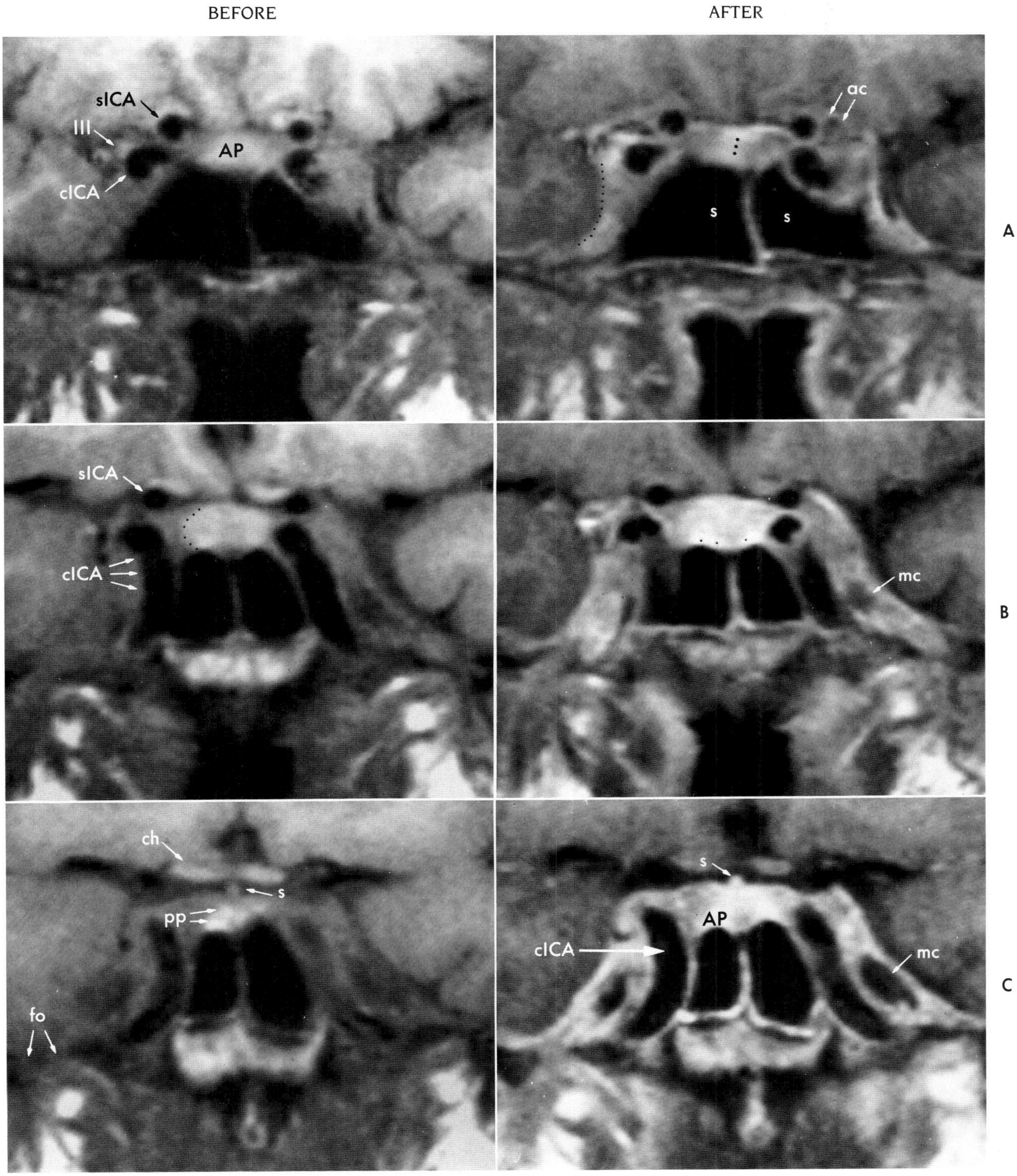

Figure 18-6 For legend see opposite page.

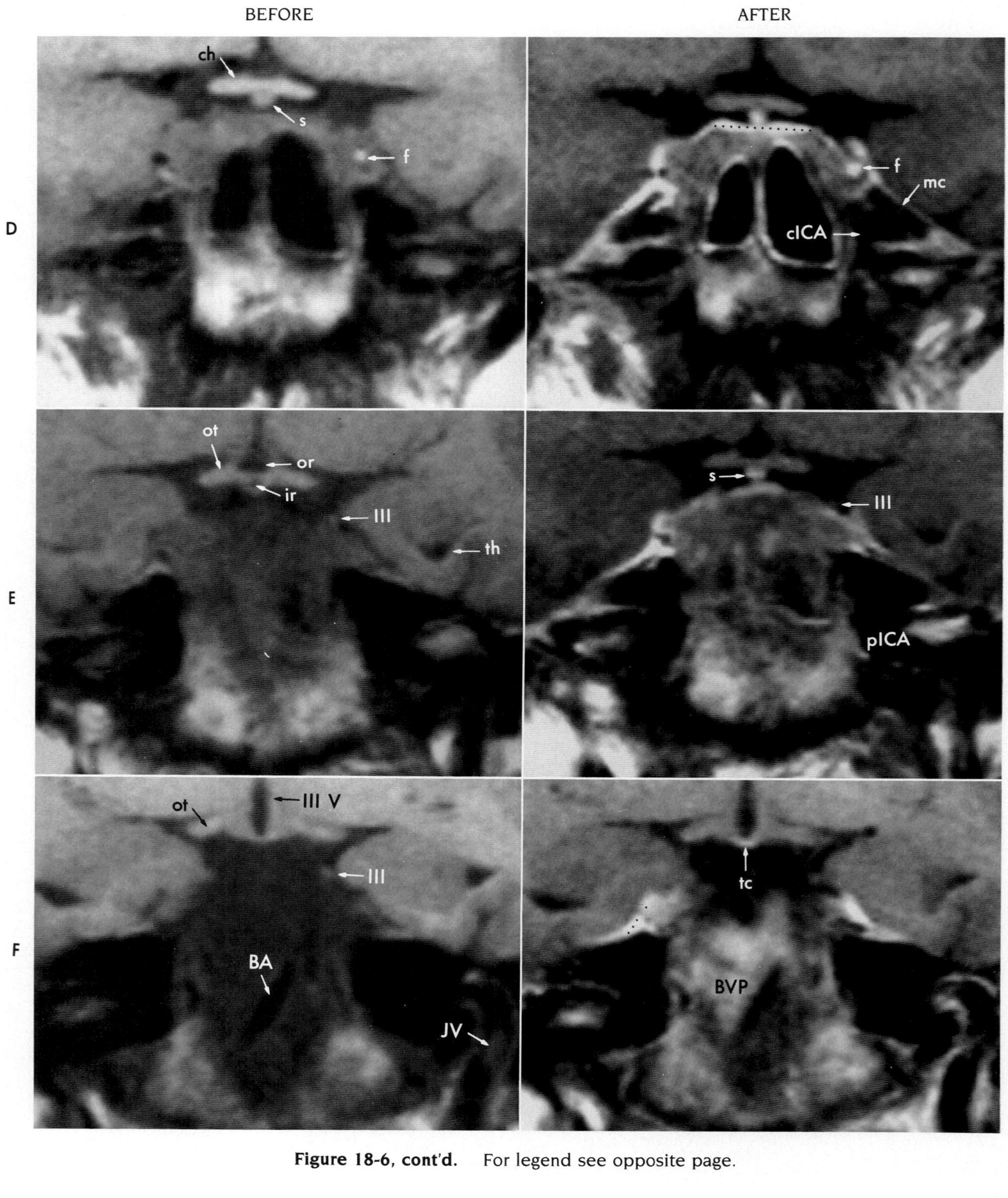

Figure 18-6, cont'd. For legend see opposite page.

Figure 18-6, cont'd. **Section D,** MR image before Gd-enhancement, shows the optic chiasm (*ch*) above the infundibular stalk (*s*) in the suprasellar (chiasmatic) cistern. A small lobule of hyperintense fat (*f*) is seen in the left cavernous sinus. Enhancement defines the dura of the diaphragma sellae (*horizontal black dots*). The cavernous internal carotid artery (*c*ICA), cavernous sinus fat (*f*), and Meckel's cave (*mc*) are again identified.
Section E, MR image before Gd enhancement shows cranial nerve III (III), optic tract (*ot*), infundibular recess (*ir*), and optic recess (*or*) of the third ventricle below the cistern of the lamina terminalis. The temporal horn (*th*) of the lateral ventricle is now seen. Enhancement defines the infundibular stalk (*s*). A flow void represents the petrous internal carotid artery (*p*ICA). Cranial nerve III (III) is less well defined on the enhanced images.
Section F, MR image before Gd enhancement shows the third ventricle (III V) surrounded inferiorly and laterally by the hypothalamus, the optic tract (*ot*), cranial nerve III (III), and the basilar artery (BA), and jugular vein (JV). Enhancement shows the absence of a blood-brain barrier in the tuber cinereum (*tc*). The dura of the petroclinoid ligament is marked by a line of small black dots. The basilar venous plexus (BVP) on the clivus shows enhancement. (Courtesy Methodist Hospital, Houston.)

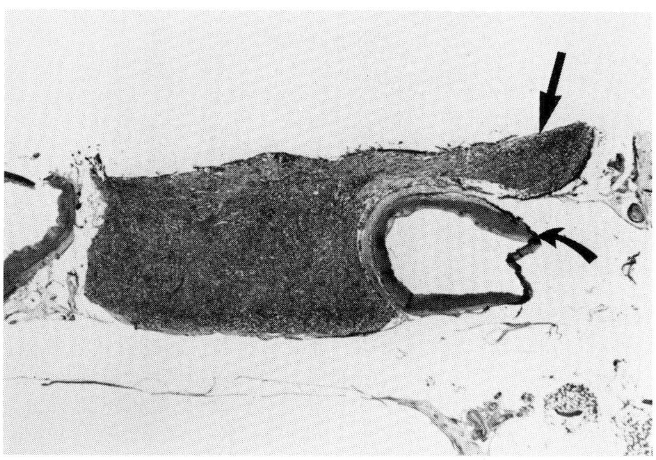

Figure 18-7 Coronal histologic section of an autopsy specimen shows a normal variation in position of the cavernous internal carotid artery (*curved arrow*). Note that a tonguelike extension of pituitary tissue extends over the carotid artery (*straight arrow*). (From Latchaw RE: MR *and* CT *imaging of the head, neck, and spine,* ed 2, vol 2, St Louis, 1991, Mosby–Year Book.)

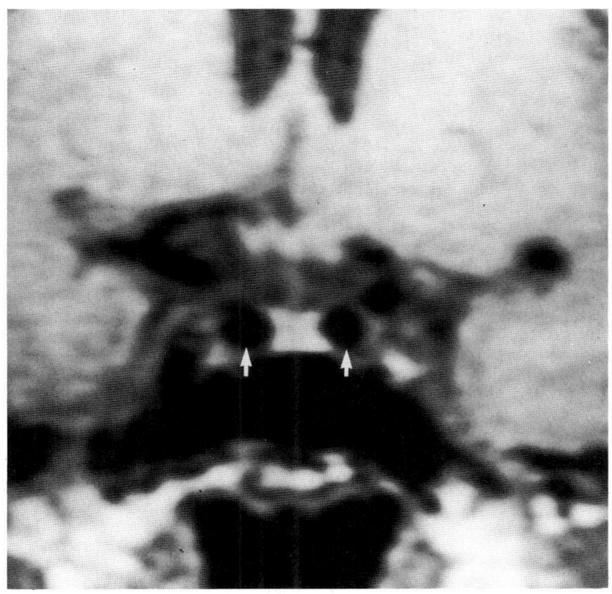

Figure 18-8 Coronal MR image (TR/TE, 600/20) through the floor of the pituitary fossa. Note the normal but unusually medial positions of both cavernous internal carotid arteries (*arrows*). (From Latchaw RE: MR *and* CT *imaging of the head, neck, and spine,* ed 2, vol 2, St Louis, 1991, Mosby–Year Book.)

CT, the lateral wall is defined between the enhancing cavernous sinus medially and the temporal lobe laterally.[25] On MRI, the lateral wall and adjacent cerebrospinal fluid (CSF) are defined as a band of low signal intensity. The medial wall of the cavernous sinus, which is much thinner, is not demonstrated on CT and is rarely shown on MRI unless dynamic imaging with IV Gd contrast enhancement is employed (Figure 18-6).[10,20] On either CT or MRI, masses within the cavernous sinus are usually recognized by unilateral sinus enlargement; small masses that do not change the contour of the cavernous sinus are more difficult to discern.

Suprasellar (Chiasmatic) Cistern

Above the pituitary fossa lies an expansion of the subarachnoid space, the suprasellar cistern. This cistern contains the optic nerves, chiasm, and tracts; the circle of Willis; and the pituitary infundibulum. Familiarity with its complex anatomy is helpful in identifying suprasellar pathology by either CT or MRI.

Coronal Plane (Figures 18-6 and 18-9)

The *optic nerve* leaves the orbit through the optic canal medial to the anterior clinoid process. Intracranially, the optic nerve courses medially and posteriorly to join its contralateral companion, forming the *optic chiasm* in the suprasellar cistern. The vertical dimension of the optic chiasm is variable but is generally less than 0.6 mm. The *pituitary infundibulum* runs anteriorly and inferiorly from the hypothalamus to the posterior lobe of the pituitary gland and is located immediately behind the chiasm. The A1 segments of the anterior cerebral arteries and

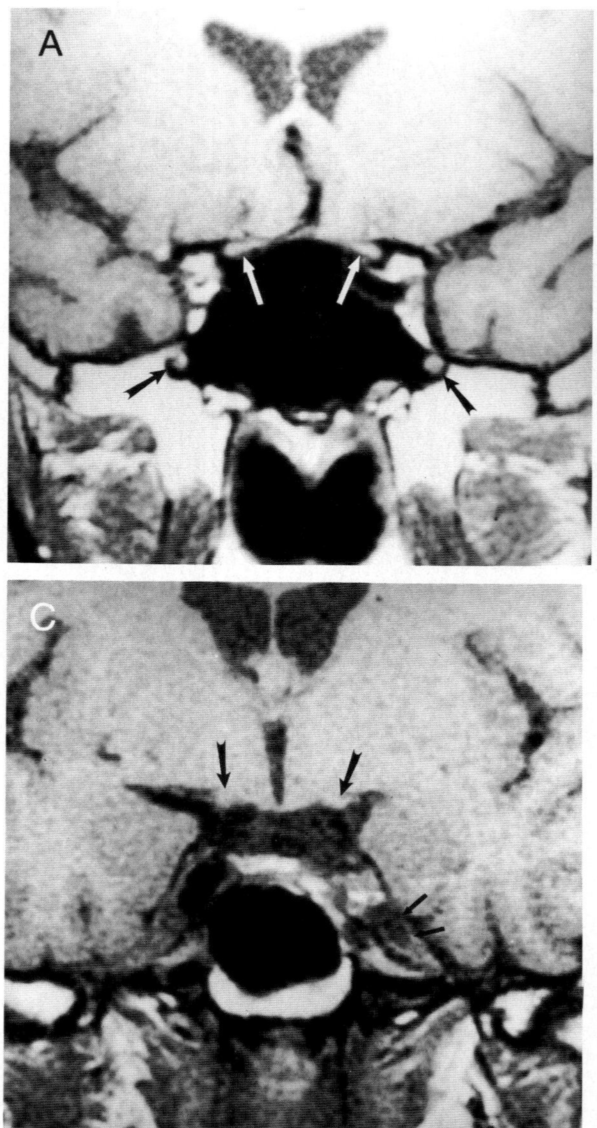

Figure 18-9 Serial coronal scans. **A,** Coronal MR image (TR/TE, 800/20) at the level of the optic canals. The optic nerve (*white arrow*) passes through the canal medial to the anterior clinoid process. The clinoid process has high signal intensity because it contains marrow fat. The clinoid blends with fat in the superior orbital fissure. Note cranial nerve V_2 as it passes through the foramen rotundum bilaterally (*black arrows*). **B,** Coronal MR image (800/20) at the level of the infundibulum. The optic nerves join to form the chiasm, which is located just anterior to the infundibular stalk. The A1 segment of the carotid artery lies immediately above the chiasm (*arrow*) and appears as a signal void. **C,** Coronal MR image (800/20) at the level of the dorsum sellae. The optic tracts (*large arrows*) are visualized. The hypothalamus can be seen between these tracts as it forms the roof of the suprasellar cistern and the floor of the third ventricle. Note that Meckel's cave, which contains the rootlets of cranial nerve V, is well seen on the patient's left (*small arrows*). (From Latchaw RE: MR *and CT imaging of the head, neck, and spine,* ed 2, vol 2, St Louis, 1991, Mosby–Year Book.)

the anterior communicating artery are usually located just above the chiasm. The *optic tracts* extend posteriorly and laterally from the chiasm to the lateral geniculate nuclei.

Axial Plane (Figure 18-10)

It is helpful to think of the suprasellar cistern as a six-pointed star. The anterior point of the star enters the interhemispheric fissure, which contains the anterior cerebral arteries. The anterolateral points are directed toward the sylvian fissures, which contain the proximal middle cerebral vessels. The posterolateral points of the star enter the perimesencephalic cisterns, which contain the proximal parts of the anterior choroidal, posterior cerebral, and superior cerebellar arteries, as well as the basal vein of Rosenthal. The posterior point defines the interpeduncular cistern. More ventral axial sections show the optic nerves leaving the orbit and joining to form the chiasm at a point just anterior to the infundibulum. An axial section through the midportion of the cistern shows the optic nerves, tracts, and chiasm. On axial sections through the superior aspect of the cistern, the diverging optic tracts are seen. On this same section, one finds the slitlike third ventricle. The mamillary bodies and interpeduncular cistern can also be identified on superior axial sections. These anatomic details are available on both CT and MR images, but the superior contrast resolution of MRI makes it the preferred modality for studying these structures. Short TR, SE images are preferred over long TR sequences because they are less subject to CSF flow artifacts.

Sagittal Plane (Figures 18-3, C and D, and 18-11)

The optic chiasm is usually centered directly over the pituitary gland. In 5% to 10% of people, the intracranial segment of the optic nerve is short, and the chiasm is centered directly over the tuberculum sellae *(prefixed chiasm).* In 15% of individuals, the intracranial portions of the optic nerves are longer than usual, and the chiasm overlies the dorsum sellae *(postfixed chiasm).* These normal anatomic variations become important when an anterior, subfrontal, surgical approach to the sella or suprasellar cistern is contemplated. This approach to the sella can be blocked by short optic nerves (prefixed chiasm) or by a large, bony tuberculum. Resection of the bony tuberculum sellae will then usually provide adequate exposure.[26] Figure 18-11 illustrates the MR appearance of a prefixed, central, and postfixed chiasm on sagittal MR images.[27]

On *parasagittal scans,* there may be partial-volume averaging of the pituitary gland and the cavernous carotid artery (Figure 18-12). This should not be mistaken for intrasellar pathology. Occasionally, the optic nerve, chiasm, and tract can herniate into the sella. It has been shown that no correlation exists between this finding and visual disturbances.[28]

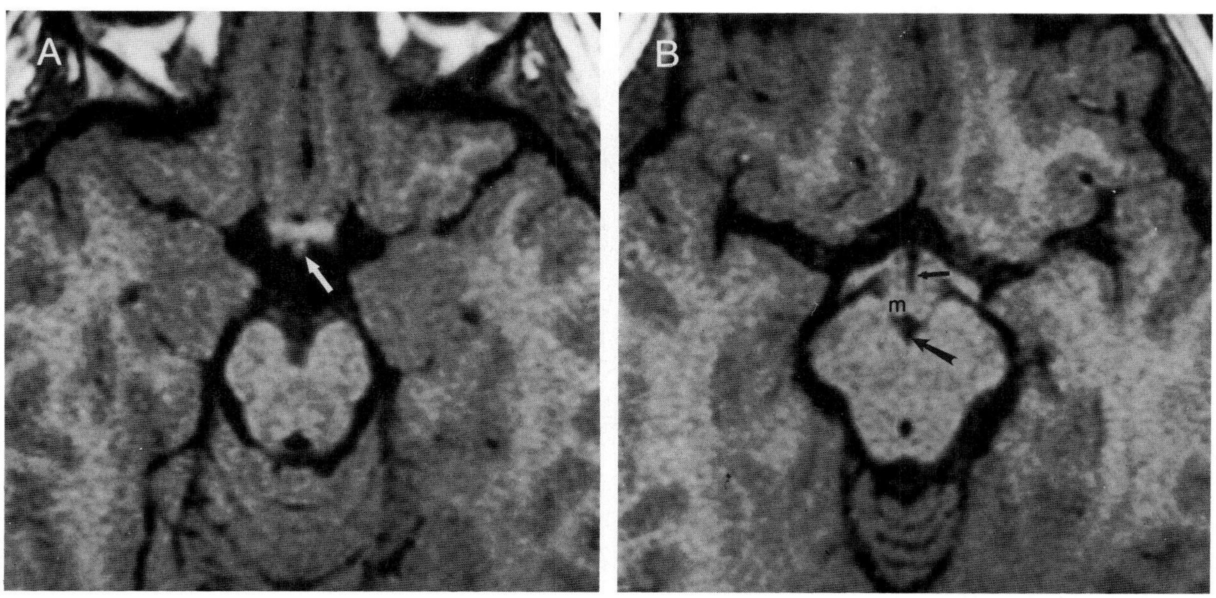

Figure 18-10 Normal axial scans. **A,** Axial MR image (TR/TE, 600/20) of the middle suprasellar cistern. The optic chiasm is immediately anterior to the infundibulum (*white arrow*). **B,** Axial MR image (600/20) of the superior aspect of the suprasellar cistern. The optic tracts are separated by the slitlike third ventricle (*small arrow*). The mamillary bodies (*m*) are located just anterior to the interpeduncular cistern (*large arrow*). (From Latchaw, RE: *MR and CT imaging of the head, neck, and spine,* ed 2, vol 2, St Louis, 1991, Mosby–Year Book.)

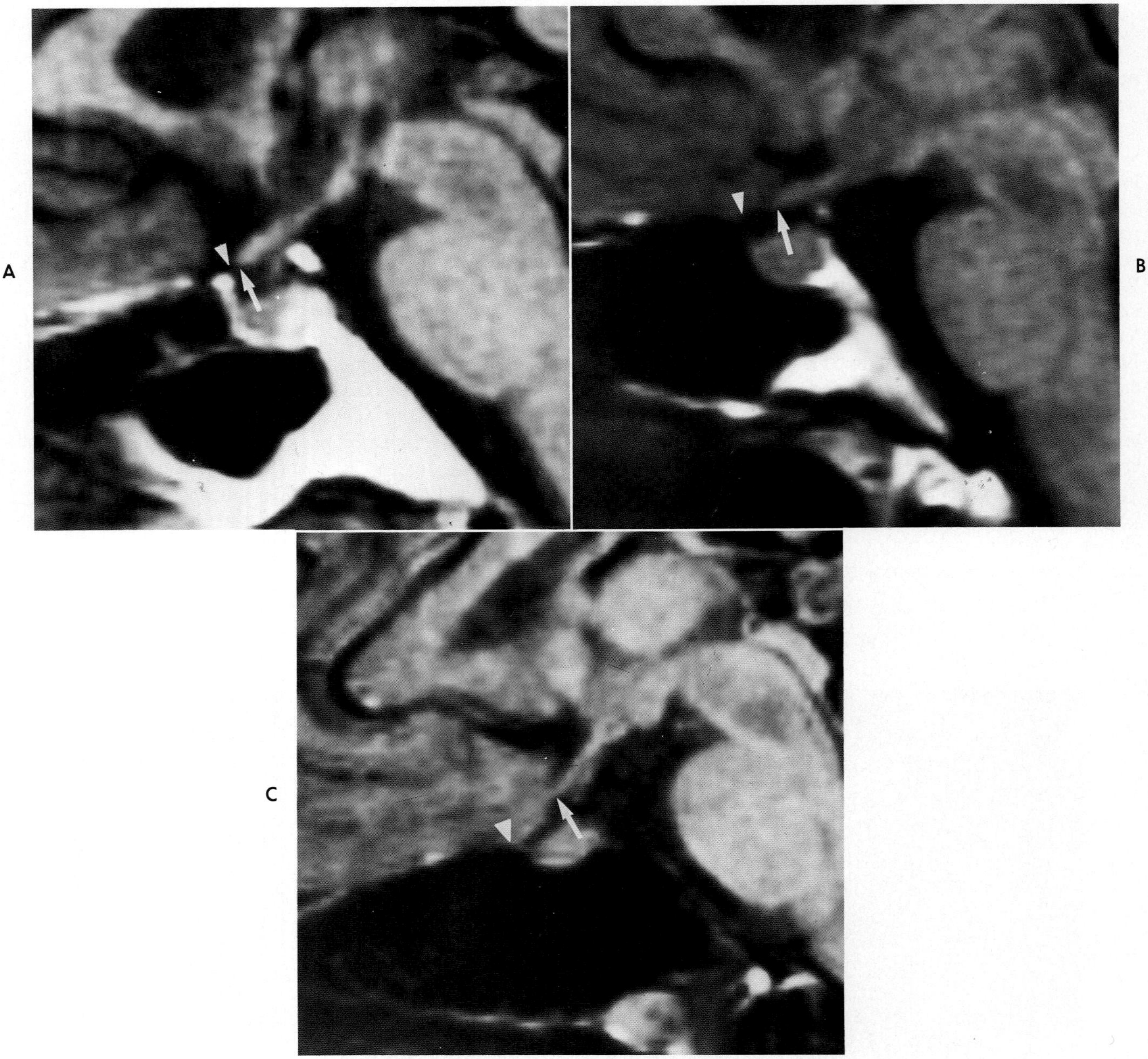

Figure 18-11 Midline sagittal MR images (TR/TE, 600/20) show the relationship between the tuberculum sellae (*arrowhead*) and the anterior border of the optic chiasm (*arrow*) when the chiasm is in a prefixed **(A)**, central **(B)**, or postfixed **(C)** position. (Reproduced with permission from Doyle AJ: AJNR 11:553-555, 1990.)

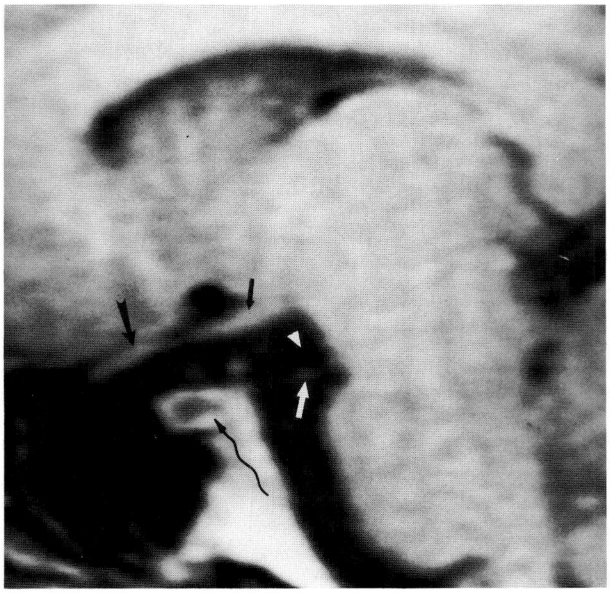

Figure 18-12 Parasagittal MR image (TR/TE, 600/20) shows the optic nerve (*large black arrow*), optic tract (*small black arrow*), third nerve (*small white arrow*), and the signal void of the posterior communicating artery (*white arrowhead*) just above the third cranial nerve. Low signal intensity in the pituitary fossa (*wavy arrow*) is caused by partial-volume averaging from the adjacent carotid artery. (From Latchaw RE: MR *and* CT *imaging of the head, neck, and spine,* ed 2, vol 2, St Louis, 1991, Mosby–Year Book.)

REFERENCES

1. David PC, Hoffman JC Jr, Spencer T, et al: MR imaging of pituitary adenoma: CT, clinical, and surgical correlation, *AJNR* 8:107-112, 1987.
2. Kulkarni MV, Lee KF, McArdle CB, et al: 1.5-T MR imaging of pituitary microadenomas: technical considerations and CT correlation, *AJNR* 9:5-11, 1988.
3. Sakamoto Y, Takahashi M, Korogi Y, et al: Normal and abnormal pituitary glands: gadopentetate dimeglumine–enhanced MR imaging, *Radiology* 178:441-445, 1991.
4. Rhoton AL, Harris FS, Renn WH: Microsurgical anatomy of the sellar region and cavernous sinus, *Clin Neurosurg* 24:54-85, 1971.
5. Johnson DM, Hopkins RJ, Hanafee WN, et al: The unprotected parasphenoidal carotid artery studied by high-resolution computed tomography, *Radiology* 155:137-141, 1985.
6. Renn WH, Rhoton AL: Microsurgical anatomy of the sellar region, *J Neurosurg* 43:288-298, 1975.
7. Dolinskas CA, Simeone FA: Transsphenoidal hypophysectomy: postsurgical CT findings, *AJNR* 6:45-50, 1985.
8. Carin M, Bergstrom K, Grimelius L, et al: A parallel study of the roentgen anatomy of the sella turcica and the histopathology of the pituitary gland in 205 autopsy specimens, *Neuroradiology* 21:55-65, 1981.
9. Dubois PJ, Orr DP, Hoy RJ, et al: Normal sellar variations in frontal tomograms, *Radiology* 131:105-110, 1979.
10. Hirsch WL, Hryshko FG, Sekhar LN, et al: Comparison of MR imaging, CT, and angiography in the evaluation of the enlarged cavernous sinus, *AJNR* 9:907-915, 1988.
11. Taptas JN: The so-called cavernous sinus: a review of the controversy and its implications for neurosurgeons, *Neurosurgery* 11:712-717, 1982.
12. Daniels DL, Pojunas KW, Kilgore DP, et al: MR of the diaphragma sellae, *AJNR* 7:765-769, 1986.
13. Sage MR, Blumbergs PC, Mulligan BP, et al: The diaphragma sellae: its relationship to the configuration of the pituitary gland, *Radiology* 145:703-708, 1982.
14. Bedford MA: The cavernous sinus, *Br J Ophthalmol* 50:41-46, 1966.
15. Parkinson D, West M: Lesions of the cavernous plexus region. In Youmans JR, editor: *Neurological surgery,* ed 2, Philadelphia, 1982, WB Saunders.
16. Parkinson D: Surgical anatomy of the cavernous sinus. In Wilkins RH, Rengachary SS, editors: *Neurosurgery,* New York, 1984, McGraw-Hill.
17. Kaplan HA, Browder J, Krieger AJ: Intracavernous connections of the cavernous sinuses, *J Neurosurg* 45:166-168, 1976.
18. Daniels DL, Pech P, Mark L, et al: Magnetic resonance imaging of the cavernous sinus, *AJNR* 6:187-192, 1985.
19. Daniels D, Czervionke LF, Bonneville JF, et al: MR imaging of the cavernous sinus: value of spin echo and gradient recalled echo images, *AJNR* 9:947-952, 1988.
20. Scotti G, Yu CY, Dillon WP, et al: MR imaging of cavernous sinus involvement by pituitary adenomas, *AJNR* 9:657-664, 1988.
21. Sekhar LN, Burgess J, Akin O: An anatomical study of the cavernous sinus emphasizing operative approaches and the related vascular and neural reconstruction, *Neurosurgery* 21:806-816, 1987.
22. Tshuha M, Aoki H, Okamura T: Roentgenological investigation of cavernous sinus structure with special reference to paracavernous cranial nerves, *Neuroradiology* 29:462-467, 1987.
23. Sekhar LN, Moller AR: Operative management of tumors involving the cavernous sinus, *J Neurosurg* 64:879-889, 1986.
24. Umansky F, Nathan H: The lateral wall of the cavernous sinus, *J Neurosurg* 56:228-234, 1982.
25. Moore T, Ganti SR, Mawad M, et al: CT and angiography of primary extradural juxtasellar tumors, *AJNR* 145:491-496, 1985.
26. Patterson RH: Subfrontal approach to the pituitary gland. In Wilkins RH, Rengachary SS, editors: *Neurosurgery,* New York, 1984, McGraw-Hill.
27. Doyle AJ: Optic chiasm position on MR images, *AJNR* 11:553-555, 1990.
28. Kaufman B, Tomsak RL, Kaufman BA, et al: Herniation of the suprasellar visual system and third ventricle into empty sellae: morphologic and clinical considerations, *AJNR* 10:65-76, 1989.

Index

*This index does not include illustrations for Chapters 1, 3, 6, 9, 11, and 13. Illustration indexes appear at the end of each of these chapters.

D

E

F

T

U

V

W

X

Z

Animal Models of
MOVEMENT DISORDERS

Animal Models of MOVEMENT DISORDERS

Edited by

Mark LeDoux

ELSEVIER
ACADEMIC
PRESS

AMSTERDAM • BOSTON • HEIDELBERG • LONDON
NEW YORK • OXFORD • PARIS • SAN DIEGO
SAN FRANCISCO • SINGAPORE • SYDNEY • TOKYO

Elsevier Academic Press
30 Corporate Drive, Suite 400, Burlington, MA 01803, USA
525 B Street, Suite 1900, San Diego, California 92101-4495, USA
84 Theobald's Road, London WC1X 8RR, UK

This book is printed on acid-free paper. ∞

Library of Congress Cataloging-in-Publication Data
APPLICATION SUBMITTED

British Library Cataloguing in Publication Data
A catalogue record for this book is available from the British Library

ISBN: 0-12-088382-1

DVD-ROM ISBN: 0-12-088383-4

For all information on all Elsevier Academic Press publications
visit our Web site at www.books.elsevier.com

Printed in the United States of America
04 05 06 07 08 09 9 8 7 6 5 4 3 2 1

Table of Contents

Preface

Scientists generate animal models in order to answer hypothesis-driven questions regarding biochemical, cellular and neural networks potentially involved in the pathophysiology of movement disorders. Researchers may also study spontaneous mutants exhibiting motor aberrations to identify novel genes or reach a better understanding of motor systems by pinpointing sites of functional abnormality within neural tissue. Both are included in the pages that follow. Therefore, a more fitting title for this book could have been "Animal Models of Movement Disorders AND Spontaneous Mutants with Motor Dysfunction."

Although not quite encyclopedic, this text explores nearly all human movement disorders and many animals relevant to their understanding. A genuine effort was made to integrate clinical delineation of disease phenotypes with investigations of non-human animals. Most scientists have recognized that animals are essential for unraveling complex neural disease mechanisms. Accordingly, new models appear almost weekly in major neuroscience journals. More specifically, interest in animal models of movement disorders is growing at an exponential rate. Thus, the time has come to review past accomplishments and gather directives for the future.

In line with Online Mendelian Inheritance in Man (OMIM™) and recommendations from The Council of Biology Editors, this book uses the non-possessive forms of eponymic terms. The first section provides conceptual, clinical and technical foundations for the subsequent sections on individual movement disorders. In general, "clinical" chapters precede chapters dealing with animal models. A central feature of this production is the accompanying DVD that contains an extraordinary collection of human and animal videos pertinent to the study of movement disorders and motor systems.

Deepest gratitude goes to our patients for allowing us to video their movements, analyze their deoxyribonucleic acid and measure their responses to a variety of treatments. Patients provide an inspiration at the bench and are the ultimate benefactors of good science. Patients also remind us that motor dysfunction rarely occurs in isolation and movement disorders cannot be successfully treated with unitary goals in mind.

Many thanks go to the outstanding roster of contributing authors. Despite hectic lives filled with writing grants, managing laboratories, reviewing manuscripts and caring for patients, these leaders in neuroscience were able to find the time and energy required to generate marvelous additions to the movement disorders literature. Their work should not go unnoticed.

The Elsevier team played a fundamental role in the success of this undertaking. The Publishing Editor, Hilary Rowe, got the ball rolling and kept the project on schedule. Erin LaBonte-McKay showed amazing fortitude and persistence throughout. Daniel Stone and Cindy Ahlheim performed unfailingly in the production phases of the text and DVD, respectively.

Special thanks go to Rita, Natalie and Christian for their patience with my various scientific adventures.

List of Contributors

Tetsuo Ashizawa, Department of Neurology, John Sealy Chair of Neurology, The University of Texas Medical Branch (UTMB), Galveston, TX

P.C. Baier, Department of Clinical Neurophysiology, Georg-August University Gottingen, Gottingen, Germany

Lore Becker, Institut für Diabetesforschung, Munich

David J. Bennett, Professor, Division of Neuroscience, University of Alberta, Edmonton, Alberta, Canada

Brett Berke, Department of Biological Sciences, University of Iowa, Iowa City, IA

Ranjita Betarbet, Center for Neurodegenerative Disease, Emory University, Atlanta, GA

Kailash P. Bhatia, Senior Lecturer and Consultant Neurologist, Sobell Department of Motor Neuroscience and Movement Disorders, Institute of Neurology, UCL, National Hospital for Neurology and Neurosurgery, Queen Square, London, UK

Francesco Bibbiani, NINDS, NIH, Bethesda, MD

David T. Blake, Keck Center for Neuroscience, University of California San Francisco, San Francisco, CA

David R. Borchelt, Department of Pathology, Johns Hopkins School of Medicine, Baltimore, MD

Prodip Bose, Department of Neuroscience, University of Florida Health Science Center, Gainsville, FL

D. Cristopher Bragg, Department of Neurology, Harvard Medical School, Massachusetts General Hospital, Boston, MA

Allison Brashear, Department of Neurology, Indiana University School of Medicine, Indianapolis, IN

Xandra O. Breakefield, Department of Neurology, Harvard Medical School, Massachusetts General Hospital, Boston, MA

Susan Bressman, Albert Einstein College of Medicine, Phillips Ambulatory Care Center, Beth Israel Medical Center, New York, NY

Kathleen Burke, School of Medicine, Child Study Center, Yale University, New Haven, CT

Nancy N. Byl, Department of Physical Therapy, University fo California San Francisco, Graduate Program, San Francisco, CA

Guy A. Caldwell, Department of Biological Sciences, The University of Alabama, Tuscaloosa, AL

Kim A. Caldwell, Biological Sciences, The University of Alabama, Tuscaloosa, AL

Songsong Cao, Biological Sciences, The University of Alabama, Tuscaloosa, AL

M. Angela Cenci, Department of Physiological Sciences, Section of Basal Ganglia Pathophysiology, Lund University, Lund, Sweden

Marie-Françoise Chesselet, Department of Neurology, University of California Los Angeles, Los Angeles, CA

Carlo Colosimo, Viale dell'Universita', Rome, Italy

Mai Dang, Department of Molecular and Integrative Physiology, Beckman Institute for Advanced Science and Technology, University of Illinois at Urbana-Champaign, Urbana, IL

Julie A. Dennis, Elizabeth Macarthur Agricultural Institute, Camden, NSW Australia

Didier Devys, Department of Molecular Pathology, Institut de Génétique et de Biologie Moléculaire et Cellulaire, Illkirch Cedex, CU de Strasbourg, France

Paula Dietrich, Department of Physiology, University of Tennessee Health Science Center, Memphis, TN

Ioannis Dragatsis, Assistant Professor, Department of Physiology, University of Tennessee Health Science Center, Memphis, TN

Ian D'Souza, Department of Medicine, Division of Gerontology and Geriatric Medicine, University of Washington School of Medicine, Seattle, WA

Rodger J. Elble, Department of Neurology, Southern Illinois University School of Medicine, Springfield, IL

Craig Evinger, Departments of Neurobiology and Behavior and Ophthalmology, State University of New York–Stony Brook, Stony Brook, NY

Pierre-Olivier Fernagut, UCLA Department of Neurology, Reed Neurological Research Center, Los Angeles, CA

Hubert H. Fernandez, Department of Clinical Neurosciences, Division of Parkinson's Disease and Movement Disorders, Brown University, Providence, RI

John K. Fink, Department of Neurology, University of Michigan; and Geriatric Research Education and Clinical Center, Ann Arbor Veterans Affairs Medical Center, Ann Arbor, MI

Sheila M. Fleming, Department of Neurology, University of California Los Angeles, CA

Colin F. Fletcher, The Genomics Institute, Novartis Research Foundation, San Diego, CA

Lyle Fox, Department of Biological Sciences, University of Iowa, Iowa City, IA

Stephen C. Fowler, Department of Pharmacology & Toxicology, University of Kansas, Lawrence, KS

Joseph H. Friedman, Department of Clinical Neurosciences, Division of Parkinson's Disease and Movement Disorders, Brown University, Providence, RI

Felix Geser, Department of Neurology, University Hospital, Innsbruck, Austria

Imad Ghorayeb, UMR-CNRS, Bordeaux Cedex, France

Monica Gorassini, Center for Neuroscience, University of Alberta, Edmonton, Alberta, Canada

J. Timothy Greenamyre, Center for Neurodegenerative Disease, Emory University, Atlanta, GA

Philip J. Harvey, Center for Neuroscience, University of Alberta, Edmonton, Alberta, Canada

Simon J. R. Heales, Neurometabolic Unit, National Hospital & Division of Neurochemistry, Institute of Neurology (UCL), Queen Square, London, UK

Peter J. Healy, "The Laurels," Braidwood, New South Wales, Australia

Dominique Helmlinger, Department of Molecular Pathology, Institut de Génétique et de Biologie Moléculaire et Cellulaire, Illkirch Cedex, CU de Strasbourg, France

Ellen J. Hess, Departments of Neurology and Neuroscience, Johns Hopkins University School of Medicine, Baltimore, MD

Ralph Hillman, Department of Biology, Temple University, Philadelphia, PA

Gregg E. Homanics, Departments of Anesthesiology and Pharmacology, University of Pittsburgh School of Medicine, Pittsburgh, PA

Keith Hyland, Horizon Molecular Medicine, Atlanta, GA

Iyare Izevbaye, Biological Sciences, The University of Alabama, Tuscaloosa, AL

Vernice Jackson-Lewis, Department of Neurology, Columbia University, New York, NY

H. A. Jinnah, Department of Neurology, Johns Hopkins Hospital, Baltimore, MD

Anita J. Jurkowski, Center for Aging and Human Development, Brain Imaging and Analysis Center, Psychological and Brain Sciences, Duke University Medical Center, Duke University, Durham, NC

Iris S. Kassem, Department of Neurobiology and Behavior, State University of New York–Stony Brook, Stony Brook, NY

Michael D. Kaytor, Department of Laboratory Medicine and Pathology, and Institute of Human Genetics, University of Minnesota, Minneapolis, MN

Jason E. Kralic, Departments of Pharmacology and Psychiatry and Bowles Center for Alcohol Studies, University of North Carolina at Chapel Hill, Chapel Hill, NC

Mark LeDoux, Departments of Neurology and Anatomy & Neurobiology, Division of Movement Disorders, University of Tennessee Health Science Center, Memphis, TN

Jada Lewis, Department of Neuroscience, Mayo Clinic Jacksonville, Jacksonville, FL

Yuqing Li, Department of Molecular and Integrative Physiology, Beckman Institute for Advanced Science and Technology, University of Illinois at Urbana-Champaign, Urbana, IL

David Lieberman, Department of Neurology, Johns Hopkins Hospital, Baltimore, MD

Gary S. Linn, Department of Psychiatry, New York University School of Medicine, New York; and Program in Cognitive Neuroscience and Schizophrenia, Nathan S. Kline Institute for Psychiatric Research, Orangeburg, NY

Irene Litvan, Department of Neurology, Raymond Lee Lebby Professor of Parkinson Disease Research, University of Louisville School of Medicine, Louisville, KY

Paul J. Lombroso, School of Medicine, Child Study Center, Yale University, New Haven, CT

Elan D. Louis, Assistant Professor of Neurology, College of Physicians and Surgeons, Columbia University, New York, NY

Martin Lundblad, Department of Physiological Sciences, Section of Basal Ganglia Pathophysiology, Lund University, Lund, Sweden

J. Lawrence Marsh, Developmental Biology Center, Developmental and Cell Biology, University of California–Irvine, Irvine, CA

Eileen McGowan, Department of Neuroscience, Mayo Clinic Jacksonville, Jacksonville, FL

T. L. McKerchar, Department of Human Development, University of Kansas, Lawrence, KS

Michael Merzenich, Keck Center for Neuroscience, UC San Francisco, San Francisco, CA

A. Leslie Morrow, Departments of Pharmacology and Psychiatry and Bowles Center for Alcohol Studies, University of North Carolina at Chapel Hill, Chapel Hill, NC

Robert Naquet, CNRS Institut Alfred Fessard, Gif sur Yvette, Cedex

Richard Nass, Department of Anesthesiology, Center for Molecular Neuroscience, Vanderbilt University Medical Center, Nashville, TN

Parvoneh Poorkaj Navas, Department of Psychiatry and Behavioral Sciences; and Department of Medicine, Division of Medical Genetics, University of Washington, Seattle, WA

Todd K. O'Buckley, Departments of Pharmacology and Psychiatry and Bowles Center for Alcohol Studies, University of North Carolina at Chapel Hill, Chapel Hill, NC

Justin D. Oh, Psychology Department, Central Michigan University, Mount Pleasant, MI

Chihiro Ohye, Functional and Gamma Knife Surgery Center, Hidaka Hospital, Takasaki, Gunma, Japan

Harry T. Orr, Department of Laboratory Medicine and Pathology; and Institute of Human Genetics, University of Minnesota, Minneapolis, MN

Jessica L. Osterman, Departments of Pharmacology and Psychiatry and Bowles Center for Alcohol Studies, University of North Carolina at Chapel Hill, Chapel Hill, NC

Leo J. Pallanck, School of Medicine, Washington University, Seattle, WA

Massimo Pandolfo, Chef de Service, Service de Neurologie, Université Libre de Bruxelles—Hôpital Erasme Brussels, Belgium

Robert G. Pendleton, Department of Biology, Temple University, Philadelphia, PA

Haixiang Peng, Novartis Research Foundation, The Genomics Institute, San Diego, CA

I-Feng Peng, Department of Biological Sciences, University of Iowa, Iowa City, IA

Dianne M. Perez, Department of Molecular Cardiology, The Cleveland Clinic, Cleveland, OH

Susan L. Perlman, Department of Neurology, David Geffen School of Medicine at UCLA, Los Angeles, CA

Joel S. Perlmutter, Departments of Neurology, Radiology, Neurobiology and Physical Therapy, Washington University School of Medicine, St. Lous, MO

Jeremy Petravicz, Department of Neurology, Harvard Medical School, Massachusetts General Hospital, Boston, MA

Ronald F. Pfeiffer, Department of Neurology, University of Tennessee Health Science Center, Memphis, TN

James O. Phillips, Department of Otolaryngology, National Primate Research Center, University of Washington; and Division of Ophthalmology, Department of Surgery, Children's Hospital and Regional Medical Center, Seattle, WA

Michael R. Pranzatelli, Departments of Neurology and Pediatrics, National Pediatric Myoclonus Center, Southern Illinois School of Medicine, Springfield, IL

Stefan-M. Pulst, Departments of Medicine and Neurobiology, UCLA, Cedars-Sinai Medical Center, Los Angeles, CA

Shirley Rainier, Department of Neurology, University of Michigan, Ann Arbor, MI

Jayaraman Rao, Department of Neurology and Neurosciences, Carl Baldridge Chair for Parkinson's Research, Louisiana State University School of Medicine, New Orleans, LA

Angelika Richter, Department of Pharmacology & Toxicology, School of Veterinary Medicine, Hannover, Germany

Farrel R. Robinson, Department of Biological Structure, University of Washington, Seattle, WA

Christopher A. Ross, Department of Pathology, Johns Hopkins Medical Institute, Baltimore, MD

Perminder S. Sachdev, School of Psychiatry, University of New South Wales & Neuropsychiatric Institute, The Prince of Wales Hospital, Sydney, NSW

Rachel Saunders-Pullman, Albert Einstein College of Medicine, Neurology, Beth Israel Medical Center, New York, NY

Gerard D. Schellenberg, Division of Neurogenetics, Department of Neurology, University of Washington, Seattle, WA

Gabriele Schilling, Department of Pathology, Johns Hopkins Medical Institute, Baltimore, MD

Peter R. Schofield, Garvan Institute of Medical Research, Sydney, New South Wales, Australia

Nutan Sharma, Department of Neurology, Harvard Medical School, Massachusetts General Hospital, Boston, MA

Todd B. Sherer, Center for Neurodegenerative Disease, Emory University, Atlanta, GA

Carmen Silva-Barrat, Laboratory de Biologie du Vieillissement, Unité d'Explorations Fonctionnelles, Ivry sur Seine Cedex, France

Harvey S. Singer, Department of Neurology, Johns Hopkins Hospital, Baltimore, MD

Richard Jay Smeyne, Department of Developmental Neurobiology, Saint Jude Children's Research Hospital, Memphis, TN

Constance Smith-Hicks, Department of Neurology, Johns Hopkins Hospital, Baltimore, MD

Mark Stacy, Department of Medicine, Neurology, Duke University, Durham, NC

Nadia Stafanova, Department of Neurology, Medical University of Innsbruck, Innsbruck, Austria

David G. Standaert, Department of Neurology, Harvard Medical School, Massachusetts General Hospital, Boston, MA

S.H. Subramony, Department of Neurology, University of Mississippi Medical Center, Jackson, MS

Samer D. Tabbal, Department of Neurology, School of Medicine, Washington University, St. Louis, MO

Kwok-Keung Tai, The Parkinson's and Movement Disorder Institute, Long Beach, CA

Floyd J. Thompson, Department of Neuroscience, McKnight Brain Institute, University of Florida, Gainesville, FL

Leslie M. Thompson, Departments of Psychiatry and Human Behavior and Biological Chemistry, University of California–Irvine, Irvine, CA

François Tison, UMR-CNRS, Bordeaux Cedex

Claudia Trenkwalder, University of Göettingen, Medical Director, Paracelsus-Elena-Klinik, Center of Parkinsonism and Movement Disorders, Kassel, Germany

Daniel D. Truong, The Parkinson's and Movement Disorder Institute, Fountain Valley, CA

Atsushi Ueda, Department of Biological Sciences, University of Iowa, Iowa City, IA

Suvi Vartiainen, Department of Neurobiology, Functional Genomics and Bioinformatics Laboratory, University of Kuopio, Kuopio

Hans Weiher, Institut fur Diabetesforschung, Munich, Germany

Avery H. Weiss, Division of Ophthalmology, Department of Surgery, Children's Hospital and Regional Medical Center, Seattle, WA

Gregor Karl Wenning, Department of Neurology, Medical University of Innsbruck, Innsbruck, Austria

Alexander J. Whitworth, Washington University, School of Medicine, Health Sciences J-113, Box 357730, Seattle, WA

Peter A. Windsor, University of Sydney, Camden, New South Wales, Australia

Garry Wong, Department of Neurobiology, Functional Genomics and Bioinformatics Laboratory, University of Kuopio, Kuopio

Chun-Fang Wu, Department of Biological Sciences, University of Iowa, Iowa City, IA

T. J. Zarcone, Schiefelbusch Institute for Life Span Studies, University of Kansas, Lawrence, KS

CHAPTER

A1

Classification and Clinical Features of Movement Disorders

ANITA J. JURKOWSKI and MARK STACY

The sensorimotor system is the primary means of interaction with the world. Incoming (sensory) information is processed in the nervous system, and in animals it may be measured by behavioral (usually motor) responses. Central to this merging of sensory and motor function are the structures of the basal ganglia: the substantia nigra, the caudate, putamen, globus pallidus, and subthalamic nucleus. Disturbances in the basal ganglia therefore lead to altered amplitude, rate, or content of movement, and may produce symptoms classified as a movement disorder. This chapter will review the functional architecture of the basal ganglia from a phylogenetic standpoint, and briefly review neuronal loops involved in cognitive, affective, and motor behaviors. In addition, this chapter will cover hypokinetic and hyperkinetic movement disorders with emphasis on etiology, historical and physical findings, pathogenesis, and treatment. Parkinson disease is the prototypical movement disorder associated with hypokinesia, or slowness of movement. The major hyperkinetic movement disorders are associated with excessive or increased involuntary movements and include the dyskinesias, tremors, dystonias, choreas, ballismus, myoclonus, stereotypies, and tic disorders.

The key to diagnosing and treating movement disorders is to recognize abnormal clinical phenomenology. Hypokinetic movement disorders are associated with slow movement and are also commonly termed the Parkinsonian disorders. The hypokinetic disorders include idiopathic Parkinson disease (PD), Parkinsonism plus syndromes (such as progressive supranuclear palsy), and secondary causes of Parkinsonism (e.g., drug-induced Parkinsonism or Parkinsonism from a concurrent central nervous system lesion). Hyperkinetic movement disorders are associated with increased involuntary movements including tremor, chorea, athetosis, ballism, dystonia, myoclonus, stereotypies, and tics. In several hereditary movement disorders such as Huntington disease, Wilson disease, and spinocerebellar ataxia (SCA), hypokinetic and hyperkinetic movements may appear at different stages of the disease process and, in some patients, may coexist.

Parkinsonism and several other movement disorders result, either in whole or part, from disordered sensorimotor processing in the basal ganglia, a collection of nuclei in the midbrain, diencephalon, and proximal telencephalon. Although specific anatomic locations cannot be linked to all movement disorders, abnormalities in some areas are associated with specific symptoms. While it is well accepted that Parkinson disease is associated with depigmentation of the substantia nigra, and hemiballismus is associated with lesions in or near the subthalamic nucleus, anatomic localization for other movement disorders is less clear. It is not surprising that progress in the understanding of etiologic, pathogenic, and potential therapies for these conditions are linked to well-defined animal models.

I. FUNCTIONAL NEUROANATOMY OF THE BASAL GANGLIA

Historically, the basal ganglia comprise the "extrapyramidal" pathway, a term coined by S.A.K. Wilson, to designate a motor system that is not pyramidal (corticospinal) or cerebellar. While lesions in the corticospinal pathway are associated with weakness, increased tone (spasticity), and pathologically increased reflexes, and cerebellar changes produce impaired coordination with decreased muscle tone, basal ganglia degeneration may exhibit a wide range of changes in muscle tone and additional alterations in the speed and amplitude of movement. The major nuclei designated as a part of the basal ganglia include the striatum (caudate and putamen), globus pallidus, subthalamic nucleus, and substantia nigra. Other cell populations are striatum-derived limbic structures such as nucleus accumbens, olfactory tubercle, and parts of the amygdala.

Although the basal ganglia were once thought to be exclusively involved in motor control, it is now accepted that the extrapyramidal system processes motor, sensory, emotional, and cognitive information through a series of topographically organized feed-forward loops from diverse cortical areas to basal ganglia and back again. Alexander and Crutcher (1990) demonstrated that in addition to motor control the basal ganglia process sensory, cognitive, and affective information that aid movement selection through five parallel closed loops (motor, oculomotor, dorsolateral prefrontal, lateral orbitofrontal, and limbic). Recent evolutionary evidence suggests that a series of open loops, once thought to be entirely segregated, allows integration of information across the closed loops in the selection of behavioral output (Joel and Weiner 1994). The open loops allow topographically organized areas of the striatum to influence other areas of the cortex that do not project to it through the closed loops. Thus, motivational information from the medial frontal cortex and sensory information from the parietal cortex can exert an effect on storage information in the dorsolateral prefrontal cortex.

The striatum receives a number of inputs from various parts of the central nervous system. The major striatal input arises from cell layer V of the cerebral cortex. These corticostriatal projections release the excitatory neurotransmitter glutamate. The second major striatal input arises from the dopamine-containing neurons in the pars compacta of the substantia nigra (SNpc). Serotonergic fibers from the raphe nuclei in the brainstem also project to the striatum. The most important receptive nuclei for these afferent pathways are the caudate and putamen. These striatal nuclei are primarily involved with convergence and integration of the various inputs, and besides gaiting motor behavior, may also play a role in depression and obsessive-compulsive disorder.

Neurons in the caudate and putamen include large "aspiny" acetylcholinergic interneurons, and medium-sized "spiny" gamma-aminobutyric-acid (GABA-ergic) output neurons. These output neurons also release the excitatory neuropeptides, substance P and enkephalin. There are two anatomically distinct areas within the striatum. The matrix comprises 80% of the striatum, and receives input from layers III and V of the cerebral cortex, and some thalamic nuclei. The striosomes represent the remaining 20% of these nuclei and receive dopaminergic information from the substantia nigra, and layer V of the cortex (Parent 1996). Both of these structures connect with the ventral lateral and ventral anterior nuclei of the thalamus. The ventral lateral nucleus projects to the motor cortex, while the ventral anterior nucleus provides axons to the premotor cortex. In addition, a direct loop connects the globus pallidus, the centromedian nucleus of the thalamus, and the putamen, and an indirect loop projects to the subthalamic nucleus (STN). The STN connects with both pallidal segments and with the substantia nigra by excitatory glutamatergic transmission, and is the output of the globus pallidus. In addition to its connections with the thalamic nuclei, the striatum provides feedback to the Substantia nigra pars reticulata (SNpr).

II. EVOLUTION (PHYLOGENY) OF THE BASAL GANGLIA

The basal ganglia circuitry appears to be remarkably similar across the phylogenetic spectrum (Reiner et al., 1998). From amphibians through mammals the division of direct and indirect motor control circuits, reciprocal striatopallidal projections, and descending midbrain efferents exists. The most preserved of all connections across these tetrapods are the SNpc and ventral tegmental dopaminergic projections to the striatum. This extensive change in the size of the basal ganglia reflects corresponding growth in modality-specific sensory thalamocortical circuits, prefrontal cortical executive functioning areas, and motor planning areas, in addition to the major corticostriatal circuits. Comparative anatomic studies identify an increase in basal ganglia cell number and expansion of the structures caudally and laterally in amphibians, perhaps reflecting a substrate change necessary to allow transition to primarily land-dwelling animals. Another change seen in comparative studies of reptiles and birds reflects a progression of basal ganglia output from the midbrain tectum in reptiles to the increasing output to the cortex in birds and mammals. In addition, the mammalian cortical output allows multimodal integration of information for a more diverse behavioral repertoire.

III. CLINICAL DIAGNOSIS OF MOVEMENT DISORDERS

Investigators gathering historical information from a clinical evaluation of movement disorders should gather data pertaining to age of onset, symptom progression, type of involuntary movement, aggravating factors, and relieving factors (e.g., anxiety, stress, sleep, alcohol, food, and medications). Almost all involuntary movements, except for segmental myoclonus, tics, and hemifacial spasm, disappear during sleep. In addition past medical history, recent travel history, family history, toxins/chemical exposure, and information regarding medications are important. Dopamine receptor-blocking drugs, such as traditional antipsychotic and antiemetic medications, are associated with Parkinsonism and tardive dyskinesia; other agents such as corticosteroids and medications for obstructive pulmonary disease are known to produce tremor.

Neurological examination should include assessment of language, memory, and other higher cortical functions. Frontal release signs such as Myerson's sign are seen commonly in Parkinson disease. Cranial nerve examination with special attention to extraocular movements (vertical saccades) is important, especially when differentiating Parkinson disease from progressive supranuclear palsy, or when searching for early signs of Huntington disease. Facial expression and speech pattern should be noted. Motor examination including muscle tone and power, sensory testing, and assessment of deep tendon and plantar reflexes is also important. Testing for rapid alternating movement, posture, and gait is necessary. In addition, emphasis on postures or movements that increase patient symptoms is helpful in defining particular syndromes (Stacy and Jankovic 1997).

IV. PARKINSON DISEASE

James Parkinson first described Parkinson disease (PD), a neurodegenerative disorder with an incidence range from 4.9 to 26 per 100,000 and prevalence of approximately 200 per 100,000, in 1817 in his monograph *Essay on the Shaking Palsy*. Parkinson termed the disease "paralysis agitans" and reported resting tremor, festinant gait, flexed posture, dysarthria, dysphagia, insomnia, and constipation as the hallmarks of the condition. Charcot subsequently used the term "Parkinson's disease," and differentiated the resting tremor of PD from the cerebellar outflow action tremor seen in multiple sclerosis. He also noted that tremor was not always present in all PD cases, and that cognitive decline may also be a part of the disease. In 1893 researchers discovered that the substantia nigra was abnormal in those afflicted with PD. Subsequent examinations of the brains of patients dying with idiopathic PD demonstrated depigmentation of the substantia nigra in the midbrain, associated with a loss of dopamine-producing cells (Duvoisin 1992).

In 1957, after demonstrating a reversal of the reserpine effects (depletion of central monoamines) in rabbits and mice, Carlsson reported that approximately 80% of all brain-derived dopamine was localized within the basal ganglia. Hornykiewicz and Birkmeyer and Barbeau independently reported therapeutic benefit from levodopa, and PD became the first disease treated by neurotransmitter replacement (Duvoisin 1992). In 1983 an effort led by Langston determined that a group of intravenous narcotic users developed a profound Parkinsonian syndrome after self-injecting 1-methyl-4-phenyl-1,2,26-tetrahydropyridine (MPTP), a meperidine analog (Ballard et al. 1985). The discovery of this compound led to the creation of animal models, and served as the observation leading to the Deprenyl and Tocopherol Antioxidant Therapy for Parkinson Disease (DATATOP) clinical trial, the initial study of the Parkinson Study Group.

A. Clinical Features of Parkinson Disease

The four cardinal signs of Parkinsonism include resting tremor, rigidity, bradykinesia, and postural instability. Tremor in PD usually occurs at rest, with the hand in a pronating-supinating ("pill-rolling") manner at approximately 4–7 Hertz frequency. The tremor in PD may also involve the chin, jaw, tongue, and legs. In addition, symptoms of PD usually present unilaterally, and will almost always maintain some asymmetry in severity of symptoms. [Video Segment 1]

Rigidity is an increase of muscle tone in which steady resistance occurs against passive movements. If the patient has tremor, a ratcheting or cogwheeling may also be noticed. Rigidity may be increased by asking the patient to perform a voluntary act in another part of the body contralateral to the limb being assessed; for example, closing and opening a contralateral fist while passively rotating the patient's wrist. Bradykinesia (slowness of movement) or hypokinesia (poverty of movement) are central to PD symptomatology. On examination, the patient may exhibit slowness with decreased amplitude in rapid succession movements when performing finger tapping, hand clasping, wrist pronation-supination, and heel tapping. In the advanced disease, the patient shows early and frequent arrests of movement while performing these tasks. Postural instability or loss of postural reflexes often occurs in moderate to severe cases of PD and is characterized by propulsion or retropulsion and a tendency to fall. A clinician can test for these responses by pulling the patient backward while he or she stands with feet together (i.e., the Pull Test).

Most of the other signs in PD are manifestations of these cardinal characteristics either alone or in combination: lack of facial expression (hypomimia), drooling, hypophonia, dysarthria, dysphagia, lack of associated movement such as arm-swing when walking, micrographia, shuffling gait, difficulty standing and turning when walking, difficulty turning in bed, start hesitation, and freezing and festination of gait. Besides motor symptoms, PD patients often develop depression, passive attitude, and dementia (Stacy 1999). Sensory symptoms such as pain, burning, coldness, or numbness are reported by about half of PD patients.

B. Pathogenesis of Parkinson Disease

Pathogenesis of PD remains unclear. The cause of this disease may be a complex interaction between genetic and largely unidentified environmental factors. Most cases of PD are sporadic but mutations may be found in rare, familial cases of PD. Both sporadic and familial cases may have a final common pathway of abnormal protein handling in the ubiquitin-proteosome system, and impairment of the host's defense to inflammation and oxidative stress, which subsequently leads to neuronal cell death in the SNpc. Among familial forms of PD, parkin gene mutation is the most common (Sathornsumetee and Stacy in press).

Lewy bodies, the pathognomonic feature of PD, are eosinophilic neuronal inclusions, most often found in the SNpc, but also present in the basal ganglia, cerebral cortex, and spinal cord. Lewy bodies consist of α-synuclein and other proteins, such as tau (microtubule-associated protein seen in neurofibrillary tangles) and synphilin-1. Lewy body formation may represent an epiphenomenon, a direct neuronal toxicity from the protein aggregates, or it may result from impaired cellular segregation of cytotoxic proteins.

C. Pharmacological Treatment of Parkinson Disease

Pharmacological therapies in PD may be classified into two main categories: presynaptic strategy (levodopa/carbidopa, catechol *O*-methyltransferase [COMT]-inhibitors, selegiline, and amantadine) attempts to maintain physiological nigrostriatal synaptic concentrations of dopamine, and post-synaptic strategy (pergolide, bromocriptine, pramipexole, ropinirole, cabergoline, and apomorphine) bypasses degenerating nigrostriatal neurons by stimulating striatal neurons directly. In addition anticholinergics may help modify acetylcholine neurotransmission, which counteracts the dopaminergic transmission system (Stacy 2000a).

Levodopa, a dopamine precursor, is converted to dopamine by the enzyme dopa-decarboxylase. Ingestion and bloodstream metabolism of levodopa to dopamine leads to activation of the area postrema, potentially causing nausea and even vomiting. Carbidopa or benserazide, dopa-decarboxylase inhibitors, do not cross the blood-brain barrier and when given with levodopa, block the conversion of dopa to dopamine, limiting these peripheral side effects. Frequently, patients with PD will notice "wearing-off" or end-of-dose deterioration in mobility, thought to result from the reduced clinical effectiveness of levodopa over short periods. A typical patient may also notice dyskinesias or involuntary movements related to peak plasma levodopa levels ("peak-dose dyskinesia"). [Video Segment 2] Treatment of these motor fluctuations is based on smoothing out the plasma concentration curves of levodopa or by the addition of COMT-inhibitors. Amantadine is an antiviral medication with anticholinergic efficacy and may increase dopamine release, block dopamine reuptake, and stimulate dopamine receptors. Selegiline, a monoamine oxidase (MAO)-B inhibitor, is reported to delay the need for levodopa use and perhaps delay the progression of PD. A long-term follow-up analysis of levodopa-treated patients reported less symptomatic progression, but more dyskinesias in subjects not randomized to selegiline (Parkinson Study Group 1996).

Dopamine agonists (DA), including apomorphine, bromocriptine, pergolide, pramipexole, and ropinirole, were effectively demonstrated as monotherapy and in combination with levodopa. Clinical studies using single photon emission computed tomography (SPECT) and positron emission tomography (PET) scanning to measure changes in radioactive tracers in PD patients randomized to DA versus levodopa consistently reported reduced loss of striatal dopamine in the DA-treated group when compared to the levodopa-treated group. However, criticism of these studies concerns the differential metabolic changes induced by DA versus levodopa on the regulation of the dopamine transporter, the concomitant use of other agents such as selegiline in some trials, and the non-randomized use of supplemental levodopa (Stacy 2003).

D. Surgical Treatment of Parkinson Disease

Surgical treatments for PD consist of ablative procedures (thalamotomy, pallidotomy, and subthalamotomy) and deep brain stimulation (DBS) in the thalamus, globus pallidus interna (GPi) and subthalamic nucleus (STN). Because the DBS procedure appears to be safer, and appears to have more long-term benefits, this approach is recommended more often than the ablative surgery (Krack et al. 2003). [Video Segment 3]

E. Differential Diagnosis

Approximately 12% of patients referred to movement disorder clinics in tertiary care medical centers with a diagnosis of PD actually have Parkinsonism-Plus syndromes. These idiopathic disorders share similarities with PD, but exhibit additional ophthalmic, motor, autonomic, or cognitive abnormalities. Other conditions that lead to misdiagnosis include drug-induced Parkinsonism, and hereditary neurodegenerative conditions (Huntington disease, Wilson disease, pantothenate kinase-associated neurodegeneration (i.e., Hallervorden-Spatz disease), olivopontocerebellar and spinocerebellar atrophies, familial basal ganglia calcification, familial Parkinsonism with peripheral neuropathy, and neuroacanthocytosis (Stacy and Jankovic 1992b).

Two PD-Plus syndromes are associated with increased axial or appendicular tone and with profound bradykinesia. Progressive supranuclear palsy (PSP) is associated with bradykinesia, rigidity, dysarthria, and dysphagia, and also exhibits more pronounced postural instability, axial rigidity, spastic speech, and dementia. The primary means of distinguishing PSP from PD is the development of vertical ocular gaze paresis, impaired convergence, and the appearance of staring due to upper lid retraction (Stacy 2002b). [Video Segment 4]

A similar disorder, cortico-basal ganglionic degeneration (CBGD), recently debated as a variant of the same pathophysiology of PSP, is associated with marked asymmetry in symptoms. At its most dramatic presentation, a CBGD patient claims to no longer be able to willfully control movement in an affected limb ("alien limb" phenomenon). [Video Segment 5] In each of these disorders, resting tremor is most often not present and patients usually do not respond to anti-Parkinsonian therapies. Primary cognitive changes are present and affected by the associated visual disturbances: changes often manifest as visual attention and scanning impairments. Depression and dementia are more prominent as the disease progresses, including agitation, irritability, apathy, and extreme emotional lability (Gibb et al. 1989).

Multiple system atrophy (MSA) exhibits symptoms overlapping with PD such as postural instability, bradykinesia, and muscular rigidity, but additional symptoms include orthostatic hypotension, thermoregulatory disturbances, and urinary and sexual dysfunction. Three categories of MSA disorders are characterized by the predominant symptomatology because this disorder involves multiple systems. Shy-Drager manifests as a predominant autonomic dysfunction with primary changes in blood pressure, pulse rate, sweating, intestinal motility, bladder, and sexual function (Stacy and Jankovic 1992b). Olivopontocerebellar atrophy manifests as a predominant cerebellar ataxia disorder with primary changes in muscle coordination and tremor. Symptoms affect gait, stance, and limbs causing balance problems, erectile dysfunction, and palsy of the vocal cord region, resulting in impaired articulation and swallowing. Striatonigral degeneration manifests as prominent pyramidal symptomatology with severely impaired speech, swallowing, and balance. In MSA, Parkinsonian medications, particularly dopaminergic therapy with levodopa and/or dopamine agonists, can be effective in the short term, but often are poorly tolerated in more advanced stages of the disease. [Video Segment 6]

V. ESSENTIAL TREMOR

A. Clinical Features of Essential Tremor

Essential tremor (ET) has prominent action/kinetic tremor, characteristically present when the patient maintains a position (postural tremor). The tremor in ET is typically a flexion-extension movement, whereas supination-pronation oscillation is more characteristic of Parkinson disease. ET is of a faster frequency (6–12 Hz) than PD tremor (4–7 Hz) and, when fully developed, usually involves the head, neck, jaw, tongue, and voice (Louis 2001). Furthermore, ET patients do not have Parkinsonian features such as hypomimia, shuffling gait, lack of arm swing or rigidity; although mild cogwheeling may be present. Action or postural tremor often interferes with handwriting, holding a spoon, using a drinking cup, and manipulating utensils and tools. The tremor is exacerbated during voluntary movement, emotional and physical stress, and diminishes with rest or ethyl alcohol. ET should be differentiated from other action tremors such as the accentuated physiological tremor seen in anxiety, thyrotoxicosis, alcohol withdrawal, and drug-induced tremor (from agents such as bronchodilators [β2 agonists], various CNS stimulants, lithium, and sodium valproate). Cerebellar kinetic (intention) tremor is most apparent during a goal-directed limb movement and may be demonstrated by finger-to-nose and heel-to-shin maneuvers. [Video Segments 7–9]

B. Treatment of Essential Tremor

The mainstay treatments for ET are beta-blockers and primidone. Some patients have shown benefit with benzodiazepines, acetazolamide, gabapentin, and topiramate. In medically intractable cases, botulinum toxin injections, and occasionally surgical procedures, such as DBS in the ventral intermediate nucleus (VIM) of the thalamus, or thalamotomy, may produce remarkably gratifying benefits (Louis 2001; Connor 2002; Ondo et al. 2000; Brin et al. 2001; Schuurman et al. 2000).

VI. HUNTINGTON DISEASE AND OTHER CHOREIFORM DISORDERS

A. Clinical Features of Huntington Disease

The typical presentation of a patient with Huntington disease (HD) is gradual onset of chorea, dementia, and behavioral abnormalities in a young adult. HD is the most common inherited form of chorea and is transmitted in an autosomal dominant pattern caused by an expansion of unstable trinucleotide (CAG)/polyglutamine (polyG) repeats within the huntingtin gene on chromosome 4. Initially, the patient may develop facial twitching and grimacing, shoulder shrugging, finger twitching (piano-playing movements), slight trunk twisting, or an extra step or kick when walking. The typical age of onset is in the late thirties and early forties.

In the juvenile form of HD, patients may present with rigidity, bradykinesia, dystonic postures, ataxia, seizures, pyramidal tract dysfunction, and mental retardation instead of chorea. This akinetic-rigid form (Westphal variant) is seen most often during the first or second decade of life, and is associated with high numbers of CAG triplet repeats. Gene amplification has been demonstrated during spermatogenesis via an unknown mechanism (Illarioshkin et al. 1994; Mahant et al. 2003). [Video Segments 11–12]

In approximately 85% of HD patients, regardless of age, chorea is the predominant movement disorder, and in the remaining 10 to 15% of patients, the motor disorder is characterized by bradykinesia, rigidity, and resting tremor. These Parkinsonian features are typically found in the juvenile variant and in the advanced stages of HD. In the terminal stage of HD, dysarthria, dysphagia, and respiratory difficulties become the most disabling and life-threatening problems. As the disease progresses, patients experience memory difficulties, inability to concentrate, confusion, and forgetfulness. Depression is common and suicide is a frequent cause of death. Other psychiatric disturbances include paranoia, hallucinations, and other delusional and psychotic symptoms.

B. Pathogenesis of Huntington Disease

Pathologic changes in the brains of HD patients include generalized atrophy with neuronal degeneration in the cortex and severe loss of small interneurons in the corpus striatum. Marked atrophy of the caudate is the pathological hallmark of HD and can be detected in coronal sections of the affected brain on MRI or CT scans. In addition, huntingtin (polyG) nuclear inclusions and dystrophic neuritis are demonstrated (Bates et al. 2003).

C. Treatment of Huntington Disease

Clinicians individualize the treatment for HD to the needs of the patient, depending on the most prominent signs and symptoms. No known treatment prevents, halts, or cures the disorder, although several clinical trials of putative neuroprotective agents were carried out recently. Riluzole and ramecemide were shown to improve motor function. Studies of the potential neuroprotective benefit of minocycline (an apoptotic/caspase inhibitor) and creatine in early symptomatic HD are in progress (Huntington Study Group 2001).

D. Differential Diagnosis

Besides Huntington disease, other less common hereditary choreas include benign familial chorea, familial paroxysmal choreoathetosis, and neuroacanthocytosis. Other forms of hereditary neurodegeneration that share the same pathogenesis of polyG aggregation and may be confused with HD include dentatorubropallidoluysian atrophy (DRPLA) and spinocerebellar ataxia (SCA) types 1, 2, 3, 6, 7, and 17 (Stacy and Jankovic 1992).

If the patient lacks a family history for a choreic or psychiatric disorder, then the clinician should consider the following disorders: senile chorea, tardive dyskinesia, central nervous system (CNS) vasculitis, subdural hematoma, Wilson disease, pantothenate kinase-associated neurodegeneration, Sydenham chorea, antiphospholipid antibody syndrome, Creutzfeldt-Jakob disease, and various toxic and metabolic disorders. The specific toxins causing chorea include oral contraceptives, levodopa, CNS stimulants, neuroleptics, phenytoin, carbamazepine, ethosuximide, and other drugs. Metabolic-endocrine disorders associated with chorea include chorea gravidarum, thyrotoxicosis, hypoparathyroidism, hypernatremia, Addison disease, and chronic hepatocerebral degeneration, among others (Stacy and Jankovic 1992b).

VII. DYSTONIA

Dystonia, defined as a sustained, involuntary contraction of muscles producing an abnormal posture, may be generalized (legs plus other parts of the body), segmental (multifocal), focal, or unilateral. The adult onset torsion dystonias are usually sporadic and proximal in distribution (e.g., torticollis). Distal dystonia, often seen in children and adolescents, is commonly inherited and may progress to generalized dystonia. Cranial dystonia (e.g., Meige syndrome, blepharospasm, oromandibular dystonia), cervical dystonia (e.g., various combinations of rotational torticollis, anterocollis, and retrocollis), and focal task-specific dystonias (e.g., writer's cramp) represent useful terms for categorizing the location of these abnormal involuntary movements. Unilateral dystonia (i.e., hemidystonia) is usually associated with a structural lesion in the contralateral striatum, such as an infarction, porencephalic cyst, arteriovenous malformation, or posttraumatic encephalomalacia (Stacy 2003). [Video Segments 13–18]

A. Clinical Features of Dystonia

A clinician can make a diagnosis of primary dystonia only if no other neurologic dysfunction exists (e.g., cognitive, pyramidal, sensory, or cerebellar deficits), and only after eliminating secondary causes of dystonia. At the initial evaluation, the clinician should obtain data from the patient about age of onset, initial and subsequent areas of involvement, course and progression, family history of dystonia, tremor, or other movement disorders, possible birth injury, developmental milestones, exposure to neuroleptic medication, consanguinity, or Jewish ancestry. The clinical expression of primary dystonia is highly variable even within families, with some patients demonstrating severe problems and requiring extensive assistance with daily activities, while others exhibit only mild symptoms (e.g., writer's cramp).

B. Genetics of Dystonia

Although no consistent structural or biochemical abnormality associated with primary dystonia has been found, researchers have long recognized the importance of genetic etiology. DYT1 is perhaps the most common type of genetically determined generalized dystonia, with a single GAG deletion in the (TOR1A) gene encoding torsinA. It is inherited in an autosomal dominant pattern with 30 to 40% penetration and it accounts for approximately 90% of primary dystonia in Ashkenazi Jews. Bressman and colleagues (2002) performed genetic screening of 267 patients with primary dystonia and found that the clinical feature most highly correlated with carrier status of DYT1 GAG deletion in patients was onset of dystonia before age twenty-six. Several other types of adult onset primary dystonias were identified including an X-linked inherited DYT3, which is found only in the Philippines (Lubag disease). Lubag disease was assigned a gene locus of Xq13, while other autosomal dominant inherited DYT6, DYT7, and DYT13 dystonias are associated with gene mutations on chromosomes 8, 18, and 1, respectively (de Carvalo et al. 2002).

One type of inherited dystonia that deserves special emphasis is dopa-responsive dystonia (DRD), formerly designated as DYT5. It is an autosomal dominant, childhood-onset dystonia that is due to mutations in the gene for GTP cyclohydrolase I. This disorder is more common in girls (2.5:1), and is frequently associated with Parkinsonian features; therefore, it may be difficult to differentiate this condition from juvenile PD. Most patients report a dramatic improvement with levodopa. Maximum benefit occurs within several days of levodopa therapy, and when combined with a dopa-decarboxylase inhibitor (carbidopa), patients may be maintained on as little as 50 mg/day (Nygaard et al. 1991).

The myoclonus-dystonia syndrome is an autosomal dominant disorder that has genetic heterogeneity and is associated with mutations of genes on chromosomes 7, 9, 11, and 18. This syndrome is characterized by the early onset of dystonia or startle-insensitive myoclonus, normal lifespan, rare seizures, no cognitive disability, ataxia or other neurological deficits, and a dramatic response to alcohol.

C. Pathogenesis of Dystonia

The pathophysiology of dystonia is not well understood. Neurophysiological assessments reveal abnormal co-contraction of agonist and antagonist muscles with prolonged bursts and overflow to extraneous muscles. Spinal and brainstem reflex abnormalities, including reduced reciprocal inhibition and prolonged stretch reflexes, are often observed. Transcranial magnetic stimulation studies and neuronal recordings during stereotactic surgery for dystonia suggest that primary dystonia is associated with a functional disturbance of the basal ganglia, particularly in the striatal control of the globus pallidus (Vitek 2002). Researchers suggest that dystonic muscle contraction is associated with changes in rate and pattern for neuronal firing, somatosensory responsiveness, and perhaps hyper-synchronization of neuronal activity. These changes cause altered thalamic control of cortical motor planning and executive areas, and abnormal regulation of brainstem and spinal cord inhibitory interneuronal mechanisms.

D. Treatment of Dystonia

High-dose anticholinergic therapy was found to be effective in ameliorating dystonia, particularly in younger patients. Other agents such as baclofen, benzodiazepines, carbamazepine, and tetrabenazine are reported to benefit some dystonic patients (Adler and Kumar 2000; Jankovic and Orman 1988). In addition, all childhood onset dystonia patients deserve a trial of levodopa. Intramuscular injection of botulinum toxin is the most effective treatment for focal dystonia, and may be used in a limited setting for patients with generalized dystonia. Intrathecal baclofen provides symptomatic benefit only for some patients who fail on oral medications (Walker et al. 2000). DBS at the internal segment of globus pallidus is effective in primary dystonia (particularly DYT1 dystonia), the myoclonus-dystonia syndrome, and complex cervical dystonia (Vitek et al. 2004).

VIII. WILSON DISEASE

A. Clinical Features of Wilson Disease

Wilson disease (WD) is an autosomal recessive disorder of copper metabolism with usual onset in children and young adolescents. The characteristic features are facial and generalized dystonia, rigidity, postural instability, dysarthria, drooling, sardonic facial grin, seizures, cerebellar incoordination, tremor, behavioral changes, deterioration in school performance, and evidence of hepatic dysfunction. An adult patient may present with Parkinsonian features, choreoathetosis, and a violent postural ("wing-beating") tremor. The clinical hallmark of the disorder is a brownish-yellow ring at the corneal rim (Kayser-Fleischer ring), which is due to copper deposits in the cornea (Jankovic and Stacy 1998).

The diagnosis of Wilson disease still depends primarily on evaluating clinical and laboratory evidence of abnormal copper metabolism. Laboratory studies reveal decreased serum ceruloplasmin (less than 20 mg/dl) and increased 24-hour urinary copper excretion (more than 100 mg/ml). In WD patients with signs and symptoms only of hepatic dysfunction, liver biopsy may reveal hepatic copper concentration of more than 100 μg/gm of dry liver. Brain MRI may show signal abnormalities on proton density and T-2 weighted images in bilateral putamen and thalami.

B. Pathogenesis of Wilson Disease

Wilson disease is due to an inherited defect in copper excretion into the bile by the liver. Several mutations of ATP7B copper-transporting ATPase gene on chromosome 13 were discovered, indicating genetic heterogeneity of WD (Tanzi et al. 1993). Researchers postulate that most symptoms result from excess copper deposits in tissues, particularly in the brain and liver. The pattern of mitochondrial enzyme defects suggests that free-radical formation and oxidative damage, probably mediated via mitochondrial copper accumulation, are important in WD pathogenesis.

C. Treatment of Wilson Disease

The goal of therapy for WD is to reduce copper intake through a low-copper diet and to increase copper excretion. D-penicillamine is the agent most often used for acute chelating therapy in WD. Trientine, an avid copper-chelating agent, may be considered for patients who cannot tolerate D-penicillamine (Brewer et al. 2003). Zinc is now the recommended therapy for long-term management of WD (Anderson et al. 1998). Orthotopic liver transplantation was reported to be effective to ameliorate neurologic progression of medically intractable WD (Bax et al. 1998).

IX. MYOCLONUS

A. Clinical Features of Myoclonus

Myoclonus is a brief, jerklike contraction of a single muscle or muscle group that occurs as an isolated event or may occur in a repetitive regular or irregular manner. Myoclonus may be associated with dementias (e.g., Creutzfeldt-Jakob disease, subacute sclerosing panencephalitis, and Alzheimer disease), lipidoses (e.g., Tay-Sachs and Niemann-Pick diseases), leukodystrophies (e.g., Krabbe and Pelizaeus-Merzbacher diseases), cerebellar degenerations (e.g., Ramsay-Hunt syndrome), epilepsy syndromes (e.g., Unverricht-Lundborg disease, Lafora body disease, and neuronal ceroid lipofuscinosis), Friedreich ataxia, hypoxic and other metabolic encephalopathies (e.g., uremic and hepatic), remote effects of cancer (e.g., infantile myoclonus associated with neuroblastoma), exposure to drugs or toxins (e.g., levodopa, lead, mercury, strychnine, methylphenidate, and amphetamines), and a variety of other disorders. Negative myoclonus, or asterixis, manifests as a sudden loss of postural tone, and has been described in various metabolic or toxic encephalopathies and in certain diencephalic lesions. Segmental or spinal myoclonus is characterized by a rhythmic contraction of a group of muscles in a particular segment, such as an arm, a leg, or the abdominal muscles. Examples include palatal myoclonus, ocular myoclonus, and hiccups. Palatal myoclonus has been described in patients with lesions involving the dentato-rubro-olivary pathway (Mollaret triangle) (Sathornsumetee and Stacy in press). [Video Segment 19]

B. Treatment of Myoclonus

Serotonin precursors (e.g., 5-hydroxytryptophan), clonazepam, and sodium valproate have produced clinical improvement of myoclonus in some patients. In segmental myoclonus, presynaptic depleting agents such as tetrabenazine and drugs used for treatment of generalized myoclonus may be beneficial. Several new antiepileptic drugs such as levetiracetam and zonisamide may also be useful in some cases of generalized and segmental myoclonus.

X. TOURETTE SYNDROME AND TIC DISORDERS

A. Clinical Features of Tourette Syndrome

Tourette syndrome (TS) is characterized by chronic waxing and waning motor and vocal tics and usually begins between the ages of twelve and fifteen years and affects boys more frequently than girls. About half of the patients start with simple motor tics such as frequent eye blinking, facial grimacing, head jerking, shoulder shrugging, or with simple vocal tics such as throat clearing, sniffing, grunting, snorting, hissing, barking, and other noises. Most patients then develop more complex tics and mannerisms such as squatting, hopping, skipping, hand shaking, compulsive touching of things, people, or self, and other stereotypical movements. The tics may change from one form to another. Although described as a lifelong condition, up to one third of patients eventually achieve spontaneous remission during adulthood. Coprolalia, echolalia, and echopraxia are the most dramatic symptoms of TS, but are present in a minority of patients. In addition to the motor and vocal tics described earlier, many patients have behavioral disorders including obsessive-compulsive disorder, attention deficit-hyperactivity disorder, self-destructive behavior, depression, and sexual disturbances (Stacy 1999, Kurlan et al. 2002, Leckman 2002). [Video Segments 20–21]

B. Pathogenesis of Tourette Syndrome

The etiopathogenesis of TS is poorly understood. It is likely a complex interaction between genetic and environmental factors. Several candidate genes have been assessed in patients with TS. Perinatal injuries, drug abuse, and recurrent streptococcal infections with postinfectious autoimmune response are among possible risk factors for the development of TS.

C. Treatment of Tourette Syndrome

Tics most often respond to dopamine receptor-blocking drugs but sometimes will benefit from α-2 adrenergic agonists such as guanfacine and clonidine. Botulinum toxin injection has been shown to decrease premonitory sensory urges in patients with simple motor tics. The obsessive-compulsive symptoms often respond to sertraline, paroxetine, or the tricyclic antidepressant clomipramine (Jankovic 2001).

XI. DRUG-INDUCED MOVEMENT DISORDERS

Since the introduction of chlorpromazine in 1952, the beneficial effects of antipsychotic medications have been clearly established. However, a variety of movement disorders may be observed in patients treated with the traditional major tranquilizers and some anti-emetic drugs, commonly grouped as dopamine receptor-blocking drugs (DRBD) (Stacy and Jankovic 1991).

A. Clinical Features of Drug-Induced Movement Disorders

The most dramatic early side effect of neuroleptic therapy is an acute dystonic reaction, usually in the form of torticollis, oromandibular dystonia, or dystonic posturing of the limbs or trunk. Up to 10% of patients who take neuroleptic drugs develop these highly distressing symptoms, usually after only one or two doses, but this reaction is reported after as long as two weeks of therapy. This acute dystonic reaction is most often seen in young male patients and is dramatically reversed by intravenous or oral administration of benztropine or other anticholinergic agents.

Parkinsonism is seen in 20 to 40% of patients treated with DRBDs and usually occurs within the first three months of drug exposure; these symptoms are disturbingly common in long-term psychiatric care institutions. [Video Segment 22] Akathisia (an urge to move) and motor restlessness of the legs, manifested by continual shifting, tapping, crossing and uncrossing of the legs, and marching in place is seen in approximately 10% of patients during the early phase of neuroleptic administration. The mechanism of this paradoxical hyperactivity is unknown, but may be related to selective blockade of the mesocortical dopamine system rather than the nigrostriatal system. Tardive dyskinesia (TD) is a drug-induced movement disorder that persists beyond two to six months after discontinuation of an offending DRBD. The most common movement disorder seen in this condition is stereotypy. These movements are usually patterned and repetitive, such as chewing, lip smacking, rocking or thrusting movements of the trunk and pelvis, and shoulder shrugging (Stacy et al. 1993). Respiratory dyskinesia can produce grunting vocalizations, hyperventilation, and shortness of breath. Other tardive movement disorders include dystonia, akathisia, Parkinsonism, tremor, myoclonus, chorea, and tics (Stacy and Jankovic 1991, 1992a). Recognition of stereotypic movements and one other movement disorder in the adult population almost always suggests the diagnosis of TD, and the need to identify the offending medication. [Video Segment 23]

Neuroleptic malignant syndrome (NMS), which manifests as a severe form of rigidity, fever, and unresponsiveness, is a potentially fatal idiosyncratic reaction to DRBD (Castillo et al. 1989). Patients should be monitored for autonomic stress, including temperature elevations, tachycardia, elevated creatine kinase (CK) levels, and mental stupor. Specific treatment must be individualized to each patient's presentation of symptoms and severity, but in general dantrolene, levodopa, and dopamine agonists have been useful in treating the signs of muscle rigidity and hyperthermia (Fleischacker et al. 1990).

Catatonia is a neuropsychiatric syndrome characterized by a combination of psychosocial withdrawal and various movement disorders. The diagnosis of catatonia has not been standardized but instead relies on a spectrum of typical clinical features that combine an alteration of behavior with stereotypic movement disorders. Cardinal signs are immobility, mutism, and withdrawal with secondary features including staring, rigidity, posturing or grimacing, negativism, waxy flexibility (or catalepsy), echophenomenon, stereotypy, and verbigeration (Gelenberg 1976). [Video Segments 24–27] Malignant catatonia is generally characterized by the additional features of hyperthermia, autonomic instability, and rigidity often severe enough to lead to death through rhabdomyolysis, renal failure, and cardiovascular collapse (Mann et al. 1986). Many authors contend that neuroleptic malignant syndrome may represent an extreme end of a continuum of catatonic symptoms, but that careful history for timing of neuroleptic exposure may be helpful in separating these entities (Shill and Stacy 2000). Catatonia is most often seen with affective disorders. Medical conditions are increasingly becoming recognized as causes of a catatonic syndrome.

Pathologic substrate for catatonia is largely unknown. When it is produced by anatomical derangement, abnormalities are most often seen in the thalamus, subthalamus, and substantia nigra. From a biochemical standpoint, changes in dopamine and GABA have been pursued as potentially important in the pathogenesis of catatonia.

Evaluation for etiology of catatonia is outlined in our report and should include full psychiatric history, possible medication and drug exposure, metabolic work-up, cerebrospinal fluid for infectious etiologies, neuroimaging, and electroencephalography (Stacy 2003). Treatment is aimed at addressing any underlying medical conditions that may produce the syndrome and once this is done, directly treating the catatonia itself. Historically, treatment types have been varied, but more recent studies suggest excellent efficacy for both high-dose intravenous benzodiazepines and electroconvulsive therapy (ECT). The mechanism for action of ECT is unknown but it likely affects a variety of neurotransmitter systems.

B. Treatment of Drug-Induced Movement Disorders

Therapeutic approaches to treatment for drug-induced movement disorders are highly individualized beyond reduction or cessation of the offending drug. Approaches have included the use of dopamine depleting agents, such as tetrabenazine for stereotypy and tremor symptoms, and botulinum toxin for focal dystonia. In patients who require DRBD for controlling their psychiatric symptoms, atypical antipsychotics with partial D2 receptor agonistic activity (aripiprazole) or with modest (clozapine) or mild (quetiapine) antagonistic effect on D2 receptors should be considered (Stacy and Jankovic 1991).

XII. HEMIBALLISM

Ballism refers to extremely large amplitude flinging choreic movements. The name is derived from the Greek word for jump or throw. Hemiballism is the more common name for this disorder as it is typically unilateral in presentation, contralateral to the lesion in the subthalamic nucleus (Postuma and Lang 2003). [Video Segment 28]

XIII. HEMIFACIAL SPASM

Hemifacial spasms are unilateral involuntary contractions involving muscles of facial expression. Incidence is less than 1 in 100,000 with prevalence rates higher in women than men, and an average age of onset in the fourth or fifth decade. The spasms last but a few minutes and come in bursts, often triggered by facial behaviors such as eating, speaking, or changes in head position. Typically, the first muscles involved are in the periorbital region, preceded by facial weakness, and within months spreading to ipsilateral facial muscles. These twitches continue in sleep. Blink reflexes are expressed normally. Hemifacial spasms occur when the facial nerve is compressed at the root entry zone, usually by the anterior or posterior inferior cerebellar or vertebral artery. Treatment of choice is botulinum toxin injections, but clonazepam is also prescribed (Sathornsumetee and Stacy in press). [Video Segment 29]

XIV. SUMMARY

Interactions between sensory and motor processing within the structures of the basal ganglia, cerebellum, and interconnected sensorimotor structures provide smooth movements and efficient control between component movements, while disturbances within these structures lead to the hyperkinetic and hypokinetic movement disorders just discussed. Although much has been learned through clinical observation and research investigation into these various syndromes, continued progress is needed. Collaboration between the clinicians who observe, diagnose, and treat these movement disorders and the scientists who investigate the etiology, development, and intervention of the disease states has always been key to driving progress in treating these fascinating medical conditions. This chapter and the accompanying videos serve to anchor scientists with a basic understanding of the different types of movement disorders encountered in a Neurology clinic.

Video Legends

SEGMENT 1 A 42-year-old man with newly diagnosed PD. In this brief exam, he exhibits resting tremor of his right hand, bradykinesia (slow movement) and hypokinesia (decreased amplitude of movement) on the right side of his body, and has absent arm swing and a flexed upper extremity posture typical of PD.

SEGMENT 2 A 56-year-old woman with advanced PD. She has marked lower extremity dyskinesia as her Levodopa "kicks in." Note the trick she uses to cope with these movements that occur every two to three hours. Note how abruptly the movements stop, as she develops mild tremor. In addition, note how the tremor in her right hand diminishes with a change to a new posture, and then re-emerges at this new "resting" position or arm extension.

SEGMENT 3 A 56-year-old man with a long history of PD with mild bradykinesia and moderate to severe resting and action tremor of the right hand. Because he had incomplete tremor response to medications, he underwent implantation of a left thalamic deep brain stimulator. Note his abrupt benefit when he activates the stimulator with a small magnet.

SEGMENT 4 A 72-year-old man with a four-year history of progressive Parkinsonism manifested by falling, vision difficulties and difficulty eating. He reports little to no benefit from anti-PD medications. On examination, he exhibits typical midline (facial) dystonia. With ambulation, he takes long strides and makes pivoting (as opposed to *en bloc*) turns. This is highly suggestive of Progressive Supranuclear Palsy.

SEGMENT 5 A 66-year-old woman with apraxia and Parkinsonism not responsive to anti-PD medications. Although she is still able to perform simple tasks, she relies increasingly on her right hand. She is able to mimic gestures of the examiner, but cannot make finger movements with her left hand if she is asked to close her eyes. These are findings highly suggestive of Corticobasal Degeneration.

SEGMENT 6 A 54-year-old man with progressive bradykinesia, blepharospasm (marked by the use of dark sunglasses), and dystonic posturing of his left arm. He also had severe orthostatic hypotension. He responded briefly to anti-PD agents, but these medications worsened his dystonia. He has many features suggestive of Multiple System Atrophy.

SEGMENT 7 A 42-year-old woman with Huntington disease. She exhibits facial, trunk and limb chorea, bradykinesia, inability to maintain tongue protrusion (serpentine tongue), "hung-up," reflexes with pendular leg movements after the initial brisk tendon response. Her gait is quite typical of the wide-based, lurching walk seen in this disorder.

SEGMENT 8 An 8-year-old girl with Juvenile Huntington disease (i.e., Westphal Variant). On genetic testing, she had greater than 50 CAG repeats typical of this condition. Rather than chorea, these children exhibit dystonic postures, bradykinesia, a gait disorder, and, with disease progression, generalized seizures.

SEGMENT 9 Primary writing tremor—a task-specific movement disorder that shows pathophysiological overlap with the task-specific dystonias.

SEGMENT 10 A 37-year-old man with orthostatic tremor. He exhibits a rapid postural tremor when at rest. When standing, he reports some cramping pain in his legs. The tremor is elicited by having the patient stand on his toes, and lean against the wall.

SEGMENT 11 A young woman who suffered a mild birth injury, most likely secondary to hypoxia. She has a typical action tremor associated with hypoxic cerebellar injury.

SEGMENT 12 A man who is applying for disability because of a tremor limiting the function of his right hand. Note the disappearance of the tremor in the right hand when he is asked to open and close the left hand. He has a non-organic tremor.

SEGMENT 13 A 19-year-old girl with DYT1 dystonia confirmed by genetic testing.

SEGMENT 14 A 44-year-old man with cranial (blepharospasm and oromandibular) and cervical dystonia.

SEGMENT 15 A 60-year-old woman with oromandibular dystonia that produces involuntary jaw opening.

SEGMENT 16 A 15-year-old girl sent by her school for oppositional behavior, because she would not hold her pen correctly. She has a task-specific dystonia, writer's cramp.

SEGMENT 17 A 32-year-old man with an unusual occupational dystonia. He experienced dystonic extension of the thumb and first finger of his right hand during only one activity–picking up cards or chips as a blackjack dealer in a Las Vegas Casino.

SEGMENT 18 A 74-year-old woman who developed left foot dystonia after suffering a small infarction in the right globus pallidus.

SEGMENT 19 A 49-year-old woman who, six months earlier, was in good health. Her family reported increasingly erratic behavior in the month prior to admission. She was able to provide some history during her admission processing, but rapidly declined to the point where she was unable to communicate. Electroencephalography showed some burst-suppression activity and marked disruption of her sleep/wake cycle. Brain biopsy confirmed a clinical diagnosis of Creutzfeldt-Jacob disease. This video segment demonstrates both spontaneous and action myoclonus of her trunk, face and limbs {1:23:54 to 1:24:34:10}.

SEGMENT 20 A 13-year-old boy with mild facial tics.

SEGMENT 21 A 76-year-old man with a long history of Tourette syndrome. In this long segment, he tries to describe the sensory "premonition" reported by some patients before the motor action.

SEGMENT 22–25 A 19-year-old woman who developed malignant catatonia, thought secondary to viral meningitis.

SEGMENT 22 After a three-week hospitalization at a community hospital, she was transferred to a tertiary care facility. In this clip she exhibits stereotypic movements of her face and a highly atypical tremor of her face and limbs. She then underwent four sessions of electroconvulsive therapy and began a rapid recovery.

SEGMENT 23 Two weeks after electroconvulsive therapy. Note clinical improvement.

SEGMENT 24 After discharge, an additional one month later. This segment shows improving bradykinesia and bradyphrenia (slow thinking).

SEGMENT 25 Complete recovery. This patient went on to make a full recovery, got married, and returned to full time employment as a journalist.

SEGMENT 26 This is an elderly, long-term resident of a state psychiatric hospital. He exhibits bradykinesia, postural changes, and decreased arm swing with walking associated with long-term dopamine-receptor-blocking drug exposure.

SEGMENT 27 A 56-year-old woman with tremor and stereotypic movements of her mouth. Her risk factors for the involuntary mouth movements are previous tooth extractions and exposure to dopamine-receptor-blocking drugs. Her tremor is suggestive of a tardive tremor in that it is asymmetric and occurs at both rest and with action. However, she is also taking valproic acid, a known tremorogenic medication.

SEGMENT 28 A 43-year-old man who, as a teenager, sustained a traumatic brain injury. During a thalamotomy procedure in the 1960's, he suffered an infarction of the left subthalamic nucleus. This iatrogenic subthalamotomy resulted in chronic right upper extremity hemiballismus.

SEGMENT 29 Hemifacial spasm. The patient reports that his symptoms began after a difficult dental extraction.

References

Adler, C.H., and R. Kumar. 2000. Pharmacological and surgical options for the treatment of cervical dystonia. *Neurology* 55:S9–S14.

Alexander, G.E., and M.D. Crutcher. 1990. Functional architecture of basal ganglia circuits: neural substrates of parallel processing. *Trends Neurosci.* **13**:266–271.

Anderson, L.A., S.L. Hakojarvi, and S.K. Boudreaux. 1998. Zinc acetate treatment in Wilson's disease. *Ann Pharmacotherapy* **32**:78–87.

Ballard, P.A., J.W. Tetrud, and J.W. Langston. 1985. Permanent human parkinsonism due to 1-methyl-4-phenyl-1,2,26-tetrahydropyridine (MPTP): seven cases. *Neurology* **35**:949–956.

Bates, G. 2003. Huntingtin aggregation and toxicity in Huntington's disease. *Lancet* **361**:1642–1644.

Bax, R.T., A. Hassler, W. Luck, H. Hefter, I. Kuageloh-Mann, P. Neuhaus, P. Emmrich. 1998. Cerebral manifestation of Wilson's disease successfully treated with liver transplantation. *Neurology* **51**:863–865.

Bressman, S.B., D. Raymond, K. Wendt, et al. 2002. Diagnostic criteria for dystonia in DYT1 families. *Neurology* **59**:1780–1782.

Brewer, G.J., P. Hedera, K.J. Kluin, et al. 2003. Treatment of Wilson disease with ammonium tetrathiomolybdate: III. Initial therapy in a total of 55 neurologically affected patients and follow-up with zinc therapy. *Arch Neurol* **60**:379–385.

Brin, M.F., K.E. Lyons, J. Doucette, et al. 2001. A randomized, double masked, controlled trial of botulinum toxin type A in essential hand tremor. *Neurology* **56**:1523–1528.

Castillo, E., R.T. Rubin, and E. Holsboer-Trachler. 1989. Clinical differentiation between lethal catatonia and neuroleptic malignant syndrome. *Am J Psychiatry* **146**:324–328.

de Carvalho Aguiar, P.M., and L.J. Ozelius. 2002. Classification and genetics of dystonia. *Lancet Neurol* **5**:316–325.

Connor, G.S. 2002. A double-blind placebo-controlled trial of topiramate treatment for essential tremor. *Neurology* **59**:132–134.

Duvoisin, R.C. 1992. A brief history of parkinsonism. *Neurol Clin N Am* **10**:301–316.

Fleishschacker, W.W., B. Unterweger, J.M. Kane, and H. Hinterhuber. 1990. The neuroleptic malignant syndrome and its differentiation from lethal catatonia. *Acta Psychiatr Scand* **81**:3–5.

Gelenberg, A.J. 1976. The catatonic syndrome. *Lancet* **1**:1339–1341.

Gibb, W.R.G., P.J. Luthert, and C.D. Marsden. 1989. Corticobasal degeneration. *Brain* **112**:1171–1192.

Huntington Study Group. 2001. A randomized, placebo-controlled trial of coenzyme Q10 and remacemide in Huntington's disease. *Neurology* **57**:397–404.

Illarioshkin, S.N., S. Igarashi, O. Onodera, et al. 1994. Trinucleotide repeat length and rate of progression in Huntington's disease. *Ann Neurol* **36**:630–635.

Jankovic, J., and J. Orman. 1988. Tetrabenazine therapy of dystonia, chorea, tics and other dyskinesias. *Neurology* **38**:391–394.

Jankovic, J., and M. Stacy. 1998. Movement Disorders. In *Textbook of Clinical Neurology*. Ed. C. Goetz and E. Pappert. pp. 655–679. Philadelphia: W.B. Saunders.

Jankovic, J. 2001. Tourette's syndrome. *N Eng J Med* **345**:1184–1192.

Joel, D., and J. Weiner. 1994. The organization of the basal ganglia-thalamocortical circuits: open interconnected rather than closed segregated. *Neuroscience* **63**:363–379.

Krack, P., A. Batir, N. van Blercom, et al. 2003. Five-year follow-up of bilateral stimulation of the subthalamic nucleus in advanced Parkinson's disease. *N Eng J Med* **349**:1925–1934.

Kurlan, R., P.G. Como, B. Miller, et al. 2002. The behavioral spectrum of tic disorders: a community-based study. *Neurology* **50**:414–420.

Leckman, J.F. 2002. Tourette's syndrome. *Lancet* **360**:1577–1586.

Louis, E.D. 2001. Clinical practice: essential tremor. *N Eng J Med* **345**: 887–891.

Mahant, N., E.A. McCusker, K. Byth, and S. Graham. 2003. Huntington's disease: clinical correlates of disability and progression. *Neurology* **61**:1085–1092.

Mann, S.C., S.N. Caroff, H.R. Bleir, R.E. Antelo, and H. Un. 1986. Lethal catatonia. *Am J Psychiatry* **143**:1374–1381.

Nygaard, T.G., C.D. Marsden, and S. Fahn. 1991. Dopa-responsive dystonia: long-term treatment response and prognosis. *Neurology* **41**: 174–181.

Ondo, W., C. Hunter, K.D. Vuong, et al. Gabapentin for essential tremor: a multiple-dose, double-blind, placebo-controlled trial. *Mov Disord* 2000; **15**:678–682.

Parent, A. 1996. *Carpenter's Human Neuro-anatomy*, Ninth Edition. pp. 795–863. Baltimore: Williams & Wilkins.

Parkinson Study Group. 1996. Impact of deprenyl and tocopherol treatment on Parkinson's disease in DATATOP patients requiring levodopa. Parkinson Study Group. *Ann Neurol* **39(1)**:37–45.

Postuma, R.B., and A.E. Lang. 2003. Hemiballism: revisiting a classic disorder. *Lancet Neurol* **2**:661–668.

Reiner, A., L. Medina, and C.L. Veenman. 1998. Structural and functional evolution of the basal ganglia in vertebrates. *Brain Research Reviews* **28**:235–285.

Sathornsumetee, S., and M. Stacy. (In press) Movement Disorders. In *Adult Neurology*. Ed. C. Bloom. St. Louis: Mosby.

Shill, H., and M. Stacy. 2000. Malignant catatonia secondary to sporadic encephalitis. *J Neurol Neurosurg Psychiatry* **69**:402–403.

Schuurman, P.R., D.A. Bosch, P.M. Bossuyt, et al. 2000. A comparison of continuous thalamic stimulation and thalamotomy for suppression of severe tremor. *N Eng J Med* **342**:461–468.

Stacy, M., F. Cardoso, and J. Jankovic. 1993. Tardive stereotypy and other movement disorders in tardive dyskinesias. *Neurology* **43**:937–941.

Stacy, M., and J. Jankovic. 1991. Tardive dyskinesia. *Curr Opin Neurol Neurosurg* **4**:343–349.

Stacy, M., and J. Jankovic. 1992a. Tardive tremor. *Mov Disord* **7**:53–57.

Stacy, M., and J. Jankovic. 1992b. Differential diagnosis of Parkinson's disease and the parkinsonism plus syndromes. *Neurol Clin N Am* **10**:341–358.

Stacy, M., and J. Jankovic. 1997. Movement Disorders. In *Adult Neurology. Second Edition*. Ed. C. Bloom. pp. 267–282. St. Louis: Mosby.

Stacy, M. 1999. Gilles de la Tourette's Syndrome and other tic disorders. In *Current Pediatric Therapy*, Vol 16. Ed. F.D. Burg, E.R. Wald, J.R. Ingelfinger, and R.A. Polin. pp. 389–390. Philadelphia: W.B. Saunders.

Stacy, M. 1999. Managing late complications of Parkinson's disease. *Med Clin North Am* **83**:469–481.

Stacy, M. 2000a. Pharmacotherapy for advanced Parkinson's disease. *Pharmacotherapy* 20;9S–16S.

Stacy, M. 2000b. Progressive Supranuclear Palsy. In *Parkinson's Disease and Movement Disorders*. Ed. C.H. Adler and J.E. Ahlskog. pp. 229–234. Totowa, NJ: Humana Press.

Stacy, M. 2003. Dopamine Agonists. In *Handbook of Parkinson's Disease*, Third Edition. Ed. R. Pahwa, K. Lyons, W. Koller. New York: Marcel-Dekker.

Tanzi, R.E., K. Petrukin K, and I. Chernov. 1993. The Wilson's disease gene is a copper transporting ATPase with homology to the Menke's disease gene. *Nat Genet* **5**:344–350.

Vitek, J.L. 2002. Pathophysiology of dystonia: a neuronal model. *Mov Disord* **17**:S49–62.

Vitek, J.L., M.S. Okun, D.V. Raju, B.L. Walter, J.L. Juncos, M.R. DeLong, K. Heilman, W.M. McDonald. 2004. Pseudobulbar crying induced by stimulation in the region of the subthalamic nucleus. *J Neurol Neurosurg Psychiatry* **75**:921–923.

Walker, R.H., F.O. Danisi, D.M. Swope, et al. 2000. Intrathecal baclofen for dystonia: benefits and complications during six years of experience. *Mov Disord* **15**:1242–1247.

CHAPTER

A2

Animal Models and the Science of Movement Disorders

MARK LeDOUX

I. SCIENTIFIC APPLICATION OF ANIMAL MODELS

What is a thought except a movement that is not connected to a motor neuron? (Walle Nauta)

An integrated approach of rigorous clinical, *in vitro*, and whole animal research is the optimal means to advance our understanding of movement disorders and closely related neurological diseases. The choice of model system (e.g., patients, mice, flies, or cultured cells) is dictated by experimental hypotheses, resource availability, finances, time constraints, and ethical principles. In the context of movement disorders research, there are two ultimate goals: (1) superior diagnosis and treatment of patients and (2) advanced understanding of biological systems. As with many scientific and engineering endeavors, you only understand how a system works if you can fix it when it is broken. Hence, critical insights into the normal control of movement have come from the study of movement disorders. Furthermore, study of motor systems and movement disorders has contributed enormously to the fields of neurodevelopment, neurodegeneration, robotics, artificial neural networks, and computational neuroscience.

A. Alternatives and Complements to Animal Models

1. Human Studies

Research activities targeting a particular movement disorder, whether it is Tourette syndrome, blepharospasm or myoclonus, must begin and end with patients. Patients provide the material and motivation for scientific investigation. Skilled clinicians initially described the primary features, secondary manifestations, and pathological hallmarks of each type of movement disorder without access to powerful modern tools of science such as magnetic resonance imaging (MRI) and the polymerase chain reaction (PCR). Even in the twenty-first century, neurologists diagnose nearly all patients with movement disorders at the bedside. Parkinson disease, cervical dystonia, essential tremor, Friedreich ataxia, and Huntington disease can be easily diagnosed, in most instances, without computed tomography, electrophysiological studies, or genetic testing. For example, identifying an expansion of CAG trinucleotide repeats in the IT15 gene serves only to confirm a clinical diagnosis of Huntington disease. In contrast, there are no highly sensitive and specific confirmatory tests for patients with idiopathic Parkinson disease, cervical dystonia, and essential tremor. Experienced clinicians must therefore be an integral component of translational research for movement disorders. One or two incorrect phenotypic classifications of research subjects can doom linkage analysis to failure. At the other end of the research spectrum, a pharmaceutical company would not want to include patients with essential tremor in a therapeutic trial of a new dopamine agonist for Parkinson disease.

Patients with movement disorders and their phenotypically normal family members serve as the fundamental source of materials for investigation. Acquisition of whole blood for subsequent DNA extraction from lymphocytes has served as the beginning to many major discoveries in the neurosciences. At this early stage, detailed and accurate phenotypic descriptions are essential for each DNA sample. Strong consideration should also be given to the establishment of lymphoblastoid or fibroblast cell lines. Fibroblasts are acquired via a skin punch biopsy and lymphocytes from whole blood. Cell lines provide a mechanism for biochemical analysis. More importantly, cell lines serve as a virtually unlimited source of DNA and RNA for future genetic and molecular studies.

Biomarker and other biochemical studies may require cerebrospinal fluid, serum, or urine from patients with movement disorders. Appropriately matched controls are essential for valid interpretations of experimental results. In addition, simply storing patient samples in a −80°C freezer may be inadequate for downstream applications; preprocessing steps such as centrifugation and degassing may be necessary.

Microarray, quantitative real-time reverse transcription (RT)-PCR, immunohistochemical, and biochemical analyses of high-quality human postmortem tissue have contributed significantly to our understanding of movement disorders. With fresh-frozen brain, researchers have quantified catecholamines, indoleamines, and other components of the metabolome in specific neuronal populations with high-pressure liquid chromatography. More recently, laser capture microdissection has been used to analyze transcript levels in particular cell types. Towards these ends, several nonprofit research foundations devoted to the study of movement disorders have established brain repositories, and several well-known brain banks maintain tissues from patients with well-characterized movement disorders. Study of human postmortem tissues can be used to formulate hypotheses for testing in animals.

Integration of electrophysiological, behavioral, and functional imaging data from patients with movement disorders can be used to identify responsible neural networks, monitor disease progression, establish phenotypes, and quantify the effects of various treatments. Available functional imaging tools include positron emission tomography (PET), magnetic resonance spectroscopy, functional MRI, single photon emission computed tomography, and magnetoencephalography. Fluoro-dopa PET, for example, can monitor progression in Parkinson disease. Electrophysiological approaches commonly employed by neurologists in clinical research include electromyography, nerve conduction studies, evoked potentials, and transcranial magnetic stimulation. Behavioral paradigms are often combined with functional imaging and/or electrophysiological measurements to define the neural subsystems responsible for specific phenotypic components of a particular movement disorder (Rothwell and Huang 2003). Psychometric test batteries, neurological rating scales (e.g., Unified Parkinson Disease Rating Scale, Toronto Western Spasmodic Torticollis Rating Scale, Unified Huntington Disease Rating Scale), and daily living assessment surveys are typically employed in clinical research trials. At a practical level, many of the techniques and approaches used in clinics and hospitals can be applied to research with animal models. Moreover, insights from human studies can serve as a source of inspiration for more focused mechanistic studies in animals.

Experimental procedures involving human subjects are governed by institutional review boards (IRBs) in accordance with principles contained in the World Medical Association Declaration of Helsinki and Department of Health and Human Services Regulations for Protection of Human Subjects (45 CFR 46) and similar Food and Drug Administration Regulations (21 CFR 50 and 56). At most medical schools and other academic research institutions, human research protocols must be submitted to a local IRB. Before any human subject research project is initiated, the project must first be reviewed and approved by the appropriate IRB and then conducted in full compliance with federal regulations. These requirements apply to both clinical trial research and the use of biological materials from patients, such as DNA, cerebrospinal fluid, and urine. Patient confidentiality must be maintained in all human studies, in accordance with standards established in the Health Insurance Portability and Accountability Act (HIPAA) of 1996.

2. Bioinformatics and Computational Biology

The National Institutes of Health released working definitions of bioinformatics and computational biology on July 17, 2000.

Bioinformatics: Research, development, or application of computational tools and approaches for expanding the use of biological, medical, behavioral, or health data, including those to acquire, store, organize, archive, analyze, or visualize such data.

Computational Biology: The development and application of data-analytical and theoretical methods, mathematical modeling, and computational simulation techniques to the study of biological, behavioral, and social systems.

Bioinformatic and computational biological approaches complement and, in some cases, can replace experiments with animals, including humans. Scientists should avoid reinventing the wheel. In a similar vein, scientists should try to maximize the impact of their painstakingly earned research dollars. Along these lines, most experiments should begin on the Internet and in the library. Unfortunately, too many examples exist of the scientific community largely ignoring novel and enlightened discoveries for years to decades.

A virtually endless collection of bioinformatic resources is available on the World Wide Web. In the United States, at least, scientists are most familiar with the Web site maintained by the National Center for Biotechnology Information (NCBI; http://www.ncbi.nlm.nih.gov/). The NCBI maintains and almost continuously updates a large number of databases and bioinformatic tools. NCBI Entrez is a system for searching numerous linked databases including PubMed, Online Mendelian Inheritance in Man (OMIM), nucleotide sequences, three-dimensional macromolecular structures, and protein sequences. Important NCBI tools include BLAST (Basic Local Alignment Search Tool), electronic PCR, and CD (Conserved Domain) Search. Using a strictly *in silico* approach, a researcher can establish a predicted function, structure, and familial classification of a protein encoded by a recently cloned gene with a few clicks of a mouse.

Computational modeling of neural networks relevant to the study of human movement disorders depends on a scaffolding of neuroanatomical and neurophysiological data acquired from animals, particularly mammals. In some scenarios, however, only a basic outline of mammalian neuronal connections is needed because artificial neural networks can be programmed to exhibit considerable self-organizing behavior. In other cases, questions regarding normal and disordered motor control derived from computer simulations can be answered with animal models. Progress in fully understanding complex biological motor control systems will require integration of systems-oriented engineering with experimental neuroscience. This type of work may to contribute to both our understanding of movement disorders and the evolution of biomimetic robotics.

3. Microbes

In the context of neuroscience research, microbes such as *Escherichia coli* and *Saccharomyces cerevisiae* are most commonly used as either protein expression systems or genetic tools (e.g., bacterial artificial chromosomes [BACs]; yeast artificial chromosomes [YACs]). These microbes can, however, be used in hypothesis-driven experiments to explore the molecular pathophysiology of movement disorders and neurodegeneration. As a case in point, Rankin and co-workers (2001) used *E. coli* to show that the E3 ubiquitin ligase activity of parkin, a protein mutant in autosomal recessive juvenile Parkinsonism, is an intrinsic function of the parkin protein and does not require post-translational modifications. In addition, some protein-protein interactions can be studied with yeast two-hybrid systems; alternative approaches must be used for bait proteins with strong intracellular targeting signals, extracellular domains and interactions that are dependent on post-translational modification.

When novel mutant genes are identified in patients with movement disorders, the next step is to generate recombinant proteins for functional and biochemical studies. The choice of expression system (e.g., bacteria, yeast, baculovirus/insect cells, or mammalian cells) depends on planned downstream applications. Bacterial expression systems can produce large quantities of protein rapidly. The major disadvantage of bacterial expression systems is that proteins are not post-translationally modified (i.e., no glycosylation or phosphorylation). In some circumstances, mammalian expression systems must be used to assure that proteins undergo correct post-translational modifications.

In most instances, recombinant proteins are first used to generate antibodies. Purely biochemical approaches can be used to analyze a variety of protein functions and characteristics such as enzymatic activity. Western blotting can characterize post-translational modifications of the protein. Recombinant proteins are also required for crystallography.

4. Cell Culture

Scientists can culture cells taken from original tissue, primary cultures, cell lines, or cell strains. Late embryonic rat hippocampus and human tumor specimens are examples of original tissues. Numerous continuous cell lines are widely available to researchers. Each continuous cell line exhibits phenotypic features that may be suitable for particular experimental applications. Mammalian cell lines commonly used for transfection experiments, for example, include 293F (human embryonic kidney), CHO-K1 (Chinese hamster ovary), COS-1 (monkey kidney), HeLa (human cervical cancer), and Jurkat (human lymphocyte).

Cell cultures are particularly suited to certain kinds of studies related to (1) morphogenesis, (2) cell adhesion and matrix interaction, (3) invasiveness, (4) signal transduction, (5) secretion, (6) protein synthesis, (7) apoptosis, (8) membrane trafficking, (9) RNA processing, (10) drug actions, and (11) transcriptional events. Several other areas of research and development such as (1) viral production, (2) *in vitro* assays of new pharmaceuticals, and (3) antibody and recombinant protein production depend heavily on cell culture techniques. Theoretically, cell cultures are less subject to the variations seen in animal studies that are due to diurnal variations in endocrine status, experimental stress, and homeostatic interactions among major organ systems.

Cell cultures offer several practical and theoretical advantages over experiments with animals. In many situations, cell cultures can reduce or eliminate the need for experimental animals. Cell cultures are particularly useful for automated applications requiring high-throughput screening of test compounds such as those generated by combinatorial chemistry. Cell cultures provide a relatively uniform physicochemical environment for comparison of treatment groups and, in most applications, markedly reduce reagent needs. Cultured cells are also particularly suitable for the study of individual genes since DNA transfer techniques are more easily applied to dissociated cells than intact tissues.

Despite the potential of cell cultures, there are numerous limitations to their application. A substantial investment in time and money is required to generate enough cells for certain types of applications. Cell culture also requires specialized equipment and can be fraught with technical difficulties. For instance, cells are quite susceptible to infection by a variety of microorganisms. Over time, cells may lose many of the characteristics of the tissue from which they were derived. In particular the two-dimensional culture plate for the nervous system is a poor representative of the complex three-dimensional synaptic interactions characteristic of the brain.

Scientists often employ cell cultures in toxicity assays of new pharmaceuticals, food products, cosmetics, and household chemicals. Although *in vitro* assays are useful for an initial screening of these compounds, they cannot entirely replace *in vivo* methods. For example, the liver converts some otherwise harmless compounds into potent toxins. Many toxins also show extraordinary tissue specificity that cannot be adequately evaluated, even with an array of cell types. Most of the common side effects associated with pharmaceuticals are systemic and, therefore, impossible to detect with plates of cultured cells. For instance, the dopamine agonists that are used to treat Parkinson disease can cause nausea and orthostatic hypotension.

B. The Ethical Care and Use of Animals

The first step in the use of animals for biomedical research is to consider the following basic principles: (1) the potential societal benefit of the research should outweigh concerns about possible subject burden; (2) an acceptable species should be chosen for the hypothesis at hand; (3) pain, distress, and suffering should be minimized; and (4) the smallest number of animals required to generate reliable scientific results should be employed in the planned experiments. The proper care and treatment of animals used in scientific research require understanding of both the subjects and experimental plan. Experiments should be designed in the context of the unique husbandry needs, physiological profiles, pharmacological agent sensitivities, life spans, and nutritional requirements that each species demands.

Institutional Animal Care and Use Committees (IACUCs) govern the appropriate conduct of animal experimentation at research institutions, and two federal laws direct the IACUCs: the Animal Welfare Act of 1966 and the Health Research Extension Act of 1985. The head of the respective institution must appoint each IACUC, and the IACUC must manage their animal care and use programs in accordance with federal guidelines, policies, and regulations. For federally funded projects, universities are required to implement their animal care and use programs as described in their Assurance of Compliance to the National Institutes of Health. IACUCs are specifically required to heed the following guidelines: (1) review all proposed animal use; (2) approve, require modifications in, or deny approval of proposed animal use; and (3) conduct continuing reviews of all approved ongoing activities. All activities must be submitted to and approved in writing by the IACUC before any activity may be initiated.

In the United States, general policies and procedures designed to ensure the humane, ethical, and scientifically appropriate use of vertebrate animals are provided in the United States Public Health Service Policy on Humane Care and Use of Laboratory Animals (National Institutes of Health, http://grants.nih.gov/grants/olaw/olaw.htm) and the *Guide for the Care and Use of Laboratory Animals* (National Academy of Sciences, http://www.nap.edu/catalog/5140.html). Guidelines for animal euthanasia are detailed in the 2000 Report of the American Veterinary Medical Association Panel on Euthanasia (http://www.avma.org/resources/euthanasia.pdf). The Association for Accreditation and Assessment of Laboratory Animal Care (AAALAC) is a private nonprofit organization that evaluates institutions that use animals in research. Those that exhibit excellence in animal care and use are awarded accreditation. The accreditation process includes a detailed internal review conducted by the institution applying for accreditation. Next, AAALAC evaluators review the internal reports and conduct their own comprehensive assessment. An institution must be re-evaluated every three years to maintain its accredited status.

C. The Value of Animal Models

The field of movement disorders research is difficult to imagine without animal models. Neuroscience research in general, and motor systems science in particular, are critically dependent on experimentation with animals. The profound complexity of normal and abnormal neural networks cannot be reproduced in either the test tube or culture dish. Attempts to identify molecular, genetic, and neurophysiological defects in animal models of movement disorders have forced scientists to make more focused analyses of normal neural function and, as a result, significant advances have been made in motor systems physiology. For example, animal models of Parkinson disease and dystonia have contributed to our understanding of basal ganglia and cerebellar local area networks, respectively.

Normal motor behavior is the final product of massive neural computation performed by tissues with precise three-dimensional organizations and connectivity patterns. Similar to an electronics technician searching for a defective transistor on a circuit board, clinicians and scientists engaged in movement disorders research identify neuronal populations causally associated with specific forms of abnormal motor behavior. Studies of this type are a critical first step in defining targets for stereotactic neurosurgical procedures. Animal models have been crucial for identifying the subthalamic nucleus (STN), globus pallidus pars interna, and ventral intermediate nucleus of the thalamus as appropriate targets for deep brain stimulation in patients with Parkinson disease, dystonia, and essential tremor, respectively. *In vivo* studies have also been critical for characterizing the neurophysiological underpinnings of spasticity and task-specific dystonias and, as a consequence, rehabilitation of these disorders has markedly improved over the past few years.

Mutant proteins and neurotoxins associated with movement and neurodegenerative disorders tend to produce cell-type-specific effects. Moreover, the effects of a toxin like 1-methyl-4-phenyl-1,2,3,6-tetrahydropyridine (MPTP) require complex interactions between neurons and glia. Cultures of multiple cell types, organotypic cultures, and glial-neuronal co-cultures are typically inadequate for assessing either the toxicity of proteins (e.g., polyglutamine tracts) and small molecules (e.g., manganese, MPTP) since they cannot reproduce the connectivity, three-dimensional structure, and extracellular milieu of the central nervous system. Furthermore, neuronal cells, glial cells, or both must be harvested from animals; they do not arise from thin air!

Animals are also needed for the seemingly less elegant aspects of movement disorders research. Studies of device compatibility, pharmacokinetics, and drug safety are highly dependent on the availability of animals. Mammalian models are often essential for evaluating the efficacy of candidate compounds that target receptors and pathways downstream of causal defects. One obvious example is the pre-clinical testing of a dopamine agonist in the rodent 6-hydroxydopamine (6-OHDA) model of Parkinson disease. In contrast, fruit flies and roundworms may be useful for high-throughput screening of compounds that target principal upstream molecular events.

D. Practical Application and Limitations of Animal Models

Movement disorders research with animal models, like all research endeavors, is ultimately a search for cause and effect. Common sense and basic scientific principles should be applied to both experimental design and data interpretation. Unfortunately, excitement over a new finding can sometimes precipitate a claim of causality when none is present. To illustrate, a unique motor phenotype in a transgenic mouse should not be attributed to the foreign gene unless the phenotype can be reproduced in at least one additional line of mice; the transgene could easily have created an insertional mutation.

Scientists should also exercise caution when tempted to generalize experimental findings in animals to human disorders. Unlike a population of neurology patients from a variety of racial and ethnic backgrounds, animals used for research studies are often inbred. Furthermore, unlike the real world that patients and their treating physicians must face each day, the laboratory environment is highly controlled. In contrast to a patient with Huntington disease, an R6/2 transgenic mouse eats the same food each day and does not have to worry about bills, groceries, or finding a ride to the doctor's office. It is not surprising that so many promising treatments derived from placebo-controlled trials in inbred lines of mice fail to pan out in the clinic.

Although vertebrate animals share a great deal of genetic common ground, they are not all the same. Rodents and primates, for example, often exhibit striking species specificity in their susceptibility to neurotoxins and infectious organisms. Therefore, a potential dopaminergic neurotoxin should not be dismissed simply because it did not produce cell death in one line of rats. The pharmacokinetic profiles of pharmaceuticals will also vary widely among animals and humans: drug dosing cannot be extrapolated from one species to another simply based on body mass. Finally, as a reminder, many human genes have no orthologs in invertebrate species and, as such, the intracellular milieu in flies and worms may differ from humans in important ways. Scientists should be careful when extrapolating the results of molecular manipulations in invertebrates to human disorders.

II. CHOICE OF THE APPROPRIATE ANIMAL MODEL

The decision to utilize an animal model should be intimately incorporated with the choice of species. Some of the more commonly used animal species in movement disorders research are presented in table 1. In many laboratories, scientists become both comfortable and skilled with a particular species and, consequently, experimental hypotheses are often constrained by the limitations of their "pet" animal. Thus, collaborative efforts should be encouraged among laboratories specializing in the maintenance and manipulation of different vertebrate and invertebrate animal models. Even within species, strain selection may be critical to the success of an experiment. For example, in the context of motor systems and movement disorders research, mouse strain shows dramatic effects on morphine-induced locomotion (Murphy et al. 2001) and sensitivity to the dopaminergic neurotoxin MPTP (Hamre et al. 1999).

TABLE 1 Selected Invertebrate and Vertebrate Species Potentially Useful in the Study of Movement Disorders

Common name	Species name	Developmental period to maturity	Life span	Major advantages
Roundworm	*Caenorhabditis elegans*	3 d	2–3 wks	inexpensive, translucent, can be frozen for long-term storage
Fruit fly	*Drosophila melanogaster*	9 d	2 wks	inexpensive, highly amenable to genetic manipulation
Zebrafish	*Danio rerio*	3 mo	5 yrs	translucent vertebrate
Mouse	*Mus musculus*	6 wks	2–3 yrs	genetic similarity to humans
Rat	*Rattus norvegicus*	10 wks	2–3 yrs	large enough for most physiological studies relevant to human diseases
Monkey	*Macaca mulatta*	4 yrs	25 yrs	neuroanatomical, physiological, and genetic likeness to humans
Human	*Homo sapiens*	16 yrs	80 yrs	the real deal

A. Worms

Caenorhabditis elegans, commonly known as the roundworm, is a nematode. Its thin unsegmented body is small (1–1.5 mm), transparent, and tapered at each end. *C. elegans* consists of approximately 1,000 cells and about 20,000 genes. Newly hatched worms contain precisely 556 cells; each of these cells develops through a series of well-described mitotic divisions. More amazingly, exactly 131 cells in the developing embryo die by apoptosis. *C. elegans* was the first multicellular eukaryote to have its complete genome sequenced.

C. elegans normally lives in soil and eats bacteria such as *E. coli*. Worms contain rudimentary feeding, neural, and reproductive systems. *C. elegans* is quite easy to grow and can be frozen for long-term storage. Worms can even be maintained in 96-well plates for high-throughput analyses and genetic manipulations. For instance, worms parceled out among a large set of 96-well plates can be fed bacteria that express target-gene dsRNA for large-scale RNA interference (RNAi) experiments (Kamath and Ahringer 2003).

B. Flies

The fruit fly, *Drosophila melanogaster*, has played an influential role in genetics for almost a century. More recently, flies have been used to study neurodegeneration in Huntington (Apostol et al. 2003), Parkinson (Greene et al. 2003), and Alzheimer (Greeve et al. 2004) diseases. Defining pathological features such as Lewy bodies and amyloid plaques have been reproduced in *Drosophila. Drosophila* may be particular useful for the screening of candidate drugs for the prevention of neurodegenerative diseases and identification of genetic modifiers of disorders governed by classical Mendelian inheritance patterns.

The *Drosophila* life cycle begins when eggs are laid. Eggs develop into larvae that develop into pupae that develop into adult flies. Females can lay one hundred eggs in a day. At 25°C, the time from fertilization to the appearance of adult flies is about ten days. Female fruit flies can store sperm from several males; therefore, virgin females must be used for genetic crosses. *Drosophila* has three pairs of autosomes plus X- and Y-chromosomes. The entire *Drosophila* genome has been sequenced and contains approximately 13,600 predicted genes. Over half of the genes associated with human diseases have homologs in *Drosophila*.

Several powerful genetic tools and numerous online resources are available to the scientist interested in modeling human disorders with *Drosophila*. Transposable P-elements include the gene for the transposase enzyme that simplifies integration of DNA constructs within the *Drosophila* genome. The GAL4-UAS (upstream-activating sequence) system allows for precise spatial control of foreign gene expression, and tight temporal control of gene expression can be achieved with Tet-On transactivators. Online resources for *Drosophila* researchers include the Berkeley Drosophila Genome Project (http://www.bdgp.org/), FlyBase (http://flybase.bio.indiana.edu/), FlyBrain (http://flybrain.neurobio.arizona.edu/Flybrain/html/index.html), and the WWW Virtual Library: *Drosophila* (http://www.ceolas.org/VL/fly/).

C. Zebrafish

The zebrafish is indigenous to the rivers of India, northern Pakistan, and surrounding countries. This very inexpensive vertebrate has recently gained popularity as a model system for cardiovascular development since its embryogenesis is similar to that of higher vertebrates, including humans. Adult zebrafish are approximately one inch long. About two hundred eggs are laid in a single nesting and the transparent embryos develop into mature adults in three to four months. Females can lay eggs each week.

The large number of offspring, vertebrate physiological systems (e.g., cardiovascular, gastrointestinal, and neural), and embryo transparency make the zebrafish a useful organism to study developmental genetics. Zebrafish have 25 chromosomes and a 1.7 Mb genome. A preliminary draft of the zebrafish genome was published in 2001. Zebrafish may be superior to both worms and flies for whole organism high-throughput screening of drugs and environmental toxins because both *C. elegans* and *Drosophila* have tough cuticles that represent a diffusion barrier for many compounds. Adult zebrafish simply absorb compounds orally from tank water.

D. Mice

In recent years, mice have served as the foremost hosts for analyzing the role of genes in the production of human disease. Increasingly powerful methods for controlling the temporal and spatial expression of specific genes in mice have become standard practice at most major academic medical centers and universities. Transgenic and embryonic stem (ES) cell core facilities are the breeding grounds for many a grant application. These facilities typically offer services such as ES cell injection into blastocysts, ES cell electroporation, and DNA injection into zygotes.

Adult male mice weigh 20–40 grams. Females reach puberty in about two months. Litter sizes range from 5–10 but can be highly variable, particularly with inbred strains and genetically manipulated lines including transgenics and knock-outs. The phrase "reproductive fitness" encompasses parameters such as litter size, age at first mating, frequency of litters, and total number of litters per lifetime. Inbred strains show important differences in reproductive fitness, a fact that must be borne in mind when designing certain types of experiments.

The mouse genome has been sequenced. The vast majority of human genes have orthologs in mice and vice versa. Several human-mouse conserved synteny maps are available on the World Wide Web to explore these genetic relationships. Some of the numerous Web sites devoted to mouse genomics include http://www.informatics.jax.org/, http://www.mgu.har.mrc.ac.uk/, http://genome.ucsc.edu/, http://www.sanger.ac.uk/Projects/M_musculus/, and http://www.ncbi.nlm.nih.gov/genome/guide/mouse/. Highlighting the importance of mouse genomics is the fact that labs throughout the world have generated over 8,000 genetically engineered lines of mice to date.

E. Rats

Adult rats weigh about 300–440 grams and their brains are approximately four-fold heavier than those of mice (2 versus 0.45 grams). Rats are, in general, large enough so that procedures like vascular cannulation, mini-osmotic pump implantation, chronic neural recordings, and surgical procedures on major organ systems can be accomplished with relative ease. For these reasons, rats have long been the animal of choice for studies of cerebral ischemia and cardiovascular physiology.

Most rat strains are reliably fertile and females have litters of eight to fourteen pups. Pups can be weaned at twenty-one days of age and are capable of breeding another 1.5–2 months later. Common outbred strains of rats include Wistar, Long-Evans, Zucker, and Sprague-Dawley whereas Fisher, Lewis, Brown Norway, and SHR are frequently used inbred strains.

Rats have been used to model most neurological diseases (e.g., stroke, traumatic brain injury, epilepsy, and multiple sclerosis). In the field of movement disorders research, rat models have contributed significantly to the study of Parkinson disease, dystonia, spasticity, myoclonus, and tremor. Although dystonia and Parkinsonism may, at first glance, "look" different in primates and rats, more thoughtful characterization of the visuals will expose the prominent similarities in both normal and pathological movements among mammalian species. In this regard, Cenci and colleagues (2002) present legitimate arguments that the neuroanatomical and biomechanical underpinnings of movement are very similar among rats and primates.

F. Primates

Primates have played a central role in motor systems and movement disorders research because of their very close neuroanatomical and neurophysiological similarity to humans. Innumerable important electrophysiological-behavioral paradigms related to hand kinematics and binocular vision simply cannot be performed in other species. Studies of vergence mechanisms, for example, would not be practical in lateral-eyed rodents and rabbits. Primate models of movement disorders can also faithfully reproduce the clinical features of the corresponding human condition. The primate MPTP model, for example, exhibits all four cardinal signs of human Parkinson disease: resting tremor, rigidity, postural instability, and bradykinesia. Scientists could demonstrate marked reduction in specific neurological signs such as resting tremor and rigidity with lesions of the subthalamic nucleus (STN) in the primate MPTP model, and this evidence helped form an experimental foundation for the highly successful application of STN deep brain stimulation in patients with Parkinson disease (Wichmann et al. 1994).

Although most primate research in the neurosciences has employed rhesus macaques, other macaque species and non-macaque primates may be applied quite suitably to a variety of hypotheses relevant to the study of movement disorders. Advantages of rhesus macaques include their substantial physical size, intelligence, and the large body of existing neuroanatomical data. Thus, it is likely that rhesus macaques will remain the primate of choice for combined behavioral-electrophysiological studies of the oculomotor system, higher-order visual processing, and fine-motor control of the digits. Another Old World monkey, the cynomolgus macaque, is genetically and behaviorally akin to the rhesus monkey, although it is smaller. Cynomolgus macaques are typically less expensive than rhesus monkeys and have been used to model Parkinson disease. The African green monkey or vervet, another Old World monkey, has also been used for motor systems research and as an MPTP model of Parkinson disease.

Although New World primates are not as closely related to humans as Old World primates, such primates as squirrel monkeys, owl monkeys, and marmosets have several attractive features in the context of movement disorders research. First, New World monkeys are small, relatively inexpensive, and more economical to house and feed than macaques. Second, unlike Old World monkeys, New World monkeys do not carry the herpes B virus and, as such, pose much less risk to caretakers. Third, several New World monkeys, particularly marmosets, have great reproductive capacity such that colony numbers can be readily increased in response to research demands. Because large breeding colonies of squirrel monkeys, owl monkeys, and marmosets are maintained in the United States, importation from South and Central America is not necessary.

III. EXPERIMENTAL APPROACHES

A. Top-down Approach

As depicted in Figure 1, the "top-down approach" to movement disorders research is a practical way to envision the complex interrelationships between patients, clinics, laboratories, and animal models. The patient is, quite fittingly, the "top" priority in this schematic. In the context of movement disorders attributable to mutant genes, most scientists would describe the central aspects of the top-down approach as "reverse genetics." In reverse genetics, genes are mutated in defined ways and then scientists examine the effects of these alterations on phenotype. As shown in Figure 1, it is often necessary to move directly from a human phenotype to a "non-genetic" animal model. Idiopathic Parkinson disease is a notable example of this situation. Although mutations in the genes for α-synuclein, parkin, and DJ-1 have received a great deal of attention, only a very small percentage of patients with Parkinson disease harbor mutations in these genes. Irrespective of genetics, the defining phenotypic feature of Parkinson disease is loss of dopaminergic neurons in the substantia nigra pars compacta (SNpc). The MPTP and 6-OHDA models reproduce many of the key pathological and behavioral features of Parkinson disease and have been employed in hypothesis-driven functional experiments for years.

In many neurological disorders, phenotypic expansion occurs once causal genes are identified. Examples of this phenomenon have been common in the field of dystonia research. For years, scientists had recognized the classic phenotype of Segawa syndrome (i.e., lower extremity action dystonia in young girls that improves dramatically with L-dopa) prior to identifying causal mutations in the gene that encodes the enzyme GTP cyclohydrolase I. Subsequent clinical-genetic correlative studies have shown that Parkinsonism, spasticity, and cervical dystonia can also be associated with mutations in the same gene. Phenotypic expansion has also occurred since identification of the mutant genes accountable for Oppenheim dystonia and the myoclonus-dystonia syndrome.

Either positional cloning or "quantitative" genetics can be used to discover disease-related genes. If the gene is novel, analysis of its transcript(s) and encoded protein(s) is the next step in the top-down approach. Because these and most subsequent experiments are best performed in animals, an important early step in the top-down approach is to identify orthologs in other species.

Movement disorders research can cover the entire spectrum of science and, as such, holds promise for investigators with expertise in almost any plane of analysis. At one end of the spectrum, the psychosocial and public health consequences of movement disorders are substantial and poorly understood. At the other end of the spectrum, we still do not know the three-dimensional structures of many proteins relevant to the study of movement disorders. Animal models are frequently needed to address hypotheses that fall between these extremes. Through the application of animal models, behaviorists, physiologists, neurochemists, and molecular biologists can all contribute to our understanding of movement disorders and motor systems.

B. Bottom-up Approach

The "bottom-up" approach begins with animals, most commonly rodents. The bottom-up approach as outlined in Figure 2 includes forward genetics as its starting point. A spontaneous mutation may manifest itself as a gait abnormality in a breeding colony of rats, for example. On closer

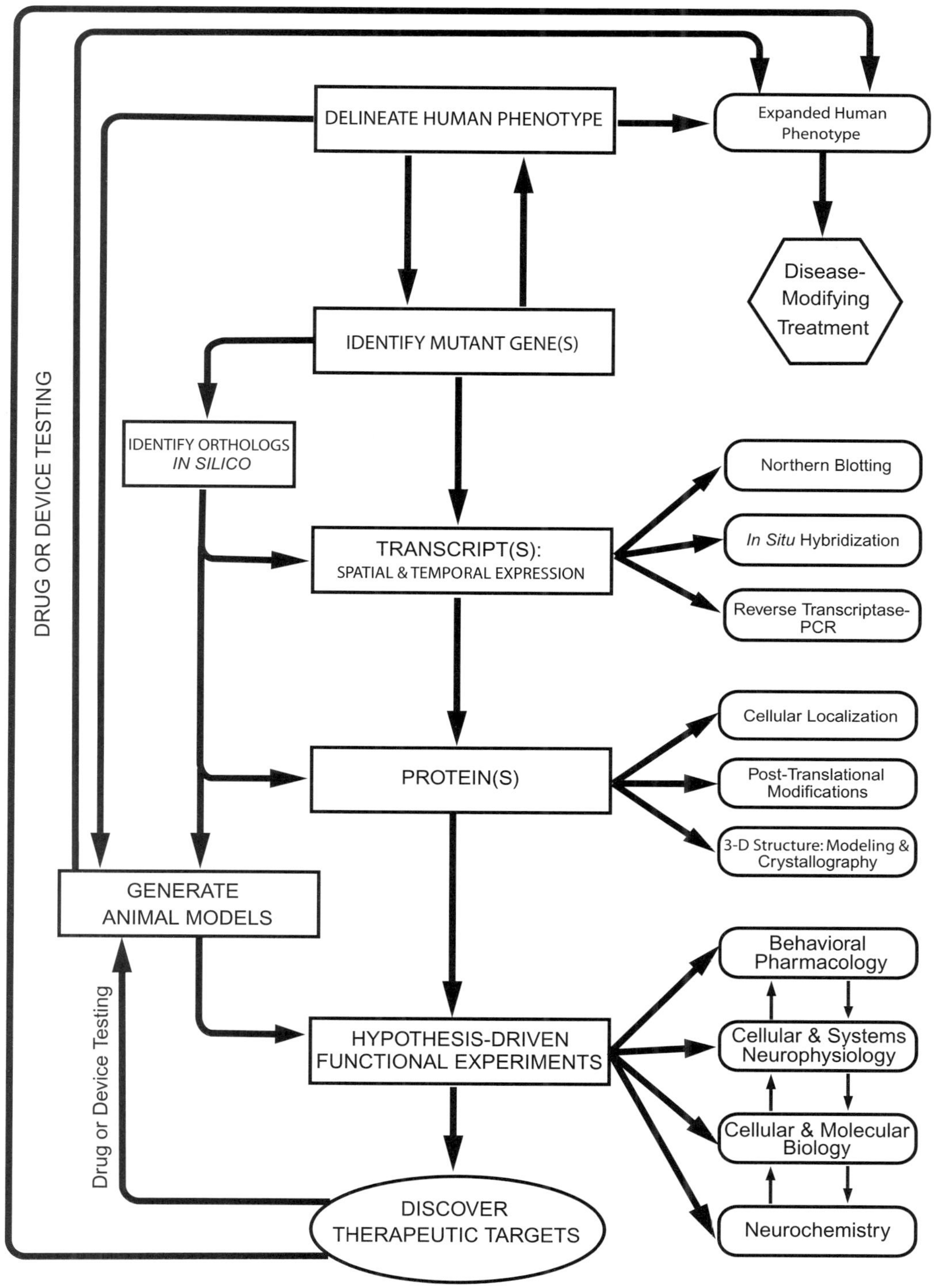

FIGURE 1 Top-Down Approach to the Study of Movement Disorders with Animal Models.

inspection, the mutant rats may exhibit ataxia, dystonia, neuropathy, or musculoskeletal defects. Alternatively, mutations can be purposefully generated with chemical agents or gene trap vectors. Various screens are then applied in an effort to detect a phenotype. The behavioral, neurochemical, or pathological phenotype of the mutant animals may be compatible with a human movement or neurodegenerative disorder and, accordingly, could be a useful model.

Several genes initially identified in mice as causally linked to neurological dysfunction were subsequently iden-

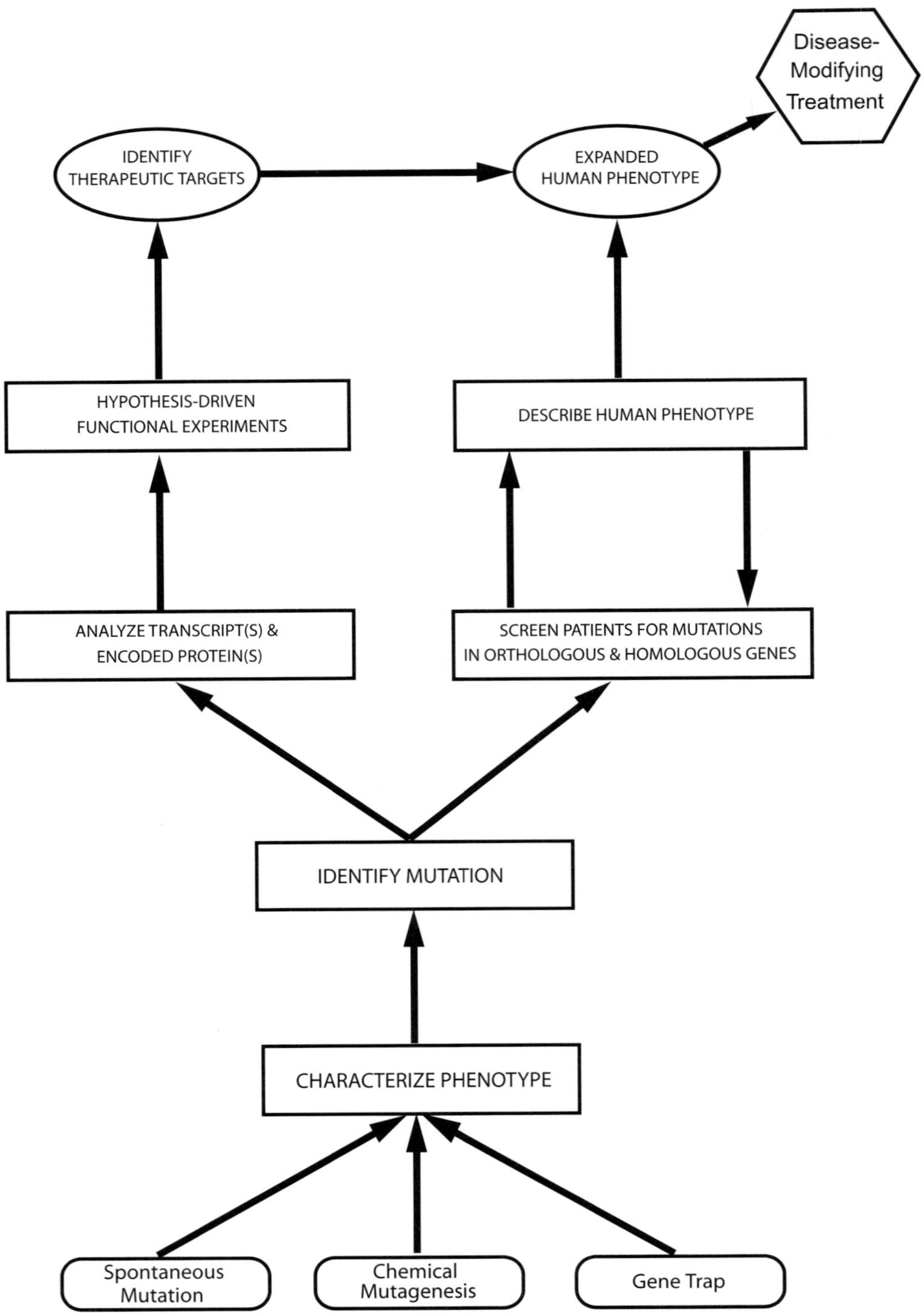

FIGURE 2 Bottom-Up Approach to the Study of Movement Disorders with Animal Models.

tified in patients with phenotypically similar conditions. Examples include reelin in reeler mice, the α-1 subunit of the voltage-gated calcium channel in leaner mice, and the β-subunit of the glycine receptor in spastic mice. A major advantage of the bottom-up approach may be the identification of genes potentially associated with rare, sporadic, or recessive movement disorders in which more classical genetic approaches are typically not possible.

IV. DISORDER-SPECIFIC ANIMAL MODELS

A partial compilation of disorder-specific animal models is provided in tables 2 and 3. Table 2 contains basic information on both engineered and spontaneous genetic models. Table 3 provides a list of models generated pharmacologically, via neurotoxin administration or through the creation of discrete neural lesions. Criteria for inclusion of tremor

TABLE 2 Selected Genetic Models of Movement Disorders

Disorder	Species	Description	Genetic & molecular characteristics	Key phenotypic features	References
Parkinson Disease	mouse	quaking	spontaneous deletion of 1.17 Mb of Ch. 17 affecting the qk gene, parkin co-regulated (PACRG) gene, & promoter and 1st 5 exons of the parkin (PRKN) gene	central & peripheral dysmyelination, action tremor, seizures	Sidman et al. 1964; Lockhart et al. 2004
	mouse	parkin knock-out	homozygotes do not express parkin	SNpc intact, no gross movement disorder, defects on some behavioral paradigms, increased striatal extracellular dopamine	Goldberg et al. 2003
	mouse	α-synuclein knock-out	homozygotes do not express α-synuclein	no gross movement disorder, SNpc intact, reduced striatal dopamine, increased dopamine release with paired-pulse stimuli	Abeliovich et al. 2000
	mouse	wild-type human α-synuclein transgenic	murine platelet-derived growth factor promoter	nuclear & cytoplasmic inclusions in cortex, hippocampus & SNpc, rotarod deficits at 1 yr	Masliah et al. 2000
	mouse	wild-type & A53T human α-synuclein transgenic	murine Thy-1 promoter	transgene not expressed in SNpc, prominent degeneration of brainstem & spinal cord motoneurons, motor abnormalities by 3 wks of age	van der Putten et al. 2000
	mouse	A53T α-synuclein transgenic	human A53T α-synuclein variant under direction of the mouse prion protein promoter	adult mice (>8 mo) develop progressive paresis & intracytoplasmic inclusions	Giasson et al. 2002
	fly	human wild-type, A30P & A53T α-synuclein transgenic lines	tissue expression requires transcriptional activation by GAL4	age-dependent loss of dopaminergic neurons, Lewy body-like inclusions & locomotor impairment in all lines	Feaney & Bender 2002
	worm	human wild-type & A53T α-synuclein transgenic lines	both pan-neuronal & motor neuron promoters were used	dopamine cell loss & motor deficits with both wild-type & A53T human α-synuclein	Lakso et al. 2003
Dystonia	mouse	dystonia musculorum mouse	spontaneous mutation in the *Bpag1* gene, which encodes a neural isoform of the human bullous pemphigoid antigen, a hemidesmosomal protein	severe generalized dystonia, abnormal central & peripheral myelination	Duchen 1976
	mouse	leaner	splice site mutation near 3′ end of the *Cacna1a* gene that encodes the α_{1A} pore-forming subunit of the voltage-gated P/Q-type calcium channel	severe generalized dystonia; ataxia	Yoon 1969
	mouse	tottering	missense mutation in the pore-forming domain of the α_{1A}-subunit of the voltage-gated P/Q-type calcium channel	paroxysmal dystonia superimposed on mild baseline ataxia	Fletcher et al. 1996

(continues)

TABLE 2 *(continued)*

Disorder	Species	Description	Genetic & molecular characteristics	Key phenotypic features	References
	mouse	α_{1A}-subunit knock-out mice	*Cacna1a* gene encodes the α_{1A} pore-forming subunit of the high voltage-gated P/Q-type calcium channel	severe generalized dystonia; without intervention die by 3–4 wks of age	Jun et al. 1999; Fletcher et al. 2001
	mouse	Wriggle mouse sagami	a point mutation the *Pmca2* gene, a plasma membrane Ca2+-ATPase	deaf by 1 month of age; complex movement disorder that includes dystonia	Takahashi & Kitamura 1999
	mouse	*med*^{J} mice	4 bp splice site deletion in *Scn8A* which encodes the Nav1.6 sodium channel	head tremor, axial dystonia, muscle weakness	Hamann et al. 2003
	mouse	torsinA knock-out	mouse torsinA null mutation	early neonatal death	Dauer & Goodchild 2004
	rat	genetically dystonic rat	unknown	severe progressive generalized dystonia, olivocerebellar functional abnormalities	Lorden et al. 1984
Huntington Disease	mouse	"R6/2 mice," 5′ end of human IT15 with >200-repeats	transgene includes human promoter, CAG repeat unstable	locomotor & behavioral defects by 6 wks	Mangiarini et al. 1996
	mouse	72-repeat full-length human huntingtin transgenic	YAC containing full-length human huntingtin gene & endogenous promoter was modified with a 72 CAG repeat expansion in exon 1	mild hyperkinetic movement disorder by 7 months, degeneration of medium spiny neurons	Hodgson et al. 1999
	mouse	82-, 44-, or 18-repeat N-terminal human huntingtin transgenics	transgene includes mouse prion protein promoter	82-repeat huntingtin mice exhibit early behavioral & motor abnormalities, intranuclear inclusions	Schiling et al. 1999
	mouse	100-repeat human huntingtin transgenic	transgenic construct containing bases 316–3210 of human huntingtin cDNA with a 100 CAG repeat insertion under control of the rat neuron-specific enolase promoter	behavioral abnormalities & nuclear inclusions by 3–6 months in hemizygous mice	Laforet et al. 2001
	mouse	Hdh(Q92) & Hdh(Q111) mice	knock-in mice with targeted insertion of a chimeric human–mouse exon 1 with 90 & 109 CAG repeats	late-onset neurodegeneration & motor abnormalities	Wheeler et al. 2000
	fly	22 & 108 polyglutamine transgenics	22 or 108 polyQ peptides flanked by very short amino acid sequences under control of the GAL4-UAS system	128 polyQ peptide markedly reduced fly viability, toxicity of polyQ peptides depends on protein context	Marsh et al. 2000
	worm	128-, 88-, & 19-repeat N-terminal human huntingtin transgenic	polyQ fused to fluorescent marker proteins & expressed in six touch receptor neurons	expanded polyQs produced touch insensitivity in young animals	Parker et al. 2001
Tremor	Pietrain pig	campus syndrome	unknown	high-frequency (14–15 Hz) tremor, myopathy	Richter et al. 1995
	mouse	trembler	AD missense mutation in peripheral myelin protein gene (PMP-22)	axial action tremor, seizures, progressive quadriparesis, severe peripheral demyelination	Suter et al. 1992

(continues)

TABLE 2 *(continued)*

Disorder	Species	Description	Genetic & molecular characteristics	Key phenotypic features	References
	mouse	vibrator	AR intronic insertional mutation-phosphatidylinositol transfer protein alpha	action tremor, brainstem & spinal cord degeneration	Hamilton et al. 1997
	mouse	shiverer	AR mutation in the myelin base protein gene, *Mbp*	generalized tremor worse with locomotion, severe CNS & moderate PNS myelin deficiency	Roach et al. 1985
	mouse	jimpy	X-linked mutation in gene for myelin-associated proteolipid protein	action tremor of hind limbs, severe CNS myelin deficiency	Dautigny et al. 1986
	mouse	$GABA_A$ receptor α-1 subunit knockout	homozygotes do not express the $GABA_A$ receptor α-1 subunit	action tremor with both postural & kinetic components	Kralic et al. 2002
	rat	zitter	AR, 8-bp deletion at a splice donor site of *Atrn* (attraction)	generalized tremor, spongiform CNS pathology	Kuramoto et al. 2001
Myoclonus	mouse	cystatin B knock-out (progressive myoclonic epilepsy)	*Cstb* knock-out	myoclonus, ataxia, apoptosis of cerebellar granule cells	Pennacchio et al. 1998
	mouse	β3 subunit of $GABA_A$ receptor knock-out	*Gabrb3* knock-out	myoclonus, hyperactivity, locomotor deficits, occasional seizures, cleft palate	Homanics et al. 1997
	baboon	*Paio paio*—reticular reflex myoclonus	unknown	reticular reflex myoclonus, epilepsy	Rektor et al. 1993
Tourette Syndrome/Tics	mouse	transgenic model of co-morbid Tourette syndrome & obsessive-compulsive disorder (OCD)	mice express cholera toxin A1 subunit within cortical-limbic dopamine D1-receptor expressing neurons	tics, OCD-like behaviors	Nordstrom & Burton 2002
Paroxysmal Movement Disorders	mouse	fibroblast growth factor 14 (FGF14)-deficient mice	FGF14 knock-out; N-β-gal inserted after exon 1	ataxia, young animals exhibit paroxysmal dystonia	Wang et al. 2002
	hamster	model of paroxysmal non-kinesigenic dyskinesia	unknown	paroxysmal attacks of generalized dystonia precipitated by environmental stressors	Loscher et al. 1989
	mouse	transgenic hyperexplexia mouse	mutant human glycine receptor α-1 subunit 271Q	hyperexplexia	Becker et al. 2002
	cow	bovine hyperexplexia	nonsense mutation in exon 2 of the glycine receptor α-1 gene	hyperexplexia	Pierce et al. 2001
PSP/CBGD	mouse	mutant tau transgenic	mice overexpress human P301L mutant tau	motor, behavioral, & pathological abnormalities present by 4.5 months in homozygous animals	Lewis et al. 2000
Multiple System Atrophy	mouse	wild-type human α-synuclein transgenic (line M)	murine Thy-1 promoter	human α-synuclein expression in glial cells	Rockenstein et al. 2002
	mouse	transgenic overexpression of α_{1B}-adrenergic receptors	isogenic α_{1B}-receptor promoter	parkinsonism, seizures, granulovacuolar neuro-degeneration, oligodendroglial & neuronal inclusions	Zuscik et al. 2000

(continues)

TABLE 2 *(continued)*

Disorder	Species	Description	Genetic & molecular characteristics	Key phenotypic features	References
	mouse	wild-type human α-synuclein expressed in oligodendroglia	proteolipid protein promoter	glial cytoplasmic inclusions, hyper-phosphorylation of α-synuclein at S129	Kahle et al. 2002
Ataxia	rat	shaker	X-linked	ataxia, generalized tremor, Purkinje cell degeneration	Clark et al. 2000
	mouse	lurcher	G-to-A transitions that change a highly conserved alanine to a threonine residue in transmembrane domain III of the glutamate receptor ionotropic delta 2 (*Grid2*)	heterozygotes ataxic, homozygotes die shortly after birth	Zuo et al. 1997
	mouse	Purkinje cell degeneration (*pcd*)	homozygous mutations in *Agtpbp1*, ATP/GTP binding protein 1	moderately severe ataxia beginning at 3–4 weeks, rapid degeneration of Purkinje cells during 3rd postnatal week	Fernandez-Gonzalez et al. 2002
	mouse	SCA1 knock-in	insertion of expanded CAG tract into the mouse Sca1 locus	intergenerational repeat instability, impaired rotarod performance, no inclusion formation	Lorenzetti et al. 2000
	fly	SCA1 transgenic	full-length human *SCA1* gene	genetic modifiers of neurodegeneration involved in RNA processing & transcriptional regulation	Fernandez-Funez et al. 2000
	mouse	SCA7 transgenic	rhodopsin promoter	photoreceptor dysfunction	Helmlinger et al. 2004
	mouse	Friedreich ataxia, heterozygous knock-in	230-GAA frataxin gene repeat mice crossed with frataxin knock-out mice	double heterozygous mice with 30% of wild-type frataxin levels, no motor abnormalities	Miranda et al. 2002
	mouse	SCA2 transgenic	full-length human ataxin-2 with Q22 or Q58, Purkinje cell specific promoter (*Pcp2*)	decreased stride-length & impaired rotarod performance in Q58 transgenics	Huynh et al. 2000
Spasticity	mouse	spastin knock-out	deletion of SPG4 exons 5 to 7	gait abnormality & impaired rotarod performance in older mice	Fassier et al. 2003
	mouse	paraplegin knock-out	deletion of SPG7	impaired rotarod performance at 6 months, mitochondrial & axonal pathology	Ferreirinha et al. 2001
	mouse	cell adhesion molecule (CAM) L1 knock-out	deletion of the *L1CAM* gene	abnormal corticospinal tract development	Cohen et al. 1998

SCA, spinocerebellar ataxia.

TABLE 3 Selected Pharmacological and Neural Lesion Models of Movement Disorders

Disorder	Species	Description of lesion	Key features	References
Parkinson Disease	mouse, rat, monkey	6-OHDA	spontaneous rotation towards lesioned side, dopamine receptor agonists produce rotation towards unlesioned side	Mendez & Finn 1975
	roundworm	6-OHDA; dopaminergic neurons express GFP under control of the dopamine transporter	dopamine cell loss	Nass et al. 2002
	monkey	intravenous MPTP	SNpc cell loss, all cardinal features of Parkinson disease	Burns et al. 1983
	mouse	systemic MPTP	Parkinsonism, SNpc cell loss	Gupta et al. 1986
	rat	systemic administration of rotenone	bradykinesia, rigidity, Lewy body-like inclusions	Betarbet et al. 2000
	mouse	chronic systemic administration of the herbicide paraquat and fungicide maneb	reduced locomotor activity & coordination, neuronal loss in the SNpc	Thiruchelvam et al. 2003
Parkinson Disease: Dyskinesias	rat	unilateral 6-OHDA lesions followed by daily injections of either L-dopa or the dopamine agonist bromocriptine	L-dopa-treated animals develop axial, limb, & orolingual dyskinesias	Lundblad et al. 2002
	monkey	L-dopa treatment of MPTP lesioned monkeys	5-HT_{1A} receptor agonist sarizotan reduced L-dopa-induced dyskinesias	Bibbiani et al. 2001
Dystonia	mouse	injection of kainic acid into cerebellar cortex	generalized dystonia	Pizoli et al. 2002
	mouse	systemic administration of L-type calcium channel agonists	generalized dystonia	Jinnah et al. 2002
	rat	injection of sigma receptor ligands into the red nucleus	dystonia	Walker et al. 1988
	rat	partial unilateral 6-OHDA lesion of the SNpc & partial unilateral denervation of the orbicularis oculi muscle	blepharospasm	Schicatano et al. 1997
	cat	unilateral injection of serotonin into the facial motor nucleus	unilateral blepharospasm, hemifacial spasm	LeDoux et al. 1998
	monkey	electrolytic lesions—medial midbrain tegmentum	contraversive torticollis	Foltz et al. 1959
	monkey	lesions of mesencephalic tegmentum	ipsiversive torticollis	Battista et al. 1976
	monkey (marmoset)	6-OHDA lesion ascending nigrostriatal pathway	ipsiversive torticollis that resolved with apomorphine	Sambrook et al. 1979
Huntington Disease	rat	intrastriatal injection of kainic acid	enhanced locomotor & stereotypy responses to amphetamine	Coyle & Schwarcz 1976
	rat	intrastriatal injection of quinolinic acid	hyperactivity, weight loss	Sanberg et al. 1989
Tremor	mouse, rat, rabbit, cat, monkey	harmaline	generalized 8–14 Hz tremor, accentuated by movement, ataxia	Montigny & Lamarre 1973
	primate	ventromedial tegmental lesions involving parvocellular red nucleus, cerebellothalamic fibers, & nigrostriatal fibers	Holmes tremor	Ohye et al. 1988
	rat	oxotremorine (a muscarinic agonist)	high-amplitude, high-frequency generalized tremor	Miwa et al. 2000
	monkey	lesions of dentate and/or superior cerebellar penduncle	intention tremor	Walker & Botterell 1937; Vilis & Hore 1977

(continues)

TABLE 3 *(continued)*

Disorder	Species	Description of lesion	Key features	References
Myoclonus	rat	urea infusions	reticular reflex myoclonus	Muscatt et al. 1986
	rat	mechanically induced cardiac arrest	auditory stimulus-induced myoclonus	Truong et al. 2000
Tourette Syndrome/Tics	rat	sera from patients with Tourette syndrome infused into ventrolateral striatum bilaterally	significant increase in oral stereotypies	Taylor et al. 2002
Multiple System Atrophy	mouse	sequential systemic administration of 3-nitroproprionic acid & MPTP	marked reduction in spontaneous nocturnal locomotor activity	Stefanova et al. 2003
Ataxia	monkey	muscimol injections into the ventrolateral corner of the cerebellar posterior interpositus nucleus	hypermetric upward & hypometric downward saccades	Robinson 2000
	monkey	muscimol injections into dentate & lateral interposed cerebellar nuclei	degradation of natural unconstrained arm/hand/digit movements	Goodkin & Thach 2003
Spasticity	rat	cord transection at the S2 sacral level	tail hypertonia, hyperreflexia, & clonus	Bennett et al. 1999
	rat	mid-thoracic spinal cord contusion injury	paraparesis, cystic central cord cavitation	Thompson et al. 2001
Drug-Induced Movement Disorders	rat	akathisia modeled by treating rats in a well-habituated environment with neuroleptic drugs	increased emotional defecation	Sachdev & Saharov 1998
	monkey	re-exposure to the neuroleptic fluphenazine decanoate	acute oral-buccal-lingual dyskinesias, acute cervical dystonia	Linn et al. 2001
	rat	chronic haloperidol treatment	slowed rhythm during water licking	Fowler & Wang 1998
	monkey (marmoset)	haloperidol treatment for one year followed by alternating three-month drug-free & treatment periods	tardive oral-buccal-lingual dyskinesias & appendicular tardive chorea	Klintenberg et al. 2002
Restless Legs Syndrome/ Periodic Limb Movements	rat	bilateral 6-OHDA lesions of A11 dopaminergic diencephalic neurons	increased standing time & standing episodes in lesioned rats	Ondo et al. 2000
	rat	none	periodic hind limb movements were detected in a subset of aged rats	Baier et al. 2002
	cat	bilateral NMDA lesions of the retrorubral nucleus & ventral mesopontine junction	rhythmic leg movements or myoclonic twitches developed in all lesioned animals	Lai & Siegel 1997

GFP, green fluorescent protein; OHDA, hydroxydopamine; NMDA, *N*-methyl-D-aspartic acid; SNpc, substantia nigra pars compacta.

and ataxia models were most problematic since secondary etiologies for these disorders are so common. For example, a search for the word "ataxia" with JAXMice generated over one hundred results. In addition, a virtually endless list of drugs can produce ataxia in animals. Nearly all drugs used to treat epilepsy (e.g., phenytoin, carbamazepine, gabapentin, valproic acid, and phenobarbital) can cause ataxia when used at the high end of their dosage ranges. In tables 2 and 3, no attempt was made to list either every species used to model the effects of a particular drug or every minor variation in genetically engineered mice (e.g., different promoters, polyglutamine tract lengths). Harmaline, for instance, has been shown to produce a tremor in mice, rats, cats, primates, rabbits, and ungulates. Additional models of movement disorders can be found on the World Wide Web at sites maintained by BioMedNet (http://research.bmn.com/mkmd; Mouse Knock-out and Mutation Database) and the Jackson Laboratories (http://jaxmice.jax.org/models/index.html; Research Models).

Acknowledgments

MSL has been supported by grants from the National Institutes of Health (K08 NS 01593 & R01 EY12232), Dystonia Medical Research Foundation, and Center for Genomics and Bioinformatics at the University of Tennessee Health Science Center.

References

Abeliovich, A., Y. Schmitz, I. Farinas, D. Choi-Lundberg, W.H. Ho, P.E. Castillo, N. Shinsky, et al. 2000. Mice lacking alpha-synuclein display functional deficits in the nigrostriatal dopamine system. *Neuron* **25**:239–252.

Apostol, B.L., A. Kazantsev, S. Raffioni, K. Illes, J. Pallos, L. Bodai, N. Slepko, et al. 2003. A cell-based assay for aggregation inhibitors as therapeutics of polyglutamine-repeat disease and validation in *Drosophila*. *Proc Natl Acad Sci U S A* **100**:5950–5955.

Baier, P.C., J. Winkelmann, A. Hohne, M. Lancel, and C. Trenkwalder. 2002. Assessment of spontaneously occurring periodic limb movements in sleep in the rat. *J Neurol Sci* **198**:71–77.

Betarbet, R., T.B. Sherer, G. MacKenzie, M. Garcia-Osuna, A.V. Panov, and J.T. Greenamyre. 2000. Chronic systemic pesticide exposure reproduces features of Parkinson's disease. *Nat Neurosci* **3**:1301–1306.

Battista, A.F., M. Goldstein, T. Miyamoto, and Y. Matsumoto. 1976. Effect of centrally acting drugs on experimental torticollis in monkeys. *Adv Neurol* **14**:329–338.

Becker, L., J. von Wegerer, J. Schenkel, H.U. Zeilhofer, D. Swandulla, and H. Weiher. 2002. Disease-specific human glycine receptor alpha1 subunit causes hyperexplexia phenotype and impaired glycine- and GABA(A)-receptor transmission in transgenic mice. *J Neurosci* **22**: 2505–2512.

Bennett, D.J., M. Gorassini, K. Fouad, L. Sanelli, Y. Han, and J. Cheng. 1999. Spasticity in rats with sacral spinal cord injury. *J Neurotrauma* **16**:69–84.

Bibbiani, F., J.D. Oh, and T.N. Chase. 2001. Serotonin 5-HT1A agonist improves motor complications in rodent and primate parkinsonian models. *Neurology* **57**:1829–34.

Burns, R.S., C.C. Chiueh, S.P. Markey, M.H. Ebert, D.M. Jacobowitz, and I.J. Kopin. 1983. A primate model of parkinsonism: selective destruction of dopaminergic neurons in the pars compacta of the substantia nigra by *N*-methyl-4-phenyl-1,2,3,6-tetrahydropyridine. *Proc Natl Acad Sci U S A* **890**:4564–4550.

Cenci, M.A., I.Q. Whishaw, and T. Schallert. 2002. Animal models of neurological deficits: how relevant is the rat? *Nat Rev Neurosci* **3**:574–579.

Clark, B.R., M. LaRegina, and D.L. Tolbert. 2000. X-linked transmission of the shaker mutation in rats with hereditary Purkinje cell degeneration and ataxia. *Brain Res* **858**:264–273.

Cohen, N.R., J.S. Taylor, L.B. Scott, R.W. Guillery, P. Soriano, and A.J. Furley. 1998. Errors in corticospinal axon guidance in mice lacking the neural cell adhesion molecule L1. *Curr Biol* **8**:26–33.

Coyle, J.T., and R. Schwarcz. 1976. Lesion of striatal neurones with kainic acid provides a model for Huntington's chorea. *Nature* **263**:244–246.

Dauer, W., and R. Goodchild. 2004. Mouse models of torsinA dysfunction. *Adv Neurol* **94**:67–72.

Dautigny, A., M.G. Mattei, D. Morello, P.M. Alliel, D. Pham-Dinh, L. Amar, D. Arnaud, D. Simon, J.F. Mattei, J.L. Guenet, and P. Avner. 1986. The structural gene coding for myelin-associated proteolipid protein is mutated in jimpy mice. *Nature* **321**:867–869.

Duchen, L.W. 1976. Dystonia musculorum—an inherited disease of the nervous system in the mouse. *Adv Neurol* **14**:353–365.

Fassier, C., A. Tarrade, D. Charvin, et al. 2003. Generation and characterization of mouse models of spastic paraplegia caused by mutation of SPG4 gene. *Am J Hum Genet* **73**:547 (Abstract).

Feany, M.B., and W.W. Bender. 2000. A *Drosophila* model of Parkinson's disease. *Nature* **404**:394–398.

Fernandez-Funez, P., M.L. Nino-Rosales, B. de Gouyon, W.C. She, J.M. Luchak, P. Martinez, E. Turiegano, et al. 2000. Identification of genes that modify ataxin-1-induced neurodegeneration. *Nature* **408**:101–106.

Fernandez-Gonzalez, A., A.R. La Spada, J. Treadaway, H.C. Higdon, B.S. Harris, R.L. Sidman, J.L. Morgan, and J. Zuo. 2002. Purkinje cell degeneration (pcd) phenotypes caused by mutations in the axotomy-induced gene, Nna1. *Science* **295**:1904–1906.

Ferreirinha, F., A. Quattrini, V. Valsecchi, A. Errico, A. Ballabio, and E. Rugarli. 2001. Mice lacking paraplegin, a mitochondrial AAA protease involved in hereditary spastic paraplegia, show axonal degeneration and abnormal mitochondria. *Am J Hum Genet* **69**(suppl):196 (Abstract).

Fletcher, C.F., C.M. Lutz, T.N. O'Sullivan, J.D. Shaughnessy, R. Hawkes, W.N. Frankel, N.G. Copeland, and N.A. Jenkins. 1996. Absence epilepsy in tottering mutant mice is associated with calcium channel defects. *Cell* **87**:607–617.

Fletcher, C.F., A. Tottene, V.A. Lennon, S.M. Wilson, S.J. Dubel, R. Paylor, D.A. Hosford, et al. 2001. Dystonia and cerebellar atrophy in Cacna1a null mice lacking P/Q calcium channel activity. *FASEB J* **15**:1288–1290.

Foltz, E.L., L.M. Knopp, and A.A. Ward Jr. 1959. Experimental spasmodic torticollis. *Neurosurg* **16**:55–67.

Fowler, S.C., and G. Wang. 1998. Chronic haloperidol produces a time- and dose-related slowing of lick rhythm in rats: implications for rodent models of tardive dyskinesia and neuroleptic-induced parkinsonism. *Psychopharmacology (Berl)* **137**:50–60.

Giasson, B.I., J.E. Duda, S.M. Quinn, B. Zhang, J.Q. Trojanowski, and V.M. Lee. 2002. Neuronal alpha-synucleinopathy with severe movement disorder in mice expressing A53T human alpha-synuclein. *Neuron* **34**:521–533.

Goldberg, M.S., S.M. Fleming, J.J. Palacino, C. Cepeda, H.A. Lam, A. Bhatnagar, E.G. Meloni, et al. 2003. Parkin-deficient mice exhibit nigrostriatal deficits but not loss of dopaminergic neurons. *J Biol Chem* **278**:43628–43635.

Goodkin, H.P., and W.T. Thach. 2003. Cerebellar control of constrained and unconstrained movements. I. Nuclear inactivation. *J Neurophysiol* **89**: 884–895.

Greene, J.C., A.J. Whitworth, I. Kuo, L.A. Andrews, M.B. Feany, and L.J. Pallanck. 2003. Mitochondrial pathology and apoptotic muscle degeneration in *Drosophila* parkin mutants. *Proc Natl Acad Sci U S A* **100**: 4078–4083.

Greeve, I., D. Kretzschmar, J.A. Tschape, A. Beyn, C. Brellinger, M. Schweizer, R.M. Nitsch, and R. Reifegerste. 2004. Age-dependent neurodegeneration and Alzheimer-amyloid plaque formation in transgenic *Drosophila*. *J Neurosci* **24**:3899–3906.

Gupta, M., B.K. Gupta, R. Thomas, V. Bruemmer, J.R. Sladek Jr, and D.L. Felten. 1986. Aged mice are more sensitive to 1-methyl-4-phenyl-1,2,3,6-tetrahydropyridine treatment than young adults. *Neurosci Lett* **70**:326–331.

Hamann, M., M.H. Meisler, and A. Richter. 2003. Motor disturbances in mice with deficiency of the sodium channel gene Scn8a show features of human dystonia. *Exp Neurol* **184**:830–838.

Hamilton, B.A., D.J. Smith, K.L. Mueller, A.W. Kerrebrock, R.T. Bronson, V. van Berkel, M.J. Daly, et al. 1997. The vibrator mutation causes neurodegeneration via reduced expression of PITP alpha: positional complementation cloning and extragenic suppression. *Neuron* **18**:711–722.

Hamre, K., R. Tharp, K. Poon, X. Xiong, and R.J. Smeyne. 1999. Differential strain susceptibility following 1-methyl-4-phenyl-1,2,3,6-tetrahydropyridine (MPTP) administration acts in an autosomal dominant fashion: quantitative analysis in seven strains of *Mus musculus*. *Brain Res* **828**:91–103.

Helmlinger, D., G. Abou-Sleymane, G. Yvert, S. Rousseau, C. Weber, Y. Trottier, J.L. Mandel, and D. Devys. 2004. Disease progression despite early loss of polyglutamine protein expression in SCA7 mouse model. *J Neurosci* **24**:1881–1887.

Hodgson, J.G., N. Agopyan, C.A. Gutekunst, B.R. Leavitt, F. LePiane, R. Singaraja, D.J. Smith, et al. 1999. A YAC mouse model for Huntington's disease with full-length mutant huntingtin, cytoplasmic toxicity, and selective striatal neurodegeneration. *Neuron* **23**:181–192.

Homanics, G.E., T.M. DeLorey, L.L. Firestone, J.J. Quinlan, A. Handforth, N.L. Harrison, M.D. Krasowski, et al. 1997. Mice devoid of gamma-aminobutyrate type A receptor beta3 subunit have epilepsy, cleft palate, and hypersensitive behavior. *Proc Natl Acad Sci U S A* **94**:4143–4148.

Huynh, D.P., K. Figueroa, N. Hoang, and S.M. Pulst 2000. Nuclear localization or inclusion body formation of ataxin-2 are not necessary for SCA2 pathogenesis in mouse or human. *Nat Genet* **26**:44–50.

Jinnah, H.A., J.P. Sepkuty, T. Ho, S. Yitta, T. Drew, J.D. Rothstein, and E.J. Hess. 2000. Calcium channel agonists and dystonia in the mouse. *Mov Disord* **15**:542–551.

Jun, K., E.S. Piedras-Renteria, S.M. Smith, D.B. Wheeler, S.B. Lee, T.G. Lee, H. Chin, et al. 1999. Ablation of P/Q-type Ca(2+) channel currents, altered synaptic transmission, and progressive ataxia in mice lacking the alpha(1A)-subunit. *Proc Natl Acad Sci U S A* **96**:15245–15250.

Kahle, P.J., M. Neumann, L. Ozmen, V. Muller, H. Jacobsen, W. Spooren, B. Fuss, et al. 2002. Hyperphosphorylation and insolubility of alpha-synuclein in transgenic mouse oligodendrocytes. *EMBO Rep* **3**:583–588.

Kamath, R.S., and J. Ahringer. 2003. Genome-wide RNAi screening in *Caenorhabditis elegans*. *Methods* **30**:313–321.

Klintenberg, R., L. Gunne, and P.E. Andren. 2002. Tardive dyskinesia model in the common marmoset. *Mov Disord* **17**:360–365.

Kralic, J.E., E.R. Korpi, T.K. O'Buckley, G.E. Homanics, and A.L. Morrow. 2002. Molecular and pharmacological characterization of GABA(A) receptor alpha1 subunit knockout mice. *J Pharmacol Exp Ther* **302**: 1037–1045.

Kuramoto, T., K. Kitada, T. Inui, Y. Sasaki, K. Ito, T. Hase, S. Kawagachi, et al. 2001. Attractin/mahogany/zitter plays a critical role in myelination of the central nervous system. *Proc Natl Acad Sci U S A* **98**:559–564.

Laforet, G.A., E. Sapp, K. Chase, C. McIntyre, F.M. Boyce, M. Campbell, B.A. Cadigan, et al. 2001. Changes in cortical and striatal neurons predict behavioral and electrophysiological abnormalities in a transgenic murine model of Huntington's disease. *J Neurosci* **21**:9112–9123.

Lai, Y.Y., and J.M. Siegel. 1997. Brainstem-mediated locomotion and myoclonic jerks. I. Neural substrates. *Brain Res* **745**:257–264.

Lakso, M., S. Vartiainen, A.M. Moilanen, J. Sirvio, J.H. Thomas, R. Nass, R.D. Blakely, and G. Wong. 2003. Dopaminergic neuronal loss and motor deficits in *Caenorhabditis elegans* overexpressing human alpha-synuclein. *J Neurochem* **86**:165–172.

LeDoux, M.S., J.F. Lorden, J.M. Smith, and L.E. Mays. 1998. Serotonergic modulation of eye blinks in cat and monkey. *Neurosci Lett* **253**: 61–64.

Lewis, J., E. McGowan, J. Rockwood, H. Melrose, P. Nacharaju, M. Van Slegtenhorst, K. Gwinn-Hardy, et al. 2000. Neurofibrillary tangles, amyotrophy and progressive motor disturbance in mice expressing mutant (P301L) tau protein. *Nat Genet* **25**:402–405.

Linn, G.S., K. Lifshitz, R.T. O'Keeffe, K. Lee, and J. Camp-Lifshitz. 2001. Increased incidence of dyskinesias and other behavioral effects of re-exposure to neuroleptic treatment in social colonies of *Cebus apella* monkeys. *Psychopharmacology (Berl)* **153**:285–294.

Lockhart, P.J., C.A. O'Farrell, and M.J. Farrer. 2004. It's a double knock-out! The quaking mouse is a spontaneous deletion of parkin and parkin co-regulated gene (PACRG). *Mov Disord* **19**:101–104.

Lorden, J.F., T.W. McKeon, H.J. Baker, N. Cox, and S.U. Walkley. 1984. Characterization of the rat mutant dystonic (dt): a new animal model of dystonia musculorum deformans. *J Neurosci* **4**:1925–1932.

Lorenzetti, D., K. Watase, B. Xu, M.M. Matzuk, H.T. Orr, and H.Y. Zoghbi. 2000. Repeat instability and motor incoordination in mice with a targeted expanded CAG repeat in the Sca1 locus. *Hum Mol Genet* **9**:779–785.

Loscher, W., J.E. Fisher Jr., D. Schmidt, G. Fredow, D. Honack, and W.B. Iturrian. 1989. The sz mutant hamster: a genetic model of epilepsy or of paroxysmal dystonia? *Mov Disord* **4**:219–232.

Lundblad, M., M. Andersson, C. Winkler, D. Kirik, N. Wierup, and M.A. Cenci. 2002. Pharmacological validation of behavioural measures of akinesia and dyskinesia in a rat model of Parkinson's disease. *Eur J Neurosci* **15**:120–132.

Mangiarini, L., K. Sathasivam, M. Seller, B. Cozens, A. Harper, C. Hetherington, M. Lawton, et al. 1996. Exon 1 of the HD gene with an expanded CAG repeat is sufficient to cause a progressive neurological phenotype in transgenic mice. *Cell* **87**:493–506.

Marsh, J.L., H. Walker, H. Theisen, Y.Z. Zhu, T. Fielder, J. Purcell, and L.M. Thompson. 2000. Expanded polyglutamine peptides alone are intrinsically cytotoxic and cause neurodegeneration in *Drosophila*. *Hum Mol Genet* **9**:13–25.

Masliah, E., E. Rockenstein, I. Veinbergs, M. Mallory, M. Hashimoto, A. Takeda, Y. Sagara, et al. 2000. Dopaminergic loss and inclusion body formation in alpha-synuclein mice: implications for neurodegenerative disorders. *Science* **287**:1265–1269.

Mendez, J.S., and B.W. Finn. 1975. Use of 6-hydroxydopamine to create lesions in catecholamine neurons in rats. *J Neurosurg* **42**: 166–173.

Miranda, C.J., M.M. Santos, K. Ohshima, J. Smith, L. Li, M. Bunting, M. Cossee, et al. 2002. Frataxin knockin mouse. *FEBS Lett* **512**:291–297.

Miwa, H., K. Nishi, T. Fuwa, and Y. Mizuno. 2000. Differential expression of c-fos following administration of two tremorgenic agents: harmaline and oxotremorine. *Neuroreport* **11**:2385–2390.

Motigny, C.D., and Y. Lamarre. 1973. Rhythmic activity induced by harmaline in the olivo-cerebello-bulbar system of the cat. *Brain Res* **53**:81–95.

Murphy, N.P., H.A. Lam, and N.T. Maidment. 2001. A comparison of morphine-induced locomotor activity and mesolimbic dopamine release in C57BL6, 129Sv and DBA2 mice. *J Neurochem* **79**:626–635.

Muscatt, S., J. Rothwell, J. Obeso, N. Leigh, P. Jenner, and C.D. Marsden. 1986. Urea-induced stimulus-sensitive myoclonus in the rat. *Adv Neurol* **43**:553–563.

Nass, R., D.H. Hall, D.M. Miller, and R.D. Blakely. 2002. Neurotoxin-induced degeneration of dopamine neurons in *Caenorhabditis elegans*. *Proc Natl Acad Sci U S A* **99**:3264–3269.

Nordstrom, E.J., and F.H. Burton. 2002. A transgenic model of comorbid Tourette's syndrome and obsessive-compulsive disorder circuitry. *Mol Psychiatry* **7**:617–625.

Ohye, C., T. Shibazaki, T. Hirai, H. Wada, Y. Kawashima, M. Hirato, and M. Matsumura. 1988. A special role of the parvocellular red nucleus in lesion-induced spontaneous tremor in monkeys. *Behav Brain Res* **28**: 241–243.

Ondo, W.G., Y. He, S. Rajasekaran, and W.D. Le. 2000. Clinical correlates of 6-hydroxydopamine injections into A11 dopaminergic neurons in rats: a possible model for restless legs syndrome. *Mov Disord* **15**:154–158.

Parker, J.A., J.B. Connolly, C. Wellington, M. Hayden, J. Dausset, and C. Neri. 2001. Expanded polyglutamines in *Caenorhabditis elegans* cause axonal abnormalities and severe dysfunction of PLM mechanosensory neurons without cell death. *Proc Natl Acad Sci U S A* **98**:13318–13323.

Pennacchio, L.A., D.M. Bouley, K.M. Higgins, M.P. Scott, J.L. Noebels, and R.M. Myers. 1998. Progressive ataxia, myoclonic epilepsy and cerebellar apoptosis in cystatin B-deficient mice. Nat Genet **20**: 251–258.

Pierce, K.D., C.A. Handford, R. Morris, B. Vafa, J.A. Dennis, P.J. Healy, and P.R. Schofield. 2001. A nonsense mutation in the alpha1 subunit of the inhibitory glycine receptor associated with bovine myoclonus. *Mol Cell Neurosci* **17**:354–363.

Pizoli, C.E., H.A. Jinnah, M.L. Billingsley, and E.J. Hess. 2002. Abnormal cerebellar signaling induces dystonia in mice. *J Neurosci* **22**:7825–7833.

Rankin, C.A., C.A. Joazeiro, E. Floor, and T. Hunter. 2001. E3 ubiquitin-protein ligase activity of Parkin is dependent on cooperative interaction of RING finger (TRIAD) elements. *J Biomed Sci* **8**:421–429.

Rektor, I., M. Svejdova, C. Silva-Barrat, and C. Menini. 1993. The cholinergic system-dependent myoclonus of the baboon *Papio papio* is a reticular reflex myoclonus. *Mov Disord* **8**:28–32.

Richter, A., J. Wissel, B. Harlizius, D. Simon, L. Schelosky, U. Scholz, W. Poewe, and W. Loscher. 1995. The "campus syndrome" in pigs: neurological, neurophysiological, and neuropharmacological characterization of a new genetic animal model of high-frequency tremor. *Exp Neurol* **134**:205–213.

Roach, A., N. Takahashi, D. Pravtcheva, F. Ruddle, and L. Hood. 1985. Chromosomal mapping of mouse myelin basic protein gene and structure and transcription of the partially deleted gene in shiverer mutant mice. *Cell* **42**:149–155.

Robinson, F.R. 2000. Role of the cerebellar posterior interpositus nucleus in saccades I. Effect of temporary lesions. *J Neurophysiol* **84**:1289–1302.

Rockenstein, E., M. Mallory, M. Hashimoto, D. Song, C.W. Shults, I. Lang, and E. Masliah. 2002. Differential neuropathological alterations in transgenic mice expressing alpha-synuclein from the platelet-derived growth factor and Thy-1 promoters. *J Neurosci Res* **68**:568–578.

Rothwell, J.C., and Y.-Z. Huang. 2003. Systems-level studies of movement disorders in dystonia and Parkinson's disease. *Curr Opin Neurobiol* **13**:691–695.

Sachdev, P.S., and T. Saharov. 1998. Effects of specific dopamine D1 and D2 receptor antagonists and agonists and neuroleptic drugs on emotional defecation in a rat model of akathisia. *Psychiatry Res* **81**:323–332.

Sambrook, M.A., A.R. Crossman, and P. Slater. 1979. Experimental torticollis in the marmoset produced by injection of 6-hydroxydopamine into the ascending nigrostriatal pathway. *Exp Neurol* **63**:583–593.

Sanberg, P.R., S.F. Calderon, M. Giordano, J.M. Tew, and A.B. Norman. 1989. The quinolinic acid model of Huntington's disease: locomotor abnormalities. *Exp Neurol* **105**:45–53.

Schicatano, E.J., M.A. Basso, and C. Evinger. 1997. Animal model explains the origins of the cranial dystonia benign essential blepharospasm. *J Neurophysiol* **77**:2842–2846.

Schilling, G., M.W. Becher, A.H. Sharp, H.A. Jinnah, K. Duan, J.A. Kotzuk, H.H. Slunt, et al. 1999. Intranuclear inclusions and neuritic aggregates in transgenic mice expressing a mutant N-terminal fragment of huntingtin. *Hum Mol Genet* **8**:397–407.

Sidman, R.L., M.M. Dickie, and S.H. Appel. 1964. Mutant mice (quaking and jimpy) with deficient myelination in the central nervous system. *Science* **144**:309–311.

Stefanova, N., Z. Puschban, P.O. Fernagut, E. Brouillet, F. Tison, M. Reindl, K.A. Jellinger, et al. 2003. Neuropathological and behavioral changes induced by various treatment paradigms with MPTP and 3-nitropropionic acid in mice: towards a model of striatonigral degeneration (multiple system atrophy). *Acta Neuropathol (Berl)* **106**:157–166.

Suter, U., A.A. Welcher, T. Ozcelik, G.J. Snipes, B. Kosaras, U. Francke, S. Billings-Gagliardi, et al. 1992. Trembler mouse carries a point mutation in a myelin gene. *Nature* **356**:241–244.

Takahashi, K., and K. Kitamura. 1999. A point mutation in a plasma membrane Ca(2+)-ATPase gene causes deafness in wriggle mouse Sagami. *Biochem Biophys Res Commun* **261**:773–778.

Taylor, J.R., S.A. Morshed, S. Parveen, M.T. Mercadante, L. Scahill, B.S. Peterson, R.A. King, et al. 2002. An animal model of Tourette's syndrome. *Am J Psychiatry* **159**:657–660.

Thiruchelvam, M., A. McCormack, E.K. Richfield, R.B. Baggs, A.W. Tank, D.A. Di Monte, and D.A. Cory-Slechta. 2003. Age-related irreversible progressive nigrostriatal dopaminergic neurotoxicity in the paraquat and maneb model of the Parkinson's disease phenotype. *Eur J Neurosci* **18**:589–600.

Thompson, F.J., R. Parmer, P.J. Reier, D.C. Wang, and P. Bose. 2001. Scientific basis of spasticity: insights from a laboratory model. *J Child Neurol* **16**:2–9.

Truong, D.D., A. Kanthasamy, B. Nguyen, R. Matsumoto, and P. Schwartz. 2000. Animal models of posthypoxic myoclonus: I. Development and validation. *Mov Disord* **15**(Suppl 1):26–30.

van der Putten, H., K.H. Wiederhold, A. Probst, S. Barbieri, C. Mistl, S. Danner, S. Kauffmann, et al. 2000. Neuropathology in mice expressing human alpha-synuclein. *J Neurosci* **20**:6021–6029.

Vilis, T., and J. Hore. 1977. Effects of changes in mechanical state of limb on cerebellar intention tremor. *J Neurophysiol* **40**:1214–1224.

Walker, A.E., and E.H. Botterell. 1937. The syndrome of the superior cerebellar peduncle in the monkey. *Brain* **60**:329–341.

Walker, J.M., R.R. Matsumoto, W.D. Bowen, D.L. Gans, K.D. Jones, and F.O. Walker. 1988. Evidence for a role of haloperidol-sensitive sigma-"opiate" receptors in the motor effects of antipsychotic drugs. *Neurology* **38**:961–965.

Wang, Q., M.E. Bardgett, M. Wong, D.F. Wozniak, J. Lou, B.D. McNeil, C. Chen, et al. 2002. Ataxia and paroxysmal dyskinesia in mice lacking axonally transported FGF14. *Neuron* **35**:25–38.

Wheeler, V.C., J.K. White, C.A. Gutekunst, V. Vrbanac, M. Weaver, X.J. Li, S.H. Li, et al. 2000. Long glutamine tracts cause nuclear localization of a novel form of huntingtin in medium spiny striatal neurons in HdhQ92 and HdhQ111 knock-in mice. *Hum Mol Genet* **9**:503–513.

Wichmann, T., H. Bergman, and M.R. DeLong. 1994. The primate subthalamic nucleus. III. Changes in motor behavior and neuronal activity in the internal pallidum induced by subthalamic inactivation in the MPTP model of parkinsonism. *J Neurophysiol* **72**:521–530.

Yoon, C.H. 1969. Disturbances in developmental pathways leading to a neurological disorder of genetic origin, "leaner," in mice. *Dev Biol* **20**:158–181.

Zuscik, M.J., S. Sands, S.A. Ross, D.J. Waugh, R.J. Gaivin, D. Morilak, and D.M. Perez. 2000. Overexpression of the alpha1B-adrenergic receptor causes apoptotic neurodegeneration: multiple system atrophy. *Nat Med* **6**:1388–1394.

Zuo, J., P.L. De Jager, K.A. Takahashi, W. Jiang, D.J. Linden, and N. Heintz. 1997. Neurodegeneration in lurcher mice caused by mutation in delta2 glutamate receptor gene. *Nature* **388**:769–773.

CHAPTER

A3

Generation of Transgenic and Gene-Targeted Mouse Models of Movement Disorders

MAI DANG and YUQING LI

In recent years, human genetic linkage studies have yielded a tremendous amount of information about the genetics of many movement disorders. Mutations have been identified in genes responsible for Parkinson disease (SNCA), Huntington disease (IT15), dystonia (TOR1A), and Rett syndrome (MECP2), among others (Amir et al. 1999; Higgins et al. 1997; Ozelius et al. 1997; Polymeropoulos et al. 1997; Research 1993; Tanzi et al. 1993). Clinical symptoms are well characterized for most movement disorders. Pathological states of the brain such as region-specific neurodegeneration and cytological events such as protein aggregation have been correlated with some disorders. The functions of most implicated proteins in movement disorders are unknown and only speculations of possible functions are gathered from sequence homology analyses. As a result, the mechanisms these mutant proteins work through to cause the pathology are also largely unknown. Furthermore, in many cases it has yet to be determined if the gene of interest acts alone or in concert with other genetic or environmental modifiers to cause the disorder.

For elucidating protein function and a mutant protein's role in producing neurological pathology, a mouse model can provide essential information. Other systems, such as yeast, worm, fly, and zebrafish, have proven to be useful genetic tools that are sometimes created and manipulated more easily. The complex mammalian physiology of a mouse that closely mimics that of humans clearly gives mouse models a distinct advantage. Also, genetically altering a mouse is now made easier with the human and mouse genome deciphered, which allows for rapid identification of the sequence of any gene of interest. In addition, a large number of available inbred mouse strains and a variety of well-developed methods of genetic manipulations, including gene targeting that can be performed efficiently only in mice, make mouse models useful for modeling human movement disorders.

The many techniques available for modifying the genome of a mouse allow for the study of a variety of genetic inheritance patterns. A gain-of-function mutation's effect on physiology can be exaggerated by the overexpression of the mutated protein. A transgenic model is suitable also for modeling disorders in which extra copies of a gene are implicated. Alternatively, a gene can be removed or knocked out to study the developmental pattern of the organism in the absence of the protein, which can either mimic a loss-of-function mutation or create a system for the study of the protein's function. A dominant disorder seen in some diseases can be faithfully replicated by knocking in a mutation into one allele. Furthermore, with each gene alteration method, various strategies have been devised to allow for greater freedom in altering the gene's expression. Inducible systems for transgenic and conditional expression of the gene alteration for knock-out and knock-in are examples. In this chapter, we will review the different methods and strategies available for making mouse models. Aspects of mouse strain selection and behavioral analysis for phenotyping a mouse model of a movement disorder will also be discussed.

I. TRANSGENIC MOUSE MODELS

Transgenic mouse models containing an overexpression of a normal or mutated gene can be used to determine aberrant development in the presence of the overexpression. Transgenic mice are made by injection of the implicated normal or mutated gene into fertilized oocytes for random insertion into the genome (Gordon et al. 1980). This technique can also be used to ablate tissues of specific brain regions to model disorders in which tissue specific degeneration has been observed (Nirenberg and Cepko 1993; Palmiter et al. 1987).

A. The Transgenic Method

Generating a transgenic mouse starts with a DNA construct containing a promoter, the wild-type or mutated gene or cDNA, and a polyadenylation (polyA) tail to signal transcription termination (Figure 1). Promoter selection is an important choice to make because it determines the level, tissue specificity, and temporal pattern of the transgene's expression. If remaining faithful to endogenous expression in regards to tissue and temporal specificity is desired, the gene's natural promoter is often used. For example, the well-characterized R6/2 Huntington mouse model uses the human huntingtin gene promoter to mimic the native tissue specificity and temporal expression pattern (Carter et al. 1999). Whole brain expression has been achieved with the Thy1 promoter or the MoPrP.Xho promoter of the murine prion protein, which have been used in both Huntington and Parkinson models (Lee et al. 2002; Luthi-Carter et al. 2000; Sommer et al. 2000). An extensive list of neuron-specific promoters has been compiled (Okabe 1999).

Following the selected promoter in the DNA construct is the gene either in its entirety with introns and regulatory sequences or just the cDNA coding sequence. The simplest option of coding region for the construct is the normal or mutated human cDNA that may have been isolated after the gene was cloned. If using a mouse gene is desired, the cDNA or complete gene must be isolated from a library and site-directed mutagenesis performed to introduce any desirable mutations. cDNA has been used successfully to generate several transgenic mouse lines for movement disorders research (Lee et al. 2002; Schilling et al. 1999). However,

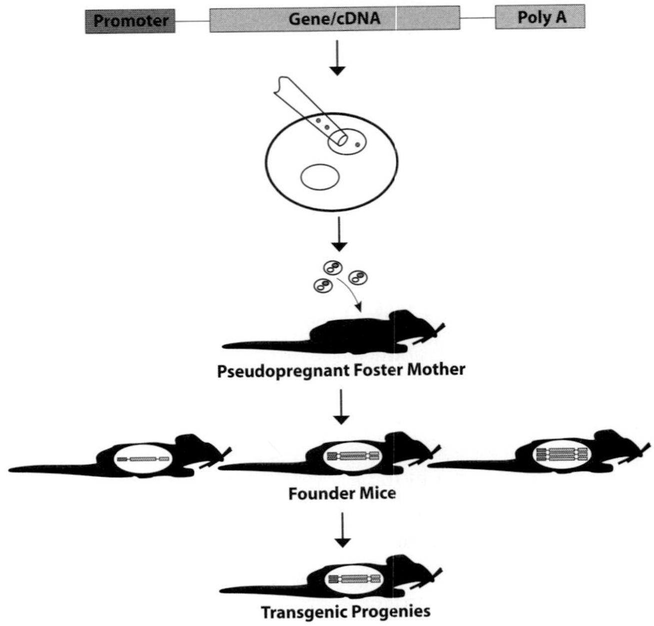

FIGURE 1 (See color version on DVD) Transgenic mouse construction. A DNA sequence (genomic fragment or cDNA) to be transcribed is placed after a selected promoter and followed by a polyadenylation tail. The cloned DNA fragments are injected into the pronuclei of many fertilized oocytes that are then reimplanted into pseudopregnant foster mothers. Mice developed from injected eggs are called founders. Different copy numbers of the transgene may be found in each founder mouse. Mice carrying the transgene in all cells including egg or sperm cells can be bred to transmit the transgene to subsequent generations.

the difference in efficiency of expression between cDNA and the entire gene should be considered. Expression of a protein has been shown to be more efficient with the use of the entire gene than that of the cDNA (Brinster et al. 1988). In one study with the metallothionein gene, the presence of intron 1 was identified as the factor that contributed to this efficiency (Palmiter et al. 1991). It has been proposed that introns may contribute enhancers or other transcriptional initiators (Oka et al. 1997) or provide sequences that assist opening of chromosomal domains for more efficient transcription (Svaren and Chalkley 1990).

The finished construct is amplified in bacteria, and the insert containing promoter, coding region, and polyA is isolated and purified. The purified fragment is then injected into the pronuclei of extracted fertilized oocytes harvested from a superovulated mouse mated one day prior to the extraction. Injected zygotes are returned to pseudopregnant mother mice. The nuclei take up one or multiple copies of the construct, which are then randomly incorporated into the genome. Multiple copies are usually taken up in a tandem head-to-tail array.

Mice that develop from these injected fertilized eggs are called founder mice. Each founder mouse may vary greatly in expression pattern of the transgene and ultimately exhibit different phenotypes. Three major aspects of the integration of DNA in transgenic mouse-making cause this variability: (1) the oocyte development stage at which integration takes place, (2) the genomic site of incorporation, and (3) the incorporated copy number. First, if integration of the construct into the chromosome happens when the cell is at the one-cell zygote stage, all tissues in the mouse will express the transgene. If the incorporation does not occur until after the cell divides, a mosaic expression pattern will result whereby some tissues will contain the altered gene while others will not. A meta-analysis of 262 transgenic mouse lines showed that about one third of the founder mice of these lines are mosaics, suggesting integration of injected DNA was incorporated after the first round of mitosis (Wilkie et al. 1986). This late incorporation results in only a subset of tissues in the mouse containing the transgene. If germline cells in founder mice differentiated from embryonic stem (ES) cells with the transgene, offspring will receive the mutation. Otherwise the transgene expression will not appear in progeny.

Second, incorporation of the transgene into random sites leads to possible positional effects. Positional effect has long been seen in chromosomal rearrangement (Wilson et al. 1990). The proximity of the newly transported gene to promoter, enhancer, and silencer sequences greatly affects the expression of the relocated gene(s). Positional effects can also greatly influence the expression of transgenes. If incorporation of the transgene occurs downstream of a strong endogenous promoter that directs expression in an undesirable tissue type, the transgene may be expressed there. This ectopic expression can complicate development in unexpected and indefinable ways. Conversely, if the transgene is inserted near a silencer, the ultimate goal to express the mutated gene can be defeated when expression is inhibited.

While endogenous genetic elements can act on the transgene expression pattern, random insertion can be just as deleterious to the endogenous genes. If the transgene is inserted within the coding region or regulatory sequence of an endogenous gene, it could disrupt the expression of this gene and at worst, completely eliminate the gene's expression. This event could lead to a secondary phenotype that may mask the true phenotype of the transgene's overexpression.

Third, with the standard transgenic protocol, the number of copies incorporated is uncontrollable and has been estimated to be anywhere from two to fifty. In some cases, the number of copies relates proportionally to the severity of the phenotype (Dal Canto and Gurney 1997). This uncertainty and that arising from the position of insertion make the generation of multiple lines of founder mice necessary. Each line's phenotype should be well characterized and compared to each other with consideration for the number of copies that were incorporated.

To avoid these potentially troublesome features of transgenic mouse making, investigators have developed methods that involve the following: additional DNA sequences to more tightly control positional effect, homologous recombination for single copy incorporation, and various vectors that allow for large DNA fragments to be cloned. Adding scaffold/matrix-attachment regions (Gutierrez-Adan and Pintado 2000) and locus control regions (reviewed in Li et al. 1999) has been shown to lessen the unpredictability in expression of transgenic DNA constructs. To eliminate the effect of potential silencers preventing transgene expression, co-integration of a highly expressed gene has been used to ensure the expression of the desired transgene (Clark et al. 1992). In addition, homologous recombination (see section III) has been employed to integrate a single copy of a transgene at a selected site (Bronson et al. 1996). With this method, investigators select an endogenous gene that is constitutively expressed as the incorporation site for the transgene linked to its own promoter. Although this method greatly improves the likelihood that the transgene will be expressed, gene targeting requires culturing of ES cells and injection of ES cells into blastocysts that increases the complexity of the mouse making process.

While the use of the entire gene enhances expression efficiency, manipulations of large genes can be troublesome with traditionally used vectors that have a limit of forty kilobases. To eliminate this problem, yeast artificial chromosomes (YACs) have been employed as cloning vectors for genomic fragments of up to two megabases (reviewed in Giraldo and Montoliu 2001; Picciotto and Wickman 1998). With this method, the YACs contain all functional elements for their survival as artificial chromosomes in yeast cells and carry all the promoter elements necessary for the desired expression pattern of the transgene. A plasmid with the desired transgene and a selectable marker flanked by two arms of sequences homologous to the yeast vector is introduced into the yeast cells. The gene fragment is then exchanged with the homologous portion of the fragment in YACs. The recombined YACs now containing the transgene are isolated, purified, and injected into the pronuclei of fertilized oocytes. The efficiency of uptake and expression of the transgene in YACs is generally seen to be similar to that of standard DNA constructs. A transgenic mouse model of Huntington disease has been created using YACs that contain the full-length human gene, including all regulatory elements. The gene was engineered to contain either 46 CAG or 72 CAG repeats. Mutant human huntingtin protein was reportedly expressed in the same tissues as the endogenous mouse protein (Hodgson et al. 1999).

Drawbacks to the use of YACs include the need to adhere to stringent requirements for intact YAC isolation that must be free of contaminating yeast proteins that may interfere with transfection. In addition, a high likelihood of the shearing of these large fragments exists for YACs during injection into the pronucleus. YACs also have resulted in frequent chimerism and clonal instability, leading to unwanted changes to the gene (Monaco and Larin 1994). Alternatives to YACs have been developed and are based on the use of bacterial artificial chromosomes (BACs) and P1-derived artificial chromosomes (PACs) that can host genomic fragments up to 100 kilobases and 300 kilobases, respectively. BACs and PACs do not exhibit the same level of chimerism as seen in YACs and are not as susceptible to shearing since they exist as supercoiled circular plasmids (Giraldo and Montoliu 2001; Monaco and Larin 1994).

B. Inducible Transgenic Systems

Widespread alteration in a gene's expression pattern from the beginning of development may disrupt normal growth to a severity that produces unhealthy animals, which could complicate analyses or even render the animals of no use. Also, compensatory mechanisms may occur during development that mask the effects of the transgene. In these cases, control over the time of transgene expression is necessary. Several systems have been developed to meet that need. The Tet system is the most widely used. Two variations of this system have been devised that differ in whether or not the gene is expressed constitutively and when exposed to an exogenous compound. The original strategy is the Tet-off system (Figure 2). In this system, an additional mouse line is produced to express tetracycline-controlled *trans*-activator (tTA) in the tissue(s) of interest. tTA is a fusion protein containing a *tet* repressor from *E. coli* transposon *Tn*10 and the activating domain of virion protein 16 of herpes simplex virus (Gossen and Bujard 1992). The transgenic mouse is made by injecting a construct with the gene of interest behind a tet-op promoter. When crossed with the tTA mouse line, tTA is expressed and activates the tet-op promoter, inducing expression of the transgene. When exposed to tetracycline (Tet) or doxycycline (Dox), a tetracycline analog, Tet/Dox binds tTA, preventing binding to the promoter and functionally inhibiting the transcription of the gene of interest (Shockett et al. 1995; Furth et al. 1994). A successful example of this inducible strategy can be seen in a conditional model of Huntington disease. The tet-responsive promoter was designed to drive the expression of chimeric mouse/human exon 1 with a 94-CAG repeat. Animals expressing the transgene showed progressively severe clasping of limps and tremors before an early death. Interestingly, with exposure to doxycycline treatment, expression of the transgene carrying the repeats was inhibited and the motor abnormalities reversed (Yamamoto et al. 2000).

The major disadvantage of the Tet-off system is that even if investigators do not want the gene expressed until later in development, the animal must be exposed to Tet or Dox from conception. The prolonged application of Tet or Dox could result in side effects. One example of this is a study where investigators demonstrated impaired spatial memory and fear conditioning in animals after long-term Dox exposure (Mayford et al. 1996). In addition, clearance of Tet or Dox in the tissue types being studied must be carefully considered.

The reverse system, TET-on, eliminates these problems. Rather than using an activator, a mutant form of tTA that is a Tet repressor (rtTA) is used. Expression of rtTA inhibits the transcription of the gene of interest, and upon exposure to Tet or Dox, the repression is lifted, allowing for gene transcription (Gossen et al. 1995). Gene expression can be achieved within a few hours, and complete induction after twenty-four hours can often be observed. Other inducible

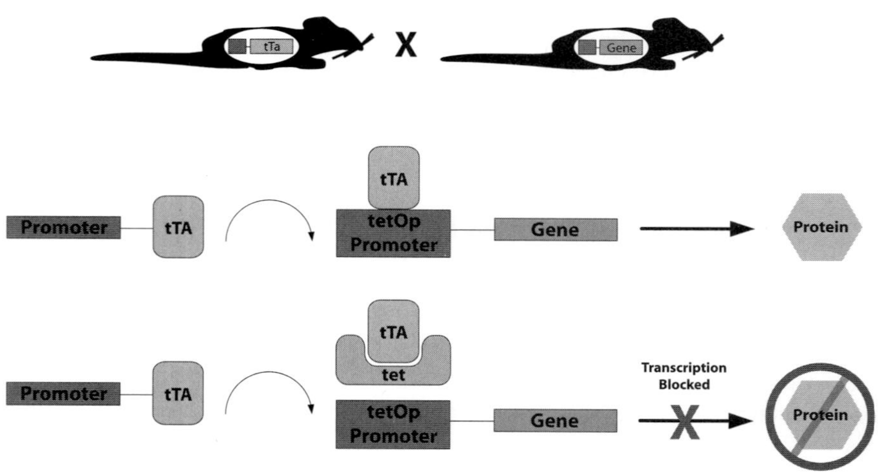

FIGURE 2 (See color version on DVD) Tet-off inducible system. A mouse carrying a Tet transactivator gene (tTA) driven by a selected promoter is crossed with a transgenic mouse with the gene of interest positioned behind the tetOp promoter. The tTA protein is expressed and binds to the tetOp promoter to induce transcription of the gene. When exogenous Tet (or Dox) is introduced into the mouse, Tet binds to tTA, and transcription is blocked.

systems have been developed using either steroids or interferon-α as the triggering agents (Kelly et al. 1997; Kuhn et al. 1995).

C. Tissue-Specific Ablation

In several movement disorders, neurodegeneration of specific neuronal types is observed, such as the dopaminergic neurons in Parkinson disease and striatal neurons in Huntington disease. A model that mimics neurodegeneration without regard for the genetics of the disorder can also be achieved with the transgenic approach. A widely used method of genetic ablation of specific tissues relies on the diphtheria toxin A-chain gene (DTA). The toxin gene's expression is controlled by the tissue-specific promoter it is linked to (Breitman et al. 1987; Palmiter et al. 1987). When expressed, the toxin causes cell death. A variation on this technique has been developed that allows for inducibility of the toxin. The promoter of tTA selects for the tissue type and the tet-op promoter drives DTA expression (Lee et al. 1998). Another conditional ablation method uses the human interleukin 2 receptor that is controlled by a desired promoter. Application of the recombinant immunotoxin anti-Tac(Fv)-PE40 kills the tissue through binding with the interleukin receptor. This method was used to create a striatal cholinergic interneuron ablation in mice that displayed an interesting acute abnormal turning behavior that was affected by dopamine actions (Kaneko et al. 2000). In another study, cerebellar Golgi cells were ablated. In these mice, severe compound motor coordination was observed leading to the conclusion that the interaction between GABA inhibition and NMDA receptor activation is necessary for normal compound movements (Watanabe et al. 1998). Yet another system of inducible ablation uses the herpes simplex virus thymidine kinase (HSV-TK) that is placed under the expression control of a chosen promoter. HSV-TK is innocuous, but can convert ganciclovir to a toxic product that disrupts DNA replication in dividing cells. In one study the GFAP promoter directed the expression of HSV-TK to cerebellar astrocytes. Early postnatal exposure to ganciclovir resulted in severe ataxia in these mice (Delaney et al. 1996).

II. GENE TARGETING

The discovery and elucidation of homologous recombination in mammalian cells and the establishment of culture conditions for ES cells have allowed the development of gene targeting methods (Smithies et al. 1984; Folger et al. 1982; Evans and Kaufman 1981). Disorders caused by loss-of-function mutations can be replicated by knocking out genes that functionally eliminate protein expression. In gene targeting, creating a mouse that contains a desired mutation involves introducing the mutation to the endogenous allelic genes through homologous recombination rather than introducing the mutated gene to the fertilized egg, as is done with transgenic methods. Uncertainties that arise from positional effects and ectopic expression patterns and levels are, for the most part, eliminated with gene targeting.

A. Gene Targeting Method

Gene targeting relies on homologous recombination whereby a piece of DNA containing the mutated gene fragment flanked by large stretches of unaltered DNA is introduced into the ES cell through electroporation which is then incorporated into the genome at a targeted site. With the help of endogenous recombinases, the flanking unaltered sequences that line up with the homologous chromosomal DNA switch places with the genomic segment, taking along the mutated fragment between the arms. A wild-type allelic fragment is thus replaced with an altered version from the DNA construct. Incorporation of the transgene in these ES cells mainly occurs randomly, but in one out of every 10^5 to 10^7 ES cells, homologous recombination occurs (Vasquez et al. 2001). The efficiency of homologous recombination depends on several factors. The first factor is the similarity between the construct DNA and its corresponding endogenous counterpart (te Riele et al. 1992). Using DNA for the construct that comes from the same mouse strain as the ES cells is one way to achieve high similarity. Another consideration is the length of the homologous arms, which generally should be several kilobases long on each end (Thomas et al. 1992). Longer homologous sequences will result in homologous recombination at high frequencies. DNA methylation status and chromatin structure have also been shown to affect the efficiency of homologous recombination (Liang and Jasin 1995; Ramdas and Muniyappa 1995). Finally, the sequence itself often determines not only if the exchange will be made, but also where the recombination will occur. Hotspots, defined as specific sequences that promote recombinase interaction with the nucleotide to induce homologous recombination, have been identified in some genes (reviewed in Smith 1994). Our lab's experience with a Tor1a knock-in targeting construct produced at least two populations of targeted ES cells in which recombination occurred at different locations. In the majority of the selected ES cells, the exchange took place within 1.5 kilobases from the site of the major gene alteration, while in a small portion the recombination occurred beyond that point (Dang and Li, unpublished data). We attributed this deviation to a hotspot located in the sequence within the 1.5 kilobases from the site of gene alteration.

Selection for ES cells that have incorporated the exogenous DNA fragment is achieved by adding to the construct a positive selector, an antibiotic resistant gene. The gene is inserted with its own promoter to allow for selection of cells carrying the transgene. Commonly used is the neomycin resistant gene driven by a ubiquitous 3-phosphoglycerate kinase (PGK) promoter, together referred to as a neo cassette (Adra et al. 1987). Transfected ES cells that survive the antibiotic selection carry the transgene. Colonies of these ES cells must then be screened by Southern blot analysis or polymerase chain reaction (PCR) to determine whether the altered gene was inserted randomly or was targeted to the desired site. Because of the infrequency of homologous recombination, a large number of colonies (from fifty to one thousand) must be picked and screened to improve the likelihood of finding one containing the targeted transgene. To minimize the effort of this search, a negative selector can be included in the construct that will eliminate cells that randomly incorporate the transgene. The most frequently used negative selectors are the herpes simplex virus thymidine kinase or diphtheria toxin genes that are placed in the construct outside the region where recombination will occur (Zimmer and Reynolds 1994; Yagi et al. 1993). Homologous recombination will cause the splicing and removal of the negative selector, while random insertion will not. ES cells containing the marker are eliminated, thereby resulting in a cell culture enriched with ES cells containing the targeted gene.

The construct design determines the type of genetic alteration. The simplest construct carries a fragment of the gene containing an antibiotic gene that replaces a coding region of the gene of interest. Although recombination efficiency is sensitive to the homologous sequence, it is not affected by the deletion of large segments of a gene (Mombaerts et al. 1991). The removal of a coding region will interfere with transcription and protein expression, disrupting the production of the protein. This construct design is used to generate a complete knock-out model.

This knock-out method was demonstrated in the generation of α-synuclein null mice (Abeliovich et al. 2000). The gene-targeting event replaced the first two exons, encoding amino acids 1–41 and upstream untranslated sequences, with a neo cassette. Western blot analysis showed α-synuclein protein expression was eliminated. RT-PCR analyses with one set of primers specific for a 5′ sequence and another set for the 3′ end also showed complete elimination of α-synuclein mRNA.

Alternatively, to improve the likelihood that transcriptional readthrough will be halted, a STOP sequence can be added after the antibiotic gene. The STOP sequence, constructed by Lakso and colleagues, contains a false translation signal, a splice donor site, and its own poly(A) tail (Lakso et al. 1992). Dauer and colleagues generated α-synuclein null mice using the STOP sequence, targeted to replace sequences upstream of the start ATG of the gene. Transcript and protein analyses confirmed that the complete elimination of α-synuclein expression was attained (Dauer et al. 2002).

To knock in a mutation, site-directed mutagenesis through high-fidelity PCR is an easy way to alter the gene in the construct. The positive selector is placed in an intron away from potential splice signals. Inserting the antibiotic resistant gene into the largest intron decreases the likelihood of hitting a splice signal.

Several Huntington mouse models have been created using the knock-in approach. In one, 71- and 94-CAG repeats were targeted to exon 1 of the mouse huntingtin gene, *Hdh*, to produce two different lines (Levine et al. 1999). In this study, these two knock-in lines were compared to the R6/2 transgenic line. Interestingly, initial analyses showed that although the overexpressed transgenic mice expressed behavioral abnormalities, the knock-ins did not. These observations suggest that replicating the genotype may not produce a replication of phenotype. An exaggerated expression of the mutation of interest may be needed for the human phenotype to be expressed in mice. Another knock-in model using a similar design to that of Levine and colleagues showed unexpected genetic instability in germline mice. Two of the three analyzed progenies of a mutant mouse carrying 77-CAG repeats had a different repeat length from their parent. One carried an additional 8-CAG and the other a 1-CAG repeat (Shelbourne et al. 1999).

Detailed descriptions and protocols for steps in genetic manipulation of a mouse are presented in "Manipulating the Mouse Embryo" (Nagy et al. 2003), which should be consulted before proceeding with a gene-targeting project. In brief, once the construct is made and a genotyping method is devised to identify genomes that have homologously taken up the construct, the plasmid is linearized and purified for transfection into ES cells. ES cells are grown in strict conditions to prevent differentiation. Electroporation is done to introduce the transgene to genomic DNA. Selection using the chosen antibiotic is performed and individual colonies are isolated and expanded. A portion is frozen down for subsequent steps and the other portion is used for screening. Clones containing the targeted transgene are then expanded and injected into 3.5-day-old blastocysts from mice with a coat color different from that of the strain from which the ES cells were extracted. The injected blastocysts are then returned to pseudopregnant foster mothers (Figure 3). Alternatively, the aggregation method can be performed whereby clumps of ES cells are incubated with eight-cell-stage embryos that will incorporate the cell aggregates into their nuclei. This method does not require an expensive injection setup and is a reasonable alternative to the eye-straining, time-intensive injections of blastocysts. However, for successful incorporation of ES cells, stringent procedural conditions must be established and maintained.

Pups developed from these chimeric fertilized eggs will have a mosaic coat color pattern. Mice containing a greater percentage of the ES cell strain color are the more useful animals, since in these mice there is a greater likelihood that their germ cells differentiated from the altered ES cells. In addition, since the majority of established ES cell lines are

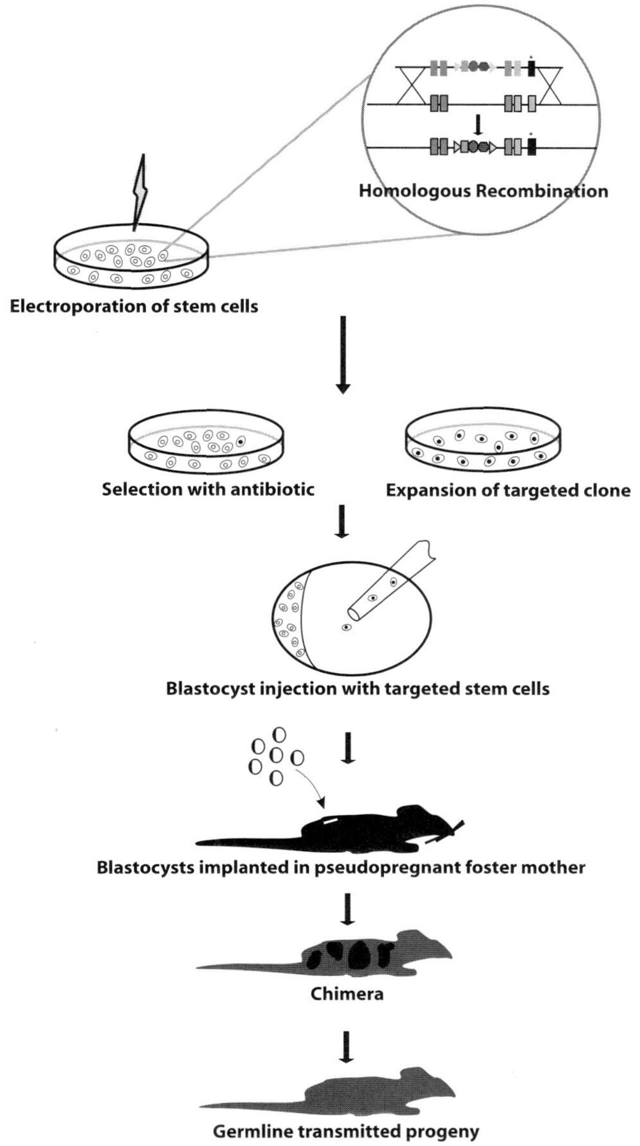

FIGURE 3 (See color version on DVD) Gene-targeting procedure to generate a knock-out or knock-in mouse. A DNA sequence is cloned with alterations and a positive selector (antibiotic resistant gene), all flanked by several kilobases of homologous sequence. Many copies of the DNA construct are introduced to stem cells through electroporation. The DNA construct is integrated into the genome at the site of interest by homologous recombination. With antibiotics, stem cells that had incorporated the altered DNA fragment carrying the antibiotic resistant gene are selected. Targeted clones are distinguished from cells carrying randomly inserted DNA constructs using PCR or Southern blot analysis. Targeted clones are expanded, and multiple stem cells of those clones are injected into blastocysts. Injected blastocysts are reimplanted into pseudopregnant foster mothers. Chimeric mice are produced displaying a mosaic coat pattern with two colors coming from mouse strains that contributed blastocysts and stem cells. Chimeras containing the transgene in germ cells can transmit the genetic alteration to progeny.

of the XY karyotype, the chimera gender ratio is usually biased towards males. Chimeras are then mated with animals of the strain from which the donor blastocysts were retrieved. Offspring of this breeding that have the color of the blastocyst donor strain do not carry the transgene. Pups with a homogeneous hybrid color (e.g., agouti or gray) have potential germline transmission. Southern or PCR analysis is performed to determine the presence of the targeted gene.

B. Conditional Gene Targeting

As with transgenic mice, compensatory mechanisms during development may compensate for the mutant gene and mask the true phenotype of the model. In other cases widespread deletion of a gene may be lethal. Reports of lethal knock-outs are not uncommon. A viable solution to this problem is to produce a conditional mutant mouse that harbors the knock-out only in specific tissues, allowing other tissues to develop normally to support life. Tissue specific gene alteration is also useful for knock-in models in order to identify an isolated brain region where the mutated protein may be important in producing a phenotype.

A tissue specific conditional mouse model requires the generation of an additional line of mice. Well-developed systems for tissue specific expression of targeted genes utilize recombinases that direct recombination of specific sequences (Ryding et al. 2001). Cre (causes recombination) is a recombinase from the P1 bacteriophage that recognizes loxP (locus of crossover) sites, exchanges one for the other, and as a result loops out one loxP and the sequence originally in between the loxPs (Sauer and Henderson 1988). Another recombinase commonly used is the Flp integrase of *Saccharomyces cerevisiae* that recombines FRT sites (McLeod et al. 1986). LoxP and FRT are 34-base-pair sequences consisting of two 13-base-pair palindromes with an asymmetrical 8-base-pair sequence in between. Depending on the orientation of the sequences, the recombinases can cause a variety of DNA exchange patterns, including deletion, duplication, integration, inversion, or translocation. With more than one system for mediating recombination, a construct can contain one recombinatorial system that directs conditional removal of exons of the protein of interest, while the other removes antibiotic resistant genes that are no longer needed after ES cell transfection.

For tissue specificity, Cre/Flp recombinase expression is placed under the control of a tissue specific promoter. To generate a Cre or Flp mouse line, a protein that expresses exclusively in the tissue(s) of interest is identified. Developmental expression pattern during the embryonic period and adulthood is carefully determined to ensure that the gene is expressed only in the desired tissue(s). The selected gene's promoter then drives the expression of Cre or Flp. Alternatively, tissue and temporal specificity can be achieved by knocking in Cre or Flp immediately after the selected promoter. We have successfully targeted Cre to the Emx1 locus to mediate hippocampus and cerebral cortex-specific recombination (Guo et al. 2000b; Jin et al. 2000). To confirm the expression pattern of the Cre produced in a particular line, a very useful ROSA26 Cre indicator mouse can be bred with the Cre line that will cause staining of tissues where Cre was expressed (Soriano 1999). The ROSA26 Cre reporter mouse contains a transgene with a neo cassette and polyA tail flanked by loxP followed by a lacZ gene and a polyA tail. Upon exposure to Cre, the loxP recombines and the neo cassette and transcriptional terminator, polyA, are removed, resulting in the expression of β-galactosidase. Tissues can then be stained for β-galactosidase activity and, accordingly, the site(s) of Cre activity can be identified.

Alternatively, existing lines of Cre/Flp mice can be sought and used if their Cre expression pattern is suitable for the project. Many lines of published Cre mice express the recombinase in specific tissues in the brain and may be important lines for animal models for movement disorders research. However, very few mice lines express Cre in just one brain region. The leakiness of some lines is its disadvantage, but variable expression levels can be evaluated to determine if the ectopic expression is tolerable in the project. For example, in the L7/pcp2-cre mice, Cre expression is specific to cerebellar Purkinje cells (Barski et al. 2000), while in the αCamKII-cre mice, Cre is expressed at high levels in the hippocampus, cortex, and amygdala, but it is expressed at low levels in the striatum, thalamus, and hypothalamus (Casanova et al. 2001; Barski et al. 2000). For a thorough list of published Cre transgenic lines, see the compilation created by the Nagy lab at www.mshri.on.ca/nagy/.

The construct design for a conditional knock-out involves placing loxP or FRT sequences on either side of a number of exons, that when deleted, eliminate the stability or function of the expressed protein (Figure 4). For a conditional knock-in of a mutated gene to model a dominant mutation, loxP or FRT is placed at each end of a neo cassette that is followed by a polyA and/or STOP sequence. Heterozygotes of chimera offspring will have one active wild-type allele of the gene. The allele with the transgene will not be functional since transcription was interrupted. Once that offspring is crossed with a Cre or Flp mouse, the neo cassette is removed, eliminating the transcriptional termination and allowing full expression of the mutated gene. A more thorough discussion of strategies for using conditional systems is available elsewhere (Torres and Kuhn 1997).

The Cre/loxP approach was used to knock out *Hdh* in the forebrain. An *Hdh* construct containing loxP sequences inserted near exon 1 was used to eliminate the promoter, exon 1, and a portion of the following intron. This *Hdh* loxP line was crossed with two αCamKII-cre lines. One expressed Cre in the forebrain and testis at embryonic day fifteen and the other at postnatal day five. Animals with huntingtin conditionally knocked out exhibited a progressive degenerative neuronal phenotype along with sterility (Dragatsis et al. 2000).

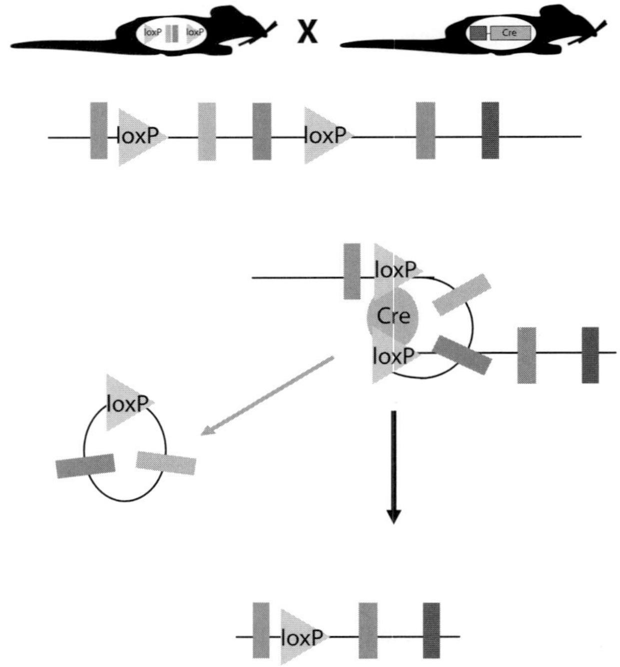

FIGURE 4 (See color version on DVD) Conditional Cre/loxP system. A standard strategy to create a knock-out mouse involves crossing a mouse expressing Cre in specific tissues and a mouse carrying the gene of interest with regions to be excised flanked by loxP sequences. In progeny containing the double transgene, Cre protein recombines DNA at the loxP sites and removes the sequence within the loxPs. The resulting gene with deleted segments encodes a nonfunctional protein.

To generate a line in which the transgene expression can be controlled for both tissue and temporal specificity, an inducible system is coupled with the Cre/loxP or Flp/FRT system. In an example of one system, Cre can be fused with the ligand-binding domain of a mutated estrogen receptor that allows for the localization of the expressed fused protein in the cytosol (Metzger and Chambon 2001). Upon exposure to tamoxifen, but not endogenous steroids, the Cre is released from the complex and enters the nucleus where it performs the recombination. Another strategy developed for this use is the tetracycline-regulated expression of Cre to create an inducible conditional model (Saam and Gordon 1999).

III. PHENOTYPING

A. Genetic Background

Proteins in an organism do not work in isolation, but rather operate as parts of complex pathways. When investigators analyze and compare the phenotype of genetically altered mice, we must carefully consider strain selection. The genetic background of each inbred mouse strain may contribute polymorphisms or mutations that could be allelic modifiers capable of contributing to a phenotype (Nadeau 2001). The affects of strain difference contributing to phenotype has been well-documented (Zielenski et al. 1999). Our lab has reported an example of strain differences in the neurodevelopment of an Emx-1-deficient condition. Emx-1 knock-outs in a C57BL/6 background developed a normal corpus callosum in our study (Guo et al. 2000a). This result contrasted the findings of two other groups who reported that in a 129 strain, the gene deficiency resulted in loss of the corpus callosum (Yoshida et al. 1997; Qiu et al. 1996). In addition, knock-out lethality has been shown to be rescued when the mutation was introduced into another inbred strain. An eye-opening case involved the epidermal growth-factor receptor knock-out that was lethal during embryonic development in the CF-1 mouse strain, but survived for up to three weeks after birth in the CD-1 strain (Threadgill et al. 1995).

Strain contribution to behavioral tests has received a great deal of attention in recent years since behavioral analysis has shown variable performance levels among wild-type animals of different inbred strains (Crawley et al. 1997; Gerlai 1996). This characteristic strain difference is highly relevant to movement disorders models. Some strains, such as C57/BL6 and CBA, are reported to outperform other strains tested on all motor behavioral tests, while strains such as 129/Sv perform the worst on many of the tests (Dunnett 2003). This difference becomes a problem when animals that are known to already perform poorly on a test are evaluated using that test to determine differences between wild-type and experimental genotypes. This issue can be avoided easily with transgenic mouse generation, but it becomes a greater problem in gene-targeting studies whereby widely used ES cells come from the 129/Sv line that is poorly suited for motor behavioral tests. In addition, mice produced in gene-targeting experiments are generally produced on mixed backgrounds. To further complicate the phenotyping of these mice, a study of environmental factors on motor behavioral skills has shown that mice carried by foster mothers of various strains demonstrated varying performance success on motor behavioral tests (Francis et al. 2003). Backcrossing germline transmitted pups to introduce the mutation into suitable inbred strains to equalize the baseline can alleviate these concerns. Our Emx1-deficient mice were backcrossed into the inbred C57BL/6J strain for ten generations before anxiety and depression-behavioral tests were performed. This study revealed an involvement of Emx1 in the emotional response (Cao and Li 2002).

B. Behavioral Analysis

The expected behavioral phenotype of a mouse model for movement disorders is initially determined in reference to the symptoms seen in patients. When a researcher sees a phenotype resembling patient symptoms by simply observing the animals, concerns about the potential relevance of this model to the human disease are mostly eliminated. However, when the disorder is less severe, or more quantitative analysis is desired, the researcher can perform a battery of motor behavioral tests to reveal and evaluate the phenotype. A thorough discussion of mouse phenotyping methods and detailed protocols are described elsewhere (Carter et al. 2001; Crawley 2000). Another useful resource is the SHIRPA battery available at http://www.mgu.har.mrc.ac.uk/facilities/mutagenesis/mutabase/shirpa_summary.html, which outlines a battery of tests in three stages ranging from a rapid neurological screen to more detailed testing based on the system being studied.

The following is an example of a test series for motor behavioral studies arranged by our lab to test our Tor1a knock-ins and tissue specific knock-outs made to model early-onset dystonia. First, a semi-quantitative test devised by Fernagut and colleagues is performed to evaluate general postural and limb flexion, hindlimb clasping, and righting (Fernagut et al. 2002). A rating scale from 1 to 3 is established based on the level of departure from the predetermined performance of wild-type mice. Grip strength is evaluated using a grip strength apparatus that contains metal bars animals can grab onto and generate a reading of the grip force. The highest of ten readings is recorded (Cabe et al. 1978). The rotarod test is performed to evaluate motor coordination and balance. A rotating rod is set to accelerate slowly. Mice are placed on the rotating rod and the latency to fall is recorded (Carter et al. 2001). In the beam crossing test, mice are made to walk across a raised beam with an enclosed dark box at the end. Latency to crossing, number of falls, and foot slips off the edge are recorded. In subsequent trials, the beam shape (square and round) and size (28 mm, 12 mm, and 5 mm) are changed to challenge the animal (Carter et al. 2001). Finally, the pawprint test is performed to evaluate the precision and coordination of gait. Mice are trained to run down a narrow corridor with a piece of white absorbent paper on the bottom. Mouse paws are dipped in ink (different colors for hind and back paws), and the animal is released to run over the paper. The footprint is scored for stride and stance length and the degree to which the forepaw and hindpaw prints overlap (Carter et al. 2001).

Behavioral studies must be performed on a large enough quantity of mice for subsequent statistical analysis. Generating a large number of mice is both time-consuming and costly, and using naïve mice for the initial run of each test can be impractical. For researchers to overcome this limitation, they can employ a test battery whereby the same group of animals is used for a series of tests. It has been suggested that initial tests be done with one group of animals and if differences are seen, subsequent studies to confirm the differences can be done on naïve animals for each test (Paylor 2003). If a battery of tests is to be performed, test order and inter-test interval must be considered. Typically, the test order is determined according to the amount of stress each test will inflict on the mice, starting with the least and continuing to the most emotionally and physically invasive tests. Studies done in Paylor's lab showed that even when tests are arranged according to the level of stress induced, behavioral performance on some tests can be affected. The performance of wild-type C57BL/6J male mice on the rotarod and open-field experiments was altered when animals were previously used in another experiment. Interestingly, while this strain showed an effect, others such as the 129S6/SvEvTac did not.

IV. CONCLUSIONS

It is not an easy task to assess whether or not the generated mouse line is a suitable model for the disorder being studied. The major question is whether or not human symptoms can be replicated by replicating the known genetic aberration. Two considerations must be made in answering this question. The first concerns whether the altered protein is suspected to act alone or in concert with another factor to cause the phenotype in humans. For example, the DYT1 mutation of early-onset dystonia has only a 30–40% penetrance, suggesting the mutation does not act alone to produce the phenotype (Ozelius et al. 1997). Making a knock-in model of this genotype may not necessarily result in phenotypic expression until the appropriate secondary factor(s) is identified and allowed to work in conjunction with the known altered protein. Second, although similarities are plentiful, differences that do exist between mice and humans may have significant effects on the system being studied and may alter the way a phenotype is expressed. Biochemical and developmental pathway variations and differences in absolutes rates of physiological and pathological processes complicate mouse model analyses, and some may indeed not model human disorders (Erickson 1989). In addition, differences between human and mouse brain development have been uncovered that may affect the relevance of mouse models for some human diseases. Examples include the finding that Wnt7a, an important gene in early development, although highly conserved, showed significant differences in spatial and temporal expression in the midbrain and telencephalon of humans and mice (Fougerousse et al. 2000). Also, neuronal migration patterns vary between humans and mice (Rao and Wu 2001). Differences between the development of mice and humans could affect the expected phenotype and also justify cautionary measures that should be taken when applying mouse findings to humans.

Ideally, a model that genetically mimics the known aberration seen in patients should mimic the behavioral phenotype seen in these patients. However, tissue pathology and cellular abnormalities are themselves phenotypes that may be explored to yield interesting information about the disorder, and these cannot be ignored. From observing such cellular dysfunction as aggregation of α-synuclein or huntingtin, researchers can now study the mechanism of aggregation formation and its relationship to neurodegeneration leading to apparent motor abnormalities. The usefulness of a model must be defined partly on the ability of the model to mimic the behavioral phenotype of the disorder as well as the presence of other features that allow further understanding of the disorder at other biological levels. Furthermore, regardless of the initially detected behavioral phenotype, a mouse model can also be introduced into various mouse strains to identify modifiers. Environmental factors that may affect a phenotype or the pathophysiology of a model can be tested. Complex interactions between numbers of genes can also be evaluated by crossing several mouse lines. The quantity and type of knowledge that can be extracted from a mouse model depend partly on the inherent nature of the mouse physiology and the changes caused by the genetic alteration. It also depends on the imagination of the researcher in seeking out potential uses for the mouse model. The flexibility and virtually limitless material offered by genetically modified mouse lines ensure that mouse models will continue to play a significant role in the understanding of human disorders.

Acknowledgment

We thank Tony Vo for the illustrations in the figures.

References

Abeliovich, A., Y. Schmitz, I. Farinas, D. Choi-Lundberg, W.H. Ho, P.E. Castillo, et al. 2000. Mice lacking alpha-synuclein display functional deficits in the nigrostriatal dopamine system. *Neuron* **25**:239–252.

Adra, C.N., P.H. Boer, and M.W. McBurney. 1987. Cloning and expression of the mouse pgk-1 gene and the nucleotide sequence of its promoter. *Gene* **60**:65–74.

Amir, R.E., I.B Van den Veyver., M. Wan, C.Q. Tran, U. Francke, and H.Y. Zoghbi. 1999. Rett syndrome is caused by mutations in X-linked MECP2, encoding methyl-CpG-binding protein 2. *Nat Genet* **23**: 185–188.

Barski, J.J., K. Dethleffsen, and M. Meyer. 2000. Cre recombinase expression in cerebellar Purkinje cells. *Genesis* **28**:93–98.

Breitman, M.L., S. Clapoff, J. Rossant, L.C. Tsui, L.M. Glode, I.H. Maxwell, and A. Bernstein. 1987. Genetic ablation: targeted expression of a toxin gene causes microphthalmia in transgenic mice. *Science* **238**:1563–1565.

Brinster, R.L., J.M. Allen, R.R. Behringer, R.E. Gelinas, and R.D. Palmiter. 1988. Introns increase transcriptional efficiency in transgenic mice. *Proc Natl Acad Sci U S A* **85**:836–840.

Bronson, S.K., E.G. Plaehn, K.D. Kluckman, J.R. Hagaman, N. Maeda, and O. Smithies. 1996. Single-copy transgenic mice with chosen-site integration. *Proc Natl Acad Sci U S A* **93**:9067–9072.

Cabe, P.A., H.A. Tilson, C.L. Mitchell, and R. Dennis. 1978. A simple recording grip strength device. *Pharmacol Biochem Behav* **8**:101–102.

Cao, B.J., and Y. Li. 2002. Reduced anxiety- and depression-like behaviors in Emx1 homozygous mutant mice. *Brain Res* **937**:32–40.

Carter, R.J., A.J. Morton, and S.B. Dunnett. 2001. Locomotor Behavior. In *Current Protocols in Neuroscience*. Crawley, J.N.E.A. (ed.) Mississauga, Ontario, Canada: Wiley.

Carter, R.J., L.A. Lione, T. Humby, L. Mangiarini, A. Mahal, G.P. Bates, et al. 1999. Characterization of progressive motor deficits in mice transgenic for the human Huntington's disease mutation. *J Neurosci* **19**: 3248–3257.

Casanova, E., S. Fehsenfeld, T. Mantamadiotis, T. Lemberger, E. Greiner, A.F. Stewart, and G. Schutz. 2001. A CamKIIalpha iCre BAC allows brain-specific gene inactivation. *Genesis* **31**:37–42.

Clark, A.J., A. Cowper, R. Wallace, G. Wright, and J.P. Simons. 1992. Rescuing transgene expression by co-integration. *Biotechnology (N Y)* **10**:1450–1454.

Crawley, J. 2000. *What's Wrong with My Mouse?* New York: Wiley-Liss.

Crawley, J.N., J.K. Belknap, A. Collins, J.C. Crabbe, W. Frankel, N. Henderson, et al. 1997. Behavioral phenotypes of inbred mouse strains: implications and recommendations for molecular studies. *Psychopharmacology (Berl)* **132**:107–124.

Dal Canto, M.C., and M.E. Gurney. 1997. A low expressor line of transgenic mice carrying a mutant human Cu,Zn superoxide dismutase (SOD1) gene develops pathological changes that most closely resemble those in human amyotrophic lateral sclerosis. *Acta Neuropathol (Berl)* **93**:537–550.

Dauer, W., N. Kholodilov, M. Vila, A.C. Trillat, R. Goodchild, K.E. Larsen, et al. 2002. Resistance of alpha-synuclein null mice to the parkinsonian neurotoxin MPTP. *Proc Natl Acad Sci U S A* **99**:14524–14529.

Delaney, C.L., M. Brenner, and A. Messing. 1996. Conditional ablation of cerebellar astrocytes in postnatal transgenic mice. *J Neurosci* **16**:6908–6918.

Dragatsis, I., M.S. Levine, and S. Zeitlin. 2000. Inactivation of Hdh in the brain and testis results in progressive neurodegeneration and sterility in mice. *Nat Genet* **26**:300–306.

Dunnett, S.B. 2003. Assessment of motor impairments in transgenic mice. In *Mouse Behavioral Phenotyping Short Course*. Crawley, J. (ed.) New Orleans: Society for Neuroscience.

Erickson, R.P. 1989. Why isn't a mouse more like a man? *Trends Genet* **5**:1–3.

Evans, M.J., and M.H. Kaufman. 1981. Establishment in culture of pluripotential cells from mouse embryos. *Nature* **292**:154–156.

Fernagut, P.O., E. Diguet, N. Stefanova, M. Biran, G.K. Wenning, P. Canioni, et al. 2002. Subacute systemic 3-nitropropionic acid intoxication induces a distinct motor disorder in adult C57Bl/6 mice: behavioural and histopathological characterisation. *Neuroscience* **114**: 1005–1017.

Folger, K.R., E.A. Wong, G. Wahl, and M.R. Capecchi. 1982. Patterns of integration of DNA microinjected into cultured mammalian cells: evidence for homologous recombination between injected plasmid DNA molecules. *Mol Cell Biol* **2**:1372–1387.

Fougerousse, F., P. Bullen, M. Herasse, S. Lindsay, I. Richard, D. Wilson, et al. 2000. Human-mouse differences in the embryonic expression patterns of developmental control genes and disease genes. *Hum Mol Genet* **9**:165–173.

Francis, D.D., K. Szegda, G. Campbell, W.D. Martin, and T.R. Insel. 2003. Epigenetic sources of behavioral differences in mice. *Nat Neurosci* **6**:445–446.

Furth, P.A., L. St. Onge, H. Boger, P. Gruss, M. Gossen, A. Kistner, et al. 1994. Temporal control of gene expression in transgenic mice by a tetracycline-responsive promoter. *Proc Natl Acad Sci U S A* **91**:9302–9306.

Gerlai, R. 1996. Gene-targeting studies of mammalian behavior: is it the mutation or the background genotype? *Trends Neurosci* **19**:177–181.

Giraldo, P., and L. Montoliu. 2001. Size matters: use of YACs, BACs and PACs in transgenic animals. *Transgenic Res* **10**:83–103.

Gordon, J.W., G.A. Scangos, D.J. Plotkin, J.A. Barbosa, and F.H. Ruddle. 1980. Genetic transformation of mouse embryos by microinjection of purified DNA. *Proc Natl Acad Sci U S A* **77**:7380–7384.

Gossen, M., and H. Bujard. 1992. Tight control of gene expression in mammalian cells by tetracycline-responsive promoters. *Proc Natl Acad Sci U S A* **89**:5547–5551.

Gossen, M., S. Freundlieb, G. Bender, G. Muller, W. Hillen, and H. Bujard. 1995. Transcriptional activation by tetracyclines in mammalian cells. *Science* **268**:1766–1769.

Guo, H., J.M. Christoff, V.E. Campos, X.L. Jin, and Y. Li. 2000a. Normal corpus callosum in Emx1 mutant mice with C57BL/6 background. *Biochem Biophys Res Commun* **276**:649–653.

Guo, H., S. Hong, X.L. Jin, R.S. Chen, P.P. Avasthi, Y.T. Tu, et al. 2000b. Specificity and efficiency of Cre-mediated recombination in Emx1-Cre knock-in mice. *Biochem Biophys Res Commun* **273**:661–665.

Gutierrez-Adan, A., and B. Pintado. 2000. Effect of flanking matrix attachment regions on the expression of microinjected transgenes during preimplantation development of mouse embryos. *Transgenic Res* **9**:81–89.

Higgins, J.J., L.T. Pho, and L.E. Nee. 1997. A gene (ETM) for essential tremor maps to chromosome 2p22-p25. *Mov Disord* **12**:859–864.

Hodgson, J.G., N. Agopyan, C.A. Gutekunst, B.R. Leavitt, F., LePiane, R. Singaraja, et al. 1999. A YAC mouse model for Huntington's disease with full-length mutant huntingtin, cytoplasmic toxicity, and selective striatal neurodegeneration. *Neuron* **23**:181–192.

Huntington's Disease Collaborative Research Group, The. 1993. A novel gene containing a trinucleotide repeat that is expanded and unstable on Huntington's disease chromosomes. *Cell* **72**:971–983.

Jin, X.L., H. Guo, C. Mao, N. Atkins, H. Wang, P.P. Avasthi, et al. 2000. Emx1-specific expression of foreign genes using "knock-in" approach. *Biochem Biophys Res Commun* **270**:978–982.

Kaneko, S., T. Hikida, D. Watanabe, H. Ichinose, T. Nagatsu, R.J. Kreitman, et al. 2000. Synaptic integration mediated by striatal cholinergic interneurons in basal ganglia function. *Science* **289**:633–637.

Kelly, E.J., E.P. Sandgren, R.L. Brinster, and R.D. Palmiter. 1997. A pair of adjacent glucocorticoid response elements regulate expression of two mouse metallothionein genes. *Proc Natl Acad Sci U S A* **94**: 10045–10050.

Kuhn, R., F. Schwenk, M. Aguet, and K. Rajewsky. 1995. Inducible gene targeting in mice. *Science* **269**:1427–1429.

Lakso, M., B. Sauer, B. Mosinger, Jr., E.J. Lee, R.W. Manning, S.H. Yu, et al. 1992. Targeted oncogene activation by site-specific recombination in transgenic mice. *Proc Natl Acad Sci U S A* **89**:6232–6236.

Lee, M.K., W. Stirling, Y. Xu, X. Xu, D. Qui, A.S. Mandir, et al. 2002. Human alpha-synuclein-harboring familial Parkinson's disease-linked Ala-53 → Thr mutation causes neurodegenerative disease with alpha-synuclein aggregation in transgenic mice. *Proc Natl Acad Sci U S A* **99**:8968–8973.

Lee, P., G. Morley, Q. Huang, A. Fischer, S. Seiler, J.W. Horner, et al. 1998. Conditional lineage ablation to model human diseases. *Proc Natl Acad Sci U S A* **95**:11371–11376.

Levine, M.S., G.J. Klapstein, A. Koppel, E. Gruen, C. Cepeda, M.E. Vargas, et al. 1999. Enhanced sensitivity to N-methyl-D-aspartate receptor activation in transgenic and knockin mouse models of Huntington's disease. *J Neurosci Res* **58**:515–532.

Li, Q., S. Harju, and K.R. Peterson. 1999. Locus control regions: coming of age at a decade plus. *Trends Genet* **15**:403–408.

Liang, F., and M. Jasin. 1995. Studies on the influence of cytosine methylation on DNA recombination and end-joining in mammalian cells. *J Biol Chem* **270**:23838–23844.

Luthi-Carter, R., A. Strand, N.L. Peters, S.M. Solano, Z.R. Hollingsworth, A.S. Menon, et al. 2000. Decreased expression of striatal signaling genes in a mouse model of Huntington's disease. *Hum Mol Genet* **9**:1259–1271.

Mayford, M., M.E. Bach, Y.Y. Huang, L. Wang, R.D Hawkins, and E.R. Kandel. 1996. Control of memory formation through regulated expression of a CaMKII transgene. *Science* **274**:1678–1683.

McLeod, M., S. Craft, and J.R. Broach. 1986. Identification of the crossover site during FLP-mediated recombination in the *Saccharomyces cerevisiae* plasmid 2 microns circle. *Mol Cell Biol* **6**:3357–3367.

Metzger, D., and P. Chambon. 2001. Site- and time-specific gene targeting in the mouse. *Methods* **24**:71–80.

Mombaerts, P., A.R. Clarke, M.L. Hooper, and S. Tonegawa. 1991. Creation of a large genomic deletion at the T-cell antigen receptor beta-subunit locus in mouse embryonic stem cells by gene targeting. *Proc Natl Acad Sci U S A* **88**:3084–3087.

Monaco, A.P., and Z. Larin. 1994. YACs, BACs, PACs and MACs: artificial chromosomes as research tools. *Trends Biotechnol* **12**:280–286.

Nadeau, J.H. 2001. Modifier genes in mice and humans. *Nat Rev Genet* **2**:165–174.

Nagy, A., M. Gertsenstein, K. Vintersten, and R. Behringer. 2003. *Manipulating the Mouse Embryo*. Cold Spring Harbor, New York: Cold Spring Harbor Laboratory Press.

Nirenberg, S., and C. Cepko. 1993. Targeted ablation of diverse cell classes in the nervous system in vivo. *J Neurosci* **13**:3238–3251.

Oka, T., I. Komuro, I. Shiojima, Y. Hiroi, T. Mizuno, R. Aikawa, et al. 1997. Autoregulation of human cardiac homeobox gene CSX1: mediation by the enhancer element in the first intron. *Heart Vessels* **Suppl**:10–14.

Okabe, S. 1999. Gene Expression in Transgenic Mice Using Neural Promoters. In *Current Protocols in Neuroscience*. Crawley, J.N.E.A. (ed.) Mississauga, Ontario, Canada: Wiley.

Ozelius, L.J., J. Hewett, P. Kramer, S.B. Bressman, C. Shalish, D. de Leon, et al. 1997. Fine localization of the torsion dystonia gene (DYT1) on human chromosome 9q34: YAC map and linkage disequilibrium. *Genome Res* **7**:483–494.

Palmiter, R.D., E.P. Sandgren, M.R. Avarbock, D.D. Allen, and R.L. Brinster. 1991. Heterologous introns can enhance expression of transgenes in mice. *Proc Natl Acad Sci U S A* **88**:478–482.

Palmiter, R.D., R.R. Behringer, C.J. Quaife, F. Maxwell, I.H. Maxwell, and R.L. Brinster. 1987. Cell lineage ablation in transgenic mice by cell-specific expression of a toxin gene. *Cell* **50**:435–443.

Paylor, R. 2003. High-throughput screening strategies. In *Mouse Behavioral Phenotyping Short Course*. Crawley, J.N. (ed.) New Orleans: Society for Neuroscience.

Picciotto, M.R., and K. Wickman. 1998. Using knockout and transgenic mice to study neurophysiology and behavior. *Physiol Rev* **78**:1131–1163.

Polymeropoulos, M.H., C. Lavedan, E. Leroy, S.E. Ide, A. Dehejia, A. Dutra, et al. 1997. Mutation in the alpha-synuclein gene identified in families with Parkinson's disease. *Science* **276**:2045–2047.

Qiu, M., S. Anderson, S. Chen, J.J. Meneses, R. Hevner, E. Kuwana, et al. 1996. Mutation of the Emx-1 homeobox gene disrupts the corpus callosum. *Dev Biol* **178**:174–178.

Ramdas, J., and K. Muniyappa. 1995. Recognition and alignment of homologous DNA sequences between minichromosomes and single-stranded DNA promoted by RecA protein. *Mol Gen Genet* **249**:336–348.

Rao, Y., and J.Y. Wu. 2001. Neuronal migration and the evolution of the human brain. *Nat Neurosci* **4**:860–862.

Ryding, A.D., M.G. Sharp, and J.J. Mullins. 2001. Conditional transgenic technologies. *J Endocrinol* **171**:1–14.

Saam, J.R., and J.I. Gordon. 1999. Inducible gene knockouts in the small intestinal and colonic epithelium. *J Biol Chem* **274**:38071–38082.

Sauer, B., and N. Henderson. 1988. Site-specific DNA recombination in mammalian cells by the Cre recombinase of bacteriophage P1. *Proc Natl Acad Sci U S A* **85**:5166–5170.

Schilling, G., M.W. Becher, A.H. Sharp, H.A. Jinnah, K. Duan, J.A. Kotzuk, et al. 1999. Intranuclear inclusions and neuritic aggregates in transgenic mice expressing a mutant N-terminal fragment of huntingtin. *Hum Mol Genet* **8**:397–407.

Shelbourne, P.F., N. Killeen, R.F. Hevner, H.M. Johnston, L. Tecott, M. Lewandoski, et al. 1999. A Huntington's disease CAG expansion at the murine Hdh locus is unstable and associated with behavioural abnormalities in mice. *Hum Mol Genet* **8**:763–774.

Shockett, P., M. Difilippantonio, N. Hellman, and D.G. Schatz. 1995. A modified tetracycline-regulated system provides autoregulatory, inducible gene expression in cultured cells and transgenic mice. *Proc Natl Acad Sci U S A* **92**:6522–6526.

Smith, G.R. 1994. Hotspots of homologous recombination. *Experientia* **50**:234–241.

Smithies, O., M.A. Koralewski, K.Y. Song, and R.S. Kucherlapati. 1984. Homologous recombination with DNA introduced into mammalian cells. *Cold Spring Harb Symp Quant Biol* **49**:161–170.

Sommer, B., S. Barbieri, K. Hofele, K. Wiederhold, A. Probst, C. Mistl, et al. 2000. Mouse models of alpha-synucleinopathy and Lewy pathology. *Exp Gerontol* **35**:1389–1403.

Soriano, P. 1999. Generalized lacZ expression with the ROSA26 Cre reporter strain. *Nat Genet* **21**:70–71.

Svaren, J., and R. Chalkley. 1990. The structure and assembly of active chromatin. *Trends Genet* **6**:52–56.

Tanzi, R.E., K. Petrukhin, I. Chernov, J.L. Pellequer, W. Wasco, B. Ross, et al. 1993. The Wilson disease gene is a copper transporting ATPase with homology to the Menkes disease gene. *Nat Genet* **5**:344–350.

te Riele, H., E.R. Maandag, and A. Berns. 1992. Highly efficient gene targeting in embryonic stem cells through homologous recombination with isogenic DNA constructs. *Proc Natl Acad Sci U S A* **89**:5128–5132.

Thomas, K.R., C. Deng, and M.R. Capecchi. 1992. High-fidelity gene targeting in embryonic stem cells by using sequence replacement vectors. *Mol Cell Biol* **12**:2919–2923.

Threadgill, D.W., A.A. Dlugosz, L.A. Hansen, T. Tennenbaum, U. Lichti, D. Yee, et al. 1995. Targeted disruption of mouse EGF receptor: effect of genetic background on mutant phenotype. *Science* **269**:230–234.

Torres, R.M., and R. Kuhn. 1997. *Laboratory Protocols for Conditional Gene Targeting*. New York: Oxford University Press.

Vasquez, K.M., K. Marburger, Z. Intody, and J.H. Wilson. 2001. Manipulating the mammalian genome by homologous recombination. *Proc Natl Acad Sci U S A* **98**:8403–8410.

Watanabe, D., H. Inokawa, K. Hashimoto, N. Suzuki, M. Kano, R. Shigemoto, et al. 1998. Ablation of cerebellar Golgi cells disrupts synaptic integration involving GABA inhibition and NMDA receptor activation in motor coordination. *Cell* **95**:17–27.

Wilkie, T.M., R.L. Brinster, and R.D. Palmiter. 1986. Germline and somatic mosaicism in transgenic mice. *Dev Biol* **118**:9–18.

Wilson, C., H.J. Bellen, and W.J. Gehring. 1990. Position effects on eukaryotic gene expression. *Annu Rev Cell Biol* **6**:679–714.

Yagi, T., S. Nada, N. Watanabe, H. Tamemoto, N. Kohmura, Y. Ikawa, and S. Aizawa. 1993. A novel negative selection for homologous recombinants using diphtheria toxin A fragment gene. *Anal Biochem.* **214**:77–86.

Yamamoto, A., J.J. Lucas, and R. Hen. 2000. Reversal of neuropathology and motor dysfunction in a conditional model of Huntington's disease. *Cell* **101**:57–66.

Yoshida, M., Y. Suda, I. Matsuo, N. Miyamoto, N. Takeda, S. Kuratani, and S. Aizawa. 1997. Emx1 and Emx2 functions in development of dorsal telencephalon. *Development* **124**:101–111.

Zielenski, J., M. Corey, R. Rozmahel, D. Markiewicz, I. Aznarez, T. Casals, et al. 1999. Detection of a cystic fibrosis modifier locus for meconium ileus on human chromosome 19q13. *Nat Genet* **22**:128–129.

Zimmer, A., and K. Reynolds. 1994. Gene targeting constructs: effects of vector topology on co-expression efficiency of positive and negative selectable marker genes. *Biochem Biophys Res Commun* **201**:943–949.

CHAPTER

A4

Genetics of Spontaneous Mutations in Mice

HAIXIANG PENG and COLIN F. FLETCHER

A variety of strategies, which employ genetic, chemical, or physical manipulations, are used to create models of human disease. Although these strategies are applied to a variety of species, the mouse in particular has proven to be an invaluable experimental resource, in large part because of the sophisticated genetic techniques and resources that have been available. The recent publication of the assembled mouse genome sequence has significantly advanced the field of mouse genetics. As a result, new resources are now available that greatly expedite the construction or isolation of mouse models of movement disorders.

Genetic approaches come in two categories. Those that begin with manipulation of specific genes, followed by phenotype assessment, are referred to as "gene-driven," "targeted," or "reverse" genetics, and are covered elsewhere in this volume. The classical approach of first searching for the deviant phenotype, and then identifying the underlying genetic mutation solely by its chromosomal position, is known as "forward" genetics. These mutations are generally referred to as "spontaneous," but they also include induced mutations that result from mutagen treatments that are not targeted to specific genes, for example, X-rays, transposons, or chemical mutagens. Once considered a Herculean task, positional cloning is now a fairly straightforward process. For example, this approach had often relied on the detection of rare, spontaneously occurring mutations, thus requiring large breeding colonies, such as the Jackson Laboratory's production facility. Screeners now use chemical mutagenesis to increase the mutation rate, enabling the efficient recovery of phenodeviants from smaller colonies. Genetic mapping of mutations had also been hampered by the lack of polymorphic markers for the inbred strains. One benefit of the genome sequencing effort has been the identification of a large collection of such markers. Finally, the laborious process of physical cloning, sequencing, and gene identification in these intervals is obsolete, as these chromosomal regions can now simply be browsed with a few mouse clicks. Spurred by these advances, there are now a large number of active mutagenesis and screening programs. A logical synthesis of the "targeted" and "forward" approaches has also emerged: it is a strategy that combines random mutagenesis with molecular screening to identify mutations in specific genes. These methods offer the promise of improving the availability of "knockout" alleles, and also providing point mutation alleles. This review will discuss the resources available for, and issues involved in, identification of new locomotor mutants in the mouse.

TABLE 1 A Selected List of Cloned Spontaneous Locomotor Mutants

Mutant name	Gene symbol	Gene name
ataxia	*Usp14*	ubiquitin specific protease 14
purkinje cell degeneration	*Agtpbp1*	ATP/GTP binding protein 1
swaying	*Wnt1*	wingless-related MMTV integration site 1
rostral cerebellar malformation	*Unc5c*	unc-5 homolog C
jittery	*Atcay*	ataxia, cerebellar, Cayman type homolog
tottering	*Cacna1a*	calcium channel, voltage-dependent, P/Q type, alpha 1A subunit
cerebellar deficient folia	*Catna2*	alpha N-catenin
motor neuron degeneration	*Cln8*	ceroid-lipofuscinosis, neuronal 8
motor endplate disease	*Scn8a*	sodium channel, voltage-gated, type VIII, alpha
staggerer	*Rora*	RAR-related orphan receptor alpha
ducky	*Cacna2d2*	calcium channel, voltage-dependent, alpha 2/delta subunit 2
dystonia	*Dst*	dystonin
jerker	*Espn*	espin
lurcher	*Grid2*	glutamate receptor, ionotropic, delta 2
weeble	*Inpp4a*	inositol polyphosphate-4-phosphatase, type I
opisthotonos	*Itpr1*	inositol 1,4,5-triphosphate receptor 1
vertigo	*Kcnq1*	potassium voltage-gated channel, subfamily Q, member 1
myodystrophy	*Large*	like glycosyltransferase
robotic	*Mllt2h*	homolog of human MLLT2
shaker	*Myo7a*	myosin VIIa
harlequin	*Pdcd8*	programmed cell death 8
vibrator	*Pitpn*	phosphatidylinositol transfer protein
muscular dysgenesis	*Cacna1s*	calcium channel, voltage-dependent, L type, alpha 1S
arrested development of righting response	*Clcn1*	chloride channel 1
spastic	*Glrb*	glycine receptor, beta subunit
spasmodic	*Glra1*	glycine receptor, alpha 1 subunit
kreisler	*Mafb*	v-maf musculoaponeurotic fibrosarcoma oncogene family, protein B
dreher	*Lmx1a*	LIM homeobox transcription factor 1 alpha
stargazer	*Cacng2*	calcium channel, voltage-dependent, gamma subunit 2

I. MUTANT RESOURCES

The so-called "classical" mouse locomotor mutations comprise a fascinating and diverse collection of mutant strains (Green 1989; Blake et al. 2003). These strains express various phenotypes, such as ataxia, dystonia, startle defects, loss of righting reflex, or motor neuron defects. A select list of cloned mutants, presented in table 1, is meant to illustrate some of the important points about spontaneous alleles. First, unlike targeted mutations, which are usually designed to be null alleles, spontaneous mutations can have a variety of effects on gene function. For example, these can be nonsense mutations that truncate the open reading frame, splice site mutations that cause exon skipping, transposon insertions that decrease transcription, missense mutations that change single amino acids, or promoter/enhancer mutations that alter expression patterns. Thus, in addition to nulls, alleles can include gain of function (neomorphic), partial

TABLE 2 ENU Mutagenesis Programs

Program	Web address
The Sloan-Kettering Mouse Project	http://mouse.ski.mskcc.org/
Neuroscience Mutagenesis Facility	http://www.jax.org/nmf/
Tennessee Mouse Genome Consortium	http://www.tnmouse.org/
Mouse Mutagenesis Center for Developmental Defects	http://www.mouse-genome.bcm.tmc.edu/ENU/MutagenesisProj.asp
Center for Functional Genomics	http://genome.northwestern.edu/a
Mouse Heart, Lung, Blood, and Sleep Disorders Center	http://pga.jax.org//index.html
Riken Mutagenesis Project	http://www.gsc.riken.go.jp/Mouse/
ENU-Mouse Mutagenesis Screen Project	http://www.gsf.de/ieg/groups/enu-mouse.html
Harwell Mutagenesis Programme	http://www.mgu.har.mrc.ac.uk/
Centre for Modeling Human Disease	http://www.cmhd.ca/
McLaughlin Research Institute	http://www.montana.edu/wwwmri/enump.html
The Medical Genome Centre	http://jcsmr.anu.edu.au/group_pages/mgc/

loss of function (hypomorphic), and dominant negative (antimorphic) alleles. In many cases, different alleles can give rise to distinct phenotypes. This can occur because the mutations have different effects, for example, nonsense versus missense mutation, or because mutations affect different specific domains or functions of the protein. A collection of mutations in a particular gene, referred to as an "allelic series," can provide insight into the biological role(s) of a gene that is not available from a single engineered null allele. A corollary of this point is that successful modeling of human disease requires the appropriate mouse allele. The most common explanation for the difference between a human and a mouse phenotype, for mutations in a given gene, is that the mutations have different effects on gene function. Typically, a targeted null mouse allele will be a poor model of a dominant human missense mutation. In cases where the mutations are equivalent it is rare to find differences in the phenotypes.

A second point is that positional cloning of mutations is an unbiased approach to gene function that can identify a locomotor-related gene in the absence of any assumptions by the investigator. In fact, the list in table 1 includes genes that one would not have anticipated to play a role in locomotor function. Using the criteria of biochemical function or gene expression to select genes for targeting, in expectation of a locomotor phenotype, does not appear to be very successful and certainly does not work for novel or poorly annotated genes.

In summary, this collection of classical mutations suggests that isolation of novel ataxic strains should be an informative and useful undertaking. These mutants have severe and overt phenotypes, in part because they were isolated by simple visual observation. This suggests that more quantitative or complex screens could uncover more subtle phenotypes.

II. MUTAGENESIS SCREENS

Currently a number of chemical mutagenesis screens are being performed, some of which include specific locomotor assays (Brown and Peters 1996; Hrabe de Angelis and Balling 1998; Kasarskis et al. 1998; Schimenti and Bucan 1998; Hardisty et al. 1999; Justice et al. 1999; Anderson 2000; Hrabe de Angelis et al. 2000; Nolan et al. 2000; Rathkolb et al. 2000; Soewarto et al. 2000; Nelms and Goodnow 2001; Brown and Hardisty 2003). Several screens are being performed with the aim of freely distributing mice to investigators, while others are operated as collaborations. Information can be found at the Web addresses listed in table 2.

Mutagenesis is accomplished by injecting male mice with *N*-ethyl-*N*-nitrosourea (ENU), an alkylating agent that acts as a potent mutagen *in vivo*. ENU is particularly potent in spermatogonial stem cells, thus giving rise to transmittable mutations (Russell and Montgomery 1982; Shelby and Tindall 1997; Justice et al. 2000; Noveroske et al. 2000; Weber et al. 2000). ENU forms 12 adducts with DNA. While these adducts are not mutations *per se*, they allow incorrect base pairing, which results in base changes after DNA replication. In mice, approximately 80% affect A:T base pairs, changing the pair to T:A or G:C. The majority of changes results in missense mutations, with splice site and nonsense mutations also being found. The mutagenesis rate for functional mutations can be as high as 1/175–700 gametes per locus. Thus, approximately 2,000 pedigrees need to be screened to ensure with greater than 95% confidence that a mutation would be recovered in any particular gene.

Injected male mice are subsequently bred to wild-type females to produce heterozygous animals (referred to as the G1 generation) that harbor upwards of fifty functional mutations. These G1 animals can be immediately screened for dominant mutations. To recover recessive mutations, breeding of two more generations is required. This can consist of mating, recovering G2 offspring, and backcrossing the G2 animals to the G1 parent. Since each G2 animal inherits half of the mutations from the G1, usually several female G2 animals are backcrossed to their G1 sire. In this way, one in eight G3 animals is expected to be homozygous for a mutation at any particular locus, and each G3 harbors as many as six homozygous mutations. Alternatively, G2 animals can be intercrossed, with one in four G3 expected to be homozygous for a given mutation, although each then harbors half the total number of mutations. The animals generated from the original founding G1 parent are referred to as a pedigree. Although the highest efficiency is accomplished by screening fewer G3s and more total pedigrees, often enough G3s are screened to recover two or more phenodeviants in a pedigree. This screening ensures success in breeding the next generation and is thought to reduce the number of false positives. Usually, inheritability of the deviant phenotype is confirmed when the G3 deviants are bred to wild type animals, offspring are intercrossed, and deviants are recovered in the next generation.

Scientists have developed several variations to this basic breeding scheme. One simple alternative is to mate two unrelated G1s together to produce G2 animals for intercrossing. This scheme preserves the advantage of reduced husbandry in the intercross and increases the mutagenic load. Another variation is breeding on mixed backgrounds. For the dominant screens, F1 hybrids are produced. This breeding strategy provides a fixed genetic background for screening and improves the efficiency of sperm freezing. Furthermore, the deviant G1 can then be immediately backcrossed to one of the parental lines for genetic mapping. For a recessive screen, another background can be introduced during G2 production, allowing the G1 × G2 mating to be a mapping backcross. Other alternatives allow the selection of mutations localized to a particular chromosomal region. Strains harboring deletions can be mated to mutagenized mice to uncover recessive alleles in the deletion interval (Rinchik et al. 1990; Justice et al. 1997; Rinchik and Carpenter 1999). The most sophisticated variation is the use of marked chromosome inversion strains (Justice et al. 1999). In this scheme, mutagenized mice are bred to strains that harbor a chromosome inversion marked with a dominant visible phenotype. Offspring are mated to a strain that carries the inversion and another dominant mutation in trans. In this way multiple offspring that carry the mutagenized chromosome and the marked inversion can be generated and identified. These mice are then intercrossed. Homozygous inversion mice die *in utero*, leaving two classes of offspring—homozygous mice carrying the mutagenized chromosome and heterozygous mice carrying the inversion and mutagenized chromosomes. The pedigree can be assumed to harbor an embryonic lethal mutation if the homozygous mutagenized mice are missing. If these mice are born, then a large cohort can be produced for screening. This regional screen, while limiting the percent of the genome that is interrogated, has the advantage of providing multiple mice known to be homozygous for the mutagenized chromosome.

The success of a screening program relies on the quality of the phenotypic screen. Unlike the usual behavioral assay that is performed at a single time point with cohorts of mutant and wild type animals, these screens are continuously performed over the course of months. Because each pedigree produces a few litters per month, it may take several months to complete the screening of twenty to thirty G3s per pedigree. Furthermore, one or two mutants may be among those thirty G3s. Therefore, the screen must be rigorous enough to reliably detect rare outliers and still have a low false positive rate. To control for variation over time and observer bias, it is useful to obtain and track quantitative measures for any screen. To that end, many of the screens for locomotor deviants use open field arenas equipped with infrared beams or video tracking to measure locomotor parameters such as total distance, velocity, ambulatory events, and rearing events. These parameters have proven to be very stable over the course of three years of screening ENU pedigrees. Equally important is the fact that the population shows a normal distribution (Figure 1), which simplifies the statistical treatment. Also, it appears that evaluating outlier mice based on a combination of parameters is quite informative. For example, ataxic mice often show reduced rearing behavior. Hyperactive mice, however, also show decreased rearing. Thus, a combination of decreased rearing and low total distance can be used to define hypoactive/ataxic animals (Figure 2). It is evident from the number of locomotor mutant strains described on various Web sites that these kinds of mutations occur relatively frequently. Heritable locomotor mutants are recovered at the Genomics Institute of the Novartis Research Foundation (GNF) at a rate of one per fifty pedigrees screened.

Once phenodeviant mice from a pedigree are proven heritable, a cohort of animals can be used for secondary assays, such as the rotarod or pole test paradigms, to further define the mutant phenotype. Finally, histological analysis can be used to diagnose neuronal or myopathic disease.

III. SENSITIZED SCREENS

An open question remains as to what extent unintentional biases affect the sorts of phenodeviants that are recovered from a screen. Such biases might include effects of the mouse strain background, which would arise from the particular collection of gene variants or predisposing mutations that are present in that genome. For example, the wheels mutation has been recovered in the dominant screen at Harwell, but never at GSF, and this may be due to the dif-

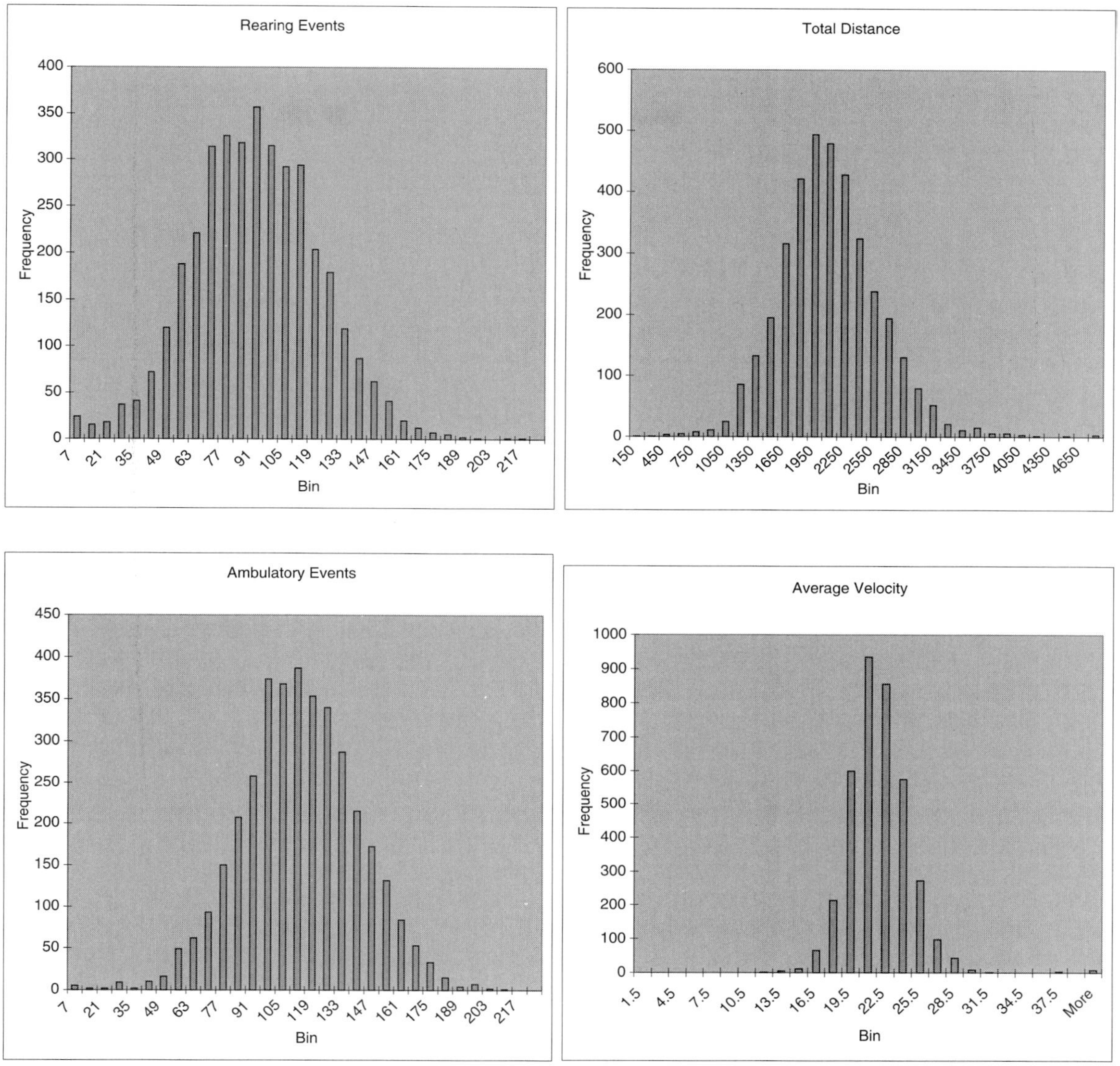

FIGURE 1 Activity parameters for 3,694 G3 animals. Histograms are presented for each parameter, rearing events (upper left), total distance (upper right), ambulatory events (lower left), and average velocity (lower right). Frequency is plotted in the Y axis and animals are binned in the X axis with maximum values for every second bin indicated. Importantly, the population parameters show normal distributions.

ferent strains used in each screen. Interestingly, the baseline levels of locomotor activity varied significantly among inbred strains (http://aretha.jax.org/pub-cgi/phenome/mpdcgi?rtn=docs/home). This discrepancy suggests the presence of genetic variants in the strains that will influence locomotor phenotype. At the least, baseline behavior must be considered in terms of whether outliers might or might not be detectable in specific assays. Moreover, it is known that genetic modifiers exist in strains, and these alleles can significantly modify certain mutant phenotypes, e.g., *Mom* (multiple intestinal neoplasia modifier), and *Scnm1* (sodium channel modifier) (MacPhee et al. 1995; Buchner et al. 2003). Therefore, mutagenesis of a variety of strains possibly may yield additional phenodeviants.

Similarly, it may be useful to sensitize a screen for particular phenotypes by intentionally incorporating predisposing mutations in the mutagenized strain. This process can be accomplished with transgenes or knockout alleles. For example, if the pedigrees carried an APP or SOD transgene, one could screen for ENU mutations that ameliorated or exacerbated the behavioral deficits. In this way screens can be tailored to explore specific disease pathways. One could also sensitize a screen by using chemical or other challenges to induce locomotor deficits. Obvious candidates include

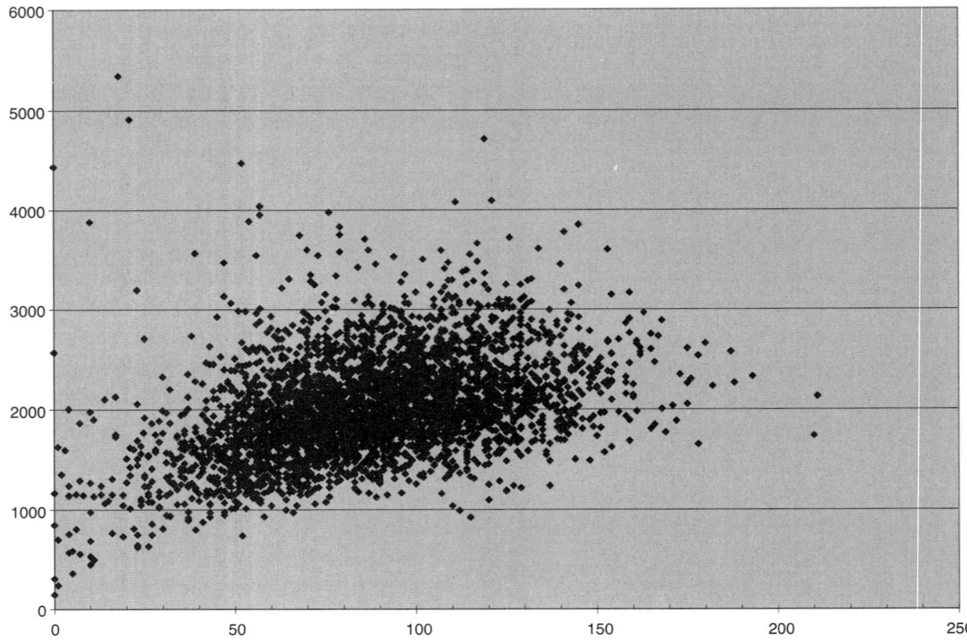

FIGURE 2 Total distance by rearing events. Plotting total distance (Y axis) by rearing events (X axis) reveals several classes of outlier animals. Ataxic animals usually show low rearing and low total distance (lower left, <50 rearings, <1,000 beam breaks). Hyperactive locomotion may be associated with normal rearing (>50 rearing events, >3,000 beam breaks) or low rearing (<50 rearing events, >3,000 beam breaks).

cocaine, amphetamines, MPTP, and harmaline. In fact, as screening programs mature, one might expect that more complex and specific screening protocols will be developed.

IV. MAPPING RESOURCES

The ultimate goal of the screening program is to identify genes that play a role in locomotor behavior and this goal is accomplished by meiotic recombination mapping of the mutant locus. The specific mapping strategy will differ depending on whether the mutagenized mice were produced on a pure or mixed strain background. For mice on a pure background, the affected animals are simply bred to another strain and the progeny are intercrossed or backcrossed to an affected parent. Offspring are then genotyped using molecular markers that distinguish the two strains and the inheritance pattern of the markers is compared to the phenotypes of the progeny. If the mutagenized strain was C57BL/6, for example, then affected animals are presumed to be homozygous C57BL/6 at the mutant locus. A linked molecular marker will show a similar inheritance pattern, with a homozygous C57BL/6 genotype only in affected animals as well, while unlinked markers will have varied genotypes. For linked markers, meiotic recombination will decrease the fidelity of the co-inheritance of genotype with frequency of nonconcordance increasing in a manner roughly proportional to physical distance. From this analysis one can define a physical interval that must contain the mutant gene. By analyzing several hundred progeny from a mapping cross, a region of 0.5–1.0 megabases can be identified, which might contain five to ten genes.

Molecular polymorphisms commonly used in the mouse include restriction fragment length polymorphisms (RFLPs), simple sequence length polymorphisms (SSLPs) and single nucleotide polymorphisms (SNPs). RFLPs are single nucleotide changes that alter restriction fragment cleavage sites, and are usually detected as a difference in fragment sizes by Southern blot analysis. SSLPs are differences in the length of simple sequence repeats, usually CA repeats, and are detected using flanking primers to amplify fragments containing the repeat (Dietrich et al. 1992). SNPs are single nucleotide differences, and are detected by various PCR amplification and primer extension strategies, as well as by direct sequencing. In the past, distantly related strains were used in order to facilitate the discovery of RFLPs and SSLPs at sufficient density for fine mapping. The rationale for using related inbred strains as mapping partners is to reduce strain background effects on the phenotype. The advent of high density SNP collections makes use of these strains feasible (Lindblad-Toh et al. 2000; Wade et al. 2002; Wiltshire et al. 2003). SNPs are highly amenable to automation and high throughput analysis, and occur at a high frequency between mouse strains, with an estimated 3×10^6

SNPs between inbred strains. Information about these markers is readily available from various databases, including the Center for Inherited Disease Research (CIDR) (http://www.cidr.jhmi.edu/mouse/mouse.html), the Broad Institute (http://www.broad.mit.edu/cgi-bin/mouse/index), the Jackson Laboratory (http://aretha.jax.org/pub-cgi/phenome/mpdcgi?rtn=projects/details&id=146), Roche Bioscience (http://mousesnp.roche.com/), the National Center for Biotechnology Information (http://www.ncbi.nlm.nih.gov/SNP/MouseSNP.html), and GNF (http://snp.gnf.org/).

Analysis of the distribution of SNP and SSLP polymorphisms in the mouse genome has revealed very discrete regions of high or low polymorphism densities between strain pairs (Wade et al. 2002; Wiltshire et al. 2003). These "hot" or "cold" regions have SNP densities of 1/1000 bp and 1/50,000 bp, respectively, on average. In some cases these intervals can be tens of megabases long and they encompass 30–40% of the genome. Because some of the strains are derived from related ancestors, the regions of near identity were probably common to the original founder mice. The implication for mutation mapping is that a locus might fall into a region of low marker density, thus hampering gene localization. The solution is simply to examine the SNP distribution in other strains and pick a mapping partner better suited for the locus in question.

Once a mutation is localized, one can examine the assembled genomic sequence to identify the genes contained in the interval (http://genome.ucsc.edu/, http://www.ensembl.org/) (Mural et al. 2002; Waterston et al. 2002). Genes have been identified and annotated with high confidence as a result of cross species comparison and full-length cDNA sequencing and annotation efforts. For example, detailed annotation information about cDNAs characterized as part of the RIKEN functional annotation of the mouse project (FANTOM) can be retrieved from http://fantom.gsc.riken.go.jp/ (Okazaki et al. 2002). Additional information about the candidate genes can be garnered from large-scale expression analyses across some fifty tissues using microarrays. The results of these analyses are available at the UCSC Web site, the RIKEN Web site, and the GNF Web site (http://expression.gnf.org/cgi-bin/index.cgi) (Su et al. 2002; Bono et al. 2003). At the very least, expression data can eliminate from consideration genes that are not expressed in the affected tissue.

Evaluation of candidate genes by sequencing candidate genes is straightforward, given that the ENU induced point mutations are likely to be found in coding sequence or splice sites. Point mutations are unlikely to act at a distance, although promoter or enhancer mutants might be found. Anecdotal evidence suggests that base changes occur on the order of 1/200–800 kilobases, with the bulk of these occurring in non-coding DNA. Approximately 10–20% of base changes are thought to cause functional mutations, so the typical interval should contain only one mutation in a coding sequence that results in an amino acid change. Of course, only a single allele will be recovered, and if the mutation is not obviously deleterious (e.g., a missense mutation not located in a highly conserved motif versus say a termination codon) then the evidence that the particular base change is a causative mutation is weakened. The solution is typically to create a transgenic strain expressing the wild type cDNA and breed it to the mutant strain. If the mutation identification is correct, the phenotype will be "rescued." Specifically, homozygous mutant animals that carry the transgene will have the normal phenotype because the cDNA supplies the wild type protein. Alternatively, one could create a targeted null allele and show that heterozygous animals with null/ENU compound alleles are affected. Molecular screening of an ENU library could also furnish additional alleles. Methods to accomplish these goals are described in the next section.

V. GENE-DRIVEN APPROACHES

A. Gene Trap

In contrast to the phenotypic screening, genotype-driven approaches are sequence driven and can involve targeted mutations through homologous recombination in embryonic stem (ES) cells. However, this approach is not suitable for the recovery of large numbers of mutations on a genome-wide basis. Instead, a gene trap strategy is a more systematic approach. Generally, in the gene trap approach a fragment of DNA (transgene) coding for a reporter or selectable marker gene is used as a mutagen. The mutagen is randomly inserted into ES cells to disrupt endogenous gene function and that insertion generates loss-of-function mutations by nonhomologous recombination and leaves a sequence tag at the mutated locus. As a result, rapid molecular characterization of the mutated locus can be achieved (Friedrich and Soriano 1993).

Different gene trap strategies are possible depending on the design of trapping vectors (for review, see Cecconi and Meyer 2000). In some cases, the vector is a reporter gene that lacks a functional promoter and so relies on the chance of integration next to an appropriate *cis*-acting sequence element that can activate its transcription. The reporter or marker gene is designed to be expressed only after it inserts within an intron, an exon, or a promoter. Only when it integrates at such positions can it acquire the expression element that it (intentionally) lacks and thus select for integrations into genes. The construct consists of a splice acceptor sequence upstream of the β-galactosidase (*lacZ*) gene and the neomycin resistance gene (*neo*) followed by a polyadenylation signal. When the transgene integrates into an intron of the endogenous gene, the splice acceptor sequence directs splicing of the transgene to the upstream exons of the endogenous gene during transcription from the endogenous promoter. Fusion transcripts from insertion of these vectors mimic endogenous gene expression at the insertion locus, which can be selected by visualizing *lacZ* activity (Frohman et al. 1988; Gossler et al. 1989). Other approaches have used a reporter gene coupled to a suitable promoter and a splice donor sequence, but lacking a downstream polyadenylation signal. Here, integration is intended to permit transgene expression with the help of the splice donor sequence, which helps the transgene to be spliced to downstream host exons in order to acquire a poly (A) tail. This strategy enables targeting of genes that are transcriptionally silent in ES cells.

Trapping vectors can be introduced into the genome by either electroporation or retroviral infection after genetic manipulation (for review, see Friedrich and Soriano 1993). Hundreds of potentially mutated ES cell lines expressing β-gal can easily be established and identified *in vitro*. Upon transfer to a pseudo-pregnant recipient, the ES cells participate in normal development of the chimeric embryo and contribute to all cell types, including the germ line (Robertson et al. 1986). The activity of β-gal can be detected in whole embryos and in sectioned postnatal tissues by a chemical reaction that leads to blue coloring of positive cells. When germline chimeras are obtained, they will be used as a source for heterozygous mice carrying the inserted trapping vector. The location of the tagged genes can be identified by the use of an anchored PCR procedure, that is, rapid amplification of cDNA ends (RACE)-PCR, a simple, automatable procedure (Frohman et al. 1988; Chowdhury et al. 1997; Townley et al. 1997). Using this strategy, the phenotypic consequences of the gene trap mutation can be studied and the spatial and temporal expression patterns of the endogenous genes during embryogenesis and adulthood can also be revealed.

Already, several large-scale gene trap screens have been carried out with various new vectors. These screens aim to generate libraries of gene trap line and sequences of the tagged genes. Four public resources of mutagenized ES cells are generated from trap insertions; these resources include more than eight thousand ES cell lines and are freely available to researchers.

The goal of the BayGenomics Gene Trap Project, California, USA (http://baygenomics.ucsf.edu), is to use gene trap vectors to inactivate ~2,500 genes per year in ES cells. As of March 2004, 8,700 identified cell lines have been obtained from the combined screens by the Skarnes and Tessier-Lavigne laboratories. The Gene Trap Project of the German Human Genome Project (http://tikus.gsf.de), which was organized by a German consortium, consists of both a gene trap (Wiles et al. 2000) and an ENU mutagenesis program (Soewarto et al. 2000). The gene trap library was constructed using four different β-geo gene trap and promoter trap vectors, introduced into ES cells through electroporation and retroviral infection. As of March 2004, 7,800 sequenced clones have been produced. The University of Manitoba Institute of Cell Biology, Winnipeg, Canada (http://www.escells.ca), projects to develop an ES cell library of 20,000–40,000 defined gene mutations based on promoter-trap vectors with a deposit of 300 clones per month. Today it contains 6,600 cell lines. The center for Modeling Human Disease (CMHD), Toronto, Canada (http://www.cmhd.ca), is carrying out ENU-based phenotypic screens, and gene trap based expression and genotypic screens using a poly (A) trap vector. Expression profiles have been generated for more than 7,800 clones. The other gene trap approach is led by Lexicon Genetics, TX, USA (http://www.lexgen.com/omnibank/omnibank_ebiology.php), which is based on using poly (A) gene trapping automated in the 96-well format and has the potential to represent insertional mutations for most of the mammalian genes in mouse ES cells (Zambrowicz et al. 1998). Today, more than 200,000 trap insertions in ES cells have been deposited in the Lexicon Genetics "OmniBank."

B. ENU Libraries

The molecular screening of ENU mutagenized mice or ES cells has also become an important topic (Beier 2000; Chen et al. 2000a; Chen et al. 2000b; Munroe et al. 2000; Coghill et al. 2002; Vivian et al. 2002; Chen et al. 2003). The basic strategy is to create a library by collecting genomic DNA from several thousand mutagenized G1 mice. At the same time, sperm is harvested from the mice and cryopreserved. The genomic DNA is screened by PCR amplification and sequencing, so that mice heterozygous for mutations in a particular gene of interest can be identified. Live mice are recovered by thawing the frozen sperm and performing *in vitro* fertilization. Mice are then intercrossed to generate homozygous mutants and phenotyping is performed. If a large enough library were to be constructed, one could conceivably recover a series of mutations in any particular gene.

Alternatively, ES cells can be treated with ENU *in vitro* and then single cell clones can be expanded and arrayed for cryopreservation and DNA extraction. In this case a little more effort is required to recover live mice, but the library could be substantially larger. Furthermore, other mutagens, such as chlorambucil, that are less effective *in vivo* could be used to treat the ES cells. Similar to the mouse ENU library, the limiting factors are the cost and effort of screening the DNA for heterozygous point mutations.

This approach has been embraced by investigators working in other species, for example, the *Arabadopsis* and zebrafish communities (Till et al. 2003). In these cases, the method is referred to as TILLING (targeting induced local lesions in genomes). Heterozygous mutation detection is accomplished using Cel 1 endonuclease which cleaves at mismatched DNA bases pairs (Oleykowski et al. 1999; Kulinski et al. 2000; Yang et al. 2000). In brief, target genomic DNA, spanning exons of interest, is amplified by PCR from mutagenized individuals. If the target region contains a point mutation in one allele, two fragments are produced that differ by a single base pair. Fragments are then melted and reannealed, so that mismatch-containing heteroduplex fragments are produced (and the two parental fragments). Following Cel 1 treatment, cleaved fragments indicate the presence of a potential mutation. Web-based programs are now available to assist in the design and analysis of such screens. One is CODDLE (codons optimized to discover deleterious mutations, http://www.proweb.org/coddle/), which selects coding regions that are most likely to contain missense and nonsense mutations based on sequence composition and chosen mutagen. The potential effect of missense mutations that are discovered can then be evaluated with PARSESNP (Project Aligned Related Sequences and Evaluate SNPs, http://www.proweb.org/parsesnp/), which evaluates amino acid changes based on a protein homology model (Taylor and Greene 2003).

VI. CONCLUSIONS

Once predicted to signal the end of genetics, the publication of the assembled mouse genome sequence has instead prompted a revival of classical genetic approaches. In part, this revival is due to recognition of the "phenotype gap" that defines the disparity between the number of genes revealed by the sequence and the size of the mutant collection. Despite over 1,200 mouse mutations in the mouse locus catalog (http://www.informatics.jax.org), this number represents only a small fraction of the total number of mammalian genes. The complete sequence also had been a terrifically enabling resource for the identification of "random" (spontaneous and induced) mutant loci. As a result, a large number of projects are under way that have the stated aim of producing mutations in every single gene (Nadeau et al. 2001). Investigators who are interested in motor systems are likely to be inundated with a host of new mutants over the coming years. Given the tremendous insights provided by the classical mutants cloned to date, one can expect that the new mutants will yield a wealth of new data. The essential players will be identified and as phenotype screens mature and evolve, they should reveal the interactions between genes, through the use of modifier and sensitized screens. Furthermore, the full depth of the "phenome" will be mined through the recovery of allelic series of mutations in specific genes. This process will most likely be accomplished by genotype-driven screens of libraries of mutations. Ultimately, this should yield a greater understanding of the biology of motor behavior and also provide models of human disease. These models will be essential for identifying, designing, and validating therapeutic strategies.

References

Anderson, K. 2000. Finding the genes that direct mammalian development: ENU mutagenesis in the mouse. *Trends Genet* **16**:99–102.

Beier, D. 2000. Sequence-based analysis of mutagenized mice. *Mamm Genome* **11**:594–597.

Blake, J., J. Richardson, C. Bult, J. Kadin, and J. Eppig. 2003. MGD: The Mouse Genome Database. *Nucleic Acids Res* **31**:193–195.

Bono, H., K. Yagi, T. Kasukawa, I. Nikaido, N. Tominaga, R. Miki, Y. Mizuno, Y. Tomaru, H. Goto, H. Nitanda, et al. 2003. Systematic expression profiling of the mouse transcriptome using RIKEN cDNA microarrays. *Genome Res* **13**:1318–1323.

Brown, S., and R. Hardisty. 2003. Mutagenesis strategies for identifying novel loci associated with disease phenotypes. *Semin Cell Dev Biol* **14**:19–24.

Brown, S.D., and J. Peters. 1996. Combining mutagenesis and genomics in the mouse—closing the phenotype gap. *Trends Genet* **12**:433–435.

Buchner, D.A., M. Trudeau, and M.H. Meisler, 2003. SCNM1, a putative RNA splicing factor that modifies disease severity in mice. *Science* **301**:967–969.

Cecconi, F., and B.I. Meyer. 2000. Gene trap: a way to identify novel genes and unravel their biological function. *FEBS Lett* **480**:63–71.

Chen, Y., J. Schimenti, and T. Magnuson. 2000a. Toward the yeastification of mouse genetics: chemical mutagenesis of embryonic stem cells. *Mamm Genome* **11**:598–602.

Chen, Y., J. Vivian, and T. Magnuson. 2003. Gene-based chemical mutagenesis in mouse embryonic stem cells. *Methods Enzymol* **365**: 406–415.

Chen, Y., D. Yee, K. Dains, A. Chatterjee, J. Cavalcoli, E. Schneider, J. Om, R. Woychik, and T. Magnuson. 2000b. Genotype-based screen for ENU-induced mutations in mouse embryonic stem cells. *Nat Genet* **24**:314–317.

Chowdhury, K., P. Bonaldo, M. Torres, A. Stoykova, and P. Gruss. 1997. Evidence for the stochastic integration of gene trap vectors into the mouse germline. *Nucleic Acids Res* **25**:1531–1536.

Coghill, E., A. Hugill, N. Parkinson, C. Davison, P. Glenister, S. Clements, J. Hunter, R. Cox, and S. Brown. 2002. A gene-driven approach to the identification of ENU mutants in the mouse. *Nat Genet* **30**:255–256.

Dietrich, W., H. Katz, S.E. Lincoln, H.S. Shin, J. Friedman, N.C. Dracopoli, and E.S. Lander. 1992. A genetic map of the mouse suitable for typing intraspecific crosses. *Genetics* **131**:423–447.

Friedrich, G., and P. Soriano. 1993. Insertional mutagenesis by retroviruses and promoter traps in embryonic stem cells. *Methods Enzymol* **225**: 681–701.

Frohman, M.A., M.K. Dush, and G.R. Martin. 1988. Rapid production of full-length cDNAs from rare transcripts: amplification using a single gene-specific oligonucleotide primer. *Proc Natl Acad Sci U S A* **85**: 8998–9002.

Gossler, A., A.L. Joyner, J. Rossant, and W.C. Skarnes. 1989. Mouse embryonic stem cells and reporter constructs to detect developmentally regulated genes. *Science* **244**:463–465.

Green, M.C. 1989. Catalog of mutant genes and polymorphic loci. In *Genetic Variants and Strains of the Laboratory Mouse*, M.F. Lyon, and A.G. Searle, eds., pp. 12–403. Oxford: Oxford University Press.

Hardisty, R., P. Mburu, and S. Brown. 1999. ENU mutagenesis and the search for deafness genes. *Br J Audiol* **33**:279–283.

Hrabe de Angelis, M., and R. Balling. 1998. Large scale ENU screens in the mouse: genetics meets genomics. *Mutat Res* **400**:25–32.

Hrabe de Angelis, M.H., H. Flaswinkel, H. Fuchs, B. Rathkolb, D. Soewarto, S. Marschall, S. Heffner, et al. 2000. Genome-wide, large-scale production of mutant mice by ENU mutagenesis. *Nat Genet* **25**:444–447.

Justice, M., D. Carpenter, J. Favor, A. Neuhauser-Klaus, D.A.M. Hrabe, D. Soewarto, A. Moser, et al. 2000. Effects of ENU dosage on mouse strains. *Mamm Genome* **11**:484–488.

Justice, M., J. Noveroske, J. Weber, B. Zheng, and A. Bradley. 1999. Mouse ENU mutagenesis. *Hum Mol Genet* **8**:1955–1963.

Justice, M., B. Zheng, R. Woychik, and A. Bradley. 1997. Using targeted large deletions and high-efficiency N-ethyl-N-nitrosourea mutagenesis for functional analyses of the mammalian genome. *Methods* **13**:423–436.

Kasarskis, A., K. Manova, and K. Anderson. 1998. A phenotype-based screen for embryonic lethal mutations in the mouse. *Proc Natl Acad Sci U S A* **95**:7485–7490.

Kulinski, J., D. Besack, C.A. Oleykowski, A.K. Godwin, and A.T. Yeung 2000. CEL I enzymatic mutation detection assay. *Biotechniques* **29**:44–46, 48.

Lindblad-Toh, K., E. Winchester, M.J. Daly, D.G. Wang, J.N. Hirschhorn, J.P. Laviolette, K. Ardlie, D.E. Reich, E. Robinson, P. Sklar, et al. 2000. Large-scale discovery and genotyping of single-nucleotide polymorphisms in the mouse. *Nat Genet* **24**:381–386.

MacPhee, M., K.P. Chepenik, R.A. Liddell, K.K. Nelson, L.D. Siracusa, and A.M. Buchberg. 1995. The secretory phospholipase A2 gene is a candidate for the Mom1 locus, a major modifier of ApcMin-induced intestinal neoplasia. *Cell* **81**:957–966.

Munroe, R., R. Bergstrom, Q. Zheng, B. Libby, R. Smith, S. John, K. Schimenti, V. Browning, and J. Schimenti. 2000. Mouse mutants from chemically mutagenized embryonic stem cells. *Nat Genet* **24**:318–321.

Mural, R.J., M.D. Adams, E. W. Myers, H.O. Smith, G.L. Miklos, R. Wides, A. Halpern, P.W. Li, G.G. Sutton, J. Nadeau, et al. 2002. A comparison of whole-genome shotgun-derived mouse chromosome 16 and the human genome. *Science* **296**:1661–1671.

Nadeau, J.H., R. Balling, G. Barsh, D. Beier, S.D. Brown, M. Bucan, S. Camper, G. Carlson, N. Copeland, J. Eppig, et al. 2001. Sequence interpretation. Functional annotation of mouse genome sequences. *Science* **291**:1251–1255.

Nelms, K., and C. Goodnow. 2001. Genome-wide ENU mutagenesis to reveal immune regulators. *Immunity* **15**:409–418.

Nolan, P., J. Peters, M. Strivens, D. Rogers, J. Hagan, N. Spurr, I. Gray, et al. 2000. A systematic, genome-wide, phenotype-driven mutagenesis programme for gene function studies in the mouse. *Nat Genet* **25**:440–443.

Noveroske, J., J. Weber, and M. Justice. 2000. The mutagenic action of N-ethyl-N-nitrosourea in the mouse. *Mamm Genome* **11**:478–483.

Okazaki, Y., M. Furuno, T. Kasukawa, J. Adachi, H. Bono, S. Kondo, I. Nikaido, et al. 2002. Analysis of the mouse transcriptome based on functional annotation of 60,770 full-length cDNAs. *Nature* **420**:563–573.

Oleykowski, C.A., C.R. Bronson Mullins, D.W. Chang, and A.T. Yeung. 1999. Incision at nucleotide insertions/deletions and base pair mismatches by the SP nuclease of spinach. *Biochemistry* **38**:2200–2205.

Rathkolb, B., T. Decker, E. Fuchs, D. Soewarto, C. Fella, S. Heffner, W. Pargent, et al. 2000. The clinical-chemical screen in the Munich ENU Mouse Mutagenesis Project: screening for clinically relevant phenotypes. *Mamm Genome* **11**:543–546.

Rinchik, E., and D. Carpenter. 1999. N-ethyl-N-nitrosourea mutagenesis of a 6- to 11-cM subregion of the Fah-Hbb interval of mouse chromosome 7: completed testing of 4557 gametes and deletion mapping and complementation analysis of 31 mutations. *Genetics* **152**:373–383.

Rinchik, E., D. Carpenter, and P. Selby. 1990. A strategy for fine-structure functional analysis of a 6- to 11-centimorgan region of mouse chromosome 7 by high-efficiency mutagenesis. *Proc Natl Acad Sci U S A* **87**:896–900.

Robertson, E., A. Bradley, M. Kuehn, and M. Evans. 1986. Germ-line transmission of genes introduced into cultured pluripotential cells by retroviral vector. *Nature* **323**:445–448.

Russell, L., and C. Montgomery. 1982. Supermutagenicity of ethylnitrosourea in the mouse spot test: comparisons with methylnitrosourea and ethylnitrosourethane. *Mutat Res* **92**:193–204.

Schimenti, J., and M. Bucan. 1998. Functional genomics in the mouse: phenotype-based mutagenesis screens. *Genome Res* **8**:698–710.

Shelby, M., and K. Tindall. 1997. Mammalian germ cell mutagenicity of ENU, IPMS and MMS, chemicals selected for a transgenic mouse collaborative study. *Mutat Res* **388**:99–109.

Soewarto, D., C. Fella, A. Teubner, B. Rathkolb, W. Pargent, S. Heffner, S. Marschall, et al. 2000. The large-scale Munich ENU-mouse-mutagenesis screen. *Mamm Genome* **11**:507–510.

Su, A.I., M.P. Cooke, K.A. Ching, Y. Hakak, J.R. Walker, T. Wiltshire, A.P. Orth, et al. 2002. Large-scale analysis of the human and mouse transcriptomes. *Proc Natl Acad Sci U S A* **99**:4465–4470.

Taylor, N.E., and E.A. Greene. 2003. PARSESNP: A tool for the analysis of nucleotide polymorphisms. *Nucleic Acids Res* **31**:3808–3811.

Till, B.J., S.H. Reynolds, E.A. Greene, C.A. Codomo, L.C. Enns, J.E. Johnson, C. Burtner, et al. 2003. Large-scale discovery of induced point mutations with high-throughput TILLING. *Genome Res* **13**:524–530.

Townley, D.J., B.J. Avery, B. Rosen, and W.C. Skarnes. 1997. Rapid sequence analysis of gene trap integrations to generate a resource of insertional mutations in mice. *Genome Res* **7**:293–298.

Vivian, J., Y. Chen, D. Yee, E. Schneider, and T. Magnuson. 2002. An allelic series of mutations in Smad2 and Smad4 identified in a genotype-based screen of N-ethyl-N-nitrosourea-mutagenized mouse embryonic stem cells. *Proc Natl Acad Sci U S A* **99**:15542–15547.

Wade, C.M., E.J. Kulbokas 3rd, A.W. Kirby, M.C. Zody, J.C. Mullikin, E.S. Lander, et al. 2002. The mosaic structure of variation in the laboratory mouse genome. *Nature* **420**:574–578.

Waterston, R.H., K. Lindblad-Toh, E. Birney, J. Rogers, J.F. Abril, P. Agarwal, R. Agarwal, et al. 2002. Initial sequencing and comparative analysis of the mouse genome. *Nature* **420**:520–562.

Weber, J., A. Salinger, and M. Justice. 2000. Optimal N-ethyl-N-nitrosourea (ENU) doses for inbred mouse strains. *Genesis* **26**:230–233.

Wiles, M.V., F. Vauti, J. Otte, E.M. Fuchtbauer, P. Ruiz, A. Fuchtbauer, H.H. Arnold, et al. 2000. Establishment of a gene-trap sequence tag library to generate mutant mice from embryonic stem cells. *Nat Genet* **24**:13–14.

Wiltshire, T., M.T. Pletcher, S. Batalov, S.W. Barnes, L.M. Tarantino, M.P. Cooke, H. Wu, et al. 2003. Genome-wide single-nucleotide polymorphism analysis defines haplotype patterns in mouse. *Proc Natl Acad Sci U S A* **100**:3380–3385.

Yang, B., X. Wen, N.S. Kodali, C.A. Oleykowski, C.G. Miller, J. Kulinski, D. Besack, et al. 2000. Purification, cloning, and characterization of the CEL I nuclease. *Biochemistry* **39**:3533–3541.

Zambrowicz, B.P., G.A. Friedrich, E.C. Buxton, S.L. Lilleberg, C. Person, and A.T. Sands. 1998. Disruption and sequence identification of 2,000 genes in mouse embryonic stem cells. *Nature* **392**:608–611.

CHAPTER

A5

Assessment of Movement Disorders in Rodents

H.A. JINNAH and ELLEN J. HESS

The neurology subspecialty field of movement disorders encompasses a wide range of abnormal motor syndromes. In general this field does not include motor seizures resulting from epilepsy, or weakness associated with dysfunction of the corticospinal or neuromuscular motor systems. Instead, it includes motor abnormalities such as tremor, Parkinsonism, choreoathetosis, dystonia, ataxia, and others (table 1). Well-accepted clinical criteria have been developed for diagnosing each of these conditions (Barbeau et al. 1981; Elble 1998). These criteria are essential, because there are few diagnostic tests to reliably discriminate one movement disorder from another.

In parallel with the development of clinical criteria for diagnosis, there has been growing interest in elucidating the pathogenesis of movement disorders and to facilitate the discovery of treatments. Ethical and technical issues preclude the use of human subjects for many important experiments, so researchers have shown considerable interest in animal models. Among the many potential species of animals to consider as animal models, non-human primates are attractive because they are most closely related to humans. In fact, researchers have developed non-human primate models for most common movement disorders. Unfortunately, a number of factors limit more widespread use of primates. These factors include a constrained supply, expenses involved in maintaining and studying the animals, the need for specialized centers and highly trained personnel, and complex ethical issues related to the collection of wild animals or the breeding of captive animals. In addition, primates are of little value for studying genetically determined movement disorders. Because of the many limitations inherent in primate research, the majority of research in animal models has focused on other species, particularly small rodents such as rats or mice.

The interest in small animal models has led to an enormous increase in the numbers of both genetic and pharmacologic rodent models for a wide variety of movement disorders. Behavioral tests also have proliferated for assessing abnormal motor behavior in these models. In this chapter, we review several basic concepts about animal modeling in general, some of the most commonly employed tests of motor function, and general strategies for selecting the most appropriate tests for specific purposes.

I. BASIC CONCEPTS OF ANIMAL MODELING

Many investigators expect a good animal model to reproduce all the key features of the human disease being modeled. Such expectations are neither realistic nor

TABLE 1 Description of Common Movement Disorders

Term	Definition
Ataxia	Dysmetria, dyssynergia, and dysdiadochokinesis not due to weakness or superimposed involuntary movements
Athetosis	Writhing movements with characteristics that fall between dystonia and chorea; usually involve distal rather than proximal muscles
Chorea	Continuous but ever changing and semi-random relatively fast, fluid, or jerky movements
Dyskinesia	Non-specific term for any abnormal involuntary movement; certain subtypes have more specific meaning, such as tardive dyskinesia associated with neuroleptics
Dystonia	Simultaneous contraction of agonist and antagonist muscles, often patterned, typically leading to twisting movements or abnormal postures
Epileptic seizure	A sudden change in behavior associated with abnormal EEG activity
Hyperkinetic syndrome	Motor syndrome described by increased movements
Hypokinetic syndrome	Motor syndrome described by reduced frequency and speed of movements
Myoclonus	Sudden, rapid, random, non-rhythmic, shock-like movement
Parkinsonism	Hypokinetic motor syndrome with reduced spontaneous activity, slowed movements, rigid increase in muscle tone, and resting tremor
Paroxysmal dyskinesia	Non-epileptic attacks of abnormal movement superimposed on a normal or near-normal baseline; individual movements may be dystonic, choreic, or other
Stereotypy	Repetitive fragments of semi-purposeful movements
Tremor	Rhythmic oscillation caused by alternating or synchronous contractions of reciprocal muscles

necessary. In fact, many useful animal models do not reproduce all the key features of the human condition, and some do not reproduce any. Instead of judging a model by how completely it mimics the human disease, models are traditionally judged by two main criteria, reliability and validity (Geyer and Markou 1995; Jinnah et al. submitted).

Reliability refers to the ability of the model to provide consistent results under different conditions (table 2). Validity refers to the conceptual framework underlying the model. Animal models for movement disorders achieve validity in one of three ways. The most intuitive model is one that has face validity, in that it has a motor syndrome that superficially resembles a human movement disorder. An example of a model with face validity for tremor involves the administration of harmaline to rodents (Wilms et al. 1999). Treated rodents demonstrate 8–15 Hz oscillations occurring at rest and exaggerated by movement. The harmaline model has been extremely valuable in investigating the involvement of olivary neurons and the cerebellum in the genesis of tremor.

Another way in which a model can achieve validity is by etiology. The first targeted model developed for a specific neurobehavioral disorder involved introduction of mutations into the *hprt* gene as a model for Lesch-Nyhan disease (Hooper et al. 1987; Kuehn et al. 1987). These mice provide an example of an etiologic model for Lesch-Nyhan disease, because the human disorder is associated with mutations in the same gene. These mice are, by definition, genetic models for the human condition. However, these mice do not exhibit dystonia or other behavioral abnormalities analogous to those occurring in the human disease (Edamura and Sasai 1998; Finger et al. 1988; Jinnah et al. 1991; Jinnah et al. 1992; Kasim and Jinnah 2002). It seems counterintuitive that an animal model for Lesch-Nyhan disease could be

TABLE 2 Criteria for Judging Animal Models

Criteria	Definition
Reliability	The model provides consistent results
Validity	
Face validity	The model exhibits a motor syndrome that meets typical criteria used to define the syndrome in humans
Etiologic validity	The model was derived from a cause known to cause the motor syndrome in humans
Predictive validity	The model predicts a key feature of the human motor syndrome, such as response to treatment

accepted as a good model because of the absence of an analogous neurobehavioral phenotype. However, this model has been very valuable for investigating the relationship between the gene defect and dysfunction of dopaminergic pathways in the basal ganglia (Dunnett et al. 1989; Finger et al. 1988; Hyland et al. 2004; Jinnah et al. 1999; Jinnah et al. 1992; Jinnah et al. 1994; Smith and Friedmann 2000; Visser et al. 2002). What makes this model and other etiologic models good, even in the absence of an analogous behavioral phenotype, is their utility in elucidating important elements of the pathogenesis of the disease (Aguzzi et al. 1994; Cenci et al. 2002; Elsea and Lucas 2002; Erickson 1989).

Perhaps the least intuitive type of animal model is the one with predictive validity. These models are useful for predicting some feature of the disease, such as treatment response. Though the predictive models may resemble their human disease the least (and sometimes not at all), they have the potential to be the most useful for guiding therapy. One of the best examples of a predictive model is the Porsolt forced swimming test for evaluating antidepressants (Geyer and Markou 1995). In this model, a rat is placed in a tank of water with no escape. The proportion of time the animal spends floating motionless in comparison to making efforts to escape provides a powerful predictor of antidepressant efficacy. This predictive power exists despite the complete lack of obvious face or etiologic validity.

A valid animal model does not require all three types of validity to be useful. The harmaline model for tremor has face validity but it does not have etiologic validity, because harmaline is not recognized as a common cause for tremor in humans. By contrast, the *hprt* knock-out mouse models for Lesch-Nyhan disease have etiologic validity, but they do not have face validity because they do not suffer from analogous neurobehavioral defects. The Porsolt forced swimming test has neither face nor etiologic validity. All of these models are useful for investigating different aspects of the diseases they model (Figure 1). In short, a good model is not one that merely *mimics* a human disease, but rather one that is *useful* for exploring pathogenesis or treatments.

The type of model being studied will determine the way in which it is best evaluated. In the models with face validity, investigators must evaluate the motor syndrome in a manner that allows for direct comparisons to the clinical motor syndrome. Since the validity of these models is based on their resemblance to a human disorder, the motor syndrome must be evaluated with far more rigor than other models. Hypotheses concerning the nature of the defect introduced usually drive the evaluation of models with etiologic validity. Because etiology determines the validity of these models, the existence of an overt motor phenotype resembling the human condition is less important.

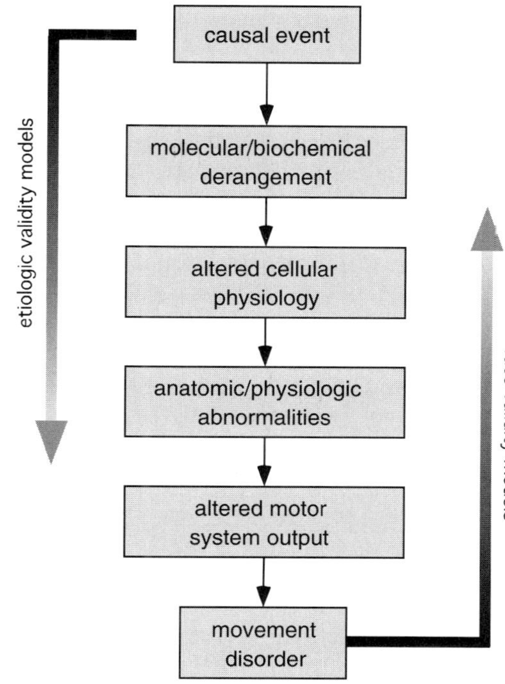

FIGURE 1 The role of animals as models for human disease. Models with etiologic validity are most useful for studying early steps in the pathogenesis of the corresponding human disease, but may not reproduce an analogous behavioral phenotype. Models with face validity are most useful for studying the behavioral phenotype and late steps in the pathophysiology of the disease, even though they may not suffer from the same cause as the human disease.

II. SPECIFIC TESTS FOR MOTOR ABNORMALITIES

This section describes some of the most commonly used tests for motor dysfunction. At the outset, it is important to emphasize that these tests are deceptively simple. Although the equipment required is not expensive and the protocols are relatively easy to perform, a meaningful interpretation of the results is not always straightforward (Crawley 2000; Wahlsten 2001). For example, there are several very simple tests to assess locomotor behavior in rodents. The results of these tests may be affected by the time of day, the duration of habituation, whether the animal had been tested in the same cage before, whether other animals had been tested in the same cage, the gender of other animals tested, the species of other animals tested, the lighting conditions, the level and variations of ambient noise, the number and types of other behavioral tests performed prior, and more. Individuals with training in behavioral sciences can best manage the understanding of these variables and how they affect the results (Crawley 2000; Wahlsten 2001).

A. Observational Methods

The simplest test for assessing motor dysfunction is the "eyeball test," or direct observation. Experienced individuals can often provide an accurate preliminary assessment for the basis for an abnormal motor syndrome by observation alone. These assessments should not be accepted at face value, but are useful for guiding the selection of further confirmatory tests. It is often suggested that the "eyeball test" is too subjective to merit any serious consideration. However, when properly performed, observations can be quantified and subjected to rigorous statistical methods. Observation-based assessments have served as one of the most important tools in the investigations of nearly every movement disorder in humans (Cohen and Spina 1996; Comella et al. 2003). In many cases, quantified observations have provided the only means to measure an abnormal behavior.

The methods for quantifying direct observations in rodents fall into two categories. The first category involves rating scales for severity. These scales must be customized for each condition. An example of a rating scale developed to assess dystonia in mice is provided in table 3 (Jinnah et al. 2000). Severity rating scales should not be based on purely subjective criteria such as 1 = mild, 2 = moderate, 3 = severe. Instead, it is more useful to specify criteria that aid in determining a score. Such criteria increase the reliability of the scale, particularly if different individuals or different laboratories will apply it. Wherever possible, an observer blinded to the experimental condition should apply the scales to avoid observer bias.

Several limitations exist with the severity scales. The first limitation is that these scales presume the nature of the disorder being evaluated is known, and they do not assist in defining it. For example, investigators could readily apply the dystonia rating scale (table 3) to animals with another motor syndrome such as myotonia, even though dystonia and myotonia are not the same disorder. The second limitation is that the scales assume that the disorder being studied reflects a continuum of severity rather than a change in quality. This assumption can be difficult to verify. For example, dystonia is provoked with low or moderate doses of L-type calcium channel activators, but epileptic seizures are provoked with extreme doses (Jinnah et al. 2000). This change in the quality of motor behavior from dystonia to seizures does not mean that epilepsy should be rated on the same scale as dystonia. The final limitation is that the results obtained are discontinuous and therefore most appropriately evaluated with non-parametric statistical measures, which are generally considered less sensitive to small differences than parametric statistics. Despite these limitations, rating scales for severity offer a simple and powerful method for certain applications.

The second category of methods for quantifying observations involves recording behavior inventories. This method provides estimates of the frequency of specific target behaviors and is therefore best suited for the description of complex patterns of behavior. In brief, a predetermined list of target behaviors is formulated from preliminary observations. Each target behavior is then recorded as being present or absent during a specified time under defined conditions. The result is a large matrix of data indicating the frequency of each behavior.

The behavior inventory methods have seen their fullest development in analyzing variations in normal motor behaviors (McNamara et al. 2003) and the complex stereotyped movements seen in animals treated with psychostimulants (Kelley 1998). The behavior inventory method is ideal for the application to complex movement disorders in rodents, where the problems of description and quantification are very similar to those of stereotyped behaviors. However, this method has been applied only recently for this purpose, and experience is limited.

The most direct manner of presenting data from observational studies is in raw tabular format, but this approach can make it difficult to convey an overview of broader patterns of behavior and what differences are most important. A more meaningful way of presenting data from behavior

TABLE 3 Rating Scale for Severity of Dystonia

Score	Functional disability	Description
0	None	Normal motor behavior
1	Inconsequential	Slightly slowed or abnormal motor behavior
2	Mild	Limited ambulation unless disturbed, transient abnormal postures, and/or infrequent falls
3	Moderate	Limited ambulation even when disturbed, frequent abnormal postures, frequent falls but upright most of the time
4	Severe	Almost no ambulation, sustained abnormal postures, not upright most of the time

Motor Disorders Score Sheet

Experiment	
Animal Group	
Animal number	
Date	
Time	

Body part	Movement	Time bin (minutes)					
		10	20	30	40	50	60
face	tonus						
	clonus						
	tremor						
neck	tremor						
	twisting						
	bobbing						
	wagging						
	sustained extension						
	sustained flexion						
trunk	tremor						
	twisting						
	sustained extension						
	sustained flexion						
limbs	tremor						
	twisting						
	clonus						
	sustained extension						
	sustained flexion						
locomotion	increased spontaneous						
	decreased spontaneous						
	slowed						
	speeded						
	listing						
	circling						
	rearing						
	falls onto flank						
	falls onto back						
	other notes						

FIGURE 2 Behavior inventory data recording sheet. This sample sheet is arranged according to body part affected. An animal is observed for sixty seconds at ten-minute intervals for an hour. The presence or absence of any of the target behaviors is recorded in an all-or-none fashion. Recording sheets for six or more animals are combined to provide group averages. Suggested target behaviors are shown, but the recording sheet can be modified by adding or subtracting items to suit specific applications.

inventories is to cluster certain behaviors into subgroups based on specific criteria. For example, a behavior inventory formed the basis for evaluating L-dopa induced dyskinesias in rodents with partial lesions of the nigrostriatal dopamine pathways (Winkler et al. 2002). In this study, different types of abnormal movements were grouped according to the body part involved to permit anatomical correlations with the affected subregions of the caudoputamen. Similar methods were used to assess paroxysmal dyskinesias in the lethargic mouse mutant and the complex movement disorder syndrome of the stargazer mouse mutant (Khan et al. 2004; Khan and Jinnah 2002). In the latter study, different types of abnormal movements were combined according to class of movement to demonstrate differences between these mutants and others with similar syndromes. Figures 2 and 3 show examples of behavior recording sheets

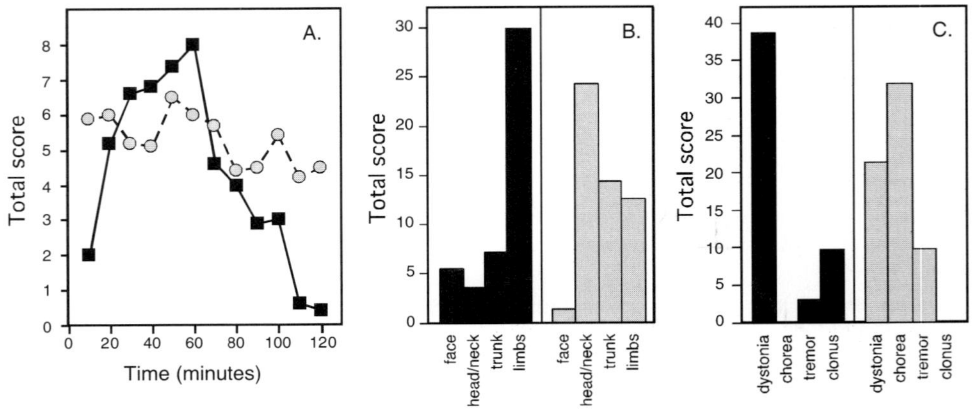

FIGURE 3 Behavior inventory data summary. Sample summary for mutant mice exhibiting two different movement disorder syndromes. The score is obtained from averages of a simple arithmetic sum from six of each mutant. Tottering mice (closed symbols) exhibit paroxysmal dystonia whereas stargazer mice (open symbols) exhibit a more continuous choreoathetoid syndrome. The paroxysmal nature of the motor syndrome in tottering mice in comparison to the more constant motor syndrome in stargazer mice becomes evident when the total abnormal movement scores are expressed as a function of time (A). The anatomic profiles of abnormal movements can be more readily identified by expressing the total abnormal movement scores as a function of body part affected (B); abnormal movements are more apparent in the limbs of tottering mice but in axial structures in stargazer mice. The type of movement disorder can be predicted by expressing abnormal movement scores according to movement class (C); tottering mice exhibit a predominantly dystonic disorder while stargazer mice exhibit a mixed disorder with chorea and dystonia. A subscore for Parkinsonism was not included because these mutants do not display any of the component behaviors.

and summary data that could be applied for movement disorders.

The behavior inventories provide a simple and powerful approach for describing complex abnormal movements, but they also have some limitations. One limitation is that the method generates a very large amount of raw data that can be difficult to summarize in meaningful ways. Several vendors have developed software and portable recording instruments to facilitate the observational sciences (table 4). Another limitation is that, like the severity scales, the data are also discontinuous and therefore best evaluated with non-parametric statistical measures. A further limitation is that this method provides a measure of frequency, and subtle differences in severity may not be apparent. For example, an animal with a very mild tremor achieves the same score as another with a very severe tremor if the tremor is continuously present throughout the recording interval in both. In this situation, investigators might consider combinations of severity scales and inventories, although data analysis becomes progressively more complicated.

B. Gross Activity Levels

Multiple methods are available for assessing gross levels of motor activity (Pierce and Kalivas 1997). The simplest methods involve drawing a series of parallel lines or a grid on the floor of a large open cage. An animal is placed into the cage, and the number of lines crossed in a specified time is manually recorded. A variety of different instruments have been developed to automate this task, including force transducing platforms, telemetry, or video recording-based methods (table 4). The most popular automated apparatus applies infrared beams within the test cage, and a computer records the number and pattern of beams interrupted. Most vendors also offer software to further refine the nature of the movements based on the pattern and frequency of beam crosses. Such derived variables include total distance traveled, forward locomotion, local behaviors, patterns of behavior, and the proportion of time spent in the center versus the perimeter of the cage. Significantly, all of these measures are derived variables based on multiple assumptions, and their reliability is not assured in all instances.

If a severe reduction in spontaneous movements occurs, then tests developed for akinesia or catalepsy might be more sensitive to subtle changes because they lower the "floor effect" that might present a problem for the other methods. These tests all involve recording the time required for an animal to move in a manner that reaches specific predetermined criteria. The simplest tests involve placing the animal in an open cage in the center of a circle, and recording the time the animal takes to place one or all limbs outside the circle. To encourage movement in animals with severe akinesia, investigators may place the animals in an unnatural position with one or both forelimbs resting on a block (Bristow et al. 1997). Normal animals will withdraw their paws and run away immediately. Those with severe akine-

TABLE 4 Vendors for Equipment Used in Motor Disorders Research

Vendor	Activity chamber	Rotarod	Video tracking	Grip meter	Other
AccuScan Instruments accuscan-usa.com	yes	yes	yes	no	foot misstep
Clever Systems www.cleversysinc.com	yes	no	yes	no	detailed kinematics observation recording
Columbus Instruments colinst.com	yes	yes	yes	yes	foot mis-step
Coulbourn Instruments coulbourn.com	yes	yes	yes	no	
Data Sciences International www.datasci.com	no	no	no	no	wireless telemetry
MED Associates med-associates.com	yes	yes	yes	no	
Mouse Specifics mousespecifics.com	no	no	no	no	detailed kinematics wireless telemetry
Noldus noldus.com	no	no	yes	no	observation recording
PanLab panlab-sl.com	yes	yes	yes	no	observation recording
Peak Performance www.peakperform.com	no	no	no	no	detailed kinematics
San Diego Instruments sd-inst.com	yes	yes	yes	yes	
TSE Systems tse-systems.de	yes	yes	yes	no	wireless telemetry
Ugo Basile ugobasile.com	yes	yes	yes	yes	

sia will leave their paws on the block for varying lengths of time, and the measured variable is the time elapsed before the animal withdraws its paw from the block. As an alternative, mice may be placed head down on a steeply inclined wire mesh (Puglisi-Allegra and Cabib 1988). Normal mice typically turn around quickly and climb to the top of the apparatus. Those with akinesia will remain in the head-down position and/or take more time to reach the top of the grid.

C. Coordinated Motor Function

A great number of tests have been developed to assess coordinated motor activity in rodents (Carter et al. 2001; Crawley 2000). The beam-walking test has been popular because it is simple to perform and the apparatus can be constructed from materials available in almost any laboratory. For this test, investigators observe the animal while it traverses a narrow beam, usually approximately a meter long. A bright light is placed at the starting point and a darkened escape box is placed at the finish to encourage the animal to traverse the beam. After a few training runs, normal mice can rapidly run across the top of a beam as narrow as 10 mm without falling. Task difficulty can be modified by using beams of varying width, or by using rounded dowels. Mice with impairments in motor coordination exhibit a variety of abnormalities including gripping the sides of the beam rather than walking on the top, frequently hesitating or traversing the beam more slowly, misstepping leading to a foot slipping transiently off the side of the beam, and falling from the beam. These problems can be translated into a number of different measures such as the number of foot grips, the number of foot slips, the time required to traverse the beam, and the number of falls. While these items can all be scored by direct observation, videotape recordings are preferable because some movements occur so quickly in normal or minimally impaired mice that they are readily missed.

In another simple test of coordinated motor function, stepping patterns are analyzed during ambulation (Carter et al. 2001; Crawley 2000). A mouse is trained first to walk down a wide runway, again using a bright light at the start and a dark box at the finish. Next, a piece of white paper is placed on the runway. To record the stepping pattern, the forepaws are painted with one color and the rear paws are painted with another color. The result is a record of the footprints as the animal walks on the paper. Obvious abnormalities can be seen directly, but a full analysis involves calculating several parameters such as stance width, stride length, overlap between ipsilateral forelimb and hind limb, and step variability. This test is deceptively simple, because multiple potential difficulties can arise. These difficulties include several technical challenges such as training the animal to reliably traverse the runway, objectively selecting a representative record with enough clearly identifiable steps to measure, the mess often associated with multiple trials, and the labor involved in analyzing the traces. This test is also limited to the spatial characteristics of stepping, since it is not readily suited for analysis of temporal characteristics, such as a slowed gait. Finally, this test has never been critically evaluated for different movement disorders. It may therefore be capable of detecting abnormalities, but these abnormalities do not provide unequivocal information concerning the nature of the movement disorder. It is nevertheless a valuable technique when other instrumentation is not available.

Semi-automated methods have also been developed to analyze stepping patterns in rodents (table 4). These methods involve videotaping mice walking on a runway, with computer-assisted analysis of both spatial and temporal aspects of the stepping pattern. In one strategy an animal is videotaped from below while it walks on a clear runway. A bright light is directed into the edge of the runway, causing a reflecting pattern that amplifies each footfall. In another strategy, the animal is videotaped from both sides, and its feet and limbs are labeled with a colored marker. Such tests can provide extraordinarily detailed information about subtle motor defects that could not be detected with other methods (Miklyaeva et al. 1995; Whishaw et al. 1991). These methods have the potential to provide enough information to discriminate among different movement disorders and provide measures of severity, but they have not yet been explored in detail for this purpose. A more widespread use of these systems has been discouraged because of their relatively focused application and high cost.

One of the most popular tests for coordinated motor function is the rotarod, which assesses the ability of mice to walk on a rotating bar (Carter et al. 2001; Crawley 2000; Jones and Roberts 1968). For this test, mice are placed on top of a wide bar, which is rotated at progressively increasing speeds. Mice with impairments in coordinated motor function fall from the bar more readily than normal animals. Depending on the instrument, falls are recorded manually or automatically; and results are expressed as the duration the animal stays on the bar or the maximum speed achieved. Although this test is easy to perform, the results can be difficult to interpret because the specificity of the rotarod for motor incoordination is poor. Impaired performance on the rotarod can be ascribed to weakness, nearly any hyperkinetic or hypokinetic movement disorder, impaired motor learning, convulsive and nonconvulsive seizures, lack of motivation, anxiety level, ill health, and other factors. Nevertheless, this test is widely used because of its simplicity, its sensitivity to even mild deficits, and the relatively low cost of the apparatus (table 4).

Most of the preceding tests of motor function address gross motor control, but several techniques exist for addressing fine motor control, such as reaching and grasping in rodents (Whishaw et al. 1998; Whishaw et al. 1991). The best characterized of these tests involves training a rodent to perform a reaching task to grasp a food pellet. Different levels of difficulty can be achieved by changing the size and shape of the barrier between the animal and the food pellet, the distance to the pellet, and the size of the pellet. Basic parameters that are easy to record may include the success rate for reaching and/or the time required for successful reaching. Videotape recording with kinematic analysis provides the most sophisticated means of detecting subtle abnormalities.

D. Muscle Tone

The assessment of muscle tone is critical to several movement disorders, such as Parkinson disease and dystonia. The main challenge is to distinguish among the main subtypes of increased muscle tone: rigidity, dystonia, and spasticity (Sanger et al. 2003). Tone assessment is challenging in rodents, because it must be evaluated by passive limb manipulation in the awake state with muscles fully relaxed. The struggling movements made by awake rodents frequently complicate this evaluation.

Despite these difficulties, objective assessments can be made when blinded examiners provide subjective assessments according to criteria normally used to distinguish tonal abnormalities (table 5). In one recent example, examiners distinguished between spasticity and dystonia in neonatal rabbits subjected to prenatal hypoxia/ischemia as models for cerebral palsy (Derrick et al. 2004). The most rigorous assessments might combine force-transducing instruments with the standard criteria (Fischer et al. 2002). When the type of tonal abnormality is uncharacterized, it is preferable to use a generic term (e.g., hypertonia) rather than a more specific term (e.g., rigidity or spasticity) for which there is no supportive evidence.

TABLE 5 Discrimination of Increased Muscle Tone

	Spasticity	Rigidity	Dystonia
Effect of increased speed of passive movement	Resistance increases with increasing speed	Resistance not influenced by speed	Resistance not influenced by speed
Effect of rapidly reversing direction of passive movement	Resistance is delayed	Resistance is immediate	Resistance is immediate
Abnormal postures when awake	Only in severe cases	Not common	Frequent
Abnormal postures when asleep	Only in severe cases	Not common	Not common
Effect of voluntary activity with opposite limb	Minor increase in resistance	Minor increase in resistance	Significant increase in resistance and abnormal postures
Effect of task difficulty with opposite limb	Minor increase in resistance	Minor increase in resistance	Significant increase in resistance and abnormal postures

E. Motor Strength

Movement disorders generally exclude abnormal motor behavior resulting from motor weakness. An assessment of strength is often necessary, however, because motor weakness may mimic certain movement disorders. For example, subtle weakness may result in poor performance on tests of coordinated motor function, leading to the misleading suggestion of cerebellar ataxia. More severe weakness may result in reduced ambulation or even akinesia, resembling Parkinsonism.

A simple screen for motor weakness involves closely inspecting body posture, which is best appreciated on videotape of a lateral view (Whishaw et al. 1998). Normal mice walk with 3–5 mm of clearance between the ventral body and the floor. Weak mice often walk with their ventral surface closer to the floor, and sometimes dragging on the floor. This screen provides only a crude estimate for weakness, but it can be useful to guide the selection for more specific tests of strength, if detected early. Another simple test is to place the animal on an inverted wire mesh grid, and measure the time it takes to fall (Hamann et al. 2003). This method also provides only a crude estimate, as the results are also influenced by motor coordination and other factors (Khan et al. 2004).

Scientists have developed a variety of instruments to estimate strength in rodents (table 4). Gripping bars measure forelimb grasp strength (Connolly et al. 2001; Tilson and Cabe 1978). For this test, the mouse is held by its tail and lowered towards a bar that is attached to a force transducer. The test takes advantage of the tendency of rodents suspended by the tail to grab and cling to the nearest available object. When the animal has grasped the bar, it is pulled away and the average force generated over several trials provides an estimate of forelimb grip strength. A related test measures the grip strength of all four limbs. For this test, the mouse is placed on a wire mesh grid attached to a force transducer. The animal is then pulled from the grid, and the force generated when the mouse grabs the mesh provides an estimate of the strength of all four limbs. Neither the grip bars nor wire mesh tests are completely specific for motor strength. The results can be influenced by coordination, motivational changes, and other variables.

F. Reflexes

A variety of simple reflexes may also be useful in characterizing an abnormal motor syndrome (Crawley 2000). The righting reflex, for example, is simple to perform and may provide the only means of assessment if the motor syndrome is severe enough to preclude the use of other tests. For this test, the examiner positions the animal by holding the tail with one hand and holding the dorsal neck skin with the other hand. The animal is inverted and placed immediately on a flat table, and the examiner records the time required for all four paws to contact the surface. This reflex changes with early development, but by adulthood normal animals can right themselves in less than a second.

Among the many other reflexes that could be tested, the hindlimb grasping reflex, deserves a special mention. To evaluate this reflex, a mouse is picked up by its tail and slowly lowered towards a support over five to ten seconds. Normal mice anticipate the support by reaching out with both forelimbs and extending both hind limbs posteriorly. The procedure should be conducted quickly, since mice suspended by their tails for long periods will begin to struggle, twist, and even flex their trunks so that they climb up their own tails with their forepaws. They should also be lowered slowly, as certain strains are susceptible to a vestibular reflex that leads to brief tonic extensor spasms of the trunk and limbs. The reflex is judged abnormal when the hind limbs adduct close to the body and paws clasp together. Although this reflex is usually evaluated qualitatively, grades of severity have been used (e.g., 0 = normal, 1 = one or both paws adduct but do not clasp, 2 = clasping of hind paws, 3 = clasping of all four limbs). It is important to emphasize that the hind limb grasping reflex is a very non-specific marker of neurologic dysfunction. It provides no indication of Parkinsonism, dystonia, chorea, or stereotypy.

G. Electrophysiological Methods

A review of the electrophysiological correlates and procedures for movement disorders in rodents is beyond the scope of this chapter. Only a few specific examples can be provided. Electroencephalography (EEG) is particularly helpful when the motor disorder appears in discrete attacks. For example, EEG helps discriminate paroxysmal dyskinesias from epileptic seizures (Khan and Jinnah 2002; Loscher et al. 1989). Electromyography (EMG) can assist when a movement disorder might be confused with a neuromuscular disorder. The motor syndromes of action dystonia and neurotonia or myotonia may be indistinguishable without EMG (Jinnah et al. 2000; Shirakawa et al. 2002; Zielasek et al. 2000). Nerve conduction studies (NCS) can also help characterize tremor in rodents, because neuropathy is very commonly expressed as tremor in rodents (Wilms et al. 1999). EMG and NCS are also useful when weakness must be excluded as an underlying cause of a motor syndrome

H. Video Kinematics

Video kinematics represents a computer-driven variation of the "eyeball test" for direct observations. In this method animals performing a specific task, such as locomotion, are videotaped at high frame rates. Specific body parts such as a joint or distal part of a limb are marked either physically or via software analysis of the videotapes. The frequency, speed, directions, coordination, variability, and many other variables can be calculated with remarkable precision from the movements of the markers. This method has the potential to provide a "gold standard" for movement disorders, because it can both identify and quantify most of the basic abnormalities that define individual movement disorders. The video kinematics method has been used to characterize the gait of normal rodents, or asymmetries resulting from cortical or nigrostriatal lesions (Clarke and Still 1999; Clarke and Still 2001; Miklyaeva et al. 1995; Whishaw et al. 1991). It has also been used to characterize ataxia in the lurcher mouse (Fortier et al. 1987), but it is not yet widely applied in other movement disorders for two reasons. The equipment is relatively expensive and labor-intensive, precluding the testing of large numbers of animals.

III. GLOBAL STRATEGIES FOR ASSESSING MOVEMENT DISORDERS

Although there are many simple tests for motor disorders, devising a strategy for selecting the best tests for specific purposes is more challenging. Many available methods have been demonstrated to provide precise and reliable results for evaluating abnormal motor behavior. Unfortunately, experience with these methods has led to an increasing awareness that they are not adequate for application to most movement disorders. Most methods can detect functional disability, but they generally cannot define the nature of the motor syndrome.

A frequently recommended strategy is to conduct a large battery of motor and non-motor tests to provide a comprehensive assessment of the behavioral phenotype. Unfortunately, the comprehensive battery strategy has limited utility for most movement disorders. As a result, a hypothesis-driven or observation-driven strategy for selecting the most helpful behavioral tests may be more appropriate. The following section describes these three main strategies; suggested test batteries for specific movement disorders are provided later.

A. Comprehensive Battery Strategy

The comprehensive battery strategy has already been reviewed several times in detail and will be described only briefly here (Crawley 2000; Crawley and Paylor 1997; Rogers et al. 1997; van der Staay and Steckler 2001). The comprehensive evaluation begins with a brief but broad-based observation of simple behaviors. The observations are typically not quantified, although statistical methods can be applied to uncover certain broad patterns of behaviors (Rogers et al. 1999). Instead, the purpose of this initial step is to identify defects that might influence the selection of subsequent tests. For example, simple screens for visual impairment might steer the investigator away from tests that require good eyesight. Several standardized lists of what to look for have been developed. The Irwin and SHIRPA batteries contain hundreds of items, while others have suggested shorter and more focused lists (Crawley 2000). Following the initial observational screen, a battery of secondary tests is applied addressing specific domains (Figure 4). These tests encompass sensory, cognitive, psychological, ingestive, and motor functions. A third round of tests may then proceed, focusing on any abnormalities uncovered in preceding steps.

The obvious advantage of the comprehensive battery strategy is that the assessment is less likely to miss unanticipated abnormalities that might not be detected with a more focused selection of specific tests. An example is provided by the subtle phenotype displayed by mice with targeting disruption of the D5 dopamine receptor (Holmes et al. 2001). This approach also suffers a number of disadvantages. First, it is best suited for large laboratories specializing in behavioral analysis where all the necessary equipment is available for each test in the battery. It is simply not feasible for most laboratories to purchase all of the necessary

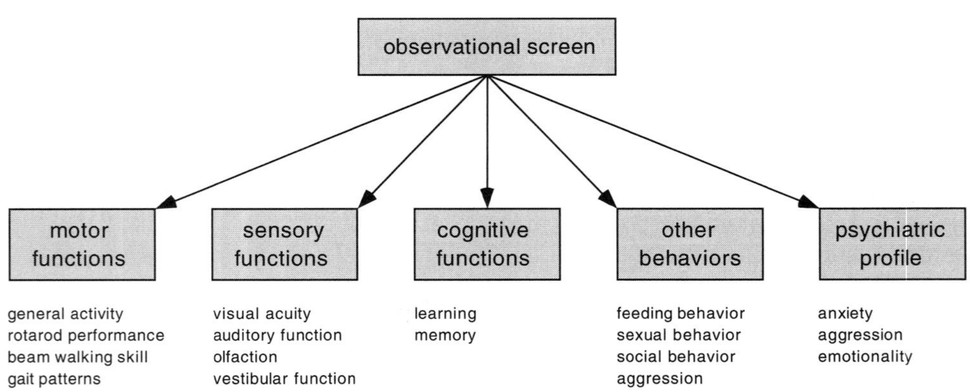

FIGURE 4 The comprehensive battery strategy for assessing abnormal motor behavior.

equipment and develop the technical expertise to use it. Second, this strategy may waste valuable resources by directing efforts towards many tests that may not provide informative results and other tests that may be redundant. For example, the value of performing multiple tests for coordinated motor function rather than a single "best" test remains unproven. Third, the comprehensive battery philosophy is at variance with general trends to focus questions on more hypothesis-driven experimentation rather than broad "fishing expeditions" that may yield results of uncertain significance.

The most serious limitation of the comprehensive battery strategy is that it is not adequate for assessing most movement disorders. The batteries provide excellent assessments of cognitive and psychiatric functions, but relatively weak assessments for motor functions. The tests of motor function in these batteries address functional disability, but they do not help determine the nature of the motor disorder. None of the tests in these batteries incorporates methods that allow the investigator to confidently discriminate Parkinsonism, choreoathetosis, dystonia, or cerebellar ataxia. The value of applying multiple sophisticated measures of motor dysfunction is not clear when the nature of the disorder being studied cannot be determined.

B. Hypothesis-Driven Strategy

A hypothesis-driven approach provides an alternative strategy that has proven successful in many recent studies. In this approach, the selection of tests is guided by known or suspected etiologic mechanisms, or by the human condition being modeled (Figure 5).

One example involves the rodent models for Parkinsonism, which typically focus on identifying abnormalities similar to the human condition or focus on tests thought to be most sensitive for revealing defects associated with its pathogenesis. For example, chronic treatment of rats with rotenone leads to overt motor abnormalities analogous to those of human Parkinsonism, including reduced spontaneous mobility, slowed movements, and flexed postures (Betarbet et al. 2002; Hirsch et al. 2003; Orth and Tabrizi 2003). In this model, observational studies combined with a few tests for gross motor activity and function are adequate. On the other hand, several transgenic and knock-out mouse models focusing on the α-synuclein or parkin genes have resulted in motor phenotypes bearing less obvious resemblances to the human condition (Orth and Tabrizi 2003). In this situation, a hypothesis-driven approach would point to tests more sensitive for subtle motor defects or tests known to be sensitive to dysfunction of basal ganglia dopamine systems.

The advantage of this strategy is that the results obtained have more direct relevance to the human condition being modeled. The obvious disadvantage is that the focused selection of specific tests may result in some important aspect of the behavioral phenotype being overlooked. In addition, the hypothesis-driven approach is obviously not suited for neurotoxicological studies where the outcome is uncertain or transgenic and knock-out mouse models where the functions of the gene product are unknown. In these cases, the comprehensive battery or observation-driven strategies are more appropriate.

C. Observation-Driven Strategy

In some cases, a manipulation provokes an obvious motor phenotype that was not predicted. The manipulation may involve a surgical intervention, drug administration, or gene alteration. In these cases, an observation-driven approach for evaluating the motor syndrome is most appropriate (Figure

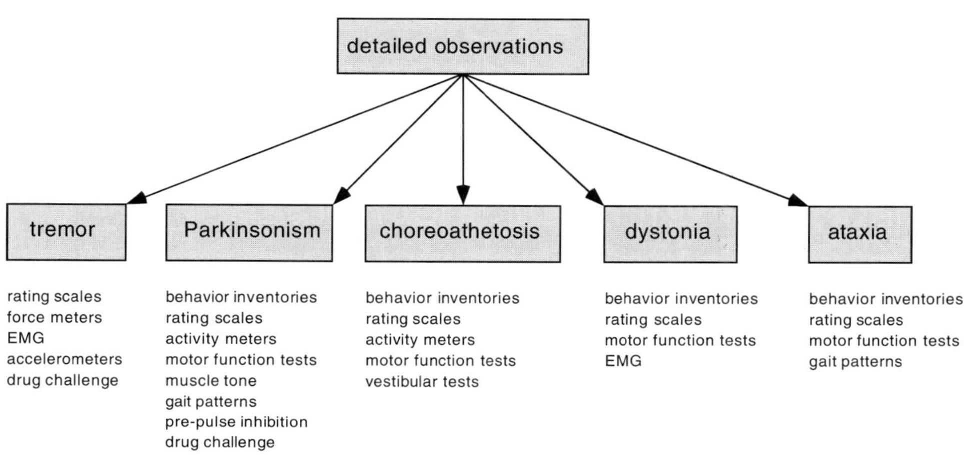

FIGURE 5 Alternative hypothesis-driven or observation-driven strategies for assessing abnormal motor behavior.

5). This approach requires careful observations of the motor syndrome in relation to known motor syndromes of humans, followed by specific tests to confirm or refute similarities.

One example of the observation-driven strategy involves ion channels and dystonia. Administration of an L-type calcium channel activator was shown to provoke a motor syndrome resembling generalized dystonia in mice (Jinnah et al. 2000). Other studies demonstrated that mice carrying mutations in genes encoding P/Q-type calcium channels and related subunits exhibited paroxysmal or generalized dystonia (Campbell and Hess 1999; Fletcher et al. 2001; Khan and Jinnah 2002). These studies have helped point to a link between dystonia and calcium channels that had not been appreciated in prior studies of human dystonia. Further studies have shown that derangements in intracellular calcium handling can also lead to dystonia (Matsumoto et al. 1996; Street et al. 1997). Taken together, these studies establish a strong link between calcium handling and dystonia in mice, and similar defects have been uncovered only recently in human dystonia (Giffin et al. 2002; Sethi and Jankovic 2002).

This strategy has the advantage of providing a focused assessment of a motor syndrome that can be directly compared to a human condition. It is also attractive because it can be possible to establish a previously unrecognized link between the manipulation performed and a human motor disorder. The observation-driven strategy shares the same disadvantage as the hypothesis-driven strategy: it is more likely to miss some important aspect of the behavioral phenotype than the comprehensive approach. It can also be difficult to establish the etiologic relevance of the manipulation to a human condition.

IV. SUGGESTED TEST BATTERIES FOR SPECIFIC MOVEMENT DISORDERS

A. Tremor

Tremor is defined as a rhythmic oscillation of a body part (Barbeau et al. 1981; Deuschl and Krack 1998). Clinically, tremor can be divided into two major types: resting and action. Action tremors can be classified into two major subtypes: postural and kinetic. A resting tremor occurs when an individual is awake but the involved limb is fully relaxed. A postural tremor occurs when the limb is held in a fixed posture, and a kinetic tremor emerges when the limb is moving. A resting tremor is characteristic of Parkinsonism, whereas postural and kinetic tremors are typical of the more common essential tremor.

Most coarse tremors in rodents can be identified by observation. The observations should focus on the tremor type and body parts affected. It is useful to remember that a tremor occurring when an animal is standing is more appropriately classified as a postural tremor than as a resting tremor. Severity scales can be useful to document changes under different experimental conditions.

A variety of instruments can facilitate more precise measurements and detection of very subtle tremors. Such instruments include accelerometers, force-transducing platforms, and EMG (Fowler et al. 2001; Wilms et al. 1999). These instruments can measure many important physiological aspects of tremor, including frequency, amplitude, and force. The functional consequences of the tremor can be assessed with any of the tests for coordinated motor function, such as the rotarod.

In primates, tremor is most often associated with dysfunction of motor systems of the brain (Wilms et al. 1999). Resting tremor is thought to result from dysfunction of the basal ganglia and its connections, while postural and kinetic tremors are thought to result from dysfunction of the cerebellum and its connections. In rodents, tremor may also result from dysfunction of the basal ganglia or cerebellum. The drug harmaline has provided one of the most thoroughly characterized models for tremor in rodents (Wilms et al. 1999). Many mice and rats also have inherited tremor, with several exhibiting pathology in the cerebellum or its connections. Many others have selective defects of central or peripheral myelination, a pathology not commonly associated with tremor in primates (Wilms et al. 1999). In view of the strong association between tremor and peripheral nerve dysfunction in rodents, NCS and histological studies of peripheral nerves are warranted.

B. Parkinsonism

Parkinsonism is a hypokinetic motor syndrome characterized by a resting tremor, reduced spontaneous movements, slowed movements with reduced dexterity, rigid increase in muscle tone, flexed posture, and gait impairment with reduced postural reflexes (Marsden 1994). The initial assessment of a mouse model for Parkinsonism should again begin with observations to document the presence or absence of these features. The many components that define Parkinsonism make it most suited for the behavioral inventories to define the extent of the syndrome, though severity scales could also be applied. If tremor occurs, it can be evaluated as described in the preceding section. However, resting tremor is not commonly observed in rodents, and it is even absent in most primate models of Parkinsonism (Wilms et al. 1999). With the possible exception of tremor, all of the other major features of Parkinsonism can be observed in rodents.

Reduced spontaneous movements and slowed movements are best documented by tests for gross levels of activity, such as activity chambers. Gross functional disability can be determined by tests for coordinated motor function, but difficulties with fine dexterous movements may require more precise evaluation of functions such as reaching skills or beam walking tests (Drucker-Colin and Garcia-Hernandez 1991; Walsh and Wagner 1992). Muscle tone can be assessed using subjective measures or force-transducing instruments. Some additional tests might be warranted because of their known sensitivity for defects in the function of the basal ganglia, and particularly the dopamine systems. Pre-pulse inhibition may be sensitive to even minor defects in basal ganglia dopamine systems (Geyer and Swerdlow 1998; Ralph et al. 1999). Models of unilateral Parkinsonism can be evaluated with rotometers, which have been reviewed extensively elsewhere (Kelly 1977; Miller and Beninger 1991). In some cases where no apparent overt motor defect attributable to basal ganglia dopamine systems can be detected, pharmacological challenges may be useful to reveal subclinical defects (Jinnah et al. 1992).

A major challenge investigators face when evaluating Parkinsonism in rodents is the exclusion of generally poor health. An unhealthy rodent exhibits many of the other behavioral aspects suggestive of Parkinsonism, such as reduced spontaneous movements, slowed movements, hunched posture, and impaired gait.

C. Choreoathetosis

Chorea is a hyperkinetic motor syndrome characterized by irregular, unsustained, fluidly changing movements (Barbeau et al. 1981; O'Brien 1998). Movements may be quick and jerky, or subtle and writhing. Subtle writhing movements are considered athetotic, and the frequent combination of chorea and athetosis has led to the common use of the term choreoathetosis. In its mildest form, choreoathetosis has the appearance of fidgeting. In more severe forms, choreoathetosis takes the form of a dramatic and continual dance.

The complex motor syndrome of choreoathetosis has not been well described in rodents. Mice with mutations of the *it15* gene have been produced as etiologic models for Huntington's disease. These mutants have been extremely valuable for studying the pathogenesis of the disease and for screening for treatments, but most of the strains do not exhibit a motor syndrome that is readily classified as choreoathetoid (Bates 2003; Bates and Hockly 2003; Carter et al. 1999; Gutekunsk et al. 2000). However, many elements can be recognized that resemble the syndrome in other settings. For example, some researchers have argued that the motor syndrome exhibited by rodents treated with high doses of psychostimulants such as amphetamine resembles choreoathetosis. The psychostimulant syndrome includes a hyperkinetic gait (locomotor hyperactivity with circling, spinning, and reverse locomotion), frequent twitch-like movements of the trunk or limbs, and other dyskinetic or stereotypical movements (head bobbing, repetitive licking, or biting). Rodents with inherited or acquired vestibular defects also exhibit a complicated hyperkinetic motor syndrome with many features that suggest choreoathetosis. These mice exhibit a hyperkinetic gait with circling and spinning, frequent and chaotic movements of the head and neck in both the vertical and horizontal planes, and occasional writhing movements of the trunk (Khan et al. 2004). In rodents, the vestibular syndrome has been labeled the waltzing syndrome, in view of its resemblance to dancing.

At face value, the overall appearance of a psychostimulant-intoxicated rodent or one with a vestibular defect does not clearly resemble choreoathetosis of humans. However, the defining characteristics of any motor syndrome must be interpreted in the proper ethological perspective. Specifically, choreoathetoid movements that are so prominent in the upper limbs of bipedal humans are unlikely to be evident in a quadripedal rodent. It is possible that choreoathetosis might be expressed predominantly as a hyperkinetic gait in rodents, although such comparisons are difficult to make with certainty. Rodents treated with psychostimulants and those with vestibulopathy have traditionally been described as having "dyskinetic" motor behavior rather than choreoathetosis because of uncertainties regarding their relationship with the human disorder.

Observation-based behavioral inventories are ideally suited for characterizing the complex components that define choreoathetosis and similar dyskinetic motor syndromes in rodents. Tests for gross motor activity are useful for documenting the hyperkinetic state. Tests for coordinated motor function help measure motor disability. Because of the frequent associations between the choreoathetoid dyskinetic syndrome and vestibular disease in rodents, further tests of vestibular function are warranted when the syndrome occurs. Several behavioral and physiological tests for vestibular function in rodents have been described elsewhere (Khan et al. 2004).

D. Dystonia

Dystonia is a motor syndrome characterized by co-contractions of agonist-antagonist muscle pairs, abnormally sustained contractions, and overflow of contractions to nearby muscles. These problems lead to tonically sustained movements, twisting movements, and sometimes unusual postures (Fahn 1988). Unlike chorea, the movements tend to be stiffer, more sustained, and frequently repetitive. Dystonia has many different manifestations, making it difficult to provide a summary description and proposed test batteries that would be appropriate for all types. Dystonia may be restricted to a limited group of muscles, such as the frequent and exaggerated eye blinking associated with blepharospasm (Schicatano et al. 1997), to life-threatening dystonia affecting the entire body that impairs all basic functions such as ambulation, grooming, and ingestive behaviors (Lorden et al. 1984).

Because of the many potential manifestations of dystonia, observation-based behavior inventories or rating scales provide the most appropriate starting place. Tests for gross or fine motor disability can then be tailored to the problem observed. A major challenge in assessing dystonia in rodents is the close superficial resemblance of the motor syndrome to several other disorders. For example, the autonomous muscle contractions of myotonia can result in sustained muscle contractions, co-contraction of antagonistic muscle groups, and even odd postures (Shirakawa et al. 2002). Autonomous firing of peripheral nerves in neurotonia or neuromyotonia can result in similar behavioral phenomena (Zielasek et al. 2000). Also, defects in spinal inhibitory interneurons have been associated with behavioral manifestations that could be readily mistaken for dystonia (Simon 1997). These disorders are not considered to be forms of dystonia in humans or rodents, even though the motor manifestations may be quite similar. The exclusion of all three of these disorders requires careful EMG and/or NCS, which provide electrophysiological signatures that help to discriminate each.

In addition to excluding disorders that may mimic dystonia, EMG can help identify the basic underlying defects in dystonia: co-contraction of antagonistic muscle pairs and sustained contractions (Jinnah et al. 2000). The main difficulty is discriminating dystonic movements from the frequent struggling movements displayed by rodents restrained for physiological measures. Chronically implanted surface electrodes, and wireless telemetry systems offer alternatives and are just now beginning to be applied in small rodents (Biedermann et al. 2000; Scholle et al. 2001; Schumann et al. 2002; Whelan 2003).

E. Ataxia

The term ataxia probably should be avoided in descriptions of abnormal motor syndromes in rodents, because it has different meanings in different contexts. General neurologists and neuroscientists often use the term as a synonym for clumsiness secondary to any motor defect. In the field of movement disorders, the term ataxia is reserved for a motor syndrome characterized by imprecise timing and distancing of simple movements (dysmetria) and poor temporal and spatial coordination of more complex movements (dysdiadochokinesis) that cannot be attributed to another motor disorder (Massaquoi and Hallet 1998). The term ataxia is not usually applied by specialists in motor control when poor coordination is known to result from weakness or intervening involuntary movements such as dystonia. The use of the term among specialists implies dysfunction of cerebellar input or output.

True cerebellar ataxia must be interpreted with an ethological perspective. In bipedal primates, ataxia of the upper limbs leads to obvious defects in reaching and other fine motor skills. Ataxia of the trunk and lower limbs leads to a characteristic swaggering gait with frequent falls. In quadripedal rodents, these problems are much less evident. The forelimbs are used much less for fine motor tasks, so gross motor incoordination is more difficult to identify. A swaggering gait and falls are much less likely with support being provided by four limbs instead of two. In fact, the motor syndrome in mice with complete loss of output from the cerebellar cortex resulting from degeneration of Purkinje cells is relatively subtle (Fortier et al. 1987; Grusser-Cornehls et al. 1999; Mullen et al. 1976). The supporting stance is widened, although this may be sufficiently subtle that investigators can identify it only by viewing the animal from directly above. Falls are infrequent, but the gait has a jerky quality caused by the poor timing of the limbs during stepping. Falls may occur, but the animal can right itself quickly in the absence of concurrent motor defects.

Functional disability resulting from ataxia can be detected via any of the tests for gross or fine motor coordination such as the rotarod or beam-walking tests. No validated tests are specific for cerebellar ataxia. Footprint analysis may offer the best tool, because several relevant variables can be quantified such as stance width and step variability. Another promising approach involves determining an "ataxia index" which is derived from lateral movements in relation to forward movements during locomotion (Matsukawa et al. 2003). Further characterization of both of these methods may be required to discriminate true cerebellar ataxia from the step variability and lateral movements that may occur in other movement disorders, such as dystonia and choreoathetosis.

A major challenge facing investigators evaluating rodents with cerebellar ataxia is its reliable discrimination from other motor defects that produce impaired coordinated motor behavior. A review of the literature reveals a large number of rodent motor syndromes labeled as ataxia that reflect other motor disorders. Dystonia, in particular, is frequently confused with cerebellar ataxia (Jinnah et al. 2000; Sotelo and Guenet 1988). Table 6 provides a brief list of some readily identifiable differences that help to discriminate dystonia from cerebellar ataxia.

V. SUMMARY

Detailed assessments of abnormal motor syndromes in rodents are a challenging but necessary task facing many investigators interested in elucidating pathogenesis and discovering new treatments for movement disorders. Currently a large number of tests are available for motor function, as well as several strategies for selecting the most appropriate tests for specific purposes; but the development of more refined techniques for discriminating among the many different types of movement disorders is still needed.

TABLE 6 Discriminating Ataxia from Dystonia

	Ataxia	Dystonia
Morphology	Clumsiness not due to weakness or superimposed involuntary movement	Twisting pattern movements with sustained abnormal postures
Falling	Imprecise and inaccurate foot placement	Propelled to side by stiffened or twisting limbs
Righting after Falls	Rapid	Slow
Muscle Tone	Normal or decreased	Increased
Resting Postures	Normal	Abnormal
Mortality	Normal	Increased

Acknowledgments

This work was supported by grants from the National Institutes of Health (NS40470 and NS33592).

References

Aguzzi, A., S. Brandner, U. Sure, D. Ruedi, and S. Isenmann. 1994. Transgenic and knock-out mice: models of neurological disease. *Brain Pathol* **4**:3–20.

Barbeau, A., R.C. Duvoisin, F. Gerstenbrand, J.P.W.F. Lakke, and C.D. Marsden. 1981. Classification of extrapyramidal disorders. *J Neurol Sci* **51**:311–327.

Bates, G. 2003. Huntingtin aggregation and toxicity in Huntington's disease. *Lancet.* **361**:1642–1644.

Bates, G.P., and E. Hockly. 2003. Experimental therapeutics in Huntington's disease: are models useful for therapeutic trials? *Curr Opin Neurol* **16**:465–470.

Betarbet, R., T.B. Sherer, and J.T. Greenamyre. 2002. Animal models of Parkinson's disease. *Bioessays* **24**:308–318.

Biedermann, F., N.P. Schumann, M.S. Fischer, and H.Ch. Scholle. 2000. Surface EMG recordings using a miniaturised matrix electrode: a new technique for small animals. *J Neurosci Meth* **97**:69–75.

Bristow, L.J., N. Collinson, G.P. Cook, N. Curtis, S.B. Freedman, J.J. Kulagowski, P.D. Leeson, S. Patel, C.I. Ragan, M. Ridgill, K.L. Saywell, and M.D. Tricklebank. 1997. L-745,870, a subtype selective dopamine D_4 receptor antagonist, does not exhibit a neuroleptic-like profile in rodent behavioral tests. *J Pharmacol Exp Ther* **283**:1256–1263.

Campbell, D.B., and E.J. Hess. 1999. L-type calcium channels contribute to the tottering mouse dystonic episodes. *Mol Pharmacol* **55**:23–31.

Carter, R.J., L.A. Lione, T. Humby, L. Mangiarini, A. Mahal, G.P. Bates, S.B. Dunnett, and A.J. Morton. 1999. Characterization of progressive motor deficits in mice transgenic for the human Huntington's disease mutation. *J Neurosci* **19**:3248–3257.

Carter, R.J., A.J. Morton, and S.B. Dunnet. 2001. Motor coordination and balance in rodents. In *Current Protocols in Neuroscience* pp. 8.12.1–8.12.14. New York: John Wiley & Sons Inc.

Cenci, M.A., I.Q. Whishaw, and T. Schallert. 2002. Animal models of neurological deficits: how relevant is the rat? *Nature Rev Neurosci* **3**:574–579.

Clarke, K.A., and J. Still. 1999. Gait analysis in the mouse. *Physiol Behav* **66**:723–729.

Clarke, K.A., and J. Still. 2001. Development and consistency of gait in the mouse. *Physiol Behav* **73**:159–164.

Cohen, G., and M.B. Spina. 1989. The Huntington Study Group. 1996. Unified Huntington's disease rating scale: reliability and consistency. *Mov Disord* **11**:136–142.

Comella, C.L., S. Leurgans, J. Wuu, G.T. Stebbins, and T. Chmura. 2003. Rating scales for dystonia: a multicenter trial. *Mov Disord* **18**:303–312.

Connolly, A.M., R.M. Keeling, S. Mehta, A. Pestronk, and J.R. Sanes. 2001. Three mouse models of muscular dystrophy: the natural history of strength and fatigue in dystrophin-, dystrophin/utrophin-, and laminin α2-deficient mice. *Neuromusc Disord* **11**:703–712.

Crawley, J.N. 2000. *What's wrong with my mouse: behavioral phenotyping of transgenic and knockout mice.* New York: Wiley-Liss.

Crawley, J.N., and R. Paylor. 1997. A proposed test battery and constellations of specific behavioral paradigms to investigate the behavioral phenotypes of transgenic and knockout mice. *Horm Behav* **31**:197–211.

Derrick, M., N.L. Luo, J.C. Bregman, T. Jilling, X. Ji, K. Fisher, C.L. Gladson, D.J. Beardsley, G. Murdoch, S.A. Back, and S. Tan. 2004. Preterm fetal hypoxia-ischemia causes hypertonia and motor deficits in the neonatal rabbit: a model for human cerebral palsy? *J Neurosci* **24**:24–34.

Deuschl, G., and P. Krack. 1998. Tremors: differential diagnosis, neurophysiology, and pharmacology. In *Parkinson's disease and movement disorders.* Ed. J. Jankovic, and E. Tolosa. pp. 419–452. Baltimore: Williams & Wilkins.

Drucker-Colin, R., and F. Garcia-Hernandez. 1991. A new motor test sensitive to aging and dopaminergic function. *J Neurosci Meth* **39**:153–161.

Dunnett, S.B., D.J.S. Sirinathsinghji, R. Heavens, D.C. Rogers, and M.R. Kuehn. 1989. Monoamine deficiency in a transgenic (Hprt-) mouse model of Lesch-Nyhan syndrome. *Brain Res* **501**:401–406.

Edamura, K., and H. Sasai. 1998. No self-injurious behavior was found in HPRT-deficient mice treated with 9-ethyladenine. *Pharmacol Biochem Behav* **61**:175–179.

Elble, R.J. 1998. Motor control and movement disorders. In *Parkinson's disease and movement disorders.* Ed. J. Jankovic, and E. Tolosa. pp. 15–45. Baltimore: Williams & Wilkins.

Elsea, S.H., and R.E. Lucas. 2002. The mousetrap: what we can learn when the mouse model does not mimic the human disease. *ILAR J* **43**:66–79.

Erickson, R.P. 1989. Why isn't a mouse more like a man? *Trends Genet* **5**:1–3.

Fahn, S. 1988. Concept and classification of dystonia. *Adv Neurol* **50**:1–8.

Finger, S., R.P. Heavens, D.J.S. Sirinathsinghji, M.R. Kuehn, and S.B. Dunnett. 1988. Behavioral and neurochemical evaluation of a transgenic mouse model of Lesch-Nyhan syndrome. *J Neurol Sci* **86**:203–213.

Fischer, D.A., B. Ferger, and K. Kuschinsky. 2002. Discrimination of morphine- and haloperidol-induced muscular rigidity and akinesia/catalepsy in simple tests in rats. *Behav Brain Res* **134**:317–321.

Fletcher, C.F., A. Tottene, V.A. Lennon, S.M. Wilson, S.J. Dubel, R. Paylor, D.A. Hosford, L. Tessarollo, M.W. McEnery, D. Pietrobon, N.G.

Copeland, and N.A. Jenkins. 2001. Dystonia and cerebellar atrophy in *Cacna1a* null mice lacking P/Q calcium channel activity. *FASEB J* **March 5**.

Fortier, P.A., A.M. Smith, and S. Rossignol. 1987. Locomotor deficits in the mutant mouse, Lurcher. *Exp Brain Res* **66**:271–286.

Fowler, S.C., B.R. Birkestrand, R. Chen, S.J. Moss, E. Vorontsova, G. Wang, and T.J. Zarcone. 2001. A force-plate actometer for quantitating rodent behaviors: illustrative data on locomotion, rotation, spatial learning, stereotypies, and tremor. *J Neurosci Meth* **107**:107–124.

Geyer, M.A., and A. Markou. 1995. Animal models for psychiatric disorders. In *Psychopharmacology: the fourth generation of progress.* Ed. F.E. Bloom, and D.J. Kupfer. pp. 787–798. New York: Raven Press.

Geyer, M.A., and N.R. Swerdlow. 1998. Measurement of startle response, prepulse inhibition, and habituation. In *Current Protocols in Neuroscience*. pp. 8.7.1–8.7.15. New York: John Wiley & Sons Inc.

Giffin, N.J., S. Benton, and P.J. Goadsby. 2002. Benign paroxysmal torticollis of infancy: four new cases and linkage to CACNA1A mutation. *Dev Med Child Neurol* **44**:490–493.

Grusser-Cornehls, U., C. Grusser, and J. Baurle. 1999. Vermectomy enhances parvalbumin expression and improves motor performance in weaver mutant mice: an animal model for cerebellar ataxia. *Neurosci* **91**:315–326.

Gutekunsk, C.A., F. Norflus, and S.M. Hersch. 2000. Recent advances in Huntington's disease. *Curr Opin Neurol* **13**:445–450.

Hamann, M., M.H. Meisler, and A. Richter. 2003. Motor disturbances in mice with deficiency of the sodium channel gene *Scn8a* show features of human dystonia. *Exp Neurol* **184**:830–838.

Hirsch, E.C., G. Hoglinger, E. Rousselet, T. Breidert, K. Parin, J. Feger, M. Ruberg, A. Prigent, C. Cohen-Salmon, and J.M. Launay. 2003. Animal models of Parkinson's disease in rodents induced by toxins: an update. *J Neural Transm Suppl* **65**:89–100.

Holmes, A., T.R. Hollon, T.C. Gleason, Z. Liu, J. Dreiling, D.R. Sibley, and J.N. Crawley. 2001. Behavioral characterization of dopamine D5 receptor null mutant mice. *Behav Neurosci* **115**:1129–1144.

Hooper, M., K. Hardy, A. Handyside, S. Hunter, and M. Monk. 1987. HPRT-deficient (Lesch-Nyhan) mouse embryos derived from germline colonization by cultured cells. *Nature* **326**:292–295.

Hyland, K., S. Kasim, K. Egami, L.A. Arnold, and H.A. Jinnah. 2004. Tetrahydrobiopterin and brain dopamine loss in a genetic mouse model of Lesch-Nyhan disease. *J Inher Metab Dis* In press.

Jinnah, H.A., F.H. Gage, and T. Friedmann. 1991. Amphetamine-induced behavioral phenotype in a hypoxanthine-guanine phosphoribosyltransferase-deficient mouse model of Lesch-Nyhan syndrome. *Behav Neurosci* **105**:1004–1012.

Jinnah, H.A., E.J. Hess, M.S. LeDoux, N. Sharma, M.G. Baxter, and M.R. DeLong. In press. Rodent models for dystonia research: workshop summary. *Mov Disord.*

Jinnah, H.A., M.D. Jones, B.E. Wojcik, J.D. Rothstein, E.J. Hess, T. Friedmann, and G.R. Breese. 1999. Influence of age and strain on striatal dopamine loss in a genetic mouse model of Lesch-Nyhan disease. *J Neurochem* **72**:225–229.

Jinnah, H.A., P.J. Langlais, and T. Friedmann. 1992. Functional analysis of brain dopamine systems in a genetic mouse model of Lesch-Nyhan syndrome. *J Pharmacol Exp Ther* **263**:596–607.

Jinnah, H.A., J.P. Sepkuty, T. Ho, S. Yitta, T. Drew, J.D. Rothstein, and E.J. Hess. 2000. Calcium channel agonists and dystonia in the mouse. *Mov Disord* **15**:542–551.

Jinnah, H.A., B.E. Wojcik, M.A. Hunt, N. Narang, K.Y. Lee, M. Goldstein, J.K. Wamsley, P.J. Langlais, and T. Friedmann. 1994. Dopamine deficiency in a genetic mouse model of Lesch-Nyhan disease. *J Neurosci* **14**:1164–1175.

Jones, B.J., and D.J. Roberts. 1968. The quantitative measurement of motor inco-ordination in naive mice using an accelerating rotarod. *J Pharm Pharmacol* **20**:302–304.

Kasim, S., and H.A. Jinnah. 2002. Thresholds for self-injurious behavior in a genetic mouse model of Lesch-Nyhan disease. *Pharmacol Biochem Behav* **73**:583–592.

Kelley, A.E. 1998. Measurement of rodent stereotyped behavior. In *Current Protocols in Neuroscience.* pp. 8.8.1–8.8.13. New York: John Wiley & Sons Inc..

Kelly, P.H. 1977. Drug-induced motor behavior. In *Handbook of psychopharmacology: drugs, neurotransmitters, and behavior.* Ed. L.L. Iversen, S.D. Iversen, and S.H. Snyder. pp. 295–331. New York: Plenum Press.

Khan, Z., J. Carey, M. Lehar, D. Lasker, and H.A. Jinnah. 2004. Abnormal motor behavior and vestibular dysfunction in the stargazer mouse mutant. *Neuroscience* **127**:785–796.

Khan, Z., and H.A. Jinnah. 2002. Paroxysmal dyskinesias in the lethargic mouse mutant. *J Neurosci* **22**:8193–8200.

Kuehn, M.R., A. Bradley, E.J. Robertson, and M.J. Evans. 1987. A potential animal model for Lesch-Nyhan syndrome through introduction of HPRT mutations into mice. *Nature* **326**:295–298.

Lorden, J.F., T.W. McKeon, H.J. Baker, N. Cox, and S.U. Walkley. 1984. Characterization of the rat mutant dystonic (*dt*): a new animal model of dystonia musculorum deformans. *J Neurosci* **4**:1925–1932.

Loscher, W., J.E. Fisher, D. Schmidt, G. Fredow, D. Honack, and W.B. Iturrian. 1989. The sz mutant hamster: a genetic model of epilepsy or of paroxysmal dystonia? *Mov Disord* **4**:219–232.

Marsden, C.D. 1994. Parkinson's disease. *J Neurol Neurosurg Psychiatry* **57**:672–681.

Massaquoi, S.G., and M. Hallet. 1998. Ataxia and other cerebellar syndromes. In *Parkinson's disease and movement disorders.* Ed. J. Jankovic and E. Tolosa. pp. 623–686. Baltimore: Williams & Wilkins.

Matsukawa, H., A.M. Wolf, S. Matsushita, R.H. Joho, and T. Knopfel. 2003. Motor dysfunction and altered synaptic transmission at the parallel fiber-Purkinje cell synapse in mice lacking potassium channels Kv3.1 and Kv3.3. *J Neurosci* **23**:7677–7684.

Matsumoto, M., T. Nakagawa, T. Inoue, E. Nagata, K. Tanaka, H. Takano, O. Minowa, J. Kuno, S. Sakakibara, M. Yamada, H. Yoneshima, A. Miyawaki, Y. Fukuuchi, T. Furuichi, H. Okano, K. Mikoshiba, and T. Noda. 1996. Ataxia and epileptic seizures in mice lacking type 1 inositol 1,4,5-triphosphate receptor. *Nature* **379**:168–171.

McNamara, F.N., J.J. Clifford, O. Tighe, A. Kinsella, J. Drago, D.T. Croke, and J.L. Waddington. 2003. Congenic D1A dopamine receptor mutants: ethologically based resolution of behavioural topography indicates genetic background as a determinant of knockout phenotype. *Neuropsychopharmacol* **28**:86–99.

Miklyaeva, E.I., D.J. Martens, and I.Q. Whishaw. 1995. Impairments and compensatory adjustments in spontaneous movement after unilateral dopamine depletion in rats. *Brain Res* **681**:23–40.

Miller, R., and R.J. Beninger. 1991. On the interpretation of asymmetries of posture and locomotion produced with dopamine agonists in animals with unilateral depletion of striatal dopamine. *Prog Neurobiol* **36**:229–256.

Mullen, R.J., E.M. Eicher, and R.L. Sidman. 1976. Purkinje cell degeneration, a new neurological mutation in the mouse. *Proc Nat Acad Sci U S A* **73**:208–212.

O'Brien, C.F. 1998. Chorea. In *Parkinson's disease and movement disorders.* Ed. J. Jankovic, and E. Tolosa. pp. 357–364. Baltimore: Williams & Wilkins.

Orth, M., and S.J. Tabrizi. 2003. Models of Parkinson's disease. *Mov Disord* **18**:729–737.

Pierce, C., and P. Kalivas. 1997. Locomotor behavior. In *Current Protocols in Neuroscience.* pp. 8.1.1–8.1.8. New York: John Wiley & Sons Inc.

Puglisi-Allegra, S., and S. Cabib. 1988. The D2 dopamine receptor agonist LY171555 induces catalepsy in the mouse. *Pharmacol Biochem Behav* **30**:765–768.

Ralph, R.J., G.B. Varty, M.A. Kelly, Y.M. Wang, M.G. Caron, M. Rubinstein, D.K. Grandy, M.J. Low, and M.A. Geyer. 1999. The dopamine D2, but not D3 or D4, receptor subtype is essential for the disruption of prepulse inhibition produced by amphetamine in mice. *J Neurosci* **19**:4627–4663.

Rogers, D.C., E.M.C. Fisher, S.D.M. Brown, J. Peters, A.J. Hunter, and J.E. Martin. 1997. Behavioral and functional analysis of mouse phenotype: SHIRPA, a proposed protocol for comprehensive phenotype assessment. *Mamm Genome* **8**:711–713.

Rogers, D.C., D.N.C. Jones, P.R. Nelson, C.M. Jones, C.A. Quilter, T.L. Robinson, and J.J. Hagan. 1999. Use of SHIRPA and discriminant analysis to characterise marked differences in the behavioural phenotype of six inbred mouse strains. *Behav Brain Res* **105**:207–217.

Sanger, T.D., M.R. Delgado, D. Gaebler-Spira, M. Hallet, J.W. Mink, and F. Task. 2003. Classification and definition of disorders causing hypertonia in childhood. *Pediatrics* **111**:89–97.

Schicatano, E.J., M.A. Basso, and C. Evinger. 1997. Animal model explains the origins of the cranial dystonia benign essential blepharospasm. *J Neurophysiol* **77**:2842–2846.

Scholle, H.Ch., N.P. Schumann, F. Biedermann, D.F. Stegeman, R. Grae, K. Roeleveld, N. Schilling, and M.S. Fisher. 2001. Spatiotemporal surface EMG characteristics from rat triceps brachii muscle during treadmill locomotion indicate selective recruitment of functionally distinct muscle regions. *Exp Brain Res* **138**:26–36.

Schumann, N.P., F.H.W. Biedermann, B.U. Kleine, D.F. Stegeman, K. Roeleveld, R. Hackert, and H.Ch. Scholle. 2002. Multi-channel EMG of the M. triceps brachii in rats during treadmill locomotion. *Clin Neurophysiol* **113**:1142–1151.

Sethi, K.D., and J. Jankovic. 2002. Dystonia in spinocerebellar ataxia type 6. *Mov Disord* **17**:150–153.

Shirakawa, T., K. Sakai, Y. Kitagawa, A. Hori, and G. Hirose. 2002. A novel murine myotonia congenita without molecular defects in the *CLC-1* and the *SCN4A*. *Neurology* **59**:1091–1094.

Simon, E.S. 1997. Phenotypic heterogeneity and disease course in three murine strains with mutations in genes encoding for alpha 1 and beta glycine receptor subunits. *Mov Disord* **12**:221–228.

Smith, D., and T. Friedmann. 2000. Characterization of the dopamine defect in primary cultures of dopaminergic neurons from hypoxanthine phosphoribosyltransferase knockout mice. *Mol Ther* **1**:486–491.

Sotelo, C., and J.L. Guenet. 1988. Pathologic changes in the CNS of dystonia musculorum mutant mouse: an animal model for human spinocerebellar ataxia. *Neurosci* **27**:403–424.

Street, V.A., M.M. Bosma, V.P. Demas, M.R. Regan, D.D. Lin, L.C. Robinson, W.S. Agnew, and B.L. Tempel. 1997. The type 1 inositol triphosphate receptor gene is altered in the opisthotonus mouse. *J Neurosci* **17**:635–647.

Tilson, H.A., and P.A. Cabe. 1978. Assessment of chemically-induced changes in the neuromuscular function of rats using a new recording grip meter. *Life Sci* **23**:1365–1370.

van der Staay, F.J., and T. Steckler. 2001. Behavioural phenotyping of mouse mutants. *Behav Brain Res* **125**:3–12.

Visser, J.E., D.W. Smith, S.S. Moy, G.R. Breese, T. Friedmann, J.D. Rothstein, and H.A. Jinnah. 2002. Oxidative stress and dopamine deficiency in a genetic mouse model of Lesch-Nyhan disease. *Dev Brain Res* **133**:127–139.

Wahlsten, D. 2001. Standardizing tests of mouse behavior: reasons, recommendations, and reality. *Physiol Behav* **73**:695–704.

Walsh, S.L., and G.C. Wagner. 1992. Motor impairments after methamphetamine-induced neurotoxicity in the rat. *J Pharmacol Exp Ther* **263**:617–626.

Whelan, P.J. 2003. Electromyogram recordings from freely moving animals. *Methods* **30**:127–141.

Whishaw, I.Q., F. Haun, and B. Kolb. 1998. Analysis of behavior in laboratory rodents. In *Modern Techniques in Neuroscience*. Ed. U. Windhorst, and H. Johansson. pp. 1243–1275. Berlin: Springer-Verlag.

Whishaw, I.Q., S.M. Pellis, B.P. Gorny, and V.C. Pellis. 1991. The impairments in reaching and the movements of compensation in rats with motor cortex lesions: an endpoint, videorecording, and movement notation analysis. *Behav Brain Res* **42**:77–91.

Wilms, H., J. Sievers, and G. Deuschl. 1999. Animal models of tremor. *Mov Disord* **14**:557–571.

Winkler, C., D. Kirik, A. Bjorklund, and M.A. Cenci. 2002. L-dopa-induced dyskinesias in the intrastriatal 6-hydroxydopamine model of Parkinson's disease: relation to motor and cellular parameters of nigrostriatal function. *Neurobiol Dis* **10**:165–186.

Zielasek, J., R. Martini, U. Suter, and K.V. Toyka. 2000. Neuromyotonia in mice with hereditary myelinopathies. *Muscle Nerve* **23**:696–701.

C H A P T E R

A6

Response Dynamics: Measurement of the Force and Rhythm of Motor Responses in Laboratory Animals

STEPHEN C. FOWLER, T.L. McKERCHAR, and T.J. ZARCONE

Through the use of force transducers and computer technology we have developed three behavioral paradigms that permit high-resolution measurement of the force and rhythm of motor behavior expressed by tongue, forelimb, or the whole body of rats or mice. In the lick-force-rhythm task, significant effects of environmental, pharmacological, neurotoxic, genetic, and age-related manipulations on tongue movements were reviewed. With respect to the fore limbs of rats, the press-while-licking task afforded measures of tremor induced by low doses (below the threshold dose for visible whole-body tremor) of harmaline and physostigmine. Regarding behaviors assessed at the whole body level, effects of tremorogenic drugs and indirect-acting dopamine agonists (e.g., amphetamine) were quantified in a force-plate actometer, a new instrument that records both the spatial location of an animal and its movements at that location. This instrument revealed that the focused stereotypy induced in rats by amphetamine is characterized by a near-10 Hz rhythm of head movements while locomotion is completely suppressed. In separate experiments with the force-plate actometer, harmaline and physostigmine produced demonstrably different types of whole-body tremor in rats. Finally, the versatility of the force-plate approach to quantifying motor behavior was demonstrated with dopamine D2 receptor knock-out mice and inbred mice. The experimental methods described here are broadly applicable to the development of laboratory animal models of movement disorders.

I. BACKGROUND

Like all scientific initiatives, the work reported here relied on methods and findings brought forth by other scientists. More specifically, the contributions of Notterman and Mintz (1965) were a defining node that importantly influenced the evolution of concepts and methods embodied in the approach to the measurement of motor behavior reported here. One of the foundational assumptions of their book *Dynamics of Response* (Notterman and Mintz 1965) was that any behavioral response had a measurable duration (i.e., the time interval between the beginning and the end of the response) and an amplitude property (e.g., force, millivolts, etc.) that could be measured with the tools of the physical sciences. At the time of Notterman and Mintz's seminal work, the behaviorists were rapidly developing a powerful technology for behavioral measurement based on counting electric switch closures by animals that had learned to operate switches ("operant lever pressing") to obtain rewards. Switch closure rates became the central dependent variable for characterizing behavior and behavioral alterations induced by independent variables of interest, such as schedules of reinforcement, drugs, or brain lesions. Switch closures were treated as events that were equal to one another. Notterman and Mintz (1965) showed that these events were not equal because, instead of using switches to sense the animal's behavior they used a force-transducer and an analog computer to measure the peak forces and durations of individual responses made by rats. The resulting analyses showed that both the duration and force of rats' operant responses varied in important ways that were governed by both environmental and physiological variables. For example, they showed that extinction (the termination of expected reward) led to a rapid rise in peak force and duration of responses while response rate declined. Although the Notterman-Mintz approach to behavioral measurement defined the physical properties of operant responding, the operant method was incomplete as viewed from a biobehavioral perspective because it could not measure the behavior of the organism when it was not interacting with the switch or force transducer. The methods described here address this problem by arranging the contingencies of reward delivery so that continuous or nearly continuous contact with a force sensor is required for delivery of reward (i.e., the press-while-licking task and the lick-force-rhythm-task). A third behavioral measurement technique described here, the force-plate actometer, does not use operant behavior technology, but its development, nevertheless, grew out of the theme of continuous measurement of the physical attributes of behavior. The force-plate actometer uses force-transducer technology to measure an animal's spontaneous movements with unprecedented spatial and temporal resolution (Fowler et al. 2001).

Characterized in anatomical terms, the work reviewed here describes the motor behavior of the tongue (lick-force-rhythm task), the forelimb (press-while-licking task), and the whole body (the force-plate actometer). The empirical results concern the motor effects of drugs that have implications for neurology (tremor, rhythmic behaviors), drug abuse (effects of stimulants), and behavioral neuroscience (neurotransmitter receptors associated with specific behavioral alterations). Thorough reviews of these areas were not undertaken, because the emphasis here is on measurement methods. A related chapter (Fowler et al. this volume) describes the motor effects of antipsychotic drugs, with special emphasis on the motor effects of the atypical antipsychotic drug clozapine in the press-while-licking and lick-force-rhythm procedures.

II. MEASURING TREMOR DURING SUSTAINED FORELIMB FORCE IN UNRESTRAINED RATS

A. Overview

Initially, we developed the behavioral procedures and analytical methods presented in this section on forelimb tremor in an effort to quantify in rats the Parkinsonian-like side effects of the classical (typical), dopamine-receptor-blocking antipsychotic drugs (Fowler et al. 1990). The aim was to measure changes in response initiation, force control, and tremor in response to haloperidol treatment; haloperidol is the prototypical high potency antipsychotic drug that frequently induces extrapyramidal side effects (EPS). In addition, muscarinic anticholinergic drugs were included in the experimental analyses to determine if these agents could ameliorate haloperidol-induced motor effects in rats as they do in human patients. Over time, experiments included reference drugs to establish further parallels between drug-induced motor alterations in rats and humans. The reference drugs with motor response implications included pentobarbital (Kallman and Fowler 1994), scopolamine (Stanford and Fowler 1997), physostigmine (Stanford and Fowler 1997), harmaline (Stanford and Fowler 1998), and sodium dantrolene (Stanford and Fowler 2002). The effects of these reference drugs will be the focus of this chapter. Data indicative of the force- and/or tremor-modulating effects of both typical and atypical antipsychotic drugs will be reviewed in a separate chapter (Fowler et al. this volume). In addition to the findings with drug treatments, this chapter will summarize the effect of variation in force requirements for reinforcement (Stanford et al. 2000) as well as the behavioral effects of unilateral 6-hydroxydopamine (OHDA)-induced lesions of the substantia nigra compacta (Skitek 1998), a popular rodent model of Parkinson disease.

The motor control task that we devised for rats required them to use a designated forelimb to press downward on a force transducer operandum and to lick a liquid reinforcer at the same time (Fowler et al. 1990). This motor task is directly analogous to the task of a human operating a common water fountain that gives water only when the human exerts force against a spring-loaded valve. If the human continuously maintains the required force on the water fountain valve above a set force criterion governed by the spring constant in the valve, water will flow continuously. In the experiments with rats, the manually operated valve was replaced by a silent isometric force transducer, and a computer program that controlled access to the liquid continuously monitored and recorded the force and activated a solenoid that brought the reward within reach of the rat's tongue. The dipper presenting the liquid reinforcer had sufficient volume to induce the rat to hold and drink continuously for several seconds. This interval of continuous

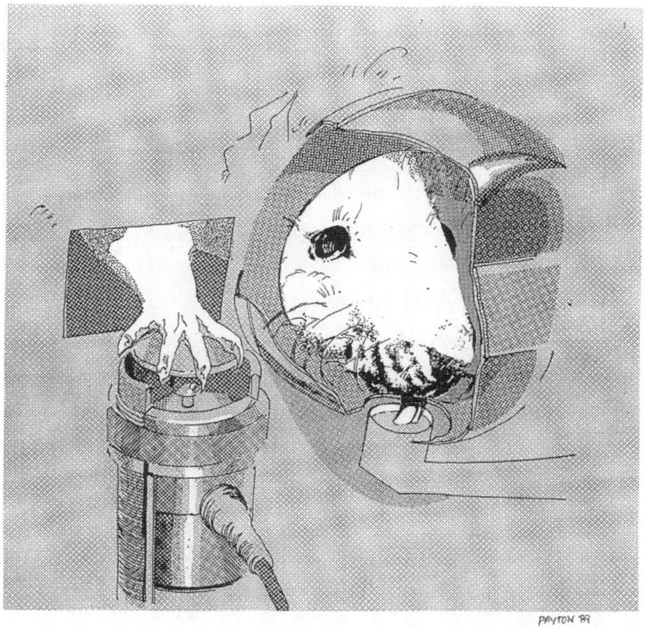

FIGURE 1 Line drawing of a rat performing the press-while-licking task. The rat's right forepaw is exerting a downward force on a disk that is mounted on the shaft of a force transducer. In this task, access to the reward was contingent upon a rat's maintaining forelimb force above an experimenter-selected criterion. If force fell below this force criterion, the dipper dropped back into the reward reservoir (not shown). Reprinted from Fowler (1999).

forelimb force provided time series of force variation suitable to successfully apply Fourier analysis (power spectrum analysis) to detect and quantify any tremor in the forelimb performance.

B. Methods Summary

1. Apparatus for the Press-While-Licking Task

The portion of the apparatus that engages the rat's behavior is shown in Figure 1. Dimensional details have been reported (Fowler et al. 1990). The location of the operandum in relation to the dipper ensures that only the experimenter-designated forelimb can gain access to the reward. This latter point is important for experiments employing unilateral forelimb treatments, such as unilateral brain lesions or direct treatments (e.g., injection of a pro-inflammatory substance into the forepaw) of a designated forelimb. Thus, the spatial arrangement depicted in Figure 1 limits the effective behavioral response to the forelimb sustaining the treatment because the animal cannot successfully switch to the unaffected limb or other body part such as the snout. Motivation to use the affected forelimb remains high because potential alternative routes to the reward have been eliminated. Another important consideration involves the positioning of the operandum so that the rat's forelimb is not braced against the sides of the operandum-access aperture. Such bracing may attenuate variation in the limb's force emission compared to unrestricted movement, and thereby compromise the measurements.

The sampling rate of the analog force signal was 100 samples/s in most studies. This digitizing rate is sufficient to capture faithfully the frequencies of force variation up to 50 Hz. In practice, the force signal from the transducer should be electronically filtered with a high pass cutoff of 100 Hz. If electronic filtering is not used then initial exploratory studies should be undertaken with a range of sampling rates (e.g., 100, 200, and 400 samples/s) to verify that no frequency aliases are contaminating the power spectra that are obtained with the 100 samples/s rate (see Marple 1987, for a discussion of aliases). In addition, the investigator should recall that mechanical systems have characteristic natural frequencies of oscillation, where the frequency is determined by the mass and stiffness of the system. Moreover, the natural frequency that is of interest here is that of the assembled system with the operandum in place, not that of the force transducer specifications per se. Adding an operandum to the shaft of the transducer increases the mass of the system and lowers the natural frequency. In most cases the natural frequency of the transducer-operandum system can be measured with an oscilloscope. With the oscilloscope leads attached to the transducer output, the operandum can be struck sharply with an object, and the "ringing" of the system can be observed as sinusoidal oscillations on the oscilloscope. During this test, care should be taken to apply forces that fall within the transducer's specified range to prevent permanent damage to the transducer. We have used Model 31a load cells with a range of 0–250 gram equivalent weights supplied by Sensotec (Columbus, OH). Our operandum, an aluminum disk 18 mm in diameter, weighs 1 gram. Our measurements show that the natural frequency of the transducer-operandum ensemble is above 100 Hz.

The sensing shaft of the Sensotec Model 31a is mounted in the center of a diaphragm spring element. This design makes the sensor relatively insensitive to off-axis loading effects. In other words, a given force applied near the periphery of the operandum disk will produce the same measurement as a force applied to the center of the disk. Although considerably less expensive than the Model 31a, beam-type force transducers are not recommended for measuring biobehavioral forces because the beam-type transducers allow measurable force to vary considerably depending on the point on the beam where a given force is applied. For example, if one uses a beam-type force sensor with a 4-cm-long beam (measured from the center of the strain-gauge sensing region to the distal tip of the beam), then a 20 g force applied at the distal tip of the beam would register 20 g, but the same 20 g force applied at a point 3 cm from the center of the strain gauge would be detected as a 15 g force. This amount of error (25%) based on the point of the rat's application of force to the beam is unacceptably large.

2. Training Procedures

Operant behavior training procedures shape the performance of operandum-pressing while licking. Depending on whether food (sweetened milk) or water is used as a reward, the male rats are placed on a restricted feeding or watering schedule that permits a weight gain of 2–3 grams per week, which is consistent with good health and provides high levels of motivation to work for the reward. The method of successive approximations (e.g., Reynolds 1968) brings the animal from an initial "naïve" state to the final required skill of pressing and licking at the same time. A skilled trainer can successfully accomplish the training during the course of five to seven daily sessions of ten to fifteen minutes per day. Once the rat begins to gain one or two seconds of access to the reward while maintaining contact with the operandum, a computer program takes over the training, which typically lasts another fifteen to thirty sessions of eight minutes each on separate days. The data are then checked for stability over the current and preceding two days. If performance has stabilized, then the experimental manipulations are begun the next day.

In the studies reviewed here, the volume of liquid reward in the dipper was 0.5 ml. With this volume of reward, rats were required to lick for six to nine seconds to empty the dipper. Although not explicitly trained to do so, the rat learned that it could obtain further reinforcement beyond the first dipperful only by lessening the force on the operandum to let the dipper fall back into the liquid reservoir for refilling. In the majority of studies conducted by our group after 1995, the force level required to present the dipper was 20 g and the force must drop below 6.7 g to deactivate the dipper solenoid. This inequality of dipper-raising and dipper-lowering force was successfully instituted to encourage relatively discrete responses with unambiguous start and end points. Identification of separate responses enabled the type of quantitative approaches to data analysis that are described next.

3. Dependent Variables and Quantitative Methods

Figure 2 shows a force-time record for one response of a rat that learned to completely release the transducer each time the dipper was emptied. The inset axes show the power spectrum for the hold segment of the response. The force-time data for each response were divided into three separate segments to make the portion of the signal analyzed for tremor phenomena conform to the assumptions of spectral analysis. These segments were the start, hold, and discarded segments. A key assumption in spectral analyses is that the

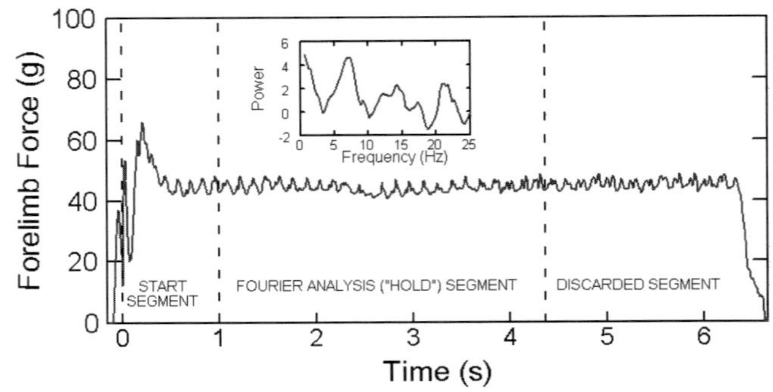

FIGURE 2 A force-time waveform and corresponding power spectrum (inset axes) of the hold segment of the forelimb force applied to the force-sensing operandum in the press-while-licking task shown in Fig. 1. The prominent oscillation visible in the force-time data and appearing at 7 Hz in the power spectrum was caused by the rat's licking behavior that was mechanically transmitted through the forelimb to the transducer. Reprinted from Fowler et al. (1994).

data are statistically stationary (the mean and variance are stable across time). The first second of a response contained large non-stationary force transients associated with the rat positioning itself in accord with task parameters. Thus, this start segment was not spectrally analyzed, but other information from this start segment, such as peak force attained (i.e., the maximum force reached in this segment), often served as a dependent variable. The hold segment was taken as the 3.36 seconds of data after the one second start segment. This value was chosen for three reasons. First, its length (336 sequential time points 0.01 seconds apart) was compatible with a prime factor fast Fourier analysis (Alligator Technologies, Costa Mesa, CA). Second, experience showed that almost every well-trained rat produced responses lasting longer than 4.36 seconds; therefore, ending the hold segment 4.36 seconds after response initiation eliminated from the analysis those non-stationary components of the time series that were associated with release of the operandum. Third, power spectral functions for each response were averaged for each rat, and this need to average functions meant that the time series length had to be held constant so that all Fourier functions contained the same number of frequency estimates (i.e., the number of frequency estimates in each function was determined by series length). The discarded segment generally was not analyzed based on the assumption that its stationary component contained little information beyond that contained in the hold segment.

Inspection of the force-time record and the power spectrum presented in Figure 2 indicates a prominent rhythmic process with a frequency near 7 Hz. We know from measurements of licking taken with a submersible force transducer attached to the reward dipper (unpublished observations) that this 7 Hz rhythm reflects the rat's lick rhythm. This means that lick rhythm can be estimated from the same force records used to measure forelimb tremor. The presence of licking-related power in the spectrum implies that tremor analyses based on the power spectrum should exclude force variation caused by licking. This was done by selecting the power in the 10–25 Hz frequency band as a reflection of tremor uncontaminated by licking. Thus, the dependent variable that we have used to reflect forelimb tremor is the integrated power in the 10–25 Hz frequency band per response.

Other measures of behavior in this task were time on task, averaged response force, and duration of the response. Time on task was the total amount of time in an eight minute session that the rat's forelimb was in contact with the operandum; contact was defined by force exceeding 1 g of weight. Time on task gives an estimate of the rat's motivation to continue responding in the presence of drugs at and doses that suppress this learned behavior. Averaged response force was computed as ensemble averages for the first 4.36 seconds of response that lasted at least 4.36 seconds (one second start segment plus 3.36 seconds hold segment, but no discarded segment). Alignment of the responses for time averaging was based on the time point when force first rose above 1 g. Response duration was the interval of time from the beginning of the start segment to the point in time when force fell to 6.7 g.

C. Results of Behavioral, Pharmacological, and Direct CNS Manipulations

1. Manipulation of Behavior-Controlling Variables

a. Variation in Required Force

A parametric study of variation in the forces required to raise and lower the dipper showed that forelimb tremor power in the 10–25 Hz frequency band increased with increasing force requirement (Stanford et al. 2000). These data were seen as congruent with results for human subjects that showed increased tremor with increased force requirement (Homberg et al. 1986). Experiments with human subjects also suggested that power spectral analysis of sustained isometric force (Homberg et al. 1986), as well as isotonic force (McAuley et al. 1997) yielded tremor estimates that paralleled those measured via electromyography (EMG). Thus, forelimb-force measurements in the rat preparation described here are likely to reflect tremor processes that are homologous to those in humans and are accessible to study without resorting to EMG techniques, which generally require surgery in rats when chronic measurements are sought.

b. Practice Effects

The work by Stanford et al. (2000) produced two additional noteworthy findings. First, two weeks of performance on the forelimb task under relatively high force requirements led to significant reductions in tremor, which were likely the result of growth in the muscles used to perform the task. The practice-related change in tremor is important because it suggests that experimental analyses of treatments that may affect tremor need to take account of the practice effects so as not to confound them with the treatments of interest. The second finding was that the 7 Hz peak in the power spectrum (inset axes in Figure 2) remained at 7 Hz despite changes in force requirement and consequent changes in tremor power. This result further supports our conclusion that the 7 Hz rhythm reflects tongue movements and is not related to forelimb tremor.

2. Pharmacological Manipulations, Excluding Antipsychotic Drugs

a. Pentobarbital

Table 1 summarizes the effects of tremor-inducing drugs and reference drugs on performance in the press-while-licking task. Effects of the sedative-hypnotic barbiturate pentobarbital were studied in a group of ten male rats trained on the task (Kallman and Fowler 1994). Pentobarbital was seen as a positive control for sedative effects at a 10 mg/kg dose that is well below that required to produce ataxia. While pentobarbital at 10 mg/kg significantly reduced task engagement, it did not affect the power in the 10–25 Hz frequency band of the power spectrum. However, pentobarbital did significantly slow lick rhythm (nine of ten rats exhibited a demonstrable slowing and one rat showed no difference between vehicle and drug).

b. Sodium Dantrolene

Dantrolene was examined in this task because of this drug's capacity to decrease muscle spasticity by acting on the muscle contractile process (literature briefly summarized in Stanford and Fowler 2002). Consistent with its primarily peripheral site of action, dantrolene had no effect on task engagement, but it significantly reduced tremor below normal physiological levels observed after saline control injections. The drug significantly reduced average hold force, but peak force of the start segment was non-significantly lowered. No effect on lick rhythm was detected. The pattern of results for dantrolene reflects intact motivation to perform in the context of reduced muscle tone.

c. Harmaline

Harmaline is a well-known tremorogenic agent used to model some aspects of essential tremor in human patients (Elble 1998). Little background on this drug is given here because much pertinent information is reviewed elsewhere in this volume. The effects of harmaline on rat forelimb tremor were evaluated in two separate studies that used the same apparatus (Stanford and Fowler 1998; Wang 2000), but

TABLE 1 Summary of the Effects of Reference Drugs on Tremor and Other Response Parameters Measured in Rats Performing the Press-While-Licking Task

	Drugs and Doses Used					
Dependent variable	**Pentobarbital 10.0[1]**	**Dantrolene 5, 7.5, 10**	**Harmaline 0.5, 1.0**	**Harmaline 4.0**	**Physostigmine 0.05, 0.10**	**Scopolamine 0.1, 0.2**
Time on Task	<[2]	O	O	<	<, <	<
Tremor Band Power	O	<	>	>	>, >	<
Response Duration	O	n.r.	>	>	n.r., O	n.r.
Peak Force	O	O	n.r.	n.r.	>, n.r.	<
Hold Force	n.r.[3]	<	O	n.r.	O, n.r.	<
Lick Rhythm	<	O	<	<	O, >	O
Citation[4]	(a)	(e)	(c)	(d)	(b), (d)	(b)

Notes:
1. doses are in mg/kg.
2. <, O, > indicate significant decrease, no change, and significant increase compared to no drug, respectively.
3. n.r. means not reported.
4. key to citations: (a) Kallman and Fowler 1994; (b) Stanford and Fowler 1997; (c) Stanford and Fowler 1998; (d) Wang 2000; (e) Stanford and Fowler 2002.

different doses, as shown in table 1. A sample force-time recording and corresponding power spectrum from Wang (2000) are shown in Figure 3. Although obvious tremor was present in the response shown, not all responses in the same rat displayed tremor. This intermittency of tremor expression evoked by harmaline is well known among experimentalists but is often not reported, and the mechanism(s) for the intermittency is (are) currently unknown. Interpretation of data from various studies is often hampered by the lack of information on how the irregular emergence and subsidence of harmaline tremor is or is not incorporated into the data analysis strategy. We have chosen to average together all the available data from a session of forelimb responding to obtain power spectrum estimates of the amount of tremor induced by a drug. These two studies obtained congruent results in that harmaline significantly increased tremor, lengthened average response duration (the time between the onset of the dipper-raising force and the dipper-lowering force), and slowed lick rhythm (see table 1). The primary difference between the two sets of results was that 4.0 mg/kg harmaline reduced time on task (Wang 2000), but 0.5 and 1.0 mg/kg did not (Stanford and Fowler 1998). In the latter study the doses of harmaline were below the threshold for inducing frank, whole-body tremor. According to data presented by Wang and Fowler (2001), a dose of 4.0 mg/kg is near the threshold for evoking whole-body tremor and suppresses spontaneous locomotion. Thus, 4.0 mg/kg of harmaline interferes with the expression of both learned and unlearned behaviors.

The data collected from rats performing the press-while-licking task show that low doses of harmaline have multiple behavioral effects beyond evoking tremor. The harmaline-related slowing of lick rhythm is particularly interesting not only because it is a rhythmic behavior affected by harmaline, but also because harmaline-slowed lick rhythm is half the frequency of the evoked tremor in the forelimb (see the power spectra in Figure 3). This relationship between lick rhythm and tremor frequency was also seen for averaged power spectra presented in Stanford and Fowler (1998). These observations raise the possibility that harmaline-induced brain processes that produce tremor (i.e., over-excitation of the inferior olive) also have an entraining effect on lick rhythm.

In regard to the response-duration-lengthening effect of harmaline, it is not clear whether the response prolongation is the result of the slower and/or less efficient licking or the result of increased latency to respond to the sensory cues associated with the empty dipper. In a separate apparatus that measured force and rhythm of licking without a forelimb response requirement (the lick-force-rhythm task described below), Moss (2001) demonstrated that harmaline reduced lick peak force. This finding supports the interpretation that licking is probably less efficient after harmaline treatment compared to undrugged conditions; that is, the rat takes longer under harmaline to empty the dipper because it licks with a lower rhythm and less efficiently than in the non-drugged condition.

d. Physostigmine

The acetylcholinesterase inhibitor physostigmine is a tremorogenic agent, inducing whole-body tremor at doses near or above 0.2 mg/kg (Brimblecomb and Pinder 1972). At lower doses (0.05 and 0.1 mg/kg), the tremorogenic effect has also been documented through the use of the

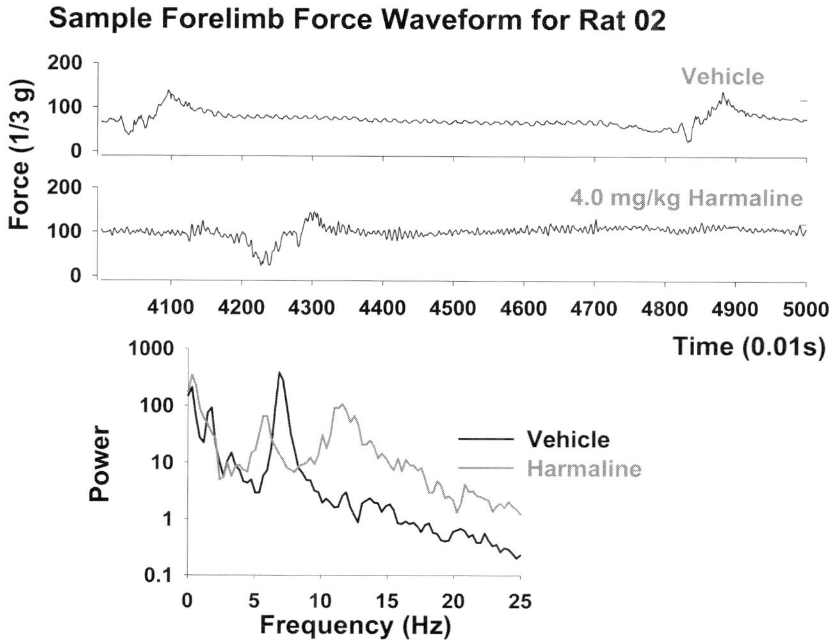

FIGURE 3 Sample data from a rat performing the press-while-licking task after a saline control injection or after treatment with the tremorogenic drug harmaline. Harmaline induced a 12 Hz tremor and shifted the lick rhythm from the saline value of 7 Hz to the lower 6 Hz rhythm. Data from Wang (2000).

press-while-licking task (Stanford and Fowler 1997; Wang 2000). Figure 4 shows sample force recordings for vehicle and 0.1 mg/kg physostigmine treatments and corresponding power spectra. The impression given by these two responses is supported by group data as summarized in table 1. In both studies, physostigmine decreased time on task and increased tremor power in the 10–25 Hz band. With respect to the other dependent variables listed in table 1, the results were not available uniformly for both studies, except for lick rhythm, which was observed to be unchanged or increased by physostigmine. No evidence supported a substantial reduction in lick rhythm by physostigmine as there was for harmaline.

e. Scopolamine

Mohanakumar et al. (1990) had suggested that tremor induced by physostigmine was primarily mediated by serotonergic mechanism partly because anticholinergic drugs did not block the observer-rated tremor in their experiments. To gain more information on this issue at physostigmine doses lower than those generally used to induce tremor, we investigated the ability of low doses of scopolamine to antagonize physostigmine's effects in the press-while-licking paradigm. As shown in table 1, scopolamine by itself produced force-lowering and tremor-reducing effects without influencing lick rhythm. Scopolamine and physostigmine in combination were found to be mutually antagonistic as measured by time on task, peak force, hold force, and tremor power (data not shown here; Stanford and Fowler 1997). Thus, forelimb tremor induced by low doses of physostigmine operates substantially via cholinergic mechanisms.

3. Unilateral Neurotoxic Lesions of the Substantia Nigra Pars Compacta

Skitek (1998) studied the effects of unilateral 6-OHDA injection into the substantia nigra pars compacta (SNpc) in rats trained in the press-while-licking task. Of the rats that sustained major depletions of dopamine (DA) in the affected striatum (depletions of DA > 75%), three sustained the depletion ipsilateral to the trained forelimb and six sustained the lesion contralateral to the trained forelimb. Assessment of performance began on the day after surgery and lasted for twenty-eight consecutive days. Both ipsilesional and contralesional groups showed significantly reduced time on task, and by the end of the assessment period the ipsilesional group had recovered to 50% of their pre-lesion baseline; however, the rats in the contralesional group showed no recovery and task engagement times remained near 5% of control value. The inability of the contralesional group to perform the task was an impediment to measuring the nature of their motor deficits; nevertheless, these rats occasionally made one or more responses of sufficient duration to analyze with the methods described

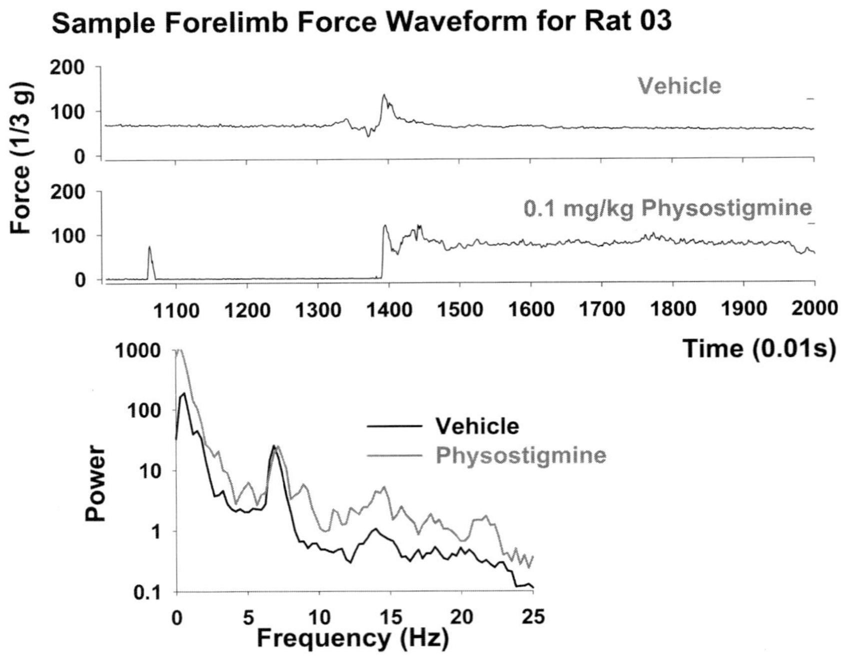

FIGURE 4 Force-time data from a representative rat responding in the press-while-licking task after saline or the indicated dose of the cholinesterase inhibitor physostigmine. The power spectrum of the force-time measurements in the lower set of axes shows that physostigmine increased power in the 10–25 Hz frequency band which is reflective of forelimb tremor. Power in the 7 Hz region, which is indicative of the lick rhythm, was slightly increased in this example. Data from Wang (2000).

above. Peak force increased in the ipsilesional group, but was not changed or decreased in rats of the contralesional group. In regard to force during the hold segment, the ipsilesional group exhibited increases, whereas the contralesional group had lower forces. While the ipsilesional group showed increased tremor as measured by the power in the 10–25 Hz frequency band, this increase may have been primarily the result of the higher forces in this group. The contralesional rats also displayed increased tremor, but the result was difficult to assess statistically because of the few individuals that made responses of a sufficient duration to analyze spectrally. Examination of the force recordings of the few, mostly shorter duration responses of the contralesional group suggested the presence of irregular high frequency tremor and marked forelimb dyscontrol. These initial observations suggest that the press-while-licking task may help characterize rodent models of Parkinson disease, but the inability of the rats with major DA depletion to perform the task suggests that procedural modifications will be necessary to make it practically applicable in the unilateral 6-OHDA Parkinson disease model.

D. Summary

The press-while-licking task provides several concurrent measures of motor performance in rats. In the same preparation one can quantify behavior expressed by the tongue and by a single designated forelimb. The method appears to be particularly well suited for characterizing tremor induced by low doses of tremorogenic compounds such as harmaline and physostigmine. In another chapter (Fowler et al. this volume) the task was used to distinguish successfully between the typical antipsychotic drug haloperidol and the atypical antipsychotic drug clozapine. Another potential use of this method by behavioral neuroscientists is in the context of electrophysiological recording of neuronal activity during ongoing behavior. The press-while-licking task has distinct motor-related conditions that the rat senses, such as the beginning or end of a response. These conditions could be used to construct peri-event histograms of neuronal units that are influenced by these specific motor activities.

III. DIRECT LICK-FORCE-RHYTHM MEASUREMENTS IN RATS AND MICE

A. Overview

Quantitative characterization of rodents' licking probably began with the observations of Stellar and Hill (1952), who arranged a low-current contact circuit for the electronic detection of individual tongue contacts as rats licked water from a sipper tube. They reported that lick rhythm, usually specified in Hz (cycles per second), was 5–7 Hz. Their emphasis was on the constancy of this lick rhythm despite large variations in thirst. Since this early observation, it has become clear that lick rhythm is not constant, but instead is influenced by many environmental and pharmacological factors (Fowler and Mortell 1992; Das and Fowler 1995; Weijnen 1998). For example, the distance between the rat's mouth and the liquid dispensed substantially and reliably affects lick rhythm (Weijnen 1998; Fowler and Wang 1998). Vrtunski and Wolin (1974) were the first to record the force of licking in rats and to show that the force of individual tongue contacts with the water dispenser exhibited measurable variability. Under some circumstances, lick peak force varies systematically during the intervals between successive water drop deliveries (Fowler and Mortell 1992). Although rat licking has been studied extensively in the context of research on variables that affect food and water intake (e.g., Davis et al. 2001), that will not be the focus here. Instead, the lick response will be viewed as a highly coordinated motor behavior that is responsive to pharmacological or neural manipulations. In addition, the extension of the lick-force-rhythm task to mice will also be described as a method capable of revealing genetic influences on behavior.

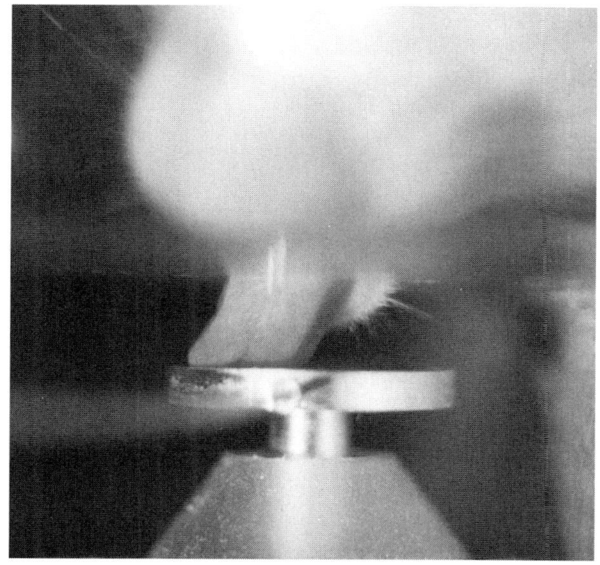

FIGURE 5 Photograph of a rat's tongue licking a force-sensing disk through which water was delivered by a peristaltic pump. For this photograph, the distance from the inside of the access port (where the rat's nose can be seen out of focus) to the top of the disk was 5 mm. The disk itself was 18 mm in diameter. Also see Figure 6.

B. Methods Summary

1. Apparatus and Procedures for Lick-Force-Rhythm Measurement

Figure 5 provides a close-up photograph of a rat licking. The spatial layout of the essential components of the apparatus is shown in Figure 6. Although the apparatus has been described in detail (Fowler and Mortell 1992; Fowler and Wang 1998), it may be useful here to point out key aspects of the apparatus design that contribute to reliable measurements. The lick sensor is a Model 31a Sensotec load cell with a 1 g aluminum disk attached to a sensing shaft. In the center of the 18 mm diameter disk is a 0.56 mm hole through which the liquid is pumped for access by the rat or mouse. The upper surface of the disk contains a 1 mm deep concavity so dispensed liquid will remain on the top of the disk. Liquid is delivered to the disk via small bore plastic tubing (i.e., the tubing pressure fits over a 24 gauge needle) attached to the output of a peristaltic pump. The pump is controlled by the computer program that continuously records the lick-force-time waveforms at 100 samples per second. As indicated in Figure 6, the load cell sits on top of a micrometer that precisely measures the distance between the rat's mouth and the lick disk. A rat accesses the liquid (e.g., water or milk) by placing its head inside a transparent plastic enclosure (see Figure 6) with a 12 mm diameter round hole in the bottom plane. The lick disk is centered below this access hole. The drip ring and drip deflector cone ensure that any excess liquid does not flow into the transducer, which is not waterproof. In practice, the risk of overflow is confined to calibration procedures; during data collection the probability of overflow is very low because the rat or mouse must strike the transducer with the tongue to activate liquid delivery.

Unlike methods based on rodents drinking from a sipper tube that is elevated several centimeters above the cage floor, the current technique places a sensor and liquid source near the plane of the floor that supports the rat or mouse. This arrangement was selected for four reasons. First, it is more natural in mammalian biology for the rodent to lift the liquid upward into the mouth than to drink from a raised tube; ingestive reflexes evolved before sipper tubes were invented. Second, our method eliminates variation in pressure at the lick orifice that is present in sipper tubes attached to containers that allow changes in water column height as the liquid is consumed within and between sessions. Third, attaching a force transducer to a conventional sipper tube substantially raises the mass of the tube-liquid-transducer ensemble, and thereby reduces the system's capacity to resolve peak force of tongue contacts. A fourth reason relates to the ease of calibrating the distance between the rat's mouth and the lick sensor; this is easily accomplished with a vertically mounted micrometer, but is mechanically problematic with the sipper tube arrangement.

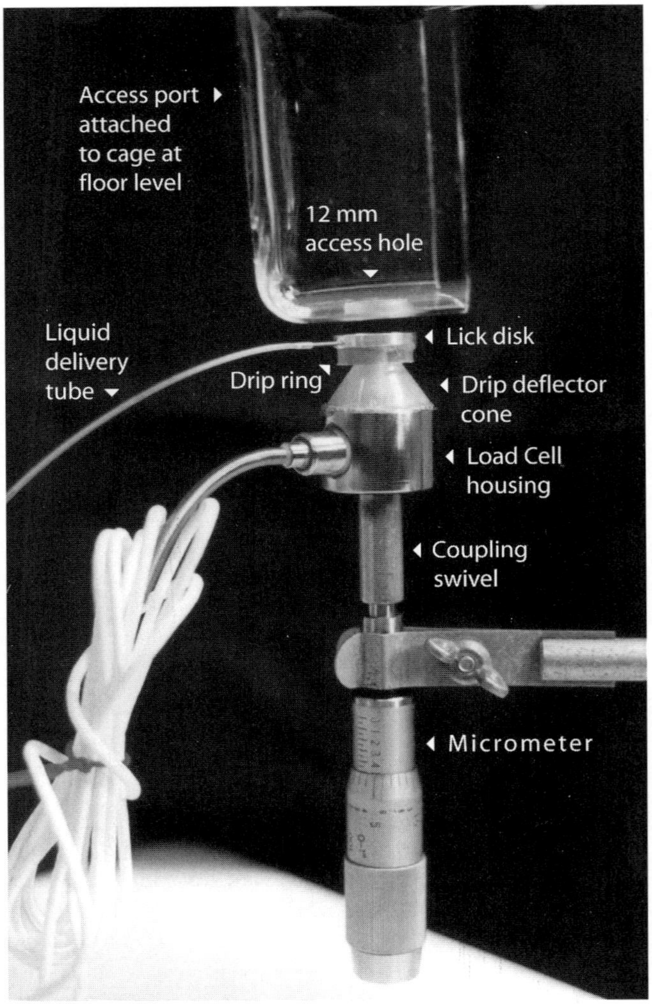

FIGURE 6 Photograph showing the parts of the sensor/positioner ensemble used to measure tongue dynamics in rats or mice. The liquid delivery tube was connected to a peristaltic pump controlled by a computer that was used to record the force-time data.

Thirsty male Sprague Dawley rats readily acquire the response of approaching and licking water from the disk. Most rats produce at least a few licks within the first two-minute session. Subsequent two-minute sessions are needed before rats lick continuously during the whole session. A two-minute session was purposefully chosen because it represents a time period too brief for appreciable satiety effects to occur, and at the same time it provides, in the undrugged rat, about 650 tongue contacts for analysis. In addition, a two-minute session was chosen because, in a period this brief, blood or brain levels of most drugs given intraperitoneally (ip), subcutaneously, or intramuscularly would be nearly constant during the session (i.e., elimination kinetics are relatively slow compared to two minutes). For rats a 2.0 gram weight force threshold was used to define the occurrence of a lick, and 24 licks were required to activate the pump that delivered 0.10 ml water over a period of 1.85 seconds. Resolution of the force measurements was to the nearest 0.2 g.

In one experiment that used Fischer 344 male rats (Stanford et al. 2003), other parameters were selected for a typical session because the Fischer rats took about twenty times longer to master the task than Sprague Dawley rats. Parameters for the rat experiments described here are listed in Table 2.

2. Dependent Variables and Data Analysis for Lick-Force-Rhythm

The entire two-minute session was recorded, split into eleven contiguous segments 10.24 seconds in duration, and spectrally analyzed. The resulting power spectra were averaged together for each rat, and the frequency or lick rhythm was read from these functions by a peak-finding computer program written by the authors. This method for measuring lick rhythm used the entire force recording, not just recordings above 2 g. As a consequence, lick rhythm could be estimated when tongue contacts fell below 2 g. Peak force was measured for every tongue contact above 2 g. The mean or median of these values served as the peak force variable for each rat for each session. The number of licks was simply a count of the tongue contacts 2 g or above during a two-minute session. It is important to note that lick rhythm and number of licks are non-redundant measures of the licking. Lick rhythm is the rhythmicity of behavior irrespective of the total number of licks; the rhythm can be estimated from as few as ten consecutive licks. An instance of this non-redundancy can be seen in table 5 for the drug pilocarpine at the 4.0 mg/kg dose; the number of licks declined significantly from a saline control level of 682 to 613, but lick rhythm increased significantly from a control level of 5.75 Hz to 6.11 Hz under the influence of pilocarpine 4.0 mg/kg.

C. Experimental Manipulations Affecting Tongue Dynamics in Rats

1. Behavioral Variables

a. Distance Manipulation

The effect of manipulating the distance between the inside surface of the access port and the lick disk is illustrated here by previously unreported data gathered in an experiment described by Fowler and Wang (1998). Prior to drug treatment, forty-eight male Sprague Dawley rats received twenty-one daily two-minute sessions with the distance set at 2 mm. The distance was then manipulated in the following sequence of daily sessions: 2 mm, 4 mm, 2 mm, 6 mm, 2 mm, 8 mm. All rats made substantial numbers of licks at the 2 mm, 4 mm, and 6 mm distances, but only half of the rats were able to make any licks above 2 g at 8 mm.

TABLE 2 Group Mean Effects of the Distance Manipulation on Three Parameters of Tongue Dynamics During Water Licking in 48 Male Sprague Dawley Rats

Variable	Descriptive statistic	Distance (mm)			Test statistic	
		2	4	6	F(2,94)	p
Rhythm (Hz)	Mean	5.74	5.61	5.44	37.671	<.001
	SEM	0.03	0.03	0.04		
Peak Force (g)	Mean	13.7	7.4	4.3	462.597	<.001
	SEM	0.4	0.2	0.1		
Number of Licks	Mean	641.4	558.6	277.7	271.053	<.001
	SEM	6.4	10.6	20.4		

TABLE 3 Practice Effects for 12 Male Sprague Dawley Rats Given Daily 2-min Sessions in the Lick-Force-Rhythm Task for 105 Consecutive Days. Data Shown Are for the Average Performance for the First and Fifteenth Weeks

Variable	Descriptive statistic	Week 1	Week 15	Paired t-test	p_t	Pearson correlation	p_r
Rhythm (Hz)	Mean	5.71	5.77	1.510	NS*	0.835	<0.001
	SEM	0.06	0.07				
Peak Force (g)	Mean	13.6	10.7	−5.117	<0.001	0.796	<0.001
	SEM	0.9	0.9				
Number of Licks	Mean	548.8	673.3	5.709	<0.001	0.535	NS
	SEM	18.2	11.5				

*NS means not significant.

Thus, the data for 2 mm, 4 mm, and 6 mm were used in the statistical analysis, which consisted of one-way repeated measures analyses of variance performed separately for lick rhythm, lick force, and number of licks. These data are shown in table 2. Each variable exhibited a significant decrease as a function of increased distance. Therefore, ensuring precise experimental control of lick distance is essential for obtaining reproducible results with these methods of quantitating tongue dynamics.

b. Practice Effects

How stable are these measures across time in the same group of rats? To address this question, data were taken from a control group (n = 12) referred to in Fowler and Wang (1998). For these data "Week 1" was the first week of lick measurement at 2 mm after the initial three weeks of baseline training. "Week 15" was the performance for the last week of 105 consecutive days of two-minute lick sessions. Between Week 1 and Week 15 the rats received acute doses of scopolamine, trihexyphenidyl, ritanserin, or quipazine in the doses shown for these drugs in table 5. Week 15 and the two days prior were drug free. Data for the practice effects are shown in table 3. Lick rhythm remained stable across this fifteen-week period, and the individual differences in lick rhythm also were stable as reflected by the significant positive correlation between Week 1 and Week 15 rhythms. However, both mean peak force and number of licks in two minutes exhibited significant practice-related changes. Over time, peak force decreased significantly while number of licks increased significantly (see table 3). Mean peak force in Week 1 was significantly correlated with this measure in Week 15, reflecting relatively enduring individual differences in peak force. In contrast, number of licks in Week 1 was not significantly predictive of number of licks in Week 15. Overall, significant practice effects were apparent for peak force and number of licks, but not for lick rhythm. Individual differences across the practice interval were most reproducible for lick rhythm and least reproducible for number of licks.

c. Age Effects

Figure 7 shows representative force recordings from one young (six months) and one old (twenty-four months) male Fischer 344 rat (Stanford et al. 2003). The lower rhythm of

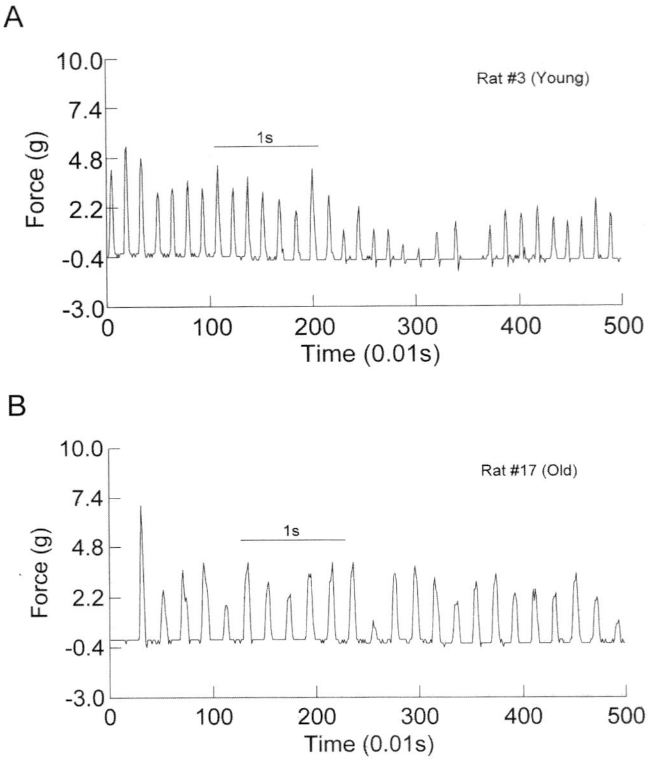

FIGURE 7 Sample force-time waveforms from a young (~6 mo.) and an old (about 24 mo.) male Fischer 344 rat. The lick rhythm of the older rat (Panel B) was substantially slower than the rhythm of the younger rat (Panel A). Reprinted from Stanford et al. (2003).

the older rat is apparent. On a group-mean basis (n = 12 young and n = 12 old rats), the old rats had significantly lower lick rhythm than the young rats (see the baseline data in table 5). This lower lick rhythm in old rats was accompanied by higher peak force and more licks in a six-minute period compared to the younger rats. The lick peak force of the Fischer 344 rats was dramatically lower than the same measure for Sprague Dawley rats. As shown in table 4, session length and force threshold for registering a lick were less stringent than the same parameters for the Sprague Dawley rats because the Fischer 344 rats learned and performed the licking less avidly than the Sprague Dawley rats despite closely comparable motivational and measurement conditions for both rat strains. These data suggest that the lick-force-rhythm methods described here will be informative in biobehavioral studies of aging.

2. Pharmacological Manipulations

The drugs listed in tables 4 and 5 were selected for study as reference drugs in experiments where antipsychotic drugs were the agents of primary interest (see Chapter M3, this volume). Antipsychotic drugs are well known to have motor effects in human patients (e.g., acute dystonia, neuroleptic-induced Parkinsonism, and tardive dyskinesia; e.g., Tarsy 1989). Yet the low-dose, laboratory modeling of these clinical symptoms has been problematic. Given that the side effects of antipsychotic drugs used in the clinical setting frequently involve orolingual organs, we have proposed that high-precision measurement of orolingual function in rats may provide insights into the side effect liability of antipsychotic drugs during preclinical testing (e.g., Fowler and Wang 1998). As part of this effort, we characterized the behavioral effects of a number of reference drugs, and these drugs are the focus of this section. Most of these reference drugs were selected on the basis of documented effects on the neurotransmitter receptors that are shared by antipsychotic drugs with a broad spectrum of receptor affinities, such as clozapine (Leysen et al. 1993; Schotte et al. 1996). Harmaline was tested in the lick-force-rhythm paradigm because of its lick-rhythm-slowing effect at low doses observed in the press-while-licking task (Stanford and Fowler 1998). The effects of ibogaine were assessed because of its structural and functional similarity to harmaline (e.g., O'Hearn and Molliver 1993; Deecher et al. 1992).

a. Dopaminergic Agonists

To date we have examined the effects on lick dynamics of two indirect-acting dopamine agonists, amphetamine and nomifensine. Both drugs are believed to act at the dopamine transporter to block the reuptake of dopamine, thereby raising the extracellular concentration of dopamine. Amphetamine similarly affects norepinephrine and serotonin neurotransmission, while nomifensine is much less active in influencing reuptake in serotonin systems. As shown in table 5, amphetamine dose had a biphasic effect on number of licks in two minutes, where 0.5 mg/kg increased number of licks and 2.0 mg/kg decreased this measure. However, across the dose range sampled (generally below the focused stereotypy-inducing dose in an acute dosing regimen) neither force nor rhythm was significantly affected by amphetamine. The results for nomifensine (see table 5, bottom two rows) were similar to those of amphetamine in that number of licks was decreased by the 3.0 mg/kg in dose both the young and old Fischer 344 rats, while neither peak force nor rhythm was affected. In light of the limited number of doses used in the nomafensine study (Stanford et al. 2003), the question of whether nomifensine can induce an increase in number of licks, as amphetamine did, must await further experimentation. Overall, these data, though scant, suggest that indirect-acting dopamine agonists do not strongly modulate peak force or rhythm of licking.

b. Cholinergic Agonists and Antagonists

Pilocarpine is a direct-acting muscarinic cholinergic agonist that can induce salivation, pupillary constriction, and sweating at relatively low doses, with seizures and death

TABLE 4 Summary of Experimental Conditions and Drugs Studied for Their Effects on Tongue Dynamics in Rats. The Ordering of the Citations and Drugs Studied Is the Same as in the Subsequent Table 5, which Lists Selected Results from These Experiments

Citation[1]	Rat type[2]	N	Force threshold (g)[3]	Licks/ pump cycle	Cycle duration (s)	Volume delivered (ml)	Distance (mm)	Session time (min)	Drug or treatment
(a)	MSD	21	2	24	1.85	0.10	2	2	Amphetamine
(a)	MSD	21	2	24	1.85	0.10	2	2	Ketanserin
(b)	MSD	12	2	24	1.85	0.10	2	2	Ritanserin
(a)	MSD	21	2	24	1.85	0.10	2	2	Morphine
(a)	MSD	21	2	24	1.85	0.10	2	2	Physostigmine
(a)	MSD	21	2	24	1.85	0.10	2	2	Pilocarpine
(a)	MSD	21	2	24	1.85	0.10	2	2	Prazosin
(b)	MSD	12	2	24	1.85	0.10	2	2	Quipazine
(b)	MSD	12	2	24	1.85	0.10	2	2	Scopolamine
(b)	MSD	12	2	24	1.85	0.10	2	2	Trihexyphenidyl
(c)	MSD	12 & 10	2	12	1.0	0.06	2	2	Unilateral SNpc[4] 6-OHDA[5]
(d)	MSD	12	2	24	1.85	0.10	2	2	Harmaline
(d)	MSD	12	2	24	1.85	0.10	2	2	Ibogaine
(e)	MSD	13	2	24	1.85	0.10	2	2	3-AP[6]
(d)	MSD	12 & 24	2	24	1.85	0.10	2	2	3-AP+ Harmaline+ Nicotinamide
(f)	MF344 young	12	1	12	0.9	0.05	2	6	Nomafensine
(f)	MF344 old	12	1	12	0.9	0.05	2	6	Nomafensine

Notes: 1. key to citations: (a) Fowler et al. 1997; (b) Fowler and Wang 1998; (c) Skitek et al. 1999; (d) Moss 2001; (e) Moss et al. 2001; (f) Stanford et al. 2003.

2. MSD means male Sprague Dawley 3–6 months old; MF344 means male Fischer 344.

3. Force threshold refers to the force on the lick disk required to advance the count for water delivery.

4. SNpc means substantia pars compacta.

5. 6-OHDA is 6-hydroxydopamine, a neurotoxin for dopamine and norepinephrine neurons.

6. 3-AP means 3-acetylpyridine, a neurotoxin that preferentially destroys neurons in the inferior olive.

occurring at higher doses. As shown in table 5, low doses of pilocarpine significantly affected tongue dynamics. At 1.0 mg/kg, pilocarpine increased number of licks, reduced peak force, and increased lick rhythm. Although the 4.0 mg/kg dose significantly reduced number of licks, it further decreased peak force, and further increased rhythm. The acetylcholinesterase inhibitor physostigmine significantly reduced number of licks and peak force, but it did not affect lick rhythm. The muscarinic antagonists scopolamine and trihexyphenidyl interfered with licking by decreasing the number of licks and reducing the peak force measure of performance. Both muscarinic antagonists tended to increase the lick rhythm, with this effect being statistically significant, but small, for trihexyphenidyl. It is interesting that among the drugs (aside from the neurotoxins 3-AP and 6-OHDA) listed in table 5, the muscarinic cholinergic agonists *and* antagonists were the only ones to increase lick rhythm. Given that agonists and antagonists produced similar patterns of effects on lick dynamics, no straightforward interpretation of these results is apparent at this time. However, this information allows one to rule out cholinergic factors by themselves in cases where drugs with multiple pharmacological effects produce rhythm slowing (see Chapter M3, this volume).

c. *Noradrenergic Drugs*

Prazosin is a selective α_1 noradrenergic antagonist with both peripheral and central effects. This drug was selected for study as a reference drug for two reasons. First, atypical antipsychotic drugs, such as clozapine, have a substantial α_1 antagonist effect (Leysen et al. 1993). Second, norepinephrine acts in an excitatory fashion at α_1 sites on hypoglossal motor neurons (Parkis et al. 1995; Volgin et al. 2001).

Thus, antagonism of α_1 receptors would be expected to alter tongue dynamics as well as other physiological processes modulated by these receptors. As shown in table 5, prazosin substantially and significantly reduced number of licks, peak force, and rhythm.

TABLE 5 Selected Results for the Drugs and Conditions Listed in Table 4. The Drug Data Presented Are for One or Two Doses of Each Drug that Produced Significant Effects on Number of Licks Without Abolishing the Rhythmic Quality of Licking

Drug and citation[1]	Doses (mg/kg)	Vehicle or baseline: N licks	Vehicle or baseline: Peak force (g)	Vehicle or baseline: Rhythm (Hz)	Data for the indicated dose: Dose[2] (m/kg)	Data for the indicated dose: N licks	Data for the indicated dose: Peak force (g)	Data for the indicated dose: Rhythm (Hz)
Amphetamine (a)	0.25, 0.5, 1, 2	692	14.6	5.78	0.5	700*[3]>	15.0	5.82
		692	14.6	5.78	2.0	660*<	14.9	5.73
Ketanserin (a)	1, 2, 4, 8	690	14.4	5.78	8.0	624*<	9.4*<	5.45*<
Ritanserin (b)	0.5, 1, 2, 4	641	10.7	5.75	4.0	610*<	9.0*<	5.60*<
Morphine (a)	1, 2, 4, 8	673	14.3	5.78	8.0	483*<	12.1*<	5.31*<
Physostigmine (a)	0.025, 0.05, 0.1, 0.2	684	13.9	5.79	0.20	499*<	10.9*<	5.80
Pilocarpine (a)	0.5, 1, 2, 4	682	14.3	5.75	1.0	715*>	13.0*<	6.03*>
		682	14.3	5.75	4.0	613*<	8.4*<	6.11*>
Prazosin (a)	1, 2, 4, 8	691	14.6	5.81	8.0	324*<	5.0*<	4.87*<
Quipazine (b)	0.5, 1, 2, 4	662	11.5	5.75	2.0	655	13.7*>	5.78
Scopolamine (b)	0.05, 0.1, 0.2	660	12.8	5.75	0.10	554*<	9.0*<	5.96
Trihexyphenidyl (b)	0.15, 0.3, 1.0	659	11.9	5.73	1.0	565*<	10.1	5.84*>
6-OHDA Unilateral Lesion	Mean dopamine depletion was 92.4%	574	13.2	5.67	8 μg in 4 μl	468*<	7.0*<	5.39*<
Harmaline (d)	0.5, 1, 2, 4	630	11.7	5.65	2.0	390*<	9.3*<	4.80*<
Ibogaine (d)	1.5, 3, 6	590	11.4	5.55	6.0	410*<	9.2*<	4.85*<
3-AP (e)	12.5, 25, 50	600	11.0	5.70	50.0	440*<	7.5*<	5.55
3-AP+ Harmaline+ Nicotinamide (d)[4]	3-AP: 75 harmaline: 15 Nicotin amire: 300	540	11.6	5.50	—	370*<	8.1*<	6.10*>
Young Rats Nomafensine (f)	1, 3	450	2.7	6.20	3.0	250*<	2.3	5.90
Old Rats Nomafensine (f)	1, 3	650	3.3	5.25	3.0	425*<	2.9	5.30

Notes: 1. key to citations: (a) Fowler et al. 1997; (b) Fowler and Wang 1999; (c) Skitek et al. 1999; (d) Moss 2001; (e) Moss et al. 2001; (f) Stanford et al. 2003.

2. The listing of more than one dose per drug indicates a biphasic effect for some of the measures of tongue dynamics.

3. *significant ($p < 0.05$) dose effect and/or different from control; >,< represent increase or decrease, respectively.

4. In this experiment rats that survived the neurotoxic treatment of the inferior olive were treated with harmaline (2.0 mg/kg), and these rats exhibited the expected rhythm slowing seen in unlesioned rats.

d. Serotonergic Agonists and Antagonists

Quipazine is a broad-spectrum serotonin receptor agonist (e.g., Sanchez and Arnt 2000). In the lick-force-rhythm paradigm, quipazine significantly elevated peak force of licking, but it did not affect number of licks or lick rhythm (see table 5). Ritanserin and ketanserin are $5\text{-HT}_{2a/c}$ antagonists with similar affinities for the 5-HT_{2a} receptor (about 3 nanomolar) but ketanserin has about fifty-fold less affinity for the 5-HT_{2c} site than ritanserin. Both ketanserin and ritanserin significantly decreased lick force and lick rhythm as well as number of licks (see table 5). Recent data (Zhan et al. 2002) suggest that 5-HT_{2a} receptors are the predominant 5-HT receptor subtype on hypoglossal motor neurons. Therefore, behavioral results for the serotonin-modulating drugs shown in table 5 are consistent with these observations at the cellular level. Also consistent with these observations is the report by Berry and Hayward (2003) showing that the rat genioglossus (tongue protrusor) muscle exhibits increased electromyographic activity in response to the intravenous administration of the serotonin precursor 5-hydroxytryptophan.

e. Opiates

We assessed the effects of morphine in the lick-force-rhythm paradigm because we suspected that the well-known respiratory depressive effect of mu-receptor agonists would manifest itself through the anatomical and physiological linkage between brainstem respiratory centers and the motor neurons of the hypoglossal nucleus (Li et al. 2003; Greer et al. 1995). Additional evidence (e.g., Back and Gorenstein 1994) also suggests that mu opioid receptors are located on hypoglossal motor neurons. Thus, it was expected that morphine would significantly affect lick dynamics. As shown in table 5 this expectation was confirmed. Number of licks, peak force, and rhythm were all significantly reduced by morphine with the effects becoming observable at 4.0 mg/kg (data for the 4.0 mg/kg dose not shown in table 5).

f. Tremorogenic Agents

As a consequence of finding that low doses of harmaline decreased lick rhythm as measured in the press-while-licking task (Stanford and Fowler 1998; and replicated by Wang 2000), this drug was also studied in the lick-force-rhythm task to rule out the possibility that the expression of harmaline-induced lick-rhythm slowing was somehow dependent upon concurrent tongue and fore limb usage. For the licking-only task, the data shown in table 5 indicate that harmaline slowed lick rhythm, reduced peak force, and reduced number of licks at doses below the threshold for producing whole-body tremor (Moss 2001). Thus, the slowing of lick rhythm occurred in experimental contexts with and without skilled use of a forelimb, indicating that harmaline-related rhythm slowing does not depend upon concurrent fore limb activation. It should be recalled that the baseline lick rhythm is higher in the press-while-licking task than in the lick-force-rhythm task (~6.7 Hz compared to ~5.7 Hz, respectively). The lower rhythm in the lick-force-rhythm task is the result of the 2 mm distance between the access orifice and the lick disk compared to no distance constraint in the press-while-licking task. Data presented by Skitek et al. (1999) suggested that even with the 2 mm distance, rats begin a session by licking at about 7 Hz and adjust to the lower 5.7 Hz rhythm within five or six licks. Regardless of the experimental context, harmaline, in the 2.0 to 4.0 mg/kg dose range, slowed lick rhythm by about 1 Hz. Like harmaline, ibogaine decreased number of licks, decreased peak force, and slowed lick rhythm (Moss 2001). The potency of ibogaine in the lick-force-rhythm test was about half that of harmaline, and the log dose-effect functions for lick rhythm were parallel, suggesting that both drugs were possibly operating through the same pharmacological mechanisms (Moss 2001).

3. Neurotoxic Manipulations

a. 6-OHDA Unilaterally in the SNpc

The lick-force-rhythm task was used to assess the effects of unilateral 6-OHDA injected into the SNpc (Skitek et al. 1999). Destruction of dopamine cell bodies by unilateral injection of 6-OHDA is perhaps the world's most popular rodent model of Parkinson disease, where the severity of basal ganglia dysfunction is measured by the amount and/or direction of compulsive locomotor rotation induced by amphetamine or apomorphine (originally developed by Ungerstedt and Arbuthnott 1970). In the lick-force-rhythm task, rats with substantial dopamine depletion on the lesioned side exhibited significant impairments in the number of licks, peak force, and lick rhythm compared to unlesioned controls (see table 5). Rats that sustained modest dopamine depletion (mean of 20.1%) were not impaired. These results show that Parkinson-like motor symptoms were apparent in non-locomotor systems in rats and are consistent with the orolingual impairments observed in human Parkinson disease patients.

b. 3-Acetylpyridine

The neurotoxin 3-acetylpyridine (3AP) preferentially targets the inferior olive (IO) neurons (the source of the climbing fiber inputs to the Purkinje cells of the cerebellum) and tends to spare neurons in other brain regions (Balaban 1985; Welsh 2002). Lesioning the IO with 3AP is done in two different ways. The simplest method is to use ip injections of 3AP in doses that produce partial lethality in a group of recipient rats (e.g., Moss et al. 2001). A second method (Llinas et al. 1975) involves administering 3AP, harmaline, and nicotinamide sequentially (i.e., 3AP followed by harmaline 3 hours later and nicotinamide following harmaline by 1.5 hours). The rationale underlying the use of the combination of three drugs is that 3AP's toxic effects are exacerbated selectively in the IO because of harmaline's excitatory selectivity for IO neurons, while the nicotinamide is an antagonist of 3AP and terminates the toxin's effects before non-IO neurons are fatally damaged. Moss (2001) compared both methods and reported 54% lethality with the single drug method (3AP alone at 50 mg/kg) and 33% lethality with the three-drug method (3AP at 75 mg/kg). Survivors of both methods exhibited reductions in numbers of licks and peak force, *but not significant rhythm slowing*. One difference appeared between the two methods: the three-drug method significantly increased lick rhythm compared to pre-treatment conditions in the same rats. This speeding of lick rhythm was unexpected, and it suggests that the IO may have been exerting (directly or indirectly) modulatory control over another pertinent brainstem locus, possibly the hypoglossal nucleus. Both lesioning methods left intact the basic rhythmicity of licking behavior. Therefore, it appears that the IO is not the site of the oscillator that produces the lick rhythm. This conclusion is conditional upon the assumption that the 3AP lesioning of the IO was effectively complete. Recent evidence using postmortem immunostaining targeting neuron-specific enolase showed that the three-drug method resulted in 96% destruction of the IO neurons with no detectable damage to neurons in other nuclei (Welsh 2002). Thus, the assumption that the three-drug 3AP method is selective for IO neurons appears sound. In the rats with heavy loss of IO neurons, harmaline was observed to slow lick rhythm (Moss 2001). This observation further supports the conclusion that the IO is not the primary origin of the oscillatory control of the tongue.

c. Summary of Pharmacological Effects on Lick Dynamics

Although the foregoing data on the pharmacology of lick dynamics in rats demonstrated robust effects of drugs on the three measured parameters (number of licks in two minutes, peak force, and lick rhythm) the pattern of results did not suggest selectivity. Apparently, many different neurotransmitters and their receptors participate in the control of rat tongue dynamics, probably both directly and indirectly at many levels of the neuraxis. The data show that the three measures emphasized here each reflect a different dimension of the control of tongue dynamics; instances can be cited where number of licks was increased but neither force nor rhythm was changed (i.e., amphetamine). Rhythm can increase while force is decreased (pilocarpine, scopolamine, trihexyphenidyl). For many of the drugs, a decrease in one measure was accompanied by a decrease in the other two measures (i.e., ketanserin, ritanserin, morphine, prazosin, 6-OHDA lesion, harmaline, and ibogaine). The serotonin agonist quipazine significantly increased peak force without affecting number of licks or lick rhythm. If the drug effects are viewed in terms of size of effect, instead of statistical significance per se, then the drugs that had the largest slowing effect on lick rhythm were prazosin, harmaline, and ibogaine. These drugs have cerebellar involvement for their expression (prazosin: Parfitt et al. 1988; harmaline and ibogaine: O'Hearn and Molliver 1993, 1997), and modulation of cerebellar circuitry may play a role in the strong rhythm-slowing effect of these three drugs. In addition, Parkis et al. (1995) have shown that alpha-1 noradrenergic receptors (the receptors that prazosin blocks) are importantly involved in the excitability of hypoglossal motor neurons. The rhythm-slowing exhibited by prazosin is thus consistent with a direct action on the motor neurons that drive the tongue.

D. Tongue Dynamics in Mice

With the increasing availability of methods to manipulate CNS-related mouse genes, scientists have shown a corresponding growing interest in the behavioral consequences of such gene manipulations (Crawley 2000). In mice, the expression of behavioral consequences of experimental manipulations always has a motor component. Therefore, our laboratory has begun the process of adapting our rat-based tongue dynamics measurement procedures to mice (Wang and Fowler 1999; Fowler et al. 2002a, b) in order to contribute to this rapidly expanding field (Table 6).

TABLE 6 Comparison of Group Mean Parameters of Tongue Dynamics in Inbred and Genetically Altered Mice

Citation	Mouse type	Number of mice	Number of licks	Peak force (g)	Rhythm (Hz)	Age at testing (wk)	Supplier
(a)[1]	CD-1	24	760 ± 25	3.5 ± 0.10	8.30 ± 0.10	12	CRL
(a)	BALB/c	16	560 ± 20	2.0 ± 0.06	8.50 ± 0.10	12	JAX[4]
(a)	C57BL/6	16	350 ± 15[2]	1.8 ± 0.04[3]	7.30 ± 0.10[2]	12	JAX
(b)	Wt on C57BL/6 background	12	431 ± 29	1.9 ± 0.12	7.49 ± 0.17	12	Dr. Wright's Laboratory
(b)	NT3 over-expression	12	399 ± 23	1.6 ± 0.06[5]	7.36 ± 0.10	12	Dr. Wright's Laboratory
(c)	Wt control for D2 knockout[6]	6	475 ± 21	2.0 ± 0.04	6.87 ± 0.16	20	JAX
(c)	+/– heterozygous D2 knockout	6	431 ± 71	1.7 ± 0.06	6.79 ± 0.21	23	JAX
(c)	–/– homozygous D2 knockout	6	485 ± 62	2.0 ± 0.08	6.38 ± 0.14	23	JAX
(c)	129Sv	6	671 ± 30	1.4 ± 0.03	8.06 ± 0.14	16	JAX
(c)	C3H	6	541 ± 21	1.7 ± 0.07	7.79 ± 0.26	16	JAX
(c)	C57BL/6	6	500 ± 45	2.1 ± 0.22	7.05 ± 0.14	16	JAX

Notes: 1. key to citations: (a) Fowler and Wang 1999; (b) Fowler et al. 2002a; (c) Fowler et al. 2002b.
2. C57BL/6 significantly different from CD-1 and BALB/c.
3. C57BL/6 significantly different from CD-1.
4. JAX means Jackson Laboratories.
5. NT3 over-expressing mouse significantly different from Wt control.
6. The Wt controls for the D2 knockout mouse experiments were congenic at ten generations on the C57BL/6 background.

The CD-1 mouse is an outbred stock derived from Swiss-Webster laboratory mice; they are supplied by Charles River Laboratories. The BALB/c and C57BL/6 mice are commonly used inbred strains supplied by Jackson Laboratories. The C57BL/6 mouse is of special interest because it frequently serves as the background strain for the expression of knocked out or added genes, and this mouse was the first to have its genome sequenced (Waterson et al. 2002). Data on tongue dynamics in these three types of male mice are shown in Figure 8. Statistical analyses supported the graphic differences depicted in figure 8; that is, all but one of the pair-wise group comparisons were significant by the Tukey HSD test. The exception was the lack of a rhythm difference between the CD-1 and BALB/c mice. Moreover, the large difference (non-overlapping sample distributions) between the BALB/c and C57BL/6 mice in lick rhythm suggests the possibility of potentially identifying the allelic differences responsible for this difference in the control of lick rhythm.

In two additional studies that used the C57BL/6 mouse as a background strain or as a pure inbred control, we found the C57BL/6 mouse to have a lick rhythm near 7.0 Hz (Fowler et al. 2002a, b). Mice that over-express neurotrophin-3 (Wright et al. 1997) had significantly lower tongue force than controls, but lick rhythm was not affected by this genetic manipulation (Fowler et al. 2002a). In a separate study (Fowler et al. 2002b), mice lacking the dopamine D2 receptor had a lick rhythm of 6.38 Hz compared to wild-type controls that had a rhythm of 6.87 Hz. However, this difference was not statistically significant, owing to the relatively small sample size (n = 6 in each of the two groups); therefore, the experiment should be repeated with a somewhat larger group size. Thus, it is probably premature to reach any conclusion regarding the role of the D2 receptor in the modulation of lick rhythm. In the study of the D2 knock-out mice, three pure inbred strains were also studied. These were 129x1/SvJ, C3H/HeJ, and C57BL/6J mice that produced group mean (n = 6) lick rhythms of 8.06 Hz, 7.79 Hz, and 7.05 Hz, respectively (table 6). The C57BL/6 mice showed lower rhythms than the 129x1/Sv and C3H/HeJ mice, and the rhythm for the C57BL/6J mice was consistent with the data shown for this strain in Figure 8.

Overall, these data on mice show that the lick-force-rhythm paradigm is a useful method for characterizing behavioral/functional differences among genetically defined mice. Moreover, the data in Figure 8 show that each of the three parameters of tongue dynamics provides non-redundant information about behavioral performance. For example, the BALB/c and CD-1 mice have similar rhythms but different numbers of licks in two minutes. Another instance of this non-redundancy is the closely similar peak forces of the BALB/c and C57BL/6 mice while these two strains have markedly different lick rhythms.

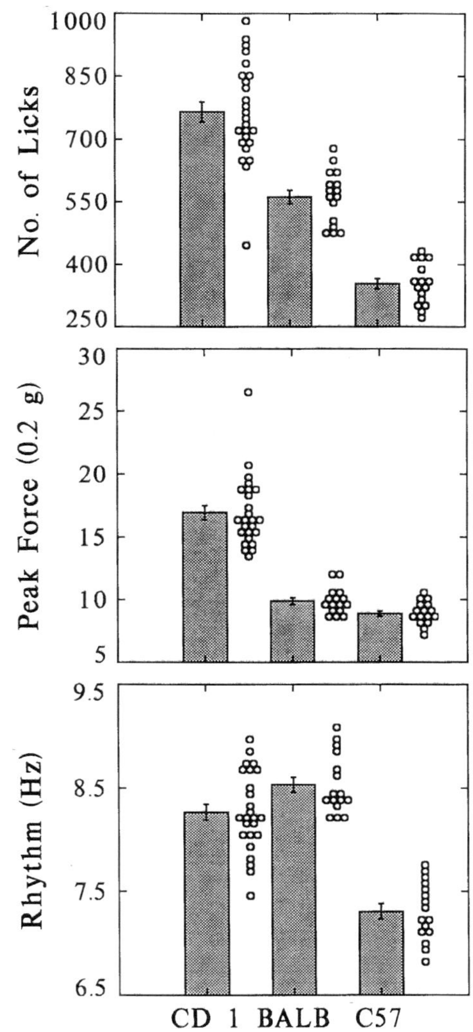

FIGURE 8 Group means (bars with +/− 1 SEM) and individual subject data (open circles) for number of licks, peak force, and rhythm for the indicated three types of mice. The liquid dispensed through the force-sensing disk was sweetened condensed milk diluted with tap water (two parts water to one part milk product). The lick rhythms of BALB/c and C57BL/6 mice appear to form distinctly different populations, suggesting that the lick rhythm is attributable to genetic differences between these two inbred strains of mice. Reprinted from Wang and Fowler (1999).

E. Summary

Of particular interest in the foregoing results is the general finding that lick rhythm is not constant in either rats or mice. Instead, lick rhythm can be influenced in a graded fashion by behavioral, pharmacological, neurotoxic, and genetic variables. In addition, the three measures of tongue dynamics (i.e., number of licks, peak force, and rhythm) can vary independently of one another depending on the type of the experimental manipulation. While the pharmacological manipulations showed that drugs from several different classes substantially affect tongue dynamics, the studies with the neurotoxin 3-AP suggested that the origin of the lick rhythm is probably not in the IO. Stanford et al. (2003) showed that lick rhythm slows with age in Fischer 344 rats. Thus, the lick-force-rhythm measurement methods described here should be useful in analyses aimed at understanding the decline in motor systems associated with aging. Finally, the finding that C57BL/6 mice have a distinctly lower lick rhythm than BALB/c and CD-1 mice shows that genetic influences on motor behavior can be quantified with the methods presented here, and that these methods should be useful in phenotyping knock-out and transgenic mice.

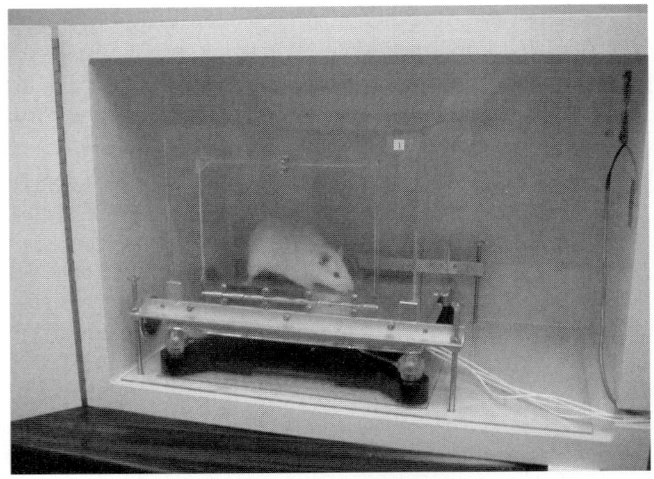

FIGURE 9 Male Sprague Dawley rat in a force-plate actometer. The surface on which the rat is standing is supported by four force transducers, one at each of the four corners of the force plate. Two of the force transducer housings can be seen as the cylindrically shaped objects below and to the right and left of the hinged chamber door. The cage confining the rat to the plate is elevated 2 mm above the force-sensing plate so that the rat is the only mass on the plate. When combined with suitable software, the force-plate actometer allows for the determination of the rat's center of force at any instant, and at the same time provides a continuous recording of the variations in vertical force caused by the rat's movements. Extensive details on this instrument are given in a recent paper (Fowler et al. 2001).

IV. THE FORCE PLATE ACTOMETER AS A METHOD TO MEASURE MOTOR BEHAVIOR IN RATS AND MICE

A. Overview

Whereas the foregoing sections on forelimb tremor and lick-force-rhythm described methods and results aimed at high precision characterization of movements of specific body parts, this section describes our approach to quantifying motor behavior of the whole body. Contemporary suppliers of behavioral instrumentation provide a range of options for recording and quantifying whole body movements. Photobeam actometers and video tracking systems are especially popular for measuring locomotor activity of rodents. However, these approaches have limited spatial and temporal resolution. For example, photobeam actometers sense the location of a rodent by recording the position of the infrared emitter-detector pairs that are blocked by the animal's body at any given time. In the higher resolution systems these sensors are spaced about 2.5 cm apart. This lack of spatial resolution results in the inability of these systems to quantify small-amplitude movements such as tremor or focused stereotypies induced by amphetamine. While video tracking systems offer generally higher spatial resolution than the photobeam systems, the video-based approaches, as most commonly implemented, are limited to 30 frames/s in temporal resolution. The low sampling rate makes the systems inadequate for recording tremor or focused stereotypies (a state of little or no locomotion accompanied by rhythmic head movements), and the 30 Hz sampling rate is not convenient for synchronizing the behavioral data with electrophysiological recording instruments that one may want to use to identify physiological correlates of behavior, such as neuronal activity. In order to bypass these and other limitations of the light-based systems, we have developed a new approach to measuring whole-body behavior in rodents: the force-plate actometer (Fowler et al. 2001). With this system an animal's movements are sensed by four force transducers that support a low-mass, rigid floor to which a test subject is confined by a transparent chamber (see Figure 9). The force-plate actometer has allowed us to quantify successfully a wide range of movement characteristics of rats and mice. These include total locomotor activity (e.g., Fowler et al. 2001, 2002a, b), spatial pattern of locomotion (Fowler et al. 2003), gait disturbances (Stanford et al. 2003), rotation around the center of the floor (Fowler et al. 2001), tremor (Wang and Fowler 2001), amphetamine-induced focused stereotypies (Fowler et al. 2003), wall rears (Fowler et al. 2002b), and ataxia (Zarcone et al. 2003). Presented below are illustrative data on focused stereotypies in rats, whole-body tremor in rats and mice, and ethanol-induced ataxia in mice.

B. Methods Summary

1. Apparatus

The force-plate apparatus for rodents has been described thoroughly elsewhere (Fowler et al. 2001). The force plate embodies the physical principle of moments applied to forces in a plane. This principle can be illustrated by considering one dimension and then two dimensions. Think of a rigid, horizontal rod supported by two force transducers, one at each end of the rod. Imagine that the apparatus is viewed from the side and that the transducer on the left is labeled "L" and the one on the right is labeled "R." The two force transducers can be calibrated to read zero force thereby canceling out the weight of the rod itself. If a mouse is placed on the mid-point of the horizontal rod, then each transducer will bear exactly half of the mouse's weight and will accordingly report this value. As the mouse moves from the mid-point of the rod toward transducer L, the force registered by L will increase while correspondingly the force on transducer R will diminish. If the position of each transducer is fixed and the distance between the transducers is known, then force information can be used to calculate the position of the force (mouse) on the rod. This principle can be generalized to a square plane with a force transducer located in fixed positions at each of the four corners of the square. In this case, the position of the mouse on the plane is expressed in a Cartesian coordinate system with the center of the square at $x = 0$, $y = 0$. At any given instant, the x-y coordinates of a force on the plane can be calculated from the forces registered by the four transducers located at the corners of the square. This is the center of force, and it is independent of the magnitude of the force. Instead of a mouse on the rod in the above exercise, imagine a rat ten times the mass of the mouse; the relative force differences will give the position of the rat regardless of its weight. Two fundamental quantities become available in the four-transducer system: the position of the center of force, expressed in spatial coordinates, and the magnitude of the vertical applied force (termed Fz), expressed in force units. By sampling the readings of the four force transducers very rapidly (e.g., at 50 samples/s) changes in position of the center of force and in the Fz can be used to track the activity of a mouse or rat (or other small terrestrial animal). It is important to note that vertical changes in Fz are detected in the absence of any change in spatial position in the plane (i.e., the plane is the force-plate). The implication of this latter point is that "in-place" activities, such as tremor in a non-locomoting mouse or head movements in a stationary rat, can be recorded and analyzed with signal processing methods.

The force-plate actometers used to collect the data reported below measured 28 cm × 28 cm for the sensing surface. This size was a compromise (smaller than commercially available actometers for rats and larger than those sold for mice). The plate itself was made from 5 mm thick aluminum honeycomb epoxyed between two 0.125 mm thick aluminum "skins," and the mass was about 100 grams. The force transducers were Sensotec Model 31a load cells with a range of 0–250 gram equivalent weights. The analog-to-digital sampling rate was 50 samples/s and the interface board was a LabMaster supplied by Scientific Solutions (Mentor, OH). As a matter of convenience, the forces were expressed as gram equivalent weights, instead of newtons, because of the calibration method, which used standard gram masses. Another reason for expressing forces in gram-force units was that the sum of the forces on the four transducers, taken over an interval of several seconds, was equal to a mouse's or rat's body weight, which is usually expressed in grams, not newtons. Thus, using force units that were easily related to the animal subject's weight facilitated communication. The actometers were located in sound-attenuating polyvinylchloride chambers (Med Associates, Georgia, VT) to reduce effects of extraneous acoustic energy. Most recordings were conducted in nearly total darkness; the only source of light was from the wide-angle peep hole in the front door and the two 5 cm diameter louvered air intakes.

The grid ataxia procedure used to assess ethanol-induced ataxia was carried out in a specially designed force-plate actometer that had two parallel horizontal sensing planes. The upper plane was a grid and the second plane, 1 cm below the first, was a smooth floor as in the force-plate actometers just described. Both the upper and lower planes were supported by force transducers to form two separate force plates. The upper plane was constructed of parallel lightweight aluminum tubing 2 mm in diameter and spaced 1 cm apart. It weighed about 55 grams. While walking on this grid, a mouse sometimes had foot slips such that the limb or limbs involved in the slip struck the lower plane, which measured and recorded the force, duration, and location of these slips. This is similar to the grid ataxia test described used extensively by Crabbe et al. (1996), except the instrument described here has substantially greater spatial and temporal resolution and is capable of recording tremor if present. Because the floor plate that registered the magnitude and duration of the slips also provided information about the spatial location of the slips, it may be reasoned, though erroneously, that the grid itself did not need to be instrumented with force transducers. However, sensors were required on the grid as a way of distinguishing between a mouse that was nearly motionless and one that was active but made no slips (unlikely for the ethanol dose used, but possible for other drugs or types of mice).

2. Dependent Variables and Quantitative Methods

All dependent variables were derived from the spatial coordinates as a function of time and the vertical or Fz force as a function of time. These quantities were combined in a variety of ways that provided meaningful neurobehavioral descriptors. To quantify the basic rhythmic frequencies of tremor or focused stereotypies, the Fz time series were subjected to Fourier analysis (power spectrum analysis) as implemented by AutoSignal™ 1.50 (SYSTAT Software, Inc., Richmond, CA). For these Fourier analyses the time series length was 20.48 s (1024 samples) for the focused stereotypy analyses and 40.96 s (2048 samples) for the tremor analyses. The CS_2-Hanning data window was applied to the time series prior to Fourier analysis. Spatial plots of the center of force trajectories over time were made from the distance between successive center-of-force coordinates that were 0.1 s apart in time. The graphics were done with SYSTAT 10.0 (SYSTAT Software, Inc., Richmond, CA). Custom programs written in Turbo Pascal in our laboratory managed the data acquisition process, while FreePascal (University of Freiburg, Germany) was used to write utility programs needed to put the raw data in a format that enabled input into SYSTAT. Excel (Microsoft, Redmond, WA) formatting was necessary for taking advantage of AutoSignal's automation feature for Fourier analysis.

With respect to the grid-ataxia chamber, our method, like Crabbe and colleagues' (1996) procedure, allowed the number of slips to be assessed in relation to the total amount of movement on the grid so that number of slips as a measure of ataxia was not confounded with distance traveled. Thus, the ataxia score was expressed as a ratio of number of slips (detected by the smooth floor) to distance traveled detected by the grid. This ratio was log transformed to normalize the data for statistical tests. Custom software written in Turbo Pascal was used to process the data from the floor to quantify the number, peak force, and duration of slips.

C. Results of Pharmacological and Genetic Manipulations

1. Stimulants: Amphetamine- and Cocaine-Induced Focused Stereotypies

Amphetamine produces a rise in extracellular concentrations of brain dopamine and concomitant behavioral manifestations in rats and other species. At relatively low doses (up to 1.2 mg/kg, ip) amphetamine increases locomotor movements, and at intermediate to high doses (1.5 to 6.0 mg/kg) the locomotor behavior ceases and gives way to a stationary posture accompanied by highly repetitive, rapid head movements (see video clip for this chapter). This latter, non-locomotor, phase of stimulation is referred to as focused stereotypy. The stereotypy phase can last for over an hour and is usually followed by a period of locomotor stimulation (Schiorring 1971). At very high doses (>10.0 mg/kg) amphetamine can induce intense oral behaviors and self-injury (Lara-Lemus et al. 1997). Amphetamine-induced focused stereotypies are of interest because the hyper-dopaminergic state underlying the behavior has been theoretically linked to schizophrenia (e.g., Robinson and Becker 1986), L-dopa-induced dyskinesias observed in Parkinson disease patients (Graybiel et al. 2000), and addiction to CNS stimulants (Robinson and Berridge 1993).

Instrument-based measurement of focused stereotypies has heretofore been problematic because instruments, such as photobeam actometers, designed to quantify locomotion are unable to characterize adequately the small spatial amplitude of the focused stereotypies. The force-plate actometer permits a robust measurement of both locomotor behavior and focused stereotypies in the same rat at the same time (Fowler et al. 2003). Figure 10 gives two illustrative examples of our quantitative characterization of locomotion and focused stereotypy in separate rats receiving either 5.0 mg/kg amphetamine or 24 mg/kg cocaine immediately before a one-hour session. Power spectra of Fz (the multiphasic functions shown in Figure 10) indicate that both drugs induced a near 10 Hz rhythm and no locomotion (as shown by the dots enclosed in the squares adjacent to each spectral function). A rat's head movements produce the near 10 Hz rhythm. It is readily apparent by inspection that the duration of action for cocaine induction of focused stereotypy is much shorter than the duration of action of amphetamine. This is congruent with the well-known more rapid elimination pharmacokinetics of cocaine compared to amphetamine. The cocaine data also show an easily discernable phase of locomotor stimulation following the focused stereotypy phase. The same pattern occurs for amphetamine, but the locomotor stimulation phase manifests itself after the first hour and cannot be seen in this plot. During the focused stereotypy phase of behavioral stimulation, the near 10 Hz dominant frequency of the power spectrum shifts to the right (examine Figure 10 and sight along the dashed line marking 10 Hz) for both amphetamine and cocaine. Parametric data for amphetamine show that this within-session frequency shift is a reliable phenomenon; fifteen out of sixteen rats treated with 5.0 mg/kg amphetamine exhibited the frequency shift (Fowler et al. 2003). Moreover, after repeated dosing (every three days for five dosing cycles) the rhythm of the head movements shifted to significantly lower frequencies, while the within-session upward shift of the head movement rhythm continued to be expressed (Fowler et al. 2003). These frequency-change analyses have not yet been conducted for cocaine.

What these frequency-shift phenomena and the 10 Hz rhythm imply about CNS function remains to be elucidated. A recently published paper suggests several speculative possibilities (Fowler et al. 2003). From a methodological perspective, the foregoing analyses show that the force-plate actometer affords a new arena for a quantitative experimental analysis of CNS-stimulant-induced behaviors. Another chapter in this volume reports on the ability of the antipsychotic drug clozapine to modulate the head-movement rhythm of amphetamine-induced focused stereotypies.

2. Tremorogenic Drugs: Harmaline and Physostigmine

Tremor is an important symptom of prevalent neurological disorders such as essential tremor and Parkinson

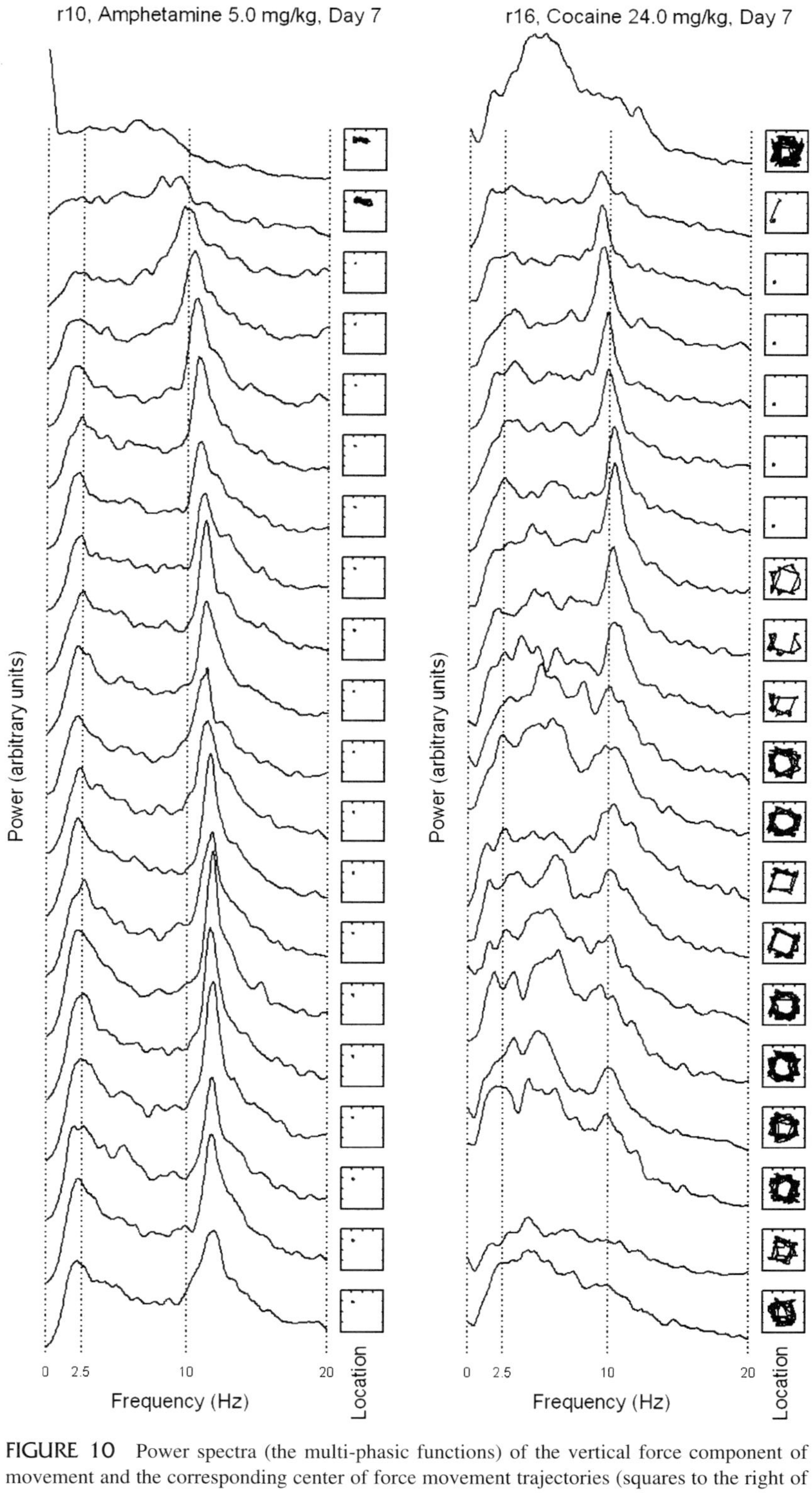

FIGURE 10 Power spectra (the multi-phasic functions) of the vertical force component of movement and the corresponding center of force movement trajectories (squares to the right of each function) for two separate male Sprague Dawley rats treated with the indicated drugs a few seconds before being placed in the actometer for a one-hour session. Each power spectrum and the plot of movement trajectory were for a three-minute period with time proceeding from top to bottom. Each power spectrum is the average function for nine separate power spectra computed for nine equal-length force time series covering the three-minute period. The peak in the power spectra near 10 Hz reflects the head movements during focused stereotypies induced by amphetamine (left side) or cocaine (right side). As shown by the movement trajectories, lack of locomotion or "the stationary phase" (Schiorring 1971) was associated with the presence of the peaks near 10 Hz in the power spectra. Also evident in this figure is the shorter duration of action of cocaine compared to amphetamine.

disease, yet noninvasive, quantitative studies of pertinent laboratory investigations in animals have been relatively rare. In sufficient doses, both harmaline (e.g., Llinas and Volkind 1973; Lorden et al. 1985; Stanford and Fowler 1998) and physostigmine (e.g., Gothoni et al. 1983) induce whole-body tremor. Harmaline-induced tremor has been used to model essential tremor (Deuschl and Elble 2000). Whether or not physostigmine tremor in rodents usefully models a disease state is debatable, but its mechanism of action is quite different from that of harmaline. Harmaline acts on the inferior olive to produce excessive stimulation of the cerebellar Purkinje cells via their climbing fiber inputs that originate in the inferior olive. Physostigmine inhibits acetylcholinesterase leading to excess acetylcholine in peripheral and CNS cholinergic systems, including the basal ganglia. Detailed quantitative analyses in the force-plate actometer have shown that the two types of tremors differed in that harmaline produced a more narrow-band focus of energy than did physostigmine (Wang and Fowler 2001). Both drugs produced tremor with a peak frequency in the power spectrum near 10 Hz in rats, but the shapes of the power spectral functions lacked the prominent power seen near 2.5 Hz for the CNS-stimulant-induced head movements described in the previous section. At doses sufficient to produce whole-body tremor, both harmaline and physostigmine suppressed locomotion (Wang and Fowler 2001).

Another prominent difference between harmaline and physostigmine whole-body tremor is observed when attention is directed to the temporal pattern of tremor as seen in the time series recording of Fz. Harmaline tremor is well known to express intermittently with relatively high intensity tremor episodes of many seconds interspersed with periods of no tremor. In contrast, physostigmine tremor is continuously expressed but at a generally lower intensity than that produced by harmaline. When data for an entire recording session are combined into a single averaged power spectrum, this difference in tremor induced by harmaline and physostigmine is difficult to appreciate because of averaging. For harmaline, periods of intense tremor lasting twenty to thirty seconds are averaged together with periods of no tremor; for physostigmine, continuous low-level tremor is averaged together with brief episodes (two to three seconds) of high amplitude tremor. Therefore, the averaged power spectra of the Fz recordings for both drugs are similar in terms of total tremor power estimated for all the data recorded over fifteen or thirty minutes. This averaging problem can be addressed by comparing the two types of tremors in terms of the *minimum* tremor expressed during a recording session. Data in Figure 11 show the results of a minimum tremor analysis for the first exposure to harmaline at 16 mg/kg and physostigmine at 0.5 mg/kg. It is clear from inspection of the records that the harmaline treatment produced a more nearly tremor-free state than did physostigmine. The amount of force variation in the minimum tremor records presented in Figure 11 for the eight harmaline-treated rats was comparable to non-drugged rats in a stationary posture (data not shown). To ensure that these minimum-tremor data did not simply reflect the animal's state after the respective drugs had been eliminated from the body, the episodes of minimum tremor were selected for examination only if they were followed by at least one episode of high intensity tremor lasting at least two to three seconds.

A satisfactory explanation for the apparent randomly alternating bouts of tremor and the absence of tremor in the harmaline-treated animals has remained elusive. However, Fowler et al. (2002a) have suggested that (1) the harmaline tremor is induced when an organism initiates voluntary movements (like the cerebellar intention tremor described by clinical neurologists), and (2) the tremor state is aversive. The aversiveness of the body shaking (and probably vertigo sensations as well) punishes attempts to move, and the harmaline-treated animal learns to avoid movements while in the harmaline state. This hypothesis about harmaline tremor could be used to explain (1) the apparently random intermittency of tremor during the first exposure to the drug, (2) the tremor tolerance both within and across recording sessions, (3) the non-tolerating locomotor suppression, and (4) the low levels of Fz variation during the "silent" periods when tremor is temporarily absent. A corollary of this hypothesis is that the putative learning that occurs does not especially depend on the cerebellum because it is likely dysfunctional due to the overexcitation of Purkinje cells produced by the excess release of glutamate from the climbing fiber terminals.

3. Motor Effects of D2 Dopamine Receptor Deficiency in Knock-out Mice

This section summarizes the successful use of the force-plate actometer to identify specific motor impairments in mice lacking the D2 dopamine receptor. The mice originated in the laboratory of E. Borrelli (Baik et al. 1995), and the initial report suggested that these mice had "Parkinson-like" motor impairments, including hypoactivity and difficulty initiating movements. Our laboratory studied the D2 knockouts on a congenic (n = 10 generations of backcross) C57BL/6 background to minimize any contribution of the 129Sv stem-cell-donor strain. In addition to confirming that the D2 knockout mice were hypoactive compared to wild-type controls, two additional new findings emerged from the force-plate actometer data. The D2 knockouts were more responsive to harmaline challenge than wild-type controls, and they exhibited longer duration "wall rears" (Fowler et al. 2002a).

The harmaline challenge consisted of one 30-minute session of recording immediately after an ip injection of 15 mg/kg harmaline dihydrochloride. Data for the whole session were Fourier analyzed, and integrated power in the

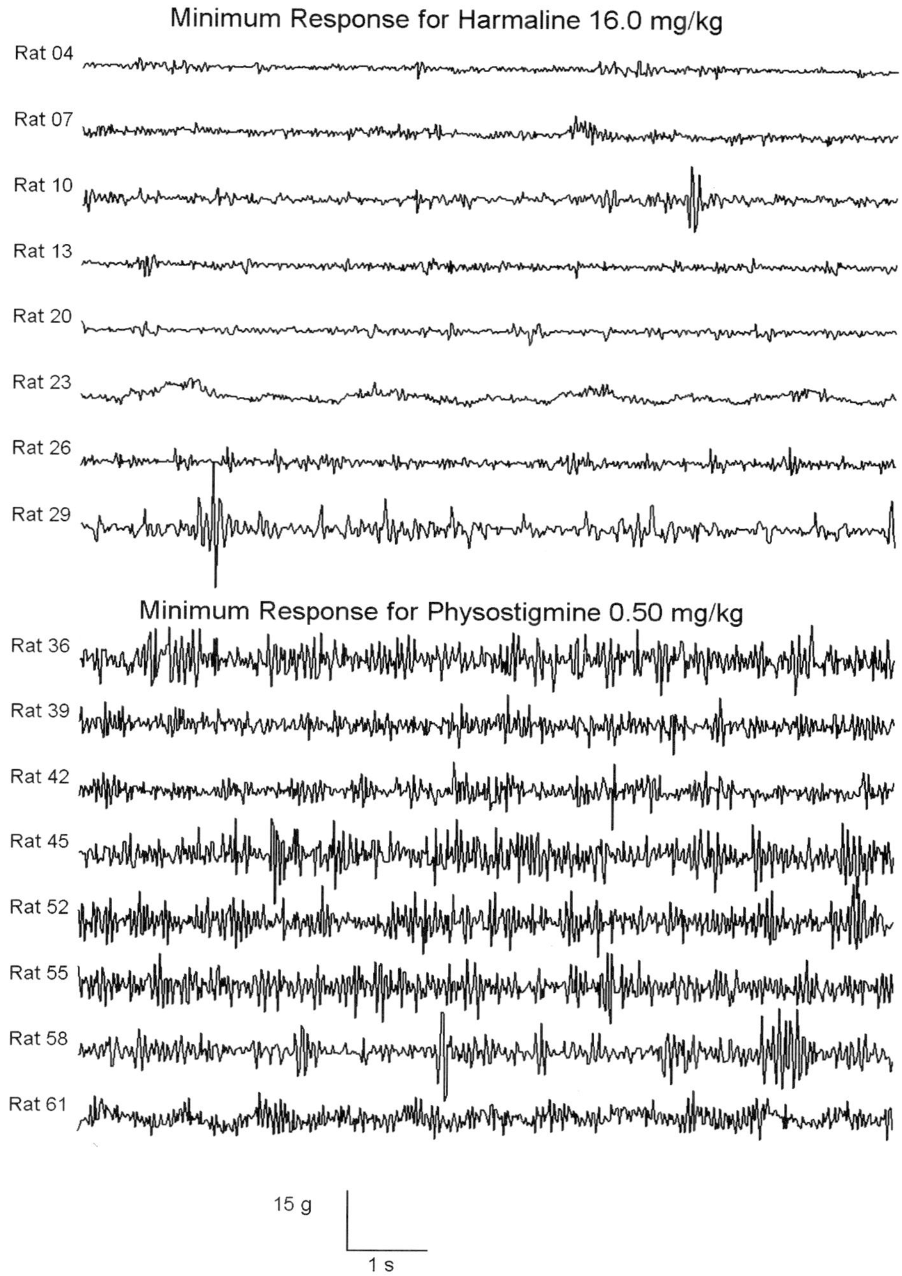

FIGURE 11 Minimum tremor recordings for eight rats that were treated with harmaline and eight separate rats treated with physostigmine. These are previously unpublished data from an experiment reported by Wang and Fowler (2001). Data were recorded in force-plate actometers, one of which is shown in Fig. 9. During the intermittent periods of loss of tremor in harmaline-treated rats, the amount of tremor was substantially less than the lowest level of tremor exhibited by rats treated with physostigmine.

5–15 Hz frequency served as the dependent variable. This integrated score was sensitive to both the intensity and duration of tremor expression. The main finding was that the D2 knockouts exhibited a much more enduring expression of tremor than controls (Fowler et al. 2002a). This result is illustrated by one wild-type and one D2 knock-out in Figure 12. For D2 knock-outs, the amplitude of the tremor response was indistinguishable from that of controls, but D2 knock-outs exhibited greatly diminished time in the non-tremor state. The interpretation offered for this result was that D2

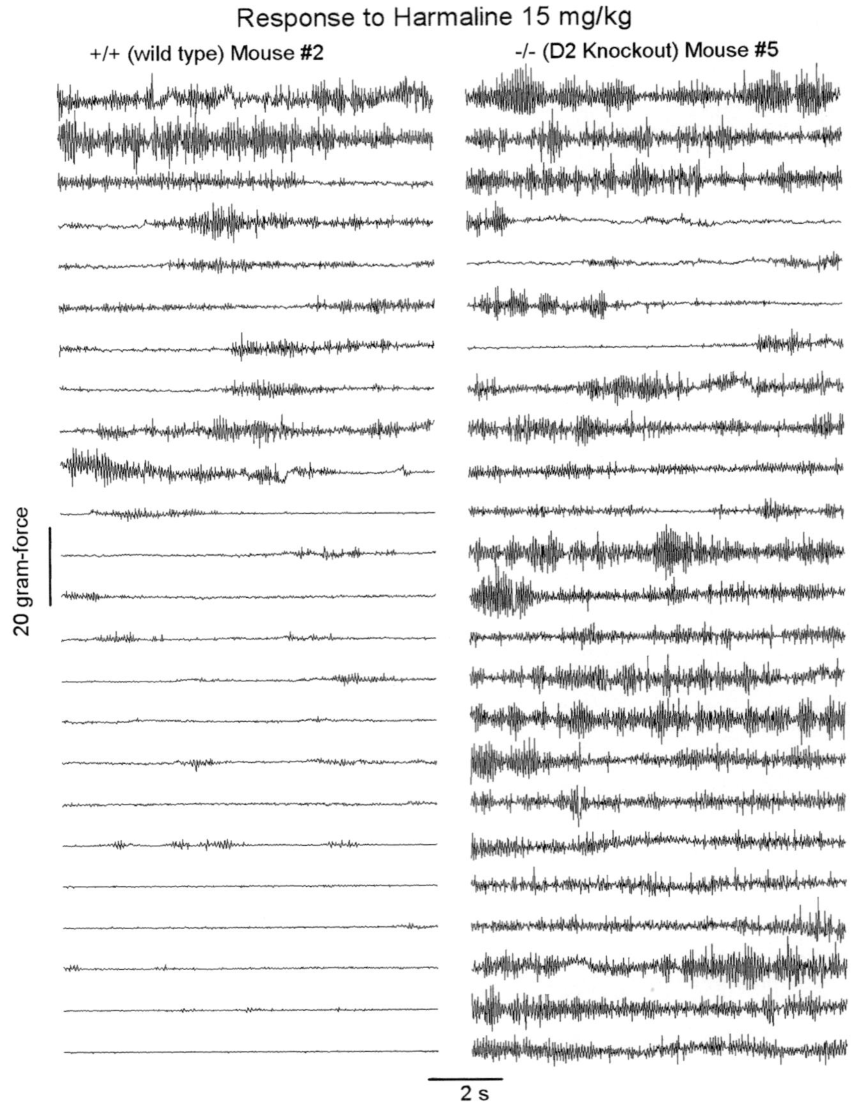

FIGURE 12 Representative tremor response to harmaline by a wild-type control and by a D2 dopamine receptor knock-out mouse. These are previously unpublished individual-subject data from research reported by Fowler et al. (2002). Although tremor amplitudes were similar for both types of mice, the tremor response was expressed by D2 knock-outs for a much larger proportion of the recording session than was the case for wild-type control mice.

knock-outs had difficulty learning that attempts to move brought on the tremor (Fowler et al. 2002a). This interpretation was made more plausible by the finding that D2 knock-outs were markedly slow in acquiring a rewarded-operant response, a result that supports the assertion that D2 knock-outs have an associative deficiency for this kind of learning (Fowler et al. 2002a).

A wall rear is a discrete response characterized by a mouse's raising its fore limbs from the floor and reaching upward to place its fore limbs on the wall. In a force-plate actometer, wall rears are detected as negativities in the Fz record resulting from the offloading of a portion of the animal's body weight from the floor to the wall via the fore limbs leaning against the wall. The response is considered to be discrete because it can be assigned a beginning time and an ending time. Theoretically, a mouse must initiate a response and then terminate it. The duration of a wall rear (ending time minus the beginning time) is probably governed by a number of factors, and it is sensible to assume that one of the factors is the motor execution time to return to an all-fours posture after the initial portion of the rear has been fully expressed. We developed an algorithm to count

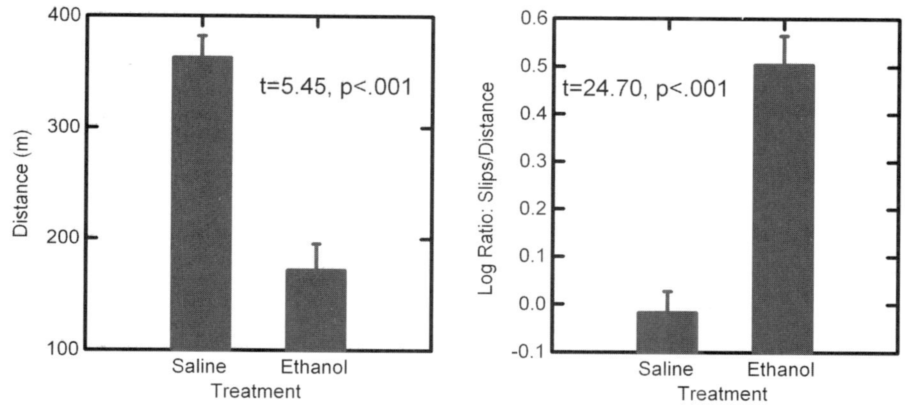

FIGURE 13 Group means (+/– 1 SEM) for eight C57BL/6 mice after saline or 2 g/kg ethanol treatment. Data were collected in a grid/ataxia chamber in which foot slips while walking on a grid were detected by a force plate located 1 cm below the grid.

the number of wall rears and measure their duration and magnitude (Fowler et al. 2002a). Essentially, a negativity of 3.3 gram force defined the start of a wall rear and 0.6 gram force defined the end. The time between these force criteria was the duration of the wall rear. Compared to wild-type controls and several comparison strains (BALB/cJ, C3H/HeJ, C57BL/6J), the D2 knock-outs had markedly longer duration of wall rears. This result was interpreted to confirm the hypothesis that the absence of the D2 dopamine receptors produces Parkinson-like slowing of discrete motor responses.

4. Ethanol-Induced Ataxia in C57BL/6 Mice in the Grid-Ataxia Force Plate

To validate the ability of the grid-ataxia instrument to detect drug-induced ataxia, C57BL/6 mice (n = 8) were studied for thirty minutes in the instrument after either saline or ethanol 2 g/kg injection (ip). The order of ethanol experience was counterbalanced across the two sessions. Two noteworthy results emerged from the statistical analysis. First, distance traveled on the grid was significantly reduced under ethanol compared to saline treatment (see Figure 13). When tested in a solid floor apparatus, C57BL/6 mice generally exhibit increased locomotor activity after moderate-dose (2 g/kg) ethanol treatment (Crawley et al. 1997). Unpublished data from our laboratory confirm this moderate, but significant, hyperactivity that occurs in the first fifteen minutes after treatment with 2 g/kg ethanol. The ethanol-related reduction in distance traveled on the grid was probably a reflection of the impaired ability to ambulate, which can be appreciated by examining the ratio of foot slips as shown in Figure 13, right panel. Ethanol significantly decreased distance traveled on the grid and at the same time greatly increased the number of slips. These data validate the grid-ataxia actometer as a quantitative method for measuring ethanol-induced ataxia and suggest that the method should be sensitive to other manipulations that disturb the motor capabilities of mice.

D. Summary

The data presented here show that the force-plate actometer is a versatile instrument for measuring motor behavior. Its high spatial and temporal resolution, combined with the physical principles on which it is based, allow for measurement of locomotion, stimulant-induced focused stereotypies, and whole-body tremor. In addition, characteristics of specific responses such as wall rears can be counted and quantitated in terms of force and duration of each wall-rear event. When combined with a second force-sensing plane configured as a grid, the force-plate measurement concepts can be used to quantify ataxia induced by drugs. In the interest of brevity, some demonstrated uses of the force-plate actometer were not described here; these uses include the measurement of rotations around the center of the chamber, which is the main dependent variable in the unilateral dopamine depletion model of Parkinson disease (Fowler et al. 2001), as well as the detection and quantification of jumps induced in BALB/c mice by high dose (10.0 mg/kg) treatment with amphetamine (unpublished observations). Finally, it should be noted that many additional behavioral measurement problems can be addressed with this methodology. If the behavior of interest has distinctive spatial and temporal properties that are terrestrially expressed (i.e., these methods will not work if the behavior is occurring in air or water) it should be possible to develop computer algorithms to extract these patterns from the force-plate data and thereby quantify such behaviors.

V. CONCLUSIONS

Electro-mechanical instrumentation continues to be a fundamental component of hypothesis-driven research in the life and behavioral sciences. Instrumentation allows the embodiment of the conceptual schemes that constitute the hypotheses of interest. In addition, new instrumentation that broadens and deepens scientists' powers of observation and measurement often opens up fruitful new lines of investigation. As Abelson (1986) has succinctly stated, "Instruments shape research, determine what discoveries are made, and perhaps, even select the types of individuals likely to succeed as scientists" (p. 182).

The instruments and methods described here made possible several new observations that may contribute to ongoing analyses of animal models of movement disorders. For example, in the lick-force-rhythm task, harmaline and ibogaine were shown to slow the lick rhythm of rats at low doses that do not produce visually observed whole-body tremor. When the effects of harmaline were studied in the same low dose range in the press-while-licking task, again the drug slowed the lick rhythm and it induced measurable forelimb tremor in rats, while failing to produce visually detectable tremor. Studied at higher doses (above 4.0 mg/kg, ip), harmaline produced marked whole-body tremor while greatly suppressing locomotor behavior in the force-plate actometer. These data show that harmaline has a spectrum of motor effects in addition to inducing whole-body tremor. The methods presented here should make possible new experimental analyses aimed at understanding the pharmacological and neural mechanism of tremor and orolingual function.

Another example of potential new directions involves the use of these methods to examine changes in motor systems with advancing age. Not only have Stanford et al. (2003) shown that lick rhythm in rats slows with age, but they have also reported that older rats exhibit altered patterns of gait as measured in the force-plate actometer (Stanford et al. 2002).

The observation that the focused stereotypies induced by amphetamine are frankly rhythmic, with a frequency near 10 Hz, was an unexpected finding enabled by the high spatial and temporal resolution of the force-plate actometer. The distinctive rhythmic pattern of this drug-induced behavior makes it possible to quantitatively separate the locomotor stimulation and focused stereotypy responses to amphetamine. Moreover, Fowler et al. (2003) reported that the rhythm of the rats' head movements shifted to reliably lower frequencies as repeated doses were given and as the stationary phase of the amphetamine increased in duration. These repeated-dosing effects, known as sensitization, are of interest to researchers working on the problem of L-dopa-related dyskinesias in Parkinson disease (e.g., Graybiel et al. 2000) and to scientists who have established links between brain neuroplasticity and sensitizing doses of amphetamine or cocaine (Kolb et al. 2003). Thus, the force-plate actometer should facilitate research involving animal motor behavior in a variety of research contexts.

Acknowledgments

This work was supported by MH43429, DA12508, and HD002528.

Video Legend

At relatively low doses (up to 1.2 mg/kg, ip), amphetamine increases locomotor movements. At intermediate to high doses (1.5 to 6.0 mg/kg), the locomotor behavior ceases and gives way to a stationary posture accompanied by highly repetitive, rapid head movements.

References

Abelson, P.H. 1986. Instrumentation and computers. *American Scientist* **74**:182–192.

AutoSignal (Version 1.5) [Computer Software]. 2000. Richmond, California: SYSTAT Software.

Back, S.A., and C. Gorenstein. 1994. Differential response of neutral endopeptidase 24.11 ("enkephalinase"), and cholinergic and opioidergic markers to hypoglossal axotomy. *J Comp Neurol* **340**:149–160.

Baik, J.H., R. Picetti, A. Saiardi, G. Thiriet, A. Dierich, A. Depaulis, M. Le Meur, and E. Borrelli. (1995). Parkinsonian-like locomotor impairment in mice lacking dopamine D2 receptors. *Nature (London, U.K.)* **377**: 424–428.

Balaban, C.D. 1985. Central neurotoxic effects of intraperitoneally administered 3-acetylpyridine, harmaline and niacinamide in Sprague-Dawley and Long-Evans rats: a critical review of central 3-acetylpyridine neurotoxicity. *Brain Res* **356**:21–42.

Berry, R.B., and L.F. Hayward. 2003. Selective augmentation of genioglossus electromyographic activity by L-5-hydroxytryptophan in the rat. *Pharmacol Biochem Behav* **74**:877–882.

Brimblecombe, R.W., and R.M. Pinder. 1972. *Tremors and Tremorogenic Agents*. Bristol, U.K.: Scientechnica.

Crabbe, J.C., T.J. Phillips, E.J. Gallaher, L.I. Crawshaw, and S.R. Mitchell. 1996. Common genetic determinants of the ataxic and hypothermic effects of ethanol in BXD/Ty recombinant inbred mice: genetic correlations and quantitative trait loci. *J Pharmacol Exp Ther* **277**:624–632.

Crawley, J.N. 2000. *What's Wrong with My Mouse?* New York: Wiley-Liss.

Das, S., and S.C. Fowler. 1995. Acute and subchronic effects of clozapine on licking in rats: tolerance to disruptive effects on number of licks, but no tolerance to rhythm slowing. *Psychopharmacology (Berlin, Ger.)* **120**:249–255.

Davis, J.D., G.P. Smith, B. Singh, and D.L. McCann. 2001. The impact of sucrose-derived unconditioned and conditioned negative feedback on the microstructure of ingestive behavior. *Physiol Behav* **72**:393–402.

Deecher, D.C., M. Teitler, D.M. Soderlund, W.G. Bornmann, M.E. Kuehne, and S.D. Glick. 1992. Mechanisms of action of ibogaine and harmaline congeners based on radioligand binding studies. *Brain Res* **571**: 242–247.

Deuschl, G., and R.J. Elble. 2000. The pathophysiology of essential tremor. *Neurology* **54**:S14–S20.

Elble, R.J. 1998. Animal models of action tremor. *Mov Disord* **13** (Suppl. 3):35–39.

Fowler, S.C., and C. Mortell. 1992. Low doses of haloperidol interfere with rat tongue extensions during licking: a quantitative analysis. *Behav Neurosci* **106**:386–395.

Fowler, S.C., J. Blosser, C. Hayes, E. Skitek, and G. Wang. Comparison of typical and atypical neuroleptics and reference drugs on rats' tongue dynamics during licking. *Soc Neurosci Abs* 27: abstract no. 939.8.

Fowler, S.C., K.H. Davison, and J.A. Stanford. 1994. Unlike haloperidol, clozapine slows and dampens rats' forelimb force oscillations and decreases force output in a press-while-licking behavioral task. *Psychopharmacology* **116**:19–25.

Fowler, S.C., and G. Wang. 1998. Chronic haloperidol produces a time- and dose-related slowing of lick rhythm in rats: implications for rodent models of tardive dyskinesia and neuroleptic-induced parkinsonism. *Psychopharmacology (Berlin, Ger.)* **137**:50–60.

Fowler, S.C., R.M. Liao, and P. Skjoldager. 1990. A new rodent model for neuroleptic-induced pseudo-parkinsonism: low doses of haloperidol increase forelimb tremor in the rat. *Behav Neurosci* **104**:449–456.

Fowler, S.C., B.R. Birkestrand, R. Chen, S.J. Moss, E. Vorontsova, G. Wang, and T.J. Zarcone. 2001. A force-plate actometer for quantitating rodent behaviors: illustrative data on locomotion, rotation, spatial patterning, stereotypies, and tremor. *J Neurosci Methods* **107**:107–124.

Fowler, S.C., T.J. Zarcone, R. Chen, M.D. Taylor, and D.E. Wright. 2002a. Low grip strength, impaired tongue force and hyperactivity induced by overexpression of neurotrophin-3 in mouse skeletal muscle. *Int J Dev Neurosci* **20**:303–308.

Fowler, S.C., T.J. Zarcone, E. Vorontsova, and R. Chen. 2002b. Motor and associative deficits in D2 dopamine receptor knockout mice. *Int J Dev Neurosci* **20**:309–321.

Fowler, S.C., B. Birkestrand, R. Chen, E. Vorontsova, and T. Zarcone. 2003. Behavioral sensitization to amphetamine in rats: changes in the rhythm of head movements during focused stereotypies. *Psychopharmacology (Berlin, Ger.)* **170**:167–177.

Gothoni, P., M. Lehtinen, and M. Fincke. 1983. Drugs for Parkinson's disease reduce tremor induced by physostigmine. *Naunyn-Schmiedeberg's Arch Pharmacol* **323**:205–210.

Graybiel, A.M., J.J. Canales, and C. Capper-Loup. 2000. Levodopa-induced dyskinesias and dopamine-dependent stereotypies: a new hypothesis. *Trends Neurosci* **23**:S71–S77.

Greer, J.J., J.E. Carter, and Z. al-Zubaidy. 1995. Opioid depression of respiration in neonatal rats. *J Physiol (Cambridge, U.K.)* **485(Pt 3)**: 845–855.

Homberg, V., K. Reiners, H. Hefter, and H.J. Freund. 1986. The muscle activity spectrum: spectral analysis of muscle force as an estimator of overall motor unit activity. *Electroencephalogr Clin Neurophysiol* **63**: 209–222.

Kallman, M.J., and S.C. Fowler. 1994. Assessment of chemically induced alterations in motor functions. In *Principles of Neurotoxicology*. Ed. L.W. Chang. Vol. 26. pp. 373–396. New York: Marcel Dekker.

Kolb, B., G. Gorny, Y. Li, A.-N. Samaha, T. Robinson. 2003. Amphetamine or cocaine limits the ability of later experience to promote structural plasticity in the neocortex and nucleus accumbens. *Proceedings of the National Academy of Sciences.* **100**:10523–10528.

Leysen, J.E., P.M. Janssen, A. Schotte, W.H. Luyten, and A.A. Megens. 1993. Interaction of antipsychotic drugs with neurotransmitter receptor sites in vitro and in vivo in relation to pharmacological and clinical effects: role of 5HT2 receptors. *Psychopharmacology (Berlin, Ger.)* **112**:S40–S54.

Lara-Lemus, A., M. Perez de la Mora, J. Mendez-Franco, M. Palomero-Rivero, and R. Drucker-Colin. 1997. Effects of REM sleep deprivation on the d-amphetamine-induced self-mutilating behavior. *Brain Res* **770**:60–64.

Li, Y.M., L. Shen, J.H. Peever, and J. Duffin. 2003. Connections between respiratory neurons in the neonatal rat transverse medullary slice studied with cross-correlation. *J Physiol (Cambridge, U.K.)* **549**:327–332.

Llinas, R., and R.A. Volkind. 1973. The olivo-cerebellar system: functional properties as revealed by harmaline-induced tremor. *Exp Brain Res* **18**: 69–87.

Llinas, R., K. Walton, D.E. Hillman, and C. Sotelo. 1975. Inferior olive: its role in motor learning. *Science* **190**:1230–1231.

Lorden, J.F., G.A. Oltmans, T.W. McKeon, J. Lutes, and M. Beales. 1985. Decreased cerebellar 3′, 5′-cyclic guanosine monophosphate levels and insensitivity to harmaline in the genetically dystonic rat (dt). *J Neurosci* **5**:2618–2625.

Marple, S.L. 1987. *Digital Spectral Analysis: With Applications*. Englewood Cliffs, New Jersey: Prentice-Hall.

McAuley, J.H., J.C. Rothwell, and C.D. Marsden. 1997. Frequency peaks of tremor, muscle vibration and electromyographic activity at 10 Hz, 20 Hz and 40 Hz during human finger muscle contraction may reflect rhythmicities of central neural firing. *Exp Brain Res* **114**:525–541.

Mohanakumar, K.P., N. Mitra, and D.K. Ganguly. 1990. Tremorogenesis by physostigmine is unrelated to acetylcholinesterase inhibition: evidence for serotoninergic involvement. *Neurosci Lett* **120**:91–93.

Moss, S.J. 2001. *Tongue Dynamics in the Rat after Treatment with Agents Known to Affect the Olivo-Cerebellar Pathway*. Unpublished Doctoral Dissertation, University of Kansas, Lawrence.

Moss, S.J., G. Wang, R. Chen, R. Pal, and S.C. Fowler. 2001. 3-Acetylpyridine reduces tongue protrusion force but does not abolish lick rhythm in the rat. *Brain Research* **920**:1–9.

Notterman, J.M., and D.E. Mintz. 1965. *Dynamics of Response*. New York: Wiley.

O'Hearn, E., and M.E. Molliver. 1993. Degeneration of Purkinje cells in parasagittal zones of the cerebellar vermis after treatment with ibogaine or harmaline. *Neuroscience (Oxford, U.K.)* **55**:303–310.

O'Hearn, E., and M.E. Molliver. 1997. The olivocerebellar projection mediates ibogaine-induced degeneration of Purkinje cells: a model of indirect, trans-synaptic excitotoxicity. *J Neurosci* **17**:8828–8841.

Parfitt, K.D., R. Freedman, and P.C. Bickford-Wimer. 1988. Electrophysiological effects of locally applied noradrenergic agents at cerebellar Purkinje neurons: receptor specificity. *Brain Res* **462**:242–251.

Parkis, M.A., D.A. Bayliss, and A.J. Berger. 1995. Actions of norepinephrine on rat hypoglossal motoneurons. *J Neurophysiol* **74**:1911–1919.

Reynolds, G.S. 1968. *A Primer of Operant Conditioning*. Glenview, Illinois: Scott Foresman.

Robinson, T.E., and J.B. Becker. 1986. Enduring changes in brain and behavior produced by chronic amphetamine administration: a review and evaluation of animal models of amphetamine psychosis. *Brain Res* **396**:157–198.

Robinson, T.E., and K.C. Berridge. 1993. The neural basis of drug craving: an incentive-sensitization theory of addiction. *Brain Res Brain Res Rev* **18**:247–291.

Sanchez, C., and J. Arnt. 2000. In-vivo assessment of 5-HT2A and 5-HT2C antagonistic properties of newer antipsychotics. *Behav Pharmacol* **11**:291–298.

Schiorring, E. 1971. Amphetamine induced selective stimulation of certain behaviour items with concurrent inhibition of others in an open-field test with rats. *Behaviour* **39**:1–17.

Schotte, A., P.F. Janssen, W. Gommeren, W.H. Luyten, P. Van Gompel, A.S. Lesage, K. De Loore, and J.E. Leysen. 1996. Risperidone compared with new and reference antipsychotic drugs: in vitro and in vivo receptor binding. *Psychopharmacology (Berlin, Ger.)* **124**:57–73.

Skitek, E.B. 1998. *Quantitative analysis of motor abnormalities in a rat model of Parkinson's disease*. Unpublished Master's Thesis, University of Kansas, Lawrence.

Skitek, E.B., S.C. Fowler, and R.E. Tessel. 1999. Effects of unilateral striatal dopamine depletion on tongue force and rhythm during licking in rats. *Behav Neurosci* **113**:567–573.

Stanford, J.A., and S.C. Fowler. 1997. Scopolamine reversal of tremor produced by low doses of physostigmine in rats: evidence for a cholinergic mechanism. *Neurosci Lett* **225**:157–160.

Stanford, J.A., and S.C. Fowler. 1998. At low doses, harmaline increases forelimb tremor in the rat. *Neurosci Lett* **241**:41–44.

Stanford, J.A., and S.C. Fowler. 2002. Dantrolene diminishes forelimb force-related tremor at doses that do not decrease operant behavior in the rat. *Exp Clin Psychopharmacol* **10**:385–391.

Stanford, J.A., E. Vorontsova, and S.C. Fowler, 2000. The relationship between isometric force requirement and forelimb tremor in the rat. *Physiol Behav* **69**:285–293.

Stanford, J.A., E. Vorontsova, S.P. Surgener, G.A. Gerhardt, and S.C. Fowler. 2003. Aged Fischer 344 rats exhibit altered orolingual motor function: relationships with nigrostriatal neurochemical measures. *Neurobiol Aging* **24**:259–266.

Stellar, E., and J.H. Hill. 1952. The rat's rate of drinking as a function of water deprivation. *J Comp Physiol Psychol* **45**:96–102.

SYSTAT (Version 10.0) [Computer Software]. 2000. Richmond, California: SYSTAT Software.

Tarsy, D. 1989. Neuroleptic-induced movement disorders. In *Disorders of Movement: Clinical, Pharmacological, and Physiological Aspects*. Ed. N.P. Quinn and P.G. Jenner. pp. 361–393. San Diego: Academic Press.

Ungerstedt, U., and G.W. Arbuthnott. 1970. Quantitative recording of rotational behavior in rats after 6-hydroxy-dopamine lesions of the nigrostriatal dopamine system. *Brain Res* **24**:485–493.

Volgin, D.V., M. Mackiewicz, and L. Kubin. 2001. Alpha(1B) receptors are the main postsynaptic mediators of adrenergic excitation in brainstem motoneurons, a single-cell RT-PCR study. *J Chem Neuroanat* **22**:157–166.

Vrtunski, P., and L.R. Wolin. 1974. Measurement of licking response execution in the rat. *Physiol Behav* **12**:881–886.

Wang, G. 2000. Quantification of harmaline and physostigmine's tremorogenic effects and clozapine's antitremor effect in rats. Unpublished Doctoral Dissertation, University of Kansas, Lawrence.

Wang, G., and S.C. Fowler. 1999. Effects of haloperidol and clozapine on tongue dynamics during licking in CD-1, BALB/c and C57BL/6 mice. *Psychopharmacology (Berlin, Ger.)* **147**:38–45.

Wang, G., and S.C. Fowler. 2001. Concurrent quantification of tremor and depression of locomotor activity induced in rats by harmaline and physostigmine. *Psychopharmacology (Berlin, Ger.)* **158**:273–280.

Waterston, R.H., K. Lindblad-Toh, E. Birney, J. Rogers, J.F. Abril, P. Agarwal, R. Agarwala, et al. [Mouse Genome Sequencing Consortium]. 2002. Initial sequencing and comparative analysis of the mouse genome. *Nature (London, U.K.)* **420**:520–562.

Weijnen, J.A. 1998. Licking behavior in the rat: measurement and situational control of licking frequency. *Neurosci Biobehav Rev* **22**:751–760.

Welsh, J.P. 2002. Functional significance of climbing-fiber synchrony: a population coding and behavioral analysis. *Ann N Y Acad Sci* **978**: 188–204.

Wright, D.E., L. Zhou, J. Kucera, and W.D. Snider. 1997. Introduction of a neurotrophin-3 transgene into muscle selectively rescues proprioceptive neurons in mice lacking endogenous neurotrophin-3. *Neuron* **19**: 503–517.

Zarcone, T.J., M. Caruso, E. Vorontsova, and S.C. Fowler. 2003. Quantitation of drug-induced ataxia or tremor in mice by a grid-actometer comprised of two parallel force plates. In *Abstract Viewer/Itinerary Planner* Program No. 864.10. Society for Neuroscience, Washington, D.C.

Zhan, G., F. Shaheen, M. Mackiewicz, P. Fenik, and S.C. Veasey. 2002. Single cell laser dissection with molecular beacon polymerase chain reaction identifies 2A as the predominant serotonin receptor subtype in hypoglossal motoneurons. *Neuroscience (Oxford, U.K.)* **113**:145–154.

C H A P T E R

A7

Behavior in *Drosophila*: Analysis and Control

RALPH HILLMAN and ROBERT G. PENDLETON

Behavioral observations of *Drosophila*, both informal and formal, are as old as some of the early genetic studies of this organism. In the "fly room" in T.H. Morgan's laboratory, scientists observed that larvae burrowed deep into the medium, but that immediately before metamorphosis they moved out of the medium and pupated in relatively dry areas above the food. Scientists also saw that adult flies tended to congregate at the top of the culture bottles rather than near the food at the bottom of the bottle. While the reports of phenomena such as these were anecdotal, the early observations clearly showed that the flies possessed behavioral characteristics, and these characteristics soon became a matter of investigation. Such investigations of behavior and of the control of behavior, both at the genetic and environmental levels, have consisted of both observational and experimental reports for a large number of larval and adult behavior patterns. These range from simple patterns such as locomotion and geotaxis to complex patterns such as courtship and mating behavior. Moreover, since the genetics of *Drosophila* has been studied extensively, the appearance of these specific behavioral patterns in adults and larvae has almost immediately led to investigations of their genetic control. Application of *Drosophila* to the study of movement disorders research must begin with a detailed understanding of fly behavioral genetics.

I. MATING BEHAVIOR

Sturtevant (1915) reported the first detailed study of a behavioral characteristic when he described mating behavior in *Drosophila* and investigated the control of mating in a number of eye color and morphological mutants that had been isolated in Morgan's laboratory at Columbia. As described by Sturtevant, the basic pattern of behavior in all *Drosophila* species involves courting by the male together with response and receptivity by the female. The process begins with the male approaching the female. If the female does not move away, the male extends and vibrates the wing nearest the female's head. The male faces the female and continues the sequence of vibrations several times, moving around the female but always facing her. During this procedure, the male, as he circles the female, extends and vibrates the wing closest to the female's head, producing what is essentially a "song." If the female remains in place, the male will extend his genitalia and begin to lick the female's posterior end. If the female is receptive, she will extend her ovipositor, sometimes extruding a droplet that causes nearby males to begin courtship. For copulation to take place, the female must open her genitalia and spread her wings. The male then mounts the female and inserts his penis. If the female does not extend her genitalia and spread her wings, mounting and copulation cannot occur.

Sturtevant's original observations in *Drosophila melanogaster* are interesting for several reasons. First, he reported that females rejected yellow-bodied males more often than they did wild-type males. His data also suggested that other cues were involved in the response to the mating process. The investigation of differences in mating behavior was further studied by Bastock (1956) who concluded that the reduced attractivity of yellow-bodied males was a result of their demonstrating fewer and shorter bouts of courtship behavior than those demonstrated by control males. She found that yellow-bodied males had lower success in mating under both light and dark conditions, ruling out visual cues for the initiation of courtship. These data indicated that the residual genotype was important in the behavioral process. There were also indications that neurological changes resulted in aberrant behavior. These changes are supported by observations that the mutation, *yellow*, acts in the same neurological pathway as does *fruitless* (see below and Drapeau et al. 2003), a mutation that results in males courting other males rather than females.

The report by Sturtevant that females showed receptivity during the latter stages of courtship by extruding a droplet that resulted in increased male courtship behavior has led to a series of investigations on the role of volatile compounds in the behavioral process. The role of olfactory stimulation in male courtship behavior was studied by Averhoff and Richardson (1974) and Shorey and Bartell (1970). The importance of olfactory stimulation is supported by the observations that males will court isolated female abdomens. Moreover, Savarit et al. (1999) reported that washing the abdomen with heptane to eliminate organic compounds results in the loss of male courtship behavior. The evidence indicates that the olfactory response is an evolutionary phenomenon that has been selected for in the mating process. The assumption here is that the pheromones have evolved to insure conspecific mating because apparently the molecular attractions are species specific.

Further investigations of mating and courtship behavior have proceeded in several directions. Studies have shown that in addition to genetic control, environmental and physiological influences work on both female receptivity and male courtship. These influences involve, among others, interactions between female and male behavior. For example, Tompkins et al. (1982) showed that female movement during courtship was necessary for males to complete courtship. The courtship index (CI) was defined "as the percentage of time during which the male performed any of the courtship behaviors" (Tompkins et al. 1980). Using a temperature sensitive paralytic mutation, *shibire* (*shi*), in the females, the investigators reported that males courted the mobile females at the permissive temperature but did not court the immobile females at the restrictive temperature. Investigators also noted that while female movement is important for courtship behavior, copulation is more likely to occur for those females who slow down at the end of the male courtship sequence. In fact, one aspect of female rejection is a rapid movement away from the male prior to the end of courtship.

Body size, age, experience, and the environment also affect courtship behavior and female receptivity in *Drosophila*. Lefranc and Bundgaard (2000) have shown that copulation duration and fecundity in *Drosophila melanogaster* are both dependent upon the size of the males and females. Small females mate faster but are less fecund than medium and large size females, while medium size males are more fecund than either large or small males. On the other hand, Partridge et al. (1987) and Ewing (1961) reported that large male size was important for courtship success in both *Drosophila melanogaster* and *Drosophila pseudoobscura*. In both species, larger males have a distinct advantage. The age and experience of the flies are also factors affecting courtship behavior and female receptivity. The age of males was shown to be important by Kosuda (1985) who reported that older *Drosophila melanogaster* males were consistently less active than were younger males. Koref-Santibanez (2001) found that in *Drosophila pavani* and *Drosophila gaucha* female receptivity decreases with experience while male activity increases with experience. In addition, *Drosophila gaucha* males show increased activity as they age whereas young *Drosophila parvani* females and old *Drosophila gaucha* females are less receptive. Observations of virgin versus postcopulatory females in experiments with *Drosophila melanogaster* have shown that females after copulation are less receptive than virgin females.

Drosophila melanogaster and *Drosophila pseudoobscura* coexist in nature but rarely inbreed. These two species show differences in the timing of their mating behavior. *Drosophila pseudoobscura* tends to mate just before darkness while *Drosophila melanogaster* has a peak of mating before dusk (Tauber et al. 2003). These reports show that mating behaviors are species specific and have led to discussions of the relation between mating behavior, circadian rhythms, speciation, and evolution (Rosato and Kyriacou 2001; Doi et al. 2001). (For a fuller discussion of circadian rhythms and their effect on behavior, see below.)

In a series of experiments Sakai et al. (2002) showed that the wavelength of light was important in triggering male sexual behavior. *Drosophila melanogaster* males are able to perform under both normal light and dark conditions. Their behavior, however, is reduced under ultraviolet and blue light. The importance of visual stimuli on male mating behavior has been shown by the observations of Tompkins et al. (1982) and Markow and Manning (1980), both of whom investigated mating behavior in flies carrying mutations that resulted in partial or complete loss of vision. Tompkins studied three mutations, *optomotor-blind*, *tan*, and *glass*, and showed that males carrying these genotypes had a much longer period of courtship before copulation than did wild-type flies. Markow and Manning compared the relative mating success of wild-type and *no-receptor-potential* mutant (blind) flies and showed that males with serious visual deficiencies had a lowered probability for successfully completing courtship. These data, together with those of Tompkins et al. (1982), indicate a synergistic relationship between female movement and the male's ability to discern this movement.

The genetic control of courtship and mating behavior in *Drosophila* has been a focal point for investigation since Sturtevant's original paper in 1915. A complete review of the earlier work may be found in Hall (1994). He has reviewed the literature on the genetic control of mating behavior in terms of its behavioral, physiological, and neurological aspects. While this current review is too brief to encompass all of the work leading up to more recent investigations, several points that Hall emphasized are relevant for this discussion. For example, any mutation in *Drosophila* that affects the frequency of male wing vibrations (the mating song) will have a major effect on the length and success of courtship before copulation. Mutations that result in reduced locomotor activity, visual and olfactory abnormalities of males and females, as well as learning and memory mutations all affect the mating process. For a listing and discussion of these mutations see the reviews by Hall (1994) and Yamamoto (1997) and the description of the mutations in Flybase@flybase.bio.indiana.edu.

One of the most interesting of these mutations, *fruitless* (*fru*), results in male bisexual behavior. Mutant males will court both males and females but most are incapable of copulation. The inability to copulate appears to be related to a neurological change that affects the formation of a male specific abdominal muscle. Since the male must bend his abdomen in order to insert his penis into the female genitalia, the anatomical abnormality prevents bending, and copulation does not occur. Evidence also shows that *fru* affects terminal arborizations of a number of abdominal muscle motor neurons, indicating a general neurological effect of the mutation as well.The *fru* males produce normal amounts of both sperm and seminal fluid, but those few males that do copulate appear to have difficulty transferring sperm and seminal fluid to the female. There is evidence that this inability to transfer semen is related to abnormalities of the serotonergic neurons in the reproductive organs (Lee et al. 2001).

Sex determination genes also affect mating behavior. Genotypical female (XX) adults carrying a hypomorphic *sex-lethal* (*Sxl*) mutation or a null *transformer* (*tra*) mutation court males, but these mutant females are themselves not attractive to males. Certain complications, however, must be taken into account in any study of behavioral changes caused by sex-determining genes. Both *Sxl* and *tra* are early acting genes in a cascade of gene effects resulting in male and female sex determination. Mutations further down in the cascade, e.g., *double-sex* (*dsx*) and *intersex* (*ix*), have little or no effect on behavior. Also, there is evidence that *tra*, in addition to its control of *dsx* activity, influences the expression of *fru* and *dissatisfaction* (*dsf*), both of which are involved in male courtship. Both of these genes have been implicated in the inability of the male to bend his abdomen at copulation, thus leading to low fecundity and a reduction of egg laying in the courted female (Yamamoto et al. 1998).

II. PHOTOTROPISM

As stated above, two of the earliest observations on behavior in *Drosophila melanogaster* were the burrowing of larvae into food and the positive attraction of adults to light. These observations led to a series of experiments that indicated that the two behavior patterns, negative phototropism in the larvae and positive phototropism in the adult, were common to all of the *Drosophila* species tested. The early literature concerned with the experimental designs used to study these behavior patterns has been reviewed by Rockwell and Seiger (1973). The recent experiments testing adult phototaxis has involved a T-maze (Jacob et al. 1977) or a Y-maze in which the flies are given a choice of a light or dark pathway or of pathways illuminated by monotonic and nonmonotonic light of different wavelengths. In addition to orientation toward light, visual fixation has been studied in wild-type adult flies. Bulthoff et al. (1982) reported that flies, given free choice, alternate between fixation and nonfixation of an inaccessible visual object. Competitive vision leading to random orientation between objects may explain a lack of pattern discrimination in adult flies.

Recent experiments have examined the physiological and genetic control of the adult response to light. Jacob et al. (1977) assayed wild-type and mutant flies. They found that wild-type flies had a significant response to visible light but a lesser response to ultraviolet light at 307 nm. *Drosophila* carrying a series of mutations that affected the optic apparatus showed reduced response to low doses of both yellow light and ultraviolet light when compared to the response of wild-type flies. A number of investigators (Stark 1975; Harris et al. 1976; Hu and Stark 1977, 1980; Heisenberg and Buchner 1977; Miller et al. 1981; Coombe 1984; Schaffel and Willmund 1985; Chou et al. 1996) have associated the phototropic behavioral responses to monochromatic light to specific mutations and to the presence and absence of specific photopigments in the eye. In an early investigation, Willmund and Fischbach (1977) related aberrant phototropic behavior after long exposure to blue light to mutations resulting in defects of the receptor cells in the ommatidia. These investigators have related a series of visually stimulated behavioral characteristics as diverse as fast walking and courtship to the presence and absence of specific photopigments.

The diverse behavioral responses by adult *Drosophila melanogaster* to light may be explained, in part, by the fact that the phototropic response itself is under polygenic control (Hirsch 1959; Hadler 1964a, 1964b). Hirsch was able to show specific chromosome influences on the phototropic response, using a Y-maze that he designed. Hadler, using a modification of Hirsch's Y-maze, was able to take flies with a neutral response to light and select for both positive and negative responses in the Y-maze. Dobzhansky et al. (1974) selected for phototropism in *Drosophila pseudoobscura*, using lights of different wavelengths and intensities. They observed that flies selected for photonegativity in the Y-maze responded negatively to white light and to visible light at low wavelengths but positively to red light above 670 nm. In a series of related experiments comparing the sibling species *Drosophila pseudoobscura* and *Drosophila persimilis*, Polivanov (1975) found that he could select for both positive and negative phototropism (as well as geotropism) within several generations.

The response to light by *Drosophila* larvae, on the other hand, appears to be consistent. The phototropic response has been shown to depend upon the larval stage (instar) of the organism and is intimately related to foraging behavior in the first and second instars and wandering behavior in preparation for pupation and metamorphosis in the late third larval instar. One method designed to measure the light response of larvae is the use of a petri dish containing clear agar. Prior to coating with agar, the outside of the bottom of the dish is quartered, and alternate quarters are painted black. In a darkroom the plate is placed on a platform over a hole through which light shines from below. No other light should enter the dish. A specific number of synchronized larvae at a specific developmental stage are then placed in the center of the dish. After a period of time (depending upon the experiment) the number of larvae in the dark and light quarters is counted. This procedure can be repeated for a number of trials, and the mean phototropic behavior (index) calculated.

Studies have shown that the response of larvae to light depends upon wavelength. Warrick et al. (1999) reported that larvae are repelled by, and are most responsive to, light at 500 nm, 420 nm, and 380 nm. This response is in contrast to the response of adults, which are attracted to 350 nm and wavelengths in the 515 nm to 550 nm range (Schumperli 1973; Miller et al. 1981).

III. LOCOMOTION RELATED TO FORAGING

In assessing the effect of light on foraging behavior, an investigator must be aware that other factors influence the locomotor activity of larvae. For example, Sokolowski et al. (1997) showed that locomotor paths were affected by genetic factors and larval density. Two alleles at the *foraging* (*for*) locus were selected: one a rover allele; the second, a sitter allele. Selection experiments showed that these two alleles controlled the path lengths for foraging and could respond to selection based on larval density. The role of genetics in the control of behavior may also be seen in the foraging response of larvae and the locomotor response of adults. Busto et al. (1999) showed that light-induced locomotion in adults and larvae is under the control of different genes affecting vision. It is clear, however, that this is not the complete explanation. Hassan et al. (2000) reported that certain mutations that affect adult vision also interfere with larval responses. Moreover, in a study of mutant and isofemale larvae, Warrick et al. (1999) showed that different mutant and isofemale lines had different locomotor responses to different wavelengths.

Care should always be taken, therefore, in obtaining measurements of foraging behavior and locomotor activity. Both of these behaviors have been shown to be under polygenic control. Shaver et al. (2000) reported that seven loci on the *Drosophila* second chromosome affect larval locomotion and two others affect foraging behavior. Connolly (1966) found that he could select for active and inactive lines from a heterogeneous Pacific strain of *Drosophila melanogaster*. A report by Shaver et al. (1998) illustrated additional complexities involved in measuring locomotor behavior in relation to olfactory responses in adult and larval *Drosophila*. Using *rover* and *sitter* alleles at the *for* locus in larval and adult stages, these investigators found that the olfactory response leading to changes in locomotor activity in mutant larvae was unchanged, but that the locomotor activity in adults was affected. In the adult mutant flies the locomotor response to yeast odors was affected but not the response to propionic acid, ethyl acetate, or acetone.

IV. OLFACTION

The measurement of olfactory responses in larval *Drosophila* is based on the attraction and/or the repulsion of larvae to specific chemical odorants. Washed larvae of a specific age are placed in the center of an agar-coated (1.2% to 1.4% agar) petri dish. Filter paper discs impregnated with the odor to be tested are placed along the periphery of the dish and the behavior of the larvae is noted. In this way a number of olfactants may be tested, both on wild-type larvae and on larvae from flies that have been treated with mutagens (Heimbeck et al. 1999). Smith (1996) has reported on a number of mutations that affect behavior in response to olfactory stimulants. These include defects in response to benzaldehyde and other aldehydes; isoamyl acetate, ethyl acetate, and other short chain acetates; ketones; and propionic acid. Evidence supports the presence of fifty-seven genes encoding a series of odorant receptors on the antennae and maxillary palps of the flies (Vosshall et al. 2000). The discrimination of odor is under the control of these genes that are responsible for the olfactory receptors and their neurological connections within the antennal glomeruli of the insect brain (Heimbeck et al. 1999; Vosshall et al. 2000).

One aspect of olfactory-induced behavior in *Drosophila* is that the response of the organism to specific olfactory stimulants may be learned. Scherer et al. (2003), using larval response as the test object, reported that when they paired odorants with positive (fructose) or negative (quinine) reinforcers, the larvae show associative learning between odorant and reinforcer. In a series of experiments using an apparatus that they described, Wuttke and Tompkins (2000) measured larval response to benzaldehyde, ethyl acetate, and propionic acid. Wuttke and Tompkins determined that adaptation to the odorants depended on concentration and dosage. They also showed that flies recovered from adaptation, and that this recovery depended on the transient receptor potential (TRP) calcium channel in adults but was independent of the TRP channel in larvae. [For a review of the neurobiology of olfaction in cyclorrhaphous larvae, including a list of olfactory agents, see Cobb (1999).]

While olfactory responses in adult *Drosophila* have been associated with specific receptors on specific structural elements in the fly, behavioral traits such as locomotion and geotaxis are more difficult to trace neurologically. The measurement of geotropic behavior is relatively simple. A known number of flies of a specific genotype, either wild-type or mutant, and of the same sex and age are placed in a cylinder, usually a plugged 28.5 by 95 mm vial. A line is drawn 80 mm from the bottom of the vial and the flies are allowed to acclimate. They are then shaken to the bottom of the vial, and after a determined time, the number of flies above the line is counted. After several trials, the numbers of flies above the line are averaged. This measure of climbing ability is used as the geotactic index. Care must be taken that the subjects tested do not have problems with their locomotor ability since it has been noted that locomotion and geotropism are closely related.

V. GEOTROPISM

Adult *Drosophila* collected from wild populations as well as those in laboratory collections are generally geotropically neutral. Several laboratories, however, have investigated strains showing geotropic behavior using selection techniques and have reported that the response is under polygenic control. Hostetter and Hirsch (1967) selected a series of positive and negative lines for geotropic behavior and subjected these lines to complementation tests. They determined that there was variability in the polygenic control between these lines. Walton (1968) selected for and investigated both positive and negative geotropic lines and confirmed that the responses were under polygenic control. In hybridization tests between the selected lines, his data suggested that the factors controlling positive phototrapism were primarily partial dominants while primarily recessive factors controlled negative phototropism. Experiments analyzing genetic control in both *Drosophila melanogaster* and *Drosophila pseudoobscura* have shown that the genes responsible for the geotropic behavior patterns are located on all of the chromosomes, the X-chromosome as well as the autosomes. Woolf et al. (1978) investigated sex-linked effects in *Drosophila pseudoobscura* and found factors favoring both positive and negative geotropism on the X-chromosome. Hirsch (1959), Pyle (1978), and Ricker and Hirsch (1988), studying both positive and negative lines in *Drosophila melanogaster*, showed that the three large chromosomes all contained factors that directed both positive and negative responses. Most recently, Toma et al. (2002), using cDNA microarrays, identified several genes that contribute to the polygenic control of this behavioral pattern. One point of interest concerning polygenic inheritance is the response of flies to selection for geotropism. Kessler et al. (1982) studied selection for and against geotaxis for over nineteen generations. Starting with a line that showed positive geotropic behavior, they found that they could decrease geotropism by the sixth generation of selection, after which the flies remained geotropically neutral. This correlates with the fact that six generations of brother-sister matings result in approximately ninety-five percent homozygosity in the selected lines.

VI. CLIMBING AND OTHER LOCOMOTOR BEHAVIOR

Multiple factors also affect other behavioral patterns. For example, Ganetzky and Flanagan (1978) investigated climbing ability as a measure of locomotor activity in older flies. The experiments were based on the casual observation that older flies showed less movement in culture bottles. They reported that on a time scale, an abrupt fifty percent decrease occurred in locomotor activity in older flies in both the Oregon-R and Canton-S strains of *Drosophila melanogaster*. Moreover, they found that the time of the decrease was later in Oregon-R flies than in the Canton-S flies and that this time difference correlated with the difference in life span between the two strains.

While Ganetzky and Flanagan reported that the abrupt loss of activity could be related to the life span of the flies, LeBourg (1987) found that the level of spontaneous locomotor activity did not influence the life span of either males or females. In addition, LeBourg et al. (1984) reported that spontaneous locomotor activity was independent of female fecundity and life span, and they hypothesized that the measure of this activity was a measure of the fitness of the flies. These observations on the relationship between age and locomotion have been confirmed. LeBourg (1983) reported that young flies show patterns of movement that result in dispersion while old flies tend to move in close relation to their release point. LeBourg and Lints (1984) investigated the sex of flies in relation to age and activity. They reported that females were more active than males at all ages and confirmed the observations that activity in both sexes decreased in older flies.

Observations by Ganetzky and Flanagan (1978) suggested the importance of the role of genotype in regulating locomotor activity, reporting differences in the aging effect on locomotion in two strains of their flies. Fernandez et al. (1999) investigated the relationship between genetics, aging, and locomotion and found that the aging effect differed in different strains of *Drosophila*. Their evidence indicated that genetics, aging, and locomotor activity had interwoven effects. In addition, aging affects behavior patterns other than climbing activity and locomotion. Fresquet and Medioni (1993) studied a conditioning effect in *Drosophila* and reported on the relationship between aging and conditioning. They trained individual flies to respond to olfactory stimulants related to a white negative reinforcer and a black non-reinforcer. The response measured was the Proboscis Extension Response (PER), which is regulated by tarsal receptors. The investigators found that training subjects to acquire conditional expression (e.g., the expression of the PER) under the influence of the negative reinforcer was more effective in younger flies. Because there is ample evidence that aging is under quantitative genetic control (Nuzhdin et al. 1997; Curtsinger and Khazaeli 2002), and because motor responses and memory (see below) are subject to polygenic control, investigating the interaction between age and conditioning as well as age and locomotion is extremely difficult.

VII. TEMPERATURE AND HUMIDITY

Drosophila also show strong response to both temperature and humidity. Sayeed and Benzer (1996), using a device that they designed, found that wild-type flies had a temperature gradient preference that peaked at 24°C and a response that resulted in flies aggregating at 22°C as opposed to 30°C. The investigators also tested two mutants of *Drosophila* that responded abnormally to temperature gradients. The first, *bizarre* (*biz*), was a sex-linked mutation that was isolated by countercurrent methodology. Flies carrying this mutation did not respond to temperature. The second was *spineless-aristapedia* (ss^a), a mutation in which the arista and the third antennal segment are changed into a leg. This latter mutation results in loss of the temperature preference. Ablation experiments removing parts of the antenna demonstrate that temperature receptors are present on the third antennal segment. Removal of the arista had no effect; removal of the third segment eliminated the response. Response to humidity was also shown to be associated with receptors on the antennal segments. Wild-type flies, when given a choice of wet or dry conditions, chose dry conditions in almost all cases. Flies that had intact third segments but from which the arista had been removed lost the humidity response and chose both wet and dry conditions at random. Temperature receptors are therefore found on the third antennal segment while humidity receptors are present on the arista. Zars (2001) confirmed the presence of a low temperature receptor on the antenna and also reported a high temperature receptor at a second unknown location in *Drosophila*.

VIII. NEURAL CONTROL OF BEHAVIOR IN *DROSOPHILA*

Scott et al. (2001) investigated gustatory and olfactory receptors in larvae and adults and traced their connections to the central nervous system. Gustatory receptors in larvae are found in the terminal organ and in the ventral pits. Olfactory receptors are found in the terminal organ and in the dorsal organ. These receptors send impulses to the antennal lobe (from the dorsal and terminal organ) and to the subesophageal ganglion (from the terminal organ and the mouth parts). In the adult fly, gustatory receptors are found in a number of organs including the proboscis, pharynx, wings, legs, and female genitalia. Olfactory receptors are found on the antennae. The olfactory neurons carry impulses to the antennal lobe of the adult brain while gustatory neurons carry impulses to the subesophageal ganglion where they synapse with neurons that mediate behavioral responses.

The role of the central nervous system in controlling behavior has been studied by a number of investigators. Two behavioral patterns, locomotion and olfaction, have been the main areas of investigation. Neural regulation of locomotor patterns was shown to be associated with the central complex of the *Drosophila* brain (for a review see Strauss 2002). Strauss and Heisenberg (1993) reported a high correlation between behavioral impairment and structural defects in the central complex. Varnam et al. (1996) investigated larval locomotor behavior associated with genes affecting the central complex and found normal motor control in these mutant larvae, ruling out a motor deficit for the behavioral change. Strauss et al. (1992) reported that a mutation causing a structural defect in the protocerebral bridge in the *Drosophila* brain slowed adult walking speed and occasionally resulted in a spastic stage.

The mushroom bodies and the pars intercerebralis in the central nervous system were also shown to control behavior. Changes in olfactory-related behavior have been related to changes in the mushroom bodies. Heisenberg et al. (1985)

studied two mutations affecting mushroom body structure and found that these mutations impaired olfactory conditioning. deBelle and Heisenberg (1994, 1996) reported that both genetic defects and treatment with hydroxyurea cause the loss of mushroom body Kenyon cell fibers, which in turn causes an inability of adult flies to respond to associative odor learning. In addition, a distinction has been found between olfactory memory acquisition and memory recall. Dubnau et al. (2001) and McGuire et al. (2001) have shown that synaptic transmission in the mushroom body is necessary for olfactory memory recall but not for memory acquisition and storage. Also, male-female sex behavior has been associated with a feminizing transgene that is expressed in the pars intercerebralis (Sylvain et al. 2000). Adult transgenic males act as females when the transgene is present in a cluster of pars intercerebralis cells. In all of these observations the behavioral change is associated with a structural or mutational change in a specific structure in the central nervous system.

Certain molecular changes in the brain, in addition to structural changes, influence behavioral patterns. Memory and learning are influenced by mutations in *dunce* (*dnc*) and *rutabaga* (*rut*), genes that are associated with the cAMP cascade (Tully 1984; Zhong and Wu 1991). These mutations result in changed levels of cAMP in the mutant flies. The *dnc* mutants lack phosphodiesterase activity leading to increased levels of cAMP, while *rut* mutants lack adenyl cyclase resulting in decreased cAMP. A third mutant, *cAMP-dependent protein kinase 1* (*Pka-C1*) affects protein kinase A activity, interfering with cAMP activity. The cAMP system, and its relation to olfactory learning, has been traced to the mushroom bodies in the brain (Davis et al. 1995; Connolly et al. 1996). Both *dnc* and *rut*, and a third mutation, *amnesiac* (*amn*), lead to changes in olfactory memory. Mutations in the latter gene affect pituitary adenylate cyclase-activating polypeptide, a neurotransmitter in both *Drosophila* and mammals, whose absence results in memory loss in both of these groups of organisms (Hashimoto et al. 2002).

There are neurophysiological effects other than those on neurotransmitters that affect behavior. Wang et al. (1997, 2002) studied mutations that affected Na^+ and K^+ channels and caused changes in locomotor activity. Mutations in the Na^+ channel associated with the mutant gene *paralytic* (*para*) caused paralysis at high temperatures (29°C) while a series of mutations in the K^+ channel caused muscular contractions, shaking, and quivering in adults and changes in locomotion in larvae. A mutation in *narrow abdomen* (*na*), a gene that controls Ca^{+2} channel activity, affected sensitivity to anesthetics and resulted in reversal of locomotor activity under light and dark conditions. This mutation affects ion channels related to voltage-gated sodium and calcium channels in the neuropile of the optic lobe and central complex (Nash et al. 2002). Physiological changes related to feeding drugs and alcohol to flies were also shown to affect behavior. Alcohol treatment results in increased walking behavior and locomotion up to those concentrations where sedation sets in (Singh and Heberlein 2000; Parr et al. 2001). McClung and Hirsh (1998) reported changes in grooming behavior and in locomotion associated with exposure to cocaine. A relationship between these drugs and the neurotransmitter pathway controlled by dopamine and the catecholamines has been reported (Bainton et al. 2000; reviewed in Rothenfluh and Heberlein 2002). In all of these experimental procedures it should be noted that anesthetizing *Drosophila* by either chilling them or administering CO_2 or ether affects behavior (Greenspan 1997). Barron (2000), investigating the effect of anesthesia on copulation latency, reported that CO_2 increased copulation latency more than did chilling the flies.

External factors that affect the physiology and molecular biology of *Drosophila* are clearly reflected in behavioral changes by the organism. Further, it is reasonable to conclude that "normal" behavior is also associated with the physiology and biochemistry of the fly, and that these latter characteristics are controlled by the genotype of the organism, a genotype that functions in both an internal and external environment. Behavior is a phenotype in the same sense that morphology, physiology, and biochemistry are phenotypes, all of which are a result of the interactions of the genotype with the environment. Mutations that cause a change in response to environmental conditions will cause changes in physiology and molecular biology and can thus be expected to be reflected in behavioral changes.

IX. CIRCADIAN RHYTHM

A further example of behavior controlled by a genetic response to external stimuli is the role of genes in the response by *Drosophila* to cycles of light and dark, the circadian rhythm. The genetic control of circadian rhythm and the changes that result in the response due to mutations are well documented (for a review of the genetic control of circadian rhythms see Hall 1998). The first gene that was isolated and found to be responsible for rhythmic activity in *Drosophila* was *period* (*per*), whose mutant alleles can cause either an increase or a decrease in the periodicity of activity. Mutations in *per*, together with a number of other mutant genes regulating rhythmic behavior, have been shown to be correlated with changes in the molecular biology of the fly (Hall 2003). These mutations affect circadian transcriptional control, protein stability, and other physiological parameters affecting rhythmic activity. Their products affect morphological characteristics as well as regulatory events in specific tissues and at specific times in development (Ceriani et al. 2002). Two of these mutations, *timeless* (*tim*) and *Disconnected* (*Disco*), were shown to be basic for the control of rhythmic activity. Mutations in *Disco* affect a number of morphological structures including neuronal connections apparently responsible for control in the central nervous system (Helfrich-Forster 1998). There is an apparent feedback loop involving *tim* and *per* together with two other genes, *Clock* (*Clk*) and cycle (*cyc*). These latter two genes code for transcription factors regulating *tim* and *per* activity (Rutilla et al. 1998; Stanewsky 2002; Ashmore et al. 2003).

Circadian activity, as well as the effects of external and physiological changes on behavior, has been classically measured by changes in locomotor activity. Other behaviors, however, are also affected by changes in circadian rhythms. Feeding behavior, olfaction, and sexual behavior are all under rhythmic control. Sakai and Ishida (2001) reported that female mating activity was controlled by *per* and *tim*, and Petersen et al. (1988) reported that periodicity controlled by *per* was different in different species of *Drosophila*. This difference in the timing of periodic locomotor behavior, which then leads to separable periods of courtship and sexual behavior, was postulated to be a mechanism of sexual isolation between species, possibly leading to evolutionary change (Tauber et al. 2003).

X. SUMMARY

All aspects of behavior are clearly under the genetic control of the physiology and morphology of the organism. Also, activity is complex and not due to a single behavioral response but to a number of genetically controlled responses (Sokolowski 2001). For example, mating behavior depends on locomotion, vision, mechanical stimulation, and olfaction, all of which are under genetic control. Circadian rhythms are influenced by at least eight major genes and a number of "minor" genes that affect locomotion, mating behavior, and eclosion time (Hall 2003). All of the latter behaviors are, in turn, controlled by complex physiological and molecular interactions. Memory and learning are influenced by mutations in three genes, *dnc*, *rut*, and *Pka-C1*, which affect the cAMP cascade. These mutations all affect activity in the mushroom body (Davis et al. 1995), supporting the role of the mushroom body and its connections in controlling complex behavioral patterns.

There are obvious complications in all organisms that result in problems for studying the control of behavioral and motor patterns. *Drosophila*, however, still possess important advantages for these studies. The central nervous system is amenable to study. While it is complex, it is still possible to sort out changes within the brain and the peripheral nervous system. More importantly, however, is the wealth of knowledge associated with the genetic control of behavioral responses in *Drosophila*. The genetic manipulations resulting in mutagenesis and transgenesis have become standard, and it is probable that deliberate interference with gene activity and intentional interference with physiological processes in *Drosophila* can lead to a fuller understanding of behavioral and motor functions in "higher" organisms.

References

Ashmore, L.J., S. Sathyanarayanan, D.W. Silvestue, M.M. Emersor, P. Schutland, and A. Sehgal. 2003. Novel insight into the regulation of the timeless protein. *J Neurosci* **23**:7810–7819.

Averhoff, W.W., and R.H. Richardson. 1974. Pheromonal control of mating patterns in *Drosophila melanogaster. Behav Genet* **4**:207–225.

Bainton, R.J., L.T. Tsai, C.M. Sinah, M.S. Moore, W.S. Neckameyer, and U. Heberlein. 2000. Dopamine modulates acute responses to cocaine, nicotine, and ethanol in *Drosophila. Curr Biol* **10**:187–194.

Barron, A.B. 2000. Anaesthetizing *Drosophila* for behavioral studies. *J Insect Physiol* **46**:439–442.

Bastock, M. 1956. A gene mutation which changes a behavior pattern. *Evolution* **10**:421–439.

Bulthoff, H., et al. 1982. Recurrent inversion of visual orientation in the walking fly, *Drosophila melanogaster. J Comp Physiol* **148**:471–481.

Busto, M., B. Iyengar, and A.R. Campos. 1999. Genetic dissection of behavior: modulation of locomotion by light in the *Drosophila melanogaster* larva requires genetically distinct visual system functions. *J Neurosci* **19**:3337–3344.

Ceriani, M.F., J.B. Hogenesch, M. Yanovsky, S. Panda, M. Straume, and S.A. Kay. 2002. Genome-wide expression analysis in *Drosophila* reveals genes controlling circadian behavior. *J Neurosci* **22**:9305–9319.

Chou, W.H., J.C. Hall, D.B. Wilson, C.L. Wideman, S.M. Townson, L.U. Chadwell, and S.G. Britt. 1996. Identification of a novel *Drosophila* opsin reveals specific patterning of the R7 and R8 photoreceptor cells. *Neuron* **17**:1101–1115.

Cobb, M. 1999. What and how do maggots smell? *Biol Rev* **74**:425–459.

Connolly, K. 1966. Locomotor activity in *Drosophila*. II. Selection for active and inactive strains. *Anim Behav* **14**:444–449.

Connolly, J.B., I.J. Roberts, J.D. Armstrong, K. Kaiser, M. Forte, T. Tully, and C.J. O'Kane. 1996. Associative learning disrupted by impaired Gs signaling in *Drosophila* mushroom bodies. *Sci* **274**:2104–2107.

Coombe, P.E. 1984. The role of retinula cell types in fixation behavior of walking *Drosophila melanogaster. J Comp Physiol A* **155**:661–672.

Curtsinger, J.W., and A.A. Khazael. 2002. Lifespan, QTLs, age specificity, and pleiotropy in *Drosophila. Mech Aging and Devel* **123**:81–93.

Davis, R.L., J. Cherry, B. Dauwalder, P.L. Han, and E. Skowlakis. 1995. The cyclic AMP system and *Drosophila* learning. *Mol Cell Biochem* **149/150**:271–278.

deBelle, J.S., and Heisenberg, M. (1994). Associative odor learning in *Drosophila* abolished by chemical ablation of mushroom bodies. *Sci* **263**:692–695.

deBelle, J.S., and M. Heisenberg. 1996. Expression of *Drosophila* mushroom body mutations in alternative genetic backgrounds: a case study of the *mushroom body miniature* gene (*mbm*). *Proc Natl Acad Sci U S A* **93**:9875–9880.

Dobzhansky, T., C.L. Judson, and O. Paulousky. 1974. Behavior in different environments of populations of *Drosophila pseudoobscura* selected for phototaxis and geotaxis. *Proc Natl Acad Sci U S A* **71**,:1974–1976.

Doi, M., M. Matsuda, M. Tomaru, H. Matsubayashi, and Y. Oguma. 2001. A locus for female discrimination behavior causing sexual isolation in *Drosophila. Proc Natl Acad Sci U S A* **98**:6714–6719.

Drapeau, M.D., A. Radovic, P.J. Wittkopp, and A.D. Long. 2003. A gene necessary for normal male courtship, *yellow*, acts downstream of *fruitless* in the *Drosophila melanogaster* larval brain. *J Neurobiol* **55**:53–72.

Dubrau, J., L. Grady, T. Kitamoto, and T. Tully. 2001. Disruption of neurotransmission in *Drosophila* mushroom body blocks retrieval but not acquisition of memory. *Nature* **411**:476–480.

Ewing, A. 1961. Body size and courtship behavior in *Drosophila melanogaster*. *Anim Behav* **9**:93–99.

Fernandez, J.R., M.D. Grant, N.M. Tulli, L.M. Karkowski, and G.E. McClearn. 1999. Differences in locomotor activity across the lifespan of *Drosophila melanogaster*. *Exp Gerontol* **34**:621–631.

Fresquet, N., and J. Medioni. 1993. Effects of aging on visual discrimination learning in *Drosophila melanogaster*. *Q J Exp Psychol B* **46**: 399–412.

Gantezky, B., and J.R. Flanagan. 1978. On the relationship between senescence and age-related changes in two wild-type strains of *Drosophila melanogaster*. *Exp Gerontol* **13**:189–196.

Greenspan, R.J. 1997. A kinder, gentler genetic analysis of behavior: dissection gives way to modulation. *Curr Opin Neurobiol* **7**:805–811.

Hadler, N.M. 1964a. Genetic influence on phototaxis in *Drosophila melanogaster*. *Biol Bull* **126**:264–273.

Hadler, N.M. 1964b. Heritability and phototaxis in *Drosophila melanogaster*. *Genetics* **50**:1269–1277.

Hall, J.C. 1994. The mating of a fly. *Sci* **264**:1702–1714.

Hall, J.C. 1998. Genetics of biological rhythms in *Drosophila*. In *Adv In Genet*. Vol. **38**:135–184. Eds. J.C. Hall, J.C. Dunlap, T. Friedmann, F. Giannelli, NY: Academic Press.

Hall, J.C. 2003. Genetics and molecular biology of rhythms in *Drosophila* and other species. In *Advances in Genetics*, Vol. **38**. Editors: J.C. Hall, J.C. Dunlap, T. Friedmann, F. Gianelli. New York: Academic Press.

Harris, W.A., W.S. Stark, and J.A. Walker. 1976. Genetic dissection of the photoreceptor system in the compound eye of *Drosophila melanogaster*. *J Physiol* **256**:415–439.

Hashimoto, H., N. Shirtani, and A. Baba. 2002. Higher brain functions of PACAP and a homologous *Drosophila* memory gene *amnesiac*: insights from knockouts and mutants. *Biochem Biophys Res Commun* **297**:427–431.

Hassan, J., M. Busto, B. Iyengar, and A.R. Campos. 2000. Behavioral characterization and genetic analysis of the *Drosophila melanogaster* larval response to light as revealed by a novel individual assay. *Behav Genet* **30**:59–69.

Heimbeck, G., V. Bugnon, N. Gendre, C. Haberlin, and R.F. Stocker. 1999. Smell and taste perception in *Drosophila melanogaster* larvae: toxin expression studies in chemosensory neurons. *J Neurosci* **19**:6599–6609.

Heisenberg, M. 1994. Central brain function in insects: genetic studies on the mushroom bodies and central complex in *Drosophila*. Ed. Schildberger, K., and Elsner N. In *Neural basis of behavioral adaptations*. pp. 61–79. Stuttgart: Fisher.

Heisenberg, M., and E. Buchner. 1977. Role of retinula cell types in visual behavior of *Drosophila melanogaster*. *J Comp Physiol A* **117**: 127–162.

Heisenberg, M., A. Borst, S. Wagner, and D. Byeys. 1985. *Drosophila* mushroom body mutants are deficient in olfactory learning. *J Neurogenet* 2:1–30.

Helfrich-Forster, C. 1998. Robust circadian rhythmicity of *Drosophila melanogaster* requires the presence of lateral neurons: a brain–behavioral study of *disconnected* mutants. *J Comp Physiol* **182**: 435–453.

Hirsch, J. 1959. Studies in experimental behavior genetics II. Individual differences in geotaxis as a function of chromosome variations in synthesized *Drosophila* populations. *J Comp Physiol Psychol* **52**: 304–308.

Hostetter, R.C., and J. Hirsch. 1967. Genetic analysis of geotaxis in *Drosophila melanogaster*: complementation between forward and reverse selection lines. *J Comp Physiol Psychol* **63**:66–70.

Hu, K.G., and W.S. Stark. 1977. Specific receptor input into spectral preference in *Drosophila*. *J Comp Physiol A* **121**:241–252.

Hu, K.G., and W.S. Stark. 1980. The roles of *Drosophila ocelli* and compound eyes in phototaxis. *J Comp Physiol A* **135**:85–95.

Jacob, K.G., R. Willmund, E. Folkers, K.-F. Fischbach, and H. Ch. Spatz. 1977. T-maze phototaxis of *Drosophila melanogaster* and several mutants in the visual systems. *J Comp Physiol* **116**:209–225.

Kessler, S., R.F. Rockwell, and L. Levine. 1982. Effects of selection for decreased movement through the *Drosophila* geotaxis maze *J Hered* **73**:381–382.

Koref-Santibanez, S. 2001. Effects of age and experience on mating activity in the sibling species *Drosophila pavani* and *Drosophila gaucha*. *Behav Genet* **31**:287–297.

Kosacla, K. 1985. The aging effect on male mating activity in *Drosophila melanogaster*. *Behav Genet* **15**:297–303.

Le Bourg, E. 1983. Patterns of movement and aging in *Drosophila melanogaster*. *Arch Gerontol Geriatr* **2**:299–306.

Le Bourg, E., and F.A. Lints. 1984. A longitudinal study of the effects of age on spontaneous locomotor activity in *Drosophila melanogaster*. *Gerontol* **30**:79–86.

Le Bourg, E. 1987. The rate of living theory. Spontaneous locomotor activity, aging, and longevity in *Drosophila melanogaster*. *Exp Gerontol* **22**:359–369.

Le Bourg, E., F.A. Lints, and C.V. Lints. 1984. Does a relationship exist between spontaneous locomotor activity, fitness, and lifespan in *Drosophila melanogaster*. *Exp Gerontol* **19**:205–210.

Lee, G., A. Villella, B.J. Taylor, and J.C. Hall. 2001. New reproductive anomalies in *fruitless*-mutant *Drosophila* males: extreme lengthening of mating durations and infertility correlated with defective serotonergic innervation of reproductive organs. *J Neurobiol* 47:121–149.

Lefranc, A., and J. Bundgaard. 2000. The influence of male and female body size on copulation duration and fecundity in *Drosophila melanogaster*. *Hered* **132**:243–247.

Markow, T.A., and M. Manning. 1980. Mating success of photoreceptor mutants of *Drosophila melanogaster*. *Behav Neural Biol* **29**:276–280.

McClung, C., and J. Hirsch. (1998). Stereotypic behavioral responses to free-base cocaine and the development of behavioral sensitization in *Drosophila*. *Curr Biol* **8**:109–112.

McGuire, S.E., P.T. Le, and R.L. Davis. 2001. The role of *Drosophila* mushroom body signaling in olfactory memory. *Sci* **293**:1330–1333

Miller, G.V., K.N. Hansen, and W.S. Stark. 1981. Phototaxis in *Drosophila*: R1-6 input and interaction among ocellar and compound eye receptors. *J Insect Physiol* **27**:813–819.

Nash, H.A., R.L. Scott, B.C. Lear, and R. Allada. 2002. An unusual cation channel mediates photic control of locomotion in *Drosophila*. *Curr Biol* **12**:2153–2158.

Nuzhdin, S.V., E.G. Pasyukova, C.L. Dilda, Z.B. Deng, and T.F. MacKay. 1997. Sex-specific quantitative trait loci affecting longevity in *Drosophila melanogaster*. *Proc Natl Acad Sci U S A* **94**:9734–9739.

Parr, J., A. Large, X. Wang, S.C. Fowler, K.L. Ratzlaff, D.M. Ruden. 2001. The inebri–actometer: a device for measuring the locomotor activity of *Drosophila* exposed to ethanol vapor. *J Neurosci Methods* **107**:93–99.

Partridge, L., A. Hoffman, and J.S. Jones. 1987. Male size and mating success in *Drosophila melanogaster* and *Drosophila pseudoobscura* under field conditions. *Anim Behav* **35**:468–476.

Petersen, G., J.C. Hall, and M. Rosbash. 1988. The *period* gene of *Drosophila* carries species-specific behavioral instructions. *The EMBO J* **7**:3939–3947.

Polivanov, S. 1975. Response of *Drosophila persimilis* to phototactic and geotactic selection. *Behav Genet* **5**:255–267.

Pyle, D. 1978. A chromosome substitution analysis of geotactic maze behavior in *Drosophila melanogaster*. *Behav Genet* **8**:53–64.

Ricker, J.P., and J. Hirsch. 1988. Genetic changes occurring over 500 generations in lines of *Drosophila melanogaster* selected divergently for geotaxis. *Behav Genet* **18**:13–25.

Rockwell, R.F., and M.B. Seiger. 1973. A comparative study of photoresponse in *Drosophila pseudoobscura* and *Drosophila persimilis*. *Behav Genet* **3**:163–174.

Rosato, E., and C.P. Kyriacou. 2001. Flies, clocks, and evolution. *Philos Trans R Soc Lond Biol Sci* **356**:1769–1778.

Rothenfluh, A., and U. Heberlein. 2002. Drugs, flies, and videotape: the effects of ethanol and cocaine on *Drosophila* locomotion. *Curr Opin Neurobiol* **12**:639–645.

Rutila, J.E., V. Suri, M. Le, W.V. So, M. Rosbash, and J.C. Hall. 1998. Cycle is a second bHLH–PAS clock protein essential for circadian rhythmicity and transcription of *Drosophila period* and *timeless*. *Cell* **93**:805–814.

Sakai, Y., and N. Ishida. 2001. Circadian rhythms of female mating activity governed by clock genes. *Proc Natl Acad Sci U S A* **98**:9221–9225.

Sakai, T., K. Isono, M. Tomaru, A. Fukatami, and Y. Oguma. 2002. Light wavelength dependency of mating activity in the *Drosophila melanogaster* species subgroup. *Genes Genet Syst* **77**:187–195.

Savarit, F., G. Sureau, M. Cobb, and J.F. Ferveur. 1999. Genetic elimination of known pheromones reveals the fundamental chemical basis of mating and isolation in *Drosophila*. *Proc Natl Acad Sci U S A* **96**:9015–9020.

Sayeed, O., and S. Menzer. 1966. Behavioral genetics of thermosensation and hydrosensation in *Drosophila*. *Proc Natl Acad Sci U S A* **93**:6074–6084.

Schaffel, E., and R. Willmund. 1985. Visual signals in the courtship of *Drosophila melanogaster* mutant analysis. *Insect Physiol* **31**:899–907.

Schumperli, R.A. 1973. Evidence for colour through spontaneous phototactic choice behavior. *J Comp Physiol A* **86**:77–94.

Scherer, S., R.F. Stocker, and B. Gerber. 2003. Olfactory learning in individually assayed *Drosophila* larvae. *Learn Mem* **10**:217–225.

Scott, K., R. Brady Jr., A. Grauchik, P. Morozov, A. Rzhetsky, C. Zuker, and R. Axel. 2001. A chemosensory gene family encoding candidate gustatory and olfactory receptors in *Drosophila*. *Cell* **104**:661–673.

Shaver, S.A., C.J. Varnam, A.J. Hilliker, and M.B. Sokolowski. 1998. The foraging gene affects adult but not larval olfactory-related behavior in *Drosophila melanogaster*. *Behav Brain Res* **95**:23–29.

Shaver, S.A., C.A. Riedl, T.L. Parkes, M.B. Sokolowski, and A.J. Hilliker. 2000. Isolation of larval behavioral mutants in *Drosophila melanogaster. J Neurogent* **14**:193–205.

Shorey, H.H., and R.J. Bartell. 1970. Role of a volatile female sex pheromone in stimulating male courtship in *Drosophila melanogaster*. *Anim Behav* **18**:159–164.

Singh, C.M., and U. Heberlein. 2000. Genetic control of acute ethanol-induced behavior in *Drosophila*. *Alcohol Clin Exp Res* **24**:1127–1136.

Smith, D.P. 1996. Olfactory mechanisms in *Drosophila melanogaster*. *Curr Opin Neurobiol* **6**:500–505.

Sokolowski, M. 2001. *Drosophila*: genetics meets behavior. *Nat Rev Genetics* **2**:879–890.

Sokolowski, M.B., H.S. Pereira, and K. Hughes. 1997. Evolution of foraging behavior in *Drosophila* by density-dependent selection. *Proc Natl Acad Sci U S A* **94**:7373–7377.

Stanewsky, R. 2002. Clock mechanisms in *Drosophila*. *Cell Tissue Res* **309**:11–26.

Stark, W.S. 1975. Spectral sensitivity of visual response alterations mediated by interconversions of native and intermediate photopigments in *Drosophila*. *J Comp Physiol A* **96**:343–356.

Strauss, R. 2002. The central complex and the genetic dissection of locomotor behavior. *Curr Opin Neurobiol* **12**:833–838.

Strauss, R., and M. Heisenberg. 1993. A higher control center of locomotor behavior in the *Drosophila* brain. *J Neurosci* **13**:1852–1861.

Strauss, R., U. Hanesch, M. Kinkelin, R. Wolf, and M. Heisenberg. 1992. *No-Bridge* of *Drosophila melanogaster*: portrait of a structural brain mutant of the central complex. *J Neurogen* **8**:125–155.

Sturtevant, A.H. 1915. Experiments in sexual recognition and the problem of sexual selection in *Drosophila*. *J Anim Behav* **5**:351–366.

Sylvain, G., G. Jean-Francois, and F. Jean-Rene. 2000. Genetic identification of neurons controlling a sexually dimorphic behavior. *Curr Biol* **10**:667–670.

Tauber, E., H. Roe, R. Costa, J.M. Hennessy, and C.P. Kyriacou. 2003. Temporal mating isolation driven by a behavioral gene in *Drosophila*. *Curr Biol* **13**:140–145.

Toma, D.P., K.P. White, J. Hirsch, and R.J. Greenspan. 2002. Identification of genes involved in *Drosophila melanogaster* geotaxis, a complex behavioral trait. *Nat Genet* **31**:349–353.

Tompkins, L., J.C. Hall, and L.M. Hall 1980. Courtship-stimulating volatile compounds from normal and mutant *Drosophila*. *J Insect Physiol* **26**:689–697.

Tompkins, L., A.C. Gross, J.C. Hall, D.A. Gailey, and R.W. Siegel. 1982. The role of female movement in the sexual behavior of *Drosophila melanogaster. Behav Genet* **12**:295–307.

Tully, T. 1984. *Drosophila* learning: behavior and biochemistry. *Behav Genet* **14**:527–557.

Vosshall, L.B., A.M. Wong, and R. Axel. 2000. An olfactory sensory map in the fly brain. *Cell* **102**:147–159.

Walton, P.D. 1968. The genetics of geotaxis in *Drosophila melanogaster*. *Can J Genet Cytol* **10**:673–687.

Wang, J.W., A.W. Sylwester, D. Reed, D.A. Wu, D.R. Soll, and C.F. Wu. 1997. Morphometric description of the wandering behavior in *Drosophila* larvae: aberrant locomotion in the Na^+ and K^+ channel mutants revealed by computer-assisted motion analysis. *J Neurogent* **11**:231–254.

Wang, J.W., D.R. Soll, and C.F. Wu. 2002. Morphometric description of the wandering behavior in *Drosophila* larvae: a phenotypic analysis of K^+ channel mutants. *J Neurogenet* **16**:45–63.

Warrick, J.M., M.F. Vakil, and L. Tompkins. 1999. Spectral sensitivity of wild-type and mutant *Drosophila melanogaster* larvae. *J Neurogenet* **13**:145–156.

Willmund, R., and K.F. Fischbach. 1977. Light induced modification of phototactic behavior of *Drosophila melanogaster* wildtype and some mutants in the visual system. *J Comp Physiol* **118**:261–271.

Woolf, C.M., H.M. Sasmor, and T.A. Markow. 1978. Positive and negative geotaxis: sex-linked traits in *Drosophila pseudoobscura*. *Behav Genet* **8**:65–71.

Wuttke, M.S., and L. Tompkins. 2000. Olfactory adaptation in *Drosophila* larvae. *J Neurogent* **14**:43–62.

Yamamoto, D., J.M. Jallon, and A. Komatsu. 1997. Genetic dissection of sexual behavior in *Drosophila melanogaster*. *Ann Rev Entomol* **42**:551–585.

Yamamoto, D., K. Fujitani, K. Vsui, H. Ito, and Y. Nakano. 1998. From behavior to development: genes for sexual behavior define the neuronal sexual switch in *Drosophila*. *Mech Devel* **73**:135–146.

Zars, T. 2001. Two thermosensors in *Drosophila* have different behavioral functions. *J Comp Physiol* [A] **187**:235–242.

Zhong, Y., and C-F. Wu, 1991. Altered synaptic plasticity in *Drosophila* memory mutants with a defective cyclic AMP cascade. *Sci* **251**: 198–201.

CHAPTER

A8

Use of *C. elegans* to Model Human Movement Disorders

GUY A. CALDWELL, SONGSONG CAO, IYARE IZEVBAYE, and KIM A. CALDWELL

"Ye have made your way from the worm to man, and much within you is still worm."

(F. Nietzsche, *Thus Spake Zarathustra*)

The recent completion of the human genome sequence not only represents a most significant milestone for our species and the science of biology, but is also a scientific cornerstone in our biomedical foundation for understanding the molecular basis of inherited disorders (Lander et al. 2001; Venter et al. 2001). Greater than 11,000 genetic loci for Mendelian traits have been identified, yet only approximately 1500 of these have known mutations associated with them at this time. As the fields of bioinformatics and molecular genomics continue to expand, an exponentially increasing number of genetic contributions to disease etiology will be discerned.

As disease susceptibility is further defined by specific changes in DNA via single-nucleotide polymorphisms and with expression changes delineated by microarray analyses, we will increasingly mark our respective genomes with uncharacterized factors. These molecular "tags" for specific characteristics, many of which will be linked to poorly understood cellular processes, hasten the need for subsequent discovery. The current and growing challenge to biomedicine lies in determining the functional significance of genetic alterations in the context of both normal and disease mechanisms. In this regard applying comparative genomics, via simple animal models, toward investigating functional relationships conserved through evolution among organisms represents a rapid route toward a comprehensive understanding of cellular malfunction.

I. *C. ELEGANS:* WHY THE WORM?

Starting in the early 1960s, Sydney Brenner championed the establishment of the nematode *Caenorhabditis elegans* as a model system for investigating embryonic and neuronal development (Wood 1988). Brenner's vision was centered upon the premise that the simplicity of *C. elegans* anatomy and genetics, coupled with its ease of culturing, manipulating, and rapidly generating (three days from fertilized egg to adult), would render it experimentally accessible for discerning more complex issues of development (Brenner 1974). Notably, although males can result from rare chromosomal non-disjunction events, *C. elegans* is primarily found as a hermaphrodite. The ability of this animal to self-fertilize is especially advantageous for purposes of laboratory propagation and in designing genetic crosses.

Literally hundreds of isogenic animals can be obtained from a single worm in the course of several days, making stock expansion trivial. Moreover, these microscopic worms (~1 mm as an adult) can be stored frozen, much like bacterial and yeast cultures, and revived to replenish stocks even after several years.

II. TOOLS OF THE WORM TRADE

The greatest strength of *C. elegans* as an animal model system is its use for screening purposes—be those genetic, genomic, or chemical. Several technical advances in *C. elegans* research have placed this nematode directly in the forefront of modern biological analysis. Both green fluorescent protein (GFP)-expression analyses and double-stranded ribonucleic acid (dsRNA)-mediated inhibition of gene function (RNA interference-RNAi) were developed and popularized in *C. elegans* (Chalfie et al. 1994; Fire et al. 1998). In late 1998, *C. elegans* truly ushered in the genomic era for metazoan species, as it became the first animal to have its complete genome sequence released (*C. elegans* Sequencing Consortium 1998). This milestone enabled rapid and comprehensive molecular analyses to join powerful traditional genetic resources—all in the context of a multicellular organism. These new tools augmented existing and unique resources for this animal, such as a defined neuronal connectivity and fully mapped cell lineage (Bargmann 1998).

While traditional genetic mutagenesis and screening for suppressors and enhancers of increasingly discerning phenotypes will remain a staple in the technical repertoire of worm researchers (Jorgensen and Mango 2002), the advent of RNAi has revolutionized *C. elegans* phenotypic analysis. RNAi is a method by which a native intracellular mechanism that specifically degrades mRNA can be induced by the presence of double-stranded RNA (dsRNA) that corresponds to a segment of any given gene (Fire et al. 1998). RNAi directed against specific target genes can be performed in *C. elegans* by several means that are distinguished by the manner in which dsRNA is introduced into animals: (1) microinjecting dsRNA (Fire et al. 1998), (2) soaking through the cuticle (Tabara et al. 1998), or (3) feeding worms bacteria producing a specific dsRNA (Timmons et al. 2001). Parental hermaphrodites are typically treated for RNAi and their progeny exhibit altered phenotypes that are scored in these cases. Additionally, heritable RNAi, in stable transgenic lines that contain vectors expressing either heat-shock or specific promoter-controlled expression of dsRNA, offers an alternate means to introduce RNAi into specific *C. elegans* cell types (Tavernarakis et al. 2000). This latter approach offers the advantage of generating a stable strain of RNAi-producing animals allowing for multigenerational analyses (assuming lethality is not the RNAi phenotype being induced!). One caveat to generating these strains is the difficulty of cloning inverted repeat segments of genes into the appropriate expression vectors, as bacteria typically reject or induce rearrangements of such fragments. Additional concerns are the ability of RNAi to spread across tissue boundaries, thus making cell-specific effects difficult to interpret, and reports that RNAi may be less effective in neurons. While the latter concern is debated, a range of mutants in the systemic RNAi mechanism are being identified and will likely resolve such issues in the near future (Simmer et al. 2002; Feinberg and Hunter 2003).

Worms eat bacteria. In laboratory environs, this translates into *C. elegans* dining on lawns of *E. coli.* The utility of RNAi feeding has been exploited in high-throughput screening for both embryonic and post-embryonic phenotypes using chromosomal libraries of *individually* cloned genes that can produce dsRNA to target nearly every predicted open-reading frame in *C. elegans* (Kamath et al. 2001, 2003). These data sets include a variety of phenotypic information ranging from overt lethality and visible uncoordination to time-lapse digital videos of mitotic defects in embryogenesis. While these large-scale RNAi screens have yielded much important information, it is vital to recognize that in most cases these data represent a preliminary analysis and merely set the stage for subsequent, more detailed studies or secondary screens. Nevertheless, the ability to rapidly knock down the activity of large sets of individual genes is extraordinarily powerful, especially considering the homology that exists in this organism with respect to many conserved gene families among metazoans.

The leadership role that *C. elegans* has taken in the genomics field goes beyond genome sequencing and harkens back to the formation of some of the initial bioinformatics databases for any species. This rich tradition has expanded into the twenty-first century with the development of a variety of pooled resources. Mature database information (wormbase.org) contains a wealth of genetic mutational data, RNAi screen results, knock-out strains, protein interaction data, gene expression patterns and microarray analyses. These valuable resources are freely accessible to the scientific community (Kim et al. 2001; Harris et al. 2003). For example, the combined data from hundreds of microarray experiments by different investigators has enabled worm researchers to chart gene topology maps, wherein co-expressed genes can be cataloged and coordinated with data on RNAi phenotypes or other mutants to stimulate more rapid functional analysis of novel genes. This type of combined integrated analysis is currently unique to this animal model and allows rapid exploration of experimental leads.

Multicolored GFP variants for labeling and co-localization studies and a new calcium-sensitive GFP (chameleon) have expanded the range of reporter gene applications in this transparent nematode (Miller et al. 1999; Kerr et al. 2000). Moreover, recent advances in short-term cell culturing techniques for *C. elegans* have enabled worm researchers to couple GFP technology with fluorescence-activated cell-sorting (FACS) methods (Christensen et al. 2002). This advance allows cell cultures from specific mutant populations of animals to be amenable to separation, thus facilitating mRNA isolation for refined microarray experiments. In this manner, *C. elegans* researchers are identifying genetic factors contributing to everything from synaptic specificity to aging.

Clearly, the valuable attributes of this microscopic worm are vast. As the realm of modern post-genomic analysis expands, this tiny nematode is once again leading the way. Large-scale projects are in the works to acquire crystal structures for every protein comprising this animal and to discern all putative protein-protein interactions within its cells (Walhout et al. 2000; Adams et al. 2003). It is very likely that *C. elegans* is already the best understood animal on our planet and will continue to be so for years to come. Perhaps the ultimate validation of *C. elegans* as an exceptionally useful model organism has come just recently; Sidney Brenner's insight has been appropriately rewarded by the scientific community with his receipt of the 2002 Nobel Prize in Medicine, along with fellow worm pioneers, John Sulston and H. Robert Horvitz.

III. AS THE WORM TURNS: APPLICATION OF *C. ELEGANS* TO MOVEMENT DISORDERS RESEARCH

While numerous and significant technical inroads have been made in recent years, the complexity of the mammalian nervous systems is generally intractable to detailed mechanistic analysis of many features associated with the development of movement disorders.

The anatomically transparent, genetically malleable nematode roundworm, however, is ideal for the analysis of neurological dysfunction (Wood 1988). Whereas the human brain contains 10^{11} neurons, *C. elegans* has only 302 neurons (even adult fruit flies are estimated to have greater than 100,000 neurons). Despite this simplicity, the nematode nervous system contains all of the hallmarks of neuronal function in higher organisms (Bargmann 1998). These include ion channels and transporters, neurotransmitters (serotonin, dopamine, acetylcholine, GABA), neuropeptides, synaptic junction components, and axon pathfinding cues (netrins, which were first discovered in worms).

C. elegans is capable of complicated behaviors, many of which are directly associated with specific neurotransmitters and neuromuscular responsiveness. These include locomotive uncoordination, egg-laying, pharyngeal pumping, chemotaxis, thermosensation, defecation, mechanosensory response, and more (Wood 1988). The availability of numerous molecular markers and a complete neuronal "wiring diagram" for *C. elegans,* wherein the connections between each and every neuron and muscle have been mapped via serial reconstruction of electron micrographs, represents an unprecedented resource for any animal model system (White et al. 1976). Perhaps a common misconception in modeling neurological disease mechanisms in invertebrates is the assumption that a "movement disorder" must involve a similarly discernable phenotypic characteristic, such as a convulsion or uncoordinated locomotion. While this is certainly true in some cases, many times less direct or overt changes in cellular malfunction may illuminate the functional aspects of disease mechanism. For example, a deficit leading to a tremor in a human might manifest itself as altered egg-laying or defecating in a worm. The conservation of underlying cellular function remains paramount in discerning the validity of such comparisons.

The ability to rapidly perturb behaviors or assess cellular activity, in the context of an intact animal with defined neuronal processes, is highly advantageous for directly linking genetic abnormality to anatomical structure and protein function. In this regard, multiple investigators and biotechnology companies are currently exploiting *C. elegans* for the insights it may provide into disease mechanisms related to human movement disorders. Here we attempt to provide an overview of some recent work in the development of worm models for probing the function of gene products implicated in specific movement disorders.

IV. DYSTONIA: MOVEMENT ON THE WORM FRONT

Dystonia is a term used to describe a series of clinically similar neurological movement disturbances characterized by involuntary muscle contractions, which force certain parts of the body into abnormal, sometimes painful, movements or postures. Dystonia can affect any part of the body including the arms and legs, trunk, neck, eyelids, face, or vocal cords. Classification of dystonia is typically performed in association with age of onset, physical location of symptoms, and etiology or cause (Bressman 2003). Dystonia is a complex disorder from both a clinical and molecular perspective and interplay between environmental factors and genetic predisposition is clearly at work in the establishment of symptomatic features.

Early-onset generalized torsion dystonia is the most severe and common form of primary hereditary dystonia and is characterized by twisting contortions and muscle contractions that begin in childhood, typically beginning in the legs or trunk and moving to other body parts with age. This autosomal dominant disorder (DYT1) is associated with specific deletions in a gene (*TOR1A*), encoding a protein termed torsinA (Ozelius et al. 1997, 1999; Leung et al. 2001). Individual carriers of DYT1 deletions have 30–40% chance of exhibiting disease symptoms (Bressman 2003). Evolutionary conservation of the *DYT1* gene family, termed torsins, is evident in the genomes of all completely sequenced metazoan species to date including mice, zebrafish, fruit flies, and nematodes, and provides a framework for comparative genomic analysis in animal models.

C. elegans contains three predicted torsin-related protein coding sequences in its genome. These include the *tor-1*, *tor-2*, and *ooc-5* genes (Basham and Rose 1999, 2001; Caldwell et al. 2003a). While all three gene products share significant sequence similarity with human torsins, *C. elegans tor-1* and *tor-2* lie adjacent to each other on chromosome IV of *C. elegans*. This is intriguing for two reasons: (1) the genes encoding human torsinA and a related protein, torsinB, are also adjacently positioned on human chromosome 9q34 (Ozelius et al. 1997); and (2) *C. elegans* genes often lie in operons (Blumenthal et al. 2002). This conservation of genomic positioning implies these genes may have arisen via a tandem duplication of a common evolutionary precursor. The worm *tor-1* and *tor-2* genes lie in the same direction, separated by just 348 bases of sequence; whereas human torsinA and torsinB lie adjacent but in opposite orientations (Ozelius et al. 1997; Caldwell et al. 2003a). As operons are common in *C. elegans,* the small intergenic distance between the nematode *tor-1* and *tor-2* genes suggests that they may be present within a single co-expressed operon unit and may function together (Blumenthal et al. 2002). Two additional gene products of unknown function also lie just 161 bases downstream from *tor-2* and have been shown to be part of a putative polycistronic expression unit (Blumenthal et al. 2002). To date, correctly spliced and isolated cDNA sequences have been obtained only for the *tor-2* and *ooc-5* gene products (Caldwell et al. 2003a). Despite exhaustive efforts to isolate the *tor-1* cDNA, it remains elusive, perhaps suggesting this open-reading frame may be one of the many abundant pseudogenes found in the worm genome (Caldwell, G.A., unpublished observations; Mounsey et al. 2002).

Although causative mutations for early-onset torsion dystonia have been known for years, a cellular activity associated with torsinA could be inferred only from several lines of convergent evidence. Phylogenetic analysis of the torsin protein family indicates these proteins share distant sequence similarity with the large and diverse family of AAA+/HSP/Clp-ATPase proteins (Neuwald et al. 1999; Ozelius et al. 1999; Vale 2000). As this group includes such functionally divergent gene products as the molecular motor protein dynein, cellular proteases, transcriptional regulators, proteosome subunits, and molecular chaperones, no definitive activity for torsins could be discerned by primary sequence analysis alone. While the predicted *tor-1* and *tor-2* proteins of *C. elegans* end with a sequence (NDEL) reminiscent of an ER-retention signal, no such motif is present on either the *OOC-5* protein or human torsinA, although both of these proteins have also been shown to exhibit ER localization (Basham and Rose 2001; Kustejdo et al. 2000; Caldwell et al. 2003a).

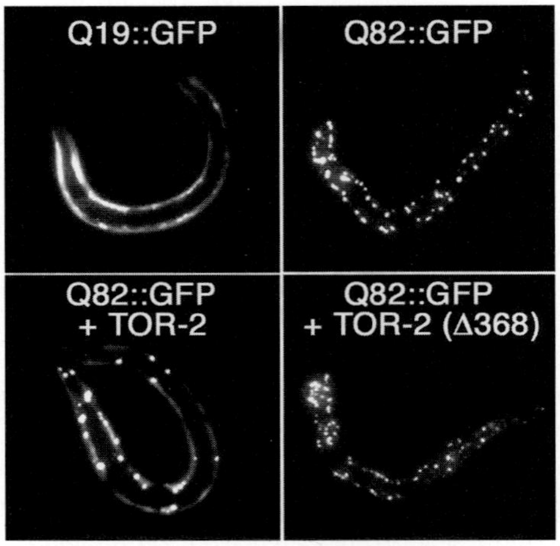

FIGURE 1 *C. elegans* strains containing integrated transgenes expressing polyglutamine-GFP fusions with and without TOR-2 or mutant TOR-2 (Δ368) protein. Suppression of protein aggregation is evident in the presence of wild-type torsin, whereas the mutant is incapable of this activity.

The experimental advantages of *C. elegans* have demonstrated the first direct evidence of a cellular activity associated with torsins in an animal model system (Caldwell et al. 2003a). Using an *in vivo* assay for investigating states of intracellular polyglutamine repeat-induced protein aggregation in living animals (Satyal et al. 2000), it was shown that ectopic overexpression of a *C. elegans* torsin homolog, *tor-2,* causes a dramatic and sustained reduction of polyglutamine-dependent protein aggregation in a manner similar to that previously reported for molecular chaperones (Figure 1). The same suppressive effects on aggregation were evident following overexpression of human torsinA in transgenic nematodes. The suppressive effects of *tor-2* overexpression persisted as animals aged, whereas a mutant torsin (Δ368) engineered to mimic a deletion found in dystonia was incapable of ameliorating aggregate formation (Figure 1; Caldwell et al. 2003a). These data conclusively demonstrate that torsins can mediate protein folding *in vivo.* Consistent with putative chaperone function, both human torsinA and endogenous *C. elegans tor-2* are co-immunolocalized with markers of the endoplasmic reticulum (Kustedjo et al. 2000; Caldwell et al. 2003a). Additional studies involving torsin overexpression in both cell cultures and in *C. elegans* demonstrated that torsins can reduce the formation of aggregates of human α-synuclein, a gene product linked to familial forms of Parkinson disease (McLean et al. 2002; Izevbaye and Caldwell, unpublished observations).

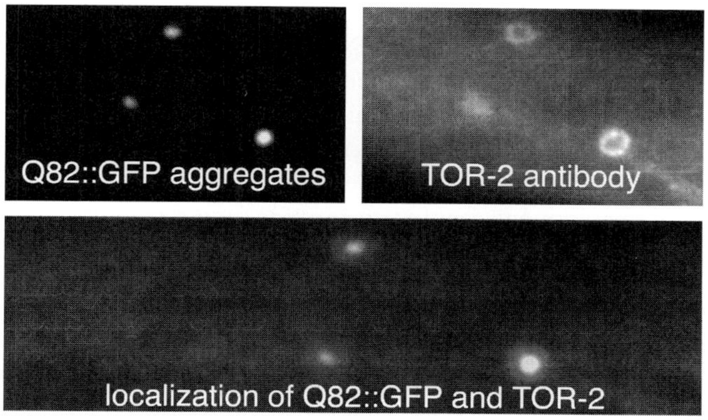

FIGURE 2 Immunolocalization of TOR-2 in transgenic *C. elegans* overexpressing polyglutamine aggregates (Q82::GFP) and torsin. Animals exhibit strong torsin localization to sites of protein aggregation when stained with antibody recognizing TOR-2.

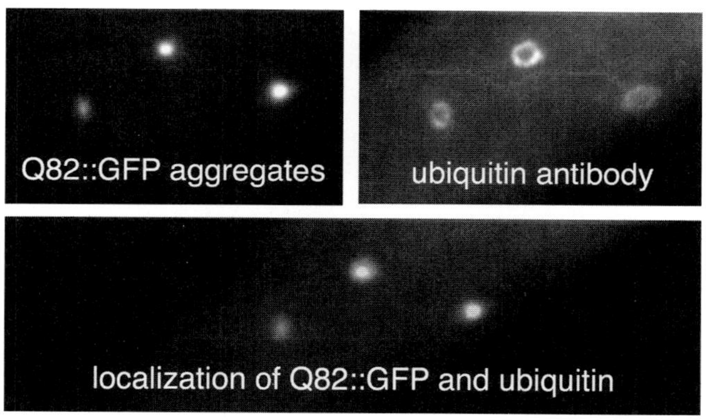

FIGURE 3 Immunolocalization of ubiquitin in transgenic *C. elegans* overexpressing polyglutamine aggregates (Q82::GFP) and torsin. Animals exhibit strong ubiquitin localization to sites of protein aggregation when stained with antibody recognizing polyubiquitin.
Video. Transgenic *C. elegans* expressing a polyglutamine fusion to GFP (Q82::GFP) in the body wall of muscle cells. Aggregates of fluorescent protein are readily apparent.

Antibody staining of transgenic *C. elegans* using antibodies specific to *tor-2* indicated this protein was highly localized to sites of protein aggregation (Figure 2), along with ubiquitin (Figure 3), a protein degradation-targeting signal (Caldwell et al. 2003). Walker et al. (2003a) also found torsin/ubiquitin localization when examining torsinA localization in brain tissue from genetically confirmed cases of Huntington disease (HD) and spinocerebellar ataxia type III. This co-localization is similar to that of ubiquitin-containing cellular inclusions termed "aggresomes" (Kopito 2000). Postmortem tissues from patients with Parkinson disease (PD) uncovered intense immunoreactivity for torsinA in protein aggregates termed Lewy bodies (Shashidharan et al. 2000a; Shashidharan et al. 2000b). Using FRET (fluorescence resonance energy transfer), Sharma et al. (2001) also demonstrated that torsinA is in close physical proximity to α-synuclein, the principal component of Lewy bodies. Given the existing links between protein degradation machinery and genes implicated in PD (Ciechanover and Brundin 2003; Cookson 2003), it is intriguing to consider that torsin proteins may partially mediate cellular "quality control" processes that monitor protein misfolding or aggregation and these processes may significantly influence neuronal activity. Thus, human and worm torsin proteins can function as molecular chaperones in preventing the aggregation of misfolded proteins (McLean et al. 2002; Caldwell et al. 2003). While these data are compelling in support of a putative role for torsins in the cellular management of protein misfolding, dystonia is not known as a disease of protein aggregation, and no such pathological consequences are associated with torsin malfunction. Given the low penetrance of symptoms in mutant DYT1 carriers, environmental factors or subtle causes of stress may evoke altered cellular responses that exceed a hypothetical threshold of susceptibility that results in the disease state.

The expression of human torsins in the dopaminergic neurons of the substantia nigra suggests that dystonia may also be a manifestation of cellular malfunction in dopamine release or signaling (Augood et al. 1999, 2003). Dopamine neurons are also implicated in dystonia by virtue of the enzyme GTP cyclohydrolase I (GTPCH), an essential enzymatic component in the synthesis of the tyrosine hydroxylase co-factor tetrahydrobiopterin. Mutations in GTPCH are linked to an autosomal dominant form of dystonia where, unlike the case for DYT1 and other dystonias, patients respond dramatically to L-dopa treatment (Ichinose et al. 1994). These same neurons are acutely susceptible to oxidative stress and oxidative damage and specific proteins within these neurons may represent a possible cause of neuronal malfunction associated with dystonia. Hewett et al. (2003) have demonstrated that torsinA in cell cultures appeared to be up-regulated in response to oxidative stress. Likewise, overexpression of either worm *tor-2* or human torsinA results in significant neuroprotection from the oxidative stress associated with dopamine-specific toxicity in *C. elegans* (Cao and Caldwell, unpublished observations).

Further investigation into a role for torsins in preventing cellular stress will depend on discerning the consequences of aberrant torsin activity and identifying additional neuroprotective co-factors that may enhance normal torsin function (Caldwell et al. 2004). While no neuronal function or expression is reported for *C. elegans ooc-5*, mutants in this torsin homolog exhibit defects in nuclear rotation and spindle positioning in early worm embryogenesis (Basham and Rose 1999, 2001). The application of *C. elegans* genetics toward isolating genetic suppressors or enhancers of either the *ooc-5* phenotype or protein aggregation may reveal novel gene products in torsin function and clarify components in the functional pathway leading to early-onset torsion dystonia (Caldwell et al. 2004). Candidate effectors from such genetic screens can be quickly examined for putative neuronal expression patterns and phenotypically examined by RNAi to lead to a more rapid evaluation of potential mechanistic interactions between proteins.

These combined insights notwithstanding, the precise cellular function of torsin proteins remains undefined and the pathophysiology of dystonia is a mystery (Walker and Shashidharan 2003b). The absence of obvious neurodegeneration in dystonia argues that more subtle causes of cellular dysfunction produce disease symptoms. Furthering our understanding of the molecular basis of dystonia will depend upon revealing the functional properties and interactions of torsins. In this regard, a variety of animal models for both normal and mutant torsin protein activity are a fundamental prerequisite for future investigation. The powerful assay systems that now exist for assessing torsin activity in *C. elegans* establish this nematode as a prime resource for identifying torsin effector molecules and genetic components linked to dystonia. The clinical similarities between different forms of inherited dystonias suggest an underlying commonality of cellular dysfunction. The recent identification of the *DTT12* gene encoding a Na^+/K^+-ATPase linked to rapid-onset dystonia parkinsonism may represent a point of functional convergence that can be evaluated in *C. elegans*, as this protein is highly conserved (de Carvalho Aguiar et al. 2004). This microscopic worm may lead the way to identifying conserved genetic factors responsible for this family of debilitating disorders, and provide possible clues to therapeutic avenues for preventing their incapacitating effects.

V. TO PROTECT AND SERVE: *C. ELEGANS* AND PARKINSON DISEASE

PD is a slowly progressive neurodegenerative disease characterized by resting tremors, postural instability, slow movement, rigidity, and difficulty initiating movements. By the time symptoms appear, over 70% of the dopaminergic neurons projecting from the *substantia nigra pars compacta* to the striatum are lost, resulting in a greater than 90% reduction in striatal dopamine. In addition, the formation of Lewy bodies, eosinophilic cytoplasmic inclusions characteristically found in post-mortem brains from PD patients, occurs in the surviving dopaminergic neurons.

PD is likely a heterogeneous group of related disorders with numerous etiological factors contributing to its pathogenesis. These include oxidative stress from toxin exposure and free radical formation, mitochondrial dysfunction, and inflammation (Halliwell 1992; Grunblatt et al. 2000). Age is also noted as the most consistent risk factor with 3% of the population above the age of sixty-five affected (Lang and Lozano 1998). Many rare genetic mutations are identified in familial cases of PD, including α-synuclein (or PARK1) located on chromosome 4q21, parkin (PARK2) on 6q25–27, DJ-1 (PARK7) on 1p36, and ubiquitin terminal hydrolase (PARK5) on 4p14, and PINK1 (PARK6) on 1p35–36 (Kruger et al. 1998; Polymeropoulos et al. 1997; Gasser 1998; Kitada et al. 1998; Bonifati et al. 2003; Valente et al. 2004). These genes suggest potential mechanisms for the development of PD. α-synuclein, a 140 amino acid protein, is the predominant aggregate-forming component of Lewy bodies (Spillantini et al. 1997). It is a pre-synaptic protein of uncertain function implicated in dopamine-dependent oxidative stress toxicity; this cellular stress leads to neurodegeneration (Goedert 2001; Xu et al. 2002). Additional gene products implicated in PD are components of the ubiquitin proteasome pathway (UPS), a major cellular mechanism that provides defense against misfolded proteins. Combined, these genetic facts infer that a considerable link exists between cellular mechanisms of protein degradation and disease susceptibility (Ciechanover and Brundin 2003).

Many disease models elucidate the pathogenesis of PD and help identify therapeutic targets. An ideal model should not only replicate all the features observed in the human disease (e.g., chronically progressive neurodegeneration, age-dependent motor deficits, presence of Lewy bodies in surviving neurons, and responsiveness to L-dopa) but should also be amenable to both genetic and biochemical dissection and high-throughput drug screening. Though multiple models recapitulate many of these features, some are more suited to studying specific aspects of the disease process. However, no single model meets all these criteria and valuable insights may be gathered from a variety of sources.

Numerous cell culture models are particularly important in the biochemical analysis of α-synuclein and parkin expression and their interaction with respiratory chain function, oxidative stress, and various cellular components associated with essential processes [e.g. Endoplasmic Reticulum-Associated Degradation (ERAD) and the Unfolded Protein Response (UPR)] (Cookson 2003; Ciechanover and Brundin 2003). While cell culture experiments represent rapid and simple access to experimental results, they fall short in recapitulating the postmitotic factors at play in dopaminergic neurons of intact, developed animals. Thus, omnipresent questions of unregulated and transient gene expression artifacts are unresolved in such systems (Danda et al. 2000; Hsu et al. 2000; Tanaka et al. 2001).

Toxin-induced rodent models for PD typically involve the administration of one of three chemicals, specifically MPTP, 6-OHDA, or rotenone. This exposure causes acute dopaminergic neuronal cell death in mice or rats (Bloem et al. 1990; Adams and Odunze 1991). The toxins act by inhibiting mitochondrial complex I. Though these models generally do not form Lewy bodies (except for rotenone-induced models) they encapsulate the clinical characteristics of PD. These models also highlight the role of the immune system and inflammation in PD and have contributed immensely to present development of drug and surgical therapies (Bloem et al. 1990). Transgenic mice expressing wild-

TABLE 1 *C. elegans* Genes Involved in Catecholamine Regulation and Transport

Gene (with open reading frame #)	Protein	Reference
cat-1 (W01C8.6)	Vesicular monoamine transporter (VMAT)	Duerr et al., 1998
cat-2 (B0432.5a)	Tyrosine hydroxylase (TH)	Lints and Emmons, 1999
bas-1 (C05D2.4)	Aromatic l-amino acid decarboxylase (AAAD)	Loer and Kenyon, 1993
cat-4 (unidentified)	GTP cyclohydrolase I (GTPCH)	Loer and Kenyon, 1993
dat-1 (T23G5.5)	Dopamine transporter (DAT)	Jayanthi et al., 1998
R13G10.2	Monoamine oxidase (MOA)	Sulston et al., 1992
C48D5.1	Nurr1 homolog (NHR)	BLAST search
K01C8.3	Dopa decarboxylase (DDC)	BLAST search
F01F1.9	Aldehyde dehydrogenase (ALD-D)	BLAST search
H13N06.5	Catecholamines up (Catsup)	BLAST search

type or various mutant forms of α-synuclein also exhibited motor deficits but lacked the selective dopaminergic neurodegeneration and Lewy bodies characteristic of PD (Goedert et al. 2001). While such rodent models are useful, and are generally preferred for more clinically relevant analyses, they remain limited by the complex genetics of mammals.

In contrast, invertebrate models open the door to powerful genetic analyses that can provide significant insights into disease mechanisms. A transgenic *Drosophila* model for PD expressing either wild-type or mutant α-synuclein showed age-dependent motor impairment. Furthermore, dopaminergic neurodegeneration with cytoplasmic aggregates that closely resembled Lewy bodies at the ultrastructural level were observed (Feany and Bender 2000). These results closely capture the essential features of PD and also characterize gene expression profiles through the life cycle of these model animals to identify changes that presage disease development (Scherzer et al. 2003).

C. elegans is a recently emerging tool for the study of PD (Wintle and Van Tol 2001). As a simple metazoan system, it can complement the findings from higher eukaryotic models. Worms are genetically tractable and can be easily manipulated to characterize biological components implicated in PD (e.g., aging, apoptosis, necrosis). Most significantly, as *C. elegans* is amenable to high-throughput screening for drug development, it represents a potentially powerful tool for revealing therapeutic aspects of PD.

C. elegans hermaphrodites possess four bilaterally symmetric pairs of dopamine neurons [two pairs of CEP and one pair of ADE neurons in the head region and one pair of PDE neurons in a posterior lateral position (White et al. 1976)]. These neurons function primarily in mechanosensory transmission and while deficits do not produce motor impairment akin to what have been described in humans, these neurons contain the full complement of components required for dopamine neurotransmission (table 1; Sulston et al. 1992; Loer et al. 1993; Jayanthi et al. 1998; Lints et al. 1999; Duerr et al. 1999; Sawin et al. 2000). The dopamine transporter (DAT) plays a particularly important role in dopaminergic neuronal toxicity. It serves as the transporter for both dopamine and the toxins 6-OHDA and MPTP (Adams et al. 1991; Du et al. 2001). Transporter expression in non-neuronal cells produces susceptibility to otherwise neuronal-specific toxins, thereby indicating this protein is necessary and sufficient for uptake (Javitch et al. 1985; Kitayama et al. 1992; Pifl et al. 1993; Glinka et al. 1997).

A *C. elegans* model for the study of PD was constructed in which transgenic worms were generated that expressed GFP driven by the promoter of the *C. elegans dat-1* gene (Nass et al. 2002). In this system, the morphology of dopamine neurons was easily visualized by fluorescence microscopy and could be scored over short times in these intact, anatomically transparent, animals. This model was used to examine 6-OHDA-induced neurodegeneration and demonstrated, like other models, that this process depended on *dat-1* mediated transport, but involved *ced-3* and *ced-4* independent pathways. This data differs slightly from studies performed in cell cultures that implicate apoptosis as a pathway to neurodegeneration (Tanaka et al. 2001). While this is not a disease model in the strictest sense, it serves as a marker of dopaminergic neuronal integrity and offers the opportunity to identify molecular determinants of toxin-induced neurodegeneration via genetic screens for suppressors and enhancers of 6-OHDA sensitivity. In addition, similar studies may be performed with genetic mutants in characterized cell death pathways (e.g., necrosis, apoptosis). These methodologies may lead to the delineation of a dopaminergic neuronal cell death pathway. The potential also exists to identify additional factors that evoke unknown environmental insults leading to oxidative stress in PD. In this regard, worms are also a useful model for high-throughput screening for chemicals and genes that may function in neuroprotection.

Molecular pathways and markers of aging are well characterized in *C. elegans* (Braeckman et al. 2001; Herndon et al. 2002; Lithgow et al. 2002), thus positioning the nematode as a powerful tool for investigations of aging in PD. Numerous factors are associated with this process. Aging brains show reduced mitochondrial respiration in the *substantia nigra* (DiMonte 1991) and dopamine levels also decrease with age in various parts of the mammalian brain (Goicoechea et al. 1997). Fruit flies also exhibit an age-dependent decline in dopaminergic transmission (Neckameyer et al. 2000). Neurons are postulated to become more susceptible to oxidative stress with aging (Parkes et al. 1998). Oxidative damage to proteins, specifically in dopamine neurons, may represent a small but significant "seed" source of misfolded proteins that lead to subsequent toxicity or aggregation (Pattison et al. 2001; Tavernarakis and Driscoll 2002; Beal 2003). Taken together, some current theories of aggregate diseases attribute the age-related neurodegeneration to toxicity from time-dependent accumulation and progression of protein aggregation.

Using numerous long-lived mutants and recently characterized aging phenotypes and molecular markers in this animal, investiagors have an opportunity with *C. elegans* to assess the specific contribution of aging to neurodegeneration. In 6-OHDA experiments, scientists can investigate the age-related neuronal susceptibility to oxidative stress of both wild-type and long-lived mutants. A powerful approach for identifying factors associated with age-related decline is to combine gene-specific targets defined by microarray experimentation and RNAi methodologies for knocking down putative effector genes in aging pathways. For example, resistance to oxidative stress or additional age-related cellular changes in neurotransmission may be identified (Murphy et al. 2003; Lee et al. 2003).

In recent phase II clinical trials coenzyme Q (CoQ), a component of the mitochondrial respiratory chain, showed multiple beneficial effects on PD patients (Beal 2003). In *C. elegans*, animals defective in the *clk-1* gene (which normally produces a mitochondrial polypeptide involved in the synthesis of CoQ) exhibit an exogenous CoQ-required increase in longevity (Larsen and Clarke 2002). CoQ is involved in mitochondrial respiratory transport and fatty acid oxidation and it functions as an antioxidant (Trumpower et al. 1981; Frerman et al. 1988; Ernster et al. 1995). Exogenous CoQ, while retaining its antioxidant activity, does not completely repair the mitochondrial functions of *clk-1* animals (Felkai et al. 1999). Oxidative stress experiments comparing neurodegeneration in wild-type versus post-larval CoQ-replete animals and CoQ-deficient animals may potentially reveal mechanisms of actions for toxins. Furthermore, contributions from anti-oxidant effects of CoQ on mitochondrial dysfunction could be studied with *clk-1* mutations (Jonassen et al. 2001).

Another *C. elegans* model related to PD involved transgenic animals expressing wild-type and mutant human α-synuclein controlled by various *C. elegans* neuronal promoters: pan-neuronal, dopaminergic, and motor neuron-specific promoters (Lakso et al. 2003). Though evidence of dopaminergic neuron loss emerged in this model, it seemed limited to a developmental defect and not necessarily to age-related neurodegeneration. Furthermore, α-synuclein aggregation was either absent or rarely occurred. Motor deficits occurred, but mainly in animals expressing α-synuclein in the non-dopaminergic motor neurons. Despite these incongruent data, the model may prove useful for investigating dopamine-dependent neurotoxic effects related to α-synuclein (Xu et al. 2002). For example, comparative effects of neurodegeneration mediated by reactive oxygen species within dopamine-deficient *C. elegans* mutants and wild-type animal backgrounds may provide insights into the recently revealed effects that α-synuclein overexpression may have on PD-related progression (Singleton et al. 2003).

Expression of α-synuclein-specific aggregates in other cell types, such as the readily visualized and well-studied body wall muscles of *C. elegans*, would be a useful tool because *C. elegans* neurons are notoriously small for conclusive evaluation of factors that may affect protein misfolding and degradation. Forward and reverse genetic screens with such a model would help correlate the contribution of specific gene products with the course of aging (Herndon et al. 2002; Tavernarakis and Driscoll 2002). For example, the worm homologs of PD-associated genes (table 2) such as the E3 ligase parkin or recently identified DJ-1 gene, could be assessed and would establish a system for rapidly assessing co-factors for α-synuclein effects (Kitada et al. 1998; Bonifati et al. 2003). Coupling primary tests or screens in body wall muscles to assays for secondary effects in loss or gain of neuroprotection in worm dopamine (or other) neurons may point to novel genetic factors influencing Parkinson's pathology. The complete set of chromosomal RNAi libraries for *C. elegans* is being used to assess phenotypes for specific gene families associated with cellular processes such as the ERAD and UPR pathways. This assessment represents an initial foray into genomic-scale analysis of putative PD-related gene effectors in *C. elegans* (Izevbaye, Hamanic and Caldwell and Caldwell, unpublished observations). Worm models of this type allow rapid examination of gene-specific effects over time, as animals age, since the established molecular markers of *C. elegans* aging are currently evaluated in body wall muscle cells (Herndon et al. 2002).

C. elegans has only begun to be exploited for elucidating multiple aspects of PD pathology. This model system is poised for functional analyses of both ectopic and endogenous factors of the disease. Harnessing the powerful genetic,

TABLE 2 *C. elegans* Genes Exhibiting Amino Acid Sequence Similarity to Gene Products Implicated in Human Movement Disorders

Human disease	Human gene	*C. elegans* ORF #	BLASTp (*P* value)
Amyotrophic lateral sclerosis	SOD1	C15F1.7	3.8e–45
Angelman syndrome	UBE3A	Y48G8AL.1	6.4e–150
		Y65BR.4a	5.1e–41
Ataxia telangiectasia	ATM	Y48G1BL.2	4.7e–64
Dentatorubral-pallidoluysian atrophy	ATROPHIN-1	F42A6.7	1.2e–68
Early-onset torsion dystonia	DYT1	Y37A1B.13 (*tor-2*)	2.3e–63
		C18E9.11 (*ooc-5*)	5.0e–59
		Y37A1B.12 (*tor-1*)	9.6e–56
Friedreich ataxia	FRATAXIN (FRDA)	F59G1.7 (*frh-1*)	2.5e–25
Dopa-responsive dystonia	GCH1 (DYT5)	F32G8.6	1.1e–92
Rapid-onset dystonia parkinsonisn	ATP1A3 (DYT12)	B03G5.3 (eat-6)	0
Parkinson disease	PARKIN	K08E3.7	8.8e–57
	UCH-L1	F46E10.8	1.6e–30
	DJ-1	B0432.2	5.5e–46
		C49G7.11	3.1e–36
	PINK1	EEED8.9	2.1e–53
Spinocerebellar ataxia type-1	SCA-1	K04F10.1	3.0e–20
Spinocerebellar ataxia type-2	SCA-2	D2045.1 (*atx-2*)	7.9e–16
Spinocerebellar ataxia type-3	SCA-3	F28F8.6	5.2e–41
Spinocerebellar ataxia type-6	SCA-6	T02C5.5 (*unc-2*)	0
Wilson disease	WND	Y76A2A.2	1.1e–248

genomic, proteomic, and bioinformatic tools of worm biology to discern the molecular nature of PD and related movement disorders will likely reveal significant mechanistic insights for years to come.

VI. POLYGLUTAMINE-RELATED DISEASES: WORMING OUT THE AGGRAVATION OF AGGREGATION

Polyglutamine (polyQ) diseases are neurological disorders grouped together with a common feature—they all result from glutamine residues expanding within proteins; a repeated codon (CAG) in the corresponding genes causes this expansion. At least nine degenerative disorders are caused by polyQ expansions in otherwise unrelated proteins (Zoghbi and Orr 2000). These disorders include Huntington's disease (huntingtin), spinal and bulbar muscular atrophy (SBMA; androgen receptor), dentatorubral and pallidoluysian atrophy (DRPLA; atrophin-1), and a number of spinocerebellar ataxias (SCA; ataxins). All of these mutant proteins seem to undergo conformational changes and eventually form misfolded protein aggregates within cells. Controversy has risen about the role of this aggregration in the neuronal loss associated with these disorders (Michalik and Van Broeckhoven 2003). While neuronal loss is a consistent feature among these diseases, it occurs only in specific regions of the brain in each disorder. Nevertheless, there are some brain regions in common, including the basal ganglia, brainstem nuclei, cerebellum, and spinal motor nuclei (Ross 1995). The pathological features present in these regions are the hallmarks of polyQ disorders, which distinguish them from other neurodegenerative disorders, such as Alzheimer disease and Parkinson disease.

Although investigators have rigorously studied these disorders, a plethora of unanswered questions still remain: (1) what are the exact molecular mechanisms underlying polyQ-induced protein aggregation? (2) what is the subcellular localization of polyQ aggregates? (3) what is the mechanism by which specific proteins (e.g., molecular chaperones) protect cells from aggregates? and (4) arguably most importantly, does aggregation have a protective role in, or toxic effect on neuronal loss (Michalik and Van Broeckhoven 2003)? To solve these mysteries, researchers have developed polyQ-protein related models in several different systems, including *C. elegans*, *Drosophila*, mice, and cell culture.

The many advantages of *C. elegans* biology described previously can be applied to the study of polyQ disorders. The worm model can be used to assess the functional consequences of genetic perturbation of putative polyQ effector genes. The obvious disadvantage of using worms could be an inability to translate pathogenesis to vertebrates if it arises from factors specific to more complex animals. Most of the primary responsible proteins for these disorders are not native to *C. elegans*; thus the information derived from ectopic experimentation in this simple system might not precisely reflect what occurs in vertebrates. Nevertheless, current *C. elegans* models have successfully reproduced specific aspects of the disease conditions and have thus far validated this animal as a very useful model system for studying polyQ-related dysfunction. Here we review the current knowledge gained from *C. elegans* concerning the general properties of polyQ aggregates, the relationship between polyQ aggregates and toxic effects, and modifiers of polyQ aggregate formation and cytotoxicity. Finally, we outline a few suggestions for future research directions in this area.

As pathologically diverse as different polyQ disorders are, they all involve intracellular polyQ aggregates that form in the respective affected brain regions. The tendency toward aggregation of proteins containing extended polyQ tracts is demonstrated in a variety of systems, both *in vivo* and *in vitro*. The first reports of polyQ aggregation in *C. elegans* came from two seminal papers (Faber et al. 1999; Satyal et al. 2000). Faber and colleagues (1999) showed that expression of human huntingtin (Htn) fragments containing 2, 23, or 95 polyglutamine repeats did not result in any detected aggregation in ASH sensory neurons. In contrast, fragments containing 150 polyglutamine repeats (Htn-Q150) resulted in protein aggregates, specifically in the cytoplasm (nuclear protein aggregates were not detected). These results suggested that a length threshold for polyQ-containing proteins to aggregate in ASH neurons was exceeded in the case of the 150Q fragment. Satyal et al. (2000) directed expression of polyQ-induced protein aggregation to the body wall muscle cells of *C. elegans*. With fusion of GFP to either 19 polyQ repeats (Q19-GFP) or 82 polyQ repeats (Q82-GFP), discernable differences in fluorescent protein aggregate formation could be visualized using fluorescent microscopy. In stark contrast to the diffuse and soluble fluorescence observed in Q19-GFP fusion, expression of a Q82-GFP fusion resulted in visibly distinct aggregates of GFP (see video). These aggregates were insoluble under mild denaturing conditions, but soluble under higher concentration of denaturant, indicating that the aggregates formed do not involve covalent linkages. These aggregates were also localized to cytoplasm in a perinuclear location (Satayl et al. 2000).

Both of these reports appear partly contradictory to studies from other systems with respect to the intracellular localization of aggregates. Human neuronal cell lines showed that the primary site of aggregation for huntingtin fragment was the nucleus (Saudou et al. 1998). Investigators obtained similar results in mice, wherein aggregates also formed in the nucleus when ataxin-1 was expressed in Purkinje cells (Davies et al. 1997). However, polyQ aggregation is not always exclusively nuclear and has sometimes been detected in the cytoplasm (DiFiglia et al. 1997; Onodera et al. 1997; Paulson et al. 1997). Several factors could explain the discrepancies between *C. elegans* and other model systems. First, localization studies in transgenic mice were usually done in postmortem tissues, and physiological changes after the death of the animals may account for some differences. Second, the subcellular localization could depend on the local context of the protein; thus different disease models expressing different proteins in different animals (or cells) might yield different results, even when using the same protein. Moreover, if a slightly different gene fragment is fused with polyQ, it might change the protein subcellular localization as well. Interestingly, studies in cell culture have identified a conserved Nuclear Export Signal (NES) sequence in huntingtin that is present among several vertebrate species, but no Nuclear Localization Signal (NLS) has been identified (Xia et al. 2003). Another plausible explanation could be that *C. elegans* cells, particularly neurons, are relatively small compared to mammalian cells and, consequently, the scale of aggregation is smaller. Therefore, microscopically discernable aggregates in the nucleus may not be visible without electron microscopy. Finally, species-specific differences in expression levels could also account for the observed differences.

Previous studies have established 35 to 40 polyQ repeats as the threshold for disease-related symptoms to emerge in humans (Huntington Disease Collaborative Research Group 1993; Duyao et al. 1993). Taking advantage of the short lifespan of *C. elegans*, Morley et al. (2002) determined that the threshold for polyQ aggregation was dynamic and influenced by aging. At day three, the threshold was 40, whereas at days four and five, the threshold shifted to 33 or 35, while at days nine and ten, the threshold shifted to 29. This finding is in line with the well-documented clinical onset of Huntington's disease being in reverse correlation with the length of polyQ expansion. These researchers also found that the lifespan-extending mutation in *C. elegans*, *age-1*, delayed the onset of polyQ aggregation, thereby suggesting that polyQ aggregation may at least partly share a common pathway with cellular mechanisms affecting the aging process in this animal.

An issue that is under extensive scrutiny in the protein aggregation field is whether or not polyQ aggregates have a causal effect on neurotoxicity or are protective in nature (Michalik and Van Broeckhoven 2003). Seemingly contradictory data have arisen on both sides of this debate. Morley et al. (2002) expressed polyQ repeats tagged with GFP in the body wall muscle of *C. elegans* and found that the motility of the worms is affected when aggregates form. While this suggests that toxicity is directly correlated to the polyQ aggregation, these experiments could not distinguish between the aggregates themselves causing the toxicity or aggregates being a byproduct of the toxicity.

To better mimic human disease conditions, polyQ toxicity studies in worms have also been extended to neurons. The polyQ-induced neuronal toxicity appeared in both sensory neuron ASH and mechanosensory neuron PLM (Faber et al. 1999; Parker et al. 2001). Expression of Htn-Q150 led to progressive ASH neurodegeneration but no cell death. Progressive cell death and enhanced neurodegeneration were observed in ASH neurons only when a sub-threshold dose of a toxic OSM-10::GFP fusion was co-expressed. These results suggest that other factors likely play a role in the pathogenesis of polyQ diseases in humans, wherein in a different onset age the same length of polyQ repeats may result. Interestingly, Htn-Q95, which greatly exceeds the canonical threshold, did not result in aggregation and neurodegeneration. However, Parker et al. (2001) demonstrated that a Htn-Q88 fusion formed aggregates in PLM neurons wherein the touch sensitivity of these mechanosensory cells was altered. Interestingly, in the Htn-150 expression experiments aggregate formation preceded the neurodegeneration (Faber et al. 1999). Similar results were obtained in PLM neurons where neuronal dysfunction also preceded cell death (Parker et al. 2001). More interestingly, the ASH neuronal death depended on *ced-3* caspase function, indicating the cell death observed was apoptotic. Taken with studies in other model systems, researchers can conclude that differences in cell, tissue, and species specificity have an impact on determining a strict threshold for polyQ aggregation. The findings in worms are generally consistent with the findings in human disease conditions: polyQ length, progressive degeneration, and neurotoxicity are accompanied by aggregation. Therefore, *C. elegans* appears to be a suitable model for assessing polyQ toxicity and has proven useful for identifying factors influencing the process.

To better understand the mechanism underlying polyQ aggregation and cytotoxicity, and to more effectively prevent and control polyQ diseases, investigators have devoted much effort to searching for the modifiers of polyQ aggregation. Studies in *C. elegans* have found proteins that specifically interact with the huntingtin fragment containing polyQ expansion. Genetic screening for specific suppressors of polyQ toxic effects identified an evolutionarily conserved protein of unknown function, PQE-1 (Faber et al. 2002). Loss of *polyQ enhancer-1* (*pqe-1*) gene function strongly and specifically exacerbated neurodegeneration and cell death, whereas overexpression of a *pqe-1* cDNA protected *C. elegans* neurons from the toxic effects of expanded Htn-polyQ fragments. The enhanced cell death in *pqe-1* was unchanged in *pqe-1;ced-3* double mutants, indicating the *pqe-1* does not play a direct role in the apoptotic cell death pathway.

Although *pqe-1* contains a glutamine/proline-rich domain, direct interaction between *pqe-1* and Htn-Q150 was not detected (Faber et al., 2002). These results suggest that *pqe-1* does not directly bind to Htn-Q150 but potentially protects neurons by binding Q-rich cellular targets, shielding them from inappropriate interactions with expanded huntingtin fragments. Alternatively, *pqe-1* may actually bind to soluble or aggregate forms of Htn-Q150 in the nucleus; however, these are not microscopically discernable. These hypotheses are not necessarily mutually exclusive. Since binding is dependent only upon its Q-rich domain, *pqe-1* should not discriminate between Htn-Q150 and other Q-rich nuclear proteins, despite the fact that the binding kinetics might be different. Nevertheless, the fact that nuclear localized PQE-1 can suppress neurodegeneration suggests that neurotoxicity is more likely associated with the nucleus, as several known Q-rich cellular targets affected by polyQ are transcription factors (Faber et al. 1998; McCampbell et al. 1998; Nucifora et al. 2001). Notably, Q-rich transcription factors were not identified in genetic screening for effectors of polyQ toxicity. This may not be surprising, as transcription factors like CBP and Sp1 have such an essential role that worms with mutations in them will not be viable.

In another screen using the yeast two-hybrid system to identify interactors with huntingtin, Holbert et al. (2003) identified the *C. elegans* gene K08E3.3b. The gene product encoded by this gene is an SH3 domain protein with a human homolog termed Cdc42-interacting protein 4 (CIP4). CIP4 is a protein involved in Cdc42 and Wiskott-Aldrich syndrome protein-dependent signal transduction. Cdc42 is a Rho family member that controls the actin cytoskeleton while CIP4 is a downstream target of Cdc42 (Aspenstrom 1997). Interaction between huntingtin fragment and K08E3.3b was augmented with the expansion of polyQ repeats. This finding links Huntington disease to Rho GTPase-regulated signaling pathway, possibly because the expansion of polyQ repeats in Htn initiates an inappropriate interaction between huntingtin and CIP4 and causes the disruption in the Cdc42 signaling pathway through CIP4, followed by disorganization of the neuronal cytoskeleton. In support of this theory, CIP4 accumulated in HD brain tissues and the overexpression of CIP4 in striatal neurons induced cell death (Aspenstrom 1997).

Other general modifiers for aggregation or cytotoxicity are also identified in *C. elegans*. In one study, yeast chaperone Hsp104 reduced formation of aggregates and cytotoxicity induced by polyglutamine expansion (Q82) in body wall muscle cells, while mutant Hsp104, Ydj1 (DnaJ family), Ssa1 (Hsp70 family), and Hsp82 (Hsp90 family) did not show any effect (Satyal et al. 2000). As noted previously in experiments designed to discern a potential activity for dystonia-related proteins, *C. elegans tor-2*, *ooc-5*, and torsinA (human), which all belong to the AAA+ protein family, reduced the formation of protein aggregates induced by Q82 upon their overexpression (Caldwell et al. 2003). Co-localization of polyglutamine aggregates with torsins by immunostaining suggests that *tor-2* has a direct role in protein aggregation (Caldwell et al. 2003a; Walker et al. 2003). The reproducible identification of chaperone proteins as effectors of aggregated polyQ proteins is expected from genetic screens or genomic microarray experiments, given the general role the proteins have in mediating protein folding. Furthermore, since polyQ aggregates are often found ubiquitinated, one might expect to find modifiers in the UPS or ERAD pathways to be putative partners in regulating aggregate formation and degradation (Caldwell et al. 2003a; Holbert et al. 2003).

C. elegans is a great model organism for genetics and it should be fully utilized to screen for more genetic modifiers. One technical hurdle for researchers is that many suppressors for cytotoxicity could not be identified by forward genetics due to the lethality associated with essential genes. *C. elegans* can play a unique role in identifying additional evolutionarily conserved proteins of unknown function that may be involved in these mechanisms, through applying large-scale RNAi screening technology with bacterial feeding libraries (Kamath et al. 2002). With RNAi weaker phenotypes of genes can be detected, in addition to null mutants. Thus, investigators can identify genes whose partial loss of function is enough to exacerbate neurodegeneration and cell death while the whole organism is still viable. Likewise, isolating potential enhancers can provide information about the molecular mechanism of polyQ cytotoxicity and about potential drug targets.

The local context of specific polyQ-containing disease proteins has a great impact on pathogenesis (Chen et al. 2003; Emamian et al. 2003). However, in *C. elegans*, most models are based on huntingtin-polyQ-containing fragments (Faber et al. 1999; Parker et al. 2001). Undoubtedly, these models can reveal the common mechanisms in the pathogenesis of all polyQ diseases, but to fully understand each disease, models expressing each specific polyglutamine disease protein should be generated and evaluated individually. Moreover, the extensive tissue specific promoters, localization signals, and markers available for *C. elegans* research can be used to identify contextual features associated with disease gene expression. Current *C. elegans* models also constitutively express polyQ proteins. Although these models show the progressive feature of cytotoxicity, it is unclear whether it is because older animals are simply exposed to polyQ proteins for a longer time, and overloaded over time, or whether older animals are intrinsically more susceptible to polyQ proteins because they cannot handle a variety of stresses that accumulate with aging. Therefore, inducible models such as those for amyloid-beta peptide expression in *C. elegans* could be generated to precisely control the temporal expression of polyQ proteins (Drake et al. 2003).

The research field for polyQ-related diseases was established approximately twelve years ago, and scientific advances have occurred during this time. However, many critical questions concerning the exact mechanism of polyQ aggregation, the role of local protein context, the role of aggregates in neurotoxicity, and nuclear versus cytoplasmic aggregate-related cytotoxicity, all remain elusive. *C. elegans* as a model organism has proved useful for studying polyQ diseases and will continue to influence this field. The research capacity of this organism is far from complete, given its powerful genetic tools and amenable features; *C. elegans* polyQ disease research has a long "to-do list"!

VII. AN ELEGANT SOLUTION: TOWARD THE FUTURE OF WORM MOVEMENT DISORDERS RESEARCH

In the case of movement disorders, disease progression is nearly inexorably linked with time. Symptoms are exacerbated with aging and consequences for rapid cellular decline increase with extended environmental exposure in postmitotic neurons. It is readily apparent that factors that increase lipid and protein oxidation and induce misfolding have negative consequences for cellular health. Defining the primary versus secondary effects of specific stressors is of paramount importance to our mechanistic understanding of movement disorders and our ability to effectively intervene with these processes pharmacologically (Cheichanover and Brundin 2003). Perhaps, unlike any other model system, *C. elegans* is best poised to address questions directly related to the aging process. With a wealth of existing age-related mutations and recent microarray and RNAi data pinpointing longevity target genes in worms, the functional implications associated with these genes can be rapidly assessed in models of protein aggregation or neurodegeneration (Lee et al. 2003; Murphy et al. 2003).

Surprisingly, as this review points out, the number of *C. elegans* models for movement disorders is limited and much more is possible in this realm. For instance, researchers have just begun to take on the challenges of modeling ALS (amyotrophic lateral sclerosis), specific ataxias, or other age-related neurodegenerative diseases in worms (Kiehl et al. 2000; Link 2001; Odea et al. 2001; Driscoll and Gerstbrein 2003). Table 2 contains only a partial list of the growing number of genes in *C. elegans* that share significant sequence similarity to gene products with direct links to movement disorders. With the completion of the human genome project, the potential is great to rapidly translate the results of human genetic mapping studies directly into functional analyses in *C. elegans* and will likely exponentially increase the number of worm disease models in the coming years.

C. elegans offers an animal model that is a truly comprehensive approach toward discerning the molecular basis of disease processes. Simultaneously, investigators can apply traditional genetic, modern genomic, and high-throughput chemical screening to this system as a multi-variable and inclusive assault on movement disorders. The ultimate goal of this research is to find treatments or cures for these disorders. Therefore, along with continuing studies to decipher the molecular mechanisms of these diseases, developing *C. elegans*-based assays for direct screening of small molecules is a worthwhile focus for future studies to increase the pipeline of therapeutic candidates. In the end, perhaps the wisest approach is to modestly defer to nature and "let the animal tell us what is happening." As the name *C. elegans* implies, this simple yet elegant animal may provide graceful solutions to complex problems of movement disorders.

Acknowledgments

We would like to thank all our colleagues and collaborators in this field who have contributed to the body of work represented herein and offer our sincere apologies to those we may have inadvertently overlooked. Special thanks to Cody Locke for generating the polyglutamine-containing worm video and Christopher Gelwix for his thoughts on some of the subject matter in this review. Movement disorders research in the Caldwell lab is supported by grants from the Bachmann-Strauss Dystonia & Parkinson Foundation, Dystonia Medical Research Foundation, Michael J. Fox Foundation for Parkinson Research, Parkinson Disease Foundation, National Parkinson Foundation, and the National Institute for Neurological Disorders and Stroke. We also acknowledge additional support from an Undergraduate Science Program Grant from the Howard Hughes Medical Institute to the University of Alabama.

Video Legend

A Q82-GFP fusion construct resulted in visibly distinct aggregates of GFP in *C. elegans*.

References

Adams, J.D., and I.N. Odunze. 1991. Biochemical mechanisms of MPTP toxicity. *Biochem Pharmaco* **41**:1099–1105.

Adams, M.W., H.A. Dailey, L.J. DeLucas, M. Luo, J.H. Prestegard, J.P. Rose, and B.C. Wang. 2003. The Southeast Collaboratory for Structural Genomics: a high-throughput gene to structure factory. *Acc Chem Res* **36**:191–198.

Aspenstrom, P. 1997. A Cdc42 target protein with homology to the non-kinase domain of FER has a potential role in regulating the actin cytoskeleton. *Curr Biol* **7**:479–487.

Augood, S.J., Z. Hollingsworth, D.S. Albers, L. Yang, J.C. Leung, X.O. Breakefield, and D.G. Standaert. 2003. Dopamine transmission in DYT1 dystonia. In *Dystonia 4: Advances in Neurology*. Ed. S. Fahn, M.A. Hallet, and M.R. De Long. Lippincott Williams & Wilkins Publishers, 94. Philadelphia, pp. 53–60.

Augood, S.J., D.M. Martin, L.J. Ozelius, X.O. Breakefield, J.B. Penney, Jr, and D.G. Standaert. 1999. Distribution of the mRNAs encoding torsinA and torsinB in the normal adult human brain. *Ann Neurol* **46**:761–769.

Auluck, P.K., H.Y. Chan, J.Q. Trojanowski, V.M. Lee, and N.M. Bonini. 2002. Chaperone suppression of alpha-synuclein toxicity in a *Drosophila* model for Parkinson's disease. *Science* **295**:865–868.

Bargmann, C.I. 1998. Neurobiology of the *Caenorhabditis elegans* genome. *Science* **282**:2028–2033.

Basham, S.E., and L.S. Rose. 1999. Mutations in *ooc-5* and *ooc-3* disrupt oocyte formation and the reestablishment of asymmetric PAR protein localization in two-cell *Caenorhabditis elegans* embryos. *Dev Biol* **215**:253–263.

Basham, S.E., and L.S. Rose. 2001. The *Caenorhabditis elegans* polarity gene *ooc-5* encodes a torsin-related protein of the AAA+ ATPase superfamily. *Development* **28**:4645–4656.

Beal, M.F. 2003. Mitochondria, oxidative damage and inflammation in Parkinson's disease. *Ann N Y Acad Sci* **991**:120–131.

Bloem, B.R., I. Irwin, O.F. Buruma, J. Hann, F.A. Roos, J.W. Tetrud, and J.W. Langston. 1990. The MPTP model: versatile contributions to the treatment of idiopathic Parkinson's disease. *J Neurol Sci* **97**:273–293.

Blumenthal, T., D. Evans, C.D. Link, A. Guffanti, D. Lawson, J. Thierry-Mieg, D. Thierry-Mieg, et al. 2002. A global analysis of *Caenorhabditis elegans* operons. *Nature* **417**:851–854.

Bonifati, V., P. Rizzu, M.J. van Baren, O. Schaap, G.J. Breedveld, E. Krieger, M.C. Dekker, et al. 2003. Mutations in the DJ-1 gene associated with autosomal recessive early-onset parkinsonism. *Science* **299**:256–259.

Braeckman, B.P., K. Houthoofd, and J.R. Vanfleteren. 2001. Insulin-like signaling, metabolism, stress resistance and aging in *C. elegans*. *Mech Ageing Dev* **122**:673–693.

Brenner, S. 1974. The genetics of *Caenorhabditis elegans*. *Genetics* **77**:71–94.

Bressman, S.B. 2003. Dystonia genotypes, phenotypes and classification. In *Dystonia 4: Advances in Neurology*. Ed. S. Fahn, M.A. Hallet, and M.R. De Long. pp. 101–107. Philadelphia: Lippincott Williams & Wilkins Publishers.

C. elegans Sequencing Consortium. 1998. Genome sequence of the nematode *Caenorhabditis elegans*: a platform for investigating biology. *Science* **282**:2012–2018.

Caldwell, G.A., S. Cao, C.C. Gelwix, E.G. Sexton, J.P. Bevel, and K.A. Caldwell. 2003. Suppression of polyglutamine-induced protein aggregation in *C. elegans* by torsin proteins. *Hum Mol Genet* **12**: 307–319.

Caldwell, G.A., S. Cao, C.C. Gelwix, E.G. Sexton, and K.A. Caldwell. 2004. An animal model to discern torsin function: suppression of protein aggregation in *C. elegans*. In *Dystonia 4: Advances in Neurology*. Ed. S. Fahn, M.A. Hallet, and M.R. De Long. pp. 79–85. Philadelphia: Lippincott Williams & Wilkins Publishers.

de Carvalho Aguiar, P., K.J. Sweadner, J.T. Penniston, J. Zaremba, L. Liu, M. Caton, G. Linazasoro et al. 2004. Mutations in the Na^+/K^+-ATPase 23 Gene *ATP1A3* are Associated with Rapid-Onset Dystonia Parkinsonism. *Neuron* **43**:169–175.

Chen, H.K., P. Femandez-Funez, S.F. Acevedo, Y.V. Lam, M.D. Kaytor, M.H. Femandez, A. Aitken, et al. 2003. Interaction of Akt-phosphorylated ataxin-1 with 14-3-3 mediates neurodegeneration in spinocerebellar ataxia type 1. *Cell* **113**:457–468.

Chalfie, M., Y. Tu, G. Euskirchen, W.W. Ward, and D.C. Prasher. 1994. Green fluorescent protein as a marker for gene expression. *Science* **263**:802–805.

Christensen, M., A. Estevez, X. Yin, R. Fox, R. Morrison, M. McDonnell, C. Gleason, et al. 2002. A primary culture system for functional analysis of *C. elegans* neurons and muscle cells. *Neuron* **33**:503–514.

Ciechanover, A., and P. Brundin. 2003. The ubiquitin proteosome system in neurodegenerative diseases: sometimes the chicken, sometimes the egg. *Neuron* **40**:427–446.

Cookson, M. 2003. Pathways to Parkinsonism. *Neuron* **37**:7–10.

Danda, S., J.F. Bishop, M.A. Eglitis, Y. Yang, and M.M. Mouradian. 2000. Enhanced vulnerability to oxidative stress by alpha-synuclein mutations and C-terminal truncation. *Neuroscience* **97**:279–284.

Davies, S.W., M. Turmaine, B.A. Cozens, M. Difiglia, A.H. Sharp, C.A. Ross, E. Scherzinger, et al. 1997. Formation of neuronal intranuclear inclusions underlies the neurological dysfunction in mice transgenic for the HD mutation. *Cell* **90**:537–548.

DiFiglia, M., E. Sapp, K.O. Chase, S.W. Davies, G.P. Bates, J.P. Vonsattel, and N. Aronin. 1997. Aggregation of huntingtin in neuronal intranuclear inclusions and dystrophic neurites in brain. *Science* **277**: 1990–1993.

Di Monte, D.A. 1991. Mitochondrial DNA and Parkinson's disease. *Neurology* **41**:38–42.

Drake, J., C.D. Link, and D. Butterfield. 2003. Oxidative stress precedes fibrillar deposition of Alzheimer's disease amyloid beta-peptide (1–42) in a transgenic *Caenorhabditis elegans* model. *Neurobiol Aging* **24**:415–420.

Driscoll, M., and B. Grestbrein. 2003. Dying for a cause: invertebrate genetics takes on human neurodegeneration. *Nat Rev Genet* **4**:181–194.

Du, Y., Z. Ma, S. Lin, R.C. Dodel, F. Gao, K.P. Bales, L.C. Triarhou, et al. 2001. Minocycline prevents nigrostriatal dopaminergic neurodegeneration in the MPTP model of Parkinson's disease. *Proc Natl Acad Sci U S A* **98**:14669–14674.

Duerr, J.S., D.L. Frisby, J. Gaskin, A. Duke, K. Asermely, D. Huddleston, L.E. Eiden, and J.B. Rand. 1999. The *cat-1* gene of *Caenorhabditis elegans* encodes a vesicular monoamine transporter required for specific monoamine-dependent behaviors. *J Neurosci* **19**:72–84.

Duyao, M., C. Ambrose, R. Myers, A. Novelletto, F. Persichetti, M. Frontali, S. Folstein, et al. 1993. Trinucleotide repeat length instability and age of onset in Huntington's disease. *Nat Genet* **4**:387–392.

Emamian, E.S., M.D. Kaytor, L.A. Duvick, T. Zu, S.K. Tousey, H.Y. Zoghbi, H.B. Clark, and H.T. Orr. 2003. Serine 776 of ataxin-1 is critical for polyglutamine-induced disease in SCA1 transgenic mice. *Neuron* **38**:375–387.

Ernster, E.D. 1995. Biochemical, physiological and medical aspects of ubiquinone function. *Biochim Biophys Acta* **1271**:195–204.

Faber, P.W., G.T. Barnes, J. Srinidhi, J. Chen, J.F. Gusella, and M.E. MacDonald. 1998. Huntingtin interacts with a family of WW domain proteins. *Hum Mol Genet* **7**:1463–1474.

Faber, P.W., J.R. Alter, M.E. MacDonald, and A.C. Hart. 1999. Polyglutamine-mediated dysfunction and apoptotic death of a *Caenorhabditis elegans* sensory neuron. *Proc Natl Acad Sci U S A* **96**:179–184.

Faber, P.W., C. Voisine, D.C. King, E.A. Bates, and A.C. Hart. 2002. Glutamine/proline-rich PQE-1 proteins protect *Caenorhabditis elegans* neurons from huntingtin polyglutamine neurotoxicity. *Proc Natl Acad Sci U S A* **99**:17131–17136.

Feany, M.B., and W.W. Bender. 2000. A *Drosophila* model of Parkinson's disease. *Nature* **404**:394–398.

Feinberg, E.H., and C.P. Hunter. 2003. Transport of dsRNA into cells by the transmembrane protein SID-1. *Science* **301**:1545–1547.

Felkai, S., J.J. Ewbank, J. Lemieux, J.C. Labbe, G.G. Brown, and S. Hekimi. 1999. CLK-1 controls respiration, behavior and aging in the nematode *Caenorhabditis elegans. EMBO J* **18**:1783–1792.

Fire, A., S. Xu, M.K. Montgomery, S.A. Kostas, S.E. Driver, and C.C. Mello. 1998. Potent and specific genetic interference by double-stranded RNA in *Caenorhabditis elegans. Nature* **391**:806–881.

Frerman, F.E. 1988. AcylCoA dehydrogenase, electron transport flavoproteins and electron transport flavoprotein dehydrogenase. *Biochem Soc Trans* **16**:416–418.

Gasser, T. 1998. Genetics of Parkinson's disease. *Clin Genet* **54**:259–265.

Glinka, Y., M. Gassen, and M.B. Youdim. 1997. Mechanism of action of 6-OHDA neurotoxicity. *J Neural Transmission Suppl* **5**:55–66.

Goedert, M. 2001. Alpha-synuclein and neurodegenerative diseases. *Nat Rev Neurosci* **2**:492–501.

Goicoechea, C., M. Ormazabal, M. Alfaro, and M. Martin. 1997. Age-related changes in nociception, behavior and monoamine levels in rats. *Gen Pharm* **28**:116–331.

Grunblatt E., S. Mandel, and M.B. Youdim. 2000. Neuroprotective strategies in Parkinson's disease using the models of 6-OHDA and MPTP. *Ann NY Acad Sci* **899**:262–273.

Halliwell, B. 1992. Reactive oxygen species and the central nervous system. *J Neurochem* **59**:1609–1623.

Harris, T.W., R. Lee, E. Schwarz, K. Bradnam, D. Lawson, W. Chen, D. Blasier, et al. 2003. WormBase: a cross-species database for comparative genomics. *Nucleic Acids Res* **31**:133–137.

Herndon, L.A., P.J. Schmeissner, J.M. Dudaronek, P.A. Brown, K.M. Listner, Y. Sakano, M.C. Paupard, et al. 2002. Stochastic and genetic factors influence tissue-specific decline in ageing *C. elegans. Nature* **419**:808–814.

Hewett, J., C. Gonzalez-Agosti, D. Slater, P. Ziefer, S. Li, D. Bergeron, D.J. Jacoby, et al. 2000. Mutant torsinA, responsible for early-onset torsion dystonia, forms membrane inclusions in cultured neural cells. *Hum Mol Gen* **9**:1203–1313.

Holbert, S., A. Dedeoglu, S. Humbert, F. Saudou, R.J. Ferrante, and C. Neri. 2003. Cdc42-interacting protein 4 binds to huntingtin: neuropathologic and biological evidence for a role in Huntington's disease. *Proc Natl Acad Sci U S A* **100**:2712–2717.

Hsu, L.J., Y. Sagara, A. Arroyo, E. Rockenstein, A. Sisk, M. Mallory, J. Wong, et al. 2000. Alpha-synuclein promotes mitochondrial deficit and oxidative stress. *Am J Pathol* **157**:401–410.

Huntington's Disease Collaborative Research Group. 1993. A novel gene containing a trinucleotide repeat that is expanded and unstable on Huntington's disease chromosomes. *Cell* **72**:971–983.

Ichinose, H., T. Ohye, E. Takahashi, N. Seki, T. Hori, M. Segawa, Y. Nomura, et al. 1994. Hereditary progressive dystonia with marked diurnal fluctuation caused by mutations in the GTP cyclohydrolase I gene. *Nat Genet* **8**:236–242.

Javitch, J., R.J. D'Amato, S.M. Strittmatter, and S.H. Snyder. 1985. Parkinsonism-inducing neurotoxin, N-MPTP: uptake of the metabolite N-methyl-4-phenylpyridine by dopamine neurons explains selective toxicity. *Proc Natl Acad Sci U S A* **82**:2173–2177.

Jayanthi, L.D., S. Apparsundaram, D. Malone, E. Ward, D.M. Miller, M. Eppler, and R.D. Blakely. 1998. The *C. elegans* gene T23G5.5 encodes an antidepressant and cocaine sensitive dopamine transporter. *Mol Pharmacol* **545**:601–609.

Jonassen, T., P.L. Larsen, and C.F. Clarke. 2001. A dietary source of coenzyme Q is essential for growth of longlived *C. elegans clk-1* mutants. *Proc Natl Acad Sci U S A* **2**:421–426.

Jorgensen, E.M., and S.E. Mango. 2002. The art and design of genetic screens: *Caenorhabditis elegans. Nat Rev Genet* **3**:356–369.

Kamath, R.S., M. Martinez-Campos, P. Zipperlen, A.G. Fraser, and J. Ahringer. 2001. Effectiveness of specific RNA-mediated interference through ingested double-stranded RNA in *Caenorhabditis elegans. Genome Biol* **2**:1–10.

Kamath, R.S., A.G. Fraser, Y. Dong, Y. Durbin, G. Poulin, R. Durbin, M. Cotta, et al. 2003. Systematic functional analysis of the *Caenorhabditis elegans* genome using RNAi. *Nature* **421**:231–237.

Kerr, R., V. Lev-Ram, G. Baird, P. Incent, R.Y. Tsien, and W.R. Schafer. 2000. Optical imaging of calcium transients in neurons and pharyngeal muscle of *C. elegans. Neuron* **26**:583–594.

Kiehl, T.R., H. Shibata, and S.M. Pulst. 2000. The ortholog of human ataxin-2 is essential for early embryonic patterning in *C. elegans. J Mol Neurosci* **15**:231–241.

Kim, S.K., J. Lund, M. Kiraly, K. Duke, M. Jiang, J.M. Stuart, A. Eizinger, et al. 2001. A gene expression map for *Caenorhabditis elegans. Science* **293**:2087–2092.

Kitada, T., S. Asakawa, N. Hattori, H. Matsumine, Y. Yamamura, S. Minoshima, M. Yokochi, et al. 1998. Mutations in the parkin gene cause autosomal recessive juvenile parkinsonism. *Nature* **392**:605–608.

Kitayama, S., S. Shimada, and G.R. Uhl. 1992. Parkinsonism-inducing neurotoxin MPP+; uptake and toxicity in nonneuronal COS cells expressing dopamine transporter cDNA. *Ann Neurol* **32**:109–111.

Kopito, R.R. 2000. Aggresomes, inclusion bodies and protein aggregation. *Trends Cell Biol* **10**:524–530.

Kruger, R., W. Kuhn, T. Muller, D. Woitalla, M. Graeber, S. Kosel, H. Przuntek, et al. 1998. Ala30Pro mutation in the gene encoding α-synuclein gene identified in families with Parkinson's disease. *Nat Genet* **28**:106–108.

Kustedjo, K., M.H. Bracey, and B.F. Cravatt. 2000. TorsinA and its torsion dystonia-associated mutant forms are lumenal glycoproteins that exhibit distinct subcellular localizations. *J Biol Chem* **275**: 27933–27939.

Lakso, M., S. Vartiainen, A. Moilanen, J. Sirvio, J.H. Thomas, R. Nass, R.D. Blakely, and G. Wong. 2003. Dopaminergic neuronal loss and motor deficits in *C. elegans* overexpressing human α-synuclein. *J Neurochem* **86**:165–172.

Lander, E.S., L.M. Linton, B. Birren, C. Nusbaum, M.C. Zody, J. Baldwin, K. Devon, et al. 2001. Initial sequencing and analysis of the human genome. *Nature* **409**:860–921.

Lang, A.E., and A.M. Lozano. 1998. Parkinson's disease. First of two parts. *N Engl J Med* **339**:1044–1053.

Larsen, P.L., and C.F. Clarke. 2002. Extension of life-span in *Caenorhabditis elegans* by a diet lacking coenzyme Q. *Science* **295**:120–123.

Lee, S.S., R.Y.N. Lee, A.G. Fraser, R.S. Kamath, J. Ahringer, and G. Ruvkun. 2002. A systematic RNAi screen identifies a critical role for mitochondria in *C. elegans* longevity. *Nat Gene* **33**:40–48.

Leung, J.C., C. Klein, J. Friedman, P. Vieregge, H. Jacobs, D. Doheny, C. Kamm, et al. 2001. Novel mutation in the *TOR1A (DYT1)* gene in atypical early onset dystonia and polymorphisms in dystonia and early onset parkinsonism. *Neurogenetics* **3**:133–143.

Link, C.D. 2001. Transgenic invertebrate models of age-associated neurodegenerative diseases. *Mech Ageing Dev* **122**:1639–1649.

Lithgow, G.J., and G.A. Walker. 2002. Stress resistance as a determinant of *C. elegans* lifespan. *Mech Ageing Dev* **123**:765–771.

Lints, R., and S.W. Emmons. 1999. Patterning of dopaminergic neurotransmitter identity among *C. elegans* ray sensory neurons by a TGFB family signaling pathway and a *Hox* gene. *Development* **126**: 5819–5831.

Loer, C.M., and C.J. Kenyon. 1993. Serotonin-deficient mutants and male mating behavior in the nematode *C. elegans*. *J Neurosci* **13**:5407–5417.

McCampbell, A., J.P. Taylor, A.A. Taye, J. Robitschek, M. Li, J. Walcott, D. Merry, et al. 2000. CREB-binding protein sequestration by expanded polyglutamine. *Hum Mol Genet* **9**:2197–2202.

McLean, P.J., H. Kawamata, S. Saadat, J. Hewett, N. Sharma, K. Ueda, X.O. Breakefield, and B.T. Hyman. 2002. TorsinA and heat shock proteins act as molecular chaperones: suppression of α-synuclein aggregation. *J Neurochem* **83**:846–854.

Michalik, A., and C. Van Broeckhoven. 2003. Pathogenesis of polyglutamine disorders: aggregation revisited. *Hum Mol Genet* **12**:R173–186.

Miller, D.M., III, N. Desai, D. Hardin, D.W. Piston, G.H. Patterson, J. Fleenor, S.Q. Xu, and A. Fire. 1999. A two-color GFP expression system for *C. elegans*. *BioTechniques* **26**:914–921.

Morley, J.F., H.R. Brignull, J.J. Weyers, and R.I. Morimoto. 2002. The threshold for polyglutamine-expansion protein aggregation and cellular toxicity is dynamic and influenced by aging in *Caenorhabditis elegans*. *Proc Natl Acad Sci U S A* **99**:10417–10422.

Mounsey, A., P. Bauer, and I.A. Hope. 2002. Evidence suggesting that a fifth of annotated *Caenorhabditis elegans* genes may be pseudogenes. *Genome Res* **12**:770–775.

Murphy, C.T., S.A. McCarroll, C.I. Bargmann, A. Fraser, R.S. Kamath, J. Ahringer, H. Li, and C. Kenyon. 2003. Genes that act downstream of DAF-16 to influence the lifespan of *Caenorhabditis elegans*. **424**:277–284.

Nass, R., D.H. Hall, D.M. Miller, and R.D. Blakely. 2002. Neurotoxin-induced degeneration of dopamine neurons in *Caenorhabditis elegans*. *Proc Natl Acad Sci U S A* **99**:3264–3269.

Neckamayer, W., S. Woodrome, B. Holt, and A. Mayer. 2000. Dopamine and senescence in *D. melanogaster*. *Neurobiol Aging* **1**:145–152.

Neuwald A.F., L. Aravind, J.L. Spouge, and E.V. Koonin. 1999. AAA+: a class of chaperone-like ATPases associated with the assembly, operation, and disassembly of protein complexes. *Genome Res* **9**:27–43.

Nucifora, F.C.J., M. Sasaki, M.F. Peters, H. Huang, J.K. Cooper, M. Yamada, H. Takahashi, et al. 2001. Interference by huntingtin and atrophin-1 with cbp-mediated transcription leading to cellular toxicity. *Science* ••:2423–2428.

Oeda, T., S. Shimohama, N. Kitagawa, R. Kohno, T. Mura, H. Shibasaki, and N. Ishii. 2003. Oxidative stress causes abnormal accumulation of familial amyotrophic lateral sclerosis-related mutant SOD1 in transgenic *Caenorhabditis elegans*. *Hum Mol Genet* **19**:2013–2023.

Onodera, O., J.R. Burke, S.E. Miller, S. Hester, S. Tsuji, A.D. Roses, and W.J. Strittmatter. 1997. Oligomerization of expanded-polyglutamine domain fluorescent fusion proteins in cultured mammalian cells. *Biochem Biophys Res Comm* **238**:599–605.

Ozelius, L.J., J.W. Hewett, C.E. Page, S.B. Bressman, P.L. Kramer, C. Shalish, D. de Leon, et al. 1997. The early-onset torsion dystonia gene *(DYT1)* encodes an ATP-binding protein. *Nat Genet* **17**:40–48.

Ozelius, L.J., C.E. Page, C. Klein, J.W. Hewett, M. Mineta, J. Leung, C. Shalish, et al. 1999. The *TOR1A (DYT1)* gene family and its role in early onset torsion dystonia. *Genomics* **62**:377–384.

Parker, J.A., J.B. Connolly, C. Wellington, M. Hayden, J. Dausset, and C. Neri. 2001. Expanded polyglutamines in *Caenorhabditis elegans* cause axonal abnormalities and severe dysfunction of PLM mechanosensory neurons without cell death. *Proc Natl Acad Sci U S A* **98**:13318–13323.

Parkes, T.L., A.J. Elia, D. Dickinson, A.J. Hilliker, J.P. Phillips, and G.L. Boulianne. 1998. Extension of *Drosophila* life span by overexpression of human SOD1 in motorneurons. *Nature Genetics* **19**:171–174.

Pattison, D.I., R.T. Dean, and M.J. Davies. 2001. Oxidation of DNA, protein and lipids by DOPA protein-bound DOPA, and related catecholamines. *Toxicology* **177**:23–37.

Paulson, H.L., M.K. Perez, Y. Trottier, J.Q. Trojanowski, S.H. Subramony, S.S. Das, P. Vig, et al. 1997. Intranuclear inclusions of expanded polyglutamine protein in spinocerebellar ataxia type 3. *Neuron* **19**:333–344.

Peters, M.F., F.C. Nucifora, Jr., J. Kushi, H.C. Seaman, J.K. Cooper, W.J. Herring, V.L. Dawson, et al. 1999. Nuclear targeting of mutant Huntingtin increases toxicity. *Mol Cell Neurosci* **14**:121–128.

Pifl, C., B. Giros, and M.G. Caron. 1993. Dopamine transporter expression confers cytotoxicity to low doses of the parkinsonism-inducing neurotoxin 1-MPP. *J Neurosci* **13**:4246–4253.

Polymeropoulos, M.H., C. Lavedan, E. Leroy, S.E. Ide, A. Dehejia, A. Dutra, B. Pike, et al. 1997. Mutation in the α-synuclein gene identified in families with Parkinson's disease. *Science* **276**:2045–2047.

Ross, C.A. 1995. When more is less: pathogenesis of glutamine repeat neurodegenerative diseases. *Neuron* **15**:493–496.

Satyal, S.H., E. Schmidt, K. Kitagawa, N. Sondheimer, S. Lindquist, J.M. Kramer, and R.I. Morimoto. 2000. Polyglutamine aggregates alter protein-folding homeostasis in *Caenorhabditis elegans*. *Proc Natl Acad Sci U S A* **97**:5750–5755.

Saudou, F., S. Finkbeiner, D. Devys, and M.E. Greenberg. 1998. Huntingtin acts in the nucleus to induce apoptosis but death does not correlate with the formation of intranuclear inclusions. *Cell* **95**:55–66.

Sawin, E.R., R. Ranganathan, and H.R. Horvitz. 2000. *C. elegans* locomotory rate is modulated by the environment through a dopaminergic pathway and by experience through a serotonergic pathway. *Neuron* **26**:619–631.

Scherzer, C.R., R.V. Jensen, S.R. Gullans, and M.B. Feany. 2003. Gene expression changes presage neurodegeneration in a *Drosophila* model of PD. *Hum Mol Genet* **12**:2457–2466.

Sharma, N., J. Hewett, L.J. Ozelius, V. Ramesh, P.J. McLean, X.O. Breakefield, and B.T. Hyman. 2001. A close association of torsinA and alpha-synuclein in Lewy bodies: a fluorescence resonance energy transfer study. *Am J Pathol* **159**:339–344.

Shashidharan, P., P.F. Good, A. Hsu, D.P. Perl, M.F. Brin, and C.W. Olanow. 2000a. TorsinA accumulation in Lewy bodies in sporadic Parkinson's disease. *Brain Res* **877**:379–381.

Shashidharan, P., B.C. Kramer, R.H. Walker, C.W. Olanow, and M.F. Brin. 2000b. Immunohistochemical localization and distribution of torsinA in normal human and rat brain. *Brain Res* **853**:197–206.

Simmer, F., M. Tijsterman, S. Parrish, S.P. Koushika, M.L. Nonet, A. Fire, J. Ahringer, and R.H. Plasterk. 2002. Loss of the putative RNA-directed RNA polymerase RRF-3 makes *C. elegans* hypersensitive to RNAi. *Curr Biol* **12**(15):1317–1319.

Singleton, A.B., M. Farrer, J. Johnson, A. Singleton, S. Hague, J. Kachergus, M. Hulihan, et al. 2003. Alpha-synuclein locus triplication causes Parkinson's disease. *Science* **302**:841.

Spillantini, M.G., M.L. Schmidt, V.M. Lee, J.Q. Trojanowski, R. Jakes, and M. Goedert. 1997. Alpha-synuclein in Lewy bodies. *Nature* **388**: 839–840.

Sulston, J., Z. Du, K. Thomas, R. Wilson, L. Hillier, R. Staden, N. Halloran, et al. 1992. The *C. elegans* genome sequencing project: A beginning. *Nature* **356**:37–41.

Tabara H., A. Grishok, and C.C. Mello. 1998. RNAi in *C. elegans*: soaking in the genome sequence. *Science* **282**:430–431.

Tanaka, Y., S. Engelender, S. Igarashi, R.K. Rao, T. Wanner, R.E. Tanzi, A.L. Sawa, et al. 2001. Inducible expression of mutant alpha-synuclein decreases proteasome activity and increases sensitivity to mitochondria-dependent apoptosis. *Hum Mol Gen* **10**:919–926.

Tavernarakis, N., and M. Driscoll. 2002. Caloric restriction and lifespan: a role for protein turnover? *Mech Aging Dev* **123**:215–229.

Tavernarakis, N., S. Wang, M. Dorovokov, A. Ryazanov, and M. Driscoll. 2000. Heritable and inducible genetic interference by double stranded RNA encoded by transgenes. *Nature Genetics* **24**:180–183.

Timmons, L., D.L. Court, and A. Fire. 2001. Ingestion of bacterially expressed dsRNAs can produce specific and potent genetic interference in *Caenorhabditis elegans*. *Gene* **263**:103–112.

Trumpower, B. 1981. New concepts on the role of ubiquinone in the mitochondrial respiratory chain. *J Bioenerg Biomem* **13**:1–24.

Vale, R.D. 2000. AAA proteins. Lords of the ring. *J Cell Biol* **150**:F13–F19.

Valente, F.M., P.M. Abou-Sleiman, V. Caputo, M.M.K. Muquit, K. Harvey, S. Gispert, Z. Ali, et al. 2004. Hereditary Early-Onset Parkinsonism Disease caused by mutations in *PINK1*. *Science* **304**:1158–1160.

Venter, J.C. M.D. Adams, E.W. Myers, P.W. Li, R.J. Mural, G.G. Sutton, H.O. Smith, et al. 2001. The sequence of the human genome. *Science* **291**:1304–1351.

Walhout, A.J., R. Sordella, X. Lu, J.L. Hartley, G.F. Temple, M.A. Brasch, N. Thierry-Mieg, and M. Vidal. 2000. Protein interaction mapping in *C. elegans* using proteins involved in vulval development. *Science* **287**:116–122.

Walker, R.H., P.F. Good, and P. Shashidharan. 2003a. TorsinA immunoreactivity in inclusion bodies in trinucleotide repeat diseases. *Mov Disord* **18**:1041–1044.

Walker, R.H., and P. Shashidharan. 2003b. Developments in the molecular biology of *DYT1* dystonia. *Mov Disord* **18**:1102–1107.

White, J.G., E. Southgate, J.N. Thomson, and S. Brenner. 1976. The structure of the ventral nerve cord of *Caenorhabditis elegans*. *Philos Trans R Soc Lond B Biol Sci* **275**:327–348.

Wintle, R.F., and H.H.M. Van Tol. 2001. Dopamine signaling in *Caenorhabditis elegans*–potential for parkinsonism research. *Parkinsonism and Related Disorders* **7**:177–183.

Wood, W.B. 1988. *The Nematode Caenorhabditis elegans.* Cold Spring Harbor, New York: Cold Spring Harbor Laboratory Press.

Xia, J., D.H. Lee, J. Taylor, M. Vandelft, and R. Truant. 2003. Huntingtin contains a highly conserved nuclear export signal. *Hum Mol Genet* **12**:1393–1403.

Xu, J., S. Kao, G.J.S. Lee, W. Song, L. Jin, and B.A. Yankner. 2002. Dopamine-dependent neurotoxicity of α-synuclein: A mechanism for selective neurodegeneration in PD. *Nat Med* **8**:600–606.

Zoghbi, H.Y., and H.T. Orr. 2000. Glutamine repeats and neurodegeneration. *A Rev Neurosci* **23**:217–247.

CHAPTER

B1

The Phenotypic Spectrum of Parkinson Disease

RONALD F. PFEIFFER

In 1817, James Parkinson, a physician and sometime political provocateur, penned a treatise in which by his own admission, "mere conjecture takes the place of experiment" and in which "analogy is the substitute for anatomical examination" (Parkinson 1817). A mere six cases formed the basis for his description of a previously unrecognized disease process that he labeled "the shaking palsy." Even more astounding is the fact that of the six cases that comprise the clinical material for the manuscript, Dr. Parkinson actually examined only three, and one of these was quickly lost to follow-up after the individual had an abscess drained! Apparently, he merely encountered two individuals and spoke with one the street, while another was "only seen at a distance."

Despite the shortcomings of his available clinical material, Parkinson was able to compose an elegant clinical description of the disease process that now bears his name. He focused on the tremor and gait disturbances characteristic of the condition, perhaps because he could not actually examine half of his reported cases, and he also took note of many (though not all) of the other motor and even non-motor features of the illness. Although his methods of case ascertainment might not meet muster for publication in a neurological journal today, his remarkable description of the clinical features of what is today called Parkinson disease (PD) is both fascinating and instructive for anyone interested in this condition.

This chapter will briefly summarize some of the epidemiological, genetic, and pathophysiological characteristics of PD, but will primarily focus on the clinical features of the illness and, thus, provide a frame of reference for comparison with the various animal models of PD presented in other chapters in this text.

I. EPIDEMIOLOGY OF PARKINSON DISEASE

Parkinson disease is the second most common neurodegenerative disorder, trailing only Alzheimer disease. In the general population, the prevalence of PD is approximately 100 in 100,000. However, PD is an age-related illness and in individuals age sixty-five or older its prevalence mushrooms to 1–2%. The average age of symptom onset is sixty to sixty-five, but approximately 10% of PD patients develop symptoms before age forty. Investigators have never identified a uniform etiology for PD and it has become increasingly clear in recent years that there is probably no single cause and that PD is, in fact, not a disease in the strict sense, but rather a syndrome with multiple

TABLE 1 Possible Environmental Factors in Parkinson Disease

Agriculture-Related Factors
- Rural living
- Farming
- Gardening
- Well water drinking
- Pesticide/herbicide/fungicide exposure

Occupation-Related Factors
- Metal exposure
- Wood pulp/paper manufacturing
- Teaching
- Health care work
- Social science, law, and library work
- Construction work
- Carpentry
- Cleaning
- Iron ore mining
- Chemical manufacturing
- Organic solvent exposure
- Glue, paint, lacquer exposure
- Wood preservative exposure
- Carbon monoxide exposure

Infectious Factors
- *Nocardia*

Other Factors
- Head trauma
- High fat diet
- Emotional stress
- Heavy physical work
- General anesthesia

etiologies: some environmental, some genetic, and perhaps the majority a combination of the two.

Various environmental factors are hypothesized to be operative in the development of PD. Rural living with its agricultural chemical exposure, certain industrial environments, and even occupations such as the teaching and medical professions are reported to confer an increased risk for development of PD. Marras and Tanner (2004) recently reviewed the epidemiology of PD and the reported potential (though not proven) associations are listed in table 1.

II. GENETICS OF PARKINSON DISEASE

Modern molecular genetic techniques have helped investigators identify a growing number of mutations that produce a phenotypic picture of PD. It is also quite clear, however, that the vast majority of individuals with PD does not possess one of these mutations and that additional factors, perhaps susceptibility genes, remain to be discovered. A detailed discussion of the genetic aspects of PD lies beyond the scope of this chapter, but excellent reviews of the subject have been published (Warner and Schapira. 2003; Wszolek and Farrer 2003; Cordato and Chan 2004; Pankratz and Foroud 2004; Wszolek et al. 2004). Table 2 contains information derived from these reviews.

TABLE 2 Genetic Factors in Parkinson Disease

Locus	Chromosome	Gene	Inheritance	Lewy bodies
PARK 1	4	α-synuclein	AD	Yes
PARK 2	6	parkin	AR	No
PARK 3	2	?	AD	Yes
PARK 4	4	?	AD	Yes
PARK 5	4	UCH-L1	AD	?
PARK 6	1	?	AR	?
PARK 7	1	DJ-1	AR	?
PARK 8	12	?	AD	No

AD = autosomal dominant, AR = autosomal recessive.

III. PATHOPHYSIOLOGY OF PARKINSON DISEASE

Investigators have long considered the progressive destruction of nigrostriatal dopaminergic neurons with consequent striatal dopamine deficiency as the pathological hallmark of PD. The presence of Lewy bodies in surviving dopaminergic neurons in the substantia nigra is also considered central to the pathologic confirmation of PD. In recent years it has become evident, however, that neither of these dogmas is absolutely true. While nigrostriatal dopaminergic cellular loss is certainly a central feature of the disease process, the damage is not confined to this pathway and neuronal loss in other locations within the central nervous system has clearly been identified. Moreover, damage in PD is not even confined to the central nervous system. Neuronal loss and even dopamine deficiency are documented within the enteric nervous system of the gastrointestinal tract (Singaram et al. 1995). Peripheral cardiac sympathetic denervation is also identified in the setting of PD (Goldstein 2003).

Even the Lewy body is no longer sacrosanct in that the parkin mutation that results in an autosomal recessive form of young-onset PD is not accompanied by the presence of Lewy bodies (Mouradian 2002).

IV. CLINICAL FEATURES OF PARKINSON DISEASE

A. Premonitory Features

Although the diagnosis of PD ultimately rests on the individual developing the classic clinical features of the illness described in the following sections, when individuals with incipient PD are carefully interrogated they often reveal a variety of other non-specific, sometimes ill-defined manifestations of the illness that may appear in the months, and even years, prior to classic clinical features emerging. These premonitory features, because they do not directly point toward the presence of basal ganglia dysfunction, may prompt an extensive and fruitless search for other disease processes and lead to initiating inappropriate treatment that is rectified only after the more classic clinical features coalesce and facilitate diagnosis.

Stiffness and soreness, often in one shoulder, may provide the first inkling to the individual that something is amiss. However, rather than prompt a diagnosis of PD, such symptoms often trigger suspicion of other clinical entities, such as rotator cuff injury, arthritis, and especially bursitis. The individual may be treated with anti-inflammatory medications and even steroid injections into the symptomatic shoulder. Absence of response to such treatment and eventual emergence of more specific PD features ultimately allow correct diagnosis. This is actually not a trivial mode of symptomatic presentation in PD. The shoulder discomfort may lead to reduced use of the limb and this, in turn, may lead to development of a frozen shoulder. In one study, shoulder discomfort was the first symptom in 8% of PD patients and preceded the emergence of more typical PD features by as much as two years (Nutt et al. 1992).

A sense of undue fatigue and diminished energy may also herald the onset of clinical PD (Hoehn and Yahr 1967). Clinicians may sometimes simply attribute this symptom to advancing age, but other conditions, such as depression, thyroid dysfunction, and even myasthenia gravis, may also be erroneously suspected. The development of paresthesias or dysesthesias may prompt investigation of possible peripheral neuropathy, whereas stiffness and soreness in muscles, along with muscle cramps, may lead to suspicion of conditions such as fibromyalgia. Autonomic symptoms (discussed more fully in paragraphs below) may also appear before the individual develops the motor features of PD. Thus, patients may present with dizziness, constipation, urinary dysfunction, seborrheic dermatitis, or sweating abnormalities. Impaired olfaction, with consequent impairment of taste, may also antedate motor features of PD (Furtado and Wszolek 2004).

Another phenomenon the individual with incipient PD may describe is a sense of internal, though not outwardly visible, tremulousness. This may be difficult for the patient to describe and is often misinterpreted by both patient and physician as anxiety or nervousness. This sensation of internal tremulousness can be quite uncomfortable for the patient. The subsequent appearance of visible tremor ultimately clarifies the situation.

TABLE 3 Cardinal Features of Parkinson Disease

Tremor
Rigidity
Bradykinesia
Postural Instability

B. Cardinal Features

Neurological texts traditionally identify four cardinal features as being at the core of PD: tremor, rigidity, bradykinesia, and postural instability (Table 3). Postural instability has not always been included in this list, and this is understandable, since it typically does not develop until the more advanced stages of the illness. It has been suggested that gait impairment be added to the list of cardinal features (Giladi 2002), but only time will tell if this "promotion" will be embraced.

1. Tremor

Tremor is the feature of PD that is most readily recognized by the lay public and the one that most often prompts its diagnosis. It is the initially identified clinical feature in 50–70% of PD patients, but may never develop at all in up to 15% (Jankovic 2003; Pal et al. 2002). As tremor first emerges, it may be only intermittent and even fleeting and it may be brought out or accentuated by stress, fatigue, or anxiety.

The tremor of PD is classically described as being present at rest, disappearing with movement. While this is usually true, it is not invariably so. Particularly in the early stages of PD, tremor may also (or even exclusively) be present when the limb is held in a posture against gravity or when performing voluntary tasks. Throughout the course of PD, individuals may also display upper extremity postural tremor that appears after a brief latency when the arms are outstretched. This is sometimes referred to as "reemergent" tremor (Jankovic et al. 1999). Both of these situations can lead to diagnostic confusion with essential tremor or other conditions, but the concomitant presence of rest tremor and additional Parkinsonian features clarifies the situation.

Parkinsonian rest tremor is relatively slow, with a frequency that may range from 3 to 7 Hz, but is usually 4 or 5 Hz (Hallett 2003). When tremor first develops it is typically unilateral, most frequently appearing in an upper extremity. The classic clinical picture in the individual with emerging PD is intermittent rest tremor in one hand, often initially involving the thumb and one or more fingers in an oscillating motion labeled "pill-rolling" tremor. With time and advancement of the disease process, the tremor usually becomes bilateral, but it remains asymmetric and more prominent in the initially affected side. Tremor amplitude also tends to increase with disease progression. In advanced PD, however, tremor may actually diminish in prominence and sometimes virtually disappear (Toth et al. 2004). Although tremor in PD most frequently involves the arms, it may also be present in the legs. Distal portions of the limbs are typically affected first, with subsequent proximal progression. Although tremor of the lips, tongue, and jaw may develop in PD, head tremor is distinctly unusual and its presence suggests a diagnosis of essential tremor rather than PD. Parkinsonian tremor disappears when individuals are soundly asleep, but may reappear in light stages of sleep (Comella 2003) or as the person awakens, sometimes prompting patients and family members (and even Parkinson in his 1817 essay) to report the presence of tremor during sleep.

The pathophysiological basis of tremor in PD is not entirely clear. In animal models lesioning of the nigrostriatal tract alone does not produce Parkinsonian tremor (Pechadre et al. 1976). This may explain why tremor often responds incompletely to dopaminergic medication in the treatment of PD. Some investigators have suggested a thalamic origin to Parkinsonian tremor, due to disinhibition of pacemaker cells in the thalamus (Jankovic 2003; Findley and Gresty 1984; McAuley 2003) but others discount this origin (Hallett 2003).

2. Rigidity

Rigidity is characterized by increased muscle tone that produces abnormal resistance to passive movement. The resistance is velocity-independent in that the speed of passive movement does not significantly affect the degree of resistance to the movement (Dewey 2000), and it is equal in agonist and antagonist muscles. The term, "lead-pipe" rigidity is sometimes used to describe this constant resistance to movement. A ratchety quality may be superimposed on the resistance to movement, which has given rise to the term "cogwheel" rigidity. The basis for the cogwheeling phenomenon has not been clearly defined. Attribution of cogwheeling to superimposed tremor seems doubtful, since cogwheeling may be present in individuals who have no tremor (Pal et al. 2003). Cogwheeling has, perhaps, received an inordinate amount of attention and emphasis in the literature and is actually not present in most individuals with PD.

While rigidity may not be evident initially, it eventually develops in virtually all PD patients and may account for the sense of muscle stiffness patients experience. When rigidity is very mild it may not be readily apparent upon routine examination of the involved limb, but it may be brought out by having the patient move the opposite limb in some repetitive pattern, such as opening and closing the hand.

Clinicians sometimes experience difficulty distinguishing rigidity from several other phenomena that produce increased muscle tone. Spasticity, due to upper motor neuronal dysfunction, is characterized by velocity-dependent increased muscle tone. Unlike Parkinsonian rigidity, the resistance to movement that constitutes spasticity rapidly melts away with continued application of force, much as a pocket knife will snap shut after initially resisting closure (the "clasp-knife" phenomenon). Moreover, spasticity is accompanied by other signs of upper motor neuron dysfunction such as hyperreflexia and Babinski responses. Gegenhalten, or paratonia, sometimes displayed by individuals with dementia, is characterized by resistance to movement that adjusts to the force applied, making it appear that the patient is either helping or actively hindering the examiner. Some individuals with advanced essential tremor and consequent coarse, prominent postural tremor may display resistance to limb movement secondary to the tremor itself, which can be mistakenly identified as rigidity (Findley et al. 1981).

3. Bradykinesia

The terminology employed for what, in many respects, embodies the essence of Parkinsonism can be very confusing. Three terms—bradykinesia, akinesia, and hypokinesia—can be found in the literature and are often used interchangeably to describe the same phenomenon, although in their strictest sense they have somewhat different meanings: bradykinesia means slow movement; akinesia means absence of movement; and hypokinesia means poverty of or reduced amplitude of movement. In the clinical literature bradykinesia is probably the most frequently-employed term.

Bradykinesia is ultimately the most disabling component of PD and the cardinal feature that most closely correlates with nigrostriatal dopaminergic cell loss and dopamine deficiency. It also, perhaps not surprisingly, is the feature most responsive to dopaminergic therapy. Some degree of bradykinesia eventually develops in virtually all PD patients (Selby 1990).

While slowness of movement is an integral component of bradykinesia, it is not its sole manifestation. Bradykinesia also entails difficulty or delay in initiating movement, difficulty in arresting movement once it has been initiated, difficulty performing repetitive movements, and difficulty performing simultaneous or sequential movements. On neurological examination clinicians quantify bradykinesia by globally assessing spontaneous movement and by having the patient perform repetitive movements such as tapping the fingers, opening and closing the hands, pronating and supinating the hands, and tapping the feet. In addition to slowness, these movements are characterized by progressive fatigue or reduced amplitude; hesitations and transient arrests may also disturb and distort the repetitive movements. In everyday living bradykinesia manifests not only by overall slowness in volitional movement, but also by reduced frequency and fluidity of spontaneous movements such as crossing the legs when sitting, swinging the arms when walking, and making gestures during conversation. Individuals with bradykinesia also experience difficulty with tasks such as brushing the teeth, shampooing the hair, using a screwdriver, stirring liquids, and mixing or beating ingredients when cooking. Bradykinesia also causes the reduced blink rate evident in many PD patients and plays a role in other secondary features of PD, such as micrographia, reduced facial expression, and speech changes, which are described below.

From a neurophysiological standpoint bradykinesia is characterized by reduced kinesthetic perception, which results in underestimation of movement, and by insufficient bursts of muscle activity that result in undershooting the target and necessitate subsequent corrective bursts (Hallett 2003).

4. Postural Instability

Postural instability is a somewhat confusing label for the fourth of the cardinal features of PD. Perhaps this is appropriate, since postural instability stands somewhat apart from the other three cardinal features already discussed in that it develops late in the course of PD. The term, postural instability, refers to a loss of righting reflexes with consequent balance impairment and potential falling. Postural instability appears to be the consequence of loss or diminution of the normal anticipatory responses or reflexes that appear following postural perturbations or the expectation of such (Hallett 2003).

Postural instability is tested in the clinic by performing the "pull test" in which the patient is suddenly pulled backward by the examiner, who is standing behind the patient (and prepared to catch the patient should the patient fall). If the patient can maintain balance by taking only one or, at most, two backward steps, the test is considered normal. With mild postural instability the patient may take three or more steps, but can ultimately recover balance. With more advanced impairment the patient may backpedal after the "pull" without ever completely recovering balance until the examiner intercedes or a wall is reached. Ultimately, individuals with severe impairment of righting reflexes may not take any steps at all after being pulled backward, but instead topple backward like a falling tree unless caught by the examiner.

Individuals who have developed postural instability as part of their PD are at risk for frequent falling and the injuries that may accompany such falling. Unfortunately, postural instability responds poorly, if at all, to dopaminergic medication, prompting speculation that the pathophysiological basis for the phenomenon is outside the nigrostriatal system. The exact location, however, has not been determined.

TABLE 4. Secondary Features of Parkinson Disease

Micrographia
Speech and Voice Abnormalities
Gait Disturbances
Reduced armswing
Stooped posture
Small, shuffling steps
Festination
Freezing phenomena
Masked face

C. Secondary Features

In addition to the four cardinal features discussed above, PD is also characterized by a number of secondary features that, while distinctive, reflect contributions in varying proportions from the four cardinal PD features. Several of the more prominent secondary features will be highlighted in the paragraphs that follow (see Table 4).

1. Micrographia

Changes in handwriting frequently develop in individuals with PD and are occasionally the presenting feature. The earliest change may be a slight diminution in the size of the letters after prolonged writing, such as at the end of long sentences. This "writing fatigue" is reminiscent of the fatigability with progressive reduction in amplitude seen when individuals with PD perform repetitive movements such as finger tapping. With disease progression, the handwriting develops a more pervasive small, cramped quality, with the letters sometimes running together, once again especially at the end of sentences. Hesitation in initiating writing may also occur. Difficulty writing in a straight line, with a tendency for the script to gradually go uphill or downhill, may evolve. Many patients find it easier to print rather than write in cursive as their PD progresses. When asked to write a sentence, the PD patient may economize movement by breaking the sentence up into several short lines, rather than extending a single line across the page. Handwriting difficulty in PD may ultimately progress to the point of illegibility.

Difficulties similar to those noted with handwriting also develop with drawing. Micrographia in PD is primarily the consequence of the combined effects of rigidity and bradykinesia; sometimes a tremulous quality is also evident in the handwriting.

2. Speech and Voice Abnormalities

Impairment of speech or voice eventually develops in over 75% of persons with PD (Ramig et al. 2002). Investigators have described a rather extensive array of changes. The voice typically becomes softer and speech less forceful. Articulation may become imprecise. The combination of reduced volume and impaired articulation is labeled hypokinetic dysarthria. A hoarse, or breathy, quality to the voice may become evident, and speech often has a monotonous or monopitch quality.

PD patients may experience difficulty initiating speech, displaying a form of vocal "start hesitation." Individuals with more advanced PD may also display a tendency toward progressively more rushed and rapid speech toward the end of sentences; this abnormality has been likened to the festination of gait displayed by some with PD and the term, festination of speech, has been coined for it (Selby 1990).

Speech and voice abnormalities in PD are the result of rigidity and bradykinesia affecting the tongue, lips, pharyngeal, and laryngeal musculature. Respiratory changes also play a role in Parkinsonian speech impairment in that airflow abnormalities, probably due to rigidity and bradykinesia of respiratory musculature, cause less air expenditure during phonation (Mueller 1971).

3. Gait Disturbances

Both patients and physicians sometimes confuse, or perhaps it is more accurate to say they fuse, the gait disturbances and the postural instability of PD. While these features often coincide, they also occur independently; moreover, the pathophysiological mechanisms underlying the two are almost certainly different.

The earliest gait-related abnormality that develops in PD is often first observed not by the patient, but by family members or acquaintances and consists of reduced robustness of the arm-swinging that normally accompanies walking. The reduction is usually unilateral at first, subsequently becoming bilateral with disease progression. As PD advances, the arms tend to be held in a somewhat flexed position close against the body during walking. When this position is unilateral, clinicians may misinterpret it as hemiparesis and search for cerebrovascular disease or neoplasia.

Changes in gait pattern also become evident during the course of PD. Steps become shorter (stride length is reduced) and the feet are not adequately lifted off the ground, producing a shuffling quality to the gait. The shuffling may be unilateral or bilateral, and sometimes the examiner can more easily hear the foot dragging or shuffling over the carpet than see it. The inability to adequately elevate the feet also predisposes the individual with PD to tripping over obstacles that generally don't pose difficulty, such as door jambs. The gait in PD remains narrow-based, unlike the wide-based gait that develops in individuals with normal pressure hydrocephalus, vascular Parkinsonism, or cerebellar dysfunction.

As the changes in gait evolve, patients with PD also begin to display changes in posture, which becomes stooped. The knees also become slightly flexed and patients tend to lean slightly forward as they walk. In advanced PD these abnormalities can culminate in a tendency to shuffle increasingly faster with prolonged walking, with the patient eventually breaking into a shuffle-run. This phenomenon is called gait festination. With the advent of effective symptomatic therapy with levodopa, full-blown gait festination has become rare.

Other gait abnormalities may appear in more advanced PD. Gait freezing, in which one or both feet suddenly become immobile, as if held to the ground by a magnet or glued in place, can be an especially aggravating problem for the PD patient. When this phenomenon occurs as the individual attempts to start walking, the term "start hesitation" is employed. Similar freezing can emerge during, or immediately following, turning. Freezing phenomena may also occur while walking is under way, especially in narrow or crowded environments or when passing through doorways. Such gait freezing is typically momentary, but occasionally may be more prolonged. Patients prone to freezing may develop maneuvers or tricks to break out of prolonged freezing episodes. Such tricks may include imagining one is climbing a step or stepping over an object, marching to imagined music or a cadence, or occasionally even more unusual maneuvers such as crouching down and breaking into a run, like a runner starting a race.

The pathophysiological basis for the gait abnormalities of PD is not entirely clear. Rigidity and bradykinesia certainly play a role, but other factors may also operate. The basis for freezing phenomena is also unclear, although disruption of, or inability to efficiently initiate, anticipatory postural adjustments may be responsible (Giladi 2002).

4. Other Abnormalities

PD patients may also display a number of additional motor difficulties. Reduced facial expression, sometimes referred to as a masked face, is due to rigidity and bradykinesia of facial musculature, coupled with reduced blinking frequency. The staring, unsmiling facial expression of the PD patient may be misinterpreted as anger, especially by children. Individuals with PD also frequently experience difficulty turning over in bed, which can lead to discomfort and may be one source of insomnia in the setting of PD. Eye movement abnormalities may also develop in PD. Saccadic hypometria, especially for memory-guided voluntary saccades, is the most characteristic abnormality (Kennard and Nachev 2004). Reduced upgaze is often noted, but this is not specific for PD. Apraxia of eyelid opening is occasionally seen in PD, but it is more often encountered in Parkinsonism-plus syndromes.

TABLE 5 Non-Motor Features of Parkinson's Disease

Non-Motor Features
Behavioral Dysfunction
Depression
Anxiety
Obsessionality
Dementia
Psychosis
Autonomic Dysfunction
Gastrointestinal dysfunction
Excess saliva
Dysphagia
Gastroparesis
Intestinal dysfunction
Anorectal dysfunction
Urological dysfunction
Irritative symptoms
Obstructive symptoms
Sphincter bradykinesia
Sexual dysfunction
Cardiovascular dysfunction
Thermoregulatory dysfunction
Respiratory dysfunction
Sleep-Related Dysfunction
Insomnia
REM sleep behavior disorder
Excessive daytime sleepiness
Sleep apnea
Sensory Dysfunction
Visual dysfunction
Impaired contrast sensitivity
Impaired color vision
Visuo-cognitive impairment
Olfactory impairment
Disordered sensation
Pain syndromes
Musculoskeletal
Radicular
Painful dystonia
Central pain
Akathisia
Sensorimotor dysfunction
Oculomotor dysfunction
Fatigue

D. Non-Motor Features

Although PD is commonly conceptualized as consisting purely of motor dysfunction, it has been quite clear, even dating back to Parkinson's original description, that non-motor features may play an important, and sometimes even dominant, role in the condition (Table 5). Recognizing these non-motor features is important, because treatment often entails approaches distinct from dopaminergic therapy.

1. Behavioral Abnormalities

A number of behavioral changes may develop in the setting of PD. Depression is the most frequently encountered psychological problem in PD patients. Reported prevalence figures vary considerably, but some degree of depression appears to be present in approximately 50% of PD patients, although moderate to severe depression is present in approximately only 5% (Burke et al. 2004; Tandberg et al. 1996). Depression may antedate the appearance of motor dysfunction in some patients. Anxiety, including panic attacks, may also become problematic for PD patients, sometimes in conjunction with depression but also independently (Fernandez and Simuni 2004). Anxiety may also appear as a wearing-off phenomenon in individuals on dopaminergic therapy. Obsessive-compulsive features have also been noted in individuals with PD (Bruneau 2004)). Cognitive impairment, sometimes progressing to frank dementia, is yet another facet of behavioral dysfunction in PD. The prevalence of dementia in PD is reported at between 20 to 40% (Kavanagh and Marder 2004), and it is more common in older individuals with advanced PD. Psychosis may also develop in patients with PD, typically as a complication of dopaminergic medication (Molho and Factor 2004).

2. Autonomic Dysfunction

While autonomic dysfunction is a well-known component of multiple system atrophy, it is less widely recognized that patients with PD may experience a broad array of abnormalities indicative of autonomic impairment (Siddiqui et al. 2002). Although autonomic dysfunction is usually associated with more advanced PD, it can appear early in the course of the illness, occasionally even prior to motor dysfunction.

Gastrointestinal dysfunction is the most widely recognized element of autonomic dysfunction in PD (Pfeiffer 2003; Pfeiffer and Quigley 2004). Excess saliva is often present and sometimes very troubling to PD patients. The excess is not due to overproduction of saliva, but rather the result of decreased swallowing frequency. Some degree of dysphagia develops in many PD patients. The disordered swallowing can be due to dysfunction at oral, pharyngeal, or esophageal levels (Leopold 2004). Aspiration is a potentially serious complication of dysphagia in PD. Gastroparesis, or impaired gastric emptying, may also develop in the setting of PD, and can produce a sense of bloating, early satiety, and nausea (Gurevich et al. 2004). Since levodopa is absorbed in the small intestine, delayed gastric emptying can also delay and diminish levodopa absorption. Bowel dysfunction is the most widely recognized gastrointestinal derangement in PD. It is less widely recognized that the bowel dysfunction may take on two forms: delayed or slowed colonic transit resulting in decreased bowel movement frequency; and defecatory dysfunction with increased straining and incomplete evacuation due to impaired coordination and relaxation of the anal sphincters and pelvic musculature (Pfeiffer 2004). Gastrointestinal dysfunction in PD appears to be due to central nervous system dysfunction combined with the documented loss of dopaminergic neurons and formation of Lewy bodies in the enteric nervous system within the gastrointestinal tract itself (Singaram et al. 1995; Wakabayashi et al. 1990).

Urinary dysfunction also develops frequently in PD. Symptoms of bladder irritability, with urinary frequency and urgency, develop in 57 to 83% of persons with PD (Singer 2004). Obstructive urinary symptoms, such as hesitancy and weak urinary stream, are much less frequent, but do occur. Sphincter dysfunction in the form of delayed relaxation, sometimes labeled sphincter bradykinesia, is also described (Pavlakis et al. 1983).

Sexual dysfunction, yet another manifestation of autonomic impairment in PD, has been more extensively studied in men but also may develop in women with PD (Waters and Smolowitz 2004). A majority of PD patients report decreased sexual activity. Decreased libido is documented in both men and women, and erectile dysfunction is common in men with PD. In addition to autonomic dysfunction, depression and motor disability contribute to sexual dysfunction in PD.

Cardiovascular sympathetic dysfunction in the form of orthostatic hypotension is widely recognized as a prominent component of multiple system atrophy. Orthostatic hypotension can also develop in PD, sometimes as a complication of antiparkinson medication, but also as part of the disease process itself. Unlike multiple system atrophy, where the defect producing cardiovascular dysfunction lies predominantly within the central nervous system, patients with PD and orthostatic hypotension demonstrate diffuse or localized loss of cardiac sympathetic innervation on cardiac scanning, indicating peripheral autonomic involvement (Goldstein 2003; Goldstein 2004).

Abnormalities of thermoregulatory function also occur in PD (LeDoux 2004). Paroxysmal perspiration, sometimes profuse, may develop and preferentially involves the head, neck, and upper trunk. Most often this occurs as a wearing-off phenomenon, but may also develop during periods of prominent dyskinesia. Sometimes it occurs without any obvious trigger.

3. Sleep Disturbances

Investigators have identified a variety of sleep disturbances in persons with PD. Insomnia is the most common sleep disturbance in PD and is characterized by sleep fragmentation with frequent awakening. Multiple factors may be responsible, including discomfort from immobility, medication effects, restless legs symptoms, depression, and even frequent nocturia (Moro-de-Casillas and Riley 2004). REM sleep behavior disorder is a fascinating and potentially dangerous parasomnia that clinicians now recognize to develop quite frequently in individuals with PD and other synucleinopathies, sometimes months or even years before typical PD motor features emerge. This disorder is characterized by absence of the muscle atonia that typically accompanies dreaming. Individuals with REM sleep behavior disorder can still move while dreaming and, thus, may punch, kick, scream, jump out of bed, or even take off running as they act out their dreams. The potential for injury (both for the patient and for the spouse) during these episodes is obvious. The pathophysiological basis for REM sleep behavior disorder in PD is uncertain, but dysfunction at the level of the pedunculopontine nucleus and the laterodorsal tegmental nucleus in the brainstem is suspected (Stevens and Comella 2004). Researchers have recently suggested that obstructive sleep apnea may also occur more frequently in PD than in the normal population (Carlucci and Hauser 2004).

4. Disorders of Sensation

Non-motor dysfunction in PD even extends to several of the primary senses. Abnormalities in both vision and olfaction have been clearly identified in PD and may be due to involvement of dopaminergic neuronal populations distinct from the nigrostriatal system. Pain and other subtle abnormalities of sensation also frequently appear in individuals with PD, although their pathophysiological basis is uncertain.

Individuals with PD frequently report blurred vision, especially when reading. Although formal studies actually have demonstrated subtle group differences in visual acuity between PD patients and controls, routine visual acuity testing in individual patients is often unremarkable (Repka et al. 1996). However, a number of other abnormalities of visual function occur in PD that may account for the vague visual symptoms patients experience (Rodnitzky 2004). Convergence insufficiency may produce difficulty viewing close objects clearly. Impaired sensitivity to visual contrast, which measures the minimal contrast necessary to distinguish objects from each other, is also consistently identified in patients with PD and is attributed to retinal dopamine deficiency. Impaired color vision, especially of the tritan (blue-yellow) axis, also occurs in PD. Finally, abnormalities of visuo-cognitive function have been identified with sophisticated testing of PD patients (Bodis-Wollner and Antal 2004).

Impaired function of another primary sensory modality, olfaction, is also firmly delineated in the setting of PD. Elevated threshold for detecting odors, reduced ability to identify odors, and impaired odor recognition memory are all identified in PD (Furtado and Wszolek 2004). Although researchers recently reported that olfactory impairment is not present in individuals with PD due to the parkin mutation (Khan et al. 2004), impairment is documented in some other types of familial Parkinsonism (Markopoulou et al. 1997). Neuronal loss with Lewy body formation in the olfactory bulb is documented in PD and may be the basis for the impaired olfactory ability, although simple reduced ability to sniff vigorously may also play a role (Sobel et al. 2001).

Although routine neurological examination does not demonstrate objective sensory impairment in PD, individuals with PD frequently describe subjective sensory symptoms such as pain, numbness, tingling, and even burning paresthesias. These "primary sensory symptoms" were documented in 43% of PD patients in one study (Snider et al. 1976). Experimental evaluation with refined experimental testing techniques has demonstrated objective abnormalities of proprioception and sensorimotor integration in persons with PD (Zia et al. 2000; Klockgether et al. 1995). Painful or unpleasant sensations often plague PD patients; their presence has been reported in 38–54% of individuals and may derive from several mechanisms (Ford and Pfeiffer 2004). Pain may be musculoskeletal in origin, the consequence of rigidity and bradykinesia. Changes in posture may predispose patients with PD to pain of radicular origin. Painful dystonia, sometimes due to antiparkinson medication but sometimes part of the disease process itself, may also occur. Although mercifully rare, pain of central nervous system origin, often bizarre in both location and character, can be a tremendously troubling and treatment-resistant problem for those afflicted. Akathisia, an internal sense of restlessness that is uncomfortable though perhaps not painful in the classical sense, is typically seen in individuals receiving neuroleptic medication for schizophrenia, but may also appear in persons with PD.

E. Treatment Complications

Long-term treatment of PD with levodopa may be complicated by the emergence of some additional features of motor dysfunction that are distinctive and occasionally devastating. When treatment is initiated, the duration of benefit from a dose of levodopa is prolonged and patients experience no waning of benefit, even if they take a scheduled dose late. In fact, one or even several doses may be completely missed without any loss of benefit. With the passage of time and progression of the disease process, however, a different picture emerges. The duration of benefit derived from a dose of levodopa diminishes and patients may note reemergence of their Parkinsonian features before their next dose of medication is due. This has been termed the "wearing-off" phenomenon. Initially this phenomenon occurs rather predictably at the end of a dose interval, but eventually more unpredictable and precipitous fluctuations may develop that bear no identifiable relationship to the timing of levodopa administration. These more chaotic fluctuations are called "on-off" motor responses and can be tremendously disabling for affected individuals.

The development of involuntary movements, typically choreiform in character but occasionally dystonic, represents another complication of levodopa therapy that may emerge after several years of treatment, often in conjunction with the "wearing off" phenomenon. These movements typically appear as the benefit of a levodopa dose reaches its peak and are, therefore, labeled "peak-dose dyskinesia." More rarely, they may appear shortly after taking a dose of levodopa, just as benefit becomes evident, and then disappear as full benefit from the dose is achieved, only to reemerge as the benefit from the dose wears off. This phenomenon is labeled "biphasic dyskinesia." Dyskinetic movements may be magnified by stress or anxiety; this can sometimes be brought out in the clinic by having the patient count backwards by threes or some other interval. An unusual facet of dyskinesia is that the patient is often completely unaware of the involuntary movements; family members may first bring them to the attention of the physician.

V. SUMMARY

In some respects PD is like a Russian babushka, or nesting, doll. On the surface it is characterized by the cardinal features of tremor, rigidity, bradykinesia, and postural instability. Hidden within this façade, however, are multiple layers of complexity in the form of secondary motor features, non-motor features, and treatment-related motor complications. In assessing and developing animal models for PD, researchers must recognize this phenotypic heterogeneity. The perfect animal model that duplicates all the clinical features of PD does not yet exist, and given the complexity of the human disease process, perhaps it is unreasonable to expect one.

Video Legends

SEGMENT 1 This patient with PD was on no symptomatic treatment at the time of videotaping. Her examination demonstrates tremor (rest tremor and "re-emergent" tremor), bradykinesia (diminished spontaneous movement and impaired repetitive and alternating movements), slight postural instability, stooped posture, gait characterized by small, shuffling steps with a hint of festination, and transient freezing (start hesitation and at doorways).

SEGMENT 2 Patient with PD demonstrates Levodopa-induced dyskinesia, which is accentuated by stress in the form of counting backwards.

References

Bodis-Wollner, I., and A. Antal, 2004. Primary visual and visuo-cognitive deficits in Parkinson's disease. In *Parkinson's Disease and Non-Motor Dysfunction*. Ed. R.F. Pfeiffer and I. Bodis-Wollner. In Press. Totowa, New Jersey: Humana Press.

Bruneau, M-A. 2004. Obsessionality in Parkinson's disease. In *Parkinson's Disease and Non-Motor Dysfunction*. Ed. R.F. Pfeiffer and I. Bodis-Wollner. In Press. Totowa, New Jersey: Humana Press.

Burke, W.J., S.P. Wengel, and D. Bohac. 2004. Depression in Parkinson's disease. In *Parkinson's Disease and Non-Motor Dysfunction.* Ed. R.F. Pfeiffer and I. Bodis-Wollner. In Press. Totowa, New Jersey: Humana Press.

Carlucci, C.M., and R.A. Hauser. 2004. Sleep apnea and Parkinson's disease. In *Parkinson's Disease and Non-Motor Dysfunction.* Ed. R.F. Pfeiffer and I. Bodis-Wollner. In Press. Totowa, New Jersey: Humana Press.

Comella, C.L. 2003. Sleep disturbances in Parkinson's disease. *Curr Neurol Neurosci Rep* **3**:173–180.

Cordato, D.J., and D.K.Y. Chan. 2004. Genetics and Parkinson's disease. *J Clin Neurosci* **11**:119–123.

Dewey, R.B. Jr. 2000. Clinical features of Parkinson's disease. In *Parkinson's Disease and Movement Disorders: Diagnosis and Treatment Guidelines for the Practicing Physician.* Ed. C.H. Adler and J.E. Ahlskog. pp. 71–84. Totowa, New Jersey: Humana Press.

Fernandez, H.H., and T. Simuni. 2004. Anxiety in Parkinson's disease. In *Parkinson's Disease and Non-Motor Dysfunction.* Ed. R.F. Pfeiffer and I. Bodis-Wollner. In Press. Totowa, New Jersey: Humana Press.

Findley, L.J., M.A. Gresty, and G.M. Halmagyi. 1981. Tremor and cogwheel phenomena and clonus in Parkinson's disease. *J Neurol Neurosurg Psychiatry* **44**:534–546.

Findley, L.J., and M.A. Gresty. 1984. Tremor and rhythmical involuntary movements in Parkinson's disease. In *Movement Disorders: Tremors.* Ed. L.J. Findley and R. Capildeo. pp. 295–304. New York: Oxford University Press.

Ford, B., and R.F. Pfeiffer, 2004. Pain syndromes and disorders of sensation in Parkinson's disease. In *Parkinson's Disease and Non-Motor Dysfunction.* Ed. R.F. Pfeiffer and I. Bodis-Wollner. In Press. Totowa, New Jersey: Humana Press.

Furtado, S., and Z.K. Wszolek. 2004. Olfactory dysfunction in Parkinson's disease. In *Parkinson's Disease and Non-Motor Dysfunction.* Ed. R.F. Pfeiffer and I. Bodis-Wollner. In Press. Totowa, New Jersey: Humana Press.

Giladi, N. 2002. Gait disturbances. In *Parkinson's Disease. Diagnosis and Clinical Management.* Ed. S.A. Factor and W.J. Weiner. pp. 57–65. New York: Demos.

Goldstein, D.S. 2003. Dysautonomia in Parkinson's disease: neurocardiological abnormalities. *Lancet Neurol* **2**:669–676.

Goldstein, D.S. 2004. Cardiovascular autonomic dysfunction in Parkinson's disease. In *Parkinson's Disease and Non-Motor Dysfunction.* Ed. R.F. Pfeiffer and I. Bodis-Wollner. In Press. Totowa, New Jersey: Humana Press.

Gurevich, T., A.D. Korczyn, and N. Giladi. 2004. Gastric dysfunction in Parkinson's disease. In *Parkinson's Disease and Non-Motor Dysfunction.* Ed. R.F. Pfeiffer and I. Bodis-Wollner. In Press. Totowa, New Jersey: Humana Press.

Hallett, M. 2003. Parkinson revisited: pathophysiology of motor signs. *Adv Neurol* **91**:19–28.

Hoehn, M.M., and M.D. Yahr. 1967. Parkinsonism: onset, progression and mortality. *Neurology* **17**:427–442.

Jankovic, J., K.S. Schwartz, and W. Ondo. 1999. Re-emergent tremor of Parkinson's disease. *J Neurol Neurosurg Psychiatry* **67**:646–650.

Jankovic, J. 2003. Pathophysiology and clinical assessment of parkinsonian symptoms and signs. In *Handbook of Parkinson's Disease, Third Edition.* Ed. R. Pahwa, K.E. Lyons, and W.C. Koller. pp. 71–106. New York: Marcel Dekker.

Kavanagh, P., and K. Marder. 2004. Dementia in Parkinson's disease. In *Parkinson's Disease and Non-Motor Dysfunction.* Ed. R.F. Pfeiffer and I. Bodis-Wollner. In Press. Totowa, New Jersey: Humana Press.

Kennard, C., and P. Nachev. 2004. Oculomotor dysfunction in Parkinson's disease. In *Parkinson's Disease and Non-Motor Dysfunction.* Ed. R.F. Pfeiffer and I. Bodis-Wollner. In Press. Totowa, New Jersey: Humana Press.

Khan, N.L., R. Katzenschlager, H. Watt, K.P. Bhatia, N.W. Wood, N. Quinn, and A.J. Lees. 2004. Olfaction differentiates parkin disease from early-onset parkinsonism and Parkinson disease. *Neurology* **62**:1224–1226.

Klockgether, T., M. Borutta, H. Rapp, S. Spieker, and J. Dichgans. 1995. A defect of kinesthesia in Parkinson's disease. *Mov Disord* **10**:460–465.

LeDoux, M.S. 2004. Thermoregulatory dysfunction in Parkinson's disease. In *Parkinson's Disease and Non-Motor Dysfunction.* Ed. R.F. Pfeiffer and I. Bodis-Wollner. In Press. Totowa, New Jersey: Humana Press.

Leopold, N.A. 2004. Dysphagia in Parkinson's disease. In *Parkinson's Disease and Non-Motor Dysfunction.* Ed. R.F. Pfeiffer and I. Bodis-Wollner. In Press. Totowa, New Jersey: Humana Press.

Markopoulou, K., K.W. Larsen, E.K. Wszolek, M.A. Denson, A.E. Lang, R.F. Pfeiffer, and Z.K. Wszolek. 1997. Olfactory dysfunction in familial parkinsonism. *Neurology* **49**:1262–1267.

Marras, C., and C.M. Tanner. 2004. Epidemiology of Parkinson's disease. In *Movement Disorders: Neurologic Principles and Practice, Second Edition.* Ed. R.L. Watts and W.C. Koller. pp. 177–195. New York: McGraw-Hill.

McAuley, J.H. 2003. The physiological basis of clinical deficits in Parkinson's disease. *Prog Neurobiol* **69**:27–48.

Molho, E.S., and S.A. Factor. 2004. Psychosis in Parkinson's disease. In *Parkinson's Disease and Non-Motor Dysfunction.* Ed. R.F. Pfeiffer and I. Bodis-Wollner. In Press. Totowa, New Jersey: Humana Press.

Moro-de-Casillas, M.L., and D.E. Riley. 2004. Insomnia in Parkinson's disease. In *Parkinson's Disease and Non-Motor Dysfunction.* Ed. R.F. Pfeiffer and I. Bodis-Wollner. In Press. Totowa, New Jersey: Humana Press.

Mouradian, M.M. 2002. Recent advances in the genetics and pathogenesis of Parkinson's disease. *Neurology* **58**:179–185.

Mueller, P.B. 1971. Parkinson's disease: motor-speech behavior in a selected group of patients. *Folia Phoniatr* **23**:333–346.

Nutt, J.G., J.P. Hammerstad, and S.T. Gancher. 1992. *Parkinson's Disease. 100 Maxims.* St. Louis: Mosby Year Book.

Pal, P.K., A. Samii, and D.B. Calne. 2002. Cardinal features of early Parkinson's disease. In *Parkinson's Disease. Diagnosis and Clinical Management.* Ed. S.A. Factor and W.J. Weiner. pp. 41–56. New York: Demos.

Pankratz, N., and T. Foroud. 2004. Genetics of Parkinson's disease. *NeuroRx* **1**:235–242.

Parkinson, J. 1817. *An Essay on the Shaking Palsy.* London: Sherwood, Neely, and Jones.

Pavlakis, A.J., M.B. Siroky, I. Goldstein, and R.J. Krane. 1983. Neurourologic findings in Parkinson's disease. *J Urol* **129**:80–83.

Pechadre, J.C., I. Larochelle, and L.J. Porier. 1976. Parkinsonian akinesia, rigidity and tremor in the monkey. Histopathological and neuropharmacological study. *J Neurol Sci* **28**:147–157.

Pfeiffer, R.F. 2003. Gastrointestinal dysfunction in Parkinson's disease. *Lancet Neurol* **2**:107–116.

Pfeiffer, R.F. 2004. Intestinal dysfunction in Parkinson's disease. In *Parkinson's Disease and Non-Motor Dysfunction.* Ed. R.F. Pfeiffer and I. Bodis-Wollner. In Press. Totowa, New Jersey: Humana Press.

Pfeiffer, R.F., and E.M.M. Quigley. 2004. Gastrointestinal dysfunction in diseases of the cerebral hemispheres and movement disorders. In *Neurogastroenterology.* Ed. E.M.M. Quigley and R.F. Pfeiffer. pp. 59–81. Philadelphia: Butterworth Heinemann.

Ramig, L.O., S. Countryman, C. Fox, and S. Sapir. 2002. Speech, voice, and swallowing disorders. In *Parkinson's Disease. Diagnosis and Clinical Management.* Ed. S.A. Factor and W.J. Weiner. pp. 75–86. New York: Demos.

Repka, M. X., M.C. Claro, D.N. Loupe, and S.G. Reich. 1996. Ocular motility in Parkinson's disease. *J Pediatr Ophthalmol Strabismus* **33**: 144–147.

Rodnitzky, R. 2004. Visual dysfunction in Parkinson's disease. In *Parkinson's Disease and Non-Motor Dysfunction.* Ed. R.F. Pfeiffer and I. Bodis-Wollner. In Press. Totowa, New Jersey: Humana Press.

Selby, G. 1990. Clinical features. In *Parkinson's Disease*. Ed. G. Stern. pp. 333–388. Baltimore: The Johns Hopkins University Press.

Siddiqui, M.F., S. Rast, M.J. Lynn, A.P. Auchus, and R.F. Pfeiffer. 2002. Autonomic dysfunction in Parkinson's disease: a comprehensive symptom survey. *Parkinsonism Relat Disord* **8**:277–284.

Singaram, C., W. Ashraf, E.A. Gaumnitz, C. Torbey, A. Sengupta, R. Pfeiffer, and E.M.M. Quigley. 1995. Dopaminergic defect of enteric nervous system in Parkinson's disease patients with chronic constipation. *Lancet* **346**:861–864.

Singer, C. 2004. Urological dysfunction in Parkinson's disease. In *Parkinson's Disease and Non-Motor Dysfunction.* Ed. R.F. Pfeiffer and I. Bodis-Wollner. In Press. Totowa, New Jersey: Humana Press.

Snider, S.R., S. Fahn, W.P. Isgreen, and L.J. Cote. 1976. Primary sensory symptoms in parkinsonism. *Neurology* **26**:423–429.

Sobel, N., M.E. Thomason, I. Stappen, C.M. Tanner, J.W. Tetrud, J.M. Bower, E.V. Sullivan, and J.D.E. Gabrieli. 2001. An impairment in sniffing contributes to the olfactory impairment in Parkinson's disease. *Proc Natl Acad Sci USA* **98**:4154–4159.

Stevens, S., and C. Comella. 2004. REM sleep behavior disorder in Parkinson's disease. In *Parkinson's Disease and Non-Motor Dysfunction.* Ed. R.F. Pfeiffer and I. Bodis-Wollner. In Press. Totowa, New Jersey: Humana Press.

Tandberg, E., J.P. Larsen, D. Aarsland, and J.L. Cummings. 1996. The occurrence of depression in Parkinson's disease. A community-based study. *Arch Neurol* **53**:175–179.

Toth, C., M. Rajput, and A.H. Rajput. 2004. Anomalies of asymmetry of clinical signs in parkinsonism. *Mov Disord* **19**:151–157.

Wakabayashi, K., K. Takahashi, E. Ohama, and F. Ikuta. 1990. Parkinson's disease: an immunohistochemical study of Lewy body-containing neurons in the enteric nervous system. *Acta Neuropathol* **79**:581–583.

Warner, T.T., and A.H.V. Schapira. 2003. Genetic and environmental factors in the cause of Parkinson's disease. *Ann Neurol* **53**(suppl 3):S16–S25.

Waters, C., and J. Smolowitz, 2004. Impaired sexual function in Parkinson's disease. In *Parkinson's Disease and Non-Motor Dysfunction.* Ed. R.F. Pfeiffer and I. Bodis-Wollner. In Press. Totowa, New Jersey: Humana Press.

Wszolek, Z.K., and M. Farrer. 2003. Genetics. In *Handbook of Parkinson's Disease.* Third Edition. Ed. R. Pahwa, K.E. Lyons, and W.C. Koller. pp. 325–337. New York: Marcel Dekker.

Wszolek, Z.K., K. Markopoulou, and B.A. Chase. 2004. Genetics of Parkinson's disease and parkinsonian disorders. In *Movement Disorders: Neurologic Principles and Practice, Second Edition* Ed. R.L. Watts and W.C. Koller. pp. 163–176. New York: McGraw-Hill.

Zia, S., F. Cody, and D. O'Boyle. 2000. Joint position sense is impaired by Parkinson's disease. *Ann Neurol* **47**:218–228.

CHAPTER

B2

MPTP-Induced Nigrostriatal Injury in Nonhuman Primates

JOEL S. PERLMUTTER and SAMER D. TABBAL

MPTP-induced injury to dopaminergic neurons of the nigrostriatal pathways of nonhuman primates has been an important model for parkinsonism and, more recently, also for dystonia. In particular, the nonhuman primate model provides behavioral responses that closely mimic human parkinsonism, including response to medication. This may reflect the close similarities between basal ganglia anatomy and pharmacology of nonhuman primates and humans. These advantages have led to the use of this model system to investigate pathophysiology of nigrostriatal denervation and to develop and test new therapeutic interventions. This chapter reviews the different methods of MPTP administration, the behavioral responses to MPTP, the pathophysiological consequences of this denervation, and the use of this model to investigate new treatments for parkinsonism.

I. BACKGROUND

The initial report of a chemist developing a parkinsonian condition after exposure to the neurotoxin 1-methyl-4-phenyl-1,2,3,6-tetrahydropyridine (MPTP) was published more than twenty years ago (Langston & Ballard 1983). Soon thereafter, Dr. William Langston and associates (Langston et al. 1983; Ballard et al. 1985) identified MPTP as the proximate cause of acute parkinsonism in people exposed to this designer drug. Pathological identification of selective loss of dopaminergic neurons in people exposed to MPTP confirmed the specificity of this neurotoxin (Burns et al. 1983; Langston et al. 1984) and established the notion that MPTP could provide a convenient animal model of parkinsonism (Burns et al. 1983). The most obvious choice of an animal for such studies included nonhuman primates that have similar basal ganglia anatomy and could potentially exhibit motor behaviors with great similarity to human parkinsonism. This nonhuman primate model has included investigations of basal ganglia pathophysiology, pharmacology, pharmacotherapy, and surgical interventions. These types of studies have been variably addressed with different modes of MPTP delivery, each with its own advantages and disadvantages. In this chapter, we will first review the modes of MPTP delivery, describe the behavioral responses to MPTP, and finally review how this model has been used for investigations.

II. MPTP DELIVERY

Researchers may vary the delivery of MPTP by site of administration and timing of the delivery. The first reports included subcutaneous or intravenous administration of MPTP either in a single dose, daily dose, or weekly dose until a specific behavioral goal was achieved (Schwartzman et al. 1985a,b; Hartvig et al. 1986; Irwin et al. 1990; Gerlach et al. 1990; Perez-Otano et al. 1992; Blanchet et al. 1998b). These systemic modes of delivery typically produce bilateral parkinsonism with bradykinesia, rigidity, flexed posture, and variable tremor (Burns 1983; Langston 1984; Jenner 1984; Chiueh 1985; Doudet 1985). The tremor appears to be species dependent and has been most often described as a postural or action tremor rather than the more characteristic resting tremor of human Parkinson disease (PD) (Burns 1983; Langston 1984; Jenner et al. 1984; Chiueh et al. 1985; Doudet et al. 1985). The advantage of systemic delivery includes ease of administration, but it frequently produces severely bilaterally affected animals that require intense care.

Alternatively, Bankiewicz first reported that intracarotid administration of MPTP produced a unilateral lesion of the striatonigral system with subsequent development of contralateral clinical manifestations (Bankiewicz et al. 1986). This unilateral model has two key advantages. First, animals can typically care for themselves, at least after the acute stage, which may include sedation, decreased appetite, and generally depressed activity. Second, unilateral intracarotid delivery limits delivery of MPTP to just one side of the brain, thereby potentially permitting the use of the other side of the brain as an internal control (Brooks et al. 1987). However, some data suggest that this non-injected side is not entirely unaffected (Todd et al. 1996).

Subsequently, these modes of administration were modified to attempt to produce an animal model of parkinsonism that more closely mimics the pathological insult of idiopathic human PD, based upon the assumption that human PD does not represent a single "hit" followed by age-related decline in the nigrostriatal dopaminergic pathways. These other modes include relatively low doses of systemic MPTP to produce mild bilateral nigrostriatal deficits with an additional intracarotid infusion of MPTP to make one side more severely affected (Oiwa et al. 2003). This approach more closely mimics human PD in the sense that most people with idiopathic PD have asymmetric involvement (Hughes et al. 1992; Rajput et al. 1991). In the same fashion, others have used repeated low doses of MPTP (usually with subcutaneous or intravenous administration) to mimic the progressive nature of PD (Blanchet et al. 1998b).

Each of these modes of MPTP has its own advantages and disadvantages. The correct mode depends upon the nature of the experiment for which the animal model will be used. Of course, this will depend largely upon the behavioral manifestations produced by the MPTP-induced brain damage.

III. BEHAVIORAL RESPONSES TO MPTP

Systemic rather than intracarotid or intrastriatal administration of MPTP produces bilateral clinical manifestations. These effects may be severe at first and then gradually diminish over time. Clinical manifestations include bradykinesia, akinesia (or lack of spontaneous activity), flexed posturing, and tremor. A few reports have also documented paradoxical kinesia, which is the abrupt onset of rather fast movement when a severely affected animal is confronted with a sudden threat such as the approach of an investigator (Degryse and Colpaert 1986). This response is well known in human PD and adds to the clinical validity of the animal model. However, in animals exposed to MPTP that have severe bilateral clinical manifestations, these motor deficits may gradually reduce over the course of one to two years (Oiwa et al. 2003). For some longitudinal research studies, this reduction can be a major limiting factor or potential confound.

Unilateral internal carotid administration of MPTP produces reduction of dopaminergic neurons and reduction of striatal dopamine content on only one side of the brain. MPTP was administered this way in a wide variety of nonhuman primates including baboons (Todd et al. 1996), rhesus macaques (Chen et al. 1991), marmosets (Jenner et al. 1984), nemestrina (Barrio et al. 1990), and cynomologous macaques (Joyce et al. 1986). The original intent was to provide a model of Parkinsonism with its attendant clinical features produced by striatal dopamine deficiency. However, many investigators described an acute phase beginning within one day of MPTP administration before more typical parkinsonian manifestations developed. Upon further evaluation, this early, transient phase appears to have features similar to human dystonia with abnormal extensor-type posturing of the upper and lower limbs contralateral to the side of MPTP administration (Perlmutter et al. 1997a). This may be associated with ipsiversive (with respect to the side of MPTP injection) spontaneous rotation of the animal. This transient dystonic phase may last several weeks and then is followed by stable parkinsonism lasting at least one to two years (Perlmutter et al. 1997a). Interestingly, dystonia may be an early manifestation of PD, especially in young onset PD (Lucking et al. 2000; Bonifati et al. 2001; Khan et al. 2003; Fishman and Oyler 2002; Lohmann et al. 2003). Thus intracarotid administration of MPTP may provide a model of transient dystonia as well as chronic, stable parkinsonism.

The behavioral responses to MPTP appear to be age-dependent, whether given systemically or via the intracarotid route (Degryse et al. 1986; Ovadia et al. 1995; Irwin et al. 1997; Narabayashi et al. 1987). Younger immature or adolescent animals may have no or little behavioral response to MPTP. At least in adolescent animals, repeated exposures may produce a behavioral deficit suggesting that sensitivity to MPTP reflects an age-dependence of the nigrostriatal damage induced by MPTP (Guttman 1988; Ovadia 1995; Burns 1991; Doudet 1998). The pathophysiology of this age-related sensitivity remains to be determined.

Some researchers have also used this model of nigrostriatal injury to assess its effects on cognitive function. For example, cognitive and oculomotor impairments may develop before onset of motor deficits in MPTP monkeys (Slovin et al. 1999). More specifically, spatial working memory may be impaired by MPTP and then improved by selective nicotinic receptor agonists (Schneider et al. 2003). Another study has investigated the effects of MPTP-induced dopamine depletion on the function of mesial frontal areas with priopriocepive-guided limb movements (Escola et al. 2002).

IV. RESEARCH APPLICATIONS

A. Basal Ganglia Pathophysiology

MPTP-induced striatal dopamine depletion in primates provides a model to measure the effects on basal ganglia physiology (DeLong et al. 1990). Electrophysiological studies can be divided into those that evaluated neuronal activity of various nuclei with the animals at quiet rest and those that measured animals during various tasks. For example, DeLong and associates (Bergman et al. 1994; Wichmann et al. 1994) found that spontaneous activity in the subthalamic nucleus was increased in MPTP-treated monkeys (Bergman et al. 1990). Similarly, neuronal firing rate was increased in internal pallidum (GPi) and decreased in external pallidum (GPe) in MPTP-treated monkeys (Filion and Tremblay 1991). These firing rates became normal after administering the mixed D1 and D2 agonist apomorphine or a selective D2 agonist (Filion et al. 1991).

Numerous investigators have done physiological and electrophysiological studies with MPTP-treated nonhuman primates while the animal was active. For example, MPTP-treated nonhuman primates have prolonged reaction times measured by EMG and prolonged time to reach and manipulate food rewards (Schultz et al. 1989). Furthermore, independence of pallidal neurons may diminish after MPTP-induced parkinsonism as demonstrated by increased synchrony of firing between pallidal neurons (Nini et al. 1995). Tonically active neurons in striatum also increase their synchrony with firing of pallidal neurons after MPTP in vervet monkeys (Raz et al. 2001). Dopamine replacement therapy normalizes firing rates in GPe and GPi in vervet monkeys trained to perform a button-pressing task and also reverses the abnormal MPTP-induced synchronization of pallidal neuronial firing (Heimer et al. 2002). Other studies found that responses to reversible lesions using focal injections of the GABA agonist muscimol into centromedial GPi or the lateral area of the sensorimotor subthalamic nucleus ameliorated parkinsonian motor behaviors in behaving animals, suggesting that these areas might be good targets for ablative or deep brain stimulation (Baron et al. 2002).

Another approach to assessing basal ganglia function is to measure by autoradiography changes in markers of neuronal activity such as 2-deoxyglucose (2-DG). For example, after systemic MPTP administration, 2-DG uptake increased in the globus pallidus but not in substantia nigra pars reticulata, suggesting that MPTP affects selected components of basal ganglia pathways (Mitchell et al. 1986). Intracarotid infusion of MPTP altered 2-DG uptake in the brain only ipsilateral to the MPTP infusion (Palombo et al. 1990). Autoradiographic studies also have included evaluations of mRNA expression for comodulators within basal ganglia pathways such as those that affect the direct and indirect pathways (Wade and Schneider, 2001). For example time-dependent changes in striatal mRNA expression for substance P and Met-enkephalin occur after MPTP administration in marmosets (Perez-Otano et al. 1992; Jolkkonen 1995), but levodopa administration reverses changes only in substance P mRNA expression, which is primarily associated with the direct pathway. In contrast, concentrations of other comodulators such as cholecystokinin and neurotensin do not appear to change after MPTP (Taquet et al. 1988; Taylor et al. 1991).

Autoradiographic studies can be done *in vivo* using positron emission tomography (PET), which permits repeated measurements in a single subject. Although conventional PET measurements have limited resolution compared to *ex vivo* or *in vitro* autoradiography, new microPET techniques are narrowing these margins (Tai et al. 2003). Nevertheless, PET studies of either [18F]fluorodeoxyglucose (FDG), oxygen metabolism, or blood flow as markers of neuronal activity have provided insights into the effects of nigrostriatal damage produced by MPTP in primates. For example, blood flow, oxygen extraction, and glucose utilization increase in globus pallidus but decrease in striatum after systemic MPTP (Brownell et al. 2003). However, an older study found that striatal blood flow decreased after unilateral intracarotid MPTP (Doudet et al. 1993). Differences in anesthesia and experimental conditions may account for these discrepancies (Hershey et al. 2000).

PET measurements may also be used to evaluate the integrity of presynaptic neurons in MPTP-treated monkeys. The most commonly used tracer for such studies is [18F]fluorodopa (FD). Uptake of FD, mainly reflects decarboxylase activity in presynaptic neurons and may provide an index of these dopaminergic neurons (Chiueh et al. 1987; Barrio et al. 1990; Martin and Perlmutter 1994). For example, FD PET suggests that increased dopamine turnover may compensate for nigrostriatal neuronal loss after low doses of MPTP that do not produce clinical symptoms in monkeys (Doudet et al. 1998). Development of unilateral clinical parkinsonism requires about 50% reduction of FD uptake after intracarotid infusion of MPTP into monkeys (Barrio et al. 1990). Comparisons of FD PET measurements with *in vitro* measures of decarboxylase activity in MPTP treated monkeys indicate the complicated relationship between changes in activity in the substantia nigra and those that occur in striatum (Yee et al. 2000).

Other tracers also may be used to measure presynaptic dopaminergic terminals and these can be divided into those that mark presynaptic dopamine transporter sites, vesicular transport sites, or also reflect decarboxylase activity like FD. Various cocaine-like analogs bind to dopamine transport sites and have been used with PET or single photon emission tomography (Hantraye et al. 1992) to demonstrate loss of uptake after MPTP administration in monkeys. Vesicular monoamine transport sites can be labeled with [11C]dihydrotetrabenzine ([11C]DTBZ) and may be less prone to regulation than dopamine transport sites (Wilson et al. 1996) although no peer-reviewed reports have been published on MPTP-treated monkeys. Finally, [18F]6-fluoro-l-m-tyrosine (FMT) uptake, like FD, mainly reflects the decarboxylase activity of residual dopaminergic neurons. Its imaging characteristics may have some benefits compared to FD, but direct comparisons have not been made. Nevertheless, application of this tracer has been useful; FMT uptake correlates with severity of tremor and post-mortem dopamine levels in hemiparkinsonian monkeys (Eberling et al. 2000).

In general, these PET tracers are important for potential application to studies in humans with PD. Of course, before the tracers can be used in a human study, the PET measure must be validated; a strategy that is likely to use nonhuman primates to determine how well the PET measure reflects nigrostriatal neuronal counts, striatal dopamine content, or both under the conditions proposed for the human study.

B. Pharmacology

Initial studies in monkeys with MPTP-induced nigrostriatal lesions investigated the effects of striatal denervation upon striatal dopamine receptors. Studies varied by the types of dopamine receptors measured and the methods used for the measurements (Falardeau et al. 1988). These approaches led to substantial variation in findings (Falardeau et al. 1988; Lau and Fung 1986). For example, one initial study found that qualitative *ex vivo* binding of radiolabeled spiperone, a D2-family antagonist, was higher after intracarotid MPTP (Joyce et al. 1986) but another found no change after systemic MPTP (Jenner et al. 1984). However, *in vitro* methods using homogenates, *ex vivo* methods using tissue slices incubated in baths containing radioligand, and *in vivo* methods using intravenous administration of radioligand with subsequent autoradiographic analysis found varying results. These results, could reflect methodological variations due to availability of specific binding sites for radioligands, measurements of nonspecific binding, selectivity of radioligands, or other factors (Perlmutter and Raichle 1986).

PET studies of radiolabeled spiperone in a human with intravenous MPTP-induced parkinsonism revealed elevated binding compared to age-matched normals (Perlmutter et al. 1987), but measures in other humans with idiopathic PD or MPTP-treated monkeys found varying results with some having decreased, some unchanged, and some with elevated D_2-like striatal receptor binding (Decamp et al. 1999; Doudet et al. 2000). These disparate findings led to a longitudinal study of radioligand binding in nonhuman primates with intracarotid MPTP administration that were not treated with dopaminergic medications (Todd et al. 1996). MPTP decreased ipsilateral striatal dopamine content by more than 90%, which did not change with time. Receptor binding, however, demonstrated time-dependence. D_2-like receptor binding in caudate and putamen initially decreased about 30% then increased two- to seven-fold over the first three months and returned toward baseline levels by sixteen months. Relative levels of D_2 mRNA were unchanged over this period. D_4 mRNA was not detected. In contrast, D_3 mRNA levels increased six-fold by two weeks and then decreased. At the peak period of increase in specific binding sites, all D_2-like receptors were in a low affinity agonist binding state, implying an increase in uncoupled-D_2 but not -D_3 receptor protein. In this animal model, there is a dissociation of the normal steady state relationships between receptor number, dopamine content, and messenger RNA levels. This dissociation suggests that MPTP lesion-induced changes are complex and include translational or posttranslational mechanisms. Interestingly, the transient phase of decreased striatal D_2-like binding corresponded with transient dystonia whereas stable chronic parkinsonism persisted despite first increased and then decreased D_2 striatal binding (Perlmutter et al. 1997a). These findings may explain some of the disparities found in the literature in people with idiopathic PD. These findings also provide an important model of dystonia since the reduced striatal D_2 binding during the transient dystonic phase in the nonhuman primates closely matches the decreased striatal binding of D_2-like radioligands in humans with primary cranial or hand dystonia (Perlmutter et al. 1997b; Perlmutter and Mink 2004). Changes in D_1-like receptors have been less revealing. Autoradiographic studies in nonhuman primates have not identified consistent changes in D_1-like striatal binding after MPTP (Grondin et al. 1999b; Decamp et al. 1999). Other changes in basal ganglia pharmacology have been found in MPTP-treated animals. For example, intracerebral microdialysis found increased GABA in the external pallidum (Robertson et al. 1991). Reductions in pallidal glutamic acid decarboxylase (GAD) activity also may be a key feature in the development of parkinsonian manifestations (Schneider and Wade, 2003). Treatment with antisense oligonucleotides to GAD mRNA reverses the parkinsonism, suggesting new avenues for treatment (Schneider and Wade 2003).

C. Therapeutic Interventions

Because the behavior of MPTP-treated nonhuman primates closely mimics human PD, it seems reasonable to use this model to evaluate various therapeutic interventions. Initially, researchers assessed a variety of drug interventions. This assessment was particularly useful because these animals not only responded positively to standard clinical interventions like levodopa (Burns et al. 1983; Jenner et al. 1984; Bankiewicz et al. 1986), but they also developed dopa-induced involuntary movements including choreiform dyskinesias and dystonia similar to responses in humans with PD (Kuoppamaki et al. 2002). This faithful model of human response to levodopa set the stage to evaluate a variety of selective dopaminergic agonists to determine whether they also would provide benefit and whether they posed a risk of producing dyskinesias or dystonia (Smith et al. 2002). For example, MPTP monkeys were used to determine that D_1 antagonists reduce dopa-induced dyskinesias but worsen parkinsonism (Grondin et al. 1999a). Another study suggests that D_3 receptor binding decreases in the striatum of MPTP-treated monkeys with dyskinesias (Bezard et al. 2003) and administering a D_3 partial agonist decreases the levodopa-induced dyskinesias without diminishing the dopa-induced motor benefit. Subsequent administration of a D_3 antagonist produces recurrent dyskinesias. Another study found that quetiapine, a D_2/D_3 and $5HT_{2A/C}$ antagonist reduces dopa-induced dyskinesias in MPTP-treated monkeys (Oh et al. 2002). Other studies identified changes in electrophysiological properties of various basal ganglia nuclei induced by different dopamine agonists in MPTP-treated monkeys (Boraud et al. 2001).

Investigators also evaluated the mode of dopaminergic drug delivery. For example, studies in rodents suggested that pulsatile levodopa produced more changes in basal ganglia function than continuous delivery (Engber et al. 1991); raising the question of whether these changes in basal ganglia function underlie development of dopa-induced dyskinesias. Although the rat model was convenient, relatively inexpensive, and could use small amounts of drug, it lacked the behavioral aspects that permit direct comparisons with human responses to levodopa. Newer rodent models with dopa-induced dyskinesias are now available but still are not directly analogous to human behavior like the nonhuman primate model. Therefore, tests of delivery modes have utilized monkeys treated with MPTP (Smith et al. 2003) as well as with different dopamine agonists with short and long lasting effects (Maratos et al. 2003).

In these nonhuman primate studies, researchers have tested the effects of nondopaminergic drugs on Parkinsonism, dopa-induced dyskinesias, and dopa-induced dystonia (Nash et al. 2000; Henry et al. 2001; Fox et al. 2002; Iravani et al. 2003; Chassain et al. 2003). For example, initial studies in nonhuman primates suggested that NMDA antagonists like amantadine reduce dopa-induced dyskinesias (Blanchet et al. 1998a) and AMPA antagonists may have a similar effect (Konitsiotis et al. 2000). This model also permits evaluation of the effects of drug injections into specific basal ganglia nuclei (Nandi et al. 2002; Graham et al. 1990). A variety of other similar studies such as remacemide (Greenamyre et al. 1994) or rasagiline (Kupsch et al. 2001) have been done in monkeys prior to testing in humans. Finally, studies have explored the effects of intraventricular and intra-putamenal delivery of drugs that do not cross the blood-brain barrier such as dopamine receptor agonists, cholinergic antagonists, the glutamate receptor antagonist MK801, and a 5-HT receptor agonist (Close and Elliott 1991).

Drug-treatment of MPTP-treated monkeys also provides an opportunity to study the pathophysiology underlying drug-induced involuntary movements. Initially, investigators found that levodopa produced marked changes in 2-DG uptake throughout many brain regions in MPTP-treated monkeys but little change in 2-DG uptake in normal animals (Porrino et al. 1987). Varying the severity of the MPTP lesion demonstrates the importance of lesion severity on subsequent development of dopa-induced dyskinesias (Di Monte et al. 2000). Another group used this model to investigate regional metabolic changes that correspond with development of dyskinesias (Mitchell et al. 1990, 1992). During the dyskinetic responses to levodopa, investigators injected animals with 2-DG to measure the uptake in various brain regions during dyskinesias and compared the 2-DG uptake in animals that had not developed dyskinesias to animals that had developed dopa-induced dystonia. Two main issues hamper the interpretation of these studies. First, animals with dopa-induced dystonia also had dopa-induced dyskinesias, making it difficult to isolate these different drug-induced responses. Second, 2-DG uptake can be affected by the behavior of the animal during the uptake phase as well as by the brain's response to the drug, making it difficult to distinguish these two factors. This so-called chicken-egg problem limits unambiguous interpretation of some of these studies.

However, in more recent studies investigators have sought to identify specific biochemical or physiological changes in the basal ganglia associated with levodopa treatment (Heimer et al. 2002) or development of dyskinesias (Henry et al. 2003; Quik et al. 2002; Calon et al. 2002). For example, firing rates of neurons in GPi decreased after administration of different dopamine agonists (apomorphine, a mixed D_1/D_2 agonist; SKF 38393, a partial D_1 agonist; and piribidel, a D_2/D_3 agonist) in relation to reduced parkinsonian manifestations, but firing pattern changes distinguished those MPTP-treated animals that developed drug-induced dyskinesias from normal animals that did not (Bourad et al. 2001).

The MPTP primate model also has provided an opportunity to investigate surgical interventions. For example, lesioning the STN in MPTP-treated monkeys demonstrated reduction of parkinsonism (Bergman et al. 1990). This strategy was tested due to the earlier observation that spontaneous activity in STN neurons was increased in MPTP monkeys compared to normal animals. Further, others found that direct lesions of the subthalamic nucleus alleviated parkinsonism in MPTP monkeys (Aziz et al. 1992). Similarly, lesions of the pars reticulata of the substantia nigra may reduce contralateral bradykinesia and akinesia in MPTP monkeys (Wichmann et al. 2001). A recent study investigated the effects of high frequency stimulation of the STN and found that it increased firing in internal pallidum, consistent with the notion that deep brain stimulation drives rather than inhibits output neurons (Hashimoto et al. 2003). Researchers also used the MPTP model to investigate tissue graft viability (Starr et al. 1999; Howel et al. 2000), administration of growth factors (Palfi et al. 2002; Emborg et al. 2001; Kordower et al. 2000), or gangliosides such as GM1 that may partially restore striatal dopaminergic terminals from MPTP damage in monkeys (Pope-Coleman et al. 2000).

Finally, investigators used MPTP-induced nigrostriatal injury in primates as a model to test interventions that could potentially slow or halt the ongoing pathological insult of human PD. This model assumes that the pathological mechanisms of MPTP-induced damage are similar to those that produce human PD. The advantage of an animal study, however, is that it permits careful evaluation of mechanisms and effects of the intervention. For example, a study of rasagiline and selegiline, MAO-B inhibitors that decrease MPTP-induced nigrostriatal damage, may also reduce the cell size of dopaminergic neurons, raising questions about potential toxicity (Kupsch et al. 2001).

V. LIMITATIONS OF THE MODEL

Although MPTP administration in nonhuman primates provides a good behavioral, physiological, and pharmacological model of human idiopathic PD, several limitations must be considered. First, the etiology of this form of parkinsonism, regardless of timing of MPTP administration is not the same as human PD. There are proposed similarities in the potential biochemical mechanism, with MPP+ inhibition of the complex I in the respiratory chain, but whether this is truly critical for the etiopathology of PD remains to be determined. Second, some differences exist in the pathological changes in brain. For example, the typical gradient of selective loss of striatal dopamine content in human PD is not seen in MPTP-treated primates (Pifl et al. 1988) and dopaminergic cells not typically involved in PD may be affected after MPTP (Gibb et al. 1986). Furthermore, acute administration of MPTP does not produce pathological inclusions in dopaminergic neurons similar to Lewy bodies seen in humans with idiopathic PD that are widely recognized as the pathologic hallmark of PD, however, protracted administration of MPTP in older squirrel monkeys did cause Lewy-like bodies in amygdala-parahippocampus; but these inclusions had structural differences from Lewy bodies (Forno et al. 1995). Therefore, investigators must carefully assess the purpose of the study before assuming that use of the MPTP-induced nigrostriatal injury in nonhuman primates is the proper model. Nevertheless, many important advances in understanding both parkinsonism and dystonia have been made with MPTP-treated nonhuman primates.

Acknowledgments

Supported by the Greater St. Louis Chapter of the American Parkinson Disease Association (APDA), The APDA Center for Advanced PD Research at Washington University, NIH grants (NS41248; NS41509), the Barnes-Jewish Hospital Fund, the Ruth Kopolow Fund, the Elliot H. Stein Family Fund, and the Sam & Barbara Murphy Fund.

References

Aziz, T.Z., D. Peggs, E. Agarwal, M.A. Sambrook, and A.R. Crossman. 1992. Subthalamic nucleotomy alleviates Parkinsonism in the 1-methyl-4-phenyl-1,2,3,6-tetrahydropyridine (MPTP)-exposed primate. *British J Neurosurg* **6(6)**:575–582.

Ballard, P.A., J.W. Tetrud, and J.W. Langston. 1985. Permanent human Parkinsonism due to 1-methyl-4-phenyl-1,2,3,6-tetrahydropyridine (MPTP): seven cases. *Neurology* **35**:949–956.

Bankiewicz, K., E. Oldfield, C. Chiueh, J. Doppman, D. Jacobowitz, and I. Kopin. 1986. Hemiparkinsonism in monkeys after unilateral internal carotid artery infusion of 1-methyl-4-phenyl-1,2,3,6-tetrahydropyridine (MPTP). *Life Sci* **39**:7–16.

Baron, M.S., T. Wichmann, D. Ma, and M.R. DeLong. 2002. Effects of transient focal inactivation of the basal ganglia in parkinsonian primates. *J Neurosci* **22**:592–599.

Barrio, J.R., S.C. Huang, W.P. Melega, D.C. Yu, J.M. Hoffman, J.S. Schneider, N. Satyamurthy, J.C. Mazziotta, and M.E. Phelps. 1990. 6-[18F]fluoro-L-dopa probes dopamine turnover rates in central dopaminergic structures. *J Neurosci Res* **27**:487–493.

Bergman, H., T. Wichmann, and M.R. DeLong. 1990. Reversal of experimental Parkinsonism by lesions of the subthalamic nucleus. *Science* **249**:1436–1438.

Bergman, H., T. Wichmann, B. Karmon, and M.R. DeLong. 1994. The primate subthalamic nucleus. II. Neuronal activity in the MPTP model of Parkinsonism. *J Neurophysiol* **72**:507–520.

Bezard, E., S. Ferry, U. Mach, H. Stark, L. Leriche, T. Boraud, C. Gross, and P. Sokoloff. 2003. Attenuation of levodopa-induced dyskinesia by normalizing dopamine D3 receptor function. *Nat Med* **9**:762–767.

Blanchet, P.J., S. Konitsiotis, and T.N. Chase. 1998a. Amantadine reduces levodopa-induced dyskinesias in parkinsonian monkeys. *Mov Disord* **13**:798–802.

Blanchet, P.J., S. Konitsiotis, K. Hyland, L.A. Arnold, K.D. Pettigrew, and T.N. Chase. 1998b. Chronic exposure to MPTP as a primate model of progressive Parkinsonism: a pilot study with a free radical scavenger. *Exp Neurol* **153**:214–222.

Bonifati, V., G. De Michele, C.B. Lucking, A. Durr, E. Fabrizio, G. Ambrosio, N. Vanacore, M. De Mari, R. Marconi, L. Capus, M.M. Breteler, T. Gasser, B. Oostra, N. Wood, Y. Agid, A. Filla, G. Meco, and A. Brice; Italian PD Genetics Study Group, French PD Genetics Study Group, European Consortium on Genetic Susceptibility in PD. 2001. The parkin gene and its phenotype. Italian PD Genetics Study Group, French PD Genetics Study Group and the European Consortium on Genetic Susceptibility in Parkinson's Disease. *Neurol Sci* **22**:51–52.

Boraud, T., E. Bezard, B. Bioulac, and C.E. Gross. 2001. Dopamine agonist-induced dyskinesias are correlated to both firing pattern and frequency alterations of pallidal neurones in the MPTP-treated monkey. *Brain* **124**:546–557.

Brooks, B.A., E. Eidelberg, and W.W. Morgan. 1987. Behavioral and biochemical studies in monkeys made hemiparkinsonian by MPTP. *Brain Res* **419**:329–332.

Brownell, A.L., K. Canales, Y.I. Chen, B.G. Jenkins, C. Owen, E. Livni, M. Yu, F. Cicchetti, R. Sanchez-Pernaute, and O. Isacson. 2003. Mapping of brain function after MPTP-induced neurotoxicity in a primate Parkinson's disease model. *Neuroimage* **20**:1064–1075.

Burns, R.S. 1991. Subclinical damage to the nigrostriatal dopamine system by MPTP as a model of preclinical Parkinson's disease: a review. *Acta Neurolog Scand* (Suppl). **136**:29–36.

Burns, R.S., C.C. Chiueh, S.P. Markey, M.H. Ebert, D.M. Jacobowitz, and I. Kopin. 1983. A primate model of Parkinsonism: selective destruction of dopaminergic neurons in the pars compacta of the substantia nigra by N-methyl-4-phenyl-1,2,3,6-tetrahydropyridine. *Proc Natl Acad Sci U S A* **80**:4546–4550.

Calon, F., M. Goulet, P.J. Blanchet, J.C. Martel, M.F. Piercey, and P.J. Bédard. 1995. Levodopa or D2 agonist induced dyskinesia in MPTP monkeys: correlation with changes in dopamine and $GABA_A$ receptors in the striatopallidal complex. *Brain Res* **680**:43–52.

Calon, F., M. Morissette, O. Ghribi, M. Goulet, R. Grondin, P.J. Blanchet, P.J. Bedard, and P.T. Di. 2002. Alteration of glutamate receptors in the striatum of dyskinetic 1-methyl-4-phenyl-1,2,3,6-tetrahydropyridine-treated monkeys following dopamine agonist treatment. *Prog Neuro Psych Pharm Biol Psych* **26**:127–138.

Chassain, C., A. Eschalier, and F. Durif. 2003. Antidyskinetic effect of magnesium sulfate in MPTP-lesioned monkeys. *Exp Neurol* **182**:490–496.

Chen, S.D., X.D. Zhou, D.L. Xu, G.W. Li, Q.M. Tang, and X.R. Xu. 1991. Hemiparkinsonism in monkeys following unilateral common carotid artery infusion of MPTP. A study of behavior, biochemistry and histology. *Chinese Med Journal* **104**:758–763.

Chiueh, C.C., R.S. Burns, S.P. Markey, D.M. Jacobowitz, and I.J. Kopin. 1985. Primate model of Parkinsonism: selective lesion of nigrostriatal neurons by 1-methyl-4-phenyl-1,2,3,6-tetrahydropyridine produces an extrapyramidal syndrome in rhesus monkeys. *Life Sci* **36(3)**: 213–218.

Chiueh, C.C., G. Firnau, R.S. Burns, C. Nahmias, R. Chirakal, I.J. Kopin, and E.S. Garnett. 1987. Determination and visualization of damage to striatal dopaminergic terminals in 1-methyl-4-phenyl-1,2,3,6-tetrahydropyridine-induced Parkinsonism by [18F]-labeled 6-fluoro-L-dopa and positron emission tomography. *Adv Neurol* **45**:167–169.

Close, S.P, and P.J. Elliott. 1991. Procedure for assessing the behavioral effects of novel anti-parkinsonian drugs in normal and MPTP-treated marmosets following central microinfusions. *J Pharm Methods* **25**: 123–131.

Decamp, E., T. Wade, and J.S. Schneider. 1999. Differential regulation of striatal dopamine D(1) and D(2) receptors in acute and chronic parkinsonian monkeys. *Brain Res* **847**:134–138.

Degryse, A.D., and F.C. Colpaert. 1986. Symptoms and behavioral features induced by 1-methyl-4-phenyl-1,2,3,6-tetrahydropyridine (MPTP) in an old Java monkey [Macaca cynomolgus fascicularis]. *Brain Res Bull* **16**:561–571.

DeLong, M.R. 1990. Primate models of movement disorders of basal ganglia origin. *Trends Neurosci* **13**:281–285.

Di Monte, D.A., A. McCormack, G. Petzinger, A.M. Janson, M. Quik, and W.J. Langston. 2000. Relationship among nigrostriatal denervation, Parkinsonism, and dyskinesias in the MPTP primate model. *Mov Disord* **15**:459–466.

Doudet, D., C. Gross, P. Lebrun-Grandie, and B. Bioulac. 1985. MPTP primate model of Parkinson's disease: a mechanographic and electromyographic study. *Brain Res* **335**:194–199.

Doudet, D.J., R.J. Wyatt, E. Cannon-Spoor, R. Suddath, C.A. McLellan, and R.M. Cohen. 1993. 6-[18F]fluoro-L-dopa and cerebral blood flow in unilaterally MPTP-treated monkeys. *J Neural Transpl Plast* **4**:27–38.

Doudet, D.J., G.L. Chan, J.E. Holden, E.G. McGeer, T.A. Aigner, R.J. Wyatt, and T.J. Ruth. 1998. 6-[18F]Fluoro-L-dopa PET studies of the turnover of dopamine in MPTP-induced Parkinsonism in monkeys. *Synapse* **29**:225–232.

Doudet, D.J., J.E. Holden, S. Jivan, E. McGeer, and R.J. Wyatt. 2000. *In vivo* PET studies of the dopamine D2 receptors in rhesus monkeys with long-term MPTP-induced Parkinsonism. *Synapse* **38**:105–113.

Eberling, J.L., P. Pivirotto, J. Bringas, and K.S. Bankiewicz. 2000. Tremor is associated with PET measures of nigrostriatal dopamine function in MPTP-lesioned monkeys. *Exp Neurol* **165**:342–346.

Eidelberg, E., B.A. Brooks, W.W. Morgan, J.G. Walden, and R.H. Kokemoor. 1986. Variability and functional recovery in the N-methyl-4-phenyl-1,2,3,6-tetrahydropyridine model of Parkinsonism in monkeys. *Neuroscience* **18**:817–822.

Emborg, M.E., P. Shin, B. Roitberg, J.G. Sramek, Y. Chu, G.T. Stebbins, J.S. Hamilton, P.D. Suzdak, J.P. Steiner, and J.H. Kordower. 2001. Systemic administration of the immunophilin ligand GPI 1046 in MPTP-treated monkeys. *Exp Neurol* **168**:171–182.

Engber, T.M., Z. Susel, S. Kuo, C.R. Gerfen, and T.N. Chase. 1991. Levodopa replacement therapy alters enzyme activities in striatum and neuropeptide content in striatal output regions of 6-hydroxydopamine lesioned rats. *Brain Res* **552**:113–118.

Escola, L., T. Michelet, G. Douillard, D. Guehl, B. Bioulac, and P. Burbaud. 2002. Disruption of the proprioceptive mapping in the medial wall of parkinsonian monkeys. *Ann Neurol* **52**:581–587.

Falardeau, P., P.J. Bédard, and T. Di Paolo. 1988. Relation between brain dopamine loss and D_2 dopamine receptor density in MPTP monkeys. *Neurosci Lett* **86**:225–229.

Filion, M., and L. Tremblay. 1991. Abnormal spontaneous activity of globus pallidus neurons in monkeys with MPTP-induced Parkinsonism. *Brain Res* **547**:142–151.

Filion, M., L. Tremblay, and P.J. Bedard. 1991. Effects of dopamine agonists on the spontaneous activity of globus pallidus neurons in monkeys with MPTP-induced Parkinsonism. *Brain Res* **547**:152–161.

Fishman, P.S., and G.A. Oyler. 2002. Significance of the parkin gene and protein in understanding Parkinson's disease. *Curr Neurol Neurosci Rep* **2**:296–302.

Forno, L.S., L.E. DeLanney, I. Irwin, and J.W. Langston. 1995. Ultrastructure of eosinophilic inclusion bodies in the amygdala-parahippocampal region of aged squirrel monkeys treated with 1-methyl-4-phenyl-1,2,3,6-tetrahydropyridine, a dopaminergic neurotoxin. *Neurosci Lett* **184**:44–47.

Fox, S.H., B. Henry, M. Hill, A. Crossman, and J. Brotchie. 2002. Stimulation of cannabinoid receptors reduces levodopa-induced dyskinesia in the MPTP-lesioned nonhuman primate model of Parkinson's disease. *Mov Disord* **17**:1180–1187.

Gagnon, C., P.J. Bédard, and T. Di Paolo. 1990. Effect of chronic treatment of MPTP monkeys with dopamine D-1 and/ or D-2 receptor agonists. *Eur J Pharmacol* **178**:115–120.

Gerlach, M., M. Gotz, A. Dirr, A. Kupsch, B. Janetzky, W. Oertel, J. Sautter, J. Schwarz, H. Reichmann, and P. Riederer. 1996. Acute MPTP treatment produces no changes in mitochondrial complex activities and indices of oxidative damage in the common marmoset ex vivo one week after exposure to the toxin. *Neurochem Intl* **28**:41–49.

Gibb, W.R., A.J. Lees, P. Jenner, and C.D. Marsden. 1986. The dopamine neurotoxin 1-methyl-4-phenyl-1,2,3,6-tetrahydropyridine (MPTP) produces histological lesions in the hypothalamus of the common marmoset. *Neurosci Lett* **65**:79–83.

Graham, W.C., R.G. Robertson, M.A. Sambrook, and A.R. Crossman. 1990. Injection of excitatory amino acid antagonists into the medial pallidal segment of a 1-methyl-4-phenyl-1,2,3,6-tetrahydropyridine (MPTP) treated primate reverses motor symptoms of Parkinsonism. *Life Sci* **47**:PL91–PL97.

Greenamyre, J.T., R.V. Eller, Z. Zhang, A. Ovadia, R. Kurlan, and D.M. Gash. 1994. Antiparkinsonian effects of remacemide hydrochloride, a glutamate antagonist, in rodent and primate models of Parkinson's disease. *Ann Neurol* **35(6)**:655–661.

Grondin, R., V.D. Doan, L. Gregoire, and P.J. Bedard. 1999a. D1 receptor blockade improves L-dopa-induced dyskinesia but worsens Parkinsonism in MPTP monkeys. *Neurology* **52**:771–776.

Grondin, R., M. Goulet, M. Morissette, P.J. Bedard, and T. Di Paolo. 1999b. Dopamine D1 receptor mRNA and receptor levels in the striatum of MPTP monkeys chronically treated with SKF-82958. *Eur J Pharmacol* **378**:259–263.

Guttman, M., V.W. Yong, S.U. Kim, D.B. Calne, W.R. Martin, M.J. Adam, and T.J. Ruth. 1988. Asymptomatic striatal dopamine depletion: PET scans in unilateral MPTP monkeys. *Synapse* **2**:469–473.

Hantraye, P., A.L. Brownell, D. Elmaleh, R.D. Spealman, U. Wullner, G.L. Brownell, B.K. Madras, and O. Isacson. 1992. Dopamine fiber detection by [11C]-CFT and PET in a primate model of Parkinsonism. *Neuroreport* **3**:265–268.

Hartvig, P., N.G. Lindquist, S.M. Aquilonius, R. d'Argy, K. Bergstrom, U. Bondesson, S.A. Eckernas, P. Gullberg, B.S. Larsson, B. Lindberg, et al. 1986. Distribution of 1-methyl-4-phenyl-1,2,3,6-tetrahydropyridine in experimental animals studied by positron emission tomography and whole body autoradiography. *Life Sci* **38**:89–97.

Hashimoto, T., C.M. Elder, M.S. Okun, S.K. Patrick, and J.L. Vitek. 2003. Stimulation of the subthalamic nucleus changes the firing pattern of pallidal neurons. *J Neurosci* **23**:1916–1923.

Heimer, G., I. Bar-Gad, J.A. Goldberg, and H. Bergman. 2002. Dopamine replacement therapy reverses abnormal synchronization of pallidal neurons in the 1-methyl-4-phenyl-1,2,3,6-tetrahydropyridine primate model of Parkinsonism. *J Neuroscience* **22**:7850–7855.

Henry, B., S.H. Fox, A.R. Crossman, and J.M. Brotchie. 2001. Mu- and delta-opioid receptor antagonists reduce levodopa-induced dyskinesia in the MPTP-lesioned primate model of Parkinson's disease. *Exp Neurol* **171**:139–146.

Henry, B., S. Duty, S.H. Fox, A.R. Crossman, and J.M. Brotchie. 2003. Increased striatal pre-proenkephalin B expression is associated with dyskinesia in Parkinson's disease. *Exp Neurol* **183**:458–468.

Hershey, T., K.J. Black, J.L. Carl, and J.S. Perlmutter. 2000. Dopa-induced blood flow responses in non-human primates. *Exp Neurol* **166**:342–349.

Howel, L.L., L.D. Byrd, A.M. McDonough, P.M. Iuvone, and R.A. Bakay. 2000. Behavioral evaluation of hemiparkinsonian MPTP monkeys following dopamine pharmacological manipulation and adrenal co-graft transplantation. *Cell Transpl* **9**:609–622.

Hughes, A.J., Y. Ben-Shlomo, S.E. Daniel, and A.J. Lees. 1992. What features improve the accuracy of clinical diagnosis in Parkinson's disease: a clinicopathologic study. *Neurology* **42**:1142–1146.

Iravani, M.M., M.J. Jackson, M. Kuoppamaki, L.A. Smith, and P. Jenner. 2003. 3,4-methylenedioxymethamphetamine (ecstasy) inhibits dyskinesia expression and normalizes motor activity in 1-methyl-4-phenyl-1,2,3,6-tetrahydropyridine-treated primates. *J Neurosci* **23(27)**: 9107–9115.

Irwin, I., L.E. DeLanney, L.S. Forno, K.T. Finnegan, D.A. Di Monte, and J.W. Langston. 1990. The evolution of nigrostriatal neurochemical changes in the MPTP-treated squirrel monkey. *Brain Res* **531**:242–252.

Irwin, I., L. Delanney, P. Chan, M.S. Sandy, D.A. Di Monte, and J.W. Langston. 1997. Nigrostriatal monoamine oxidase A and B in aging squirrel monkeys and C57BL/6 mice. *Neurobiol Aging* **18**:235–241.

Jenner, P., N.M. Rupniak, S. Rose, E. Kelly, G. Kilpatrick, A. Lees, and C.D Marsden. 1984. 1-Methyl-4-phenyl-1,2,3,6-tetrahydropyridine-induced Parkinsonism in the common marmoset. *Neurosci Letts* **50**:85–90.

Jolkkonen, J., P. Jenner, and C.D. Marsden. 1995. L-dopa reverses altered gene expression of substance P but not enkephalin in the caudate-putamen of common marmosets treated with MPTP. *Brain Res Mol Brain Res* **32**:297–307.

Joyce, J.N., J.F. Marshall, K.S. Bankiewicz, I.J. Kopin, and D.M. Jacobowitz. 1986. Hemiparkinsonism in a monkey after unilateral internal carotid artery infusion of 1-methyl-4-phenyl-1,2,3,6-tetrahydropyridine (MPTP) is associated with regional ipsilateral changes in striatal dopamine D-2 receptor density. *Brain Res* **382**:360–364.

Khan, N.L., E. Graham, P. Critchley, A.E. Schrag, N.W. Wood, A.J. Lees, K.P. Bhatia, and N. Quinn. 2003. Parkin disease: a phenotypic study of a large case series. *Brain* **126**:1279–1292.

Klintenberg, R., P. Svenningsson, L. Gunne, and P.E. Andren. 2002. Naloxone reduces levodopa-induced dyskinesias and apomorphine-induced rotations in primate models of Parkinsonism. *J Neural Transm* **109(10)**: 1295–1307.

Konitsiotis, S., P.J. Blanchet, L. Verhagen, E. Lamers, and T.N. Chase. 2000. AMPA receptor blockade improves levodopa-induced dyskinesia in MPTP monkeys. *Neurology* **54**:1589–1595.

Kordower, J.H., M.E. Emborg, J. Bloch, S.Y. Ma, Y. Chu, L. Leventhal, J. McBride, E.Y. Chen, S. Palfi, B.Z. Roitberg, W.D. Brown, J.E. Holden, R. Pyzalski, M.D. Taylor, P. Carvey, Z. Ling, D. Trono, P. Hantraye, N. Deglon, and P. Aebischer. 2000. Neurodegeneration prevented by lentiviral vector delivery of GDNF in primate models of Parkinson's disease. *Science* **290**:767–773.

Kuoppamaki, M., G. Al-Barghouthy, M. Jackson, L. Smith, B.Y. Zeng, N. Quinn, and P. Jenner. 2002. Beginning-of-dose and rebound worsening in MPTP-treated common marmosets treated with levodopa. *Mov Disord* **17**:1312–1317.

Kupsch, A., J. Sautter, M.E. Gotz, W. Breithaupt, J. Schwarz, M.B. Youdim, P. Riederer, M. Gerlach, and W.H. Oertel. 2001. Monoamine oxidase-inhibition and MPTP-induced neurotoxicity in the non-human primate: comparison of rasagiline (TVP 1012) with selegiline. *J Neural Transm* **108**:985–1009.

Langston, J.W., and P.A. Ballard, Jr. 1983. Parkinson's disease in a chemist working with 1-methyl-4-phenyl-1,2,5,6-tetrahydropyridine. *N Engl J Med* **309**:310.

Langston, J.W., P. Ballard, J.W. Tetrud, and I. Irwin. 1983. Chronic Parkinsonism in humans due to a product of meperidine analog synthesis. *Science* **219**:979–980.

Langston, J.W., L.S. Forno, C.S. Rebert, and I. Irwin. 1984. Selective nigral toxicity after systemic administration of 1-methyl-4-phenyl-1,2,5,6-tetrahydropyrine (MPTP) in the squirrel monkey. *Brain Res* **292(2)**: 390–394.

Lau, Y.-S., and Y.K. Fung 1986. Pharmacological effects of 1-methyl-4-phenyl-1,2,3,6-tetrahydropyridine (MPTP) on striatal dopamine receptor system. *Brain Res* **369**:311–315.

Lavoie, B., A. Parent, and P.J. Bedard. 1991. Effects of dopamine denervation on striatal peptide expression in parkinsonian monkeys. *Can J Neurol Sci* **18**:373–375.

Lohmann, E., M. Periquet, V. Bonifati, N.W. Wood, G. De Michele, A.M. Bonnet, V. Fraix, E. Broussolle, M.W. Horstink, M. Vidailhet, P. Verpillat, T. Gasser, D. Nicholl, H. Teive, S. Raskin, O. Rascol, A. Destee, M. Ruberg, F. Gasparini, G. Meco, Y. Agid, A. Durr, A. Brice; French Parkinson's Disease Genetics Study Group; European Consortium on Genetic Susceptibility in Parkinson's Disease. 2003. How much phenotypic variation can be attributed to parkin genotype? *Ann Neurol* **54**:176–185.

Lucking, C.B., A. Durr, V. Bonifati, J. Vaughan, G. De Michele, T. Gasser, B.S. Harhangi, G. Meco, P. Denefle, N.W. Wood, Y. Agid, and A. Brice. 2000. Association between early-onset Parkinson's disease and mutations in the parkin gene. French Parkinson's Disease Genetics Study Group. *N Engl J Med* **342**:1560–1567.

Maratos, E.C., M.J. Jackson, R.K. Pearce, C. Cannizzaro, and P. Jenner. 2003. Both short- and long-acting D-1/D-2 dopamine agonists induce less dyskinesia than L-dopa in the MPTP-lesioned common marmoset (Callithrix jacchus). *Exp Neurol* **179**:90–102.

Mitchell, I.J., A.J. Cross, M.A. Sambrook, and A.R. Crossman. 1986. Neural mechanisms mediating 1-methyl-4-phenyl-1,2,3, 6-tetrahydropyridine-induced Parkinsonism in the monkey: relative contributions of the striatopallidal and striatonigral pathways as suggested by 2-deoxyglucose uptake. *Neurosci Lett* **63**:61–65.

Mitchell, I.J., R. Luquin, S. Boyce, C.E. Clarke, R.G. Robertson, M.A. Sambrook, and A.R. Crossman. 1990. Neural mechanisms of dystonia: evidence from a 2-deoxyglucose uptake study in a primate model of dopamine agonist-induced dystonia. *Mov Disord* **5**:49–54.

Mitchell, I.J., S. Boyce, M.A. Sambrook, and A.R. Crossman. 1992. A 2-deoxyglucose study of the effects of dopamine agonists on the parkinsonian primate brain. Implications for the neural mechanisms that mediate dopamine agonist-induced dyskinesia. *Brain* **115**: 809–824.

Nandi, D., T.Z. Aziz, N. Giladi, J. Winter, and J.F. Stein. 2002. Reversal of akinesia in experimental Parkinsonism by GABA antagonist microinjections in the pedunculopontine nucleus. *Brain* **125**:2418–2430.

Narabayashi, H. 1987. Similarity and dissimilarity of MPTP models to Parkinson's disease: importance of juvenile Parkinsonism. *Eur Neurol* **26**:24–29.

Nash, J.E., S.H. Fox, B. Henry, M.P. Hill, D. Peggs, S. McGuire, Y. Maneuf, C. Hille, J.M. Brotchie, and A.R. Crossman. 2000. Antiparkinsonian actions of ifenprodil in the MPTP-lesioned marmoset model of Parkinson's disease. *Exp Neurol* **165**:136–142.

Nini, A., A. Feingold, H. Slovin, and H. Bergman. 1995. Neurons in the globus pallidus do not show correlated activity in the normal monkey, but phase-locked oscillations appear in the MPTP model of Parkinsonism. *J Neurophysiol* **74**:1800–1805.

Oh, J.D., F. Bibbiani, and T.N. Chase. 2002. Quetiapine attenuates levodopa-induced motor complications in rodent and primate parkinsonian models. *Exp Neurol* **177**:557–564.

Oiwa, Y., J.L. Eberling, D. Nagy, P. Pivirotto, M.E. Emborg, and K.S. Bankiewicz. 2003. Overlesioned hemiparkinsonian nonhuman primate model: correlation between clinical, neurochemical and histochemical changes. *Frontiers Bioscience* **8**:155–166.

Ovadia, A., Z. Zhang, and D.M. Gash. 1995. Increased susceptibility to MPTP toxicity in middle-aged rhesus monkeys. *Neurobiol Aging* **16**: 931–937.

Palfi, S., L. Leventhal, Y. Chu, S.Y. Ma, M. Emborg, R. Bakay, N. Deglon, P. Hantraye, P. Aebischer, and J.H. Kordower. 2002. Lentivirally delivered glial cell line-derived neurotrophic factor increases the number of striatal dopaminergic neurons in primate models of nigrostriatal degeneration. *J Neurosci* **22**:4942–4954.

Palombo, E., L.J. Porrino, K.S. Bankiewicz, A.M. Crane, L. Sokoloff, and I.J. Kopin. 1990. Local cerebral glucose utilization in monkeys with hemiparkinsonism induced by intracarotid infusion of the neurotoxin MPTP. *J Neurosci* **10**:860–869.

Perez-Otano, I., M.T. Herrero, M.R. Luquin, J.A. Obeso, and J. Del Rio. 1992. Chronic MPTP treatment reduces substance P and met-enkephalin content in the basal ganglia of the marmoset. *Brain Res* **585**:156–160.

Perlmutter, J.S., and M.E. Raichle. 1986. *In vitro* or *in vivo* receptor binding: where does the truth lie? *Ann Neurol* **19**:384–385.

Perlmutter, J.S., M.R. Kilbourn, M.E. Raichle, and M.J. Welch. 1987. MPTP induced up-regulation of in vivo dopaminergic radioligand-receptor binding in man. *Neurology* **37**:1575–1579.

Perlmutter, J.S., M.K. Stambuk, J. Markham, K.J. Black, L. McGee-Minnich, J. Jankovic, and S.M. Moerlein. 1997a. Decreased [^{18}F]spiperone binding in putamen in idiopathic focal dystonia. *J Neurosci* **17**:834–842.

Perlmutter, J.S., L.W. Tempel, K.J. Black, D. Parkinson, and R.D. Todd. 1997b. MPTP induces dystonia and Parkinsonism: clues to the pathophysiology of dystonia. *Neurology* **49**:1432–1438.

Perlmutter, J.S., and J.W. Mink 2004. Dysfunction of dopaminergic pathways in dystonia. In *Dystonia 4*. Ed S. Fahn. *Adv Neurol* **94**:163–170.

Pifl, C., G. Schingnitz, and O. Hornykiewicz. 1988. The neurotoxin MPTP does not reproduce in the rhesus monkey the interregional pattern of striatal dopamine loss typical of human idiopathic Parkinson's disease. *Neurosci Lett* **92**:228–233.

Pope-Coleman, A., J.P. Tinker, and J.S. Schneider. 2000. Effects of GM1 ganglioside treatment on pre- and postsynaptic dopaminergic markers in the striatum of parkinsonian monkeys. *Synapse* **36**:120–128.

Porrino, L.J., R.S. Burns, A.M. Crane, E. Palombo, I.J. Kopin, and L. Sokoloff. 1987. Local cerebral metabolic effects of L-dopa therapy in1-methyl-4-phenyl-1,2,3,6-tetrahydropyridine-induced Parkinsonism in monkeys. *Proc Natl Acad Sci U S A* **84**:5995–5999.

Quik, M., S. Police, J.W. Langston, and D.A. Di Monte. 2002. Increases in striatal preproenkephalin gene expression are associated with nigrostriatal damage but not L-dopa-induced dyskinesias in the squirrel monkey. *Neurosci* **113**:213–220.

Rajput, A.H., B. Rozdilsky, and A. Rajput. 1991. Accuracy of clinical diagnosis in Parkinsonism—a prospective study. *Can J Neurol Sci* **18**:275–278.

Raz, A., V. Frechter-Mazar, A. Feingold, M. Abeles, E. Vaadia, and H. Bergman. 2001. Activity of pallidal and striatal tonically active neurons is correlated in mptp-treated monkeys but not in normal monkeys. *J Neurosci* **21**:RC128.

Robertson, R.G., W.C. Graham, M.A. Sambrook, and A.R. Crossman. 1991. Further investigations into the pathophysiology of MPTP-induced Parkinsonism in the primate: an intracerebral microdialysis study of gamma-aminobutyric acid in the lateral segment of the globus pallidus. *Brain Res* **563**:278–280.

Schneider, J.S., and T.V. Wade. 2003. Experimental Parkinsonism is associated with increased pallidal GAD gene expression and is reversed by site-directed antisense gene therapy. *Mov Disord* **18**:32–40.

Schneider, J.S., J.P. Tinker, F. Menzaghi, and G.K. Lloyd. 2003. The subtype-selective nicotinic acetylcholine receptor agonist SIB-1553A improves both attention and memory components of a spatial working memory task in chronic low dose 1-methyl-4-phenyl-1,2,3,6-tetrahydropyridine-treated monkeys. *J Pharmacol Exp Therap* **306**:401–406.

Schultz, W., A. Studer, R. Romo, E. Sundstrom, G. Jonsson, and E. Scarnati. 1989. Deficits in reaction times and movement times as correlates of hypokinesia in monkeys with MPTP-induced striatal dopamine depletion. *J Neurophysiol* **61**:651–668.

Schwartzman, R.J., and G.M. Alexander. 1985. Changes in the local cerebral metabolic rate for glucose in the 1-methyl-4-phenyl-1,2,3,6-tetrahydropyridine (MPTP) primate model of Parkinson's disease. *Brain Res* **358**:137–143.

Slovin, H., M. Abeles, E. Vaadia, I. Haalman, Y. Prut, and H. Bergman. 1999. Frontal cognitive impairments and saccadic deficits in low-dose MPTP-treated monkeys. *J Neurophysiol* **81**:858–874.

Smith, L.A., B.C. Tel, M.J. Jackson, M.J. Hansard, R. Braceras, C. Bonhomme, C. Chezaubernard, S. Del Signore, S. Rose, and P. Jenner. 2002. Repeated administration of piribedil induces less dyskinesia than L-dopa in MPTP-treated common marmosets: a behavioural and biochemical investigation. *Mov Disord* **17**:887–901.

Smith, L.A., M.J. Jackson, M.J. Hansard, E. Maratos, and P. Jenner. 2003. Effect of pulsatile administration of levodopa on dyskinesia induction in drug-naive MPTP-treated common marmosets: effect of dose, frequency of administration, and brain exposure. *Mov Disord* **18**:487–495.

Starr, P.A., T. Wichmann, C. van Horne, and R.A. Bakay. 1999. Intranigral transplantation of fetal substantia nigra allograft in the hemiparkinsonian rhesus monkey. *Cell Transpl* **8**:37–45.

Tai, Y.C., A.F. Chatziioannou, Y. Yang, R.W. Silverman, K. Meadors, S. Siegel, D.F. Newport, J.R. Stickel, and S.R. Cherry. 2003. MicroPET II: design, development and initial performance of an improved microPET scanner for small-animal imaging. *Phys Med Biol* **48**: 1519–1537.

Taquet, H., M. Nomoto, S. Rose, P. Jenner, F. Javoy-Agid, A. Mauborgne, J.J. Benoliel, C.D. Marsden, J.C. Legrand, Y. Agid, et al. 1988. Levels of Met-enkephalin, Leu-enkephalin, substance P and cholecystokinin in the brain of the common marmoset following long term 1-methyl-4-phenyl-1,2,3,6,-tetrahydropyridine treatment. *Neuropeptides* **12**: 105–110.

Taylor, M.D., M.L. de Ceballos, S. Rose, P.N. Chong, P. Jenner, and C.D. Marsden. 1991. Neuropeptide levels in the basal ganglia of aged common marmosets following prolonged treatment with MPTP. *J Neural Trans* **3**:99–108.

Todd, R.D., and J.S. Perlmutter. 1998. Mutational and biochemical analysis of dopamine in dystonia: evidence for decreased dopamine D2 receptor inhibition. *Mol Neurobiol* **16**:135–147.

Todd, R.D., J. Carl, S. Harmon, K.L. O'Malley, and J.S. Perlmutter. 1996. Dynamic changes in striatal dopamine D2 and D3 receptor protein and mRNA in response to MPTP denervation in baboons. *J Neurosci* **16**: 7776–7782.

Wade, T.V., and J.S. Schneider. 2001. Expression of striatal preprotachykinin mRNA in symptomatic and asymptomatic 1-methyl-4-phenyl-1,2,3,6-tetrahydropyridine-exposed monkeys is related to parkinsonian motor signs. *J Neurosci* **21**:4901–4907.

Wichmann, T., H. Bergman, and M.R. DeLong. 1994. The primate subthalamic nucleus. I. Functional properties in intact animals. *J Neurophysiol* **72**:494–506.

Wichmann, T., M.A. Kliem, and M.R. DeLong. 2001. Antiparkinsonian and behavioral effects of inactivation of the substantia nigra pars reticulata in hemiparkinsonian primates. *Exp Neurol* **167**:410–424.

Wilson, J.M., A.I. Levey, A. Rajput, L. Ang, M. Guttman, K. Shannak, H.B. Niznik, O. Hornykiewicz, C. Pifl, and S.J. Kish. 1996. Differential changes in neurochemical markers of striatal dopamine nerve terminals in idiopathic Parkinson's disease. *Neurology* **47**:718–726.

Yee, R.E., S.C. Huang, D.B. Stout, I. Irwin, K. Shoghi-Jadid, D.M. Togaski, L.E. DeLanney, J.W. Langston, N. Satyamurthy, K.F. Farahani, M.E. Phelps, and J.R. Barrio. 2000. Nigrostriatal reduction of aromatic L-amino acid decarboxylase activity in MPTP-treated squirrel monkeys: in vivo and in vitro investigations. *J Neurochem* **74**:1147–1157.

CHAPTER

B3

From Man to Mouse: The MPTP Model of Parkinson Disease

VERNICE JACKSON-LEWIS and RICHARD JAY SMEYNE

In 1817 Dr. James Parkinson first described the syndrome that we know today as Parkinson disease (PD) in a paper entitled "An Essay on the Shaking Palsy" (Parkinson 1817). PD is a debilitating neurological disorder that strikes approximately 1–2% of the adult population older than fifty years of age (new incidence is 20 per 100,000 persons) (de Rijk et al. 1995). Current estimates from the American Parkinson Disease Foundation put the number of American citizens suffering from this disease at greater than one million persons. The costs of treatment of PD can be staggering. At an average per patient cost of $6,000 per year—for drugs, physicians, and loss of pay to patient and family members—(Whetten-Goldstein et al. 1997), the total cost of the disease may approach $6,000,000,000 per year; of which 85% is borne by private and government (e.g., Social Security, Medicare) insurance. In fact, more individuals present with PD than with multiple sclerosis, muscular dystrophy, and amyotropic lateral sclerosis (Lou Gehrig disease) combined (The Parkinsons Web, 1997). Since the population of the world is, on average, getting progressively older (United States Census Bureau, 1996), the number of people suffering from this disease should increase substantially within the next several decades. Furthermore, PD is an incurable disease with an average life expectancy after diagnosis of over fifteen years, thus there should be an even larger burden on both the social and financial resources of families, insurance companies, and the federal government than is present today.

I. BACKGROUND

Parkinson disease is characterized by a loss of the pigmented cells located in the midbrain substantia nigra pars compacta (SNpc). The loss of these cells results in a reduction in afferent fibers that project to the striatum. PD symptoms first manifest when approximately 60% of the SNpc neurons have already died (German et al. 1989). Because the progression of cell loss is thought to occur over a somewhat protracted period of time in a defined spatiotemporal manner (Damier et al. 1999; Nurmi et al. 2001), the onset of Parkinson disease symptoms is often insidious.

The underlying cause for the vast majority of PD cases is unknown. Controversy still exists as to how much of the disease results from a strict genetic causation, a purely environmental factor, or the more parsimonious combination of the two risk factors (Duvoisin 1999; Williams et al. 1999; Gasser 2001). Empirical evidence suggests that less than 10% of all diagnosed Parkinsonism has a strict familial etiology (Payami and Zareparsi 1998). A small number of familial parkinsonian patients appear to have polymorphisms in the α-synuclein gene (Polymeropoulos et al. 1997), suggesting that this aggregating protein (Spillantini et al. 1997) may play a role in Lewy body formation that ultimately results in substantia nigra cell death (Nussbaum and Polymeropoulos, 1997). A second autosomal recessive locus coding for the parkin protein maps to the long arm of chromosome 6 (6q25.2-q27). Mutations in this gene cause a form of juvenile onset PD. Other genes that are associated with PD include loci at human chromosome 2p13 and 4p (Gasser, 2001). The PD linked to this locus more closely resembles that of idiopathic PD, although like the α-synuclein protein, this unknown protein has very low penetrance. However, at this time no mutations in these proteins are reported in idiopathic PD (Hu et al. 1999; Scott et al. 1999).

Because the vast majority of PD patients have no direct tie to any identified genetic mutation, important information regarding the pathophysiology of PD may be gleaned through the study of animal models. Several animal models have examined the mechanism(s) underlying the pathophysiology of experimental PD, including surgical and chemical models. One of the earliest models made use of a lesion of nigrostriatal pathway in which fibers emanating from the substantia nigra proceedings to the striatum rostrally through the medial forebrain bundle (Faull and Mehler 1978; Levine et al. 1983; Brecknell et al. 1995). In addition to the physical lesion studies, chemical lesions have also modeled Parkinson disease. In these studies, animals were injected with 6-OHDA, a neurotoxin that when injected into the striatum causes a retrograde degeneration of dopaminergic neurons in the SNpc (reviewed in Olney et al. 1990; Schwarting and Huston 1996; Deumens et al. 2002; Hirsch et al. 2003). A third model of experimental PD utilizes the properties of selective neurotoxins, the most famous of which is the loss of SNpc neurons following administration of 1-methyl-4-phenyl-1,2,3,6-tetrahydropyridine (MPTP).

II. MPTP

The discovery of MPTP has provided a useful model of Parkinsonism that appears to recapitulate the pathology of the disease seen in humans. The identification of MPTP may be one of the few cases in which a specific neurotoxin was discovered in humans first, followed by development of an animal model. The story first started around 1976 when a chemistry student named Barry Kidston was synthesizing a "designer" heroin, MPPP, for recreational use. Although generally successful, at one point he hurried the catalysis of the procedure and instead of producing MPPP, he synthesized a neurotoxin that a team from the National Institutes of Mental Health later found to be MPTP. After IV injection of the incorrectly designed drug, Kidston quickly exhibited a severe bradykinesia. Following a rapid hospitalization and initial diagnosis as a catatonic schizophrenic, physicians eventually suspected that he had an acute form of Parkinson disease. Kidston's symptomatic recovery after he was administered L-dopa confirmed suspicions. Because this was an isolated case, the details never attained public prominence, but this changed in the early 1980s after a number of northern California heroin users were identified who presented at various emergency rooms with symptoms indistinguishable from those of Parkinson disease (Burns et al. 1985; Langston 1985). The potential threat of a public health risk that could have been epidemic, brought the case of these "frozen addicts" to public awareness (Langston 1985). A complete history of these cases is presented in the book *The Case of the Frozen Addicts* (Langston and Palfreman 1996) as well as in the NOVA documentary of the same name (original broadcast date: February 18, 1986).

In the subsequent years since MPTP was identified in humans as a Parkinsonian agent, researchers have demonstrated that MPTP exerts its neurotoxic effects in a number of other primates (Kopin and Markey 1988; Jenner 2003; Wichmann and DeLong 2003), as well as in cats, and in several rodents. In rodents, only specific strains of mice are sensitive to the administration of MPTP (Sundstrom et al. 1987; Riachi and Harik 1988; Mitra et al. 1994; Hamre et al. 1999). MPTP structurally resembles several known environmental agents, including well-known herbicides such as paraquat (Di Monte et al. 1986) and garden insecticides and fish toxins such as rotenone (McNaught et al. 1996) that induce dopamine cell degeneration (Brooks et al. 1999; Betarbet et al. 2000; Thiruchelvam et al. 2000; Chun et al. 2001). As such, it is possible, although as of yet unproven, that the genetic pathways and mechanisms that underlie the toxin-induced cell death of each of these compounds may interact.

There are many points systemically where MPTP can affect the dopaminergic system (Figure 1). In this chapter, we will discuss each step in the MPTP toxification pathway.

Step 1. Introduction of MPTP into the CNS

MPTP, in and of itself, is not toxic. The enzyme MAO-B metabolizes MPTP to the unstable 1-methyl-4-phenyl-2, 3-dihydropyridium ($MPDP^+$) that then rehydrogenates or deprotonates to generate MPTP or the corresponding pyridium species, MPP^+, respectively (Figure 2). At the point of interface with the periphery, exogenous compounds can either enter or be excluded from the CNS by the blood-brain barrier (BBB). The BBB is composed on tight-junctioned endothelial cells that make up the microvasculature of the brain in tight opposition with the end feet of glial processes. Endothelial cells of the microvasculature contain monoamine oxidases, and several studies have correlated levels of monoamine oxidases with MPTP-induced neuronal loss (Kalaria et al. 1987; Riachi et al. 1988). Since MPP^+

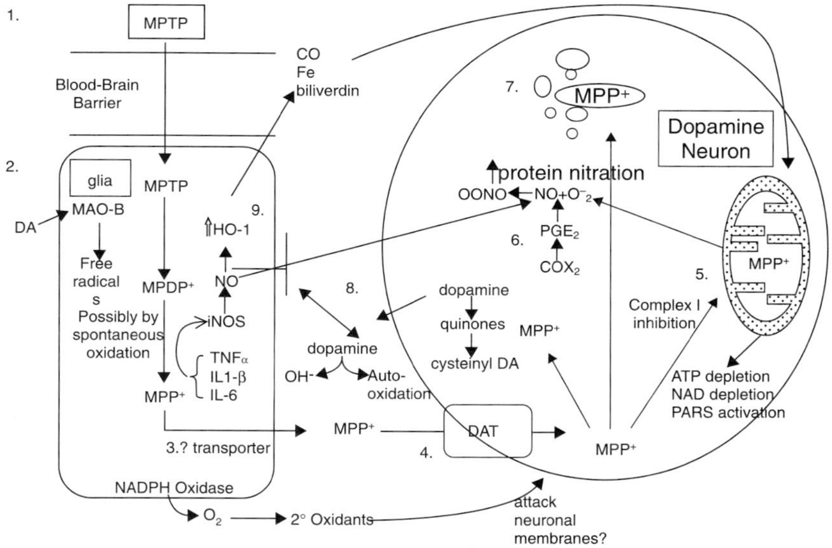

FIGURE 1 Proposed mechanism of MPTP action in the substantia nigra and striatum. The numbers represent each step in the toxification process outlined in this chapter.

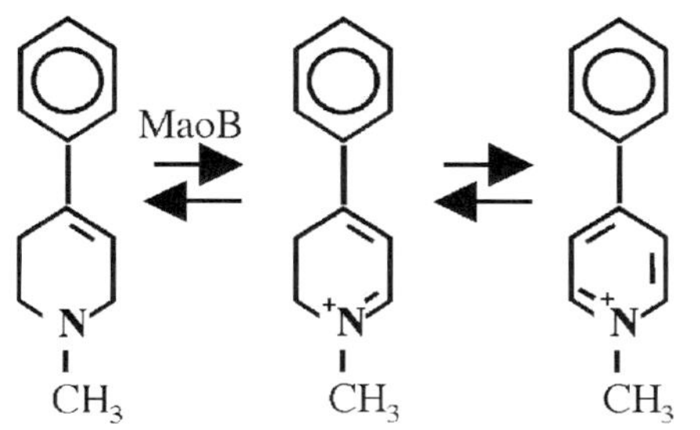

MPTP **MPDP+** **MPP+**

FIGURE 2 The protoxin MPTP is converted by monoamine oxidase B (MaoB) through intermediates to the toxin MPP$^+$.

cannot be transported through the BBB (Riachi et al. 1990), this level of toxification/detoxification can provide a first line of defense against exogenous agents.

Step 2. Role of Glia in the Toxification of MPTP

MPTP that is not deprotonated to MPP$^+$ rapidly enters the brain and is taken up into glial cells by a number of mechanisms including monoamine (Brooks et al. 1989) and glutamate (Hazell et al. 1997) transporters or pH-dependent antiporters (Kopin 1992; Marini et al. 1992). Glia, like endothelial cells, also contain large pools of monoamine oxidases and also convert MPTP from its protoxin form to MPP$^+$ (Ransom et al. 1987), in a manner dependent on the presence of MAO-B. A study by Brooks et al. (1989) provided additional support for the role of glial cells in dopaminergic neuronal toxicity, demonstrating that administration of fluoxetine (a serotonergic uptake inhibitor) immediately before systemic injection of MPTP attenuated neurotoxicity. Because fluoxetine did not alter the neurotoxicity of injected MPTP, the site of activation was proven to be extraneuronal, lending credence to the observation that the primary step in MPTP toxicity occurred in the astrocyte.

Once converted to MPP$^+$ in the astrocyte, MPP$^+$ stimulates the up-regulation of TNF-alpha, interleukin-1-beta (IL-1β) and interleukin-6 (IL-6) (Youdim et al. 2002; Teismann et al. 2003a) and these, in turn, up-regulate inducible nitric oxide synthese (iNOS) (Hunot et al. 1999). Of the three NOS isoforms present in the brain, endothelial NOS (eNOS), found mainly in the vasculature of the brain, does not contribute to MPTP toxicity (Wu and Przedborski, personal communication). In addition, since neuronal NOS (nNOS) knock-out mice show partial protection against the disastrous effects of MPTP administration (Przedborski et al. 1996) in the substantia nigra pars compacta (SNpc), another NOS isoform must also contribute to the neurotoxicity of MPTP. iNOS, a NOS isoform that is minimally expressed in the brain in non-pathological conditions, is highly expressed in the substantia nigra in both Parkinson disease (PD) and in mice (most likely in the microglia) following MPTP treatment (Hunot et al. 1996; Liberatore et al. 1999; Wu et al. 2002; Wu et al. 2003). iNOS produces large amounts of nitric oxide (NO), which is an uncharged, lipophilic molecule (Lancaster 1996) that can freely pass through membranes and travel distances greater than the length of a neuron, up to 300 microns, to do its damage remotely. Thus, under pathological conditions or following MPTP treatment, neurons in the vicinity of the NO molecule are at risk for possible attack by glial-derived reactive nitrogen–related species. Because minocycline, a second-generation tetracycline antibiotic, can block iNOS induction (Wu et al. 2002), this step in the toxification process of MPTP presents a point where potential therapeutics may have a significant impact.

Step 3. Release of MPP^+ from Glia

MPP^+ is a polar compound and as such cannot freely exit glial cells. The question of how this compound exits the cell is currently under investigation. Investigators speculate that a specific transporter may actively move this polar molecule out of the glia (Russ et al. 1996; Inazu et al. 2003), however, at present, the specific mechanism remains unknown.

Step 4. Transport of MPP^+ into the Dopaminergic Neuron

Once released into the extracellular space, upon encountering neurons, MPP^+ is taken up into the cell preferentially by the dopamine transporter (DAT). *In situ* analysis has shown that the midbrain contains the highest concentration of dopamine transporters/cell (Cerruti et al. 1993). For this reason, as well as for the selectivity of dopaminergic neurons to many exogenous compounds, the DAT may be a control point in determining differential susceptibility to agents that are known to damage midbrain neurons (Kitayama et al. 1993; Le Couteur et al. 1997) (but see also the study by Higuchi et al. 1995). Two groups demonstrated the absolute necessity for the DAT in MPTP toxicity when they examined mice carrying null mutations of the DAT (Gainetdinov et al. 1997; Bezard et al. 1999). In these studies, MPTP-susceptible strains of mice carrying null mutations of the DAT were completely protected from MPTP toxicity.

Step 5. Effects of MPP^+ on Mitochondria within Dopaminergic Neurons

Once in the cell, MPP^+ has several paths: it can enter into mitochondria (step 5) where it interferes with complex I of the electron transport chain (Nicklas et al. 1987; Lander and Schork 1994) or it can be sequestered into cytoplasmic vesicles through the vesicular monoamine transporter (see step 7) (Liu et al. 1992; Del Zompo et al. 1993). Both of these steps have been implicated in processes that either protect or kill the dopaminergic neurons.

MPP^+ enters the mitochondria by the diffusion of this lipophilic cation through the mitochondrial inner membrane. The uptake of MPP^+ into mitochondria is not passive but is actively driven by an electrical gradient within the membrane (a Km of about 5 mM). This active transport was supported by experiments in which valinomycin plus K^+, which collapses the electrochemical mitochondrial gradient, abolished MPP^+ uptake, while agents that specifically collapsed the proton gradient had no effect on MPP^+ uptake (Ramsay et al. 1986; Ramsay and Singer 1986).

Once in the mitochondria, MPP^+ has been implicated in significant alterations of mitochondrial function. MPP^+ inhibits cellular respiration by blocking the mitochondrial electron transport enzyme NADH:ubiquinone oxidoreductase (complex I) (Nicklas et al. 1985; Suzuki et al. 1990) leading to a reduction in cellular ATP. Although this appears to be the major step in blocking mitochondrial function, studies also demonstrate that MPP^+ can directly inhibit complexes III (ubiquinol:ferrocytochrome c oxidoreductase) and IV (ferrocytochrome c:oxygen oxidoreductase or cytochrome c oxidase) of the electron transport chain (Mizuno et al. 1988a,b). The loss of cellular energy has several consequences, including the generation of the oxygen free radicals that rearrange to form hydrogen peroxide. Further catalysis leads to the formation of hydroxyl radicals.

The energy depletion due to MPP^+'s interference with complex I-III has led to a number of potential therapies. One of the most interesting is the use of Coenzyme Q10 supplementation, as several studies show that orally administering this enzyme can slow the progression of idiopathic PD (Beal 2003; Muller et al. 2003; Shults 2003).

Step 6. Role of Nitration within Dopaminergic Neurons

Although complex I inhibition by MPP^+ is known to reduce the energy production within dopaminergic neurons, it is possible, if not likely, that this is not the direct cause of the observed neuronal death. The damage done within SNpc neurons likely results from compounds generated in the cell, secondary to energy depletion. The formation of the superoxide radical is one example of this process. To establish the role of the superoxide radical in the MPTP neurotoxic cascade of events, a study by Cleeter et al. (1992), showed that MPP^+ inhibits mitochondrial complex 1 activity, which causes an excessive amount of superoxide radicals to form within the neuronal cytosol. Further support came from a study by Przedborski et al. (1992), which demonstrated that over-expression of the copper-zinc form of superoxide dismutase in mice is neuroprotective against the damaging effects of MPTP. Moreover, research by Wu et al. (2003), using the fluorescent tag hydroethidium, provided an *in vivo* demonstration of the presence of the superoxide radical in the MPTP neurotoxic process.

NO, produced in the glial cells, can enter the cytosol of the neuron via simple membrane diffusion. Neither the superoxide radical nor NO are particularly damaging by themselves; however, when the two interact, peroxynitrite ($OONO^-$), one of the most destructive oxidizing molecules, is formed (Ischiropoulos and al-Mehdi 1995; Przedborski et al. 2000; Przedborski and Vila 2003). This fast-moving molecule as a single entity is hard to detect, however, its handiwork, the nitration of the tyrosine residues of a number of cellular components that include enzymes, transmitters, proteins, fatty acids, and DNA (Radi et al. 2002), can readily be documented.

While many molecules are affected by peroxynitrite, this chapter concentrates on intracellular proteins that are affected both in PD as well as in the MPTP mouse model. One potential target is tyrosine hydroxylase (TH), which is the rate-limiting enzyme in catecholamine synthesis. The most densely packed TH-positive cell area in the brain is the SNpc, which projects its dense TH-positive fibers to the striatum (Grofova 1979). Because the cell-body rich SNpc contains primarily the soluble form of the TH enzyme, TH is often used as a faithful phenotypic marker for dopaminergic neuron numbers as well as an indicator of dopaminergic neuron loss (Jackson-Lewis et al. 1995).

TH is a tetrameric enzyme composed of four identical subunits. Each subunit carries catalytic activity, and catalytic domains have been localized to the carboxy terminals between leucine residue 188 and phenylalanine residue 456. While rodent (rat and mouse) TH contains seventeen tyrosine residues of which fifteen are in the catalytic domain, human TH, although similar, contains only fifteen tyrosine residues of which fourteen are in the catalytic domain (Saadat et al. 1988; Daubner et al. 1993). Tyrosine residues are the keys to the inactivation and nitration of TH, as they are the targets of nitration. At present, researchers speculate that Tyr225 is the most important residue because it lies within the sequence that is targeted for nitration (Przedborski and Jackson-Lewis 1998).

In PD, clinical symptoms appear when about 60–70% of the TH-positive cells in the SNpc have degenerated (Fahn and Przedborski 2000). In addition to the cell loss, brains of Parkinsonian patients show deficits in TH enzyme activity (Ara et al. 1998). Both *in vitro* and *in vivo* studies demonstrate that peroxynitrite impairs TH activity. In mice treated with MPTP, TH nitration seems to occur as early as three hours after MPTP administration. Immunoprecipitation studies using striata from MPTP-treated mice confirm that TH is indeed the nitrated protein. Furthermore, transgenic mice that overexpress human SOD do not show any detectable levels of nitrated striatal TH following MPTP treatment (Ara et al. 1998). Mice deficient in iNOS show less ventral midbrain nitrotyrosine, a fingerprint for tyrosine nitration, after MPTP administration than in their wild-type counterparts (Liberatore et al., 1999). Thus, the inactivation of TH via its nitration following exposure to both peroxynitrite and MPTP is important to the development of PD in humans and to the MPTP neurotoxic process in mice.

Dopamine (DA) is a relatively unstable molecule that is subjected to hydroxyl radical attack (Slivka and Cohen 1985) and autooxidizes in the extracellular space (Hirrlinger et al. 2002). In addition, dopamine can be nitrated within the neuron (LaVoie and Hastings 1999) and therefore may contribute to the degeneration of the cells that contain it as a transmitter. Here, DA is oxidized to DA quinone, which then undergoes a nucleophilic addition via the sulfhydryl group from cysteine, forming 5-cysteinyl-DA (Graham 1978). In pathological situations, the up-regulation of the cyclooxygenase-2 (COX-2) enzyme facilitates the oxidation of DA to 5-cysteinyl-DA (Hastings 1995; O'Banion 1999). The relationship of 5-cysteinyl-DA to neurodegeneration in PD as well as to the degeneration of DA neurons seen in the MPTP mouse model was recently investigated using a combination of immunocytochemistry (PD brains) or a combination of immunocytochemistry and HPLC (MPTP studies). In both PD brains and ventral midbrain from MPTP-treated mice, COX-2 enzyme activity and protein levels were significantly higher than in controls. Robust COX-2 immunostaining was also noted in both the human and mouse brains where the enzyme appeared to be confined to the cytosol of dopaminergic neurons (Teismann et al. 2003b). Furthermore, inhibition of the COX-2 response to MPTP prevented the rise in protein cysteinyl dopamine that occurred in mice following the administration of MPTP (Teismann et al. 2003b).

Peroxynitrite is formed from NO and the superoxide radical inside the neuron, and as such poses a serious threat to intracellular components such as mitochondria. For example, the nitration of manganese SOD (MnSOD), the primary mitochondrial antioxidant, was detected both *in vitro* (Quijano et al. 2001) and during inflammatory responses *in vivo* (MacMillan-Crow et al. 1996; Aulak et al. 2001). Here, nitration was proven to be site-specific in that it is tyrosine 34 (Tyr^{34}) among the tyrosine residues that is nitrated. In the MPTP mouse model, over-expression of human MnSOD localized to mitochondria prevented the accumulation of 3-nitrotyrosine, the faithful fingerprint of peroxynitrite-mediated nitration (Klivenyi et al. 1998). Several other mitochondrial components such as NADH: ubiquinone reductase (Complex I) (Riobo et al. 2001), cytochrome c (Cassina et al. 2000), aconitase, ATPase and VDAC (voltage dependent anion channel) (Radi et al. 2002) are nitrated following exposure to peroxynitrite. Whether these are nitrated in PD and in the MPTP mouse model has yet to be determined.

Step 7. Sequestration of MPP^+ within the Dopaminergic Neuron

The vesicular monoamine transporter VMAT2, is a proton-dependent transporter that sequesters monoamine neurotransmitters from free cytoplasmic space into synaptic vesicles (Miller et al. 1999a). Like the monoamines, MPP^+ can be transported by the VMAT into these vesicles, and as such, can be prevented from entering the mitochondria where it can inhibit complex I. Investigators postulate that this sequestration may be a mechanism for attenuating the effects of any number of monoaminergic toxins. Support for this hypothesis comes from analyses in mice containing partial or complete deletions of VMAT2 and from human studies of VMAT expression. In parkinsonian humans, immunocytochemical localization of VMAT demonstrates reduced expression in striatum, paralleling the reductions seen in DAT. In fact, the relative expression of VMAT2, compared to that of DAT, may allow one to predict if and which dopamine neurons may be lost in PD (Miller et al. 1999b). In animal studies, mice heterozygous for VMAT2 and exposed to MPTP were examined for markers of dopaminergic neuron toxicity, including striatal dopamine content, the levels of DAT protein, as well as for a secondary marker of neurotoxicity, the expression of glial fibrillary acidic protein (GFAP) mRNA. In all parameters measured, VMAT2 +/- mice were more sensitive to MPTP-induced toxicity than their wild-type littermates (Gainetdinov et al. 1998). Further examination of these mice revealed that heterozygous VMAT2 mice, in addition to the loss of striatal markers, also had increased SNpc cell loss following administration of MPTP (Takahashi et al. 1997). These studies suggested an important role for VMAT2 in potentiating the effects of MPTP. Conversely, cells transfected to overexpress a greater density of VMAT2 were converted from MPP^+ sensitive to MPP^+ resistant cells (Liu et al. 1992). These studies suggested an important role for VMAT2 in potentiating or allaying the effects of MPTP.

Alpha-synuclein is another molecule relevant to the development of PD in humans and to the neurotoxic process in the MPTP mouse model of PD that is susceptible to nitration because of the presence of tyrosine residues. Historically, synucleins are vertebrate-specific cytosolic proteins that contain about 127–140 residues that have a unique 11-residue repeat that occurs in five to seven copies, accounting for roughly half of their structure and no structural domains. Four proteins, alpha, beta, and gamma synuclein and synoretin make up this family of proteins. Only two proteins in this family, alpha and beta, are synthesized in relatively large amounts in the brain and are highly expressed in presynaptic nerve terminals (Schluter et al. 2003). Synucleins account for about 1% of brain proteins and to date their functions are still unknown. Mutations in alpha-synuclein are associated with a familial form of PD (Polymeropoulos et al. 1997) that is readily indistinguishable from the more common sporadic form of the disease. The interaction between WT alpha-synuclein and mutant alpha-synuclein may enhance the ability of the different alpha-synucleins to interact with other cellular proteins to form aggregates (Conway et al. 1998).

One of the hallmarks of PD is the presence of Lewy bodies within neurons in the SNpc. Lewy bodies are both ubiquitin and alpha-synuclein positive. Since alpha-synuclein is the only synuclein present in Lewy bodies, it has to be determined whether this molecule is toxic or whether it is just a by-product of cellular metabolism in a pathological situation. A number of cellular proteins have been found to be nitrated in PD tissues (Ischiropoulos and al-Mehdi 1995), which was taken as evidence that nitrating agents such as peroxynitrite engaged in nitration reactions here. Specific antibodies that recognize nitrated alpha-synuclein have demonstrated that alpha-synuclein is the protein that is nitrated in Lewy bodies in a number of disease states including PD (Giasson et al. 2000a,b). Furthermore, alpha-synuclein inclusions in tissues from PD patients were strongly labeled with antibodies that recognize the faithful fingerprint of peroxynitrite-induced nitration, 3-nitrotyrosine (Souza et al. 2000). Both *in vitro* studies and the MPTP mouse model were used to prove that tyrosine residues in the alpha-synuclein molecule are indeed the targets of nitration and that peroxynitrite is indeed the culprit. In HEK 293 cells transfected to overexpress human alpha-synuclein and that were exposed to peroxynitrite, a nitrated band that corresponded to the molecular mass of alpha-synuclein was noted (Przedborski et al. 2001). In the MPTP mouse model, immunoprecipitation studies using striatum and ventral midbrain from treated mice showed that alpha-synuclein was nitrated as early as four hours after MPTP administration. In contrast, beta-synuclein was not nitrated in either situation (Przedborski et al. 2001).

Step 8. Release of Dopamine from Intracellular Stores

A second consequence of the depletion of cellular ATP is the release of dopamine from intracellular stores (Schmidt et al. 1984; Ofori and Schorderet 1987; Rollema et al. 1988; Lau et al. 1991; Schmidt et al. 1999). Once released into the extracellular space, the enzymatic oxidation of dopamine results in the rapid formation of hydroxyl radicals. It is clear that the presence of free radicals can lead to membrane damage and subsequent cell death. That dopamine rapidly auto-oxidizes and contributes to neurotoxicity always leads to the controversial topic of L-dopa therapy in PD. Simply stated, one can question whether the therapy that best treats the symptoms of PD may also exacerbate the disease. In support of this hypothesis, Whone and colleagues showed that the progression of PD using PET scanning was greater in patients treated with L-dopa than those treated with the dopamine agonist ropinirole (Whone et al. 2003). However, other studies do not support this hypothesis (Fornai et al. 2000; Melamed et al. 2000), and for this reason, the question of L-dopa toxicity has yet to be resolved.

While the above question is still not settled, the formation of hydroxyl radicals apart from direct dopamine oxidation can also modulate several other processes that can lead to cell death, including the fragmentation of DNA (Walkinshaw and Waters 1995) and inhibition of Na+, K+-ATPase activity (Khan et al. 2003). Additional sites of hydroxyl radical formation may occur as a result of interactions with neuromelanin (D'Amato et al. 1986) as well as with cellular iron (Jellinger 1999), each of which could contribute to its neurotoxicity.

Step 9. A Second Role for Glial Cells?

Based upon our hypothesis of the mechanism(s) of MPTP-induced cell death (Figure 1), a dramatic interplay occurs between neurons and the non-neuronal milieu. As discussed earlier in this chapter (step 2), the astrocytes are necessary for the bioactivation of MPTP into its toxic metabolite, MPP^+. The glial cells, in addition to their toxifying function, also are believed to play a significant role in neuronal protection. A recent report, using *in vitro* chimeric cell cultures, has demonstrated that the toxicity of MPTP is determined by the response of the glial cells following MPP^+ intoxication (Smeyne et al. 2001) and numerous *in vitro* studies support this data (Di Monte et al. 1992; Forno et al. 1992; Di Monte et al. 1996).

Glial cells contribute directly to the toxic effects of MPTP through several mechanisms, including the mediation of free radical formation and damage by induction of nitric oxide synthase (iNOS) (Hirsch et al. 1998; McGeer and McGeer 1998; McNaught and Jenner 1999). Administration of MPTP leads to a rapid gliosis (Schneider and Denaro 1988), which subsequently increases production and releases iNOS (Zietlow et al. 1999). In a model of iNOS action that extends the role of glia, Hirsch and Hunot (2000) suggest that MPTP acts directly on the induction of cytokines that activates iNOS. iNOS is then released from the glial cells to directly damage the dopaminergic neurons. Thus, differential expression of iNOS may underlie some of the strain specific responses to MPTP seen in mice, and, perhaps, the differential sensitivity to different environmental toxins in humans.

In addition to inducing and modulating cytokines, dopamine in the extracellular space can induce a number of different molecules that are involved in oxidative stress. One of these molecules, hemeoxygenase-1 (Fernandez-Gonzales et al. 2000), the rate limiting enzyme in heme degradation, plays a critical role in heme and iron homeostasis (Schipper et al. 1998b; Maines 2000). Several isoforms of hemeoxygenase have been identified (reviewed in Elbirt and Bonkovsky 1999), each of which converts heme to bilirubin and carbon monoxide, while at the same time releasing iron into the cellular milieu (Maines 1997). Further support for the importance of this molecule is that hemeoxygensase-1 is elevated in astrocytes of Parkinsonian patients (Schipper et al. 1998a). In addition, the brains of hemeoxygenase-1 null mice show excessive iron deposits, increased sensitivity to oxidative stress, and chronic inflammation (Poss and Tonegawa 1997). Moreover, astrocytes in the striatum of MPTP-treated mice show increases in hemeoxygensase-1 as early as six hours after the administration of MPTP (Fernandez-Gonzales et al. 2000). On the flip-side, over-expression of hemeoxygensase-1 leads to a reduced damage in the presence of free radicals (Maines 1997) which is why investigators have postulated the induction of hemeoxygensase-1 as a potential therapy for PD. However, based on the breakdown of heme, which leads to the formation of biliverdin and carbon monoxide as well as free iron, it is possible that in the specific environment of the SNpc, hemeoxygensase-1 can act counterintuitively and lead to further neurotoxicity (Hansen 1994; Schipper 1999). The breakdown products of heme induced by hemeoxygensase-1 also may act as mitochondrial toxins, leading to a feed-forward loop that eventually leads to cell death.

In addition to participating in cellular toxicity, astrocytes, either in the substantia nigra or striatum, may also act as a protective agent through several mechanisms, including their ability to act as "cellular buffers" and by producing neurotrophic factors. Several studies show that astrocytes can aid in neuronal protection thorough the synthesis and release of the free-radical scavenger glutathione and/or its precursors glutamate, cysteine, and glycine (Drukarch et al. 1998; Dringen et al. 1999). Unlike neurons, glia can generate this neuroprotectant through the biochemical pathways that use cysteine and cystine to produce GSH (Sagara 1993 #1117; Wang and Cynader, 2000). Since GSH levels are lower in the SNpc of PD patients, the local astrocytes in the substantia nigra may serve this important function. The efficiency of glial cells in producing or in maintaining levels of glutathione in different strains of mice (Hatakeyama et al. 1996) may be an important factor in the pathogenesis of dopaminergic neuron loss in experimental models of PD and may provide a therapeutic target for neuroprotection.

In addition to providing the precursors for redox modulating compounds such as glutathione, astrocytes also produce a number of neurotrophic factors (Schaar et al. 1993, 1994; Nakajima et al. 2001). Several neurotrophins support dopaminergic neurons following MPTP or MPP^+ intoxication (Nagatsu et al. 2000). These factors include BDNF (Spina et al. 1992; Frim et al. 1994; Tsukahara et al. 1995), GDNF (Cheng et al. 1998; Date et al. 1998), FGF (Otto and Unsicker 1994), and EGF (Hadjiconstantinou et al. 1991). Neurotrophins act to prevent cell death through a number of mechanisms including interference with the intrinsic cell death programs (Schabitz et al. 2000; Heaton et al. 2003) and modulating oxidative stress (Spina et al. 1992; Kirschner et al. 1996; Skaper et al. 1998; Gong et al. 1999; Petersen et al. 2001).

III. CONCLUSIONS

The discovery that MPTP, which is structurally similar to a number of commonly used herbicides and pesticides, can induce specific loss of substantia nigra neurons in many vertebrate species, from humans to mice, has lead to the development of a useful model of Parkinson disease. In mice, MPTP demonstrates differential toxicity that is dependent on the strain of animal examined (Sonsalla and Heikkila 1988; Muthane et al. 1994; Hamre et al. 1999). This finding supports the hypothesis that the loss of substantia nigra neurons in Parkinson disease may result from a genetic sensitivity to a number of environmental agents (Veldman et al. 1998; Stoessl 1999). In a recent study, the chromosomal loci containing the genetic sequences responsible for this sensitivity was identified on the telomeric end of mChr.1 (Cook et al. 2003). Further studies into the genetic and biochemical pathways involved in MPTP toxicity will lead to a better understanding of idiopathic Parkinson disease and provide clues to novel targets for therapeutic interventions.

References

Ara, J., S. Przedborski, A.B. Naini, V. Jackson-Lewis, R.R. Trifiletti, J. Horwitz, and H. Ischiropoulos. 1998. Inactivation of tyrosine hydroxylase by nitration following exposure to peroxynitrite and 1-methyl-4-phenyl-1,2,3,6-tetrahydropyridine (MPTP). *Proc Natl Acad Sci U S A* **95**:7659–7663.

Aulak, K.S., M. Miyagi, L. Yan, K.A. West, D. Massillon, J.W. Crabb, and D.J. Stuehr. 2001. Proteomic method identifies proteins nitrated in vivo during inflammatory challenge. *Proc Natl Acad Sci U S A* **98**:12056–12061.

Beal, M.F. 2003. Mitochondria, oxidative damage, and inflammation in Parkinson's disease. *Ann N Y Acad Sci* **991**:120–131.

Betarbet, R., T.B. Sherer, G. MacKenzie, M. Garcia-Osuna, A.V. Panov, and J.T. Greenamyre. 2000. Chronic systemic pesticide exposure reproduces features of Parkinson's disease. *Nat. Neurosci* **3**:1301–1306.

Bezard, E., C.E. Gross, M.C. Fournier, S. Dovero, B. Bloch, and M. Jaber. 1999. Absence of MPTP-induced neuronal death in mice lacking the dopamine transporter. *Exp Neurol* **155**:268–273.

Brecknell, J.E., S.B. Dunnett, and J.W. Fawcett. 1995. A quantitative study of cell death in the substantia nigra following a mechanical lesion of the medial forebrain bundle. *Neurosci* **64**:219–227.

Brooks, A.I., C.A. Chadwick, H.A. Gelbard, D.A. Cory-Slechta, and H.J. Federoff. 1999. Paraquat elicited neurobehavioral syndrome caused by dopaminergic neuron loss. *Brain Res* **823**:1–10.

Brooks, W.J., M.F. Jarvis, and G.C. Wagner. 1989. Astrocytes as a primary locus for the conversion MPTP into MPP+. *J Neural Transm* **76**:1–12.

Burns, R.S., P. LeWitt, M.H. Ebert, H. Pakkenberg, and I.J. Kopin. 1985. The clinical syndrome of striatal dopamine deficiency; parkinsonism induced by MPTP. *N Engl J Med* **312**:1418–1421.

Cassina, A.M., R. Hodara, J.M. Souza, L. Thomson, L. Castro, H. Ischiropoulos, B.A. Freeman, and R. Radi. 2000. Cytochrome c nitration by peroxynitrite. *J Biol Chem* **275**:21409–21415.

Cerruti, C., D.M. Walther, M.J. Kuhar, and G.R. Uhl. 1993. Dopamine transporter mRNA expression is intense in rat midbrain neurons and modest outside midbrain. *Mol Brain Res* **18**:181–186.

Cheng, F.C., D.R. Ni, M.C. Wu, J.S. Kuo, and L.G. Chia. 1998. Glial cell line-derived neurotrophic factor protects against 1-methyl-4-phenyl-1,2,3,6-tetrahydropyridine (MPTP)-induced neurotoxicity in C57BL/6 mice. *Neurosci Lett* **252**:87–90.

Chun, H.S., G.E. Gibson, L.A. DeGiorgio, H. Zhang, V.J. Kidd, and J.H. Son. 2001. Dopaminergic cell death induced by MPP(+), oxidant and specific neurotoxicants shares the common molecular mechanism. *J Neurochem* **76**:1010–1021.

Cleeter, M.W., J.M. Cooper, and A.H. Schapira. 1992. Irreversible inhibition of mitochondrial complex I by 1-methyl-4-phenylpyridinium: evidence for free radical involvement. *J Neurochem* **58**:786–789.

Conway, K.A., J.D. Harper, and P.T. Lansbury. 1998. Accelerated *in vitro* fibril formation by a mutant alpha-synuclein linked to early-onset Parkinson disease. *Nat Med* **4**:1318–1320.

Cook, R., L. Lu, J. Gu, R.W. Williams, and R.J. Smeyne. 2003. Identification of a single QTL, Mptp1, for susceptibility to MPTP-induced substantia nigra pars compacta neuron loss in mice. *Mol Brain Res* **110**:279–288.

D'Amato, R.J., Z.P. Lipman, and S.H. Snyder. 1986. Selectivity of the parkinsonian neurotoxin MPTP: toxic metabolite MPP+ binds to neuromelanin. *Science* **231**:987–989.

Damier, P., E.C. Hirsch, Y. Agid, and A.M. Graybiel. 1999. The substantia nigra of the human brain. II. Patterns of loss of dopamine-containing neurons in Parkinson's disease. *Brain* **122**:1437–1448.

Date, I., M. Aoi, S. Tomita, F. Collins, and T. Ohmoto. 1998. GDNF administration induces recovery of the nigrostriatal dopaminergic system both in young and aged parkinsonian mice. *Neuroreport* **9**:2365–2369.

Daubner, S.C., D.L. Lohse, and P.F. Fitzpatrick. 1993. Expression and characterization of catalytic and regulatory domains of rat tyrosine hydroxylase. *Protein Sci* **2**:1452–1460.

de Rijk, M.C., M.M. Breteler, G.A. Graveland, A. Ott, D.E. Grobbee, F.G. van der Meche, and A. Hofman. 1995. Prevalence of Parkinson's disease in the elderly: the Rotterdam Study. *Neurology* **45**:2143–2146.

Del Zompo, M., M.P. Piccardi, S. Ruiu, M. Quartu, G.L. Gessa, and A. Vaccari. 1993. Selective MPP+ uptake into synaptic dopamine vesicles: possible involvement in MPTP neurotoxicity. *Br J Pharm* **109**:411–414.

Deumens, R., A. Blokland, and J. Prickaerts. 2002. Modeling Parkinson's disease in rats: an evaluation of 6-OHDA lesions of the nigrostriatal pathway. *Exp Neurol* **175**:303–317.

Di Monte, D., M.S. Sandy, G. Ekstrom, and M.T. Smith. 1986. Comparative studies on the mechanisms of paraquat and 1-methyl-4-phenylpyridine (MPP+) cytotoxicity. *Biochem Biophys Res Commun* **137**:303–309.

Di Monte, D.A., J.E. Royland, I. Irwin, and J.W. Langston. 1996. Astrocytes as the site for bioactivation of neurotoxins. *Neurotoxicology* **17**:697–703.

Di Monte, D.A., E.Y. Wu, I. Irwin, L.E. Delanney, and J.W. Langston. 1992. Production and disposition of 1-methyl-4-phenylpyridinium in primary cultures of mouse astrocytes. *Glia* **5**:48–55.

Dringen, R., B. Pfeiffer, and B. Hamprecht. 1999. Synthesis of the antioxidant glutathione in neurons: supply by astrocytes of CysGly as precursor for neuronal glutathione. *J Neurosci* **19**:562–569.

Drukarch, B., E. Schepens, J.C. Stoof, C.H. Langeveld, and F.L. Van Muiswinkel. 1998. Astrocyte-enhanced neuronal survival is mediated by scavenging of extracellular reactive oxygen species. *Free Rad Biol Med* **25**:217–220.

Duvoisin, R.C. 1999. Genetic and environmental factors in Parkinson's disease. *Adv Neurology* **80**:161–163.

Elbirt, K.K., and H.L. Bonkovsky. 1999. Heme oxygenase: recent advances in understanding its regulation and role. *Proc Assoc Am Physicians* **111**:438–447.

Fahn, S., and S. Przedborski. 2000. Parkinsonism. In *Merritt's Neurology*, 10th Edition Ed. L.P. Rowland. pp 679–693. Philadelphia: Lippincott Williams and Wilkins.

Faull, R.L., and W.R. Mehler. 1978. The cells of origin of nigrotectal, nigrothalamic and nigrostriatal projections in the rat. *Neuroscience* **3**:989–1002.

Fernandez-Gonzales, A., I. Perez-Otano, and J.I. Morgan. 2000. MPTP selectively induces heme oxygenase-1 expression in striatal astrocytes. *Eur J Neurosci* **12**:1573–1583.

Fornai, F., G. Battaglia, M. Gesi, F.S. Giorgi, F. Orzi, F. Nicoletti, and S. Ruggieri. 2000. Time-course and dose-response study on the effects of chronic L-dopa administration on striatal dopamine levels and dopamine transporter following MPTP toxicity. *Brain Res* **887**: 110–117.

Forno, L.S., L.E. DeLanney, I. Irwin, D. Di Monte, and J.W. Langston. 1992. Astrocytes and Parkinson's disease. *Prog Brain Res* **94**:429–436.

Frim, D.M., T.A. Uhler, W.R. Galpern, M.F. Beal, X.O. Breakefield, and O. Isacson. 1994. Implanted fibroblasts genetically engineered to produce brain-derived neurotrophic factor prevent 1-methyl-4-phenylpyridinium toxicity to dopaminergic neurons in the rat. *Proc Natl Acad Sci U S A* **91**:5104–5108.

Gainetdinov, R.R., F. Fumagalli, S.R. Jones, and M.G. Caron. 1997. Dopamine transporter is required for in vivo MPTP neurotoxicity: evidence from mice lacking the transporter. *J Neurochem* **69**: 1322–1325.

Gainetdinov, R.R., F. Fumagalli, Y.M. Wang, S.R. Jones, A.I. Levey, G.W. Miller, and M.G. Caron. 1998. Increased MPTP neurotoxicity in vesicular monoamine transporter 2 heterozygote knockout mice. *J Neurochem* **70**:1973–1978.

Gasser, T. 2001. Genetics of Parkinson's disease. *J Neurol* **248**:833–840.

German, D.C., K. Manaye, W.K. Smith, D.J. Woodward, and C.B. Saper. 1989. Midbrain dopaminergic cell loss in Parkinson's disease: computer visualization. *Ann Neurol* **26**:507–514.

Giasson, B.I., R. Jakes, M. Goedert, J.E. Duda, S. Leight, J.Q. Trojanowski, and V.M. Lee. 2000a. A panel of epitope-specific antibodies detects protein domains distributed throughout human alpha-synuclein in Lewy bodies of Parkinson's disease. *J Neurosci Res* **59**:528–533.

Giasson, B.I., J.E. Duda, I.V. Murray, Q. Chen, J.M. Souza, H.I. Hurtig, H. Ischiropoulos, J.Q. Trojanowski, and V.M. Lee. 2000b. Oxidative damage linked to neurodegeneration by selective alpha-synuclein nitration in synucleinopathy lesions. *Science* **290**:985–989.

Gong, L., R.J. Wyatt, I. Baker, and J.M. Masserano. 1999. Brain-derived and glial cell line-derived neurotrophic factors protect a catecholaminergic cell line from dopamine-induced cell death. *Neurosci Lett* **263**: 153–156.

Graham, D.G. 1978. Oxidative pathways for catecholamines in the genesis of neuromelanin and cytotoxic quinones. *Mol Pharmacol* **14**:633–643.

Grofova, I. 1979. Extrinsic connections of the neostriatum. In *The Neostriatum*. Ed. I. Divac and R.G.E. Oberg . pp 37–51. Oxford: Pergamon Press.

Hadjiconstantinou, M., J.G. Fitkin, A. Dalia, and N.H. Neff. 1991. Epidermal growth factor enhances striatal dopaminergic parameters in the 1-methyl-4-phenyl-1,2,3,6-tetrahydropyridine-treated mouse. *J Neurochem* **57**:479–482.

Hamre, K., R. Tharp, K. Poon, X. Xiong, and R.J. Smeyne. 1999. Differential strain susceptibility following 1-methyl-4-phenyl-1,2,3,6-tetrahydropyridine (MPTP) administration acts in an autosomal dominant fashion: quantitative analysis in seven strains of Mus musculus. *Brain Res* **828**:91–103.

Hansen, T.W. 1994. Bilirubin in the brain. Distribution and effects on neurophysiological and neurochemical processes. *Clin Pediatr (Phila)* **33**:452–459.

Hastings, T.G. 1995. Enzymatic oxidation of dopamine: the role of prostaglandin H synthase. *J Neurochem* **64**:919–924.

Hatakeyama, S., Y. Hayasaki, M. Masuda, A. Kazusaka, and S. Fujita. 1996. Mechanism for mouse strain differences in the protective effect of Sudan III against the *in vivo* genotoxicity of 7,12-dimethylbenz[a]anthracene. *Tox Lett* **89**:231–239.

Hazell, A.S., Y. Itzhak, H. Liu, and M.D. Norenberg. 1997. 1-Methyl-4-phenyl-1,2,3,6-tetrahydropyridine (MPTP) decreases glutamate uptake in cultured astrocytes. *J Neurochem* **68**:2216–2219.

Heaton, M.B., M. Paiva, I. Madorsky, J. Mayer, and D.B. Moore. 2003. Effects of ethanol on neurotrophic factors, apoptosis-related proteins, endogenous antioxidants, and reactive oxygen species in neonatal striatum: relationship to periods of vulnerability. *Dev Brain Res* **140**:237–252.

Higuchi, S., T. Muramatsu, H. Arai, M. Hayashida, H. Sasaki, and J.Q. Trojanowski. 1995. Polymorphisms of dopamine receptor and transporter genes and Parkinson's disease. *J Neural Transn* **10**:107–113.

Hirrlinger, J., J.B. Schulz, and R. Dringen. 2002. Effects of dopamine on the glutathione metabolism of cultured astroglial cells: implications for Parkinson's disease. *J Neurochem* **82**:458–467.

Hirsch, E.C., and S. Hunot. 2000. Nitric oxide, glial cells and neuronal degeneration in parkinsonism. *TIPS* **21**:163–165.

Hirsch, E.C., S. Hunot, P. Damier, and B. Faucheux. 1998. Glial cells and inflammation in Parkinson's disease: a role in neurodegeneration?. *Ann Neurol* **44**:S115–120.

Hirsch, E.C., G. Hoglinger, E. Rousselet, T. Breidert, K. Parain, J. Feger, M. Ruberg, A. Prigent, C. Cohen-Salmon, and J.M. Launay. 2003. Animal models of Parkinson's disease in rodents induced by toxins: an update. *J Neural Transm* Suppl:89–100.

Hu, C.J., S.M. Sung, H. Liu, and J.G. Chang. 1999. No mutation of G209A in the alpha-synuclein gene in sporadic Parkinson's disease among Taiwan Chinese. *Eur Neurol* **41**:85–87.

Hunot, S., F. Boissiere, B. Faucheux, B. Brugg, A. Mouatt-Prigent, Y. Agid, and E.C. Hirsch. 1996. Nitric oxide synthase and neuronal vulnerability in Parkinson's disease. *Neuroscience* **72**:355–363.

Hunot, S., N. Dugas, B. Faucheux, A. Hartmann, M. Tardieu, P. Debre, Y. Agid, B. Dugas, and E.C. Hirsch. 1999. FcepsilonRII/CD23 is expressed in Parkinson's disease and induces, in vitro, production of nitric oxide and tumor necrosis factor-alpha in glial cells. *J Neurosci* **19**:3440–3447.

Inazu, M., H. Takeda, and T. Matsumiya. 2003. Expression and functional characterization of the extraneuronal monoamine transporter in normal human astrocytes. *J Neurochem* **84**:43–52.

Ischiropoulos, H., and A.B. al-Mehdi. 1995. Peroxynitrite-mediated oxidative protein modifications. *FEBS Lett* **364**:279–282.

Jackson-Lewis, V., M. Jakowec, R.E. Burke, and S. Przedborski. 1995. Time course and morphology of dopaminergic neuronal death caused by the neurotoxin 1-methyl-4-phenyl-1,2,3,6-tetrahydropyridine. *Neurodegeneration* **4**:257–269.

Jellinger, K.A. 1999. The role of iron in neurodegeneration: prospects for pharmacotherapy of Parkinson's disease. *Drugs Aging* **14**:115–140.

Jenner, P. 2003. The contribution of the MPTP-treated primate model to the development of new treatment strategies for Parkinson's disease. *Parkinsonism Relat Disord* **9**:131–137.

Kalaria, R.N., M.J. Mitchell, and S.I. Harik. 1987. Correlation of 1-methyl-4-phenyl-1,2,3,6-tetrahydropyridine neurotoxicity with blood-brain barrier monoamine oxidase activity. *Proc Natl Acad Sci U S A* **84**: 3521–3525.

Khan, F.H., T. Sen, and S. Chakrabarti. 2003. Dopamine oxidation products inhibit Na+, K+-ATPase activity in crude synaptosomal-mitochondrial fraction from rat brain. *Free Radic Res* **37**:597–601.

Kirschner, P.B., B.G. Jenkins, J.B. Schulz, S.P. Finkelstein, R.T. Matthews, B.R. Rosen, and M.F. Beal. 1996. NGF, BDNF and NT-5, but not NT-3 protect against MPP+ toxicity and oxidative stress in neonatal animals. *Brain Res* **713**:178–185.

Kitayama, S., J.B. Wang, and G.R. Uhl. 1993. Dopamine transporter mutants selectively enhance MPP+ transport. *Synapse* **15**:58–62.

Klivenyi, P., D. St Clair, M. Wermer, H.C. Yen, T. Oberley, L. Yang, and M. Flint Beal. 1998. Manganese superoxide dismutase overexpression attenuates MPTP toxicity. *Neurobiol Dis* **5**:253–258.

Kopin, I.J. 1992. Features of the dopaminergic neurotoxin MPTP. *Ann NY Acad Sci* **648**:96–104.

Kopin, I.J., and S.P. Markey. 1988. MPTP toxicity: implications for research in Parkinson's disease. *Annu Rev Neurosci* **11**:81–96.

Lancaster, J.R., Jr. 1996. Diffusion of free nitric oxide. *Methods Enzymol* **268**:31–50.

Lander, E.S., and N.J. Schork. 1994. Genetic dissection of complex traits. *Science* **265**:2037–2048.

Langston, J.W. 1985. The case of the tainted heroin. *The Sciences* **25**:34–40.

Langston, J.W., and J. Palfreman. 1996. *The Case of the Frozen Addicts*. New York: Vintage Books.

Lau, Y.S., Y.K. Fung, K.L. Trobough, J.R. Cashman, and J.A. Wilson. 1991. Depletion of striatal dopamine by the N-oxide of 1-methyl-4-phenyl-1,2,3,6-tetrahydropyridine (MPTP). *Neurotoxicology* **12**:189–199.

LaVoie, M.J., and T.G. Hastings. 1999. Peroxynitrite- and nitrite-induced oxidation of dopamine: implications for nitric oxide in dopaminergic cell loss. *J Neurochem* **73**:2546–2554.

Le Couteur, D.G., P.W. Leighton, S.J. McCann, and S. Pond. 1997. Association of a polymorphism in the dopamine-transporter gene with Parkinson's disease. *Movement Dis* **12**:760–763.

Levine, M.S., C.D. Hull, R.S. Fisher, N.A. Buchwald, and A. Heller. 1983. Effects of neonatal destruction of the medial forebrain bundle in the cat: long-term neurochemical, locomotor, and regulatory deficits. *Exp Neurol* **81**:340–358.

Liberatore, G.T., V. Jackson-Lewis, S. Vukosavic, A.S. Mandir, M. Vila, W.G. McAuliffe, V.L. Dawson, T.M. Dawson, and S. Przedborski. 1999. Inducible nitric oxide synthase stimulates dopaminergic neurodegeneration in the MPTP model of Parkinson disease. *Nat Med* **5**:1403–1409.

Liu, Y., D. Peter, A. Roghani, S. Schuldiner, G.G. Prive, D. Eisenberg, N. Brecha, and R.H. Edwards 1992. A cDNA that suppresses MPP+ toxicity encodes a vesicular amine transporter. *Cell* **70**:539–551.

MacMillan-Crow, L.A., J.P. Crow, J.D. Kerby, J.S. Beckman, and J.A. Thompson. 1996. Nitration and inactivation of manganese superoxide dismutase in chronic rejection of human renal allografts. *Proc Natl Acad Sci U S A* **93**:11853–11858.

Maines, M.D. 1997. The heme oxygenase system: a regulator of second messenger gases. *Annu Rev Pharmacol Toxicol* **37**:517–554.

Maines, M.D. 2000. The heme oxygenase system and its functions in the brain. *Cell Mol Biol (Noisy-le-grand)* **46**:573–585.

Marini, A.M., R.H. Lipsky, J.P. Schwartz, and I.J. Kopin 1992. Accumulation of 1-methyl-4-phenyl-1,2,3,6-tetrahydropyridine in cultured cerebellar astrocytes. *J Neurochem* **58**:1250–1258.

McGeer, P.L., and E.G. McGeer. 1998. Glial cell reactions in neurodegenerative diseases: pathophysiology and therapeutic interventions. *Alz Dis Assoc Dis* **12** Suppl 2:S1–6.

McNaught, K.S., U. Thull, P.A. Carrupt, C. Altomare, S. Cellamare, A. Carotti, B. Testa, P. Jenner, and C.D. Marsden. 1996. Effects of isoquinoline derivatives structurally related to 1-methyl-4-phenyl-1,2,3,6-tetrahydropyridine (MPTP) on mitochondrial respiration. *Biochem Pharmacol* **51**:1503–1511.

McNaught, K.S.P., and P. Jenner. 1999. Altered glial function causes neuronal death and increases neuronal susceptibility to 1-methyl-4-phenylpyridium and 6-hydroxydopamine induced toxicity in astrocytic/ventral mesencephalic co-cultures. *J Neurochem* **73**:2469–2476.

Melamed, E., D. Offen, A. Shirvan, and I. Ziv. 2000. Levodopa—an exotoxin or a therapeutic drug? *J Neurol* **247** Suppl 2:II135–139.

Miller, G.W., R.R. Gainetdinov, A.I. Levey, and M.G. Caron. 1999a. Dopamine transporters and neuronal injury. *TIPS* **20**:424–429.

Miller, G.W., J.D. Erickson, J.T. Perez, S.N. Penland, D.C. Mash, D.B. Rye, and A.I. Levey. 1999b. Immunochemical analysis of vesicular monoamine transporter (VMAT2) protein in Parkinson's disease. *Exp Neurol* **156**:138–148.

Mitra, N., K.P. Mohanakumar, and D.K. Ganguly. 1994. Resistance of golden hamster to 1-methyl-4-phenyl-1,2,3,6-tetrahydropyridine: relationship with low levels of regional monoamine oxidase B. *J Neurochem* **62**:1906–1912.

Mizuno, Y., N. Sone, K. Suzuki, and T. Saitoh. 1988a. Studies on the toxicity of 1-methyl-4-phenylpyridinium ion (MPP+) against mitochondria of mouse brain. *J Neurol Sci* **86**:97–110.

Mizuno, Y., N. Sone, K. Suzuki, and T. Saitoh. 1988b. Studies on the toxicity of 1-methyl-4-phenylpyridinium ion (MPP+) against mitochondria of mouse brain. *J Neurol Sci* **86**:97–110.

Muller, T., T. Buttner, A.F. Gholipour, and W. Kuhn. 2003. Coenzyme Q10 supplementation provides mild symptomatic benefit in patients with Parkinson's disease. *Neurosci Lett* **341**:201–204.

Muthane, U., K.A. Ramsay, H. Jiang, V. Jackson-Lewis, D. Donaldson, S. Fernando, M. Ferreira, and S. Przedborski. 1994. Differences in nigral neuron number and sensitivity to 1-methyl-4-phenyl-1,2,3,6-tetrahydropyridine in C57/bl and CD-1 mice. *Exp Neurol* **126**:195–204.

Nagatsu, T., M. Mogi, H. Ichinose, and A. Togari. 2000. Changes in cytokines and neurotrophins in Parkinson's disease. *J Neural Transm* Suppl:277–290.

Nakajima, K., H. Hida, Y. Shimano, I. Fujimoto, T. Hashitani, M. Kumazaki, T. Sakurai, and H. Nishino. 2001. GDNF is a major component of trophic activity in DA-depleted striatum for survival and neurite extension of DAergic neurons. *Brain Res* **916**:76–84.

Nicklas, W.J., I. Vyas, and R.E. Heikkila. 1985. Inhibition of NADH-linked oxidation in brain mitochondria by 1-methyl-4-phenyl-pyridine, a metabolite of the neurotoxin, 1-methyl-4-phenyl-1,2,5,6-tetrahydropyridine. *Life Sci* **36**:2503–2508.

Nicklas, W.J., S.K. Youngster, M.V. Kindt, and R.E. Heikkila. 1987. MPTP, MPP+ and mitochondrial function. *Life Sci* **40**:721–729.

Nurmi, E., H.M. Ruottinen, J. Bergman, M. Haaparanta, O. Solin, P. Sonninen, and J.O. Rinne. 2001. Rate of progression in Parkinson's disease: a 6-[18F]fluoro-L-dopa PET study. *Mov Disord* **16**:608–615.

Nussbaum, R.L., and M.H. Polymeropoulos. 1997. Genetics of Parkinson's disease. *Hum Mol Gen* **6**:1687–1692.

O'Banion, M.K. 1999. COX-2 and Alzheimer's disease: potential roles in inflammation and neurodegeneration. *Expert Opin Investig Drugs* **8**:1521–1536.

Ofori, S., and M. Schorderet. 1987. Effects of 1-methyl-4-phenyl-1,2,3,6-tetrahydropyridine (MPTP) on dopamine synthesis and release in the rabbit retina *in vitro*. *Neuropharm* **26**:1607–1610.

Olney, J.W., C.F. Zorumski, G.R. Stewart, M.T. Price, G.J. Wang, and J. Labruyere. 1990. Excitotoxicity of L-dopa and 6-OH-dopa: implications for Parkinson's and Huntington's diseases. *Exp Neurol* **108**:269–272.

Otto, D., and K. Unsicker. 1994. FGF-2 in the MPTP model of Parkinson's disease: effects on astroglial cells. *Glia* **11**:47–56.

Parkinson, J. 1817. *An essay on shaking palsy*. London: Sherwood, Neeley and Jones.

Payami, H., and S. Zareparsi. 1998. Genetic epidemiology of Parkinson's disease. *J Ger Psych Neurol* **11**:98–106.

Petersen, A.A., K.E. Larsen, G.G. Behr, N. Romero, S. Przedborski, P. Brundin, and D. Sulzer. 2001. Brain-derived neurotrophic factor inhibits apoptosis and dopamine-induced free radical production in striatal neurons but does not prevent cell death. *Brain Res Bull* **56**:331–335.

Polymeropoulos, M.H., C. Lavedan, E. Leroy, S.E. Ide, A. Dehejia, A. Dutra, B. Pike, H. Root, J. Rubenstein, R. Boyer, E.S. Stenroos, S. Chandrasekharappa, A. Athanassiadou, T. Papapetropoulos, W.G. Johnson, A.M. Lazzarini, R.C. Duvoisin, G. Di Iorio, L.I. Golbe, and R.L. Nussbaum. 1997. Mutation in the alpha-synuclein gene identified in families with Parkinson's disease. *Science* **276**:2045–2047.

Poss, K.D., and S. Tonegawa 1997. Heme oxygenase 1 is required for mammalian iron reutilization. *Proc Natl Acad Sci U S A* **94**:10919–10924.

Przedborski, S., and V. Jackson-Lewis. 1998. Mechanisms of MPTP toxicity. *Mov Disord* 13 Suppl **1**:35–38.

Przedborski, S., and M. Vila. 2003. The 1-methyl-4-phenyl-1,2,3,6-tetrahydropyridine mouse model: a tool to explore the pathogenesis of Parkinson's disease. *Ann N Y Acad Sci* **991**:189–198.

Przedborski, S., V. Jackson-Lewis, R. Yokoyama, T. Shibata, V.L. Dawson, and T.M. Dawson. 1996. Role of neuronal nitric oxide in 1-methyl-4-phenyl-1,2,3,6-tetrahydropyridine (MPTP)-induced dopaminergic neurotoxicity. *Proc Natl Acad Sci U S A* **93**:4565–4571.

Przedborski, S., V. Jackson-Lewis, R. Djaldetti, G. Liberatore, M. Vila, S. Vukosavic, and G. Almer. 2000. The parkinsonian toxin MPTP: action and mechanism. *Rest Neurol Neurosci* **16**:135–142.

Przedborski, S., V. Kostic, V. Jackson-Lewis, A.B. Naini, S. Simonetti, S. Fahn, E. Carlson, C.J. Epstein, and J.L. Cadet. 1992. Transgenic mice with increased Cu/Zn-superoxide dismutase activity are resistant to N-methyl-4-phenyl-1,2,3,6-tetrahydropyridine-induced neurotoxicity. *J Neurosci* **12**:1658–1667.

Przedborski, S., Q. Chen, M. Vila, B.I. Giasson, R. Djaldatti, S. Vukosavic, J.M. Souza, V. Jackson-Lewis, V.M. Lee, and H. Ischiropoulos. 2001. Oxidative post-translational modifications of alpha-synuclein in the 1-methyl-4-phenyl-1,2,3,6-tetrahydropyridine (MPTP) mouse model of Parkinson's disease. *J Neurochem* **76**:637–640.

Quijano, C., D. Hernandez-Saavedra, L. Castro, J.M. McCord, B.A. Freeman, and R. Radi. 2001. Reaction of peroxynitrite with Mn-superoxide dismutase. Role of the metal center in decomposition kinetics and nitration. *J Biol Chem* **276**:11631–11638.

Radi, R., A. Cassina, R. Hodara, C. Quijano, and L. Castro. 2002. Peroxynitrite reactions and formation in mitochondria. *Free Radic Biol Med* **33**:1451–1464.

Ramsay, R.R., and T.P. Singer. 1986. Energy-dependent uptake of N-methyl-4-phenylpyridinium, the neurotoxic metabolite of 1-methyl-4-phenyl-1,2,3,6-tetrahydropyridine, by mitochondria. *J Biol Chem* **261**:7585–7587.

Ramsay, R.R., J. Dadgar, A. Trevor, and T.P. Singer. 1986. Energy-driven uptake of N-methyl-4-phenylpyridine by brain mitochondria mediates the neurotoxicity of MPTP. *Life Sci* **39**:581–588.

Ransom, B.R., D.M. Kunis, I. Irwin, and J.W. Langston. 1987. Astrocytes convert the parkinsonism inducing neurotoxin, MPTP, to its active metabolite, MPP+. *Neurosci Lett* **75**:323–328.

Riachi, N.J., and S.I. Harik. 1988. Strain differences in systemic 1-methyl-4-phenyl-1,2,3,6-tetrahydropyridine neurotoxicity in mice correlate best with monoamine oxidase activity at the blood-brain barrier. *Life Sci* **42**:2359–2363.

Riachi, N.J., W.D. Dietrich, and S.I. Harik. 1990. Effects of internal carotid administration of MPTP on rat brain and blood-brain barrier. *Brain Res* **533**:6–14.

Riachi, N.J., S.I. Harik, R.N. Kalaria, and L.M. Sayre. 1988. On the mechanisms underlying 1-methyl-4-phenyl-1,2,3,6-tetrahydropyridine neurotoxicity. II. Susceptibility among mammalian species correlates with the toxin's metabolic patterns in brain microvessels and liver. *JPET* **244**:443–448.

Riobo, N.A., E. Clementi, M. Melani, A. Boveris, E. Cadenas, S. Moncada, and J.J. Poderoso. 2001. Nitric oxide inhibits mitochondrial NADH: ubiquinone reductase activity through peroxynitrite formation. *Biochem J* **359**:139–145.

Rollema, H., W.G. Kuhr, G. Kranenborg, J. De Vries, and C. Van den Berg. 1988. MPP+-induced efflux of dopamine and lactate from rat striatum have similar time courses as shown by *in vivo* brain dialysis. *JPET* **245**:858–866.

Russ, H., K. Staust, F. Martel, M. Gliese, and E. Schomig. 1996. The extraneuronal transporter for monoamine transmitters exists in cells derived from human central nervous system glia. *Eur J Neurosci* **8**: 1256–1264.

Saadat, S., A.D. Stehle, A. Lamouroux, J. Mallet, and H. Thoenen. 1988. Predicted amino acid sequence of bovine tyrosine hydroxylase and its similarity to tyrosine hydroxylases from other species. *J Neurochem* **51**:572–578.

Schaar, D.G., B.A. Sieber, C.F. Dreyfus, and I.B. Black. 1993. Regional and cell-specific expression of GDNF in rat brain. *Exp Neurol* **124**:368–371.

Schaar, D.G., B.A. Sieber, A.C. Sherwood, D. Dean, G. Mendoza, L. Ramakrishnan, C.F. Dreyfus, and I.B. Black. 1994. Multiple astrocyte transcripts encode nigral trophic factors in rat and human. *Exp Neurol* **130**:387–393.

Schabitz, W.R., C. Sommer, W. Zoder, M. Kiessling, M. Schwaninger, and S. Schwab. 2000. Intravenous brain-derived neurotrophic factor reduces infarct size and counterregulates Bax and Bcl-2 expression after temporary focal cerebral ischemia. *Stroke* **31**:2212–2217.

Schipper, H.M. 1999. Glial HO-1 expression, iron deposition and oxidative stress in neurodegenerative diseases. *Neurotox Res* **1**:57–70.

Schipper, H.M., A. Liberman, and E.G. Stopa. 1998a. Neural heme oxygenase-1 expression in idiopathic Parkinson's disease. *Exp Neurol* **150**:60–68.

Schipper, H.M., R. Vininsky, R. Brull, L. Small, and J.R. Brawer. 1998b. Astrocyte mitochondria: a substrate for iron deposition in the aging rat substantia nigra. *Exp Neurol* **152**:188–196.

Schluter, O.M., F. Fornai, M.G. Alessandri, S. Takamori, M. Geppert, R. Jahn, and T.C. Sudhof. 2003. Role of alpha-synuclein in 1-methyl-4-phenyl-1,2,3,6-tetrahydropyridine-induced parkinsonism in mice. *Neurosci* **118**:985–1002.

Schmidt, C.J., L.A. Matsuda, and J.W. Gibb. 1984. *In vitro* release of tritiated monoamines from rat CNS tissue by the neurotoxic compound 1-methyl-phenyl-tetrahydropyridine. *Eur J Pharm* **103**:255–260.

Schmidt, J., K. Mertz, and J.I. Morgan. 1999. Regulation of heme oxygenase-1 expression by dopamine in cultured C6 glioma and primary astrocytes. *Mol Brain Res* **73**:50–59.

Schneider, J.S., and F.J. Denaro. 1988. Astrocytic responses to the dopaminergic neurotoxin 1-methyl-4-phenyl-1,2,3,6-tetrahydropyridine (MPTP) in cat and mouse brain. *J Neuropath Exp Neurol* **47**:452–458.

Schwarting, R.K., and J.P. Huston. 1996. The unilateral 6-hydroxydopamine lesion model in behavioral brain research. Analysis of functional deficits, recovery, and treatments. *Prog Neurobiol* **50**: 275–331.

Scott, W.K., L.H. Yamaoka, J.M. Stajich, B.L. Scott, J.M. Vance, A.D. Roses, M.A. Pericak-Vance, R.L. Watts, M. Nance, J. Hubble, W. Koller, M.B. Stern, A. Colcher, F.H. Allen, Jr., B.C. Hiner, J. Jankovic, W. Ondo, N.G. Laing, F. Mastaglia, C. Goetz, E. Pappert, G.W. Small, D. Masterman, J.L. Haines, and T.L. Davies. 1999. The alpha-synuclein gene is not a major risk factor in familial Parkinson disease. *Neurogenetics* **2**:191–192.

Shults, C.W. 2003. Coenzyme Q10 in neurodegenerative diseases. *Curr Med Chem* **10**:1917–1921.

Skaper, S.D., M. Floreani, A. Negro, L. Facci, and P. Giusti. 1998. Neurotrophins rescue cerebellar granule neurons from oxidative stress-mediated apoptotic death: selective involvement of phosphatidylinositol 3-kinase and the mitogen-activated protein kinase pathway. *J Neurochem* **70**:1859–1868.

Slivka, A., and G. Cohen. 1985. Hydroxyl radical attack on dopamine. *J Biol Chem* **260**:15466–15472.

Smeyne, M., O. Goloubeva, and R.J. Smeyne. 2001. Strain-dependent susceptibility to MPTP and MPP+-induced Parkinsonism is determined by glia. *Glia* **74**:73–80.

Sonsalla, P.K., and R.E. Heikkila. 1988. Neurotoxic effects of 1-methyl-4-phenyl-1,2,3,6-tetrahydropyridine (MPTP) and methamphetamine in several strains of mice. *Prog Neuropsychopharmacol Biol Psychiatry* **12**:345–354.

Souza, J.M., B.I. Giasson, Q. Chen, V.M. Lee, and H. Ischiropoulos. 2000. Dityrosine cross-linking promotes formation of stable alpha-synuclein polymers. Implication of nitrative and oxidative stress in the pathogenesis of neurodegenerative synucleinopathies. *J Biol Chem* **275**:18344–18349.

Spillantini, M.G., M.L. Schmidt, V.M. Lee, J.Q. Trojanowski, R. Jakes, and M. Goedert. 1997. Alpha-synuclein in Lewy bodies. *Nature* **388**:839–840.

Spina, M.B., S.P. Squinto, J. Miller, R.M. Lindsay, and C. Hyman. 1992. Brain-derived neurotrophic factor protects dopamine neurons against 6-hydroxydopamine and N-methyl-4-phenylpyridinium ion toxicity: involvement of the glutathione system. *J Neurochem* **59**:99–106.

Stoessl, A.J. 1999. Etiology of Parkinson's disease. *Can J Neurol Sci* **26** Suppl 2:S5–12.

Sundstrom, E., I. Stromberg, T. Tsutsumi, L. Olson, and G. Jonsson. 1987. Studies on the effect of 1-methyl-4-phenyl-1,2,3,6-tetrahydropyridine (MPTP) on central catecholamine neurons in C57Bl/6 mice. Comparison with three other strains of mice. *Brain Res* **405**:26–38.

Suzuki, K., Y. Mizuno, and M. Yoshida. 1990. Effects of 1-methyl-4-phenyl-1,2,3,6-tetrahydropyridine (MPTP)-like compounds on mitochondrial respiration. *Adv Neurol* **53**:215–218.

Takahashi, N., L.L. Miner, I. Sora, H. Ujike, R.S. Revay, V. Kostic, V. Jackson-Lewis, S. Przedborski, and G.R. Uhl. 1997. VMAT2 knockout mice: heterozygotes display reduced amphetamine-conditioned reward, enhanced amphetamine locomotion, and enhanced MPTP toxicity. *Proc Natl Acad Sci U S A* **94**:9938–9943.

Teismann, P., K. Tieu, O. Cohen, D.K. Choi, du C Wu, D. Marks, M. Vila, V. Jackson-Lewis, and S. Przedborski. 2003a. Pathogenic role of glial cells in Parkinson's disease. *Mov Disord* **18**:121–129.

Teismann, P., K. Tieu, D.K. Choi, D.C. Wu, A. Naini, S. Hunot, M. Vila, V. Jackson-Lewis, and S. Przedborski. 2003b. Cyclooxygenase-2 is instrumental in Parkinson's disease neurodegeneration. *Proc Natl Acad Sci U S A* **100**:5473–5478.

The Parkinsons Web. 1997. http://neuro-chief-e.mgh.harvard.edu:80/parkinsonsweb/Main/pdmain.html#mainmenu.

Thiruchelvam, M., E.K. Richfield, R.B. Baggs, A.W. Tank, and D.A. Cory-Slechta. 2000. The nigrostriatal dopaminergic system as a preferential target of repeated exposures to combined paraquat and maneb: implications for Parkinson's disease. *J Neurosci* **20**:9207–9214.

Tsukahara, T., M. Takeda, S. Shimohama, O. Ohara, and N. Hashimoto 1995. Effects of brain-derived neurotrophic factor on 1-methyl-4-phenyl-1,2,3,6-tetrahydropyridine-induced parkinsonism in monkeys. *Neurosurgery* **37**:733–739.

United States Census Bureau. 1996. Population Projections of the United States by Age, Sex, Race, and Hispanic Origin: 1993 to 2050.

Veldman, B.A., A.M. Wijn, N. Knoers, P. Praamstra, and M.W. Horstink 1998. Genetic and environmental risk factors in Parkinson's disease. *Clin Neurol Neurosurg* **100**:15–26.

Walkinshaw, G., and C.M. Waters. 1995. Induction of apoptosis in catecholaminergic PC12 cells by L-dopa. Implications for the treatment of Parkinson's disease. *J Clin Invest* **95**:2458–2464.

Wang, X.F., and M.S. Cynader. 2000. Astrocytes provide cysteine to neurons by releasing glutathione. *J Neurochem* **74**:1434–1442.

Whetten-Goldstein, K., F. Sloan, E. Kulas, T. Cutson, and M. Schenkman. 1997. The burden of Parkinson's disease on society, family, and the individual. *J Am Ger Soc* **45**:479–485.

Whone, A.L., R.L. Watts, A.J. Stoessl, M. Davis, S. Reske, C. Nahmias, A.E. Lang, O. Rascol, M.J. Ribeiro, P. Remy, W.H. Poewe, R.A. Hauser, and D.J. Brooks. 2003. Slower progression of Parkinson's disease with ropinirole versus levodopa: The REAL-PET study. *Ann Neurol* **54**:93–101.

Wichmann, T., and M.R. DeLong. 2003. Pathophysiology of Parkinson's disease: the MPTP primate model of the human disorder. *Ann N Y Acad Sci* **991**:199–213.

Williams, A.C., M.L. Smith, R.H. Waring, and D.B. Ramsden. 1999. Idiopathic Parkinson's disease: a genetic and environmental model. *Adv Neurol* **80**:215–218.

Wu, D.C., P. Teismann, K. Tieu, M. Vila, V. Jackson-Lewis, H. Ischiropoulos, and S. Przedborski. 2003. NADPH oxidase mediates oxidative stress in the 1-methyl-4-phenyl-1,2,3,6-tetrahydropyridine model of Parkinson's disease. *Proc Natl Acad Sci U S A* **100**:6145–6150.

Wu, D.C., V. Jackson-Lewis, M. Vila, K. Tieu, P. Teismann, C. Vadseth, D.K. Choi, H. Ischiropoulos, and S. Przedborski. 2002. Blockade of microglial activation is neuroprotective in the 1-methyl-4-phenyl-1,2,3,6-tetrahydropyridine mouse model of Parkinson disease. *J Neurosci* **22**:1763–1771.

Youdim, M.B., E. Grunblatt, Y. Levites, G. Maor, and S. Mandel. 2002. Early and late molecular events in neurodegeneration and neuroprotection in Parkinson's disease MPTP model as assessed by cDNA microarray; the role of iron. *Neurotox Res* **4**:679–689.

Zietlow, R., S.B. Dunnett, and J.W. Fawcett. 1999. The effect of microglia on embryonic dopaminergic neuronal survival *in vitro*: diffusible signals from neurons and glia change microglia from neurotoxic to neuroprotective. *Eur J Neurosci* **11**:1657–1667.

CHAPTER

B4

Rotenone Rat and Other Neurotoxin Models of Parkinson Disease

TODD B. SHERER, RANJITA BETARBET, and J. TIMOTHY GREENAMYRE

Parkinson disease (PD) is a progressive neurodegenerative disease marked by motor and non-motor abnormalities. The hallmark pathological features of PD are selective nigrostriatal dopaminergic degeneration and formation of filamentous, cytoplasmic inclusions called Lewy bodies, containing α-synuclein and ubiquitin. Brains of PD patients show evidence of extensive oxidative damage and microglial activation. Additionally, PD patients are characterized by systemic mitochondrial dysfunction, marked by inhibition of complex I of the mitochondrial electron transport chain. The pathogenesis of idiopathic PD is believed to involve an interaction between genetic and environmental factors. Specifically, PD has been associated with pesticide exposure and rural living. Two recently developed animal models of PD investigate the involvement of environmental exposures in PD pathogenesis. In the rotenone model of PD, rats are exposed, chronically and systemically, to low doses of rotenone, a commonly used pesticide and specific mitochondrial complex I inhibitor. Because of its lipophilic nature, rotenone crosses biological membranes easily, independent of transporters. Despite causing uniform mitochondrial inhibition throughout the brain, rotenone treatment reproduces many features of PD including motor abnormalities, selective nigrostriatal dopaminergic degeneration, and formation of α-synuclein, ubiquitin-positive aggregates in nigral neurons. In the paraquat model of PD, mice exposed to paraquat, an environmental toxin, demonstrate selective nigrostriatal dopaminergic degeneration accompanied by aggregation of α-synuclein in nigral neurons. Thus, the rotenone and paraquat models of PD provide useful systems to understand PD pathogenesis and screen potential therapeutic strategies.

I. BACKGROUND

PD is a late-onset neurodegenerative disease affecting at least 1% of the population over the age of fifty-five. The symptoms of PD include tremor, rigidity, and slowness of movement. These symptoms are attributed, for the most part, to loss of striatal dopamine resulting from degeneration of the nigrostriatal dopaminergic pathway (Wooten 1997). The pathological hallmark of idiopathic PD is the presence of α-synuclein, ubiquitin-positive, filamentous cytoplasmic aggregates, known as Lewy bodies in dead or dying neurons of the substantia nigra (Spillantini et al. 1997). The exact role of these aggregates in the neurodegenerative process of PD remains to be determined.

The pathogenesis of PD is not completely understood but may involve an interaction between genetic and environmental factors (Sherer et al. 2002a). Although more than ten genetic loci are associated with PD, only four genes have been reported so far. Mutations in α-synuclein, parkin, ubiquitin carboxy-terminal hydroxylase LI (UCHLI), and DJ-1 are all associated with familial forms of PD (Bonifati et al. 2003; Hattori et al. 1998; Kitada et al. 1998; Leroy et al. 1998; Polymeropoulos et al. 1997). The role that these proteins play in the more common, sporadic, form of PD is unclear. However, the finding that α-synuclein is a major constituent of Lewy bodies in sporadic PD cases that do not have α-synuclein mutations suggests a role for α-synuclein in the pathogenesis of idiopathic PD (Spillantini et al. 1997). Investigators also believe environmental factors may play a role in PD etiology, as PD occurrence has been associated with pesticide exposure and rural living (Gorell et al. 1998; Menegon et al. 1998). Most likely, both genetic and environmental factors are important.

PD pathogenesis is also associated with mitochondrial dysfunction and oxidative stress (Jenner 1998; Schapira 1999). PD patients demonstrate systemic reductions in mitochondrial activity in tissues ranging from the brain to skeletal muscle and platelets (Cardellach et al. 1993; Haas et al. 1995; Mizuno et al. 1989; Parker et al. 1989; Schapira et al. 1989). Mitochondrial function may result in oxidative stress and the brains of PD patients demonstrate evidence of oxidative damage. Current research has focused on determining the role of oxidative stress and use of antioxidant therapies in PD.

The accumulation of α-synuclein, ubiquitin, and other proteins into Lewy bodies in PD has suggested a role for altered proteasome activity in PD. The proteasome normally degrades misfolded or oxidatively damaged cellular proteins; reduced proteasome function can cause protein aggregates to form (McNaught et al. 2002b). In fact, proteasomal function is reduced in PD brain (McNaught et al. 2003; McNaught and Jenner 2001). The exact role of decreased proteasomal function in PD is an area of active research.

The inflammatory response, including microglial activation, is also implicated in PD. Microglia are the resident immune cells of the central nervous system and become activated in response to injury. Under certain conditions, activated microglia may play either a protective or toxic role following injury. The brains of individuals with PD show clear evidence of microglial activation in substantia nigra (Banati et al. 1998; Mirza et al. 2000).

Animal models of PD seek to reproduce as many features of the disease as possible. These characteristics include:

1. Selective nigrostriatal dopaminergic degeneration
2. α-synuclein aggregation and Lewy body formation
3. Reduced proteasomal function
4. Pesticide exposure
5. Systemic mitochondrial impairment
6. Oxidative damage
7. Microglial activation

In this chapter, we will discuss results obtained from two recently developed models of PD. In the rotenone model of PD, rats were exposed chronically and systemically, to low doses of rotenone, a commonly used pesticide and complex I inhibitor. Rotenone exposure reproduces many features of PD including selective nigrostriatal dopaminergic degeneration, α-synuclein aggregation, microglial activation, and oxidative damage (Betarbet et al. 2000; Sherer et al. 2003c). In the paraquat model of PD, mice are exposed chronically to paraquat, an environmental toxin and potent oxidative stressor. Paraquat treatment causes selective death of dopaminergic nigral neurons and formation of fibrillar α-synuclein-positive aggregates in nigral neurons (McCormack et al. 2002). Both the rotenone and paraquat models of PD substantiate the potential role of environmental toxins in PD.

II. PATHOLOGICAL FEATURES OF PARKINSON DISEASE

A. Selective Nigrostriatal Dopaminergic Degeneration

The cardinal feature of PD is relatively selective neurodegeneration of the nigrostriatal dopaminergic pathway, a neuronal circuit that controls motor activity. The symptoms of PD, including tremor, rigidity, and bradykinesia, are believed to result from depletion of striatal dopamine and the resultant changes in motor circuitry (Wooten 1997). For this reason, dopamine replacement therapy has been the gold standard for treating PD symptoms. Investigators have hypothesized that neurodegeneration of the nigrostriatal pathway begins in dopaminergic terminals in the striatum and progressively affects nigral cell bodies. Roughly 80% of dopaminegric nigral neurons must be lost before the onset of symptoms. Intrinsic neurons of the striatum and other basal ganglia nuclei are markedly less affected in PD.

B. Lewy Bodies Containing Aggregated α-Synuclein and Ubiquitin

Another important pathological feature of PD is the development of filamentous, cytoplasmic inclusions called Lewy bodies. Lewy bodies are composed of aggregated proteins and are found in dopaminergic nigral neurons, as well as in other brain regions including the cortex and magnocellular basal forebrain nuclei (Braak et al. 1995). The list of proteins found in Lewy bodies is expanding but includes ubiquitin, parkin, neurofilament, and α-synuclein (Dev et al. 2003), Considerable interest is shown in the role of α-synuclein in PD because α-synuclein is a component of Lewy bodies and because mutations in α-synuclein can cause familial PD (Polymeropoulos et al. 1997; Spillantini et al. 1997).

Experimental models of PD also demonstrate the importance of α-synuclein in PD pathogenesis. In mice and *Drosophila* overexpressing mutant α-synuclein there is evidence of selective dopaminergic degeneration (Feany and Bender 2000; Masliah et al. 2000). The reason all transgenic α-synuclein mice do not show selective nigrostriatal dopaminergic degeneration is unclear (Lee et al. 2002; van der Putten et al. 2000).

C. Reduced Proteasome Activity in Parkinson Disease

The formation of cytoplasmic protein aggregates in PD brain has lead researchers to a proposed role for decreased proteasomal function in PD pathophysiology. Under normal conditions, the proteasome degrades damaged proteins, including those affected by oxidative stress. Proteins are targeted to the proteasome through several pathways including a ubiquitination pathway. Since Lewy bodies, the protein aggregates found in PD, contain accumulations of ubiquitin, proteasomal function was investigated in PD brain. Additionally, a number of proteins that mutated in familial forms of PD, such as UCHL1 and parkin, normally function in the ubiquitin proteasomal system (Leroy et al. 1998; Zhang et al. 2000). Reduced proteasomal function was observed in substantia nigra of brains of PD patients (McNaught et al. 2003; McNaught and Jenner 2001). This decreased proteasomal activity may result from reduced expression of proteasomal subunits (McNaught et al., 2002a). Researchers reported that inhibiting proteasome function caused nigral cell loss (McNaught et al. 2002b). The exact role of reduced proteasomal activity and its relation to aggregation of α-synuclein in PD pathogenesis remain unclear.

D. Environmental Factors and Parkinson Disease

The discovery that accidental ingestion of 1-methyl-4-phenyl-1,2,3,6-tetrahydropyridine (MPTP) caused an acute Parkinsonism in humans provided important evidence for the role of environmental factors in PD (Langston et al. 1983). MPTP was subsequently found to reproduce features of PD in experimental models. Mice and primates treated with MPTP demonstrate selective dopaminergic degeneration and some evidence supports increased levels and aggregation of α-synuclein in brains of MPTP-treated animals (Beal et al. 1998; Kowall et al. 2000; Przedborski et al. 2001). Epidemiological studies have repeatedly associated occupational exposure to pesticides with an increased risk of developing PD (Menegon et al. 1998). Similarly, drinking well water in rural areas is also associated with increased risk of PD (Gorell et al. 1998). To date, however, no specific class of environmental toxin has been conclusively linked with PD.

E. Mitochondria in Parkinson Disease

After discovering that MPTP caused a Parkinson-like syndrome, researchers investigated the mechanism through which MPTP was toxic to cells. They discovered that MPP^+, the active metabolite of MPTP, acted as an inhibitor of complex I of the mitochondrial electron transport chain (Nicklas et al. 1985). Several laboratories have since determined that a selective defect occurs in complex I in brains of PD patients (Mizuno et al. 1989; Schapira et al. 1989). Subsequently, a modest reduction in complex I activity, systemically, was discovered in PD patients in tissues including skeletal muscle and platelets (Blin et al. 1994; Cardellach et al. 1993; Haas et al. 1995; Parker et al. 1989). Additionally, certain polymorphisms in complex I genes encoded in the mitochondrial genome influence the risk of developing PD (van der Walt et al. 2003). Mitochondrial dysfunction, associated with PD, can have adverse effects on cell physiology, including bioenergetic defects and oxidative damage.

F. Oxidative Stress in Parkinson Disease

The brains of PD patients are characterized by oxidative damage including lipid peroxidation, elevated protein carbonyl levels, and increased oxidative DNA damage (Alam et al. 1997; Dexter et al. 1989; Floor and Wetzel 1998; Yoritaka et al. 1996). Brains of PD patients also demonstrate decreased expression of certain antioxidant enzymes (Pearce et al. 1997). Whether mitochondrial impairment directly accounts for this oxidative damage is unknown. Experimental models of PD also suggest a role for oxidative stress in PD pathophysiology. Brains of mice treated with MPTP demonstrate elevated levels of reactive oxygen species (ROS), oxidative damage to lipids, and increased 3-nitrotyrosine levels (Cassarino et al. 1997; Hasegawa et al. 1990; Lotharius and O'Malley 2000; Matthews et al. 1999). Antioxidants and spin trap agents attenuate MPTP toxicity (Beal et al. 1998; Matthews et al. 1999).

Additionally, an interaction occurs between α-synuclein aggregation and oxidative damage. Oxidatively modified α-synuclein may be more prone to aggregation than native protein (Souza et al. 2000). Oxidative modifications to α-synuclein occur in brains of MPTP-treated mice (Przedborski et al. 2001). Importantly, there is selective and specific nitration of α-synuclein in PD (Giasson et al. 2000). Cells overexpressing mutant α-synuclein are more prone to cell death from oxidative stressors (Kanda et al. 2000; Ko et al. 2000).

G. Glial Cells in Parkinson Disease

The inflammatory response may play a central role in PD pathogenesis. Brains of PD patients are marked by limited reactive astrocytosis but profound activation of microglia (Banati et al. 1998; Mirza et al. 2000). Microglia are the brain's resident immune cells. In response to injury, microglia alter their morphology and produce potentially neurotoxic ROS. PD is characterized by extensive microglial activation in the substantia nigra (Banati et al. 1998; Mirza et al. 2000). Activated microglia may contribute to oxidative damage seen in PD brain through activation of NADPH oxidase, an enzyme expressed in activated microglia that produces superoxide radicals (Wu et al. 2003). Furthermore, many years after MPTP exposure in humans, there is evidence for ongoing microglial activation in substantia nigra (Langston et al. 1999). In MPTP-treated mice, extensive microglial activation occurs and inhibiting microglial activation may lessen MPTP toxicity under some conditions (Czlonkowska et al. 1996). On balance, however, the role of microglial activation in PD is unclear.

III. THE ROTENONE MODEL OF PARKINSON DISEASE

A. Mitochondrial Impairment in the Rotenone Model

To model the systemic defect in complex I reported in PD, researchers have used rotenone exposure. Rotenone is a commonly used pesticide and potent, specific inhibitor of mitochondrial complex I. Although MPP^+ is a mitochondrial toxin, it is not well suited to mimic the systemic mitochondrial impairment that occurs in PD. MPP^+ is a substrate for the dopamine transporter and depends on expression of the dopamine transporter to gain access to cells (Javitch and Snyder 1984). Thus, MPP^+ inhibits complex I activity solely in dopaminergic neurons. Rotenone, on the other hand, because of its lipophilic nature, crosses biological membranes easily and independent of transporters. As a result, systemic rotenone exposure inhibits complex I uniformly throughout brain (Betarbet et al. 2000). This model system addresses whether the nigrostriatal dopaminergic pathway is intrinsically sensitive to complex I impairment.

B. Routes of Administration and Animal Strains

Most studies using the rotenone model of PD use chronic treatment regimens. Rotenone gains access to the brain whether given intravenously, subcutaneously, or intraperitoneally (Alam and Schmidt 2002; Betarbet et al. 2000; Sherer et al. 2003c). Researchers have exposed various strains of rats to rotenone, including Wistar, Sprague-Dawley, and Lewis. Lewis rats show the most consistent responses to rotenone exposure and to another mitochondrial toxin, 3-nitropropionic acid (Betarbet et al. 2000; Ouary et al. 2000). The most extensively studied rotenone model of PD involves chronic exposure of Lewis rats to rotenone by implanting subcutaneous osmotic minipumps (Sherer et al. 2003c). Similar results are obtained whether rotenone is given intravenously or subcutaneously (Betarbet et al. 2000; Sherer et al. 2003c).

C. Rotenone Treatment Reproduces Many Behavioral Symptoms of Parkinson Disease

PD is characterized by motor impairment including slowness of movement, tremor, postural problems, rigidity, and freezing behaviors. Investigators believe these symptoms stem from the depletion of striatal dopamine resulting from nigrostriatal dopaminergic degeneration (Wooten 1997). Most of the above behaviors were observed to varying extents in rotenone-treated animals. Rotenone-infused animals demonstrated reduced locomotor activity, hunched posture, and in some cases rigidity and freezing behavior (Betarbet et al. 2000; Sherer et al. 2003c). Specifically, rotenone-treated animals show decreased rearing, line crossing, and head dips in open field tests and increased catalepsy. In this study, behavioral deficits in rotenone-treated animals correlated with striatal dopamine loss (Alam and Schmidt, 2002). However, detailed studies on the effects of dopamine replacement on the behavioral deficits in rotenone-treated rats have not been conducted yet.

D. Selective Nigrostriatal Dopaminergic Degeneration in the Rotenone Model

One of the pathological hallmarks of PD is selective nigrostriatal dopaminergic degeneration. An initial study examining the effects of rotenone on the nigrostriatal dopaminergic system demonstrated that direct stereotaxic injection of rotenone into the medial forebrain bundle damaged the nigrostriatal dopaminergic system, marked by reduced dopamine levels in the striatum (Heikkila et al. 1985). Stereotaxic injections of rotenone did not cause selective dopaminergic depletion, as serotonin levels were reduced in striatum as well. However, only one dose of rotenone was administered so effects of lower doses of rotenone were unknown (Heikkila et al. 1985). Direct stereotaxic administration of rotenone also does not examine the effects of systemic rotenone infusion (and systemic mitochondrial impairment) on other brain regions. Never-

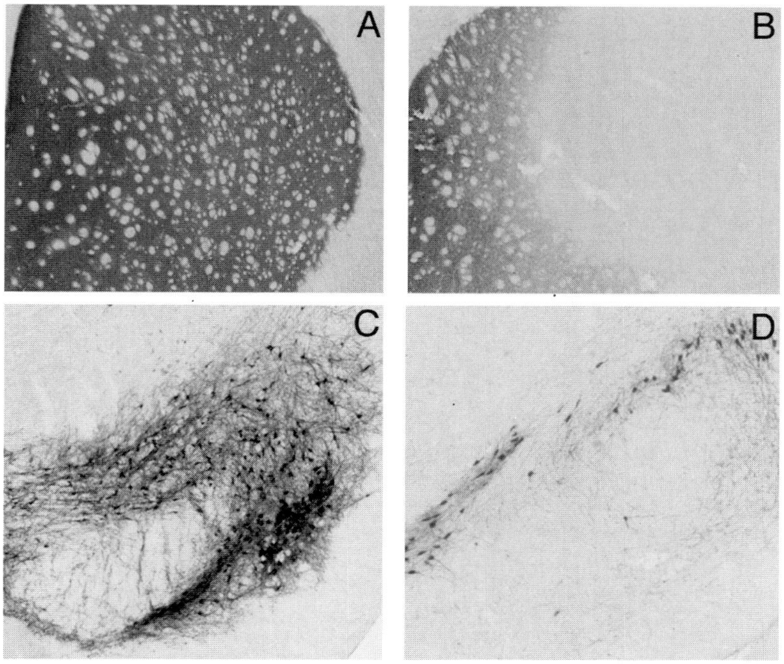

FIGURE 1 Rotenone-induced loss of tyrosine hydroxylase (TH) immunoreactivity in the nigrostriatal pathway. TH immunocytochemistry in striatum of vehicle-infused (A) and rotenone-infused (B) animals. TH immunocytochemistry in nigra of vehicle-treated (C) and rotenone-treated (D) rats. Rotenone-treated animal received 3.0 mg/kg/day rotenone, subcutaneously, for five days.

theless, this study demonstrates that rotenone could be toxic to the nigrostriatal dopaminergic pathway.

More recent studies have used systemic, low dose rotenone infusion in rats. Chronic rotenone treatment, in most cases, replicates the selective nigrostriatal dopaminergic degeneration that occurs in PD. While chronic exposure to rotenone at high doses (12 mg/kg/day) failed to cause selective dopaminergic neurodegeneration (Ferrante et al. 1997), chronic systemic low dose (2–3 mg/kg/day) rotenone exposure caused highly selective nigrostriatal dopaminergic degeneration (Figure 1). Dopaminergic degeneration began in dopaminergic striatal terminals before affecting nigral cell bodies. The effects of rotenone were selective as intrinsic striatal neurons (including DARPP-32$^+$ neurons, GABAergic neurons and cholinergic neurons) and neurons of other basal ganglia neurons remained relatively unaffected. Even dopaminergic neurons from neighboring dopaminergic brain regions (ventral tegmental area and nucleus accumbens) were relatively spared (Betarbet et al. 2000; Sherer et al. 2003c). In other examples of rotenone infusion, chronic injections of rotenone (IP or SC) altered striatal dopamine metabolism in both rats and mice (Alam and Schmidt 2002; Thiffault et al. 2000). Rotenone treatment did not affect norepinephrine and serotonin levels in rats, demonstrating the selectivity of rotenone toxicity (Alam and Schmidt 2002).

Chronic rotenone treatment, if given intravenously through the femoral vein, however, caused less selective neuronal degeneration in which small percentages of intrinsic striatal neurons were lost. In this study, striatal dopaminergic terminals were the neuronal population that was most sensitive to chronic rotenone exposure. Researchers also found that rotenone toxicity was selective within dopaminergic neuronal populations. Despite the loss of nigral dopaminergic neurons, dopaminergic neurons of the ventral tegmental area remained unaffected (Hoglinger et al. 2003b). Reasons for the discrepancy between rotenone administration following femoral vein cannulation and other routes of rotenone administration are unclear.

In vitro evidence also demonstrates that rotenone toxicity selects for midbrain dopaminergic neurons. In a rat brain slice model, short-term rotenone exposure damaged nigral dopaminergic neurons to a greater extent than hypothalamic A11 dopaminergic neurons (Bywood and Johnson 2003). Dopaminergic neurons were also the most sensitive neurons to rotenone treatment in mixed neuron/glia mesencephalic cultures (Gao et al. 2002). However, in neuronal-enriched mesencephalic cultures, rotenone exposure was equally toxic to all neuronal populations (Hoglinger et al. 2003a).

In summary, under most conditions chronic rotenone treatment reproduced the selective nigrostriatal dopaminergic degeneration observed in PD. Rotenone treatment

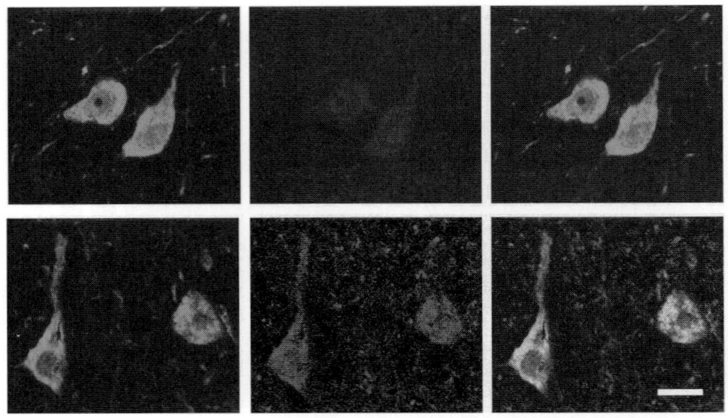

FIGURE 2 (See color version on DVD) Cytoplasmic α-synuclein aggregates in dopaminergic nigral cells of rotenone-treated animals. Nigral sections from control and rotenone-treated animals were double-stained with antibodies against tyrosine hydroxylase (green) and α-synuclein (red). There were increased levels and aggregation of α-synuclein in tyrosine hydroxylase-positive nigral neurons in rotenone-treated animals.

altered dopamine metabolism and caused progressive nigrostriatal dopaminergic degeneration beginning in striatal terminals. Other non-dopaminergic neural pathways, including other basal ganglia nuclei, remained relatively spared.

E. Oxidative Stress in the Rotenone Model

Researchers believe oxidative stress plays an important role in PD pathogenesis. Oxidative damage occurs when ROS interacts with proteins, lipids, or DNA, causing the structure or function of the molecule to alter. A major source of ROS is mitochondrial oxidative metabolism through the electron transport chain. Sites of electron leak in the electron transport chain for production of ROS exist in complex I and complex III. Results from studies with isolated mitochondria indicate that partial inhibition of complex I, produced by rotenone exposure, elevates ROS production (Hensley et al. 1998; Kushnareva et al. 2002). Other *in vitro* studies show that rotenone is an oxidative stressor to intact cells, and antioxidant treatment diminishes rotenone toxicity (Barrientos and Moraes 1999; Li et al. 2003; Seaton et al. 1997; Sherer et al. 2003b). Chronic rotenone exposure causes oxidative damage to accumulate in proteins and DNA and renders cells vulnerable to secondary oxidative stressors (Sherer et al. 2002b).

Rotenone treatment appears to induce oxidative damage *in vivo* as well. Chronic systemic rotenone exposure caused selective oxidative damage, measured by protein carbonyl levels, across brain regions with the largest effects in dopaminergic brain regions including midbrain and olfactory bulb (Betarbet et al. 2002; Sherer et al. 2003b). Additionally, mitochondria isolated from rotenone-infused animals show elevated superoxide production compared to mitochondria isolated from vehicle-treated animals (Cormier et al. 2003). The causal relationship between rotenone-induced oxidative damage and neurodegeneration *in vivo* remains to be determined.

F. α-Synuclein and Ubiquitin Aggregation in the Rotenone Model

Another pathological hallmark of PD is the formation of filamentous cytoplasmic aggregates containing ubiquitin and α-synuclein, among other proteins (Spillantini et al. 1997). Following chronic rotenone exposure in rats, nigral neurons accumulated cytoplasmic inclusions containing ubiquitin and α-synuclein (Figure 2). Ultrastructurally, these inclusions resembled Lewy bodies with a homogeneous dense core surrounded by fibrillar elements (Betarbet et al. 2000). It appears that rotenone-treated animals also accumulate high molecular weight species of α-synuclein in nigra similar to that observed in α-synuclein transgenic mice and PD brain (Betarbet et al. 2002; Lee et al. 2002).

In vitro evidence also demonstrated that rotenone treatment caused α-synuclein aggregation. Chronic rotenone exposure caused accumulation of insoluble endogenous α-synuclein and ubiquitin in the cytoplasm (Sherer et al. 2002b). In cells overexpressing α-synuclein, rotenone treatment caused α-synuclein aggregation through a mechanism that required the continued presence of rotenone (Lee et al. 2001). Additionally, rotenone caused α-synuclein fibrillization in a cell free system (Uversky et al. 2001). Interestingly, cells overexpressing α-synuclein were more sensitive to rotenone toxicity, perhaps providing a link between mitochondrial impairment and α-synuclein aggregation in causing cell death (Lehmensiek et al. 2002). However, a recent study demonstrated that α-synuclein overexpression protected cells from rotenone toxicity (Jensen et al. 2003).

G. Decreased Proteasomal Function in the Rotenone Model of Parkinson Disease

One pathway that targets misfolded or oxidatively damaged proteins for degradation is the ubiquitin-proteasome system (UPS). This pathway involves covalent attachment of ubiquitin to protein substrates, which are then catalytically degraded by the 26S proteasome. 20S proteasome mediates the degradation of nonubiquitinated short peptides (McNaught and Jenner 2001). As mentioned previously, a defective protein degradation pathway is also implicated in PD pathogenesis due to proteinaceous cytoplasmic inclusions in affected neurons that are rich in ubiquitin and α-synuclein. Indeed, impaired proteasomal activity and reduced expression of proteasomal subunits are reported in nigral but not in cortical or striatal post-mortem tissue (McNaught et al. 2003) from sporadic PD patients.

Rotenone-infused rats also demonstrate selective alterations in proteasome function. 20S proteasomal enzymatic activities were significantly and selectively reduced in the ventral midbrain regions (VMB) in rotenone-infused rats. Furthermore, ubiquitin-conjugated proteins, an indicator of proteins marked for degradation, were markedly increased in VMB, suggesting impairment of the 26S proteasome degradation pathway (Betarbet et al. 2003).

Impaired proteasomal function could be due to complex I inhibition-induced changes in bioenergetics such as ATP production and complex I inhibition-induced increases in free radical production resulting in oxidatively damaged proteins. Acute *in vitro* studies using ventral mesencephalic primary cultures implied that rotenone-induced impairment of proteasomal function is primarily due to ATP depletion and not from free radical production (Hoglinger et al. 2003a). However chronic exposure to low levels of rotenone, while minimally affecting bioenergetics, significantly increases the levels of oxidative stress, which may have a greater role in neuronal degeneration (Betarbet et al. 2003; Sherer et al. 2002b). In fact, investigators have demonstrated that rotenone causes oxidative modification to proteasomal subunits, which decreases proteasomal activity (Shamoto-Nagai et al. 2003). Increased levels of oxidatively damaged proteins, observed following rotenone-infusion, could impair the proteasomal pathway, by either "clogging-up" the UPS or by oxidatively modifying the proteasomal subunits themselves.

H. Glial Responses in the Rotenone Model of Parkinson Disease

Brains of individuals dying of PD are characterized by selective and extensive microglial activation in the nigrostriatal pathway with minimal reactive astrocytosis (Banati et al. 1998; Mirza et al. 2000). This glial response is replicated following chronic rotenone treatment. In rotenone-treated rats, extensive microglial activation occurs in the substantia nigra and striatum with less activation in the cortex. Reactive astrocytosis in response to rotenone infusion was minimal and limited to a thin rim around the lesion in a small subset of rotenone-treated rats. Interestingly, rotenone-induced microglial activation preceded apparent neurodegeneration, suggesting that microglial activation may play a causal role in rotenone toxicity (Sherer et al. 2003a).

In vitro studies provide additional evidence for a causal role for microglial activation in rotenone toxicity. The fact that rotenone was substantially more toxic to dopaminergic neurons in mixed neuron-glia cultures was attributed to microglial activation and production of ROS (Gao et al. 2002). Additionally, selective rotenone toxicity to dopaminergic neurons was synergistic with the inflammogen, lipopolysaccharide (Gao et al. 2003). Further studies are needed to investigate the exact role of microglial activation in the rotenone model *in vivo*.

IV. THE PARAQUAT MODEL OF PARKINSON DISEASE

Although PD is associated with pesticide exposure, no specific environmental toxin is linked directly to PD. Because of its structural similarity to MPP^+, paraquat has generated substantial interest. Investigators studying a Taiwanese population determined a relationship between cumulative lifetime exposure to paraquat and development of PD (Liou et al. 1997). For these reasons, researchers have investigated the effects of paraquat on the central nervous system in model systems. The most extensively studied paraquat model of PD involves chronic, systemic exposure of mice to paraquat through intraperitoneal injections. In this model, mice are given paraquat once per week for three weeks (McCormack et al. 2002).

A. Selective Nigrostriatal Dopaminergic Degeneration in the Paraquat Model

Systemic paraquat exposure reproduced some characteristics of the selective dopaminergic degeneration observed in PD. Mice exposed to paraquat showed selective degeneration of dopaminergic neurons of the substantia nigra

(Brooks et al. 1999; McCormack et al. 2002). GABAergic neurons of the substantia nigra pars compacta were spared and no evidence appeared of degenerating neurons in the hippocampus (McCormack et al. 2002). Systemic paraquat exposure, however, did not replicate the striatal dopamine depletion that is characteristic of PD. Perhaps, there is a compensatory increase in tyrosine hydroxylase activity in surviving dopaminergic neurons to maintain striatal dopamine levels (McCormack et al. 2002). In rats exposed to paraquat, however, there was irreparable striatal dopamine depletion (Liou et al. 1996). Additionally, paraquat was toxic to dopaminergic neurons in organotypic midbrain cultures. However, the selectivity of the effects of paraquat on dopaminergic cells was not examined in the cultures (Shimizu et al. 2003).

B. Behavioral Changes Following Paraquat Treatment

Paraquat exposure was associated with behavioral changes similar to those seen in PD patients. Paraquat-treated mice showed reduced ambulatory activity. Intranigral injection of paraquat caused rotational behavior following apomorphine administration similar to that seen in unilateral 6-hydroxydopamine-lesioned animals (Liou et al. 1996, 2001). Apomorphine-induced rotational behavior was attenuated by (−)-deprenyl, a selective type B monoamine oxidase inhibitor, further demonstrating that dopamine depletion caused paraquat-induced behavioral changes (Liou et al. 2001).

C. Environmental Factors

One potential reason that no particular environmental toxin has been linked to PD is that an individual's cumulative exposures may be an important risk factor for PD. In other words, individuals may be exposed to multiple agents throughout their lifetimes that interact and result in the development of PD. Studies in the paraquat model of PD have provided evidence for this hypothesis. A combinational treatment of paraquat with maneb (manganese ethylenebis-dithiocarbamate), another environmental toxin, caused more substantial dopaminergic cell loss in the substantia nigra and loss of tyrosine hydroxylase immunoreactivity in the striatum than following exposure to either compound alone. The effects of paraquat, in combination with maneb, were selective as dopaminergic neurons of the nucleus accumbens and ventral tegmental area were spared. Additionally, combined treatment with paraquat and maneb caused greater behavioral deficits than exposure to either compound alone (Thiruchelvam et al. 2000a,b).

D. α-Synuclein Aggregation in Paraquat-Treated Animals

Paraquat exposure elevated α-synuclein protein levels in the frontal cortex and midbrain as early as two days following treatment. Paraquat treatment also caused α-synuclein aggregation in midbrain neurons determined by thioflavine S staining (Manning-Bog et al. 2002). *In vitro* evidence suggests that paraquat causes α-synuclein fibril formation in a dose-dependent manner (Uversky et al. 2001). The exact role of α-synuclein aggregates in paraquat toxicity is unknown, but it is interesting that mice overexpressing either wild-type or mutant α-synuclein were resistant to paraquat toxicity. In these transgenic mice, paraquat still caused α-synuclein aggregates to form, but dopaminergic neurons were spared (Manning-Bog et al. 2003). The paraquat model of PD may help uncover the exact neurotoxic and possibly neuroprotective role of α-synuclein aggregate formation in PD.

E. Paraquat Effects on Proteasomal Activity

Because paraquat caused protein aggregates to form, another focus of interest is whether paraquat affects proteasomal function. The evidence on this topic remains inconclusive. Paraquat exposure may decrease or have no effect on proteasome activity depending on the cell type studied (Ding and Keller 2001; Grune et al. 1996). Investigators have yet to determine whether paraquat alters proteasomal activity *in vivo*.

F. Glial Responses

Paraquat exposure also caused a selective gliosis that replicated some characteristics of the glial reaction in PD (Liou et al. 1996). Paraquat treatment was associated with reactive astrocytosis and activated microglia in the midbrain but not in the cortex and cerebellum (McCormack et al. 2002). The exact role of gliosis in paraquat toxicity has not been thoroughly studied as of this writing.

G. Paraquat as an Oxidative Stressor

Investigators have hypothesized that paraquat toxicity depends on oxidative damage. *In vitro*, paraquat treatment caused oxidative damage, including ROS production, glutathione depletion, and lipid peroxidation. Antioxidant treatment prevented paraquat toxicity (Chun et al. 2001; Li and Sun 1999; Mollace et al. 2003; Osakada et al. 2003; Schmuck et al. 2002; Yang and Sun 1998a; Yang and Sun 1998b). *In vivo*, directly injecting paraquat into the substantia nigra caused lipid peroxidation (Mollace et al. 2003). The source of this oxidative damage may be paraquat itself, as paraquat can undergo redox cycling and become a reac-

TABLE 1 The Rotenone and Paraquat Models Reproduce Features of PD

Parkinson disease	Rotenone model	Paraquat model
Selective nigrostriatal dopaminergic degeneration	Dopaminergic cell loss begins in striatum followed by nigral death	Loss of dopaminergic nigral cells without substantial loss of striatal dopamine
α-Synuclein aggregation	Fibrillar aggregates in nigral cells	Thioflavin S-positive aggregates in nigral cells
Environmental toxin	Used as a pesticide and to kill nuisance fish in lakes	Commonly used pesticide
Mitochondrial inhibition	Classical complex 1 inhibitor causes systemic mitochondrial impairment	May inhibit complex 1 directly or through oxidative damage
Oxidative damage	Selective oxidative damage to dopaminergic brain regions	Known oxidative stressor from *in vitro* studies
Microglial activation	Selective microglial activation in striatum and nigra	Reactive astrocytosis and microglial activation
Proteasomal activity	Selective reductions in nigral lysates	Inconclusive *in vitro* data. Not examined *in vivo* as of yet.

tive radical. This redox cycling may involve an interaction with complex I of the mitochondrial electron transport chain (Fukushima et al. 1995). Investigators must still determine whether paraquat-induced oxidative damage causes paraquat toxicity *in vivo*.

H. Mitochondrial Function in the Paraquat Model

Due to its structural similarity to MPP^+, paraquat may act as a direct inhibitor of mitochondrial complex I. In fact, mitochondria isolated from rats previously exposed to paraquat show decreased complex I activity (Tawara et al. 1996). However, not much evidence demonstrates that paraquat directly binds to and inhibits complex I—as is the case with rotenone and MPP^+. At high concentrations (1 mM), paraquat competed with tritiated dihydrorotenone for rotenone-binding sites in complex I in isolated brain mitochondria (Richardson et al. 2003). However, it is unclear whether the high concentrations of paraquat needed in this study to determine paraquat binding to complex I were relevant to paraquat toxicity *in vivo*. Paraquat may also inhibit mitochondrial function through an oxidative mechanism and not through direct binding to mitochondrial complexes. For example, paraquat-induced oxidative damage may adversely affect mitochondrial components and impair mitochondria. Additional studies are needed to determine the mechanisms of paraquat-induced mitochondrial dysfunction.

V. SUMMARY

The recently developed rotenone and paraquat models of PD provide novel systems in which to study mechanisms underlying the pathogenesis of the disease. Rats treated with rotenone demonstrate many features of PD including motor abnormalities, selective nigrostriatal dopaminergic degeneration, oxidative stress, microglial activation, α-synuclein aggregation, and selective reductions in proteasomal activity (table 1). Mice chronically exposed to paraquat demonstrate selective dopaminergic nigral cell loss, reactive gliosis, and formation of α-synuclein-positive inclusions (table 1). These models substantiate the involvement of pesticide exposures in PD. Future studies will evaluate therapeutic strategies for neuroprotection in these models of PD.

References

Alam, A., and W.J. Schmidt. 2002. Rotenone destroys dopaminergic neurons and induces parkinsonian symptoms in rats. *Behavioural Brain Research* **136**:317–324.

Alam, Z.I., S.E. Daniel, A.J. Lees, D.C. Marsden, P. Jenner, and B. Halliwell. 1997. A generalised increase in protein carbonyls in the brain in Parkinson's but not incidental Lewy body disease. *J Neurochem* **69**:1326–1329.

Banati, R.B., S.E. Daniel, and S.B. Blunt. 1998. Glial pathology but absence of apoptotic nigral neurons in long-standing Parkinson's disease. *Mov Disord* **13**:221–227.

Barrientos, A., and C.T. Moraes. 1999. Titrating the effects of mitochondrial complex I impairment in the cell physiology. *J Biol Chem* **274**: 16188–16197.

Beal, M.F., R.T. Matthews, A. Tieleman, and C.W. Shults. 1998. Coenzyme Q10 attenuates the 1-methyl-4-phenyl-1,2,3,tetrahydropyridine (MPTP) induced loss of striatal dopamine and dopaminergic axons in aged mice. *Brain Res* **783**:109–114.

Betarbet, R., T.B. Sherer, J.H. Kim, M. Baptista, M.R. Cookson, and J.T. Greenamyre. 2002. Rotenone models of Parkinson's disease: altered alpha-synuclein expression following chronic inhibition of complex I. *Society for Neuroscience Abstract*, **386**:316.

Betarbet, R., T.B. Sherer, S. Lund, and J.T. Greenamyre. 2003. Rotenone models of Parkinson's disease: altered proteasome activity following sustained inhibition of complex I. *Society for Neuroscience Abstract.*

Betarbet, R., T.B. Sherer, G. MacKenzie, M. Garcia-Osuna, A.V. Panov, and J.T. Greenamyre. 2000. Chronic systemic pesticide exposure reproduces features of Parkinson's disease [In Process Citation]. *Nat Neurosci* **3**:1301–1306.

Blin, O., C. Desnuelle, O. Rascol, M. Borg, H. Peyro Saint Paul, J.P. Azulay, F. Bille, D. Figarella, F. Coulom, J.F. Pellissier, et al. 1994. Mitochondrial respiratory failure in skeletal muscle from patients with

Parkinson's disease and multiple system atrophy. *J Neurol Sci* **125**: 95–101.

Bonifati, V., P. Rizzu, M.J. van Baren, O. Schaap, G.J. Breedveld, E. Krieger, M.C. Dekker, F. Squitieri, P. Ibanez, M. Joosse, et al. 2003. Mutations in the DJ-1 gene associated with autosomal recessive early-onset parkinsonism. *Science* **299**:256–259.

Braak, H., E. Braak, D. Yilmazer, C. Schultz, R.A. de Vos, and E.N. Jansen. 1995. Nigral and extranigral pathology in Parkinson's disease. *J Neural Transm Suppl* **46**:15–31.

Brooks, A.I., C.A. Chadwick, H.A. Gelbard, D.A. Cory-Slechta, and H.J. Federoff. 1999. Paraquat elicited neurobehavioral syndrome caused by dopaminergic neuron loss. *Brain Res* **823**:1–10.

Bywood, P.T. and S.M. Johnson. 2003. Mitochondrial complex inhibitors preferentially damage substantia nigra dopamine neurons in rat brain slices. *Exp Neurol* **179**:47–59.

Cardellach, F., M.J. Marti, J. Fernandez-Sola, C. Marin, J.B. Hoek, E. Tolosa, and A. Urbano-Marquez. 1993. Mitochondrial respiratory chain activity in skeletal muscle from patients with Parkinson's disease. *Neurology* **43**:2258–2262.

Cassarino, D.S., C.P. Fall, R.H. Swerdlow, T.S. Smith, E.M. Halvorsen, S.W. Miller, J.P. Parks, W.D. Parker, Jr., and J.P. Bennett, Jr. 1997. Elevated reactive oxygen species and antioxidant enzyme activities in animal and cellular models of Parkinson's disease. *Biochim Biophys Acta* **1362**:77–86.

Chun, H.S., G.E. Gibson, L.A. DeGiorgio, H. Zhang, V.J. Kidd, and J.H. Son. 2001. Dopaminergic cell death induced by MPP(+), oxidant and specific neurotoxicants shares the common molecular mechanism. *J Neurochem* **76**:1010–1021.

Cormier, A., C. Morin, R. Zini, J.P. Tillement, and G. Lagrue. 2003. Nicotine protects rat brain mitochondria against experimental injuries. *Neuropharmacology* **44**:642–652.

Czlonkowska, A., M. Kohutnicka, I. Kurkowska-Jastrzebska, and A. Czlonkowski. 1996. Microglial reaction in MPTP (1-methyl-4-phenyl-1,2,3,6-tetrahydropyridine) induced Parkinson's disease mice model. *Neurodegeneration* **5**:137–143.

Dev, K.K., K. Hofele, S. Barbieri, V.L. Buchman, and H. van der Putten. 2003. Part II: alpha-synuclein and its molecular pathophysiological role in neurodegenerative disease. *Neuropharmacology* **45**:14–44.

Dexter, D.T., C.J. Carter, F.R. Wells, F. Javoy-Agid, Y. Agid, A. Lees, P. Jenner, and C.D. Marsden. 1989. Basal lipid peroxidation in substantia nigra is increased in Parkinson's disease. *J Neurochem* **52**:381–389.

Ding, Q., and J.N. Keller. 2001. Proteasome inhibition in oxidative stress neurotoxicity: implications for heat shock proteins. *J Neurochem* **77**:1010–1017.

Feany, M.B., and W.W. Bender. 2000. A *Drosophila* model of Parkinson's disease [see comments]. *Nature* **404**:394–398.

Ferrante, R.J., J.B. Schulz, N.W. Kowall, and M.F. Beal. 1997. Systemic administration of rotenone produces selective damage in the striatum and globus pallidus, but not in the substantia nigra. *Brain Res* **753**:157–162.

Floor, E., and M.G. Wetzel. 1998. Increased protein oxidation in human substantia nigra pars compacta in comparison with basal ganglia and prefrontal cortex measured with an improved dinitrophenylhydrazine assay. *J Neurochem* **70**:268–275.

Fukushima, T., T. Tawara, A. Isobe, N. Hojo, K. Shiwaku, and Y. Yamane. 1995. Radical formation site of cerebral complex I and Parkinson's disease. *J Neurosci Res* **42**:385–390.

Gao, H.M., J.S. Hong, W. Zhang, and B. Liu. 2002. Distinct role for microglia in rotenone-induced degeneration of dopaminergic neurons. *J Neurosci* **22**:782–790.

Gao, H.M., J.S. Hong, W. Zhang, and B. Liu. 2003. Synergistic dopaminergic neurotoxicity of the pesticide rotenone and inflammogen lipopolysaccharide: relevance to the etiology of Parkinson's disease. *J Neurosci* **23**:1228–1236.

Giasson, B.I., J.E. Duda, I.V. Murray, Q. Chen, J.M. Souza, H.I. Hurtig, H. Ischiropoulos, J.Q. Trojanowski, and V.M. Lee. 2000. Oxidative damage linked to neurodegeneration by selective alpha-synuclein nitration in synucleinopathy lesions. *Science* **290**:985–989.

Gorell, J.M., C.C. Johnson, B.A. Rybicki, E.L. Peterson, and R.J. Richardson. 1998. The risk of Parkinson's disease with exposure to pesticides, farming, well water, and rural living. *Neurology* **50**:1346–1350.

Grune, T., T. Reinheckel, and K.J. Davies. 1996. Degradation of oxidized proteins in K562 human hematopoietic cells by proteasome. *J Biol Chem* **271**:15504–15509.

Haas, R.H., F. Nasirian, K. Nakano, D. Ward, M. Pay, R. Hill, and C.W. Shults. 1995. Low platelet mitochondrial complex I and complex II/III activity in early untreated Parkinson's disease. *Ann Neurol* **37**:714–722.

Hasegawa, E., K. Takeshige, T. Oishi, Y. Murai, and S. Minakami. 1990. 1-Methyl-4-phenylpyridinium (MPP+) induces NADH-dependent superoxide formation and enhances NADH-dependent lipid peroxidation in bovine heart submitochondrial particles. *Biochem Biophys Res Commun* **170**:1049–1055.

Hattori, N., H. Matsumine, S. Asakawa, T. Kitada, H. Yoshino, B. Elibol, A.J. Brookes, Y. Yamamura, T. Kobayashi, M. Wang, et al. 1998. Point mutations (Thr240Arg and Gln311Stop) [correction of Thr240Arg and Ala311Stop] in the Parkin gene. *Biochem Biophys Res Commun* **249**:754–758.

Heikkila, R.E., W.J. Nicklas, I. Vyas, and R.C. Duvoisin. 1985. Dopaminergic toxicity of rotenone and the 1-methyl-4-phenylpyridinium ion after their stereotaxic administration to rats: implication for the mechanism of 1-methyl-4-phenyl-1,2,3,6-tetrahydropyridine toxicity. *Neurosci Lett* **62**:389–394.

Hensley, K., Q.N. Pye, M.L. Maidt, C.A. Stewart, K.A. Robinson, F. Jaffrey, and R.A. Floyd. 1998. Interaction of alpha-phenyl-N-tert-butyl nitrone and alternative electron acceptors with complex I indicates a substrate reduction site upstream from the rotenone binding site. *J Neurochem* **71**:2549–2557.

Hoglinger, G.U., G. Carrard, P.P. Michel, F. Medja, A. Lombes, M. Ruberg, B. Friguet, and E.C. Hirsch. 2003a. Dysfunction of mitochondrial complex I and the proteasome: interactions between two biochemical deficits in a cellular model of Parkinson's disease. *J Neurochem* **86**:1297–1307.

Hoglinger, G.U., J. Feger, A. Prigent, P.P. Michel, K. Parain, P. Champy, M. Ruberg, W.H. Oertel, and E.C. Hirsch. 2003b. Chronic systemic complex I inhibition induces a hypokinetic multisystem degeneration in rats. *J Neurochem* **84**:491–502.

Javitch, J.A., and S.H. Snyder. 1984. Uptake of MPP(+) by dopamine neurons explains selectivity of parkinsonism-inducing neurotoxin, MPTP. *Eur J Pharmacol* **106**:455–456.

Jenner, P. 1998. Oxidative mechanisms in nigral cell death in Parkinson's disease. *Mov Disord* **13**:24–34.

Jensen, P.J., B.J. Alter, and K.L. O'Malley. 2003. Alpha-synuclein protects naive but not dbcAMP-treated dopaminergic cell types from 1-methyl-4-phenylpyridinium toxicity. *J Neurochem* **86**:196–209.

Kanda, S., J.F. Bishop, M.A. Eglitis, Y. Yang, and M.M. Mouradian. 2000. Enhanced vulnerability to oxidative stress by alpha-synuclein mutations and C-terminal truncation. *Neuroscience* **97**:279–284.

Kitada, T., S. Asakawa, N. Hattori, H. Matsumine, Y. Yamamura, S. Minoshima, M. Yokochi, Y. Mizuno, and N. Shimizu. 1998. Mutations in the parkin gene cause autosomal recessive juvenile parkinsonism [see comments]. *Nature* **392**:605–608.

Ko, L., N.D. Mehta, M. Farrer, C. Easson, J. Hussey, S. Yen, J. Hardy, and S.H. Yen. 2000. Sensitization of neuronal cells to oxidative stress with mutated human alpha-synuclein. *J Neurochem* **75**:2546–2554.

Kowall, N.W., P. Hantraye, E. Brouillet, M.F. Beal, A.C. McKee, and R.J. Ferrante. 2000. MPTP induces alpha-synuclein aggregation in the substantia nigra of baboons. *Neuroreport* **11**:211–213.

Kushnareva, Y., A.N. Murphy, and A. Andreyev. 2002. Complex I-mediated reactive oxygen species generation: modulation by cytochrome c and NAD(P)+ oxidation-reduction state. *Biochem J* **368**:545–553.

Langston, J.W., P. Ballard, J.W. Tetrud, and I. Irwin. 1983. Chronic Parkinsonism in humans due to a product of meperidine-analog synthesis. *Science* **219**:979–980.

Langston, J.W., L.S. Forno, J. Tetrud, A.G. Reeves, J.A. Kaplan, and D. Karluk. 1999. Evidence of active nerve cell degeneration in the substantia nigra of humans years after 1-methyl-4-phenyl-1,2,3,6-tetrahydropyridine exposure. *Ann Neurol* **46**:598–605.

Lee, H.J., S.Y. Shin, C. Choi, Y.H. Lee, and S.J. Lee. 2001. Formation and removal of alpha-synuclein aggregates in cells exposed to mitochondrial inhibitors. *J Biol Chem* **27**:5411–5417.

Lee, M.K., W. Stirling, Y. Xu, X. Xu, D. Qui, A.S. Mandir, T.M. Dawson, N.G. Copeland, N.A. Jenkins, and D.L. Price. 2002. Human alpha-synuclein-harboring familial Parkinson's disease-linked Ala-53 → Thr mutation causes neurodegenerative disease with alpha-synuclein aggregation in transgenic mice. *Proc Natl Acad Sci U S A* **99**:8968–8973.

Lehmensiek, V., E.M. Tan, J. Schwarz, and A. Storch. 2002. Expression of mutant alpha-synucleins enhances dopamine transporter-mediated MPP+ toxicity in vitro. *Neuroreport* **13**:1279–1283.

Leroy, E., R. Boyer, G. Auburger, B. Leube, G. Ulm, E. Mezey, G. Harta, M.J. Brownstein, S. Jonnalagada, T. Chernova, et al. 1998. The ubiquitin pathway in Parkinson's disease. *Nature* **395**:451–452.

Li, N., K. Ragheb, G. Lawler, J. Sturgis, B. Rajwa, J.A. Melendez, and J.P. Robinson. 2003. Mitochondrial complex I inhibitor rotenone induces apoptosis through enhancing mitochondrial reactive oxygen species production. *J Biol Chem* **278**:8516–8525.

Li, X., and A.Y. Sun. 1999. Paraquat induced activation of transcription factor AP-1 and apoptosis in PC12 cells. *J Neural Transm* **106**:1–21.

Liou, H.H., R.C. Chen, T.H. Chen, Y.F. Tsai, and M.C. Tsai. 2001. Attenuation of paraquat-induced dopaminergic toxicity on the substantia nigra by (-)-deprenyl *in vivo*. *Toxicol Appl Pharmacol* **172**:37–43.

Liou, H.H., R.C. Chen, Y.F. Tsai, W.P. Chen, Y.C. Chang, and M.C. Tsai. 1996. Effects of paraquat on the substantia nigra of the wistar rats: neurochemical, histological, and behavioral studies. *Toxicol Appl Pharmacol* **137**:34–41.

Liou, H.H., M.C. Tsai, C.J. Chen, J.S. Jeng, Y.C. Chang, S.Y. Chen, and R.C. Chen. 1997. Environmental risk factors and Parkinson's disease: a case-control study in Taiwan. *Neurology* **48**:1583–1588.

Lotharius, J., and K.L. O'Malley. 2000. The parkinsonism-inducing drug 1-methyl-4-phenylpyridinium triggers intracellular dopamine oxidation. A novel mechanism of toxicity. *J Biol Chem* **275**:38581–38588.

Manning-Bog, A.B., A.L. McCormack, J. Li, V.N. Uversky, A.L. Fink, and D.A. Di Monte. 2002. The herbicide paraquat causes up-regulation and aggregation of alpha-synuclein in mice: paraquat and alpha-synuclein. *J Biol Chem* **277**:1641–1644.

Manning-Bog, A.B., A.L. McCormack, M.G. Purisai, L.M. Bolin, and D.A. Di Monte. 2003. Alpha-synuclein overexpression protects against paraquat-induced neurodegeneration. *J Neurosci* **23**:3095–3099.

Masliah, E., E. Rockenstein, I. Veinbergs, M. Mallory, M. Hashimoto, A. Takeda, Y. Sagara, A. Sisk, and L. Mucke. 2000. Dopaminergic loss and inclusion body formation in alpha-synuclein mice: implications for neurodegenerative disorders. *Science* **287**:1265–1269.

Matthews, R.T., P. Klivenyi, G. Mueller, L. Yang, M. Wermer, C.E. Thomas, and M.F. Beal. 1999. Novel free radical spin traps protect against malonate and MPTP neurotoxicity. *Exp Neurol* **157**:120–126.

McCormack, A.L., M. Thiruchelvam, A.B. Manning-Bog, C. Thiffault, J.W. Langston, D.A. Cory-Slechta, and D.A. Di Monte. 2002. Environmental risk factors and Parkinson's disease: selective degeneration of nigral dopaminergic neurons caused by the herbicide paraquat. *Neurobiol Dis* **10:**119–127.

McNaught, K.S., R. Belizaire, O. Isacson, P. Jenner, and C.W. Olanow. 2003. Altered proteasomal function in sporadic Parkinson's disease. *Exp Neurol* **179**:38–46.

McNaught, K.S., R. Belizaire, P. Jenner, C.W. Olanow, and O. Isacson. 2002a. Selective loss of 20S proteasome alpha-subunits in the substantia nigra pars compacta in Parkinson's disease. *Neurosci Lett* **326**:155–158.

McNaught, K.S., L.M. Bjorklund, R. Belizaire, O. Isacson, P. Jenner, and C.W. Olanow. 2002b. Proteasome inhibition causes nigral degeneration with inclusion bodies in rats. *Neuroreport* **13**:1437–1441.

McNaught, K.S., and P. Jenner. 2001. Proteasomal function is impaired in substantia nigra in Parkinson's disease. *Neurosci Lett* **297**:191–194.

Menegon, A., P.G. Board, A.C. Blackburn, G.D. Mellick, and D.G. Le Couteur. 1998. Parkinson's disease, pesticides, and glutathione transferase polymorphisms [see comments]. *Lancet* **352**:1344–1346.

Mirza, B., H. Hadberg, P. Thomsen, and T. Moos. 2000. The absence of reactive astrocytosis is indicative of a unique inflammatory process in Parkinson's disease. *Neuroscience* **95**:425–432.

Mizuno, Y., S. Ohta, M. Tanaka, S. Takamiya, K. Suzuki, T Sato, H. Oya, T. Ozawa, and Y. Kagawa. 1989. Deficiencies in complex I subunits of the respiratory chain in Parkinson's disease. *Biochem Biophys Res Commun* **163**:1450–1455.

Mollace, V., M. Iannone, C. Muscoli, E. Palma, T. Granato, V. Rispoli, R. Nistico, D. Rotiroti, and D. Salvemini. 2003. The role of oxidative stress in paraquat-induced neurotoxicity in rats: protection by non peptidyl superoxide dismutase mimetic. *Neurosci Lett* **335**:163–166.

Nicklas, W.J., I. Vyas, and R.E. Heikkila. 1985. Inhibition of NADH-linked oxidation in brain mitochondria by 1-methyl-4-phenyl-pyridine, a metabolite of the neurotoxin, 1-methyl-4-phenyl-1,2,5,6-tetrahydropyridine. *Life Sci* **36**:2503–2508.

Osakada, F., A. Hashino, T. Kume, H. Katsuki, S. Kaneko, and A. Akaike. 2003. Neuroprotective effects of alpha-tocopherol on oxidative stress in rat striatal cultures. *Eur J Pharmacol* **465**:15–22.

Ouary, S., N. Bizat, S. Altairac, H. Menetrat, V. Mittoux, F. Conde, P. Hantraye, and E. Brouillet. 2000. Major strain differences in response to chronic systemic administration of the mitochondrial toxin 3-nitropropionic acid in rats: implications for neuroprotection studies. *Neuroscience* **97**:521–530.

Parker, W.D., Jr., S.J. Boyson, and J.K. Parks. 1989. Abnormalities of the electron transport chain in idiopathic Parkinson's disease. *Ann Neurol* **26**:719–723.

Pearce, R.K., A. Owen, S. Daniel, P. Jenner, and C.D. Marsden. 1997. Alterations in the distribution of glutathione in the substantia nigra in Parkinson's disease. *J Neural Transm* **104**:661–677.

Polymeropoulos, M.H., C. Lavedan, E. Leroy, S.E. Ide, A. Dehejia, A. Dutra, B. Pike, H. Root, J. Rubenstein, R. Boyer, et al. 1997. Mutation in the alpha-synuclein gene identified in families with Parkinson's disease [see comments]. *Science* **276**:2045–2047.

Przedborski, S., Q. Chen, M. Vila, B.I. Giasson, R. Djaldatti, S. Vukosavic, J.M. Souza, V.V. Jackson-Lewis, V.M. Lee, and H. Ischiropoulos. 2001. Oxidative post-translational modification of alpha-synuclein in the 1-methyl-4-phenyl-1,2,3,6-tetrahydropyridine (MPTP) mouse model of Parkinson's disease. *J Neurochem* **76**:637–640.

Richardson, J.R., T.B. Sherer, J.T. Greenamyre, and G.W. Miller. 2003. Mechanism of complex I inhibition by MPP+ and paraquat. *Society for Neuroscience Abstract.*

Schapira, A.H. 1999. Mitochondrial involvement in Parkinson disease, Huntington disease, hereditary spastic paraplegia and Friedreich's ataxia. *Biochim Biophys Acta* **1410**:159–170.

Schapira, A.H., J.M. Cooper, D. Dexter, P. Jenner, J.B. Clark, and C.D. Marsden. 1989. Mitochondrial complex I deficiency in Parkinson's disease [letter] [see comments]. *Lancet* **1**:1269.

Schmuck, G., E. Rohrdanz, Q.H. Tran-Thi, R. Kahl, and G. Schluter. 2002. Oxidative stress in rat cortical neurons and astrocytes induced by paraquat *in vitro*. *Neurotox Res* **4**:1–13.

Seaton, T.A., J.M. Cooper, and A.H. Schapira. 1997. Free radical scavengers protect dopaminergic cell lines from apoptosis induced by complex I inhibitors. *Brain Res* **777**:110–118.

Shamoto-Nagai, M., W. Maruyama, Y. Kato, K. Isobe, M. Tanaka, M. Naoi, and T. Osawa. 2003. An inhibitor of mitochondrial complex I, rotenone, inactivates proteasome by oxidative modification and induces aggregation of oxidized proteins in SH-SY5Y cells. *J Neurosci Res* **74**:589–597.

Sherer, T.B., R. Betarbet, and J.T. Greenamyre. 2002a. Environment, mitochondria, and Parkinson disease. *Neuroscientist* **8**:192–197.

Sherer, T.B., R. Betarbet, J.H. Kim, and J.T. Greenamyre. 2003a. Selective microglial activation in the rat rotenone model of Parkinson disease. *Neurosci Lett* **341**:87–90.

Sherer, T.B., R. Betarbet, A.K. Stout, S. Lund, M. Baptista, A.V. Panov, M.R. Cookson, and J.T. Greenamyre. 2002b. An in vitro model of Parkinson's disease: linking mitochondrial impairment to altered alpha-synuclein metabolism and oxidative damage. *J Neurosci* **22**:7006–7015.

Sherer, T.B., R. Betarbet, C.M. Testa, B.B. Seo, J.R. Richardson, J. Kim, G.W. Miller, T. Yagi, A. Yagi-Matsuno, and J.T. Greenamyre. 2003b. Mechanisms of toxicity in rotenone models of Parkinson Disease. *J Neurosci* **23**:10756–10764.

Sherer, T.B., J.H. Kim, R. Betarbet, and J.T. Greenamyre. 2003c. Subcutaneous rotenone exposure causes highly selective dopaminergic degeneration and alpha-synuclein aggregation. *Exp Neurol* **179**:9–16.

Shimizu, K., K. Matsubara, K. Ohtaki, and H. Shiono. 2003. Paraquat leads to dopaminergic neural vulnerability in organotypic midbrain culture. *Neurosci Res* **46**:523–532.

Souza, J.M., B.I. Giasson, Q. Chen, V.M. Lee, and H. Ischiropoulos. 2000. Dityrosine cross-linking promotes formation of stable alpha-synuclein polymers. Implication of nitrative and oxidative stress in the pathogenesis of neurodegenerative synucleinopathies. *J Biol Chem* **275**:18344–18349.

Spillantini, M.G., M.L. Schmidt, V.M. Lee, J.Q. Trojanowski, R. Jakes, and M. Goedert. 1997. Alpha-synuclein in Lewy bodies. *Nature* **388**:839–840.

Tawara, T., T. Fukushima, N. Hojo, A. Isobe, K. Shiwaku, T. Setogawa, and Y. Yamane. 1996. Effects of paraquat on mitochondrial electron transport system and catecholamine contents in rat brain. *Arch Toxicol* **70**:585–589.

Thiffault, C., J.W. Langston, and D.A. Di Monte. 2000. Increased striatal dopamine turnover following acute administration of rotenone to mice. *Brain Res* **885**:283–288.

Thiruchelvam, M., B.J. Brockel, E.K. Richfield, R.B. Baggs, and D.A. Cory-Slechta. 2000a. Potentiated and preferential effects of combined paraquat and maneb on nigrostriatal dopamine systems: environmental risk factors for Parkinson disease? *Brain Res* **873**:225–234.

Thiruchelvam, M., E.K. Richfield, R.B. Baggs, A.W. Tank, and D.A. Cory-Slechta. 2000b. The nigrostriatal dopaminergic system as a preferential target of repeated exposures to combined paraquat and maneb: implications for Parkinson's disease. *J Neurosci* **20**:9207–9214.

Uversky, V.N., J. Li, and A.L. Fink. 2001. Pesticides directly accelerate the rate of alpha-synuclein fibril formation: a possible factor in Parkinson disease. *FEBS Lett* **500**:105–108.

van der Putten, H., K.H. Wiederhold, A. Probst, S. Barbieri, C. Mistl, S. Danner, S. Kauffmann, K. Hofele, W.P. Spooren, M.A. Ruegg, et al. 2000. Neuropathology in mice expressing human alpha-synuclein. *J Neurosci* **20**:6021–6029.

van der Walt, J.M., K.K. Nicodemus, E.R. Martin, W.K. Scott, M.A. Nance, R.L. Watts, J.P. Hubble, J.L. Haines, W.C. Koller, K. Lyons, et al. 2003. Mitochondrial polymorphisms significantly reduce the risk of Parkinson disease. *Am J Hum Genet* **72**:804–811.

Wooten, G.F. 1997. Neurochemistry and neuropharmacology of Parkinson disease. In *Movement Disorders: Neurologic Principles and Practice*. Ed. R.L. Watts and Koller. pp. 153–160. New York: McGraw-Hill,

Wu, D.C., P. Teismann, K. Tieu, M. Vila, V. Jackson-Lewis, H. Ischiropoulos, and S. Przedborski. 2003. NADPH oxidase mediates oxidative stress in the 1-methyl-4-phenyl-1,2,3,6-tetrahydropyridine model of Parkinson disease. *Proc Natl Acad Sci U S A* **100**:6145–6150.

Yang, W., and A.Y. Sun. 1998a. Paraquat-induced free radical reaction in mouse brain microsomes. *Neurochem Res* **23**:47–53.

Yang, W.L., and A.Y. Sun. 1998b. Paraquat-induced cell death in PC12 cells. *Neurochem Res* **23**:1387–1394.

Yoritaka, A., N. Hattori, K. Uchida, M. Tanaka, E.R. Stadtman, and Y. Mizuno. 1996. Immunohistochemical detection of 4-hydroxynonenal protein adducts in Parkinson disease. *Proc Natl Acad Sci U S A* **93**: 2696–2701.

Zhang, Y., J. Gao, K.K. Chung, H. Huang, V.L. Dawson, and T.M. Dawson. 2000. Parkin functions as an E2-dependent ubiquitin- protein ligase and promotes the degradation of the synaptic vesicle-associated protein, CDCrel-1. *Proc Natl Acad Sci U S A* **97**:13354–13359.

CHAPTER

B5

Drosophila Models of Parkinson Disease

LEO J. PALLANCK and ALEXANDER J. WHITWORTH

Our knowledge of the molecular mechanisms of Parkinson disease (PD) has been dramatically advanced by the recent identification of genes underlying relatively rare heritable forms of this disorder (Hardy et al., 2003). These breakthroughs may provide a window into the mechanisms underlying the more common sporadic form of PD. However, our current understanding of the functions of these genes and the mechanisms by which their mutational alteration results in neuronal death is limited. One approach to this problem that has great potential is classical genetic analysis in the fruit fly *Drosophila melanogaster* to identify the genetic pathways leading to pathology in fly models of this disease. This review will describe the features that make *Drosophila* useful in studies of the genes implicated in PD and how these studies have begun to contribute to our understanding of the pathogenesis of this disorder.

I. BACKGROUND

For nearly a century, studies of *Drosophila* genetic and molecular pathways have provided pivotal advances in our understanding of many fundamental biological processes, such as chromosome structure and segregation, regulation of gene expression, and mechanisms of development (Ashburner and Novitski 1976). These studies, together with more recent genome sequencing efforts, have made it clear that gene sequence and gene function are highly conserved between flies and humans (Rubin et al. 2000). This conservation has contributed enormously to our current understanding of human biology and the pathogenesis of particular human diseases. For example, the *Drosophila* counterparts to a number of tumor suppressor and proto-oncogenes (*wingless, Notch,* and *patched*) have provided a wealth of understanding about the pathways involved in cancer. While much of the insight into human disease mechanisms derived from genetic studies of *Drosophila* has been a byproduct of investigations of fundamental biological questions, the increasing appreciation of the usefulness of *Drosophila* to address questions of human pathogenesis has led more recently to overt efforts to model specific human diseases. In particular over the past several years, researchers have invested significant effort in developing *Drosophila* models of neurological diseases, such as Alzheimer's disease, polyglutamine diseases, and Parkinson disease (Muqit and Feany 2002; Shulman et al. 2003). The extensive degree of conservation of neuronal function and development at the cellular level between *Drosophila* and higher vertebrates, coupled with the paucity of treatments for many neurological diseases, makes *Drosophila* an ideal system to advance our understanding of neurological disease mechanisms. Such an advance may ultimately yield preventative treatments for these disorders.

The relatively recent completion and annotation of the genome sequence of *Drosophila melanogaster* (Adams et al. 2000) and the availability of Internet-accessible homology search algorithms make identifying candidate *Drosophila* disease homologs trivial. After identifying a sequence predicted to encode a *Drosophila* homolog of a human gene implicated in disease, researchers can search the EST database for corresponding cDNA sequences to validate the existence of the candidate gene (http://www.fruitfly.org/EST/index.shtml). These gene identification strategies indicate that the *Drosophila* genome encodes homologs of four out of the five genes currently implicated in PD. In particular, the *Drosophila* genome encodes excellent homologs of the *parkin*, *DJ-1*, *UCH-L1*, and *PINK1* genes (table 1). There appears to be only a single *Drosophila* homolog of the *parkin*, *PINK1* and *UCH-L1* genes, but two closely related *DJ-1* homologs exist in *Drosophila*. Only the human *α–synuclein* gene appears to lack a clear *Drosophila* counterpart. However, the dominant, toxic gain-of-function mechanism by which α–synuclein is thought to act in dopamine neuron death validates the use of a transgenic approach using the human *α–synuclein* gene to study α–synuclein pathogenesis in *Drosophila* (see below). The existence of *Drosophila* homologs of four of the five genes implicated in heritable forms of PD implies that the pathways regulated by these genes are likely to be well conserved in *Drosophila*.

II. TECHNIQUES AVAILABLE IN *DROSOPHILA*

Investigators have used both mutational and transgenic approaches to create and study *Drosophila* models of neurological disease. The mutational approach involves creating mutations in *Drosophila* counterparts of human disease genes, whereas the transgenic approach involves introducing and expressing a human disease gene in *Drosophila*. Researchers typically use the former approach when the corresponding human disease results from a loss-of-function mutation in a particular gene, whereas they often use the latter approach when the corresponding human disease appears to result from a dominant toxic gain-of-function mutational mechanism. In this section we describe the methodology involved in the mutational and transgenic approaches.

Numerous techniques can be employed to generate mutations in a particular *Drosophila* gene of interest. Many of the classical methods for recovering mutations in defined genes in *Drosophila* require a predictable phenotype that can be readily identified. However, several methods are now available that allow the recovery of mutations in defined genes irrespective of the mutant phenotype. One particularly powerful approach involves transposon mutagenesis. A number of specifically engineered transposons have been designed that can be used for insertional mutagenesis in *Drosophila*. The Berkeley Drosophila Genome Project is using these transposons in an effort to generate mutations in most *Drosophila* genes as a service to the *Drosophila* research community. Primarily as a result of these efforts, greater than 50% of the predicted *Drosophila* genes are estimated to have associated transposon insertions (Hiesinger and Bellen 2004). For those *Drosophila* genes that do not currently have associated transposon alleles, several methods can be used to selectively recover such alleles following mobilization of a transposon. One method uses plasmid rescue in *E. coli* of genomic sequences flanking *P* element transposon insertions and testing these sequences for hybridization to a cDNA corresponding to the desired target gene (Hamilton et al. 1991). A second method selectively identifies desired *P* element insertions by using PCR primers specific to sequences within the *P* element and target gene (Ballinger and Benzer 1989). Only DNA from flies containing a *P* element insert in or near the gene of interest will be amplified. In this way, hundreds of flies bearing different inserts can be simultaneously screened to identify the rare individual with an appropriate insertion. Although frequencies of *P* element mutagenesis are somewhat locus

TABLE 1 Drosophila Homologs of Genes Implicated in Parkinson Disease

Gene	Mode of inheritance	Mechanism of pathology	*Drosophila* homolog(s)	amino acid identity to human protein
alpha synuclein	autosomal dominant	gain of function	none	N/A
UCH-L1	autosomal dominant	loss of function?	*UCH*	45%
parkin	autosomal recessive	loss of function	*park*	42%
DJ-1	autosomal recessive	loss of function	CG6646	56%
			CG1349	52%
PINK1	autosomal recessive	loss of function	CG4523	43%

dependent, recent estimates provided by the Berkeley *Drosophila* Genome Project indicate that the vast majority of genes in *Drosophila* can serve as targets for *P* element mutagenesis (Spradling et al. 1999), and a large number of examples are now available of the successful use of transposon mutagenesis to selectively inactivate particular genes.

A more recently developed method to target genes for mutagenesis in *Drosophila* involves a homologous recombination methodology similar to that used in making mouse knock-outs (Rong and Golic, 2000). Briefly, in this method a targeting construct is generated that bears an inactivating mutation in the gene of interest and a site for the rare cutting endonuclease *I-Cre*I flanked by target sites for the yeast flp recombinase. Co-expression of *I-Cre*I and flp recombinase in transgenic flies with the engineered targeting construct causes the targeting construct to be excised as a linear extra-chromosomal fragment. That fragment then recombines with the homologous chromosomal locus, possibly through a double strand break repair mechanism. A more recent iteration of gene-targeting, called ends-out targeting (Gong and Golic 2003), significantly simplifies the molecular engineering required to produce the targeting construct and should therefore make this methodology quite attractive to *Drosophila* researchers.

Another approach that is used with increasing frequency in place of traditional genetic analysis in *Drosophila* is RNA interference (RNAi) (Kalidas and Smith 2002). This approach capitalizes on the finding that double-stranded RNA (dsRNA) molecules corresponding in sequence to endogenous transcripts can trigger the degradation of the endogenous transcript. For this approach a transgenic construct bearing an inverted repeat sequence corresponding to the target transcript must be created. Using the GAL4 system (see below), researchers can achieve targeted expression of the dsRNA in any desired tissue simply by conducting the appropriate cross. One reason this approach has become popular is the speed with which researchers can create a transgenic line bearing an RNAi construct relative to more traditional genetic approaches. However, the many studies involving RNAi approaches indicate that this method effects only partial gene inactivation. Thus, a phenotype resulting from RNAi is typically equivalent to a hypomorphic loss-of-function mutation (Andrews et al. 2002). This feature of RNAi can be an advantage or a limitation depending on the context of the experiment and the goals of the experimenter.

One of the most powerful and versatile tools available in *Drosophila* is the ability to generate transgenic constructs that can be used to drive the expression of a chosen gene in a tissue-specific manner by exploiting a yeast transcriptional activation mechanism. The GAL4/UAS system uses the yeast transcriptional activator GAL4 expressed under the temporal and spatial control of endogenous enhancer/promoter elements, to drive the expression of a specific transgene (Brand and Perrimon 1993). The transgene is cloned in a vector containing a minimal promoter coupled with upstream activator sequences (UAS) that are specifically recognized by the GAL4 transcription factor. Upon binding of GAL4 to the UAS sites, expression of the transgene is induced in a tissue-specific manner dependent on the endogenous enhancer/promoter elements controlling GAL4 expression. Many different GAL4 lines are now available that drive expression in a wide variety of tissues (e.g., nervous system, muscle tissue or ubiquitously). This technique has been used with great effect to determine the *in vivo* consequence of misexpression or overexpression of fly genes and has been adapted to study the ectopic expression of human genes and their disease-causing aberrant forms.

The single greatest advantage of using *Drosophila* to model human disease may be the ability to conduct relatively unbiased genetic screens for mutations in other genes that suppress or enhance the phenotypes associated with the disease model. This approach has the potential to identify cellular factors that act in the same or parallel pathways to the disease gene, as well as factors that normally act to antagonize these pathways and maintain cellular balance. In addition, important protective cellular mechanisms may be identified that are induced in response to pathogenic insult. The power of such screening approaches cannot be overstated; human counterparts corresponding to suppressors identified from screens using *Drosophila* define potential targets for therapeutic intervention. It is primarily the feasibility of conducting such high-throughput screens that sets *Drosophila* apart from vertebrate models of disease.

A large number of approaches are available for conducting genetic modifier screens in *Drosophila*. One of the most commonly used approaches involves crossing a collection of 2,400 enhancer *P* (*EP*) element insertions (Rørth 1996) into a disease model background and investigating the effects of these insertions on the disease model phenotypes. The *EP* transposons have been engineered to drive overexpression of sequences flanking the transposon in a GAL4-dependent fashion. Thus, when used in conjunction with a particular GAL4 line, these transposons might suppress or enhance the disease model phenotype as a result of insertional inactivation of the genes they reside in or as a result of overexpression of flanking genes. These potential effects can be easily distinguished in subsequent studies. This modifier screening approach is compatible with a variety of phenotypes and could be used to identify modifiers of behavioral, morphological, or recessive lethal phenotypes. A particularly useful attribute of this screening method is that the insertion location of all of the *EP* lines has been determined and thus modifier genes are readily identified. Use of the *EP* collection in a modifier screening context has proven extremely valuable in studies to identify modifiers of polyglutamine and tau pathology in *Drosophila* (Fernandez-Funez et al. 2000; Shulman and Feany 2003).

III. THE NEUROANATOMY AND FUNCTION OF DOPAMINE NEURONS IN *DROSOPHILA*

An extremely important feature of *Drosophila* that makes it useful for studying mechanisms of PD is its well-characterized and relatively simple dopamine neuron system. All of the *Drosophila* dopamine-producing neurons have been identified, and their development has been traced throughout the fly life cycle of this organism. Thus, investigators can readily identify genetic perturbations affecting the number, morphology, or locations of dopamine neurons in *Drosophila*.

During embryonic and larval brain development, dopamine is expressed in approximately eighty cells. Many of these cells are grouped together into three symmetrical clusters in the two lobes of the brain, with the remaining dopamine neurons distributed singly along the length of the ventral ganglion. These dopamine neurons are retained in the central nervous system of adult flies and are primarily grouped together into six major clusters. These six clusters are arranged symmetrically about the midline with the neuronal cell bodies residing at the periphery of the brain and their axons projecting toward the center (Nassel and Elekes 1992). As shown in Figure 1A, on the anterior side of the brain, there is a small cluster of approximately five dopamine neurons, designated the protocerebral anterior lateral (PAL), and a larger cluster of approximately sixty dopamine neurons with characteristically small cell bodies, designated the protocerebral anterior medial (PAM). Four additional clusters of dopamine neurons are on the posterior side of the brain: two medial clusters, designated the protocerebral posterior medial (PPM) 2 and 3, and two lateral clusters, named the protocerebral posterior lateral (PPL) 1 and 2. The PPM2/3 and PPL2 clusters typically have five to eight neurons while the PPL1 cluster contains approximately twelve neurons (Figure 1B). In addition to these clusters, there are also a small number of dopamine neurons that are not arranged into clusters, such as the protocerebral posterior medial 1 (PPM1), the deutocerebral 1 (D1), and a number of ventral unpaired medial (VUM) neurons.

To date, most studies of dopamine neuron integrity in *Drosophila* models of PD have used antiserum against tyrosine hydroxylase (TH), an enzyme required for dopamine biosynthesis, to image dopamine neurons. However, several different immunocytochemical methods have been utilized to conduct these imaging studies. Most of the studies conducted to date have used thick sections of paraffin-embedded CNS samples to analyze dopamine neuron integrity. More recently, confocal microscopy of whole mount brain samples has been applied to image the CNS dopamine neurons. One potential advantage of the confocal microscopic imaging approach is that it provides more detailed analysis of these neurons in intact brains. This method allows a better visualization of the three-dimensional arrangement of the neurons across the whole brain and might facilitate studies of more subtle aspects of dopamine neuron dysfunction, such as axonal projection and synaptic defects (for example see Figure 1C).

In addition to the spatial distribution of dopamine neurons in *Drosophila*, researchers have also studied the functional effects of dopamine depletion and dopamine neuron perturbation. Genetic or pharmacological depletion of dopamine in *Drosophila* results in a variety of characteristic phenotypes. Mutations affecting the *Dopa decarboxylase* gene result in decreased learning ability, while mutations in the TH-encoding gene *pale* cause a dose-dependent loss of general locomotor ability (Tempel et al., 1984, Pendleton et al. 2002a). Systemically administering chemical inhibitors of TH synthesis, such as 3-iodo-tyrosine, caused developmental delay, decreased fertility, and inhibition of a simple learning paradigm (Neckameyer 1996, 1998). However, it is unclear from these studies whether these phenotypes result from loss of dopamine signaling in the nervous system or from a non-neuronal requirement for dopamine. The *Drosophila pale* gene encodes two alternatively spliced isoforms of TH; one isoform is neuronally expressed while the other is expressed in the developing mesoderm and required for cuticle hardening and pigmentation (Friggi-Grelin 2003b).

To address the specific roles of dopamine neurons in the *Drosophila* nervous system, authors of a recent report used the GAL4/UAS system to express tetanus toxin in TH-expressing neurons to block dopamine neuron signaling (Friggi-Grelin 2003a). Tetanus toxin cleaves the synaptic vesicle protein synaptobrevin, and this cleavage was previously shown to block evoked neurotransmitter release in *Drosophila*. *Drosophila* expressing tetanus toxin in the pattern of TH are viable, display normal locomotion, and have a wild-type appearance. The only phenotype displayed by these flies is a hyperexcitable response to a startle stimulus. Vigorous tapping of vials containing flies expressing tetanus toxin in dopamine neurons causes the flies to fall and whirl erratically, failing to immediately right themselves. This result suggests that one of the functions of dopamine signaling in the *Drosophila* nervous system is to negatively control excitability behavior. This phenotype provides a useful reference point for the behavioral analysis of *Drosophila* models of PD.

IV. *DROSOPHILA* MODELS OF PARKINSON DISEASE

The first *Drosophila* model of Parkinson disease was created by Mel Feany and Welcome Bender using a transgenic approach to express human α–synuclein in the

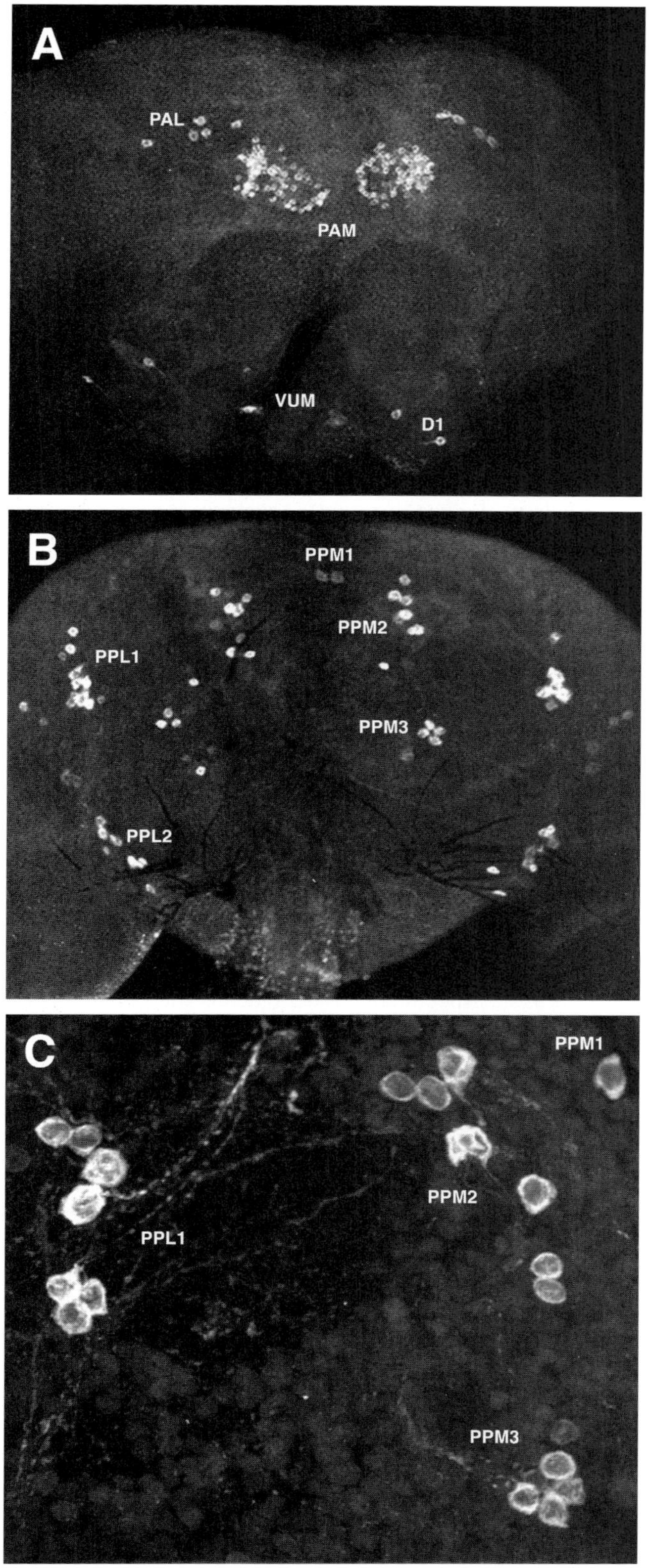

FIGURE 1 Tyrosine hydroxylase staining showing the distribution of dopamine neurons in the adult brain. (A) The anterior side contains a large group of dopamine neurons (PAM), a small cluster (PAL), and several single neurons (VUM and D1). (B) The posterior side consists of several clusters symmetrically arranged either medially (PPM1/2/3) or laterally (PPL1/2). (C) A projected image of a z-series stack of images of the posterior clusters showing punctate tyrosine hydroxylase staining in the axonal projections.

Drosophila nervous system (Feany and Bender 2000). Transgenic expression of wild-type and mutationally altered forms of human α–synuclein (corresponding to the A30P and A53T mutations responsible for heritable forms of PD in humans) throughout the *Drosophila* nervous system caused an age-dependent loss of TH-staining of a subset of dopamine neurons in paraffin sections of *Drosophila* CNS samples. To investigate whether the loss of TH staining represents loss of dopamine neurons and not simply loss of TH expression, investigators conducted additional experiments with transgenic lines co-expressing α–synuclein and β–galactosidase. Results of these experiments revealed that β–galactosidase and α–synuclein staining were also absent in a subset of dopamine neurons from aged flies relative to controls, leading the authors to conclude that α–synuclein expression induces the death of a subset of the *Drosophila* dopamine neurons in the CNS. The number of serotonergic neurons and gross brain morphology in α–synuclein expressing flies were reportedly unaffected, indicating that the toxic effects of α–synuclein expression are relatively specific to dopamine neurons in the CNS. However, expression of α–synuclein in the *Drosophila* compound eye was found to induce a retinal degeneration phenotype, demonstrating that α–synuclein toxicity is not entirely restricted to dopamine neurons. Although both wild-type and mutationally altered forms of α–synuclein induced dopamine neuron loss, it was unclear from this study whether the mutationally altered forms of α–synuclein produced differential toxicity relative to wild type.

Pan-neuronal expression of α–synuclein in the *Drosophila* CNS also produced in neuronal protein aggregates closely resembling the size, morphology, and composition of the Lewy bodies seen in humans suffering from idiopathic PD, and an accompanying locomotor defect. While young α–synuclein expressing flies display a normal geotactic response, quickly climbing to the top of a vial after being tapped down, climbing ability attenuates significantly in older α–synuclein expressing flies. Climbing ability also decays in aged wild-type flies, but the rate of decay was found to be significantly accelerated in all of the α–synuclein expressing flies tested, particularly the A30P mutational derivative of α–synuclein. The appearance of this locomotor defect paralleled the loss of dopamine neurons and the onset of aggregate formation, suggesting a mechanistic connection between aggregate formation, neuron loss, and locomotor dysfunction. This initial work provided the foundation for all of the subsequent studies of α–synuclein pathogenesis described below.

Perhaps the most significant feature of the α–synuclein transgenic model of PD is its amenability to genetic screens for suppressors and enhancers of the retinal degeneration phenotype to gain insight into α–synuclein pathogenesis. While these screens are undoubtedly in progress in a number of laboratories, such screens require considerable time and effort, and all of the current studies that have made use of the α–synuclein transgenic fly model of PD have explored the effects of candidate modifiers of α–synuclein toxicity. One of the first such studies explored the possible suppressive effects of chaperone protein expression on dopamine neuron loss in α–synuclein expressing flies (Auluck et al. 2002). These studies were prompted by previous work showing that chaperone expression was able to suppress the deleterious effects of transgenic polyglutamine protein expression in *Drosophila*. The authors of this study showed that the loss of TH–positive neurons resulting from α–synuclein expression in the nervous system was abrogated by co-overxpression of HSP70. Moreover, co-expression of a dominant-negative form of HSP70 enhanced the loss of TH staining resulting from α–synuclein expression. Interestingly, pan-neuronal expression of the dominant-negative form of HSP70 in wild-type flies completely lacking α–synuclein also resulted in loss of TH-positive neurons. Consistent with these observations, feeding α–synuclein transgenic flies geldanamycin, which induces HSP70 expression, had a suppressive effect on dopamine neuron loss (Auluck and Bonini 2002).

These results suggest several possible models by which HSP70 exerts its effect. HSP70 may act directly on α–synuclein to prevent it from assuming a toxic conformation. Consistent with this model, the authors of this study also showed that Lewy bodies from human postmortem tissue stain positively for the presence of molecular chaperones. However, HSP70 overexpression did not detectably influence the appearance of Lewy body-like aggregates, indicating that HSP70 has a subtle effect on α–synuclein conformation or acts primarily on soluble oligomeric forms of α–synuclein. An alternative model consistent with the effect of reduced HSP70 activity on dopamine neuron integrity in the complete absence of α–synuclein is that α–synuclein toxicity ensues from sequestering HSP70 into an inactive form. Finally, these findings are also consistent with a general effect of HSP70 on dopamine neuron viability that is independent of any interaction between HSP70 and α–synuclein. Further experiments will be required to resolve these matters.

Using the transgenic α–synuclein fly model investigators have also explored a possible modifying role of the parkin ubiquitin protein ligase in α–synuclein pathogenesis. These experiments were premised on work showing that vertebrate parkin can recognize and ubiquitinate an unusual *O*-glycosylated form of α–synuclein, suggesting that α–synuclein is a pathogenic substrate of parkin. To investigate this possibility, Yang et al. (2003) co-expressed α–synuclein and human parkin in *Drosophila* and found that the dopamine neuron death triggered by ectopic expression of human α–synuclein protein could be mitigated by parkin. Co-overexpression of the green fluorescent protein had no effect on α–synuclein mediated dopamine neuron death, indicating that parkin is specifically required to suppress dopamine neuron death. A more recent related study by Haywood and Staveley (2004) showed that co-expression of *Drosophila* parkin and human α–synuclein in dopamine and serotonergic neurons suppressed the locomotor defect associated with expression of α–synuclein alone. Further, these authors showed that expression of *Drosophila* parkin rescues the α–synuclein induced retinal degeneration phenotype. Together, these studies show that increased expression of both human and *Drosophila* parkin suppresses α–synuclein toxicity *in vivo*.

To investigate the mechanism by which parkin mediates attenuation of α–synuclein toxicity, Yang et al. (2003) performed immunocytochemical studies on brain sections from flies expressing α–synuclein alone or in combination with human parkin. Results of this analysis revealed a reduction in the abundance of α–synuclein positive grain-like structures and ubiquitin-positive Lewy body-like neurites observed in flies expressing α–synuclein alone. By contrast, western blot analysis revealed no difference in the total abundance of α–synuclein protein between flies co-expressing human parkin and α–synuclein and in flies expressing α–synuclein alone. This observation suggests that parkin acts specifically to degrade aberrant α–synuclein deposits. However, this finding appears contradictory to the observation that at least most of the cases of Parkinson disease resulting from loss of parkin function do not display aggregates of α–synuclein-positive Lewy bodies. If parkin acts to prevent the formation of α–synuclein positive inclusions, then we should expect to see Lewy bodies in great abundance in humans with PD resulting from loss of parkin function.

One possible model that would explain these discordant findings is that parkin may be involved in both forming and breaking down Lewy body inclusions. Perhaps low levels of parkin activity are sufficient to support Lewy body inclusions, whereas higher levels of parkin activity lead to rapid destruction of aberrant α–synuclein species. An alternative model suggests that overexpression of human parkin in *Drosophila* may activate endogenous *Drosophila* stress pathways that direct degradation or disassembly of protein aggregates. Further work will be required to distinguish between these models.

Another useful feature of Drosophila models of PD is the ability to use these models in genomic studies to identify pathways involved in pathogenesis. A recent genomic study of the α–synuclein transgenic fly model of PD identified fifty-one *Drosophila* transcripts that displayed an altered abundance relative to control flies (Scherzer et al. 2003). Importantly, these transcripts were unaffected in transgenic flies expressing the neurodegeneration-inducing tau protein, indicating that the abundance of these fifty-one transcripts are specifically altered in response to α–synuclein expression. The fifty-one transcripts that display altered abundance in the α–synuclein transgenic flies encode proteins involved in lipid metabolism, energy production, and membrane transport, potentially implicating these pathways in α–synuclein pathogenesis. Interestingly, a recent study of α–synuclein pathogenesis in yeast identified lipid metabolism and vesicle transport components as a major category of genetic modifiers of α–synuclein toxicity (Willingham et al. 2003). Together, these two studies suggest an evolutionarily conserved pathway of PD pathogenesis involving lipid metabolic and vesicle trafficking defects. Additional work will be required to validate the functional significance of these pathways to dopamine neuron degeneration.

While the pioneering work of Feany and Bender convincingly established the relevance of the *Drosophila* system to studies of PD pathogenesis, one feature of the α–synuclein transgenic fly model of PD remains unclear. That feature is the relationship of the geotactic climbing defect to dopamine neuron loss. In the original report by Feany and Bender (2000), this phenotype was associated with pan-neuronal expression of α–synuclein, thus leaving open the possibility that the phenotype derives from dysfunction of any one of a number of neuron types. A more recent study confirmed the climbing defect in α–synuclein expressing flies using a GAL4 driver that is expressed in dopamine and serotonergic neurons (Haywood and Staveley 2004), thus narrowing the range of neuron types that could underlie this phenomenon.

Several studies, however, raise questions about the relevance of the integrity of dopamine neurons to the locomotor phenotype, and indeed the relevance of α–synuclein to this phenotype. For instance, a subsequent study using the same α–synuclein transgenic lines created in the original study of Feany and Bender recapitulated the geotactic climbing defect in the complete absence of a GAL4 driver (Pendleton et al. 2002b). Moreover, these authors showed that the climbing defect could be rescued by dietary supplementation of L-dopa. While this result is consistent with dopamine neuron dysfunction in the α–synuclein transgenic lines, it is unclear how α–synuclein mediates dopamine neuron loss in the absence of a GAL4 driver. Another study using the same α–synuclein transgenic lines failed to detect an age-related geotactic climbing defect upon pan-neuronal expression of α–synuclein (Auluck et al. 2002). While these discordant results cannot be completely reconciled, the recent finding that dopaminergic neuron dysfunction results in a hyperexcitable phenotype upon vigorous mechanical disturbance suggests that technical differences in how climbing assays are performed may partially explain the lack of correspondence in these studies. Climbing studies employing vigorous rapping of vials might induce a startle response that would manifest as a climbing defect in response to DA neuron loss, whereas studies using a more mild approach might fail to induce the startle response.

Another transgenic model of PD was created in *Drosophila* by expressing the putative human G-protein coupled receptor Pael-R in the *Drosophila* nervous system (Yang et al. 2003). Pael-R was previously identified as a vertebrate binding partner of parkin and is an *in vitro* substrate of vertebrate parkin that accumulates in an insoluble fraction when overexpressed in cell lines (Imai et al. 2001). Pan-neuronal expression of Pael-R in *Drosophila* reduces the number of neurons that stain positively for TH without accompanying overt degeneration of other neuronal cell types. Pael-R mediated loss of TH staining was attenuated by co-expression of human parkin and exacerbated by inhibiting the activity of endogenous fly parkin using RNA interference. In contrast to the apparent selectivity of parkin towards α–synuclein inclusions, co-expression of parkin with Pael-R resulted in a net reduction of Pael-R levels, suggesting that parkin acts to degrade all forms of Pael-R or that all of the Pael-R expressed in *Drosophila* is in an aberrant conformation recognized by parkin.

While the above results are suggestive, a number of questions remain unexplained. For example, is Pael-R specifically toxic to dopamine neurons or would dopamine neuron toxicity ensue from the overexpression of any one of a number of putative vertebrate G-protein coupled receptors? Another issue that was not addressed was whether the apparent cell death triggered by Pael-R expression in *Drosophila* involves the unfolded stress pathway (as suggested in the original study linking Pael-R to parkin) or activation of an endogenous G-protein coupled receptor pathway. Given the genetic tools available in *Drosophila*, these matters should be relatively straightforward to address.

While researchers believe the α–synuclein mutations responsible for PD pathogenesis are dominant toxic gain-of-function mutations, four of the five known genes associated with heritable forms of PD appear to involve loss-of-function mutations. Thus, the creation of *Drosophila* models of these loss-of-function forms of PD will likely require the use of mutational approaches to perturb the functions of *Drosophila* homologs of these genes. The recent mutational analysis of the *Drosophila parkin* gene represents an example of this approach.

As mentioned above, the *Drosophila parkin* gene encodes a protein with a high degree of sequence similarity to the human parkin protein. Moreover, the characteristic domain structure of human parkin is uniquely conserved in

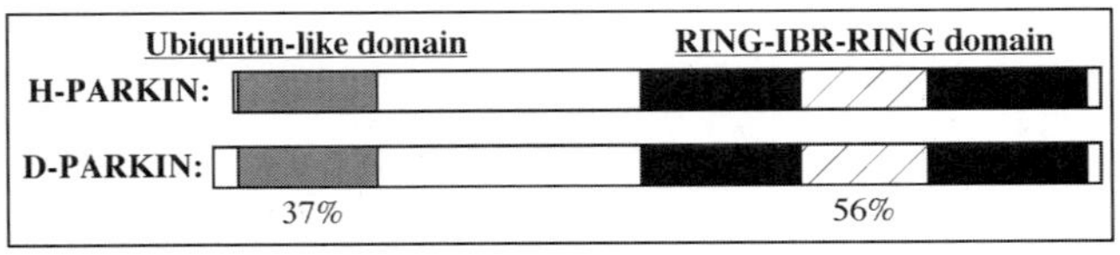

FIGURE 2 The domain organization of human and *Drosophila* parkin is conserved. Schematic depiction of conserved domains in human parkin (H-PARKIN) and *Drosophila* parkin (D-PARKIN). Differentially shaded boxes correspond to N-terminal ubiquitin-like, RING and IBR domains of parkin. Percentages refer to amino acid identities within the ubiquitin-like and RING-IBR-RING domains, respectively.

the *Drosophila* parkin ortholog (Figure 2). To explore the biological role of *parkin*, we and others created a collection of *parkin* mutations using a *P* element mutagenesis strategy (Greene et al. 2003; Pesah et al. 2004). This work resulted in the recovery of *P* element transposon insertions immediately flanking *parkin*, as well as deletions that completely remove *parkin*. Further, missense and nonsense alleles of the *parkin* gene were recovered from a noncomplementation screen of the parkin deletion mutations (Greene et al. 2003).

Flies completely lacking the *parkin* gene are semi-viable and display significantly shortened life span and partial pupal lethality. *Drosophila parkin* mutants do not appear to display an obvious loss of dopaminergic neurons in the CNS, possibly reflecting the short life span, the lack of evolutionary conservation of pathogenic parkin substrates in *Drosophila* dopamine neurons (e.g., Pael-R, α–synuclein), or technical limitations in the methodology used to document dopamine neuron integrity in previously published work. By contrast, *parkin* mutants exhibit dramatic and widespread apoptotic degeneration of flight muscle tissue and male sterility owing to a defect in spermatid development. Ultrastructural analysis of flight muscle and spermatids from *Drosophila parkin* mutants demonstrated a severe disruption of mitochondrial integrity in both tissue types. Moreover, mitochondrial pathology appears to be the earliest detectable phenotype in *Drosophila parkin* mutants and clearly precedes the onset of apoptosis in the flight muscle by at least several days (Greene et al. 2003).

In addition to the muscle and germline defects, a recent report indicates that *parkin* mutants also display decreased mass with respect to wild-type flies and a corresponding decrease in the size of at least some cells in the mutants (Pesah et al. 2004). The origin of decreased mass and cell size will require further investigation, although recent work implicating parkin in cyclin E turnover and tumorigenesis leads the authors to speculate that the phenotypes may indicate cell cycle dysfunction.

The reason remains unclear why the primary cell types affected by loss of parkin function differ in humans and *Drosophila*. However, phenotypic differences resulting from mutations in orthologous genes in different species often belie significant underlying molecular pathway conservation. Indeed, increasing evidence suggests that the mechanisms that cause flight muscle degeneration and germline dysfunction in *Drosophila parkin* mutants may be similar to the mechanisms that cause dopamine neuron loss in humans. The fact that mitochondrial pathology is a major feature of both muscle degeneration and spermatid individualization failure in *Drosophila parkin* mutants suggests a role for parkin in mitochondrial integrity. Previous work strongly supports the involvement of mitochondrial dysfunction in PD pathogenesis and recent studies of the vertebrate parkin protein suggest a role for parkin in mitochondrial integrity. For example, overexpression of vertebrate parkin was found to protect PC12 cells from ceramide-mediated cell death by delaying mitochondrial swelling and cytochrome *c* release (Darios et al. 2003). More recently, studies of a mouse *parkin* knock-out model have established that the knockouts display diminished mitochondrial function and reduced abundance of particular mitochondrial proteins (Palacino et al. 2004). Perhaps most importantly, a recent study of leukocytes from human parkin patients revealed a dramatic reduction mitochondrial complex I activity relative to age-matched controls (Muftuoglu et al. 2004). Although the mechanism by which parkin prevents mitochondrial dysfunction is currently unknown the finding that parkin distributes with mitochondrial-containing subcellular fractions in vertebrates (Darios et al. 2003) and flies (our data, not show raises the possibility of a direct effect of parkin on mitochondrial function.

Another feature that may connect flight muscle degeneration in *Drosophila* parkin mutants and dopamine neuron loss in humans is the potentially unique sensitivity of these cell types to oxidative stress. A significant body of literature supports the involvement of oxidative stress pathway dysfunction in Parkinson disease (Jenner 2003). Likewise, the exquisitely high metabolic demand of insect flight muscle may make this cell type particularly vulnerable to oxidative stress. In support of this hypothesis, *Drosophila* parkin mutants were recently found to be significantly more sensitive to the free radical generator paraquat (Pesah et al. 2004).

Our studies of parkin mutants are consistent with this observation but also imply that parkin mutants are sensitive to a wide range of chemical agents, including mercaptoethanol, dithiothreitol, rotenone, and a variety of other compounds, suggesting that parkin may be involved in the response to a wide range of cellular stresses. Nevertheless, oxidative stress resulting from loss of parkin function may be the primary factor triggering dopamine neuron loss in humans and flight muscle degeneration in flies. Important future goals will be to determine the *Drosophila* parkin substrate(s) and the pathways regulated by these substrates that are responsible for flight muscle and germline pathology and to evaluate the relevance of these factors to dopamine neuron loss in humans. The genetic tools available in *Drosophila*, coupled with emerging proteomic methodology that can help identify *Drosophila* parkin substrates, should lead to a rapid delineation of these pathways.

V. SUMMARY

The *Drosophila* system provides a unique opportunity to evaluate the functions of genes implicated in Parkinson disease and to identify mechanisms relevant to this disorder in a relatively unbiased fashion. While significant progress has already been made, PD modeling in *Drosophila* is still relatively new and the reagents and methodologies for conducting these studies are still in their infancy. There are currently *Drosophila* homologs of three genes identified from linkage studies of PD patients for which we await a description of the mutant phenotype. Given the pace of identification of genes responsible for heritable forms of PD and the number of genetic loci that have thus far been identified, there will clearly be much to keep us busy in the coming years.

References

Adams, M.D., S.E. Celniker, R.A. Holt, C.A. Evans, J.D. Gocayne, P.G. Amanatides, S.E. Scherer, et al. 2000. The genome sequence of Drosophila melanogaster. *Science* **287**:2185–2195.

Ashburner, M., and E. Novitski. 1976. *The Genetics and Biology of Drosophila*. London: Academic Press.

Auluck, P.K., and N.M. Bonini. 2002. Pharmacological prevention of Parkinson disease in Drosophila. *Nat Med* **8**:1185–1186.

Auluck, P.K., H.Y. Chan, J.Q. Trojanowski, V.M. Lee, and N.M. Bonini. 2002. Chaperone suppression of alpha-synuclein toxicity in a *Drosophila* model for Parkinson's disease. *Science* **295**:865–868.

Ballinger, D.G., and S. Benzer. 1989. Targeted gene mutations in *Drosophila. Proc Natl Acad Sci U S A* **86**:9402–9406.

Brand, A.H., and N. Perrimon. 1993. Targeted gene expression as a means of altering cell fates and generating dominant phenotypes. *Development* **118**:401–415.

Darios, F., O. Corti, C.B. Lucking, C. Hampe, M.P. Muriel, N. Abbas, W.J. Gu, et al. 2003. Parkin prevents mitochondrial swelling and cytochrome c release in mitochondria-dependent cell death. *Hum Mol Genet* **12**: 517–526.

Feany, M.B., and W.W. Bender. 2000. A *Drosophila* model of Parkinson's disease. *Nature* **404**:394–398.

Fernandez-Funez, P., M.L. Nino-Rosales, B. de Gouyon, W.C. She, J.M. Luchak, P. Martinez, E. Turiegano, et al. 2000. Identification of genes that modify ataxin-1-induced neurodegeneration. *Nature* **408**:101–106.

Friggi-Grelin, F., H. Coulom, M. Meller, D. Gomez, J. Hirsh, and S. Birman. 2003a. Targeted gene expression in Drosophila dopaminergic cells using regulatory sequences from tyrosine hydroxylase. *J Neurobiol* **54**:618–627.

Friggi-Grelin, F., M. Iche, and S. Birman. 2003b. Tissue-specific developmental requirements of Drosophila tyrosine hydroxylase isoforms. *Genesis* **35**:175–184.

Gong, W.J., and K.G. Golic. 2003. Ends-out, or replacement, gene targeting in Drosophila. *Proc Natl Acad Sci U S A* **100**:2556–2561.

Greene, J.C., A.J. Whitworth, I. Kuo, L.A. Andrews, M.B. Feany, and L.J. Pallanck. 2003. Mitochondrial pathology and apoptotic muscle degeneration in *Drosophila* parkin mutants. *Proc Natl Acad Sci U S A* **100**: 4078–4083.

Hamilton, B.A., M.J. Palazzolo, J.H. Chang, K. VijayRaghavan, C.A. Mayeda, M.A. Whitney, and E.M. Meyerowitz. 1991. Large scale screen for transposon insertions into cloned genes. *Proc Natl Acad Sci U S A* **88**:2731–2735.

Hardy, J., M.R. Cookson, and A. Singleton. 2003. Genes and parkinsonism. *Lancet Neurol* **2**:221–228.

Haywood, A.F., and B.E. Staveley. 2004. Parkin counteracts symptoms in a *Drosophila* model of Parkinson's disease. *BMC Neurosci* **5**:14.

Hiesinger, P.R., and H.J. Bellen. 2004. Flying in the face of total disruption. *Nat Genet* **36**:211–212.

Imai, Y., M. Soda, H. Inoue, N. Hattori, Y. Mizuno, and R. Takahashi. 2001. An unfolded putative transmembrane polypeptide, which can lead to endoplasmic reticulum stress, is a substrate of Parkin. *Cell* **105**: 891–902.

Jenner, P. 2003. Oxidative stress in Parkinson's disease. *Ann Neurol* 53 Suppl 3:S26–36; discussion S36–28.

Kalidas, S., and D.P. Smith. 2002. Novel genomic cDNA hybrids produce effective RNA interference in adult Drosophila. *Neuron* **33**:177–184.

Muftuoglu, M., B. Elibol, O. Dalmizrak, A. Ercan, G. Kulaksiz, H. Ogus, T. Dalkara, and N. Ozer. 2004. Mitochondrial complex I and IV activities in leukocytes from patients with parkin mutations. *Mov Disord* **19**:544–548.

Muqit, M.M., and M.B. Feany. 2002. Modelling neurodegenerative diseases in *Drosophila*: a fruitful approach? *Nat Rev Neurosci* **3**: 237–243.

Nassel D.R., and K. Elekes. 1992. Aminergic neurons in the brain of blowflies and Drosophila: dopamine- and tyrosine hydroxylase-immunoreactive neurons and their relationship with putative histaminergic neurons. *Cell Tissue Res* **267**:147–167.

Neckameyer, W.S. 1996. Multiple roles for dopamine in Drosophila development. *Dev Biol* **176**:209–219.

Neckameyer, W.S. 1998. Dopamine and mushroom bodies in Drosophila: experience-dependent and -independent aspects of sexual behavior. *Learn Mem* **5**:157–165.

Palacino, J.J., D. Sagi, M.S. Goldberg, S. Krauss, C. Motz, M. Wacker, J. Klose, and J. Shen. 2004. Mitochondrial dysfunction and oxidative damage in parkin-deficient mice. *J Biol Chem* **279**:18614–18622.

Pendleton, R.G., F. Parvez, M. Sayed, and R. Hillman. 2002. Effects of pharmacological agents upon a transgenic model of Parkinson's disease in *Drosophila* melanogaster. *J Pharmacol Exp Ther* **300**:91–96.

Pendleton, R.G., A. Rasheed, T. Sardina, T. Tully, and R. Hillman. 2002a. Effects of tyrosine hydroxylase mutants on locomotor activity in Drosophila: a study in functional genomics. *Behav Genet* **32**:89–94.

Pesah, Y., T. Pham, H. Burgess, B. Middlebrooks, P. Verstreken, Y. Zhou, M. Harding, H. Bellen, and G. Mardon. 2004. Drosophila parkin mutants have decreased mass and cell size and increased sensitivity to oxygen radical stress. *Development* **131**:2183–2194.

Rong, Y.S., and K.G. Golic. 2000. Gene targeting by homologous recombination in *Drosophila. Science* **288**:2013–2018.

Rorth, P. 1996. A modular misexpression screen in *Drosophila* detecting tissue-specific phenotypes. *Proc Natl Acad Sci U S A* **93**:12418–12422.

Rubin, G.M., M.D. Yandell, J.R. Wortman, G.L. Gabor Miklos, C.R. Nelson, I.K. Hariharan, M. Fortini, et al. 2000. Comparative genomics of the eukaryotes. *Science* **287**:2204–2215.

Scherzer, C.R., R.V. Jensen, S.R. Gullans, and M.B. Feany. 2003. Gene expression changes presage neurodegeneration in a *Drosophila* model of Parkinson's disease. *Hum Mol Genet* **12**:2457–2466.

Shulman, J.M., and M.B. Feany. 2003. Genetic modifiers of tauopathy in Drosophila. *Genetics* **165**:1233–1242.

Shulman, J.M., L.M. Shulman, W.J. Weiner, and M.B. Feany. 2003. From fruit fly to bedside: translating lessons from Drosophila models of neurodegenerative disease. *Curr Opin Neurol* **16**:443–449.

Spradling, A.C., D. Stern, A. Beaton, E.J. Rhem, T. Laverty, N. Mozden, S. Misra, and G.M. Rubin. 1999. The Berkeley Drosophila Genome Project gene disruption project: single P-element insertions mutating 25% of vital Drosophila genes. *Genetics* **153**:135–177.

Tempel, B.L., M.S. Livingstone, and W.G. Quinn. 1984. Mutations in the dopa decarboxylase gene affect learning in Drosophila. *Proc Natl Acad Sci U S A* **81**:3577–3581.

Willingham, S., T.F. Outeiro, M.J. DeVit, S.L. Lindquist, and P.J. Muchowski. 2003. Yeast genes that enhance the toxicity of a mutant huntingtin fragment or alpha-synuclein. *Science* **302**:1769–1772.

Yang, Y., I. Nishimura, Y. Imai, R. Takahashi, and B. Lu. 2003. Parkin suppresses dopaminergic neuron-selective neurotoxicity induced by Pael-R in Drosophila. *Neuron* **37**:911–924.

CHAPTER

B6

Phenotypical Characterization of Genetic Mouse Models of Parkinson Disease

SHEILA M. FLEMING and MARIE-FRANÇOISE CHESSELET

Parkinson disease (PD) is a debilitating disease primarily characterized by the loss of dopaminergic (DA) neurons in the substantia nigra and the development of Lewy body inclusions. Patients suffer from sensorimotor impairments, including bradykinesia, tremor, and rigidity that worsen over time. Mutations in the genes encoding α-synuclein, parkin, DJ-1, and UCHL1, can cause familial forms of PD (Bonifati et al. 2003; Kitada et al. 1998; Kruger et al. 1998; Leroy et al. 1998; Polymeropoulos et al. 1997; Singleton et al. 2003; Wintermeyer et al. 2000). Although familial PD is rare, these findings provide a new approach for the study of PD and mark the beginning of a whole new generation of animal models of PD.

Investigators need a careful phenotypical characterization to make the most use of these models. The hope for genetic mouse models of PD is that they will recapitulate the early and late stages of the disease, anatomically and behaviorally, provide insights into the mechanisms causing degeneration, and contribute to developing treatments that prevent or slow disease progression. In this chapter, we describe several new sensorimotor tests that are sensitive to subtle and progressive alterations in the nigrostriatal dopamine system and are abnormal in genetic mouse models of PD. A characterization of a behavioral profile in these mice makes the tests useful for determining optimal time points for molecular studies and for the preclinical testing of therapeutic interventions.

I. OVERVIEW OF TRANSGENIC MOUSE MODELS OF PARKINSON DISEASE

A. α-Synuclein Mice

The presynaptic protein α-synuclein is linked to both familial and sporadic PD. α-synuclein is a major component of Lewy bodies, the pathological hallmark of idiopathic PD, and researchers have found specific mutations in α-synuclein that cause familial PD (Kruger et al. 1998; Polymeropoulos et al. 1997; Spillantini et al. 1997). Furthermore, increased levels of normal α-synuclein due to gene duplication also lead to early-onset PD in affected families (Singleton et al. 2003).

Transgenic mice overexpressing wild-type or mutant α-synuclein show varying degrees of pathological accumulation of α-synuclein within the brain depending on the promoter used. The first transgenic α-synuclein mice overexpressed the human wild-type α-synuclein under the PDGFβ promoter (Masliah et al. 2000). These mice have increased α-synuclein expression throughout the brain and show α-synuclein inclusions in the neocortex, hippocampus, olfactory bulb, and substantia nigra. At twelve months of age these mice have significantly reduced tyrosine hydroxylase (TH) activity and striatal DA content and display motor impairments on the rotarod. Transgenic mice overexpressing human wildtype and α-synuclein under the Thy-1 promoter have expression levels throughout the brain that are tenfold higher than human levels (Rockenstein et al. 2002). These mice have extensive accumulation of human wildtype and α-synuclein in the neocortex, hippocampus, thalamus, and substantia nigra with no abnormal-synuclein accumulation in the spinal cord, neuromuscular junction, or glial cells (Rockenstein et al. 2002).

In contrast, transgenic mice with the human A53T mutation controlled by the Thy 1 promoter have α-synuclein expression throughout most of the brain and spinal cord with the exception of the substantia nigra (van der Putten et al. 2000). These mice show degeneration in spinal roots and neuromuscular junctions and have α-synuclein inclusions in the spinal cord and brainstem. Behaviorally, they display rotarod deficits as early as forty days of age.

Similarly, transgenic mice with the A30P mutation under the Thy 1 promoter have expression throughout the brain and an abnormal accumulation of α-synuclein in the cortex, hippocampus, cerebellum, substantia nigra, and striatum (Kahle et al. 2000). No overt behavioral impairments were observed in these mice. Under the mouse prion promoter, A53T, α-synuclein expression occurs throughout the brain and spinal cord and inclusions are found in the brainstem, cerebellum, and caudate putamen (Giasson et al. 2002). These mice have a severe motor phenotype consisting of decreased movement, weight loss, hindlimb paralysis, and an inability to feed that eventually leads to death.

Transgenic mice with the A30P mutation under the mouse prion promoter show α-synuclein expression throughout the brainstem and spinal cord and abnormal accumulation of insoluble α-synuclein in midbrain, brainstem, and cerebellum (Lee et al. 2002). These mice, too, have a severe progressive motor phenotype that results in death. Under the control of the TH promoter, overexpression of the wild-type or mutated forms of α-synuclein caused α-synuclein expression in catecholaminergic cells without loss of TH positive neurons in the substantia nigra or striatal projections, and no detectable behavioral impairments (Matsuoka et al. 2001; Rathke-Hartlieb et al. 2001). However, in doubly-mutated transgenic mice (both A30P and A53T mutations) under the TH promoter, striatal dopamine was reduced by sixteen months of age and amphetamine induced locomotor activity and motor coordination were impaired (Richfield et al. 2002). Although none of the transgenic mice completely recapitulates the features of human PD, some of the models do have nigrostriatal DA alterations consistent with PD.

B. Parkin Knock-Out Mice

Parkin is an E3 ubiquitin ligase; mutations that cause a loss of parkin function are associated with early onset autosomal recessive PD (Kitada et al. 1998; Lucking et al. 2000; Periquet et al. 2003). Exon 3 deletion in parkin eliminates the parkin protein. In mice expressing this mutation (Goldberg et al. 2003; Itier et al. 2003) no overt loss of TH positive neurons occurs in the substantia nigra or their projections to the striatum, but subtler nigrostriatal DA alterations were uncovered. These parkin "knock-out" mice have increased extracellular striatal DA, reduced synaptic excitability in striatal medium spiny neurons, and sensorimotor impairments (Goldberg et al. 2003). Similarly, in a separate study, another line of mice with a similar mutation had inhibited amphetamine-induced DA release, inhibited glutamate transmission, reduced DA transporter protein, and motor and cognitive deficits (Itier et al. 2003). Despite the lack of accumulation of parkin substrates such as CDCrel-1, synphilin-1, or α-synuclein in parkin knock-out mice, their DA phenotype makes them useful in the study of PD.

Although the DA phenotypes of these genetic mouse models of PD are not as profound as some of the toxin models, they may provide insight into the early stages of the disease. In PD, there is a presymptomatic phase where patients experience more subtle sensorimotor abnormalities that are difficult to detect until the severity of the disease increases (Di Paola and Uitti 1996). Animals with known genetic mutations associated with PD can be thoroughly assessed behaviorally and anatomically at various ages to uncover potential mechanisms that may ultimately contribute to DA cell death. However, this brief overview of existing genetic mouse models of PD underscores the fact that, although a few models have profound behavioral anomalies likely related to PD (Masliah et al. 2000; Richfield et al. 2002), the majority of mice do not show anomalies in traditional tests such as open field, locomotor activity, or rotarod, or when these are abnormal, the anomalies appear late in life (Masliah et al. 2000; Richfield et al. 2002). This problem seriously limits the usefulness of the mice for preclinical drug testing. A battery of more sensitive sensorimotor tests is clearly necessary to accurately assess the behavior of these mice.

II. SENSORIMOTOR TESTS FOR DOPAMINE DEFICITS

Excellent non-drug-induced behavioral measures exist for the unilateral 6-hydroxydopamine (6-OHDA) rat model of PD. These measures include tests for limb-use asymmetry, movement initiation, somatosensory neglect, and reaching abilities, among others (Schallert et al. 1982, 1983,

1992; Schallert and Tillerson 2000; Whishaw et al. 1986). The tests discern varying degrees of nigrostriatal DA neuron loss and are used extensively to evaluate the efficacy of various types of transplants and viral vectors (Connor et al. 1999, 2001; Kozlowski et al. 2000; Luo et al. 2002; Mignon et al. 2003; Yang et al. 2002). As in the battery of tests used in rats, rating scales similar to those that assess patients with PD are frequently used in nonhuman primate models of PD (Imbert et al. 2000). With the development of new genetic mouse models of PD, sensitive and reliable sensorimotor tests are needed to accurately assess the function of mice with bilateral deficits.

The most common tests used in mice include activity in the open field and the rotarod test for coordination (for review see Sedelis et al. 2001). Although both of these tests are automated, relatively easy to use, and provide information on sensorimotor function, they often lack the sensitivity needed to detect subtle alterations in the nigrostriatal DA system. For example, parkin-deficient mice with subtle alterations in DA function do not display impairments on the rotarod but do display motor impairments on a challenging beam test (Goldberg et al. 2003). In addition, mice treated with moderate doses of the neurotoxin 1-methyl-4-phenyl-1,2,3,6-tetrahydropyridine (MPTP) do not show impairments on the rotarod but do show significant alterations in gait and impairments on an inverted grid test (Tillerson et al. 2002). Therefore, studies that use only the rotarod for phenotypic assessment may miss more subtle impairments. The best approach to behavioral characterization is one that includes a battery of tests that detect different aspects of sensory and motor function, including subtle changes in the nigrostriatal DA system (Fleming et al. 2003; Goldberg et al. 2003; Sedelis et al. 2001; Tillerson et al. 2002).

III. SENSORIMOTOR TESTS IN GENETIC MOUSE MODELS OF PARKINSON DISEASE

Our laboratory has developed a battery of sensorimotor tests to characterize genetic mouse models of PD. The battery includes tests of motor performance and coordination (the challenging beam test), response to sensory stimuli, spontaneous exploratory activity, spontaneous shredding behavior (bin cotton use), and gait analysis. We have assessed several different lines of transgenic mice with varying levels of nigrostriatal dysfunction (table 1) including parkin knock-out mice (Goldberg et al. 2003), α-synuclein knock-out mice (Abeliovich et al. 2000), and mice overexpressing the human wild-type α-synuclein under the Thy-1 promoter (Rockenstein et al. 2002).

The battery of tests described in this chapter assesses sensorimotor function in mice. However, whenever researchers characterize genetic mouse models of disease, they must also examine the animal. Researchers should monitor body weight and temperature throughout testing and note any

TABLE 1 Sensorimotor Impairments in Genetic Mouse Models

Mouse	Parkin knockout			α-synuclein overexpressor				α-synuclein knock-out			
Age (months)	2–4	7–9	18	2	4	6	8	2	4	6	8
Beam											
Errors	↑	↑	↑	↑	↑	↑↑	↑↑	=	↑	=	↑
Time	↓	=	=	↑	↑	↑	↑↑	=	=	=	=
Steps	=	=	=	↑	↑	↑	↑↑	=	=	=	=
Sensory Neglect	↑	↑	=	=	=	↑	=	=	=	=	=
Spontaneous											
Activity											
Rearing	=	↓	=	↓	=	=	=	↑	↑	↑	↑
Forelimb Steps	=	=	=	↓	=	↓	=	↑	=	↑	↑
Hindlimb Steps	=	=	=	↓↓	↓↓	↓↓	↓↓	↑	=	=	↑
Grooming	=	=	=	=	=	=	↓	↑	=	↑	↑
Bin Cotton Use		↓			↓		↓↓				↓
Stride Length							=				↓

Summary of Behavioral Results in Various Sensorimotor Tests (Goldberg et al. 2003; Fleming et al. 2003).

↑ = increased compared to age-matched control mice, = profoundly increased compared to age-matched controls and/or compared to their earlier ages. ↓ = decreased compared to age-matched controls, ↓↓ = profoundly decreased compared to age-matched controls and/or compared to their earlier ages, = represents not significantly different from age-matched control mice.

abnormal behaviors, for example if the mouse removes vibrissae or clasps its hind limbs when it is picked up by the tail. Basic neurological assessments are described elsewhere in detail (Crawley 2000; Crawley and Paylor 1997; Fernagut et al. 2003).

A. Challenging Beam Traversal

After injury or disease, both humans and animals use compensatory strategies to perform tasks accurately, making it difficult for investigators to detect impairments, especially in the early stages of the disease (LeVere 1988; Schallert 1988; Whishaw 2000). Therefore, it is important to challenge the animals to the limit of their abilities to uncover early effects of the mutations. In traditional beam-walking tests, animals must traverse several different beams of narrowing widths (Drucker-Colín et al. 1991). Time to traverse and slips along the beam both indicate alterations in DA function (Dluzen et al. 1995, 2001; Drucker-Colín et al. 1991). With this evidence in mind, we recently designed a challenging beam test that is highly sensitive to subtle sensorimotor dysfunction (Fleming et al. 2003; Goldberg et al. 2003). The test shows some selectivity for PD-causing mutations, as knock-in mouse models of Huntington disease do not display impairments on this test (Fleming et al. 2003; Hickey et al. 2003) at an age when they show other motor anomalies (Menalled et al. 2003). Instead of using several different beams as in previous studies, we constructed one tapered beam. The beam is made of Plexiglas (Plastics Zone Inc., Woodland Hills, CA) and consists of four sections (25 cm each, 1 meter total length), each section having a different width. The beam starts at a width of 3.5 cm and gradually narrows to 0.5 cm by 1 cm increments. Animals are trained to traverse the length of the beam starting at the widest section and ending at the narrowest, most difficult, section. Training is relatively easy and is done over two days. For training and testing, the beam must be placed approximately 10 cm off the ground and the narrow end must lead directly to the home cage. On the first day of training, the animal is placed on the widest part of the beam and the home cage is positioned in close proximity to the animal. As the animal begins to approach the home cage, the cage is gradually moved to the narrow end of the beam. After two assisted trials, animals can typically traverse the entire length of the beam unassisted. Animals then must complete five unassisted runs across the entire length of the beam. On the second day of training, animals must run five trials across the beam. On the day of the test, investigators increase task difficulty by placing a mesh grid (1 cm squares) of corresponding width over the beam surface, leaving approximately a 1 cm space between the grid and the beam surface. Animals are then videotaped and scored while they traverse the grid-surfaced beam for a total of five trials (see Video 1).

1. Analysis of the Challenging Beam Traversal Test

An experimenter blind to genotype should view the videotapes in slow motion and rate for errors (slips through the grid), number of steps made by each animal, and time to traverse across five trials. An error is counted when, during a forward movement, a limb (forelimb or hindlimb) slips through the grid and is visible between the grid and the beam surface. An individual animal can make a maximum of four slips per step. By scoring each limb slip individually, the experimenter can measure the severity of the error. For instance, an animal that slips with three or all four limbs through the grid during a step receives a higher error per step score than an animal that slips only one limb through the grid during a step. Slips should not be counted if the animal is not moving forward or if the animal's head is oriented to the left or right of the beam. Error-per-step scores, time to traverse and number of steps are calculated for wild-type and transgenic mice and averaged across all five trials. Error-per-step scores, time to traverse, and number of steps can also be broken down by beam width, illustrating where on the beam transgenic mice may be different from wild-type controls.

2. Challenging Beam Data

We have shown that parkin knock-out, α-synuclein overexpressing, and α-synuclein knock-out mice display significant impairments on the challenging beam test (table 1). α-synuclein overexpressing mice display more profound deficits that were progressive compared to both parkin and α-synuclein knock-out mice.

B. Response to Sensory Stimuli

Sensory neglect or sensory inattention was first shown to be associated with nigrostriatal damage in rats (Ljungberg and Ungerstedt 1976; Marshall and Gotthelf 1979). Marshall et al. (1971) presented rats treated with the neurotoxin 6-OHDA with various sensory stimuli and measured their responsiveness to each stimulus. Stimuli were presented to various parts of the body including the snout. Subsequently, it has been shown that sensory neglect can be reversed by DA agonists (table 2; Marshall and Gotthelf 1979) and is correlated with DA cell damage in the substantia nigra (table 2; Lees et al. 1985). Similarly, a somatosensory test was designed by Schallert et al. (1982, 1983, 2000; Schallert and Tillerson, 2000) to assess nigrostriatal DA dysfunction in the unilateral 6-OHDA rat. In the first phase of the test, small adhesive stickers are placed on the rat's forelimbs (radial/ulnar region) so that both forelimbs are simultaneously stimulated. Contact and removal times are measured for each fore limb. Typically, animals are consistently slower to contact and remove the stimulus from the contralateral

TABLE 2 Reversal of Sensorimotor Impairments with Dopamimetic Treatments

Behavioral tests	Animal	Model	Reversal			Reference
			L-dopa	APO/AMP	Grafts/viral vectors (DA or TH)	
Beam Walking	Aged vs. Young Rats	Haloperidol	Y	Y	Y	1, 2
Inverted Grid Walking	Aged mice	MPTP, Faults correlated with striatal DA content	Y			3
Sensory Neglect	Rats	6-OHDA, Neglect correlated with nigrostriatal DA neurons		Y	Y	4, 5, 6, 7, 8, 9
	Mice	MPTP				10
Locomotor Activity	Mice	MPTP	Y	N		11, 12, 13, 14
	Mice	6-OHDA		Y		15
	Rats	6-OHDA		Y		16
Bin Cotton Use	Mice	DA-deficient			Y	17
		MPTP				18, 19
Stride Length	Mice	MPTP, Correlated with striatal DA content	Y			3
	Mice	Reserpine	Y			20
	Rats	6-OHDA				21

Summary of reversal or improvement in motor function by L-dopa, apomorphine (APO), amphetamine (AMP), dopamine-producing grafts, or viral vectors expressing tyrosine hydroxylase following lesions of nigrostriatal dopaminergic system or dopamine antagonist treatment. Citation (ref): 1. Drucker-Colin et al. 1991; 2. Garcia-Hernandez et al. 1993; 3. Tillerson et al. 2002; 4. Lees et al. 1985; 5. Schallert et al. 1983; 6. Schallert et al. 1982; 7. Marshall and Gotthelf 1979; 8. Ljungberg and Ungerstedt 1976; 9. Dunnett et al. 1987; 10. Weihmuller et al. 1988; 11. Archer and Fredriksson 2003; 12. Archer et al. 2003; 13. Fredriksson et al. 1990; 14. Sundstrom et al. 1990; 15. Protais et al. 1983; 16. Breese et al. 1984; 17. Szczypka et al. 2001; 18. Sedelis et al. 2000; 19. Hofele et al. 2001; 20. Fernagut et al. 2002; 21. Schallert et al. 1978.

(impaired) side. For the second phase, a somatosensory threshold is established by systematically altering the size of the stimuli. Direct-acting DA agonists can reverse impairments in somatosensory detection (table 2; Schallert and Tillerson 2000; Schallert et al. 1982).

Because genetic mouse models of PD have bilateral deficits, we developed a sensory test adapted from Marshall et al. (1971) and Schallert et al. (1982). In this test, we measure response times to sensory stimuli placed on the snout. Small adhesive stimuli (Avery adhesive-backed labels) are placed on the snout of the mouse and time to make contact and remove the stimulus is recorded. To remove the stimulus, an animal raises both forelimbs towards its face and removes the stimulus with both forepaws. Typically, wild-type mice will make contact and remove a stimulus within ten seconds. Each animal receives two trials and the trials are alternated between mice. All testing is performed in the animal's home cage with cage mates and bedding temporarily removed during testing as both can interfere with stimulus removal. If an animal does not remove the stimulus within sixty seconds then the experimenter removes it, and the trial for the next mouse is initiated. If the animal does not remove the stimulus on either trial, then the size of the stimulus can be systematically increased until the animal makes contact and removes it (Goldberg et al. 2003).

1. Analysis of Sensory Response

Stimulus contact and removal times can be analyzed when animals remove the stimulus in under sixty seconds. If the animal requires larger stimuli to contact and remove the stimulus, then a rank score corresponding to the size of the stimulus can be given to the stimulus and an analysis with nonparametric statistics can be used.

2. Sensory Response Data

Both parkin knock-out and α-synuclein overexpressing mice displayed sensory response impairments whereas α-synuclein knock-out mice did not (table 1). Parkin mice showed impairments as early as two months of age whereas α-synuclein overexpressing mice did not develop sensorimotor impairments until six months of age, suggesting a more progressive phenotype in the α-synuclein overexpressing mice.

C. Spontaneous Activity

Although activity measures are affected by habituation (Sedelis et al. 2001) and differences can be masked with repeated testing, they have been used extensively in MPTP-treated mice (Sedelis et al. 2001). Hypoactivity in MPTP-treated mice is DA-dependent and can be reversed by L-dopa (table 2; Fredriksson et al. 1990). Spontaneous activity is easily measured using automated activity chambers equipped with photobeam sensors, but it can also be measured without automation. In this case, animals are placed in a small transparent cylinder (height: 15.5 cm and diameter: 12.7 cm) and their spontaneous behaviors are videotaped for three minutes. The cylinder is placed on a piece of glass and a mirror is situated at an angle beneath the cylinder to permit a clear view of motor movements along the ground and along the walls of the cylinder. Four different activity parameters including the number of rears, forelimb and hindlimb steps, and time spent grooming are measured (see Video 2).

1. Analysis of Spontaneous Activity

Videotapes should be viewed and rated in slow motion by an experimenter blind to genotype and experimental manipulation. The experimenter counts forelimb and hindlimb steps when an animal moves either both forelimbs or both hindlimbs across the floor of the cylinder. A rear is counted when an animal makes a vertical movement with both forelimbs removed from the ground. The experimenter also measures time spent grooming within the three minutes.

2. Spontaneous Activity Data

In this test, α-synuclein overexpressing mice showed significantly reduced spontaneous activity that persisted over time including educations in rearing, forelimb and hindlimb stepping, and grooming (table 1). Parkin knock-out mice showed decreased rearing at seven months of age, however, decreased rearing was not observed in the other ages tested. In contrast to both α-synuclein overexpressing and parkin knock-out mice, α-synuclein knock-out mice displayed significant increases in spontaneous activity that were persistent over time and included increases in rearing, forelimb and hindlimb stepping, and grooming (table 1; Fleming et al. 2003). Interestingly, Huntington disease knock-in mice also display increased rearing at an early age similar to α-synuclein knock-out mice (Menalled et al. 2002; 2003) indicating that rearing is one the earliest motor behaviors to be affected by various forms of basal ganglia dysfunction. However, in contrast to rearing, grooming was never affected in Huntington disease knock-in models, suggesting that anomalies in this behavior may be more specifically related to nigrostriatal dysfunction (Menalled et al. 2002, 2003).

D. Bin Cotton Use

Orofacial shredding is an important motor behavior involved in nest building, a natural mouse behavior related to thermoregulation and pup survival (Broida and Svare 1982; Crawley 2000; Lynch 1980). Both male and female mice shred material to build nests, and researchers have analyzed shredding behavior to assess nigrostriatal sensorimotor function in rodents (Hofele et al. 2001; Sedelis et al. 2000; Szczypka et al. 2001; Upchurch and Schallert 1983). The behavior requires orofacial and forelimb movements, where animals pull the nesting material apart with their forelimbs and teeth and then break down the material in their mouths and incorporate it into their bedding. These movements are dopamine dependent, are significantly reduced with dopamine antagonists (table 2; Upchurch and Schallert 1983), and impairments can be reversed with increased DA production (table 2; Szczypka et al. 2001). When experimenters place the nesting material in the feeder bin of the cage, animals must rear up and pull the nesting material from the feeder. This adjustment makes the test more challenging than if the nesting material was just placed on the floor of the cage. However, in the case where animals do not pull and shred the nesting material at all, researchers must perform an additional test where nesting material is placed on the cage floor, making it more accessible, and then measure the amount of cotton shredded.

1. Analysis of Bin Cotton Use

Experimenters measure shredding behavior by placing preweighed cotton into the feeder of each mouse's cage for each day of testing. Nests should be removed before placing new cotton into the feeder. Experiments measure the percent of bin cotton use daily for each mouse and compare the amounts between transgenic and wild-type mice.

2. Bin Cotton Use Data

Parkin, α-synuclein overexpressing, and α-synuclein knock-out mice displayed varying levels of impairments in bin cotton use (table 1). α-synuclein overexpressing mice display severe impairments at four and eight months of age. Both parkin and α-synuclein knock-out mice displayed significant but more subtle impairments in bin cotton use when tested at eight to nine months of age. When cotton was placed in the bottom of the cage and not in the feeder all animals shredded the cotton, and this behavior ruled out loss of nesting instinct.

E. Gait Analysis

Alterations in gait are a major cause of disability in PD patients (Rao et al. 2003). PD patients typically move in short shuffling steps that can cause falls and injury (Rao et al. 2003). Researchers can easily measure gait in rodents. In MPTP-treated mice shorter stride lengths correlate with reduced DA content in the striatum and can be reversed with L-dopa (table 2; Eilam et al. 1998; Tillerson et al. 2002). To measure gait, experimenters train animals to walk through a narrow alley leading into their home cage. Once the animals are trained, paper is placed along the alley floor and the animals' forelimbs and/or hindlimbs are brushed with different colors of non-toxic paints. Animals are then placed at the beginning of the alley. As they walk into their home cage they leave their paw prints on the paper underneath (Barlow et al. 1996; Fernagut et al. 2002; Schallert et al. 1978; Tillerson et al. 2002). Stride length is determined by measuring the distance between paw prints. Only strides made while continuously walking (no stopping) should be included in the analysis and the first and last stride lengths should be excluded from the analysis because animals tend to make irregular steps at the beginning and end of the test. Several parameters can be recorded including stride length, stride width, and maximum stride difference (variability between stride lengths).

Gait analysis data showed that α-synuclein knock-out mice had significantly shorter stride lengths compared to wild-type mice (table 1) at eight months of age. In contrast, α-synuclein overexpressing mice at eight months of age did not have significantly altered hindlimb gait compared to wild-type mice. Parkin knock-out mice were not tested on gait. In comparison, Huntington disease knock-in mice show gait impairments, but only at a much later age than rearing and locomotor impairments (Menalled et al. 2003).

F. Additional Motor Tests

In addition to the tests described here, other tests have been developed that are highly sensitive in MPTP mice and would be useful when phenotyping genetic mouse models of PD. These include the inverted grid test (Tillerson et al. 2002, 2003) and the pole test (Matsuura et al. 1997; Ogawa et al. 1985, 1987; Sedelis et al. 2001). For the inverted grid test, animals are placed upside down on a grid approximately 20 cm above the ground for thirty seconds. In this test, moderate doses of MPTP in mice caused shortened forelimb step length, increased time spent against the wall, and increased forelimb faults compared to controls. These parameters correlate with dopaminergic markers in the striatum that are reversible with L-dopa. For the pole test, researchers placed animals head up on the top of a pole and measured the time to orient the body downward and time to descend. MPTP-treated mice display slower times in both parameters compared to controls and, similar to the inverted grid test, the impairments are reversed by L-dopa (Matsuura et al. 1997; Ogawa et al. 1985, 1987). In addition, Huntington disease knock-in mice display significant impairments in the pole test (Hickey et al. 2003), indicating it is a useful test for basal ganglia dysfunction.

G. Cognitive Tests

In PD patients, motor impairments are the primary symptoms used to diagnose the disorder, but patients also suffer from cognitive impairments and depression (Kuzis et al. 1997; Rao et al. 2003; Uekermann et al. 2003). Cognitive impairments often precede motor impairments and researchers may benefit from analyzing these types of impairments when studying the early stages of PD. Cognitive impairments have been modeled in primate models of PD (Schneider and Roeltgen 1993) and to a lesser extent in rodent models. In primates impairments manifest as delayed matching to sample, and problems with visual discrimination and object retrieval tasks, while rodents show delayed alternation in the T-maze (Tanila et al. 1998) and impaired habit learning in the cross maze (Packard and McGaugh 1996), suggesting cognitive tests could help characterize phenotypes for the genetic mouse models of PD.

H. Specificity of Behavioral Impairments in Models of Parkinson Disease

As indicated in table 2, the alterations in sensorimotor function found in the genetic mouse models of PD are similar to those observed in animals with a selective loss of nigrostriatal DA neurons induced by toxin injections and the changes are reversible by DA agonists. However, sensorimotor function can also be altered in other disease models including Huntington disease (Carter et al. 1999; Menalled et al. 2002, 2003) and ataxia telangiectasia (Barlow et al. 1996; Eilam et al. 1998). In the course of our studies we noticed that anomalies in beam traversal are more selective for PD than Huntington disease knock-in models. Interestingly, PD and Huntington disease models show opposite changes in rearing and locomotor activity at the early stages, but as Huntington disease knock-in mice age, they begin to show defects similar to PD mice. These results agree with clinical data showing pervasive akinesia in patients with Huntington disease (Curra et al. 2000; Jahanshahi et al. 1993; Thompson et al. 1988). Furthermore, some studies demonstrated deficits in dopamine function in Huntington disease mouse models, further blurring the line between both diseases (Hickey et al. 2002). This illustrates the major advantage of genetic disease models, where the effects of the mutation in the whole organism can be mimicked, as opposed to toxin models, which produce selective lesions of one pathway, where many more pathways are affected during the disease in humans (Braak et al. 2003; Gesi et al. 2000; Patt and Gerhard 1993).

IV. CONCLUSIONS

Although the cause of most cases of PD remains unknown, the recently discovered familial forms of the disease have created a new approach for studying PD. Researchers continue to generate mice engineered with genetic mutations similar to those found in familial PD for assessing the long-term effects of these mutations *in vivo*. Researchers must characterize the behavior of these mice to validate their role as a model of PD and to determine optimal therapeutic targets.

Acknowledgments

We gratefully acknowledge Yves Mignon for his assistance with the video files and Jonathan Salcedo for his help with rating. In addition, we thank Ehud Gruen and Cynthia Chavira for all of their work with the mouse colony. Funded by Morris K. Udall Parkinson Disease Research Center of Excellence at UCLA (P50NS38367) and NIH/NIEHS (U54ES12078).

Video Legends

Spontaneous Activity in the Cylinder:
Animals are placed in a clear plastic cylinder and are videotaped from underneath the cylinder to permit viewing of forelimb and hindlimb movements.

SEGMENT 1 A wild-type (littermate control) mouse in the cylinder at four months of age.

SEGMENT 2 An alpha-synuclein-overexpressing mouse in the cylinder at four months of age. Notice the lack of hindlimb stepping compared to the wild-type mouse in segment 1.

Challenging Beam Traversal:
Animals are placed on a tapered beam and time to traverse, number of steps and errors are recorded as the animal moves along the beam.

SEGMENT 1 A wild-type (littermate control) mouse on the challenging beam at four months of age.

SEGMENT 2 An alpha-synuclein-overexpressing mouse on the challenging beam at four months of age. Notice the increased number of errors (slips) and amount of time to traverse compared to the wild-type mouse in segment 1.

SEGMENT 3 The same wild-type mouse as in segment 1, now at six months of age.

SEGMENT 4 The same alpha-synuclein-overexpressing mouse as in segment 2, now at six months of age. Notice the increased number of errors (slips) and time to traverse compared to segment 2.

References

Abeliovich, A., Y. Schmitz, I. Farinas, D. Choi-Lundberg, W.H. Ho, P.E. Castillo, N., Shinsky, et al. 2000. Mice lacking alpha-synuclein display functional deficits in the nigrostriatal dopamine system. *Neuron* **25(1)**: 239–252.

Archer, T., and A. Fredriksson. 2003. An antihypokinesic action of alpha2-adrenoceptors upon MPTP-induced behaviour deficits in mice. *J Neural Transm* **110(2)**:183–200.

Archer, T., T. Palomo, R. McArthur, and A. Fredriksson. 2003. Effects of acute administration of DA agonists on locomotor activity: MPTP versus neonatal intracerebroventricular 6-OHDA treatment. *Neurotox Res* **5(1–2)**:95–110.

Barlow, C., S. Hirotsune, R. Paylor, M. Liyanage, M. Eckhaus, F. Collins, Y. Shiloh, et al. 1996. Atm-deficient mice: a paradigm of ataxia telangiectasia. *Cell* **86(1)**:159–171.

Bonifati, V., P. Rizzu, M.J. van Baren, O. Schaap, G.J. Breedveld, E. Krieger, M.C. Dekker, et al. 2003. Mutations in the DJ-1 gene associated with autosomal recessive early-onset Parkinsonism. *Science* **299(5604)**:256–259.

Braak, H., K. Del Tredici, U. Rub, R.A. de Vos, E.N. Jansen Steur, and E. Braak. 2003. Staging of brain pathology related to sporadic Parkinson's disease. *Neurobiol Aging* **24(2)**:197–211.

Breese, G.R., A.A. Baumeister, T.J. McCown, S.G. Emerick, G.D. Frye, K. Crotty, and R.A. Mueller. 1984. Behavioral differences between neonatal and adult 6-hydroxydopamine-treated rats to dopamine agonists: relevance to neurological symptoms in clinical syndromes with reduced brain dopamine. *J Pharmacol Exp Ther* **231(2)**:343–354.

Broida, J., and B. Svare. 1982. Strain-typical patterns of pregnancy-induced nest building in mice: maternal and experiential influences. *Physiol Behav* **29(1)**:153–157.

Carter, R.J., L.A. Lione, T. Humby, L. Mangiarini, A. Mahal, G.P. Bates, S.B. Dunnett, and A.J. Morton. 1999. Characterization of progressive motor deficits in mice transgenic for the human Huntington's disease mutation. *J Neurosci* **19(8)**:3248–3257.

Connor, B., D.A. Kozlowski, T. Schallert, J.L. Tillerson, B.L. Davidson, and M.C. Bohn. 1999. Differential effects of glial cell line-derived neurotrophic factor (GDNF) in the striatum and substantia nigra of the aged Parkinsonian rat. *Gene Ther* **6(12)**:1936–1951.

Connor, B., D.A. Kozlowski, J.R. Unnerstall, J.D. Elsworth, J.L. Tillerson, T. Schallert, and M.C. Bohn. 2001. Glial cell line-derived neurotrophic factor (GDNF) gene delivery protects dopaminergic terminals from degeneration. *Exp Neurol* **169(1)**:83–95.

Crawley, J.N. 2000. *What's Wrong With My Mouse? Behavioral Phenotyping of Transgenic and Knockout Mice.* New York: Wiley-Liss.

Crawley, J.N., and R. Paylor. 1997. A proposed test battery and constellations of specific behavioral paradigms to investigate the behavioral phenotypes of transgenic and knockout mice. *Horm Behav* **31(3)**:197–211.

Curra, A., R. Agostino, P. Galizia, F. Fittipaldi, M. Manfredi, and A. Berardelli. 2000. Sub-movement cueing and motor sequence execution in patients with Huntington's disease. *Clin Neurophysiol* **111(7)**: 1184–1190.

Di Paola, R., and R.J. Uitti. 1996. Early detection of Parkinson's disease. Implications for treatment. *Drugs Aging* **9(3)**:159–168.

Dluzen, D.E., B. Liu, C.Y. Chen, and S.E. DiCarlo. 1995. Daily spontaneous running alters behavioral and neurochemical indexes of nigrostriatal function. *J Appl Physiol* **78(4)**:1219–1224.

Dluzen, D.E., X. Gao, G.M. Story, L.I. Anderson, J. Kucera, and J.M. Walro. 2001. Evaluation of nigrostriatal dopaminergic function in adult +/+ and +/– BDNF mutant mice. *Exp Neurol* **170(1)**:121–128.

Drucker-Colin, R., and F. Garcia-Hernandez. 1991. A new motor test sensitive to aging and dopaminergic function. *J Neurosci Methods* **39(2)**: 153–161.

Dunnett, S.B., I.Q. Whishaw, D.C. Rogers, and G.H. Jones. 1987. Dopamine-rich grafts ameliorate whole body motor asymmetry and sensory neglect but not independent limb use in rats with 6-hydroxydopamine lesions. *Brain Res* **415(1)**:63–78.

Eilam, R., Y. Peter, A. Elson, G. Rotman, Y. Shiloh, Y. Groner, and M. Segal. 1998. Selective loss of dopaminergic nigrostriatal neurons in brains of Atm-deficient mice. *Proc Natl Acad Sci U S A* **95(21)**: 12653–12656.

Fernagut, P.O., E. Diguet, B. Labattu, and F. Tison. 2002. A simple method to measure stride length as an index of nigrostriatal dysfunction in mice. *J Neurosci Methods* **113(2)**:123–130.

Fernagut, P.O., S. Chalon, E. Diguet, D. Guilloteau, F. Tison, and M. Jaber. 2003. Motor behaviour deficits and their histopathological and functional correlates in the nigrostriatal system of dopamine transporter knockout mice. *Neuroscience* **116(4)**:1123–1130.

Fleming, S.M., M.S. Levine, E. Masliah, and M.-F. Chesselet. 2003. Early and persistent motor abnormalities in transgenic mice expressing wild-type human α-synuclein and mice lacking α-synuclein. *Abstract Viewer/Itinerary Planner*. Washington D.C.: Society for Neuroscience.

Fredriksson, A., A. Plaznik, E. Sundstrom, G. Jonsson, and T. Archer. 1990. MPTP-induced hypoactivity in mice: reversal by L-dopa. *Pharmacol Toxicol* **67(4)**:295–301.

Garcia-Hernandez, F., M.T. Pacheco-Cano, and R. Drucker-Colin. 1993. Reduction of motor impairment by adrenal medulla transplants in aged rats. *Physiol Behav* **54(3)**:589–598.

Gesi, M., P. Soldani, F.S. Giorgi, A. Santinami, I. Bonaccorsi, and F. Fornai. 2000. The role of the locus ceruleus in the development of Parkinson's disease. *Neurosci Biobehav Rev* **24(6)**:655–668.

Giasson, B.I., J.E. Duda, S.M. Quinn, B. Zhang, J.Q. Trojanowski, and V.M. Lee. 2002. Neuronal alpha-synucleinopathy with severe movement disorder in mice expressing A53T human alpha-synuclein. *Neuron* **34(4)**:521–533.

Goldberg, M.S., S.M. Fleming, J.J. Palacino, C. Cepeda, H.A. Lam, A. Bhatnagar, E.G. Meloni, et al. 2003. Parkin-deficient mice exhibit nigrostriatal deficits but not loss of dopaminergic neurons. *J Biol Chem* **278(44)**:43628–43635.

Hickey, M.A., G.P. Reynolds, and A.J. Morton. 2002. The role of dopamine in motor symptoms in the R6/2 transgenic mouse model of Huntington's disease. *J Neurochem* **81(1)**:46–59.

Hickey, M.A., S.E. Thomasian, E. Gruen, S. Zeitlin, X.J. Li, K.F. Faull, M.S. Levine, and M.-F. Chesselet. 2003. Antioxidant treatment and behavioral characterization of a knock-in mouse model of Huntington's disease. *Abstract Viewer/Itinerary Planner*. Washington D.C.: Society for Neuroscience.

Hofele, K., M. Sedelis, G.W. Auburger, S. Morgan, J.P. Huston, and R.K. Schwarting. 2001. Evidence for a dissociation between MPTP toxicity and tyrosinase activity based on congenic mouse strain susceptibility. *Exp Neurol* **168(1)**:116–122.

Imbert, C., E. Bezard, S. Guitraud, T. Boraud, and C.E. Gross. 2000. Comparison of eight clinical rating scales used for the assessment of MPTP-induced Parkinsonism in the Macaque monkey. *J Neurosci Methods* **96(1)**:71–76.

Itier, J.M., P. Ibanez, M.A. Mena, N. Abbas, C. Cohen-Salmon, G.A. Bohme, M. Laville, et al. 2003. Parkin gene inactivation alters behaviour and dopamine neurotransmission in the mouse. *Hum Mol Genet* **12(18)**:2277–2291.

Jahanshahi, M., R.G. Brown, and C.D. Marsden. 1993. A comparative study of simple and choice reaction time in Parkinson's, Huntington's and cerebellar disease. *J Neurol Neurosurg Psychiatry* **56(11)**:1169–1177.

Kahle, P.J., M. Neumann, L. Ozmen, V. Muller, H. Jacobsen, A. Schindzielorz, M. Okochi, et al. 2000. Subcellular localization of wild-type and Parkinson's disease-associated mutant alpha-synuclein in human and transgenic mouse brain. *J Neurosci* **20(17)**:6365–6373.

Kitada, T., S. Asakawa, N. Hattori, H. Matsumine, Y. Yamamura, S. Minoshima, M. Yokochi, et al. 1998. Mutations in the parkin gene cause autosomal recessive juvenile Parkinsonism. *Nature* **392(6676)**: 605–608.

Kozlowski, D.A., B. Connor, J.L. Tillerson, T. Schallert, and M.C. Bohn. 2000. Delivery of a GDNF gene into the substantia nigra after a progressive 6-OHDA lesion maintains functional nigrostriatal connections. *Exp Neurol* **166(1)**:1–15.

Kruger, R., W. Kuhn, T. Muller, D. Woitalla, M. Graeber, S. Kosel, H. Przuntek, et al. 1998. Ala30Pro mutation in the gene encoding alpha-synuclein in Parkinson's disease. *Nat Genet* **18(2)**:106–108.

Kuzis, G., L. Sabe, C. Tiberti, R. Leiguarda, and S.E. Starkstein. 1997. Cognitive functions in major depression and Parkinson disease. *Arch Neurol* **54(8)**:982–986.

Lee, M.K., W. Stirling, Y. Xu, X. Xu, D. Qui, A.S. Mandir, T.M. Dawson, et al. 2002. Human alpha-synuclein-harboring familial Parkinson's disease-linked Ala-53 → Thr mutation causes neurodegenerative disease with alpha-synuclein aggregation in transgenic mice. *Proc Natl Acad Sci U S A* **99(13)**:8968–8973.

Lees, G.J., R.R. Kydd, and J.J. Wright. 1985. Relationship between sensorimotor neglect and the specificity, degree, and locus of mesotelencephalic dopaminergic cell loss following 6-hydroxydopamine. *Psychopharmacology (Berl)* **85(1)**:115–122.

Leroy, E., R. Boyer, G. Auburger, B. Leube, G. Ulm, E. Mezey, G. Harta, et al. 1998. The ubiquitin pathway in Parkinson's disease. *Nature* **395(6701)**:451–452.

LeVere, T.E. 1988. Neural system imbalances and the consequences of large brain injuries. In *Brain Injury and Recovery, Theoretical and Controversial Issues* Ed. S. Finger, T.E. LeVere, C.R. Almi, and D.G. Stein. New York: Plenum Press.

Ljungberg, T., and U. Ungerstedt. 1976. Sensory inattention produced by 6-hydroxydopamine-induced degeneration of ascending dopamine neurons in the brain. *Exp Neurol* **53(3)**:585–600.

Lucking, C.B., A. Durr, V. Bonifati, J. Vaughan, G. De Michele, T. Gasser, B.S. Harhangi, et al. 2000. Association between early-onset Parkinson's disease and mutations in the parkin gene. French Parkinson's Disease Genetics Study Group. *N Engl J Med* **342(21)**: 1560–1567.

Luo, J., M.G. Kaplitt, H.L. Fitzsimons, D.S. Zuzga, Y. Liu, M.L. Oshinsky, and M.J. During. 2002. Subthalamic GAD gene therapy in a Parkinson's disease rat model. *Science* **298(5592)**:425–429.

Lynch, C.B. 1980. Response to divergent selection for nesting behavior in Mus musculus. *Genetics* **96(3)**:757–765.

Marshall, J.F., B.H. Turner, and P. Teitelbaum. 1971. Sensory neglect produced by lateral hypothalamic damage. *Science* **174(8)** 523–525.

Marshall, J.F., and T. Gotthelf. 1979. Sensory inattention in rats with 6-hydroxydopamine-induced degeneration of ascending dopaminergic neurons: apomorphine-induced reversal of deficits. *Exp Neurol* **65(2)**: 398–411.

Masliah, E., E. Rockenstein, I. Veinbergs, M. Mallory, M. Hashimoto, A. Takeda, Y. Sagara, et al. 2000. Dopaminergic loss and inclusion body formation in alpha-synuclein mice: implications for neurodegenerative disorders. *Science* **287(5456)**:1265–1269.

Matsuoka, Y., M. Vila, S. Lincoln, A. McCormack, M. Picciano, J. LaFrancois, X. Yu, et al. 2001. Lack of nigral pathology in transgenic mice expressing human alpha-synuclein driven by the tyrosine hydroxylase promoter. *Neurobiol Dis* **8(3)**:535–539.

Matsuura, K., H. Kabuto, H. Makino, and N. Ogawa. 1997. Pole test is a useful method for evaluating the mouse movement disorder caused by striatal dopamine depletion. *J Neurosci Methods* **73(1)**:45–48.

Menalled, L.B., J.D. Sison, Y. Wu, M. Olivieri, X.J. Li, H. Li, S. Zeitlin, and M.F. Chesselet. 2002. Early motor dysfunction and striosomal distribution of huntingtin microaggregates in Huntington's disease knock-in mice. *J Neurosci* **22(18)**:8266–8276.

Menalled, L.B., J.D. Sison, I. Dragatsis, S. Zeitlin, and M.F. Chesselet. 2003. Time course of early motor and neuropathological anomalies in a knock-in mouse model of Huntington's disease with 140 CAG repeats. *J Comp Neurol* **465(1)**:11–26.

Mignon, L., P. Vourc'h, M. Romero-Ramos, N. Dunkelman, M.A. El-Kalay, and M.-F. Chesselet. 2003. Pluripotent stem cells from adult muscle survive and express a neuronal phenotype after transplantation into a rat model of Parkinson's disease. *Abstract Viewer/Itinerary Planner*. Washington D.C.: Society for Neuroscience.

Ogawa, N., Y. Hirose, S. Ohara, T. Ono, and Y. Watanabe. 1985. A simple quantitative bradykinesia test in MPTP-treated mice. *Res Commun Chem Pathol Pharmacol* **50(3)**:435–441.

Ogawa, N., K. Mizukawa, Y. Hirose, S. Kajita, S. Ohara, and Y. Watanabe. 1987. MPTP-induced parkinsonian model in mice: biochemistry, pharmacology and behavior. *Eur Neurol* **26 Suppl 1**:16–23.

Packard, M.G., and J.L. McGaugh. 1996. Inactivation of hippocampus or caudate nucleus with lidocaine differentially affects expression of place and response learning. *Neurobiol Learn Mem* **65(1)**:65–72.

Patt, S., and L. Gerhard. 1993. A Golgi study of human locus ceruleus in normal brains and in Parkinson's disease. *Neuropathol Appl Neurobiol* **19(6)**:519–523.

Periquet, M., M. Latouche, E. Lohmann, N. Rawal, G. De Michele, S. Ricard, H. Teive, et al. 2003. Parkin mutations are frequent in patients with isolated early-onset Parkinsonism. *Brain* **126(Pt 6)**: 1271–1278.

Polymeropoulos, M.H., C. Lavedan, E. Leroy, S.E. Ide, A. Dehejia, A. Dutra, B. Pike, et al. 1997. Mutation in the alpha-synuclein gene identified in families with Parkinson's disease. *Science* **276(5321)**:2045–2047.

Protais, P., J.J. Bonnet, and J. Costentin. 1983. Pharmacological characterization of the receptors involved in the apomorphine-induced polyphasic modifications of locomotor activity in mice. *Psychopharmacology (Berl)* **81(2)**:126–134.

Rao, G., L. Fisch, S. Srinivasan, F. D'Amico, T. Okada, C. Eaton, and C. Robbins. 2003. Does this patient have Parkinson disease? *JAMA* **289(3)**:347–353.

Rathke-Hartlieb, S., P.J. Kahle, M. Neumann, L. Ozmen, S. Haid, M. Okochi, C. Haass, and J.B. Schulz. 2001. Sensitivity to MPTP is not increased in Parkinson's disease-associated mutant alpha-synuclein transgenic mice. *J Neurochem* **77(4)**:1181–1184.

Richfield, E.K., M.J. Thiruchelvam, D.A. Cory-Slechta, C. Wuertzer, R.R. Gainetdinov, M.G. Caron, D.A. Di Monte, and H.J. Federoff. 2002. Behavioral and neurochemical effects of wild-type and mutated human alpha-synuclein in transgenic mice. *Exp Neurol* **175(1)**:35–48.

Schallert, T. 1988. Aging-dependent emergence of sensorimotor dysfunction in rats recovered from dopamine depletion sustained early in life. *Ann N Y Acad Sci* **515**:108–120.

Schallert, T., S.M. Fleming, J.L. Leasure, J.L. Tillerson, and S.T. Bland. 2000. CNS plasticity and assessment of forelimb sensorimotor outcome in unilateral rat models of stroke, cortical ablation, Parkinsonism, and spinal cord injury. *Neuropharmacology* **39(5)**:777–787.

Schallert, T., D. Norton, and T.A. Jones. 1992. A clinically relevant unilateral rat model of parkinsonian akinesia. *J Neural Transplant Plast* **3**: 332–333.

Schallert, T., and J.L. Tillerson. 2000. Intervention strategies for degeneration of DA neurons in Parkinsonism: Optimizing behavioral assessment of outcome. In *Central Nervous System Diseases* Ed. D.F. Emerich, R.L. Dean III, and P.R. Sandberg. Totowa: Humana Press.

Schallert, T., M. Upchurch, N. Lobaugh, S.B. Farrar, W.W. Spirduso, P. Gilliam, D. Vaughn, and R.E. Wilcox. 1982. Tactile extinction: distinguishing between sensorimotor and motor asymmetries in rats with unilateral nigrostriatal damage. *Pharmacol Biochem Behav* **16(3)**: 455–462.

Schallert, T., M. Upchurch, R.E. Wilcox, and D.M. Vaughn. 1983. Posture-independent sensorimotor analysis of inter-hemispheric receptor asymmetries in neostriatum. *Pharmacol Biochem Behav* **18(5)**:753–759.

Schallert, T., I.Q. Whishaw, V.D. Ramirez, and P. Teitelbaum. 1978. Compulsive, abnormal walking caused by anticholinergics in akinetic, 6-hydroxydopamine-treated rats. *Science* **199(4336)**:1461–1463.

Schneider, J.S., and D.P. Roeltgen. 1993. Delayed matching-to-sample, object retrieval, and discrimination reversal deficits in chronic low dose MPTP-treated monkeys. *Brain Res* **615(2)**:351–354.

Sedelis, M., K. Hofele, G.W. Auburger, S. Morgan, J.P. Huston, and R.K. Schwarting. 2000. MPTP susceptibility in the mouse: behavioral, neurochemical, and histological analysis of gender and strain differences. *Behav Genet* **30(3)**:171–182.

Sedelis, M., R.K. Schwarting, and J.P. Huston. 2001. Behavioral phenotyping of the MPTP mouse model of Parkinson's disease. *Behav Brain Res* **125(1–2)**:109–125.

Singleton, A.B., M. Farrer, J. Johnson, A. Singleton, S. Hague, J. Kachergus, M. Hulihan, et al. 2003. alpha-Synuclein locus triplication causes Parkinson's disease. *Science* **302(5646)**:841.

Spillantini, M.G., M.L. Schmidt, V.M. Lee, J.Q. Trojanowski, R. Jakes, M. Goevdert. 1997. Alpha-synuclein in Lewy bodies. Nature 388(6645):839–840.

Sundstrom, E., A. Fredriksson, and T. Archer. 1990. Chronic neurochemical and behavioral changes in MPTP-lesioned C57BL/6 mice: a model for Parkinson's disease. *Brain Res* **528(2)**:181–188.

Szczypka, M.S., K. Kwok, M.D. Brot, B.T. Marck, A.M. Matsumoto, B.A. Donahue, and R.D. Palmiter. 2001. Dopamine production in the caudate putamen restores feeding in dopamine-deficient mice. *Neuron* **30(3)**:819–828.

Tanila, H., M. Bjorklund, and P. Riekkinen, Jr. 1998. Cognitive changes in mice following moderate MPTP exposure. *Brain Res Bull* **45(6)**:577–582.

Thompson, P.D., A. Berardelli, J.C. Rothwell, B.L. Day, J.P. Dick, R. Benecke, and C.D. Marsden. 1988. The coexistence of bradykinesia and chorea in Huntington's disease and its implications for theories of basal ganglia control of movement. *Brain* **111(Pt 2)**:223–244.

Tillerson, J.L., W.M. Caudle, M.E. Reveron, and G.W. Miller. 2002. Detection of behavioral impairments correlated to neurochemical deficits in mice treated with moderate doses of 1-methyl-4-phenyl-1,2,3,6-tetrahydropyridine. *Exp Neurol* **178(1)**:80–90.

Tillerson, J.L., and G.W. Miller. 2003. Grid performance test to measure behavioral impairment in the MPTP-treated-mouse model of Parkinsonism. *J Neurosci Methods* **123(2)**:189–200.

Uekermann, J., I. Daum, S. Peters, B. Wiebel, H. Przuntek, and T. Muller. 2003. Depressed mood and executive dysfunction in early Parkinson's disease. *Acta Neurol Scand* **107(5)**:341–348.

Upchurch, M., and T. Schallert. 1983. A behavior analysis of the offspring of "haloperidol-sensitive" and "haloperidol-resistant" gerbils. *Behav Neural Biol* **39(2)**:221–228.

van der Putten, H., K.H. Wiederhold, A. Probst, S. Barbieri, C. Mistl, S. Danner, S. Kauffmann, et al. 2000. Neuropathology in mice expressing human alpha-synuclein. *J Neurosci* **20(16)**:6021–6029.

Weihmuller, F.B., M. Hadjiconstantinou, and J.P. Bruno. 1988. Acute stress or neuroleptics elicit sensorimotor deficits in MPTP-treated mice. *Neurosci Lett* **85(1)**:137–142.

Whishaw, I.Q., W.T. O'Connor, and S.B. Dunnett. 1986. The contributions of motor cortex, nigrostriatal dopamine, and caudate-putamen to skilled forelimb use in the rat. *Brain* **109(Pt 5)**:805–843.

Whishaw, I.Q. 2000. Loss of the innate cortical engram for action patterns used in skilled reaching and the development of behavioral compensation following motor cortex lesions in the rat. *Neuropharmacology* **39(5)**:788–805.

Wintermeyer, P., R. Kruger, W. Kuhn, T. Muller, D. Woitalla, D. Berg, G. Becker, et al. 2000. Mutation analysis and association studies of the UCHL1 gene in German Parkinson's disease patients. *Neuroreport* **11(10)**:2079–2082.

Yang, M., N.D. Stull, M.A. Berk, E.Y. Snyder, and L. Iacovitti. 2002. Neural stem cells spontaneously express dopaminergic traits after transplantation into the intact or 6-hydroxydopamine-lesioned rat. *Exp Neurol* **177(1)**:50–60.

CHAPTER

B7

Utility of 6-Hydroxydopamine Lesioned Rats in the Preclinical Screening of Novel Treatments for Parkinson Disease

M. ANGELA CENCI and MARTIN LUNDBLAD

Parkinson disease (PD) is one of the most common neurodegenerative disorders, affecting about 1% of people over sixty years of age (for review see Bezard et al. 2001; Dauer and Przedborski 2003; Fahn 2003). The disease got its name from the English neurologist James Parkinson, who first described it in 1817 as a "shaking palsy." The characteristic motor symptoms of PD consist of resting tremor, rigidity, hypo- and bradykinesia, and postural abnormalities (Gelb et al. 1999). These symptoms are caused by the depletion of dopamine (DA) in the target structures of nigral DA neurons, whose progressive degeneration represents the pathological hallmark of PD (Dauer and Przedborski 2003; Fahn 2003). Positron emission tomography (PET) studies in human patients have shown that the severity of Parkinsonian motor symptoms is inversely related to the levels of ^{18}F-fluorodopa (FD) uptake in the motor part of the striatum, that is, the putamen (Morrish et al. 1996; Brooks 2003).

The motor symptoms of PD may be accompanied by autonomic disturbances affecting the cardiovascular system, gastrointestinal and urinary tracts, as well as sweat and thermoregulation (Jost 1995; Schrag et al. 2000). Moreover, PD patients show a high incidence of depression and cognitive impairment (Brown and Marsden 1984; Schrag et al. 2000). These non-motor symptoms are related to the degeneration of brain structures other than the nigrostriatal DA neurons (Ito et al. 2002; Brooks 2003). Although neuronal loss is massive in the substantia nigra pars compacta (SNpc), the neurodegenerative process in PD involves some additional brain stem structures, such as the locus ceruleus, the dorsal nucleus of the vagus nerve, and the reticular formation in the pons and the midbrain (Duyckaerts et al. 2003; Mayer 2003). Neurodegeneration may also be pronounced in the cortex and basal forebrain, accounting for the high liability to cognitive decline in PD patients (Girotti and Soliveri 2003; Kovari et al. 2003). The motor symptoms of PD represent a major source of disability for the vast majority of patients (Schrag et al. 2000), calling for DA replacement therapy early on during the course of the disease.

I. THE PHARMACOLOGICAL TREATMENT OF PARKINSON DISEASE AND ITS COMPLICATIONS

Pharmacological DA replacement with the DA precursor, L-dihydroxyphenylalanine (L-dopa) is the most effective treatment for the motor symptoms of PD. Common L-dopa preparations contain a peripheral dopa-decarboxylase inhibitor (i.e., carbidopa or benserazide), which helps reduce the risk of side effects that are due to the extracerebral conversion of L-dopa to DA, such as nausea and hypotension. All patients in the initial stages of PD respond to L-dopa with a pronounced symptomatic improvement. The therapeutic benefit produced by L-dopa is, however, hampered by the gradual development of motor fluctuations and dyskinesia. Researchers have estimated that these motor complications affect greater than 50% of PD patients within only five years of initiating L-dopa pharmacotherapy (Obeso et al. 2000). With time, especially in patients with young onset PD (Quinn et al. 1987), motor complications often increase in severity and challenge the possibility of providing an optimal drug therapy (Marsden et al. 1981; Nutt 1992; Quinn 1998).

The most common form of motor fluctuation results from a decrease in duration of the LDOPA response. In the first years of the disease, L-dopa intake every four hours is sufficient to produce a stable and smooth motor improvement during the whole day. As the disease progresses the improvement produced by intake of L-dopa (the so called "on" state) lasts for only two to three hours, and is followed by pronounced akinesia, rigidity, and tremor (the "off" state). This type of fluctuation is called "end-of-dose deterioration" or "wearing-off phenomenon." PD patients may also exhibit unpredictable and sudden fluctuations between "on" and "off" states, as well as dose failure episodes, that is, inexplicable lack of responses to the intake of L-dopa (for a classification see Quinn 1998; Fahn 2003).

In the complicated stage of PD, the patients usually exhibit abnormal involuntary movements (dyskinesia). Dyskinesias appear in three temporal patterns in relation to the intake of antiparkinsonian medications. "On"-phase dyskinesias manifest themselves when plasma (and brain) levels of L-dopa and DA are highest, and they represent the most common pattern. Dyskinesias can however appear also at low L-dopa/DA levels ("off" phase dyskinesia), and when L-dopa/DA levels are rising and falling, that is at the beginning and the end of the L-dopa action cycle (biphasic dyskinesia) (Marsden et al. 1981; Luquin et al. 1992; Nutt 1992; Quinn 1998). While large individual variability occurs in the phenomenology of dyskinesia at any point during the dopaminergic drug cycle, certain types of dyskinetic movements are more commonly seen during specific phases. "On"-phase dyskinesias are typically characterized by choreiform and choreo-dystonic movements that appear spontaneously but are provoked or exaggerated by mental stress, speaking, and physical activity (Marsden et al. 1981; Luquin et al. 1992; Nutt 1992; Durif et al. 1999). "On"-phase dyskinesias can affect virtually any muscle group, but predominate in the upper body (Luquin et al. 1992; Nutt 1992). Biphasic dyskinesias typically manifest as stereotypic, repetitive, or ballistic movements, and/or dystonia, which most commonly affect the legs and feet. In the "off" phase, dystonic posturing, typically affecting the lower limbs, is the predominant type of dyskinesia (Marsden et al. 1981; Luquin et al. 1992; Nutt 1992; Quinn 1998). Dyskinesias constitute a cosmetic problem, but they may also be a cause of disability as they interfere with the execution of any physiological motor activity.

Pharmacological treatments that either prevent the occurrence of dyskinesia or reduce their severity once they have developed would clearly have an important role in PD (Bezard et al. 2001). At present, the only pharmacological treatment for alleviating dyskinesia is the noncompetitive *N*-methyl-D-aspartate (NMDA) receptor antagonist, amantadine (for review see Blanchet et al. 2003), which is not well tolerated by all patients. Lesions or electrical stimulation in the deep basal ganglia nuclei, such as the subthalamic nucleus and the pars interna of the globus pallidus, represent an effective palliative treatment for dyskinesia in the most severe cases (Benabid et al. 2000; Lang 2000). There are also indications that co-treatment with L-dopa and long-acting DA receptor agonists, such as cabergoline, may lead to a gradual reduction of dyskinesias and expand the therapeutic window of L-dopa (Hadj Tahar et al. 2000; Odin et al. 2003).

II. DEVISING NEW TREATMENTS FOR PARKINSON DISEASE THROUGH RESEARCH ON ANIMAL MODELS

The current problem for treating PD lies in the lack of therapies that can provide a long-term benefit in the absence of disabling complications. Devising novel efficacious treatments for the future is an important goal for both preclinical and clinical investigators in the Parkinson field. New therapeutic options can be classified in three main categories: (1) *neuroprotective treatments*, which aim at halting the neurodegenerative process at the basis of PD. For example, investigators are attempting to counteract the degeneration of DA neurons through intracerebral delivery of trophic factors (Gill et al. 2003; Grondin et al. 2003) or systemic administration of antioxidants (Shults 2002; Mandel et al. 2003); (2) *restorative treatments*, which aim at restoring the integrity of the damaged nigrostriatal system by intracerebral transplant of DA-producing cells (Lindvall and Hagell 2000; Bjorklund et al. 2003), or by delivery of viral vectors encoding DA-synthesizing enzymes (Kirik et al. 2002a); (3) *symptomatic treatments*, which aim at improving the symptoms of the disease or the motor complications that result from traditional L-dopa pharmacotherapy (for review see Brotchie 1997; Bezard et al. 2001; Tuite and Riss 2003). All these research lines critically depend on the availability of suitable animal models of PD. Different animal models may be best suited for different applications. The ideal model for testing the efficacy of neuroprotective treatments would be one where the etiopathological features and time course of DA cell degeneration resemble as much as possible the neurodegenerative process in PD. In reality, no perfect etiopathological model for PD exists, since the etiology of this disease is unknown (Mandel et al. 2003). Different models reproduce slightly different features of the cell death process. Intoxication with 1-methyl-4-phenyl-1,2,5,6-tetrahydropyridin (MPTP) or 6-hydroxydopamine mainly reproduces aspects of energy failure and oxidative damage (for review see Dauer and Przedborski 2003; Mandel et al. 2003). Novel promising models reproduce aspects of protein aggregation and failure of protein degradation (Kirik et al. 2002b; Kirik et al. 2003; McNaught et al. 2001). When the aim of experiments is to devise purely symptomatic or restorative treatments for PD, the way DA cells die may not be so crucial, as long as the model presents with stable DA denervation that is sufficiently severe for motor deficits to appear. Indeed, restorative or symptomatic interventions aim at restoring function when the nigrostriatal DA system has already undergone a considerable degree of damage. Costs and labor are important aspects for investigators to consider when selecting a model for large-scale pharmacological screening experiments. Finally, adequate behavioral testing routines are a critical issue for the preclinical screening of any type of intervention. Even when studying neuroprotection researchers must evaluate both the anatomical integrity of the nigrostriatal system and the behavioral recovery produced by the treatment, as the relationship between anatomical and functional measures of treatment outcome is not always clear and straightforward (Rosenblad et al. 2000; Cenci et al. 2002). An important example is provided by the neuroprotective effect of intranigral GDNF infusion in 6-hydroxydopamine (6-OHDA) lesioned rats, which can preserve the integrity of nigral DA cell bodies but does not achieve a significant recovery of behavioral deficits (Rosenblad et al. 2000). Adequate symptomatic models of Parkinsonian-like motor deficits or treatment-related motor complications in animals should reproduce the main functional features of the corresponding human symptom and show a similar response to the effects of manipulations that either exacerbate or ameliorate the symptom (Cenci et al. 2002).

III. THE 6-HYDROXYDOPAMINE (OHDA) LESION MODEL OF PARKINSONISM IN THE RAT

At the end of the sixties, Ungerstedt and collaborators reported that the catecholamine-selective neurotoxin, 6-OHDA could be injected at the origin of the ascending nigrostriatal DA pathway to produce a nearly complete depletion of DA in the ipsilateral side of the brain (Ungerstedt 1968). Rats sustaining unilateral injections of the toxin showed a postural asymmetry at rest and exhibited turning behavior when challenged with direct or indirect DA agonists (Ungerstedt 1976). Since this seminal description, rats with unilateral 6-OHDA lesions have been the most commonly used animal model of PD. This model is cost-effective and non-laborious. Since the lesion is unilateral, the animals are not disabled in their daily activities and do not need to be force-fed after the surgery. Moreover, the side contralateral to the lesion serves as a within-animal control for behavioral, cellular, molecular, or biochemical studies. Injections of the toxin at the origin of the nigrostriatal DA bundle produces large (>97%) DA depleting lesions, which model a very advanced stage of PD. Injections of 6-OHDA in the terminal field of the nigrostriatal pathway produce partial and more slowly progressing lesions that are particularly suitable for testing the effects of neuroprotective interventions (Sauer and Oertel 1994; Kirik et al. 1998).

Drug-induced rotation is the most widely used test in studies using unilaterally 6-OHDA lesioned rats. After challenge with direct or indirect DA receptor agonists, a rat will turn in the direction opposite to the side where DA receptor stimulation is greater. Indirect DA receptor agonists, such as amphetamine, produce DA release from intact nigrostriatal terminals. This treatment will therefore cause a unilaterally 6-OHDA lesioned rat to rotate away from the intact side of the brain, that is, in the same direction as the 6-OHDA lesion (ipsiversive rotation). In contrast, administering direct DA receptor agonists will cause a rat to rotate away from the 6-OHDA lesioned side (contraversive rotation), where striatal DA receptors are supersensitive because of the denervation. Drug-induced rotation is the most commonly used test to assess the extent of unilateral DA denervating lesions, and the relationship between rotational rates and degree of striatal DA depletion or nigral DA cell loss was established in several studies (Schmidt et al. 1982; Carman et al. 1991). Rotational tests are also a well-established procedure to monitor the effects of interventions that promote the sparing of intrinsic DA fibers (neuroprotective treatments) or the new growth of DA fibers from intrastriatal grafts (for review see Schwarting and Huston 1996). Contraversive rotation is also extensively used to predict antiparkinsonian efficacy in drug screening experiments. Indeed, all conventional antiparkinsonian agents have agonistic properties at DA receptors, and cause contralateral rotation in unilaterally 6-OHDA lesioned rats. However, antiparkinsonian compounds that do not exert their effect by stimulating DA receptors would not necessarily cause contralateral rotation (see, for example, Fenu et al. 1997).

Drug-induced rotation tests have many advantages. They are not laborious since they are automated and do not require rats to be pretrained. They provide an outcome measure (number of turns) that is objective and exhibits a wide dynamic range. They can be repeated on several occasions during long-term experiments and yet maintain a high degree of reliability (provided that the inter-trial interval is sufficiently long to avoid sensitization and conditioning phenomena (Schwarting and Huston 1996). These tests do have some limitations. Drug-induced rotation is an artificial behavior of uncertain classification, which lacks any obvious counterpart in humans (for review see Cenci et al. 2002). This may pose interpretational problems in a number of applications. In particular, contralateral rotation per se cannot distinguish between dyskinetic and anti-akinetic effects of antiparkinsonian drug treatments (Lundblad et al. 2002). Moreover, when neuroprotective or restorative interventions in the rat are evaluated, the reversal of lesion-induced rotational patterns may not be accompanied by improvements in more complex and physiologically relevant behaviors (Abrous et al. 1993; Isacson 1995; Metz and Whishaw 2002). Finally, rotational behavior depends on mesolimbic systems involved in the control of locomotion in the rat, such as ventral striatal-ventral pallidal circuits (Kelly and Moore 1976; Swerdlow and Koob 1984; Brundin et al. 1987), and these systems do not seem to be implicated in the pathophysiology of Parkinsonian motor symptoms (Brooks 2003).

For these reasons, many laboratories have made increasing efforts to devise, characterize, and validate more articulate behavioral testing routines for 6-OHDA lesioned rats.

IV. TESTS OF PHYSIOLOGICAL MOTOR BEHAVIOR

Investigators have applied many tests with success for evaluating physiological motor performance in 6-OHDA-lesioned rats. Qualitative assessments of motor behavior in 6-OHDA-lesioned rats have revealed motor patterns that are reminiscent of Parkinsonian motor features in humans (Miklyaeva et al. 1995; Whishaw et al. 2002), including tremor (for review see Cenci et al. 2002). Although qualitative observations are extremely important for interpreting the significance of one's models, such observations offer limited possibilities in the screening of new treatments, where quantitative measures of efficacy are needed. Some of the tests that provide quantitative measures of adaptive, sensorimotor behavior are listed in Table 1. Different tests evaluate different behavioral features and may differ greatly on several crucial aspects, for example, dynamic range, need for animal pretraining or aversive motivation, and feasibility of repeated testing during long-term experiments. The dynamic range is the range of numerical values that the test's outcome variable can have between the two end points represented by total motor impairment and a normal performance. A sufficiently large dynamic range is required to compare degrees of motor improvement (or motor disability) produced by different interventions. Most of the tests listed in Table 1 detect an altered motor performance even after pathological conditions that are different from PD, such as ischemic brain damage. Because of this potential lack of specificity, the researcher must verify the relevance of testing paradigms to PD by showing some relationship between the magnitude of the behavioral deficit in rats and the extent of striatal DA depletion and an improvement in the test's outcome measure(s) after L-dopa treatment.

In the following chapter we shall present the tests that are used in our laboratory for evaluating the therapeutic efficacy of antiparkinsonian drug treatment in the rat. We first provide methodological information and then discuss the range of applicability and the pros and cons of each test in the light of our experience. Although devised and optimized through research in the 6-OHDA lesion model, the tests described below are also suitable for application to other models of unilateral Parkinsonism in the rat (Kirik et al. 2002b).

A. The Stepping Test

Originally described by Schallert and collaborators (Schallert et al. 1992), the stepping test assesses a rat's ability to adjust its steps in response to experimenter-imposed lateral movements. The test does not require any special equipment other than a table surface (approx. 90–100 cm in length). This test has been renamed and modified in different studies, for example, the bracing test (Schallert and Tillerson 2000); akinesia test (Olsson et al. 1995; Lindner et al. 1996); forepaw adjusting steps (Chang et al. 1999). Here we describe the methodology that is used in our laboratory. The experimenter firmly holds a rat by lifting up its hindlimbs and one forelimb, but letting the unrestrained paw contact the table surface. Then, the experimenter moves the rat sideways (in the forehand direction) across the table at a predefined speed (0.9 m in five seconds), counting the number of adjusting steps that the animal performs to catch up with the translocation of the body. The animals are habituated to the handling associated with this test for a few days. The test is then applied twice daily on three consecutive days to reach a stable baseline performance before the experimenter evaluates the effect of different interventions.

The function specifically measured by this test is a rat's ability to use its forelimb to maintain center of gravity when rapid weight shifts are imposed. Parkinsonian-like motor features, such as akinesia and postural abnormalities, negatively affect this ability. Rats with unilateral 6-OHDA lesions show a dramatic deficit in this test, dragging the forelimb contralateral to the lesion across the table and making either very few or no adjusting steps. A clear inverse relationship exists between the extent of DA-denervation on the side of the striatum ipsilateral to the lesion and the performance of the contralateral forelimb (Kirk et al. 2001). Investigators have obtained validation of this test as a method for antiparkinsonian drug screening by showing that

TABLE 1 Quantitative Tests Evaluating Sensorimotor Function in 6-OHDA Lesioned Rats

Test name	Task or function measured	Original description (or review)	Type of lesion	Improved by L-DOPA or DA agonists
Reaction time	Lever pressing after visual cue	Arnolric et al. (1995) *Eur J Neurosci* 7:972–980	Bilateral 6-OHDA	Yes (chronic treatment)
Reaction time	Head orientation to eccentric visual cues	Carli et al. (1985) *Nature* 313:679–682	Unilateral 6-OHDA	Not known
Reactive capacity	Release of a lever to escape footshock	Spirduse et al. (1985) *Brain Res* 335:45–54	Unilateral 6-OHDA	Not known
Sensorimotor orientation	Head onentation to body touch	Marshall et al. (1980) *Comp Phys Psy* 94:833–846	Unilateral 6-OHDA	Yes
Disengage behaviour	Switching between eating behavior and orientation to somatosensory stim.	Schallert and Hall (1988) *Behav Brain Res* 30:15–24	Unilateral 6-OHDA	Not known
Muscle tone (rigidity)	Hinding resistance to passive movement EMG recordings	Wolfarth et al. (1996) *Neuroscience* 74:985–996	Bilateral 6-OHDA	Not known
Tremor	Tremulous jaw movements	Salamone et al. (1998) *Prog Neurobiol* 56:591–611	Bilateral 6-OHDA	Yes
Foot print analysis	Gait pattern and stride length	Schallert et al. (1978) *Science* 199:1461–1463	Bilateral 6-OHDA	Not known
Rotarod test	General locomotor coordination	Rozas et al. (1997) *Brain Res Protoc* 2:75–84	Unilateral 6-OHDA	Yes
Videomonitored rotarod	Rating scales of postures and movements during rotarod stepping	Whishaw et al. (2003) *J Neurosci Meth* 126:13–23	Unilateral 6-OHDA	Not known
The staircase test	Independent limb use for reaching and grasping food pellets	Montoya et al. (1991) *J Neurosci Meth* 36:219–228	Unilateral 6-OHDA	No
The pasta matrix test	Retrieving pieces of straight uncooked pasta arranged in a matrix	Ballermann et al. (2001) *J Neurosci Meth* 106:39–45	Unilateral 6-OHDA	No
Forelimb akinesia test	Independent limb use of movement initiation	Schallert et al. (1992) 3:332–333	Unilateral 6-OHDA	Yes
Stepping (bracing) test	Adjusting steps induced by a passive, lateral translocation of the body	Olsson et al. (1995) *J Neurosci* 15:3863–3875 Rodter et al. (2000) *Cell Transplant* 9:197–214	Unilateral 6-OHDA Bilateral 6-OHDA	Yes Not known
Postural adjustment	Capacity to maintain balance when a rat is pushed laterally by the investigator	Rodter et al. (2000) *Cell Transplant* 9:197–214	Bilateral 6-OHDA	Not known
Cylinder test	Independent forelimb use for weight shifting during vertical exploration	Schallert et al. (2000) *Neuropharmacology* 39:777–787	Unilateral 6-OHDA	Yes

the performance of the affected forelimb is significantly improved after treatment with L-dopa and DA-receptor agonists (Olsson et al. 1995; Lindner et al. 1996; Chang et al. 1999; Lundblad et al. 2002). The improvement induced by these treatments is maintained even when the rats develop dyskinesia (Figure 1). Indeed, the fact that the rat is firmly held by the investigator during the test counteracts the disabling effect of dyskinesia on the coordination of limb movements (Winkler et al. 2002). This issue constitutes a potential problem for drug-screening studies, because it implies that the test could not distinguish between truly beneficial treatments and treatments that relieve akinesia at the expense of producing abnormal movements and postures. Another potential caveat of the test lies in the need for direct, close, and continuous physical interaction between the animal and the investigator. This requirement implies that the experimenter's proficiency conditions the reproducibility of the test. In our experience, experimenters must handle the rat as gently and consistently as possible among all testing sessions. Any methodological inconsistency may cause a rat to perceive stress or fear, and thus attempt to escape from the hands of the experimenter. Rapid, self-initiated steps may cause the experimenter to overestimate the effects of the tested treatment (or to underestimate the effects of the lesion). A stable baseline performance must therefore be established in each rat prior to testing any intervention. The test lends itself to repeated applications during long-term experiments, although experimenters should check regularly for changes in baseline performance during the course of the experiment. For this purpose, a blind cross-over design is recommended, whereby experimenters examine rats after the injection of either the tested drug or its vehicle on consecutive days (see, for example, Winkler et al. 2002).

B. The Staircase Test

Originally introduced by Montoya and collaborators (Montoya et al. 1991), the staircase test evaluates a rat's ability to use its forelimbs to reach for small objects and pick them up. The test is also called the "paw-reaching test." The test apparatus consists of a narrow Plexiglas box (285 × 90 × 60 mm) accommodating a double staircase, which is positioned along the sides of a central platform. This platform provides a support for the rat's body. The rat must stretch its forelimbs down each side of the platform to retrieve food pellets that are loaded on each stair. The central platform is sufficiently high to prevent the forelimbs from crossing over between the two sides. In our test apparatus, the staircases are baited with ten sugar pellets per step (Noyes Inc., England), on four steps on each side. The outcome measures provided by the test are the number of pellets taken and the number of pellets eaten, which can amount to a maximum count of forty per paw. If the rat drops

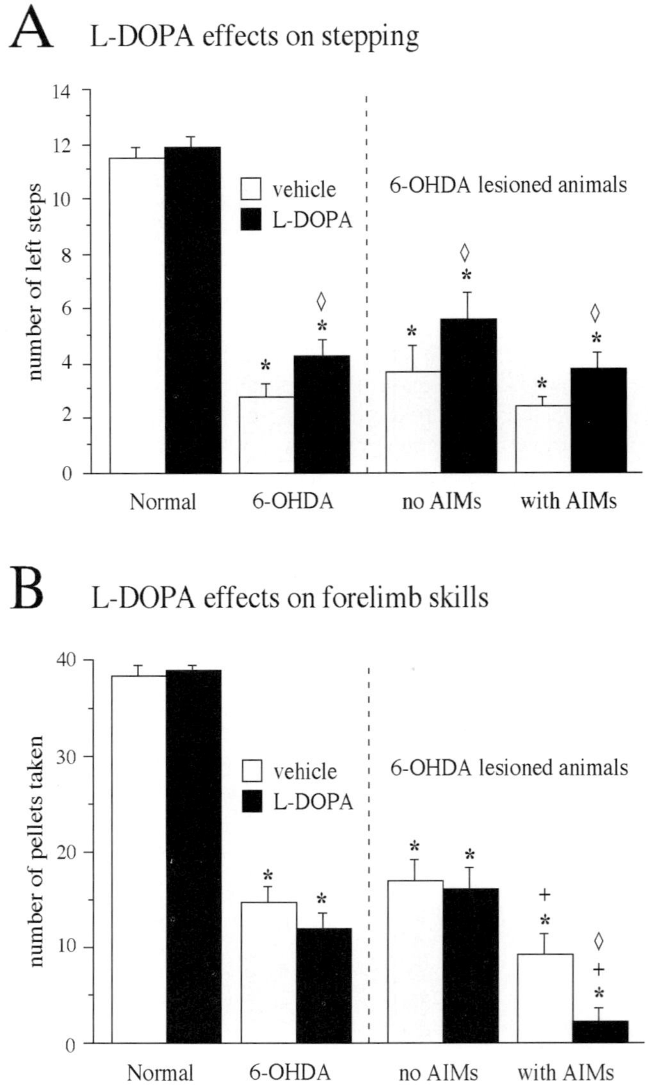

FIGURE 1 Stepping test and staircase test: effects of 6-OHDA lesions and L-dopa treatment. These data were collected from a large (n = 52) group of rats with unilateral 6-OHDA lesions ("6-OHDA"). The lesioned rats or a group of non-lesioned controls ("Normal") had been treated chronically with a dose of L-dopa that was just above threshold to produce a significant improvement in the stepping test (6 mg/kg methyl L-dopa, combined with 15 mg/kg benserazide; single daily ipsilateral [ip] injections). The left-hand panel in A shows that the 6-OHDA lesion reduced the number of steps performed with the contralateral paw to about 25% of normal values, and that L-dopa treatment enhanced the level of performance to about 40% of normal. In the right-hand panel, the same 6-OHDA lesioned rats are divided in two subgroups based on the presence or absence of dyskinesia ("with AIMs" and "no AIMs," respectively). This analysis shows that the motor improvement produced by L-dopa in this test is not affected by the presence of dyskinesia. In B, the same rats were examined for their performance in the staircase test. The left-hand panel in B shows that the number of pellets taken with the paw contralateral to the lesion was reduced to approximately 40% of normal values in the 6-OHDA lesioned rats, and that it was not improved at all by L-dopa treatment. The right-hand panel in B shows that rats exhibiting dyskinesia in response to L-dopa ("with AIMs") actually performed worse in this test after the the drug was administered, compared to vehicle. These tests were performed between forty-five and sixty minutes after the injection of L-dopa. * $p < 0.05$ vs. normal controls; $p < 0.05$ vs performance of the same rats after vehicle; (in B) + $p < 0.05$ vs. 6-OHDA lesioned rats without AIMs sustaining the same (vehicle or L-dopa) treatment (from Winkler et al. 2002). (Reproduced by permission of Elsevier Publishing Ltd.)

a pellet after taking it up, the pellet will fall down in a compartment of the box that is not accessible to the rat. This allows the investigator to estimate the success rate in the test, as defined by the ratio between "pellets eaten" and "pellets taken." DA denervation affects all components of the performance of the contralateral paw, that is, attempt, motor coordination, and success (Montoya et al. 1991; Barneoud et al. 1995; Barneoud et al. 2000). There is a close relationship between the number of pellets taken and eaten on the side contralateral to the lesion and the degree of DA depletion in the lesioned striatum (Barneoud et al. 1995; Kirik et al. 1998). Moreover, the test is highly sensitive to even mild DA-depleting lesions. Indeed, partial DA denervating lesions that are targeted on the dorsal striatum and do not result in either apomorphine-induced rotation or stepping deficits cause a significant impairment in the staircase test (Barneoud et al. 2000). These features make the test suitable for monitoring the effects of manipulations that either deplete or restore DA terminals in the striatum in a graded way. Improved performance in the staircase test depends on a precise anatomical restoration of the DA input to the critical striatal region, as obtained by such approaches as intrastriatal delivery of GDNF (Kirik et al. 2001). Interventions that attain only a partial anatomical restoration of the nigrostriatal DA pathway, such as transplants of fetal ventral mesencephalic neurons, have a limited ability to improve performance in this test (Abrous et al. 1993; Nikkhah et al. 2001). Likewise, pharmacological DA replacement with L-dopa does not significantly improve performance in this test, if results are expressed as the number of pellets taken or eaten (Winkler et al. 2002). L-dopa treatment may however increase the likelihood that the rat successfully retrieves pellets by the paw contralateral to the lesion, as reflected by the ratio between pellets eaten and pellets taken (Lundblad and Cenci unpublished). When treatment with L-dopa induces dyskinesia, the rat's performance in the staircase test is dramatically worsened compared to baseline levels (Figure 2). These results can easily be explained by the fact that dyskinesias disrupt the precision and coordination of limb movements (Hagell and Widner 1999).

The staircase test is usually referred to as a test of skilled forelimb use, although it also depends on the rat's ability to learn a new and complex motor pattern. Indeed, it may take ten consecutive days of testing for a normal rat to reach a stable and optimal performance in this test (Lundblad and Cenci unpublished). The staircase test provides several advantages: it has a good dynamic range and it assesses a physiological type of motor behavior that has a clear adaptive value for the animal. As stated above, the performance in this test is very sensitive to the effects of interventions

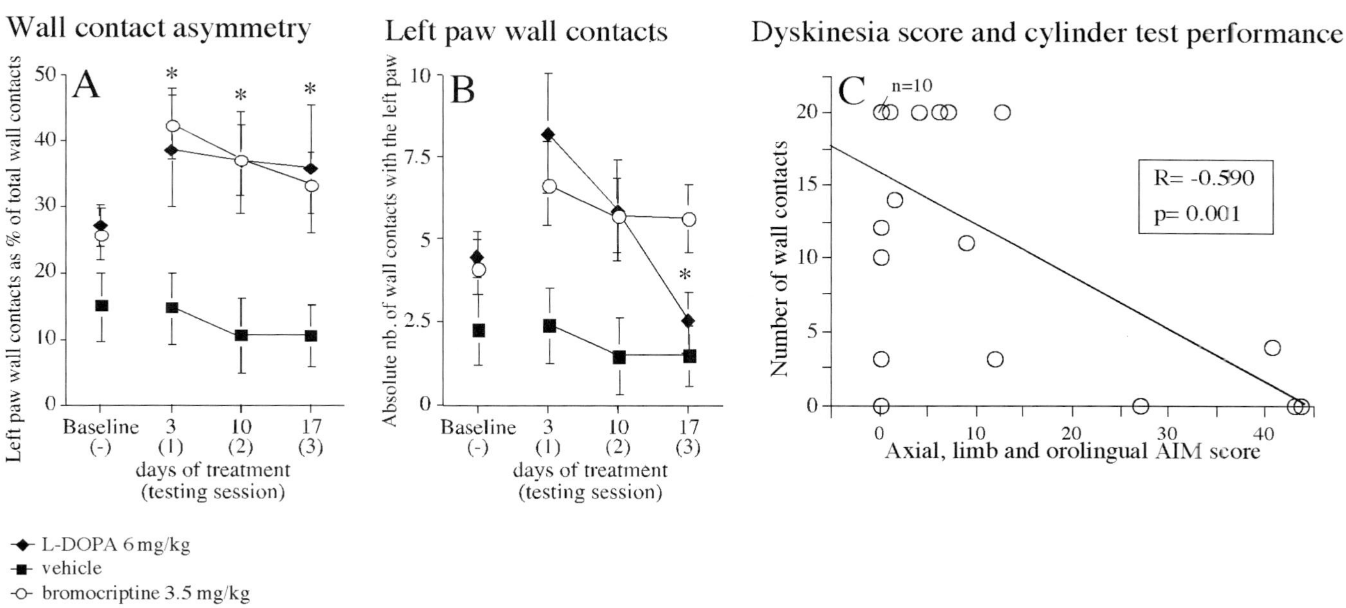

FIGURE 2 Effects of anti-Parkinsonian drug treatment on the rat's performance in the cylinder test. The cylinder test was executed both before ("baseline") and during a three-week course of treatment with either L-dopa (6 mg/kg/day combined with benserazide, 15 mg/kg; n = 14), bromocriptine (3.5 mg/kg/day; n = 14), or vehicle (n = 8). Limb use asymmetry (i.e., the percentage of wall contacts performed with the Parkinsonian [left] paw) is shown in A, while the absolute number of wall contacts performed with this paw is shown in B. Animals affected by severe L-dopa-induced dyskinesia (grade 4 AIMs) performed zero wall contacts and were therefore excluded from the computation of a percentage value in A. The plot in C shows that an inverse relationship exists between the absolute number of wall contacts performed in the cylinder test and the rats'AIM scores. * $p < 0.05$ vs. vehicle (From Lundblad et al. 2002). (Reproduced by permission of Blackwell Publishing Ltd.)

that cause depletion or restoration of striatal DA fiber terminals. A potential disadvantage of the test lies in its complexity. The performance in this test depends not only on the animals' fine motor skills but also on learning and motivational components. Indeed, rats that learn the test prior to the 6-OHDA lesion show a much milder degree of impairment post-lesion (Lundblad and Cenci unpublished).

A regimen of partial food deprivation lasting for a few days before and during the test is necessary in order for the rat to perform in the test. Researchers should consider the need for food deprivation of animals when planning complex experiments that require multiple testing with and without drug treatments. For example, we have found that a lower dose of L-dopa is required to produce appreciable dyskinetic effects when the drug is administered to food-deprived rats. Indeed, L-dopa competes with dietary amino acids for transport across the blood-brain barrier (Pincus and Barry 1987).

C. The Cylinder Test

The cylinder test, which was originally described by Schallert and Tillerson (2000), assesses the independent use of each forelimb in the context of a naturally occurring behavior. The test takes advantage of rats' innate drive to explore a novel environment by standing on their hind limbs and using their forelimbs to lean on the enclosing walls. To perform this test, rats are put individually in a glass cylinder (21 cm diameter, 34 cm height) and video recorded for five minutes. The rats are not habituated to the cylinder prior to filming. Investigators then use the video recordings to count the number of supporting wall contacts the rat executes with the right and the left paw. Only supporting wall contacts are counted, that is, appositions of the paw to the walls of the cylinder with fully extended digits. We usually count up to a maximum of twenty wall contacts per session. To stimulate rats that show little or no tendency to explore, we apply the following maneuvers in this given order: (1) turn the room light on and off two to three times, and then leave it off with only a red light bulb as a source of illumination, (2) mildly shake the cylinder for two to three seconds (red light on), and (3) take the rat out of the cylinder for less than thirty seconds and then put it back.

Researchers use the results from the cylinder test to compute a limb-use asymmetry score, either by expressing the performance of the contralateral limb as a percentage of the total performance (Lundblad et al. 2002), or by subtracting the percentage of wall contacts executed by the impaired limb from the percentage of the non-impaired limb (Picconi et al. 2003). A rat with unilateral 6-OHDA lesions uses the paw contralateral to the lesion in about 10–30% of all supporting wall contacts, whereas a normal rat uses the right and the left paw indifferently in this test (Figure 2). The dynamic range of this test is therefore relatively narrow (from approximately 20% to 50%). Another potential disadvantage of the test lies in the fact that it cannot be repeated too often, or else the rat will lose interest in exploring the novel environment and will not perform at all. In our hands, a testing frequency of one session per week over two months may still be feasible, but additional repetitions of the tests will compromise its sensitivity (Lundblad et al. 2002).

Despite these potential caveats, the cylinder test offers some notable advantages: it is very rapid in its execution, it does not require any particular experience on the part of the investigator, nor does it require pretraining of the animals. The test provides a true measure of spontaneous forelimb use as the movements exhibited by the rat in the testing cylinder are identical to those performed in the home cage. The performance in the cylinder test is improved by treatment with L-dopa and bromocriptine (Figure 2A) and it is disrupted by the appearance of dyskinesia (Figure 2B). The dependence on an intact nigrostriatal system, the improvement produced by antiparkinsonian medications, and the sensitivity of the outcome measure to the disrupting effect of L-dopa-induced dyskinesia fully validate the cylinder test as a method for the preclinical screening of antiparkinsonian treatments in the rat.

D. The Rotarod Test

The rotarod test is widely used to generally assess motor performance in rats and mice (Zausinger et al. 2000; Luesse et al. 2001; Jeong et al. 2003; Karl et al. 2003). The test measures a rat's ability to maintain itself on a rod that turns at accelerating speeds. Rozas and Labandeira Garcia (Rozas et al. 1997; Rozas and Labandeira Garcia 1997) were the first to report that performance in this test is disrupted after unilateral 6-OHDA lesions and improved after treatment with DA receptor agonists, a finding that was confirmed in our laboratory (Lundblad et al. 2003; Picconi et al. 2003). The same authors introduced a simple formula to express rotarod performance as the integral of time spent on the rod at different rotational speeds (Rozas et al. 1997). Thanks to this formula, the rotarod test has gained an extremely wide dynamic range, and is very sensitive to detecting graded improvements or graded deterioration of motor function after different types of interventions.

The following description explains how the test is applied in our laboratory. Our rotarod apparatus is a Rotamex 4/8 from Columbus Instruments (Ohio, USA). We pretrain the rats during three sessions on three consecutive days, where each session includes two separate testing trials. In the testing trials the animals are placed on the testing rod at an initial speed of 4 rotations per minute (rpm). Then the rod speed increased gradually to 44 rpm over ninety seconds. We tap the animals on their tails several times in each session, because we have found that this action helps them stay more alert in the test. The time spent on the rod is

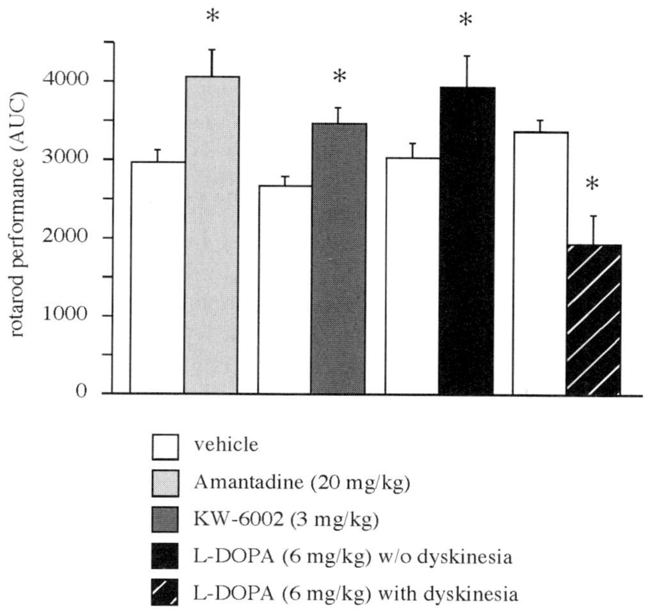

FIGURE 3 Effects of anti-Parkinsonian drug treatment and dyskinesia on the performance of unilaterally 6-OHDA lesioned rats in the rotarod test. The first three pairs of bars from the left show that the overall performance in the rotarod test (area under the curve [AUC]; see text) is significantly improved after acute administration of the following anti-Parkinsonian drugs: amantadine (20 mg/kg ip., light gray), the A2a receptor antagonist KW-6002 (3 mg/kg p.o., dark gray), and L-dopa (6 mg/kg combined with 12 mg/kg benserazide ip, black solid bars). Investigators assess the improvement each drug produces by comparing the performance of the same animals after administering the corresponding vehicle (empty bars). The last pair of bars (to the right) shows the L-dopa-treated animals after several weeks of chronic treatment with this drug, causing severe dyskinesia to develop (black striped bars). The dyskinetic movements interfere with the rats'ability to perform in the rotarod test, and the AUC value is now dramatically reduced after the injection of L-dopa compare to vehicle. All experiments were carried out using a randomized cross-over design, whereby the same rats were tested after the injection of a drug or its corresponding vehicle over two consecutive days. An experimentally blinded investigator tested animals. $^{*}p < 0.05$ vs. vehicle.

recorded automatically for each animal, and the average performance in the two consecutive trials is used for within-animal comparisons. Between the two testing trials, all animals are allowed to remain on the rod over twenty-five seconds at a lower range of rotating speeds (from 4 rpm to 14 rpm). We have found that this intermediate session has a positive effect on the animals' willingness to perform in the test (probably because the rats learn that they can remain on the rod despite its accelerating rotation). By the last of these three pretraining sessions, all animals reach a stable baseline performance and they can be used to evaluate the effects of antiparkinsonian treatments. For this purpose, we recommend a blind cross-over design whereby rats are examined after the injection of either the tested drug or its vehicle on two consecutive days of testing (see Lundblad et al. 2003).

Rotarod performance is affected by virtually any abnormality of the motor system. However, the test has fulfilled all the essential criteria for validation in the field of preclinical Parkinson research. Indeed, performance in this test depends on an intact nigrostriatal DA system, and is improved by treatment with L-dopa and other antiparkinsonian agents (Lundblad et al. 2003). Moreover, the treatment-induced improvement is compromised when the animal develops severe dyskinesia (Lundblad et al. 2003; Picconi et al. 2003) (see Figure 3). According to our experience, the rotarod test is the most sensitive method for screening drugs that aim to improve Parkinsonian disability without causing dyskinesia (Figure 3). The rotarod test also helps assess anti-dyskinetic treatments in the rat. Indeed, the test can be used to determine whether candidate anti-dyskinetic drugs attain a functionally meaningful and specific reduction of dyskinesia as opposed to a general motor depressant effect. Another advantage of the rotarod test lies in the fact that its sensitivity is not lost upon repeated application in long-term experiments. The test requires relatively high accuracy and consistency on the part of the investigator, perhaps not as high as in the stepping test, but certainly higher than in the cylinder and staircase tests. Indeed, any stressful situation severely compromises the rat's "willingness" to perform in the rotarod test.

V. EVALUATION OF DYSKINESIA IN THE RAT

Although L-dopa is still the most effective treatment for PD, its ability to provide symptomatic relief is compromised by a development of motor fluctuations and dyskinesia in the majority of the patients (Obeso et al. 2000). Novel treatments for PD will be successful to the extent that they can either retard or prevent the development of these complications. Chase and collaborators described and successfully implemented a rat model of L-dopa-induced wearing-off fluctuations and dose failure episodes (Papa et al. 1994; Papa et al. 1995).

Traditionally, experimental studies of L-dopa-induced dyskinesia were carried out only in nonhuman primates. Our group has made systematic and serial observations in unilaterally 6-OHDA-lesioned rats treated with L-dopa, and reported that these animals do exhibit a range of abnormal movements and postures affecting the orofacial region, the limbs, and the trunk. These abnormal involuntary movements (AIMs) are asymmetric and mainly affect the side of the body contralateral to the lesion. Rat AIMs present many functional and phenomenological analogies to L-dopa-induced dyskinesia in PD patients. On a phenomenological level, these movements are complex and involve many different muscle groups. They include tonic torsion of the upper trunk and the neck, associated with repetitive head movements and rapid flexion movements of the forelimb

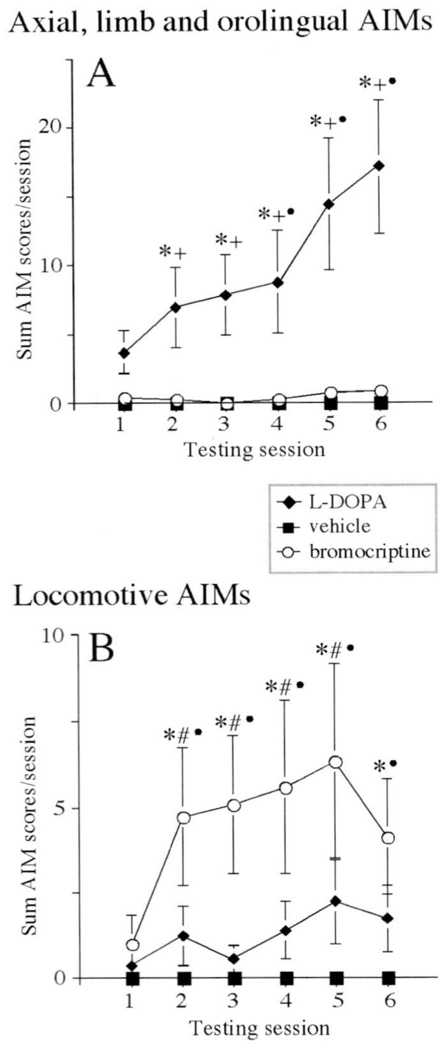

FIGURE 4 Gradual induction of abnormal involuntary movements (AIMs) during a course of chronic treatment with L-dopa or bromocriptine. The latter compound is the prototype of a class of anti-Parkinsonian agents that do not induce dyskinesia in nonhuman primate models of PD if administered de novo (i.e., without prior treatment with L-dopa). In this experiment, L-dopa, bromocriptine, or vehicle was given by single daily ip injections to L-dopa-naïve rats that had sustained unilateral 6-OHDA lesions. The treatment was given for three weeks and ratings of AIMs were carried out twice a week. The daily dose of L-dopa and bromocriptine used in this experiment produced a similar improvement in the cylinder test (see Figure 2) and a similar number of rotations on the first, acute administration. Only L-dopa treatment produced a gradual development of abnormal movements affecting the forelimb, the upper trunk, and the orofacial region, whereas bromocriptine did not significantly induce this type of dyskinesia (A). However, treatment with bromocriptine induced increasingly pronounced locomotive AIMs (B). This set of data indicates that locomotive AIMs (hence contralateral rotation) do not provide a specific measure of dyskinesia in the rat. $p < 0.05$ vs: *, vehicle; +, bromocriptine; #, L-dopa; •, testing session 1 in the same group (from Lundblad et al. 2002). (Reproduced by permission of Blackwell Publishing Ltd.)

(Video Segment 1), which are reminiscent of the choreiform "on" dyskinesias seen in patients. On a functional level, these movements are involuntary and disabling (Lee et al. 2000; Lundblad et al. 2002; Winkler et al. 2002; Lundblad et al. 2003) as are L-dopa-induced dyskinesias in PD patients (Hagell and Widner 1999). Moreover, rat AIMs are alleviated by pharmacological agents that have anti-dyskinetic efficacy in nonhuman primate models of L-dopa-induced dyskinesia and/or in PD patients (Lundblad et al. 2002; Dekundy et al. 2003), and they are not induced by antiparkinsonian treatments that have low dyskinetic potential in primates (Lundblad et al. 2002; Lundblad et al. 2003).

The rat model of dyskinesia has proven very powerful for studying the cellular and molecular underpinnings of this movement disorder (Cenci et al. 1998; Andersson et al. 1999; Johansson et al. 2001; Westin et al. 2001; Picconi et al. 2003) and is now used in an increasing number of laboratories for different applications (Mura et al. 2002; Steece-Collier et al. 2003; Delfino et al. 2004; Stefanova et al. 2004). The following description explains our laboratory's methods for recording dyskinesia. Our standard L-dopa treatment for inducing dyskinetic movements consists of single daily intraperitoneal injections of L-dopa for two to three weeks, followed by two to four injections per week to maintain stable dyskinesia scores over long-term experiments (see Lee et al. 2000; Westin et al. 2001). In most experiments we recommend including a control group of 6-OHDA lesioned rats receiving intraperitoneal injections of physiological saline. With a daily dose of 6–10 mg/kg/day L-dopa (combined with 15 mg/kg/day benserazide), approximately 50 to 80% of the treated rats develop AIMs by the end of the treatment period (Cenci et al. 1998; Andersson et al. 1999; Picconi et al. 2003). The latency for the first appearance of dyskinetic movements may vary between one and thirteen days among individual rats (Cenci et al. 1998). The incidence of dyskinesia can be boosted and its latency shortened using higher doses of L-dopa (Stefanova et al. 2004). The investigator who rates the AIMs is kept unaware of the rats' group membership and pharmacological treatment (experimentally blind). To quantify drug-induced AIMs, experimenters place rats individually in transparent cages and observe them for one minute of every twentieth minute, between 20 and 180 minutes after the injection of L-dopa.

Rat AIMs are classified into four subtypes, based on their topographic distribution: *axial AIMs*, i.e., dystonic postures or choreiform twisting of the neck and upper body towards the side contralateral to the lesion (Video Segment 1); *limb AIMs*, or abnormal, purposeless movements of the forelimb and digits contralateral to the lesion (Video Segment 2); *orolingual AIMs*, or empty jaw movements and contralateral tongue protrusion (Video Segment 3); *locomotive AIMs*, or increased locomotion with contralateral side bias (Video Segment 4). Each of these four subtypes is scored on a severity scale from 0 to 4 (1 = present during less than half of the observation time; 2 = present during more than half of the observation time; 3 = present all the time but suppressible by outer stimuli; 4 = present all the time and not suppressible). Although locomotive AIMs (contralateral rotation) are part of the dyskinetic syndrome expressed by unilaterally 6-OHDA lesioned rats, we have found out that this measure per se is not a specific predictor of dyskinesia as it may simply result from increased locomotor activity in rats that have a sensorimotor asymmetry. In fact, treatments producing either no or very mild dyskinesia may induce pronounced contralateral rotation, and hence high locomotive AIM scores, in unilaterally 6-OHDA lesioned rats (Figure 4).

The relative representation of different AIM subtypes differs among animals, but is very consistent in the same rat upon repeated testing. Lee et al. (2000) reported that different AIM subtypes are preferably associated with different postures, since locomotion requires full contact of a rats' paws with the floor and is not expressed when a rat sits on its hindlimbs. On the other hand, intense locomotor activity can mask adventitious movements of the limbs and paws. For this reason, we sometimes used maneuvers that allowed us to rate locomotive AIMs in animals that did not spontaneously express locomotion, and to rate dyskinetic limb movements in rats engaged in intense rotation (Cenci et al. 1998; Lee et al. 2000). To examine for locomotive AIMs, we gently lifted up the animal by its tail and forced it to contact the floor of the cage with the forepaws, which activated locomotor behavior. Conversely, to obtain ratings of abnormal limb movements in a "rotating" rat, we gently held and lifted up the upper part of the rat's body, while its hind paws remained in contact with the floor of the cage. This maneuver freed the rat's forelimbs from supporting floor contacts and facilitated the expression of forelimb AIMs. In this way, the theoretical maximum score that one animal could accumulate in one testing session was 144 (maximum score per observation point = 16; number of observation points per session = 9). In our latest studies we have ceased to apply these maneuvers as they do not add to the sensitivity of the test and introduce an unnecessary source of stress and variability.

To increase the sensitivity of the test, we have instead introduced an additional scale based on the amplitude of the dyskinetic limb and axial movements (box 1). This scale can be applied simultaneously with the scale described above (which is based on the duration, frequency, and persistence of the dyskinetic movements). Moreover, Steece-Collier and collaborators (2003) have recently introduced a valuable modification of the rat AIM scale where dystonic and hyperkinetic movements of the trunk and the forelimb are scored separately, each on a severity scale from 0 to 3. This improved method allows investigators to detect differential effects of treatments on dystonic versus hyperkinetic subtypes of dyskinesia, which may have a different pathophysiological substrate (Bezard et al. 2001). In particular, Steece-Collier and colleagues have reported improvements in L-dopa-induced dystonia but exacerbation of limb hyperkinesias after intracerebral neural grafting (Steece-Collier et al. 2003).

VI. OUR ADVICE ABOUT THE DYSKINESIA TEST

We are often approached by colleagues asking for practical advice about how to set up the rat dyskinesia test in their laboratories. A matter of concern pertains to the confidence with which the rat dyskinetic movements can be distinguished from naturally occurring behaviors. Overt dyskinesia that includes severe dystonic postures of the trunk and ample flexion-extension movements of the forelimb are unequivocally abnormal, and do not require any particular familiarity with the rat behavioral repertoire to be detected and rated. Some mild, "borderline" forms of dyskinetic movements, however, may require some experience to be detected and scored in a consistent way. Incipient dyskinesia of the forelimb may go unnoticed, as it may either appear to be an oscillatory movement of low amplitude (resembling tremor) or may manifest as a repeated stepping movement of the limb against the floor (A1 in box 1). However, ignoring this type of dyskinesia would not necessarily affect the experiment's outcome in a negative way, because we have noticed (Cenci and Lundblad unpublished data) that rats exhibiting these mild dyskinetic movements have not yet developed those molecular adaptations that constitute the hallmark of L-dopa-induced dyskinesia in both rodents and nonhuman primates, such as striatal upregulation of FosB and opioid precursor mRNA (for review see Cenci et al. 2002). A more difficult case occurs with stereotypic "gnawing-like" movements, which are by themselves not abnormal but may represent a rat equivalent of the biphasic dyskinesias caused by low-intermediate levels of DA in patients (see above). We are presently characterizing L-dopa-induced gnawing stereotypies with the specific aim of establishing their relationship to plasma and brain L-dopa levels. Thus far, when we encountered this type of behavior during the AIM ratings, we scored only the limb and orolingual components that showed abnormal, myoclonic, or jerky features and/or lack of symmetry.

Among the four AIM subtypes that we have described in the rat, orolingual dyskinesia is probably the most difficult subtype to rate, as it can be either overestimated or overlooked. Orolingual movements that lack specificity are movements that resemble swallowing or chewing without jaw opening in a rat that does not exhibit any other sign of dyskinesia. In particular, rats normally express these sorts of movements when they are either falling asleep or waking up. In these situations, the orolingual movements should never be scored as AIMs. Stress-induced orolingual

BOX 1 Dyskinesia Amplitude Scale

In most cases, rats display dyskinetic movements of varying amplitudes. We chose to give an amplitude score that reflects the most severe movements.

I. Amplitude of Forelimb Dyskinesia (Scale A1 to A4)

A1. Small Movements of the Paw Around a Fixed Position

There are two variants of A1: (1) while being apposed to the snout, the paw exhibits lateral translocations and circular movements. This type of behavior should be differentiated from tremor, which affects the paw contralateral to the lesion when it is at rest (i.e., in a non weight-bearing position; see video films published as an electronic link to Cenci, Whishaw, and Schallert 2002). Tremor is however not exacerbated but improved by L-dopa treatment. Moreover, a close apposition of the paw to the snout is not seen in the rat limb tremor. (2) The paw is engaged in fast and repetitive stepping-like movements with a fluttering character, that is, the paw is repetitively lifted up and down the cage floor, as if the rat were about to start going without being able to do it. Strictly speaking, this latter variant does not consist of "small movements of the paw," since the distal limb is obviously moved as well. However, we have found that this type movement represents an incipient form of forelimb dyskinesia in the same way as does the movement described above at (1).

A2. Low Amplitude Movements with Visible Translocation of the Distal Limb

Low-amplitude translocation of the limb either sideways or up-and-down (or in combination, resembling a circular movement). Practically, this means that the paw loses contact with the snout and reaches almost halfway to the floor.

A3. Notable Translocation of the Whole Limb (Both Distal and Proximal Limb)

Flexion-extension of the forelimb on the sagittal plane, or abduction-adduction on the frontal plane. More often, the movement is circular, and therefore implies both a sagittal and a frontal component. Like A4, grade A3 implies visible contraction of shoulder muscles, but the amplitude of the movement is not maximal.

A4. Vigorous Limb Movements of Maximal Amplitude and Speed with Conspicuous, Visible Contraction of Both Proximal Limb Muscles (at the Shoulder) and Extensor Muscles (Those on the Back Side of the Paw)

This practically means: (1) if the movement is circular, the limb is translocated around almost half of the circumference around the body (The movement is circular around the shoulder, but may be accompanied by flexion of the distal limb, and paw and digit movements). (2) If the movement is performed in the sagittal plane the limb is lifted up to form an angle >90° with respect to the body.

II. Amplitude of Axial Dystonia (Scale X1 to X4)

The amplitude of the axial subtype of dyskinesia is determined by the degree of deviation of the head and neck (X1, X2) or torsion of the upper trunk (X3, X4) with respect to the longitudinal axis of the rat's body.

X1. Sustained Deviation of the Head and Neck, at ~30° Angle

Make sure that the deviation is actively maintained (consistent and sustained), and exclude that the rat is simply looking at objects that are located on the side contralateral to the lesion.

X2. Sustained Deviation of the Head and Neck, Angle ≤60°

X3. Sustained Torsion of the Upper Trunk, at >60° Angle to ≤90° (Rat in Bipedal Position)

X4. Sustained Torsion of the Upper Trunk at >90° Angle, Causing the Rat to Lose Balance (from a Bipedal Position)

movements can also occur. We have noticed that even normal rats, when they are repeatedly exposed to stressful situations, can exhibit bursts of orolingual movements of considerable magnitude. To verify that a rat's orolingual movements have a dyskinetic character, we pay particular attention to the speed, magnitude, and perseverance of the movement and to its lack of symmetry. Facial grimaces should engage jaw muscles contralateral to the lesion more than the ipsilateral muscles. Tongue protrusion should be consistently directed toward the side contralateral to the lesion. One type of movement that is clearly abnormal is repetitive biting on the fur or the skin along the forelimb contralateral to the lesion. We have never seen this sort of movement in 6-OHDA rats injected with either saline or antiparkinsonian agents that do not cause dyskinesia (e.g., bromocriptine or A2a antagonists), nor have we seen it in normal rats injected with high doses of L-dopa.

In general, when the investigator is uncertain about the dyskinetic nature of a certain movement, it may help to remember that stress aggravates all forms of dyskinesia (Marsden et al. 1981; Luquin et al. 1992; Nutt 1992; Durif et al. 1999). To induce stress in a controlled way during the testing sessions we use the tail pinch stimulus, which is a well-established stressor in rodents (Antelman et al. 1975;

Rowland and Antelman 1976). We manually pinch the mid part of the rat's tail for ten seconds in a non-painful manner (i.e., the pinch does not cause the rat to squeak). This maneuver, however, should not be used indiscriminately and inconsistently. We would approve the use of tail pinch to verify or exclude the presence of dyskinesia in the following cases: (1) when the researcher is uncertain about whether or not gnawing- or grooming-like movements are part of a dyskinetic syndrome; (2) in rats that have previously shown dyskinesias but suddenly appear inactive on a certain monitoring period (however, one need not keep applying this maneuver if AIM scores have returned to 0 on two consecutive observation points at ≥100 minutes post L-dopa-injection); (3) in non-dyskinetic rats at the peak of the effect of L-dopa (i.e., at sixty and eighty minutes post injection). Tail pinch should not be applied to increase the AIM score in a rat that is already dyskinetic.

VII. CONCLUDING REMARKS

Thanks to the efforts of many investigators, a wide repertoire of behavioral testing methods have now been devised and characterized to permit a preclinical screening of anti-Parkinsonian treatments in the rat. Our laboratory has contributed to the characterization and validation of the first testing method that specifically rates L-dopa-induced abnormal involuntary movements (dyskinesia) in the rat. Since new treatments for PD will be successful to the extent that they can alleviate akinesia without producing abnormal movements and postures, the availability of a dyskinesia model in the rat represents a considerable methodological and conceptual advance. As we have illustrated in this chapter, different behavioral tests evaluate different aspects of a rat's motor function, they show different relationships to the degree of brain DA depletion, and exhibit different sensitivities to the anti-akinetic effect of L-dopa and to the disrupting effect of L-dopa-induced dyskinesia. Thus, the power and predictive validity of the 6-OHDA lesion model will be considerably increased by implementing different testing methods in the same study, or series of studies. A clear example of this concept is provided in the field of intra-cerebral transplantation. The first studies of fetal nigral grafts in the rat 6-OHDA model reported complete restoration of drug-induced rotational asymmetries. Later implementation of more articulate testing routines, however, showed that intra-cerebral grafts have a limited capacity to restore complex and physiologically more relevant behaviors (Herman et al. 1986; Mandel et al. 1990; Abrous et al. 1993). The need for articulate behavioral testing is further highlighted by the necessity to differentiate anti-akinetic treatments that restore normal motor patterns from those that also induce abnormal movements and postures. Moreover, if investigators specifically design aim at evaluating novel treatments for L-dopa-induced dyskinesia, they must combine ratings of dyskinesia with assessments of adaptive motor behavior in the same study. Indeed, clinically useful treatments against dyskinesia should eliminate abnormal movements and postures without compromising the therapeutic effect of L-dopa. Dyskinesias can indeed be reduced by treatments that have a general motor depressant effect and thus interfere with the anti-akinetic effect of L-dopa, but these treatments would obviously not bear any promise for a better management of PD. Thanks to the advances made in the behavioral analysis of 6-OHDA lesioned rats, investigators can now evaluate both anti-dyskinetic and anti-akinetic treatments for PD in the rat in a clinically relevant way.

Video Legends

SEGMENT 1 Axial dystonia/dyskinesia. After treatment with L-DOPA, rats with a unilateral 6-OHDA lesion show torsional movements and twisted postures of the trunk and the neck toward the side contralateral to the lesion. When the dystonic posture of the upper trunk is very severe it may cause the animal to lose balance and fall down to the floor, making one or more rotational movements before regaining a bipedal sitting position (note that the asymmetric body posture precedes and accompanies the rotational movement).

SEGMENT 2 Limb dyskinesia. After administration of L-DOPA, the forelimb contralateral to the lesion is engaged in hyperkinetic, fluttering movements involving both the proximal and distal forelimb and the digits. Note the random (chorea-like) variation in the direction, amplitude and frequency of the movements. The movements are purposeless and not part of the normal motor repertoire of the rat.

SEGMENT 3 Orolingual dyskinesia. These video recordings show empty, asymmetric jaw movements, associated with rapid twitching of orofacial muscles, and protrusion of the tongue towards the side contralateral to the lesion. These movements are induced by L-dopa and are not part of the grooming and gnawing behavior that is normal for a rat.

SEGMENT 4 Locomotive dyskinesia. In this sequence, the animal shows persistent hyperactive locomotion with a contralateral side bias. In our rating scale, locomotive AIM scores are given only when all four limbs contact the floor to perform an active turn (passive turns caused by side falling are not scored).

References

Abrous, D.N., A.R. Shaltot, E.M. Torres, and S.B. Dunnett. 1993. Dopamine-rich grafts in the neostriatum and/or nucleus accumbens: effects on drug-induced behaviors and skilled paw-reaching. *Neuroscience* **53**:187–197.

Andersson, M., A. Hilbertson, and M.A. Cenci. 1999. Striatal fosB expression is causally linked with l-dopa-induced abnormal involuntary movements and the associated upregulation of striatal prodynorphin mRNA in a rat model of Parkinson's disease. *Neurobiol Dis* **6**:461–474.

Antelman, S.M., H. Szechtman, P. Chin, and A.E. Fisher. 1975. Tail pinch-induced eating, gnawing, and licking behavior in rats: dependence on the nigrostriatal dopamine system. *Brain Res* **99**:319–337.

Barneoud, P., E. Descombris, N. Aubin, and D.N. Abrous. 2000. Evaluation of simple and complex sensorimotor behaviors in rats with a partial lesion of the dopaminergic nigrostriatal system. *Eur J Neurosci* **12**: 322–336.

Barneoud, P., S. Parmentier, M. Mazadier, J.M. Miquet, A. Boireau, P. Dubedat, and J.C. Blanchard. 1995. Effects of complete and partial lesions of the dopaminergic mesotelencephalic system on skilled forelimb use in the rat. *Neuroscience* **67**:837–848.

Benabid, A.L., A. Benazzouz, P. Limousin, A. Koudsie, P. Krack, B. Piallat, and P. Pollak. 2000. Dyskinesias and the subthalamic nucleus. *Ann Neurol* **47**:S189–192.

Bezard, E., J.M. Brotchie, and C.E. Gross. 2001. Pathophysiology of levodopa-induced dyskinesia: potential for new therapies. *Nat Rev Neurosci* **2**:577–588.

Bjorklund, A., S.B. Dunnett, P. Brundin, A.J. Stoessl, C.R. Freed, R.E. Breeze, M. Levivier, et al. 2003. Neural transplantation for the treatment of Parkinson's disease. *Lancet Neurol* **2**:437–445.

Blanchet, P.J., L.V. Metman, and T.N. Chase. 2003. Renaissance of amantadine in the treatment of Parkinson's disease. *Adv Neurol* **91**: 251–257.

Brooks, D.J. 2003. PET studies on the function of dopamine in health and Parkinson's disease. *Ann N Y Acad Sci* **991**:22–35.

Brotchie, J.M. 1997. Novel approaches to the symptomatic treatment of Parkinsonian syndromes: alternatives and adjuncts to dopamine-replacement. *Curr Opin Neurol* **10**:340–345.

Brown, R.G., and C.D. Marsden. 1984. How common is dementia in Parkinson's disease? *Lancet* **2**:1262–1265.

Brundin, P., R.E. Strecker, E. Londos, and A. Bjorklund. 1987. Dopamine neurons grafted unilaterally to the nucleus accumbens affect drug-induced circling and locomotion. *Exp Brain Res* **69**:183–194.

Carman, L.S., F.H. Gage, and C.W. Shults, 1991. Partial lesion of the substantia nigra: relation between extent of lesion and rotational behavior. *Brain Res* **553**:275–283.

Cenci, M.A., C.S. Lee, and A. Björklund. 1998. L-dopa-induced dyskinesia in the rat is associated with striatal overexpression of prodynorphin- and glutamic acid decarboxylase mRNA. *Eur J Neurosci* **10**:2694–2706.

Cenci, M.A., I.Q. Whishaw, and T. Schallert. 2002. Animal models of neurological deficits: how relevant is the rat? *Nat Rev Neurosci* **3**:574–579.

Chang, J.W., S.R. Wachtel, D. Young, and U.J. Kang. 1999. Biochemical and anatomical characterization of forepaw adjusting steps in rat models of Parkinson's disease: studies on medial forebrain bundle and striatal lesions. *Neuroscience* **88**:617–628.

Dauer, W., and S. Przedborski. 2003. Parkinson's disease: mechanisms and models. *Neuron* **39**:889–909.

Dekundy, A., M.A. Cenci, and W. Danysz. 2003. Clinically proven anti-dyskinetic agents are effective in a rat model of L-dopa-induced dyskinesia. In *2003 Abstract Viewer/Itinerary Planner*. pp. 757–751. Washington, D.C.: Society for Neuroscience.

Delfino, M.A., A.V. Stefano, J.E. Ferrario, I.R.E. Taravini, M.G. Murer, and O.S. Gershanik. 2004. Behavioural sensitization to different dopamine agonists in a parkinsonian rodent model of drug-induced dyskinesias. *Behav Brain Res* **152**:297–306.

Durif, F., M. Vidailhet, B. Debilly, and Y. Agid. 1999. Worsening of levodopa-induced dyskinesias by motor and mental tasks. *Mov Disord* **14**:242–245.

Duyckaerts, C., M. Verny, and J.J. Hauw. 2003. Recent neuropathology of parkinsonian syndromes. *Rev Neurol* (Paris) **159**:3S11–18.

Fahn, S. 2003. Description of Parkinson's disease as a clinical syndrome. *Ann N Y Acad Sci* **991**:1–14.

Fenu, S., A. Pinna, E. Ongini, and M. Morelli. 1997. Adenosine A2A receptor antagonism potentiates L-dopa-induced turning behavior and c-fos expression in 6-hydroxydopamine-lesioned rats. *Eur J Pharmacol* **321**: 143–147.

Gelb, D.J., E. Oliver, and S. Gilman. 1999. Diagnostic criteria for Parkinson disease. *Arch Neurol* **56**:33–39.

Gill, S.S., N.K. Patel, G.R. Hotton, K. O'Sullivan, R. McCarter, M. Bunnage, D.J. Brooks, et al. 2003. Direct brain infusion of glial cell line-derived neurotrophic factor in Parkinson disease. *Nat Med* **9**: 589–595.

Girotti, F., and P. Soliveri. 2003. Cognitive and behavioral disturbances in Parkinson's disease. *Neurol Sci* 24 Suppl **1**:S30–31.

Grondin, R., Z. Zhang, Y. Ai, D.M. Gash, and G.A. Gerhardt. 2003. Intracranial delivery of proteins and peptides as a therapy for neurodegenerative diseases. *Prog Drug Res* **61**:101–123.

Hadj Tahar, A., L. Gregoire, E. Bangassoro, and P.J. Bedard. 2000. Sustained cabergoline treatment reverses levodopa-induced dyskinesias in Parkinsonian monkeys. *Clin Neuropharmacol* **23**:195–202.

Hagell, P., and H. Widner. 1999. Clinical rating of dyskinesias in Parkinson's disease: use and reliability of a new rating scale. *Mov Disord* **14**:448–455.

Herman, J.P., K. Choulli, M. Geffard, D. Nadaud, K. Taghzouti, and M. Le Moal. 1986. Reinnervation of the nucleus accumbens and frontal cortex of the rat by dopaminergic grafts and effects on hoarding behavior. *Brain Res* **372**:210–216.

Isacson, O. 1995. Behavioral effects and gene delivery in a rat model of Parkinson's disease. *Science* **269**:856–857.

Ito, K., A. Nagano-Saito, T. Kato, Y. Arahata, A. Nakamura, Y. Kawasumi, K. Hatano, et al. 2002. Striatal and extrastriatal dysfunction in Parkinson's disease with dementia: a 6-[18F]fluoro-L-dopa PET study. *Brain* **125**:1358–1365.

Jeong, S.W., K. Chu, K.H. Jung, S.U. Kim, M. Kim, and J.K. Roh. 2003. Human neural stem cell transplantation promotes functional recovery in rats with experimental intracerebral hemorrhage. *Stroke* **34**:2258–2263.

Johansson, P.A., M. Andersson, K.E. Andersson, and M.A. Cenci. 2001. Alterations in cortical and basal ganglia levels of opioid receptor binding in a rat model of L-dopa-induced dyskinesia. *Neurobiol Dis* **8**:220–239.

Jost, W.H. 1995. Disorders of autonomic regulation in Parkinson syndrome. *Fortschr Neurol Psychiatr* **63**:194–205.

Karl, T., R. Pabst, and S. von Horsten. 2003. Behavioral phenotyping of mice in pharmacological and toxicological research. *Exp Toxicol Pathol* **55**:69–83.

Kelly, P.H., and K.E. Moore. 1976. Mesolimbic dopaminergic neurones in the rotational model of nigrostriatal function. *Nature* **263**:695–696.

Kirik, D., C. Rosenblad, and A. Björklund. 1998. Characterization of behavioral and neurodegenerative changes following partial lesions of the nigrostriatal dopamine system induced by intrastriatal 6-hydroxydopamine in the rat. *Exp Neurol* **152**:259–277.

Kirik, D., B. Georgievska, C. Rosenblad, and A. Bjorklund. 2001. Delayed infusion of GDNF promotes recovery of motor function in the partial lesion model of Parkinson's disease. *Eur J Neurosci* **13**:1589–1599.

Kirik, D., L.E. Annett, C. Burger, N. Muzyczka, R.J. Mandel, and A. Bjorklund. 2003. Nigrostriatal alpha-synucleinopathy induced by viral vector-mediated overexpression of human alpha synuclein: a new primate model of Parkinson's disease. *Proc Natl Acad Sci U S A* **100**:2884–2889.

Kirik, D., B. Georgievska, C. Burger, C. Winkler, N. Muzyczka, R.J. Mandel, and A. Bjorklund. 2002a. Reversal of motor impairments in Parkinsonian rats by continuous intrastriatal delivery of L-dopa using rAAV-mediated gene transfer. *Proc Natl Acad Sci U S A* **99**: 4708–4713.

Kirik, D., C. Rosenblad, C. Burger, C. Lundberg, T.E. Johansen, N. Muzyczka, R.J. Mandel, and A. Bjorklund. 2002b. Parkinson-like neurodegeneration induced by targeted overexpression of alpha-synuclein in the nigrostriatal system. *J Neurosci* **22**:2780–2791.

Kovari, E., G. Gold, F.R. Herrmann, A. Canuto, P.R. Hof, C. Bouras, and P. Giannakopoulos. 2003. Lewy body densities in the entorhinal and anterior cingulate cortex predict cognitive deficits in Parkinson's disease. *Acta Neuropathol* (Berl) **106**:83–88.

Lang, A.E. 2000. Surgery for levodopa-induced dyskinesias. *Ann Neurol* **47**:S193–199; discussion S199–202.

Lee, C.S., M.A. Cenci, M. Schulzer, and A. Bjorklund. 2000. Embryonic ventral mesencephalic grafts improve levodopa-induced dyskinesia in a rat model of Parkinson's disease. *Brain* **123**:1365–1379.

Lindner, M.D., M.A. Plone, J.M. Francis, and D.F. Emerich. 1996. Validation of a rodent model of Parkinson's Disease: evidence of a therapeutic window for oral Sinemet. *Brain Res Bull* **39**:367–372.

Lindvall, O., and P. Hagell. 2000. Clinical observations after neural transplantation in Parkinson's disease. *Prog Brain Res* **127**:299–320.

Luesse, H.G., J. Schiefer, A. Spruenken, C. Puls, F. Block, and C.M. Kosinski. 2001. Evaluation of R6/2 HD transgenic mice for therapeutic studies in Huntington's disease: behavioral testing and impact of diabetes mellitus. *Behav Brain Res* **126**:185–195.

Lundblad, M., E. Vaudano, and M.A. Cenci. 2003. Cellular and behavioural effects of the adenosine A2a receptor antagonist KW-6002 in a rat model of L-dopa-induced dyskinesia. *J Neurochem* **84**:1398–1410.

Lundblad, M., M. Andersson, C. Winkler, D. Kirik, N. Wierup, and M.A. Cenci. 2002. Pharmacological validation of behavioural measures of dyskinesia and akinesia in a rat model of Parkinson's disease. *Eur J Neurosci* **15**:120–132.

Luquin, M.R., O. Scipioni, J. Vaamonde, O. Gershanik, and J.A. Obeso. 1992. Levodopa induced dyskinesias in Parkinson's disease: clinical and pharmacological classification. *Mov Disord* **7**:117–124.

Mandel, R.J., P. Brundin, and A. Bjorklund. 1990. The importance of graft placement and task complexity for transplant-induced recovery of simple and complex sensorimotor deficits in dopamine denervated rats. *Eur J Neurosci* **2**:888–894.

Mandel, S., E. Grunblatt, P. Riederer, M. Gerlach, Y. Levites, and M.B. Youdim. 2003. Neuroprotective strategies in Parkinson's disease: an update on progress. *CNS Drugs* **17**:729–762.

Marsden, C.D., J.D. Parkes, and N. Quinn. 1981. Fluctuations in disability in Parkinson's disease—clinical aspects. In *Movement Disorders*. Ed. C.D. Marsden and S. Fahn. pp. 96–122. London: Butterworths.

Mayer, R.J. 2003. From neurodegeneration to neurohomeostasis: the role of ubiquitin. *Drug News Perspect* **16**:103–108.

McNaught, K.S., D.P. Perl, A.L. Brownell, and C.W. Olanow. 2004. Systemic exposure to proteasome inhibitors causes a progressive model of Parkinson's Disease. *Ann Neurol* **56**:149–162.

Metz, G.A., and I.Q. Whishaw. 2002. Drug-induced rotation intensity in unilateral dopamine-depleted rats is not correlated with end point or qualitative measures of forelimb or hindlimb motor performance. *Neuroscience* **111**:325–336.

Miklyaeva, E.I., D.J. Martens, and I.Q. Whishaw. 1995. Impairments and compensatory adjustments in spontaneous movement after unilateral dopamine depletion in rats. *Brain Res* **681**:23–40.

Montoya, C.P., L.J. Campbell-Hope, K.D. Pemberton, and S.B. Dunnett. 1991. The "staircase test": a measure of independent forelimb reaching and grasping abilities in rats. *J Neurosci Methods* **36**:219–228.

Morrish, P.K., G.V. Sawle, and D.J. Brooks. 1996. An [18F]dopa-PET and clinical study of the rate of progression in Parkinson's disease. *Brain* **119 (Pt 2)**:585–591.

Mura, A., M. Mintz, and J. Feldon. 2002. Behavioral and anatomical effects of long-term L-dihydroxyphenylalanine (L-dopa) administration in rats with unilateral lesions of the nigrostriatal system. *Exp Neurol* **177**: 252–264.

Nikkhah, G., G. Falkenstein, and C. Rosenthal. 2001. Restorative plasticity of dopamine neuronal transplants depends on the degree of hemispheric dominance. *J Neurosci* **21**:6252–6263.

Nutt, J.G. 1992. Dyskinesia induced by levodopa and dopamine agonists in patients with Parkinson's disease. In *Drug-induced Movement Disorders*. Ed. A.E. Lang and W.J. Weiner. pp. 281–314. Mount Kisko: Futura Publishing Co., Inc.

Obeso, J.A., C.W. Olanow, and J.G. Nutt. 2000. Levodopa motor complications in Parkinson's disease. *Trends Neurosci* **23**:S2–7.

Odin, P., A. Storch, U. Pollzer, G. Werner, R. Renner, M. Shing, A. Ludolph, and C. Oehlwein. 2003. High dose dopamine agonists. *Acta Neurol Scand* 108.

Olsson, M., G. Nikkhah, C. Bentlage, and A. Bjorklund. 1995. Forelimb akinesia in the rat Parkinson model: differential effects of dopamine agonists and nigral transplants as assessed by a new stepping test. *J Neurosci* **15**:3863–3875.

Papa, S.M., T.M. Engber, A.M. Kask, and T.N. Chase. 1994. Motor fluctuations in levodopa treated Parkinsonian rats: relation to lesion extent and treatment duration. *Brain Res* **662**:69–74.

Papa, S.M., R.C. Boldry, T.M. Engber, A.M. Kask, and T.N. Chase 1995. Reversal of levodopa-induced motor fluctuations in experimental Parkinsonism by NMDA receptor blockade. *Brain Res* **701**:13–18.

Picconi, B., D. Centonze, K. Hakansson, G. Bernardi, P. Greengard, G. Fisone, M.A. Cenci, and P. Calabresi. 2003. Loss of bidirectional striatal synaptic plasticity in L-dopa-induced dyskinesia. *Nat Neurosci* **6**:501–506.

Pincus, J.H., and K.M. Barry. 1987. Plasma levels of amino acids correlate with motor fluctuations in parkinsonism. *Arch Neurol* **44**:1006–1009.

Quinn, N., P. Critchley, and C.D. Marsden. 1987. Young onset Parkinson's disease. *Mov Disord* **2**:73–91.

Quinn, N.P. 1998. Classification of fluctuations in patients with Parkinson's disease. *Neurology* **51**:S25–29.

Rosenblad, C., D. Kirik, and A. Bjorklund. 2000. Sequential administration of GDNF into the substantia nigra and striatum promotes dopamine neuron survival and axonal sprouting but not striatal reinnervation or functional recovery in the partial 6-OHDA lesion model. *Exp Neurol* **161**:503–516.

Rowland, N.E., and S.M. Antelman. 1976. Stress-induced hyperphagia and obesity in rats: a possible model for understanding human obesity. *Science* **191**:310–312.

Rozas, G., and J.L. Labandeira Garcia. 1997. Drug-free evaluation of rat models of parkinsonism and nigral grafts using a new automated rotarod test. *Brain Res* **749**:188–199.

Rozas, G., M.J. Guerra, and J.L. Labandeira-Garcia. 1997. An automated rotarod method for quantitative drug-free evaluation of overall motor deficits in rat models of parkinsonism. *Brain Res Brain Res Protoc* **2**:75–84.

Sauer, H., and W.H. Oertel. 1994. Progressive degeneration of nigrostriatal dopamine neurons following intrastriatal terminal lesions with 6-hydroxydopamine: a combined retrograde tracing and immunocytochemical study in the rat. *Neuroscience* **59**:401–415.

Schallert, T., and J.L. Tillerson. 2000. Intervention strategies for degeneration of dopamine neurons in parkinsonism: optimizing behavioral assessment of outcome. In *Central Nervous System Diseases: Innovative Models of CNS Diseases from Molecule to Therapy*. Ed. D.F. Emerich, R.L. Dean III, and P.R. Sanberg. pp. 131–151. Totowa, New Jersey: Humana Press.

Schallert, T., D. Norton, and T.A. Jones. 1992. A clinically relevant unilateral model of Parkinsonian akinesia. *J Neurotranspl Plasticity* **3**:332–333.

Schmidt, R.H., M. Ingvar, O. Lindvall, U. Stenevi, and A. Björklund. 1982. Functional activity of substantia nigra grafts reinnervating the striatum: neurotransmitter metabolism and [$_{14}$C] 2-deoxy-D-glucose autoradiography. *J Neurochem* **38**:737–748.

Schrag, A., M. Jahanshahi, and N. Quinn. 2000. What contributes to quality of life in patients with Parkinson's disease? *J Neurol Neurosurg Psychiatry* **69**:308–312.

Schwarting, R.K.W., and J.P. Huston. 1996. The unilateral 6-hydroxydopamine lesion model in behavioural brain research. Analysis of functional deficits, recovery and treatments. *Prog Neurobiol* **50**:275–331.

Shults, C. 2002. Effects of coenzyme Q10 in early Parkinson's disease, evidence for slowing of the functional decline (the QE2 study). *Mov Dis* 17/Suppl. **5**:S14.

Steece-Collier, K., T.J. Collier, P.D. Danielson, R. Kurlan, D.M. Yurek, and J.R. Sladek, Jr. 2003. Embryonic mesencephalic grafts increase levodopa-induced forelimb hyperkinesia in Parkinsonian rats. *Mov Disord* **18**:1442–1454.

Stefanova, N., M. Lundblad, F. Tison, W. Poewe, M.A. Cenci, and G.K. Wenning. 2004. Effects of pulsatile L-dopa treatment in the double lesion rat model of striatonigral degeneration (multiple system Atrophy). *Neurobiol Dis* **15**:630–639.

Swerdlow, N.R., and G.F. Koob. 1984. The neural substrates of apomorphine-stimulated locomotor activity following denervation of the nucleus accumbens. *Life Sci* **35**:2537–2544.

Tuite, P., and J. Riss. 2003. Recent developments in the pharmacological treatment of Parkinson's disease. *Expert Opin Investig Drugs* **12**: 1335–1352.

Ungerstedt, U. 1968. 6-Hydroxy-dopamine induced degeneration of central monoamine neurons. *Eur J Pharmacol* **5**:107–110.

Ungerstedt, U. 1976. 6-hydroxydopamine-induced degeneration of the nigrostriatal dopamine pathway: the turning syndrome. *Pharmacol Ther* [B] **2**:37–40.

Westin, J.E., M. Andersson, M. Lundblad, and M.A. Cenci. 2001. Persistent changes in striatal gene expression induced by long-term L-dopa treatment in a rat model of Parkinson's disease. *Eur J Neurosci* **14**: 1171–1176.

Whishaw, I.Q., O. Suchowersky, L. Davis, J. Sarna, G.A. Metz, and S.M. Pellis. 2002. Impairment of pronation, supination, and body coordination in reach-to-grasp tasks in human Parkinson's disease (PD) reveals homology to deficits in animal models. *Behav Brain Res* **133**: 165–176.

Winkler, C., D. Kirik, A. Bjorklund, and M.A. Cenci. 2002. L-dopa-induced dyskinesia in the intrastriatal 6-hydroxydopamine model of Parkinson's disease: relation to motor and cellular parameters of nigrostriatal function. *Neurobiol Dis* **10**:165–186.

Zausinger, S., E. Hungerhuber, A. Baethmann, H. Reulen, and R. Schmid-Elsaesser. 2000. Neurological impairment in rats after transient middle cerebral artery occlusion: a comparative study under various treatment paradigms. *Brain Res* **863**:94–105.

CHAPTER

B8

Motor Complications in Primate Models of Parkinson Disease

FRANCESCO BIBBIANI and JUSTIN D. OH

Chronic levodopa treatment of Parkinson disease (PD) patients ultimately produces motor response complications (MRCs) that include response fluctuations and dyskinesias. Similarly, in MPTP-lesioned nonhuman primates, administering dopaminomimetics produces many of the features of the human motor complication syndromes. Recent nonhuman primate studies suggest that MRCs from the pulsatile nonphysiological stimulation of dopaminergic receptors on striatal spiny neurons increase the sensitivity of corticostriatal glutamatergic synaptic transmission. Changes to the glutamatergic signaling pathways and adenosinergic and serotonergic pathways both intrinsic and extrinsic to the striatal dopaminoceptive medium-spiny neurons also may contribute to the pathogenesis of motor dysfunction in advanced PD. As a result of these alterations, basal ganglia output changes in ways that favor the appearance of Parkinsonian signs and motor complications. Conceivably, safer and more effective therapies for PD can be provided by drugs that target signaling molecules within striatal neurons or those that interact extracellularly with nondopaminergic receptors such as *N*-methyl-D-aspartate (NMDA), amino-3-hydroxy-5-methyl-4-isoxazole proprionic acid (AMPA), adenosine, and serotonin.

I. PARKINSON DISEASE AND MOTOR RESPONSE COMPLICATIONS

A. Parkinson Disease and Levodopa Therapy

PD is a neurodegenerative disorder of unknown etiology that currently afflicts over one million Americans. The pathological hallmark of PD is a selective loss of dopaminergic neurons in the substantia nigra pars compacta in the midbrain that projects to the corpus striatum (Greenfield and Bonsaquet 1953). When the loss of dopamine (DA) exceeds 50–80%, Parkinsonian symptoms become clinically evident (Ehringer and Hornykiewcz 1960; Hornykiewcz 1963). The cardinal features of PD include resting tremor, rigidity, bradykinesia, and impaired postural reflexes (Parkinson 1817; Lang and Lonzano 1998).

Since Cotzias demonstrated the dramatic therapeutic effects of the dopamine precursor levodopa on the motor symptoms of PD patients (Cotzias et al. 1967), the prevailing therapeutic strategy has been to restore striatal dopaminergic transmission (Lang and Lonzano 1998). Initially, pharmacologic agents such as levodopa, the metabolic precursor of DA, or a direct DA receptor agonist that restores dopaminergic transmission, typically afford substantial symptomatic relief. But with disease progression, increasing difficulties arise. With DA agonists, the ability to provide adequate symptom suppression gradually declines; most agonists require levodopa supplementation within two years of initiation. With levodopa, the problem is not so much a loss of anti-Parkinsonian efficacy as a gain in adverse effects, especially motor response complications (Chase and Oh 2000). Elements of the motor complication syndrome eventually occur with all currently available dopaminomimetic therapies, although latency to onset is longer with the commonly used agonists (Marjama-Lyons and Koller 2001). Notwithstanding the introduction of several new dopaminomimetics since the discovery of levodopa, most Parkinsonian patients still become significantly disabled within ten years of symptom onset.

B. Motor Response Complications

Administering levodopa or other direct dopamine agonists alleviates the severity of Parkinsonian signs. Although levodopa is safe and effective, after a few years of levodopa therapy patients may experience motor complications from repetitive administration of dopaminergic drugs (Marsden 1990). The most common motor complications observed in humans are the involuntary and nonfinalized movements known as dyskinesias, and the reduced duration of the anti-Parkinsonian effect of the therapy, known as "wearing-off effect" (Shaw et al. 1980).

1. Motor Fluctuations

While patients with early PD characteristically enjoy a good response to levodopa, the combination of disease progression and chronic levodopa therapy eventually compromises this benefit in several ways (Marsden 1994). Over the years, the anti-Parkinsonian effect of each levodopa dose lasts for a progressively shorter time, requiring increasingly more frequent levodopa administration. At first, when the shortening of motor benefit occurs in a predictable and gradual fashion, patients are said to have wearing-off fluctuations. Subsequently, when the effect of an individual dose ceases in an unpredictable and abrupt manner, the term "on-off phenomenon" is used. Combined, motor fluctuations and dyskinesias are referred to as motor response complications (MRCs) and occur in over 50% of patients after five years of levodopa treatment (Marsden 1994).

2. Dyskinesias

In addition to these fluctuations in motor function, patients also develop involuntary movements called dyskinesias. When these symptoms first arise, they are usually associated with high levodopa levels and may be prevented or minimized by lowering the levodopa dose. Later on, however, the therapeutic window of levodopa narrows progressively and dyskinesias occur at a plasma levodopa level equal to that needed to induce an anti-Parkinson effect (obligatory dyskinesias). Dyskinesias are most commonly choreiform and occur when plasma levodopa levels are high (peak-dose dyskinesias) or, in the more advanced disease, throughout the levodopa-induced motor benefit (square-wave dyskinesias). They may also be more dystonic or ballistic in appearance and occur when levodopa levels are rising or falling (diphasic dyskinesias).

C. Therapeutic Strategies and Animal Models of Motor Response Complications

In an effort to find ways to prevent or relieve the long-term complications of levodopa treatment, investigators established animal models for the motor complication syndrome (Engber et al. 1989; Papa et al. 1994; Marin et al. 1996), conceptualized and began to characterize the functional consequences of the chronic nonphysiologic stimulation of striatal DA receptors (Mouradian et al. 1989), and began to exploit the therapeutic implications of these findings in primate models (Chase 1998). Recent studies have extended these findings in ways that advance our understanding of mechanisms contributing to the production of motor complication symptoms and enhance our ability to identify novel targets for palliative intervention. In addition, they have begun to delineate molecular mechanisms subserving motor memory and synaptic integration in striatal spiny neurons. Recent observations have also provided added support for the revolutionary concept that symptom relief in PD might be better achieved, not by replacing the deficient neurotransmitter, but rather by preventing or correcting the consequences of dopaminergic denervation at downstream sites. Clinical investigations over the past few decades have tested novel hypotheses generated by preclinical research with nonhuman primates and provided initial evidence for promising new therapeutic approaches. These translational studies have also begun to shed light on another problem plaguing late-stage Parkinsonian patients: the pathogenesis of the increasing motor disabilities—such as those involving speech, swallowing, and gait—that resist current dopaminomimetic therapy.

II. NONHUMAN PRIMATE MODELS OF MOTOR RESPONSE COMPLICATIONS

A. MPTP and Parkinson Disease

In 1982, several young drug addicts in California developed a severe Parkinson-like syndrome after injecting a potent synthetic drug containing 1-methyl-4-phenyl-1,2,3,6-tetrahydropyridine (MPTP) (Langston et al. 1983; Jenner 2003). Exposure to MPTP produced bradykinesia and rigidity, almost identical to signs exhibited by patients with idiopathic Parkinson disease (PD) (Ballard et al. 1985; Jenner 2003). Moreover, these symptoms showed optimal therapeutic response to dopamine and dopamine agonist.

B. MPTP and Nonhuman Primate Model of Parkinson Disease

The possibility of recreating a syndrome resembling the major characteristics of PD triggered researchers to develop an experimental animal model using systemic administration of MPTP. Previously, the commonly used animal model of PD was the 6-hydroxydopamine (6-OHDA) rat, which is an excellent model for testing and determining modes of action of new pharmacological compounds. However, the model lacks the behavioral features of idiopathic PD and the ability to develop motor complications closely resembling those commonly observed in Parkinsonian patients. With the exception of a few strains of mice, most rodents were highly resistant to MPTP administration. On the other hand, primates were sensitive to MPTP and developed a syndrome that resembled that observed in intoxicated humans (Burns et al. 1983). Nonhuman primates treated with MPTP show clear Parkinsonian features such as bradykinesia, rigidity, stooped posture and tremor, which, unlike idiopathic PD, are mostly postural. Once induced, the Parkinsonian syndrome remains stable over time and its symptoms show an excellent response to levodopa and other direct dopamine agonists.

Among nonhuman primates, several species develop Parkinsonism following exposure to MPTP, including marmosets, macaques, squirrel monkeys, and vervet monkeys. In addition to the bilateral model, a unilateral lesion can be produced by intracarotid administration of the neurotoxin resulting in an ipsilateral brain lesion and a contralateral hemiparkinsonian syndrome (Bankiewicz et al. 1986). This procedure yields faster lesioning of the brain and, since it is unilateral, might alleviate the invalidity that sometimes accompanies the bilateral model. Acute MPTP administration, however, does not consistently reproduce all clinical features of the disease and does not mimic the gradual evolution seen in the human pathology. The progressive degeneration of dopamine neurons observed in idiopathic Parkinson disease was first produced by injecting low doses of MPTP in baboons on a chronic basis (Hantraye et al. 1993) and successfully replicated in cynomolgus monkeys (Bezard et al. 1997; Blanchet et al. 1998).

Biochemical and histological investigations have shown that MPTP-induced Parkinsonism reflects the human disease as demonstrated by the selective degeneration of the nigrostriatal dopaminergic pathway (Stern 1990). The nerve cells in the ventrolateral portion of the substantia nigra pars compacta were particularly vulnerable (as observed in idiopathic PD) but the typical formation of Lewy bodies, another peculiar characteristic of idiopathic PD, was not observed in the monkey model. Inclusion bodies, found quite consistently in aged MPTP-lesioned monkeys, appear to be the pathological consequence of lesions in the experimental model and show some similarities to Lewy bodies (Forno et al. 1993).

C. MPTP and Nonhuman Primate Model of Motor Response Complications

After dopaminomimetic treatment is initiated, Parkinsonian primates develop motor response complications (MRCs) that include motor fluctuations and dyskinesias (Blanchet et al. 1996). After the MPTP lesioning cycle, which takes approximately five to six weeks adopting the chronic administration regimen of a weekly dose of 0.5 to 1 mg/kg subcutaneously, all animals are left drug-free for six to eight weeks. They are scored on a regular basis using the Laval University Disability Scale for MPTP Monkeys (Gomez-Mancilla et al. 1993), where the normal state extends from 0 to 2 points and maximal disability is 10 points. When a mild to moderate Parkinsonian syndrome stabilizes (baseline disability scores between 4 to 6 points), monkeys begin receiving chronic treatment with 0.5 to 2 tablets of carbidopa/levodopa (25/100 mg) every other day, orally administered by means of a pet piller. All monkeys develop dyskinesias within one month, which can be reproduced consistently and predictably following the same oral dose of carbidopa/levodopa (Bibbiani et al. 2001). The dyskinesias predominantly observed are of the choreiform type and, less frequently, of the dystonic variety. These movements are usually observed beginning twenty to forty minutes after administering a dopaminergic agent and are most severe midway through to the end of each therapeutic dose (peak-dose dyskinesias).

III. PATHOGENESIS OF MOTOR RESPONSE COMPLICATIONS IN NONHUMAN PRIMATES

A. Pulsatile and Nonphysiological Dopaminergic Stimulation

While the entity of nigral degeneration can definitely play a role in the onset of motor complications (Di Monte et al. 2000), it is not essential for inducing dyskinesias (Jenner 2000). Any dopaminergic agent can induce dyskinetic movements, including both D1 and D2 dopamine agonists (Jenner 2000). Their ability to induce involuntary movements is mostly attributed to their pharmacokinetic and pharmacodynamic properties: long-acting dopamine agonists are less prone to induce complications than short-acting ones. While normal motor function depends on the continuous synthesis and release of dopamine by neurons projecting from the substantia nigra to the striatum, the pulsatile stimulation resulting from the standard anti-Parkinsonian therapy is deemed responsible for the pathogenesis of motor complications (Chase 1998).

In the non-Parkinsonian brain, the nigrostriatal pathway is usually tonically active, leading to relatively constant dopaminergic stimulation of striatal dopamine receptors (Bunney et al. 1973; Schultz 1994). In the striatum of MPTP-lesioned Parkinsonian primates, dopamine synthesis from exogenous levodopa largely takes place in non-dopaminergic cells containing dopa-decarboxylase that are not equipped to store and release dopamine in a controlled fashion (Melamed et al. 1980). As a result, striatal intrasynaptic dopamine levels no longer remain constant but mirror the broad swings in plasma levodopa levels associated with the intermittent administration of this rapidly metabolized prodrug. Dopaminergic transmission is thus converted from a tonic to a phasic process (Chase et al. 1996). In Parkinsonian primates, the periodic high intensity stimulation of striatal postsynaptic dopamine receptors is believed to contribute to the development of the motor response complication syndrome (Chase et al. 1998; Verhagen Metman et al. 2000). On the other hand, when the levodopa is administered in a more continuous fashion, instead of intermittently, none of the above changes occurs (Engber et al. 1998; Gnanalingham and Robertson 1994). In a recent experiment we demonstrated that continuous release of a dopaminergic agent through a subcutaneously implantable polymeric matrix allows continuous stimulation of striatal dopaminergic receptors and prevents onset of dyskinesias for the entire treatment period (Bibbiani et al. unpublished observation). While a causative relationship between pulsatile and nonphysiological dopaminergic stimulation and the development of MRCs is generally accepted (Fahn 1999), the intricacies of the cellular mechanisms by which this occurs are only beginning to be unraveled.

B. Glutamate Striatal Plasticity

Dopamine receptors are expressed on striatal medium-sized spiny neurons that constitute the predominant neuronal population in the striatum. The close proximity of dopaminergic and glutamatergic terminals on the dendrites of medium spiny neurons (Cepeda and Levine 1998; Kotter 1994) provides the anatomical setting for functional interactions between the two transmitter systems, further raising the possibility that enhanced glutamatergic transmission may be relevant to the development of the MRC syndrome.

1. Striatal Medium Spiny Neurons

Striatal spiny neurons receive synaptic input from the dopaminergic nigrostriatal pathway and also from glutamatergic corticostriatal pathways as well as a number of other systems intrinsic and extrinsic to the striatum, including adenosinergic, adrenergic, and serotonergic pathways. Their projections provide inhibitory GABA-ergic input to the major output nuclei of the basal ganglia, the internal segment of the globus pallidus and the pars reticulata of the substantia nigra (Gerfen 1992; Graybiel et al. 1994; Kotter 1994). Medium spiny neurons may thus serve as integrative anatomical sites that process the flow of cortical and nigral information into the basal ganglia.

2. Striatal Plasticity

The striatum plays a critical role in motor learning (Graybiel et al. 1994). Long-term activity-dependent alterations in the efficacy of excitatory synaptic transmission are considered fundamental to the process of information storage in different areas of the brain. In the striatum, corticostriatal excitatory transmission can express two forms of neuronal plasticity: long-term potentiation (LTP) and long-term depression (LTD) (Calabresi et al. 1996; Calabresi et al., 1997; Calabresi et al. 2000). Both require activation of glutamate NMDA and AMPA receptors as well as DA receptors. Dopaminergic denervation induces hyperactivity of corticostriatal glutamate-mediated transmission and interferes with the normal corticostriatal synaptic plasticity. Subsequent nonphysiological dopamine replacement may further modify the corticostriatal synaptic activity in ways that lead to impaired motor performance and altered responses to dopaminomimetic therapy (Calabresi et al. 1997; Chase and Oh 2000).

3. Striatal Signaling Mechanism

Since protein phosphorylation serves as a major regulatory mechanism for glutamate receptors, the phosphorylation state of different subunits of NMDA and AMPA receptors was recently investigated in the 6-OHDA-lesioned rat. These studies indicate that nonphysiological stimulation of DA receptors on striatal spiny neurons leads to changes in the subunit phosphorylation pattern of co-expressed NMDA and AMPA glutamatergic receptors. It now appears that alterations in the phosphorylation states of striatal NMDA and AMPA receptors reflect the aberrant activation of signaling cascades linking DA and glutamate receptors expressed along the dendrites of medium spiny neurons (Chase and Oh 2000; Chase et al. 1998). More specifically, changes in the balance between specific spiny-neuron kinase and phosphatase activity appear to affect the degree and pattern of phosphorylation and thus corticostriatal synaptic activity (Chase and Oh 2000; Chase et al. 1998; Oh et al. 1997; Oh et al. 1998).

IV. PHARMACOTHERAPY OF MOTOR RESPONSE COMPLICATIONS IN MPTP NONHUMAN PRIMATES

MPTP primate research on pharmacological interventions for PD have focused on practical approaches to restore the physiologic striatal dopaminergic transmission, as well as pharmacological strategies to prevent or reverse secondary changes at downstream sites (Anderson et al. 1999), occurring as a result of their nonphysiologic dopaminergic stimulation. The enhanced striatal glutamatergic and intracellular signaling cascades and motor response complications, can be attenuated by drugs that target signaling proteins within striatal spiny neurons (Chase et al. 1998) or by pharmaceutical agents that interact extracellularly with various receptors on the striatal medium spiny neurons, including glutamatergic, serotonergic, and adenosinergic system.

A. Glutamatergic Antagonist

1. NMDA Antagonist

If enhanced NMDA receptor sensitivity plays a significant role in expressing motor response complications, then NMDA receptor blockade can be predicted to confer therapeutic benefit. Current evidence from studies in the MPTP-lesioned primates suggests this is indeed the case.

a. Competitive NMDA Antagonist

Systemic administration of some, but not all, NMDA antagonists reduces dyskinesia at doses that have no effect on the anti-Parkinson benefit from levodopa (Blanchet et al. 1995). In cynomolgus and rhesus monkeys, the competitive NMDA antagonist LY 235959, co-administered subcutaneously with a dyskinetic dose of levodopa, reduced choreic dyskinesia without diminishing the anti-Parkinsonian benefit of levodopa (Papa and Chase 1996). At the highest dose given, however, chorea suppression continued, but dystonic posturing tended to increase.

b. Noncompetitive NMDA Antagonist

Earlier studies with the noncompetitive NMDA antagonist MK-801 had led to quite different results. In cynomolgus monkeys, MK-801 blocked both the anti-Parkinson and dyskinetic effects of levodopa (Gomez-Mancilla and Bedard 1993). In squirrel monkeys, MK-801 again blocked the anti-Parkinson effect of levodopa and also converted chorea into dystonia (Rupniak et al. 1992). Studies in Parkinsonian primates further revealed that not all noncompetitive NMDA-receptor antagonists have the same effects on motor behavior, despite a generally similar subunit-nonselective profile (Papa et al. 1996). No definite anti-Parkinsonian or anti-dyskinetic activity was observed with remacemide, which is also a noncompetitive and subunit-nonselective NMDA-receptor antagonist with relatively low affinity, in MPTP-lesioned monkeys (Blanchet and Chase unpublished observation). Taken together, these findings suggest a possibility that high NMDA-receptor binding affinity might be required for the genesis of motoric effects in this model.

c. Aminoadamantanes

Amantadine is an aminoadamantane that has a long history in the treatment of PD. The NMDA antagonist property of amantadine, however, was recognized only recently (Kornhuber et al. 1991), providing a safe opportunity to evaluate the hypothesis that NMDA antagonists diminish dyskinesias in nonhuman primates. Researchers have demonstrated that in levodopa-primed Parkinsonian monkeys, co-administration of amantadine with relatively low-dose levodopa suppresses nearly all choreiform dyskinesias and substantially reduces dystonic dyskinesias, albeit at the expense of some diminution in anti-Parkinsonian efficacy (Blanchet et al. 1998). With higher-dose levodopa, the NMDA-receptor channel blocker had a smaller but still strongly suppressive effect on dyskinesias without altering the anti-Parkinsonian response. Memantine, another aminoadamantane with higher affinity for the NMDA receptor than amantadine, however, had no effect on dyskinesias in the same model although it did improve Parkinsonian symptoms (Bibbiani unpublished observation).

2. Subunit Selective NMDA Antagonist

Current MPTP primate studies suggest that selectivity for NMDA-receptor subtypes may determine the behavioral effects of NMDA antagonists, with some evidence pointing to the relative importance of the NR2B subunit for anti-dyskinetic efficacy (Blanchet et al. 1999; Chase and Oh 2000). Investigators evaluated these results by examining the motoric effects of NR2A blockade using MDL 100,453 and NR2B blockade by means of ACEA10–1244 in levodopa-treated MPTP-lesioned monkeys (Blanchet et al. 1999). Following injection of a fully effective dose of levodopa, MDL 100,453 administration produced an increase in dyskinesia scores. In contrast, ACEA10–1244 treatment did not change motor activity by itself and showed only a tendency to potentiate the anti-Parkinsonian response when given in combination with low-dose levodopa. With a high dose of levodopa, however, ACEA10–1244 displayed potent anti-dyskinetic effects without diminishing the anti-Parkinsonian benefit of levodopa. Taken together, these results suggest that augmented activity of NR2B subunits, alone or in combination with the smaller rise in NR2A subunit activity, contributes to the apparent enhancement in striatal NMDA-receptor sensitivity and thus to the plastic alterations in dopaminergic responses in levodopa-treated Parkinsonian animals.

3. AMPA Antagonist

In addition to NMDA receptors, medium spiny neurons also express glutamatergic receptors of the AMPA type. Blockade of these receptors with the AMPA antagonist, LY300164, a drug acting at an allosteric modulation site, not only potentiated the motor response to low- and medium-dose levodopa, but also decreased levodopa-induced chorea (Konitsiotis et al. 2000). In the same study, administration of CX516, an ampakine that enhances glutamatergic transmission, did not enhance motor activity, but increased dyskinesia severity. While researchers have extensively investigated the individual contribution of the AMPA receptors and the NMDA receptors, the effect produced by the simultaneous blockade on both receptors has not been fully explored. To evaluate this, we administered the NMDA antagonist amantadine and the AMPA antagonist GYKI 47261 with a dyskinetic dose of levodopa, singularly and in combination. Both antagonists were administered at the lowest effective dose in order to evaluate an eventual potentiation of their anti-dyskinetic effect. Both amantadine and GYKI 47261, when administered together with levodopa, modestly reduced dyskinesias by 20% and 22%, respectively; the combination of the two antagonists with the same dose of levodopa reduced dyskinesias by 51% (Bibbiani unpublished observation).

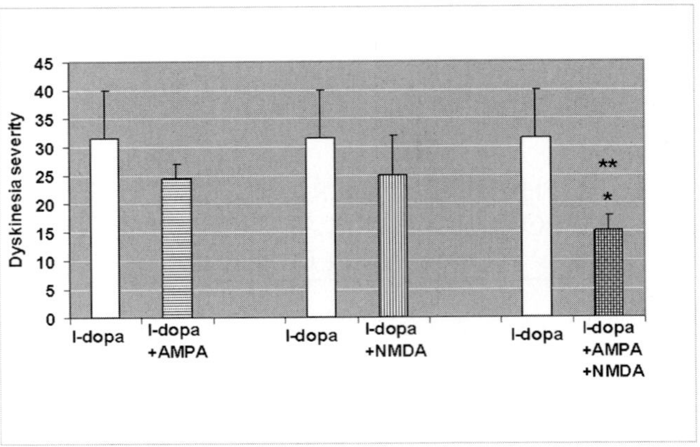

FIGURE 1 Dyskinesia severity after administration of a dyskinetic dose of levodopa, alone or in combination with the AMPA antagonist GYKI 47261 (L-dopa + AMPA [vertically hatched] bar), the NMDA antagonist Amantadine (L-dopa + NMDA [horizontally hatched] bar), and the combination of both (L-dopa + NMDA + AMPA [horizontal + vertical hatch] bar). *$p < 0.05$ for AMPA+NMDA+levodopa vs. levodopa alone; **$p < 0.05$ for AMPA+NMDA+levodopa vs. AMPA+levodopa and NMDA+levodopa (percentage of improvement).

B. Serotonergic and Adenosinergic Drugs

Investigators have implicated the contribution of serotonergic and adenosinergic mechanisms in the pathogenesis of motor dysfunction in Parkinson disease. Recent evidence from studies of MPTP-lesioned nonhuman primates suggests that serotonergic and adenosinergic signaling mechanisms in the striatum may indeed play a critical role in the development of motor response complications associated with chronic levodopa therapy. These findings strengthen the rationale for developing drugs that target these receptors as a potential drug therapy for PD motor dysfunction in humans.

1. 5-HT$_{1A}$ Receptors

5-HT$_{1A}$ receptors are expressed presynaptically on serotonergic terminals where they regulate transmitter release. In patients with advanced PD, striatal serotonergic terminals serve as an important site for the decarboxylation of exogenous levodopa to DA. It is thus conceivable that 5-HT$_{1A}$ agonists can act at striatal serotonergic terminals to modify the release of DA produced by levodopa treatment. Under such circumstances, 5-HT$_{1A}$ agonists might be expected to influence dopaminergic mechanisms in ways that affect motor function. In addition, clinical and preclinical observations suggest that an increase in serotonergic transmission can contribute to the appearance of dyskinesias. In MPTP primates, administering the 5-HT$_{1A}$ agonist sarizotan with a dyskinetic dose of levodopa produced a 75% reduction of levodopa-induced dyskinesias. The anti-dyskinetic action of the 5-HT$_{1A}$ agonist was much greater against choreiform dyskinesias than against dystonic dyskinesias. In fact sarizotan reduced choreiform dyskinesias by as much as 91%, whereas dystonic dyskinesias were not significantly altered (Bibbiani et al. 2001).

2. 5-HT$_{2A}$ Receptors

Serotonin 5-HT$_{2A}$ receptors are abundantly expressed in the central nervous system, including the striatum. Drugs that block these receptors, including atypical neuroleptics such as clozapine, ameliorate various movement disorders, including dyskinesias. In MPTP-treated PD primates, quetiapine, another atypical antipsychotic with 5-HT$_{2A/C}$ and D$_{2/3}$ antagonistic activity, had no effect on Parkinsonian dysfunction when given alone or with levodopa to Parkinsonian monkeys but it did, however, substantially reduce levodopa-induced dyskinesias (57%

reduction) when co-administered with levodopa (Oh et al. 2002).

3. Adenosine A_{2A} Receptors

Adenosine A_{2A} receptors, richly expressed on D_2 DA receptor-containing striatal medium spiny neurons, appear to activate signaling cascades that regulate co-expressed ionotropic glutamatergic receptors. In primates, once daily co-administration of an A_{2A} antagonist KW-6002 with apomorphine prevented the development of dyskinesias, which appeared in control animals seven to ten days after initiating apomorphine treatment. Animals initially given apomorphine plus KW-6002 for three weeks did not begin to manifest apomorphine-induced dyskinesias until ten to twelve days after discontinuing the A_{2A} antagonist. These results suggest that KW-6002 can attenuate the induction and expression of motor response alterations to chronic dopaminergic stimulation in Parkinsonian animals, possibly by blocking A_{2A} receptor-stimulated signaling pathways (Bibbiani et al. 2003).

V. SUMMARY

MPTP lesioning of the nigrostriatal dopamine system of nonhuman primates induces Parkinsonian signs, and subsequent treatment with levodopa produces many features of the human PD motor response complications. While MRCs associated with chronic levodopa therapy are a major cause of treatment failure, the biochemical mechanisms underlying this phenomenon remain yet unclear. Based on recent behavioral and pharmacological data, the pathogenesis of PD motor complications in MPTP primates may be influenced by increased synaptic efficacy of corticostriatal glutamatergic synaptic transmission associated with changes in medium spiny neuron signaling pathways. In addition to delivery systems that provide more continuous and physiological dopaminergic receptor stimulation, future goals of primate research in MRCs should include developing pharmacological agents that normalize striatal glutamatergic dysfunction by interacting with striatal NMDA and AMPA receptors or other surface receptors. The MPTP-lesioned nonhuman primate therefore serves as an invaluable tool for discovering more novel and salutary treatment approaches to attenuate levodopa-induced motor complications and to prevent a loss of its therapeutic efficacy during the course of the disease.

Acknowledgments

Investigations by the authors discussed herein were conducted at the Experimental Therapeutics Branch, National Institute of Neurological Disorders and Stroke, National Institutes of Health in Bethesda, MD, under Thomas N. Chase, M.D.

Video Legends

SEGMENT 1 Normal non-human primate. MPTP untreated normal untreated cynomolgus monkeys, as observed in this example, are very active, prone to climbing, very interested in the surrounding environment and quickly reach for food treats when presented.

SEGMENT 2 MPTP-lesioned non-human primate showing Parkinsonian symptoms. Following chronic MPTP administration, animals begin to exhibit PD signs. This animal appears to be much slower in moving around the cage and picking up food treats. It tends to sit still unless stimulated. Balance and movement coordination are poor compared to a normal animal.

SEGMENT 3 MPTP-lesioned and Levodopa-treated non-human primate showing dyskinesias. Chronic Levodopa therapy produces dyskinesias, as observed in patients with PD. The animal is "ON" with dyskinesias. Involuntary movements can be observed in all four limbs and as twisting of the trunk which can impair its ability to stand. Oral dyskinesias can also be observed as "chewing" movements.

References

Andersson, M., A. Hilbertson, and M.A. Cenci. 1999. Striatal fosB expression is causally linked with L-Dopa-induced abnormal involuntary movements and the associated upregulation of striatal prodynorphin mRNA in a rat model of Parkinson's disease. *Neurobiol Dis* **6**:461–474.

Ballard, P.A., J.W. Tetrud, and J.W. Langston. 1985. Permanent human Parkinsonism due to 1-methyl-4-phenyl-1,2,3,6-tetrahydropyridine (MPTP): seven cases. *Neurology* **35**:949–956.

Bankiewicz, K.S., E.H. Oldfield, C.C. Chiueh, J.L. Doppman, D.M. Jacobowitz, and I.J. Kopin. 1986. Hemiparkinsonism in monkeys after unilateral internal carotid artery infusion of 1-methyl-4-phenyl-1,2,3,6-tetrahydropyridine (MPTP). *Life Sci* **39**:7–16.

Bezard, E., C. Imbert, X. Deloire, B. Bioulac, and C.E. Gross. 1997. A chronic MPTP model reproducing the slow evolution of Parkinson's disease: evolution of motor symptoms in the monkey. *Brain Res* **766**:107–112.

Bibbiani, F., J.D. Oh, and T.N. Chase. 2001. Serotonin 5-HT1A agonist improves motor complications in rodent and primate parkinsonian models. *Neurology* **57**:829–834.

Bibbiani, F., J.D. Oh, J.P. Petzer, N. Castagnoli Jr., J.-F. Chen, M.A. Schwarzschild, and T.N. Chase. 2003. A2A antagonist prevents dopamine agonist-induced motor complications in animal models of Parkinson's disease. *Exp Neurol* **184**:285–294.

Blanchet, P.J., F. Calon, J.C. Martel, P.J. Bedard, T. Di Paolo, R.R. Walters, and M.F. Piercey. 1995. Continuous administration decreases and pulsatile administration increases behavioral sensitivity to a novel dopamine D_2 agonist (U-91356A) in MPTP-exposed monkeys. *J Pharmacol Exp Ther* **272**:854–859.

Blanchet, P.J., R. Grondin, and P.J. Bedard. 1996. Dyskinesia and wearing-off following dopamine D1 agonist treatment in drug-naive 1-methyl-4-phenyl-1,2,3,6-tetrahydropyridine-lesioned primates. *Mov Disord* **11**:91–94.

Blanchet, P.J., S. Konitsiotis, and T.N. Chase. 1998. Amantadine reduces levodopa-induced dyskinesias in Parkinsonian monkeys. *Mov Disord* **13**:798–802.

Blanchet, P.J., S. Konitsiotis, K. Hyland, L.A. Arnold, K.D. Pettigrew, T.N. Chase. 1998. Chronic exposure to MPTP as a primate model of progressive Parkinsonism: a pilot study with a free radical scavenger. *Exp Neurol* **153**:214–222.

Blanchet, P.J., S. Konitsiotis, N. Whitmore, R. Woodward, and T.N. Chase. 1999. Differing effects of N-methyl-D-aspartate receptor subtype selective antagonists on dyskinesias in levodopa-treated 1-methyl-4-

phenyl-tetrahydropyridine monkeys. *J Pharmacol Exp Ther* **290**:1034–1040.

Blanchet, P.J., L. Verhagen Metman, M.M. Mouradian, and T.N. Chase. 1996. Acute pharmacologic blockade of dyskinesias in Parkinson's disease. *Mov Disord* **11**:580–581.

Bunney, B.S., J.R. Walters, R.H. Roth, and G.K. Aghajanian. 1973. Dopaminergic neurons: effect of antipsychotic drugs and amphetamine on single cell activity. *J Pharmacol Exp Ther* **185**:560–571.

Burns, R.S., C.C. Chiueh, S.P. Markey, M.H. Ebert, D.M. Jacobowitz, and I.J. Kopin. 1983. A primate model of Parkinsonism: selective destruction of dopaminergic neurons in the pars compacta of the substantia nigra by N-methyl-4-phenyl-1,2,3,6-tetrahydropyridine. *Proc Natl Acad Sci U S A* **80**:4546–4550.

Calabresi, P., D. Centonze, and G. Bernardi. 2000. Electrophysiology of dopamine in normal and denervated striatal neurons. *Trends Neurosci* **23**:S57–S63.

Calabresi, P., A. Pisani, M.B. Mercuri, and G. Bernardi. 1996. The corticostriatal projection: from synaptic plasticity to dysfunctions of the basal ganglia. *Trends Neurosci* **19**:19–24.

Calabresi, P., A. Saiardi, A. Pisani, J.H. Baik, D. Centonze, M.B. Mercuri, G. Bernardi, and E. Borrelli. 1997. Abnormal synaptic plasticity in the striatum of mice lacking dopamine D_2 receptors. *J Neurosci* **7**:4536–4544.

Cepeda, C., and M.S. Levine. 1998. Dopamine and N-methyl-D-aspartate receptor interactions in the neostriatum. *Dev Neurosci* **20**:1–18.

Chase, T.N. 1998. Levodopa therapy: consequences of the non-physiologic replacement of dopamine. *Neurology* **50**:S17–S25.

Chase, T.N., T.M. Engber, and M.M. Mouradian. 1996. Contribution of dopaminergic and glutamatergic mechanisms to the pathogenesis of motor response complications in Parkinson's disease. *Adv Neurol* **69**:497–501.

Chase, T.N., and J.D. Oh. 2000. Striatal dopamine- and glutamate-mediated dysregulation in experimental parkinsonism. *Trends Neurosci* **23**:S86–S91.

Chase, T.N., J.D. Oh, and P.J. Blanchet. 1998. Neostriatal mechanisms in Parkinson's disease. *Neurology* **51**:S30–S35.

Chase, T.N., J.D. Oh, and S. Konitsiotis. 2000. Antiparkinsonian and antidyskinetic activity of drugs targeting central glutamatergic mechanisms. *J Neurology* **247**:S36–S42.

Cotzias, G.C., W.M., Van, and L.M. Schiffer. 1967. Aromatic amino acids and modification of parkinsonism. *N Engl J Med* **276**:374–379.

Di Monte, D.A., A. McCormack, G. Petzinger, A.M. Janson, M. Quik, and W.J. Langston. 2000. Relationship among nigrostriatal denervation, Parkinsonism, and dyskinesias in the MPTP primate model. *Mov Disord* **15**:459–466.

Ehringer, H., and O. Hornykiewcz. 1960. Distribution of noradrenaline and dopamine (3-hydroxytyramine) in the human brain and their behavior in diseases of the extrapyramidal system. *Klinische Wochenschrift* **38**:1236–1239.

Engber, T.M., Z. Susel, J.L. Juncos, and T.N. Chase. 1989. Continuous and intermittent levodopa differentially affects rotation induced by D-1 and D-2 dopamine agonists. *Eur J Pharmacol* **168**:291–298.

Fahn, S. 1999. Parkinson disease, the effect of levodopa, and the ELLDOPA trial. *Arch Neurol* **56**:529–535.

Forno L.S., L.E. DeLanney, I. Irwin, and J.W. Langston. 1993. Similarities and differences between MPTP-induced Parkinsonism and Parkinson's disease. *Neuropathologic dv Neurol* **60**:600–608.

Gerfen, C.R. 1992. The neostriatal mosaic: multiple levels of compartmental organization in the basal ganglia. *Ann Rev Neurosci* **15**:285–320.

Gnanalingham, K.K., and R.G. Robertson. 1994. The effects of chronic continuous versus intermittent levodopa treatments on striatal and extrastriatal D_1 and D_2 dopamine receptors and dopamine uptake sites in the 6-hydroxydopamine lesioned rat—an autoradiographic study. *Brain Res* **640**:185–194.

Gomez-Mancilla, B., R. Boucher, C. Gagnon, T. Di Paolo, R. Markstein, and P.J. Bédard. 1993. Effect of adding the D1 agonist CY 208–243 to chronic bromocriptine treatment. I: Evaluation of motor parameters in relation to striatal catecholamine content and dopamine receptors. *Mov Disord* **8**:144–150.

Gomez-Mancilla, B., and P.J. Bedard. 1993. Effect of nondopaminergic drugs on L-dopa-induced dyskinesias in MPTP-treated monkeys. *Clin Neuropharmacol* **16**:418–427.

Graybiel, A.M., T. Aosaki, A.W. Flaherty, and M. Kimura. 1994. The basal ganglia and adaptive motor control. *Science* **265**:1826–1831.

Greenfield, J.G., and F.D. Bosanquet. 1953. The brain stem lesions in Parkinsonism. *J Neurol Neurosurg Psychiatry* **16**:213–226.

Hantraye, P., M. Varastet, M. Peschanski, D. Riche, P. Cesaro, J.C. Willer, and M. Maziere. 1993. Stable Parkinsonian syndrome and uneven loss of striatal dopamine fibres following chronic MPTP administration in baboons. *Neuroscience* **53**:169–178.

Hornykiewicz, O. 1963. Die Topische Lokalisation und das Verhalten von Noradrenalin und Dopamin in der substantia nigra des normalen und Parkinsonkranken Menschen. *Wien Klin Wochenschr* **75**:309–312.

Jenner, P. 2000. Factors influencing the onset and persistence of dyskinesia in MPTP-treated primates. *Ann Neurol* **47**:S90–S99.

Jenner, P. 2003. The MPTP-treated primate as a model of motor complications in PD: Primate model of motor complications. *Neurology* **61**:S4–S11.

Konitsiotis, S., P.J. Blanchet, L. Verhagen E. Lamers, and T.N. Chase. 2000. AMPA receptor blockade improves levodopa-induced dyskinesia in MPTP monkeys. *Neurology* **54**:1589–1595.

Kornhuber, J., J. Bormann, M. Hubers, K. Rusche, and P. Riederer. 1991. Effects of the 1-amino-adamantanes at the MK-801-binding site of the NMDA receptor-gated ion channel: a human postmortem brain study. *Eur J Pharmacol* **206**:297–300.

Kotter, R. 1994. Postsynaptic integration of glutamatergic and dopaminergic signals in the striatum. *Prog Neurobiol* **44**:163–196.

Lang, A.E., and A.M. Lozano. 1998. Parkinson's disease. *N Engl J Med* **339**:1044–1053.

Langston, J.W., and P.A. Ballard, Jr. 1983. Parkinson's disease in a chemist working with 1-methyl-4-phenyl-1,2,5,6-tetrahydropyridine. *N Engl J Med* **309**:310.

Marin, C., S.M. Papa, T.M. Engber, M. Bonastre, E. Tolosa, and T.N. Chase. 1996. MK801 prevents levodopa-induced motor response alterations in parkinsonian rats. *Brain Res* **736**:202–205.

Marjama-Lyons, J.M., and W.C. Koller. 2001. Parkinson's disease. Update in diagnosis and symptom management. *Geriatrics* **56**:24–55, 29–30, 33–35.

Marsden, C.D. 1990. Parkinson's disease. *Lancet* **335**:948–952.

Marsden, C. 1994. Problems with long-term levodopa therapy for Parkinson's disease. *Clin Neuropharmacol* **17**:S32–S44.

Melamed, E., F. Hefti, and R.J. Wurtman. 1980. Nonaminergic striatal neurons convert exogenous L-dopa to dopamine in parkinsonism. *Ann Neurol* **8**:558–563.

Mouradian, M.M., I.J. Heuser, F. Baronti, G. Fabbrini, J.L. Juncos, and T.N. Chase. 1989. Pathogenesis of dyskinesias in Parkinson's disease. *Ann Neurol* **25**:523–526.

Oh, J.D., F. Bibbiani, and T.N. Chase. 2002. Quetiapine attenuates levodopa-induced motor complications in rodent and primate parkinsonian models. *Exp Neurol* **177**:557–564.

Oh, J.D., P.L. Del Dotto, and T.N. Chase. 1997. Protein kinase A inhibitor attenuates levodopa-induced motor response alterations in the hemi-Parkinsonian rat. *Neurosci Lett* **228**:5–8.

Oh, J.D., D. Russell, C.L. Vaughan, and T.N. Chase. 1998. Enhanced tyrosine phosphorylation of striatal NMDA receptor subunits: effects of dopaminergic denervation and levodopa administration. *Brain Res* **813**:150–159.

Papa, S.M., and T.N. Chase. 1996. Levodopa-induced dyskinesias improved by a glutamate antagonist in Parkinsonian monkeys. *Ann Neurol* **39**:574–578.

Papa, S.M., T.M. Engber, A.M. Kask, and T.N. Chase. 1994. Motor fluctuations in levodopa treated parkinsonian rats: relation to lesion extent and treatment duration. *Brain Res* **662**:69–74.

Parkinson, J. 1817. *An Essay on the Shaking Palsy*. London: Sherwood, Neely and Jones.

Rupniak, N.M., S. Boyce, M.J. Steventon, S.D. Iversen, and C.D. Marsden. 1992. Dystonia induced by combined treatment with L-Dopa and MK-801 in Parkinsonian monkeys. *Ann Neurol* **32**:103–105.

Schultz, W. 1994. Behavior-related activity of primate dopamine neurons. *Rev Neurol (Paris)* **150**:634–639.

Shaw, K.M., A.J. Lees, and G.M. Stern. 1980. The impact of treatment with levodopa on Parkinson's disease. *Q J Med* **49**:283–93.

Stern, Y. 1990. MPTP-induced Parkinsonism. *Prog Neurobiol* **34**:107–114.

Verhagen Metman, L., S. Konitsiotis, and T.N. Chase. 2000. Pathophysiology of motor response complications in Parkinson's disease: hypotheses on the why, where, and what. *Mov Disord* **15**:3–8.

CHAPTER

B9

C. elegans Models of Parkinson Disease

SUVI VARTIAINEN and GARRY WONG

C. elegans is a soil-dwelling nematode that measures ~1 mm in length. Advantageous features that make it a suitable model organism to study human neurodegenerative diseases include its body transparency for direct visualization of neurons, a reproductive cycle of three days, a life span of three weeks, and richness in posture, movement, and behavior. *C. elegans* has well-developed methods and resources for genetic manipulation including visible phenotypic markers, a completed genome sequence, a library of mutants, and the ability to perform forward and reverse genetics. *C. elegans* hermaphrodites have eight dopaminergic neurons that modify behaviors as diverse as egg-laying, sexual reproduction, response to drugs, habituation, and muscle movement. Investigators have identified two *C. elegans* dopamine receptors and studied their role in behavior. Parkinson disease models produced from the wild-type *C. elegans* can be divided into classes based on genetic mutations, chemical treatments, and transgenic manipulations. A family of uncoordinated (*unc*) mutants define postural and movement deficits. Chemical models using 6-hydroxydopamine show loss of dopamine neurons, and transgenic overexpression of human α-synuclein causes *C. elegans* to exhibit both loss of dopamine neurons and movement deficits. The models recapitulate some features of human Parkinson disease that can be seen at the biochemical, cellular, and behavioral levels. Experimental flexibility and resources to address Parkinson disease research makes *C. elegans* a unique model system.

I. *C. ELEGANS* GENERAL BIOLOGY AND NEUROBIOLOGY

C. elegans is a free-living nematode that is approximately 1 mm in length. In nature, the nematode eats essentially any organic material that can be placed through its mouth. *C. elegans* has two sexes: male and hermaphrodite. Males fertilize hermaphrodites; however, when males are not around, hermaphrodites produce their own offspring by self-fertilization. During its lifetime *C. elegans* lays approximately 300 eggs, 1000 if fertilized by the male. The reproductive life cycle is three days. Like other nematodes, *C. elegans* goes through four larval stages culminating in the fourth stage just two days after fertilization. After this stage, *C. elegans* is fully an adult and can self-produce or mate to produce the next generation of offspring. The entire life span of *C. elegans* lasts between fourteen and twenty-one days depending upon temperature and other environmental factors, and it continues to lay eggs throughout its adult life.

The body plan consists of a tube within a tube. The inner tube largely consists of an intestine for eating, digesting, and eliminating waste. The outer tube contains a hard protein cuticle. The space in between the tubes, the pseudocoelomic space, is where the reproductive organs, muscles, neurons, and other cells reside. Adult hermaphrodites and males have a total of 959 and 1031 cells, respectively. Of these, the numbers of neurons are 302 and 381, respectively. These extra male neurons are important in locating hermaphrodites and facilitating copulation. Most of the neurons reside in the head region where they form a structure termed the "nerve ring." A ventral nerve cord runs across the length of the body and also forms collateral connections to the dorsal cord. The neurons utilize most of the same neurotransmitters as higher organisms including glutamate, GABA, acetylcholine, and dopamine. In addition, *C. elegans* neurons utilize octopamine, but do appear to use epinephrine or norepinephrine. *C. elegans* hermaphrodites have eight dopaminergic neurons (White et al. 1986). There are two pairs of cephalic (CEP) neurons and one pair of anterior deirid (ADE) neurons located in the nerve ring, and one pair of posterior deirid (PDE) neurons located between the vulva and tail. In addition to these neurons, males have three pairs of dopaminergic neurons (R5A, R7A, R9A) located in the tail rays.

II. *C. ELEGANS* GENERAL MOVEMENT

C. elegans has four sets of bilateral muscles across the length of its body. The neuromuscular junction consists of synapses that utilize acetylcholine as the excitatory transmitter. On the opposite side of the worm, a coordinated release of GABA, the inhibitory neurotransmitter, opposes the excitatory actions of acetylcholine and this coordinated inhibition and excitation produce the characteristic sine wave movement of *C. elegans.* Other neurotransmitters, such as dopamine and glutamate, modulate the actions of GABA and acetylcholine. *C. elegans* is capable of forward and backward locomotion and researchers have mapped the neuronal circuits for both of these directions. Many environmental factors and cues affect the speed, direction, and duration of normal movement. These factors include the location of food, the appearance of noxious or pleasant chemical compounds, mechanical stimulation, medium of movement, and presence of other nematodes.

Movements or deficits in movements are defined in *C. elegans* in a variety of ways. By far, the most abundant class of movement deficits in *C. elegans* are in a class termed "uncoordinated." This very large class, in which over 200 separate genetic loci have been attributed, contains deficits that deviate from the normal sine wave. Uncoordinated movements can fall into several phenotypic classes and are largely self-explanatory including kinkers, coilers, slow or irregular movers, forward or backward movers, loopers, paralyzed, twitchers, shrinkers, curlers, and shakers, all with varying degrees of severity. *C. elegans* uncoordinated mutants can also contain combinations of these phenotypes. Other movement disorders have been described, but concern more specialized functions that require movement. These functions include mating, egg laying, pharyngeal pumping, eating, and defecation. Among the most peculiar of movement disorders are *C. elegans* that move only in a small circle, able only to travel a few body lengths, which typically roll over themselves in a ring. These animals have been termed rollers.

Due to interest in understanding the underlying biological basis of movement and movement disorders in *C. elegans*, investigators have developed assays to measure movement in different contexts. The simplest of measurements include postural defects. Postural assays require that the investigator observe the animal through transmitted light microscopy and determine whether the nematode deviates from the normal sinusoidal bent form. The above-mentioned coilers, curlers, and loopers all fall into this class. To measure movement deficits, investigators often employ movement assays in response to physical stimuli. Upon touch, *C. elegans* normally back up or move forward in the direction opposite the stimuli in a sinusoidal pattern. Any deviation from this prototypical pattern can be observed and scored. These deficits are termed after the response and include the shrinkers. *C. elegans* nonresponsive to touch stimulation are termed mechanically insensitive.

The thrashing assay measures how well worms can bend across their body axis in liquid media (Miller et al. 1996; Thomas and Lockery 1999). This assay consists of transferring live worms into a liquid bubble of ionic buffer. After thirty to sixty seconds, worms typically bend across their body axis from one side to the other in a rhythmic and rapid fashion. In a typical control experiment, the number of times the worm will bend and have its head cross the body axis will be ~200 times per minute (Duerr et al. 1999). This assay is easy to score, requires minimal equipment, and is reproducible. Additional parameters that can be measured in the thrashing assay include over-bending and under-bending from which the amplitude of the movement can be scored (Ackley et al. 2003). Sophisticated video equipment and computer programs to collect and interpret this information have been built and are also currently under development.

A radial assay is another measure of movement ability. In this test, worms are placed in the center of a 15 cm petri dish that has been seeded with bacteria in an even layer throughout the plate (Reiner et al. 1999). *C. elegans* typically forage on a lawn of bacteria. Investigators can track movement from the center as the worms leave a trail through the bacteria. Researchers measure and calculate the distance that worms move from the center within a given time, typically two minutes. While worms may move in circles or return to the origin, investigators can see the tracks made in the bacterial lawn, and therefore can measure the distance from the origin and actual distance. One advantage of this assay over the thrashing assay is that it takes into account actual locomotive ability, rather than whether gross movement under a physical challenge occurs. A summary of the major assay types appears in table 1.

III. *C. ELEGANS* PARKINSON DISEASE MODELS GENERATED BY GENETIC MUTATIONS

Among the earliest experiments performed on *C. elegans* were mutagenesis studies aimed at recovering visible phenotypes. From these, the scoreable phenotypes included those with movement deficits and were defined as uncoordinated (*unc*). Other deficits of neuromuscular origin were also described such as egg-laying defective (*egl*) and anterior body contraction and expulsion defective in defecation (*aex*) (Iwasaki et al. 1997). We have already mentioned the types of uncoordinated phenotypes. Slow and sluggish moving worms that could be described as bradykinetic are found in the *unc* class. Mutated genes that underlie this broad phenotypic class include neuronal voltage-sensitive calcium channels (*unc-2*), alpha-subunit of nicotinic acetylcholine receptor (un*c-29*), novel protein (*unc-31*), and syntaxin homolog (*unc-64*). Other mutated genes associated with poor backing in response to stimuli include extracellular matrix component (*unc 6*), LIM class homeoprotein (*mec-3*), and degenerin (*mec-6*). The touch-insensitive class of *C. elegans*, *mec*, of which at least eighteen are described, are also nearly universally lethargic. Admittedly, deficits in movements describe an incredibly broad class of phenotypes in *C. elegans*, and the model they represent may be nonspecific.

Parkinson disease models based on neurochemical criteria would likely be more useful. A phenotypic class of *C. elegans* that is catecholamine-defective(*cat*) was described in 1975 (Sulston et al. 1975). At least six separate genetic loci were identified using formaldehyde-induced fluorescence techniques. Later genetic mapping and cloning identified many of these genes as involved in the synthesis pathway of catecholamines. The phenotypes include dramatic loss of dopamine (>90% as measured by fluorescence techniques) (*cat-1*, *cat-2*, *cat-4*). Serotonin is also diminished in *cat-1* and *cat-4*, but is normal in *cat-2*. Cloned *cat-1* encodes a vesicular monoamine transporter (Duerr et al. 1999); *cat-2* encodes a tyrosine hydroxylase (Lints and Emmons 1999); and *cat-4* encodes GTP cyclohydrolase I, which synthesizes a cofactor for tyrosine hydroxylase (Loer and Kenyon 1993). HPLC analysis indicates that the loss of dopamine in the *cat* mutants mentioned above is 60–90% (Wintle and van Tol 2001; Nass and Blakely 2003; Sanyal et al. 2004). Despite the diminishment of dopamine, *cat-1* mutants move amazingly well. In movements off food, trashing assays, and egg-laying, they performed as well as wild-type animals (Duerr et al. 1999). They do show deficits, however, in dopamine-mediated sensory behaviors such as in movements on food, where they should slow down and graze, and in male mating success. *Cat-2* mutants move normally while *cat-4* mutants are sluggish, have enhanced foraging movements, and deficits in mating (Loer and Kenyon 1993). The mating deficits associated with *cat-4* can be rescued by adding exogenous serotonin (Loer and Kenyon 1993). Investigators describe a *bas-1* mutant that is deficient in serotonin and dopamine (Loer and Kenyon 1993), and like *cat-2* and *cat-4*, has difficulties in male turning behavior that is important for sexual reproduction. The *bas-1* gene is identified as an aromatic amino acid decarboxylase (Loer and Kenyon 1993; Wintle and van Tol 2001). A summary of these mutants appears in table 2.

Researchers have cloned two dopamine receptor genes from *C. elegans*. The *dop-1* gene resembles the mammalian D1-like receptor while the *dop-2* gene resembles the D2-like receptor (Suo et al. 2002; Suo et al. 2003; Sanyal et al. 2004). *Dop-1* mutants move like wild-type worms when on food and lack the slow down response mediated by dopamine (Sanyal et al. 2004). *Dop-1* mutants also respond to dopamine in an egg-laying assay similar to wild-type worms, altogether suggesting that other dopamine receptors mediate these behaviors. *Dop-1* mutants do respond to nonlocalized mechanical stimulation (taps to the culture plate) either by speeding up, or reversing the direction of movement. This movement is subject to habituation: the responses to repeated stimulation become blunted (Rose and Rankin

TABLE 1 Summary of Movement Assays in *C. elegans*

Type	Description	Examples
Postural	Determines deviation from sinusoidal shape	Coilers, curlers
Stimulation	Measures response to mechanical stimulation	Shrinkers, mec
Thrashing	Measures frequency or amplitude of body bend in liquid	Fast or slow
Radial	Measures distance moved from origin	Near or far

TABLE 2 Summary of *C. elegans* Parkinson Disease Models

Type	Description	Phenotype
Genetic	*cat-1*	DA and 5-HT deficient
Genetic	*cat-2*	DA deficient
Genetic	*cat-4*	DA and 5-HT deficient
Genetic	*bas-1*	DA and 5-HT deficient
Chemical	6-OHDA treated	Degeneration of DA neurons
Transgenic	Over-X α-synuclein	Loss of DA neurons, movement deficits

2001). In *dop-1* mutants, the habituation was enhanced, implicating this dopamine receptor in a type of behavioral plasticity, but also suggesting that this form of behavior could be an early indicator of lost dopamine signaling. In this context, learning and memory deficits are known to precede movement deficits in some Parkinson disease animal models.

IV. *C. ELEGANS* PARKINSON DISEASE MODELS GENERATED BY CHEMICAL TREATMENTS

Investigators have applied chemical neurotoxin treatments to *C. elegans* as a rapid and facile means to model Parkinson disease. Among neurotoxins specifically targeting dopaminergic neurons, we have used 6-hydroxydopamine (6-OHDA) (Nass et al. 2002). A key to visualizing dopaminergic neurons in this study was using GFP controlled by the *C. elegans* dopamine transporter (*dat-1*) (Nass et al. 2001). Transgenic injection of this construct permits identification of all eight hermaphrodite neurons under fluorescent microscopy in whole animals. After 6-OHDA treatment, death of CEP neurons could be seen as early as thirty minutes after the injection. Membrane blebbing could be seen within two hours. Ultrastructural studies using transmission electron microscopy confirmed overt pathology in CEP neurons and suggested an apoptotic pattern of cell death due to presence of chromatin condensation. Cell perturbations required the *C. elegans* dopamine transporter, but not a cell death pathway mediated by *C. elegans* death genes CED-3 or CED-4. We have also proposed use of other dopaminergic neuron specific toxins, such as 1-methyl-4-phenyl-1,2,3,6-tetrahydropyridine (MPTP) (Nass et al. 2001). Investigators have not yet conducted movement and dopamine-mediated behavioral studies with rigor on these models. Other neurotoxins such as rotenone or mitochondrial function inhibitors could also be tried. Though not a chemical treatment, physical ablation of dopamine neurons by laser treatment has been performed (Sawin, 1996). The ablation of all dopamine neurons appeared necessary to affect dopamine-mediated response to encountering a bacterial lawn.

V. *C. ELEGANS* PARKINSON DISEASE MODELS GENERATED BY TRANSGENIC MANIPULATIONS

Researchers have also applied transgenic approaches to *C. elegans* (Mello and Fire 1995). We have produced a transgenic Parkinson disease model in *C. elegans* using overexpression of α-synuclein (Lakso et al. 2003). The product of this gene is found in Lewy bodies, the pathological hallmark of Parkinson disease (Spillantini et al. 1997). Mutations in this gene lead to familial forms of Parkinson disease (Polymeropoulus et al. 1997). Some of the biochemical features of Parkinson disease were recapitulated in our model. For example, loss of dopaminergic neurons and processes was observed when α-synuclein was overexpressed under control of a dopaminergic neuron-specific promoter. Cellular inclusions consisting of α-synuclein protein were also observed although these events were rare. With regard to movement deficits, a thrashing assay was used. We observed that transgenic *C. elegans* overexpressing α-synuclein under a pan-neuronal promoter had thrashing values ~50% less than transgenic controls expressing only the transgenic marker. Both overexpressing wild-type (WT) and mutant α-synuclein (A53T) (Lee et al. 2002) worms displayed similar deficit values. An example of tracks left in bacteria by wild-type and transgenic *C. elegans* overexpressing α-synuclein appears in Figure 1. These transgenic worms were scored at four days of age, which is a young adult stage. In perspective, *C. elegans* has a life span of three weeks under standard laboratory conditions. Their movement slows during the last week of life and they can appear sluggish. Thus, the basal level in a thrashing assay changes depending upon the age. Whether overexpression of α-synuclein would accelerate this decline in movement remains to be determined. Transgenic *C. elegans* overexpressing α-synuclein under a pan neuronal promoter also showed deficits in a radial distance assay (unpublished observation). The score for controls ranges from 4 to 7 cm while overexpressing α-synuclein transgenic worms scored from 0 to 2 cm.

One advantage in *C. elegans* transgenics is direct expression of transgenes specifically to subsets of cells, and in particular to specific subsets of neurons. The deficits in movement that we observed in transgenic *C. elegans* overexpressing α-synuclein are likely due to pathology in motor neurons. When α-synuclein is overexpressed in dopaminergic neurons, no deficits in movement, as determined by the thrashing assay, were observed. When α-synuclein was overexpressed by the pan-neuronal promoter of either of two different motor neuron promoters, *unc-30* or *acr-2*, investigators observed movement deficits. *Unc-30*

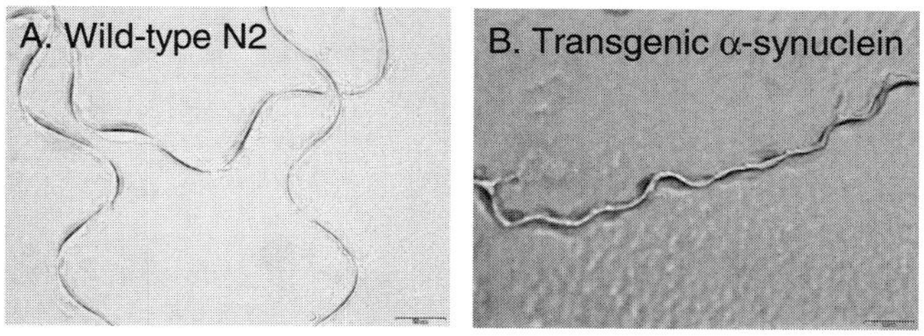

FIGURE 1 Tracks on a bacteria lawn. The tracks are left by N2 wild-type *C. elegans* (A) or a transgenic overexpressing human α-synuclein with an A53T mutation (B). The bar indicates 20 μM.

encodes a homeodomain transcription factor that is necessary and sufficient to specify cell fate of nineteen type-D GABA-ergic motor neurons (Jin et al. 1994). These motor neurons line the ventral side of *C. elegans* and inhibition by GABA in these neurons, synchronized with excitation by acetylcholine of *C. elegans* permits the sine wave movement characteristic of worms. Thus, overexpression of α-synuclein within these neurons appears sufficient to perturb movement and is highly suggestive of motor neuron pathology in α-synuclein pathology. An obvious experiment is to mark these neurons with GFP and determine whether they are still present. ACR-2 encodes a non-alpha acetylcholine receptor subunit and ectopic expression of GFP under this promoter indicates expression in most of the ventral cord motor neurons (Hallam et al. 2000). *C. elegans* overexpressing α-synuclein under control of *acr-2* promoter showed the most pronounced motor deficits with thrashing assay values of 40–50% of the controls. How expression of human α-synuclein can alter these neurons remains a matter of speculation, since *C. elegans* does not have an obvious ortholog to the human gene. Cells need not die for researchers to observe perturbations in movement. For example, transgenic worms overexpressing polyglutamine, as a model of Huntington disease, display neuronal dysfunction in the form of touch insensitivity without neuronal loss (Parker et al. 2001). General effects on gross movement can be attributed in some cases to perturbations in the neuromuscular junction, which would resemble the origin of pathology in many *unc* mutants. To address possible interacting proteins or downstream targets that contribute to perturbations in movement, we utilize RNA interference (RNAi) studies (Kamath et al. 2003). In this paradigm, phenotypically affected worms are fed bacteria that produce double-stranded RNA upon induction by isopropyl-β-thiogalactopyranoside. Through a mechanism still under intense investigation, the complementary RNA is degraded, and worms undergo a form of worm gene therapy whereby they lose genes necessary to mediate movement deficits. Identifying such genes should indicate new molecules central to the neuropathology of movement disorders. An example of postures of wild-type N2, transgenic α-synuclein, and *unc-22* RNAi-treated *C. elegans* appears in Figure 2.

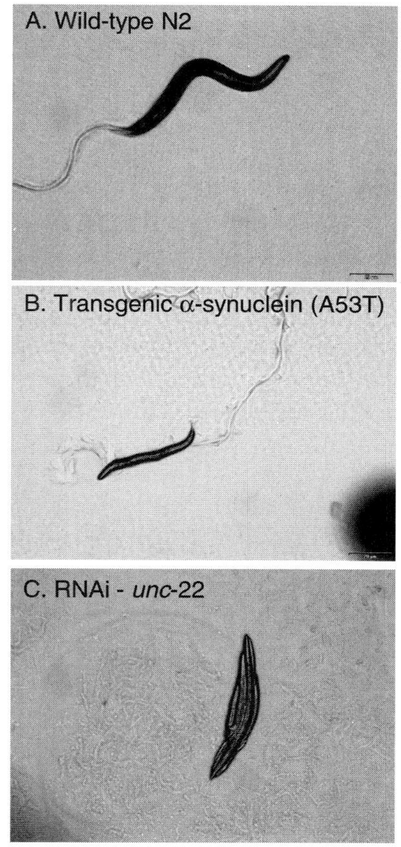

FIGURE 2 *C. elegans* moving on a bacteria lawn. (A) Wild-type N2. (B) Transgenic *C. elegans* overexpressing human α-synuclein. (C) Same as in panel B, but fed bacteria producing double-stranded RNA (RNAi) for the *unc-22* gene encoding twitching.

While the focus of pathology in Parkinson disease has been degeneration of dopaminergic neurons of the substantia nigra, other regions of the brain are affected. Investigators have shown that brain stem bulbar nuclei that send projections to premotor and motor neurons are affected in human Parkinson disease brains (Braak et al. 2000). In a transgenic mouse model overexpressing α-synuclein controlled by a general promoter, pathology is seen in brainstem and motor neurons that included axonal damage and denervation of the neuromuscular junction (van der Putten 2000). At least one approach could help to resolve whether direct pathology of motor neurons underlie movement deficits in the α-synuclein overexpressing worms: direct evaluation of motor neuron pathology in transgenic worms that would be coupled to an inducible transgene system. Such an experimental set-up would eliminate confounds such as developmental effects of the transgene and indirect effects of perturbed motor neurons.

VI. ADVANTAGES AND DISADVANTAGES OF *C. ELEGANS* PARKINSON DISEASE MODELS

The single most obvious advantage of modeling in *C. elegans* has to be its exquisite genetics. Investigators can conduct genetic manipulation, either by forward or reverse genetics, in an expedited manner due to the short generation time of three days and the flexible sexual or asexual reproduction schemes of the hermaphrodite (Jorgensen and Mango 2002). The large number of progeny (>300) produced by each hermaphrodite in its lifetime is an added bonus. Long-standing research in the field has produced hundreds of easily scored genetic markers for mapping mutations. Sequencing of the entire genome has further enhanced the utility of this animal model by providing predicted gene sequences and human orthologs. Up to 75% of human genes are estimated to have an ortholog in *C. elegans*. The "worm" sequencing project has also provided the foundation to map genes by single nucleotide polymorphisms (SNPs).

Beyond genetics, the transparency of *C. elegans* has long been recognized as a powerful tool to study development. Currently, the use of GFP to identify neuronal populations provides a means to visualize cell death events in a living model. Moreover, neuropathology can be visualized in the model using a large range of microscopy and immunohistochemical techniques (Crittenden and Kimble 1999; Miller and Shakes 1995). These events can be studied over time, which provides the next advantage: the short life span of *C. elegans*. Parkinson disease, for the most part, is an age-associated disorder. The approximate three-week life span affords investigators the opportunity to study cellular events over the life of the animal model and the possibility to conduct simple life span measurements. Practical considerations, such as the ability to freeze worm stocks, and the ability to grow at room temperature also make *C. elegans* an attractive model. From a pharmacologic perspective, *C. elegans* is useful because it is small and it can be grown in liquid culture. Thus, high-throughput drug screening in live animals can be carried out in 96- and 384-well formats (Baumeister and Ge 2002). The low cost of each animal, minimal equipment requirements, and permissive legislation further contribute to the attractiveness of *C. elegans* as a model system to study Parkinson disease.

Finally, the *C. elegans* research community has been open and willing to share resources. Sydney Brenner initiated these ideals during the early days of the field, and his post-doctoral fellows and later generations of *C. elegans* researchers have promulgated these standards. This has had an undeniable impact on the field. The tone of cooperation set forth and its impact on development of the field are likely the biggest strengths of this model system.

Why isn't everyone using *C. elegans* as a model in Parkinson disease? The strength of the model is also its weakness. The simplicity of *C. elegans*, with eight dopaminergic neurons, can go only so far to model the likely complexity of human Parkinson disease. Movements seen in humans, as well as an enormously sophisticated central nervous system, are problematic for modeling in such a simple organism. The lack of limbs or vertebra can cause one to wonder what movement is being emulated in *C. elegans*. The lack of some human gene orthologs known to be involved in the etiology of Parkinson disease also raises concerns regarding comparison of the different biological systems.

VII. RELEVANCE OF *C. ELEGANS* IN MODELING HUMAN MOVEMENT DISORDERS

Weaknesses aside, ethical questions will always arise about using humans as experimental animals, and therefore investigators must find useful model systems. *C. elegans* has been historically important in biology by opening new doors to fundamental processes in development and neuroscience. Fundamental science, with all its inherent flaws, still provides the only viable alternative to human testing. Models are therefore extremely useful.

A surprisingly limited number of worm models have been created that attempt to recapitulate features of human movement disorders, especially when one considers the number of mouse models. Even considering the number of *Drosophila* models, a paucity of invertebrate movement disorder models remains. Published models include an amyotrophic lateral sclerosis model in *Drosophila* (Elia et al. 1999), a Parkinson disease model in *Drosophila* (Feany and Bender 2000), and several polyglutamine repeat diseases including Huntington in *C. elegans* (Faber et al. 1999) and in *Drosophila* (Jackson 1998). If viewed from the perspective of movement phenotypes, an Alzheimer disease model in *C. elegans* that overexpresses beta-amyloid peptide results in a dramatic progressive paralysis (Link 1995). A more recent study has described overexpression of torsin A that serves as a model of torsion dystonia (Caldwell et al. 2003).

One could also envision tying together results from several model systems. To date, investigators have produced several transgenic mouse models overexpressing α-synuclein (Kahle et al. 2000; Kahle et al. 2002; Kirik et al. 2002; Masliah et al. 2000; Richfield et al. 2002). Investigators could perform large scale analysis by comparing microarray results or by RNA interference studies. A recent report that compared gene expression patterns during aging in *C. elegans* and *Drosophila* models indicates the feasibility of such an approach (McCarroll et al. 2004). *C. elegans* could also act as an experimental bridge between cell culture models and vertebrate models. Scientists should be able to validate intriguing results derived from *in vitro* studies in

C. elegans, an *in vivo* system. These studies could include transgenic crosses with *C. elegans* orthologs of torsin A (McLean et al. 2002; Caldwell et al 2003), dopamine transporters (Lee et al. 2001), and tyrosine kinases (Negro et al. 2002; Seo et al. 2002). Beyond α-synuclein, more human genes involved in familial Parkinson disease could also be constructed as a *C. elegans* model, either by overexpression or mutation. Parkin immediately comes to mind as a viable candidate (Lucking et al. 2000).

As scientists press forward in their search to understand the underlying biological principles that govern disease processes in movement disorders, the use of models, such as *C. elegans*, should provide new ideas and concepts at a rate that is faster, cheaper, and more ethically acceptable, than models in higher organisms.

References

Ackley, B.D., S.H. Kang, J.R. Crew, C. Suh, Y. Jin, and J.M. Kramer. 2003. The basement membrane components nidogen and type XVIII collagen regulate organization of neuromuscular junctions in the *Caenorhabditis elegans*. *J Neurosci* **23**:3577–3587.

Baumeister, R., and L. Ge. 2002. The worm in us—*Caenorhabditis* as a model of human disease. *Trends Biotech* **20**:147–148.

Braak, H., U. Rub, D. Sandmann-Keil, W.P. Gai, R.A. de Vos, E.N. Steur, K. Arai, and E. Braak. 2000. Parkinson's disease: affection of brain stem nuclei controlling premotor and motor neurons of the somatomotor system. *Acta Neuropathol* (Berl) **99**:489–495.

Caldwell, G.A., S. Cao, E.G. Sexton, C.C. Gelwix, J.P. Bevel, and K.A. Caldwell. 2003. Suppression of polyglutamine-induced protein aggregation in *Caenorhabditis elegans* by torsin proteins. *Hum Mol Genet* **12**:307–319.

Crittenden, S.L., and J. Kimble. 1999. Confocal methods for *Caenorhabditis elegans*. *Methods Mol Biol* **122**:141–151.

Duerr, J.S., D.L. Frisby, J. Gaskin, A. Duke, K. Asermely, D. Huddleston, L.E. Eiden, and J.B. Rand. 1999. The cat-1 gene of *Caenorhabditis elegans* encodes a vesicular monoamine transporter required for specific monoamine-dependent behaviors. *J Neurosci* **19**:72–84.

Elia, A.J., T.L. Parkes, K. Kirby, P. St. George-Hyslop, G.L. Boulianne, J.P. Phillips, and A.J. Hilliker. 1999. Expression of human FALS SOD in motorneurons of *Drosophila*. *Free Radic Biol Med* **26**:1332–1338.

Feany, M.B., and W.W. Bender. 2000. A *Drosophila* model of Parkinson's disease. *Nature* **404**:394–398.

Faber, P.W., J.R. Alter, M.E. MacDonald, and A.C. Hart. 1999. Polyglutamine-mediated dysfunction and apoptotic death of a *Caenorhabditis elegans* sensory neuron. *Proc Natl Acad Sci U S A* **96**:179–184.

Hallam, S., E. Singer, D. Waring, and Y. Jin. 2000. The *C. elegans* NeuroD homolog cnd-1 functions in multiple aspects of motor neuron fate specification. *Development* **127**:4239–4252.

Iwasaki, K., J. Staunton, O. Saifee, M. Nonet, and J.H. Thomas. 1997. aex-3 encodes a novel regulator of presynaptic activity in *C. elegans*. *Neuron* **18**:613–622.

Jackson, G.R., I. Salecker, X. Dong, X. Yao, N. Arnheim, P.W. Faber, M.E. MacDonald, and S.L. Zipursky. 1998. Polyglutamine-expanded human huntingtin transgenes induce degeneration of *Drosophila* photoreceptor neurons. *Neuron* **21**:633–642.

Jin, Y., R. Hoskins, and H.R. Horvitz. 1994. Control of type-D GABAergic neuron differentiation by *C. elegans* UNC-30 homeodomain protein. *Nature* **372**:780–783.

Jorgensen, E.M., and S. Mango. 2002. The art and design of genetic screens: *Caenorhabditis elegans*. *Nature Rev Genet* **3**:356–369.

Kahle, P.J., M. Neumann, L. Ozmen, V. Muller, H. Jacobsen, A. Schindzielorz, M. Okochi, et al. 2000. Subcellular localization of wild-type and Parkinson's disease-associated mutant alpha-synuclein in human and transgenic mouse brain. *J Neurosci* **20**:6365–6373.

Kahle, P.J., C. Haass, H.A. Kretzschmar, and M. Neumann. 2002. Structure/function of α-synuclein in health and disease: rational development of animal models for Parkinson's and related diseases. *J Neurochem* **82**:449–457.

Kamath, R.S., A.G. Fraser, Y. Dong, G. Poulin, R. Durbin, M Gotta, A. Kanapin, et al. 2003. Systematic functional analysis of the *Caenorhabditis elegans* genome using RNAi. *Nature* **16**:231–237.

Kirik, D., C. Rosenblad, C. Burger, C. Lundberg, T.E. Johansen, N. Muzyczka, R.J. Mandel, and A. Bjorklund. 2002. Parkinson-like neurodegeneration induced by targeted overexpression of alpha-synuclein in the nigrostriatal system. *J Neurosci* **22**:2780–2791.

Lakso, M., S. Vartiainen, A.M. Moilanen, J. Sirvio, J.H. Thomas, R. Nass, R.D. Blakely, and G. Wong. 2003. Dopaminergic neuronal loss and motor deficits in *Caenorhabditis elegans* overexpressing human alpha-synuclein. *J Neurochem* **86**:165–172.

Lee, F.J.S., F. Liu, Z.B. Pristupa, and H.B. Niznik. 2001. Direct binding and functional coupling of α-synuclein to the dopamine transporters accelerate dopamine-induced apoptosis. *FASEB J* **15**:916–926.

Lee, M.K., W. Stirling, Y. Xu, X. Xu, D. Qui, A.S. Mandir, T.M. Dawson, et al. 2002. Human alpha-synuclein-harboring familial Parkinson's disease-linked Ala-53 → Thr mutation causes neurodegenerative disease with alpha-synuclein aggregation in transgenic mice. *Proc Natl Acad Sci U S A* **99**:8968–8973.

Link, C.D. 1995. Expression of human beta-amyloid peptide in transgenic *Caenorhabditis elegans*. *Proc Natl Acad Sci U S A* **92**:9368–9372.

Lints, R., and S.W. Emmons. 1999. Patterning of dopaminergic neurotransmitter identity among *Caenorhabditis elegans* ray sensory neurons by a TGFβ family signaling pathway and a *Hox* gene. *Development* **126**: 5819–5831.

Loer, C.M., and C.J. Kenyon. 1993. Serotonin-deficient mutants and male mating behavior in the nematode *Caenorhabditis elegans*. *J Neurosci* **13**:5407–5417.

Lucking, C.B., A. Durr, V. Bonifati, J. Vaughan, G. De Michele, T. Gasser, B.S. Harhangi, et al. 2000. Association between early-onset Parkinson's disease and mutations in the parkin gene. French Parkinson's Disease Genetics Study Group. *N Engl J Med* **342**:1560–1567.

Masliah, E., E. Rockenstein, I. Veinbergs, M. Mallory, M. Hashimoto, A. Takeda, Y. Sagara, et al. 2000. Dopaminergic loss and inclusion body formation in alpha-synuclein mice: implications for neurodegenerative disorders. *Science* **287**:1265–1268.

McCarroll, S.A., C.T. Murphy, S. Zou, S.D. Pletcher, C.S. Chin, Y.N. Jan, C. Kenyon, C.I. Bargmann, and H. Li. 2004. Comparing genomic expression patterns across species identifies shared transcriptional profile in aging. *Nat Genet* **36**:197–204.

McLean, P.J., H. Kawamata, S. Shariff, J. Hewett, N. Sharma, K. Ueda, X.O. Breakefield, and B.T. Hyman. 2002. TorsinA and heat shock proteins act as molecular chaperones: suppression of alpha-synuclein aggregation. *J Neurochem* **83:**846–854.

Mello, C., and A. Fire. 1995. DNA transformation. *Methods Cell Biol* **48**: 451–482.

Miller, K.G., A. Alfonso, M. Nguyen, J.A. Crowell, C.D. Johnson, and J.B. Rand. 1996. A genetic selection for *Caenorhabditis elegans* synaptic transmission mutants. *Proc Natl Acad Sci U S A* **93**:12593–12598.

Miller, D.M., and D.C. Shakes. 1995. Immunofluorescence microscopy. *Methods Cell Biol* **48**:365–394.

Nass, R., and R.D. Blakely. 2003. The *Caenorhabditis elegans* dopaminergic system: opportunities for insights into dopamine transport and neurodegeneration. *Annu Rev Pharmacol Toxicol* **43**:521–544.

Nass, R., D.H. Hall, D.M. Miller, 3rd., and R.D. Blakely. 2002. Neurotoxin-induced degeneration of dopamine neurons in *Caenorhabditis elegans*. *Proc Natl Acad Sci U S A* **99**:3264–3269.

Nass R., D.M. Miller, and R.D. Blakely. 2001. *C. elegans*: a novel pharmacogenetic model to study Parkinson's disease. *Parkinsonism Relat Disord* **7**:185–191.

Negro, A., A.M. Brunati, A. Conella-Deana, M.L. Massimino, and L.A. Pinna. 2002. Multiple phosphylation of α-synuclein by protein tyrosine kinase Syk prevents eosin-induced aggregation. *FASEB J* **16**:210–212.

Parker, J.A., J.B. Connolly, C. Wellington, M. Hayden, J. Dausset, and C. Neri. 2001. Expanded polyglutamines in *Caenorhabditis elegans* cause axonal abnormalities and severe dysfunction of PLM mechanosensory neurons without cell death. *Proc Natl Acad Sci U S A* **98**: 13318–13323.

Polymeropoulos, M.H., C. Lavedan, E. Leroy, S.E. Ide, A. Dehejia, A. Dutra, B. Pike, et al. 1997. Mutation in the alpha-synuclein gene identified in families with Parkinson's disease. *Science* **276**:2045–2047.

Reiner, D.J., E.M. Newton, H. Tian, and J.H. Thomas. 1999. Diverse behavioural defects caused by mutations in *Caenorhabditis elegans* unc-43 CaM kinase II. *Nature* **402**:199–203.

Richfield, E.K., M.J. Thiruchelvam, D.A. Cory-Slechta, C. Wuertzer, R.R. Gainetdinov, M.G. Caron, D.A. Di Monte, and H.J. Federoff. 2002. Behavioral and neurochemical effects of wild-type and mutated human alpha-synuclein in transgenic mice. *Exp Neurol* **175**:35–48.

Rose, J.K., and C.H. Rankin. 2001. Analyses of habituation in *Caenorhabditis elegans*. *Learn Mem* **8**:63–69.

Sanyal, S., R.F. Wintle, K.S. Kindt, W.M. Nuttley, R. Arvan, P. Fitzmaurice, E. Bigras, et al. 2004. Dopamine modulates the plasticity of mechanosensory responses in *Caenorhabditis elegans*. *EMBO J* **23**: 473–82.

Sawin, E.R. 1996. Genetic and cellular analysis of modulated behaviors in *Caenorhabditis elegans*. PhD thesis, Massachusetts Institute of Technology.

Seo, J.H., J.C. Rah, S.H. Choi, J.K. Shin, K. Min, H.S. Kim, C.H. Park, et al. 2002. Alpha-synuclein regulates neuronal survival via Bcl-2 family expression and PI3/Akt kinase pathway. *FASEB J* **16**:1826–1828.

Spillantini, M.G., M.L. Schmidt, V.M. Lee, J.Q. Trojanowski, R. Jakes, and M. Goedert. 1997. Alpha-Synuclein in Lewy bodies. *Nature* **388**: 839–840.

Sulston, J., M. Dew, and S. Brenner. 1975. Dopaminergic neurons in the nematode *C. elegans*. *J Comp Neurol* **163**:215–226.

Suo, S., N. Sasagawa, and S. Ishiura. 2002. Identification of a dopamine receptor from *Caenorhabditis elegans*. *Neurosci Lett* **319**:13–16.

Suo, S., N. Sasagawa, and S. Ishiura. 2003. Cloning and characterization of a *Caenorhabditis elegans* D2-like dopamine receptor. *J Neurochem* **86**:869–878.

Thomas, J.H., and S. Lockery. 1999. Neurobiology. In *C. elegans: A Practical Approach*. Ed. I. Hope. pp. 143–176. Oxford: Oxford University Press.

van der Putten, H., K.H. Wiederhold, A. Probst, S. Barbieri, C. Mistl, S. Danner, S. Kauffmann, et al. 2000. Neuropathology in mice expressing human alpha-synuclein. *J Neurosci* **20**:6021–6029.

White, J.G., E. Southgate, J.N. Thomson, and S. Brenner. 1986. The structure of the nervous system of the nematode *Caenorhabditis elegans*. *Philos Trans R Soc Lond B Biol Sci* **314**:1–340.

Wintle, R.F., and H.H. Van Tol. 2001. Dopamine signaling in *Caenorhabditis elegans*-potential for parkinsonism research. *Parkinsonism and Related Disorders* **7**:177–183.

C H A P T E R

C1

Clinical Features and Classification of the Human Dystonias

RACHEL SAUNDERS-PULLMAN and SUSAN BRESSMAN

I. CLINICAL FEATURES AND CLASSIFICATION OF THE HUMAN DYSTONIAS

Dystonia is characterized by sustained muscle contractions causing twisting and repetitive movements and postures (Fahn 1988), which are often precipitated by action (Fahn 1988; Fahn et al. 1998). The clinical spectrum of dystonias is wide. Dystonia may start as early as infancy or present in late adulthood (Bandmann et al. 1998; Opal et al. 2002). It may be limited to a single muscle group, such as spasm of a vocal cord adductor or it may affect entire body regions, as in generalized dystonia involving legs, the trunk and both arms (table 1). The etiologies of dystonias are similarly broad. Dystonia may be due to a myriad of genetic etiologies, some of which are known, or it may be secondary to various toxic causes. Different classification schema have been devised, including a clinically oriented one (Fahn 1988; Bressman 2003; Bressman 2004), and a molecular one using the Human Genome Organization/ Genome Database (HUGO/GDB) identification for dystonia with genetic etiology (www.gene.ucl.ac.uk/nomenclature/). However, the HUGO/GDB designation lists a very diverse group of dystonias in chronologic order by year of discovery, and does not account for the majority of dystonias; therefore we will focus on the proposed clinical classification, and discuss where the HUGO/GDB designations have been integrated into this schema.

Under the clinically oriented classification, two main etiologic categories appear: primary torsion dystonia (PTD), defined as a syndrome in which dystonia is the predominant phenotypic manifestation and there is no evidence of neuronal degeneration or an acquired cause, and secondary (nonprimary) dystonia, which may be further divided into those with inherited, complex, and acquired etiologies (Bressman 2003; Bressman 2004). No consistent pathological changes have been demonstrated to date for primary dystonia. In contrast, many secondary forms of dystonia are often associated with degenerative processes, such as striatal necrosis in glutaric aciduria (Strauss et al. 2003). Although dystonia may improve with oral medications, botulinum toxin injections, and deep brain stimulation surgery, investigators have not identified a specific single treatment for primary dystonia (Jankovic 2004). Treatment of secondary dystonia is often directed at treating the underlying condition, such as copper chelation treatment in Wilson disease. As a framework for understanding animal models of dystonia, we will briefly discuss the epidemiology and pathology of the human dystonias and then more thoroughly review the clinical features of the major forms of primary dystonias and dystonia-plus syndromes.

TABLE 1 Classifications of Dystonia

A) *Age at onset* of dystonia
  Early (≤ 26 years)
  Late

B) *Distribution* of sites affected by dystonia
  Focal (single body region)
  Segmental (contiguous regions)
  Multifocal (non-contiguous regions)
    Includes Hemidystonia (ipsilateral arm and leg)
  Generalized (leg and trunk and at least one other region OR both legs +/– trunk and one other region)

C) *Etiology*
  I. Primary Dystonia (dystonia is only movement disorder except tremor, and there is no acquired/exogenous cause, degenerative disorder, or excellent response to levodopa)
    1. Early Onset (≤26 years)
      Many due to TOR1A (DYT1) GAG deletion
    2. Mixed Phenotype
      Child- or adult-onset in limb, neck, or cranial muscles, dysarthria/dysphonia common: mapped to chr 8 (DYT6) in Swiss Mennonite families
      Early-onset segmental cervical/cranial: child or adult-onset in cervical/cranial or brachial muscles mapped to chr 1p (DYT13) in an Italian family
    3. Adult cervical, cranial, or brachial-onset
      Dystonia usually localized
      Mapped to chr 18p (DYT7) in a German torticollis family; other similar families excluded from locus
      Torticollis and blepharospasm associated with a dopamine receptor D5 polymorphism
  II. Secondary dystonia (due to inherited and/or degenerative disorders or signs other than dystonia)
    1. Associated with hereditary neurological syndromes
      a. Dystonia Plus (similar to primary dystonia in that degenerative pathology not identified, dystonia a prominent sign, but signs other than dystonia do occur)
        Dopa-responsive dystonia
          GCHI mutations (previously DYT5); DYT14; Other monoamine synthetic disorders (tyrosine hydroxylase deficiency, other biopterin deficient states, and dopa-decarboxylase deficiency)
        Myoclonus—Dystonia
          Epsilon-sarcoglycan mutations (DYT 11) on chromosome 7; single family linked to 18p (DYT15)
        Rapid-onset dystonia-parkinsonism (DYT12)
      b. Other inherited disorders associated with neurodegeneration
        Autosomal Dominant
          Huntington disease; Machado-Joseph disease/SCA3 disease; Other SCA subtypes; DRPLA; Familial basal ganglia calcifications; Fronto-temporal dementias
        Autosomal Recessive
          Juvenile Parkinsonism (PARK2); Wilson; Glutaric academia; PKAN (Hallervorden-Spatz disease); Gangliosidoses; Metachromatic leukodystrophy; Homocystinuria; Hemochromatosis; Hartnup disease; Methylmalonic aciduria; Niemann-Pick, type C/Dystonic lipidosis; Ceroid-lipofuscinosis; Ataxia-telangiectasia; Neuroacanthocytosis—Chorein; Intraneuronal inclusion disease
        X-Linked Recessive
          Lubag (X-linked dystonia-parkinsonism, DYT3); Lesch-Nyhan syndrome; Deafness/Dystonia (Mohr-Tranebjaerg Syndrome)
        Mitochondrial
          MERRF/MELAS; Leber's disease
    2. Due to acquired/exogenous causes
      Perinatal cerebral injury; Encephalitis, infectious and post-infectious; Head trauma; Pontine myelinolysis; Primary antiphospholipid syndrome; Stroke; Tumor; Multiple sclerosis; Cervical cord injury or lesion; Peripheral injury; Drugs (e.g., dopamine receptor blockers);Toxins; Psychogenic
    3. Dystonia due to degenerative parkinsonian disorders of unknown/complex etiologies
      PD; PSP (Progressive Supranuclear Palsy); CBGD (Cortico basal ganglionic degeneration)
    4. Dystonia as a feature of other dyskinetic disorders)
      a. Tics
      b. Paroxysmal disorders: PKD (DYT 10/EKD1, EKD2); PNKD (DYT8); CSE (DYT9)

CSE = Choreoathetosis/spasticity, episodic; DRD = dopa-responsive dystonia; EKD = episodic kinesigenic dystonia; GCH1 = GTP cyclohydrolase1; NBIA1-neurodegeneration with brain iron accumulation; DDP = deafness dystonia peptide; DRPLA = dentatorubral-pallidoluysian atrophy; MEERF = myoclonic epilepsy associated with ragged red fibers; MELAS = mitochondrial myopathy, encephalopathy, lactic acidosis, and stroke-like episodes; PD = Parkinson disease; PKAN = pantothenate kinase; PKD (Paroxysmal kinesogenic dystonia); PNKD (Paroxysmal non-kinesogenic dystonia); SCA = spinocerebellar ataxia.

II. EPIDEMIOLOGY

Despite the greater prevalence of dystonia than other well-known neurological conditions, such as myasthenia gravis and motor neuron disease (Cockerell 1993), there are limited estimates of the frequency of dystonia in the United States and worldwide (Duffey et al. 1998). Those that do exist are most likely underestimates. Two primary reasons arise for underestimating the prevalence of dystonia: misdiagnosis and individuals with a mild form of the disease never seeking medical advice. Dystonia is often misdiagnosed because it is a clinical diagnosis with a wide spectrum of symptoms that may affect multiple body sites, leading to physician misinterpretation. Neurologists not trained in movement disorders and primary care physicians may have difficulty clinically diagnosing dystonia. Finally, while dystonia affects the lifestyles of many, in some cases it may be so mild that subjects may not present to a physician with symptomatic complaints. In previous genetic studies, Bressman and colleagues demonstrated that as many as 50% of all people with dystonia who were ascertained during family studies did not seek medical attention or were misdiagnosed (Bressman et al. 1989). Because the members of Bressman's study population were a mostly well-educated group, and all of these cases had a family member with dystonia, even 50% may be an underestimate of the cases that go undiagnosed. Evaluating primary dystonia in northern England, Duffey and colleagues showed that at least 10% of the dystonia cases diagnosed in their study had gone undiagnosed by physicians from nonmovement disorder specialties (Duffey et al. 1998).

Current prevalence estimates of dystonia range from 6.1 in 100,000 for focal dystonia in the Tottori prefecture in Japan (Nakashima et al. 1995) to 34 in 100,000 for all primary dystonia, and 29.5 in 100,000 for focal dystonia in a records-based study from Olmstead County, Minnesota (Nutt et al. 1988). Between both estimates, a clinic-based study of thirteen dystonia specialists in Europe found a total prevalence of 15.2 in 100,000, and focal dystonia 11.7 in 100,000 (Epidemiologic Study of Dystonia in Europe [ESDE] Collaborative Group 2000). However, such retrospective and clinic-based studies are limited by patients actually presenting for medical attention as well as by the correct physician diagnosis. In order to avoid these pitfalls, Muller et al. (2002) examined all patients over fifty years old who were participating in a study of cerebrovascular disease in South Tyrol, and found the prevalence of dystonia in this age group to be as high as 723 in 100,000. Such high rates of dystonia have yet to be replicated.

There are gender differences among types of focal dystonia, with dystonia more common among women for all types except writer's cramp (Epidemiologic Study of Dystonia in Europe [ESDE] Collaborative Group 1999). Gender differences are most pronounced in dopa-responsive-dystonia, where the ratio of females to males affected is between 2 : 1 to 6 : 1 (Furukawa et al. 1998b). There are also numerous examples of ethnic differences in the frequency of dystonia, and these are presumed secondary to founder effects in different populations. Several groups showed an increased frequency of early-onset dystonia in Ashkenazi Jews in the United States and Israel (Zeman and Dyken 1967; Eldridge et al. 1971; Zilber et al. 1984; Risch et al. 1995). Almasy et al. (1997) demonstrated a relative excess of adult onset cranial dystonia in those of Ashkenazi descent. Increased frequency of adult onset blepharospasm was also shown in southern Italy (Defazio 2002), and this may suggest a founder effect. Further studies of large multiethnic populations are needed, and careful analysis of phenotype may lend insight into possible genetic subtypes arising from founder effects.

III. PATHOLOGY

Investigators often observe lesions of the basal ganglia and thalamus in secondary forms of dystonia. They may also observe abnormal dopaminergic transmission along with basal ganglia lesions, or as the isolated etiology, such as in dopa-responsive dystonia. In contrast, a pathological or neurochemical substrate in primary torsin dystonia (PTD) remains to be clarified. Neurochemical abnormalities, including norepinephrine and serotonin levels are not consistently elevated or decreased in different brain regions (Zeman and Dyken 1967; Zeman 1970; Hornykiewicz et al. 1986; Zweig et al. 1988). Three studies from the same group have suggested an association between copper metabolism and PTD. Elevated globus pallidus copper and manganese were noted in three patients with focal dystonia (Becker et al. 1999) and the copper-metabolizing Menkes protein was decreased in PTD (Berg et al. 2000), with low Menkes mRNA and low copper in leukocytes in patients with cervical PTD (Kruse et al. 2001). However, no clear pathogenic mutations were identified in either copper-translocating ATPases or intracellular copper chaperones in PTD patients (Bandmann 2002) to suggest that copper genes are associated with the development of PTD. Thus the role of copper in PTD remains unclear.

A major group of childhood onset PTD arises from a mutation in the DYT1 gene. This gene encodes the torsinA protein, which is related to the class of heat shock proteins and may affect protein folding and other regulatory functions (Vale 2000; Neuwald et al.1999). Pathologic studies of DYT1 brains, although limited in number, have noted only abnormalities of unclear significance. No evidence of intracellular aggregation or degeneration was observed (Walker et al. 2002; Rostasy et al. 2003), although one study found qualitatively larger and more tightly packed dopamine neurons (Rostasy et al. 2003) and another of a DYT1 family member with Parkinsonism showed loss of pigmented substantia nigra neurons (Augood et al. 2002). Neurochemical analysis has shown slightly decreased dopamine and homovanillic acid (HVA) levels in the rostral caudate and putamen (Furukawa et al. 2000). Augood and colleagues, however, found normal striatal dopamine, HVA, and DOPAC levels but an increased ratio of striatal DOPAC to dopamine (Augood et al. 2002), and torsinA has been identified in Lewy bodies of Parkinson disease (PD) (Shashidharan et al. 2000). The significance of dopamine in the pathogenesis of DYT1 dystonia remains uncertain, as clinically DYT1 is not associated with Parkinsonism, and does not demonstrate a clear or consistent response to dopaminergic therapy as is seen in the secondary dystonias, dopa-responsive-dystonia, and dystonia associated with Parkinsonism (Bressman 2004).

IV. CLINICAL CLASSIFICATION OF DYSTONIA

To describe the heterogeneity in phenotype and etiology, researchers have used three major categories to classify dystonia: age at onset, distribution of body parts affected by dystonia, and etiology (Marsden and Harrison 1974; Marsden et al. 1976). These three factors are not independent; age of onset is often associated with site of onset and final distribution, and the genetic etiology may be associated with age of onset, such as DYT1, which frequently starts in childhood or adolescence, usually in a limb, and may spread to become generalized (Greene et al. 1995; Bressman et al. 1998). With advances in genetics, genotype has often been the major classifying factor in disease. However with dystonia, different genotypes may have overlapping phenotypes, and many forms of primary dystonia do not yet have associated genotypes, so phenotypic classification remains relevant. This chapter will focus on these different forms of classification, with greatest emphasis on etiologic classification, and when known, genetic classification among the primary and dystonia-plus etiologies (table 1).

A. Classification by Age of Onset and Distribution

In the early descriptions of dystonia, the late David Marsden emphasized age of onset as the most important feature in predicting clinical outcome, with earlier age of onset portending both greater spread to other body regions, and more severe dystonia (Marsden and Harrison 1974; Marsden et al. 1976). Among primary dystonia, younger onset (childhood and adolescence) is more likely to affect the legs and spread rostrally, and later adult-onset dystonia is more likely to start in the neck, voice, or face and is less likely to spread (Greene et al. 1995).

Stratification of age at onset has undergone several revisions. In 1984 an ad hoc committee of the Dystonia Medical Research Foundation categorized age of onset into childhood (zero to twelve years), adolescent (thirteen to twenty years) and adult (greater than twenty-one years) onset. However, as dystonia referred to a tertiary care center showed a bimodal distribution with peaks at nine and forty-five years and a nadir at twenty-seven years (Bressman et al. 1989), most recent classification schemes (Bressman 1998; Jarman and Warner 1998) have favored the dichotomous categories of early and late onset, with early onset defined as age twenty-six or less and late onset defined as twenty-seven years or greater. The latter classification is now widely accepted (Fahn et al. 1998; Nemeth 2002; Bressman 2003; Bressman 2004).

The ad hoc committee of the Dystonia Medical Research Foundation also recommended defining five subclasses of distribution of dystonia: focal, segmental, generalized, multifocal, and hemidystonia. Focal dystonia is limited to a single body region, segmental to contiguous body regions, generalized to crural involvement (one leg and the trunk or both legs with or without the trunk) plus another body region, multifocal to noncontiguous body regions, and hemidystonia to dystonia affecting ipsilateral limbs. This classification is useful for the clinical monitoring of patients and classification of families for genetics studies. For example, treatment with botulinum toxin may be targeted for focal dystonia because it is usually more practical for a single body area as dose limitations are easily reached if multiple large muscle groups are injected. However, multiple smaller muscle groups can be injected, and therefore segmental cranio-cervical dystonia may also respond, or botulinum toxin may be injected into a single symptomatic site, such as the arm, even though other body regions are affected. This classification is most limited when viewed independently, as it does not take into account the complex relationship between age of onset, sites of dystonia at onset, progression, and etiology (Greene et al. 1995; Bressman 2004).

B. Classification by Etiology

Traditionally, etiology was split into two major categories: idiopathic, where no exogenous cause or brain pathology was identified, and symptomatic dystonia, where an exogenous cause can be determined (see table 1) (Fahn 1988; Fahn et al. 1998). However, with the elucidation of dystonia genes, it became clear that idiopathic dystonia was not truly idiopathic, and this category was relabeled "primary," and symptomatic dystonia was labeled "secondary" (Fahn et al. 1998). A subcategory of secondary dystonia, dystonia-plus, genetic forms of dystonia with neurological features in addition to dystonia, but without apparent neurodegeneration, has been added (Fahn et al.

1998) to distinguish "pure" dystonic syndromes from those with dystonia plus other movement disorders, such as dopa-responsive dystonia, where Parkinsonism and spasticity may also be present. Current nomenclature refers to primary torsion dystonia when (1) dystonia is the only neurological feature (with the exception of tremor), (2) an exogenous or acquired cause cannot be historically identified (e.g., stroke, neuroleptic exposure), (3) there is no laboratory or imaging abnormality to suggest an acquired or degenerative etiology (e.g., Parkinson Disease, Wilson Disease), and (4) there is no dramatic response to levodopa, which would suggest dopa-responsive-dystonia (Bressman 2003).

Dystonia may also be classified genetically, using the Human Genome Organization/Genome Database (HUGO) designations "DYT," but this is a heterogeneous group encompassing at least fifteen different dystonia syndromes (table 2). HUGO DYT designations include different etiologic subtypes: primary dystonia, some forms of secondary dystonia, and dystonia plus (GCH1 which was previously labeled DYT5: DRD and DYT13 and DYT15: myoclonus-dystonia (M-D), as well as the paroxysmal dystonias, which

TABLE 2 Molecular Classification of Dystonia

Dystonia type	Mode of inheritance/ *OMIM*	Chromosomal location	Gene product & mutation
DYT1			
Early-onset generalized torsin dystonia	autosomal dominant *128100*	9q34	3-bp (GAG) deletion in the gene (TOR1A) that encodes torsinA
DYT2			
Autosomal recessive	autosomal recessive *224500*	unknown	Unknown
DYT3			
X-linked dystonia-Parkinsonism, "Lubag"	X-linked *314250*	Xq13.1	Disease specific nucleotide changes (DSC3) putatively regulating transcription
DYT4			
"non-DYT1" torsin dystonia Whispering dystonia in one family	autosomal dominant *128101*	unknown	Unknown
***GCH1* (previously DYT5)**			
Dopa responsive dystonia and parkinsonism; Segawa syndrome	autosomal dominant *128230*	14q22.1–q22.2	Mutations in the GTP cyclohydrclase I gene
DYT6			
Adolescent and early-onset dystonia of mixed phenotype	autosomal dominant *60269*	8	Unknown
DYT7			
Late-onset focal dystonia	autosomal dominant *602124*	18p	Unknown
DYT8			
Paroxysmal non-kinesigenic dyskinesia or dystonic choreoathetosis	autosomal dominant *118800*	2q33–q35	Unknown
DYT9			
Paroxysmal choreoathetosis with episodic ataxia and spasticity	autosomal dominant *601042*	1p21–p13.3	Unknown
DYT10			
Paroxysmal kinesiogenic dyskinesia/choreoathetosis	autosomal dominant *128200*	16p11.2–q12.1	Unknown
DYT11			
Myoclonus-dystonia syndrome	autosomal dominant *159900*	7q21–31	Different mutations in epsilon-sarcoglycan (SGCE)
DYT12			
Rapid-onset dystonia-parkinsonism	autosomal dominant *128235*	19q	Unknown
DYT13			
Early and late-onset cervical cranial dystonia	autosomal dominant *607671*	1p36.13	Unknown
DYT 14			
Dopa- responsive dystonia	autosomal dominant *607195*	14q13	Unknown
DYT 15			
Myoclonus-dystonia	autosomal dominant *607488*	18p11	Unknown

are usually not classified with dystonia, but under episodic dyskinetic syndromes with dystonic contractions (Fahn et al. 1998). Investigators have identified genes for four of the DYT subtypes: DYT1 (Ozelius et al. 1997), DYT3 (Nolte et al. 2003), DYT5 (now renamed GCH1, Ichinose et al. 1994) and DYT11 (Zimprich et al. 2001), and genetic loci have been determined for most, but not all of the other HUGO DYT subtypes. DYT2, autosomal recessive dystonia in the Spanish Roma population (Gimenez-Roldan et al. 1988), and DYT4 whispering dysphonia (Parker 1985; Ahmad et al. 1993) were described only clinically, without linkage to a particular region, and currently, additional DYT designations are not assigned without genetic examination. While some authors have described clinical subtypes under the HUGO designations, such as DYT4 comprising all adult onset PTD, or autosomal recessive primary dystonia as DYT2-like (Khan et al. 2003), these subtypes may be confusing because the genetic loci for these forms are not known, and they may eventually obtain other HUGO/GDB designations.

Despite the large number of loci, genes for most forms of primary dystonia have not been revealed, and the majority of dystonia cannot be classified with a HUGO/GDB designation. Therefore splitting dystonia into primary and secondary (including dystonia-plus) remains useful, as these criteria help to categorize and separate more types of dystonia than genetic criteria alone. Nonetheless, more specific phenotypic criteria may emerge, as essential tremor, for example may accompany cervical dystonia (Couch 1976; Bressman et al. 1996). Elucidation of genes or other biomarkers, particularly functional imaging, may further distinguish subgroups of PTD, and may facilitate better accounting of the diversity of primary dystonia.

1. Primary Torsion Dystonia

Using classification previously discussed, we will address early onset PTD, including DYT1 and non-DYT1 followed by late onset PTD.

a. Early Onset PTD

In 1911 Oppenheim originally described early onset PTD as a childhood and adolescent disorder, *dystonia musculorum deformans* (Oppenheim 1911). Schwalbe further described PTD and emphasized the familial nature of the disease (Schwalbe 1980), and later Zeman described the increased frequency among Ashkenazi Jews, which has been estimated at three to five times that in other populations (Zeman and Dyken 1967; Risch et al. 1995). Early onset PTD shows autosomal dominant transmission with reduced penetrance of 30–40% in Ashkenazi Jews and non-Ashkenazim (Zilber et al. 1984; Bressman et al. 1989; Fletcher et al. 1990; Pauls and Korczyn 1990). Initial study demonstrated linkage to 9q34 in a large non-Jewish family with early onset PTD. Through linkage disequilibrium and positional cloning, investigators determined the DYT1 locus, and identified a three base pair GAG deletion that produces the loss of a glutamic acid residue at the carboxyl end of the encoded protein torsinA (TOR1A) (Ozelius et al. 1997). The TOR1A mutation accounts for 80% of early onset PTD in Ashkenazim (Bressman et al. 1994; Bressman et al. 2000), and 16–53% in non-Ashkenazim (Valente et al. 1998; Lebre, Durr et al. 1999; Slominsky et al. 1999; Brassat et al. 2000; Bressman 2000; Zorzi et al. 2002). The increased frequency among the Ashkenazim is the result of a founder mutation estimated to have been introduced into this population in the 1600s in Lithuania or Byelorussia (Risch et al. 1995). The mutation also occurs in other populations, and was reported in eastern and western Europe, South America, and Japan (Valente et al. 1998; Slominsky et al. 1999; Major et al. 2001; Ikeuchi et al. 2002; Gatto et al. 2003): the mutation is secondary to multiple mutation events including families with de novo mutations (Klein et al. 1998a; Hjermind et al. 2002). Clinical expression among different ethnic groups is also similar (Carmona et al. 2003). The same three base pair deletion has been reported in all individuals (Ozelius et al. 1999; Leung et al. 2001; Tuffery-Giraud et al. 2001) except a family with a form of dystonia-plus, myoclonus-dystonia, who also had a mutation in the epsilon-sarcoglycan gene that caused a large proportion of familial myoclonus-dystonia (Doheny et al. 2002a; Klein et al. 2002b).

In addition to variable penetrance, the DYT1 mutation also shows tremendous variability in expression. It can be heterogeneous with regard to final distribution and severity, even among closely related family members: in some, the dystonia will remain focal and produce only mild writer's cramp, whereas in others it leads to severe generalized dystonia that progresses rapidly (Opal et al. 2002). However, common features also appear—DYT1 dystonia is usually early-onset dystonia (i.e., onset before age twenty-six), and begins in a limb (Bressman et al. 2000). Less frequently, onset may be in the neck or cranial muscles, and dystonia may remain focal in these sites (Leube et al. 1999; Bressman et al. 2000; Tuffery-Giraud et al. 2001). Although rare, late-onset dystonia has also been reported (Opal et al. 2002). Focal and segmental arm dystonia are the most common adult forms (Bressman et al. 1994; Gasser et al. 1998; Bressman et al. 2000; Opal et al. 2002). At final distribution, 95% of individuals with dystonia have at least one arm affected. Approximately 25% remain focal, 10% segmental, and 65% progress to develop generalized or multifocal dystonia. While the trunk and neck are affected in 25–35% of the cases, cranial muscles are involved in less than 15% of cases (Bressman 2003).

Investigators formulated symptomatic testing recommendations based on the study of clinical characteristics of 267 PTD patients, including 186 DYT1 carriers. Testing individuals with onset of PTD beginning before age twenty-six for the DYT1 mutation has a sensitivity of 100% and specificity of 54% (Bressman et al. 2000), although because of rare adult onset cases, testing adult PTD with a blood relative with early-onset PTD is also recommended (Bressman et al. 2000).

b. Non-DYT1 Early-Onset PTD and "Mixed"-Onset PTD

As noted, a significant proportion of non-Ashkenazim and a minority of Ashkenazi Jews do not harbor the DYT1 GAG deletion (Valente et al. 1998; Kamm et al. 1999; Slominsky et al. 1999; Brassat et al. 2000). Therefore much early-onset PTD is not DYT1, and there must be genetic heterogeneity for early-onset PTD.

Investigators have mapped two additional loci, DYT6 and DYT13, with average age of onset in adolescence. Both demonstrate autosomal dominant inheritance with incomplete penetrance. In DYT6, age of onset ranges from 5 to 38 years, and the average age of onset is 18.1 years (Almasy et al. 1997). DYT13 has a range of onset from 5 to 40 and average age of onset of 15.6 years (Valente et al. 2001a, 2001b). In contrast to DYT1, where adult onset is uncommon. Both of these disorders commonly also present in adulthood (approximately half of DYT6 cases start in childhood and half in adulthood); thus they are termed "mixed" age of onset, as both early- and late-onset dystonia occur in the families (Almasy et al. 1997; Valente et al. 2001a, 2001b).

With respect to distribution, both DYT6 and DYT13 are also different from DYT1 and are also "mixed": there is prominent cranial facial involvement, and more variability than in either the DYT1 or focal dystonia phenotypes. However, some affected individuals in DYT6 and DYT13 families may overlap with the DYT1 phenotype; e.g., as in DYT1, there are individuals in both of these kindred with early-onset focal writer's cramp (Almasy et al. 1997; Valente et al. 2001a; Valente et al. 2001b). In DYT6, onset varies from arm, cranial muscles (including larynx and tongue), neck, and leg. Most symptoms spread to other sites, although three of the fifteen cases reportedly remained focally distributed. Unlike DYT1, most disability arises from cranial and neck involvement; when the leg is involved, the dystonia tends to remain milder, and in fourteen of fifteen cases does not sufficiently limit ambulation to require an assistive device (Almasy et al. 1997). In the eleven affected DYT13 individuals, onset was in the neck, neck and cranial regions, and arm (Almasy et al. 1997; Bentivoglio, et al. 1997; Valente et al. 2001a, 2001b). In most individuals, dystonia had spread to involve cervical, cranial, and brachial muscles, although one family member had focal writer's cramp and one had focal neck dystonia. DYT6 and DYT13 vary in that leg and laryngeal involvement is less frequently reported in DYT13, although the total of affected cases in both linked families is small, and the phenotypic variation may be much greater than appreciated. Neither locus appears to account for many early-onset cases, as DYT6 was identified in two large related Amish-Mennonite families, and DYT13 in one extended Italian family; these loci have been excluded in other families with early-onset dystonia (Jarman 1998; Bressman, unpublished communication). Researchers therefore assume that multiple other as yet unidentified loci account for the many non-DYT1 early-onset cases.

c. Adult-Onset Dystonia

Most PTD is adult onset, with focal cervical dystonia constituting approximately half of prevalent cases in the aforementioned European study. While investigators calculated rates of cervical dystonia at 57 per million, rates of blepharospasm and writer's cramp were lower, at 36 per million and 14 per million, respectively (Epidemiologic Study of Dystonia in Europe [ESDE] Collaborative Group 2000). Family studies have demonstrated increased rates of dystonia among family members, suggesting a genetic etiology. With equal rates in parents, offspring, and siblings, the pattern of inheritance is consistent with autosomal dominant inheritance; however, it appears to be less penetrant than childhood-onset dystonia, with penetrance at 10–15% (Waddy et al. 1991; Maniak et al. 2003) rather than 30–40%. Therefore adult onset dystonia appears to be more complex in etiology than early-onset and the contribution and interaction of genetic and possible environmental factors is unclear. There are reported families that show higher penetrance, including families with torticollis (Bressman et al. 1996; Leube et al. 1996; Munchau et al. 2000; Defazio et al. 2003), and mixed-phenotype families (Cassetta et al. 1999). Genes in these more highly penetrant families have not yet been mapped. Adult onset DYT6 and DYT13 account for only a fraction of the cases of adult onset dystonia, as the cases thus far are limited to the reported families, and these loci have been excluded in other large adult-onset families (Jarman et al. 1999).

Investigators identified a locus for adult onset cervical dystonia, DYT7, in a northern German family (Leube et al. 1996) with seven affected individuals. All members had adult onset torticollis, although some also had brachial and cranial involvement. While investigators initially postulated that a mutation in this region may be a founder for PTD in northwest Germany and central Europe, based on allelic association for several chromosome 18 markers, others could not replicate the finding (Klein et al. 1998b), and this locus has been excluded in other European PTD families (Klein et al. 1998b; Jarman et al. 1999; Munchau et al. 2000; Defazio et al. 2003). The authors were also unable to confirm the finding using microsatellite markers, thus suggesting overall that DYT7 does not have a major founder effect (Leube and Auburger 1998).

Association studies have shown that a D5 polymorphism may be associated with adult-onset focal dystonia, in particular torticollis in British and Italian patients (Placzek et al. 2001; Brancati et al. 2003) and blepharospasm in British patients (Misbahuddin et al. 2002; Misbahuddin et al. 2004), and further studies are necessary to test this association in other dystonia populations. Other proposed etiologies of adult-onset PTD include mitochondrial complex I dysfunction (Schapira et al. 1997).

2. Secondary Dystonia

Secondary dystonias comprise those groups of dystonia that fit any of the following descriptions: (1) neurological features in addition to dystonia are present, (2) an exogenous or acquired cause can be identified (e.g., stroke, neuroleptic exposure), (3) a laboratory or imaging abnormality suggests an acquired or degenerative etiology (e.g., Parkinson Disease, Wilson Disease), or (4) a dramatic response to levodopa occurs, which would suggest dopa-responsive-dystonia (Bressman 2003). Secondary dystonias may be further subdivided by etiology into those meeting the following criteria: (1) inherited causes, (2) a group of primarily Parkinsonian disorders with complex etiologies, and (3) environmental or acquired causes (Bressman 2004). Further, dystonic phenomenology may be present with other movement disorders such as dystonic tics and paroxysmal dyskinesias. Pseudodystonias have muscle contractions that mimic dystonia, such as psychogenic dystonia and congenital torticollis, an orthopedic condition which simulates dystonia (Bressman 2004).

a. The Dystonia-Plus Syndromes

The secondary dystonias with inherited etiologies but no apparent neurodegeneration have been labeled the dystonia-plus syndromes. Because of shared features with primary and secondary dystonias, the dystonia-plus syndromes were initially in a category straddling primary and secondary dystonias (Fahn et al. 1998), although they have been reclassified as a sub-group of the secondary dystonias (Bressman 2004). Fahn et al. (1998) included three distinct syndromes in this category, myoclonus-dystonia (M-D), dopa-responsive-dystonia (DRD), and rapid-onset-dystonia-parkinsonism (RDP). The three syndromes share some features with PTD, but are different in other ways. Dystonia is present in all three conditions. Further, unlike secondary dystonia, and like PTD, none have apparent degenerative pathology. Therefore these syndromes are distinct from other inherited secondary forms of dystonia with degeneration, such as Lubag (DYT3) (Lee et al. 1991; Nolte et al. 2003). However, features other than dystonia are prominent in all: myoclonus is prominent in M-D, and Parkinsonism in RDP and DRD.

i) Dopa-responsive Dystonia Dopa-responsive-dystonia (DRD) is a syndrome characterized by childhood-onset dystonia, affecting gait more than arms, which is often diurnal, and responds dramatically to low-dose levodopa therapy (Segawa et al. 1976; Nygaard et al. 1990; Segawa and Nomura 1993). Parkinsonism, particularly bradykinesia and postural instability, as well as hyperreflexia and arm dystonia commonly occur with the leg dystonia. DRD may also present with less typical features, including isolated adult-onset Parkinsonism (Nygaard et al. 1992), focal cervical dystonia, adult-onset oromandibular dystonia (Steinberger et al. 1999) and may mimic cerebral palsy with developmental delay, scoliosis, hypotonia with proximal weakness (Nygaard et al. 1994; Kong et al. 2001), and myoclonus-dystonia (Leuzzi et al. 2002). Typically, onset is age six, although DRD has been reported in infancy, and may begin with Parkinsonism in the elderly (Nygaard et al. 1990; Segawa and Nomura 1993; Bandmann et al. 1998). While sustained response to low-dose levodopa is the norm, higher doses may be necessary (Furukawa et al. 1998b; Steinberger et al. 1999; Tassin et al. 2000).

DRD is genetically heterogeneous. The most common form of DRD is autosomal dominant with incomplete penetrance, and is secondary to mutations in the GTP cyclohydrolase 1 (GCH1) gene. There is incomplete gender-related penetrance, with girls and women manifesting two to four times more than boys and men (Nygaard et al. 1993; Ichinose et al. 1994; Furukawa et al. 1998b; Nygaard and Wooten 1998). GTPCH catalyzes the first and rate-limiting step in the synthesis of tetrahydrobiopterin (BH4), which is an essential cofactor for aromatic amino acid hydroxylases including phenylalanine and tyrosine hydroxylase, enzymes involved in the conversion of phenylalanine to tyrosine and tyrosine to levodopa, respectively. Many GTPCH mutations are unique (see www.bh4.org/biomdb1.html for a list of reported mutations) and up to 40% of patients with DRD do not have identifiable mutations in coding exons (Furukawa 2004). Other mutations, as well as deletions may account for some of the mutation negative cases (Bandmann et al. 1998; Furukawa et al. 2000a; Klein et al. 2002a), although a small amount of DRD may have another etiology (Furukawa 2004). Compound heterozygous mutations may result in a more severe form of the disease that causes developmental motor delay, with limb dystonia progressing to generalized dystonia (Furukawa et al. 1998a). Patients with autosomal recessive GTPCH deficiency usually develop severe neurological dysfunction (Niederweiser 1995). Linkage to a region proximal to GCH1 on 14q has also been reported in one family with autosomal dominant DRD (DYT14) (Grotzsch et al. 2002).

DRD may also be secondary to other metabolic defects in the dopamine synthesis pathway. Autosomal recessive mutations in the tyrosine hydroxylase (TH) gene may also produce DRD and the clinical picture may be mild or severe, with infantile Parkinsonism and motor delay (Knappskog et al. 1995; Ludecke et al. 1995; van den Heuvel et al. 1998; Furukawa et al. 2001).

Because of the heterogeneity of GTPCH1 mutations, as well as the inability to identify mutations in many individuals, clinical features and response to levodopa have remained the diagnostic gold standard for DRD. However, juvenile Parkinsonism secondary to mutations in the parkin gene may also produce young-onset dystonia-parkinsonism which may mimic DRD. Typically, JPD has slightly later onset and has more prominent early Parkinsonism and dyskinesias (Tassin et al. 2000). As outlined in table 3, diagnostic tests to distinguish JPD from classic DRD and TH deficiency include lumbar puncture with analysis of neopterin and biopterin (Brautigam et al. 1999; Furukawa et al. 1995; Furukawa and Kish 1999; Furukawa 2003), and phenylalanine loading to assess the response of liver phenylalanine hydroxylase (which is reduced in manifesting and non-manifesting GTPCH mutation carriers) (Hyland et al. 1997; Hyland et al. 1999). While most investigators have found the phenylalanine loading test highly sensitive (Hyland et al. 1997; Hyland et al. 1999; Bandmann et al. 2003), we found false negative results among manifesting gene carriers. Functional imaging may also help discriminate DRD from JPD: fluorodopa PET scanning is abnormal in JPD, but normal in DRD (Snow et al. 1993; Turjanski et al. 1993). Similarly, single-photon emission tomography using ^{123}I-β-CIT or FP-CIT to measure the dopamine transporter, is normal in DRD but shows decreased uptake in JPD (Naumann et al. 1997; O'Sullivan et al. 2001). Raclopride PET, measuring D2 dopamine-receptor binding, in contrast shows increased binding in both symptomatic and asymptomatic GTPCH1 gene carriers (Kishore et al. 1998). More recently, Bonafe et al. (2001) have demonstrated that GTPCH1 activity, biopterin, and neopterin can be measured

TABLE 3 Differential Diagnosis of Dopa-Responsive Dystonia (DRD)

	DRD (autosomal dominant)	**DYT1**	**Juvenile PD/parkin**
Age–onset, average (range)	6 years (infancy-6th decade)	13 years: range 4 years-7th decade	Adolescence (7 years-6th decade)
Gender	Female > Male	Female = Male	Male = Female
Initial signs	Leg > arm or trunk action dystonia, gait dystonic and often spastic with toe walking	Arm or leg action dystonia, occasionally trunk or neck	Foot/leg > hand/arm dystonia, rest tremor, akinesia/ rigidity
Diurnal fluctuations	Often prominent	Rare	May occur but usually not dramatic
Bradykinesia	Yes (maybe mild)	No	Yes
Postural instability	Yes	No	Yes
Response to L-dopa			
Initial	Excellent (low dose)	Inconsistent, and usually not dramatic	Excellent and low to moderate dose
Long term	Excellent		Dyskinesias, may fluctuate
CSF			
HAV	⇓	normal	⇓
Biopterin	⇓	normal	⇓
Neopterin	⇓⇓	normal	normal
F-DOPA PET	Normal	Normal	Decreased
Inheritance	AD, reduced penetrance	AD, reduced penetrance	AR
Gene	Heterozygous mutations in GCH1 in many	Heterozygous GAG deletion in DYT1	Homozygous or compound heterozygous parkin mutations
Testing	Screening for GCH1 mutations in select labs	Commercially available	Screening for some parkin mutations in select labs
Prognosis	Sustained excellent response, near complete symptom resolution in most	Progression then stabilization	Slow to moderate progression

in cytokine-stimulated fibroblasts. This test may have clinical utility in distinguishing DRD from JPD and other forms of childhood-onset PTD.

ii) Myoclonus-dystonia Myoclonus is characterized by fast lightninglike jerks. Myoclonus may be isolated, or occur in association with other movement disorders, particularly dystonia. Some patients with DYT1 and other forms of primary dystonia may have dystonic movements as brief as 100 ms and occasional myoclonic jerks may be superimposed on dystonic movements (Obeso et al. 1983). Conversely, in families with myoclonus and dystonia, myoclonus may be the primary inherited feature, and may frequently occur independently of dystonia, and this is termed myoclonus-dystonia (M-D) (Gasser 1998; Nygaard et al. 1999). Families are characterized as having M-D when one individual has prominent early-onset myoclonus (usually the first or second decade), which may or may not be associated with dystonia, and there are no other neurologic features such as ataxia or dementia. Rarely, dystonia may be the only movement disorder in a family member (Kyllerman et al. 1990; Gasser 1998; Asmus et al. 2002). The neck and arms are the most commonly involved sites, followed by the trunk and bulbar muscles, and least commonly the legs (Kyllerman et al. 1990; Gasser 1998; Nygaard et al. 1999; Asmus et al. 2002). The disorder usually plateaus in adulthood, and the myoclonus usually shows dramatic improvement with ingestion of alcohol. Psychiatric symptoms are more prominent in family members, although it is unclear whether this is secondary to the gene, or secondary to the burden of the disorder (Doheny et al. 2002a, 2002b; Saunders-Pullman et al. 2002).

Familial M-D is inherited in an autosomal dominant manner with incomplete penetrance and variable expressivity, with a maternal imprinting pattern, that is, most individuals who inherit the gene from the father manifest symptoms, whereas those who inherit from the mother usually do not. A locus on chromosome 7q21 was mapped for familial M-D (DYT11), and narrowed in additional families, and the epsilon sarcoglycan gene was identified (Nygaard et al. 1999; Asmus et al. 2001; Vidailhet et al. 2001; Zimprich et al. 2001). The sarcoglycans are a family of genes that encode components of the dystrophin-glycoprotein complex and mutations in alpha, beta, gamma, and delta sarcoglycan produce recessive muscular limb-girdle dystrophy. Epsilon sarcoglycan however, is expressed widely in the brain and is imprinted. However, the function and mechanism by which the mutated protein produces M-D remain unknown. Locus heterogeneity occurs, however, as one family with M-D did not have an SGCE mutation, and a locus on 18p was mapped (Grimes et al. 2001).

iii) Rapid-Onset Dystonia-Parkinsonism RDP (DYT 12) is a rare disorder described in three unrelated families in the United States and Ireland (Dobyns et al. 1993; Brashear et al. 1997; Webb et al. 1999; Pittock et al. 2000). It is characterized by the sudden and rapid evolution or worsening of dystonia and Parkinsonism. Onset is usually in adolescence or the early adult years. Motor features may include dystonia-Parkinsonism-hyperreflexia, or dystonia alone. The dystonia is usually tonic rather than clonic or rhythmic with prominent bulbar features of dysarthria and grimacing. The Parkinsonism is notable for bradykinesia and postural instability. Symptoms usually present extremely rapidly (hours to days) then plateau (Dobyns et al. 1993; Brashear et al. 1997; Webb, Broderick et al. 1999; Pittock et al. 2000). Psychiatric features, including, but not limited to, depression and social phobia have also been reported, as have seizures (Pittock et al. 2000, Brashear et al. 1997). The disorder is refractory to treatments, including levodopa, although the CSF dopamine metabolite homovanillic acid (HVA) is reduced in some patients (Brashear et al. 1998). β-CIT SPECT does not suggest nigral degeneration (Brashear et al. 1999), and pathology of a single case does not demonstrate nigral cell loss (Pittock et al. 2000). Linkage to chromosome 19q13 (DYT12) has been independently demonstrated by two groups (Kramer et al. 1999; Pittock et al. 2000).

V. CONCLUSION

Clinical classification of dystonia into etiologic subtypes provides a framework for understanding the diversity of dystonias and their genetic heterogeneity. Further delineation of clinical subtypes will guide in the identification of further dystonia genes, as better genotype-phenotype correlations will also improve our clinical descriptions of dystonia subtypes. Through the study of relevant animal models and the use of additional biochemical, neuropyschiatric, molecular genetic, and neuroimaging tools, greater understanding of and better treatments for dystonia will be possible.

Acknowledgments

This work was performed while Rachel Saunders-Pullman was a Pfizer/Society for Women's Health Research scholar. Susan Bressman is supported by National Institutes of Health (RO1NS26656)

References

Ahmad, F., M.B. Davis, H.M. Waddy, C.A. Oley, C.D. Marsden, and A.E. Harding. 1993. Evidence for locus heterogeneity in autosomal dominant torsion dystonia. *Genomics* **15(1)**:9–12.

Almasy, L., S. Bressman, D. de Leon, and N. Risch. 1997. Ethnic variation in the clinical expression of idiopathic torsion dystonia. *Mov Disord* **12(5)**:715–721.

Almasy, L., S.B. Bressman, D. Raymond, P.L. Kramer, P.E. Greene, G.A. Heiman, B. Ford, et al. 1997. Idiopathic torsion dystonia linked to chromosome 8 in two Mennonite families. *Ann Neurol* **42(4)**:670–673.

Asmus, F., A. Zimprich, M. Naumann, D. Berg, M. Bertram, A. Ceballos-Baumann, R. Pruszak-Seel, et al. 2001. Inherited myoclonus-dystonia syndrome: narrowing the 7q21–q31 locus in German families. *Ann Neurol* **49(1)**:121–124.

Asmus, F., A. Zimprich, S. Tezenas Du Montcel, C. Rabus, G. Deuschl, A. Kupsch, V. Ziemann, et al. 2002. Myoclonus-dystonia syndrome: epsilon-sarcoglycan mutations and phenotype. *Ann Neurol* **52(4)**: 489–492.

Augood, S.J., Z. Hollingsworth, D.S. Albers, L. Yang, J.C. Leung, B. Muller, C. Klein, et al. 2002. Dopamine transmission in DYT1 dystonia: a biochemical and autoradiographical study. *Neurology* **59(3)**: 445–448.

Bandmann, O., F. Asmus, D. Sibbing, M. Grundmann, S.G. Schwab, J. Muller, D.B. Wildenaver, et al. 2002. Copper genes are not implicated in the pathogenesis of focal dystonia. *Neurology* **59(5)**:782–783.

Bandmann, O., M. Goertz, J. Zschocke, G. Derschl, W. Jost, H. Hefter, U. Muller, et al. 2003. The phenylalanine loading test in the differential diagnosis of dystonia. Neurology **60(4)**:700–702.

Bandmann, O., E.M. Valente, P. Holmans, R.A. Surtees, J.H. Walters, R.A. Wevers, C.D. Marsden. 1998. Dopa-responsive dystonia: a clinical and molecular genetic study. *Ann Neurol* **44(4)**:649–656.

Becker, G., D. Berg, W.D. Rausch, H.K. Lange, P. Riederer, K. Reiners. 1999. Increased tissue copper and manganese content in the lentiform nucleus in primary adult-onset dystonia. *Ann Neurol* **46(2)**:260–263.

Bentivoglio, A.R., N. Del Grosso, A. Albanese, E. Cassetta, P. Tonali, M. Frontali. 1997. Non-DYT1 dystonia in a large Italian family. J *Neurol Neurosurg Psychiatry* **62(4)**:357–360.

Berg, D., A. Weishaupt, M.J. Francis, N. Miura, X.L. Yang, I.D. Goodyer, M. Naumann, et al. 2000. Changes of copper-transporting proteins and ceruloplasmin in the lentiform nuclei in primary adult-onset dystonia. *Ann Neurol* **47(6)**:827–830.

Bonafe, L., B. Thony, W. Leimbacher, L. Kierat, N. Blau. 2001. Diagnosis of dopa-responsive dystonia and other tetrahydrobiopterin disorders by the study of biopterin metabolism in fibroblasts. *Clin Chem* **47(3)**:477–485.

Brancati, F., E.M. Valente, M. Castori, N. Vanacore, M. Sessa, G. Galardi, A. Berardelli, et al. Italian Movement Disorder Study Group. 2003. Role of the dopamine D5 receptor (DRD5) as a susceptibility gene for cervical dystonia. *J Neurol Neurosurg Psychiatry* **74(5)**:665–666.

Brashear, A., I.J. Butler, L.J. Ozelius, P.I. Kramer, M.R. Farlow, X.O. Breakefield, W.B. Dobyns. 1998. Rapid-onset dystonia-parkinsonism: a report of clinical, biochemical, and genetic studies in two families. *Adv Neurol* **78**:335–339.

Brashear, A., D. DeLeon, S.B. Bressman, D. Thyagarajan, M.R. Farlow, W.B. Dobyns. 1997. Rapid-onset dystonia-parkinsonism in a second family. *Neurology* **48(4)**:1066–1069.

Brashear, A., G.K. Mulholland, Q.H. zheng, M.R. Farlow, E.R. Siemers, G.D. Hutchins. 1999. PET imaging of the presynaptic dopamine uptake sites in rapid-onset dystonia-parkinsonism (RDP). *Mov Disord* **14(1)**: 132–137.

Brassat, D., A. Camuzat, M. Vidailhet, I. Feki, P. Jedynak, P. Klap, Y. Agid, et al. 2000. Frequency of the DYT1 mutation in primary torsion dystonia without family history. *Arch Neurol* **57(3)**:333–335.

Brautigam, C., G.C. Steenbergen-Spanjer, G.F. Hoffman, C. Dionisi-Vici, L.P. van den Heuvel, J.A. Smeitink, R.A. Wevers. 1999. Biochemical and molecular genetic characterization of severe forms of tyrosine hydroxylase deficiency. *Clin Chem* **45**:2073–2078.

Bressman, S.B. 1998. Dystonia. *Curr Opin Neurol* **11(4)**:363–372.

Bressman, S.B. 2003. Dystonia: phenotypes and genotypes. *Rev Neurol* (Paris) **159(10 Pt 1)**:849–856.

Bressman, S.B. 2004. Dystonia genotypes, phenotypes, and classification. *Adv Neurol* **94**:101–107.

Bressman, S.B., D. de Leon, M.F. Brin, N. Risch, R.E. Burke, P.E. Greene, H. Shale, et al. 1989. Idiopathic dystonia among Ashkenazi Jews: evidence for autosomal dominant inheritance. *Ann Neurol* **26(5)**:612–620.

Bressman, S.B., D. de Leon, P.L. Kramer, L.J. Ozelius, M.F. Brin, P.E. Greene, S. Fahn, et al. 1994. Dystonia in Ashkenazi Jews: clinical characterization of a founder mutation. *Ann Neurol* **36(5)**:771–777.

Bressman, S.B., D. de Leon, D. Raymond, L.J. Ozelius, X.O. Breakefield, T.G. Nygaard, L. Almasy, et al. 1998. Clinical-genetic spectrum of primary dystonia. *Adv Neurol* **78**:79–91.

Bressman, S.B., C. Sabatti, D. Raymond, D. de Leon, C. Klein, P.L. Kramer, M.F. Brin, et al. 2000. The DYT1 phenotype and guidelines for diagnostic testing. *Neurology* **54(9)**:1746–1752.

Bressman, S.B., T.T. Warner, L. Almasy, R.J. Uitti, P.E. Greene, G.A. Heiman, D. Raymond, et al. 1996. Exclusion of the DYT1 locus in familial torticollis. *Ann Neurol* **40(4)**:681–684.

Carmona, J., J.A. Burguera, B. Molla, F. Mulas, P. Smeyers, F. Carratala, J.G. De Yebenes, et al. 2003. Unique origin and low penetrance of the 946delGAG mutation in Valencian DYT1 families. *Clin Genet* **64(2)**:153–159.

Cassetta, E., N. Del Grosso, A.R. Bentivoglio, E.M. Valente, M. Frontali, A. Albanese. 1999. Italian family with cranial cervical dystonia: clinical and genetic study. *Mov Disord* **14(5)**:820–825.

Cockerell, O.C., J.W. Sander, and S.D. Shorvon. 1993. Neuroepidemiology in the United Kingdom. *Journal of Neurology, Neurosurgery and Psychiatry* **56**:735–738.

Couch, J.R. 1976. Dystonia and tremor in spasmodic torticollis. *Adv Neurol* **14**:245–258.

Defazio, G., M.S. Aniello, G. Masi, V. Lucchese, D. De Candia, D. Martino. 2003. Frequency of familial aggregation in primary adult-onset cranial cervical dystonia. *Neurol Sci* **24(3)**:168–169.

Defazio, G., and P. Livrea. 2002. Epidemiology of primary blepharospasm. *Mov Disord* **17(1)**:7–12.

Dobyns, W.B., L.J. Ozelius, P.L. Kramer, A. Brashear, M.R. Farlow, T.R. Perry, L.E. Walsh, et al. 1993. Rapid-onset dystonia-parkinsonism. *Neurology* **43(12)**:2596–2602.

Doheny, D., F. Danisi, C. Smith, C. Morrison, M. Velickovic, D. De Leon, S.B. Bressman, et al. 2002a. Clinical findings of a myoclonus-dystonia family with two distinct mutations. *Neurology* **59(8)**:1244–1246.

Doheny, D.O., M.F. Brin, C.E. Morrison, C.J. Smith, R.H. Walker, S. Abbasi, B. Muller, et al. 2002b. Phenotypic features of myoclonus-dystonia in three kindreds. *Neurology* **59(8)**:1187–1196.

Duffey, P.O., A.G. Butler, M.R. Hawthorne, M.P. Barnes. 1998. The epidemiology of the primary dystonias in the north of England. *Adv Neurol* **78**:121–125.

Eldridge, R., A. Edgar, I.S. Cooper. 1971. Genetics, geography and intelligence in the torsion dystonias. *Birth Defects Orig Artic Ser* **7(1)**:167–177.

Epidemiologic Study of Dystonia in Europe (ESDE) Collaborative Group. 1999. Sex-related influences on the frequency and age of onset of primary dystonia. *Neurology* **53(8)**:1871–1873.

Epidemiologic Study of Dystonia in Europe (ESDE) Collaborative Group. 2000. A prevalence study of primary dystonia in eight European countries. *J Neurol* **247(10)**:787–792.

Fahn, S. 1988. Concept and classification of dystonia. *Adv Neurol* **50**: 1–8.

Fahn, S., S.B. Bressman, C.D. Marsden. 1998. Classification of dystonia. *Adv Neurol* **78**:1–10.

Fletcher, N.A., A.E. Harding, C.D. Marsden. 1990. A genetic study of idiopathic torsion dystonia in the United Kingdom. *Brain* **113 (Pt 2)**:379–395.

Furukawa, Y. 2003. Genetics and biochemistry of dopa-responsive dystonia: significance of striatal tyrosine hydroxylase protein loss. *Adv Neurol* **91**:401–410.

Furukawa, Y. 2004. Update on dopa-responsive dystonia: locus heterogeneity and biochemical features. *Adv Neurol* **94**:127–138.

Furukawa, Y., W.D. Graf, H. Wong, M. Shimadzu, S.J. Kish. 2001. Dopa-responsive dystonia simulating spastic paraplegia due to tyrosine hydroxylase (TH) gene mutations. *Neurology* **56(2)**:260–263.

Furukawa, Y., M. Guttman, S.P. Sparagana, J.M. Trugman, K. Hyland, P. Wyatt, A.E. Lang, et al. 2000a. Dopa-responsive dystonia due to a large deletion in the GTP cyclohydrolase I gene. *Ann Neurol* **47(4)**: 517–520.

Furukawa, Y., O. Hornykiewicz, S. Fahn, S.J. Kish. 2000b. Striatal dopamine in early-onset primary torsion dystonia with the DYT1 mutation. *Neurology* **54(5)**:1193–1195.

Furukawa, Y., and S.J. Kish 1999. Dopa-responsive dystonia: recent advances and remaining issues to be addressed. *Mov Disord* **14(5)**: 709–715.

Furukawa, Y., S.J. Kish, E.M. Bebin, R.D. Jacobson, J.S. Fryburg, W.G. Wilson, M. Shimadzu, et al. 1998a. Dystonia with motor delay in compound heterozygotes for GTP-cyclohydrolase I gene mutations. *Ann Neurol* **44(1)**:10–16.

Furukawa, Y., A.E. Lang, J.M. Trugman, T.D. Bird, A. Hunter, M. Sadeh, T. Tagawa, et al. 1998b. Gender-related penetrance and de novo GTP-cyclohydrolase I gene mutations in dopa-responsive dystonia. *Neurology* **50(4)**:1015–1020.

Furukawa, Y., K. Nishi, Y. Mizuno, H. Narabayashi. 1995. Significance of CSF biopterin and neopterin in hereditary progressive dystonia with marked diurnal fluctuation (HPD)—a clue to pathogenesis. [In Japanese] *No To Shinkei* **47(3)**:261–268.

Furukawa, Y., M. Shimadzu, O. Hornykiewicz, S.J. Kish. 1998. Molecular and biochemical aspects of hereditary progressive and dopa-responsive dystonia. *Adv Neurol* **78**:267–282.

Gasser, T. 1998. Inherited myoclonus-dystonia syndrome. *Adv Neurol* **78**:325–334.

Gasser, T., K. Windgassen, B. Bereznai, C. Kabus, A.C. Ludolph. 1998. Phenotypic expression of the DYT1 mutation: a family with writer's cramp of juvenile onset. *Ann Neurol* **44(1)**:126–128.

Gatto, E.M., M.M. Pardal, F.E. Micheli. 2003. Unusual phenotypic expression of the DYT1 mutation. *Parkinsonism Relat Disord* **9(5)**:277–279.

Gimenez-Roldan, S., G. Delgado, et al. 1988. Hereditary torsion dystonia in gypsies. *Adv Neurol* **50**:73–81.

Greene, P., U.J. Kang, S. Fahn. 1995. Spread of symptoms in idiopathic torsion dystonia. Mov Disord **10(2)**:143–152.

Grimes, D.A., D. Bulman, P.S. George-Hyslop, A.E. Lang. 2001. Inherited myoclonus-dystonia: evidence supporting genetic heterogeneity. *Mov Disord* **16(1)**:106–110.

Grotzsch, H., G.P. Pizzolato, J. Ghika, D. Schorderet, F.J. Vingerhoets, T. Landis, P.R. Burkhard. 2002. Neuropathology of a case of dopa-responsive dystonia associated with a new genetic locus, DYT14. *Neurology* **58(12)**:1839–1842.

Hjermind, L.E., L.M. Werdelin, S.A. Sorensen. 2002. Inherited and de novo mutations in sporadic cases of DYT1-dystonia. *Eur J Hum Genet* **10(3)**: 213–216.

Hornykiewicz, O., S.J. Kish, L.E. Becker, I. Farley, K. Shannak. 1986. Brain neurotransmitters in dystonia musculorum deformans. *N Engl J Med* **315(6)**:347–353.

Hyland, K., J.S. Fryburg, et al. 1997. Oral phenylalanine loading in dopa-responsive dystonia: a possible diagnostic test. *Neurology* **48(5)**: 1290–1297.

Hyland, K., T.G. Nygaard, J.M. Trugman, K.J. Swoboda, L.A. Arnold, S.P. Sparagana. 1999. Oral phenylalanine loading profiles in symptomatic and asymptomatic gene carriers with dopa-responsive dystonia due to dominantly inherited GTP cyclohydrolase deficiency. *J Inherit Metab Dis* **22(3)**:213–215.

Ichinose, H., T. Ohye, E. Takahashi, N. Seki, T. Hori, M. Segawa, Y. Nomura, et al. 1994. Hereditary progressive dystonia with marked diurnal fluctuation caused by mutations in the GTP cyclohydrolase I gene. *Nat Genet* **8(3)**:236–242.

Ikeuchi, T., Y. Nomura, M. Segawa, L.J. Ozelius, T. Shimohata, S. Tsuji. 2002. Multiple founder effects in Japanese families with primary torsion dystonia harboring the GAG deletion in the Tor1A (DYT1) gene. *Neurogenetics* **4(2)**:105–106.

Jankovic, J. 2004. Dystonia: medical therapy and botulinum toxin. *Adv Neurol* **94**:275–286.

Jarman, P.R., N. del Grosso, E.M. Valente, B. Leube, E. Cassetta, A.R. Bentivoglio, H.M. Waddy, et al. 1999. Primary torsion dystonia: the search for genes is not over. *J Neurol Neurosurg Psychiatry* **67(3)**:395–397.

Jarman, P.R., and T.T. Warner 1998. The dystonias. *J Med Genet* **35(4)**: 314–318.

Kamm, C., E. Castelon-Konkiewitz, M. Naumann, F. Heinen, M. Brack, A. Nebe, A. Ceballos-Baumann, et al. 1999. GAG deletion in the DYT1 gene in early limb-onset idiopathic torsion dystonia in Germany. *Mov Disord* **14(4)**:681–683.

Khan, N.L., N.W. Wood, K.P. Bhatia. 2003. Autosomal recessive, DYT2-like primary torsion dystonia: a new family. *Neurology* **61(12)**:1801–1803.

Kishore, A., T.G. Nygaard, R. de la Fuente-Fernandez, A.B. Naini, M. Schulzer, E. Mak, T.J. Ruth, et al. 1998. Striatal D2 receptors in symptomatic and asymptomatic carriers of dopa-responsive dystonia measured with [11C]-raclopride and positron-emission tomography. *Neurology* **50(4)**:1028–1032.

Klein, C., M.F. Brin, D. de Leon, S.A. Limborska, I.A. Ivanova-Smolenskaya, S.B. Bressman, A. Friedman, et al. 1998a. De novo mutations (GAG deletion) in the DYT1 gene in two non-Jewish patients with early-onset dystonia. *Hum Mol Genet* **7(7)**:1133–1136.

Klein, C., K. Hedrich, K. Kabakci, K. Mohrmann, K. Wiegers, O. Landt, J. Hagenah, et al. 2002a. Exon deletions in the GCHI gene in two of four Turkish families with dopa-responsive dystonia. *Neurology* **59(11)**:1783–1786.

Klein, C., L. Liu, D. Doheny, N. Kock, B. Muller, P. de Carvalho Aguiar, J. Leung, et al. 2002b. Epsilon-sarcoglycan mutations found in combination with other dystonia gene mutations. *Ann Neurol* **52(5)**: 675–679.

Klein, C., L.J. Ozelius, J. Hagenah, X.O. Breakefield, N.J. Risch, P. Vieregge. 1998. Search for a founder mutation in idiopathic focal dystonia from Northern Germany. *Am J Hum Genet* **63(6)**:1777–1782.

Klein, C., P.P. Pramstaller, C.C. Castellan, X.O. Breakefield, P.L. Kramer, L.J. Ozelius. 1998b. Clinical and genetic evaluation of a family with a mixed dystonia phenotype from South Tyrol. *Ann Neurol* **44(3)**: 394–398.

Knappskog, P.M., T. Flatmark, et al. 1995. Recessively inherited L-dopa-responsive dystonia caused by a point mutation (Q381K) in the tyrosine hydroxylase gene. *Hum Mol Genet* **4(7)**:1209–1212.

Kong, C.K., C.H. Ko, S.F. Tong, C.W. Lam. 2001. Atypical presentation of dopa-responsive dystonia: generalized hypotonia and proximal weakness. *Neurology* **57(6)**:1121–1124.

Kramer, P.L., M. Mineta, et al. 1999. Rapid-onset dystonia-parkinsonism: linkage to chromosome 19q13. *Ann Neurol* **46(2)**:176–182.

Kruse, N., D. Berg, M.J. Francis, M. Naumann, W.D. Rausch, K. Reiners, P. Rieckmann, et al. 2001. Reduction of Menkes mRNA and copper in leukocytes of patients with primary adult-onset dystonia. *Ann Neurol* **49(3)**:405–408.

Kyllerman, M., L. Forsgren, G. Sanner, G. Holmgren, J. Wahlstrom, U. Drugge. 1990. Alcohol-responsive myoclonic dystonia in a large family: dominant inheritance and phenotypic variation. *Mov Disord* **5(4)**:270–279.

Lebre, A.S., A. Durr, P. Jedynak, G. Ponsot, M. Vidailhet, Y. Agid, A. Brice. 1999. DYT1 mutation in French families with idiopathic torsion dystonia. *Brain* **122(Pt 1)**:41–45.

Lee, L.V., K.G. Kupke, F. Caballar-Gonzaga, M. Hebron-Ortiz, U. Muller. 1991. The phenotype of the X-linked dystonia-parkinsonism syndrome. An assessment of 42 cases in the Philippines. *Medicine* (Baltimore) **70(3)**:179–187.

Leube, B., and G. Auburger. 1998. Questionable role of adult-onset focal dystonia among sporadic dystonia patients. *Ann Neurol* **44(6)**:984–985.

Leube, B., K.R. Kessler, A. Ferbert, M. Ebke, G. Schwendemann, F. Erbguth, R. Benecke, et al. 1999. Phenotypic variability of the DYT1 mutation in German dystonia patients. *Acta Neurol Scand* **99(4)**: 248–251.

Leube, B., D. Rudnicki, T. Ratzlaff, K.R. Kessler, R. Benecke, G. Auburger. 1996. Idiopathic torsion dystonia: assignment of a gene to chromosome 18p in a German family with adult onset, autosomal dominant inheritance and purely focal distribution. *Hum Mol Genet* **5(10)**:1673–1677.

Leung, J.C., C. Klein, J. Friedman, P. Vieregge, H. Jacobs, D. Doheny, C. Kamm, et al. 2001. Novel mutation in the TOR1A (DYT1) gene in atypical early onset dystonia and polymorphisms in dystonia and early onset parkinsonism. *Neurogenetics* **3(3)**:133–143.

Leuzzi, V., C. Carducci, C. Carducci, F. Cardona, C. Artiola, I. Antonozzi. 2002. Autosomal dominant GTP-CH deficiency presenting as a dopa-responsive myoclonus-dystonia syndrome. *Neurology* **59(8)**:1241–1243.

Ludecke, B., B. Dworniczak, et al. 1995. A point mutation in the tyrosine hydroxylase gene associated with Segawa's syndrome. *Hum Genet* **95(1)**:123–125.

Major, T., M. Svetel, S. Romac, V.S. Kostic. 2001. DYT1 mutation in primary torsion dystonia in a Serbian population. *J Neurol* **248(11)**: 940–943.

Maniak, S., M. Sieberer, J. Hagenah, C. Klein, P. Vieregge. 2003. Focal and segmental primary dystonia in northwestern Germany—a clinico-genetic study. *Acta Neurol Scand* **107(3)**:228–232.

Marsden, C.D., and M.J. Harrison. 1974. Idiopathic torsion dystonia (dystonia musculorum deformans). A review of forty-two patients. *Brain* **97(4)**:793–810.

Marsden, C.D., M.J. Harrison, S. Bundey. 1976. Natural history of idiopathic torsion dystonia. *Adv Neurol* **14**:177–187.

Misbahuddin, A., M.R. Placzek, K.R. Chaudhuri, N.W. Wood, K.P. Bhatia, T.T. Warner. 2002. A polymorphism in the dopamine receptor DRD5 is associated with blepharospasm. *Neurology* **58(1)**:124–126.

Misbahuddin, A., M.R. Placzek, T.T. Warner. 2004. Focal dystonia is associated with a polymorphism of the dopamine D5 receptor gene. *Adv Neurol* **94**:143–146.

Muller, J., S. Kiechl, G.K. Wenning, K. Seppi, J. Willeit, A. Gasperi, J. Wissel, et al. 2002. The prevalence of primary dystonia in the general community. *Neurology* **59(6)**:941–943.

Munchau, A., E.M. Valente, M.B. Davis, V. Stinton, N.W. Wood, N.P. Quinn, K.P. Bhatia. 2000. A Yorkshire family with adult-onset cranio-cervical primary torsion dystonia. *Mov Disord* **15(5)**:954–959.

Nakashima, K., M. Kusumi, Y. Inoue, K. Takahashi. 1995. Prevalence of focal dystonias in the western area of Tottori Prefecture in Japan. *Mov Disord* **10(4)**:440–443.

Naumann, M., W. Pirker, K. Reiners, K. Lange, G. Becker, T. Brucke. 1997. [123I]beta-CIT single-photon emission tomography in DOPA-responsive dystonia. *Mov Disord* **12(3)**:448–451.

Nemeth, A.H. 2002. The genetics of primary dystonias and related disorders. *Brain* **125(Pt 4)**:695–721.

Neuwald, A.F., L. Aravind, J.L. Spouge, E.V. Koonin. 1999. AAA+: a class of chaperone-like ATPases associated with the assembly, operation, and disassembly of protein complexes. *Genome Res* **9**:27–43.

Niederweiser, A., N. Blan, M. Wang, P. Joller, M. Atares, J. Cardesa-Garcia. 1995. GTP cyclohydrolase I deficiency, a new enzyme defect causing hyperphenylalaninemia with neopterin, biopterin, dopamine and serotonin deficiencies and muscular hypotonia. *Eur J Pediatr* **126**:401–405.

Nolte, D., S. Niemann, U. Muller. 2003. Specific sequence changes in multiple transcript system DYT3 are associated with X-linked dystonia parkinsonism. *Proc Natl Acad Sci U S A* **100(18)**:10347–10352.

Nutt, J.G., M.D. Muenter, A. Aronson, L.T. Kurland, L.J. Melton 3rd. 1988. Epidemiology of focal and generalized dystonia in Rochester, Minnesota. *Mov Disord* **3(3)**:188–194.

Nygaard, T.G., D. Raymond, C. Chen, I. Nishino, P.E. Greene, D. Jennings, G.A. Heiman, et al. 1999. Localization of a gene for myoclonus-dystonia to chromosome 7q21–q31. *Ann Neurol* **46(5)**:794–798.

Nygaard, T.G., H. Takahashi, G.A. Heiman, B.J. Snow, S. Fahn, D.B. Calne. 1992. Long-term treatment response and fluorodopa positron emission tomographic scanning of parkinsonism in a family with dopa-responsive dystonia. *Ann Neurol* **32(5)**:603–608.

Nygaard, T.G., J.M. Trugman, J.G. de Yebenes, S. Fahn. 1990. Dopa-responsive dystonia: the spectrum of clinical manifestations in a large north American family. *Neurology* **40(1)**:66–69.

Nygaard, T.G., S.P. Waran, R.A. Levine, A.B. Naini, A.M. Chutorian. 1994. Dopa-responsive dystonia simulating cerebral palsy. *Pediatr Neurol* **11(3)**:236–240.

Nygaard, T.G., K.C. Wilhelmsen, N.J. Risch, D.L. Brown, J.M. Trugman, T.C. Gilliam, S. Fahn, et al. 1993. Linkage mapping of dopa-responsive dystonia (DRD) to chromosome 14q. *Nat Genet* **5(4)**:386–391.

Nygaard, T.G., and G.F. Wooten. 1998. Dopa-responsive dystonia: some pieces of the puzzle are still missing. *Neurology* **50(4)**:853–855.

O'Sullivan, J.D., D.C. Costa, S. Gacinovic, A.J. Lees. 2001. SPECT imaging of the dopamine transporter in juvenile-onset dystonia. *Neurology* **56(2)**:266–267.

Obeso, J.A., J.C. Rothwell, A.E. Lang, C.D. Marsden. 1983. Myoclonic dystonia. *Neurology* **33(7)**:825–830.

Opal, P., R. Tintner, J. Jankovic, J. Leung, X.O. Breakefield, J. Friedman, L. Ozelius. 2002. Intrafamilial phenotypic variability of the DYT1 dystonia: from asymptomatic TOR1A gene carrier status to dystonic storm. *Mov Disord* **17(2)**:339–345.

Oppenheim, H. 1911. Ueber eine eigenartige Krampfkrankheit des kindlichen und jugendlichen Alters. *Neurol Centrabl* **30**:1090–1107.

Ozelius, L.J., J.W. Hewett, C.E. Page, S.B. Bressman, P.L. Kramer, C. Shalish, D. de Leon, et al. 1997. The early-onset torsion dystonia gene (DYT1) encodes an ATP-binding protein. *Nat Genet* **17(1)**:40–48.

Ozelius, L.J., C.E. Page, C. Klein, J.W. Hewett, M. Mineta, J. Leung, C. Shalish, et al. 1999. The TOR1A (DYT1) gene family and its role in early onset torsion dystonia. *Genomics* **62(3)**:377–384.

Parker, N. 1985. Hereditary whispering dysphonia. *J Neurol Neurosurg Psychiatry* **48(3)**:218–224.

Pauls, D.L., and A.D. Korczyn. 1990. Complex segregation analysis of dystonia pedigrees suggests autosomal dominant inheritance. *Neurology* **40(7)**:1107–1110.

Pittock, S.J., C. Joyce, V. O'Keane, B. Hugle, M.O. Hardiman, F. Brett, A.J. Green, et al. 2000. Rapid-onset dystonia-parkinsonism: a clinical and genetic analysis of a new kindred. *Neurology* **55(7)**:991–995.

Placzek, M.R., A. Misbahuddin, K.R. Chaudhuri, N.W. Wood, K.P. Bhatia, T.T. Warner. 2001. Cervical dystonia is associated with a polymorphism in the dopamine (D5) receptor gene. *J Neurol Neurosurg Psychiatry* **71(2)**:262–264.

Risch, N., D. de Leon, L. Ozelius, P. Kramer, L. Almasy, B. Singer, S. Fahn, et al. 1995. Genetic analysis of idiopathic torsion dystonia in Ashkenazi Jews and their recent descent from a small founder population. *Nat Genet* **9(2)**:152–159.

Rostasy, K., S.J. Augood, J.W. Hewett, J.C. Leung, H. Sasaki, L.J. Ozelius, V. Ramesh, et al. 2003. TorsinA protein and neuropathology in early onset generalized dystonia with GAG deletion. *Neurobiol Dis* **12(1)**:11–24.

Saunders-Pullman, R., J. Shriberg, G. Heiman, D. Raymond, K. Wendt, P. Kramer, K. Schilling, et al. 2002. Myoclonus dystonia: possible association with obsessive-compulsive disorder and alcohol dependence. *Neurology* **58(2)**:242–245.

Schapira, A.H., T. Warner, M.T. Gash, M.W. Cleeter, C.F. Marinho, J.M. Cooper. 1997. Complex I function in familial and sporadic dystonia. *Ann Neurol* **41(4)**:556–559.

Schwalbe, W. 1980. Eine eigentumliche tonische Krampfform mit hysterischen Symptomen. *Medizin und Chirurgie*. Berlin: Ueniversitaets-Buchdrueckerei von Gustav Schade.

Segawa, M., A. Hosaka, F. Miyagawa, Y. Nomura, H. Imai. 1976. Hereditary progressive dystonia with marked diurnal fluctuation. *Adv Neurol* **14**:215–233.

Segawa, M., and Y. Nomura. 1993. Hereditary progressive dystonia with marked diurnal fluctuation. Pathophysiological importance of the age of onset. *Adv Neurol* **60**:568–576.

Shashidharan, P., P.F. Good, A. Hsu, D.P. Perl, M.F. Brin, C.W. Olanow. 2000. TorsinA accumulation in Lewy bodies in sporadic Parkinson's disease. *Brain Res* **877(2)**:379–381.

Slominsky, P.A., E.D. Markova, M.I. Shadrina, S.N. Illarioshkin, N.I. Miklina, S.A. Limborska, I.A. Ivanova-Smolenskaya. 1999. A common 3-bp deletion in the DYT1 gene in Russian families with early-onset torsion dystonia. *Hum Mutat* **14(3)**:269.

Snow, B.J., T.G. Nygaard, H. Takahashi, D.B. Calne. 1993. Positron emission tomographic studies of dopa-responsive dystonia and early-onset idiopathic parkinsonism. *Ann Neurol* **34(5)**:733–738.

Steinberger, D., H. Topka, D. Fischer, U. Muller. 1999. GCH1 mutation in a patient with adult-onset oromandibular dystonia. *Neurology* **52(4)**: 877–879.

Strauss, K.A., E.G. Puffenberger, D.L. Robinson, D.H. Morton. 2003. Type I glutaric aciduria, part 1: natural history of 77 patients. *Am J Med Genet* **121C(1)**:38–52.

Tassin, J., A. Durr, A.M. Bonnet, R. Gil, M. Vidailhet, C.B. Lucking, J.Y. Goas, et al. 2000. Levodopa-responsive dystonia. GTP cyclohydrolase I or parkin mutations? *Brain* **123(Pt 6)**:1112–1121.

Tuffery-Giraud, S., L. Cavalier, A. Roubertie, C, Guittard, S. Carles, P. Calvas, B. Echenne, et al. 2001. No evidence of allelic heterogeneity in the DYT1 gene of European patients with early onset torsion dystonia. *J Med Genet* **38(10)**:E35.

Turjanski, N., K. Bhatia, D.J. Burn, G.V. Sawle, C.D. Marsden, D.J. Brooks. 1993. Comparison of striatal 18F-dopa uptake in adult-onset dystonia-parkinsonism, Parkinson's disease, and dopa-responsive dystonia. *Neurology* **43(8)**:1563–1568.

Vale, R.D. 2000. AAA proteins: lords of the ring. *J Cell Biol* **150**:F13–F19.

Valente, E.M., A.R. Bentivoglio, E. Cassetta, P.H. Dixon, M.B. Davis, A. Ferraris, T. Ialongo, et al. 2001a. DYT13, a novel primary torsion dystonia locus, maps to chromosome 1p36.13—36.32 in an Italian family with cranial-cervical or upper limb onset. *Ann Neurol* **49(3)**:362–366.

Valente, E.M., A.R. Bentivoglio, et al. 2001b. Identification of a novel primary torsion dystonia locus (DYT13) on chromosome 1p36 in an Italian family with cranial-cervical or upper limb onset. *Neurol Sci* **22(1)**:95–96.

Valente, E.M., T.T. Warner, P.R. Jarman, D. Mathen, N.A. Fletcher, C.D. Marsden, K.P. Bhatia, et al. 1998. The role of DYT1 in primary torsion dystonia in Europe. *Brain* **121(Pt 12)**:2335–2339.

van den Heuvel, L.P., B. Luiten, J.A. Smeitink, J.F. de Rijk-van Andel, K. Hyland, G.C. Steenbergen-Spanjers, R.J. Janssen, et al. 1998. A common point mutation in the tyrosine hydroxylase gene in autosomal recessive L-Ddopa-responsive dystonia in the Dutch population. *Hum Genet* **102(6)**:644–646.

Vidailhet, M., J. Tassin, F. Durif, A. Nivelon-Chevallier, Y. Agid, A. Brice, A. Durr, et al. 2001. A major locus for several phenotypes of myoclonus—dystonia on chromosome 7q. *Neurology* **56(9)**:1213–1216.

Waddy, H.M., N.A. Fletcher, A.E. Harding, C.D. Marsden. 1991. A genetic study of idiopathic focal dystonias. *Ann Neurol* **29(3)**:320–324.

Walker, R.H., M.F. Brin, D. Sandu, P.F. Good, P. Shashidharan. 2002. TorsinA immunoreactivity in brains of patients with DYT1 and non-DYT1 dystonia. *Neurology* **58(1)**:120–124.

Webb, D.W., A. Broderick, A. Brashear, W.B. Dobyns. 1999. Rapid onset dystonia-parkinsonism in a 14-year-old girl. *Eur J Paediatr Neurol* **3(4)**:171–173.

Zeman, W. 1970. Pathology of the torsion dystonias (dystonia musculorum deformans). *Neurology* **20(11)**:79–88.

Zeman, W., and P. Dyken. 1967. Dystonia musculorum deformans. Clinical, genetic and pathoanatomical studies. *Psychiatr Neurol Neurochir* **70(2)**:77–121.

Zilber, N., A.D. Korczyn, E. Kahana, K. Fried, M. Alter. 1984. Inheritance of idiopathic torsion dystonia among Jews. *J Med Genet* **21(1)**:13–20.

Zimprich, A., M. Grabowski, F. Asmus, M. Naumann, D. Berg, M. Bertram, K. Scheidtmann, et al. 2001. Mutations in the gene encoding epsilon-sarcoglycan cause myoclonus-dystonia syndrome. *Nat Genet* **29(1)**:66–69.

Zorzi, G., B. Garavaglia, F. Invernizzi, F. Girotti, P. Soliveri, M. Zeviani, L. Angelini, et al. 2002. Frequency of DYT1 mutation in early onset primary dystonia in Italian patients. *Mov Disord* **17(2)**:407–408.

Zweig, R.M., J.C. Hedreen, W.R. Jankel, M.F. Casanova, P.J. Whitehouse, D.L. Price. 1988. Pathology in brainstem regions of individuals with primary dystonia. *Neurology* **38(5)**:702–706.

C H A P T E R

C2

The Genetically Dystonic Rat

MARK LeDOUX

I. THE GENETICS OF HUMAN DYSTONIA

Dystonia has been defined as a syndrome of sustained muscle contractions, frequently causing twisting and repetitive movements, or abnormal postures (Fahn et al. 1987). It is one of the more common movement disorders seen in neurological specialty clinics. Primary dystonia includes syndromes in which dystonia is the sole phenotypic manifestation with the exception that tremor can be present as well. Primary dystonia may be generalized, segmental, or focal. Primary generalized dystonias usually begin in childhood, whereas focal dystonias normally present during adult life.

Mutant genes are believed to play a major role in many cases of primary dystonia. Approximately 15% of patients with apparently sporadic primary dystonia have one or more family members affected with dystonia, tremor, or another movement disorder (Stojanovic et al. 1995). Although much less common than sporadic dystonia, at least fifteen forms of hereditary primary dystonia with clearly recognizable Mendelian inheritance patterns have been identified to date. Discovering additional genes associated with dystonia in either humans or animal models and characterizing the functions of their encoded proteins will greatly improve our understanding of this movement disorder. Three proteins clearly associated with the development of a dystonic phenotype without overt neurodegeneration are torsinA in Oppenheim dystonia (DYT1, Ozelius et al. 1977), GTP-cyclohydrolase I in dopa-responsive dystonia (DYT5, Ichinose et al. 1994), and ε-sarcoglycan in the myoclonus-dystonia syndrome (DYT11, Zimprich et al. 2001). DYT1, DYT5, and DYT11 are inherited in an autosomal dominant fashion.

Initially described in Spanish gypsies (Santangelo 1934; Gimenez-Roldan et al. 1988), autosomal recessive generalized dystonia (DYT2, MIM 224500) has also been reported in Iranian (Khan et al. 2003) and Arab-American (Moretti et al. 2001) families. The DYT2 locus and other loci may also be responsible for sporadic cases of DTY1-negative childhood-onset generalized dystonia. In other well-known autosomal recessive diseases, such as cystic fibrosis, sporadic cases are the norm rather than the exception. Thus, lessons learned from the study of a recessive dystonia in an animal model could have broad implications for sporadic human disease.

II. PHENOTYPIC CHARACTERIZATION OF THE GENETICALLY DYSTONIC RAT

A. Origins and General Features of the Model

The genetically dystonic rat (SD-dt:JFL), an autosomal recessive animal model of primary generalized dystonia, develops a dystonic motor syndrome by postnatal day 12 (P12, Lorden et al. 1984). The dystonic rat is a spontaneous mutant discovered in the Sprague-Dawley (SD) strain. The mutation is fully penetrant and there is negligible variability to its expressivity. Mutations in the coding region of the gene (TOR1A) associated with Oppenheim dystonia have been excluded in the dystonic rat (Ziefer et al. 2002). An active effort to clone the mutant gene in the dystonic rat is in progress. Dystonic rats exhibit both axial and appendicular dystonia that progresses in severity with increasing postnatal age. Neonatal dystonic rats can be reliably differentiated from normal littermates by P12. Prior to P10, normal and dystonic rats have an identical motor phenotype and display qualitatively similar motor activities in the open field (e.g., head elevation, grooming, crawling, and quadruped stability). Dystonia is reduced when the animals are at rest and disappears during sleep. Without surgical intervention, dystonic rats develop a progressive, severe, generalized dystonia that involves both the limbs and trunk and, invariably, leads to death prior to P40 despite gavage feedings and other supportive measures.

The earliest features of the dystonic rat motor syndrome are a stiff paddling gait secondary to dystonia of the hind limbs and mild twisting movements of the head upon the trunk. As the disorder progresses in severity, dystonic rats begin to fall to their sides during ambulation. In the dystonic rat, both truncal and appendicular dystonia are frequently precipitated by action, particularly attempts at locomotion. More advanced clinical signs include clasping of the paws, hyperflexion of the trunk, and dystonic "spasms" of the fore limbs, hind limbs or both.

With normally sized litters of ten to twelve pups, dystonic rats maintain body weight until at least P16 (Lorden et al. 1984). After P16, dystonic rats slowly lose weight in comparison with phenotypically normal littermates. The relative weight differences between normal and dystonic rats accelerate with increasing postnatal age. At least part of the weight loss exhibited by dystonic pups is due to competition with littermates for milk, since weight is maintained for longer periods when either litters are culled to fewer pups or dystonic rats are hand fed.

B. Motor Deficits in the Genetically Dystonic Rat

To quantitatively evaluate disease progression and the effects of various therapeutic interventions, investigators defined four motor signs characteristic of the dystonic rat motor syndrome: (1) FALL; animal lying on its flank with the fore limb and hind limb on one side of the body lifted off the mat, (2) TWIST; rotation of the head, neck, and upper thorax about the longitudinal axis of the body bringing an ear close to the mat, (3) CLASP; animal extends any two limbs and brings them into apposition, flexing the digits of one paw around those of the other, and (4) PIVOT; rotation at least 180 degrees about an adducted hind limb. The motor signs of the dystonic rat consist of relatively slow movements that culminate in briefly held postures that facilitate counting. Before and after interventions, animals were tested individually on a rubber mat and signs were counted over five-minute periods (LeDoux et al. 1993, 1995). It should be noted that pivoting is a component of normal motor development in rats, reaching its peak at P9 to P10 with virtual resolution by P15 (Altman and Sudarshan 1975). In contrast, the resolution of pivoting occurs more slowly in the dystonic rat. The frequency of falls, twists, and clasps increases with increasing age of dystonic rats. At P15, approximately forty abnormal motor signs can be counted in a five-minute period whereas the number increases to around sixty at P23 (LeDoux et al. 1993, 1995).

A collection of age-appropriate behavioral tests were also selected to characterize the dystonic rat motor syndrome: righting reflex times, climbing a 1-cm wire mesh incline, a homing task (i.e., traversing a passageway to return to the home cage), and hanging times (LeDoux et al. 1993, 1995). In addition, fifteen-minute activity scores were obtained by counting interruption of infrared light beams spaced 3 cm apart in an 18 by 28.5 cm chamber. At P12, dystonic rats show higher activity scores than their normal littermates. However, activity scores do not differ at P18, P20, or P23. Prior to P10, no reliable differences occur in climbing ability between normal and dystonic pups. After P10, the climbing ability of dystonic rats deteriorates. By P23, dystonic rats cannot ascend even the lowest inclines. Normal rats at P12 can right themselves within one second. In comparison, dystonic rats take an average of three seconds to right at P12 and, by P23, righting times average over ten seconds. Homing ability also shows a marked age-related deterioration in dystonic rats. In striking contrast, hanging times increase with increasing postnatal age in dystonic rats, which indicates that motor dysfunction in this model is not due to muscle weakness or hypotonia.

C. Morphological Analysis of Neural Tissue in the Genetically Dystonic Rat

No gross differences exist between normal and dystonic rats in terms of brain morphology. Microscopic analysis of cresyl violet, hematoxylin and eosin, Luxol fast blue, periodic acid-Schiff, and silver-stained central and peripheral nervous tissues from dystonic rats has not shown differences from normals (Lorden et al. 1984; LeDoux et al. 1998). Because striatal neurons are a central component of the basal ganglia, researchers examined the morphology of these neurons with Golgi impregnation in both dystonic and normal rats; no abnormalities were detected in the mutants (McKeon et al. 1984).

Quantitative anatomical studies in the dystonic rat have focused on olivocerebellar pathways. Dystonic rats and normal littermates do not exhibit differences in Purkinje cell number, volume of the cerebellar nuclei, soma size of cerebellar nuclear neurons, molecular layer thickness, or granular cell layer thickness, although, in vermian and paravermian tissues at P20, Purkinje cells are 5–11% smaller in dystonic rats than in normal littermates (Lorden et al. 1985, 1992). This effect is not generalized since there are no differences in the size of pyramidal neurons in the hippocampus. Furthermore, Purkinje cell dendritic arborizations are qualitatively similar between normal and dystonic rats. Therefore, these data are most consistent with a defect in Purkinje cells or their afferents rather than a generalized nutritional deficiency.

Investigators studied the inferior olivary projection to cerebellar cortex with both anterogradely and retrogradely transported horseradish peroxidase. The connectivity pattern was consistent with studies in normal rats, and cerebellar cortical terminations were normal at the level of light microscopy (Stratton 1991).

III. RESPONSE OF THE GENETICALLY DYSTONIC RAT TO PHARMACOLOGICAL AGENTS

A. Compounds Used to Evaluate Motor Subsystems

1. Physostigmine

Cholinergic systems are believed to play an important role in the pathophysiology of human dystonia. For instance, one study associated the acetylcholinesterase inhibitor physostigmine with worsening of dystonia in all seven patients tested (Stahl and Berger 1982). In normal and dystonic rats, physostigmine doses from 0.1 to 0.2 mg/kg produced increases in locomotor activity. In addition, dystonia was substantially more severe in the mutants. Lorden and colleagues (1988) suggested that physostigmine's effects may not be specific for dystonia since the compound is associated with a generalized increase in motor activity.

2. Haloperidol

Catalepsy is a condition characterized by lack of response to external stimuli and muscular rigidity; the limbs remain in whatever position they are placed. Neuroleptic drugs can induce catalepsy. Investigators used the bar test to measure the cataleptic response to haloperidol in dystonic rats and normal littermates at P8, P10, and P12 (McKeon et al. 1984). No differences occurred in median catalepsy times between normal and dystonic rats at P8 and P10. At P12, on the other hand, catalepsy times were significantly decreased in dystonic rats in comparison with littermate controls. In older dystonic rats (P16—P25), increased "runs" (i.e., rapid forward movements in which the left and right limbs are moved simultaneously) were noted following haloperidol injection. Moreover, mutant rats were less sensitive than normal littermates to the akinetic effects of haloperidol. Finally, haloperidol did not reduce the number of dystonic movements in the mutant rats (Lorden et al. 1984).

3. Morphine

To examine the specificity of haloperidol's effect on catalepsy, investigators treated both normal and dystonic rats with morphine. Although both compounds produce catalepsy, the neural circuits underlying morphine- and haloperidol-induced catalepsy are probably distinct (De Ryck et al. 1980). In contrast to the results with haloperidol, there were no differential effects of morphine on normal and dystonic rats (McKeon et al. 1984).

4. Harmaline

Harmaline produces a generalized tremor in normal rats by inducing rhythmic firing of inferior olivary neurons (Llinás and Volkind 1973). Dystonic rats do not tremor after harmaline is administered even at doses (15 mg/kg) well above that required to produce tremor in normal animals (Lorden et al. 1985).

5. Oxotremorine

To determine if the dystonic rat has a neural defect that prevents the generation of a tremor, investigators administered the centrally acting muscarinic-agonist tremorogenic agent, oxotremorine, to both normal and dystonic rats. Oxotremorine produces a tremor that is probably mediated by a neural network not critically dependent on intact climbing fibers (Miwa et al. 2000). At a dose of 0.75 mg/kg, oxotremorine produced a tremor that was similar between normal and dystonic rats (Lorden et al. 1985).

B. Compounds Used to Examine Serotonergic Systems in the Dystonic Rat

In the dystonic rat, several intersecting lines of evidence suggest the possibility of a focal defect in serotonergic systems. First, harmaline is structurally similar to serotonin. Second, the serotonergic neurotoxin, 5,7-dihydroxytryptamine prevents the behavioral effects of harmaline. Third, the responsiveness of inferior olivary neurons to harmaline coincides with maturation of serotonergic fibers in the inferior olive during the second week of postnatal development.

To examine the integrity of serotonergic systems in the dystonic rat, investigators administered a serotonergic agonist, quipazine, to normal and dystonic rats at several developmental time points. At P8, both normal and dystonic rats exhibited a high frequency forepaw tremor in response to quipazine (Michela et al. 1990). In normal rats, the response to quipazine diminishes with age. In striking contrast, dystonic rats at P16 and P25 exhibited an enhanced response to the tremorogenic effects of quipazine. In normal and dystonic rats, the response to quipazine was blocked by pretreatment with the serotonergic 5-HT_2-receptor antagonist ketanserin. Dystonic rats were also sixfold more sensitive to the ability of the 5-HT_{1A}-agonist, 8-OH-2-(di-n-propylamino)tetralin (8-OH-DPAT) to produce five out of the six components of the serotonin behavioral syndrome (forepaw treading, Straub tail, tremor, head-weaving, hindlimb abduction, and postural changes). Interestingly, dystonic rats did not tremor in response to 8-OH-DPAT. Furthermore, dystonic rats showed an impaired headshake to both a 5-HT_2 receptor agonist and mechanical stimulation of the aural pinnae. Based on these experimental results, Wieland and Lucki (1991) suggested that dystonic rats might have a defect in brainstem serotonergic systems, particularly those involved in inferior olivary innervation. Alternatively, abnormal cerebellar output in the dystonic rat could have altered dose-response curves to serotonergic agents.

C. Compounds Used to Treat Movement Disorders in Humans

Researchers analyzed the behavior of dystonic rats before and after systemically administering pharmacological agents from specific functional groups useful in dystonia and other movement disorders (Lorden et al. 1988; Bressman and Greene 2000). Benzodiapezepines are typically associated with mild clinical improvements in patients with either generalized or focal dystonia. In dystonic rats, the benzodiazepine diazepam (0.25–0.5 mg/kg) produced a dose-dependent decrease in the frequency of dystonic movements (Lorden et al. 1988). The classic dopamine agonist, apomorphine, can be a very effective treatment for "off" dystonia in patients with idiopathic Parkinson disease. At apomorphine doses of 0.5–1 mg/kg, both dystonic and normal rats showed increased activity in comparison with baseline (Lorden et al. 1984, 1988). At higher doses of apomorphine (3–5 mg/kg), both normal and mutant rats exhibited stereotypical movements such as licking and sniffing. Apomorphine was not associated with improvements in the severity or frequency of dystonic movements in the mutant. Anticholinergics often provide noticeable benefits in patients with generalized dystonia. Furthermore, anticholinergics are useful adjunctive therapy in Parkinson disease. The anticholinergic scopolamine (1 mg/kg) reduced paw clasping and falls in dystonic rats. Although rarely used in idiopathic dystonia, the α-2 adrenergic agonist clonidine has shown efficacy in patients with spasticity (Kita and Goodkin 2000). In dystonic rats, doses of clonidine from 0.05–0.3 mg/kg were associated with reduced falls and dystonic spasms. The beneficial effects of clonidine were eliminated by pretreatment with the α-2 antagonist, rauwolscine. Thus, the dystonic rat responds positively, but to a variable degree, to some agents that benefit patients with idiopathic dystonia and other movement disorders.

IV. NEUROCHEMICAL ANALYSES IN THE GENETICALLY DYSTONIC RAT

A. Noradrenergic Systems

One initial finding in the dystonic rat was an increase in the intensity of cerebellar catecholamine histofluorescence (Lorden et al. 1984). Interestingly, abnormalities in cerebellar noradrenergic systems have also been reported in several ataxic mouse mutants (Landis et al. 1975; Levitt and Noebels 1981). Consistent with catecholamine histofluorescence, norepinephrine (NE) levels are selectively increased in dystonic rat cerebellar cortex as early as P12; similar increases are not detected in dystonic rat cerebral cortex, hippocampus, or inferior olive (McKeon et al. 1986; LeDoux et al. 1994).

In the cerebellum only, dystonic rats show reduced sensitivity to the NE-depleting effects of reserpine. The biochemical response to amphetamine and the tyrosine hydroxylase inhibitor α-methyl-*p*-tyrosine are similar between dystonic rats and normal littermates. In addition, normal and dystonic rats do not show differences in levels of the major NE metabolite, 3-methoxy-4-hydroxylphenylglycol, or the number and affinity of β-adrenergic receptors. These data are compatible with increased NE storage in dystonic rat cerebellar cortex. The focal nature of the noradrenergic abnormality in the dystonic rat would argue against a primary defect in the locus ceruleus. Instead, increased NE storage in dystonic rat cerebellar cortex more likely occurs in response to altered Purkinje cell activity in the mutants. Along these lines, NE increases the frequency of inhibitory postsynaptic currents in Purkinje cells via a presynaptic mechanism (Llano and Gerschenfeld 1993).

B. Dopaminergic Systems

Because dystonic rats were less sensitive to the akinetic effects of haloperidol than their normal littermates, investigators used a series of studies to characterize dopaminergic systems in the mutants. No differences occurred in striatal or "remaining" telencephalic levels of dopamine between normal and dystonic rats (Lorden et al. 1984). Furthermore, no significant differences were found between normal and dystonic rats in striatal dopamine turnover or receptor

ERRATA

FRONTMATTER, PAGE IV

The DVD-ROM ISBN Number listed on the copyright page is incorrect.

The correct number is: 0-12-088383-X

ANIMAL MODELS OF MOVEMENT DISORDERS 0-12-088382-1
Edited by Mark LeDoux 2004, Elsevier Science (USA)

affinity. Using ^{3}H-spiroperidol as a ligand, mutant rats also showed a normal distribution and density of dopamine D_2 receptors (Beales et al. 1990).

C. Cholinergic Systems

Dystonic rats exhibit small but significant increases in cerebellar choline acetyltransferase (ChAT) activity (Lorden et al. 1988). However, there are no differences in the number or affinity of muscarinic acetylcholine receptors in the striatum (McKeon et al. 1984). Moreover, a receptor autoradiography study using the muscarinic acetylcholine ligand, ^{3}H-quinuclidinylbenzilate, failed to demonstrate differences between normal and dystonic rats. These data suggest that the responses of the dystonic rat to scopolamine and physostigmine are due to the effects of these compounds on the cerebellum (Lorden et al. 1988).

D. Serotonergic Systems

The enhanced behavioral responses of dystonic rats to both 5-HT_2 and 5-HT_{1A} agonists supported the possibility of a receptor aberration in the mutants. However, quantitative autoradiography of 5-HT_2 receptors did not demonstrate changes in the dystonic rat (Beales et al. 1990). Moreover, no differences appeared in striatal or cerebellar levels of serotonin, the serotonin metabolite, 5-hydroxyindoleacetic acid (5-HIAA) or the serotonin precursor, tryptophan, between normal and dystonic rats (Lorden et al. 1988). In contrast, there was a difference between normal and dystonic rats in the pattern of development of inferior olivary serotonergic neurotransmission (LeDoux et al. 1994). Over the developmental period from P14 to P22, the trends in inferior olivary levels of both 5-HT and 5-HIAA were quadratic in dystonic rats and linear in normal littermates.

E. GABA-ergic Systems

Profound changes in GABA-ergic markers were isolated to the cerebellar nuclei and Purkinje cells in the dystonic rat. In the cerebellar nuclei, glutamic acid decarboxylase (GAD) activity increased with increasing postnatal age in the dystonic rat (Oltmans et al. 1986; Beales et al. 1990). Opposite changes were noted in cerebellar nuclear $GABA_A$ receptors. In contrast, there were no changes in GABA levels or binding of a benzodiazepine ligand (Beales et al. 1990; Lutes et al. 1992). The distribution, size, and density of GAD-immunoreactive puncta in the cerebellar nuclei were examined in normal and dystonic rats; the only abnormality noted was a relative decrease in puncta density at P25 in dystonic rats (Lutes et al. 1992). With quantitative *in situ* hybridization, GAD_{67} mRNA was increased in Purkinje cells and decreased in the cerebellar nuclei of dystonic rats (Naudon et al. 1998). In aggregate, these findings are most compatible with increased activity of Purkinje cell GABAergic synapses within the dystonic rat cerebellar nuclei. The changes in cerebellar nuclear $GABA_A$ receptors and GAD_{67} transcript are probably compensatory responses.

F. Opioid Systems

A few bits of evidence indicate that opioid systems may play a role in the pathophysiology of dystonia. First, stimulation of rubral sigma receptors can produce dystonia in rats (Walker et al. 1988). Second, striatal pre-proenkephalin mRNA levels are intimately related to the appearance of dyskinesias in Parkinson disease (Henry et al. 2003). In the dystonic rat, however, there are no abnormalities of sigma-1 receptors, sigma-2 receptors, or striatal enkephalin mRNA (Weissman et al 1993; Naudon et al. 1998).

G. Second Messenger Systems

The second messenger, cyclic guanosine monophosphate (cGMP), together with cGMP-dependent protein kinases types I and II are expressed at high levels in cerebellar Purkinje cells (de Vente et al. 2001). Basal levels of cGMP are decreased in dystonic rat cerebellar cortex (Lorden et al. 1985). In addition, the increase in cerebellar cGMP seen in normal rats after the systemic administration of harmaline is much smaller in dystonic rats. These findings suggest that a defect in neurotransmission is present in dystonic rat cerebellar cortex.

H. Glucose Utilization

Researchers used the 2-deoxy-glucose technique to identify sites of functional abnormality in the dystonic rat. A total of sixty-two sites within the central nervous system were compared between dystonic rats and their normal littermates (Brown and Lorden 1989). Several brain regions showed marked differences between mutant and normal rats: medial cerebellar nucleus, interpositus cerebellar nucleus, lateral cerebellar nucleus, locus ceruleus, oculomotor nucleus, ventrolateral thalamus, and ventromedial thalamus. In dystonic rats, glucose utilization was higher in the cerebellar nuclei, locus ceruleus, and oculomotor nucleus and lower in the thalamic nuclei than in normal littermates.

To further explore functional relationships within sensorimotor networks, investigators calculated correlation coefficients between connected brain regions for each group of animals. Several pairs of anatomically connected regions showed differences between dystonic rats and normal littermates including the interpositus nucleus/contralateral red nucleus, fastigial nucleus/vermis, inferior olive/vermis, dorsal striatum/substantia nigra, dorsal striatum/globus pallidus, and substantia nigra/superior colliculus. Because olivocerebellar dysfunction is causally related to the dystonic rat motor syndrome, these findings indicate that abnormal cerebellar output can alter the metabolic topography of basal ganglia networks.

V. MOTORIC EFFECTS OF CEREBELLAR LESIONS IN THE GENETICALLY DYSTONIC RAT

A. Cerebellectomy (CBX)

To test the hypothesis that cerebellar dysfunction is critical to the expression of the dystonic rat motor phenotype, groups of dystonic rats and normal littermates underwent CBX at P15 (LeDoux et al. 1993). The entopeduncular nuclei were lesioned with kainic acid in a separate group of dystonic rats. Age-matched nonoperated dystonic rats served as controls. CBX included the dorsal portion of the lateral vestibular nucleus, a structure that receives direct projections from cerebellar Purkinje cells. After CBX, normal and dystonic rats could not be differentiated by behavioral observation or simple tests of motor function. Although nonoperated rats performed better than CBX rats on tests of righting and tended to perform better on a climbing task, the differences were not striking. This is in part due to the milder effects of CBX on both young animals and rodents when compared to adults and higher species, respectively. CBX rats could not, however, perform more complex motor tasks, such as narrow beam walking, that were not difficult for nonoperated rats. The group of dystonic rats with bilateral lesions of the entopeduncular nucleus showed no improvement in motor function.

After CBX, dystonic rats survive into adulthood without additional treatment. The lifespan of post-CBX dystonic rats is equivalent to that of normal littermates. Furthermore, post-CBX dystonic rats can mate and rear their offspring.

B. Selective Elimination of Cerebellar Output

The enormous amount of computation that occurs in the cerebellar cortex is ultimately expressed in the form of signals from the cerebellar nuclei and select components of the vestibular nuclear complex, particularly the dorsal portions of the lateral vestibular nuclei. Experimenters used bilateral electrolytic or excitatory amino acid lesions of the cerebellar nuclei (medial, interpositus, lateral) and dorsal portions of the lateral vestibular nucleus (dLV) to determine the structural components critical to the mutant's motor syndrome (LeDoux et al. 1995). Abnormal motor signs (falls, twists, clasps, and pivots) and motor performance (activity, climbing, righting, homing, and hanging) were quantified before surgery on P15 and again on P20. As shown in Figure 1, all lesions were associated with reductions in the frequency of abnormal motor signs. Investigators also noted significant improvements in motor performance in the

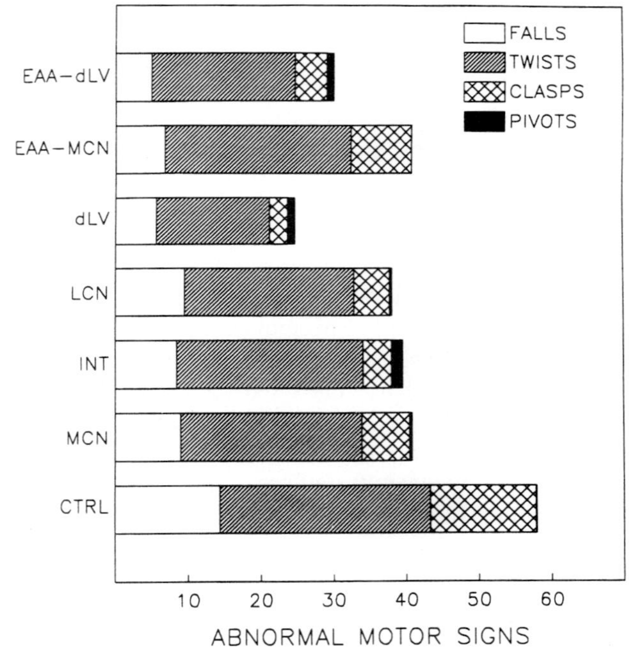

FIGURE 1 Effects of selective lesions on motor signs in the dystonic rat. The number of abnormal motor signs on P20 was counted over a five-minute observation period. All lesions had significant effects ($P < 0.01$) on the total number of motor signs. EAA, excitatory amino acid lesion; dLV, dorsal half of the lateral vestibular nucleus; MCN, medial cerebellar nucleus; INT, interpositus cerebellar nucleus; LCN, lateral cerebellar nucleus; CTRL, control. (Reprinted from *Brain Research*, vol. 697, LeDoux et al. [1995] with permission from Elsevier.)

surgically treated rats. Electrolytic lesions of the dLV were associated with the largest reductions in abnormal motor signs and greatest gains in motor performance.

VI. OLIVOCEREBELLAR NEUROPHYSIOLOGY IN THE GENETICALLY DYSTONIC RAT

Given that both neurochemical and pharmacological studies pointed to an olivocerebellar defect in the dystonic rat, researchers conducted electrophysiological studies to identify the precise site(s) of abnormality. Unfortunately, initial studies with urethane anesthesia yielded results that contradicted earlier neurochemical findings (Stratton et al. 1988). As summarized in table 1, simple-spike firing rates by Purkinje cells under urethane anesthesia were much lower in dystonic than in normal rats. With urethane anesthesia, firing rates in the medial cerebellar nucleus were twofold higher in dystonic rats than in normal littermates (Lorden et al. 1994). Clearly, this single-unit electrophysiology could not be reconciled with increased glucose utilization, increased GAD activity, and decreased muscimol binding in the cerebellar nuclei.

Electrophysiological studies in awake dystonic rats are essential to rationally explain olivocerebellar network

TABLE 1 Extracellular Single-Unit Neurophysiology in the Dystonic Rat

	Anesthesia	Mean frequency (Hz)		Reference
		Normal	Dystonic	
Medial cerebellar nucleus	Urethane	12.8 ± 2.1	23.7 ± 3.4*	Lorden et al. 1994
Cerebellar nuclei	None	36.6 ± 1.9	41.2 ± 1.9	LeDoux et al. 1998
Purkinje cells—simple spikes (preharmaline)	Urethane	35.0 ± 5.1	12.0 ± 2.1*	Stratton et al. 1988
Purkinje cells—simple spikes (preharmaline)	None	41.3 ± 2.5	46.7 ± 3.5	LeDoux & Lorden 2002
Purkinje cells—simple spikes (postharmaline)	Urethane	10.8 ± 3.1	7.0 ± 1.7	Stratton et al. 1988
Purkinje cells—simple spikes (postharmaline)	None	8.4 ± 3.6	16.1 ± 3.3*	LeDoux & Lorden 2002
Purkinje cells—complex spikes (preharmaline)	Urethane	1.3 ± 0.2	0.7 ± 0.1*	Stratton et al. 1988
Purkinje cells—complex spikes (preharmaline)	None	1.33 ± 0.06	0.78 ± 0.07*	LeDoux & Lorden 2002
Purkinje cells—complex spikes (postharmaline)	Urethane	2.92 ± 0.49	1.64 ± 0.43*	Stratton et al. 1988
Purkinje cells—complex spikes (postharmaline)	None	5.07 ± 0.36	2.97 ± 0.45*	LeDoux & Lorden 2002
Inferior olive (preharmaline)	Urethane	1.33 ± 0.13	0.45 ± 0.26*	Stratton & Lorden 1991
Inferior olive (postharmaline)	Urethane	4.19 ± 0.26	3.92 ± 0.15	Stratton & Lorden 1991

*$P < 0.05$.

abnormalities in the mutant. In comparison with normal rats (Figure 2), cerebellar nuclear cells from awake dystonic rats as young as P12 showed bursting firing patterns (Figure 3). As demonstrated in Figures 3–5, bursting activity increased with increasing postnatal age in dystonic rats (LeDoux et al. 1998). Many cerebellar nuclear cells from older dystonic rats exhibited rhythmic bursting activity that showed little modification in response to either sensory stimuli or motor activity. The bursting firing patterns displayed by cerebellar nuclear neurons from dystonic rats can be attributed to a low-threshold inactivating calcium-dependent conductance that generates rebound excitation following transient membrane hyperpolarization (Llinás and Mühlethaler 1988).

With single-unit awake recordings, there was a trend for simple-spike frequency by Purkinje cells to be higher in dystonic than in age-matched normal rats (table 1). In distinction, complex-spike frequency in Purkinje cells was markedly lower in normal than in dystonic rats, either with or without anesthesia. As demonstrated in Figure 6, Purkinje cells from dystonic rats, particularly cells from the vermis or older animals, exhibited rhythmic bursting simple-spike firing patterns. Comparison of Figures 7 and 8 highlights the striking differences in Purkinje cell spike trains between normal and dystonic rats.

As seen in table 1, inferior olivary preharmaline firing rates obtained with urethane anesthesia were compatible with complex-spike firing rates by Purkinje cells (Stratton and Lorden 1991). In contrast, no significant differences occurred in inferior olivary postharmaline firing rates between normal and dystonic rats. After the systemic administration of harmaline, complex-spike frequency increased in both normal and dystonic rats although it remained lower in the mutants. Harmaline-stimulated complex spike activity was also more rhythmic and produced greater suppression of simple spikes in normal than in dystonic rats (LeDoux and Lorden 2002). These electrophysiological findings along with earlier biochemical data indicate that a defect in the climbing fiber input to Purkinje cells is present in the dystonic rat.

VII. RELATIONSHIP TO HUMAN DYSTONIA

Twisting movements and postures like those exhibited by the dystonic rat are generally attributed to dysfunction of the basal ganglia. However, the broad phenotypic spectrum of dystonia and widespread lesion localization in secondary cases indicate that other neural structures may be pathophysiologically important (Pizoli et al. 2002; LeDoux and Brady 2003). Furthermore, multiple converging lines of experimental evidence strongly suggest that the dystonic rat's severe generalized dystonia is due to a primary abnormality within olivocerebellar structures, probably the climbing fiber synapses on cerebellar Purkinje cells (LeDoux and Lorden 2002).

Climbing fibers form a synapse on Purkinje cells in the contralateral cerebellar cortex; the collaterals of these fibers form a synapse on neurons in the cerebellar nuclei. Low spontaneous and stimulated inferior olivary firing rates would decrease complex-spike and increase simple-spike firing rates by Purkinje cells. Low complex-spike rates could explain increased NE and decreased cGMP levels within cerebellar cortex. The combination of increased Purkinje cell GABAergic and decreased climbing fiber excitatory input on neurons within the cerebellar nuclei leads to their hyperpolarization and a pathological rhythmic bursting

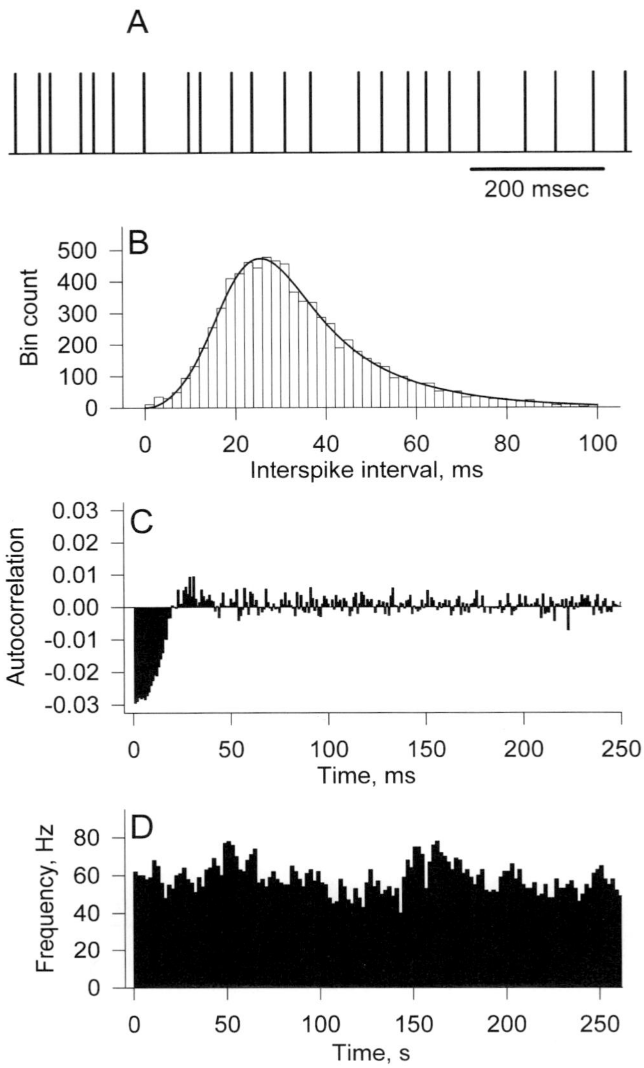

FIGURE 2 Single-unit recording from a neuron within the medial cerebellar nucleus of a P20 normal rat. (**A**) Representative portion of the spike train. Mean frequency = 29.3 Hz. (**B**) Interspike interval histogram. (**C**) Autocorrelation. (**D**) Ratemeter histogram. (Reprinted from *Neourscience*, vol. 86, LeDoux et al. [1998] with permission from Elsevier.)

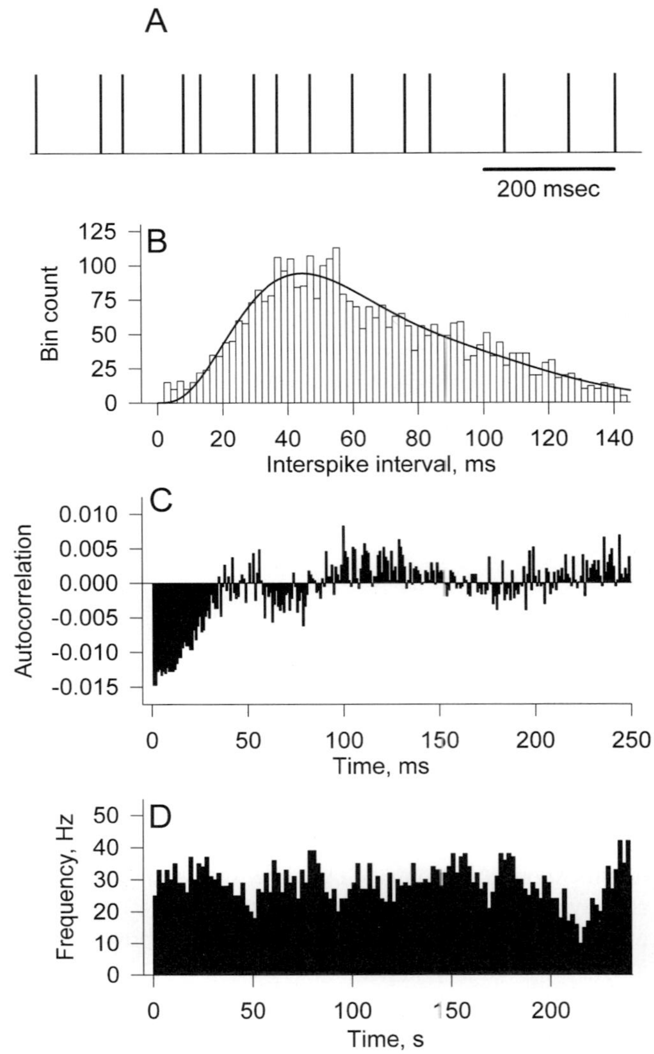

FIGURE 3 Single-unit recording from a neuron within the interpositus cerebellar nucleus of a P12 dystonic rat. (**A**) Representative portion of the spike train. Mean frequency = 14.5 Hz. (**B**) Interspike interval histogram. (**C**) Autocorrelation. (**D**) Ratemeter histogram. (Reprinted from *Neourscience*, vol. 86, LeDoux et al. [1998] with permission from Elsevier.)

firing pattern. Increased Purkinje cell GABAergic synaptic activity would also explain increased GAD activity, increased glucose utilization, and down-regulation of $GABA_A$ receptors within the cerebellar nuclei.

The beneficial effects of CBX and selective lesions of the cerebellar nuclei indicate that abnormal cerebellar output is critical to the phenotypic expression of the dystonic rat mutation. The clinically indistinguishable effects of CBX on normal and dystonic rats support this conclusion. Investigators do not know, however, exactly how the abnormal bursting activity of cerebellar neurons alters premotor systems such as rubrospinal, reticulospinal, tectospinal, and vestibulospinal pathways or the responses of these systems to cortical input.

Olivocerebellar dysfunction also plays a critical role in human dystonia. This concept receives support from a diverse assortment of research studies. First, structural lesions associated with secondary cervical dystonia are concentrated in olivocerebellar and pre-olivary structures (LeDoux and Brady 2003). Second, the genes associated with both Oppenheim dystonia and the myoclonus-dystonia syndrome are expressed at high levels in the cerebellum (Augood et al. 1998; Xiao and LeDoux 2003). Third, with positron emission tomography in patients with generalized dystonia, increased metabolic activity has been localized to the cerebellum in both movement-free and movement-related conditions (Eidelberg et al. 1998). Finally, dystonia can be either the sole or presenting feature of otherwise

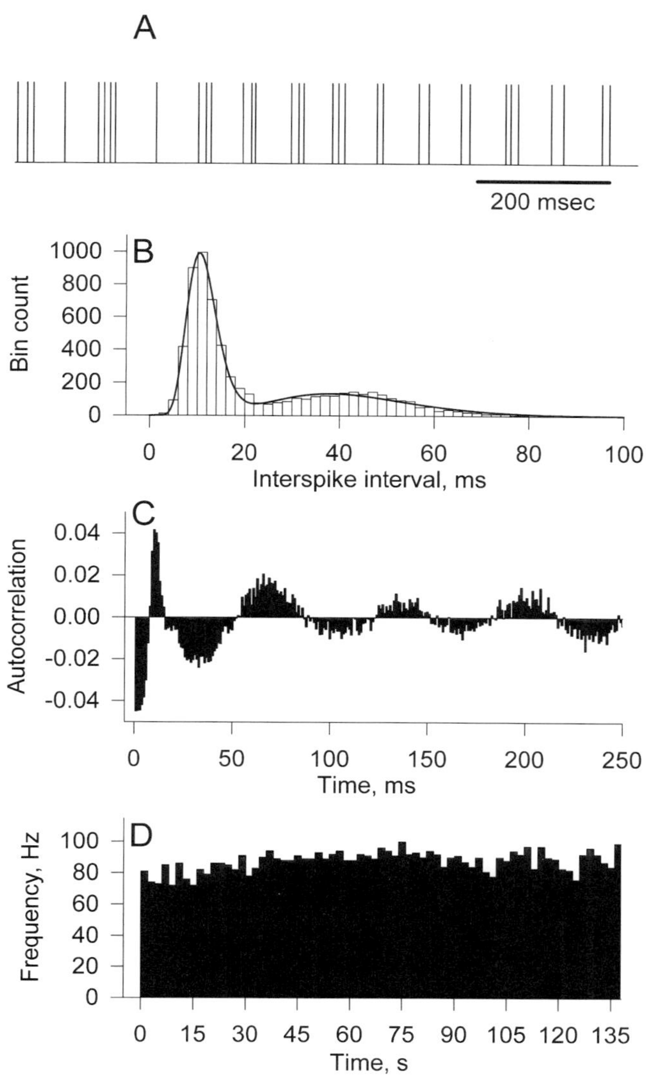

FIGURE 4 Single-unit recording from a neuron within the medial cerebellar nucleus of a P17 dystonic rat. (**A**) Representative portion of the spike train. Mean frequency = 43.1 Hz. (**B**) Interspike interval histogram. (**C**) Autocorrelation. (**D**) Ratemeter histogram. (Reprinted from *Neourscience*, vol. 86, LeDoux et al. [1998] with permission from Elsevier.)

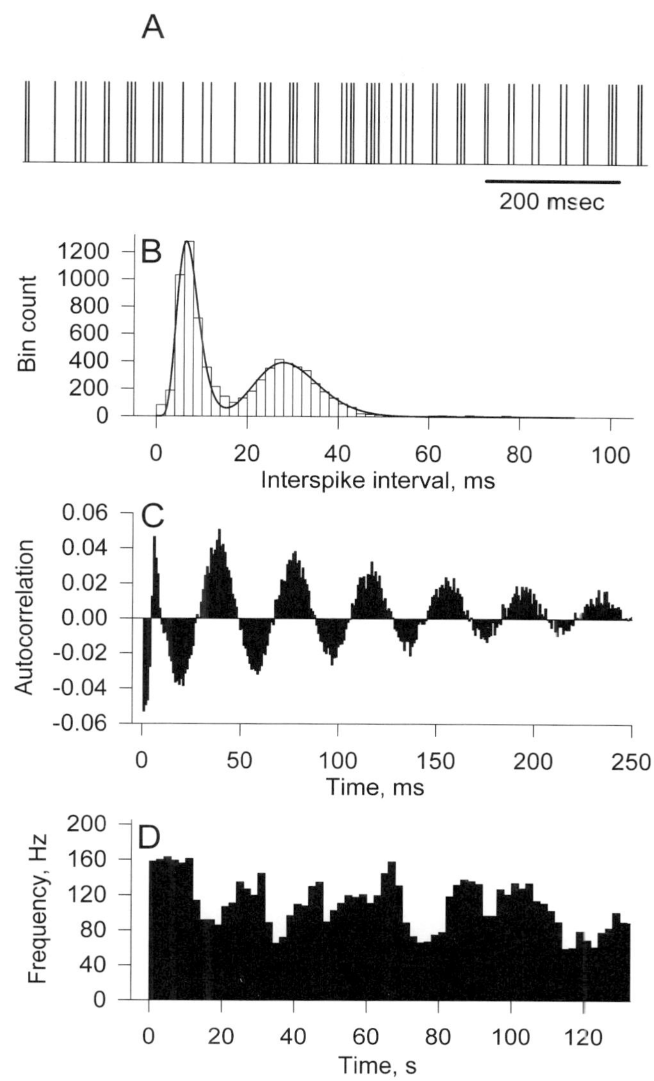

FIGURE 5 Single-unit recording from a neuron within the lateral cerebellar nucleus of a P24 dystonic rat. (**A**) Representative portion of the spike train. Mean frequency = 54.7 Hz. (**B**) Interspike interval histogram. (**C**) Autocorrelation. (**D**) Ratemeter histogram. (Reprinted from *Neourscience*, vol. 86, LeDoux et al. [1998] with permission from Elsevier.)

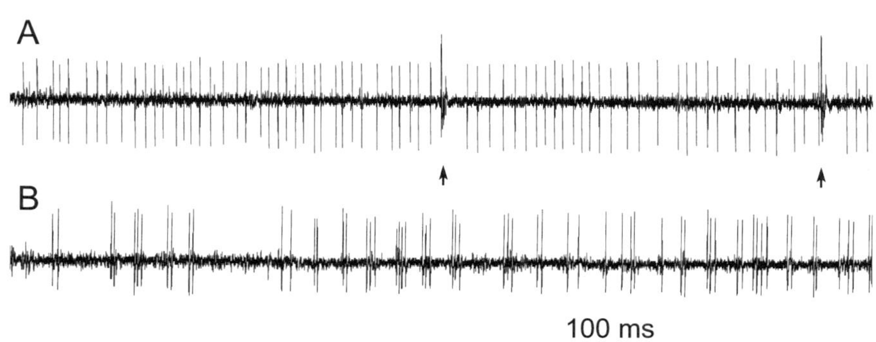

FIGURE 6 Purkinje cell spike trains from normal (**A**) and dystonic (**B**) rats. Complex spikes are identified with arrows. (Reprinted from *Experimental Brain Research*, vol. 145, LeDoux and Lorden [2002] with permission from Springer-Verlag.)

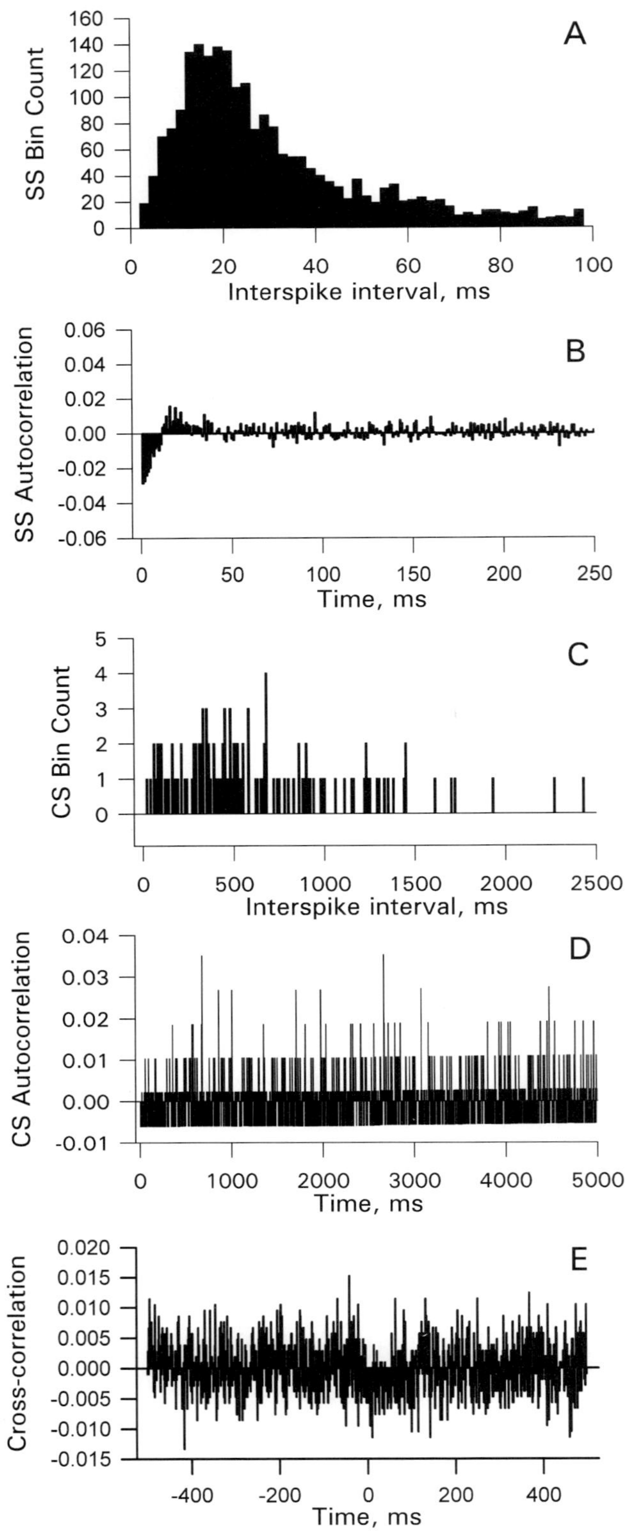

FIGURE 7 Spike train characteristics of a hemispheric Purkinje cell from a P15 normal rat. (**A**) Simple-spike interspike-interval histogram. (**B**) Simple-spike autocorrelation. (**C**) Complex-spike interspike interval histogram. (**D**) Complex-spike autocorrelation. (**E**) Cross-correlation between simple and complex spikes. (Reprinted from *Experimental Brain Research*, vol. 145, LeDoux and Lorden [2002] with permission from Springer-Verlag.)

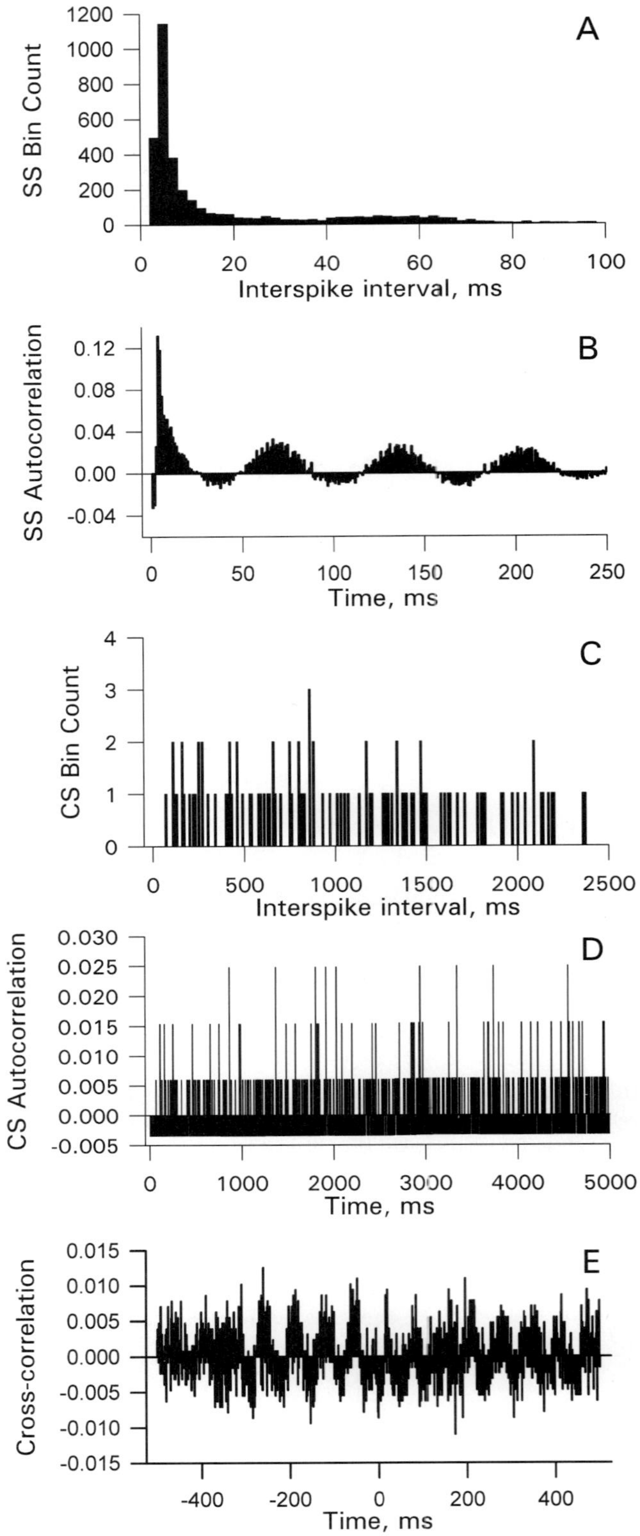

FIGURE 8 Spike train characteristics of a vermal Purkinje cell from a P16 dystonic rat. (**A**) Simple spike interspike-interval histogram. (**B**) Simple-spike autocorrelation. (**C**) Complex-spike interspike interval histogram. (**D**) Complex-spike autocorrelation. (**E**) Cross-correlation between simple and complex spikes. (Reprinted from *Experimental Brain Research*, vol. 145, LeDoux and Lorden [2002] with permission from Springer-Verlag.)

classic ataxic disorders such as ataxia with vitamin E deficiency and spinocerebellar ataxia type 6 (Arpa et al. 1999; Sethi and Jankovic 2002; Roubertie et al. 2003).

Acknowledgments

MSL has been supported by grants from the National Institutes of Health (K08 NS 01593 & R01 EY12232), Dystonia Medical Research Foundation, and Center of Genomics and Bioinformatics at the University of Tennessee Health Science Center.

Video Legends

Three rats from the same litter are used in video segments 1 to 5. Two rats from a different litter are used for segment 6. Rats are numbered on their tails. Rats #1 and #2 are dystonic. Rat #4 is normal. Rats #1 and #4 were videotaped before undergoing cerebellectomy (CBX) on P15. Rat #2 serves as a non-operated dystonic control.

SEGMENT 1 Open-field behavior of dystonic rats and a normal littermate at P15. Note the presence of both axial and appendicular dystonia. Much of the dystonic posturing is precipitated by action. The dystonic movements produce frequent falls. Rats #1 and #4 underwent CBX after acquisition of this videotape segment.

SEGMENT 2 Open-field behavior of dystonic rats at P16. Rat #1 is Postoperative Day 1 after CBX. Rat #2 is the dystonic littermate that did not undergo CBX. Rat #1 is now mildly to moderately ataxic, but does not exhibit dystonia. Rat #1's hindpaws are widely based. Rat #2's dystonia is slightly more severe.

SEGMENT 3 Open-field behavior of dystonic (#1) and normal (#4) rats after CBX. These P16 rats are Postoperative Day 1 after CBX.

SEGMENT 4 Open-field behavior of dystonic rats at P23. Rat #1 is Postoperative Day 8 after CBX. Rat #2 is the dystonic littermate that did not receive CBX. Rat #1's ataxia has improved and there is no evidence of dystonia on open-field behavior. Rat #2 demonstrates paw clasping, falls, and severe generalized dystonia.

SEGMENT 5 Open-field behavior of dystonic (#1) and normal (#4) rats after CBX. These P23 rats are Postoperative Day 8 after CBX. Both rats are ataxic but do not show signs of dystonia.

SEGMENT 6 Open-field behavior of a dystonic rat (#6; one long tail mark and one short tail mark) and non-operated normal littermate (#9; one long tail mark and four short tail marks) on P32. Rat #6 is Postoperative Day 17 after CBX. Unlike dystonic Rat #6 (post-CBX), rat #9 is able to stand on its hindpaws for environmental exploration.

References

Altman, J., and K. Sudarshan. 1975. Postnatal development of locomotion in the laboratory rat. *Anim Behav* **23**:896–920.

Arpa, J., A. Cuesta, A. Cruz-Martinez, S. Santiago, J. Sarria, and F. Palau. 1999. Clinical features and genetic analysis of a Spanish family with spinocerebellar ataxia 6. *Acta Neurol Scand* **99**:43–47.

Augood, S.J., J.B. Penney, Jr., I.K. Friberg, X.O. Breakefield, A.B. Young, L.J. Ozelivs, and D.G. Standaert. 1998. Expression of the early-onset torsion dystonia gene (DYT1) in human brain. *Ann Neurol* **43**:669–673.

Beales, M., J.F. Lorden, E. Walz, and G.A. Oltmans. 1990. Quantitative autoradiography reveals selective changes in cerebellar GABA receptors of the rat mutant dystonic. *J Neurosci* **10**:1874–1885.

Bressman, S.B., and P.E. Greene. 2000. Dystonia. *Curr Treat Options Neurol* **2**:275–285.

Brown, L.L., and J.F. Lorden. 1989. Local cerebral glucose utilization reveals widespread abnormalities in the motor system of the rat mutant dystonic. *J Neurosci* **9**:4033–4041.

De Ryck, M., T. Schallert, and P. Teitelbaum. 1980. Morphine versus haloperidol catalepsy in the rat: a behavioral analysis of postural support mechanisms. *Brain Res* **201**:143–172.

de Vente, J., E. Asan, S. Gambaryan, M. Markerink-van Ittersum, H. Axer, K. Gallatz, S.M. Lohmann, and M. Palkovits. 2001. Localization of cGMP-dependent protein kinase type II in rat brain. *Neuroscience* **108**:27–49.

Eidelberg, D., J.R. Moeller, A. Antonini, K. Kazumata, T. Nakamura, V. Dhawan, P. Spetsieris, et al. 1998. Functional brain networks in DYT1 dystonia. *Ann Neurol* **44**:303–312.

Fahn, S., C.D. Marsden, and D.B. Calne. 1987. Classification and investigation of dystonia. In *Movement Disorders 2*. Ed. C.D. Marsden, and S. Fahn. pp. 332–358. London: Butterworths.

Gimenez-Roldan, S., G. Delgado, M. Marin, J.A. Villanueva, and D. Mateo. 1988. Hereditary torsin dystonia in gypsies. *Adv Neurol* **50**:73–81.

Henry, B., S. Duty, S.H. Fox, A.R. Crossman, and J.M. Brotchie. 2003. Increased striatal pre-proenkephalin B expression is associated with dyskinesia in Parkinson's disease. *Exp Neurol* **183**:458–468.

Ichinose, H., T. Ohye, E. Takahashi, N. Seki, T. Hori, M. Segawa, Y. Nomura, et al. 1994. Hereditary progressive dystonia with marked diurnal fluctuation caused by mutations in the GTP cyclohydrolase I gene. *Nat Genet* **8**:236–242.

Khan, N.L., N.W. Wood, and K.P. Bhatia. 2003. Autosomal recessive, DYT2-like primary torsion dystonia: a new family. *Neurology* **61**: 274–275.

Kita, M., and D. Goodkin. 2000. Drugs used to treat spasticity. *Drugs* **59**: 487–495.

Landis, S.C., C. Shoemaker, W.J. Schlumpf, and F.E. Bloom. 1975. Catecholamines in mutant mouse cerebellum: fluorescence microscopic and chemical studies. *Brain Res* **93**:253–266.

LeDoux, M.S., J.F. Lorden, and J.M. Ervin. 1993. Cerebellectomy eliminates the motor syndrome of the genetically dystonic rat. *Exp Neurol* **120**:302–310.

LeDoux, M.S., J.F. Lorden, and J.M. Ervin. 1994. Inferior olive serotonin and norepinephrine levels during development in the genetically dystonic rat. *Brain Res Bull* **33**:299–305.

LeDoux, M.S., J.F. Lorden, and J. Meinzen-Derr. 1995. Selective elimination of cerebellar output in the genetically dystonic rat. *Brain Res* **696**: 91–103.

LeDoux, M.S., D.C. Hurst, and J.F. Lorden. 1998. Single-unit activity of cerebellar nuclear cells in the awake genetically dystonic rat. *Neurosci* **86**:533–545.

LeDoux, M.S., and J.F. Lorden. 2002. Abnormal spontaneous and harmaline-stimulated Purkinje cell activity in the awake genetically dystonic rat. *Exp Brain Res* **145**:457–467.

LeDoux, M.S., and K.A. Brady. 2003. Secondary cervical dystonia associated with structural lesions of the central nervous system. *Mov Disord* **18**:60–69.

Levitt, P., and J.L. Noebels. 1981. Mutant mouse tottering: selective increase of locus ceruleus axons in a defined single-locus mutation. *Proc Natl Acad Sci U S A* **78**:4630–4634.

Llano, I., and H.M. Gerschenfeld. 1993. Beta-adrenergic enhancement of inhibitory synaptic activity in rat cerebellar stellate and Purkinje cells. *J Physiol* **468**:201–204.

Llinás, R., and R.A. Volkind. 1973. The olivo-cerebellar system: functional properties as revealed by harmaline-induced tremor. *Exp Brain Res* **18**:69–87.

Llinás, R., and M. Mühlethaler. 1988. Electrophysiology of guinea-pig cerebellar nuclear cells in the *in vitro* brain stem-cerebellar preparation. *J Physiol* **404**:241–258.

Lorden, J.F., T.W. McKeon, H.J. Baker, N. Cox, and S.U. Walkley. 1984. Characterization of the rat mutant dystonic (dt): a new animal model of dystonia musculorum deformans. *J Neurosci* **4**:1925–1932.

Lorden, J.F., G.A. Oltmans, T.W. McKeon, J. Lutes, and M. Beales. 1985. Decreased cerebellar 3′,5′-cyclic guanosine monophosphate levels and insensitivity to harmaline in the genetically dystonic rat (dt). *J Neurosci* **5**:2618–2625.

Lorden, J.F., G.A. Oltmans, S. Stratton, and L.E. Mays. 1988. Neuropharmacological correlates of the motor syndrome of the genetically dystonic (dt) rat. *Adv Neurol* **50**:277–297.

Lorden, J.F., J. Lutes, V.L. Michela, and J. Ervin. 1992. Abnormal cerebellar output in rats with an inherited movement disorder. *Exp Neurol* **118**:95–104.

Lutes, J., J.F. Lorden, B.J. Davis, and G.A. Oltmans. 1992. GABA levels and GAD immunoreactivity in the deep cerebellar nuclei of rats with altered olivo-cerebellar function. *Brain Res Bull* **29**:329–336.

McKeon, T.W., J.F. Lorden, G.A. Oltmans, M. Beales, and S.U. Walkley. 1984. Decreased catalepsy response to haloperidol in the genetically dystonic (dt) rat. *Brain Res* **308**:89–96.

McKeon, T.W., J.F. Lorden, M. Beales, and G.A. Oltmans. 1986. Alterations in the noradrenergic projection to the cerebellum of the dystonic (dt) rat. *Brain Res* **366**:89–97.

Michela, V.L., S.E. Stratton, and J.F. Lorden. 1990. Enhanced sensitivity to quipazine in the genetically dystonic rat (dt). *Pharmacol Biochem Behav* **37**:129–133.

Miwa, H., K. Nishi, T. Fuwa, and Y. Mizuno. 2000. Differential expression of c-fos following administration of two tremorgenic agents: harmaline and oxotremorine. *Neuroreport* **11**:2385–2390.

Moretti, P.M., P. Hedera, J.J. Wald, and J.K. Fink. 2001. Dystonia in two siblings from a consanguineous family: further evidence for autosomal recessive primary generalized dystonia (DYT2). *Neurology* **56(S3)**: A121–122.

Naudon, L., J.M. Delfs, N. Clavel, J.F. Lorden, and M.F. Chesselet. 1988. Differential expression of glutamate decarboxylase messenger RNA in cerebellar Purkinje cells and deep cerebellar nuclei of the genetically dystonic rat. *Neuroscience* **82**:1087–1094.

Oltmans, G.A., M. Beales, and J.F. Lorden. 1986. Glutamic acid decarboxylase activity in micropunches of the deep cerebellar nuclei of the genetically dystonic (dt) rat. *Brain Res* **385**:148–151.

Ozelius, L.J., J.W. Hewett, C.E. Page, S.B. Bressman, P.L. Kramer, C. Shalish, D. de Leon, et al. 1997. The early-onset torsion dystonia gene (DYT1) encodes an ATP-binding protein. *Nat Genet* **17**:40–48.

Pizoli, C.E., H.A. Jinnah, M.L. Billingsley, and E.J. Hess. 2002. Abnormal cerebellar signaling induces dystonia in mice. *J Neurosci* **22**: 7825–7833.

Roubertie, A., B. Biolsi, F. Rivier, V. Humbertclaude, R. Cheminal, and B. Echenne. 2003. Ataxia with vitamin E deficiency and severe dystonia: report of a case. *Brain Dev* **25**:442–445.

Santangelo, G. 1934. Contributo clinico alla conoscenza delle forme familiari della dysbasia lordotica progressiva (spasmo di torsione). *G Psychiat Neuropat* **62**:52–77.

Sethi, K.D., and J. Jankovic. 2002. Dystonia in spinocerebellar ataxia type 6. *Mov Disord* **17**:150–153.

Stahl, S.M., and P.A. Berger. 1982. Bromocriptine, physostigmine, and neurotransmitter mechanisms in the dystonias. *Neurology* **32**:889–892.

Stojanovic, M., D. Cvetkovic, and V.S. Kostic. 1995. A genetic study of idiopathic focal dystonias. *J Neurol* **242**:508–511.

Stratton, S.E., J.F. Lorden, L.E. Mays, and G.A. Oltmans. 1988. Spontaneous and harmaline-stimulated Purkinje cell activity in rats with a genetic movement disorder. *J Neurosci* **8**:3327–3336.

Stratton, S.E. 1991. Neurophysiological and neuroanatomical investigations of the olivo-cerebellar system in the mutant rat dystonic (dt). Unpublished doctoral dissertation, University of Alabama at Birmingham.

Stratton, S.E., and J.F. Lorden. 1991. Effect of harmaline on cells of the inferior olive in the absence of tremor: differential response of genetically dystonic and harmaline-tolerant rats. *Neuroscience* **41**:543–549.

Walker, J.M., R.R. Matsumoto, W.D. Bowen, D.L. Gans, K.D. Jones, and F.O. Walker 1988. Evidence for a role of haloperidol-sensitive sigma-"opiate" receptors in the motor effects of antipsychotic drugs. *Neurology* **38**:961–965.

Weissman, A.D., D.J. McCann, J.F. Lorden, and T.P. Su. 1993. An absence of changes in sigma receptor subtypes in the brains of genetically dystonic (dt) rats. *Eur J Pharmacol* **250**:329–332

West, A., M. Periquet, S. Lincoln, C.B. Lucking, D. Nicholl, V. Bonifati, N. Rawal, et al. 2002. Complex relationships between Parkin mutations and Parkinson disesase. *Am J Med Genet* **8**:584–591.

Wieland, S., I. Lucki. 1991. Altered behavioral responses mediated by serotonin receptors in the genetically dystonic (dt) rat. *Brain Res Bull* **26**: 11–16.

Xiao, J., and M.S. LeDoux. 2003. Cloning, developmental regulation and neural localization of rat ε-sarcoglycan. *Brain Res Mol Brain Res* **26**: 132–143.

Ziefer, P., J. Leung, T. Razzano, C. Shalish, M.S. LeDoux, J.F. Lorden, L. Ozelius, et al. 2002. Molecular cloning and expression of rat torsinA in the normal and genetically dystonic (dt) rat. *Brain Res Mol Brain Res* **101**:132–135.

Zimprich, A., M. Grabowski, F. Asmus, M. Naumann, D. Berg, M. Bertram, K. Scheidtmann, et al. 2001. Mutations in the gene encoding epsilon-sarcoglycan cause myoclonus-dystonia syndrome. *Nat Genet* **29**:66–69.

CHAPTER

C3

Animal Models of Benign Essential Blepharospasm and Hemifacial Spasm

CRAIG EVINGER and IRIS S. KASSEM

Investigators typically use two different approaches to develop animal models of movement disorders. One method recreates the etiology of disease to determine its contribution to symptom development. For example, the hph-1, GTP cyclohydrolase deficient mouse has the same molecular dysfunction as individuals with dopa-responsive dystonia (Hyland et al. 1996; Hyland et al. 2003). The ultimate goal of etiology-based models is to identify methods to block the development of the disorder. The other approach to animal modeling recreates disease symptoms without a detailed understanding of the disease's etiology. For example, Pizoli et al. (2002) produced an animal model of generalized dystonia by injecting kainic acid into the cerebellum of normal mice. Such symptom-based models allow investigators to identify treatments that will block the symptoms of the disorder and, in some cases, discover the neural bases for the movement disorder.

I. THE BLINK SYSTEM

It is essential that the animal chosen for symptom-based model studies makes movements similar to that of affected humans. The blink system is ideal for these studies because blinks among mammals as diverse as rodents and humans are qualitatively similar (Evinger et al. 1984). For all mammals examined, upper eyelid movements result from the interactions among four forces: (1) the orbicularis oculi muscle innervated by the facial nerve generates the active lid-closing force; (2) the levator palpebrae superioris muscle innervated by the oculomotor nerve actively raises the eyelid; (3) the sympathetically innervated Mueller's muscle provides a minor lid-raising force; and (4) muscle and ligament attachments produce passive downward forces (Evinger et al. 1991; Sibony et al. 1991). Trigeminal stimulation evokes reflex blinks that are similar among mammals (Evinger et al. 1984; Manning and Evinger 1986; Gruart et al. 1995; Pellegrini and Evinger 1995; LeDoux et al. 1997; Powers et al. 1997; Peshori et al. 2001). Stimulation of the supraorbital branch of the trigeminal nerve evokes two bursts of orbicularis oculi activity, a short latency R1 and a longer latency R2. In humans, the longer latency R2 component produces most of the lid closure (Evinger et al. 1991), whereas the short latency R1 and R2 contribute equally to lid closure in rodents (Horn et al. 1993). Basal ganglia modulation of trigeminal blinks is identical for primates and rodents (Evinger et al. 1988; Basso et al. 1993; Evinger et al. 1993; Basso and Evinger 1996; Basso et al. 1996; Gnadt et al. 1997). Thus, the blink system is ideal for symptom-based animal models of lid movement disorders such as benign essential blepharospasm and hemifacial spasm.

Benign essential blepharospasm and hemifacial spasm are diseases characterized by excessive involuntary lid closure (Jankovic and Ford 1983; Hallett 2002). In both diseases, the primary cause of lid closure is spasms of the lid closing, orbicularis oculi muscle. The spasms are bilateral in benign essential blepharospasm but unilateral in hemifacial spasm. Hemifacial spasm frequently involves contraction of lower facial muscles on the same side as the affected eyelid. When lower facial muscle involvement occurs in benign essential blepharospasm, the disorder is called Meige syndrome. Despite the similarity of eyelid symptoms, the etiology of the two diseases is very different. Hemifacial spasm is a cranial nerve compression syndrome that originates from abnormal pulsatile compression of the facial nerve at its root entry zone by an aberrant artery. In contrast, the focal dystonia benign essential blepharospasm is a central disorder whose exact cause is unclear. The disease appears to involve the interaction of several factors including genetic predisposition, dopamine receptor modifications, and ocular irritation.

Despite their different etiologies, benign essential blepharospasm and hemifacial spasm illustrate the importance of using animal models to understand the neural changes that underlie these disorders. For hemifacial spasm, animal models allow investigators to explore the contribution of each of the multiple effects created by arterial compression of the facial nerve. For example, pulsatile compression produces antidromic activation of facial motoneurons as well as sensory feedback from unanticipated muscle contractions caused by orthodromic activation of facial muscles. Compression of the facial nerve can cause demyelination, possibly allowing ephaptic transmission among motor axons, as well as weakening the output to facial muscles. Each of these factors may or may not contribute to facial muscle spasms that are the hallmark of hemifacial spasm. For benign essential blepharospasm, animal models allow investigation of different central nervous system modifications that can produce lid spasms. Understanding the basis of lid spasms in these two disorders may point to common mechanisms for the two disorders or illustrate how different mechanisms can generate the same symptom.

II. BLEPHAROSPASM

Symptom-based animal models of blepharospasm have utilized brain stimulation, drug administration, and two factor approaches to produce spasms of involuntary lid closure. Although all of the animal models exhibit closure of the lid, the experimental procedures that cause involuntary closure appear only rarely to resemble processes that are likely to occur in benign essential blepharospasm. Current research in humans with focal dystonia reveals that the disorder results from or creates a significant disruption of sensorimotor processing (Feiwell et al. 1999; Ibanez et al. 1999; Murase et al. 2000; Serrien et al. 2000; Abbruzzese et al. 2001; Lim et al. 2001; Abbruzzese and Berardelli 2003; Molloy et al. 2003). Animal models that produce lid closure by electrical stimulation or systemic drug administration do not replicate sensorimotor processing deficits.

Klemm et al. (1993) reported one of the first models of involuntary lid closure by electrically stimulating premotor inputs to the facial nucleus. They implanted stimulating electrodes into the facial nucleus, parabrachial region, red nucleus, interstitial nucleus of Cajal, the sensory nucleus of V, and into the reticular nuclei, ventral reticularis pontis oralis, reticularis parvocellularis, and reticularis centralis ventralis of cats. Although stimulation parameters in this study were extreme by current standards, single pulse 50 or 10 ms duration electrical stimuli consistently produced stimulus-linked lid closure at only four sites. Single stimuli delivered to the facial nucleus, as well as to three premotor blink areas, the parabrachial region, red nucleus, or interstitial nucleus of Cajal evoked a single unilateral lid closure. Stimulus trains of 10–50 Hz at these sites produced sustained lid closure. All lid closures were ipsilateral to the stimulation sites except for the interstitial nucleus of Cajal. The result for the red nucleus is somewhat surprising because the red nucleus projects to contralateral orbicularis oculi motoneurons (Takeuchi et al. 1979; Holstege and Collewijn 1982; Takada et al. 1984; Holstege et al. 1986; Pellegrini et al. 1995; Morcuende et al. 2002). A significant distinction between lid closure produced by electrical stimulation and that of benign essential blepharospasm is that lid spasms are not tonic in blepharospasm. Dystonic as well as hemifacial lid spasms are closely spaced bursts of orbicularis oculi activity (Figure 1A), as if a series of blinks occurred too close together, holding the eyelid closed (Aramideh et al. 1994; Aramideh et al. 1995; Hallett 2002). Although the Klemm et al. (1993) study did not identify mechanisms that produce the spasms of lid closure in benign essential blepharospasm, the study suggests neural sites that may play a role in creating the spasms.

The evidence linking benign essential blepharospasm to basal ganglia dysfunction (Perimutter et al. 1997; Hallett 2002; Kerrison et al. 2003; Schmidt et al. 2003) has led investigators to modify dopamine levels to model benign essential blepharospasm. The blink system is exquisitely sensitive to dopamine concentration (Peshori et al. 2001). Elevated dopamine levels increase the rate of spontaneous blinking (Zametkin et al. 1979; Karson 1983, 1989; Bartko et al. 1990; Blin et al. 1990; Lewis et al. 1990; Elsworth et al. 1991; Taylor et al. 1999; Hallett 2000). In contrast to dopamine's effects on spontaneous blink rates, systemic treatment with the D_2/D_1 receptor agonist, apomorphine, or increasing dopamine levels lowers the excitability of trigem-

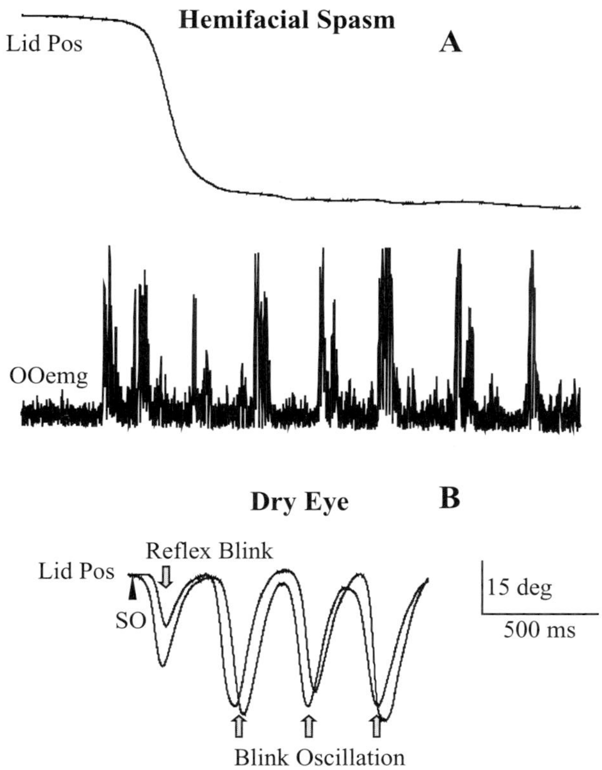

FIGURE 1 Spasms of lid closure with hemifacial spasm and blink oscillations of dry eye. (A) Position of the upper eyelid (Lid Pos) and rectified orbicularis oculi EMG (OOemg) of the affected eyelid of a hemifacial spasm patient during a lid spasm initiated by a voluntary blink. The lid closure results from bursts of orbicularis oculi contraction occurring every 76 ms on the average. Time bar = 250 ms. (B) Position of the upper eyelid of a patient with dry eye showing a reflex blink (↓) evoked by stimulation of the supraorbital nerve (▲SO) followed by a series of large amplitude blinks, blink oscillations (↑). Each trace is from a separate trial. The blink oscillations occur at an average interblink interval of 224 ms on all trials.

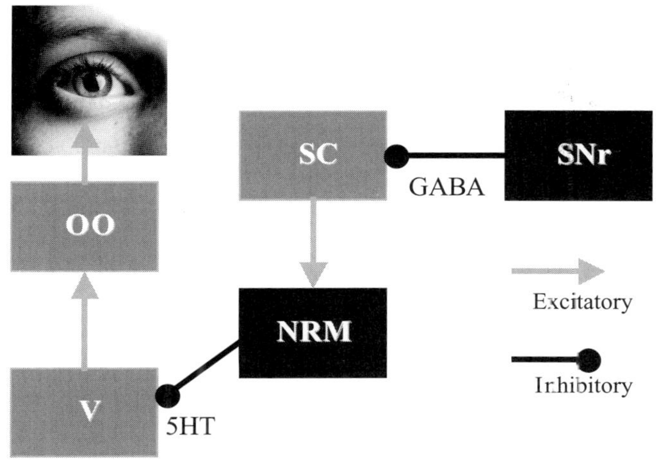

FIGURE 2 Circuit for basal ganglia modulation of trigeminal reflex blink circuits. Increasing SNr activity increases trigeminal reflex blink circuit excitability, whereas reducing SNr output decreases trigeminal reflex blink circuit excitability. Abbreviations: NRM, nucleus raphe magnus; OO, orbicularis oculi muscles; SC, intermediate layers of superior colliculus; SNr, substantia nigra pars reticulata; V, trigeminal reflex blink circuit.

inal reflex blinks (Evinger et al. 1993; Napolitano et al. 1997) and the speed of lid closure (Baker et al. 2002). Conversely, destroying dopamine neurons with catecholamine-specific toxins such as 6-hydroxydopamine (OHDA), or as a result of Parkinson disease, significantly increases the excitability of trigeminal reflex blinks (Kimura 1973; Ferguson et al. 1978; Sunohara et al. 1985; Esteban and Gimenez-Roldan 1988; Vidailhet et al. 1992; Basso et al. 1993; Rey et al. 1996; Valls-Sole et al. 1997; Goto et al. 2000; Schicatano et al. 2000; Kaneko and Sakamoto 2001). This increase in excitability can be large enough for a strong trigeminal stimulus such as touching the cornea to cause spasms of lid closure. The spasms of lid closure evoked by trigeminal stimuli in dopamine-depleted rats exhibit bursts of orbicularis oculi contraction as occurs in benign essential blepharospasm (Basso et al. 1993). As occurs in Parkinson disease, these spasms are actually reflex blepharospasm (Klawans and Erlich 1970; Esteban and Gimenez-Roldan 1988; Repka et al. 1996). Reflex blepharospasm differs from benign essential blepharospasm because reflex blepharospasm requires a significant trigeminal stimulus to elicit spasms, but they occur spontaneously in benign essential blepharospasm. Moreover, benign essential blepharospasm patients do not have Parkinson disease.

Although the circuits through which dopamine modulates spontaneous blink rate are unknown, Basso and colleagues (Basso and Evinger 1996; Basso et al. 1996) have determined how the basal ganglia regulate trigeminal reflex blink circuits (Figure 2). This circuit accounts for the reflex blepharospasm resulting from dopamine depletion (Basso et al. 1993). GABAergic substantia nigra pars reticulata (SNr) neurons inhibit neurons in the intermediate layers of the superior colliculus (SC). These neurons excite a small group of neurons in the nucleus raphe magnus (NRM). These serotonergic (5HT) NRM neurons inhibit trigeminal reflex blink circuits (V). Dopamine depletion such as occurs with Parkinson disease increases SNr inhibition of superior colliculus neurons (Wichmann and DeLong 2003). The consequent reduction of NRM excitation decreases inhibition of trigeminal blink circuit, increasing its excitability. Conversely, elevating dopamine levels in the basal ganglia increases NRM inhibition of the blink circuits and consequently reduces trigeminal blink excitability.

In addition to the reflex blepharospasm characterized in rats following 6-OHDA lesions (Basso et al. 1993), systemic injection of the catecholamine-depleting compound, Ro 4–1284, produced a "reserpine syndrome" in mice and rats that included blepharospasm (Burkard et al. 1989). The characteristics of blepharospasm in this study were unclear, but a later study (Mostofsky et al. 2000) reported that Ro

4–1284 increased blink rate. Starting with a blink rate of 0.34 blinks per minute before drug administration, ten days of Ro 4–1284 treatment increased the blink rate to 1.42 blinks per minute. Although these results appear to conflict with previous observations on the effects of dopamine on spontaneous blink rate, it is unclear whether the investigators measured spontaneous blinks increased reflex blinking from elevated trigeminal excitability caused Ro 4–1284 reductions in dopamine.

The inability to replicate benign essential blepharospasm with dopamine depletion alone, however, does not rule out a role for dopamine in this focal dystonia. Recent genetic evidence from patients with benign essential blepharospasm shows a modification in the gene for the D_5 receptor (Misbahuddin et al. 2002; Misbahuddin et al. 2004). Future animal studies need to explore the function of the D_5 receptor in blinking.

Schicatano et al. (1997) created a two-factor rat model of benign essential blepharospasm based on the common explanation for human blepharospasm: that the dystonia arises from the combination of a permissive condition and a precipitating event (Hallett 2002). Benign essential blepharospasm patients frequently come to the clinic with an initial complaint of dry eye (Elston et al. 1988). Therefore, investigators reasoned that cornea irritation might be the precipitating event for benign essential blepharospasm (Evinger et al. 2002). The normal adaptive response to dry eye or eye irritation is to increase trigeminal reflex blink excitability and generate additional large amplitude blinks in response to a single trigeminal reflex blink stimulus (Figure 1B), called blink oscillations (Evinger et al. 2002). Because blink oscillations with dry eye occur at a constant interblink interval, the trigeminal reflex blink circuit appears to oscillate in response to a single stimulus. These investigators reasoned that the spasms of lid closure were an exaggeration of the normal compensatory process evoked by dry eye or eye irritation. To create the permissive component of benign essential blepharospasm that allowed an exaggerated response to dry eye, these investigators produced a small, unilateral lesion of dopaminergic neurons in the substantia nigra pars compacta. By itself, this small 6-OHDA lesion of dopamine neurons slightly increased trigeminal reflex blink excitability but did not generate reflex blepharospasm or spasms of lid closure. To induce dry eye, the zygomatic branch of the facial nerve was crushed to eliminate approximately 30% of the orbicularis oculi innervation. The dry eye condition alone increased trigeminal reflex blink excitability and caused blink oscillations similar to that seen in human dry eye. Combining the two procedures, however, dramatically elevated trigeminal reflex blink excitability, increased spontaneous blinking, and caused long-lasting spasms of lid closure resembling benign essential blepharospasm. The striking aspect of this model was that these blepharospasm-like characteristics continued after the facial nerve regained function and eliminated the dry eye. Thus, this animal model recreated many of the characteristics of human benign essential blepharospasm.

As with most human focal dystonias (Ghika et al. 1993; Hallett 1995; Byl et al. 1996; Odergren et al. 1996; Byl and Melnick 1997; Byl et al. 1997; Bara-Jimenez et al. 1998; Berardelli et al. 1998; Tinazzi et al. 1999; Bara-Jimenez et al. 2000a; Bara-Jimenez et al. 2000b; Serrien et al. 2000; Tinazzi et al. 2000; Abbruzzese et al. 2001; Frasson et al. 2001; Sanger et al. 2001; Blake et al. 2002; Tamburin et al. 2002; Tinazzi et al. 2002; Zeuner et al. 2002; Abbruzzese and Berardelli 2003; Butterworth et al. 2003; Byl et al. 2003; McKenzie et al. 2003; Molloy et al. 2003; Tinazzi et al. 2003), data from the Schicatano animal model (Schicatano et al. 1997) suggest that benign essential blepharospasm involves sensorimotor dysfunction. The eyelid system continuously adjusts itself to ensure the integrity of the cornea. These adjustments, or motor learning, result from interactions among sensory inputs from the periphery, sensory inputs regarding eyelid movements and the intended eyelid movement. Altering any component of this triad modifies the performance of the other components. For example, reducing eyelid motility increases afferent input from the cornea from dry eye and produces an unexpectedly small sensory signal from the attempted eyelid movement. Producing LTP- and LTD-like modifications of trigeminal blink circuits (Mao and Evinger 2001) causes these sensory signals to adjust the inputs to the motor circuits in an attempt to reduce cornea afferent input and to produce a lid movement equivalent to the expected lid movement. Similarly, increasing cornea afferent input transforms the trigeminal reflex blink circuit into an oscillator. Disrupting the balance among these elements can produce involuntary spasms of lid closure in rodents (Schicatano et al. 1997) and humans (Chuke et al. 1996).

Baker and colleagues (Chuke et al. 1996; Baker et al. 1997) identified another form of blepharospasm, Bell palsy associated blepharospasm, that also appears to result from maladaptive motor learning. These investigators and others (Valls-Sole and Montero 2003) have noted that some patients with a unilateral Bell palsy develop blepharospasm-like spasms in the contralateral, unaffected eyelid. Because facial palsy reduces eyelid motility that causes cornea irritation, Bell palsy initiates two adaptive processes, an increased excitability of the trigeminal complex ipsilateral to the paralyzed eyelid and an elevated excitability of the motoneurons innervating that eyelid (Schicatano et al. 1997; Syed et al. 1999). Baker and colleagues suggested that these normally adaptive processes are exaggerated in some patients, producing spasms of lid closure in both eyelids, which only the unaffected eyelid could express. These investigators demonstrated that adding gold weights to the paralyzed eyelid to assist eyelid closure reduced the drive to increase trigeminal and motoneuron excitability and eliminated the spasms of lid closure. Similar to the Schicatano model of blepharospasm (Schicatano et al. 1997), exaggerations of a normally adaptive process caused spasms of lid closure in Bell palsy associated blepharospasm. In rare cases, the occurrence of facial palsy has been linked to the subsequent development of benign essential blepharospasm (Baker et al. 1997; Miwa et al. 2002). As with Bell palsy associated blepharospasm, these cases appeared to result from exaggerations of adaptive responses to cornea irritation and reduced eyelid motility, a sensorimotor dysfunction.

The neural basis of generating dystonic spasms of eyelid closure is unknown. Data from animal and human studies, however, suggest that the cerebellum may be crucial in this process. The cerebellum is essential for adaptive motor learning in the eyelid system (Pellegrini and Evinger 1997). The deep cerebellar neurons of the cerebellum activate orbicularis oculi motoneurons via the red nucleus (Morcuende et al. 2002) and also modulate trigeminal complex neuronal activity (Davis and Dostrovsky 1986). Thus, the cerebellum participates in sensorimotor processing and modulates blink circuits. There is significant evidence that the cerebellum is important in dystonia. A recent study (Pizoli et al. 2002) reports that a low dose injection of kainic acid into the mouse cerebellum causes a transient generalized dystonia including spasms of lid closure. These spasms result from glutamatergic modifications of Purkinje cell discharge because transgenic mice lacking Purkinje cells do not exhibit dystonic posturing following kainic acid injections into the vermis. In a genetically dystonic rat, the deep cerebellar nucleus neurons discharge in a bursting rather than a tonic pattern (LeDoux et al. 1998; LeDoux and Lorden 1998) and removal of the cerebellum eliminates dystonic posturing in these rats (LeDoux et al. 1995). Patients with benign essential blepharospasm exhibit altered cerebellar activity (Hutchinson et al. 2000; Baker et al. 2003; Kerrison et al. 2003; Schmidt et al. 2003). Thus, with dystonia, cerebellar neurons change from a tonic to an oscillatory pattern of activity, which parallels the activity of the orbicularis oculi muscle during eyelid spasms. The cerebellum may modulate the excitability of the facial nucleus and/or interact with other neural structures to create an oscillatory pattern in reflex blink circuits that can convert into spasms of lid closure when preceded by a permissive condition.

III. HEMIFACIAL SPASM

The three primary symptoms of hemifacial spasm are involuntary muscle spasms, synkinesis, and lateral spread (Sibony and Evinger 1998). The initial clinical signs of hemifacial spasm are spontaneous, unilateral spasms of the eyelid muscle that progress to the remaining ipsilateral facial muscles over a period of weeks to months. Synkinesis is an inappropriate, involuntary activation of multiple muscles that normally do not act together. For example, stimulating the supraorbital branch of the trigeminal nerve not only produces orbicularis oculi activity, it strongly activates the mentalis muscle in some patients with hemifacial spasm (Yamashita et al. 2002). Lateral spread, or abnormal muscle response, is the long latency activation of a facial muscle by percutaneous motor nerve stimulation that does not innervate that muscle. In some patients with hemifacial spasm, percutaneously stimulating the temporal branch of the facial nerve activates the orbicularis oculi, which it innervates, and at a longer latency, the mentalis muscle, which it does not normally innervate (Moller and Jannetta 1986; Ishikawa et al. 1996a; Ishikawa et al. 1996b; Ishikawa et al. 1996c; Yamashita et al. 2002).

There is general agreement that a blood vessel impinging on the facial nerve at the root entry zone is the cause of hemifacial spasm (Sibony and Evinger 1998). The aberrant arteries usually include the anterior inferior cerebellar artery, the posterior inferior cerebellar artery, or the vertebral artery. Although microvascular compression of the facial nerve is the proximate cause of hemifacial spasm, it is not sufficient to cause the disorder. Fifteen to twenty-five percent of individuals with facial nerve compression are asymptomatic (Tan et al. 1999; Fukuda et al. 2003). Nevertheless, microsurgical decompression of the facial nerve typically reduces or eliminates the spasms, synkinesis, and lateral spread of hemifacial spasm (Nielsen and Jannetta 1984; Ishikawa et al. 1997; Hatem et al. 2001). As reported in one study (Nielsen and Jannetta 1984), spasms disappeared in 64%, synkinesis was gone in 53%, and lateral spread was eliminated in 23% of hemifacial spasm patients within the first week following surgery. After two to eight months, patients showed further improvement with 90% spasm or synkinesis free. If pulsatile compression alone produced the symptoms of hemifacial spasm, then decompression surgery should eliminate symptoms immediately. Therefore, arterial compression must produce longterm changes in the facial nerve, facial motoneurons, trigeminal sensory processing, or some combination of those components.

Pulsatile arterial compression of the facial nerve can contribute to hemifacial spasm in many ways. Chronic compression at the junction of peripheral and central myelin sheaths at the root entry zone can demyelinate facial nerve axons (Nielsen 1985). Arterial compression can also injure facial axons, effectively weakening the facial muscles (Frueh et al. 1990). Facial motoneuron excitability may change because of chronic antidromic activation of facial motoneurons by pulsatile compression of axons (Moller and Jannetta 1984, 1985a, b, c) or through axotomy effects (Ferguson 1978). Orthodromic activation of muscles may alter sensory trigeminal circuits. Trigeminal receptive field reorganization may result from abnormal pairing of trigeminal sensory signals, produced by simultaneous activation of muscles that normally do not act together, e.g., mentalis and orbicularis oculi (Godde et al. 1996; Godde et al. 2000; Ziemus et al. 2000; Godde et al. 2003). Reflex blink circuit activation by trigeminal stimulation combined with antidromic depolarization of facial motoneurons may abnormally increase the synaptic strength of reflex circuit inputs to facial motoneurons. Animal models isolating each of these contributions provide a unique opportunity to determine the role of each component in hemifacial spasm.

Møller and colleagues created the first animal models of hemifacial spasm (Sen and Møller 1987; Saito and Møller 1993; Kuroki and Møller 1994a, b; Kuroki et al. 1994). In the initial model (Sen and Møller 1987; Saito and Møller 1993; Kuroki et al. 1994), the investigators electrically stimulated the seventh cranial nerve in the facial canal of rats for periods of three to thirty weeks. The stimulation paradigms varied, but the investigators gave 10 or 20 Hz stimuli for two to ten minutes each day while the rats were lightly anesthetized. To evaluate the effect of this electrical stimulation paradigm, the investigators inserted stimulating needle electrodes percutaneously around the temporal branch of the facial nerve and the supraorbital branch of the trigeminal nerve to activate these nerves. Identical electrodes were placed in the orbicularis oculi and mentalis muscles to record EMG activity. All recording experiments used light anesthesia on the rats. In twelve of the eighteen rats, stimulation of the temporal branch of the facial nerve usually produced EMG activity in the mentalis muscle with a mean latency of 6.5 ms, which the investigators characterized as lateral spread. Stimulation of the supraorbital branch of the trigeminal nerve evoked a synkinetic R1 response in both the orbicularis oculi and in the mentalis muscle with a mean latency of 6.12 ms. The investigators interpreted their data as showing that antidromic activation of the facial motoneurons produced facial motoneuron hyperexcitability that caused an abnormal muscle response and synkinesis. An alternative interpretation to these data, however, was that the stimulation of multiple muscles innervated by the facial nerve modified the inputs to the motoneurons rather than changing motoneuron excitability.

The synchronous contraction of all of the facial muscles caused by stimulation of the facial nerve produces simultaneous input to all of the second-order trigeminal complex neurons. If second-order trigeminal reflex blink neurons project weakly to other pools of motoneurons, as well as strongly to orbicularis oculi motoneurons, then weak trigeminal blink circuit inputs will arrive on motoneurons still depolarized by antidromic activation. Accepting that "neurons that fire together wire together," previously weak trigeminal blink circuit inputs to lower facial motoneurons may strengthen sufficiently to activate the motoneuron in response to supraorbital nerve stimulation. This interpretation accounts for the identical R1 latencies in the orbicularis oculi and mentalis muscles with synkinesis. Lateral spread may actually reflect the same process. Stimulation of the temporal branch of the facial nerve with percutaneous needle electrodes not only activates the facial nerve but also the cutaneous trigeminal receptors near the stimulation site. Because activation of fibers in the ophthalmic branch of the trigeminal nerve occurs with this temporal nerve stimulus, it follows that the activation of the mentalis muscle must occur at an R1 latency, slightly over 6 ms. Thus, the data from these studies (Sen and Møller 1987; Saito and Møller 1993; Kuroki et al. 1994) are consistent with a trigeminal rather than a motoneuron modification produced by facial nerve stimulation.

In a second series of studies, Kuroki and Møller examined the effect of arterial compression and demyelination on the facial nerve of rats in producing lateral spread and synkinesis (Kuroki and Møller 1994b; Kuroki et al. 1994). They tested three groups of rats. In the first group, tying a chromic suture to the facial nerve distal to the auricular branch point caused partial demyelination. In another group of rats, placing the temporal artery against the facial nerve produced pulsatile compression of the nerve. The rats with demyelination or arterial compression alone did not exhibit lateral spread or synkinesis. In a third group of rats, the temporal artery was placed over the demyelinated portion of the facial nerve following focal demyelination with a chromic suture. This latter condition replicated the basis of human hemifacial spasm in the peripheral facial nerve rather than at the root entry zone. Rats with combined arterial compression and demyelination developed lateral spread and synkinesis with latencies around 6 ms. To determine whether the lateral spread resulted from ephaptic transmission at the site of demyelination or motoneuron hyperexcitability, the investigators anesthetized the facial nerve proximal to the arterial compression. Because this procedure blocked lateral spread, the investigators interpreted their data to demonstrate that lateral spread and synkinesis resulted from changes in facial motoneuron excitability. Nevertheless, these data are equally consistent with the hypothesis that lateral spread and synkinesis result from modifications of the trigeminal input to the facial motoneurons because blocking motoneuron output prevents expression of changes in both motoneuron excitability and inputs to facial motoneurons. In a separate study, Kuroki and Møller (1994a) reported that the orbicularis oculi EMG activity ipsilateral to demyelination and nerve compression was more active than the contralateral orbicularis oculi activity in lightly anesthetized rats. Because the EMG recordings were made with needle electrodes, however, increased trigeminal sensitivity ipsilateral to nerve compression may account for these differences. Despite difficulties in drawing conclusions from these data about the effect of the stimulation procedures, Kuroki and Møller (1994b) demonstrated that demyelination is essential in the generation of the lateral spread produced by pulsatile arterial compression of the facial nerve. Although valuable in identifying stimulation parameters that can create lateral spread and synkinesis in rodents, the initial animal models did not distinguish between the multiple effects of pulsatile arterial compression in producing human hemifacial spasm.

Kassem and Evinger (2002, 2003) attempted to isolate the effect of motor axon activation from the other effects of pulsatile facial nerve compression on hemifacial spasm symptoms by chronically stimulating different branches of the facial nerve. Rats were alert during nerve stimulation, which occurred for eight hours a day. The temporal and mandibular branches of the facial nerve were synchronously stimulated at 1 Hz with intensity just sufficient to evoke EMG activity in the orbicularis oculi and lower whisker pad muscles. Prior to the start of chronic stimulation each day, rats were tested for synkinetic responses from supraorbital nerve stimulation and lateral spread of facial nerve responses by examining whether temporal or mandibular nerve stimulation elicited inappropriate orbicularis oculi and whisker pad EMG activity. The studies revealed two effects of chronic synchronous stimulation of the temporal and mandibular branches of the facial nerve.

Chronic synchronous activation of the two facial nerve branches increased the EMG activity of the whisker pad muscles in response to supraorbital nerve stimulation. This result is similar to synkinesis seen in hemifacial spasm and that reported by Møller and colleagues (Sen and Møller 1987; Saito and Møller 1993; Kuroki and Møller 1994b; Kuroki et al. 1994). Nevertheless, these rats did not exhibit lateral spread in response to temporal or mandibular nerve stimulation. This result is consistent with the hypothesis that lateral spread is actually synkinesis elicited by percutaneous stimulation of facial nerve branches. In the Kassem and Evinger studies, the facial nerve branches were stimulated with chronically implanted, insulated nerve cuffs that did not activate cutaneous trigeminal afferents. Indeed, the lateral spread reported in humans may have been synkinesis because facial nerve stimulation was done with skin electrodes overlying the facial nerve branches. This percutaneous stimulation procedure invariably activated cutaneous trigeminal afferents that can elicit a reflex response.

Chronic synchronous stimulation of the temporal and mandibular facial nerve branches also decreased the magnitude of the long latency R2 component of the blink reflex evoked by supraorbital nerve stimulation. Although depression of the R2 response is obviously inconsistent with the symptoms of hemifacial spasm, the result demonstrates that chronic activation of facial nerves can alter trigeminal reflex circuits. Comparison of the blinks evoked by stimulation of the supraorbital nerve ipsilateral and contralateral to the facial nerve branches receiving chronic stimulation demonstrated that the R2 suppression resulted from changes in the trigeminal premotor neurons rather than facial motoneurons. If a change in motoneuron excitability on the stimulated side caused reduced R2 magnitude, then R2 magnitude would be reduced regardless of which supraorbital nerve was stimulated. If the change occurred in the trigeminal complex ipsilateral to chronic stimulation, however, then both orbicularis oculi muscles would exhibit a reduced R2 response when the affected side was stimulated, but a normal R2 response when the contralateral supraorbital nerve was stimulated. Investigators obtained the latter case in these rats. Cessation of facial nerve stimulation caused a recovery of R2 amplitude elicited by supraorbital nerve stimulation ipsilateral to motor nerve stimulation. Thus, the modification of the R2 response reflects dynamic changes within trigeminal reflex blink circuits produced by stimulation of facial motor nerves.

The data from animal models suggest that a single mechanism is unlikely to produce all of the characteristics of hemifacial spasm. The different effects of pulsatile compression of the facial nerve may each contribute to one or more of the hemifacial spasm symptoms. Synchronous activation of the facial nerve by electrical stimulation (Sen and Møller 1987; Saito and Møller 1993; Kuroki et al. 1994; Kassem and Evinger 2002, 2003) or pulsatile arterial compression (Kuroki and Møller 1994b) produce synkinesis of muscle responses with trigeminal reflex blinks. The data are most consistent with the hypothesis that synchronous activation modifies the synaptic strengths of trigeminal afferents to facial motoneurons to produce synkinesis. If this interpretation is correct, then lateral spread is not a unique characteristic of hemifacial spasm, but a variant of synkinesis. Demyelination or facial nerve compression may create facial weakness that initiates compensatory motor adaptations (Sibony et al. 1991; Schicatano et al. 2002) or perhaps even ephaptic transmission that may possibly allow synkinesis and lateral spread.

None of the animal models, however, replicates the spasms of multiple facial muscles, the hallmark symptom of hemifacial spasm. Combinations of two or more neural modifications affecting both the sensory trigeminal and facial motor systems may interact to produce spasms. For example, hemifacial spasm patients exhibit hyperexcitable reflex blinks in both eyelids with stimulation of the supraorbital branch of the trigeminal nerve on the affected side, but normally excitable blinks in both eyelids following contralateral stimulation (Valls-Sole and Tolosa 1989). If trigeminal hyperexcitability alone were sufficient to produce spasms of lid closure, then both eyelids would exhibit spasms because trigeminal activation evokes a bilateral reflex blink in humans. Likewise, the proposed unilateral motoneuron hyperexcitability in hemifacial spasm (Ferguson 1978; Jannetta and Kassam 1999) is insufficient to explain unilateral spasms of lid closure. If motoneuron hyperexcitability were sufficient to produce spasms, then stimulation of either the ipsilateral or the contralateral trigeminal nerve would evoke spasms. Together, however, unilateral motoneuron hyperexcitability combined with increased trigeminal excitability may produce spasms of closure in one eyelid but not the other. The involvement of facial muscles other than the orbicularis oculi may result from synaptic modification of the trigeminal inputs to facial motoneurons produced by combined trigeminal blink circuit activity and facial motoneuron depolarization.

Although the neural mechanisms that can create unilateral spasms of lid closure are comprehensible, it is unclear how the nervous system would allow spasms to develop. The blink system normally undergoes modifications that adapt it to perform appropriately in the face of changes in the motor system, sensory inputs, or the environment (Evinger and Manning 1988; Evinger et al. 1989; Evinger et al. 2002; Schicatano et al. 2002). The nervous system increases drive to compensate for orbicularis oculi weakness and it decreases drive to counteract unexpectedly large blinks. Thus, the generation of eyelid spasms is inconsistent with these normal adaptive processes. For example, creating unexpectedly large blinks by adding weights to the upper eyelids initiates a rapid reduction in the trigeminal blink circuit drive onto orbicularis oculi motoneurons (Evinger and Manning 1988). The reduction in R2 amplitude following chronic facial nerve activation (Kassem and Evinger 2002, 2003) follows the same pattern of nervous system modification to avoid unanticipated lid movements. Thus, the convergence of facial and trigeminal modifications is insufficient to cause spasms of lid closure because the blink system modifies itself to prevent excessive blinking. The significant number of humans with pulsatile compression of the facial nerve who do not develop hemifacial spasm (Tan et al. 1999; Fukuda et al. 2003) supports this interpretation. These observations suggest that hemifacial spasm, like benign essential blepharospasm, requires a permissive condition to prevent the normal adaptive modifications that block lid spasms. Therefore, hemifacial spasm may require the confluence of several factors, synchronous activation of the facial nerve, facial nerve weakness, and a permissive condition. Finding the permissive condition for hemifacial spasm should be a goal for future animal model studies.

IV. CONCLUSIONS

Although blepharospasm and hemifacial spasm are eyelid disorders with different etiologies, the spasms of lid closure and the disruption of sensorimotor processing of both diseases are remarkably similar. In both disorders, the spasms typically result from bursts of orbicularis oculi contractions that occur too close together to allow the eyelids to open (Figure 1A). Animal models suggest that this pattern reflects an exaggeration of normal adaptive processes, a disruption of sensorimotor processing. The neural basis of the spasms may also be similar for the two disorders. Increased trigeminal responsiveness, i.e., trigeminal hyperexcitability, is present in both disorders. The cerebellum plays an important role in modulating the activity of the eyelids and becomes dysfunctional in blepharospasm patients as well as in generalized dystonia. The role of the cerebellum in hemifacial spasm remains unknown, but blepharospasm studies imply that the cerebellum may be an area worth investigating. Both diseases involve permissive and precipitating factors which when combined, result in a disorder of sensorimotor processing that allows involuntary lid closure to develop. Thus, animal models and studies of humans with hemifacial spasm or benign essential blepharospasm suggest that similar brainstem and cerebellar modifications produce symptoms of the diseases, but different mechanisms create the permissive condition that allows the symptoms to develop.

Acknowledgments

This work was supported by the National Eye Institute (EY07391) to CE and National Institute Neurological Disorders and Stroke NRSA NS4467301 to ISK.

References

Abbruzzese, G., and A. Berardelli. 2003. Sensorimotor integration in movement disorders. *Mov Disord* **18**:231–240.

Abbruzzese, G., R. Marchese, A. Buccolieri, B. Gasparetto, and C. Trompetto. 2001. Abnormalities of sensorimotor integration in focal dystonia: a transcranial magnetic stimulation study. *Brain* **124**:537–545.

Aramideh, M., B.W. Ongerboer de Visser, P.P. Devriese, L.J. Bour, and J.D. Speelman. 1994. Electromyographic features of levator palpebrae superioris and orbicularis oculi muscles in blepharospasm. *Brain* **117(Pt 1)**:27–38.

Aramideh, M., J.L. Eekhof, L.J. Bour, J.H. Koelman, J.D. Speelman, and B.W. Ongerboer de Visser. 1995. Electromyography and recovery of the blink reflex in involuntary eyelid closure: a comparative study. *J Neurol Neurosurg Psychiatry* **58**:692–698.

Baker, R.S., S.M. Radmanesh, and K.M. Abell. 2002. The effect of apomorphine on blink kinematics in subhuman primates with and without facial nerve palsy. *Invest Ophthalmol Vis Sci* **43**:2933–2938.

Baker, R.S., A.H. Andersen, R.J. Morecraft, and C.D. Smith. 2003. A functional magnetic resonance imaging study in patients with benign essential blepharospasm. *J Neuroophthalmol* **23**:11–15.

Baker, R.S., W.S. Sun, S.A. Hasan, B.R. Rouholiman, J.C. Chuke, D.E. Cowen, and J.D. Porter. 1997. Maladaptive neural compensatory mechanisms in Bell's palsy-induced blepharospasm. *Neurology* **49**:223–229.

Bara-Jimenez, W., P. Shelton, and M. Hallett. 2000a. Spatial discrimination is abnormal in focal hand dystonia. *Neurology* **55**:1869–1873.

Bara-Jimenez, W., M.J. Catalan, M. Hallett, and C. Gerloff. 1998. Abnormal somatosensory homunculus in dystonia of the hand. *Ann Neurol* **44**:828–831.

Bara-Jimenez, W., P. Shelton, T.D. Sanger, and M. Hallett. 2000b. Sensory discrimination capabilities in patients with focal hand dystonia. *Ann Neurol* **47**:377–380.

Bartko, G., E. Frecska, S. Horvath, G. Zador, and M. Arato. 1990. Predicting neuroleptic response from a combination of multilevel variables in acute schizophrenic patients. *Acta Psychiatr Scand* **82**: 408–412.

Basso, M.A., and C. Evinger. 1996. An explanation for reflex blink hyperexcitability in Parkinson's disease. II. Nucleus raphe magnus. *J Neurosci* **16**:7318–7330.

Basso, M.A., R.E. Strecker, and C. Evinger. 1993. Midbrain 6-hydroxydopamine lesions modulate blink reflex excitability. *Exp Brain Res* **94**:88–96.

Basso, M.A., A.S. Powers, and C. Evinger. 1996. An explanation for reflex blink hyperexcitability in Parkinson's disease. I. Superior colliculus. *J Neurosci* **16**:7308–7317.

Berardelli, A., J.C. Rothwell, M. Hallett, P.D. Thompson, M. Manfredi, and C.D. Marsden. 1998. The pathophysiology of primary dystonia. *Brain* **121(Pt 7)**:1195–1212.

Blake, D.T., N.N. Byl, S. Cheung, P. Bedenbaugh, S. Nagarajan, M. Lamb, and M. Merzenich. 2002. Sensory representation abnormalities that parallel focal hand dystonia in a primate model. *Somatosens Mot Res* **19**: 347–357.

Blin, O., G. Masson, J.P. Azulay, J. Fondarai, and G. Serratrice. 1990. Apomorphine-induced blinking and yawning in healthy volunteers. *Br J Clin Pharmacol* **30**:769–773.

Burkard, W.P., E.P. Bonetti, M. Da Prada, J.R. Martin, P. Polc, R. Schaffner, R. Scherschlicht, et al. 1989. Pharmacological profile of moclobemide, a short-acting and reversible inhibitor of monoamine oxidase type A. *J Pharmacol Exp Ther* **248**:391–399.

Butterworth, S., S. Francis, E. Kelly, F. McGlone, R. Bowtell, and G.V. Sawle. 2003. Abnormal cortical sensory activation in dystonia: an fMRI study. *Mov Disord* **18**:673–682.

Byl, N.N., and M. Melnick. 1997. The neural consequences of repetition: clinical implications of a learning hypothesis. *J Hand Ther* **10**:160–174.

Byl, N.N., M.M. Merzenich, and W.M. Jenkins. 1996. A primate genesis model of focal dystonia and repetitive strain injury: I. Learning-induced dedifferentiation of the representation of the hand in the primary somatosensory cortex in adult monkeys. *Neurology* **47**:508–520.

Byl, N.N., S. Nagajaran, and A.L. McKenzie. 2003. Effect of sensory discrimination training on structure and function in patients with focal hand dystonia: a case series. *Arch Phys Med Rehabil* **84**:1505–1514.

Byl, N.N., M.M. Merzenich, S. Cheung, P. Bedenbaugh, S.S. Nagarajan, and W.M. Jenkins. 1997. A primate model for studying focal dystonia and repetitive strain injury: effects on the primary somatosensory cortex. *Phys Ther* **77**:269–284.

Chuke, J.C., R.S. Baker, and J.D. Porter. 1996. Bell's Palsy-associated blepharospasm relieved by aiding eyelid closure. *Ann Neurol* **39**:263–268.

Davis, K.D., and J.O. Dostrovsky. 1986. Modulatory influences of red nucleus stimulation on the somatosensory responses of cat trigeminal subnucleus oralis neurons. *Exp Neurol* **91**:80–101.

Elston, J.S., C.D. Marsden, F. Grandas, and N.P. Quinn. 1988. The significance of ophthalmological symptoms in idiopathic blepharospasm. *Eye* **2(Pt 4)**:435–439.

Elsworth, J.D., M.S. Lawrence, R.H. Roth, J.R. Taylor, R.B. Mailman, D.E. Nichols, M.H. Lewis, and D.E. Redmond, Jr. 1991. D1 and D2 dopamine receptors independently regulate spontaneous blink rate in the vervet monkey. *J Pharmacol Exp Ther* **259**:595–600.

Esteban, A., and S. Gimenez-Roldan. 1988. Involuntary closure of eyelids in parkinsonism. Electrophysiological evidence for prolonged inhibition of the levator palpebrae muscles. *J Neurol Sci* **85**:333–345.

Evinger, C., and K.A. Manning. 1988. A model system for motor learning: adaptive gain control of the blink reflex. *Exp Brain Res* **70**:527–538.

Evinger, C., J.J. Pellegrini, and K.A. Manning. 1989. Adaptive gain modification of the blink reflex. A model system for investigating the physiologic bases of motor learning. *Ann N Y Acad Sci* **563**:87–100.

Evinger, C., K.A. Manning, and P.A. Sibony. 1991. Eyelid movements. Mechanisms and normal data. *Invest Ophthalmol Vis Sci* **32**:387–400.

Evinger, C., P.A. Sibony, K.A. Manning, and R.A. Fiero. 1988. A pharmacological distinction between the long and short latency pathways of the human blink reflex revealed with tobacco. *Exp Brain Res* **73**:477–480.

Evinger, C., M.D. Shaw, C.K. Peck, K.A. Manning, and R. Baker. 1984. Blinking and associated eye movements in humans, guinea pigs, and rabbits. *J Neurophysiol* **52**:323–339.

Evinger, C., M.A. Basso, K.A. Manning, P.A. Sibony, J.J. Pellegrini, and A.K. Horn. 1993. A role for the basal ganglia in nicotinic modulation of the blink reflex. *Exp Brain Res* **92**:507–515.

Evinger, C., J.B. Bao, A.S. Powers, I.S. Kassem, E.J. Schicatano, V.M. Henriquez, and K.R. Peshori. 2002. Dry eye, blinking, and blepharospasm. *Mov Disord* 17 Suppl **2**:S75–78.

Feiwell, R.J., K.J. Black, L.A. McGee-Minnich, A.Z. Snyder, A.M. MacLeod, and J.S. Perlmutter. 1999. Diminished regional cerebral blood flow response to vibration in patients with blepharospasm. *Neurology* **52**:291–297.

Ferguson, I.T., J.A. Lenman, and B.B. Johnston. 1978. Habituation of the orbicularis oculi reflex in dementia and dyskinetic states. *J Neurol Neurosurg Psychiatry* **41**:824–828.

Ferguson, J.H. 1978. Hemifacial spasm and the facial nucleus. *Ann Neurol* **4**:97–103.

Frasson, E., A. Priori, L. Bertolasi, F. Mauguiere, A. Fiaschi, and M. Tinazzi. 2001. Somatosensory disinhibition in dystonia. *Mov Disord* **16**:674–682.

Frueh, B.R., R.A. Preston, and D.C. Musch. 1990. Facial nerve injury and hemifacial spasm. *Am J Ophthalmol* **110**:421–423.

Fukuda, H., M. Ishikawa, and R. Okumura. 2003. Demonstration of neurovascular compression in trigeminal neuralgia and hemifacial spasm with magnetic resonance imaging: comparison with surgical findings in 60 consecutive cases. *Surg Neurol* **59**:93–99; discussion 99–100.

Ghika, J., F. Regli, and J.H. Growdon. 1993. Sensory symptoms in cranial dystonia: a potential role in the etiology? *J Neurol Sci* **116**:142–147.

Gnadt, J.W., S.M. Lu, B. Breznen, M.A. Basso, V.M. Henriquez, and C. Evinger. 1997. Influence of the superior colliculus on the primate blink reflex. *Exp Brain Res* **116**:389–398.

Godde, B., F. Spengler, and H.R. Dinse. 1996. Associative pairing of tactile stimulation induces somatosensory cortical reorganization in rats and humans. *Neuroreport* **8**:281–285.

Godde, B., J. Ehrhardt, and C. Braun. 2003. Behavioral significance of input-dependent plasticity of human somatosensory cortex. *Neuroreport* **14**:543–546.

Godde, B., B. Stauffenberg, F. Spengler, and H.R. Dinse. 2000. Tactile coactivation-induced changes in spatial discrimination performance. *J Neurosci* **20**:1597–1604.

Goto, S., K. Kihara, T. Hamasaki, S. Nishikawa, Y. Hirata, and Y. Ushio. 2000. Apraxia of lid opening is alleviated by pallidal stimulation in a patient with Parkinson's disease. *Eur J Neurol* **7**:337–340.

Gruart, A., P. Blazquez, and J.M. Delgado-Garcia. 1995. Kinematics of spontaneous, reflex, and conditioned eyelid movements in the alert cat. *J Neurophysiol* **74**:226–248.

Hallett, M. 1995. Is dystonia a sensory disorder? *Ann Neurol* **38**:139–140.

Hallett, M. 2000. Clinical physiology of dopa dyskinesia. *Ann Neurol* **47**:S147–150; discussion S150–143.

Hallett, M. 2002. Blepharospasm: recent advances. *Neurology* **59**: 1306–1312.

Hatem, J., M. Sindou, and C. Vial. 2001. Intraoperative monitoring of facial EMG responses during microvascular decompression for hemifacial spasm. Prognostic value for long-term outcome: a study in a 33-patient series. *Br J Neurosurg* **15**:496–499.

Holstege, G., and H. Collewijn. 1982. The efferent connections of the nucleus of the optic tract and the superior colliculus in the rabbit. *J Comp Neurol* **209**:139–175.

Holstege, G., J. Tan, J.J. van Ham, and G.A. Graveland. 1986. Anatomical observations on the afferent projections to the retractor bulbi motoneuronal cell group and other pathways possibly related to the blink reflex in the cat. *Brain Res* **374**:321–334.

Horn, A.K., J.D. Porter, and C. Evinger. 1993. Botulinum toxin paralysis of the orbicularis oculi muscle. Types and time course of alterations in muscle structure, physiology and lid kinematics. *Exp Brain Res* **96**: 39–53.

Hutchinson, M., T. Nakamura, J.R. Moeller, A. Antonini, A. Belakhlef, V. Dhawan, and D. Eidelberg. 2000. The metabolic topography of essential blepharospasm: a focal dystonia with general implications. *Neurology* **55**:673–677.

Hyland, K., R.S. Gunasekera, T. Engle, and L.A. Arnold. 1996. Tetrahydrobiopterin and biogenic amine metabolism in the hph-1 mouse. *J Neurochem* **67**:752–759.

Hyland, K., R.S. Gunasekara, T.L. Munk-Martin, L.A. Arnold, and T. Engle. 2003. The hph-1 mouse: a model for dominantly inherited GTP-cyclohydrolase deficiency. *Ann Neurol* 54 Suppl **6**:S46–48.

Ibanez, V., N. Sadato, B. Karp, M.P. Deiber, and M. Hallett. 1999. Deficient activation of the motor cortical network in patients with writer's cramp. *Neurology* **53**:96–105.

Ishikawa, M., J. Namiki, M. Takase, T. Ohira, A. Nakamura, and S. Toya. 1996a. Effect of repetitive stimulation on lateral spreads and F-waves in hemifacial spasm. *J Neurol Sci* **142**:99–106.

Ishikawa, M., T. Ohira, J. Namiki, Y. Ajimi, M. Takase, and S. Toya. 1996b. Abnormal muscle response (lateral spread) and F-wave in patients with hemifacial spasm. *J Neurol Sci* **137**:109–116.

Ishikawa, M., T. Ohira, J. Namiki, K. Gotoh, M. Takase, and S. Toya. 1996c. Electrophysiological investigation of hemifacial spasm: F-waves of the facial muscles. *Acta Neurochir* (Wien) **138**:24–32.

Ishikawa, M., T. Ohira, J. Namiki, M. Kobayashi, M. Takase, T. Kawase, and S. Toya. 1997. Electrophysiological investigation of hemifacial spasm after microvascular decompression: F waves of the facial muscles, blink reflexes, and abnormal muscle responses. *J Neurosurg* **86**:654–661.

Jankovic, J., and J. Ford. 1983. Blepharospasm and orofacial-cervical dystonia: clinical and pharmacological findings in 100 patients. *Ann Neurol* **13**:402–411.

Jannetta, P.J., and A. Kassam. 1999. Hemifacial spasm. *J Neurol Neurosurg Psychiatry* **66**:255–256.

Kaneko, K., and K. Sakamoto. 2001. Spontaneous blinks of Parkinson's disease patients evaluated by EMG and EOG. *Electromyogr Clin Neurophysiol* **41**:87–95.

Karson, C.N. 1983. Spontaneous eye-blink rates and dopaminergic systems. *Brain* **106(Pt 3)**:643–653.

Karson, C.N. 1989. Blinking. *Bull Soc Belge Ophtalmol* **237**:443–457.

Kassem, I.S., and C. Evinger. 2002. Effects of chronic facial nerve stimulation on the development of hemifacial spasm. *Society of Neuroscience Abstracts* **28**:463–461.

Kassem, I.S., and C. Evinger. 2003. Chronic facial nerve stimulation modifies the reflex blink. *Society of Neuroscience Abstracts* **29**:391–398.

Kerrison, J.B., J.L. Lancaster, F.E. Zamarripa, L.A. Richardson, J.C. Morrison, D.E. Holck, K.W. Andreason, et al. 2003. Positron emission tomography scanning in essential blepharospasm. *Am J Ophthalmol* **136**:846–852.

Kimura, J. 1973. Disorder of interneurons in Parkinsonism. The orbicularis oculi reflex to paired stimuli. *Brain* **96**:87–96.

Klawans, H.L., Jr., and M.A. Erlich. 1970. Observations on the mechanism of parkinsonian blepharospasm and its treatment with L-dopa. *Eur Neurol* **3**:365–372.

Klemm, W.R., G.R. Bratton, L.C. Hudson, C.J. Sherry, J. Dziezyc. 1993. A possible feline modelfor human blepharospasm. *Nevrol Res* **15**:41–45.

Kuroki, A., and A.R. Moller. 1994a. Chronic vascular irritation of the facial nerve causes facial spasm in rats. *Neurol Res* **16**:284–288.

Kuroki, A., and A.R. Moller. 1994b. Facial nerve demyelination and vascular compression are both needed to induce facial hyperactivity: a study in rats. *Acta Neurochir* (Wien) **126**:149–157.

Kuroki, A., A.R. Moller, and S. Saito. 1994. Recordings from the facial motonucleus in rats with signs of hemifacial spasm. *Neurol Res* **16**:389–392.

LeDoux, M.S., and J.F. Lorden. 1998. Abnormal cerebellar output in the genetically dystonic rat. *Adv Neurol* **78**:63–78.

LeDoux, M.S., J.F. Lorden, and J. Meinzen-Derr. 1995. Selective elimination of cerebellar output in the genetically dystonic rat. *Brain Res* **697**: 91–103.

LeDoux, M.S., D.C. Hurst, and J.F. Lorden. 1998. Single-unit activity of cerebellar nuclear cells in the awake genetically dystonic rat. *Neuroscience* **86**:533–545.

LeDoux, M.S., J.F. Lorden, A.D. Weir, and J.M. Smith. 1997. Blink reflex to supraorbital nerve stimulation in the cat. *Exp Brain Res* **116**:104–112.

Lewis, M.H., J.P. Gluck, A.J. Beauchamp, M.F. Keresztury, and R.B. Mailman. 1990. Long-term effects of early social isolation in Macaca mulatta: changes in dopamine receptor function following apomorphine challenge. *Brain Res* **513**:67–73.

Lim, V.K., E. Altenmuller, and J.L. Bradshaw. 2001. Focal dystonia: current theories. *Hum Mov Sci* **20**:875–914.

Manning, K.A., and C. Evinger. 1986. Different forms of blinks and their two-stage control. *Exp Brain Res* **64**:579–588.

Mao, J.B., and C. Evinger. 2001. Long-term potentiation of the human blink reflex. *J Neurosci* **21**:RC151.

McKenzie, A.L., S.S. Nagarajan, T.P. Roberts, M.M. Merzenich, and N.N. Byl. 2003. Somatosensory representation of the digits and clinical performance in patients with focal hand dystonia. *Am J Phys Med Rehabil* **82**:737–749.

Misbahuddin, A., M.R. Placzek, and T.T. Warner. 2004. Focal dystonia is associated with a polymorphism of the dopamine D5 receptor gene. *Adv Neurol* **94**:143–146.

Misbahuddin, A., M.R. Placzek, K.R. Chaudhuri, N.W. Wood, K.P. Bhatia, and T.T. Warner. 2002. A polymorphism in the dopamine receptor DRD5 is associated with blepharospasm. *Neurology* **58**:124–126.

Miwa, H., Kondo, T., and Y. Mizuno. 2002. Bell's palsy-induced blepharospasm. *J Neurol* **249**:452–454.

Moller, A.R., and P.J. Jannetta. 1984. On the origin of synkinesis in hemifacial spasm: results of intracranial recordings. *J Neurosurg* **61**:569–576.

Moller, A.R., and P.J. Jannetta. 1985a. Hemifacial spasm: results of electrophysiologic recording during microvascular decompression operations. *Neurology* **35**:969–974.

Moller, A.R., and P.J. Jannetta. 1985b. Microvascular decompression in hemifacial spasm: intraoperative electrophysiological observations. *Neurosurgery* **16**:612–618.

Moller, A.R., and P.J. Jannetta. 1985c. Synkinesis in hemifacial spasm: results of recording intracranially from the facial nerve. *Experientia* **41**:415–417.

Moller, A.R., and P.J. Jannetta. 1986. Physiological abnormalities in hemifacial spasm studied during microvascular decompression operations. *Exp Neurol* **93**:584–600.

Molloy, F.M., T.D. Carr, K.E. Zeuner, J.M. Dambrosia, and M. Hallett. 2003. Abnormalities of spatial discrimination in focal and generalized dystonia. *Brain* **126**:2175–2182.

Morcuende, S., J.M. Delgado-Garcia, and G. Ugolini. 2002. Neuronal premotor networks involved in eyelid responses: retrograde transneuronal tracing with rabies virus from the orbicularis oculi muscle in the rat. *J Neurosci* **22**:8808–8818.

Mostofsky, D.I., S. Yehuda, S. Rabinovitz, and R. Carasso 2000. The control of blepharospasm by essential fatty acids. *Neuropsychobiology* **41**:154–157.

Murase, N., R. Kaji, H. Shimazu, M. Katayama-Hirota, A. Ikeda, N. Kohara, J. Kimura, et al. 2000. Abnormal premovement gating of somatosensory input in writer's cramp. *Brain* **123(Pt 9)**:1813–1829.

Napolitano, A., U. Bonuccelli, and B. Rossi. 1997. Different effects of levodopa and apomorphine on blink reflex recovery cycle in essential blepharospasm. *Eur Neurol* **38**:119–122.

Nielsen, V.K. 1985. Electrophysiology of the facial nerve in hemifacial spasm: ectopic/ephaptic excitation. *Muscle Nerve* **8**:545–555.

Nielsen, V.K., and P.J. Jannetta. 1984. Pathophysiology of hemifacial spasm: III. Effects of facial nerve decompression. *Neurology* **34**: 891–897.

Odergren, T., N. Iwasaki, J. Borg, and H. Forssberg. 1996. Impaired sensory-motor integration during grasping in writer's cramp. *Brain* **119(Pt 2)**:569–583.

Pellegrini, J.J., and C. Evinger. 1997. Role of cerebellum in adaptive modification of reflex blinks. *Learn Mem* **4**:77–87.

Pellegrini, J.J., A.K. Horn, and C. Evinger. 1995. The trigeminally evoked blink reflex. I. Neuronal circuits. *Exp Brain Res* **107**:166–180.

Perimutter, J.S., M.K. Stambuk, J. Markham, K.J. Black, L. McGee-Minnich, J. Jankovic, and S.M. Moerlein. 1997. Decreased [18F]spiperone binding in putamen in idiopathic focal dystonia. *J Neurosci* **17**: 843–850.

Peshori, K.R., E.J. Schicatano, R. Gopalaswamy, E. Sahay, and C. Evinger. 2001. Aging of the trigeminal blink system. *Exp Brain Res* **136**: 351–363.

Pizoli, C.E., H.A. Jinnah, M.L. Billingsley, and E.J. Hess. 2002. Abnormal cerebellar signaling induces dystonia in mice. *J Neurosci* **22**:7825–7833.

Powers, A.S., E.J. Schicatano, M.A. Basso, and C. Evinger. 1997. To blink or not to blink: inhibition and facilitation of reflex blinks. *Exp Brain Res* **113**:283–290.

Repka, M.X., M.C. Claro, D.N. Loupe, and S.G. Reich. 1996. Ocular motility in Parkinson's disease. *J Pediatr Ophthalmol Strabismus* **33**:144–147.

Rey, R.D., N.S. Garretto, J.A. Bueri, D.D. Simonetti, O.P. Sanz, and R.E. Sica. 1996. The effect of levodopa on the habituation of the acoustic-palpebral reflex in Parkinson's disease. *Electromyogr Clin Neurophysiol* **36**:357–360.

Saito, S., and A.R. Moller. 1993. Chronic electrical stimulation of the facial nerve causes signs of facial nucleus hyperactivity. *Neurol Res* **15**:225–231.

Sanger, T.D., D. Tarsy, and A. Pascual-Leone. 2001. Abnormalities of spatial and temporal sensory discrimination in writer's cramp. *Mov Disord* **16**:94–99.

Schicatano, E.J., M.A. Basso, and C. Evinger. 1997. Animal model explains the origins of the cranial dystonia benign essential blepharospasm. *J Neurophysiol* **77**:2842–2846.

Schicatano, E.J., K.R. Peshori, R. Gopalaswamy, E. Sahay, and C. Evinger. 2000. Reflex excitability regulates prepulse inhibition. *J Neurosci* **20**: 4240–4247.

Schicatano, E.J., J. Mantzouranis, K.R. Peshori, J. Partin, and C. Evinger. 2002. Lid restraint evokes two types of motor adaptation. *J Neurosci* **22**:569–576.

Schmidt, K.E., D.E. Linden, R. Goebel, F.E. Zanella, H. Lanfermann, and A.A. Zubcov. 2003. Striatal activation during blepharospasm revealed by fMRI. *Neurology* **60**:1738–1743.

Sen, C.N., and A.R. Moller. 1987. Signs of hemifacial spasm created by chronic periodic stimulation of the facial nerve in the rat. *Exp Neurol* **98**:336–349.

Serrien, D.J., J.M. Burgunder, and M. Wiesendanger. 2000. Disturbed sensorimotor processing during control of precision grip in patients with writer's cramp. *Mov Disord* **15**:965–972.

Sibony, P.A., and C. Evinger. 1998. Normal and abnormal eyelid function. In *Walsh and Hoyt's Clinical Neuro-Ophthalmology*, 5th Edition. Ed. N.R. Miller and N.J. Newman. pp. 1509–1594. Baltimore: Williams & Wilkins.

Sibony, P.A., C. Evinger, and K.A. Manning. 1991. Eyelid movements in facial paralysis. *Arch Ophthalmol* **109**:1555–1561.

Sunohara, N., H. Tomi, E. Satoyoshi, and S. Tachibana. 1985. Glabella tap sign. Is it due to a lack of R2-habituation? *J Neurol Sci* **70**:257–267.

Syed, N.A., A. Delgado, F. Sandbrink, A.E. Schulman, M. Hallett, and M.K. Floeter. 1999. Blink reflex recovery in facial weakness: an electrophysiologic study of adaptive changes. *Neurology* **52**:834–838.

Takada, M., K. Itoh, Y. Yasui, A. Mitani, S. Nomura, and N. Mizuno. 1984. Distribution of premotor neurons for orbicularis oculi motoneurons in the cat, with particular reference to possible pathways for blink reflex. *Neurosci Lett* **50**:251–255.

Takeuchi, Y., K. Nakano, M. Uemura, K. Matsuda, R. Matsushima, and N. Mizuno. 1979. Mesencephalic and pontine afferent fiber system to the facial nucleus in the cat: a study using the horseradish peroxidase and silver impregnation techniques. Exp Neurol **66**:330–342.

Tamburin, S., P. Manganotti, C.A. Marzi, A. Fiaschi, and G. Zanette. 2002. Abnormal somatotopic arrangement of sensorimotor interactions in dystonic patients. *Brain* **125**:2719–2730.

Tan, E.K., L.L. Chan, S.H. Lim, W.E. Lim, J.B. Khoo, and K.P. Tan. 1999. Role of magnetic resonance imaging and magnetic resonance angiography in patients with hemifacial spasm. *Ann Acad Med* Singapore **28**:169–173.

Taylor, J.R., J.D. Elsworth, M.S. Lawrence, J.R. Sladek, Jr., R.H. Roth, and D.E. Redmond, Jr. 1999. Spontaneous blink rates correlate with dopamine levels in the caudate nucleus of MPTP-treated monkeys. *Exp Neurol* **158**:214–220.

Tinazzi, M., T. Rosso, and A. Fiaschi. 2003. Role of the somatosensory system in primary dystonia. *Mov Disord* **18**:605–622.

Tinazzi, M., A. Priori, L. Bertolasi, E. Frasson, F. Mauguiere, and A. Fiaschi. 2000. Abnormal central integration of a dual somatosensory input in dystonia. Evidence for sensory overflow. *Brain* **123(Pt 1)**: 42–50.

Tinazzi, M., A. Fiaschi, E. Frasson, M. Fiorio, F. Cortese, and S.M. Aglioti. 2002. Deficits of temporal discrimination in dystonia are independent from the spatial distance between the loci of tactile stimulation. *Mov Disord* **17**:333–338.

Tinazzi, M., E. Frasson, A. Polo, F. Tezzon, P. Bovi, L. Deotto, et al. 1999. Evidence for an abnormal cortical sensory processing in dystonia: selective enhancement of lower limb P37-N50 somatosensory evoked potential. *Mov Disord* **14**:473–480.

Valls-Sole, J., and E.S. Tolosa. 1989. Blink reflex excitability cycle in hemifacial spasm. *Neurology* **39**:1061–1066.

Valls-Sole, J., and J. Montero. (2003) Movement disorders in patients with peripheral facial palsy. Mov Disord **18**:1424–1435.

Valls-Sole, J., F. Valldeoriola, E. Tolosa, and M.J. Marti. 1997. Distinctive abnormalities of facial reflexes in patients with progressive supranuclear palsy. *Brain* **120(Pt 10)**:1877–1883.

Vidailhet, M., J.C. Rothwell, P.D. Thompson, A.J. Lees, and C.D. Marsden. 1992. The auditory startle response in the Steele-Richardson-Olszewski syndrome and Parkinson's disease. *Brain* **115(Pt 4)**:1181–1192

Wichmann, T., and M.R. DeLong. 2003. Pathophysiology of Parkinson's disease: the MPTP primate model of the human disorder. *Ann N Y Acad Sci* **991**:199–213.

Yamashita, S., T. Kawaguchi, M. Fukuda, K. Suzuki, M. Watanabe, R. Tanaka, and S. Kameyama. 2002. Lateral spread response elicited by double stimulation in patients with hemifacial spasm. *Muscle Nerve* **25**:845–849.

Zametkin, A.J., J.R. Stevens, and R. Pittman. 1979. Ontogeny of spontaneous blinking and of habituation of the blink reflex. *Ann Neurol* **5**:453–457.

Zeuner, K.E., W. Bara-Jimenez, P.S. Noguchi, S.R. Goldstein, J.M. Dambrosia, and M. Hallett. 2002. Sensory training for patients with focal hand dystonia. *Ann Neurol* **51**:593–598.

Ziemus, B., R. Huonker, J. Haueisen, J. Liepert, F. Spengler, and C. Weiller. 2000. Effects of passive tactile co-activation on median ulnar nerve representation in human SI. *Neuroreport* **11**:1285–1288.

CHAPTER

C4

Mouse Models of Dystonia

ELLEN J. HESS and H.A. JINNAH

Dystonia is a relatively common neurological disorder with a prevalence of at least 330 per million (Nutt et al. 1988). Dystonia is broadly characterized by simultaneous and sometimes sustained contractions of agonist and antagonist muscles. These co-contractions result in twisting movements and postures that vary among patients (Fahn and Marsden 1994; Jankovic and Fahn 1998). The variety of symptoms categorized as dystonia reflects the heterogeneous biological basis of the disorder. In fact, dystonia may arise as a result of brain injury or insult (secondary or acquired) or occur as a sporadic or inherited disorder (primary or idiopathic); most cases of dystonia are idiopathic.

Animal models of dystonia are of considerable interest as they provide experimental paradigms for elucidating the biological mechanisms underlying this movement disorder. Dystonia can be observed in mice, rats (Lorden et al. 1988), and hamsters (Richter and Loscher 1998). The dystonic rat and hamster models, which are described elsewhere in this volume, have been most intensively studied; the dystonia exhibited by the rat model is chronic, abating only when the animal is at rest, whereas the hamster exhibits episodic periods of dystonia. Functional neuroanatomical mapping studies of the hamster model have revealed abnormalities in the basal ganglia (Richter and Loscher 1998). Both the rat (LeDoux et al. 1993) and hamster models (Richter and Loscher 1998) have also clearly implicated the cerebellum and related regions such as the red nucleus and thalamus in the phenotype. These animal models have provided significant insight into the neuroanatomical regions involved in dystonia.

There are numerous mouse models of dystonia with new models being generated as quickly as human genes are identified. Mouse models of dystonia parallel findings in humans whereby the expression and etiology of the dystonia is heterogeneous. Further, dystonia in mice may arise as a primary inherited disorder or may be acquired through experimental manipulation. The similarities between the mouse and human disorders suggest that the mouse models may prove valuable for understanding the pathophysiology of dystonia.

I. GENETIC MODELS OF DYSTONIA

A. Dystonia Musculorum

1. Background

The dystonia musculorum mutant emerged spontaneously at the Institute of Animal Genetics in Edinburgh and was first described in 1963 (Duchen et al. 1963). The mutation later proved allelic with the athetoid mutant (dt^J), which had arisen at least three times at the Jackson Laboratories in Bar Harbor, Maine (Duchen 1976). Several additional alleles have emerged independently in other mouse colonies, including one in Albany, New York (dt^{Alb}) and another (dt^{Orl}) in Orleans La Source, France (Messer and Strominger 1980; Sotelo and Guenet 1988).

Dystonia musculorum mice carry a mutation in the *Bpag1* gene, which encodes a neural isoform of the human bullous pemphigoid antigen, a hemidesmosomal protein (Brown et al. 1995; Brown et al. 1994). The protein plays a role in anchoring and stabilizing the cytoskeletal network within neurons (Dalpe et al. 1998; Yang et al. 1999). The mutation causes loss of neuronal cytoskeletal organization (Dalpe et al. 1998; De Repentigny et al. 2003), axonal swelling (Duchen et al. 1964; Janota 1972) and abnormal axonal transport (De Repentigny et al. 2003) that culminates in axonal degeneration of primary sensory neurons (Duchen 1976; Duchen et al. 1963; Duchen et al. 1964; Guo et al. 1995; Janota 1972; Kothary et al. 1988; Sotelo and Guenet 1988). Additionally, investigators observe postnatal degeneration of muscle spindles that correlates with the onset of the motor disorder, but skeletal muscle appears normal (Dowling et al. 1997). *Bpag1* mRNA expression is actually much broader than that predicted by the histopathology (Dowling et al. 1997), suggesting that not all neurons are dependent on *Bpag1* for cytoskeletal maintenance. *Bpag1* is expressed in pontine, olivary, and sensory neurons that degenerate but *Bpag1* is also expressed in the optic nerve, olfactory nerve, and sympathetic ganglia, which do not degenerate. Little or no *Bpag1* is expressed in the basal ganglia, cerebellum, or postnatal motor neurons, although lesions were noted in the striatum of *dystonia musculorum* mice (Messer and Strominger 1980). These mutants also exhibit abnormal myelination in both the peripheral and central nervous system (Bernier and Kothary 1998; Saulnier et al. 2002). At this time, the mechanisms by which dysfunction of the protein and subsequent pathology cause motor dysfunction are unknown.

All strains were reported to have a similar motor phenotype with features resembling torsion dystonia in humans (Duchen et al. 1964; Messer and Gordon 1979; Messer and Strominger 1980; Richter and Loscher 1998). Their writhing and twisting movements with muscle "spasms" leading to abnormal limb postures and severe difficulty with ambulation are carefully described in many previous reports (Lalonde et al. 1994; Messer and Gordon 1979; Messer and Strominger 1980; Sotelo and Guenet 1988). However, investigators raised the possibility of a severe sensory ataxia in neuropathological studies demonstrating relatively circumscribed lesions of sensory nerves and ganglia, cerebellum, and red nucleus (Duchen et al. 1964). Some reports therefore describe the animals as ataxic (Brown et al. 1995; Janota 1972; Sotelo and Guenet 1988), but most investigators agree the motor syndrome is phenomenologically more consistent with generalized dystonia (Duchen et al. 1964; Messer and Gordon 1979; Messer and Strominger 1980; Richter and Loscher 1998).

2. Motor Disorder (Video Segment 1)

At rest, the dystonia musculorum mutants appear physically normal. Proximal movements, such as those of the shoulder or hip, are moderately abnormal. More distal movements, such as those of the elbow or knee joints, seem most abnormal. The main abnormality is stiff, twisting, and poorly controlled movements. Many movements are slow and hesitant, though others are relatively quick and fluid. The poor limb control leads to impairments in ambulation. The limbs often take abnormal trajectories during stepping, such as the hind foot retracting above the spine. Because of difficulty with limb control, the mice often ambulate with a swimming technique, in which they lie on the floor and use their limbs to paddle forward. At other times, they ambulate using an inchworm method, where the truncal muscles propel the head and shoulders forward with both fore limbs reaching out. After placing the forelimbs down, the hind limbs are drawn in towards the body. The impaired ambulation causes the animals to spend a significant proportion of time resting motionless, typically with the head and abdomen lying on the floor, the forelimbs folded back along the trunk, and the hind limbs extended caudally. Falling is infrequent since the animals maintain a widened stance with a low center of gravity, and they rarely rear onto the hind limbs. After a fall, the mouse shows an obvious delay in regaining the upright posture because of axial twisting and poor motor control.

3. Comment

The dystonia musculorum mutant demonstrates that a motor syndrome closely resembling generalized torsion dystonia in humans can occur in the mouse. Overall, the majority of abnormal movements are best characterized as dystonic, though some of the movements might also be considered choreoathetoid because they are more rapid and fluid. Though generalized, there is an anatomic gradient of involvement, with distal muscles more severely affected than proximal muscles.

B. P/Q-type Calcium Channel Mutants: Tottering, Leaner, and Knock-outs

The *Cacna1a* gene encodes the α_{1A} pore-forming subunit of the high voltage-gated P/Q-type calcium channel. Calcium channels are composed of five subunits (α_1, α_2, β, γ, and σ); however, the α_1 subunit alone is sufficient to form the structural channel and confer voltage sensitivity. These channels are characterized by voltage-sensitive activation in response to depolarization resulting in the selective increase in calcium flux into the cell. P/Q-type calcium channels are most often functionally associated with calcium-dependent neurotransmitter release (Charvin et al. 1997; Kim and Catterall 1997; Rettig et al. 1996). In humans, mutations of the *Cacna1a* gene cause spinocerebellar ataxia type 6, episodic ataxia type 2, and familial hemiplegic migraine (Ophoff et al. 1996; Zhuchenko et al. 1997); dystonia also occurs in humans carrying these mutations (Arpa et al. 1999; Giffin et al. 2002). At least four mouse models currently carry mutations in the *Cacna1a* gene that exhibit dystonia: tottering ($Cacna1a^{tg}$), leaner ($Cacna1a^{tg\text{-}la}$), and two *Cacna1a* knock-out mice.

1. Leaner Mice

a. Background

The leaner mutation arose spontaneously at the Jackson Laboratories (Yoon 1969). The leaner mutation causes a gross disruption in the α_{1A} subunit protein, resulting from a G to A point mutation of a splice donor site near the 3′ end of the gene (Doyle et al. 1997; Fletcher et al. 1996). The mutation produces aberrantly spliced mRNA species that produce a dysfunctional channel. Whole-cell recordings of leaner mutant Purkinje cells reveal an overall reduction in P/Q-type calcium current density (Dove et al. 1998; Lorenzon et al. 1998). Cell-attached patch recordings demonstrated a reduction in open-probability of leaner channels, explaining the reduction in current density (Dove et al. 1998).

b. Motor Disorder (Video Segment 2)

In leaner mice, the dystonia is chronic and extreme with episodes of increased severity that are barely detectable over the background motor dysfunction. Historically, investigators characterized leaner mice as ataxic (Heckroth and Abbott 1994; Herrup and Wilczynski 1982; Meier and MacPike 1971; Rhyu et al. 1999; Tsuji and Meier 1971; Yoon, 1969), which suggests falling due to disturbances in balance. However, when the term ataxia is applied to mice, it is often a nonspecific descriptor that encompasses a wide range of gait disturbances. Leaner mice have an extremely debilitating gait abnormality starting at ~postnatal day 18 resulting from their severe and chronic dystonia. In fact, leaner mice do not fall because they are ataxic; rather they are propelled onto their flanks because the severe dystonia causes stiff extension of the limbs on one side as they attempt to walk. After falling, the mice show a considerable delay in gaining upright posture. Limb tone is increased with a marked reduction in spontaneous activity and extremely slow and stiff movements. The dystonia is generalized with involvement of proximal and distal muscles including the jaw and tongue. Leaner mice do not generally survive past weaning because the severe dystonia limits their ability to obtain and consume both food and water. However, if leaner mice receive softened chow and adequate hydration, they can live a normal life span and even breed. As leaner mice age, the dystonia wanes but never entirely remits.

c. Pathophysiology

Neuropathological surveys demonstrate relatively circumscribed degenerative changes of the cerebellum (Heckroth and Abbott 1994; Herrup and Wilczynski 1982). These studies have revealed widespread degeneration of cerebellar granule, Purkinje, and Golgi cells that is most prominent anteromedially (Herrup and Wilczynski 1982; Meier and MacPike 1971). The degenerative process is most severe during the first few months of age, but continues throughout adulthood, leaving less than 20% of Purkinje cells by one year of age. The surviving Purkinje cells ectopically express tyrosine hydroxylase, an enzyme normally associated with catecholaminergic cells (Abbott et al. 1996; Hess and Wilson 1991). It is not yet clear how or if these abnormalities are associated with the dystonia.

2. α_{1A} Knock-outs

a. Background

Two strains of *Cacna1a* knock-out mice were generated by targeted disruption (Fletcher et al. 2001; Jun et al. 1999) resulting in the elimination of the α_{1A} subunit protein and the P/Q-type calcium channel current (Aldea et al. 2002; Fletcher et al. 2001; Jun et al. 1999). The neuropathology in these mice is very similar to leaner mice with late-onset progressive degeneration of the anterior cerebellum (Fletcher et al. 2001).

b. Motor Disorder (as Observed by the Authors)

Juvenile *Cacna1a* null mutants exhibit a motor disorder similar to that of juvenile leaner mutants, with some minor differences. In comparison to leaner mutants, the *Cacna1a* null mutants are much smaller throughout development, have more profound motor impairments, and display much less spontaneous activity. They almost uniformly perish at three to four weeks of age when the transition from suckling to eating solid food occurs in normal mice. With daily parenteral hydration and nutrition, a very small percentage of α_{1A} null mutants survive to adulthood. The adult *Cacna1a* null mutants again resemble the adult leaner mice, but they have more severe motor impairments characterized by akinesia, bradykinesia, stiff movements, and increased muscle tone. They cannot eat or drink on their own, requiring daily parenteral supplementation for survival. The motor disorder of the *Cacna1a* knock-outs, like that of leaner mice, is most consistent with generalized dystonia.

c. Pathophysiology

Investigators observed an increase in the expression of N-type and L-type calcium channels in the null mutants (Aldea et al. 2002; Fletcher et al. 2001; Jun et al. 1999; Pagani et al. 2004). This abnormality in calcium handling may play a role in the dystonia as described below in the pathophysiology section for tottering mice.

3. Tottering Mice

a. Background

Tottering is an autosomal recessive mutation that occurs spontaneously. The tottering missense mutation is located in the pore-forming domain of the P/Q-type calcium channel (Fletcher et al. 1996). Surprisingly, channel properties of tottering mice reveal only subtle changes, with a slight increase in the non-inactivating component of voltage-dependent inactivation (Wakamori et al. 1998) but a ~40% reduction in whole-cell calcium current density.

Though investigators can identify few gross neuropathological abnormalities in Nissl-stained material from the tottering brain (Green and Sidman 1962; Levitt 1988; Noebels and Sidman 1979), quantitative measures demonstrate subtle decreases in brain volume and the size of cerebellar Purkinje cells (Isaacs and Abbott 1995). Electron microscopic and Golgi-impregnated material reveal subtle abnormalities, including shrunken cerebellar Purkinje cells, abnormal Purkinje cell connectivity, and diffuse axonal swellings or torpedoes in older mice (Meier and MacPike 1971; Rhyu et al. 1999). In addition, catecholaminergic measures appear abnormal. There is apparent hyperinnervation of multiple brain regions by noradrenergic fibers, with an associated increase in tissue norepinephrine content (Levitt and Noebels 1981; Noebels 1984). Further, tyrosine hydroxylase is ectopically expressed in cerebellar Purkinje cells, with relatively normal patterns of expression in the midbrain and locus ceruleus (Abbott et al. 1996; Fletcher et al. 1996; Heckroth and Abbott 1994; Hess and Wilson 1991).

The initial report of the motor disorder described a mild baseline ataxia with intermittent attacks of more profound motor dysfunction that were originally thought to represent motor seizures (Green and Sidman 1962). However, subsequent EEG studies failed to identify any abnormal activity consistently associated with the motor attacks, and these results questioned the classification of the intermittent attacks as epileptic seizures (Kaplan et al. 1979; Noebels and Sidman 1979). Instead, several of these studies describe 6 Hz polyspike discharges in association with brief periods of behavioral inactivity suggestive of absence seizures (Heller et al. 1983; Kaplan et al. 1979; Noebels and Sidman 1979). Although tottering mice exhibit a motor disorder that was originally classified as epilepsy, recent studies suggest that the motor disorder is better described as paroxysmal dystonia.

b. Motor Disorder (Video Segment 3)

Tottering mouse motor attacks are highly stereotyped. The start of an attack is nearly always signaled by the extension of the hind limbs. This initial phase is followed by abduction at the hip and extension at the knee, ankle, and paw with a stiffly arched back, which presses the perineum against the cage bottom. The motor dysfunction then spreads to involve the forelimbs and head, with severe flexion of the neck. During this time, mice assume and maintain twisted and abnormal postures involving the entire body. In the final phase, the mice regain control of the hind limbs, often rearing, while forepaw and facial muscles continue to contract (Green and Sidman 1962). The entire episode lasts thirty to sixty minutes without loss of consciousness.

Movement disorders in humans are sometimes difficult to classify, and these disorders are even more difficult in mice, where normal and abnormal motor behaviors are not well studied. As a result, motor abnormalities in mice are often mislabeled or vaguely classified. Although investigators have described the tottering mouse motor phenotype as myoclonus, convulsions, focal motor seizures, or Jacksonian march, the episodic motor events in tottering mice are better characterized as paroxysmal dystonia rather than epilepsy for several reasons. First, the observed phenomenology, with sustained and asynchronous twisting postures, is more characteristic of dystonia than motor seizures. Second, the duration of thirty to sixty minutes is consistent with dystonia, but quite unusual for a seizure, which typically lasts for only one to sixty seconds. Third, despite apparent generalization with involvement of the entire trunk and all limbs, the motor abnormalities are not associated with epileptiform activity on EEG (Kaplan et al. 1979; Noebels and Sidman 1979).

c. Pathophysiology

The gene defect(s) in the *Cacna1a* mutants predicts that abnormalities in calcium handling likely play a role in the mutant phenotype. In fact, calcium channel expression appears to be abnormal in these mutants. Investigators observed a compensatory increase in the expression of N-type and L-type calcium in both the *Cacna1a* knock-out mice and in tottering mice (Aldea et al. 2002; Campbell and Hess 1999; Fletcher et al. 2001; Jun et al. 1999; Pagani et al. 2004; Qian and Noebels 2000; Zhou et al. 2003). Consistent with these findings, drugs that block L-type calcium channels block the paroxysmal dystonia in tottering mutant mice (Campbell and Hess 1999). Conversely, L-type calcium channel agonists induce dystonia in tottering mice (Campbell and Hess 1999). This response suggests that an upregulation in the L-type calcium channel subtype, which appears to be a secondary effect of the mutated P/Q-type calcium channel, contributes to the expression of the dystonia in tottering mice.

In tottering mice, the neuroanatomical substrates of the dystonic events were identified using markers of cell activity, such as the immediate early transcription factor c-*fos*. During a dystonic attack, the cerebellum, including granule cells, Purkinje cells, and neurons in deep cerebellar nuclei, are activated. Further, medial vestibular nuclei, deep cerebellar nuclei, red nuclei, inferior olivary complex, and ventrolateral thalamic nuclei, which are principal relay components of cerebellar circuitry, are also activated during the dystonic episodes. Dystonic events do not induce c-*fos* expression in the basal ganglia, a region involved in motor control and traditionally associated with dystonia. These findings clearly implicate the cerebellum and related nuclei in the dystonia (Campbell and Hess 1998).

Through lesion studies, investigators again implicated the cerebellum in the expression of the tottering mouse paroxysmal dystonia. A genetic approach was used to lesion Purkinje cells, the sole output neurons of the cerebellar cortex, using the *pcd* mutation. *pcd* is a recessive mutation that causes all cerebellar Purkinje cells to degenerate (Landis and Mullen 1978). The generation of *tg/tg; pcd/pcd* double mutant mice produced tottering mice that lacked Purkinje cells. These mice do not exhibit dystonia (Campbell et al. 1999), suggesting that Purkinje cells are an essential link in generating or maintaining dystonia. Further, surgical and chemical lesions of the tottering mouse cerebellum, particularly the anterior vermis, are also effective in reducing the duration and frequency of the attacks (Abbott et al. 2000).

d. Comment

These findings suggest that the cerebellum is involved in the expression of dystonia in tottering mouse mutants. Although the cerebellum itself does not directly produce or initiate movements, these results suggest that the abnormal signal can ultimately influence the expression of the motor component of dystonic episodes. This notion concurs with the rat (Lorden et al. 1988) and hamster (Richter and Loscher 1998) models of dystonia and functional imaging in humans (Ceballos-Baumann and Brooks 1998; Hutchinson et al. 2000; Kluge et al. 1998; Mazziotta et al. 1998; Odergren et al. 1998; Playford et al. 1998), where the cerebellum is also implicated.

C. Scn8A Mutants

1. Background

Investigators have identified several mutations at the mouse locus "motor endplate disease" (*med*), which encodes the gene *Scn8A*, the $Na_v1.6$ sodium channel expressed throughout the nervous system (Burgess et al. 1995). The *med* mouse mutant arose from an insertion of a truncated LINE element into exon 2 of *Scn8A*, causing abnormal splicing of exon 1 to an acceptor site within intron 2 and a frame shift that reads a premature stop codon in exon 3 (Kohrman et al. 1996a). These mice are essentially null mutants and exhibit severe neurological impairment including paralysis, progressive muscle atrophy, and death within the first month (Duchen et al. 1967). The allelic mouse mutant, jolting (*med^{jo}*), is caused by a point mutation that replaces the Ala with Thr at residue 1071 (Kohrman et al. 1996b). This mutation results in a small shift in voltage-dependent activation of the channel (Kohrman et al. 1996b) and a relatively mild phenotype consisting of widened stance, unsteady gait, and tremor of the head and neck (Dick et al. 1985). The mouse mutant *med^{J}* carries a 4 base pair deletion within the 5′ splice donor site of exon 3, causing aberrant splicing from exon 1 to exon 4 (Kohrman et al. 1996a). Most Scn8A mRNA produced in these mutants is abnormally spliced, but a small percentage of transcript is correctly spliced, resulting in very low expression of the protein (Kearney et al. 2002; Sprunger et al. 1999). When the *med^{J}* mutation is expressed on a C57BL/6J background, the phenotype is nearly identical to the severe lethal phenotype of *med* mice. However, on a mixed-strain background (C57BL/6J X C3H), many *med^{J}* mice survive to adulthood and display a phenotype with features resembling dystonia. The enhanced survival is due to the presence of a sodium channel modifier gene (*Scnm1*) in the C3H mouse strain that doubles the percentage of correctly spliced transcripts; in C57BL/6J mice, this modifier is mutated, rendering it non-functional (Buchner et al. 2003).

2. Motor Disorder (as Reported)

Adult *med^{J}* mice on a mixed-strain background (C57BL/6J X C3H) exhibit movement-induced tremor of the head and dystonic posturing. Abnormal twisting postures of the trunk and repetitive movements of the limbs are sustained over the course of seconds to minutes (Hamann et al. 2003; Messer and Gordon 1979). Mice cannot ambulate with a coordinated gait due to the persistence of the twisting and posturing. The abnormal movements of the extremities abate with sleep, but axial torsions persist. These mice also exhibit severe muscle weakness and reduced muscle mass (Hamann et al. 2003; Kearney et al. 2002; Sprunger et al. 1999). The profound movement disorder reduces spontaneous locomotor activity. The EEG is normal in these mice, ruling out a possible seizure disorder. In contrast to most other dystonias, the movement disorder of *med^{J}* mice can be suppressed with phenytoin, a sodium channel blocker (Hamann et al. 2003).

3. Pathophysiology

Many of the physiological studies have focused on the *med* and *med^{jo}* alleles. There are clear abnormalities in neuromuscular transmission in *med* mice, which do not express the $Na_v1.6$ sodium channel. The weakness in these mice results from a failure of evoked transmitter release from motor nerves; this likely causes the loss of muscle mass (Harris and Pollard 1986). A similar defect likely accounts for the weakness observed in *med*^{J} mice. Because the *med*^{jo} mice are ataxic, Purkinje cell firing rates were examined in *med* and *med*^{jo} mice. In both mutants, simple-spike firing in Purkinje cells is strikingly reduced (Dick et al. 1985; Harris et al. 1992; Raman et al. 1997). Similar defects occur in cortical pyramidal neurons, neurons of the dorsal cochlear nucleus, and spinal motor neurons (Chen et al. 1999; Garcia et al. 1998; Maurice et al. 2001), suggesting that the phenomenon is not specific to the cerebellum.

4. Comment

med^J mice exhibit a movement disorder very similar to generalized dystonia but some elements of the phenotype are uncharacteristic of dystonia. Generally, dystonia in humans abates with sleep (McGeer and McGeer 1988), whereas the *med*^{J} mice maintain twisted postures. The muscle weakness in these mice is also not common in dystonia. Overall, the mice appear to be dystonic with some atypical features. EMG, which generally reveals co-contraction of agonist and antagonist muscles in dystonia, may help to clarify the nature of the movement disorder.

D. Wriggle Mouse Sagami

1. Background

The mouse mutant known as wriggle mouse Sagami (*wri*) arose spontaneously at the Ohmura Institute for Laboratory Animals in Japan. Investigators identified the mutation in wriggle mouse Sagami as a point mutation in the *Pmca2* gene, a plasma membrane Ca2+-ATPase (Takahashi and Kitamura 1999). This mutation is allelic with deafwaddler (*dfw*), a mutant that investigators studied as a model of deafness and vestibular disorders. In fact, stereocilia of the cochlea are completely absent in wriggle mouse Sagami (Takahashi and Kitamura 1999), the cochlea and saccule degenerate, and the mice are completely deaf at one month of age (Takahashi et al. 1999). No gross changes occur within the nervous system itself, but closer inspection reveals a decrease in the number of parallel fiber Purkinje cell contacts and an increase in "bouton-like" structures of Purkinje cells (Inoue et al. 1993). Additionally, the levels of several neurotransmitters are altered in these mutants; norepinephrine and serotonin are increased (Ishikawa et al. 1989; Kumazawa et al. 1989) while GABA is increased only in the striatum (Ikeda et al. 1989). The increase in the monoamines may contribute to the motor abnormalities because ritanserin, a serotonergic antagonist, and prazosin, a noradrenergic antagonist, reduce the motor signs (Ikeda et al. 1989).

2. Motor Disorder (as Reported)

Wriggle mouse Sagami exhibits a complex motor disorder characterized by jerky movements of the head and neck, occasional limb abduction, and frequent rolling of the trunk, which makes it difficult for the mice to remain upright and to obtain food and water (Ikeda et al. 1989). These mice do not exhibit seizures nor are they weak; tone appears to be increased. Although the movements abate with sleep, the mice maintain an abnormal posture while sleeping, which is atypical of dystonia.

3. Comment

Although wriggle mouse Sagami has been presented as a dystonic mouse mutant, the presence of additional abnormalities such as vestibular defects suggests that dystonia is only a minor component of a more complex phenotype. Since vestibular defects alone may induce a variety of abnormal movements, the use of these mice as a model for dystonia must be interpreted with caution.

E. Fibroblast Growth Factor 14 (FGF14)-Deficient Mice

FGF14-deficient mice are not yet the subject of extensive research, but offer an interesting and unexpected mouse model of paroxysmal dystonia. The function of FGF14 is unknown, but it is expressed in the developing and adult nervous system. In adults, FGF14 mRNA is expressed at high levels in the basal ganglia and cerebellum with lower levels in the hippocampus and cortex (Wang et al. 2002). FGF14-deficient mice develop normally and have an intact nervous system, although the mice show decreased sensitivity to dopamine agonists, suggesting abnormalities of the basal ganglia. These mice are described as ataxic with a widened stance and abnormal gait. In addition, paroxysmal dyskinesia is observed in the younger mutants. Episodes of limb extensions with involuntary rearing and twisting that cause the mice to topple over occur several times a day and last for seven to twelve minutes (Wang et al. 2002). These episodes do not appear to be seizures as no abnormalities were detected with EEG. A video of the paroxysmal dyskinesia exhibited by the FGF14-deficient mice can be viewed at http://www.neuron.org/cgi/content/full/35/1/25/DC1/. These mice are intriguing because they implicate dysfunction of several brain regions, including the basal ganglia, cortex, and cerebellum in the motor disorder.

F. Genetic Models: Summary

The ease with which scientists can now genetically manipulate the mouse has spurred the production of mice that carry mutations in genes known to cause dystonia in humans. These genetic models have etiologic validity, but surprisingly few of these models have face validity. That is, none of the genetic models, with the exception of the α-synuclein mutants, exhibit dystonia, although most exhibit some kind of motor dysfunction (table 1).

The lack of a dystonic phenotype may be attributed to several causes. First, few models are an exact genocopy of the human mutation. Many of the mouse models were generated by transgene insertion, chemically-induced mutation, or homologous recombination to produce null mutants (knock-outs) and thus do not carry the exact mutation that causes the human disease. It is interesting to note that where dystonia is observed in the α-synuclein mutants, a transgene with the precise human point mutation was used to generate the mice (Gomez-Isla et al. 2003; Lee et al. 2002). In contrast, α-synuclein knock-out mice, which are completely deficient in α-synuclein, do not display dystonia and have very mild phenotype (Cabin et al. 2002). Thus, the mutant protein itself may be an important factor in driving the dystonic phenotype, and a precise recapitulation of human mutations in mice may be necessary to reproduce the dystonia. Clearly, the generation of more knock-in models will help to address this question.

Alternatively, the lack of a dystonic phenotype in these genetic models may be attributed to species-specific effects. The mouse brain may be sufficiently different from humans to prevent the expression of dystonia, or mice may not live long enough to fully develop the disease with the accompanying dystonia. Obviously, species-specific attributes are impossible to avoid in genetic models, but this does not mean the models should be discarded nor does it diminish the utility of the models. The genetic models have proven invaluable in understanding the molecular, cellular, and neuropathological phenotypes underlying the genetic disorders.

II. DRUG-INDUCED MODELS OF DYSTONIA

Genetic models of dystonia provide obvious parallels to human disease and are a rich source for understanding the

TABLE 1 Genotypic Models

Gene	Protein	Human disease	Mouse motor phenotype	Citations
ASA	arylsulfatase A	metachromatic leukodystrophy	Abnormal rotarod performance and progressive ataxia	(D'Hooge et al. 2001)
ATM	ATM	ataxia telangiectasia	Supersensitive to amphetamine; stride length asymmetry	(Eilam et al. 1998)
ATP7B	copper ATPase	Wilson disease	None reported	(Buiakova et al. 1999)
DYT1	torsin A	Oppenheim dystonia	Failure to feed in knock-outs; slowed habituation in knock-downs	(Dauer and Goodchild 2004)
GCDH	glutaryl-CoA dehydrogenase	glutaric acidemia	Abnormal performance on rotarod, beam walking, and prepulse inhibition	(Koeller et al. 2002)
HPH1	GTP cyclohydrolase	Dopa-responsive dystonia	Normal behavior with wasting syndrome after phenylalanine challenge	(Bode et al. 1988)
HPRT	hypoxanthine phosphoribosyl transferase	Lesch-Nyhan disease	Normal behavior but supersensitive to amphetamine	(Jinnah et al. 1991)
NPC1	NPC1 (endosomal cholesterol transporter)	Niemann-Pick type C	Hypoactivity, abnormal habituation, poor coordination, tremor, abnormal gait	(Morris et al. 1982; Voikar et al. 2002)
PARKIN	parkin	Parkinson disease	Impaired beam walking and somatosensory function	(Goldberg et al. 2003)
PLP	proteolipid protein	Pelizaeus-Merzbacher disease	Tremor, seizures	(Eicher and Hoppe 1973; Meier and MacPike 1970)
PPT1	palmitoyl protein thioesterase	infantile neuronal ceroid lipofuscinosis	Spasticity, myoclonus, seizures	(Gupta et al. 2001)
SCA3	ataxin-3	Machado-Joseph disease	Gait abnormalities, hypotonia, tremor, hypoactivity	(Cemal et al. 2002; Ikeda et al. 1996)
SNCA	α-synuclein	Parkinson disease	Rigidity, dystonia, hindlimb freezing, loss of righting reflex, paralysis	(Giasson et al. 2002; Gomez-Isla et al. 2003; Lee et al. 2002)
TH	tyrosine hydroxylase	Dopa-responsive dystonia	Mild to marked hypoactivity	(Althini et al. 2003)

pathophysiology of dystonia. However, all genetic models are fraught with the complications that accompany the development of the nervous system in the context of a mutation, including compensatory changes and cell death. In contrast, drug-induced models of dystonia provide a tool to understand the pathophysiology of dystonia on a background of normal neurological function. The etiology of the dystonia in these models may not directly reflect the etiology of the condition in humans but this does not detract from the value of the model or the knowledge gained from the model. The real value of drug-induced models is that they may help define pathophysiological defects common to many forms of dystonia. Drug-induced models complement the genetic models whereby hypotheses derived from work in genetic models may be tested for their general applicability in the drug-induced models and vice versa. Currently, there are only three well-characterized drug-induced models of dystonia in the mouse; all were developed quite recently.

A. Kainic Acid-Induced Dystonia

1. Background

Abnormal cerebellar function is implicated in human dystonia (Ceballos-Baumann and Brooks 1998; Hutchinson et al. 2000; Kluge et al. 1998; Mazziotta et al. 1998; Odergren et al. 1998; Playford et al. 1998; Eidelberg et al. 1998) as well as dystonia in mice (Campbell et al. 1999; Messer and Strominger 1980; Sprunger et al. 1999), rats (Lorden et al. 1988), and hamsters (Richter and Loscher 1998). The accumulated evidence for cerebellar involvement in dystonia suggests that artificial disruption of cerebellar signaling should produce dystonia in normal mice. Therefore, the cerebellum became an obvious target for a drug-induced model of dystonia.

2. Motor Disorder (Video Segment 4)

Low doses of the excitatory glutamate receptor agonist kainic acid microinjected into the mouse cerebellum produces dystonia in mice (Pizoli et al. 2002). Kainate microinjection results in the acute expression of gross generalized dystonia without cerebellar cell death and without inducing seizures (Pizoli et al. 2002). After kainate injection, mice display abnormal postures including a stiffly arched back, which presses the perineum against the cage bottom, a dystonic paddling motion of the hind limbs, and sustained twisted abnormal postures that involve most of the body. With moderate doses of kainate, mice assume dystonic postures after being disturbed and dystonia occurs with volitional movement. At higher doses of kainic acid, mice assume sustained abnormal postures for several minutes with involvement of the face, neck, and the rest of the body.

3. Pathophysiology

Human functional imaging and lesion experiments in animal models suggest that cerebellar activation is likely involved in the expression of dystonia. Specifically, the excitatory action of kainate within the cerebellum appears to cause the dystonia in this drug-induced model. Microinjection of kainate elsewhere in the brain does not cause dystonia, and mice lacking cerebellar Purkinje cells exhibit significantly less dystonia than intact mice (Pizoli et al. 2002). Further, cerebellar microinjection of a glutamatergic antagonist does not cause dystonia, suggesting that simply distorting cerebellar signaling is insufficient to produce dystonia. Rather, cerebellar excitation is necessary.

4. Comment

This model demonstrates that dystonia can be provoked in an animal with a normal nervous system. That is, chronic changes in physiology or wiring, which may occur in genetic models, are not necessary to produce dystonia. The model also demonstrates that dystonia occurs with abnormal cerebellar activity, which predicts abnormal activity in the cerebellum in dystonic patients. Indeed, the cerebellum exhibits hypermetabolism that exceeds any other brain region in functional imaging of DYT1 patients (Eidelberg et al. 1998) and other forms of human dystonia (Ceballos-Baumann and Brooks 1998; Hutchinson et al. 2000; Kluge et al. 1998; Mazziotta et al. 1998; Odergren et al. 1998; Playford et al. 1998).

B. Systemic 3-Nitropropionic Acid Intoxification

1. Background

3-Nitropropionic acid (3-NP) is an irreversible inhibitor of mitochondrial complex II. This toxin was first identified in China after individuals who ingested moldy sugarcane developed a movement disorder that included dystonia and chorea (Liu et al. 1992). In fact, the basal ganglia appear to be especially sensitive to the effects of this toxin; systemically administered 3-NP causes selective lesions within the basal ganglia, but not elsewhere in the brain. 3-NP intoxification is used as a model of Huntington disease in primates, rats and, more recently, mice.

Mice are relatively resistant to the effects of 3-NP, but Fernagut et al. (2002) demonstrated that an escalating dose regimen delivered to mice over the course of nearly two weeks causes cell death within the basal ganglia. Although the dose regimen is lethal in one-third of mice, in surviving mice, circumscribed lesions occur in the dorsolateral striatum and cell loss is observed in the globus pallidus pars externalis, and the substantia nigra pars reticulata and compacta.

2. Motor Disorder (as Reported)

Histopathology in the basal ganglia is accompanied by a complex motor disorder, which varies in severity. Investigators describe a motor syndrome similar to the rat 3-NP model that includes motor slowing, hindlimb dystonia, truncal dystonia, and impaired postural control (Fernagut et al. 2002).

3. Comment

In contrast to kainate-induced dystonia, which directly implicates the cerebellum, this model clearly implicates the basal ganglia in dystonia in mice. Indeed, abnormalities of the basal ganglia are often observed in neuropathological studies and neuroimaging of individuals with dystonia (Jankovic and Fahn 1998). The kainate- and 3-NP-induced dystonia models suggest that the neuroanatomical underpinnings of dystonia are likely heterogeneous, much like the disorder itself.

C. Dystonia Caused by L-Type Calcium Channel Activation

1. Background

Calcium channel agonists, particularly L-type calcium channel agonists, were good candidates for a drug-induced model of dystonia for several reasons. First, descriptions of the motor abnormality produced by systemic administration of the L-type calcium channel agonist Bay K 8644 suggest that the motor phenomenon is likely dystonia. Reports describe twisting movements, impairment locomotion, limb extension, back arching, and tonic-clonic movements (Bianchi et al. 1990; Bolger et al. 1985; Bourson et al. 1989; De Sarro et al. 1992; O'Neill and Bolger 1988; Palmer et al. 1993; Petersen 1986; Shelton et al. 1987). FPL 64179, another L-type calcium channel agonist, provokes a similar motor syndrome (Rampe et al. 1993; Zheng et al. 1991). Second, although the motor syndrome was characterized as a form of epilepsy, it does not respond to anticonvulsants such as carbamazepine, diphenylhydantion, phenobarbital, or valproic acid (Bianchi et al. 1990; De Sarro et al. 1992; Palmer et al. 1993; Shelton et al. 1987). Third, the *Cacna1a* calcium channel mutants clearly implicate calcium dysregulation, including upregulation of L- and N-type calcium channels, in the genesis of dystonia, suggesting that manipulating calcium homeostasis with drugs in normal mice might have similar effects.

2. Motor Disorder (Video Segment 5)

Low doses of systemically administered Bay K 8644 cause slowing of movements with occasional momentary abnormal limb positions. Higher doses cause abnormal severe flexion of the trunk with flexion of the head toward the abdomen, which often causes the mouse to fall. Attempts to move are accompanied by abnormal flexion, extension, or twisting movements of the trunk and limbs; muscle tone is increased. Movements are asymmetric and asynchronous. Generally, activity returns to baseline after ~120 minutes. Tonic-clonic seizures are rarely observed after systemic injection of Bay K 8644 and no EEG abnormalities are observed (Jinnah et al. 2000). However, on EMG, significant increases are observed in resting muscle activity and prolonged movement-related phasic bursting, consistent with dystonia. A similar motor syndrome is evoked by intracerebral injection of Bay K 8644 or systemic administration of FPL 64176 (Jinnah et al. 2000).

L-type calcium channel agonists also induce self-injurious behavior, including self-biting, stiff or Straub tail, and hypersensitivity to auditory stimuli (Jinnah et al. 2000). Thus, the response to Bay K 8644 is not a pure dystonic disorder, but part of a more complex neurobehavioral syndrome.

3. Pathophysiology

To determine if Bay K 8644 activates specific brain regions, the induction of c-*fos* was used as a marker of neuronal activation (Jinnah et al. 2003). Despite the extensive distribution of L-type calcium channels throughout the brain, c-*fos* induction after Bay K 8644 challenge is widespread, but not homogeneous. Particularly robust activation is noted in the striatum, cortex, hippocampus, locus ceruleus, and cerebellum. The broad distribution of activation suggests that Bay K 8644 may induce dystonia through its action at several different motor regions. Microinjections into specific brain regions will be required to determine if a single region drives the dystonia.

4. Comment

The Bay K 8644 model of dystonia is likely an example of dystonia caused by the simultaneous distortion of motor commands at several levels of motor control. Indeed, for disorders such as DYT1 dystonia, where the mutant gene product is expressed in many brain regions (Augood et al. 1999), such abnormal signaling from many brain regions may underlie the expression of dystonia.

III. SUMMARY AND CONCLUSIONS

Investigators generally use animal models to understand the mechanisms underlying a disorder in humans. Several common themes emerge from animal models of dystonia that provide clues for understanding the pathophysiology of dystonia in humans. First, the *Cacna1a*, *Scn8a*, and Bay K

8644 mouse models clearly implicate ion channel dysfunction in dystonia. Indeed, ion channel dysfunction induced by either mutation or pharmacologic intervention induces dystonia. Although ion channels are not yet associated with dystonia in humans, the purpose of animal models is to suggest novel approaches and mechanisms for human disease. As such, the suggestion that ion channel dysfunction may drive dystonia is worthy of investigation and presents a novel approach for unraveling the process of dystonia in humans. Next, although studies in humans have traditionally implicated dysfunction of the basal ganglia in dystonia (Ichinose et al. 1994; Marsden and Quinn 1990; Ondo et al. 1998; Vitek 2002), more recent functional studies in humans have consistently implicated the cerebellum as well (Ceballos-Baumann and Brooks 1998; Hutchinson et al. 2000; Kluge et al. 1998; Mazziotta et al. 1998; Odergren et al. 1998; Playford et al. 1998; Eidelberg et al. 1998). Mouse models clearly implicate dysfunction of *both* the basal ganglia and cerebellum in dystonia, whereby the models fall into three subtypes. The FGF14-deficient mice and 3-NP mouse models demonstrate that defects of the basal ganglia can induce dystonia, while *Cacna1a* mutants and kainate-induced dystonia implicate the cerebellum in dystonia. Still other models, including Bay K 8644, *Scn8a*, and *dt*, suggest that several dysfunctional brain regions may simultaneously contribute to the expression of dystonia. The concept that dystonia may arise from the basal ganglia or the cerebellum or a complex combination of motor systems appears to have broad general applicability, as both genetic and drug-induced models fall into each of these subtypes. Given the heterogeneous nature of dystonia in humans and the lessons learned from rodent models, it is reasonable to suppose that the site of dysfunction will not be consistent from patient to patient. The mouse models illustrate the complexity of the disorder and suggest that focusing on a single brain region or gene may be counterproductive to understanding general pathophysiological principles of motor dysfunction in dystonia.

Video Legends

SEGMENT 1 Dystonia musculorum mouse. This video demonstrates the typical resting posture, the characteristic stiff and twisting dystonic movements, and the peculiar strategy for ambulation.

SEGMENT 2 Leaner mouse. This clip demonstrates reduced spontaneous mobility with extremely slow and stiff twisting movements of the trunk and limbs suggestive of dystonia superimposed upon a hypokinetic motor syndrome.

SEGMENT 3 Tottering mouse. These clips show the ataxic and tremulous baseline ambulation followed by the characteristic attack that typically proceeds in a caudal to rostral direction.

SEGMENT 4 Kainate-induced dystonia. Each segment illustrates a typical dystonic posture after intracerebellar microinjection with 0.5 ml of 100 μg/ml kainic acid. Both the motor and temporal aspects of the dystonia in the video are representative of the model. A single mouse was used throughout the video including the recovery phase, which occurred two hours after the injection. Note that the mouse returned to near normal levels of locomotor activity.

SEGMENT 5 Bay K 8644-induced dystonia. These clips demonstrate the sustained twisting postures and slowed movement after systemic administration of 8 mg/kg Bay K 8644.

References

Abbott, L.C., M. Bump, A. Brandl, and S. De Laune. 2000. Investigation of the role of the cerebellum in the myoclonic-like movement disorder exhibited by tottering mice. *Mov Disord* **15 Suppl**:S53–S59.

Abbott, L.C., K.R. Isaacs, and J.A. Heckroth. 1996. Co-localization of tyrosine hydroxylase and zebrin II immunoreactivities in Purkinje cells of the mutant mice, tottering, and tottering/leaner. *Neuroscience* **71**:461–475.

Aldea, M., K. Jun, H.S. Shin, E. Andres-Mateos, L.M. Solis-Garrido, C. Montiel, A.G. Garcia, and A. Albillos. 2002. A perforated patch-clamp study of calcium currents and exocytosis in chromaffin cells of wild-type and alpha(1A) knockout mice. *J Neurochem* **81**:911–921.

Althini, S., H. Bengtsson, D. Usoskin, S. Soderstrom, A. Kylberg, E. Lindqvist, S. Chuva de Sousa Lopes, et al. 2003. Normal nigrostriatal innervation but dopamine dysfunction in mice carrying hypomorphic tyrosine hydroxylase alleles. *J Neurosci Res* **72**:444–453.

Arpa, J., A. Cuesta, A. Cruz-Martinez, S. Santiago, J. Sarria, and F. Palau. 1999. Clinical features and genetic analysis of a Spanish family with spinocerebellar ataxia 6. *Acta Neurol Scand* **99**:43–47.

Augood, S.J., D.M. Martin, L.J. Ozelius, X.O. Breakefield, J.B. Penney, Jr, and D.G. Standaert. 1999. Distribution of the mRNAs encoding torsinA and torsinB in the normal adult human brain. *Ann Neurol* **46**:761–769.

Bernier, G., and R. Kothary. 1998. Prenatal onset of axonopathy in Dystonia musculorum mice. *Dev Genet* **22**:160–168.

Bianchi, M., L.C. Rovati, P. Sacerdote, P. Mategazza, and A.E. Panerai. 1990. Effect of drugs belonging to different classes of calcium channel blockers on experimental seizures induced by the calcium channel agonist Bay K 8644. *Neurosci Res* **6**:157–162.

Bode, V.C., J.D. McDonald, J.L. Guenet, and D. Simon. 1988. hph-1: a mouse mutant with hereditary hyperphenylalaninemia induced by ethylnitrosourea mutagenesis. *Genetics* **118**:299–305.

Bolger, G.T., B.A. Weissman, and P. Skolnick. 1985. The behavioral effects of the calcium agonist Bay K 8644 in the mouse: antagonism by the calcium antagonist nifedipine. *Naunyn Schmiedebergs Arch Pharmacol* **328**:373–377.

Bourson, A., P.C. Moser, A.J. Gower, and A.K. Mir. 1989. Central and peripheral effects of the dihydropyridine calcium channel activator BAY K 8644 in the rat. *Eur J Pharmacol* **160**:339–347.

Brown, A., G. Bernier, M. Mathieu, J. Rossant, and R. Kothary. 1995. The mouse dystonia musculorum gene is a neural isoform of bullous pemphigoid antigen 1. *Nat Genet* **10**:301–306.

Brown, A., N.G. Copeland, D.J. Gilbert, N.A. Jenkins, J. Rossant, and R. Kothary. 1994. The genomic structure of an insertional mutation in the dystonia musculorum locus. *Genomics* **20**:371–376.

Buchner, D.A., M. Trudeau, and M.H. Meisler. 2003. SCNM1, a putative RNA splicing factor that modifies disease severity in mice. *Science* **301**:967–969.

Buiakova, O.I., J. Xu, S. Lutsenko, S. Zeitlin, K. Das, S. Das, B.M. Ross, et al. 1999. Null mutation of the murine ATP7B (Wilson disease) gene results in intracellular copper accumulation and late-onset hepatic nodular transformation. *Hum Mol Genet* **8**:1665–1671.

Burgess, D.L., D.C. Kohrman, J. Galt, N.W. Plummer, J.M. Jones, B. Spear, and M.H. Meisler. 1995. Mutation of a new sodium channel gene,

Scn8a, in the mouse mutant "motor endplate disease". *Nat Genet* **10**:461–465.

Cabin, D.E., K. Shimazu, D. Murphy, N.B. Cole, W. Gottschalk, K.L. McIlwain, B. Orrison, et al. 2002. Synaptic vesicle depletion correlates with attenuated synaptic responses to prolonged repetitive stimulation in mice lacking alpha-synuclein. *J Neurosci* **22**:8797–8807.

Campbell, D.B., and E.J. Hess. 1998. Cerebellar circuitry is activated during convulsive episodes in the tottering (tg/tg) mutant mouse. *Neuroscience* **85**:773–783.

Campbell, D.B., and E.J. Hess. 1999. L-type calcium channels contribute to the tottering mouse dystonic episodes. *Mol Pharmacol* **55**: 23–31.

Campbell, D.B., J.B. North, and E.J. Hess. 1999. Tottering mouse motor dysfunction is abolished on the Purkinje cell degeneration (pcd) mutant background. *Exp Neurol* **160**:268–278.

Ceballos-Baumann, A.O., and D.J. Brooks. 1998. Activation positron emission tomography scanning in dystonia. *Adv Neurol* **78**:135–152.

Cemal, C.K., C.J. Carroll, L. Lawrence, M.B. Lowrie, P. Ruddle, S. Al-Mahdawi, R.H. King, et al. 2002. YAC transgenic mice carrying pathological alleles of the MJD1 locus exhibit a mild and slowly progressive cerebellar deficit. *Hum Mol Genet* **11**:1075–1094.

Charvin, N., C. Leveque, D. Walker, F. Berton, C. Raymond, M. Kataoka, Y. Shoji-Kasai, et al. 1997. Direct interaction of the calcium sensor protein synaptotagmin I with a cytoplasmic domain of the α_1A subunit of the P/Q-type calcium channel. *EMBO J* **16**:4591–4596.

Chen, K., L.K. Sprunger, M.H. Meisler, H.J. Waller, and D.A. Godfrey. 1999. Reduced spontaneous activity in the dorsal cochlear nucleus of Scn8a mutant mice. *Brain Res* **847**:85–89.

D'Hooge, R., D. Van Dam, F. Franck, V. Gieselmann, and P.P. De Deyn. 2001. Hyperactivity, neuromotor defects, and impaired learning and memory in a mouse model for metachromatic leukodystrophy. *Brain Res* **907**:35–43.

Dalpe, G., N. Leclerc, A. Vallee, A. Messer, M. Mathieu, Y. De Repentigny, and R. Kothary. 1998. Dystonin is essential for maintaining neuronal cytoskeleton organization. *Mol Cell Neurosci* **10**:243–257.

Dauer, W., and R. Goodchild. 2004. Mouse models of torsinA dysfunction. *Adv Neurol* **94**:67–72.

De Repentigny, Y., J. Deschenes-Furry, B.J. Jasmin, and R. Kothary. 2003. Impaired fast axonal transport in neurons of the sciatic nerves from dystonia musculorum mice. *J Neurochem* **86**:564–571.

De Sarro, G., C. Ascioti, E.D. di Paola, M.J. Vidal, and A. De Sarro. 1992. Effects of anti-epileptic drugs, calcium channel blockers and other compounds on seizures induced by activation of voltage-dependent L calcium channel in DBA/2 mice. *Gen Pharmacol* **23**:1205–1216.

Dick, D.J., R.J. Boakes, and J.B. Harris. 1985. A cerebellar abnormality in the mouse with motor end-plate disease. *Neuropathol Appl Neurobiol* **11**:141–147.

Dove, L.S., L.C. Abbott, and W.H. Griffith. 1998. Whole-cell and single-channel analysis of P-type calcium currents in cerebellar Purkinje cells of leaner mutant mice. *J Neurosci* **18**:7687–7699.

Dowling, J., Y. Yang, R. Wollmann, L.F. Reichardt, and E. Fuchs. 1997. Developmental expression of BPAG1-n: insights into the spastic ataxia and gross neurologic degeneration in dystonia musculorum mice. *Dev Biol* **187**:131–142.

Doyle, J., X. Ren, G. Lennon, and L. Stubbs. 1997. Mutations in the Cacnl1a4 calcium channel gene are associated with seizures, cerebellar degeneration, and ataxia in tottering and leaner mutant mice. *Mamm Genome* **8**:113–120.

Duchen, L.W. 1976. Dystonia musculorum—an inherited disease of the nervous system in the mouse. *Adv Neurol* **14**:353–365.

Duchen, L.W., D.S. Falconer, and S.J. Strich. 1963. Dystonia musculorum, an hereditary neuropathy of mice affecting mainly sensory pathways. *J Physiol* **165**:7.

Duchen, L.W., A.G. Searle, and S.J. Strich. 1967. An hereditary motor end-plate disease in the mouse. *J Physiol* **189**:4P–6P.

Duchen, L.W., S.J. Strich, and D.S. Falconer. 1964. Clinical and pathological studies of an hereditary neuropathy in mice (dystonia musculorum). *Brain* **87**:367–378.

Eicher, E.M., and P.C. Hoppe. 1973. Use of chimeras to transmit lethal genes in the mouse and to demonstrate allelism of the two X-linked male lethal genes jp and msd. *J Exp Zool* **183**:181–184.

Eidelberg, D., J.R. Moeller, A. Antonini, K. Kazumata, T. Nakamura, V. Dhawan, P. Spetsieris, et al. 1998. Functional brain networks in DYT1 dystonia. *Ann Neurol* **44**:303–312.

Eilam, R., Y. Peter, A. Elson, G. Rotman, Y. Shiloh, Y. Groner, and M. Segal. 1998. Selective loss of dopaminergic nigro-striatal neurons in brains of Atm-deficient mice. *Proc Natl Acad Sci USA* **95**:12653–12656.

Fahn, S., and C.D. Marsden. 1994. The paroxysmal dyskinesias. In *Movement Disorders 3* Ed. C.D. Marsden and S. Fahn. pp. 310–347. Oxford: Butterworth-Heinemann.

Fernagut, P.O., E. Diguet, N. Stefanova, M. Biran, G.K. Wenning, P. Canioni, B. Bioulac, and F. Tison. 2002. Subacute systemic 3-nitropropionic acid intoxication induces a distinct motor disorder in adult C57Bl/6 mice: behavioural and histopathological characterisation. *Neuroscience* **114**:1005–1017.

Fletcher, C.F., C.M. Lutz, T.N. O'Sullivan, J.D. Shaughnessy, R. Hawkes, W.N. Frankel, N.G. Copeland, and N.A. Jenkins. 1996. Absence epilepsy in tottering mutant mice is associated with calcium channel defects. *Cell* **87**:607–617.

Fletcher, C.F., A. Tottene, V.A. Lennon, S.M. Wilson, S.J. Dubel, R. Paylor, D.A. Hosford, et al. 2001. Dystonia and cerebellar atrophy in Cacna1a null mice lacking P/Q calcium channel activity. *FASEB J* **15**:1288–1290.

Garcia, K.D., L.K. Sprunger, M.H. Meisler, and K.G. Beam. 1998. The sodium channel Scn8a is the major contributor to the postnatal developmental increase of sodium current density in spinal motoneurons. *J Neurosci* **18**:5234–5239.

Giasson, B.I., J.E. Duda, S.M. Quinn, B. Zhang, J.Q. Trojanowski, and V.M. Lee. 2002. Neuronal alpha-synucleinopathy with severe movement disorder in mice expressing A53T human alpha-synuclein. *Neuron* **34**:521–533.

Giffin, N.J., S. Benton, and P.J. Goadsby. (2002). Benign paroxysmal torticollis of infancy: four new cases and linkage to CACNA1A mutation. *Dev Med Child Neurol* **44**:490–493.

Goldberg, M.S., S.M. Fleming, J.J. Palacino, C. Cepeda, H.A. Lam, A. Bhatnagar, E.G. Meloni, et al. 2003. Parkin-deficient mice exhibit nigrostriatal deficits but not loss of dopaminergic neurons. *J Biol Chem* **278**:43628–43635.

Gomez-Isla, T., M.C. Irizarry, A. Mariash, B. Cheung, O. Soto, S. Schrump, J. Sondel, et al. 2003. Motor dysfunction and gliosis with preserved dopaminergic markers in human alpha-synuclein A30P transgenic mice. *Neurobiol Aging* **24**:245–258.

Green, M.C., and R.L. Sidman. 1962. Tottering—a neuromuscular mutation in the mouse. *J Hered* **53**:233–237.

Guo, L., L. Degenstein, J. Dowling, Q.C. Yu, R. Wollmann, B. Perman, and E. Fuchs. 1995. Gene targeting of BPAG1: abnormalities in mechanical strength and cell migration in stratified epithelia and neurologic degeneration. *Cell* **81**:233–243.

Gupta, P., A.A. Soyombo, A. Atashband, K.E. Wisniewski, J.M. Shelton, J.A. Richardson, R.E. Hammer, and S.L. Hofmann. 2001. Disruption of PPT1 or PPT2 causes neuronal ceroid lipofuscinosis in knockout mice. *Proc Natl Acad Sci USA* **98**:13566–13571.

Hamann, M., M.H. Meisler, and A. Richter. 2003. Motor disturbances in mice with deficiency of the sodium channel gene Scn8a show features of human dystonia. *Exp Neurol* **184**:830–838.

Harris, J.B., R.J. Boakes, and J.A. Court. 1992. Physiological and biochemical studies on the cerebellar cortex of the murine mutants "jolting" and "motor end-plate disease". *J Neurol Sci* **110**:186–194.

Harris, J.B., and S.L. Pollard. 1986. Neuromuscular transmission in the murine mutants "motor end-plate disease" and "jolting". *J Neurol Sci* **76**:239–253.

Heckroth, J.A., and L.C. Abbott. 1994. Purkinje cell loss from alternating sagittal zones in the cerebellum of leaner mutant mice. *Brain Res* **658**: 93–104.

Heller, A.H., M.A. Dichter, and R.L. Sidman. 1983. Anticonvulsant sensitivity of absence seizures in the tottering mutant mouse. *Epilepsia* **25**: 25–34.

Herrup, K., and S.L. Wilczynski. 1982. Cerebellar cell degeneration in the leaner mutant mouse. *Neuroscience* **7**:2185–2196.

Hess, E.J., and M.C. Wilson. 1991. Tottering and leaner mutations perturb transient developmental expression of tyrosine hydroxylase in embryologically distinct Purkinje cells. *Neuron* **6**:123–132.

Hutchinson, M., T. Nakamura, J.R. Moeller, A. Antonini, A. Belakhlef, V. Dhawan, and D. Eidelberg. 2000. The metabolic topography of essential blepharospasm: a focal dystonia with general implications. *Neurology* **55**:673–677.

Ichinose, H., T. Ohye, E. Takahashi, N. Seki, T. Hori, M. Segawa, Y. Nomura, et al. 1994. Hereditary progressive dystonia with marked diurnal fluctuation caused by mutations in the GTP cyclohydrolase I gene. *Nat Genet* **8**:236–242.

Ikeda, H., M. Yamaguchi, S. Sugai, Y. Aze, S. Narumiya, and A. Kakizuka. 1996. Expanded polyglutamine in the Machado-Joseph disease protein induces cell death in vitro and in vivo. *Nat Genet* **13**:196–202.

Ikeda, M., M. Mikuni, T. Nishikawa, and K. Takahashi. 1989. A neurochemical study of a new mutant mouse presenting myoclonus-like involuntary movement: a possible model of spontaneous serotonergic hyperactivity. *Brain Res* **495**:337–348.

Inoue, Y., Y. Matsumura, K. Inoue, R. Ichikawa, and C. Takayama. 1993. Abnormal synaptic architecture in the cerebellar cortex of a new dystonic mutant mouse, wriggle mouse Sagami. *Neurosci Res* **16**:39–48.

Isaacs, K.R., and L.C. Abbott. 1995. Cerebellar volume decreases in the tottering mouse are specific to the molecular layer. *Brain Res Bull* **36**:309–314.

Ishikawa, K., S. Shibanoki, T. Kubo, M. Kogure, Y. Imamura, N. Osawa, M. Ohmura, and K. Mikoshiba. 1989. Functional difference in monoamine transmitters in the behaviorally abnormal mouse mutant (wriggle mouse Sagami). *Neurosci Lett* **103**:343–348.

Jankovic, J., and S. Fahn. 1998. Dystonic disorders. In *Parkinson's Disease and Movement Disorders* Ed. J. Jankovic and E. Tolosa. pp. 513–551. Baltimore: Williams & Wilkins.

Janota, I. 1972. Ultrastructural studies of an hereditary sensory neuropathy in mice (dystonia musculorum). *Brain* **95**:529–536.

Jinnah, H.A., K. Egami, L. Rao, M. Shin, S. Kasim, and E.J. Hess. 2003. Expression of c-fos in the brain after activation of L-type calcium channels. *Dev Neurosci* **25**:403–411.

Jinnah, H.A., F.H. Gage, and T. Friedmann. 1991. Amphetamine-induced behavioral phenotype in a hypoxanthine-guanine phosphoribosyltransferase-deficient mouse model of Lesch-Nyhan syndrome. *Behav Neurosci* **105**:1004–1012.

Jinnah, H.A., J.P. Sepkuty, T. Ho, S. Yitta, T. Drew, J.D. Rothstein, and E.J. Hess. 2000. Calcium channel agonists and dystonia in the mouse. *Mov Disord* **15**:542–551.

Jun, K., E.S. Piedras-Renteria, S.M. Smith, D.B. Wheeler, S.B. Lee, T.G. Lee, H. Chin, et al. 1999. Ablation of P/Q-type Ca(2+) channel currents, altered synaptic transmission, and progressive ataxia in mice lacking the alpha(1A)-subunit. *Proc Natl Acad Sci USA* **96**:15245–15250.

Kaplan, B.J., T.N. Seyfried, and G.H. Glaser. 1979. Spontaneous polyspike discharges in an epileptic mutant mouse (tottering). *Exp Neurol* **66**: 577–586.

Kearney, J.A., D.A. Buchner, G. De Haan, M. Adamska, S.I. Levin, A.R. Furay, R.L. Albin, et al. 2002. Molecular and pathological effects of a modifier gene on deficiency of the sodium channel Scn8a (Na(v)1.6). *Hum Mol Genet* **11**:2765–2775.

Kim, D.K., and W.A. Catterall. 1997. Ca^{2+}-dependent and -independent interactions of the isoforms of the α_1A subunit of brain Ca^{2+} channels with presynaptic SNARE proteins. *Proc Natl Acad Sci USA* **94**: 14782–14786.

Kluge, A., B. Kettner, R. Zschenderlein, D. Sandrock, D.L. Munz, S. Hesse, and H. Meierkord. 1998. Changes in perfusion pattern using ECD-SPECT indicate frontal lobe and cerebellar involvement in exercise-induced paroxysmal dystonia. *Mov Disord* **13**:125–134.

Koeller, D.M., M. Woontner, L.S. Crnic, B. Kleinschmidt-DeMasters, J. Stephens, E.L. Hunt, and S.I. Goodman. 2002. Biochemical, pathologic and behavioral analysis of a mouse model of glutaric acidemia type I. *Hum Mol Genet* **11**:347–357.

Kohrman, D.C., J.B. Harris, and M.H. Meisler. 1996a. Mutation detection in the med and medJ alleles of the sodium channel Scn8a. Unusual splicing due to a minor class AT-AC intron. *J Biol Chem* **271**: 17576–17581.

Kohrman, D.C., M.R. Smith, A.L. Goldin, J. Harris, and M.H. Meisler. 1996b. A missense mutation in the sodium channel Scn8a is responsible for cerebellar ataxia in the mouse mutant jolting. *J Neurosci* **16**: 5993–5999.

Kothary, R., S. Clapoff, A. Brown, R. Campbell, A. Peterson, and J. Rossant. 1988. A transgene containing lacZ inserted into the dystonia locus is expressed in neural tube. *Nature* **335**:435–437.

Kumazawa, T., K. Adachi, and K. Ando. 1989. Concentrations of catecholamines and indoleamines in the central nervous system of wriggle mouse Sagami. *Comp Biochem Physiol. C.* **93**:167–169.

Lalonde, R., C.C. Joyal, and M.I. Botez. 1994. Exploration and motor coordination in dystonia musculorum mutant mice. *Physiol Behav* **56**: 277–280.

Landis, S.C., and R.J. Mullen. 1978. The development and degeneration of Purkinje cells in pcd mutant mice. *J Comp Neurol* **177**:125–144.

LeDoux, M.S., J.F. Lorden, and J. Ervin. 1993. Cerebellectomy eliminates the motor syndrome of the genetically dystonic rat. *Exp Neurol* **120**: 302–310.

Lee, M.K., W. Stirling, Y. Xu, X. Xu, D. Qui, A.S. Mandir, T.M. Dawson, et al. 2002. Human alpha-synuclein-harboring familial Parkinson's disease-linked Ala-53 $\rightarrow$Thr mutation causes neurodegenerative disease with alpha-synuclein aggregation in transgenic mice. *Proc Natl Acad Sci USA* **99**:8968–8973.

Levitt, P. 1988. Normal pharmacological and morphometric parameters in the noradrenergic hyperinnervated mutant mouse, "tottering". *Cell Tissue Res* **252**:175–180.

Levitt, P., and J.L. Noebels, 1981. Mutant mouse tottering: selective increase of locus ceruleus axons in a defined single-locus mutation. *Proc Natl Acad Sci USA* **78**:4630–4634.

Liu, X., X. Luo, and W. Hu. 1992. Studies on the epidemiology and etiology of moldy sugarcane poisoning in China. *Biomed Environ Sci* **5**:161–177.

Lorden, J.F., G.A. Oltmans, S. Stratton, and L.E. Mays. 1988. Neuropharmacological correlates of the motor syndrome of the genetically dystonic (dt) rat. In *Dystonia 2* Ed. S. Fahn. pp. 277–297. New York: Raven Press.

Lorenzon, N.M., C.M. Lutz, W.N. Frankel, and K.G. Beam. 1998. Altered calcium channel currents in Purkinje cells of the neurological mutant mouse leaner. *J Neurosci* **18**:4482–4489.

Marsden, C.D., and N.P. Quinn. 1990. The dystonias. *Brit Med J* **300**: 139–144.

Maurice, N., T. Tkatch, M. Meisler, L.K. Sprunger, and D.J. Surmeier. 2001. D1/D5 dopamine receptor activation differentially modulates rapidly inactivating and persistent sodium currents in prefrontal cortex pyramidal neurons. *J Neurosci* **21**:2268–2277.

Mazziotta, J.C., M. Hutchinson, T.D. Fife, and R. Woods. 1998. Advanced neuroimaging methods in the study of movement disorders: dystonia and blepharospasm. *Adv Neurol* **78**:153–160.

McGeer, E.G., and P.L. McGeer. 1988. The dystonias. *Can J Neurol Sci* **15**:447–483.

Meier, H., and A.D. MacPike. 1970. A neurological mutation (msd) of the mouse causing a deficiency of myelin synthesis. *Exp Brain Res* **10**: 512–525.

Meier, H., and D. MacPike. 1971. Three syndromes produced by two mutant genes in the mouse. *J Hered* **62**:297–302.

Messer, A., and D. Gordon. 1979. Changes in whole tissue biosynthesis of gamma-amino butyric acid (GABA) in basal ganglia of the dystonia (dtAlb) mouse. *Life Sci* **25**:2217–2221.

Messer, A., and N.L. Strominger. 1980. An allele of the mouse mutant dystonia musculorum exhibits lesions in red nucleus and striatum. *Neuroscience* **5**:543–549.

Morris, M.D., C. Bhuvaneswaran, H. Shio, and S. Fowler. 1982. Lysosome lipid storage disorder in NCTR-BALB/c mice. I. Description of the disease and genetics. *Am J Pathol* **108**:140–149.

Noebels, J.L. 1984. A single gene error of noradrenergic axon growth synchronizes central neurons. *Nature* **310**:409–411.

Noebels, J.L., and R.L. Sidman. 1979. Inherited epilepsy: spike-wave and focal motor seizures in the mutant mouse tottering. *Science* **204**: 1334–1336.

Nutt, J.G., M.D. Muenter, A. Aronson, L.T. Kurland, and L.J. Melton. 1988. Epidemiology of focal and generalised dystonia in Rochester, Minnesota. *Mov Disord* **3**:188–194.

O'Neill, S.K., and G.T. Bolger. 1988. Enantiomer selectivity and the development of tolerance to the behavioral effects of the calcium channel activator BAY K 8644. *Brain Res Bull* **21**:865–872.

Odergren, T., S. Stone-Elander, and M. Ingvar. 1998. Cerebral and cerebellar activation in correlation to the action-induced dystonia in writer's cramp. *Mov Disord* **13**:497–508.

Ondo, W.G., J.M. Desaloms, J. Jankovic, and R.G. Grossman. 1998. Pallidotomy for generalized dystonia. *Mov Disord* **13**:693–698.

Ophoff, R.A., G.M. Terwindt, M.N. Vergouwe, R. van Eijk, P.J. Oefner, S.M. Hoffman, J.E. Lamerdin, et al. 1996. Familial hemiplegic migraine and episodic ataxia type-2 are caused by mutations in the Ca2+ channel gene CACNL1A4. *Cell* **87**:543–652.

Pagani, R., M. Song, M. McEnery, N. Qin, R.W. Tsien, L. Toro, E. Stefani, and O.D. Uchitel. 2004. Differential expression of alpha1 and beta subunits of voltage dependent Ca2+ channel at the neuromuscular junction of normal and P/Q Ca2+ channel knockout mouse. *Neuroscience* **123**:75–85.

Palmer, G.C., M.L. Stagnitto, R.K. Ray, M.A. Knowles, R. Harvey, and G.E. Garske. 1993. Anticonvulsant properties of calcium channel blockers in mice: N-methyl-D-,L-aspartate- and Bay K 8644-induced convulsions are potently blocked by the dihydropyridines. *Epilepsia* **34**: 372–380.

Petersen, E.N. 1986. Bay K 8644 induces a reversible spasticity-like syndrome in rats. *Eur J Pharmacol* **130**:323–326.

Pizoli, C.E., H.A. Jinnah, M.L. Billingsley, and E.J. Hess. 2002. Abnormal cerebellar signaling induces dystonia in mice. *J Neurosci* **22**:7825–7833.

Playford, E.D., R.E. Passingham, C.D. Marsden, and D.J. Brooks. 1998. Increased activation of frontal areas during arm movement in idiopathic torsion dystonia. *Mov Disord* **13**:309–318.

Qian, J., and J.L. Noebels. 2000. Presynaptic Ca(2+) influx at a mouse central synapse with Ca(2+) channel subunit mutations. *J Neurosci* **20**:163–170.

Raman, I.M., L.K. Sprunger, M.H. Meisler, and B.P. Bean. 1997. Altered subthreshold sodium currents and disrupted firing patterns in Purkinje neurons of Scn8a mutant mice. *Neuron* **19**:881–891.

Rampe, D., B. Anderson, V. Rapien-Pryor, T. Li, and R.C. Dage. 1993. Comparison of the *in vitro* and *in vivo* cardiovascular effects of two structurally distinct Ca++ channel activators, BAY K 8644 and FPL 64176. *J Pharmacol Exp Ther* **265**:1125–1130.

Rettig, J., Z.-H. Sheng, D.K. Kim, C.D. Hodson, and T.P. Snutch. 1996. Isoform-specific interaction of the α_1A subunits of brain Ca^{2+} channels with the presynaptic proteins syntaxin and SNAP-25. *Proc Natl Acad Sci USA* **93**:7363–7368.

Rhyu, I.J., L.C. Abbott, D.B. Walker, and C. Sotelo. 1999. An ultrastructural study of granule cell/Purkinje cell synapses in tottering (tg/tg), leaner (tg(la)/tg(la)) and compound heterozygous tottering/leaner (tg/tg(la)) mice. *Neuroscience* **90**:717–728.

Richter, A., and W. Loscher. 1998. Pathology of idiopathic dystonia: findings from genetic animal models. *Prog Neurobiol* **54**:633–677.

Saulnier, R., Y. De Repentigny, V.W. Yong, and R. Kothary. 2002. Alterations in myelination in the central nervous system of dystonia musculorum mice. *J Neurosci Res* **69**:233–242.

Shelton, R.C., J.A. Grebb, and W.J. Freed. 1987. Induction of seizures in mice by intracerebroventricular administration of the calcium channel agonist BAY K 8644. *Brain Res* **402**:399–402.

Sotelo, C., and J.L. Guenet. 1988. Pathologic changes in the CNS of dystonia musculorum mutant mouse: an animal model for human spinocerebellar ataxia. *Neuroscience* **27**:403–424.

Sprunger, L.K., A. Escayg, S. Tallaksen-Greene, R.L. Albin, and M.H. Meisler. 1999. Dystonia associated with mutation of the neuronal sodium channel Scn8a and identification of the modifier locus Scnm1 on mouse chromosome 3. *Hum Mol Genet* **8**:471–479.

Takahashi, K., and K. Kitamura. 1999. A point mutation in a plasma membrane Ca(2+)-ATPase gene causes deafness in wriggle mouse Sagami. *Biochem Biophys Res Commun* **261**:773–778.

Takahashi, K., N. Osawa, M. Ohmura, and K. Kitamura. 1999. Evaluation of inner ear histology and auditory brainstem response in wriggle mouse Sagami. *Acta Otolaryngol* **119**:767–772.

Tsuji, S., and H. Meier. 1971. Evidence for allelism of leaner and tottering in the mouse. *Genet Res* **17**:83–88.

Vitek, J.L. 2002. Pathophysiology of dystonia: a neuronal model. *Mov Disord* **17**:S49–S62.

Voikar, V., H. Rauvala, and E. Ikonen. 2002. Cognitive deficit and development of motor impairment in a mouse model of Niemann-Pick type C disease. *Behav Brain Res* **132**:1–10.

Wakamori, M., K. Yamazaki, and H. Matsunodaira. 1998. Single tottering mutations responsible for the neuropathic phenotype of the P-type calcium channel. *J Biol Chem* **52**:34857–34867.

Wang, Q., M.E. Bardgett, M. Wong, D.F. Wozniak, J. Lou, B.D. McNeil, C. Chen, et al. 2002. Ataxia and paroxysmal dyskinesia in mice lacking axonally transported FGF14. *Neuron* **35**:25–38.

Yang, Y., C. Bauer, G. Strasser, R. Wollman, J.P. Julien, and E. Fuchs. 1999. Integrators of the cytoskeleton that stabilize microtubules. *Cell* **98**: 229–238.

Yoon, C.H. 1969. Disturbances in developmental pathways leading to a neurological disorder of genetic origin, "leaner", in mice. *Dev Biol* **20**: 158–181.

Zheng, W., D. Rampe, and D.J. Triggle. 1991. Pharmacological, radioligand binding, and electrophysiological characteristics of FPL 64176, a novel nondihydropyridine Ca2+ channel activator, in cardiac and vascular preparations. *Mol Pharmacol* **40**:734–741.

Zhou, Y.D., T.J. Turner, and K. Dunlap. 2003. Enhanced G protein-dependent modulation of excitatory synaptic transmission in the cerebellum of the Ca2+ channel-mutant mouse, tottering. *J Physiol* **547**: 497–507.

Zhuchenko, O., J. Bailey, P. Bonnen, T. Ashizawa, D.W. Stockton, C. Amos, W.B. Dobyns, et al. 1997. Autosomal dominant cerebellar ataxia (SCA6) associated with small polyglutamine expansions in the alpha 1A-voltage-dependent calcium channel. *Nat Genet* **15**:62–69.

CHAPTER

C5

The Owl Monkey Model of Focal Dystonia

DAVID T. BLAKE, NANCY N. BYL, and MICHAEL MERZENICH

I. INTRODUCTION

The owl monkey model of focal dystonia has allowed investigators to verify the hypothesis that somatic sensory abnormalities are part of the disorder. In this chapter, we will review the evidence of mechanisms underlying sensory and motor disorders and show that a common cortical abnormality may underlie both. Treatments that focus first on treating sensory deficits, and later progress to sensory-motor integration and sensory-motor deficits, have high efficacy in restoring predystonic motor function. We will also discuss how the range of documented physiological motor and sensory deficits in focal hand dystonia relate to poor motor function.

Focal dystonia is a movement disorder in which muscles are abnormally synchronized, and normal muscle antagonists may be co-active. The clinical diagnosis of focal hand dystonia involves a confluence of symptoms, including intermittent arrhythmic, involuntary contractions of the muscles of the hand while performing a target task (Cohen et al. 1989; Lockwood 1989; Marsden and Sheehy 1990; Newmark and Hochberg 1987; Rothwell et al. 1983; Sheehy and Marsden 1982; Wilson 1989), co-contraction of agonist and antagonist muscle groups along with inaccurate, inappropriately timed and sequenced movements between adjacent fingers and wrist during task performance (Chen et al. 1995), and poor hand posture outside task performance. Focal dystonia affects significant fractions of subpopulations that perform repetitive stereotyped motor actions with their hands, particularly musicians and typists. In addition, other groups such as athletes, particularly those that "powergrip" during shoulder motions, may be affected (Lagueny et al. 2002; Smith et al. 2003). These activities are characterized by either rapid, sequential, stereotyped movements or controlled movements during a voluntary co-contraction, or powergrip. For these individuals to achieve even half of their predystonic performance levels currently constitutes a substantial recovery. Investigators initiated studies of animal models to allow a closer look inside the physiology of an animal with focal hand dystonia, and to gain insight into treatment for the disorder. The initial hypothesis at the start of these studies could be reasonably stated as, "There are central sensory processing abnormalities in focal hand dystonia." The work has demonstrated unequivocally that abnormalities occur in sensory representations in focal hand dystonia, and that addressing these abnormalities as a first step in treatment can greatly benefit the patient population.

II. REVIEW OF BASIC SENSORY AND MOTOR SYSTEMS IN *AOTUS*

The ascending sensory pathways of the owl monkey include peripheral receptors, dorsal column nuclei, ventral posterolateral thalamic nucleus, and the primary somatosensory cortex, area 3b. Modality preservation occurs at the projections from each level to each adjacent level. That is, no connectivity occurs between groups of neurons that carry different types of response properties. In particular, neurons that respond to stimulation of hairy skin do not mix in functional connectivity with neurons that represent glabrous skin, neurons representing different fingertips do not mix, and neurons that respond only to deep skin stimulation do not mix with neurons that respond to light cutaneous stimulation. As a result, neurons either respond to one modality, or another, but not both. Investigators have observed modality preservation at the nucleus to which the peripheral neurons project, the dorsal columns (Gordon and Paine 1960; Kruger et al. 1961; Perl et al. 1962; McComas 1963; Winter 1965; Johnson et al. 1968; Millar and Basbaum 1975). Neurons cluster in the dorsal columns in small modules, roughly 0.5 mm in diameter, in which all neurons respond to the same stimulation modality, and are similar in positional representation on the skin surface (Dykes et al. 1982). The modality preservation also exists in the primary thalamic nucleus for the somatosensory inputs, the ventral posterolateral nucleus. Early studies that recorded single neurons confirmed this property of the thalamic nuclei (Mountcastle and Rose 1952), and both the anatomical and physiological basis of this phenomenon, the thalamic barreloid, have been described in great detail (Jones, 1985). Representational barreloids extend in the anterior-posterior direction in the primate thalamus, and within a barreloid all neurons respond to the same modality and respond to stimulation of skin surfaces within a small locus. This preservation of modality exists in area 3b as well (Mountcastle 1957; Powell and Mountcastle 1959; Paul et al. 1972; Merzenich et al. 1978; Sur et al. 1984). Modality preservation exists despite substantial divergence and convergence at each level on the way to the cerebral cortex. The representation of the manual skin surfaces in area 3b is an orderly, topographic map on a two dimensional sheet of cortical neurons. The first digit is represented most laterally, and the fifth digit most medially. The digit tips extend anterior to the map, whereas the finger bases are more posterior. The maps of the digit tips are adjacent and non-overlapping. The hairy dorsum of the hand is represented in islands surrounded by glabrous representations, and often some hairy skin surfaces are not represented at all. This segregation of inputs depending on modality allows nearly independent use of these inputs for effecting changes in motor outputs or in motor feedback, in addition to providing a substrate for independence in sensory perception (Johnson and Hsiao 1992). Modality segregation also exists in area 4, the primary motor cortex. In the motor map, the representations consist of neurons that activate different muscle groups when cortical microstimulation is applied. The output representation of the muscle groups are organized in a loosely topographic mosaic, in which independent muscle actions are represented in segregated modules, or columns (Kwan et al. 1978; Sessle and Wiesendanger 1982; Strick and Preston 1982; Gould et al. 1986; Huntley and Jones 1991; Donoghue et al. 1992; Nudo et al. 1992; Nudo et al. 1996). For example, microstimulation of different columns may activate different single digits, or cause antagonistic muscle actions. These columns are intermingled on a larger scale across the same cortical territory, so that independent motor actions may be represented a few hundred microns apart, or a few millimeters. These columns have output projections into the spinal motoneuron pools, at which antagonistic muscle groups have reciprocal inhibition (Liddle and Sherrington, 1924). A breakdown of columnar boundaries, in somatosensory or motor cortex, would result in some of the normally independent functional modules sharing signals. The interference between these processing modules results in focal dystonia and loss of motor control.

III. EXPERIMENTAL RESULTS

A. Experiment One

Researchers designed the first experiments to induce focal hand dystonia in owl monkeys by repetitive stereotyped hand motions and to assess sensory physiological normalcy (Byl et al. 1996b). Animals performed a palmar grasp in which the hand was forced open and allowed to close rapidly. Animals grasped two cylindrical hand holds, and the hand holds were forced open and closed across a distance of about 8 mm. After one to nine rounds of opening and closing, animals were rewarded with a food pellet. In this behavior, the rapid and sequential movements of the hand were not under voluntary control. The animal merely grasped and maintained contact throughout the changes in the position forced on its hand. Over five months of daily performance of 1000 to 3000 repetitions per day, the animals' performance had degraded to a speed of less than one half of early performance, and each of two animals were diagnosed with focal hand dystonia based on a confluence of symptoms associated with the disorder. Both animals' hand representations in primary somatosensory cortex, area 3b, were abnormal. The average receptive field sizes were 80 to 100 mm^2, which may be compared to averages in control subjects of approximately 8 mm^2. In a hand map of a normal animal, the digit representations are segregated. However, animals with focal hand dystonia did not have segregated representations of adjacent digits. This lack of segregation also extended to the representations of the hairy and glabrous skin, which were also blurred together.

Another normal feature of the somatotopic representation in area 3b is the cortical column. If neurons are sampled at horizontal distances exceeding 500 μm, their receptive fields are disjointed. As the distance between the neurons decreases, receptive fields may increasingly overlap. This organizational principle in the cortex allows substantial independence in the action of cortical modules across relatively short distances. In animals with focal dystonia, this distance was at least 2 mm. Put another way, cortical columns increased to 400% of their normal size, and the column area increased by a factor of 16. If this principle considers the total number of modules in the hand representation, that number must also decrease by a factor of 16.

B. Experiment Two

Investigators modified the behavior of owl monkeys in the second class of studies (Byl et al. 1997) so that hand movements were active, and not passive. Animals again grasped two cylinders and pulled them together.

After a 1.5 second period in which the cylinders lightly vibrated, the animals pulled the cylinders towards themselves, and received a pellet reward. Animals completed 300–400 trials per day for five months.

In the two animals trained in this behavior, one developed a focal hand dystonia, and the other developed a motor coping strategy. In the animal with the focal hand dystonia, digital receptive fields averaged close to 100 mm^2, similar to animals in the first experiment. In the animal without focal hand dystonia, receptive fields averaged 40 mm^2, about five times larger than normal. Investigators noted that normally segregated responses were mixed in both animals, although significantly more so in the animal with focal hand dystonia. In this study, investigators mapped the representations of the other hand in the contralateral somatosensory cortex, and observed a substantial abnormality. Digital receptive fields averaged five times larger than normal, and abnormal mixing of receptive field properties, such as combined multi-digit or combined hairy-glabrous responses were also observed. The contralateral cortex in the dystonic animal had physiological properties similar to that of the hand representation of the trained owl monkey that did not develop dystonia.

C. Experiment Three

Investigators conducted the third study (Blake et al. 2002) to compare the variability of physiological abnormalities to motor abnormalities across the hand map. The behavior of the animals was similar to the behavior from experiment two. Animals grasped a pair of vertical rods, and pulled them together using a palmar grasp. The animal felt a light vibration for more than a second, and then had to release the rod within reaction time limits after the vibration ended. Two animals developed a focal hand dystonia. In one, the animal could continue the behavior only by using digits 3 and 4. The other digits assumed an abnormal posture and were not used. The second animal developed a hyperextension of digit 4 at all joints, and performed the behavior with its other digits. In the hand maps of primary somatosensory cortex for these animals, the motor abnormalities were closely related to the physiological abnormalities. Receptive field sizes were larger on digits involved in motor dysfunction, and mixing of responses, such as combined multi-digit or combined hairy-glabrous responses, was largely limited to the digits with abnormal function. In one example, cortical columnar structure was broken down with columns ten times larger than normal only in the region of the map associated with the motor dysfunction. A control animal performed the same behavior as the two dystonic animals and also developed abnormally large cortical columns, although not as large as the dystonic animals. It also developed abnormally large receptive fields, but smaller than those of the dystonic animals. The control animal did not develop abnormal mixing of response properties that are normally segregated, such as the hairy-glabrous or multi-digit mixing in receptive fields seen in the dystonic animals. A plot of the cortical column functions appears in Figure 1. In this plot, each line represents one animal's overlap function. The receptive field overlap is the average shared receptive field fraction at different distances in the cerebral cortex. In untrained normals, this function is zero for distances greater than 0.5 mm, whereas in dystonic animals it may not be zero even at 2 mm.

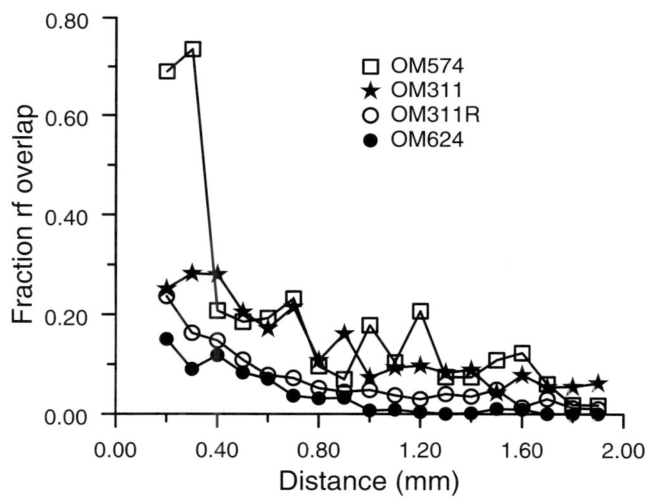

FIGURE 1 Cortical columnar functions in trained animals. Each line plots the expected receptive field overlap as a function of cortical distance in one hemisphere of one animal. In untrained normals, there is no overlap at distances exceeding 0.5 mm (Sur et al. 1980). OM574 and 311 had focal hand dystonia. OM311R is derived from the representation of the untrained hand in an animal with focal hand dystonia. OM624 had comparable training to the other animals, but did not develop hand dystonia. (From Blake et al. 2002)

D. Experiment Four

The fourth experiment (Blake et al. 2002) is a case report from an animal involved in a behavioral study unrelated to focal hand dystonia. The animal developed focal hand dystonia while learning to position its hand in a hand mold to contact two motor tips with its first and second digits. Prior to behavioral engagement, the animal had an array of microelectrodes implanted in the somatosensory cortex over the area representing the first and second digits, and also over the area for the face. In the week after the focal dystonia developed, receptive fields were three to four times larger than normal. Also, cortical substitutions began to occur. Areas of the cortex became unresponsive to skin stimulation, and then a few days later would respond to sensory stimulation of the face. Across the same period, adjacent electrodes often maintained the same receptive fields. As the dystonia progressed in time, the receptive fields grew to ten times normal size, and mixing of responses became prominent. Hairy-glabrous, multiple digit, and hand-face mixing were observed in responses on single electrodes. The border between the hand and the face became patchy, with islands of facial activity progressively invading the digital representations. The thalamus was also mapped in this animal, and receptive field sizes and mixing were also abnormal, although not as abnormal as those in the cortex.

E. Animal Model Results Summary

The results of these studies support a tight relationship between motor control and sensory processing. Sensory processing is abnormal in receptive field sizes, cortical column sizes, and mixing of response modalities that are normally segregated. In animals with focal hand dystonia, receptive fields at single sites in the primary somatosensory map average up to ten times normal size. In animals with varied dystonic severity across the hand, sensory physiological abnormalities were largest on the digits most affected. Response modalities, such as single-digit representations, or representations of glabrous or hairy skin, are mixed in the hand maps of animals with the disorder. Cortical columns are also up to four times the normal size, or sixteen times the normal area. As a result of the abnormality in cortical column size, the somatosensory system has a dramatically reduced capacity to represent independent inputs. If the hand map is $6\,\text{mm}^2$, and a cortical column is $0.25\,\text{mm}^2$, then roughly twenty-four independent sensory modules exist representing the hand. If, instead, the column size is $4\,\text{mm}^2$, as seen in animals with focal hand dystonia, only one to two independent modules can represent sensory inputs across the hand. The reduced dimension of input has an expected detrimental effect on sensory-motor processing. The impact is analogous to using one to two filters on the sensory inputs to feed into all motor control patterns. Figure 2 illustrates this concept. A normal owl monkey hand map appears on the left and a single normal column size is shown over each fingertip; independent fingertip action is clearly supported by cortical column size. Now, on the right, the same figure is superimposed with column sizes closer to those in focal hand dystonia, and the mixing of inputs to different digits is apparent.

The cortical column abnormality also appears in the contralateral hemisphere. The contralateral hemisphere was

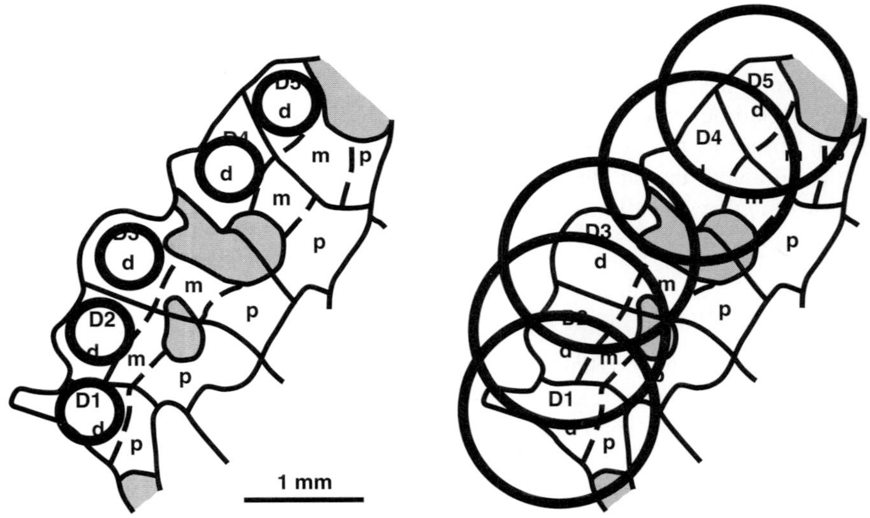

FIGURE 2 Hand maps in primary somatosensory cortex. Two copies of normal hand maps are shown on the left and right. The thumb is represented at the bottom, and the fifth digit at the top. Superimposed on each digit tip in the map on the left is a circle of the same size as the normal cortical column. On the right map, digit tips have circles superimposed on them that are the same size as cortical columns in focal hand dystonia.

never directly engaged in behavioral training, and yet enlarged receptive fields and cortical columns emerge there as a result of behavioral training and focal hand dystonia. If this same basic physiological breakdown, enlargement of cortical columns, exists in the motor cortex, it would provide a mechanism for loss of motor control, as shown in Figure 3. This figure, adapted from Donoghue et al. (1992), shows the expected result of enlarged cortical columns on the motor cortex output map. Each open circle represents flexion of the digits, and each closed circle represents extension. The darker large circles in the top figure show the expected normal cortical column, and interactions occur over about 0.5 mm. The positions representing flexion and extension are separated. But, if these columns, or interaction distances, are enlarged as seen in focal hand dystonia, flexion and extension would begin to be connected to each other. This prediction from the work in the owl monkey model suggests that columnar breakdown, and a little practice in the form of rapid stereotyped sequential movements, would cause a dramatic loss of motor function. The maps of somatosensory and motor cortex should clarify that modular independence occurs on a spatial scale of about 0.5 mm in normals. These maps are plastic (Buonomano and Merzenich 1998; Kleim et al. 1998; Nudo et al. 1996; Xerri et al. 1999; Wang et al. 1995), so that inputs that are nearby in the cortex, and occur close in time to an attended behavior, become corepresented. A violation of modular separation in motor or sensory cortex, from behaviorally driven cortical plasticity, would lead to a cascade of motor control problems.

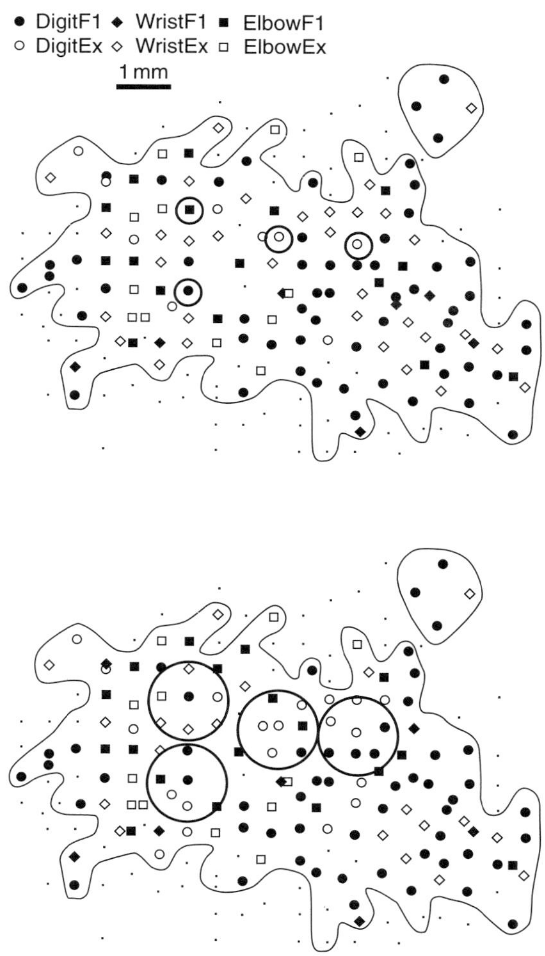

FIGURE 3 Motor maps in primary motor cortex. Two copies of normal motor maps are shown on the top and bottom. In each map, microstimulation at each site was performed, and the symbols at each location represent the muscle contractions caused. The map shows an intermingled mosaic of different muscle groups of the hand and arm. On the top map, circles are drawn of the same size as normal cortical columns, on the bottom the circles are the same size as columns observed in sensory maps of animals with focal hand dystonia. (Adapted from Donoghue et al. 1992)

IV. EFFICACY OF TREATMENTS

Several recent treatment strategies have improved sensory or motor function, or normalized sensory physiology. These strategies support the hypothesis that blurring of sensory and motor modules that are normally separated is a key component of focal hand dystonia, and that independent sensory and motor training is the most efficacious route to reestablishing normal function. This training normalizes motor modular independence, sensory modular separation, and hand function.

One treatment strategy involves sensory motor retuning (SMR), a strategy that involves splinting individual digits involved in the dystonia while the other digits are engaged in motor behavioral training (Candia et al. 2003). This process forces the independent action of adjacent digits. By forcing each digit to work independently, normal motor cortex reorganization separates modules for each digit, which predicts improved function from increased independence in motor representations. In addition, organization of somatosensory hand maps had improved, as assessed with magnetic source imaging.

Another study used a retraining strategy in which subjects read only Braille, using the digit most affected by dystonia, and the two adjacent fingers (Zeuner et al. 2002). The digits were trained individually. Several patients made significant gains in tactile discrimination, dystonia scores, and speed in hand writing after eight weeks of training. Three patients that continued training in Braille reading for a year showed continued improvement in Grating Orientation Discrimination, hand-writing speed, and self-evaluation of dystonia severity (Zeuner and Hallett 2003). In this training strategy, independent sensory function alone was isolated, and shown to have an impact on a subset of the patients. Investigators predict that independently training each digit on sensory discrimination tasks would increase the independence of the sensory representations of the digits, and aid in motor performance by providing independent sensory feedback. Finally, one study (Byl et al. 2003) used a comprehensive training plan (Byl and McKenzie 2000) that involved both independent sensory and motor training. Patients were instructed on appropriate ergonomic behaviors in the workplace and at home, and were engaged in sensory training, followed by sensory-motor training. Patients improved at all training exercises, and had nearly normal performance in their workplace pursuits at the end of training. The somatotopic organization of subjects' hand maps also improved as assessed with magnetic source imaging.

V. CONFIRMATION OF SENSORY PROCESSING DEFICITS IN HUMANS

With the documentation of sensory map abnormalities in the animal model, researchers predict that some sensory processing measures, which are sensitive to the types of perturbations seen in focal hand dystonia, would be abnormal as well. One study (Byl et al. 1996a) found abnormalities in graphesthesia and manual form perception, two percepts that require integration of somatosensory input across the skin. Two studies have found abnormally poor spatial acuity on the fingertips (Bara-Jimenez et al. 2000; Sanger et al. 2001) as assessed with a grating orientation task (Johnson and Phillips 1981). One study also found abnormal spatial localization (Bara-Jimenez et al. 2000), which is consistent with poor performance on graphesthesia and manual form perception. Temporal discrimination was also abnormal in patients with writer's cramp (Sanger et al. 2001), and patients with generalized dystonia (Tinazzi et al. 1999). In that test, patients are asked to detect the number of pulses, one or two, delivered electrically to the hand, as a function of the interval length. Patients with either writer's cramp or generalized dystonia required much longer temporal spacing to discriminate the electrical stimuli.

VI. CONFIRMATION OF SENSORY PHYSIOLOGY DEFICITS IN HUMANS

Several lines of evidence have confirmed disordered and otherwise abnormal sensory representations in somatosensory areas in humans. Studies in fMRI have found that area 1 distances from the first digit to the fifth digit are abnormally small, and are weak and disordered in other areas (Butterworth et al. 2003). Three studies from one group (Byl et al. 2000; Byl et al. 2002; McKenzie et al. 2003) used magnetic source imaging to look at the hand representation in focal hand dystonia, and found temporally abnormal evoked fields, and abnormal spatial disorganization as predicted by animal studies. A third study from another group found similar somatosensory spatial disorganization (Bara-Jimenez et al. 1998). Micro-electrode work in the human thalamus has found receptive field and map organization in patients with dystonia to be consistent with the findings in the animal studies (Lenz and Byl 1999; Hua et al. 2000). Receptive fields shifted more slowly along electrode tracks than in normal animals, which correlates with increased representational size for a point on the peripheral receptor sheet. This finding is a thalamic correlate of increased column size in primary somatosensory cortex.

VII. CONCLUSIONS

The owl monkey model of focal hand dystonia has uncovered an array of physiological abnormalities associated with the disorder. Enlarged receptive fields, enlarged columns, and a breakdown of modality separation are all now known to be part of the physiological manifestation of the disorder. Sensory testing in humans has revealed a parallel set of associated psychophysical and physiological abnormalities. Treatment strategies based in part or in whole on restoring sensory function have positively impacted patient populations. As this work progresses, the combined synergy of the human studies and animal work should serve to greatly reduce the impact of focal hand dystonia on our population.

References

Bara-Jimenez, W., M.J. Catalan, M. Hallett, and C. Gerloff. 1998. Abnormal somatosensory homunculus in dystonia of the hand. *Ann Neurol* **44**:828–831.

Bara-Jimenez, W., P. Shelton, T. Sanger, and M. Hallett. 2000. Sensory discrimination capabilities in patients with focal hand dystonia. *Ann Neurol* **47**:377–380.

Blake, D., N. Byl, S. Cheung, P. Bedenbaugh, S. Nagarajan, M. Lamb, and M. Merzenich. 2002. Sensory representation abnormalities that parallel focal hand dystonia in a primate model. *Somatosens Motor Res* **19(4)**:347–357.

Buonomano, D.V., and M.M. Merzenich. 1998. Cortical plasticity: from synapses to maps. *Ann Rev Neurosci* **21**:97–102.

Butterworth, S., S. Francis, E. Kelly, F. McGlone, R. Bowtell, and G. Sawle. 2003. Abnormal cortical sensory activation in dystonia: an fmri study. *Mov Disord* **18**:673–682.

Byl, N., F. Wilson, M. Merzenich, M. Melnick, P. Scott, A. Oakes, and A. McKenzie. 1996a. Sensory dysfunction associated with repetitive strain injuries of tendinitis and focal hand dystonia: a comparative study. *J Orthop Sports Phys Ther* **23**:234–244.

Byl, N.N., M.M. Merzenich, S. Cheung, P. Bedenbaugh, S.S. Nagarajan, and W.M. Jenkins. 1997. A primate model for studying focal dystonia and repetitive strain injury: effects on the primary somatosensory cortex. *Physical Therapy* **77**:269–284.

Byl, N.N., M.M. Merzenich, and W.M. Jenkins. 1996b. A primate genesis model of focal dystonia and repetitive strain injury: I. learning-induced dedifferentiation of the representation of the hand in the primary somatosensory cortex in adult monkeys. *Neurol* **47**:508–520.

Byl, N., and A. McKenzie. 2000. Treatment effectiveness for patients with a history of repetitive hand use and focal hand dystonia: a planned, prospective follow-up study. *J Hand Ther* **13**:289–301.

Byl, N., A. McKenzie, and S. Nagarajan. 2000. Differences in somatosensory hand organization in a healthy flutist and a flutist with focal hand dystonia: a case report. *J Hand Ther* **13**:302–309.

Byl, N., S. Nagajaran, and A. McKenzie. 2003. Effect of sensory discrimination training on structure and function in patients with focal hand dystonia: a case series. *Arch Phys Med Rehabil* **84**:1505–1514.

Byl, N., S. Nagarajan, M. Merzenich, T. Roberts, and A. McKenzie. 2002. Correlation of clinical neuromusculoskeletal and central somatosensory performance: variability in controls and patients with severe and mild focal hand dystonia. *Neural Plast* **9**:177–203.

Candia, V., C. Wienbruch, T. Elbert, B. Rockstroh, and W. Ray. 2003. Effective behavioral treatment of focal hand dystonia in musicians alters somatosensory cortical organization. *Proc Nat Acad Sci USA* **100**: 7942–7946.

Chen, R.S., C.H. Tsai, and C.S. Lu. 1995. Reciprocal inhibition in writer's cramp. *Movement Disorders* **10**:556–561.

Cohen, L.G., M. Hallett, B.D. Geller, and F. Hochberg. 1989. Treatment of focal dystonias of the hand with botulinum toxin injections. *J Neurol Neurosurgery Psych* **52**:355–363.

Donoghue, J., S. Leibovic, and J. Sanes. 1992. Organization of the forelimb area in squirrel monkey motor cortex: representation of digit, wrist, and elbow muscles. *Exp Brain Res* **89**:1–19.

Dykes, R., D. Rasmusson, D. Sretavan, and N. Rehman. 1982. Submodality segregation and receptive-field sequences in cuneate, gracile, and external cuneate nuclei of the cat. *J Neurophysiol* **47**:389–416.

Gordon, G., and C. Paine. 1960. Functional organization in nucleus gracilis of the cat. *J Physiol* **153**:331–349.

Gould, H., Jr, C.G. Cusick, T.P. Pons, and J.H. Kaas. 1986. The relationship of corpus callosum connections to electrical stimulation maps of motor, supplementary motor, and the frontal eye fields in owl monkeys. *J Comp Neurol* **247**:297–325.

Hua, S., I. Garonzik, J. Lee, and F. Lenz. 2000. Microelectrode studies of normal organization and plasticity of human somatosensory thalamus. *J Clin Neurophysiol* **17**:559–574.

Huntley, G., and E. Jones. 1991. Relationship of intrinsic connections to forelimb movement representations in monkey motor cortex: a correlative anatomic and physiological study. *J Neurophysiol* **66**: 390–413.

Johnson, J.I., W. Welker, and B.H. Pubols, Jr. 1968. Somatotopic organization of raccoon dorsal column nuclei. *J Comp Neurol* **132**:1–43.

Johnson, K.O., and S.S. Hsiao. 1992. Neural mechanisms of tactual form and texture perception. *Ann Rev Neurosci* **15**:227–250.

Johnson, K., and J. Phillips. 1981. Tactile spatial resolution. i. two-point discrimination, gap detection, grating resolution, and letter recognition. *J Neurophysiol* **46**:1177–1192.

Jones, E.G. 1985. *The Thalamus*. New York: Plenum Press.

Kleim, J.A., S. Barbay, and R.J. Nudo. 1998. Functional reorganization of the rat motor cortex following motor skill learning. *J Neurophysiol* **80**: 3321–3325.

Kruger, L., R. Siminoff, and P. Witkovsky. 1961. Single neuron analysis of dorsal column nuclei and spinal nucleus of trigeminal in cat. *J Neurophysiol* **24**:333–349.

Kwan, H., W. MacKay, J. Murphy, and Y. Wong. 1978. Spatial organization of precentral cortex in awake primates. ii. motor outputs. *J Neurophysiol* **41**:1120–1131.

Lagueny, A., P. Burbaud, J. Dubos, G. LeMasson, D. Guelh, F. Macia, C. Debras, and F. Tison. 2002. Freezing of shoulder flexion impeding boule throwing: a form of task-specific focal dystonia in petanque players. *Mov Disord* **17**:1092–1095.

Lenz, F.A., and N.N. Byl. 1999. Reorganization in the cutaneous core of the human thalamic principal somatic sensory nucleus (ventral caudal) in patients with dystonia. *J Neurophysiol* **82**:3204–3212.

Liddle, E.G.T., and C.S. Sherrington. 1924. Reflexes in response to stretch (myotatic reflexes). *Proc R Soc Lond B Biol Sci* **96**:212–242.

Lockwood, A.H. 1989. Medical problems of musicians [see comments]. *New England J Medicine* **320**:221–227.

Marsden, C.D., and M.P. Sheehy. 1990. Writer's cramp. *Trends Neurosci* **13**:148–153.

McComas, A.J. 1963. Responses of the rat dorsal column system to mechanical stimulation of the hindpaw. *J Physiol London* **166**:435–448.

McKenzie, A., S. Nagarajan, T. Roberts, M. Merzenich, and N. Byl. 2003. Somatosensory representation of the digits and clinical performance in patients with focal hand dystonia. *Am J Phys Med Rehabil* **82**:737–749.

Merzenich, M.M., J.H. Kaas, M. Sur, and C.S. Lin. 1978. Double representation of the body surface within cytoarchitectonic areas 3b and 1 in. *J Comp Neurol* **181**:41–73.

Millar, J., and A. Basbaum. 1975. Topography of the projection of the body surface of the cat to cuneate and gracile nuclei. *Exp Neurol* **49**:281–290.

Mountcastle, V.B. 1957. Modality and topographic properties of single neurons of the cat's somatic sensory cortex. *J Neurophysiol* **20**:408–434.

Mountcastle, V.B., and J.E. Rose. 1952. Activity of single neurons of the somatic sensory nuclear complex of the thalamus. *Federation Proc* **109**:11.

Newmark, J., and F.H. Hochberg. 1987. Isolated painless manual incoordination in 57 musicians. *J Neurol Neurosurgery Psych* **50**:291–295.

Nudo, R.J., W.M. Jenkins, M.M. Merzenich, T. Prejean, and R. Grenda. 1992. Neurophysiological correlates of hand preference in primary motor cortex of adult squirrel monkeys. *J Neurosci* **12**:2918–2947.

Nudo, R.J., G.W. Milliken, W.M. Jenkins, and M.M. Merzenich. 1996. Use-dependent alterations of movement representations in primary motor cortex of adult squirrel monkeys. *J Neurosci* **16**:785–807.

Paul, R.L., M.M. Merzenich, and H. Goodman. 1972. Representation of slowly and rapidly adapting cutaneous mechanoreceptors of the hand in Brodmann's areas 3 and 1 of macaca mulatta. *Brain Research* **36**: 229–249.

Perl, E., D. Whitlock, and J. Gentry. 1962. Cutaneous projection to second-order neurons of the dorsal column system. *J Neurophysiol* **25**:337–358.

Powell, T.P., and V.B. Mountcastle. 1959. Some aspects of the functional organization of the cortex of the postcentral gyrus of the monkey: a correlation of findings obtained in a single unit analysis with cytoarchitecture. *Bull Johns Hopkins Hospital* **105**:133–162.

Rothwell, J.C., J.A. Obeso, B.L. Day, and C.D. Marsden. 1983. Pathophysiology of dystonias. *Advances Neurol* **39**:851–863.

Sanger, T., D. Tarsy, and A. Pascual-Leone. 2001. Abnormalities of spatial and temporal sensory discrimination in writer's cramp. *Mov Disord* **16**: 94–99.

Sessle, B., and M. Wiesendanger. 1982. Structural and functional definition of the motor cortex in the monkey (macaca fascicularis). *J Physiol* **323**: 245–265.

Sheehy, M.P., and C.D. Marsden. 1982. Writer's cramp—a focal dystonia. *Brain* **105**:461–480.

Smith, A., C. Adler, D. Crews, R. Wharen, E. Laskowski, K. Barnes, C. ValoneBell, et al. 2003. The 'yips' in golf: a continuum between a focal dystonia and choking. *Sports Med* **33**:13–31.

Strick, P., and J. Preston. 1982. Two representations of the hand in area 4 of a primate. i. motor output organization. *J Neurophysiol* **48**:139–149.

Sur, M., M.M. Merzenich, and J.H. Kaas. 1980. Magnification, receptive-field area, and "hypercolumn" size in areas 3b and 1 of somatosensory cortex in owl monkeys. *J Neurophysiol* **44**:295–311.

Sur, M., J.T. Wall, and J.H. Kaas. 1984. Modular distribution of neurons with slowly adapting and rapidly adapting responses in area 3b of somatosensory cortex in monkeys. *J Neurophysiol* **51**:724–744.

Tinazzi, M., E. Frasson, L. Bertolasi, A. Fiaschi, and S. Aglioti. 1999. Temporal discrimination of somesthetic stimuli is impaired in dystonic patients. *Neuroreport* **10**:1547–1550.

Wang, X., M.M. Merzenich, K. Sameshima, and W.M. Jenkins. 1995. Remodelling of hand representation in adult cortex determined by timing of tactile stimulation. *Nature* **378**:71–75.

Wilson, F.R. 1989. Acquisition and loss of skilled movement in musicians. *Seminars Neurol* **9**:146–151.

Winter, D.L.N. 1965. N. gracilis of cat. Functional organization and corticofugal effects. *J Neurophysiol* **28**:48–70.

Xerri, C., M.M. Merzenich, W. Jenkins, and S. Santucci. 1999. Representational plasticity in cortical area 3b paralleling tactual-motor skill acquisition in adult monkeys. *Cerebral Cortex* **9**:264–276.

Zeuner, K., W. Bara-Jimenez, P. Noguchi, S. Goldstein, J. Dambrosia, and M. Hallett. 2002. Sensory training for patients with focal hand dystonia. *Ann Neurol* **51**:593–598.

Zeuner, K., and M. Hallett. 2003. Sensory training as treatment for focal hand dystonia: a 1-year follow-up. *Mov Disord* **18**:1044–1047.

C H A P T E R

C6

DYT1 Transgenic Mouse

NUTAN SHARMA, D. CRISTOPHER BRAGG, JEREMY PETRAVICZ,
DAVID G. STANDAERT, and XANDRA O. BREAKEFIELD

The most common type of early-onset, generalized dystonia is a GAG deletion in the DYT1 (TOR1A) gene encoding torsinA. This mutation results in loss of a glutamic acid residue near the carboxy terminus of torsinA. The function of torsinA is unknown, but it is a member of the AAA+ superfamily of chaperone proteins that serve a variety of functions within the cell, including proper folding and degrading of proteins, organelle biogenesis, and vesicle movement and release from nerve terminals.

To determine the role of the DYT1 mutation in generating a dystonic phenotype, we established multiple lines of transgenic mice that express either mutant or wild-type human torsinA controlled by the strong, constitutive CMV promoter. Western blots of brain homogenates reveal elevated expression of torsinA using a specific antibody. Transgenic mice expressing human mutant torsinA displayed normal movement during the first six months of life, but then manifested abnormal posturing in the limbs, reminiscent of dystonic movements.

I. DYT1 DYSTONIA

The most common type of early-onset generalized dystonia is DYT1 dystonia. The DYT1 mutation consists of a 3-bp deletion (GAG) in the DYT1 (TOR1A) gene that encodes the protein, torsinA (1). Symptoms of this disorder typically present before the age of twenty-one with involuntary sustained muscle contractions that cause posturing of a foot, leg, or arm. The contractions frequently, but not invariably, generalize to other body regions. No other neurological abnormalities are usually present, except for postural arm tremor. Disease severity can vary considerably within the same family. Isolated writer's cramp may be the only sign of dystonia in one family member, whereas another relative may exhibit multifocal or generalized dystonia (2). The lifespan of affected individuals is not shortened and no evidence exists of other medical problems that can be attributed to the DYT1 mutation. Rarely does onset of symptoms occur after the age of twenty-eight, suggesting a window of susceptibility during postnatal development.

DYT1 is inherited in an autosomal dominant manner (3). Offspring of a mating between a carrier and noncarrier have a 50% chance of inheriting the disease-causing mutation, but only a 30–40% chance of developing abnormalities that are detected on clinical exam. The lack of phenotypic expression in 60–70% of those who carry the DYT1 mutation is referred to as reduced penetrance. Thus, although the DYT1 mutation is necessary, it is not sufficient to cause disease. Secondary factors (environmental or genetic) must operate in conjunction with the DYT1 mutation. Numerous reports suggest the role of a modifying gene(s) or environmental agent in variable disease expression in individuals who share the same disease mutation. For example, adult and childhood forms of adrenoleukodystrophy can be caused by the same mutations in the X-ALD gene (4) (5). Three families with severe cases of autosomal recessive limb-girdle muscular dystrophy have the same mutation in the γ-sarcoglycan gene as a family with much milder symptoms (6). Sex-of-affected-parent may play a role in determining severity of disease in affected offspring, in that maternally transmitted DYT1 dystonia tends toward somewhat later onset and milder expression (7). Environmental factors, specifically childhood infection and peripheral trauma, have been posited as triggers in the expression of DYT1 dystonia. One recent, retrospective study identified varicella or mumps infection prior to the age of six years as increasing the risk that a DYT1 carrier will develop dystonia (8). However, this epidemiologic study must be repeated in a larger cohort. In addition, the pathophysiologic mechanism by which a viral infection prior to the age of six years precipitates the expression of dystonia is not clear.

In the few cases examined, no evidence exists of significant neuropathology in DYT1 dystonia. Two recent reports, utilizing different antibodies against torsinA, characterized torsinA expression in the brains of individuals with DYT1 dystonia and control brains. Both reports did not reveal any differences in the pattern of torsinA immunoreactivity with the brains of individuals with DYT1 dystonia (9) (10). However, Rostasy et al. did report a trend toward larger size of nigral dopaminergic neurons in dystonia brains versus normal brains (10).

II. THE TORSINA PROTEIN

The DYT1 gene, on chromosome 9q34, encodes the protein torsinA. TorsinA is a 332 amino acid protein of 37,800 Daltons with potential sites for glycosylation and phosphorylation. TorsinA appears to be an endoplasmic reticulum (ER) lumenal protein with an N-terminal signal sequence and potential membrane-spanning domain (1) (11) (12) (13). Its high mannose glycosylation pattern is consistent with this predominant ER localization.

Although the function of torsinA is unknown, its deduced amino acid sequence provides some clues as to its biochemical properties. Analysis of the primary amino acid sequence of torsinA reveals that it is a member of the AAA^+ ATPase gene family (14) (15). The AAA^+ ATPases are a superfamily of proteins that have in common an ATP-binding domain, an AAA^+-specific region of homology, and usually a six-membered oligomeric ring structure (16). Members of this family are typically chaperone proteins, which mediate conformational changes in target proteins. The cellular functions in which they participate are numerous, including protein folding and degradation, membrane trafficking, and vesicle fusion. Well-known members of this family include N-ethylmaleimide-sensitive factor (NSF), which is essential for vesicle recycling events throughout the cell, including those between synaptic vesicles and plasma membrane in nerve terminals (17); cytoplasmic dynein, which is a microtubule-based motor involved in organelle movement (18); and various Clp/Hsp100 proteins, which are implicated in promoting protein folding, renaturation, and degradation (19).

TorsinA monomers are predicted to form a six-membered, doughnut-like ring structure within the lumen of the ER, consistent with the structures of other members of the AAA^+ ATPase superfamily (20). TorsinA is membrane-associated and may be tethered to the ER membrane via hydrophobic sequences in the amino terminus (21) (22). The loss of the glutamic acid residue in the carboxyl terminal of one or more subunits might act to disrupt either closure of the ring or interaction with a partner protein. If the mutation prevents contact or communication between homomers, even a single defective member could render all torsinA molecules within the ring inactive, accounting for the dominant effect of the mutation. When expressed in cultured cells, the GAG-deleted, but not wild-type, torsinA forms membrane whorls, apparently derived from the ER and frequently associated with the nuclear membrane (11) (12) (23). One hypothesis regarding the pathogenesis of DYT1 dystonia is that a mutation in torsinA may result in abnormalities in membrane trafficking and downstream vesicular release from neurons. Abnormalities in vesicular release may cause deficits in neurotransmitter signaling among neurons, resulting in a dystonic phenotype.

III. DOPAMINE AND DYSTONIA

Investigators have reported data supporting the hypothesis that abnormalities in dopamine transmission play a role in the pathophysiology of DYT1 dystonia. The mRNA for torsinA is strongly expressed in dopamine neurons in normal adult human brain (24, 25). TorsinA immunoreactivity is found within axons and presynaptic terminals in adult human and nonhuman primate striatum (26). Morphologically, some of the torsinA immunoreactive terminals resemble dopamine terminals, and within the terminals torsinA immunoreactivity is found in association with vesicles (26) (26). Additional studies analyzed dopamine, its metabolites, dopamine transporters, and dopamine receptors in four postmortem DYT1 brains (27). During life, three of the individuals had carried a clinical diagnosis of dystonia and one had carried a clinical diagnosis of Parkinsonism. The tissue content of dopamine and its metabolites 3,4-dihydroxyphenylacetic acid (DOPAC) and homovanillic acid (HVA) were measured by HPLC from these cases as well as a group of controls (n = 6) matched for age and postmortem interval. In the DYT1 brains, striatal dopamine was low and DOPAC was elevated, which resulted in a significant increase in the DOPAC/dopamine ratio. The densities of the presynaptic high affinity dopamine transporter (DAT: $[H^3]$-mazindol), the vesicular transporter (VMAT2: $[H^3]$-dihydrotetrabenazine), and both the postsynaptic dopamine D1 ($[H^3]$-SCH23390) and D2 receptor ($[H^3]$-YM-09151-2) sites were measured by quantitative autoradiography. No significant differences were found in the density of DAT or VMAT2 binding; however, there was a trend towards a reduction in D1 receptor (−15%) and D2 receptor (−40%) binding. Collectively, these data are consistent with an intact nigrostriatal pathway in those with an abnormal neurological phenotype and carrying the DYT1 mutation, yet the data suggest an increase in striatal dopamine turnover coupled with a reduction in postsynaptic dopamine D1 and D2 receptor binding. A weakness of this study is the small number of cases, which reflects the very limited number of DYT1 cases currently available from brain banks and other sources. In addition, data on neurotransmitter levels from postmortem human DYT1 are limited in their ability to shed light on the pathogenesis of DYT1 dystonia in a living organism.

IV. TRANSGENIC MICE

Identification of the DYT1 gene now makes it possible to generate genetic mouse models of early onset dystonia that should bring insights into the pathophysiology of this condition. These animals will provide a more physiologically relevant picture of torsinA function than could be achieved by studies in cell culture or postmortem human tissue. In addition, phenotypic analysis of the mice should provide insight into the mechanism by which expression of the GAG-deleted torsinA protein results in dystonia in humans.

A torsinA construct containing the immediate early CMV promoter and the cDNA for either human wild-type or human mutant torsinA (Figure 1) was introduced into B6C3Fq fertilized eggs that were implanted in C57BL/6 mice (11). Investigators identified founder offspring by detecting the transgene with both Southern blot and polymerase chain reaction (PCR) analysis. Based on the strength of the transgene signal, three founder mice, one expressing human wild-type torsinA (C3-NC) and two expressing human mutant torsinA (C5-1L and C5-1R) were chosen for subsequent backcrosses to generate three distinct colonies of transgenic mice. Table 1 lists the names of the three transgenic lines and the protein expressed by each.

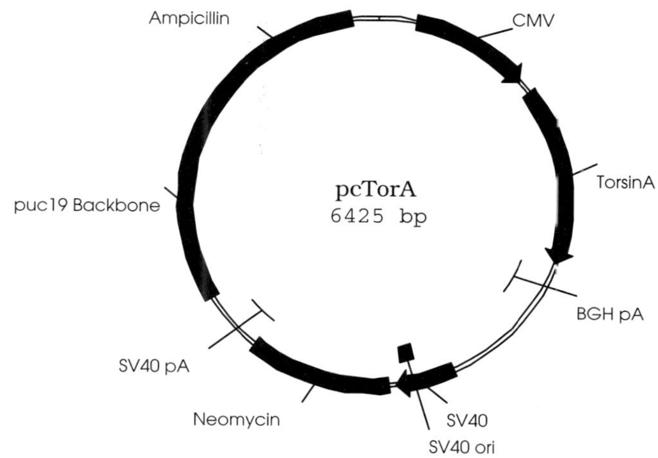

FIGURE 1 The pcTorA construct, containing either the human wild-type or GAG-deleted torsinA sequence, driven by the human CMV promoter.

TABLE 1 Nomenclature of the Three Transgenic Lines and the Protein that Each Line Expresses

Line	Protein expressed
C3-NC	Human wild-type torsinA
C5-1L	Human GAG-deleted torsinA
C5-1R	Human GAG-deleted torsinA

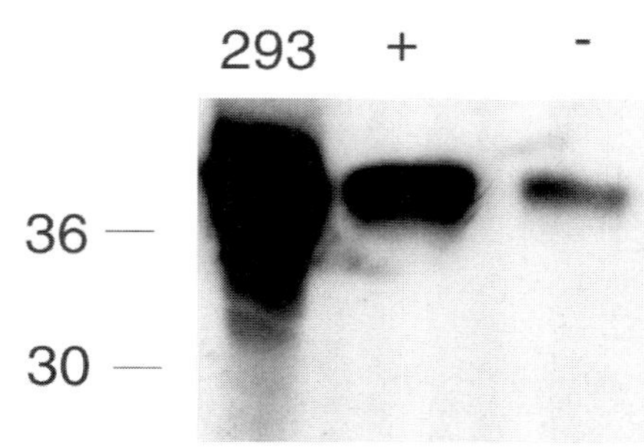

FIGURE 2 Western blot analysis of the crude nuclear pellet fraction from mice expressing human mutant torsinA (+) and wild type litter mate controls (−). 293 indicates torsinA overexpressed in HEK293 cells. Blot probed with D-M2A8 antibody to torsinA.

A. Protein Expression

Investigators analyzed crude nuclear fractions from transgenic mice, heterozygous for human wild-type or mutant torsinA and their nontransgenic littermates for torsinA expression by western blot analysis. An example of such a western blot is shown in Figure 2 in which equal amounts of brain homogenate protein of littermates from the C5-1R line was analyzed. The brain of the transgene-positive mouse (+) expresses significantly higher levels of the 37 kD torsinA protein than the brain of its nontransgenic littermate (−). Researchers have performed similar western blots in the other two lines of transgenic mice (C5-1L and C3-NC), both of which also demonstrate increased expression of the 37 kD torsinA protein in the transgene positive mouse when compared to its nontransgenic littermate.

Thus, western blot analysis confirms that the two lines of transgenic mice expressing human mutant torsinA and one line of transgenic mice expressing human wild-type torsinA have been established. Any pathologic, phenotypic, or neurochemical abnormalities that are found in one line of mice expressing human mutant torsinA should be duplicated in the second line, to ensure that the abnormality is due to expression of the mutant transgene and not to the insertion site of the transgene in the mouse genome. In addition, any pathologic, phenotypic, or neurochemical abnormalities that are found in both lines of mice expressing human mutant torsinA should not be seen in the line expressing human wild-type torsinA, to ensure that the abnormality is due to expression of the mutant protein and not simply due to overexpression of a human torsin protein in the mouse.

B. Phenotype of DYT1 Transgenic Mice

Initial phenotypic characterization of the mice involved a systematic study of posture. Founder mice, aged fourteen months, were analyzed for abnormalities in limb position when hung by the tail. Wild-type mice are known to extend their hind limbs when held in such a position, whereas other transgenic mice expressing, for example, the mutant huntingtin gene display prominent clasping of the forelimbs in front of their body (28). Figure 3 depicts the postural abnormalities seen in one of the two 14-month-old founders expressing human mutant torsinA (C5-1L) compared to the 14-month-old founder of the line expressing human wild-type torsinA (C3-NC). The mouse expressing human wild-type torsinA displayed extension of the hind limbs, which is the normal response seen in nontransgenic mice. The mouse expressing human mutant torsinA displayed marked abnormalities in posture, with the hind limbs adducted and retracted to such a marked degree that the paws are barely visible.

The accompanying digital video demonstrates the hindlimb posturing in a fourteen-month-old C57/BL6 mouse, the fourteen-month-old founder of the C3-NC line and the fourteen-month-old founder of the C5-1L line. Each mouse was held by the tail for sixty seconds and videotaped. Both the C57/BL6 mouse and the C3-NC mouse displayed similar posturing, composed of extension of the hind limbs with multiple attempts to elevate the head and climb into an upright position. In contrast, the C5-1L founder displayed marked adduction of the hind limbs, but not clasping of the fore limbs as seen in transgenic mouse models of Huntington disease (28). This abnormal posturing seen in the mouse expressing human mutant torsinA may represent a sensitive marker of abnormal motor control, tone, or both.

To quantify this postural abnormality, two- and four-month-old F2 progeny from the two transgenic lines expressing human mutant torsinA (C5-1L and C5-1R) were hung by the tail for sixty seconds and videotaped. Two observers, blinded to genotype, ranked the posture using a numerical scale in which 1 represented normal posture, 5 represented curling of the toes of one or both hind paws, and 10 represented curling of one or both entire hind limbs. An average score for mice from the same founder, with the same age and genotype, was calculated and is shown in Table 2. The four-month-old progeny of the C5-1L line display a

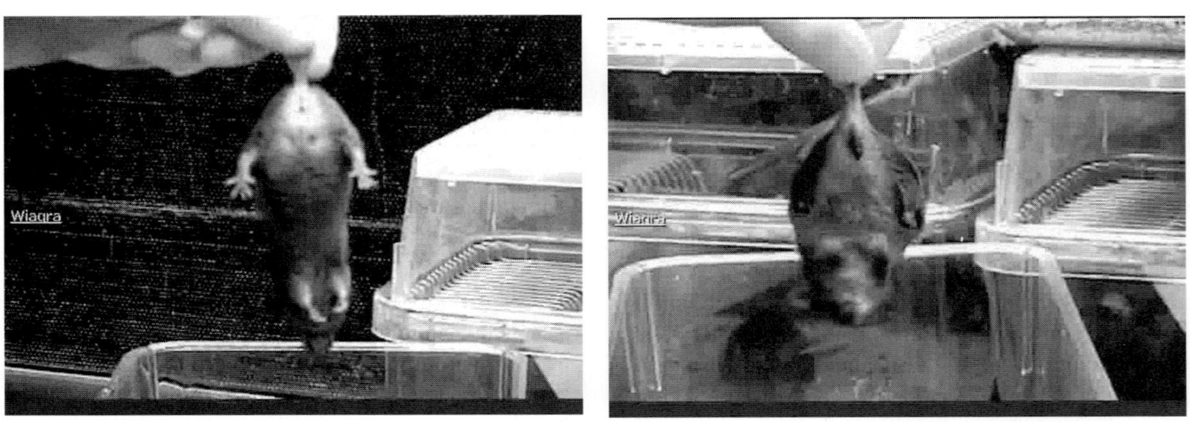

FIGURE 3 Tail hanging and resultant posture seen in the 14-month-old founder of the line expressing human wild-type torsinA (on left, C3-NC line founder) and one of the two 14-month-old founders expressing human mutant torsinA (on right, C5-1L founder). The mouse expressing human mutant torsinA displays marked abnormalities in posture.

TABLE 2 Quantitative Analysis of Abnormal Posture

Line	Genotype	Sample size	Age	Score
C5-1L	+	2	2 mo	2
	−	3	2 mo	1.5
	+	6	4 mo	**3.7**
	−	1	4 mo	**1.5**
C5-1R	+	6	2 mo	1.3
	−	2	2 mo	2.3
	+	5	4 mo	2.1
	−	1	4 mo	1.5

Progeny from two lines, both expressing human mutant torsinA, are shown. Transgenic mice (+) and their non-transgenic littermates (−) were compared at 2 and 4 months of age. Abbreviations: mo = months old.

markedly abnormal posture compared to their nontransgenic littermates (score in **bold**). Although these findings are promising, the animals were young and the sample size was small.

To perform detailed phenotypic analysis, investigators are currently back-crossing heterozygous transgenic mice to C57Bl/6J mice. They will conduct ten generations of back-crosses to generate transgenic and nontransgenic littermates in a genetically homogenous background. The resulting progeny will be used for systematic, in-depth evaluation of posture and other behavioral characteristics, including performance on a rotarod and spontaneous locomotor activity.

V. FUTURE ANALYSIS

Acquired, focal dystonia can be precipitated by either extended practice of skilled movements or damage to the neuronal circuits that are implicated in motor learning (29) (30). From these observations, investigators propose a theory that dystonia results from a failure of adaptive mechanisms that normally support the acquisition of new skills. This theory is supported by the demonstration by Dr. Eidelberg and colleagues of abnormalities in motor sequence learning in nonmanifesting human carriers of the DYT1 mutation (31). Thus, it is reasonable to study mice carrying the DYT1 mutation for abnormalities in motor learning. The most widely accepted and validated tool for the study of motor skills in the mouse is the rotarod (32). Thus, in addition to systematically evaluating posture with an emphasis on detecting abnormal postures similar to those seen in humans with dystonia, investigators will study future generations of DYT1 transgenic mice for their ability to maintain balance and remain coordinated with repeated rotarod testing.

Acknowledgments

This work was supported by the Jack Fasciana Fund for Support of Dystonia Research (XOB) and NINDS NS37409 (XOB) and NINDS NS044272-01A1 (NS).

Video Legend

Hindlimb posturing in a 14-month-old C57/BL6 mouse, the 14-month-old founder of the C3-NC line (i.e., human wild-type torsinA transgenic) and the 14-month-old founder of the C5-1L line (human GAG-deleted torsinA transgenic). Each mouse was held by the tail for 60 seconds and then video-taped. Both the C57/BL6 and the C3-NC mice display similar posturing, comprised of extension of the hindlimbs with multiple attempts to elevate the head and climb into an upright position. In contrast, the C5-1L founder displays marked adduction of the hindlimbs, but not clasping of the fore-limbs as seen in transgenic mouse models of Huntington disease.

References

1. Ozelius, L., J.W. Hewett, C.E. Page, S.B. Bressman, P.L. Kramer, C. Shalish, D. de Leon, et al. 1997. The early-onset torsion dystonia gene (DYT1) encodes an ATP-binding protein. *Nat Genet* **17**:40–48.
2. Bressman, S.B., D. de Leon, M.F. Brin, N. Risch, R.E. Burke, P.E. Greene, H. Shale, S. Fahn. 1989. Idiopathic dystonia among Ashkenazi Jews: evidence for autosomal dominant inheritance. *Ann Neurol* **26**:612–620.
3. Bressman, S., S. Fahn, L.J. Ozelius, P.L. Kramer, N.J. Risch. 2001. The DYT1 mutation and nonfamilial primary torsion dystonia. *Arch Neurol* **58**:681–682.
4. McGuinness, M.G., G.V. Raymond, C.A. Washington, H.W. Moser, and K.D. Smith. 1995. Tumor necrosis factor-alpha and X-linked adrenoleukodystrophy. *J Neuroimmunol* **61**:161–169.
5. Moser, H., A.B. Moser, K.D. Smith, A. Bergin, J. Borel, J. Shankroff, O.C. Stine, et al. 1992. Adrenoleukodystrophy: phenotypic variabilty and implications for therapy. *J Inherit Metab Dis* **15**:645–664.
6. McNally, E., M.R. Passos-Bueno, C.G. Bonnemann, M. Vainzof, E. de Sa Moreira, M.G.W. Lidov, K.B. Othmane, et al. 1997. Mild and severe muscular dystrophy caused by a single y-saracoglycan mutation. *Am J Hum Genet* **59**:1040–1047.
7. de Leon, D., S.B. Bressman, M.F. Brin, N.J. Risch, and S. Fahn. 1992. Torsion dystonia in Ashkenazi Jews: Is there evidence for an imprinted gene? *Mov Disord* **7**:297.
8. Saunders-Pullman, R., J. Shriberg, V. Shanker, and S.B. Bressman. 2004. Penetrance and expression of dystonia genes. *Adv Neurol* **94**:121–125.
9. Walker, R., M.F. Brin, D. Sandu, P.F. Good, and P. Shashidharan. 2002. TorsinA immunoreactivity in brains of patients with DYT1 and non-DYT1 dystonia. *Neurology* **58**:120–124.
10. Rostasy, K., S.J. Augood, J.W. Hewett, J.C. Leung, H. Sasaki, L.J. Ozelius, V. Ramesh, et al. 2003. TorsinA protein and neuropathology in early onset generalized dystonia with GAG deletion. *Neurobiol Dis* **12**:11–24.
11. Hewett, J., C. Gonzalez-Agosti, D. Slater, P. Ziefer, S. Li, D. Bergeron, D.J. Jacoby, et al. 2000. Mutant torsinA, responsible for early onset torsion dystonia, forms membrane inclusions in neural cells. *Hum Mol Genet* **9(9)**:1403–1413.
12. Kustedjo, K., M.H. Bracey, and B.F. Cravatt. 2000. Torsin A and its torsion dystonia-associated mutant forms are lumenal glycoproteins that exhibit distinct subcellular localizations. *J Biol Chem* **275(36)**: 27933–27939.
13. Hewett, J., P. Ziefer, D. Bergeron, T. Naismith, H. Boston, D. Slater, J. Wilbur, et al. 2003. TorsinA in PC12 cells: localization in the

endoplasmic reticulum and response to stress. *J Neurosci Res* **72**: 158–168.

14. Lupas, A., J.M. Flanagan, T. Tamura, and W. Baumeister. 1997. Self-compartmentalization proteases. *Trends Biochem Sci* **22**:399–404.
15. Neuwald, A., L. Aravind, J.L. Spouge, and E.V. Koonin. 1999. AAA+: A class of chaperone-like ATPases associated with the assembly, operation, and disassembly of protein complexes. *Genome Res* **9(1)**: 27–43.
16. Vale, R. 2001. AAA proteins: lords of the ring. *J Cell Biol* **150**:F13–F19.
17. Hanson, P.I., R. Roth, H. Morisaki, R. Jahn, and J. Heuser. 1997. Structure and conformation changes in NSf and its membrane receptor complexes visualized by quick-freeze/deep-etch electron microscopy. *Cell* **90**:523–535.
18. Asai, D., and M.P. Koonce. 2001. The dynein heavy chain: structure, mechanics and evolution. *Trends Cell Biol* **11**:196–202.
19. Wickner, S., M.R. Maurizi, and S. Gottesman. 1999. Posttranslational quality control: folding, refolding, and degrading proteins. *Science* **286**:1888–1893.
20. Breakefield, X.O., C. Kamm, and P.I. Hanson. 2001. TorsinA: movement at many levels. *Neuron* **31(1)**:9–12.
21. Kustedjo, K., S. Deechongkit, J.W. Kelly, and B.F. Cravatt. 2003. Recombinant expression, purification, and comparative characterization of TorsinA and its torsion dystonia-associated variant E-TorsinA. *Biochemistry* **42**:15333–15341.
22. Liu, Z., A. Zolkiewska, and M. Zolkiewski. 2003. Characterization of human torsinA and its dystonia-associated mutant form. *Biochem J* **374(1)**:117–122.
23. Bragg, D., D.J. Slater, and X.O. Breakefield. 2004. TorsinA and early onset torsion dystonia. In *Dystonia 4: Advances in Neurology*. Ed. S. Fahn, M. Hallet, and M.R. DeLong. pp. 87–93. Philadelphia: Lipincott, Williams, Wilkins.
24. Augood, S., J.B. Penney, I.K. Friberg, X.O. Breakefield, A.B. Young, L.J. Ozelius, and D.G. Standaert. 1998. Expression of the early-onset torsion dystonia gene (DYT1) in human brain. *Ann Neurol* **43**:669–673.
25. Augood, S., D.M. Martin, L.J. Ozelius, X.O. Breakefield, J.B. Penney, and D.G. Standaert. 1999. Distribution of the mRNAs encoding torsinA and torsinB in the normal adult human brain. *Ann Neurol* **46**:761–769.
26. Augood, S.J., C.E. Keller-McGandy, A. Siriani, J. Hewett, V. Ramesh, E. Sapp, M. Difiglia, et al. 2003. Distribution and ultrastructural localization of torsinA immunoreactivity in the human brain. *Brain Res* **986**:12–21.
27. Augood, S.J., Z. Hollingsworth, D.S. Albers, L. Yang, J.C. Leung, B. Muller, C. Klein, et al. 2002. Dopamine transmission in DYT1 dystonia: a biochemical and autoradiographic study. *Neurology* **59**:445–448.
28. Mangiarini, L., K. Sathasivam, M. Seller, B. Cozens, A. Harper, C. Hetherington, M. Lawton, et al. 1996. Exon 1 of the HD gene with an expanded CAG repeat is sufficient to cause a progressive neurological phenotype in transgenic mice. *Cell* **87**:493–506.
29. Hochberg, F., S.U. Harris, and T.R. Blattert. 1990. Occupational hand cramps: professional disorders of motor control. *Hand Clin* **6**:417–428.
30. Byl, N.N., and M. Melnick. 1997. The neural consequences of repetition: clinical implications of a learning hypothesis. *J Hand Ther* **10**: 160–174.
31. Ghilardi, M.F., M. Carbon, G. Silvestri, V. Dhawan, M. Tagliati, S. Bressman, C. Ghez, et al. 2003. Impaired Sequence Learning in Carriers of the DYT1 Dystonia Mutation. *Ann Neurol* **54**:102–109.
32. Crawley, J.N. 1999. Behavioral phenotyping of transgenic and knockout mice: experimental design and evaluation of general health, sensory functions, motor abilities, and specific behavioral tests. *Brain Res* **835**:18–26.

CHAPTER

C7

The *hph-1* Mouse

KEITH HYLAND and SIMON J.R. HEALES

The *hph-1* mouse has a deficiency of GTP cyclohydrolase that leads to decreased synthesis of tetrahydrobiopterin. This is a cofactor required for the metabolism of phenylalanine and for the synthesis of serotonin, the catecholamines, and nitric oxide. The mouse therefore provides a platform for studying the pathophysiological effects of abnormalities in these areas of metabolism. There are no overt signs of a movement disorder on spontaneous open field behavior but biochemical features suggest that this animal will be a good model for the investigation of dominantly inherited GTP cyclohydrolase deficiency (dopa-responsive dystonia; Segawa disease) and nitric oxide deficiency.

I. BACKGROUND

The *hph*-1 mouse was generated by screening *N*-ethyl-*N'*–nitrosurea treated mice for the presence of hyperphenylalaninemia (Bode et al. 1988), the intention being to produce a mouse model of phenylalanine hydroxylase (PAH) deficiency in which to study the human disease, phenylketonuria (McDonald et al. 1990). Several hyperphenylalaninemic lines were produced, with one being the *hph-1* mutant (Bode et al. 1988). In this animal, the cause of the elevated plasma phenylalanine levels was shown to be a deficiency of tetrahydrobiopterin (BH4) which acts as a cofactor for the PAH enzyme (Figure 1).

BH4 is formed in a multi-step pathway from GTP with the first and rate-limiting enzyme being GTP cyclohydrolase (GCH-1). The GCH-1 activity is low in the liver and brain from the *hph-1* mouse (McDonald et al. 1988) but investigators have yet to establish its molecular basis, as sequencing of the GCH-1 coding exons (Gutlich et al. 1994; Maeda et al. 2000) and the 5′ flanking region (Shimoji et al. 1999; Maeda et al. 2000) has failed to locate any abnormalities. However, linkage analysis has shown the mutation and GCH-1 loci to be within 8cM of each other (Montanez and McDonald 1999).

II. BIOCHEMISTRY

A. Hyperphenylalaninemia

The abnormal biochemistry in the *hph-1* mouse is directly related to the low concentrations of BH4 observed in all examined tissues. The mutant animals are hyperphenylalaninemic at birth but the elevated plasma phenylalanine levels normalize within a few weeks following a slow accumulation of BH4 in the liver to levels that are

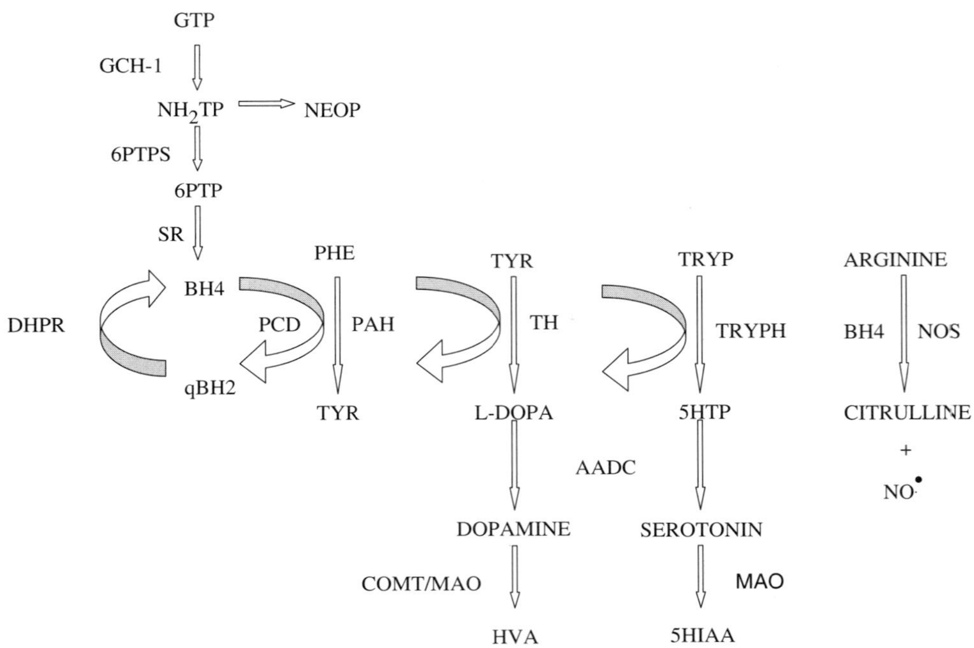

FIGURE 1 GTP, guanosine triphosphate; GCH-1, GTP cyclohydrolase; NH_2TP, dihydroneopterin triphospate; Neop, neopterin; 6PTPS, 6-pyruvoyltetrahydropterin synthase; 6PTP, 6-pyruvoyltetrahydropterin; SR, shepiapterin reductase; BH4, tetrahydrobiopterin; PCD, pterin α-carbolamine dehydratase; qBH_2, quinonoid dihydrobiopterin; PHE, phenylalanine; PAH, phenylalanine hydroxylase; TYR, tyrosine; TH, tyrosine hydroxylase; TRYP, tryptophan; TRYPH, tryptophan hydroxylase; 5HTP, 5-hydroxytryptophan; AADC, aromatic L-amino acid decarboxylase; MAO, monoamine oxidase; 5HIAA, 5-hydroxyindoleacetic acid; NOS, nitric oxide synthase; COMT, catechol O-methyltransferase; HVA, homovanillic acid; NO·, nitric oxide.

approximately 50% of those found in controls (Hyland et al. 1996). Although resting phenylalanine levels are normal after these first few weeks of life, the metabolism of phenylalanine to tyrosine in the liver remains compromised. This can be demonstrated by examining the conversion of phenylalanine to tyrosine after administering a bolus of phenylalanine (McDonald et al. 1988). After phenylalanine loading, plasma phenylalanine to tyrosine ratios remain elevated for extended periods as compared to controls, thus demonstrating a decreased capacity for phenylalanine hydroxylation.

The presence of hyperphenylalaninemia in the neonatal period may have some long-lasting effects, as elevated phenylalanine levels affect brain development and many areas of neurochemistry (Huttenlocher 2000; Surtees and Blau 2000). Investigators have yet to perform in-depth studies to investigate this feature of the *hph-1* mouse, but the above information should be considered if the animal will be used as a model system to investigate mild BH4 deficiencies.

B. Serotonin and Catecholamine Metabolism

As well as being a cofactor for PAH in the liver, BH4 is also the cofactor required to activate tryptophan hydroxylase and tyrosine hydroxylase; these respectively are the rate-limiting enzymes for the synthesis of serotonin and the catecholamine neurotransmitters (Figure 1). In the *hph-1* mouse brain, concentrations of BH4 are approximately 40% of the wild-type levels and serotonin (–22%), dopamine (–14%), norepinephrine (–5%), and their major metabolites, 5-hydroxyindoleacetic acid (–44%), homovanillic acid (–26%), and 3-methoxy-4-hydroxyphenylglycol (–10%) are all significantly decreased (Hyland et al. 1996).

C. Nitric Oxide Metabolism

Tetrahydrobiopterin is also the cofactor required for all forms of nitric oxide synthase (NOS) (Tayeh and Marletta 1989). In the presence of molecular oxygen, this enzyme catalyses the conversion of arginine to citrulline and nitric oxide (NO) (Figure 1). Investigators have described three isoforms of NOS: a calcium-independent form (iNOS), a calcium-dependent vascular endothelial constitutive form (eNOS), and a calcium-dependent neuronal constitutive form (nNOS) (Knowles and Moncada 1994). Each isoform contains a heme moiety linked to an NADPH-cytochrome P-450 reductase-like domain. Stimulation causes reducing equivalents to transfer from NADPH to flavin mononucleotide, which subsequently reduces the heme. This leads to oxygen activation, followed by oxidation of arginine to NO and citrulline.

Nitric oxide has a number of important functions within the central nervous system that are largely mediated via stimulation of guanylate cyclase to produce cyclic GMP (cGMP). Among other actions, it aids in modulating ion channels and receptors, acts as an intercellular messenger in memory formation and synaptic plasticity, and can activate protein kinases and phosphodiesterases (Bredt and Snyder 1994; Moncada et al. 1991). The low levels of BH4 in the *hph-1* brain reduce nNOS activity by 20% (Brand et al. 1995) and this is associated with a 40% decrease in cGMP level (Canevari et al. 1999); there is also a reduced concentration of citrulline (Brand et al. 1996) and a decreased affinity of the enzyme for its arginine substrate (Brand et al. 1995).

Evidence for impaired NO availability in the brain of the *hph-1* mouse also comes from studies about the activity of the enzyme glyceraldehyde-3-phosphate dehydrogenase (GAPDH). This enzyme appears to be particularly sensitive to NO, with loss of activity occurring as a result of exposure (Zhang and Snyder 1992). The sensitivity of GAPDH to NO suggests that NO may be a physiological regulator of the activity of this enzyme (Zhang and Snyder 1992). Assessment of GAPDH activity in *hph-1* brain preparations reveals an approximate fourfold increase in activity when compared to wild-type preparations, providing additional evidence that NO generation is impaired in the *hph-1* mouse brain and that NO availability regulates GAPDH activity (Heales et al. 1997).

Several studies have shown that uncoupling of the oxygen reduction and the arginine oxidation occurs if concentrations of BH4 are sub-optimal after the NOS enzyme is activated. This leads to production of superoxide anion (O_2^-) and hydrogen peroxide (Pou et al. 1992; Vasquez et al. 1998). The production of O_2^- in the presence of continued, though diminished, production of NO can form the highly damaging peroxynitrite free radical (Lipton et al. 1993). As yet it is unclear whether or not any pathological changes occur in the *hph-1* brain that are associated with the altered NO metabolism; however, researchers have used the mouse as a model to investigate how altered NO and BH4 metabolism affect endothelial function (Cosentino et al. 2001).

III. THE *HPH-1* MOUSE AS A MODEL FOR SEGAWA DISEASE (DOMINANTLY INHERITED GTP CYCLOHYDROLASE DEFICIENCY)

The primary biochemical abnormality in the *hph-1* mouse is reduced GCH-1 activity that results in lowered levels of BH4 and disturbed metabolism of NO and the serotonin and catecholamine neurotransmitters. Low levels of BH4 and homovanillic acid (the major dopamine metabolite found in human cerebrospinal fluid (CSF)) have also been demonstrated in CSF from patients with Segawa disease (Segawa 1976; Fink et al. 1989). In 1994, Ichinose and colleagues identified dominantly inherited mutations in the GCH-1 gene as the basis for the altered metabolism and the clinical phenotype (Ichinose et al. 1994). Since then investigators have identified more than eightfive independent mutations in the coding region of the GCH-I gene (Furukawa et al. 2003). Neuropathology has been unrevealing in brains from affected patients (Rajput et al. 1994) but neurohistochemistry and biochemical measurements have shown low levels of dopamine in the striatum and substantia nigra and low levels of tyrosine hydroxylase protein and activity in the striatum (Furukawa et al. 1999). As in the adult *hph-1* mouse, the BH4 deficiency in the liver from patients with dominantly inherited GCH-1 deficiency is not severe enough to lead to resting hyperphenylalaninemia. But, again if the system is stressed by giving oral phenylalanine, conversion to tyrosine is slow, as demonstrated by elevated phenylalanine to tyrosine ratios in plasma after the loading (Hyland et al. 1997).

The clinical phenotype in dominantly inherited GCH-1 deficiency is variable. Typically the first signs appear between four and six years of age with the patient developing a dystonic posture of one foot. The dystonia then spreads to the other extremities within several years. The spectrum of clinical manifestations is, however, broad and may include a total absence of symptoms, minor muscle cramps, infantile or adult onset, an early nonprogressive course, delayed attainment of motor milestones, spastic diplegia, and the occurrence of Parkinsonian-like features in later life (Nygaard 1993). Initial presentations have included adult-onset oromandibular dystonia (Steinberger et al. 1999), an apparent primary torsion dystonia that was responsive to anticholinergic agents (Jarman et al. 1997), and a phenotype that included both myoclonus and dystonia (Leuzzi et al. 2002). In most patients with typical presentation, a diurnal variation in the symptoms occurs with improvement after overnight sleep. Penetrance and phenotype are not disease allele dependent and the frequency of penetrance is threefold to fourfold higher in females, as compared to males (Nygaard 1993).

The low activities of GCH-1 in the *hph-1* mutant mark it as a candidate model to study pathogenesis in the human dominantly inherited GCH-1 deficiency. To date, researchers have not conducted formal investigations to ascertain a certain type of movement disorder in this animal, but on casual observation, no overt signs appear. Biochemically, the animals closely mimic the changes seen in the human disease, with low levels of BH4 leading to perturbed liver phenylalanine metabolism when the system is stressed and to reduced levels of serotonin, the catecholamines, and their metabolites in the brain (McDonald et al. 1988; Hyland et al. 1996). The animals also have reduced activities and amounts of tyrosine hydroxylase in striatal tissue (Hyland et al. 1996). They therefore provide a model system to study the mechanisms underlying the intrafamilial phenotypic variation, the incomplete penetrance, the diurnal variation in symptoms and the female predominance seen in human subjects with dominantly inherited GCH-1 deficiency. Examination of the mechanism of striatal tyrosine hydroxylase protein loss is also likely to provide clues to pathogenesis in this intriguing disorder.

Investigators have performed several studies that begin to investigate these unresolved issues. Comparison of GCH-1 gene expression in male and female wild-type mice clearly showed lower levels of GCH-1 mRNA within serotonergic, dopaminergic, and noradrenergic neurons in female mice, with the greatest deficit being in serotonergic neurons. In these cell types, GCH-1 expression was also lower in *hph-1* male and female mice when compared to their wild-type counterparts. However, lower levels of GCH-1 mRNA were seen only in the dopaminergic neurons of female mice when comparing expression levels between female and male mutants. These data indicate that basal levels of GCH-1 mRNA expression are heterogeneous across wild-type murine monoamine cell types and that gene expression is also modified in a sex-linked and cell-specific fashion by the *hph-1* gene locus (Shimoji et al. 1999). The mechanism for the lower GCH-1 expression in females remains unclear but further investigation might provide an explanation for the increased penetrance of disease phenotype seen in human females as compared to males with dominantly inherited GCH-1 deficiency. The influence of hormones on the BH4 synthesis has been suggested, as estrogen or estrogen analogues might have a negative effect upon BH4 metabolism (Blair 1985).

The lowered tyrosine hydroxylase protein concentration found in the striatum from patients with dominantly inherited GCH-1 deficiency and in the *hph-1* mouse could arise either because of protein instability in the face of reduced levels of the BH4 cofactor or from a decrease in GCH-1 gene expression. Administering BH4 to levels that elevate brain BH4 concentrations to above normal leads to normalization of tyrosine hydroxylase activity and protein concentration in the *hph-1* mice (Hyland et al. 1996). Preliminary studies indicate that this normalization leads to increased tyrosine hydroxylase gene expression (Hyland and Munk-Martin 2001); however, other investigations using a 6-pyruvoyltetrahydropterin synthase gene-null mouse have shown loss of tyrosine hydroxylase protein but not of tyrosine hydroxylase mRNA in the brains of these BH4 deficient animals (Sumi-Ichinose et al. 2001), suggesting that in this model system, BH4 stabilizes the tyrosine hydroxylase protein rather than affects gene expression.

IV. EVALUATION OF NOVEL TREATMENT REGIMES IN THE *HPH-1* MOUSE

The nature of the metabolic defect in the *hph-1* mouse makes it a useful model for evaluating treatment regimes for correcting the biochemical consequences of the impaired GCH-1 activity. To date, cofactor replacement has been evaluated in the *hph-1* mouse. These studies revealed that peripheral administration of BH4 leads to a transient normalization of the brain BH4 concentration. However, despite these results, no overt stimulation of monoamine metabolism occurs (Brand et al. 1996). Failure to correct monoamine metabolism following acute BH4 administration is likely due to the loss of aromatic amino acid hydroxylase proteins associated with BH4 deficiency states. In contrast, NOS expression is apparently not affected by BH4 availability, and acute administration of the cofactor stimulates brain NO metabolism (Brand et al. 1995; Canevari et al. 1999).

V. SUMMARY

In summary, the *hph-1* mouse provides an animal model system for investigating pathophysiological consequences of a partial deficiency of BH4. In particular, the biochemical features of this animal closely mimic those seen in dominantly inherited GCH-1 deficiency, and careful investigation of the model may unravel some of the intriguing questions that remain unanswered in this disorder. Overt signs of any movement disorder are absent but it is likely that specialized testing in the future will reveal abnormalities. If this is the case, the model may be suitable for the investigation of pharmacological interventions.

References

Blair, J.A. 1985. Tetrahydrobiopterin metabolism in the central nervous system. In *Biochemical and Clinical Aspects of Pteridines*. pp. 103–118. Ed. H. Wachter, H.C. Curtius, and W. Pfleiderer. Berlin: Walter de Gruyter.

Bode, V.C., J.D. McDonald, J.L. Guenet, and D. Simon. 1988. hph-1: a mouse mutant with hereditary hyperphenylalaninemia induced by ethylnitrosourea mutagenesis. *Genetics* **118**:299–305.

Brand, M.P., A. Briddon, J.M. Land, J.B. Clark, and S.J. Heales. 1996. Impairment of the nitric oxide/cyclic GMP pathway in cerebellar slices prepared from the hph-1 mouse. *Brain Res* **735**:169–172.

Brand, M.P., S.J. Heales, J.M. Land, and J.B. Clark. 1995. Tetrahydrobiopterin deficiency and brain nitric oxide synthase in the hph-1 mouse. *J Inherit Metab Dis* **18**:33–39.

Brand, M.P., K. Hyland, T. Engle, I. Smith, and S.J. Heales. 1996. Neurochemical effects following peripheral administration of tetrahydropterin derivatives to the hph-1 mouse. *J Neurochem* **66**:1150–1156.

Bredt, D.S., and S.H. Snyder. 1994. Nitric oxide: a physiologic messenger molecule. *Ann Rev Biochem* **63**:175–195.

Canevari, L., J.M. Land, J.B. Clark, and S.J. Heales. 1999. Stimulation of the brain NO/cyclic GMP pathway by peripheral administration of tetrahydrobiopterin in the hph-1 mouse. *J Neurochem* **73**:2563–2568.

Cosentino, F., J.E. Barker, M.P. Brand, S.J. Heales, E.R. Werner, J.R. Tippins, N. West, et al. 2001. Reactive oxygen species mediate endothelium-dependent relaxations in tetrahydrobiopterin-deficient mice. *Arterioscler Thromb Vasc Biol* **21**:496–502.

Fink, J.K., P. Ravin, C.E. Argoff, R.A. Levine, R.O. Brady, M. Hallett, and N.W. Barton. 1989. Tetrahydrobiopterin administration in biopterin-deficient progressive dystonia with diurnal variation. *Neurology* **39**: 1393–1395.

Furukawa, Y. 2003. Genetics and biochemistry of dopa-responsive dystonia: significance of striatal tyrosine hydroxylase protein loss. *Adv Neurol* **91**:401–410.

Furukawa, Y., T.G. Nygaard, M. Gutlich, A.H. Rajput, C. Pifl, L. DiStefano, L.J. Chang, et al. 1999. Striatal biopterin and tyrosine hydroxylase protein reduction in dopa-responsive dystonia. *Neurology* **53**:1032–1041.

Gutlich, M., I. Ziegler, K. Witter, B. Hemmens, L. Hultner, J.D. McDonald, T. Werner, et al. 1994. Molecular characterization of hph-1: a mouse mutant deficient in GTP cyclohydrolase I activity. *Biochem Biophys Res Commun* **203**:1675–1681.

Heales, S.J., J.E. Barker, V.C. Stewart, M.P. Brand, I.P. Hargreaves, P. Foppa, J.M. Land, et al. 1997. Nitric oxide, energy metabolism, and neurological disease. *Biochem Soc Trans* **25**:939–943.

Huttenlocher, P.R. 2000. The neuropathology of phenylketonuria: human and animal studies. *Eur J Pediatr* **159 Suppl 2**:S102–S106

Hyland, K., J.S. Fryburg, W.G. Wilson, E.M. Bebin, L.A. Arnold, R.S. Gunasekera, R.D. Jacobson, et al. 1997. Oral phenylalanine loading in dopa-responsive dystonia: a possible diagnostic test. *Neurology* **48**: 1290–1297.

Hyland, K., R.S. Gunasekera, T. Engle, and L.A. Arnold. 1996. Tetrahydrobiopterin and biogenic amine metabolism in the hph-1 mouse. *J Neurochem* **67**:752–759.

Hyland, K., and T.L. Munk-Martin. 2001. Tetrahydrobiopterin regulates tyrosine hydroxylase and phenylalanine hydroxylase gene expression in dominantly inherited GTP cyclohydrolase deficiency. *J Inherit Metab Dis* **24 Suppl 1**:30. 2001.

Ichinose, H., T. Ohye, E. Takahashi, N. Seki, T. Hori, M. Segawa, Y. Nomura, et al. 1994. Hereditary progressive dystonia with marked diurnal fluctuation caused by mutations in the GTP cyclohydrolase I gene. *Nat Genet* **8**:236–242.

Jarman, P.R., O. Bandmann, C.D. Marsden, and N.W. Wood. 1997. GTP cyclohydrolase I mutations in patients with dystonia responsive to anticholinergic drugs. *J Neurol Neurosurg Psychiatry* **63**:304–308.

Knowles, R.G., and S. Moncada. 1994. Nitric oxide synthases in mammals. *Biochem J* **298**:249–258.

Leuzzi, V., C. Carducci, C. Carducci, F. Cardona, C. Artiola, and I. Antonozzi. 2002. Autosomal dominant GTP-CH deficiency presenting as a dopa-responsive myoclonus-dystonia syndrome. *Neurology* **59**: 1241–1243.

Lipton, S.A., Y.B. Choi, Z.H. Pan, S.Z. Lei, H.S. Chen, N.J. Sucher, J. Loscalzo, et al. 1993. A redox-based mechanism for the neuroprotective and neurodestructive effects of nitric oxide and related nitroso-compounds. *Nature* **364**:626–632.

Maeda, T., S. Haeno, K. Oda, D. Mori, H. Ichinose, T. Nagatsu, and T. Suzuki. 2000. Studies on the genotype-phenotype relation in the hph-1 mouse mutant deficient in guanosine triphosphate (GTP) cyclohydrolase I activity. *Brain Dev* **22 Suppl 1**:S50–S53

McDonald, J.D., V.C. Bode, W.F. Dove, and A. Shedlovsky. 1990. The use of N-ethyl-N-nitrosourea to produce mouse models for human phenylketonuria and hyperphenylalaninemia. *Prog Clin Biol Res* **340C**: 407–413.

McDonald, J.D., R.G. Cotton, I. Jennings, F.D. Ledley, S.L. Woo, and V.C. Bode. 1988. Biochemical defect of the hph-1 mouse mutant is a deficiency in GTP-cyclohydrolase activity. *J Neurochem* **50**:655–657.

Moncada, S., R.M. Palmer, and E.A. Higgs. 1991. Nitric oxide: physiology, pathophysiology, and pharmacology. *Pharmacol Rev* **43**:109–142.

Montanez, C.S., and J.D. McDonald. 1999. Linkage analysis of the hph-1 mutation and the GTP cyclohydrolase I structural gene. *Mol Gene Metab* **68**:91–92.

Nygaard, T.G. 1993. Dopa-responsive dystonia. Delineation of the clinical syndrome and clues to pathogenesis. *Adv Neurol* **60**:577–585.

Pou, S., W.S. Pou, D.S. Bredt, S.H. Snyder, and G.M. Rosen. 1992. Generation of superoxide by purified brain nitric oxide synthase. *J Biol Chem* **267**:24173–24176.

Rajput, A.H., W.R. Gibb, X.H. Zhong, K.S. Shannak, S. Kish, L.G. Chang, and O. Hornykiewicz. 1994. Dopa-responsive dystonia: pathological and biochemical observations in a case. *Ann Neurol* **35**:396–402.

Segawa, M., A. Hosaka, F. Miyagawa, Y. Nomura, and H. Imai. 1976. Hereditary progressive dystonia with marked diurnal fluctuation. In *Advances in Neurology*. Ed. R. Eldredge, and S. Fahn. pp. 215–220. New York: Raven Press.

Shimoji, M., K. Hirayama, K. Hyland, and G. Kapatos. 1999. GTP cyclohydrolase I gene expression in the brains of male and female hph-1 mice. *J Neurochem* **72**:757–764.

Steinberger, D., H. Topka, D. Fischer, and U. Muller. 1999. GCH1 mutation in a patient with adult-onset oromandibular dystonia. *Neurology* **52**:877–879.

Sumi-Ichinose, C., F. Urano, R. Kuroda, T. Ohye, M. Kojima, M. Tazawa, H. Shiraishi, et al. 2001. Catecholamines and serotonin are differently regulated by tetrahydrobiopterin. A study from 6-pyruvoyltetrahydropterin synthase knockout mice. *J Biol Chem* **276**:41150–41160.

Surtees, R., and N. Blau. 2000. The neurochemistry of phenylketonuria. *Eur J Pediatr* **159 Suppl 2**:S109–S113.

Tayeh, M.A., and M.A. Marletta. 1989. Macrophage oxidation of L-arginine to nitric oxide, nitrite, and nitrate. Tetrahydrobiopterin is required as a cofactor. *J Biol Chem* **264**:19654–19658.

Vasquez-Vivar, J., B. Kalyanaraman, P. Martasek, N. Hogg, B.S. Masters, H. Karoui, P. Tordo, and K.A.J. Pritchard. 1998. Superoxide generation by endothelial nitric oxide synthase: the influence of cofactors. *Proc Natl Acad Sci USA* **95**:9220–9225.

Zhang, J., and S.H. Snyder. 1992. Nitric oxide stimulates auto-ADP-ribosylation of glyceraldehyde-3-phosphate dehydrogenase. *Proc Natl Acad Sci USA* **89**:9382–9385.

C H A P T E R

D1

Clinical and Pathological Characteristics of Huntington Disease

JAYARAMAN RAO

Huntington disease (HD) is an autosomal dominant neurodegenerative disorder that is relentlessly progressive, characterized by cognitive, behavioral, and motor dysfunctions.[1–3] The prevalence rate in the United States is approximately five cases per 100,000 and is much lower in Asia and Africa. Approximately 30,000 HD patients live in the United States and about 150,000 people are at risk of developing HD.[3,4] The mean age of onset of HD is about forty years, but may occur as early as four years[5,6] and as late as eighty years of age.

I. HUNTINGTON DISEASE GENETICS

Huntington Disease (HD) is caused by a trinucleotide (CAG) repeat expansion of the HD gene.[7] The HD protein huntingtin (*htt*) normally contains 6–35 polyglutamine (PolyQ) repeats. So far, HD has not been reported in individuals with less than 36 CAG repeats. In affected individuals, CAG repeats can vary from 36 to 180 and the age of onset and severity of the disease is inversely proportional to the length of the polyQ tract. Patients with 36–38 repeats may express a much milder form of HD, with the onset of disease at or beyond sixty years of age and may present with only mild chorea and without the cognitive, psychiatric and behavioral problems noted with a common expression of the adult form of HD associated with CAG repeats from 39–60. The presence of 60 or more repeats is common with juvenile HD.[1,3] HD is a classic example of an autosomal dominant disease. The age of onset and the severity of the disease are dictated by the extent of the mutation of the HD gene and by the sex of the parent with HD, however, environmental factors and genetic modifiers may modify the variability of clinical expression.[2]

Homozygous expression of HD is rare. Most published reports (see Squitieri et al. 2003 for an exception) suggest that homozygotes do not show more severe patterns of disease than heterozygotes. As with other autosomal dominant disorders, the phenomenon of "anticipation" has been well identified with HD.[9,10] While contractions and elongations of the trinucleotide repeats do occur with successive generation, it is much less variable if HD is inherited from the maternal side. The trinucleotide repeat length in paternal transmission is very unstable and becomes longer with each successive generation, leading to the phenomenon of "anticipation" and the appearance of the disease approximately eight years earlier in children of an affected father.[3,10]

II. MOLECULAR PATHOLOGY

A. Huntingtin (*htt*)

The HD gene is localized to chromosome 4p16.3 and comprises 67 exons and 3144 amino acids.[11] The protein *htt* consists of a series of CAG repeats coding for glutamine residues (polyQ) followed immediately by two short stretches of proline rich domain (polyP), all of which are derived from exon 1 Located downstream of the polyQ/polyP region, *htt* contains thirty-six HEAT repeats.[12,13] HEAT repeats are characterized by short amino acid repetitions within the protein structure and play an important role in protein-protein interactions.[14] Of the thirty-six HEAT repeats, ten are located close to the polyQ/polyP area at the N-terminal region, a region of *htt* that interacts with several transcription factors, receptors, and enzymes. Abnormalities of this basic architecture of *htt* induced by polyQ elongation ultimately lead to progressive degeneration of striatal and cerebral cortical neurons.[15,16]

The protein *htt* is expressed widely within the central nervous system[17–20] and in extraneural tissues.[19] Within the brain, *htt* is expressed ubiquitously, but the highest levels are found in the cerebellum, hippocampus, cerebral cortex, substantia nigra pars reticulata, and pontine nuclei.[17] Huntingtin is expressed more intensely in neurons than in glial cells. Within the neurons, *htt* is located mostly within the cytoplasm; some of *htt* within the cytoplasm is associated with membranes, but *htt* is also found in the nucleus. The role played by *htt* is currently being elucidated. The varied functions of *htt* may be accomplished by its interactions with various binding proteins located both within the cytoplasm, Golgi and endoplasmic reticular membranes, and the nucleus wherein *htt* is normally expressed intensely.[15,16] The *htt* protein appears to be necessary for normal embryogenesis, especially during gastrulation, and for normal development of hemopoietic progenitor cells, neurogenesis, endocytosis, vesicular trafficking, cytoplasmic and nuclear transport process, iron homeostasis, signal transduction, transcription regulation, and cell survival.[15,16,21]

B. Mutant Huntingtin (*mhtt*)

The clinical expression of HD is due to an expansion of a CAG tract in exon 1 that results in the aggregation of proteolytic fragments[22,23] of the N-terminal segment of the elongated polyglutamine tract within the cytoplasm and the nucleus of striatal and cortical neurons. The initial "toxic" event may be the accumulation of proteolytic fragments within the cytoplasm, wherein *HTT* is normally expressed intensely. This cytoplasmic event may facilitate the entry of proteolytic fragments into the nucleus[24] where these fragments may interfere with many transcriptional factors[25,26] and cause death of neurons. In unaffected individuals, the CAG repeats vary from six to thirty-five. An addition of just two more repeats, from thirty-six to thirty-eight, alters the hydrophobicity of the elongated polyglutamine tract and initiates aggregation of the protein within cells.[27] While the theory is widely accepted that the neurotoxic effects of the mutant allele are due to gain of function, investigators also propose that the mutant allele may actually induce loss of function of the normal allele, which may also contribute further to the pathology in HD.

C. Neuropathology

Even though *htt* is expressed less intensely in the striatum than many other regions of the brain, the most significant pathology of HD occurs in the striatum. During the early stages of the disease (grade 1) 50% of neurons in the caudate nucleus are lost and at grade 4, the most advanced stage of HD, 95% of caudate neurons are lost.[28] The earliest pathological changes (grade 0) are seen in the medial periventricular and the tail of the caudate nucleus and the dorsal putamen. As the disease progresses to grade 4, the neuronal degeneration and astrocytic processes are noted to encompass the entire striatum.[28]

Within the striatum, medium spiny neurons degenerate the most, and almost all types of interneurons[29] including the large cholinergic interneurons[30,31] are preserved. The GABA/enkephalinergic striatal neurons projecting to lateral pallidal segment appear to degenerate first, followed by GABA/substance P containing striatonigral neurons. Ultimately the GABA/substance P containing striatal neurons that project to the medial pallidal segments dies.[32] However, in both human HD and animal models of HD, the CB1 subtype of cannabinoid receptors, a system that modulates dopaminergic signaling in the basal ganglia, deteriorate in an impressive pattern as the disease progresses.[32,33]

In addition to the striatum, cortical neuronal degeneration leads to excessive thinning of the cerebral mantle of the entire brain.[34] In late stages (grade 3 or 4), very significant neuronal loss in the frontal cortex, especially the large pyramidal neurons of layers II, III, V, and VI, and significant gliosis in layers V (75%) and VI (68%) cause frontal atrophy.[35–37] In very advanced cases neurons are lost in the thalamus, substantia nigra pars reticulata, and subthalamic nucleus.[38] The juvenile HD cases may also demonstrate significant cerebellar atrophy.

III. CLINICAL MANIFESTATIONS

A. Motor Dysfunction

1. Chorea

The most common motor manifestation of HD is chorea. Chorea is defined as quick, vermicular movements, which may be superimposed on a purposeful act. Chorea is more prominent in the orofacial regions and the distal musculature of hands and feet. However, as the disease progresses truncal chorea may be severe enough to cause sudden lurching of the body that leads to frequent falls. When superimposed on akathetic movements, chorea might be missed as part of motor manifestations of fidgety behavior. Chorea can be an early manifestation[39] in HD and may be the only manifestation in late onset HD.[40] Choreic movements of the feet and toes may be present in at-risk individuals[41] and as an early manifestation of the disease. Choreiform movements of the orofacial, tongue, and oropharyngeal musculature may be severe enough to cause significant speech difficulties and dysphagia and may lead to aspiration. In patients untreated with antidopaminergic agents, chorea may be severe enough to prevent any normal voluntary and goal-directed motor activity.

2. Oculomotor Abnormalities

In terms of eye movements, HD patients have significant abnormalities of saccades, fixation, and smooth pursuit.[42,43] Early in the disease, the patients have difficulties in initiating voluntary saccades, especially on command and to maintain a steady fixation. However, as the disease progresses a more severe slowing of saccades is noted. Vertical saccadic movements are more severely involved than the horizontal saccades.[44,45] The eye movement abnormalities reflect dysfunctions of a significant area of the head of the caudate nucleus where projections from oculomotor centers of the frontal and parietal cortical areas, the thalamic and other brain stem regions converge.[46]

3. Dystonia

While chorea is the most common and widely recognized movement disorder of HD, clinicians often may not recognize the presence of dystonic movements. In one study, dystonic movements of different types and of varying degrees were present in 95% of patients.[47] The rotatory dystonic movements of the shoulder were the most common, but dystonic movements of the foot, hands, trunk torticollis and blepharospasms were noted. Cervical dystonia may even be an initial manifestation of HD.[48] Severe motor tics and myoclonus may also be present in patients with HD.[49] It should be pointed out that tardive dystonias and tardive dyskinesias induced by antidopaminergic agents may superimpose on many of these movement disorders.

4. Parkinsonism

Even though hyperkinetic movements are the cardinal features of HD, bradykinesia may coexist[39] and might even be an early manifestation of HD.[50] Bradykinesia may be present during simultaneous and sequential movements;[51] significant slowing of saccades is also noted in HD. Rigidity is one of the most prominent features of the Westphal variant of juvenile HD. The hypokinetic movements may also respond to L-dopa treatment. Investigators have proposed that the occurrence of both hypokinetic and hyperkinetic features may be due to differential involvement of the direct and indirect pathways of the basal ganglia.[39]

5. Gait Disorder

Gait dysfunction is a major and disabling feature of HD.[52] A significant decrease in gait velocity and length of each stride, spontaneous flexion of the knees, swaying of the trunk, and broad-based gait are some of the features of gait dysfunctions in HD patients. A detailed study of the dynamics of gait suggests that HD patients have random fluctuation of stride, decreased stride interval, decreased correlation of one stride to the next, and in advanced stages more severely affected stride-to-stride correlation.[53–55] These features of gait dysfunction may give patients with HD an appearance of being drunk, and this in fact has caused legal problems, hospitalization, or nursing home placements for many patients. While antidopaminergic therapy may reduce the severity of chorea, it does not seem to improve gait dysfunction.

6. Cerebellar Dysfunction

Despite the fact that *htt* is expressed most intensely in the cerebellum, severe cerebellar findings are not that common in adult-onset HD, but may be seen in juvenile HD. In contrast, many of the recently identified HD-like disorders are associated with significant cerebellar ataxia and other signs of cerebellar involvement.

B. Cognitive Manifestations

1. Dementia

Severe cognitive dysfunction reflecting both cortical and subcortical types of dementias is quite common in HD.[1,56,57] The major feature is a progressive decline of attentional and executive function, which investigators speculate is due to fronto-striatal disconnection. In addition to the striatal lesions, neurons of the pyramidal and other layers of frontal, temporal, and parietal cortical areas degenerate, resulting in a wide variety of cognitive defects as the disease progresses including problems with memory acquisition and recall, decline in verbal skills, concentration, abstract thinking, and visuospatial perceptional difficulties. Severe dementia of the Alzheimer type is not a major feature of HD unless the patient is in very advanced stages of the disease.

2. Psychiatric Problems

Psychiatric and mood dysfunctions precede motor dysfunctions and can be destructive to the lives of the patients and their family members.[58–60] Paranoid ideations, delusions, and other features of schizophrenia have been noted in 3–11% of HD patients. A significant bihemispheric decrease in metabolism is noted in PET scans of HD patients, a pattern very much similar to that seen in schizophrenics. Varieties of mood disorders are noted in 38% of HD patients, and the most common and fatal consequences are depression and suicidal tendencies. Suicide was the cause of death in 7.8% of HD patients in one study. Suicide risks are of higher frequency in HD patients,[61–63] patients at risk for HD,[64] and even in normal patients with a family history of HD.[65] The suicide rate in HD is four to six times higher than in the general population and the rate is even higher in patients over the age of fifty. Investigators have observed obsessive-compulsive disorder,[66,67] paraphilia and other sexual disorders, aggression, irritability, agitation, delirium, and mania and hypomania in patients with HD.[59,60]

C. Weight Loss and Other Hormonal Changes

A feature of HD that investigators have not given serious attention is the significant weight loss invariably noted in all patients with HD.[68,69] Significant weight loss occurs even in animal models of HD. The mechanism underlying the weight loss is not known and it is not correlated with the severity of chorea, dystonia, depressive mood, or the course of the disease.[69,70] An interesting observation is that a loss occurs in 90% of the 60,000 neurons normally found in the lateral tuberal nucleus (LTN) of the hypothalamus.[71,72] The severity of the neuronal loss in this nucleus appears to be directly correlated with the severity of the disease. HD patients with minimal motor dysfunction have the least number of losses of neurons in this nucleus.[72] This nucleus contains high levels of NMDA and AMPA receptors and the neuronal loss may be due to glutamate toxicity that may be associated with Huntington disease.[73] In early and recent literature, investigators have extensively reported alternations of prolactin levels, L-dopa induced growth hormone release, stress responsive corticotrophin releasing factor, and steroid and altered glucose metabolism.[74,75] An increased frequency of diabetes mellitus has been observed in HD[76] and even the transgenic models of HD develop diabetes mellitus with significant intranuclear inclusion and pathology similar to that noted in HD in islet cells of the pancreas.[77,78]

IV. CLINICAL PRESENTATIONS OF HUNTINGTON DISEASE

While molecular and neuropathological mechanisms are similar in all HD patients, phenotypic expression of the disease may vary dramatically.

A. Juvenile HD

About 5–7% of HD patients present before the age of twenty-one with the juvenile form of HD.[79] Juvenile HD is commonly seen in association with sixty or more CAG repeats. Unlike adult onset HD, chorea is not a major manifestation of juvenile HD, but rigidity and dystonia may be very prominent in these patients. More importantly, significant addictive, sexually aggressive, and inappropriate behavior may actually precede the motor manifestations of juvenile HD. Unlike adult onset HD, juvenile HD may also present with cerebellar ataxia and other signs of cerebellar involvement since *htt* is expressed maximally in the cerebellar granule cells. Seizures may also be seen with juvenile HD.

B. Adult-Onset HD

1. Chorea Predominant Adult-Onset Type of HD

This type of presentation is the classic presentation of HD.[1,3] The average age of onset for the disease is about forty and the average CAG counts are about forty-four. Initially the patients have vague behavioral and personality changes, but with the progression of the disease, choreic movements become more evident and become prominent throughout the duration of the illness until emaciation and aspiration lead to death after about fifteen to twenty years.

2. Dystonia Predominant Adult-Onset Type

Dystonia, bradykinesia, and not chorea, may be the most prominent presentation in a small group of adult-onset HD patients.[80]

C. Late-Onset HD

1. L-Dopa Responsive Rigid Type

A type of late onset HD presents with significant features of Parkinson disease. The combination of both hyperkinesia and bradykinesia is different from the rigid type of juvenile onset of HD in that the Parkinsonian features may improve after treatment with L-dopa. The age of onset of these patients has varied from less than fifty to mid-to-late sixties, and CAG repeats reported in these patients have varied from forty-two to forty-six.[81]

TABLE 1 HD-Like Diseases

Disease	Chromosomal localization	Protein involved	Genetic defect	Clinical spectrum	Inheritance pattern	References
HD	4p16.3	huntingtin	CAG expansion	chorea, cognitive dysfunction, bradykinesia	AD	7, 11
HDL-1	20p12	prion protein	192 bp insertion	cognitive decline, chorea, basal ganglia atrophy, ataxia	AD	83
HDL-2	16q24.3	junctophilin-3	CAG/CTG expansion	30–35% acanthocytes, chorea	AD	84–87
DRPLA	12p13.31	atrophin-1	CAG expansion	Ataxia, myoclonus, seizures, dementia, chorea	AD	88, 89, 90
Haw River Syndrome	12p13.31	atrophin-1	CAG expansion	Ataxia, seizures, chorea, dementia	AD	91
Spinocerebellar ataxia type 17	6q27	TATA-binding protein (TBP)	CAG/CAA expansion	cerebellar ataxia, dementia, chorea	AD	92, 93
Benign hereditary chorea	14q	thyroid transcription factor-1 (TITF-1)	large deletion	benign hereditary chorea, dystonia, myoclonus	AD	94
AR HDL	4p15.3	?	?	juvenile HD, chorea, ataxia, mutism	AR	95
Abbreviations	HD	Huntington disease				
	HDL	Huntington disease-like				
	DRPLA	Dentatorubropallidoluysian atrophy				
	AD	Autosomal dominant				
	AR	Autosomal recessive				

2. Chorea Only

The major clinical picture for chorea only is that of an elderly person, over sixty years of age, with thirty-six to thirty-nine CAG repeats. The patient presents with mild non-debilitating chorea and gait dysfunction, with or without very mild cognitive impairment and demonstrates a very slow disease progression over many years and a more or less normal life expectancy.[40,82]

D. Huntingtonlike Diseases

The vast majority of patients who exhibit phenotypic expression of HD have a mutation of the HD gene, but a small percentage of patients with clinical expression very similar to HD, do not exhibit *htt* mutations. This trend suggests that other gene mutations may induce a phenotypic expression of HD. These HD-like (HDL) disorders exhibit a wide range of clinical expression of basal ganglia, cortical, and cerebellar dysfunction and, in some cases, trinucleotide (CAG, CTG, or CAA) expansions in a gene other than the HD gene. All of these disorders have some degree of chorea and cognitive decline that may initially lead to a clinical diagnosis of HD (Table 1).

V. TREATMENT OF HUNTINGTON DISEASE

A. Symptomatic Therapy

Currently, only symptomatic therapy is available for HD.[96] The major goals of symptomatic therapy are to control psychosis, treat depression and suicidal tendencies, and possibly control the severity of chorea and other motor manifestations. Dopaminergic and serotonergic receptor blockade with typical and atypical antipsychotics have been the major source symptomatic therapy for HD patients. Among the drugs that are commonly used are haloperidol, risperidol, quetiapine, olanzapine, and clozaril.[97–100] Anti-dopaminergic agents appear to be ineffective in the treatment of chorea. However, long-term use of typical antipsychotics may also complicate the course of the disease by inducing either drug-induced Parkinson's disease and/or tardive dyskinesias and tardive dystonia. Severe depression is treated with SSRIs and other antidepressants.

B. Experimental Therapy

1. Anti-Glutaminergic Drugs

Based on the theory that glutamate excitotoxicity plays a major role in progressive degeneration of spiny striatal neurons,[101] several drugs that decrease glutamatergic transmission have been tried as symptomatic treatment as well as their potentials as neuroprotective agents.[102] Among these, riluzole, a drug that inhibits glutamate release and induces neuroprotection in 3-nitroproprionic acid,[103] quinolinic acid[104] and in transgenic models of HD,[105] has not demonstrated significant and sustained benefit in human clinical trials.[106–108] Remacemide and amantadine, two noncompetitive NMDA antagonists, and lamotrigine, an antiepileptic that inhibits glutamate release, might offer transient symptomatic improvement,[109,110] but do not have neuroprotective properties.

2. Mitochondrial Protectants

The theory that oxidative stress resulting from mitochondrial dysfunction[111] may play a role in striatal neuronal death in HD is reinforced by the observation that in HD patients complex II is deficient,[112,113] and that 3-nitroproprionic acid,[114,115] a specific and an irreversible inhibitor of complex II, and malonate, another complex II inhibitor, replicate several pathogenic mechanisms observed in the spiny neurons of the striatum of HD patients. A dose of 600 mg of coenzyme Q10, a mitochondrial protector, has been shown to be marginally effective in HD.[116]

3. Anti-Apoptotic Drugs

Glutamate toxicity and mitochondrial dysfunction together might ultimately induce the molecular cascades that are involved in apoptosis. Investigators have tried minocycline and doxycycline, caspase inhibitors, in transgenic models, but the results are inconclusive.[117–120]

4. Transcriptional Regulators

The histone deacetylase (HDAC) inhibitors are a promising new avenue for the treatment of HD. The earliest step of neurodegeneration might be the accumulation of the polyQ tracts in the cytoplasm followed by the entry of fragments into the nucleus, which ultimately may interfere with several transcriptional factors necessary for normal function and survival of spiny neurons of the striatum. This may lead ultimately to cell death. The HDAC inhibitors are a new class of drugs, several of which are already in clinical trials to treat different types of cancers,[121] that can reactivate the expression of suppressed genes for transcription factors and might help to prevent neurotoxicity. HDAC inhibitors have been shown to "arrest" polyQ toxicity in cell culture,[122] yeast,[123] *Drosophila*,[124] and mouse models of HD,[125] and improve motor function in the R6/2 HD mouse model.[126]

5. Restorative Therapy

Restoration of striatal dysfunction by administering growth factors, including ciliary neurotrophic factor, nerve growth factor, BDNF, NT3, or by transplanting xenografts, human fetal cells or stem cells, has provided mixed results.[127–131]

Acknowledgment

This work was supported by the Grace Benson Research Fund.

References

1. Biglan, K., and I. Shoulson. 2002. Huntington's disease. In *Parkinson's Disease and Movement Disorders*. 4th Ed. Ed. J. Jankovic, and E. Tolosa. pp. 212–227. Philadelphia: Lippincott, Williams & Wilkins.
2. Wexler, N.S., J. Lorimer, J. Porter, F. Gomez, C. Moskowitz, E. Shackell, K. Marder, et al. 2004. Venezuelan kindreds reveal that genetic and environmental factors modulate Huntington's disease age of onset. *Proc Natl Acad Sci USA* **101**:3498–3503.
3. Margolis, R.L., and C.A. Ross. 2003. Diagnosis of Huntington disease. *Clin Chem* **49**:1726–1732.
4. Murgod, U.A., Q. Saleem, A. Anand, S.K. Brahmachari, S. Jain, and U.B. Muthane. 2001. A clinical study of patients with genetically confirmed Huntington's disease from India. *J Neurol Sci* **190**:73–78.
5. Byers, R.K., and J.A. Dodge. 1967. Huntington's chorea in children. Report of four cases. *Neurology* **17**:587–596.
6. Byers, R.K., F.H. Gilles, and C. Fung. 1973. Huntington's disease in children. Neuropathologic study of four cases. *Neurology* **23**:561–569.
7. The Huntington's Disease Collaborative Research Group. 1993. A novel gene containing a trinucleotide repeat that is expanded and unstable on Huntington's disease chromosomes. *Cell* **72**:971–983.
8. Squitieri, F., C. Gellera, M. Cannella, C. Mariotti, G. Cislaghi, D.C. Rubinsztein, E.W. Almqvist, et al. 2003. Homozygosity for CAG mutation in Huntington disease is associated with a more severe clinical course. *Brain* **126**:946–955.
9. McInnis, M.G. 1996. Anticipation: an old idea in new genes. *Am J Hum Genet* **59**:973–979.
10. Ranen, N.G., O.C. Stine, M.H. Abbott, M. Sherr, A.M. Codori, M.L. Franz, N.I. Chao, A.S. Chung, et al. 1995. Anticipation and instability of IT-15 (CAG)n repeats in parent-offspring pairs with Huntington disease. *Am J Hum Genet* **57**:593–602.
11. Gusella, J.F., N.S. Wexler, P.M. Conneally, S.L. Naylor, M.A. Anderson, R.E. Tanzi, P.C. Watkins, et al. 1983. A polymorphic DNA marker genetically linked to Huntington's disease. *Nature* **306**:234–238.
12. Takano, H., and J.F. Gusella. 2002. The predominantly HEAT-like motif structure of huntingtin and its association and coincident nuclear entry with dorsal, an NF-kB/Rel/dorsal family transcription factor. BMC *Neurosci* **3**:15.
13. Andrade, M.A., and P. Bork. 1995. HEAT repeats in the Huntington's disease protein. *Nat Genet* **11**:115–116.
14. Andrade, M.A., C. Perez-Iratxeta, and C.P. 2001. Protein repeats: structures, functions, and evolution. J Struct Biol **134**:117–131.
15. MacDonald, M.E. 2003. Huntingtin: alive and well and working in middle management. *Sci* STKE 2003: pe48.

16. Harjes, P., and E.E. Wanker. 2003. The hunt for huntingtin function: interaction partners tell many different stories. *Trends Biochem Sci* **28**:425–433.
17. Landwehrmeyer, G.B., S.M. McNeil, L.St. Dure, P. Ge, H. Aizawa, Q. Huang, C.M. Ambrose, et al. 1995. Huntington's disease gene: regional and cellular expression in brain of normal and affected individuals. *Ann Neurol* **37**:218–230.
18. Sharp, A.H., S.J. Loev, G. Schilling, S.H. Li, X.J. Li, J. Bao, M.V. Wagster, et al. 1995. Widespread expression of Huntington's disease gene (IT15) protein product. *Neuron* **14**:1065–1074.
19. Strong, T.V., D.A. Tagle, J.M. Valdes, L.W. Elmer, K. Boehm, M. Swaroop, K.W. Kaatz, et al. 1993. Widespread expression of the human and rat Huntington's disease gene in brain and nonneural tissues. *Nat Genet* **5**:259–265.
20. Ferrante, R.J., C.A. Gutekunst, F. Persichetti, S.M. McNeil, N.W. Kowall, J.F. Gusella, M.E. MacDonald, et al. 1997. Heterogeneous topographic and cellular distribution of huntingtin expression in the normal human neostriatum. *J Neurosci* **17**:3052–3063.
21. Hilditch-Maguire, P., F. Trettel, L.A. Passani, A. Auerbach, F. Persichetti, and M.E. MacDonald. 2000. Huntingtin: an iron-regulated protein essential for normal nuclear and perinuclear organelles. *Hum Mol Genet* **9**:2789–2797.
22. Lunkes, A., K.S. Lindenberg, L. Ben-Haiem, C. Weber, D. Devys, G.B. Landwehrmeyer, J.L. Mandel, and Y. Trottier. 2002. Proteases acting on mutant huntingtin generate cleaved products that differentially build up cytoplasmic and nuclear inclusions. *Mol Cell* **10**: 259–269.
23. DiFiglia, M. 2002. Huntingtin fragments that aggregate go their separate ways. *Mol Cell* **10**:224–225.
24. Trushina, E., M.P. Heldebrant, C.M. Perez-Terzic, R. Bortolon, I.V. Kovtun, J.D. Badger, 2nd, A. Terzic, et al. 2003. Microtubule destabilization and nuclear entry are sequential steps leading to toxicity in Huntington's disease. *Proc Natl Acad Sci USA* **100**:12171–12176.
25. Sugars, K.L., and D.C. Rubinsztein. 2003. Transcriptional abnormalities in Huntington disease. *Trends Genet* **19**:233–238.
26. Li, S.H., and X.J. Li. 2004. Huntingtin-protein interactions and the pathogenesis of Huntington's disease. *Trends Genet* **20**:146–154.
27. Burke, M.G., R. Woscholski, and S.N. Yaliraki. 2003. Differential hydrophobicity drives self-assembly in Huntington's disease. *Proc Natl Acad Sci USA* **100**:13928–13933.
28. Vonsattel, J.P., R.H. Myers, T.J. Stevens, R.J. Ferrante, E.D. Bird, and E.P. Richardson, Jr. 1985. Neuropathological classification of Huntington's disease. *J Neuropathol Exp Neurol* **44**:559–577.
29. Cicchetti, F., L. Prensa, Y. Wu, and A. Parent. 2000. Chemical anatomy of striatal interneurons in normal individuals and in patients with Huntington's disease. *Brain Res Rev* **34**:80–101.
30. Bugiani, O., M. Tabaton, and S. Cammarata. 1984. Huntington's disease: survival of large striatal neurons in the rigid variant. *Ann Neurol* **15**:154–156.
31. Roberts, R.C., and M. DiFiglia. 1989. Short- and long-term survival of large neurons in the excitotoxic lesioned rat caudate nucleus: a light and electron microscopic study. *Synapse* **3**:363–37.
32. Glass, M., M. Dragunow, and R.L. Faull. 2000. The pattern of neurodegeneration in Huntington's disease: a comparative study of cannabinoid, dopamine, adenosine and GABA(A) receptor alterations in the human basal ganglia in Huntington's disease. *Neuroscience* **97**:505–519.
33. Denovan-Wright, E.M., and H.A. Robertson. 2000. Cannabinoid receptor messenger RNA levels decrease in a subset of neurons of the lateral striatum, cortex and hippocampus of transgenic Huntington's disease mice. *Neuroscience* **98**:705–713.
34. Rosas, H.D., A.K. Liu, S. Hersch, M. Glessner, R.J. Ferrante, D.H. Salat, A. van der Kouwe, et al. 2002. Regional and progressive thinning of the cortical ribbon in Huntington's disease. *Neurology* **58**:695–701.
35. Selemon, L.D., G. Rajkowska, and P.S. Goldman-Rakic. 2004. Evidence for progression in frontal cortical pathology in late-stage Huntington's disease. *J Comp Neurol* **468**:190–204.
36. Macdonald, V., G.M. Halliday, R.J. Trent, and E.A. McCusker. 1997. Significant loss of pyramidal neurons in the angular gyrus of patients with Huntington's disease. *Neuropathol Appl Neurobiol* **23**:492–495.
37. Macdonald, V., and G. Halliday. 2002. Pyramidal cell loss in motor cortices in Huntington's disease. *Neurobiol Dis* **10**:378–386.
38. Yohrling, G.J., G.C. Jiang, M.M. DeJohn, D.W. Miller, A.B. Young, K.E. Vrana, and J.H. Cha. 2003. Analysis of cellular, transgenic and human models of Huntington's disease reveals tyrosine hydroxylase alterations and substantia nigra neuropathology. *Brain Res Mol Brain Res* **119**:28–36.
39. Berardelli, A., J. Noth, P.D. Thompson, E.L. Bollen, A. Curra, G. Deuschl, J.G. van Dijk, et al. 1999. Pathophysiology of chorea and bradykinesia in Huntington's disease. *Mov Disord* **14**:398–403.
40. Myers, R.H., D.S. Sax, M. Schoenfeld, E.D. Bird, P.A. Wolf, J.P. Vonsattel, R.F. White, and J.B. Martin. 1985. Late onset of Huntington's disease. *J Neurol Neurosurg Psychiatry* **48**:530–534.
41. McCusker, E., F. Richards, D. Sillence, M. Wilson, and R.J. Trent. 2000. Huntington's disease: neurological assessment of potential gene carriers presenting for predictive DNA testing. *J Clin Neurosci* **7**: 38–41.
42. Starr, A. 1967. A disorder of rapid eye movements in Huntington's chorea. *Brain* **90**:545–564.
43. Leigh, R.J., S.A. Newman, S.E. Folstein, A.G. Lasker, and B.A. Jensen. 1983. Abnormal ocular motor control in Huntington's disease. *Neurology* **33**:1268–1275.
44. Lasker, A.G., and D.S. Zee. 1997. Ocular motor abnormalities in Huntington's disease. *Vision Res* **37**:3639–3645.
45. Winograd-Gurvich, C.T., N. Georgiou-Karistianis, A. Evans, L. Millist, J.L. Bradshaw, A. Churchyard, E. Chiu, and O.B. White. 2003. Hypometric primary saccades and increased variability in visually-guided saccades in Huntington's disease. *Neuropsychologia* **41**:1683–1692.
46. Jayaraman, A. 1985. Functional compartments of the cat striatum. *Neurosci Abs* **11**:199.
47. Louis, E.D., P. Lee, L. Quinn, and K. Marder. 1999. Dystonia in Huntington's disease: prevalence and clinical characteristics. *Mov Disord* **14**:95–101.
48. Ashizawa, T., and J. Jankovic. 1996. Cervical dystonia as the initial presentation of Huntington's disease. *Mov Disord* **11**:457–459.
49. Jankovic, J., and T. Ashizawa. 1995. Tourettism associated with Huntington's disease. *Mov Disord* **10**:103–105.
50. Sanchez-Pernaut, R., G. Kunig, A. del Barrio Alba, J.G. de Yebenes, P. Vontobel, and K.L. Leenders. 2000. Bradykinesia in early Huntington's disease. *Neurology* **54**:119–125.
51. van Vugt, J.P., K.K. Piet, L.J. Vink, S. Siesling, A.H. Zwinderman, H.A. Middelkoop, and R.A. Roos. 2004. Objective assessment of motor slowness in Huntington's disease: clinical correlates and 2-year follow-up. *Mov Disord* **19**:285–297.
52. Koller, W.C., and J. Trimble. 1985. The gait abnormality of Huntington's disease. *Neurology* **35**:1450–1454.
53. Thaut, M.H., R. Miltner, H.W. Lange, C.P. Hurt, and V. Hoemberg. 1999. Velocity modulation and rhythmic synchronization of gait in Huntington's disease. *Mov Disord* **14**:808–819.
54. Hausdorff, J.M., S.L. Mitchell, R. Firtion, C.K. Peng, M.E. Cudkowicz, J.Y. Wei, and A.L. Goldberger. 1997. Altered fractal dynamics of gait: reduced stride-interval correlations with aging and Huntington's disease. *J Appl Physiol* **82**:262–269.
55. Churchyard, A.J., M.E. Morris, N. Georgiou, E. Chiu, R. Cooper, and R. Iansek. 2001. Gait dysfunction in Huntington's disease: parkinsonism and a disorder of timing. Implications for movement rehabilitation. *Adv Neurol* **87**:375–385.

56. Ho, A.K., B.J. Sahakian, R.G. Brown, R.A. Barker, J.R. Hodges, M.N. Ane, J. Snowden, et al. 2003. Profile of cognitive progression in early Huntington's disease. *Neurology* **61**:1702–1706.
57. Snowden, J.S., D. Craufurd, J. Thompson, and D. Neary. 2002. Psychomotor, executive, and memory function in preclinical Huntington's disease. *J Clin Exp Neuropsychol* **24**:133–145.
58. Mendez, M.F. 1994. Huntington's disease: update and review of neuropsychiatric aspects. *Int J Psychiatry Med* **24**:189–208.
59. Rosenblatt, A., and I. Leroi. 2000. Neuropsychiatry of Huntington's disease and other basal ganglia disorders. *Psychosomatics* **41**:24–30.
60. Paulsen, J.S., R.E. Ready, J.M. Hamilton, M.S. Mega, and J.L. Cummings. 2001. Neuropsychiatric aspects of Huntington's disease. *J Neurol Neurosurg Psychiatry* **71**:310–314.
61. Schoenfeld, M., R.H. Myers, L.A. Cupples, B. Berkman, D.S. Sax, and E. Clark. 1984. Increased rate of suicide among patients with Huntington's disease. *J Neurol Neurosurg Psychiatry* **47**:1283–1287.
62. Arciniegas, D.B., and C.A. Anderson. 2002. Suicide in neurologic illness. *Curr Treat Options Neurol* **4**:457–468.
63. Di Maio, L., F. Squitieri, G. Napolitano, G. Campanella, J.A. Trofatter, and P.M. Conneally. 1993. Suicide risk in Huntington's disease. *J Med Genet* **30**:293–295.
64. Sorensen, S.A., and K. Fenger. 1992. Causes of death in patients with Huntington's disease and in unaffected first degree relatives. *J Med Genet* **29**:911–914.
65. Robins Wahlin, T.B., L. Backman, A. Lundin, A. Haegermark, B. Winblad, and M. Anvret. 2000. High suicidal ideation in persons testing for Huntington's disease. Acta Neurol Scand 102:150–161.
66. Cummings, J.L. 1995. Behavioral and psychiatric symptoms associated with Huntington's disease. *Adv Neurol* **65**:179–186.
67. Anderson, K.E., E.D. Louis, Y. Stern, and K.S. Marder. 2001. Cognitive correlates of obsessive and compulsive symptoms in Huntington's disease. *Am J Psychiatry* **158**:799–801.
68. Kremer, H.P., and R.A. Roos. 1992. Weight loss in Huntington's disease. *Arch Neurol* **49**:349.
69. Djousse, L., B. Knowlton, L.A. Cupples, K. Marder, I. Shoulson, and R.H. Myers. 2002. Weight loss in early stage of Huntington's disease. *Neurology* **59**:1325–1330.
70. Hamilton, J.M., T. Wolfson, G.M. Peavy, M.W. Jacobson, and J. Corey-Bloom. 2004. Rate and correlates of weight change in Huntington's disease. *J Neurol Neurosurg Psychiatry* **75**:209–212.
71. Braak, H., and E. Braak. 1992. Anatomy of the human hypothalamus (chiasmatic and tuberal region). *Prog Brain Res* **93**:3–14; discussion 14–16.
72. Kremer, H.P. 1992. The hypothalamic lateral tuberal nucleus: normal anatomy and changes in neurological diseases. *Prog Brain Res* **93**: 249–261.
73. Kremer, B., S.J. Tallaksen-Greene, and R.L. Albin. 1993. AMPA and NMDA binding sites in the hypothalamic lateral tuberal nucleus: implications for Huntington's disease. *Neurology* **43**:1593–1595.
74. Keogh, H.J., R.H. Johnson, R.N. Nanda, and W.R. Sulaiman. 1976. Altered growth hormone release in Huntington's chorea. *J Neurol Neurosurg Psychiatry* **39**:244–248.
75. Kremer, H.P., R.A. Roos, M. Frolich, J.K. Radder, A.C. Nieuwenhuijzen Kruseman, A. Van der Velde, and O.J. Buruma. 1989. Endocrine functions in Huntington's disease. A two-and-a-half years follow-up study. *J Neurol Sci* **90**:335–344.
76. Podolsky, S., N.A. Leopold, and D.S. Sax. 1972. Increased frequency of diabetes mellitus in patients with Huntington's chorea. *Lancet* **1**:1356–1358.
77. Hurlbert, M.S., W. Zhou, C. Wasmeier, F.G. Kaddis, J.C. Hutton, and C.R. Freed. 1999. Mice transgenic for an expanded CAG repeat in the Huntington's disease gene develop diabetes. *Diabetes* **48**:649–651.
78. Andreassen, O.A., A. Dedeoglu, V. Stanojevic, D.B. Hughes, S.E. Browne, C.A. Leech, R.J. Ferrante, et al. 2002. Huntington's disease of the endocrine pancreas: insulin deficiency and diabetes mellitus due to impaired insulin gene expression. *Neurobiol Dis* **11**:410–424.
79. Nance, M.A., and R.H. Myers. 2001. Juvenile onset Huntington's disease–clinical and research perspectives. *Ment Retard Dev Disabil Res Rev* **7**:153–157.
80. Louis, A.G.E.D., K.E. Anderson, C. Moskowitz, D.Z. Thorne, and K. Marder. 2000. Dystonia-predominant adult-onset Huntington disease: association between motor phenotype and age of onset in adults. *Arch Neurol* **57**:1326–1330.
81. Reuter, I., M.T. Hu, T.C. Andrews, D.J. Brocks, C. Clough, and K.R. Chaudhuri. 2000. Late onset levodopa responsive Huntington's disease with minimal chorea masquerading as Parkinson plus syndrome. *J Neurol Neurosurg Psychiatry* **68**:238–241.
82. James, C.M., G.D. Houlihan, R.G. Snell, J.P. Cheadle, and P.S. Harper. 1994. Late-onset Huntington's disease: a clinical and molecular study. *Age Ageing* **23**:445–448.
83. James, R.C. James, F. Xiang, J. Monaghan, D. Han, Z. Zhang, L. Edstrom, M. Anvret, and S.B. Prusiner. 2001. Huntington disease phenocopy is a familial prion disease. *Am J Hum Genet* **69**:1385–1388.
84. Margolis, R.L., E. O'Hearn, A. Rosenblatt, V. Willour, S.E. Holmes, M.L. Franz, C. Callahan, H.S. Hwang, J.C. Troncoso, and C.A. Ross. 2001. A disorder similar to Huntington's disease is associated with a novel CAG repeat expansion. *Ann Neurol* **50**:373–380.
85. Holmes, S.E., E. O'Hearn, A. Rosenblatt, C. Callahan, H.S. Hwang, R.G. Ingersoll-Ashworth, A. Fleisher, et al. 2001. A repeat expansion in the gene encoding junctophilin-3 is associated with Huntington disease-like 2. *Nat Genet* **29**:377–378.
86. Walker, R.H., A. Rasmussen, D. Rudnicki, S.E. Holmes, E. Alonso, T. Matsuura, T. Ashizawa, et al. 2003. Huntington's disease-like 2 can present as chorea-acanthocytosis. *Neurology* **61**:1002–1004.
87. Walker, R.H., J. Jankovic, E. O'Hearn, and R.L. Margolis. 2003. Phenotypic features of Huntington's disease-like 2. *Mov Disord* **18**: 1527–1530.
88. Singer, C. 1992. "Haw River syndrome" or dentato-rubro-pallido-luysian atrophy? *Arch Neurol* **49**:13–14.
89. Burke, J.R., T. Ikeuchi, R. Koide, S. Tsuji, M. Yamada, M.A. Pericak-Vance, and J.M. Vance. 1994. Dentatorubral-pallidoluysian atrophy and Haw River syndrome. *Lancet* **344**:1711–1712.
90. Burke, J.R., M.S. Wingfield, K.E. Lewis, A.D. Roses, J.E. Lee, C. Hulette, M.A. Pericak-Vance, and J.M. Vance. 1994. The Haw River syndrome: dentatorubropallidoluysian atrophy (DRPLA) in an African-American family. *Nat Genet* **7**:521–524.
91. Potter, N.T., H. Yanagisawa, and M. Yamada. 1996. Different origins of expanded repeats for Haw River syndrome and dentatorubral-pallidoluysian atrophy. *Lancet* **347**:1271.
92. Stevanin, G., H. Fujigasaki, A.S. Lebre, A. Camuzat, C. Jeannequin, C. Dode, J. Takahashi, C. San, et al. 2003. Huntington's disease-like phenotype due to trinucleotide repeat expansions in the TBP and JPH3 genes. *Brain* **126**:1599–1603.
93. Bauer, P., F. Laccone, A. Rolfs, U. Wullner, S. Bosch, H. Peters, S. Liebscher, et al. 2004. Trinucleotide repeat expansion in SCA17/TBP in white patients with Huntington's disease-like phenotype. *J Med Genet* **41**:230–232.
94. Breedveld, G.J., J.W. van Dongen, C. Danesino, A. Guala, A.K. Percy, L.S. Dure, P. Harper, et al. 2002. Mutations in TITF-1 are associated with benign hereditary chorea. *Hum Mol Genet* **11**:971–979.
95. Kambouris, M., S. Bohlega, A. Al-Tahan, and B.F. Meyer. 2000. Localization of the gene for a novel autosomal recessive neurodegenerative Huntington-like disorder to 4p15.3. *Am J Hum Genet* **66**:445–452.
96. Grimbergen, Y.A., and R.A. Roos. 2003. Therapeutic options for Huntington's disease. *Curr Opin Investig Drugs* **4**:51–54.
97. Parsa, M.A., E. Szigethy, J.M. Voci, and H.Y. Meltzer. 1997. Risperidone in treatment of choreoathetosis of Huntington's disease. *J Clin Psychopharmacol* **17**:134–135.

98. Erdemoglu, A.K., and C. Boratav. 2002. Risperidone in chorea and psychosis of Huntington's disease. *Eur J Neurol* **9**:182–183.
99. Bonelli, R.M., F.A. Mahnert, and G. Niederwieser. 2002. Olanzapine for Huntington's disease: an open label study. *Clin Neuropharmacol* **25**:263–265.
100. Paleacu, D., M. Anca, and N. Giladi. 2002. Olanzapine in Huntington's disease. *Acta Neurol Scand* **105**:441–444.
101. DiFiglia, M. 1990. Excitotoxic injury of the neostriatum: a model for Huntington's disease. *Trends Neurosci* **13**:286–289.
102. Kieburtz, K. 1999. Antiglutamate therapies in Huntington's disease. *J Neural Transm* Suppl **55**:97–102.
103. Palfi, S., R.J. Ferrante, E. Brouillet, M.F. Beal, R. Dolan, M.C. Guyot, M. Peschanski, and P. Hantraye. 1996. Chronic 3-nitropropionic acid treatment in baboons replicates the cognitive and motor deficits of Huntington's disease. *J Neurosci* **16**:3019–3025.
104. Mary, V., F. Wahl, and J.M. Stutzmann. 1995. Effect of riluzole on quinolinate-induced neuronal damage in rats: comparison with blockers of glutamatergic neurotransmission. *Neurosci Lett* **201**:92–96.
105. Schiefer, J., G.B. Landwehrmeyer, H.G. Luesse, A. Sprunken, C. Puls, A. Milkereit, E. Milkereit, and C.M. Kosinski. 2002. Riluzole prolongs survival time and alters nuclear inclusion formation in a transgenic mouse model of Huntington's disease. *Mov Disord* **17**:748–757.
106. Rosas, H.D., W.J. Koroshetz, B.G. Jenkins, Y.I. Chen, D.L. Hayden, M.F. Beal, and M.E. Cudkowicz. 1999. Riluzole therapy in Huntington's disease (HD). *Mov Disord* **14**:326–330.
107. Seppi, K., J. Mueller, T. Bodner, E. Brandauer, T. Benke, H. Weirich-Schwaiger, W. Poewe, and G.K. Wenning. 2001. Riluzole in Huntington's disease (HD): an open label study with one year follow up. *J Neurol* **248**:866–869.
108. Huntington Study Group. 2003. Dosage effects of riluzole in Huntington's disease: a multicenter placebo-controlled study. *Neurology* **61**:1551–1556.
109. Lucetti, C., G. Gambaccini, S. Bernardini, G. Dell'Agnello, L. Petrozzi, G. Rossi, and U. Bonuccelli. 2002. Amantadine in Huntington's disease: open-label video-blinded study. *Neurol Sci* 23 Suppl 2:S83–84.
110. Verhagen Metman, L., M.J. Morris, C. Farmer, M. Gillespie, K. Mosby, J. Wuu, and T.N. Chase. 2002. Huntington's disease: a randomized, controlled trial using the NMDA-antagonist amantadine. *Neurology* **59**:694–699.
111. Panov, A.V., C.A. Gutekunst, B.R. Leavitt, M.R. Hayden, J.R. Burke, W.J. Strittmatter, and J.T. Greenamyre. 2002. Early mitochondrial calcium defects in Huntington's disease are a direct effect of polyglutamines. *Nat Neurosci* **5**:731–736.
112. Gu, M., M.T. Gash, V.M. Mann, F. Javoy-Agid, J.M. Cooper, and A.H. Schapira. 1996. Mitochondrial defect in Huntington's disease caudate nucleus. *Ann Neurol* **39**:385–389.
113. Schapira, A.H. 1998. Mitochondrial dysfunction in neurodegenerative disorders. *Biochim Biophys Acta* 1**366**:225–233.
114. Vis, J.C., M.M. Verbeek, R.M. De Waal, H.J. Ten Donkelaar, and H.P. Kremer. 1999. 3-Nitropropionic acid induces a spectrum of Huntington's disease-like neuropathology in rat striatum. *Neuropathol Appl Neurobiol* **25**:513–521.
115. Napolitano, M., D. Centonze, P. Gubellini, S. Rossi, S. Spiezia, G. Bernardi, A. Gulino, and P. Calabresi. 2004. Inhibition of mitochondrial complex II alters striatal expression of genes involved in glutamatergic and dopaminergic signaling: possible implications for Huntington's disease. *Neurobiol Dis* **15**:407–414.
116. Huntington Study Group. 2001. A randomized, placebo-controlled trial of coenzyme Q10 and remacemide in Huntington's disease. *Neurology* **57**:397–404.
117. Diguet, E., R. Rouland, and F. Tison. 2003. Minocycline is not beneficial in a phenotypic mouse model of Huntington's disease. *Ann Neurol* **54**:841–842.
118. Hersch, S., K. Fink, J.P. Vonsattel, and R.M. Friedlander. 2003. Minocycline is protective in a mouse model of Huntington's disease. *Ann Neurol* **54**:841; author reply 842–843.
119. Bonelli, R.M., C. Heuberger, and F. Reisecker. 2003. Minocycline for Huntington's disease: an open label study. *Neurology* **60**:883–884.
120. Smith, D.L., B. Woodman, A. Mahal, K. Sathasivam, S. Ghazi-Noori, P.A. Lowden, G.P. Bates, and E. Hockly. 2003. Minocycline and doxycycline are not beneficial in a model of Huntington's disease. *Ann Neurol* **54**:186–196.
121. Johnstone, R.W. 2002. Histone-deacetylase inhibitors: novel drugs for the treatment of cancer. *Nat Rev Drug Discov* **1**:287–299.
122. McCampbell, A., A.A. Taye, L. Whitty, E. Penney, J.S. Steffan, and K.H. Fischbeck. 2001. Histone deacetylase inhibitors reduce polyglutamine toxicity. *Proc Natl Acad Sci USA* **98**:15179–15184.
123. Hughes, R.E., R.S. Lo, C. Davis, A.D. Strand, C.L. Neal, J.M. Olson, and S. Fields. 2001. Altered transcription in yeast expressing expanded polyglutamine. *Proc Natl Acad Sci USA* **98**:13201–13206.
124. Steffan, J.S., L. Bodai, J. Pallos, M. Poelman, A. McCampbell, B.L. Apostol, A. Kazantsev, et al. 2001. Histone deacetylase inhibitors arrest polyglutamine-dependent neurodegeneration in *Drosophila*. *Nature* **413**:739–743.
125. Ferrante, R.J., J.K. Kubilus, J. Lee, H. Ryu, A. Beesen, B. Zucker, K. Smith, et al. 2003. Histone deacetylase inhibition by sodium butyrate chemotherapy ameliorates the neurodegenerative phenotype in Huntington's disease mice. *J Neurosci* **23**:9418–9427.
126. Hockly, E., V.M. Richon, B. Woodman, D.L. Smith, X. Zhou, E. Rosa, K. Sathasivam, et al. 2003. Suberoylanilide hydroxamic acid, a histone deacetylase inhibitor, ameliorates motor deficits in a mouse model of Huntington's disease. *Proc Natl Acad Sci USA* **100**:2041–2046.
127. Alberch, J., E. Perez-Navarro, and J.M. Canals. 2004. Neurotrophic factors in Huntington's disease. *Prog Brain Res* **146**:195–229.
128. Horellou, P., and J. Mallet. 1998. Neuronal grafts for Huntington's disease. *Nat Med* **4**:669–670.
129. Gaura, V., A.C. Bachoud-Levi, M.J. Ribeiro, J.P. Nguyen, V. Frouin, S. Baudic, P. Brugieres, et al. 2004. Striatal neural grafting improves cortical metabolism in Huntington's disease patients. *Brain* **127**:65–72.
130. Hauser, R.A., S. Furtado, C.R. Cimino, H. Delgado, S. Eichler, S. Schwartz, D. Scott, et al. 2002. Bilateral human fetal striatal transplantation in Huntington's disease. *Neurology* **58**:687–695.
131. Albin, R.L. 2002. Fetal striatal transplantation in Huntington's disease: time for a pause. J *Neurol Neurosurg Psychiatry* **73**:612.

CHAPTER

D2

Transgenic Rodent Models of Huntington Disease

GABRIELE SCHILLING, CHRISTOPHER A. ROSS, and DAVID R. BORCHELT

Have you ever had an exam question where the instructor told you that there was more than one correct answer? The study of transgenic mouse models of Huntington disease (HD) is a classic example of such a situation. A number of investigators have asked whether a mouse that models this disease can be created and very few have used the same approach. The spectrum of answers provides insight into the molecular mechanisms of HD and other disorders caused by glutamine-encoding CAG repeat expansions.

I. GENETIC, CLINICAL, AND PATHOLOGICAL FEATURES OF HD

A number of neurodegenerative disorders, including HD, several types of spinocerebellar ataxia (SCA), spinobulbar muscular atrophy (SBMA), Machado-Joseph Disease (MJD), and dentato-rubral pallido-luysian atrophy (DRPLA), are caused by the expansion of polymorphic tracts of CAG repeats (coding for consecutive glutamine residues) within a diverse set of genes (La Spada et al. 1991; Huntington's Disease Collaborative Research Group 1993; Orr et al. 1993; Kawaguchi et al. 1994; Koide et al. 1994; Nagafuchi et al. 1994). Although the type of genetic mutation is similar among these disorders, the populations of affected neurons, the clinical syndromes, and the neuropathological lesions are quite distinct for each disorder [for reviews see (Ross et al. 1997; Orr 2001; Fischbeck 2001; Sieradzan and Mann 2001)]. Each of the CAG repeat disorders is associated with a distinct gene product: huntingtin for HD, ataxins for SCA-1 to 13 and MJD (ataxin-3), androgen receptor for SBMA, and atrophin-1 for DRPLA. With the exception of the androgen receptor, the normal function of the disease-associated gene is either unknown or incompletely characterized; hence many of the gene products have been given a disease-specific name. The length of the glutamine repeat correlates inversely with disease onset; the longer the repeat, the earlier the age of onset [for reviews see (Ross 1995; Ross et al. 1997)].

Like the other CAG repeat disorders, HD is progressively debilitating, ultimately leading to death over a protracted (fifteen to twenty-five year) period. The symptoms of the disease include motor dysfunction (chorea and/or rigidity), cognitive changes that progress to dementia, and psychiatric disturbances [for review see (Ross et al. 1997)]. The worldwide incidence of HD is about 1 : 10,000 people, with virtually all cases caused by mutations in the huntingtin gene. The HD gene was initially localized to the short arm of chromosome 4 by standard linkage analyses and then subsequently identified by the presence of the CAG repeat expansion in exon 1 of the huntingtin (*htt*) gene. Expansions beyond a threshold of thirty-six CAGs cause the disease (Huntington's Disease Collaborative Research Group, 1993). Studies to date suggest that HD is likely to be caused by a "gain of property" mechanism where mutant htt acquires a property that is toxic [for review see (Ross 1995)].

The pathologic features of HD have been well characterized. HD postmortem brains show substantial general atrophy, but most prevalent is the selective loss of striatal medium spiny, GABA-ergic, neurons in the caudate and putamen. Interneurons of the striatum, mostly NAPDH- and ChAT-positive, are spared. In the cortex, degeneration of neurons projecting to the basal ganglia is observed in the deeper layers—3, 5, and 6. Other less-affected areas include the globus pallidus, subthalamic nucleus, and amygdala. Pathology outside the CNS is thought to be minimal.

At the cellular level, neurons throughout the CNS contain inclusion structures that are immuno-labeled by antibodies to htt and ubiquitin (Davies et al. 1997; DiFiglia et al. 1997; Becher et al. 1998; Gutekunst et al. 1999). At initial inspection of immunostained sections, prominent inclusions are immediately visualized within nuclei of multiple neuronal populations throughout the brain. The frequency and overall distribution of nuclear inclusion pathology are largely proportional to the length of the repeat; with longer repeats, the frequency of neuronal inclusions increases and the number of affected brain regions broadens (Becher et al. 1998). The immunoreactivity of these structures to htt antibodies is restricted to those raised against the N-terminus of htt, suggesting that proteolytic activities act upon full-length mutant htt to generate aggregating fragments (Davies et al. 1997; DiFiglia et al. 1997; Becher et al. 1998; Lunkes and Mandel 1998; Gutekunst et al. 1999; Hodgson et al. 1999; Sieradzan et al. 1999). In addition to nuclear inclusions of mutant htt, neurons throughout the CNS accumulate cytoplasmic htt inclusions (Gutekunst et al. 1999). Aggregates of mutant htt appear in cytoplasm prior to nuclear inclusions, and at end-stage become much more numerous than the nuclear inclusions. Like the nuclear inclusions, cytoplasmic aggregates appear to be formed from N-terminal fragments of mutant protein (Sieradzan et al. 1999). Investigators have not identified the proteases responsible for the generation of these aggregating fragments. Caspases may be involved (Wellington et al. 1998; Wellington et al. 2002), but the fragments generated appear to be much smaller than caspase-generated fragments, implicating other proteolytic activities (Lunkes et al. 2002).

II. HUNTINGTIN BIOLOGY

Huntingtin is a large protein of 3144 amino acids in length with a molecular mass of 348 kDa (Huntington's Disease Collaborative Research Group 1993). The polyglutamine repeat begins at amino acid 18 of the protein and is closely followed by a poly-proline domain. Within the body of the protein are located several HEAT-repeat domains, which may mediate protein-protein interactions (Andrade and Bork 1995). The function of normal htt is incompletely understood. Targeted deletion of huntingtin in mice leads to early embryonic lethality (Duyao et al. 1995; Zeitlin et al. 1995). Recent studies of proteins that interact with htt have suggested a role in endocytosis and/or vesicle trafficking (Henry et al. 2002; Singaraja et al. 2002). Other studies have demonstrated interactions between htt and transcriptional regulatory proteins (McCampbell et al. 2000; Nucifora, Jr. et al. 2001; Zuccato et al. 2001; Zuccato et al. 2003).

The htt protein is widely expressed in the brain and peripheral tissues (Landwehrmeyer et al. 1995; Sharp et al. 1995; Bhide et al. 1996). Medium spiny neurons do not appear to express higher levels of htt than other neurons (Landwehrmeyer et al. 1995). Indeed, single cell PCR studies suggest that htt is more highly expressed in interneurons of the striatum than in the medium spiny neurons, which are the more vulnerable population (Fusco et al. 1999). Subcellularly, htt can be found throughout neuronal cell bodies, but may be more enriched in nerve terminals and vesicles (Sharp et al. 1995).

III. MUTANT HUNTINGTIN AGGREGATION

As indicated above, aggregates of mutant htt produce neuronal nuclear and cytoplasmic inclusions in the brains of HD patients (DiFiglia et al. 1997; Becher et al. 1998; Gutekunst et al. 1999) and in the brains of transgenic mice that express mutant versions of htt (see below). Dr. Max Perutz first predicted in 1994 that such pathologic lesions might occur when he proposed that long tracts of polyglutamine may form "polar zipper" structures, in which hydrogen bonds between the glutamines assemble in anti-parallel-sheet structures (Perutz 1994). At about the time pathologic studies were demonstrating huntingtin inclusion pathology, Scherzinger and colleagues reported that purified N-terminal fragments of mutant htt aggregate in a repeat length dependent manner (Scherzinger et al. 1997). Further studies revealed that mutant huntingtin fragments display properties similar to amyloid in that aggregation proceeds through a seeding process to form aggregates that have structures similar to amyloids (Scherzinger et al. 1999). The "polar zipper model" appeared to explain how other proteins containing nonpathologic polyglutamine domains, such as CREB-binding protein (McCampbell et al. 2000; Nucifora Jr. et al. 2001), Sp1 (Dunah et al. 2002; Li et al. 2002), TATA-binding protein (Roon-Mom et al. 2002), and TAFII130 (Shimohata et al. 2000; Dunah et al. 2002), might be recruited into aggregates of mutant htt.

Despite the initial excitement over the discovery of htt aggregates in the brains of HD patients and transgenic mouse models of HD, the role of macromolecular aggregates in the pathogenesis of disease remains controversial. For example, mutant huntingtin aggregates are generally not very frequent in the most-affected regions of the human brain, i.e., medium spiny neurons in the striatum (Gutekunst et al. 1999). As discussed below, we and others have observed that neurons in brains of some of the transgenic mouse models can carry aggregates throughout their lifespans without obvious toxicity or degeneration. In mouse models of spinocerebellar ataxia 1 (SCA1), altering mutant ataxin 1 in a manner that diminishes the formation of large inclusion structures does not abolish toxicity (Klement et al. 1998). Conversely, deleting E6-AP ubiquitin ligase in mice expressing mutant ataxin 1 decreases aggregate formation while, at the same time, increasing toxicity (Cummings et al. 1999). Thus, investigators have proposed that monomeric or oligomeric species of htt may be the toxic species, not the large inclusion structures (Klement et al. 1998; Poirier et al. 2002). By contrast, Bence and colleagues recently demonstrated that polyglutamine aggregates were associated with reductions in proteasome function in cultured cell models (Bence et al. 2001). Notably, nuclear aggregates found in most polyglutamine diseases are immunoreactive for ubiquitin, adding further fuel to the notion that aggregates of polyglutamine protein may inhibit the proteasome. Thus, whether large aggregates are less toxic structures than some misfolded intermediate (monomer or small oligomer) is controversial.

IV. MOUSE MODELS OF HD NEUROPATHOLOGY

At the time of writing, ten distinct reports of transgenic or knock-in mouse models of HD could be found in the literature (Table 1). Investigators have created mice that express N-terminal fragments of mutant huntingtin, the N-terminal third of the protein, and the full-length mutant human protein. Investigators have also modified the endogenous mouse gene to encode disease length expansions. Three different groups have expressed a fragment of mutant huntingtin, ranging from only the first exon (Mangiarini et al. 1996; Yamamoto et al. 2000), exons 1–3 (Schilling et al. 1999a), to nearly one-third of the protein (Laforet et al. 2001). Although in each model different lengths of glutamine repeat were expressed, often in different strains of mice and with different promoter elements, comparing and contrasting the neuropathology of these different models have been informative. None of the models (whether full-length human htt transgenic, truncated htt, or knock-in) shows extensive neuronal cell death in the striatum.

TABLE 1 Transgenic Mouse Models of HD

Model	Gene	Promoter & mouse strain	Behavioral phenotype	Reference
R6/2	Exon 1 of htt 115–150 Q	Human htt in C57BL/6J × CBA	Impaired rotarod performance, hind limb clasping, and premature death	Mangiarini et al. 1996
HD94	Exon –1 of htt 94Q	Tetracycline—regulated with Cam Kinase II tet-transactivator	Hind limb clasping	Yamamoto et al. 2000
N171-82Q	cDNA of exons 1–3 of human htt	Mouse prion protein in C57BL/6J × C3H/HeJ	Impaired rotarod performance, hind limb clasping, hypoactivity, and premature death	Schilling et al. 1999a
HD100	cDNA of N-terminal third of htt	Rat neuron specific enolase	Impaired motor performance	Laforet et al. 2001
HD48 & HD89	cDNA full-length human htt	Cytomegalovirus FVB/N	Circling (hyperactivity) progressing to hypoactivity	Reddy et al., 1998; Guidetti et al. 2001
YAC72 YAC 128	Yeast Artificial Chromosome of human htt gene 72Q or 128Q	Human htt FVB/N	Hyperactivity progressing to impaired rotarod performance and hypoactivity	Hodgson et al 1999; Slow et al. 2003
Hdh^{Q92} Hdh^{Q111}	Knock-in mutation of mouse genome	Mouse htt	Progressive movement disorder when normal allele is partially inactivated	Wheeler et al. 2000; Auerbach et al. 2001
Hdh4/Q72 *Hdh6/Q80*			Aggressive behavior	Shelbourne et al. 1999
CAG140 knock-in			Hyperactivity progressing to hypoactivity and gait abnormalities	Menalled et al. 2003
$Hdh^{(CAG)150}$			Motor deficits, hind limb clasping, gait abnormalities	Lin et al. 2001

However, while neurons are not lost to the same extent as occurs in the human disease, there is evidence of significant neuronal atrophy, modest losses of neurons in the cortex and hippocampus, and altered morphology (Hodgson et al. 1999; Turmaine et al. 2000; Yu et al. 2003). All of the models described to date develop, to varying extents, nuclear and cytoplasmic inclusion pathology that is characteristic of HD (Gutekunst et al. 1999). Indeed, it was the prevalence of htt immunoreactive nuclear inclusion pathology in the R6/2 mouse model that first revealed the contribution of these structures to disease pathogenesis.

Like the mice expressing truncated fragments of mutant htt, the brains of mice expressing full-length versions of mutant htt develop nuclear and cytoplasmic inclusions that are immunoreactive to antibodies against N-terminal epitopes of htt but not C-terminal epitopes (Hodgson et al. 1999; Sieradzan et al. 1999; Wheeler et al. 2000; Slow et al. 2003; Yu et al. 2003). Mice expressing full-length mutant htt, of either mouse or human origin, develop nuclear inclusion pathology in the striatum well before these structures appear in other domains of the CNS (Hodgson et al. 1999; Wheeler et al. 2000). By contrast, and paradoxically, the formation of nuclear inclusion in striatal neurons is less pronounced in mice expressing truncated fragments (Schilling et al. 1999a). Notably, in human HD, medium spiny neurons of the caudate and putamen also show less extensive nuclear inclusion pathology than other regions of the brain (Gutekunst et al. 1999).

One very exciting discovery from mouse models of HD was the demonstration that huntingtin inclusion pathology may be reversible. In a study of mice developed by expressing a mutant exon-1 fragment of htt (94Q) under the influence of a tetracycline-regulated promoter (Yamamoto et al. 2000), nuclear htt inclusions were cleared when expression of the transgene was suppressed by tetracycline analogues. These findings provide evidence that neurons can repair cellular abnormalities associated with the formation of htt aggregates. Many laboratories are pursuing small interfering RNAs [for review see (Davidson and Paulson 2004)] as a mechanism to diminish mutant htt expression and the demonstration that htt inclusion pathology can be repaired provides considerable hope that effective therapies could treat symptoms and provide real cures if started early enough.

As mentioned above, the degree of neuronal loss in the striatum of the various transgenic and knock-in models is much less significant than as occurs in the human illness. Recently, however, a new model has emerged where mutant huntingtin is expressed via viral vectors injected into the striatum of mice (de Almeida et al. 2002). In this model, significant loss of striatal neurons is evident and these animals may turn out to be useful for screening compounds that target neuronal survival.

V. GENERAL BEHAVIORAL CHARACTERISTICS OF HD MICE

In the HD mice described to date, it is fair to say that we do not have a model that completely replicates both behavioral and neuropathological aspects of human disease. Mice expressing short N-terminal fragments of mutant huntingtin have the most severe behavioral disturbances and exhibit abbreviated life spans (Mangiarini et al. 1996; Schilling et al. 1999a); a finding that seems to confirm the notion that truncated fragments of mutant huntingtin possess greater toxicity [for review see (Ross 1995)]. Behavioral abnormalities in these mice include reduced motor function, incoordination, ataxia, significant weight loss, hypoactivity, and premature death. The cause of death in these models remains to be clarified.

For the most part, mice expressing full-length versions of mutant huntingtin have less severe phenotypes or significantly later onsets. Two examples exist where full-length, mutant, huntingtin was expressed in the brains of FVB/N mice. In both cases, these animals showed a tendency to circle (Reddy et al. 1998; Hodgson et al. 1999); however, in both cases, investigators observed circling in only a subset of animals. More recently, investigators have described FVB/N mice expressing full-length human htt with 128 glutamine repeats. Like mice that express fragments of mutant htt, these mice develop deficits in motor function that can be measured by performance on a rotarod task (Slow et al. 2003). However, these mice do not show the abbreviated life spans seen in mice expressing the truncated fragments. Similarly, mice expressing the N-terminal third of mutant htt develop deficits in motor tasks but do not die prematurely (Laforet et al. 2001).

To assess motor function, we and others have used performance on the rotarod device as an outcome measure. Several of the HD mouse models display reduced performance on this task (Table 1). The major advantage of this task is that it is sensitive enough to detect small changes in motor function with relatively small cohorts (Schilling et al. 1999a). The major disadvantage is that the cellular and neurochemical basis for changes in rotarod performance is poorly characterized.

Investigators have also used direct mutagenesis of endogenous mouse huntingtin to produce animal models (Levine et al. 1999; Shelbourne et al. 1999; Wheeler et al. 2000; Lin et al. 2001). Investigators have recently reported that knock-in mice harboring extremely long glutamine repeats (150 consecutive glutamine repeats) develop overt behavioral phenotypes similar to those observed in mice expressing the truncated fragments (Lin et al. 2001). Knock-in htt mice harboring repeat lengths of 111 glutamines or less do not develop overt disturbances in motor function (Levine et al. 1999; Shelbourne et al. 1999; Wheeler et al.

2000). Other examples suggest that knock-in mice may require higher numbers of glutamines to induce overt behavioral phenotypes. A knock-in mouse model of SCA-1 has recently been described where 154 glutamines were inserted in axatin-1 (the SCA-1 gene). The resultant animals showed remarkable ataxic phenotypes, weight loss, clasping, and then death at approximately thirty-five weeks of age (Watase et al. 2002). *In vitro* studies have demonstrated that the rate of mutant htt aggregation is proportional to polyglutamine repeat length (Scherzinger et al. 1999). Whether this relationship explains why such long repeats are required to induce disease in the context of the full-length proteins expressed at levels equivalent to endogenous protein remains to be determined.

VI. TRANSGENIC RAT MODEL OF HD

More recently, transgenic rats have been created that express N-terminal fragments of mutant htt, using a fragment of the rat htt promoter to drive expression (von Horsten et al. 2003). Overall these animals bear striking resemblance to the mouse models described above. As described in the N171–82Q mice (Schilling et al. 1999a), the steady-state levels of the mutant htt fragment are lower than the full-length endogenous protein. These animals gain less weight than nontransgenic littermates as they mature, they perform worse on the rotarod task, and they die prematurely. Unlike the mouse models, the distribution of nuclear inclusion pathology is rather limited; inclusions were most frequent in the striatum and globus pallidus. One major advantage of the rat model is that the larger body size facilitates *in vivo* metabolic and structural imaging studies. Such studies reveal atrophy of the striatum and diminished glucose utilization. Similar to the mouse models, neuron loss is far less dramatic than occurs in the human disease.

VII. MECHANISMS OF TOXICITY

The data from mice expressing truncated versions of mutant huntingtin suggest that, once generated, N-terminal fragments of mutant htt are highly toxic. Some of the best evidence to suggest that fragmentation or truncation of polyglutamine proteins can play a significant role in the generation of toxic species comes from the study of transgenic mouse models for DRPLA, which is caused by a polyglutamine expansion in atrophin-1. Mice expressing mutant full-length atrophin-1 accumulate N-terminal fragments, which contain the polyglutamine domain, in nuclear compartments of affected neurons (Schilling et al. 1999b). Expression of similar N-terminal fragments of atrophin-1 in cultured cells causes toxicity and inactivation of an NLS in the N-terminus of atrophin-1 abrogates nuclear translocation and diminishes its toxicity (Nucifora et al. 2003). Truncation of atrophin-1 removes a nuclear export signal in the C-terminus of the protein, thereby targeting the mutant fragment to the nucleus (Schilling et al. 1999b; Nucifora et al. 2003).

Investigators have yet to determine whether the aggregated form of mutant huntingtin fragments, misfolded monomers, or some intermediate oligomer is the toxic species. There is no question that fragmentation of mutant htt facilitates aggregation, and the propensity to aggregate equates with toxicity. Intranuclear inclusions can trap components of the proteasome pathway (Cummings et al. 1998; Chai et al. 1999b), molecular chaperones (Cummings et al. 1998; Chai et al. 1999a; Stenoien et al. 1999), or other proteins with short stretches of polyglutamine such as the TATA-binding protein (Perez et al. 1998; Suhr et al. 2001). Investigators have suggested that the sequestration of these factors could be a mode of injury in these diseases. One example of this mode of injury is work demonstrating that a transcription regulatory factor, termed CREB-binding protein (CBP), is recruited to nuclear intraneuronal inclusions and that the transcriptional activating activity of CBP is diminished in the presence of polyglutamine-containing proteins (McCampbell et al. 2000; Steffan et al. 2000; McCampbell and Fischbeck 2001; Nucifora, Jr. et al. 2001; Steffan et al. 2001). The role of nuclear events in mutant htt toxicity has recently been bolstered by studies of mice expressing an htt-N171-82Q fragment engineered to encode a nuclear localization signal (NLS-N171-82Q); these animals accumulate mutant protein exclusively in the nucleus and develop HD-lik phenotypes (Schilling et al. 2004).

To study gene expression in pathological settings, investigators have turned to some of the newest tools in pathology, the gene arrays. These new tools facilitate molecular pathology, allowing investigators to study changes in cells at the molecular and systems level. In a study of transgenic mouse models of HD, Luthi-Carter and colleagues demonstrated reductions in the levels of expression of ~1% of the genes expressed in striatum (Luthi-Carter et al. 2000), indicating that the disease is not due to wholesale dysregulation of transcription in HD. As this technology improves, and as the database of transcriptional profiling expands, these powerful techniques may prove invaluable in deciphering the molecular events in disease pathogenesis.

VIII. CONCLUSIONS

Studies of transgenic animals that express variants of mutant htt provide insight into the pathogenesis of HD. From initial studies of the R6/2 model of HD, it became apparent that a prominent pathologic lesion in HD is the accumulation of mutant htt in both nuclear and cytoplasmic inclusions. The availability of so many different models that utilize different genetic strategies provides insight into the nature of the toxic species in HD and mechanisms of toxicity. By and large, N-terminal fragments of mutant htt appear to be more toxic than full-length proteins and more prone to aggregate into nuclear/cytoplasmic aggregates. In some models, severe behavioral abnormalities and premature death occur prior to dramatic losses of neurons, suggesting that altered or diminished neuronal function contributes to the HD phenotype.

Video Legends

HUNTINGTON DISEASE: Transgenic mice that express an N-terminal fragment of human Huntington were generated, using the mouse PrP vector. The Huntington fragment encompassed all of exon 1, exon 2, and part of exon 3. Within this fragment (termed N171), we introduced 3 glutamine repeat lengths-18Q, 44Q, or 82Q. Only mice that express N171-82Q develop phenotypes. We presently maintain two lines of N171-82Q mice, lines 81 and 6. The phenotypes of the two lines are similar with line 81 showing an earlier onset.

SEGMENT 1 Tremors in HD-N171-82Q mice. Tremors, if they appear at all, are not obvious until the animals are approaching end-stage; that is, until just prior to death.

SEGMENT 2 Hypoactivity in older HD-N171-82Q mice. The N171-82Q mouse is the smaller of the two animals in this cage. Watch the non-transgenic mouse explore this cage while the transgenic remains relatively stationary. Eventually, the transgenic will move slowly about the cage before becoming stationary once again.

SEGMENT 3 Hind limb clasping in N171-82Q mice. When suspended by the tail, N171-82Q mice clasp hind limbs together. By contrast, as shown in the second video, when a non-transgenic mouse is suspended by the tail, the hind limbs splay out in a reaching reflex.

SEGMENT 4 End-stage N171-82Q mice. The life expectancy of HD-N171-82Q mice from line 81 is four to six months. In the days just prior to death, the mice become extremely hypoactive, show a pronounced hunchback, and are poorly groomed. As death becomes imminent, the animals remain responsive to mild compression of the paws, pinna and tail.

DRPLA: Transgenic mouse models of dentatorubral pallidoluysian atrophy (DRPLA). To model DRPLA, we created transgenci mice that express the full-length human cDNA for atrophin-1 via the mouse PrP vector. We used two versions of atrophin 1 (AT), one with a 26 glutamine repeat (normal—AT26Q) and one with a 65 glutamine repeat (disease—AT65Q).

SEGMENT 1 AT26Q mice from line 84 express full-length human atrophin-1 (26Q) at levels that are 3- to 5-fold higher than endogenous mouse atrophin-1. As apposed to the AT65Q mice, these animals appear normal and show none of the abnormalities present in the mutant mice (Schilling, Wood, et al., Neuron, 1999)

SEGMENT 2 Tremors in AT65Q mice. Mice expressing AT65Q develop tremors relatively early in life. The severe tremors shown here appear by 4–6 months of age in mice from line 150 and persist throughout the lifespan of the animals. Mice from the 150 line represent the highest expressing line of AT65Q mice that we were able to maintain.

SEGMENT 3 Hyperactivity of AT65Q mice in their home cage. The AT65Q (line 150) mouse is the more active of the two animals in this cage.

SEGMENT 4 Gait disturbances in older AT65Q mice. Severe gait disturbances such as seen here begin to appear late in natural lifespan of the AT65Q (line 150) mice, after about one year.

SEGMENT 5 Seizures in DRPLA mice. The life expectancy of AT65Q mice (line 150) is highly variable. Some mice die well before one year of age and others live up to 24 months.

Mice from a second, lower expressing line (124), develop the motor symptoms seen in mice from line 150 at older ages-one year to develop severe tremors and 1.5 yrs to develop gait disturbances. Mice from line 124 have normal life-spans.

Initially, we had identified lines of AT65Q mice that express mutant atrophin-1 at higher levels than line 150. Seizures were more easily induced in these mice, as shown in the following segment. Unfortunately, we could not maintain these lines of mice that expressed higher levels; they bred poorly and died too quickly.

References

Andrade, M.A., and P. Bork. 1995. HEAT repeats in the Huntington's disease protein. *Nat Genet* **11**:115–116.

Auerbach, W., M.S. Hurlbert, P. Hilditch-Maguire, Y.Z. Wadghiri, V.C. Wheeler, S.I. Cohen, A.L. Joyner, et al. 2001. The HD mutation causes progressive lethal neurological disease in mice expressing reduced levels of huntingtin. *Hum Mol Genet* **10**:2515–2523.

Becher, M.W., J.A. Kotzuk, A.H. Sharp, S.W. Davies, G.P. Bates, D.L. Price, and C.A. Ross. 1998. Intranuclear neuronal inclusions in Huntington's disease and dentatorubral and pallidoluysian atrophy: correlation between the density of inclusions and *IT15* CAG triplet repeat length. *Neurobiol Dis* **4**:387–397.

Bence, N.F., R.M. Sampat, and R.R. Kopito. 2001. Impairment of the ubiquitin-proteasome system by protein aggregation. *Science* **292**:1552–1555.

Bhide, P.G., M. Day, E. Sapp, C. Schwarz, A. Sheth, J. Kim, A.B. Young, et al. 1996. Expression of normal and mutant huntingtin in the developing brain. *J. Neurosci.* **16**:5523–5535.

Chai Y., S.L. Koppenhafer, N.M. Bonini, and H.L. Paulson. 1999a. Analysis of the role of heat shock protein (Hsp) molecular chaperones in polyglutamine disease. *J Neurosci* **19**:10338–10347.

Chai Y., S.L. Koppenhafer, S.J. Shoesmith, M.K. Perez, and H.L. Paulson. 1999b. Evidence for proteasome involvement in polyglutamine disease: localization to nuclear inclusions in SCA3/MJD and suppression of polyglutamine aggregation in vitro. *Hum Mol Genet* **8**:673–682.

Cummings, C.J., M.A. Mancini, B. Antalffy, D.B. DeFranco, H.T. Orr, and H.Y. Zoghbi. 1998. Chaperone suppression of aggregation and altered subcellular proteasome localization imply protein misfolding in SCA1. *Nat Genet* **19**:148–154.

Cummings, C.J., E. Reinstein, Y. Sun, B. Antalffy, Y. Jiang, A. Ciechanover, H.T. Orr, et al. 1999. Mutation of the E6-AP ubiquitin ligase reduces nuclear inclusion frequency while accelerating polyglutamine-induced pathology in *SCA1* mice. *Neuron* **24**:879–892.

Davidson, B.L., and H.L. Paulson. 2004. Molecular medicine for the brain: silencing of disease genes with RNA interference. *Lancet Neurol* **3**: 145–149.

Davies, S.W., M. Turmaine, B.A. Cozens, M. DiFiglia, A.H. Sharp, C.A. Ross, Scherzinger E., et al. 1997. Formation of neuronal intranuclear inclusions underlies the neurological dysfunction in mice transgenic for the HD mutation. *Cell* **90**:537–548.

de Almeida, L.P., C.A. Ross, D. Zala, P. Aebischer, and N. Deglon. 2002. Lentiviral-mediated delivery of mutant huntingtin in the striatum of rats induces a selective neuropathology modulated by polyglutamine repeat size, huntingtin expression levels, and protein length. *J Neurosci* **22**: 3473–3483.

DiFiglia, M., E. Sapp, K.O. Chase, S.W. Davies, G.P. Bates, J.P. Vonsattel, and N. Aronin. 1997. Aggregation of huntingtin in neuronal intranuclear inclusions and dystrophic neurites in brain. *Science* **277**:1990–1993.

Dunah A.W., H. Jeong, A. Griffin, Y.M. Kim, D.G. Standaert, S.M. Hersch, M.M. Mouradian, A.B. Young, et al. 2002. Sp1 and TAFII130 transcriptional activity disrupted in early Huntington's disease. *Science* **296**:2238–2243.

Duyao, M.P., A.B. Auerbach, A. Ryan, F. Persichetti, G.T. Barnes, S.M. McNeil, P. Ge, et al. 1995. Inactivation of the mouse Huntington's disease gene homolog *Hdh*. *Science* **269**:407–410.

Fischbeck, K.H. 2001. Polyglutamine expansion neurodegenerative disease. *Brain Res Bull* **56**:161–163.

Fusco, F.R., Q. Chen, W.J. Lamoreaux, G. Figueredo-Cardenas, Y. Jiao, J.A. Coffman, D.J. Surmeier, et al. 1999. Cellular localization of huntingtin in striatal and cortical neurons in rats: lack of correlation with neuronal vulnerability in Huntington's disease. *J Neurosci* **19**:1189–1202.

Guidetti, P., V. Charles, E.Y. Chen, P.H. Reddy, J.H., Kordower W.O. Whetsell, Jr., R. Schwarcz, and D.A. Tagle. 2001. Early degenerative changes in transgenic mice expressing mutant huntingtin involve dendritic abnormalities but no impairment of mitochondrial energy production. *Exp Neurol* **169**:340–350.

Gutekunst, C.A., S.H. Li, H. Yi, J.S. Mulroy, S. Kuemmerle, R. Jones, D. Rye, et al. 1999. Nuclear and neuropil aggregates in Huntington's disease: relationship to neuropathology. *J Neurosci* **19**:2522–2534.

Henry, K.R., K.D. Hondt, J. Chang, T. Newpher, K. Huang, R.T. Hudson, H. Riezman, and S.K. Lemmon. 2002. Scd5p and clathrin function are important for cortical actin organization, endocytosis, and localization of sla2p in yeast. *Mol. Biol. Cell* **13**, 2607–2625.

Hodgson, J.G., N. Agopyan, C.A. Gutekunst, B.R. Leavitt, F. LePiane, R. Singaraja, D.J. Smith, et al. 1999. A YAC mouse model for Huntington's disease with full-length mutant huntingtin, cytoplasmic toxicity, and selective striatal neurodegeneration. *Neuron* **23**:181–192.

Huntington's Disease Collaborative Research Group. 1993. A novel gene containing a trinucleotide repeat that is expanded and unstable on Huntington's disease chromosomes. *Cell* **72**:971–983.

Kawaguchi, Y., T. Okamoto, M. Taniwaki, M. Aizawa, M. Inoue, S. Katayama, H. Kawakami, et al. 1994. CAG expansions in a novel gene for Machado-Joseph disease at chromosome 14q32.1. *Nat Genet* **8**: 221–227.

Klement, I.A., P.J. Skinner, M.D. Kaytor, H. Yi, S.M. Hersch, H. Brent Clark, H.Y. Zoghbi, and H.T. Orr. 1998. Ataxin-1 nuclear localization and aggregation: role in polyglutamine-induced disease in *SCA1* transgenic mice. *Cell* **95**:41–53.

Koide R., T. Ikeuchi, O. Onodera, H. Tanaka, S. Igarashi, K. Endo, H. Takahashi, et al. 1994. Unstable expansion of CAG repeat in hereditary dentatorubral-pallidoluysian atrophy (DRPLA). *Nat Genet* **6**:9–13.

La Spada, A.R., E.M. Wilson, D.B. Lubahn, A.E. Harding, and K.H. Fischbeck. 1991. Androgen receptor gene mutations in X-linked spinal and bulbar muscular atrophy. *Nature* **352**:77–79.

Laforet, G.A., E. Sapp, K. Chase, C. McIntyre, F.M. Boyce, M. Campbell, B.A. Cadigan, et al. 2001. Changes in cortical and striatal neurons predict behavioral and electrophysiological abnormalities in a transgenic murine model of Huntington's disease. *J Neurosci* **21**:9112–9123.

Landwehrmeyer, G.B., S.M. McNeil, L.S.I.V. Dure, P. Ge, H. Aizawa, Q. Huang, C.M. Ambrose, et al. 1995. Huntington's disease gene: regional and cellular expression in brain of normal and affected individuals. *Ann Neurol* **37**:218–230.

Levine, M.S., G.J. Klapstein, A. Koppel, E. Gruen, C. Cepeda, M.E. Vargas, E.S. Jokel, et al. 1999. Enhanced sensitivity to N-methyl-D-aspartate receptor activation in transgenic and knockin mouse models of Huntington's disease. *J Neurosci Res* **58**:515–532.

Li, S.H., A.L. Cheng, H. Zhou, S. Lam, M. Rao, H. Li, and X.J. Li. 2002. Interaction of Huntington disease protein with transcriptional activator Sp1. *Mol Cell Biol* **22**:1277–1287.

Lin, C.H., S. Tallaksen-Greene, W.M. Chien, J.A. Cearley, W.S. Jackson, A.B. Crouse, S. Ren, et al. 2001. Neurological abnormalities in a knock-in mouse model of Huntington's disease. *Hum Mol Genet* **10**:137–144.

Lunkes, A., K.S. Lindenberg, L. Ben Haiem, C. Weber, D. Devys, G.B. Landwehrmeyer, J.L. Mandel, and Y. Trottier. 2002. Proteases acting on mutant huntingtin generate cleaved products that differentially build up cytoplasmic and nuclear inclusions. *Mol Cell* **10**:259–269.

Luthi-Carter, R., A. Strand, N.L. Peters, S.M. Solano, Z.R. Hollingsworth, A.S. Menon, A.S. Frey, et al. 2000. Decreased expression of striatal signaling genes in a mouse model of Huntington's disease. *Hum Mol Genet* **9**:1259–1271.

Mangiarini, L., K. Sathasivam, M. Seller, B. Cozens, A. Harper, C. Hetherington, M. Lawton, et al. 1996. Exon 1 of the *HD* gene with an expanded CAG repeat is sufficient to cause a progressive neurological phenotype in transgenic mice. *Cell* **87**:493–506.

McCampbell A., and K.H. Fischbeck. 2001. Polyglutamine and CBP: fatal attraction? *Nat. Med.* **7**, 528–530.

McCampbell, A., J.P. Taylor, A.A. Taye, J. Robitschek, M. Li, J. Walcott, D. Merry, et al. 2000. CREB-binding protein sequestration by expanded polyglutamine. *Hum Mol Genet* **9**:2197–2202.

Menalled, L.B., J.D. Sison, I. Dragatsis, S. Zeitlin, and M.F. Chesselet. 2003. Time course of early motor and neuropathological anomalies in a knock-in mouse model of Huntington's disease with 140 CAG repeats. *J Comp Neurol* **465**:11–26.

Nagafuchi, S., H. Yanagisawa, K. Sato, T. Shirayama, E. Ohsaki, M. Bundo, T. Takeda, et al. 1994. Dentatorubral and pallidoluysian atrophy expansion of an unstable CAG trinucleotide on chromosome 12p. *Nat Genet* **6**:14–18.

Nucifora, F.C., Jr., L.M. Ellerby, C.L. Wellington, J.D. Wood, W.J. Herring, A. Sawa, M.R. Hayden, et al. 2003. Nuclear localization of a non-caspase truncation product of atrophin-1, with an expanded polyglutamine repeat, increases cellular toxicity. *J Biol Chem* **278**:13047–13055.

Nucifora, F.C., Jr., M. Sasaki, M.F. Peters, H. Huang, J.K. Cooper, M. Yamada, H. Takahashi, et al. 2001. Interference by huntingtin and atrophin-1 with CBP-mediated transcription leading to cellular toxicity. *Science* **291**:2423–2428.

Orr, H.T. 2001. Beyond the Qs in the polyglutamine diseases. *Genes Dev* **15**:925–932.

Orr, H.T., M.-Y. Chung, S. Banfi, T.J. Kwiatkowski, Jr., A. Servadio, A.L. Beaudet, A.E. McCall, et al. 1993. Expansion of an unstable trinucleotide CAG repeat in spinocerebellar ataxia type 1. *Nat Genet* **4**:221–226.

Perez, M.K., H.L. Paulson, S.J. Pendse, S.J. Saionz, N.M. Bonini, and R.N. Pittman. 1998. Recruitment and the role of nuclear localization in polyglutamine-mediated aggregation. *J Cell Biol* **143**:1457–1470.

Perutz, M. 1994. Polar zippers: their role in human disease. *Protein Sci* **3**:1629–1637.

Poirier, M.A., H. Li, J. Macosko, S. Cai, M. Amzel, and C.A. Ross. 2002. Huntingtin spheroids and protofibrils as precursors in polyglutamine fibrilization. *J Biol Chem* **277**:41032–41037.

Reddy, P.H., M. Williams, V. Charles, L. Garrett, L. Pike-Buchanan, W.O. Whetsell, Jr., G. Miller, and D.A. Tagle. 1998. Behavioural abnormalities and selective neuronal loss in HD transgenic mice expressing mutated full-length HD cDNA. *Nat Genet* **20**:198–202.

Roon-Mom, W.M., S.J. Reid, A.L. Jones, M.E. MacDonald, R.L. Faull, and R.G. Snell. 2002. Insoluble TATA-binding protein accumulation in Huntington's disease cortex. *Brain Res Mol Brain Res* **109**:1–10.

Ross, C.A. 1995. When more is less: pathogenesis of glutamine repeat neurodegenerative diseases. *Neuron* **15**:493–496.

Ross, C.A., R.L. Margolis, A. Rosenblatt, N.G. Ranen, M.W. Becher, and E. Aylward. 1997. Huntington disease and the related disorder, dentatorubral-pallidoluysian atrophy (DRPLA). *Medicine* **76**:305–338.

Scherzinger, E., R. Lurz, M. Turmaine, L. Mangiarini, B. Hollenbach, R. Hasenbank, G.P. Bates, et al. 1997. Huntingtin-encoded polyglutamine expansions form amyloid-like protein aggregates in vitro and in vivo. *Cell* **90**:549–558.

Scherzinger, E., A. Sittler, K. Schweiger, V. Heiser, R. Lurz, R. Hasenbank, H. Lehrach, and E.E. Wanker. 1999. Self-assembly of polyglutamine-containing huntingtin fragments into amyloid-like fibrils: implications for Huntington's disease pathology. *Proc Natl Acad Sci USA* **96**: 4604–4609.

Schilling, G., M.W. Becher, A.H. Sharp, H.A. Jinnah, K. Duan, J.A. Kotzuk, H.H. Slunt, et al. 1999a. Intranuclear inclusions and neuritic pathology in transgenic mice expressing a mutant N-terminal fragment of huntingtin. *Hum Mol Genet* **8**:397–407.

Schilling, G., A.V. Savonenko, A. Klevytska, J.L. Morton, S.M. Tucker, M. Poirier, A. Gale, N. Chan, V. Gonzales, H.H. Slunt, M.L. Coonfield, N.A. Jenkins, N.G. Copeland, C.A. Ross, and D.R. Borchelt. 2004. Nuclear-targeting of mutant huntingtin fragments produced Huntington disease-like phenotypes in transgenic mice. *Hum Mol Genet* **13**: 1599–1610.

Schilling, G., J.D. Wood, K. Duan, H.H. Slunt, V. Gonzales, M. Yamada, J.K. Cooper, et al. 1999b. Nuclear accumulation of truncated atrophin-1 fragments in a transgenic mouse model of DRPLA. *Neuron* **24**:275–286.

Sharp, A.H., S.J. Loev, G. Schilling, S.-H. Li, X.-J. Li, J. Bao, M.V. Wagster, et al. 1995. Widespread expression of the Huntington's disease gene (IT-15) protein product. *Neuron* **14**:1065–1074.

Shelbourne, P.F., N. Killeen, R.F. Hevner, H.M. Johnston, L. Tecott, M. Lewandoski, M. Ennis, et al. 1999. A Huntington's disease CAG expansion at the murine Hdh locus is unstable and associated with behavioural abnormalities in mice. *Hum Mol Genet* **8**:763–774.

Shimohata, T., T. Nakajima, M. Yamada, C. Uchida, O. Onodera, S. Naruse, T. Kimura, et al. 2000. Expanded polyglutamine stretches interact with $TAF_{II}130$, interfering with CREB-dependent transcription. *Nat Genet* **26**:29–35.

Sieradzan, K.A., and D.M. Mann. 2001. The selective vulnerability of nerve cells in Huntington's disease. *Neuropathol. Appl. Neurobiol.* **27**:1–21.

Sieradzan, K.A., A.O. Mechan, L. Jones, E.E. Wanker, N. Nukina, and D.M. Mann. 1999. Huntington's disease intranuclear inclusions contain truncated, ubiquitinated huntingtin protein. *Exp Neurol* 156:92–99.

Singaraja, R.R., S. Hadano, M. Metzler, S. Givan, C.L. Wellington, S. Warby, A. Yanai, et al. 2002. HIP14, a novel ankyrin domain-containing protein, links huntingtin to intracellular trafficking and endocytosis. *Hum Mol Genet* **11**:2815–2828.

Slow, E.J., J. van Raamsdonk, D. Rogers, S.H. Coleman, R.K. Graham, Y. Deng, R. Oh, et al. 2003. Selective striatal neuronal loss in a YAC128 mouse model of Huntington disease. *Hum Mol Genet* **12**:1555–1567.

Steffan, J.S., L. Bodai, J. Pallos, M. Poelman, A. McCampbell, B.L. Apostol, A. Kazantsev, et al. 2001. Histone deacetylase inhibitors arrest polyglutamine-dependent neurodegeneration in *Drosophila*. *Nature* **413**: 739–743.

Steffan, J.S., A. Kazantsev, O. Spasic-Boskovic, M. Greenwald, Y.Z. Zhu, H. Gohler, E.E. Wanker, et al. 2000. The Huntington's disease protein interacts with p53 and CREB-binding protein and represses transcription. *Proc Natl Acad Sci U S A* **97**:6763–6768.

Stenoien, D.L., C.J. Cummings, H.P. Adams, M.G. Mancini, K. Patel, G.N. DeMartino, M. Marcelli, et al. 1999. Polyglutamine-expanded androgen receptors form aggregates that sequester heat shock proteins, proteasome components and SRC-1, and are suppressed by the HDJ-2 chaperone. *Hum Mol Genet* **8**:731–741.

Suhr, S.T., M.C. Senut, J.P. Whitelegge, K.F. Faull, D.B. Cuizon, and F.H. Gage. 2001. Identities of sequestered proteins in aggregates from cells with induced polyglutamine expression. *J Cell Biol* **153**:283–294.

Turmaine, M., A. Raza, A. Mahal, L. Mangiarini, G.P. Bates, and S.W. Davies. 2000. Nonapoptotic neurodegeneration in a transgenic mouse model of Huntington's disease. *Proc Natl Acad Sci U S A* **97**:8093–8097.

von Horsten, S., I. Schmitt, H.P. Nguyen, C. Holzmann, T. Schmidt, T. Walther, M. Bader, et al. 2003. Transgenic rat model of Huntington's disease. *Hum Mol Genet* **12**:617–624.

Watase, K., E.J. Weeber, B. Xu, B. Antalffy, L. Yuva-Paylor, K. Hashimoto, M. Kano, et al. 2002. A long CAG repeat in the mouse Sca1 locus replicates SCA1 features and reveals the impact of protein solubility on selective neurodegeneration. *Neuron* **34**:905–919.

Wellington, C.L., L.M. Ellerby, C.A. Gutekunst, D. Rogers, S. Warby, R.K. Graham, O. Loubser, et al. 2002. Caspase cleavage of mutant huntingtin precedes neurodegeneration in Huntington's disease. *J Neurosci* **22**: 7862–7872.

Wellington, C.L., L.M. Ellerby, A.S. Hackam, R.L. Margolis, M.A. Trifiro, R. Singaraja, K. McCutcheon, et al. 1998. Caspase cleavage of gene products associated with triplet expansion disorders generates truncated fragments containing the polyglutamine tract. *J Biol Chem* **273**:9158–9167.

Wheeler, V.C., J.K. White, C.A. Gutekunst, V. Vrbanac, M. Weaver, X.J. Li, S.H. Li, et al. 2000. Long glutamine tracts cause nuclear localization of a novel form of huntingtin in medium spiny striatal neurons in Hdh^{Q92} and Hdh^{Q111} knock-in mice. *Hum Mol Genet* **9**:503–513.

Yamamoto, A., J.J. Lucas, and R. Hen. 2000. Reversal of neuropathology and motor dysfunction in a conditional model of Huntington's disease. *Cell* **101**:57–66.

Yu, Z.X., S.H. Li, J. Evans, A. Pillarisetti, H. Li, and X.J. Li. 2003. Mutant huntingtin causes context-dependent neurodegeneration in mice with Huntington's disease. *J Neurosci* **23**:2193–2202.

Zeitlin, S., J.-P. Liu, D.L. Chapman, V.E. Papaioannou, and A. Efstratiadis. 1995. Increased apoptosis and early embryonic lethality in mice nullizygous for the Huntington's disease gene homologue. *Nat Genet* **11**: 155–163.

Zuccato, C., A. Ciammola, D. Rigamonti, B.R. Leavitt, D. Goffredo, L. Conti, M.E. MacDonald, et al. 2001. Loss of huntingtin-mediated BDNF gene transcription in Huntington's disease. *Science* **293**:493–498.

Zuccato, C., M. Tartari, A. Crotti, D. Goffredo, M. Valenza, L. Conti, T. Cataudella, et al. 2003. Huntingtin interacts with REST/NRSF to modulate the transcription of NRSE-controlled neuronal genes. *Nat Genet* **35**:76–83.

C H A P T E R

D3

Knock-in and Knock-out Models of Huntington Disease

PAULA DIETRICH and IOANNIS DRAGATSIS

Information regarding the mechanism underlying Huntington disease (HD) has come primarily from the analysis of transgenic mice overexpressing additional copies of full-length or truncated mutant huntingtin. However, unraveling the molecular causes of neuronal dysfunction in transgenic mouse models requires caution since overexpression of the transgene (either truncated or full-length) may cause abnormalities by mechanisms other than those in HD.

From a genetic perspective, the most accurate strategy for replicating HD in the mouse is to insert pathogenic expanded CAG repeats into the mouse homolog of the HD gene (Hdh). Several groups have used such a knock-in approach by gene targeting to establish mouse models of HD. These mouse models have provided new tools to investigate the early events of the disease as well as its progression. Another important issue regarding HD pathogenesis is whether HD results from a gain-of-function mechanism or whether loss of the wild-type function contributes to the disease. Recent evidence stemming from hypomorphic and knock-out mouse models suggests that loss of wild-type protein function may also play a role in HD.

I. KNOCK-IN MOUSE MODELS

A. General Description

The strategy to generate a knock-in mouse model for HD consists in inserting a CAG expansion by gene targeting into the mouse Huntington disease homolog (Hdh) gene, which encodes huntingtin. As a result, in the knock-in mice the mutant gene is expressed under the natural Hdh promoter and in the appropriate genomic context of the mouse Hdh gene.

In mice, the Hdh gene encodes an invariable polyglutamine stretch of only seven repeats. Investigators have employed two strategies to generate knock-in mice: either replacement of the mouse Hdh exon 1 with a human exon 1 containing a long CAG expansion or targeted insertion of an expanded CAG repeat into the mouse Hdh exon 1. To date, several research groups have generated knock-in mouse models with variable stretches of CAG repeats ranging from 50 to 150. With the exception of HdhQ50 (50 CAG repeats), all other mouse models have repeat lengths of the range found in juvenile HD. A general description and a summary of the findings in knock-in mice are presented in table 1.

TABLE 1 Knock-in Mouse Models of Huntington Disease

Mouse model	No. of CAG repeats	Abnormal behavior/ time of onset	Neuropathology: NIIs and aggregates	Neuropathology: Cell death, gliosis	Other observations	References
HdhQ50	50	No (up to 6 months)	Not reported	No (up to 6 months) in HdhQ50/Q50	Increased Rrs1 mRNA (14 months)	White et al. 1997 Fossale et al. 2002
HdhQ92	92	No (up to 17 months)	Diffuse nuclear stain in striatum at 4.5 months; Microaggregates and NIIs at 12 months	No cell death; No gliosis (up to 17 months)	Increased Rrs1 mRNA (8.5 months)	Wheeler et al. 1999 Wheeler et al. 2000 Fossale et al. 2002
HdhQ111	111	Slight gait deficits at 24 months	Diffuse nuclear stain in striatum at 2.5 months; Microaggregates at 5 months; NIIs at 10 months	Cell shrinkage in striatum at 17 months; Cell death and gliosis in striatum at 24 months	Decreased expression of BDNF in cortex and striatum at 5 months; Progressive decline of cAMP in cortex and striatum starting at 3 months; Mitochondria respiratory chain deficits; Increased Rrs1 mRNA at 3 weeks	Wheeler et al. 1999 Wheeler et al. 2000 Wheeler et al. 2002 Fossale et al. 2002 Gines et al. 2003
CHL1	80	No	Rare NIIs at 22 months	No neuronal cell loss (up to 22 months); Gliosis in striatum	Seizure susceptibility	Lin et al. 2001
CHL2	150	Gait disturbances; Locomotor abnormalities and tendency to clasp upon tail suspension at 10 months for 150/+ and at 4 months for homozygous 150/150	Nuclear stain at 7 months; NIIs at 10 months	No neuronal cell loss (up to 12 months); Gliosis in striatum; No dystrophic neurites	Seizure susceptibility	Lin et al. 2001
Hdh 80	77	Not reported	Not reported	No neuronal cell loss (up to 16 months); gliosis in globus pallidus, substantia nigra, and striatum	Not reported	Ishiguro et al. 2001
Hdh 6/Q72 and Hdh 4/Q80	72 80	Aggressive behavior at 3 months	Nuclear stain at 4 months; Microaggregates at 11 months; NIIs at 21 months; Neuropil aggregates at 11 months	No cell loss; No gliosis axonal degeneration at 17 months	Impaired synaptic plasticity in hippocampus	Shelbourne et al. 1999 Usdin et al. 1999 Li et al. 2000 Li et al. 2001 Kennedy and Shelbourne 2000
Hdh $71Q^{R42}$	$71Q^{R42}$	No	Not reported	No cell loss; No gliosis	Not reported	Levine et al. 1999 Menalled et al. 2000

(continues)

TABLE 1 (*continued*)

Mouse model	No. of CAG repeats	Abnormal behavior/ time of onset	Neuropathology: NIIs and aggregates	Neuropathology: Cell death, gliosis	Other observations	References
Hdh $94Q^{R42}$	$94Q^{R42}$	Increased locomotor activity at 2 months; Decreased locomotor activity at 4 months	Nuclear microaggregates at 4–6 months in striatum; NIIs at ≥18 months	No cell loss; No gliosis	Reduced enkephalin expression in striatum; Increased sensitivity to NMDA receptor activation	Levine et al. 1999 Menalled et al. 2000 Menalled et al. 2002
Hdh 140Q	140	Increased locomotor activity at 1 month; Decreased locomotor activity at 4 months; Abnormal gait at 12 months	Nuclear microaggregates at 2 months; NIIs at 6 months; Neuropil aggregates at 4 months	Not reported	Not reported	Menalled et al. 2003

B. Behavioral Abnormalities

The motor disorders of HD include chorea (rapid involuntary movements of limbs and distal muscles) and progressively impaired coordination of voluntary movements (Sharp and Ross 1996). In patients with juvenile-onset HD, the signs and symptoms are somewhat different: they include bradykinesia, rigidity, and dystonia (involuntary movements of proximal muscles of the trunk), and chorea can be completely absent. Involuntary movements can manifest as tremors and affected children often develop epileptic seizures (Vonsatell and DiFiglia 1998).

Although initially knock-in models were disappointing due to the lack of obvious abnormal behaviors (White et al. 1997; Wheeler et al. 2000), a more detailed analysis of the mice and the generation of additional knock-in mice with longer CAG repeat expansions revealed the presence of progressive motor deficits. Motor abnormalities were only observed in knock-in models with more than 90 CAG repeats and were more severe in mice with 150 CAG repeats.

Hindlimb-clasping on tail suspension, a hallmark sign of neurological problems in transgenic HD mice (Sathasivam et al. 1999), seizure susceptibility, and impaired motor coordination and balance were observed in CAG-150 mice between ten to fifteen months of age (Lin et al. 2001) and were more prominent and of earlier onset in homozygous mice.

Investigators also observed increased and decreased locomotor activity in some knock-in models. Increased rearing activity at early age (one to two months) was reported for mice containing CAG expansions of 94 and 140 repeats (table 1). In both mouse lines, decreased rearing and overall locomotor activity occurred at around four months of age (Menalled et al. 2002; Menalled et al. 2003). A much-delayed decrease in locomotor activity was detected in another mouse line with 150 repeats (Lin et al. 2001). The discrepancy observed in locomotor behavior may be due to differences in the testing methods. For instance, the tests used to uncover the early locomotor abnormalities were performed during the dark cycle of the diurnal phase, which corresponds to the time of maximum motor activity in mice. Gait deficits, characteristic of most HD patients (Koller and Trimble 1985), were observed in HdhQ111 mice at twenty-four months of age, and in mice carrying 140 and 150 CAG repeats at twelve months and ten months of age respectively (Wheeler et al. 2002; Lin et al. 2001; Menalled et al. 2003).

Cognitive impairment, including memory and information-processing deficits, mood changes, and aggressive behavior are among the earliest symptoms of HD, occurring before other late-stage symptoms, such as movement disorders (Jason et al. 1997; Lawrence et al. 1996; Lawrence et al. 1998). Aggressive behavior was reported only in two mouse knock-in models, Hdh6/Q72 and Hdh4/Q80 (Shelbourne et al. 1999). Starting at three months of age, mutant males, and to a lesser extent, mutant females engaged in chronic aggressive behavior towards their littermates or to a newcomer. It is significant that HD patients often exhibit behavioral abnormalities such as irritability and aggression (Harper 1996), however, the fact that this abnormality was not observed in any of the other mouse knock-in models raises the possibility that mouse strain effects may influence the manifestation of this phenotype.

C. Neuropathology

1. Intranuclear Inclusions (NII) and Aggregates

a. Intranuclear Aggregates

Neuronal intranuclear inclusions (NIIs), defined as large aggregates (1–2 μm) that stain positive for huntingtin and ubiquitin, are observed in different regions of HD postmortem brains. In the majority of HD cases the most numerous inclusion-bearing neurons are found in the neocortex, most frequently in neurons of layers III, V, and VI. Inclusions are also identified in the allocortex and in the striatum within the nuclei of medium-sized neurons in the caudate and putamen. In addition, nuclear inclusions are found in the amygdala, hippocampus, and the dentate nucleus of the cerebellum. In the cortex, but not in the striatum, the frequency of intranuclear inclusions is proportional to the length of the polyglutamine expansion (Maat-Schieman et al. 1999; Sieradzan et al. 1999; Becher et al. 1998).

A common feature of all the knock-in mouse models is the age-dependent relocalization of huntingtin into the nucleus and the progressive formation of microaggregates (puncta) followed by intranuclear inclusions. Using EM48 antibody, which preferentially detects huntingtin aggregates (Gutekunst et al. 1999), immunostaining of brain sections of knock-in mice at different ages revealed that the formation of intranuclear aggregates is progressive and that the age when NIIs are formed is inversely proportional to the polyglutamine length (Figure 1 and table 2).

In knock-in mice in which the polyglutamine expansion varies from seventy to ninety-four, huntingtin aggregates are restricted to the striatum (Wheeler et al. 2000; Menalled et al. 2002; Li et al. 2000). Nuclear translocation of huntingtin is first observed in these mice between two and a half and four months of age, depending on the mouse model. On average, microaggregates or puncta become apparent between four to twelve months of age, and nuclear inclusions are observed at a later time-point, between fifteen and twenty-two months of age (table 2). No aggregates or nuclear inclusions were observed in HdhQ50 mice up to seventeen months of age (Wheeler et al. 2000). Double immunostaining of EM48 and calbindin-D, a calcium-binding protein enriched in medium spiny neurons, showed that almost all neurons containing intranuclear EM48 staining were positive for calbindin-D. On the other hand, interneurons, which contain nitric oxide synthase (NOS), parvalbumin (PARV), or vesicular acetylcholine (VAT) do not show intranuclear inclusions (Wheeler et al. 2000; Li et al. 2000). Menalled and collaborators (Menalled et al. 2002) observed that microaggregate-containing neurons in the striatum are grouped in conspicuous clusters, in particular in the dorso-lateral part of the striatum, and were usually found in areas of dense MOR-1 (μ-opioid receptor) staining. This evidence indicates that the areas containing numerous nuclear microaggregates are not distributed randomly in the striatum but are located preferentially in the striosomal compartment of the striatum.

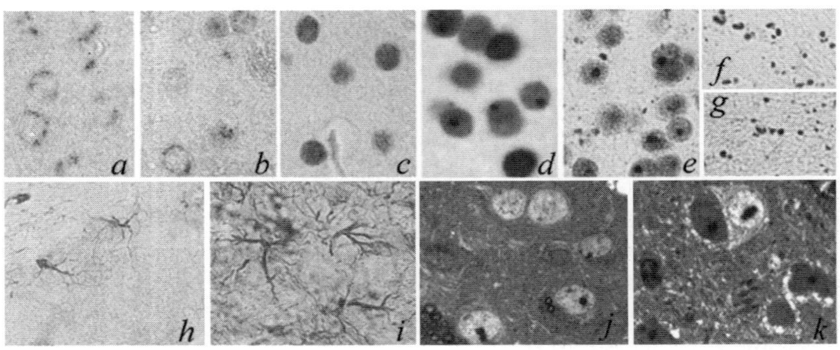

FIGURE 1 (See color version on DVD) Time-course of aggregate formation and neurodegeneration in HdhQ111 mice. Images of sections of HdhQ111 striatum prepared from mice at various ages are shown. For homozygotes, EM48 stain reveals (a) initial perinuclear reactivity (five weeks); (b) diffuse nuclear accumulation (six weeks); (c) puncta (five months); (d) N-terminal intranuclear inclusions (ten months); and (e) neuropil aggregate (seventeen months), also in terminal fields in (f) globus pallidus and (g) substantia nigra. At twenty-four months, GFAP reactivity (h and i) indicates reactive gliosis in heterozygous mutant (i) compared to wild-type (h) striatum. At twenty-four months, toluidine-blue staining (j and k) of sections from wild-type (j) and heterozygous mutant (k) striatum reveals, in the latter, darkly reactive degenerating neurons. From Wheeler et al. 2002; Early phenotypes that presage late-onset neurodegenerative disease allow testing of modifiers in Hdh CAG knock-in mice (*Hum Mol Genet* **11**:633–640; by permission of Oxford University Press).

TABLE 2 Time-course of Nuclear Aggregate Formation: Comparison between Knock-in Models

Repeat number	Age first observed (months): Nuclear staining	Microaggregates or puncta	Nuclear inclusions	References
CAG-140	NR	2	6	Menalled et al. 2003
CAG-150	NR	7	10	Lin et al. 2001
CAG-111	2.5	5	10	Wheeler et al. 2002
CAG-92	4.5	12	15	Wheeler et al. 2000
CAG-94	NR	4–6	18	Menalled et al. 2002
CAG-72-80	4	11	21	Li et al. 2000
CAG-80	NR	NR	22	Lin et al. 2001

NR = Not reported.

Similar to observations in HD and in other CAG repeat diseases (Zoghbi and Orr 2000), an increase in CAG repeats in HD knock-in mice parallels a decrease in the regional selectivity of the neuropathology. In mice carrying 111 to 150 CAG repeats in the Hdh gene, neuronal intranuclear inclusions are observed not only in the striatum but also, albeit to a lesser extent, in other brain regions, such as the neocortex (layers II/III, IV, and deep layer V), piriform cortex, hippocampus, olfactory tubercle, and cerebellum (Lin et al. 2001; Wheeler et al. 2000; Menalled et al. 2003).

The time-course for nuclear translocation of huntingtin and formation of microaggregates is similar for mice with large (111 to 150) or medium (72 to 94) expansions, although microaggregates were observed as early as two months of age in a mouse model with 140 CAG repeats (Menalled et al. 2003). In contrast, intranuclear inclusions are formed at a significantly earlier age in knock-in mice with large expansions, and when different knock-in models are compared, the time of formation of NIIs appears to be inversely proportional to the length of the CAG expansions (table 2). In mice with 111–150 CAG repeats, NIIs can already be observed at six to ten months, whereas in mice with 92–94 repeats they are apparent at fifteen to eighteen months, and even later (twenty-one to twenty-two months) for mice with 72 to 80 CAG repeats.

b. Neuropil Aggregates

Neuropil aggregates (defined as small huntingtin aggregates present in axons or dendrites) represent the vast majority of aggregates in HD brains and are distributed in different brain regions. In presymptomatic HD patients, the majority of the aggregates are neuropil aggregates and these are found in cortical layers V and VI, and to a lesser extent in layer III. At later stages, the frequency of neuropil aggregates decreases in deep layers of the cortex (probably due to neuronal loss), but increases in layer III. In the striatum, the relative frequency of neuropil versus nuclear aggregates, as well as their size, increases as the disease progresses. Analysis of the distribution of neuropil aggregates in the LGP (lateral globus pallidus), MGP (medium globus pallidus), and SN (substantia nigra) of knock-in mice containing 72 to 80 CAG repeats (Li et al. 2001) revealed that only neuropil aggregates but no intranuclear inclusions are observed in these regions. Also, neuropil aggregates are more abundant in the LGP and SN than in the MGP, suggesting that striatal neurons projecting to these two regions contain more axonal aggregates, whereas striatal neurons projecting to the internal globus pallidus form fewer aggregates in their axons. Importantly, the distribution of neuropil aggregates in this knock-in mouse model is well correlated with the brain regions that degenerate early in HD (Reiner et al. 1988; Sapp et al. 1995).

Investigators reported similar findings regarding the distribution of neuropil aggregates in the globus pallidus of Hdh 140Q mice (Menalled et al. 2003). However, in contrast to the CAG 72–80 knock-in mice, these mice also exhibit neuropil aggregates in the cortex (layer II/III and layer IV/superficial V), olfactory tubercle, piriform cortex, hippocampus, and ventral pallidum.

The formation of neuropil aggregates is also progressive. In CAG 72–80 knock-in mice (Li et al. 2001) neuropil aggregates are first seen in the LGP at seven to eight months of age, and by eleven to twelve months they are also present in the SN and become even more abundant at later ages (twenty-one to twenty-four months). However, nuclear inclusions in the striatum appear to be significantly more abundant than neuropil aggregates and are observed at an earlier age, suggesting that mutant huntingtin first accumulates in the nucleus of striatal neurons to form intranuclear inclusions and then forms aggregates in their processes. Similar to neuronal nuclear inclusions, further expansion of the CAG tract leads to earlier formation of neuropil aggregates. In mice containing a CAG 140 expansion (Menalled et al. 2003), neuropil aggregates are first observed at two months of age, predominantly in the striatum, piriform cortex, and globus pallidus. At four to six months, neuropil aggregates were also observed in the olfactory tubercle, piriform cortex, hippocampus, and ventral pallidum.

2. Gliosis and Neuronal Cell Death

The neuropathological changes in HD are characterized by neuronal cell loss and gliosis (Hedreen and Ross 1995). Selective atrophy occurs within the brain and affects the corpus striatum most severely. Selective loss of medium spiny projection neurons occurs within the striatum, but with relative preservation of interneurons. Other areas of the basal ganglia, including the globus pallidus and subthalamic areas also show atrophy. Both morphometric and cell counting studies have shown shrinkage and neuronal cell loss in the cerebral cortex, specifically in layers VI, III, and V (for a review see Sharp and Ross 1996). Up until now, investigators have reported neuronal cell loss in only one mouse knock-in line. In homozygous HdhQ111 mice (Wheeler et al. 2002), cell shrinkage in the striatum was observed at seventeen months of age, and by twenty-four months of age reported neurodegenerative changes, toluidine blue-stained neurons (indicating cell death) and reactive gliosis were observed in 50% of the mutant mice (Figure 1). Consistent with the incomplete penetrance of the phenotype, the neuronal cell loss in the striatum was low (up to 3%) although intense glial fibrillary acidic protein (GFAP) staining was observed in all cases.

Investigators observed a marked increase in reactive gliosis, with no neuronal cell loss, in ten-month-old mice carrying a 150 CAG expansion (Lin et al. 2001). Mutant mice exhibited restricted areas of intense staining in the striatum, reminiscent of patches of GFAP staining observed in HD brains. Axonal degeneration on the other hand was observed in the striatum of ten-month-old mutant mice (Yu et al. 2003).

Reactive gliosis in different brain regions were also reported for one mouse line expressing a CAG80-Hdh gene (Ishiguro et al. 2001). Immunohistochemistry for GFAP in ten-month-old mouse brains revealed an increase in glial filaments in the globus pallidus, substantia nigra, and striatum, with no obvious astrocytosis in other brain regions. In this case also, no cell loss was detected up to fifteen months of age.

Although no neuronal cell body degeneration was observed in Hdh6/Q72 and Hdh4/Q80 knock-in mice, EM examination of seventeen to twenty-seven-month-old brains (Li et al. 2001) showed neuropil degeneration in the LGP and SN regions, which also degenerate early in HD (Reiner et al. 1988).

D. Altered Cellular Functions

Compelling theories for neuronal damage in HD involve excitotoxicity and abnormal energy metabolism (DiFiglia 1990; Beal et al. 1993). The excitotoxicity theory postulates that specific subpopulations of neurons are hypersensitive to glutamate. Investigators observed increased sensitivity to *N*-methyl-D-aspartate (NMDA) receptor activation in a knock-in model with ninety-four CAG repeats (Levine et al. 1999). Striatal neuronal cells from Hdh 94Q knock-in mice (two to four months old) exhibited a more rapid and increased cell swelling than controls when exposed to NMDA. Changes in cell swelling in these knock-in mice may be due to alterations in neurophysiological properties of the cells, since a subpopulation of the striatal neurons of the mutant mice displayed more depolarized resting membrane potentials (RMPs) than controls.

Defects in gene transcription and mitochondrial function are also implicated in the process that leads to the loss of striatal neurons in HD (Tabrizi et al. 1999; Grunewald and Beal 1999). Direct measurement of respiratory chain enzyme activities has shown severe deficiency of complex II/III and a milder defect of complex IV, confined to the striatum within the HD brain.

Gines and collaborators (2003) reported a significant decrease in brain-derived neurotrophic factor (BDNF) and of phospho-CREB (the active form of CREB-cAMP-responsive binding protein) levels both in cortical and striatal neurons of HdhQ111 heterozygote and homozygote mouse brains at five months of age. As these findings indicated dominantly reduced PKA/CREB signaling, they further investigated the levels of cAMP in HD-knock-in brains. cAMP concentrations in striatal and cortical extracts were reduced as early as six to ten weeks, worsening over time. By contrast, levels of cAMP in mutant and WT in other brain areas were similar at all ages examined, even at sixteen months, indicating that the reduction of cAMP in HD knock-in mice is progressive and specific to the cortex and striatum. Studies in cultured striatal cells derived from HdhQ111 mice revealed a decrease in the synthesis of cAMP, reduced ATP and ATP/ADP ratio, reduced respiratory chain activity, and increased sensitivity to mitochondrial toxins, suggesting that striatal cells have a respiratory chain deficit. Importantly, a significant decrease in cAMP levels was also detected in postmortem HD brains.

Prior to the onset of motor abnormalities, HD patients display other symptoms, including cognitive deficits. To determine whether or not changes in synaptic function and plasticity might underlie early cognitive deficits seen in HD, Usdin and collaborators (Usdin et al. 1999) investigated the physiology of hippocampal slices from knock-in Hdh6/Q72 and Hdh4/Q80 mice. Although investigators observed no anatomical abnormalities in hippocampal preparations, synaptic plasticity was impaired, as evidenced by a significant reduction in long-term potentiation (LTP), a measure of synaptic plasticity, thought to be involved in memory. Mutant mice also showed decreased post-tetanic potentiation (PTP) and paired-pulse facilitation (PPF), suggesting that excitatory synapses in HD knock-in mutants are impaired in their ability to sustain transmission during repetitive stimulation.

E. Molecular Abnormalities

A major objective of analyzing HD models is to attempt to determine the earliest molecular changes associated with the disease. The limited availability of brain tissue from presymptomatic HD patients precludes this analysis in humans. However, analysis of HD knock-in mouse models revealed early molecular changes that precede neuropathological phenotypes. Screening of filter arrays containing human gene segments using cDNA probes prepared from the striatum of wild-type and knock-in HdhQ111 homozygote mice revealed that Rrs1 (which encodes a ribosomal regulatory protein) shows increased expression in HD mutant mice (Fossale et al. 2002). Increased expression of Rrs1 mRNA is observed in HdhQ111 mutant striatum starting at three weeks of age, and in HdhQ92 and HdhQ50 mutant striata at eight months and fourteen months, respectively. Significantly, RT-PCR analysis on HD postmortem brains also revealed increased expression of Rrs1 mRNA, demonstrating that expression of this conserved gene is increased as a consequence of mutant huntingtin in the human disease. However, while indicating that increased Rrs1 expression reflects an early disease event, further analysis is required to determine if this phenotype is a side effect of the disease mechanism or if altered ribosomal function may be part of the pathway that leads to neurodegeneration.

The striatal efferent neurons that degenerate in HD can be divided into two main classes, based on their projections and peptide content (Chesselet 1999). Neurons containing the neuropeptide enkephalin project to the external pallidum, whereas neurons containing the neuropeptides substance P and dynorphin project primarily to the internal pallidum and the substantia nigra. In presymptomatic HD carriers and patients in early stages of HD, a greater reduction of enkephalin levels in the external segment was observed compared to substance P in the internal segment of the globus pallidus (Albin et al. 1992; Sapp et al. 1995). It is not clear however, if this difference in peptide immunoreactivity is due to a difference in peptide synthesis or to a selective death of enkephalinergic neurons early in the disease.

Quantitative *in situ* hybridization revealed that, in comparison with wild-type mice, enkephalin mRNA levels were significantly reduced in four-month-old HD transgenic mice and in knock-in mice containing a chimeric mouse/human exon 1 with seventy-one or ninety-four CAG repeats (Menalled et al. 2000). The decrease in enkephalin mRNA occurred independently of changes in other mRNAs expressed by striatal neurons, such as substance P and glutamic acid decarboxilases. This analysis suggests that in HD enkephalin mRNA levels may be reduced prior to cell loss.

F. CAG Instability

The finding that expanded HD repeats exhibit striking intergenerational instability and the CAG-length-dependent pathogenic mechanism explain some of the genetic aspects of the disease. In the vast majority of transmissions from HD mothers or fathers (>80%), the expanded repeat is subtly altered, decreasing (if acquired from the mother) or increasing (if acquired from the father) by one or a few CAG units (Duyao et al. 1993; Bates et al. 1997). However, on occasion, paternal HD transmissions produce large expansions, causing the phenomenon of anticipation, where the age of onset tends to decrease in successive generations (Vonsattel and DiFiglia 1998).

Investigators also observed intergenerational CAG repeat instability in several knock-in mouse models of HD. In mice carrying CAG expansions varying from fifty to eighty (Wheeler et al. 1999; Shelbourne et al. 1999; Ishiguro et al. 2001), in about 3–4% of the mutant progeny the CAG repeats expanded (in paternal transmissions) or decreased (in maternal transmissions) with an average of three repeats. Mice carrying longer CAG tracts (HdhQ92 and HdhQ111) on the other hand, showed mutation rates of 50% and 73%, respectively (Wheeler et al. 1999). These results demonstrate that the CAG length is the primary determinant of genetic instability in mice.

In contrast to observations of HD patients, however, no apparent age-effect occurs in either female or male transmissions in knock-in mice. In addition, extreme repeat numbers are required to achieve a high frequency of CAG repeat instability in the germline of knock-in mice.

In contrast to the intergenerational instability of the expanded CAG repeats, limited length variation is seen in somatic tissues of most HD patients. Only large CAG tracts (greater than sixty-five CAGs) show extensive mosaicism in the brain and other organs of juvenile onset HD cases (Telenius et al. 1994; De Rooij et al. 1995). In these patients, regions within the brain showing the most obvious neuropathology, such as the basal ganglia and the cerebral cortex, displayed the greatest mosaicism, whereas the cerebellar cortex displayed the lowest degree of CAG instability.

Although the impact of the somatic CAG expansions is unclear, investigators have suggested that somatic increases of the mutation length may play an important role in the progression and cellular specificity of both juvenile- and adult-onset HD pathogenesis (Kennedy et al. 2003).

Investigators have also reported age-dependent and CAG-length-dependent somatic CAG repeat instability in knock-in mouse models. While little somatic instability was observed in HdhQ50 mice at fifteen months of age, mosaic expansion of the CAG tract length was observed at low/moderate levels in cortex and spleen, and extensively in the striatum and liver of HdhQ92 and HdhQ111 mice as early as nine months and five months, respectively (Wheeler et al. 1999). In a knock-in line with seventy-seven CAG repeats (Ishiguro et al. 2001), severe repeat instability was observed at ten months of age in different brain regions including the cortex, striatum, hippocampus, midbrain, thalamus, hypothalamus, pons/medulla, and olfactory bulb. Low to medium levels of instability in Hdh6/Q72 and Hdh4/Q80 mice were detected by three months of age, with a tendency for expansions smaller than five CAG repeats in non-CNS tissues as well as most regions of the brain such as the cortex, cerebellum, hippocampus, hindbrain, spinal cord, and olfactory bulbs and striatum. By nine months of age, greater CAG increases (five to thirty repeats) were detected, particularly in the cortex and striatum and by twenty-four months of age more than 80% of the striatal cells contained mutant repeat tracts that had increased in size (Kennedy and Shelbourne 2000; Kennedy et al. 2003).

II. KNOCK-OUT MOUSE MODELS

A. Targeted Disruption of the Hdh Gene

Targeted disruption of Hdh showed that huntingtin is essential during embryonic development, since homozygous embryos become developmentally retarded and disorganized, and die between days 7.5 and 10.5 of gestation (Zeitlin et al. 1995; Nasir et al. 1995; Duyao et al. 1995; Dragatsis and Zeitlin 2001). Although null embryos initiate gastrulation they do not form somites or organogenesis. Extensive apoptotic cell death in the embryonic ectoderm, a layer expressing the Hdh gene, suggests that huntingtin might be involved in processes counterbalancing the operation of an apoptotic pathway (Zeitlin et al. 1995). The fact that the homozygous knock-out embryos died in gestation was taken initially as corroborative proof that HD occurs by a gain-of-function mechanism. Three of the heterozygous knock-out mice expressing half the level of huntingtin reached adulthood and displayed no abnormalities (Zeitlin et al. 1995; Duyao et al. 1995; Dragatsis and Zeitlin 2001). In another knock-out model, a truncated N-terminal fragment of htt was expressed in heterozygous mice—these mice show increased motor activity, cognitive deficits, neuronal loss, and degeneration in the subthalamic nucleus and globus pallidus (Nasir et al. 1995; O'Kusky et al. 1999). These results suggest that the truncated protein may exert a dominant-negative effect and therefore that wild-type huntingtin may play a role in the basal ganglia.

B. Chimeras

The embryonic lethality of homozygous knock-out mice is bypassed in chimeric mice generated by injection of huntingtin null embryonic stem (ES) cells into wild-type blastocysts (Dragatsis et al. 1998). Because ES cells colonize only the embryo proper but not extra-embryonic tissues, these results suggest that the early embryonic lethality of the knock-out embryos is due to an essential role of huntingtin in extra-embryonic tissues during mouse embryonic development.

Chimeric mice are viable and survive into adulthood but tend to be smaller than control littermates and display a set of motor abnormalities, including forelimb and hindlimb clasping on tail suspension, starting as early as one month of age (Reiner et al. 2001). In general, investigators found that the severity of the motor abnormalities correlated well with the percentage of Hdh–/– cell colonization of the chimeras. However, no brain abnormalities or pathologies were observed, although Hdh–/– neurons were present throughout the brain. Interestingly, Hdh–/– cells were found to be five to ten times more abundant in the hypothalamus, midbrain, and hindbrain than in the telencephalon, thalamus, and Purkinje cell layer of the cerebellum, implying that huntingtin plays a role in the development of these regions.

C. Conditional Inactivation of Huntingtin in the Forebrain

To further investigate the function of huntingtin in the developing and postnatal brain, researchers used a conditional mutagenesis strategy using the Cre-loxP site recombination system to generate a null mutation in the mouse forebrain (Dragatsis et al. 2000). The cre gene encodes a recombinase (Cre) that catalyzes the deletion of an intervening DNA sequence located between two specific 34 bp target sequences (loxP sites) when these are in the same orientation (Sauer and Henderson 1989; Sauer 1998). To generate a conditional Hdh allele (Hdhflox) loxP sites were placed upstream from the Hdh transcription initiation site and within intron 1. Upon Cre-mediated recombination, the promoter, exon 1, and a portion of the first intron are deleted, resulting in a null allele. To inactivate the Hdh gene specifically in the forebrain, investigators used two transgenic Cre lines, expressing Cre under the control of the alpha subunit of the Calcium/calmodulin-dependent protein kinase II (CamKII) promoter: in the R1ag#5 line, cre expression and recombination starts at embryonic day 15.5 and in the L7ag#13 after postnatal day 5. Conditional mutant mice

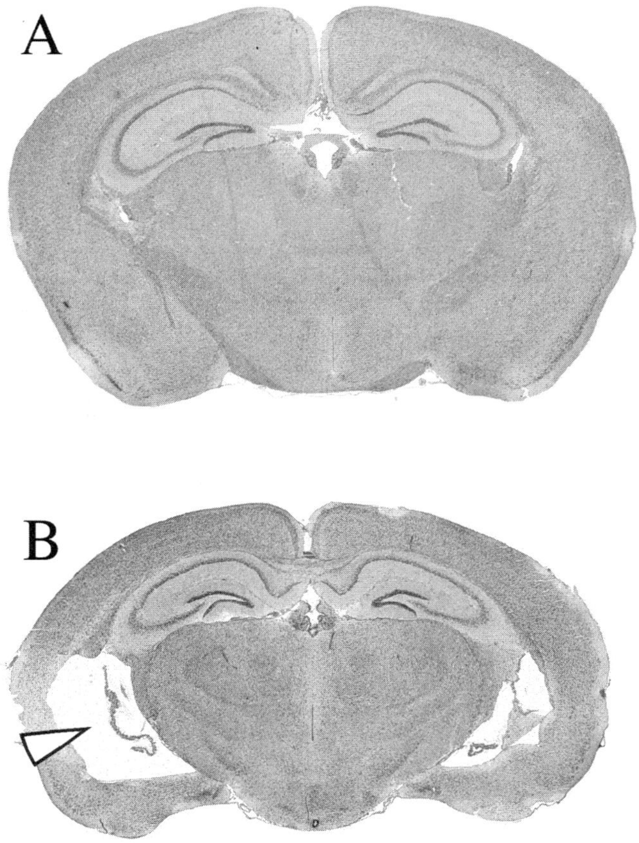

FIGURE 2 Degeneration in R1ag5 mutant brains. Hematoxylin-eosin stained coronal sections through a ten-month-old control (a) and eight-month-old R1ag5 mutant (b) brains. Degeneration adjacent to the external capsule in the caudal region is observed in R1ag5 mutant brain (arrowhead). Adapted from Dragatsis et al. 2000 (Figure 3, p. 302) by permission of Nature Publishing Group.

derived from both cre lines displayed reduced life span (thirteen months of age) and a progressive motor phenotype. Abnormal limb clasping was observed as early as postnatal day 21 in R1ag#5 mutants and postnatal day 60 in L7Ag#13 mutants, becoming progressively more severe so that by ten months all mutants exhibited body curling in the tail suspension test. Motor coordination and balance deficits were also observed at three to four months of age. In contrast, no gait deficits were observed in the mutants up to eight months of age. Extensive tissue loss was observed only in mutant mice carrying the early expressing R1ag#5 cre transgene (Figure 2B). Altered MAP2 staining was observed only in the oldest R1Ag#5 mutants, whereas gliosis was observed throughout the forebrain of both R1Ag#5 and L7Ag#13 mutants (Figure 3). These results indicate that huntingtin is required for neuronal function and survival and suggest that severe reduction of huntingtin levels (due to its sequestration into neuronal inclusions) could contribute to HD pathogenesis.

III. HD KNOCK-IN IN THE CONTEXT OF LOW HUNTINGTIN EXPRESSION

Investigators assessed the consequence of introducing the HD mutation on a background of severely reduced huntingtin levels in mice carrying a CAG expansion in hypomorphic "Hdh-neo-CAG" knock-in alleles. In an attempt to generate a model for HD in mice, a CAG expansion of fifty repeats was inserted into exon 1 of the Hdh gene (White et al. 1997). However, insertion of a PGK-neo cassette in the vicinity of the Hdh promoter gene resulted in a hypomorphic allele (HdhneoQ50) that expressed the Hdh protein

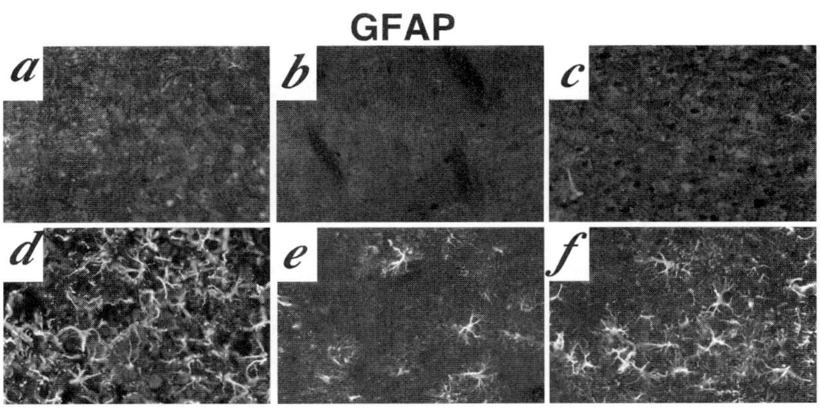

FIGURE 3 Gliosis in R1ag5 mutant brains. Immunofluorescent staining of GFAP in sagittal sections through the forebrain of an eight-month-old control (a,b,c) and eight-month-old R1ag5 mutant (d,e,f) reveals reactive astrocytosis in the entorrhinal cortex (compare d with a), striatum (compare e with b), and frontal cortex (compare f with c). Adapted from Dragatsis et al. 2000 (Figure 6, p. 304) by permission of Nature Publishing Group.

TABLE 3 Abnormal Behaviors and Neuropathology of Hypomorphic Mutants

Mouse model	Level of expression of htt	Number of CAG repeats	Abnormal behaviors	Brain abnormalities and neuropathology	Others
HdhneoQ20/null	1/10 of WT	20	Hindlimb clasping at 2 months	Enlarged lateral and third ventricles at 2 months; No cell death or gliosis	Reduced body size
HdhneoQ20/neoQ20	1/5 of WT	20	Hindlimb clasping at 2 months	None	Reduced body size
HdhneoQ20/neoQ111	1/8 of WT	20 and 111	Progressive motor dysfunction. Hindlimb clasping at 2 months. Limb stiffness or paralysis; hopping during walking; resting tremors; seizures (7–10 months); Abnormal gait at 7–10 months	Enlarged lateral and third ventricles at 2 months; No cell death or gliosis	Reduced body size; Death prior to 12 months

at one-third the level of the WT allele. Compound heterozygous mice carrying the HdhneoQ50 allele and a null allele were not viable and at late gestation displayed several brain abnormalities, most evident in the forebrain and midbrain, where ectopic masses of neurons and abnormally dilated lateral ventricles were observed (White et al. 1997).

In a subsequent work, investigators studied three lines of compound heterozygous mice in which both copies of the Hdh gene were altered, resulting in low levels of huntingtin with a normal human polyglutamine length (Q20) and/or an expanded disease-associated segment (Q111) expressing low levels of huntingtin: HdhneoQ20/neoQ20, HdhneoQ20/null, and HdhneoQ20/neoQ111 (Auerbach et al. 2001). A summary of the findings is presented in table 3. Starting at two months of age, all three lines showed movement abnormalities, with hindlimb clasping during tail suspension being most common. However, while in the HdhneoQ20/neoQ20 and HdhneoQ20/null mice the movement disorders did not worsen over time, HdhneoQ20/neoQ111 demonstrated progressively more movement problems with age. In most HdhneoQ20/neoQ111, the hindlimb clasping phenotype worsened over a period of nine months, and other abnormalities became apparent, including limb stiffness or paralysis, resting tremors, difficulties walking, and seizure-like episodes. At the most advanced stages, mice became hypokinetic. Importantly, the progressive disease phenotype and, in particular, the paralysis was not observed in the other two lines of mice, HdhneoQ20/neoQ20 and Hdh neoQ20/null, which also express very reduced levels of huntingtin but not its mutant form.

Histological examinations of brains from all three compound mutants showed that HdhneoQ20/null and HdhneoQ20/neoQ111 mice had enlarged lateral and third ventricles compared to controls. This phenotype did not worsen over time and most likely results from developmental defects associated with much-reduced levels of huntingtin expression.

Although no evidence of cell loss, apoptosis, or gliosis was detected in the striatum of HdhneoQ20/neoQ111 mice at twelve months of age, overt degeneration might occur at a much later stage and the progressive neurological phenotypes observed in these mice may be due to neuronal functional deficits. Nonetheless, these results indicate that severely reduced levels of huntingtin provide a background that sensitizes neurons to the toxic effects of mutant huntingtin.

IV. CONCLUSIONS

Knock-in mouse models have provided valuable insights into the early events and progressive alterations that are associated with HD pathogenesis. Although motor deficits are mild compared to transgenic mice and neuronal loss is limited, the cellular and molecular changes and the neuropathology of knock-in mice are similar to those observed in HD patients. The finding that accurately expressed mutant huntingtin with very long HD glutamine repeats causes overt juvenile-onset HD in humans but not in mice supports a disease process that operates in a time-dependent rather than developmental stage-dependent manner. This finding is consistent with the insidious progressive nature of HD pathology in humans and with the absence of severe phenotypes in a similar Hdh knock-in line. However, the slow progression of the disease in knock-in mice makes it possible to investigate in detail the early changes associated with the disorder.

Knock-out mouse models, on the other hand, have further given support to the hypothesis that loss of wild-type protein function may contribute to disease pathogenesis. This finding is not only important for understanding the mechanism that leads to HD pathology but also impacts the development of therapeutic strategies.

References

Albin, R.L., A. Reiner, K.D. Anderson, L.S. Dure, 4th, B. Handelin, R. Balfour, W.O. Whetsell, Jr., et al. 1992. Preferential loss of striato-external pallidal projection neurons in presymptomatic Huntington's disease. *Ann Neurol* **31**:425–430.

Auerbach, W., M.S. Hurlbert, P. Hilditch-Maguire, Y.Z. Wadghiri, V.C. Wheeler, S.I. Cohen, A.L. Joyner, et al. 2001. The HD mutation causes progressive lethal neurological disease in mice expressing reduced levels of huntingtin. *Hum Mol Genet* **10**:2515–2523.

Bates, G.P., L. Mangiarini, A. Mahal, and S.W. Davies. 1997. Transgenic models of Huntington's disease. *Hum Mol Genet* **6**:1633–1637.

Beal, M.F., B.T. Hyman, and W. Koroshetz. 1993. Do defects in mitochondrial energy metabolism underlie the pathology of neurodegenerative diseases? *Trends Neurosci* **16**:125–131.

Becher, M.W., J.A. Kotzuk, A.H. Sharp, S.W. Davies, G.P. Bates, D.L. Price, and C.A. Ross. 1998. Intranuclear neuronal inclusions in Huntington's disease and dentatorubral and pallidoluysian atrophy: correlation between the density of inclusions and IT15 CAG triplet repeat length. *Neurobiol Dis* **4**:387–397.

Chesselet, M.F. 1999. Mapping the basal ganglia. In: A.W. Toga and J.C. Mazziotta, Editors, *Brain Mapping: The Applications*, Academic Press.

De Rooij, K.E., P.A. De Koning Gans, R.A. Roos, G.J. Van Ommen, and J.T. Den Dunnen. 1995. Somatic expansion of the (CAG)n repeat in Huntington disease brains. *Hum Genet* **95**:270–274.

DiFiglia, M. 1990. Excitotoxic injury of the neostriatum: a model for Huntington's disease. *Trends Neurosci* **13**:286–289.

Dragatsis, I., Efstratiadis, A., and Zeitlin, S. (1998). Mouse mutant embryos lacking huntingtin are rescued from lethality by wild-type extraembryonic tissues. *Development* **125**, 1529–1539.

Dragatsis, I., and S. Zeitlin. 2001. A method for the generation of conditional gene repair mutations in mice. *Nucleic Acids Res* **29**:E10.

Dragatsis, I., M.S. Levine, and S. Zeitlin. 2000. Inactivation of Hdh in the brain and testis results in progressive neurodegeneration and sterility in mice. *Nat Genet* **26**:300–306.

Duyao, M., C. Ambrose, R. Myers, A. Novelletto, F. Persichetti, M. Frontali, S. Folstein, et al. 1993. Trinucleotide repeat length instability and age of onset in Huntington's disease. *Nat Genet* **4**:387–392.

Duyao, M.P., A.B. Auerbach, A. Ryan, F. Persichetti, G.T. Barnes, S.M. McNeil, P. Ge, J.P. Vonsattel, et al. 1995. Inactivation of the mouse Huntington's disease gene homolog Hdh. *Science* **269**:407–410.

Fossale, E., V.C. Wheeler, V. Vrbanac, L.A. Lebel, A. Teed, J.S. Mysore, J.F. Gusella, et al. 2002. Identification of a presymptomatic molecular phenotype in Hdh CAG knock-in mice. *Hum Mol Genet* **11**:2233–2241.

Gines, S., I.S. Seong, E. Fossale, E. Ivanova, F. Trettel, J.F. Gusella, et al. (2003). Specific progressive cAMP reduction implicates energy deficit in presymptomatic Huntington's disease knock-in mice. *Hum Mol Genet* **12**:497–508.

Grunewald, T., and M.F. Beal. 1999. Bioenergetics in Huntington's disease. *Ann N Y Acad Sci* **893**:203–213.

Gutekunst, C.A., S.H. Li, H. Yi, J.S. Mulroy, S. Kuemmerle, R. Jones, D. Rye, et al. (1999). Nuclear and neuropil aggregates in Huntington's disease: relationship to neuropathology. *J Neurosci* **19**:2522–2534.

Harper, P. 1996. *Huntington's Disease*. London: W.B. Saunders.

Hedreen, J.C., C.E. Peyser, S.E. Folstein, and C.A. Ross. 1991. Neuronal loss in layers V and VI of cerebral cortex in Huntington's disease. *Neurosci Lett* **133**:257–261.

Ishiguro, H., K. Yamada, H. Sawada, K. Nishii, N. Ichino, M. Sawada, Y. Kurosawa, et al. 2001. Age-dependent and tissue-specific CAG repeat instability occurs in mouse knock-in for a mutant Huntington's disease gene. *J Neurosci Res* **65**:289–297.

Jason, G.W., O. Suchowersky, E.M. Pajurkova, L. Graham, M.L. Klimek, A.T. Garber, and D. Poirier-Heine. 1997. Cognitive manifestations of Huntington disease in relation to genetic structure and clinical onset. *Arch Neurol* **54**:1081–1088.

Kennedy, L., E. Evans, C.M. Chen, L. Craven, P.J. Detloff, M. Ennis, and P.F. Shelbourne. 2003. Dramatic tissue-specific mutation length increases are an early molecular event in Huntington disease pathogenesis. *Hum Mol Genet* **12**:3359–3367.

Kennedy, L., and P.F. Shelbourne. 2000. Dramatic mutation instability in HD mouse striatum: does polyglutamine load contribute to cell-specific vulnerability in Huntington's disease? *Hum Mol Genet* **9**:2539–2544.

Koller, W.C., and Trimble, J. (1985). The gait abnormality of Huntington's disease. *Neurology* **35**, 1450–1454.

Lawrence, A.D., J.R. Hodges, A.E. Rosser, A. Kershaw, C. French-Constant, D.C. Rubinsztein, T.W. Robbins, and B.J. Sahakian. 1998. Evidence for specific cognitive deficits in preclinical Huntington's disease. *Brain* **121**:1329–1341.

Lawrence, A.D., B.J. Sahakian, J.R. Hodges, A.E. Rosser, K.W. Lange, and T.W. Robbins. 1996. Executive and mnemonic functions in early Huntington's disease. *Brain* **119**:1633–1645.

Levine, M.S., G.J. Klapstein, A. Koppel, E. Gruen, C., Cepeda, M.E. Vargas, E.S. Jokel, et al. 1999. Enhanced sensitivity to N-methyl-D-aspartate receptor activation in transgenic and knockin mouse models of Huntington's disease. *J Neurosci Res* **58**:515–532.

Li, H., S.H. Li, H. Johnston, P.F. Shelbourne, and X.J. Li. 2000. Amino-terminal fragments of mutant huntingtin show selective accumulation in striatal neurons and synaptic toxicity. *Nat Genet* **25**:385–389.

Li, H., S.H. Li, Z.X. Yu, P. Shelbourne, and X.J. Li. 2001. Huntingtin aggregate-associated axonal degeneration is an early pathological event in Huntington's disease mice. *J Neurosci* **21**:8473–8481.

Lin, C.H., S. Tallaksen-Greene, W.M. Chien, J.A. Cearley, W.S. Jackson, A.B. Crouse, S. Ren, et al. 2001. Neurological abnormalities in a knock-in mouse model of Huntington's disease. *Hum Mol Genet* **10**:137–144.

Maat-Schieman, M.L., J.C. Dorsman, M.A. Smoor, S. Siesling, S.G. Van Duinen, J.J. Verschuuren, J.T. den Dunnen, et al. 1999. Distribution of inclusions in neuronal nuclei and dystrophic neurites in Huntington disease brain. *J Neuropathol Exp Neurol* **58**:129–137.

Menalled, L., H. Zanjani, L. MacKenzie, A. Koppel, E. Carpenter, S. Zeitlin, and M.F. Chesselet. 2000. Decrease in striatal enkephalin mRNA in mouse models of Huntington's disease. *Exp Neurol* **162**: 328–342.

Menalled, L.B., J.D. Sison, Y. Wu, M. Olivieri, X.J. Li, H. Li, S. Zeitlin, and M.F. Chesselet. 2002. Early motor dysfunction and striosomal distribution of huntingtin microaggregates in Huntington's disease knock-in mice. *J Neurosci* **22**:8266–8276.

Menalled, L.B., J.D. Sison, I. Dragatsis, S. Zeitlin, and M.F. Chesselet. 2003. Time course of early motor and neuropathological anomalies in a knock-in mouse model of Huntington's disease with 140 CAG repeats. *J Comp Neurol* **465**:11–26.

Nasir, J., S.B. Floresco, J.R. O'Kusky, V.M. Diewert, J.M. Richman, J. Zeisler, A. Borowski, et al. 1995. Targeted disruption of the Huntington's disease gene results in embryonic lethality and behavioral and morphological changes in heterozygotes. *Cell* **81**:811–823.

O'Kusky, J.R., J. Nasir, F. Cicchetti, A. Parent, and M.R. Hayden. 1999. Neuronal degeneration in the basal ganglia and loss of pallido-subthalamic synapses in mice with targeted disruption of the Huntington's disease gene. *Brain Res* **818**:468–479.

Reiner, A., R.L. Albin, K.D. Anderson, C.J. D'Amato, J.B. Penney, and A.B. Young. 1988. Differential loss of striatal projection neurons in Huntington disease. *Proc Natl Acad Sci U S A* **85**:5733–5737.

Reiner, A., N. Del Mar, C.A. Meade, H. Yang, I. Dragatsis, S. Zeitlin, and D. Goldowitz. 2001. Neurons lacking huntingtin differentially colonize brain and survive in chimeric mice. *J Neurosci* **21**:7608–7619.

Sapp, E., P. Ge, H. Aizawa, E. Bird, J. Penney, A.B. Young, J.P. Vonsattel, and M. DiFiglia. 1995. Evidence for a preferential loss of enkephalin immunoreactivity in the external globus pallidus in low grade Huntington's disease using high resolution image analysis. *Neuroscience* **64**:397–404.

Sathasivam, K., C. Hobbs, L. Mangiarini, A. Mahal, M. Turmaine, P. Doherty, S.W. Davies, and G.P. Bates. 1999. Transgenic models of Huntington's disease. *Philos Trans R Soc Lond B Biol Sci* **354**:963–969.

Sauer, B. 1998. Inducible gene targeting in mice using the Cre/lox system. *Methods* **14**:381–392.

Sauer, B., and N. Henderson. 1989. Cre-stimulated recombination at loxP sites placed into the genome of mammalian cells. *Nucleic Acids Res* **17**:147–161.

Sharp, A.H., and C.A. Ross. 1996. Neurobiology of Huntington's disease. *Neurobiol Dis* **3**:3–15.

Shelbourne, P.F., N. Killeen, R.F. Hevner, H.M. Johnston, L. Tecott, M. Lewandoski, M. Ennis, et al. 1999. A Huntington's disease CAG expansion at the murine Hdh locus is unstable and associated with behavioural abnormalities in mice. *Hum Mol Genet* **8**:763–774.

Sieradzan, K.A., A.O. Mechan, L. Jones, E.E. Wanker, N. Nukina, and D.M. Mann. 1999. Huntington's disease intranuclear inclusions contain truncated, ubiquitinated huntingtin protein. *Exp Neurol* **156**:92–99.

Tabrizi, S.J., M.W. Cleeter, J. Xuereb, J.W. Taanman, J.M. Cooper, and A.H. Schapira. 1999. Biochemical abnormalities and excitotoxicity in Huntington's disease brain. *Ann Neurol* **45**:25–32.

Telenius H., B. Kremer, Y.P. Goldberg, J. Theilmann, S.E. Andrew, J. Zeisler, S. Adam, et al. 1994. Somatic and gonadal mosaicism of the Huntington disease gene CAG repeat in brain and sperm. *Nat Genet* **6**:409–414.

Usdin, M.T., P.F. Shelbourne, R.M. Myers, and D.V. Madison. 1999. Impaired synaptic plasticity in mice carrying the Huntington's disease mutation. *Hum Mol Genet* **8**:839–46.

Vonsattel, J.P., and M. DiFiglia. 1998. Huntington disease. *J Neuropathol Exp Neurol* **57**:369–384.

Wheeler, V.C., W. Auerbach, J.K. White, J. Srinidhi, A. Auerbach, A. Ryan, M.P. Duyao, et al. 1999. Length-dependent gametic CAG repeat instability in the Huntington's disease knock-in mouse. *Hum Mol Genet* **8**:115–122.

Wheeler, V.C., J.K. White, C.A. Gutekunst, V. Vrbanac, M. Weaver, X.J. Li, S.H. Li, et al. 2000. Long glutamine tracts cause nuclear localization of a novel form of huntingtin in medium spiny striatal neurons in HdhQ92 and HdhQ111 knock-in mice. *Hum Mol Genet* **9**:503–513.

Wheeler, V.C., C.A. Gutekunst, V. Vrbanac, L.A. Lebel, G. Schilling, S. Hersch, R.M. Friedlander, et al. 2002. Early phenotypes that presage late-onset neurodegenerative disease allow testing of modifiers in Hdh CAG knock-in mice. *Hum Mol Genet* **11**:633–640.

White, J.K., W. Auerbach, M.P. Duyao, J.P. Vonsattel, J.F. Gusella, A.L. Joyner, and M.E. MacDonald. 1997. Huntingtin is required for neurogenesis and is not impaired by the Huntington's disease CAG expansion. *Nat Genet* **17**:404–410.

Yu, Z.X., S.H. Li, J. Evans, A. Pillarisetti, H. Li, and X.J. Li. 2003. Mutant huntingtin causes context-dependent neurodegeneration in mice with Huntington's disease. *J Neurosci* **23**:2193–2202.

Zeitlin, S., J.P. Liu, D.L. Chapman, V.E. Papaioannou, and A. Efstratiadis. 1995. Increased apoptosis and early embryonic lethality in mice nullizygous for the Huntington's disease gene homologue. *Nat Genet* **11**:155—158.

Zoghbi, H.Y., and H.T. Orr. 2000. Glutamine repeats and neurodegeneration. *Annu Rev Neurosci* **23**:217–247.

CHAPTER

D4

Drosophila Models of Huntington Disease

LESLIE M. THOMPSON and J. LAWRENCE MARSH

Drosophila has emerged as a remarkably appropriate model in which to study neurodegenerative disease. As these diseases become increasingly common with increasing life expectancies, it has become imperative to develop accurate animal models in which to study the pathogenic impact of mutant gene expression and to test potential therapeutics. Ideally, this system would mimic the essential features of the specific human disease and accelerate the identification of novel and useful therapies that can translate effectively into mouse and other mammalian disease models and ultimately into human clinical trials. *Drosophila* models of polyglutamine repeat diseases are fulfilling this need and have proven to be effective tools for asking mechanistic questions regarding disease progression and for testing the therapeutic potential of drugs and other treatments. Furthermore, the ability to genetically engineer an organism that has short generation times, has extensively characterized and tractable genetics, can be propagated at relatively low cost, and allows rapid identification of the most promising compounds is an extremely useful paradigm to integrate into programs that seek to identify therapeutic strategies for neurodegenerative diseases.

I. *DROSOPHILA* AS A MODEL FOR POLYGLUTAMINE REPEAT DISEASES?

Huntington disease (HD) is a late-onset, neurodegenerative disease characterized by psychiatric disturbances, cognitive impairment, and a movement disorder; it is also associated with region-specific neuronal loss, particularly within the striatum of human brain. The causative mutation for HD is an expansion of a polymorphic CAG repeat domain within the coding region of the HD gene [1]. HD is one of a group of at least nine inherited neurodegenerative diseases that includes spinal and bulbar muscular atrophy (SBMA or Kennedy disease) and a number of spinocerebellar ataxias (SCA) that are all caused by CAG repeat expansions in the coding region of the disease gene that are translated into expanded polyglutamine (polyQ) sequences in the gene product [2,3]. All of these diseases are late onset and progressive and exhibit movement disorders. Polyglutamine repeat diseases lend themselves particularly well to modeling in *Drosophila* due to the dominant nature of the single CAG repeat gene mutation that leads to neuropathology in each case.

Can the establishment of transgenic *Drosophila* models of polyglutamine repeat disease accurately reflect the essential features of each disease? While the causative mutation is known for each of these diseases, the basis of pathology remains complex and not well understood. Here we describe efforts to develop fly models and ways in which they have been used to further clinical progress in treatment of these diseases.

A. General Characteristics of Polyglutamine Repeat Diseases

Each of the nine polyglutamine repeat diseases has several common features that are signatures of the disease process: they all are associated with the following traits:

genetically dominant (or X-linked; SBMA)
late onset
cause progressive degeneration
lead to some type of motor function loss manifested as a movement disorder or ataxia
cause early death
associated with abnormal intracellular protein aggregates
associated with transcriptional alterations

B. *Drosophila* Models Accurately Mimic the Essential Features of PolyQ Repeat Diseases

Drosophila can be engineered to express foreign genes through transposable p-element vectors containing promoters (yeast upstream activator sequence, or UAS) that are activated by the yeast GAL4 transcription factor [4,5]. Genes fused to UAS are injected into fly embryos with a helper element and integrate into the fly genome, producing transgenic lines that carry the UAS > polyQ gene. The foreign human gene is then silent until crossed to another transgenic fly that expresses the GAL4 activator protein in specific tissues, determined by the nature of the promoter driving GAL4 expression in that *Drosophila* line. These crosses can be designed such that control, nonpolyQ-expressing siblings can be compared on the basis of multiple phenotypic assays to the offspring that express the mutant transgene. Fortuitously, a large number of fly strains are available that express the GAL4 protein in different tissue specific patterns [6].

The general architecture of the fly nervous system is similar to that of mammals, with areas that separate specialized functions including learning and memory, vision, and olfaction [7–9]. Furthermore, comparative genome analysis reveals that at least 50% of fly genes have similar genes in humans [10]. Among those associated with specific human diseases, approximately 75% have a *Drosophila* ortholog [11]. Therefore selective neurodegeneration can be monitored using tools that allow one to mark and follow specific subsets of neurons as they develop and mature. Some aspects of *Drosophila* biology relevant to their use in the study of neurodegeneration are described below.

After fertilization, *Drosophila* embryogenesis spans approximately one day with neurogenesis occurring between approximately five hours and fifteen hours within the protective coverings of the egg. At this stage, precursors of the imaginal discs that will give rise to adult structures (including photoreceptor neurons as described below) are also laid down. First instar larvae (instar = larval stages) hatch from the egg and molt to the second and third stages over approximately 3.5 days. During the third larval stage, the eye imaginal discs complete their growth and the photoreceptor neurons are born. Larval development is followed by pupariation, during which time (five days) metamorphosis occurs and adult flies subsequently emerge from the pupal case. In sum, approximately ten days after the initial laying of the egg, the adult fly emerges with fully functional and formed neurons (see [12] for review).

Two extensively used measures of neurodegeneration are (a) the structure of the photoreceptor neurons of the eye [12–14] and (b) motor function, the latter phenotype described by Ralph Hillman in this book. In order to monitor photoreceptor neuron degeneration, transgenes are commonly expressed either in all neurons of the CNS and PNS from embryogenesis on, using the *elav*-GAL4 driver, or in all cells in the eye (neurons and support cells) using the *gmr*-GAL4 driver. Expression from both of these promoters is activated at the front of a morphogenetic wave that occurs in the eye disc, allowing one to expose photoreceptor neurons to toxic polyQ proteins for defined periods of time within this gradient of neurons. Typically, for the polyQ disease models, an internal degeneration of neurons is observed following expression in all neurons (*elav*-GAL4) without an external observable phenotype, while expression of transgenes with the *gmr* driver leads to both external and internal degenerative phenotypes [12–14]. For each of the polyQ disease genes that were expressed as transgenes in neurons, each of the hallmarks of the diseases were observed upon expression using these drivers. As with any model, advantages and disadvantages in their use exist. For instance, while development occurs in the egg and in the pupal case, the flies are not accessible to exogenously applied drugs.

II. SPECIFIC *DROSOPHILA* MODELS OF POLYQ DISEASE

A. Huntington Disease

The protein encoded by the HD gene is a large 350 kD protein that is ubiquitously expressed and predominantly localizes to the cytosol. The normal function of this protein is not clear, however investigators have described roles critical to proper neuronal function, intracellular trafficking, and neuronal transcription [2,15,16]. During the course of the disease, truncation of the protein and nuclear localization occur and appear to be essential for disease progression [17,18]. The formation of cytosolic and, ultimately, nuclear inclusions is a hallmark feature of the disease and is associated with these truncated forms of the protein [19]. Because of these features and because models that express full-length forms of the Huntingtin protein take an extremely long time to manifest subtle phenotypes (YAC and knock-ins), initial HD models have focused upon the expression of truncated forms of the huntingtin protein to model disease pathology [19].

Expression of a truncated mutant Htt transgene (aa1-121) in the eye showed that, as in the human disease, the age of onset and extent of the eye phenotype correlate with polyQ repeat length [20]. Furthermore, the normally cytosolic Htt protein progressively localized to the nucleus, correlating with onset of neuronal degeneration. Truncating the mutant Htt protein further results in an even more severe disease phenotype [21]. When expressed in all neurons, the expression of mutant Htt exon 1 protein with 93Qs shows progressive degeneration of photoreceptor neurons, a movement phenotype, and early death. Because of the progressive and easily assayable degeneration observed, this model has been used for chemical compound screening [21–23]. As with the subsequent polyQ disease models described below, the progressive formation of inclusions is readily observed in developing eye neurons and in developing and mature CNS neurons.

B. Spinocerebellar Ataxia 3 (Machado-Joseph Disease)

Transgenic *Drosophila* expressing a truncated form of the human SCA3/MJD protein in neurons exhibited nuclear inclusions and late-onset cellular degeneration [24]. Cell death appeared to be apoptotic based on the observation that co-expression of a viral antiapoptotic gene, P35, mitigated the pathogenesis. This suppression was not observed in models of HD [20], suggesting that while many features are shared among the different *Drosophila* disease models, some aspects of biology will be unique. Even with high levels of expression and significant cellular toxicities, tissue specific effects were observed. Expression in the nervous system caused severe consequences whereas comparable targeted expression in epithelial cells generated less toxicity, confirming an *in vivo* system where some cells are more vulnerable to polyglutamine expression. Understanding the basis of this selective susceptibility is a major unresolved aspect of polyQ pathogenesis.

C. Spinocerebellar Ataxia 1

SCA1 transgenic flies expressing full-length mutant ataxin-1 also produce a progressive degenerative phenotype [25]. Significantly, when a transgene with a normally non-pathogenic number of glutamine repeats was expressed in this system, even nonexpanded ataxin-1 causes degenerative phenotypes similar to an expanded SCA1 gene, albeit with less severe phenotypes.

D. Kennedy Disease (SBMA)

Flies engineered to express the human androgen receptor (AR) with an expanded repeat (Q52) were found to accurately mimic the human disease [26]. Particularly notable is the fact that pathogenesis depends on hormone (androgen) binding, an observation that was used to test the hypothesis that onset of SBMA can be mitigated through prevention of hormone binding. No abnormalities were found upon expression of the mutant AR in photoreceptor neurons. However, ingestion of androgen caused a ligand-dependent neurodegeneration with corresponding nuclear localization and structural alteration of the receptor.

E. PolyQ Models

Investigators tested the issue of whether polyQ chains are toxic to neurons independent of any disease gene context by engineering transgenic flies expressing various forms of polyQ peptides [27,28]. These studies show that polyQ peptides alone are intrinsically cytotoxic and cause neuronal degeneration and early adult death and that the inclusion of other amino acids modified and generally reduced toxicity. The influence of protein context is further highlighted by the insertion of an expanded polyQ repeat within a cytosolic protein, *Disheveled,* that normally contains a polyQ repeat tract [27]. When this repeat was expanded, polyglutamine-mediated phenotypes were not observed and effects on protein activity were modest.

III. RESEARCH APPLICATIONS OF *DROSOPHILA* MODELS OF POLYQ REPEAT DISEASES

A. Genetic Approaches

1. Screens

Genetic screens can identify mutations that lead to more severe (enhancers) or less severe (suppressors) phenotypes. Two types of mutations can be screened: loss-of-function alleles in which a mutation typically causes the activity of one allele to be lost, or gain-of-function alleles in which the mutation is caused by an insertion of a transposable P-element containing a UAS based enhancer and promoter (EP), resulting in ectopic activation of the gene in the presence of GAL4 drivers. Eye degeneration of a polyQ alone expressing fly model (UAS-127Q) was used in a P-element screen for modifiers of the phenotype [28]. Several modifiers were identified, highlighting a role for protein folding pathways (dHDJ1, dTPR2) and suggesting a possible association with pathways involved in cell proliferation and DNA replication (*Drosophila* homolog of human myeloid leukemia factor 1, MLF1) [29]. Using the SCA1 model to screen for suppressors and enhancers of the phenotype, several classes of modifier genes were identified. These included transcriptional regulating genes, protein modification genes, and chaperones as modifiers of mutant ataxin 1 pathology [25].

2. Candidate Gene Studies

Using the results of genetic screens and candidate genes identified through hypothesis-driven studies, investigators tested a number of emerging themes in *Drosophila*. Adequate protein folding and degradation pathways appear to be involved in the aberrant protein accumulation that characterizes many neurodegenerative diseases. Subsequent to the identification of chaperone proteins as modifiers of polyQ toxicity, studies showed that overexpression of Hsp70 reduced pathology in a fly model of SCA3 [30]; a mouse model of SCA 1 [31] confirmed the significance of chaperones that were identified in the *Drosophila* studies. DSec61α, a protein (*Drosophila* ortholog of Sec61α) involved in both protein import and endoplasmic reticulum-associated degradation, was required for polyglutamine-induced toxicity, presumably by increasing the amount of ubiquitinated protein that accumulates and cannot be accommodated by the proteasome [32]. A study using a recently developed *Drosophila* model of HD, expressing a 548 aa cDNA for Htt-Q127, provides insight into the role of non-nuclear events induced by cytoplasmic huntingtin aggregation versus nuclear aggregation induced by the ataxin 3 protein and the role of these cytoplasmic aggregates in blocking axonal transport [33].

The role of protein modification in polyQ disease has also been addressed through the genetic manipulation of components of the ubiquitin and SUMO modification pathways [34,35]. Disrupted axonal transport, an important feature of polyQ diseases, has been studied in *Drosophila* and shown to be a mechanism that can be separated from nuclear events and contribute to neurodegeneration—potentially to early neuropathology observed in HD when primarily cytosolic Htt is observed [36]. Other studies using a fly model of SCA1 have implicated phosphatidylinositol 3-kinase/AKT signaling and 14-3-3/ataxin 1 protein interactions that modulate the phosphorylation status of ataxin 1 *in vivo* [37]. Modulation of levels of these cellular proteins modifies neurodegenerative phenotypes and highlights completely novel targets for therapeutic intervention. Again, the value of invertebrate models in testing hypotheses and identifying relevant pathways is evident.

Transcriptional dysregulation has also emerged as a significant target for intervention in polyQ diseases. Studies in cultured cells and in mice showed that transcriptional regulation is altered in the presence of expanded polyQ containing proteins [2]. A significant number of transcriptional regulatory genes emerged from genetic modifier screens in flies (e.g., Sin3A, Rpd3) [25], from targeted studies showing decreased histone acetylation in the presence of mutant Htt *in vitro* (21), and from studies investigating the role of the silencing mediator of retinoid and thyroid hormone receptors (SMRTER in *Drosophila*) [38]. The hypothesis that restoration of transcriptional balance was possible by reducing the activity of histone deacetylases, enzymes that are associated with decreased gene expression, was tested genetically in *Drosophila* expressing mutant human Htt by observing that the neurodegenerative phenotype was suppressed when the dose of HDAC complex proteins was reduced. These results led to rational drug testing of HDAC inhibitors in flies [21] and mice [39,40].

A hallmark of the polyQ diseases and a number of other neurodegenerative diseases (e.g., Alzheimer disease, Parkinson disease) is the formation of visible protein aggregates. Genetic approaches to interfere with this process have proven protective and have helped to validate aggregation as a valid therapeutic target. Investigators tested synthetic peptides engineered to disrupt protein-protein interactions, including those that lead to aggregate formation, and some peptide designs significantly decreased pathology with corresponding reduction of visible inclusion formation [41]. In another study, a peptide inhibitor of aggregation, QBP1, significantly suppressed polyQ-mediated aggregation and neurodegeneration in the compound eye [42].

B. Rational Drug Development through the Use of *Drosophila*

Drosophila have proven useful in testing therapeutic strategies that target transcriptional dysregulation (HDAC inhibitors) [21], aggregation (Congo red, cystamine) [22,43], and protein folding/processing (geldanamycin) [43]. To date, the agreement between treatments that work well in polyQ disease fly models and those that are therapeutic in corresponding mouse models (e.g., HDAC inhibitors, Congo red, and cystamine) [40,44–46] has been excellent, highlighting the utility of using fly models as an intermediate *in vivo* system in translational research efforts to identify drug treatments from high throughput screens.

IV. SUMMARY

Limits exist in accurately modeling human neurodegenerative diseases in *Drosophila*. Flies have no blood-brain barrier, which prevents an assessment of drug delivery to the brain; metabolism of *Drosophila* is not identical to mammals nor do they mount a strong inflammatory response that could contribute to disease. Furthermore, the motor phenotypes that can be seen in humans may not be equivalent in flies. However, *Drosophila* models allow rapid and cost-effective screening of neuroprotective compounds without the concern of brain uptake and represent a powerful genetic model in which to understand protein-protein interactions and the impact of functionally relevant cellular pathways at an organismal level.

Video Legend

Decreased motor function in flies expressing human Huntington exon 1 (Httex1) in their nervous system. Animals on the left are controls (wild-type in this example). Those on the right are 13-day-old Huntington disease flies expressing Httex1 Q93 in all neurons, and those in the middle are their siblings who have been treated with an HDAC inhibitor SAHA (genotype = Elav > Gal4/+/Y; UAS > Httex1p93Q). Flies are negatively geotactic such that if bumped to the bottom of a vial, they immediately begin climbing upwards. Note how the sick flies have a difficult time climbing and the treated flies are better able to climb.

References

1. The Huntington's Disease Collaborative Research Group. 1993. A novel gene containing a trinucleotide repeat that is expanded and unstable on Huntington's disease chromosomes. *Cell* **72**:817–818.
2. Ross, C.A. 2002. Polyglutamine pathogenesis: emergence of unifying mechanisms for Huntington's disease and related disorders. *Neuron* **35**:819–822.
3. Zoghbi, H.Y., and H.T. Orr. 2000. Glutamine repeats and neurodegeneration. *Annu Rev Neurosci* **23**:217–247.
4. Brand, A., and N. Perrimon. 1993. Targeted gene expression as a means of altering cell fates and generating dominant phenotypes. *Development* **118**:401–415.
5. Brand, A.H., and E.L. Dormand. 1995. The GAL4 system as a tool for unravelling the mysteries of the Drosophila nervous system. *Curr Opin Neurobiol* **5**:572–578.
6. Behringer, R., and T.E. Magnuson. 2002. Editor's note. *Genesis* **34**:1–173.
7. Marin, E.C., G.S. Jefferis, T. Komiyama, H. Zhu, and L. Luo. 2002. Representation of the glomerular olfactory map in the Drosophila brain. *Cell* **109**:243–255.
8. Rein, K., M. Zockler, M.T. Mader, C. Grubel, and M. Heisenberg. 2002. The Drosophila standard brain. *Curr Biol* **12**:227–231.
9. Wong, A.M., J.W. Wang, and R. Axel. 2002. Spatial representation of the glomerular map in the Drosophila protocerebrum. *Cell* **109**: 229–241.
10. Rubin, G.M., M.D. Yandell, J.R. Wortman, G.L. Gabor Miklos, C.R. Nelson, I.K. Hariharan, M.E. Fortini, et al. 2000. The genome sequence of Drosophila melanogaster. *Science* **287**:2204–2215.
11. Reiter, L.T., L. Potocki, S. Chien, M. Gribskov, and E. Bier. 2001. A systematic analysis of human disease-associated gene sequences in Drosophila melanogaster. *Genome Res* **11**:1114–1125.
12. Marsh, J.L., J. Pallos, and L.M. Thompson. 2003. Fly models of Huntington's disease. *Hum Mol Genet* **12 Spec No 2**:R187–193.
13. Marsh, J.L., and L.M. Thompson. 2004. Can flies help humans treat neurodegenerative diseases? *Bioessays* **26**:485–496.
14. Bonini, N.M., and M.E. Fortini. 2003. Human neurodegenerative disease modeling using Drosophila. *Annu Rev Neurosci* **26**:627–656.
15. Zuccato, C., A. Ciammola, D. Rigamonti, B.R. Leavitt, D. Goffredo, L. Conti, M.E. MacDonald, et al. 2001. Loss of huntingtin-mediated BDNF gene transcription in Huntington's disease. *Science* **293**:493–498.
16. Zuccato, C., M. Tartari, A. Crotti, D. Goffredo, M. Valenza, L. Conti, T. Cataudella, et al. 2003. Huntingtin interacts with REST/NRSF to modulate the transcription of NRSE-controlled neuronal genes. *Nat Genet.*
17. Saudou, F., S. Finkbeiner, D. Devys, and M. Greenberg. 1998. Huntingtin acts in the nucleus to induce apoptosis but death does not correlate with the formation of intranuclear inclusions. *Cell* **95**:55–66.
18. Peters, M.F., F.C. Nucifora, Jr., J. Kushi, H.C. Seaman, J.K. Cooper, W.J. Herring, V.L. Dawson, et al. 1999. Nuclear targeting of mutant Huntingtin increases toxicity. *Mol Cell Neurosci* **14**:121–128.
19. Bates, G., P. Harper, and L. Jones. 2002. A novel gene containing a trinucleotide repeat that is expanded and unstable on Huntington's disease chromosomes. In *Huntington's Disease*. Oxford: Oxford University Press.
20. Jackson, G.R., I. Salecker, X. Dong, X. Yao, N. Arnheim, P.W. Faber, M.E. MacDonald, and S.L. Zipursky, 1998. Polyglutamine-expanded human huntingtin transgenes induce degeneration of Drosophila photoreceptor neurons. *Neuron* **21**:633–642.
21. Steffan, J.S., L. Bodai, J. Pallos, M. Poelman, A. McCampbell, B.L. Apostol, A. Kazantsev, et al. 2001. Histone deacetylase inhibitors arrest polyglutamine-dependent neurodegeneration in Drosophila. *Nature* **413**:739–743.
22. Apostol, B.L., A. Kazantsev, S. Raffioni, K. Illes, J. Pallos, L. Bodai, N. Slepko, et al. 2003. A cell-based assay for aggregation inhibitors as therapeutics of polyglutamine-repeat disease and validation in Drosophila. *Proc Natl Acad Sci U S A* **100**:5950–5955.
23. Pollitt, S., J. Pallos, J. Shao, A. Ma, L. Thompson, J. Marsh, and M. Diamond. 2003. A rapid cellular FRET assay of polyglutamine aggregation identifies a novel inhibitor. *Neuron* **In Press**.
24. Warrick, J.M., H.L. Paulson, G.L. Gray-Board, Q.T. Bui, K.H. Fischbeck, R.N. Pittman, and N.M. Bonini. 1998. Expanded polyglutamine protein forms nuclear inclusions and causes neural degeneration in Drosophila. *Cell* **93**:939–949.
25. Fernandez-Funez, P., M.L. Nino-Rosales, B. Gouyon, W.-C. She, J.M. Luchak, P. Martinez, E. Turleganos, et al. 2000. Identification of genes that modify ataxin-1-induced neurodegeneration. *Nature* **408**:101–106.
26. Takeyama, K., S. Ito, A. Yamamoto, H. Tanimoto, T. Furutani, H. Kanuka, M. Miura, et al. 2002. Androgen-dependent neurodegeneration by polyglutamine-expanded human androgen receptor in Drosophila. *Neuron* **35**:855–864.
27. Marsh, J.L., H. Walker, H. Theisen, Y.-Z. Zhu, T. Fielder, J. Purcell, and L.M. Thompson. 2000. Expanded polyglutamine peptides alone are intrinsically cytotoxic and cause neurodegeneration in Drosophila. *Hum Mol Gen* **9**:13–25.
28. Kazemi-Esfarjani, P., and S. Benzer. 2000. Genetic suppression of polyglutamine toxicity in Drosophila. *Science* **5459**:1837–1840.
29. Kazemi-Esfarjani, P., and S. Benzer. 2002. Suppression of polyglutamine toxicity by a Drosophila homolog of myeloid leukemia factor 1. *Hum Mol Genet* **11**:2657–2672.
30. Warrick, J.M., H.Y.E. Chan, G.L. Gray-Board, Y. Chai, H.L. Paulson, and N.M. Bonini. 1999. Suppression of polyglutamine-mediated neurodegeneration in Drosophila by the molecular chaperone HSP70. *Nat Gen* **23**:425–428.

31. Cummings, C.J., Y. Sun, P. Opal, B. Antalffy, R. Mestril, H.T. Orr, W.H. Dillmann, et al. 2001. Over-expression of inducible HSP70 chaperone suppresses neuropathology and improves motor function in SCA1 mice. *Hum Mol Gen* **10**:1511–1518.
32. Kanuka, H., E. Kuranaga, T. Hiratou, T. Igaki, B. Nelson, H. Okano, and M. Miura. 2003. Cytosol-endoplasmic reticulum interplay by Sec61alpha translocon in polyglutamine-mediated neurotoxicity in Drosophila. *Proc Natl Acad Sci U S A* **100**:11723–11728.
33. Lee, W.C., M. Yoshihara, and J.T. Littleton. 2004. Cytoplasmic aggregates trap polyglutamine-containing proteins and block axonal transport in a Drosophila model of Huntington's disease. *Proc Natl Acad Sci U S A* **101**:3224–3229.
34. Chan, H.Y., J.M., Warrick, I. Andriola, D. Merry, and N.M. Bonini. 2002. Genetic modulation of polyglutamine toxicity by protein conjugation pathways in Drosophila. *Hum Mol Genet* **11**:2895–2904.
35. Steffan, J.S., N. Agrawal, J. Pallos, E. Rockabrand, L.C. Trotman, N. Slepko, K. Illes, et al. 2004. SUMO modification of Huntingtin and Huntington's disease pathology. *Science* **304**:100–104.
36. Gunawardena, S., and L.S. Goldstein. 2001. Disruption of axonal transport and neuronal viability by amyloid precursor protein mutations in Drosophila. *Neuron* **32**:389–401.
37. Chen, H.K., P. Fernandez-Funez, S.F. Acevedo, Y.C. Lam, M.D. Kaytor, M.H. Fernandez, A. Aitken, et al. 2003. Interaction of Akt-phosphorylated ataxin-1 with 14-3-3 mediates neurodegeneration in spinocerebellar ataxia type 1. *Cell* **113**:457–468.
38. Tsai, C.C., H.Y. Kao, A. Mitzutani, E. Banayo, H. Rajan, M. McKeown, and R.M. Evans. 2004. Ataxin 1, a SCA1 neurodegenerative disorder protein, is functionally linked to the silencing mediator of retinoid and thyroid hormone receptors. *Proc Natl Acad Sci U S A* **101**:4047–4052.
39. Ferrante, R.J., J.K. Kubilus, J. Lee, H. Ryu, A. Beesen, B. Zucker, K. Smith, et al. 2003. Histone deacetylase inhibition by sodium butyrate chemotherapy ameliorates the neurodegenerative phenotype in Huntington's disease mice. *J Neurosci* **23**:9418–9427.
40. Hockly, E., V.M. Richon, B. Woodman, D.L. Smith, X. Zhou, E. Rosa, K. Sathasivam, et al. 2003. Suberoylanilide hydroxamic acid, a histone deacetylase inhibitor, ameliorates motor deficits in a mouse model of Huntington's disease. *Proc Natl Acad Sci U S A*.
41. Kazantsev, A., H. Walker, N. Slepko, J.E. Bear, E. Preisinger, J.S. Steffan, Y.-Z. Zhu, et al. 2002. A bivalent Huntingtin binding peptide suppresses polyglutamine aggregation and pathogenesis in Drosophila. *Nat Gen* **30**:367–376.
42. Nagai, Y., N. Fujikake, K. Ohno, H. Higashiyama, H.A. Popiel, J. Rahadian, M. Yamaguchi, et al. 2003. Prevention of polyglutamine oligomerization and neurodegeneration by the peptide inhibitor QBP1 in Drosophila. *Hum Mol Genet* **12**:1253–1259.
43. Auluck, P.K., and N.M. Bonini. 2002. Pharmacological prevention of Parkinson disease in Drosophila. *Nat Med* **8**:1185–1186.
44. Dedeoglu, A., J.K. Kubilus, T.M. Jeitner, S.A. Matson, M. Bogdanov, N.W. Kowall, W.R. Matson, et al. 2002. Therapeutic effects of cystamine in a murine model of Huntington's disease. *J Neurosci* **22**:8942–8950.
45. Karpuj, M.V., M.W. Becher, J.E. Springer, D. Chabas, S. Youssef, R. Pedotti, D. Mitchell, and L. Steinman. 2002. Prolonged survival and decreased abnormal movements in transgenic model of Huntington disease, with administration of the transglutaminase inhibitor cystamine. *Nat Med* **8**:143–149.
46. Sanchez, I., C. Mahlke, and J. Yuan. 2003. Pivotal role of oligomerization in expanded polyglutamine neurodegenerative disorders. *Nature* **421**:373–379.

CHAPTER

E1

Neurophysiologic Characterization of Tremor

RODGER J. ELBLE

The neurophysiologic characterization of tremor is reviewed in this chapter. The methods are applicable to studies of tremor in humans and most laboratory animals. The limitations of each method are emphasized. Detailed discussions are beyond the scope of this brief chapter, but when necessary, the reader is referred to additional references with extensive bibliographies. Reviews of animal models of human tremor disorders are found elsewhere (Elble 1998; Wilms et al. 1999).

I. KINEMATIC CHARACTERISTICS OF TREMOR

Tremor is an approximately rhythmic, roughly sinusoidal involuntary movement. This broad definition acknowledges the simple fact that no tremor is perfectly rhythmic or sinusoidal. In humans, orthostatic tremor is probably the most rhythmic form of tremor, and palatal tremor (a.k.a. palatal myoclonus) is possibly the least rhythmic. The degree of irregularity compatible with the classification of tremor is undefined, making the classification of some involuntary movements arbitrary and debatable. What is known or suspected about the underlying pathophysiology frequently influences the accepted classification. Thus, palatal tremor was called palatal myoclonus until it was proclaimed to be a tremor in 1997 by a congress of movement disorders specialists in Kiel Germany (Deuschl et al. 1998). By contrast, many movement disorders specialists prefer "rhythmic cortical myoclonus" over "cortical tremor" (Young 2002) even though rhythmic cortical myoclonus is at least as rhythmic and sinusoidal as palatal tremor. Thus, specialists with decades of experience continue to debate tremor classification.

The sinusoidal property of tremor is largely due to the mechanical smoothing produced by skeletal muscle and by joint inertia, stiffness, and damping. Thus, the body responds to tremorogenic bursts of motor unit activity like a low-pass filter. As a rule, muscles with slower twitch times and joints with greater inertia produce greater smoothing (filtering) at lower frequencies. Low-frequency tremors are smoothed less than high-frequency tremors, so low-frequency tremors are typically less sinusoidal and may appear less rhythmic, even when the percent variability in tremor period is comparable to that of higher frequency tremors.

II. TREMOR RECORDING AND MEASUREMENT

A. Motion Analysis

The neurophysiologic characterization of tremor begins with a measurement of tremor amplitude and frequency.

Commercially available motion transducers can measure the force, displacement, velocity, and acceleration of tremor (Elble and Deuschl 2002). Miniature accelerometers are the most popular devices for recording tremor because they are lightweight (<15 grams) and very sensitive (>6 mV/G; G = acceleration of gravity). However, most of these devices are sensitive to gravity, and this gravitational artifact will obscure the recording of low-amplitude tremor to the extent that the axis of sensitivity is not vertical (i.e., parallel to gravity). In fact, gravitational artifact can be an order of magnitude greater than inertial acceleration (i.e., body acceleration) when the accelerometer axis is perpendicular to gravity (Elble 2003b).

Body motion is usually a mixture of translation and rotation in three-dimensional space. In general, nine strategically positioned uniaxial accelerometers are required to measure three-dimensional translation and rotation of a body segment, and nine accelerometers must be mounted on each body segment to provide a complete recording of tremor that emerges from multiple joints (Elble 2003b). Thus, a hand-mounted triaxial accelerometer provides a very crude measure of upper extremity tremor during horizontal extension of the upper limb, and the two axes in the horizontal plane will be significantly obscured by gravitational artifact.

Gyroscopic motion transducers measure angular velocity and are not subject to gravitational artifact, but their mass and size limit their use in many situations. These devices are usually too large for small laboratory animals but have been used in studies of laboratory primates (Emborg et al. 2003). Precision potentiometers (goniometers) are suitably sensitive for recording pathologic tremor (joint rotation) in humans, but these devices are too large and encumbering for many laboratory animals. Gyroscopes and goniometers record tremor in their axis of sensitivity, and multiple devices are needed to capture rotation in two or three dimensions. Force and displacement transducers often have a recording range that necessitates intolerable restriction of motion.

Patients complain of the displacement amplitude of tremor, not the velocity or acceleration. For a sinusoidal displacement of amplitude A, the velocity and acceleration are the first and second derivatives of displacement, as given in the following equations, where ω is the frequency of oscillation in radians per second (1 cycle/s = 1 Hz = 2π radians/s) and t is time:

$$\begin{aligned} displacement &= A \sin(\omega t) \\ velocity &= A\omega \cos(\omega t) \\ acceleration &= -A\omega^2 \sin(\omega t) \end{aligned}$$

Thus, for two tremors of identical displacement amplitude but different frequencies, the tremor with the higher frequency will have a larger acceleration, as measured with an accelerometer. To the extent that tremor is rhythmic and sinusoidal, mean tremor acceleration can be converted to mean displacement amplitude by dividing mean tremor acceleration by the squared tremor frequency in radians per second.

Commercially available photogrammetric systems have precisions and accuracies suitable for studies of pathologic tremor (Bastian and Thach 1995; Cappello et al. 1997; Quintern et al. 1999). Photogrammetric systems consist of active or passive topographic markers and a set of two or more computer-controlled cameras. Active markers are usually infrared light-emitting diodes, and passive markers are small pieces of plastic that reflect stroboscopic infrared light emitted from the computer-controlled cameras. Available markers are small enough to be useful in most animal experiments (Schotland and Rymer 1993). The resolution and accuracy of these systems depend on the distance of the cameras from the body, but spatial accuracies better than 1 mm are possible. Sampling frequencies of 50 Hz or more are common and are adequate for quantifying all pathologic tremors. Photogrammetry is the best available method for studying the complex motion of multiple joints in three-dimensional space.

Computerized digitizing (graphics) tablets can be used to quantify the amplitude and frequency of tremor in handwriting and drawings (Elble et al. 1996; Elble et al. 1990). The horizontal and vertical displacement of a pen is recorded by the tablet and fed to a digital computer, and estimates of velocity and acceleration are obtained by numerical differentiation (Elble et al. 1996; Elble et al. 1990). Available digitizing tablets have accuracies better than ±0.25 mm and sampling frequencies greater than 70/s, which are suitable for measuring visible tremor in handwriting, drawings, and any other movement on the tablet surface. Digitizing tablets have not been used in animal studies of tremor but are probably adaptable to laboratory primates. A free program called VBtablet, written by Laurence Parry (profiles.yahoo.com/laurenceparry), can be downloaded from the Internet (www.bath.ac.uk/~cs1lomp/ or sourceforge.net/projects/vbtablet/) and used in Microsoft Excel to sample data from any tablet that uses the Wintab™ standard (www.pointing.com) for Microsoft Windows. Once in Excel, the sampled x-y coordinates can be analyzed with many commercially available software packages, such as Matlab (www.mathworks.com).

B. Electromyographic Recording

Normal steady muscle contractions are produced by motor unit activity containing small amounts of short-term synchronization and little or no modulation of motor unit firing frequency (Elble and Deuschl 2002). Consequently, the electromyographic interference pattern, recorded with skin or intramuscular electrodes (Figure 1), usually contains no rhythmic bursting, and the Fourier power spectrum of the

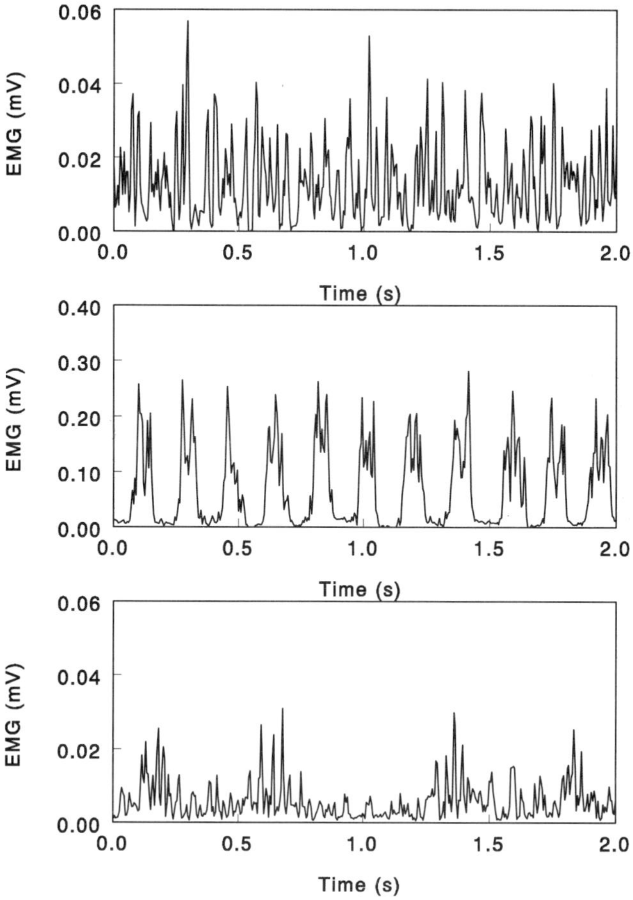

FIGURE 1 Rectified-filtered EMG of the extensor carpi radialis brevis was recorded from a normal adult (top graph) and from a patient with essential tremor (middle graph) during horizontal extension of the hand. The bottom graph is a sample of rectified-filtered EMG recorded from the nasopharynx of a patient with symptomatic palatal tremor. The bottom two graphs illustrate the rhythmic bursts of EMG seen in all pathologic tremors.

rectified-filtered interference pattern is statistically flat from 0 to 20 Hz (Figure 2, outcome 1), which is the frequency range of all pathologic tremors (Elble 2003a). The two exceptions to this normal interference pattern are the electromyographic patterns of enhanced physiologic tremor and the 8- to 12-Hz component of physiologic tremor.

The principal component of physiologic tremor is governed by the inertial and elastic properties of the body (Elble 2003c). These mechanical attributes are such that dampened oscillations of the body occur in response to pulsatile perturbations, such as those produced by irregularities in motor unit firing and by the force of blood ejection during cardiac systole (Elble and Randall 1978; Marsden et al. 1969). The frequency ω of these passive mechanical oscillations depends upon the inertia I and stiffness K of the joint, according to the equation $\omega = \sqrt{K/I}$ (Figure 3). Consequently, normal elbow tremor has a frequency of 3–5 Hz, wrist tremor 7–10 Hz, and metacarpophalangeal joint tremor 17–30 Hz (Elble and Randall 1978; Fox and Randall 1970; Stiles and Randall 1967). Furthermore, inertial loads on a joint decrease the tremor frequency, and elastic loads increase tremor frequency. Somatosensory receptors (e.g., muscle spindles) respond to these passive mechanical oscillations, but this response is usually too weak to entrain motoneurons at the frequency of tremor (Hagbarth and Young 1979; Young and Hagbarth 1980). However, fatigue, anxiety, and some medications can increase the stretch-reflex response to mechanical oscillation, producing an enhanced reflex modulation and entrainment of motor unit firing. This enhanced physiologic mechanical-reflex tremor typically has an amplitude that is five to twenty times normal, and the EMG (electromyography) interference pattern contains bursts of motor unit activity at the frequency of tremor (Hagbarth and Young 1979; Stiles 1980). These bursts are produced by entrainment of motor units with mean firing frequencies of eight to twenty-five spikes per second, and the modulation of individual motor units is such that double (paired) discharges, with interspike intervals of 10–40 ms, tend to occur during a cycle of tremor (Logigian et al. 1988). Enhanced participation of spinal and possibly long-loop stretch reflex pathways plays an important role in the entrainment of motor units.

The 8- to 12-Hz component of physiologic tremor is produced by bursts of motor unit discharge at 8–12 Hz. The frequency of this tremor is as low as 6–8 Hz in some elderly people (Elble 2003c). Most, if not all, people exhibit 8- to 12-Hz bursts of EMG during slow voluntary movements, particularly in the wrist and finger extensors during slow wrist or finger flexion (Kakuda et al. 1999; Wessberg and Vallbo 1996). Thus, 8- to 12-Hz motor unit entrainment tends to occur in everyone, but this EMG rhythm is readily detectable in only 10% of normal adults during steady postural contractions, in the absence of fatigue (Figure 2, outcome 3). It is produced by synchronous modulation of motor unit firing frequency, such that double (paired) discharges, with interspike intervals of 10–40 ms, tend to occur during a cycle of tremor (Elble and Randall 1976; Kakuda et al. 1999; Wessberg and Kakuda 1999). The mean firing frequencies of participating motor units range from eight to twenty-five spikes per second. The frequency of this tremor is independent of reflex arc length and decreases less than 1 Hz when large mass loads are attached to the limb (Elble and Randall 1976; Elble and Randall 1978; Fox and Randall 1970; Stephens and Taylor 1974). Furthermore, the stretch-reflex response to joint perturbation is too weak and too delayed to account for this entrainment (Wessberg and Vallbo 1996). Therefore, investigators believe this tremor emerges from a central source of oscillation and often refer to it as the central neurogenic component of physiologic tremor. There is experimental support for the involvement of the inferior olives, cerebellum, ventrolateral thalamus, and sensorimotor cortex in producing this tremor, but the primary source of oscillation is still unclear (Elble 2003c).

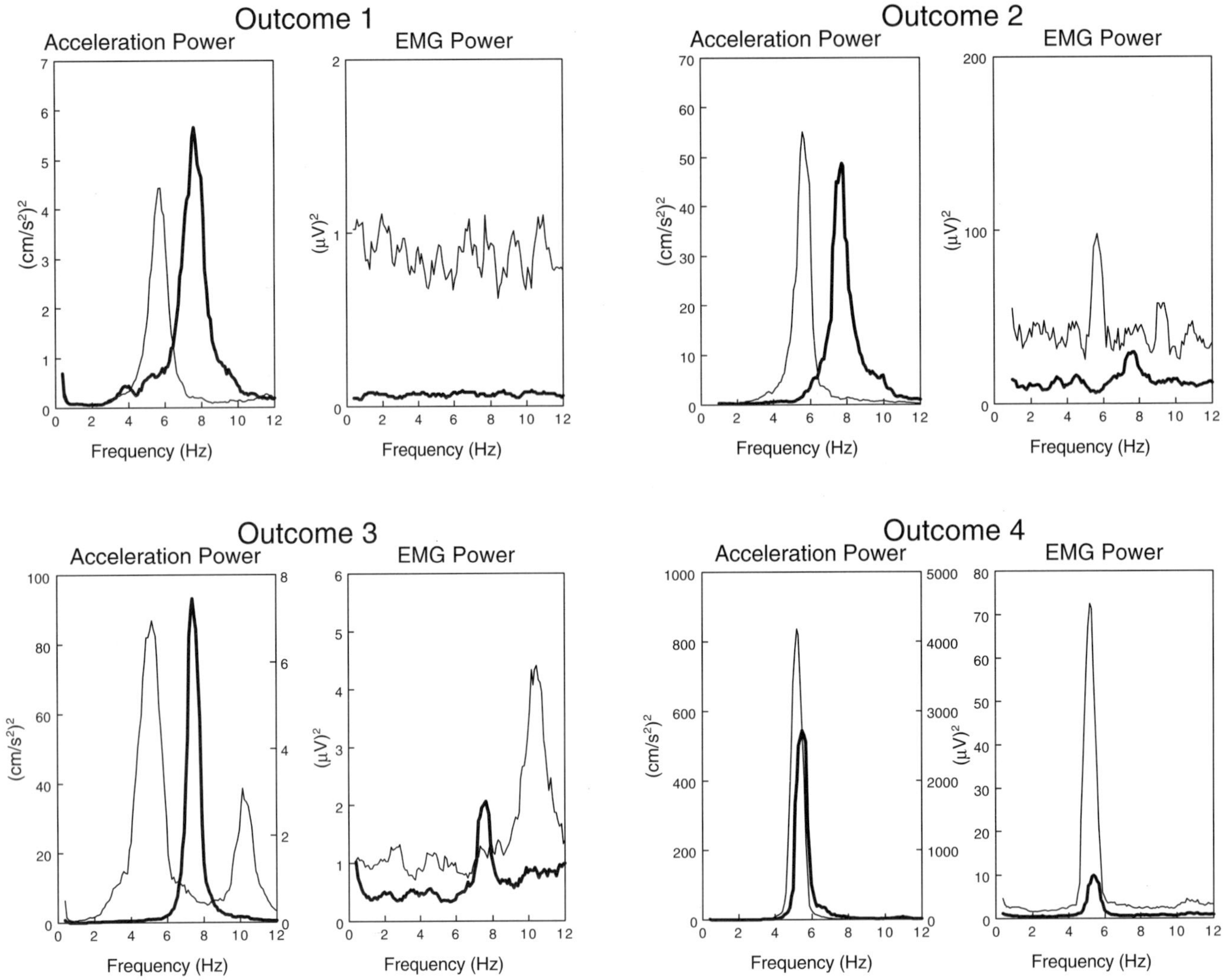

FIGURE 2 Fourier power spectra of hand acceleration and rectified-filtered extensor carpi radialis brevis EMG are shown to illustrate the four major outcomes of inertial loading. Hand tremor was recorded from the horizontally extended hand. The forearm was supported and the hand was splinted so as to limit motion to the wrist. Tremor and EMG were recorded with no mass loading (thick lines) and with a 300-gram load fastened to the hand splint (thin lines), so as to distribute the load over the distal half of the hand.

The significance of a prominent 8- to 12-Hz tremor in asymptomatic people is unclear. Identical tremor can be recorded from patients with mild essential tremor (Elble 1986) and Parkinson disease (Lance et al. 1963). Because a prominent 8- to 12-Hz tremor is found in only 10% of controls, its presence should raise the clinical suspicion of an underlying neurologic disorder. Beware that fatigue also increases this component of tremor, and so enhanced physiologic tremor can contain motor unit modulation that is mechanical-reflex, 8–12 Hz, or both (Elble and Randall 1978).

Rhythmic bursts of motor unit activity occur in all pathologic tremors (Figure 1). This EMG pattern in a rest tremor is always pathologic. It is also a pathologic sign in action tremor if enhanced physiologic tremor can be excluded. A moderate or severe pathologic tremor is easily recognized on the basis of amplitude alone, but the amplitude of mild pathologic tremor may be comparable to an enhanced physiologic tremor (Elble 1986). Unfortunately, no electrophysiologic method exists for distinguishing enhanced physiologic tremor from mild pathologic action tremor.

Investigators have described many animal models of human tremor disorders, but a thorough characterization of physiologic tremor in these laboratory animals is lacking (Elble 1998; Wilms et al. 1999). The relative contributions of central neurogenic oscillation, passive mechanical oscillation, and stretch reflex oscillation undoubtedly vary among laboratory animals and should be studied thoroughly in order to better understand the pathophysiology of tremorogenic drugs or lesions.

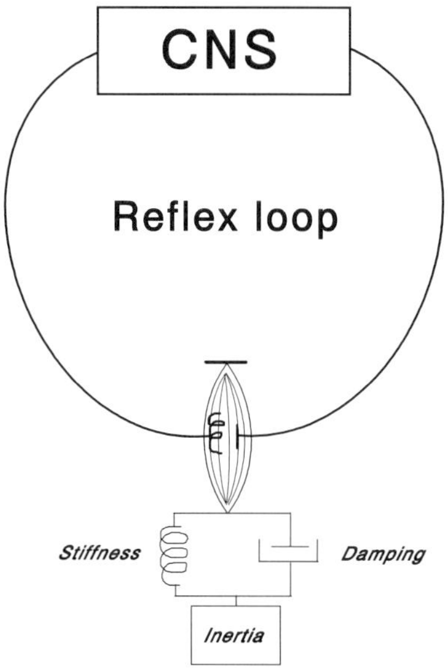

FIGURE 3 Schematic diagram of a peripheral mechanical-reflex loop. Skeletal muscle typically acts at a joint that has inertia, stiffness, and damping (viscosity). This mechanical system is usually underdamped such that pulsatile perturbation of this system produces damped joint oscillations. The stretch reflex loop has stiffness and damping that contribute to the dynamical properties of this mechanical-reflex system. The peripheral mechanical-reflex loop is also a component of longer feedback loops (e.g., transthalamocortical and transcerebellar) in the central nervous system (CNS) and may interact with sources of oscillation within the CNS.

III. NEUROPHYSIOLOGIC CHARACTERIZATION OF TREMOR

A. Distinguishing Central Neurogenic Oscillation From Mechanical-Reflex Oscillation

1. Mechanical Loading and Reflex Loop Time

Some pathologic tremors exhibit the electrophysiologic characteristics of a mechanical-reflex oscillation (e.g., cerebellar outflow tract tremors) (Elble et al. 1984; Qureshi et al. 1996), while others have the characteristics of central neurogenic oscillation (e.g., essential tremor and Parkinson tremor) (Elble and Deuschl 2002). In general, a tremor whose frequency varies predictably with mechanical load or reflex arc length (i.e., reflex latency) is produced, at least in part, by mechanical-reflex mechanisms. A tremor whose frequency is independent of mechanical load (stiffness or inertia) and reflex arc length most likely emerges from a central source of oscillation.

Inertial loads are the most commonly applied mechanical loads in tremor studies because they can be attached to a limb without restricting movement with external mechanical devices such as a manipulandum. Four outcomes are possible with inertial loading (Figure 2):

1. No entrainment of EMG activity is present with and without inertial loading, despite rhythmic oscillation of the limb, recorded with a motion transducer. The frequency of oscillation decreases when the inertial load is applied to the limb. These are the characteristics of normal mechanical-reflex tremor. The EMG Fourier power spectrum is flat because there is no significant stretch-reflex or central oscillatory entrainment of motor unit activity (Figure 2, outcome 1).
2. Motor-unit entrainment is found in the EMG (statistically significant spectral peak in the rectified-filtered EMG spectrum), and the frequency of the joint oscillation and EMG entrainment both decrease and are equal (Figure 2, outcome 2). Hence, the oscillating musculoskeletal system dictates the frequency of motor-unit entrainment through somatosensory feedback. This is the outcome in most patients with enhanced physiologic tremor and with pathologic mechanical-reflex tremors (e.g., due to cerebellar outflow tract lesions). However, this outcome also occurs when any action tremor (central or mechanical-reflex) is so irregular that the bursts of EMG simply perturb the mechanical-reflex system, resulting in an oscillation whose frequency varies predictably with mechanical load (Deuschl and Elble 2000; Deuschl et al. 1996; Elble 1991). Sustained rhythmic motor-unit entrainment by a central oscillator is needed to produce an EMG spectral peak that is frequency-invariant with mechanical loading and reflex arc length.
3. Inertial loading discloses the presence of two oscillations (Figure 2, outcome 3). In the unloaded condition, limb oscillation and EMG entrainment may have the same frequencies, but inertial loading causes the frequency of mechanical-reflex oscillation to decrease away from a second oscillation that has associated EMG entrainment. The second oscillation is interpreted as a central oscillation because its frequency does not decrease with inertial loading and bears no obvious relationship to reflex arc length. This is a common outcome in people with mild central neurogenic tremor (e.g., mild essential tremor), but identical results are obtained from those seemingly normal people that have prominent 8- to 12-Hz tremor (Elble 2003a). In some cases, EMG entrainment is also detectable for the mechanical-reflex oscillation.
4. The mechanical oscillation and EMG entrainment have the same frequency in the loaded and unloaded condition (Figure 2, outcome 4). This result is interpreted as a sign of pathologic central neurogenic oscillation. All people with moderate-severe central neurogenic tremor (e.g., essential tremor, Parkinson tremor) exhibit this outcome, although several recordings may be required if there is considerable

fluctuation in amplitude. In addition, this outcome may also occur when the frequency of a mild central neurogenic tremor is nearly the same as the mechanical resonance frequency of the joint.

Beware that the frequency of physiologic and pathologic tremors (e.g., essential tremor and Parkinson tremor) may vary with posture and movement, so posture and movement must be carefully controlled when the effect of mechanical loading on tremor frequency is being investigated. In addition, movement should be restricted to a single joint (Elble and Randall 1978).

The frequency of mechanical-reflex tremor is increasingly influenced by reflex stiffness and loop time when the sensitivity (gain) of the reflex loop increases. Meanwhile, the influence of limb inertia and stiffness decreases. Consequently, enhanced mechanical-reflex tremor and pathologic mechanical-reflex tremors have frequencies that are less dependent on limb mechanics and more dependent on reflex loop properties than normal mechanical-reflex tremor (Stiles 1980). The frequency of mechanical-reflex oscillation may change little with mechanical loading when the reflex loop gain or loop time is increased to the point of reflex oscillation (Bock and Wenderoth 1999; Stein and Oguztöreli 1976). However, the mechanical-reflex tremor frequency is still a function of reflex loop time (Bock and Wenderoth 1999) and thereby differs from oscillations of central origin.

All forms of tremor are ultimately expressed via neuronal drive to the segmental stretch reflex and limb mechanics, such that the neurophysiologic characteristics of all central neurogenic tremors result from an interaction between mechanical-reflex and central oscillation (Elble 1996). The presence of strong sensory feedback could conceivably entrain a central oscillator at the frequency of mechanical-reflex oscillation, if the natural frequencies of the central oscillator and mechanical-reflex oscillation are similar and if the strength of central oscillation is relatively weak compared to the strength of mechanical-reflex oscillation (Wenderoth and Bock 1999). In other words, a weak central oscillator could exhibit small changes in frequency with mechanical loading or reflex latency. In man, a change in frequency of less than 1 Hz indicates central neurogenic oscillation (Elble 2003a).

2. Polyelectromyography

Simultaneous recording of EMG from multiple muscles on the same or opposite sides of the body helps determine the effect of reflex arc length on tremor frequency. For example, the frequency of Parkinson tremor and essential tremor is nearly the same in different body parts, consistent with a central source of oscillation (Elble 1994; Hunker and Abbs 1990).

Polyelectromyography helps determine the degree of synchrony among muscles on the same or opposite sides of the body. The bursts of EMG activity in muscles of the same limb may be highly coherent (i.e., phase locked) in advanced pathologic tremors (Hurtado et al. 2000) but are commonly only weakly coherent or independent, particularly in physiologic tremor and mild pathologic tremors (Raethjen et al. 2000). Similarly, polyelectromyography is useful in examining the interaction between antagonistic muscles in a limb segment. Investigators have written much about random, synchronous, and alternating tremor rhythms in antagonistic muscles, but no pattern of antagonist muscle interaction has the sensitivity or specificity to be diagnostically useful (Elble and Deuschl 2002).

High coherence of the EMG rhythm among muscles of different limbs on the same and opposite sides of the body is seen only in orthostatic tremor (Figure 4). Orthostatic tremor is an unusual postural tremor that develops in the extremities and torso within seconds of assuming erect stance (Heilman 1984). Electromyography reveals rhythmic bursts of motor unit activity at a particularly high frequency of 14–18 Hz, and there is nearly perfect coherence between muscles of different limbs on the same and opposite sides of the body (Köster et al. 1999; Lauk et al. 1999). Other forms of tremor do not produce these electromyographic features.

Polyelectromyography can also help distinguish organic tremor from psychogenic tremor. Patients with psychogenic tremor cannot voluntarily oscillate the same or opposite extremity at a frequency different from the frequency of their psychogenic tremor. Attempts to do so either suppress the psychogenic tremor or cause the psychogenic tremor to shift to the frequency of voluntary repetitive movement. By contrast, the frequencies of physiologic and pathologic tremors change less than 1 Hz when the patient performs rapid repetitive movements with the same or contralateral limb (O'Suilleabhain and Matsumoto 1998). A report by McAuley and coworkers nicely illustrates this electrophysiologic approach to the diagnosis of psychogenic tremor (McAuley et al. 1998).

B. Identifying Central Sources of Oscillation

1. Single Unit Recordings

Rhythmic bursts of EMG activity occur in all forms of pathologic tremor (Das Gupta 1963; Davey et al. 1986; Dengler et al. 1989; Dengler et al. 1986; Dietz et al. 1974; Elek et al. 1991; Shahani and Young 1977). These EMG bursts are produced by the synchronous modulation of motoneurons at the tremor frequency (Elble and Deuschl 2002). The frequency modulation of motor unit activity is such that double or triple discharges (paired or grouped discharges), with interspike intervals of 10–40 ms, tend to occur

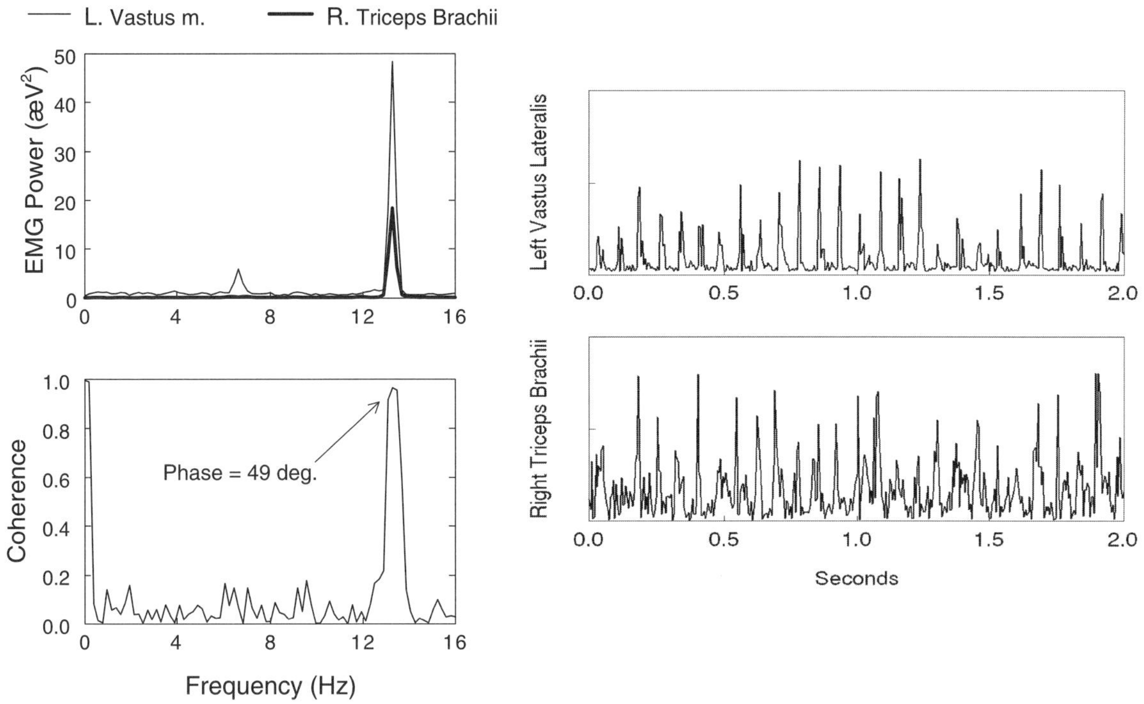

FIGURE 4 Rectified EMG recorded from the left vastus lateralis and right triceps brachii of a patient with orthostatic tremor (Patient 3 in video). The EMGs were recorded for 1 minute while the patient stood and leaned on a table with his hands so as to activate the muscles of both upper limbs. The 2-second samples of EMG illustrate the synchronous tremor rhythm in the two muscles. Spectral analysis revealed almost perfect coherence between the 13.5-Hz bursts of EMG, with a slight phase difference of 49 degrees.

during a cycle of tremor. This modulation of motor unit firing is similar to that which occurs in the 8- to 12-Hz component of physiologic tremor (Elble and Randall 1976) and in enhanced physiologic mechanical-reflex tremor (Logigian et al. 1988). Paired motor unit discharges with short interspike intervals produce stronger muscle contraction than single spikes and therefore contribute more to tremor amplitude (Elek et al. 1991; Renou et al. 1970). Thus, while some motor units fire at the frequency of tremor, most motor units fire at higher frequencies and contribute more substantially to tremor by virtue of a synchronous modulation in firing frequency.

Investigators have recorded tremor-related modulation of neuronal firing from the cerebral cortex, basal ganglia, thalamus, cerebellum, and sensory afferents of laboratory animals with various forms of tremor (Bergman et al. 1998; Bergman et al. 1994; Elble et al. 1984; Yamamoto et al. 2001), and investigators routinely perform pallidal, subthalamic and thalamic recordings in patients undergoing stereotactic surgery for tremor (Hua et al. 1998; Lemstra et al. 1999; Lenz et al. 2002; Magarinos-Ascone et al. 2000; Magnin et al. 2000; Zirh et al. 1998). Fourier spectral techniques easily quantify the strength of neuronal modulation, and investigators routinely compute the linear correlation and phase among neuronal spike trains and between neuronal modulation and other measures of tremor (e.g., movement, rectified-filtered EMG, electroencephalogram, and magnetoencephalogram) with cross-spectral (coherence and phase) techniques (Elble 2003b). There is extensive literature on spectral analysis, and the principles and mathematical methods of spectral analysis have been reviewed in the context of tremor analysis (Elble 2003b; Elble and Koller 1990; Timmer et al. 1996).

2. Electroencephalography and Magnetoencephalography

Investigators are successfully using electroencephalography (EEG) and magnetoencephalography (MEG) in the study of tremor. EEG and MEG record central tremor activity in real time and provide a macroscopic view of neural networks in tremorogenesis. Special care must be taken to maximize the signal-to-noise ratio because the tremor-related content of scalp EEG and MEG is very small. MEG has superior signal-to-noise properties and anatomical resolution. Cross-spectral (coherence and phase) analysis can identify and quantify tremor-related EEG or MEG and simultaneously recorded tremor, measured with a motion transducer or EMG. With these methods, Volkmann and coworkers found tremor-related MEG activity in the contralateral thalamus and lateral premotor, somatomotor, and somatosensory cortices (Timmermann et al. 2003; Volkmann et al. 1996). These results are consistent with the widely recognized participation of the thalamocortical loop in Parkinson tremorogenesis. Similarly, Hellwig and coworkers (Hellwig et al. 2001) found highly coherent EEG-EMG rhythmicity in patients with essential tremor. Raethjen and coworkers (Raethjen et al. 2002) demonstrated significant coherence between EEG and the central neurogenic component of physiologic tremor, but this demonstration required intracranial, epicortical EEG recording.

These studies illustrate the utility of EEG and EMG in quantifying the involvement of motor cortex in tremorogenesis. However, EEG-EMG and MEG-EMG coherence values are often 0.1 or less (Halliday et al. 2000; Timmermann et al. 2003; Volkmann et al. 1996). Spurious statistical significance is always a concern when coherencies are this small, and these small coherence values indicate that, at best, 10% of the EEG or MEG is linearly related to tremor.

EEG transients preceding the EMG bursts of tremor have been demonstrated with EEG back-averaging in patients with cortical tremor (a.k.a., rhythmic cortical myoclonus) (Elia et al. 1998; Okuma et al. 1998; Terada et al. 1997; Toro et al. 1993). Computer averaging, time locked to a series of events, is the time domain equivalent of cross-spectral analysis.

3. Resetting the Phase of Tremor

All forms of tremor have the mathematical properties of a nonlinear oscillator, and the phase of a nonlinear oscillation can be reset if the oscillator receives a pulsatile stimulus (perturbation) of sufficient strength. Elble and Koller (1990) discuss the principles of phase resetting and the related phenomenon of frequency entrainment in the context of tremor, and Winfree (2001) discusses the topic in a broader context. Researchers have studied the response of tremor to mechanical limb perturbation, electrical stimulation of peripheral nerves, and transcranial magnetic and electrical stimulation of the cerebral cortex and cerebellum (Britton et al. 1992a; Britton et al. 1993b; Elble et al. 1992; Elble and Koller 1990; Lee and Stein 1981; Manto et al. 1999; Pfeiffer et al. 1999; Rack and Ross 1986; Wu et al. 2001). The basic assumption underlying these studies was that a central oscillator should be relatively refractory to phase resetting while oscillations emerging from the stretch reflex should be more easily reset. This approach has failed because virtually all known sources of central oscillation in tremorogenesis (e.g., thalamus, inferior olive, sensorimotor cortex, spinal cord) are strongly influenced by sensory feedback and, therefore, could be reset with a reflex perturbation of adequate strength. Furthermore, a nonlinear mechanical-reflex oscillation could be so strong that stretch-reflex perturbations are not sufficient to produce phase resetting. Thus, there is no guarantee that stretch-reflex perturbations will reset a tremor that emerges from mechanical-reflex oscillation. In addition to these problems, phase resetting experiments are also plagued with random variability in tremor amplitude and frequency, which often preclude an accurate determination of steady-state phase. These limitations of phase resetting are amply illustrated in experimental studies (Britton et al. 1992a; Britton et al. 1993b; Elble et al. 1992; Elble and Koller 1990; Lee and Stein 1981; Rack and Ross 1986) and in mathematical models of tremor (Bock and Wenderoth 1999).

The demonstration of phase resetting of a tremor with stretch reflex perturbations is proof of influential somatosensory feedback on the tremor oscillator, but phase resetting does not distinguish tremors of peripheral and central origin. Parkinson tremor and essential tremor are reset by peripheral mechanical and electrical stimuli (Britton et al. 1992a; Britton et al. 1993b; Elble et al. 1992; Elble and Koller 1990; Lee and Stein 1981), but orthostatic tremor is uniquely refractory to phase resetting by these methods of stretch reflex perturbation (Britton et al. 1992b; Thompson et al. 1986). Consequently, the central oscillator of orthostatic tremor is either too strong to be reset by sensory feedback, or, less likely, it does not receive somatosensory feedback. Similarly, transcranial magnetic stimulation of the motor cortex can reset the phase of essential tremor, Parkinson postural tremor, and orthostatic tremor (Britton et al. 1993a; Pascual-Leone et al. 1994; Pfeiffer et al. 1999; Tsai et al. 1998). Such observations confirm a strong connection between the stimulated area of brain and the tremor oscillator, but they do not prove that the stimulated area is the oscillator. Absence of resetting merely proves that the stimulus was inadequate because the stimulated area was not connected to the oscillator or because the effect of stimulation on the oscillator was too weak to produce a steady-state change in the tremor rhythm.

C. Quantification of Stretch Reflex and Somatosensory Evoked Responses

Cortical tremor (also called rhythmic cortical myoclonus) is an irregular 7- to 14-Hz action tremor that occurs in patients with cortical reflex myoclonus and asterixis (Artieda et al. 1992; Ikeda et al. 1990; Oguni et al. 1995; Toro et al. 1993; Ugawa et al. 1989). More than half of these patients demonstrate an enhanced C-reflex (long-latency transcortical muscle reflex) and giant sensory evoked potentials, consistent with the presence of enhanced cortical irritability and transcortical reflexes. Despite the enhanced C-reflex, cortical tremor probably emerges from enhanced cortical rhythmicity rather than oscillation in a transcortical sensorimotor loop (Brown and Marsden 1996; Toro et al. 1993). Sudden lapses in posture (e.g., wrist flap or asterixis) are produced by EMG silent periods of 50–500 ms, called negative myoclonus. The 7- to 14-Hz action tremor can be so irregular and intermittent that it behaves like an enhanced mechanical-reflex oscillation with mass loading (see IV.A.1).

Normal rapid limb movements toward a target are decelerated with a burst of antagonist muscle contraction. Cerebellar feedforward control is critically involved in this deceleration, and loss of cerebellar feedforward control leads to delayed and inappropriately sized antagonist activity, resulting in target overshoot and limb oscillation (Diener and Dichgans 1992; Hore and Flament 1988; Hore and Vilis 1984). Similarly, in response to joint perturbations (e.g., sudden passive elbow flexion), the EMG response to muscle stretch is normal in monkeys and people with cerebellar lesions, but the subsequent activation of the antagonist muscle is inappropriately sized and delayed. Similar delays in antagonist muscle activation are seen in patients with intention tremor due to advanced essential tremor (Deuschl et al. 2000), but this antagonist muscle delay is not corrected when essential tremor is suppressed with thalamic deep brain stimulation (Zackowski et al. 2002). This result of surgery in man and additional data from laboratory primates suggest that antagonist muscle delay does not fully explain the pathophysiology of intention tremor (Elble 1998), and the degree to which antagonist delay is specific for cerebellar dysfunction has not been investigated.

IV. SUMMARY

Electrophysiologic studies help identify areas of the central and peripheral nervous system involved in tremorogenesis and define the relative contribution of central neurogenic and mechanical-reflex oscillation. The following list contains guidelines and recommendations for the neurophysiologic characterization of tremor:

1. Neurophysiologic characterization of tremor begins with a measurement of tremor amplitude and frequency at one or more anatomical sites during rest, steady posture, and voluntary movement. This process requires a motion transducer and simultaneous electromyographic recordings. The limitations of a motion transducer in quantifying complex three-dimensional motion must be considered.
2. The effect of reflex loop time and mechanical loading on tremor frequency should be determined. Motion should be restricted to a single joint when assessing the effects of mechanical loading, and the joint posture or movement must be carefully controlled. Changes in frequency greater than 1 Hz are significant.
3. Polyelectromyography can help determine the relationship of tremor frequency to reflex arc length and the coherence and phase among muscles in different body sites. Polyelectromyography is particularly useful in diagnosing orthostatic tremor and psychogenic tremor in people.
4. Single unit recordings are very useful in identifying areas of the nervous system involved in tremor, but criteria for defining the principal source of oscillation have not been developed. Most if not all tremors may emerge from widely distributed motor circuits, not from a single nucleus or cortical structure. Researchers need multi-site recordings and mathematical models to understand the manner in which tremor emerges from distributed motor networks. Simultaneous multi-site recordings are possible only in studies of laboratory animals.
5. EEG and MEG can help identify the sensory and motor pathways involved in tremorogenesis. Both provide real-time recordings of tremor activity. MEG has better resolution and has helped define tremorogenic interactions among multiple cortical and subcortical locations (Timmermann et al. 2003).
6. Reflex and evoked response methods can help quantify changes in reflex sensitivity and latency, which may be important in tremorogenesis.
7. Tremor phase resetting with peripheral and central stimulation is technically difficult to perform and analyze, making the results inconclusive in most cases.

Acknowledgments

This work was supported by the Spastic Paralysis Research Foundation of Kiwanis International, Illinois-Eastern Iowa District and by grant NS20973 from the National Institutes of Health.

Video Legends

SEGMENT 1 Early Parkinson disease with a classic pill-rolling rest tremor in the left hand.

SEGMENT 2 Moderately advanced essential tremor with typical postural and kinetic tremors in both upper limbs.

SEGMENT 3 Orthostatic tremor. The patient complains of unsteadiness while standing. Tremor was not visible, but was revealed by polyelectromyography (Figure 4).

References

Artieda, J., J. Muruzabal, R. Larumbe, C.G. de Casasola, and J.A. Obeso. 1992. Cortical mechanisms mediating asterixis. *Movement Disorders* **7**:209–216.

Bastian, A.J., and W.T. Thach. 1995. Cerebellar outflow lesions: a comparison of movement deficits resulting from lesions at the levels of the cerebellum and thalamus. *Ann Neurology* **38**:881–892.

Bergman, H., T. Wichmann, B. Karmon, and M.R. DeLong. 1994. The primate subthalamic nucleus. II. Neuronal activity in the MPTP model of parkinsonism. *J Neurophysiol* **72**:507–520.

Bergman, H., A. Raz, A. Feingold, A. Nini, I. Nelken, D. Hansel, H. Ben-Pazi, and A. Reches. 1998. Physiology of MPTP tremor. *Mov Disord* **13**:29–34.

Bock, O., and N. Wenderoth. 1999. Dependence of peripheral tremor on mechanical perturbations: modeling study. *Biological Cybernetics* **80**: 103–108.

Britton, T.C., P.D. Thompson, B.L. Day, J.C. Rothwell, L.J. Findley, and C.D. Marsden. 1992a. "Resetting" of postural tremors at the wrist with mechanical stretches in Parkinson's disease, essential tremor, and normal subjects mimicking tremor. *Annals of Neurology* **31**:507–514.

Britton, T.C., P.D. Thompson, W. van der Kamp, J.C. Rothwell, B.L. Day, L.J. Findley, and C.D. Marsden. 1992b. Primary orthostatic tremor: further observations in six cases. *Journal of Neurology* **239**:209–217.

Britton, T.C., P.D. Thompson, B.L. Day, J.C. Rothwell, L.J. Findley, and C.D. Marsden. 1993a. Modulation of postural wrist tremors by magnetic stimulation of the motor cortex in patients with PD and essential tremor and in normal subjects mimicking tremor. *Annals of Neurology* **33**:473–479.

Britton, T.C., P.D. Thompson, B.L. Day, J.C. Rothwell, L.J. Findley, and C.D. Marsden. 1993b. Modulation of postural tremors at the wrist by supramaximal electrical median nerve shocks in essential tremor, Parkinson's disease and normal subjects mimicking tremor. *Journal of Neurology, Neurosurgery and Psychiatry* **56**:1085–1089.

Brown, P., and C.D. Marsden. 1996. Rhythmic cortical and muscle discharge in cortical myoclonus. *Brain* **119**:1307–1316.

Cappello, A., A. Leardini, M.G. Benedetti, R. Liguori, and A. Bertani. 1997. Application of stereophotogrammetry to total body three-dimensional analysis of human tremor. *IEEE Transactions on Rehabilitation Engineering* **5**:388–393.

Das Gupta, A. 1963. Paired response of motor units during voluntary contraction in parkinsonism. *Journal of Neurology, Neurosurgery and Psychiatry* **26**:265–268.

Davey, N.J., P.H. Ellaway, and C.L. Friedland. 1986. Synchrony of motor unit discharge in humans with Parkinson's disease. *Journal of Physiology (London)* **377**:30P.

Dengler, R., W. Wolf, M. Schubert, and A. Struppler. 1986. Discharge pattern of single motor units in basal ganglia disorders. *Neurology* **36**:1061–1066.

Dengler, R., J. Gillespie, M. Argenta, J. Elek, W. Wolf, and A. Struppler. 1989. The impact of paired motor unit discharges on tremor. *Electromyography and Clinical Neurophysiology* **29**:113–117.

Deuschl, G., P. Krack, M. Lauk, and J. Timmer. 1996. Clinical neurophysiology of tremor. *Journal of Clinical Neurophysiology* **13**:110–121.

Deuschl, G., P. Bain, and M. Brin. 1998. Consensus statement of the Movement Disorder Society on Tremor. Ad Hoc Scientific Committee. *Mov Disord* **13**:2–23.

Deuschl, G., and R.J. Elble. 2000. The pathophysiology of essential tremor. *Neurology* **54**:S14–20.

Deuschl, G., R. Wenzelburger, K. Loffler, J. Raethjen, and H. Stolze. 2000. Essential tremor and cerebellar dysfunction clinical and kinematic analysis of intention tremor. *Brain* **123**:1568–1580.

Diener, H.-C., and J. Dichgans. 1992. Pathophysiology of cerebellar ataxia. *Movement Disorders* **7**:95–109.

Dietz, V., W. Hillesheimer, and H.-J. Freund. 1974. Correlation between tremor, voluntary contraction, and firing pattern of motor units in Parkinson's disease. *Journal of Neurology, Neurosurgery and Psychiatry* **37**:927–937.

Elble, R.J., and J.E. Randall. 1976. Motor-unit activity responsible for 8- to 12-Hz component of human physiological finger tremor. *J Neurophysiol*, **39**:370–383.

Elble, R.J., and J.E. Randall. 1978. Mechanistic components of normal hand tremor. *Electroencephalography and Clinical Neurophysiology* **44**:72–82.

Elble, R.J., M.H. Schieber, and W.T. Thach, Jr. 1984. Activity of muscle spindles, motor cortex and cerebellar nuclei during action tremor. *Brain Res* **323**:330–334.

Elble, R.J. 1986. Physiologic and essential tremor. *Neurology* **36**:225–231.

Elble, R.J., and W.C. Koller. 1990. *Tremor*. Baltimore: The Johns Hopkins University Press.

Elble, R.J., R. Sinha, and C. Higgins. 1990. Quantification of tremor with a digitizing tablet. *Journal of Neuroscience Methods* **32**:193–198.

Elble, R.J. 1991. Inhibition of forearm EMG by palatal myoclonus. *Movement Disorders* **6**:324–329.

Elble, R.J., C. Higgins, and L. Hughes. 1992. Phase resetting and frequency entrainment of essential tremor. *Experimental Neurology* **116**:355–361.

Elble, R.J. 1994. Mechanisms of physiologic tremor and relationship to essential tremor. In *Handbook of Tremor Disorders*. Ed. L.J. Findley and W.C. Koller. pp. 51–62. New York: Marcel Dekker.

Elble, R.J. 1996. Central mechanisms of tremor. *Journal of Clinical Neurophysiology* **13**:133–144.

Elble, R.J., M. Brilliant, K. Leffler, and C. Higgins. 1996. Quantification of essential tremor in writing and drawing. *Movement Disorders* **11**: 70–78.

Elble, R.J. 1998. Animal models of action tremor. *Movement Disorders* **13**: 35–39.

Elble, R.J., and G. Deuschl. 2002. Tremor. In *Neuromuscular Function and Disease: Basic, Clinical and Electrodiagnostic Aspects*. Ed. W.F. Brown, C.F. Bolton, and M. Aminoff. Vol. 2. pp. 1759–1779. Philadelphia: W. B. Saunders Co.

Elble, R.J. 2003a. Characteristics of physiologic tremor in young and elderly adults. *Clin Neurophysiol* **114**:624–635.

Elble, R.J. 2003b. Accelerometry. In *Handbook of Clinical Neurophysiology*. Ed. M. Hallett. Vol. 1. pp. 181–190. New York: Elsevier Science B. V.

Elble, R.J. 2003c. Physiologic and enhanced physiologic tremor. In *Handbook of Clinical Neurophysiology*. Ed. M. Hallett. Vol. 1. pp. 357–364. New York: Elsevier Science B. V.

Elek, J.M., R. Dengler, A. Konstanzer, S. Hesse, and W. Wolf. 1991. Mechanical implications of paired motor unit discharges in pathological and voluntary tremor. *Electroencephalography and Clinical Neurophysiology* **81**:279–283.

Elia, M., S.A. Musumeci, R. Ferri, C. Scuderi, S. Del Gracco, M. Bottitta, R. Michelucci, and C.A. Tassinari. 1998. Familial cortical tremor, epilepsy, and mental retardation: a distinct clinical entity? *Archives of Neurology* **55**:1569–1573.

Emborg, M.E., J.W. Tetrud, J. Moirano, W.W. McLaughlin, and K.S. Bankiewicz. 2003. Rest tremor in rhesus monkeys with MPTP-induced parkinsonism. *Front Biosci* **8**:a148–154.

Fox, J.R., and J.E. Randall. 1970. Relationship between forearm tremor and the biceps electromyogram. *Journal of Applied Physiology* **29**:103–108.

Hagbarth, K.-E., and R.R. Young. 1979. Participation of the stretch reflex in human physiological tremor. *Brain* **102**:509–526.

Halliday, D.M., B.A. Conway, S.F. Farmer, U. Shahani, A.J. Russell, and J.R. Rosenberg. 2000. Coherence between low-frequency activation of the motor cortex and tremor in patients with essential tremor [see comments]. *Lancet* **355**:1149–1153.

Heilman, K.M. 1984. Orthostatic tremor. *Archives of Neurology* **41**: 880–881.

Hellwig, B., S. Häussler, B. Schelter, M. Lauk, B. Guschlbauer, J. Timmer, and C.H. Lücking. 2001. Tremor-correlated cortical activity in essential tremor. *Lancet* **357**:519–523.

Hore, J., and T. Vilis. 1984. Loss of set in muscle responses to limb perturbations during cerebellar dysfunction. *J Neurophysiol* **51**:1137–1148.

Hore, J., and D. Flament. 1988. Changes in motor cortex neural discharge associated with the development of cerebellar limb ataxia. *J Neurophysiol* **60**:1285–1302.

Hua, S.E., F.A. Lenz, T.A. Zirh, S.G. Reich, and P.M. Dougherty. 1998. Thalamic neuronal activity correlated with essential tremor. *Journal of Neurology, Neurosurgery and Psychiatry* **64**:273–276.

Hunker, C.J., and J.H. Abbs. 1990. Uniform frequency of parkinsonian resting tremor in the lips, jaw, tongue and index finger. *Movement Disorders* **5**:71–77.

Hurtado, J.M., J.P. Lachaux, D.J. Beckley, C.M. Gray, and K.A. Sigvardt. 2000. Inter- and intralimb oscillator coupling in parkinsonian tremor. *Mov Disord* **15**:683–691.

Ikeda, A., R. Kakigi, N. Funai, R. Neshige, Y. Kuroda, and H. Shibasaki. 1990. Cortical tremor: a variant of cortical reflex myoclonus. *Neurology* **40**:1561–1565.

Kakuda, N., M. Nagaoka, and J. Wessberg. 1999. Common modulation of motor unit pairs during slow wrist movement in man. *J Physiol (Lond)* **520**:929–940.

Köster, B., M. Lauk, J. Timmer, M. Poersch, B. Guschlbauer, G. Deuschl, and C.H. Lucking. 1999. Involvement of cranial muscles and high intermuscular coherence in orthostatic tremor. *Ann Neurol* **45**:384–388.

Lance, J.W., R.S. Schwab, and E.A. Peterson. 1963. Action tremor and the cogwheel phenomenon in Parkinson's disease. *Brain* **86**:95–110.

Lauk, M., B. Köster, J. Timmer, B. Guschlbauer, G. Deuschl, and C.H. Lücking. 1999. Side-to-side correlation of muscle activity in physiological and pathological human tremors. *Clin Neurophysiol* **110**:1774–1783.

Lee, R.G., and R.B. Stein. 1981. Resetting of tremor by mechanical perturbations: a comparison of essential tremor and parkinsonian tremor. *Annals of Neurology* **10**:523–531.

Lemstra, A.W., L. Verhagen Metman, J.I. Lee, P.M. Dougherty, and F.A. Lenz. 1999. Tremor-frequency (3–6 Hz) activity in the sensorimotor arm representation of the internal segment of the globus pallidus in patients with Parkinson's disease. *Neuroscience Letters* **267**:129–132.

Lenz, F.A., C.J. Jaeger, M.S. Seike, Y.C. Lin, and S.G. Reich. 2002. Single-neuron analysis of human thalamus in patients with intention tremor and other clinical signs of cerebellar disease. *J Neurophysiol* **87**: 2084–2094.

Logigian, E.L., M.M. Wierzbicka, F. Bruyninckx, A.W. Wiegner, B.T. Shahani, and R.R. Young. 1988. Motor unit synchronization in physiologic, enhanced physiologic and voluntary tremor in man. *Annals of Neurology* **23**:242–250.

Magarinos-Ascone, C.M., R. Figueiras-Mendez, C. Riva-Meana, and A. Cordoba-Fernandez. 2000. Subthalamic neuron activity related to tremor and movement in Parkinson's disease. *Eur J Neurosci* **12**: 2597–2607.

Magnin, M., A. Morel, and D. Jeanmonod. 2000. Single-unit analysis of the pallidum, thalamus and subthalamic nucleus in parkinsonian patients. *Neuroscience* **96**:549–564.

Manto, M.U., F. Setta, B. Legros, J. Jacquy, and E. Godaux. 1999. Resetting of orthostatic tremor associated with cerebellar cortical atrophy by transcranial magnetic stimulation. *Arch Neurol* **56**:1497–1500.

Marsden, C.D., J.C. Meadows, G.W. Lange, and R.S. Watson. 1969. The role of the ballistocardiac impulse in the genesis of physiological tremor. *Brain* **92**:647–662.

McAuley, J.H., J.C. Rothwell, C.D. Marsden, and L.J. Findley. 1998. Electrophysiological aids in distinguishing organic tremor from psychogenic tremor. *Neurology* **50**:1882–1884.

Oguni, E., A. Hayashi, A. Ishii, H. Mizusawa, and S. Shoji. 1995. A case of cortical tremor as a variant of cortical reflex myoclonus. *European Neurology* **35**:63–64.

Okuma, Y., Y. Shimo, H. Shimura, K. Hatori, T. Hattori, S. Tanaka, T. Kondo, and Y. Mizuno. 1998. Familial cortical tremor with epilepsy: an under-recognized familial tremor. *Clinical Neurology and Neurosurgery* **100**:75–78.

O'Suilleabhain, P.E., and J.Y. Matsumoto. 1998. Time-frequency analysis of tremors. *Brain* **121**:2127–2134.

Pascual-Leone, A., J. Valls-Solé, C. Toro, E.M. Wassermann, and M. Hallett. 1994. Resetting of essential tremor and postural tremor in Parkinson's disease with transcranial magnetic stimulation. *Muscle & Nerve* **17**:800–807.

Pfeiffer, G., P. Hinse T. Humbert, and G. Riemer. 1999. Neurophysiology of orthostatic tremor: influence of transcranial magnetic stimulation. *Electromyography and Clinical Neurophysiology* **39**:49–53.

Quintern, J., I. Immisch, H. Albrecht, W. Pöllmann, S. Glasauer, and A. Straube. 1999. Influence of visual and proprioceptive afferences on upper limb ataxia in patients with multiple sclerosis. *Journal of Neurological Sciences* **163**:61–69.

Qureshi, F., A. Morales, and R.J. Elble. 1996. Tremor due to infarction in the ventrolateral thalamus. *Mov Disord* **11**:440–444.

Rack, P.M.H., and H.F. Ross. 1986. The role of reflexes in the resting tremor of Parkinson's disease. *Brain* **109**:115–141.

Raethjen, J., M. Lindemann, H. Schmaljohann, R. Schmaljohann, G. Pfister, and G. Deuschl. 2000. Multiple oscillators are causing parkinsonian and essential tremor. *Movement Disorders* **15**:84–94.

Raethjen, J., M. Lindemann, M. Dumpelmann, R. Wenzelburger, H. Stolze, G. Pfister, C.E. Elger, J. Timmer, and G. Deuschl. 2002. Corticomuscular coherence in the 6–15 Hz band: is the cortex involved in the generation of physiologic tremor? *Exp Brain Res* **142**:32–40.

Renou, G., P. Rondot, and S. Metral. 1970. Analyse de décharges itératives d'une même unité motrice dans les bouffées de tremblement. *Revue Neurologique* **122**:420–423.

Schotland, J.L., and W.Z. Rymer. 1993. Wipe and flexion reflexes of the frog. II. Response to perturbations. *J Neurophysiol* **69**:1736–1748.

Shahani, B.T., and R.R. Young. 1977. Specific abnormalities of single motor unit discharge patterns in tremor. *Neurology* **27**:354.

Stein, R.B., and M.N. Oguztöreli. 1976. Tremor and other oscillations in neuromuscular systems. *Biological Cybernetics* **22**:147–157.

Stephens, J.A., and A. Taylor. 1974. The effect of visual feedback on physiological muscle tremor. *Electroencephalography and Clinical Neurophysiology* **36**:457–464.

Stiles, R.N., and J.E. Randall. 1967. Mechanical factors in human tremor frequency. *Journal of Applied Physiology* **23**:324–330.

Stiles, R.N. 1980. Mechanical and neural feedback factors in postural hand tremor of normal subjects. *Journal of Neurophysiology* **44**:40–59.

Terada, K., A. Ikeda, T. Mima, M. Kimura, Y. Nagahama, Y. Kamioka, I. Murone, J. Kimura, and H. Shibasaki. 1997. Familial cortical myoclonic tremor as a unique form of cortical reflex myoclonus. *Mov Disord* **12**:370–377.

Thompson, P.D., J.C. Rothwell, B.L. Day, A. Berardelli, J.P.R. Dick, T. Kachi, and C.D. Marsden. 1986. The physiology of orthostatic tremor. *Archives of Neurology* **43**:584–587.

Timmer, J., M. Lauk, and G. Deuschl. 1996. Quantitative analysis of tremor time series. *Electroencephalography and Clinical Neurophysiology* **101**: 461–468.

Timmermann, L., J. Gross, M. Dirks, J. Volkmann, H.J. Freund, and A. Schnitzler. 2003. The cerebral oscillatory network of parkinsonian resting tremor. *Brain* **126**:199–212.

Toro, C., A. Pascual-Leone, G. Deuschl, E. Tate, M.R. Pranzatelli, and M. Hallett. 1993. Cortical tremor. A common manifestation of cortical myoclonus. *Neurology* **43**:2346–2353.

Tsai, C.H., J.G. Semmler, T.E. Kimber, G. Thickbroom, R. Stell, F.L. Mastaglia, and P.D. Thompson. 1998. Modulation of primary orthostatic tremor by magnetic stimulation over the motor cortex. *Journal of Neurology, Neurosurgery and Psychiatry* **64**:33–36.

Ugawa, Y., T. Shimpo, and T. Mannen. 1989. Physiological analysis of asterixis: silent period locked averaging. *Journal of Neurology, Neurosurgery and Psychiatry* **52**:89–93.

Volkmann, J., M. Joliot, A. Mogilner, A.A. Ioannides, F. Lado, E. Fazzini, U. Ribary, and R. Llinás. 1996. Central motor loop oscillations in parkinsonian resting tremor revealed by magnetoencephalography. *Neurology* **46**:1359–1370.

Wenderoth, N., and O. Bock. 1999. Load dependence of simulated central tremor. *Biological Cybernetics* **80**:285–290.

Wessberg, J., and Å.B. Vallbo. 1996. Pulsatile motor output in human finger movements is not dependent on the stretch reflex. *Journal of Physiology (London)* **493**:895–908.

Wessberg, J., and N. Kakuda. 1999. Single motor unit activity in relation to pulsatile motor output in human finger movements. *Journal of Physiology (London)* **517**:273–285.

Wilms, H., J. Sievers, and G. Deuschl. 1999. Animal models of tremor. *Movement Disorders* **14**:557–571.

Winfree, A.T. 2001. *The Geometry of Biological Time*. Interdisciplinary applied mathematics; v. 12. Springer: New York.

Wu, Y.R., P. Ashby, and A.E. Lang. 2001. Orthostatic tremor arises from an oscillator in the posterior fossa. *Mov Disord* **16**:272–279.

Yamamoto, T., M. Fukuda, and R. Llinas. 2001. Bilaterally synchronous complex spike Purkinje cell activity in the mammalian cerebellum. *Eur J Neurosci* **13**:327–339.

Young, R.R., and K.-E. Hagbarth. 1980. Physiological tremor enhanced by maneuvers affecting the segmental stretch reflex. *Journal of Neurology, Neurosurgery and Psychiatry* **43**:248–256.

Young, R.R. 2002. What is a tremor? *Neurology* **58**:165–166.

Zackowski, K.M., A.J. Bastian, S. Hakimian, J.W. Mink, J.S. Perlmutter, W.C. Koller, and W.T., Thach Jr. 2002. Thalamic stimulation reduces essential tremor but not the delayed antagonist muscle timing. *Neurology* **58**:402–410.

Zirh, T.A., F.A. Lenz, S.G. Reich, and P.M. Dougherty. 1998. Patterns of bursting occurring in thalamic cells during parkinsonian tremor. *Neuroscience* **83**:107–121.

CHAPTER

E2

Essential Tremor

ELAN D. LOUIS

Essential tremor (ET) is a progressive neurological disease characterized by a 4- to 12-Hz kinetic tremor that involves several regions of the body, including the arms and head [1–5]. Patients may have signs of more widespread cerebellar involvement (e.g., intention tremor, ataxia) [6–8], abnormalities referable to the basal ganglia (e.g., rest tremor) [9,10], and cognitive deficits [11,12]. There are both familial and nonfamilial forms of the disease [13,14], suggesting that the etiology is heterogeneous and complex. In a small number of families with apparently autosomal dominant inheritance, genetic linkage has been established to regions on chromosomes 2p and 3q [15–17], but no specific susceptibility gene has been identified yet. Animal models for action tremor, involving the administration of chemicals to laboratory animals, include the harmaline [18] and the penitrem A models [19].

I. DESCRIPTIVE EPIDEMIOLOGY

ET is the most prevalent adult-onset movement disorder [20] and the most common cause of abnormal tremor in human beings. The prevalence in some age strata is reported to be as much as twenty times higher than that of Parkinson disease [21]. Beyond these generalities, the true prevalence of the condition is not precisely known. For example, prevalence estimates in population-based studies have ranged from 0.4% to 6%, which represents a fifteen-fold difference [20–22]. From these estimates, it is often summarily stated that the prevalence of the disease in the population is approximately 1%. However, this number is certainly an underestimate as most studies have relied on screening questionnaires, a strategy that likely yields low prevalence estimates due to the high percentage of ET cases with mild tremor who screen negative [23]. In recent studies in which most or all of the individuals underwent a neurological examination, the prevalence (age ≥40 years) was in the range of 4–6% [21–23].

Both the incidence and prevalence of ET increase with advancing age [24,25], suggesting that age is a risk factor for this disease. Although cases may arise in childhood, most patients with incident and prevalent ET are in their 60s or older [20–22]. The incidence and prevalence are similar in men and women [24,25]. In several studies, the prevalence was higher in Caucasians than in African-Americans [25–27], suggesting that ethnic differences might exist. These differences could reflect different distributions of susceptibility genotypes or differences in exposure to environmental factors that might influence tremor.

II. CLINICAL CHARACTERISTICS

The predominant finding in patients with ET is a kinetic tremor (i.e., a tremor that occurs during voluntary movement), as shown in the two spirals, drawn by ET patients, in Figure 1 below. The frequency of this tremor is between 4 and 12 Hz, and is inversely related to age, with older patients tending to have tremor frequencies that are at the lower end of this spectrum [28]. The kinetic tremor occurs during a variety of different voluntary movements such as writing, pouring, drinking from a cup, eating, putting in eye drops, and other daily activities. Patients with severe ET also have a postural tremor, which can be elicited by asking the patient to hold their arms outstretched in front of the body [28]. The literature abounds in statements that define ET as a postural tremor; this is incorrect [28]. The tremor is predominantly kinetic.

The tremor most commonly affects the arms, but it may also affect additional regions of the body, especially the head (i.e., neck), voice, or both and occasionally the trunk, lower extremities, tongue, and other facial musculature [5]. The proportion of subjects with both head and arm tremor ranges from 34% to 53%, depending on the study sample [14,29–32]. In most studies, however, isolated head tremor (head tremor without accompanying arm tremor) is rare, occurring in 1–10% of patients [32].

A characteristic feature of ET is the somatotopic spread of tremor over time, from the arms to the head. Head tremor typically evolves several years after the onset of arm tremor, but the converse (arm tremor developing after the onset of isolated head tremor) is unusual and should call the diagnosis into question [32].

The hallmark feature of ET is a kinetic tremor, and this probably results from an abnormality in the cerebellum or cerebellar-thalamic outflow pathways. In addition, recent work has demonstrated that, as in other neurodegenerative diseases (e.g., Parkinson disease [PD], Alzhemier disease, and Huntington disease), involvement of the central nervous system may be diffuse, having the tendency to evolve over time. Therefore, ET patients who are sampled at different times during their disease are likely to have different clinical characteristics. There is considerable evidence that the pathological process in some patients, which in ET remains to be identified, ultimately results in diffuse cerebellar involvement, signs referable to the basal ganglia, cognitive abnormalities that may be referable to cerebellar-frontal connections, changes in personality whose basis and localization are unclear, olfactory deficits, and perhaps changes in the peripheral nervous system. Each of these clinical areas will be outlined in the succeeding paragraphs.

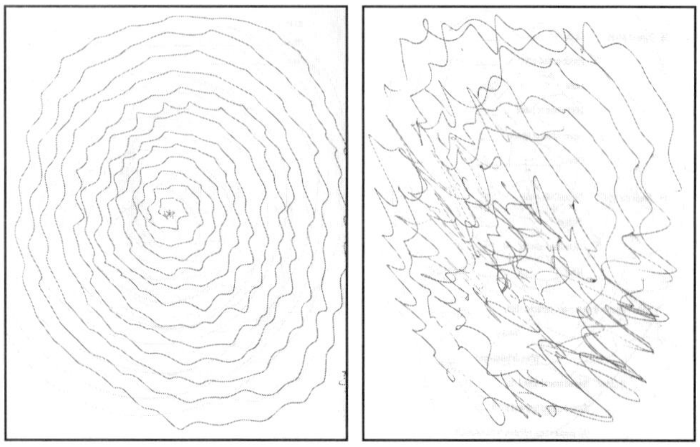

FIGURE 1 Archimedes spirals drawn by patients with mild (left) and severe (right) essential tremor.

Several studies [6–8] have demonstrated postural instability and ataxic gait in a large proportion of patients with ET, suggesting that the cerebellar involvement can become more widespread, though not as widespread as that occurring in the spinocerebellar ataxias. The diagnostic differentiation between (1) the ET patient with severe tremor who later develops gait ataxia and (2) the patient with spinocerebellar ataxia can be difficult, although the current dogma is that patients with ET do not exhibit nystagmus or scanning or dysarthric speech.

It is well known that some patients with ET develop a tremor at rest [9,33]. In one study [10], investigators studied the prevalence and clinical correlates of this tremor in a sample of ET patients who were referred to a tertiary referral center. In that study [10], 18.8% of the ET patients had a rest tremor (i.e., approximately one in five ET cases), which suggests that this type of tremor is not uncommon in ET patients who are seen at tertiary referral centers. When compared to the ET patients without rest tremor, those with rest tremor had a disease of longer duration and of greater severity. Also, their ET was more widely disseminated as evidenced by a larger proportion with head tremor. None had clinical signs of bradykinesia or rigidity, but on electrophysiological testing, they had electrophysiological features consistent with mild Parkinsonism (e.g., slow spiral speed, increased decrement of spiral speed with radius) [10]. The basis for rest tremor in patients with ET is not clear, although several possibilities exist. First, in patients with severe, longstanding, and disseminated disease, the pathological process that caused their ET may have spread into motor systems outside of the cerebellum/cerebellar outflow connections. That is, the basal ganglia and/or their connections could be involved. Interestingly, in a fluorodopa positron emission tomography (PET) study [34], uptake in the basal ganglia in ET patients was 10%–13% below that of controls, but the difference was not significant in that small study sample. A second possibility is that rest tremor may be the only clinically detectable sign of co-existing Lewy body PD that developed in these ET patients with rest tremor. Against this possibility is the observation [9] that pathological findings compatible with idiopathic PD were absent in three cases of ET with isolated rest tremor (i.e., rest tremor without other features of Parkinsonism). Second, in the PET study [34], while fluorodopa uptake in the basal ganglia was

10%–13% below normal in patients with ET, it was well above the range seen in patients with idiopathic PD, suggesting that these patients did not have PD. Finally, the severe olfactory deficit that is an early feature of patients with PD is not seen in many of the ET patients with rest tremor, suggesting that they do not have an early form of PD [35].

As in other neurodegenerative diseases, patients with ET appear to have cognitive problems. Several recent studies have demonstrated mild cognitive abnormalities in ET, and, more specifically, problems with verbal fluency, recent memory, working memory, and mental set-shifting, suggesting that the frontal cortical or frontal cortical-cerebellar pathways are involved [11,12,36–38]. These cognitive problems appear to be mild and sub-clinical.

The emerging picture of ET suggests that the pathological process involves a number of different higher order cortical domains. In addition to cognitive changes, personality changes may also occur. In one study [39], investigators administered the Tridimensional Personality Questionnaire to patients with ET and to controls. Patients with ET had higher scores on one of the three subscales of this test, namely, the harm avoidance subscale. A high harm avoidance score defines a person who is pessimistic, fearful, shy, anxious, and easily fatigued. This is an intriguing initial finding and suggests that, as in several other movement disorders (Parkinson and Huntington diseases), personality may be involved.

As in other degenerative disorders, an olfactory deficit occurs in patients with ET, which appears milder than that seen in patients with PD, although the University of Pennsylvania Smell Identification Test scores overlap in the two conditions [40]. The deficit seems to be unrelated to disease duration or severity, suggesting that, as in PD, the deficit occurs early in the disease process.

Interestingly, several studies have suggested abnormalities might occur outside of the central nervous system in patients with ET. These include a study of hearing loss in patients with ET. In that study [41], patients with ET had significantly more hearing disability, as measured by the Nursing Home Hearing Handicap Resident and Staff Assessment, than did patients with PD or normal controls. Also, a higher percentage of ET patients (16.6%) wore hearing aids than patients with PD (1.6%) or normal controls (1.6%). The authors concluded that the basis for the hearing loss might be cochlear-vestibular involvement. In another study [42], the authors showed that the peripheral silent period was shorter in patients with ET compared to normal individuals, indicating a possible role for peripheral modulation of the tremor.

Several studies have now demonstrated a mild loss of body mass index (BMI) in patients with ET [43,44]. In one study [43], investigators compared seventy-eight ET patients at a tertiary referral center to 242 controls of similar age. BMI in ET patients was $26.5 \pm 5.0\,kg/m^2$ vs. $28.2 \pm 4.8\,kg/m^2$ in controls, which was on average a 6% reduction ($p = 0.008$). Mean daily caloric intake was similar in patients and controls, suggesting that lower BMI was not due to a reduction in calories and perhaps due to increased energy expenditure in ET. In the second study [44], which was population-based, investigators compared eighty-nine ET patients who lived in the Mersin province of Turkey to eighty-nine controls in the same province. Most of the ET cases had not been previously diagnosed with ET and few were taking medications for tremor. There was a similar 5.5% reduction in BMI in these ET cases.

In summary, the old view of ET, as a simple monosymptomatic syndrome characterized by action tremor, is beginning to change. It is being replaced by a view of this entity as a disease with a complex set of clinical characteristics that evolve in a prescribed manner over time. The study of these patterns will provide clues about the underlying pathogenesis of this disease, which remains poorly understood.

A. Functional Sequelae

In the past, investigators often used the term "benign essential tremor," but this term is controversial. The large majority (as many as 90–99.5%) of ET cases who live in the population [45,46] do not seek health care, and this suggests that their tremor is of little consequence. In reality, the majority of these cases experience some functional disability resulting from their tremor. In a study of community-dwelling ET cases, the large majority (73%) reported disability, with most experiencing this disability in multiple functional domains [1]. In general, the tremor in ET is progressive [5], eventually producing disabilities with basic daily activities such as eating, writing, body care, and driving [14,47]. More than 90% of patients who come for medical attention report disability [1], and severely affected end-stage patients are physically unable to feed or dress themselves. In these patients, the tremor prevents any normal activity, resulting in a substantial loss of independence and even incapacitation [48]. Between 15% and 25% of clinic patients are forced to retire prematurely, and 60% choose not to apply for a job or promotion because of uncontrollable shaking [14,47].

B. Prognosis

As noted above, ET is clinically progressive. Clinicians have long recognized among many of their ET patients a progressive increase in tremor severity with advancing age and disease duration [2,3,5]. In our cross-sectional study of the functional correlates of tremor among ET cases [1], the correlation between tremor severity (assessed clinically using a 36-point total tremor score) and disease duration was significant ($r = 0.66$, $p < 0.001$). Also, all of the ET cases who had tremor of long duration also had high tremor scores, suggesting that longstanding disease inexorably results in a severe tremor. There have been few longitudinal studies of ET and few attempts to quantify the extent to which the tremor worsens over time. One notable exception is a prospective four-year study of ET, in which tremor amplitude was assessed electrophysiologically, and that demonstrated a 29.4% increase in tremor amplitude during the study period [49].

Although the current dogma is that the risk of mortality is not increased in patients with ET, investigators have made few attempts to study the mortality of ET. In one case-control study [24], a longitudinal retrospective study of ET patients in Rochester, Minnesota, investigators selected 266 patients and abstracted their medical records. The survival after diagnosis of ET was comparable to the expected survival for persons of similar age and sex from the West North Central region of the U.S.A (i.e., a group of historical controls) [24]. In that study, the mean age at diagnosis was fifty-eight years, and the mean length of follow-up after diagnosis was 9.7 years, suggesting that some of the cases may not have been followed into advanced age. At these advanced ages the risk of mortality in ET may rise. Further work is needed in this important area.

III. PATHOPHYSIOLOGY AND PATHOLOGY

The pathophysiology of ET is poorly understood, but several lines of evidence suggest that this disease is probably neurodegenerative. As noted above, ET is clinically progressive. In addition, the gradual development of mild incoordination and mild ataxia in some longstanding cases supports the notion that the underlying pathological process is not static, but that it becomes more pervasive, eventually extending into brain systems that produce symptoms other than tremor. Also, clinicians have observed that tremor usually begins in the arms and only later spreads to the head. These clinical findings support the notion that the underlying neuropathological changes are not static, but rather, they also develop somatotopically over time, initially involving brain regions that result in arm tremor and later, advancing into the regions that result in head tremor and more pervasive cerebellar signs, and possibly involving other systems (e.g., basal ganglia) as noted above. Finally, imaging studies ([^{1}H] magnetic resonance spectroscopic imaging, MRSI) have demonstrated a reduction in cerebellar N-acetylaspartate (NAA), often expressed as a ratio to total creatine (tCR) in ET cases [50]. NAA/tCR levels are decreased in the setting of neuronal damage or cell death [51–53], and, as such, serve as a marker for disturbed neuronal integrity. Using [^{1}H] MRSI, we demonstrated a reduction in NAA/tCR within the cerebellar cortex in ET cases, suggesting that cell damage or cell death occurs in this region of the brain in ET (table 1) [50].

TABLE 1 NAA/tCR in Different Brain Regions in ET Cases and Conrols [50]

	ET (N = 16)	Controls (N = 11)
Cerebellar Cortex	1.53 ± 0.36	1.91 ± 0.49 (p = 0.03)
Cerebellar White Matter	1.59 ± 0.26	1.64 ± 0.27
Cerebellar Vermis	1.55 ± 0.21	1.56 ± 0.29
Thalamus	2.50 ± 0.40	2.55 ± 0.53
Basal Ganglia	2.72 ± 0.70	2.62 ± 0.46

Ultimately, pathological studies are needed to more fully address the issue of pathophysiology. Despite the widespread occurrence of ET, postmortem studies are limited to fewer than twenty, with many of these published—fifty to one hundred years ago [54–62]. No consistent pathological abnormality was reported in these studies. There was, however, occasional loss of cerebellar Purkinje cells in one brain and more marked loss in three others, although quantitative cell counts were not performed [54–57]. With normal aging, Purkinje cells die at a rate of 2.5%–5% per decade [63,64], and these four cases ranged in age at the time of death from sixty-one to eighty years (mean = 70.3), making the loss of Purkinje cells difficult to interpret in the absence of age-matched control brains for comparison. Formal quantitative studies of cerebellar Purkinje or olivary neurons were not performed in any, nor were control brains studied for comparison. Moreover, in many of the cases, the diagnosis of ET is highly questionable because patients also had other involuntary movements (chorea, athetosis, Parkinsonism) or were members of families in which individuals variably expressed a mixed phenotype of action tremor with or without Parkinsonism. A concerted effort is needed to collect postmortem tissue on a larger number of ET cases, to study these cases using a standardized approach involving quantitative cell counts and immunohistochemistry, and to compare this tissue to that of control subjects of similar age.

One additional issue is that ET might represent a family of diseases rather than a single disease. The considerable pharmacological heterogeneity supports this theory, with far fewer than 50% of patients responding to most pharmacological interventions [65]. Isolated action tremor may be part of the clinical spectrum of a large number of disease entities that anatomically involve cerebellar outflow pathways or other similar systems in the brain, but which originate as the result of distinct and diverse etiologies and pathologies.

IV. ETIOLOGY: GENETIC VS. NONGENETIC CAUSES

The etiologies of ET are likely to be both genetic and nongenetic [66,67]. Differences between the genetic and nongenetic forms of the disease have not been identified, other than a possibly younger age of onset in genetic forms of the disease [45].

One important question is the magnitude of a genetic contribution to the etiology of this disease on a population level. The literature commonly states that 50% of ET cases are attributed to genetic causes. This estimate appears to be based on the proportion of cases who report a family history. However, estimates of the proportion with a family history range from as low as 17% to as high as 100% [13]. With this degree of variability, it is difficult to get a sense of the true proportion, and the commonly cited value of 50% appears highly questionable. Furthermore, the proportion of cases with a positive family history does not necessarily reflect the proportion with a genetic etiology. Most studies that examine this question have not enrolled control subjects. Many of the positive family histories could be explained by chance co-occurrence of a highly prevalent disorder rather than a genetic predisposition for tremor [13,46]. Studies suggest that as many as 18% of families may contain an affected individual, even if ascertained through an unaffected control [22].

There are additional methodologic problems with previous studies that raise further doubt about the proportion of genetic cases. Most studies have reported the percentage of probands with a family history rather than the proportion of at-risk relatives who are affected with ET, making it impossible to test consistency with genetic models or to control for characteristics of the relatives (e.g., age, gender, ethnicity, history of environmental exposures) [13]. Many studies have selected probands from clinical care settings (hospitals, clinics, tertiary referral centers) rather than from the community. ET cases who are seen in clinics and doctor's offices probably represent a very small proportion of all ET cases in the population (as few as 0.5%) [45], and these cases are five times more likely to report a positive family history than are those who never make it to clinics [68]. Clinic populations might be self-selected to over-represent familial and genetic forms of ET, and possibly autosomal dominant forms as well [68]. Finally, most studies have obtained family history information by interviewing the probands rather than by examining the relatives themselves, and the sensitivity of probands reports may be as low as 16% [69].

In the Washington Heights-Inwood Genetic Study of Essential Tremor, a population-based family study of ET that enrolled relatives of ET cases and relatives of control subjects, we found that a first-degree relative of an ET case was 4.7 times more likely to have ET than a first-degree relative of a control subject [22]. In addition, the magnitude of increased risk in relatives of ET patients versus controls was greater in relatives of ET cases with onset under fifty than in relatives of those with older onset (relative risk, RR = 10.38 vs. 4.82) [22].

In a recent twin study [66], three of five (60%) monozygotic twins were concordant for ET, compared with only three of eight (27%) dizygotic twins. Although concordance in monozygotic twins was approximately two times that in dizygotic twins, the monozygotic concordance was not 100% and the authors suggested on this basis that nongenetic factors play a role in the etiology of ET.

A. Genetics

Specific genes for ET have not yet been identified. Given the high prevalence of this disorder, one would expect that multiple genetic loci may contribute to this disease. To date, linkage has been reported on two different chromosomes, namely, 3q13 and 2p22 [15–17], demonstrating that ET is genetically heterogeneous.

In the first genetic linkage study, Gulcher and colleagues [15] reported the results of a genome scan for familial ET (FET) genes in sixteen Icelandic families containing seventy-five affected individuals. The scan revealed significant evidence for linkage to chromosome 3q13. In that study, the average age of onset was 26.7 years, and all patients had had bilateral postural tremor with or without kinetic tremor of the hands for at least five years.

In the second linkage study, Higgins and colleagues [17] reported the results of a linkage analysis in a large American family of Czech descent. Data were available on sixty-seven family members, among whom eighteen were affected. Evidence was obtained for linkage to chromosome 2p22–25 with a maximum LOD score of 5.92. For this study, the authors assumed a disease prevalence of 1%, an autosomal dominant model of inheritance, and a penetrance of 100%. The authors [16] subsequently reported that the same locus may be responsible for ET in other families, although the contribution of this or other loci to disease etiology on a population level is not known. In that study [16], all patients had bilateral postural tremor with 2–4 cm excursions in at least one arm. The mean age of onset was thirty-two years.

One interesting question is whether the mode of inheritance of ET, on a population level, is autosomal dominant, as it seems to be in these pedigrees [15–17]. There is evidence that this pattern of inheritance may not typify all families with ET. First, these large families with multiple affected individuals over several generations have been difficult to identify for genetic linkage studies. Second, some of the data from the Washington Heights-Inwood Genetic Study of Essential Tremor may not be consistent with an autosomal dominant model either. In a simple autosomal dominant model, the relative risk (RR) in second-degree relatives is expected to be one-half of the RR in first-degree relatives. For example, if the RR among first-degree relatives is 4.7, then the RR among second-degree relatives would be expected to be one-half of that (i.e., 2.35). We found a relative risk of 4.7 in first-degree relatives, but only 0.9 in second degree relatives (although confidence intervals did overlap). These findings could be consistent with a model involving multiple interacting genes (epistasis) [70]. Third, as in other highly complex diseases, genetic heterogeneity is likely, with variable modes of inheritance across families [70].

Variability within families in the age of onset and anatomical distribution of tremor has been reported, but has not been investigated systematically. A study in rural Sweden [45] is the most helpful in this regard. In that study, age at onset within families varied considerably. In some families, the age of onset ranged between twenty and sixty years and there was variable involvement of the head, arm, tongue, legs, and trunk as well. One group reported younger age of disease onset in successively younger generations [16,17], and suggested that there might be genetic anticipation in ET. However, the true age at onset, rather than age at initial recognition, may be difficult to ascertain because the disease has an insidious onset. Once families have come for medical attention, there is a greater potential for recognition of mild tremor in young cases.

Although the penetrance of ET is generally considered to be complete by age sixty-five to seventy, there are few data. One study in Sweden [45] suggested that the penetrance was complete at age seventy because the highest registered age of onset in their cohort was seventy. However, it is apparent from the authors' data that many unaffected relatives were over the age of seventy, and it is not known how many of these carried a genetic predisposition for ET. A second study of familial ET [14] similarly suggested that the penetrance was complete by age sixty-five because 46% (i.e., nearly one-half) of relatives of familial ET cases had developed tremor by that age. Assuming an autosomal dominant model of inheritance and complete penetrance, 50% of first-degree relatives of familial cases would be expected to develop the disease. However, these calculations do not account for nongenetic causes of ET among relatives. In northern Manhattan, we reported that 11.1% of control subjects' first-degree relatives had developed ET by age sixty, and 22.2% by age eighty [22]. Nongenetic causes of ET should be similar in relatives of cases and relatives of controls. Therefore, in an autosomal dominant model with complete penetrance, more than 50% of first-degree relatives of familial cases would be expected to develop the disease by advanced age. More recently, data from the Washington Heights-Inwood Genetic Study of Essential Tremor indicate that subclinical ET may be present and penetrance may not be complete even among older relatives [71]. In that study [71], data were analyzed on 201 relatives of ET cases and 212 relatives of control subjects. None of the relatives met diagnostic criteria for ET. All of the relatives were examined and videotaped and this videotape was reviewed by a neurologist specializing in movement disorders. Clinically detectable but mild tremor was present in 96.0% of the case relatives and 97.6% of control relatives, and tremor severity (as measured by a total tremor score) was higher in first-degree case relatives than in first-degree control relatives. Among first-degree relatives who were older than sixty years of age (mean age among case relatives = 72.5 years and mean age among control relatives = 71.8 years), a larger proportion of case relatives had higher total tremor scores. One possible explanation for the observed difference in distribution of tremor scores among case and control relatives is that relatives of ET cases have mild partially expressed forms of ET. The mean total tremor score was higher in relatives of ET cases than in relatives of controls among first-degree relatives but not among more distantly related (second-degree) relatives, suggesting that a genetic predisposition for tremor may have contributed to the observed difference.

B. Environmental Epidemiology

Nongenetic factors most likely contribute to the etiology of ET. The entity of non-familial ET, or "sporadic" ET, is well recognized by most clinicians, who distinguish this form of ET from "hereditary" ET [14,15,57]. In fact, in most series, the majority (>50%) of ET cases have not reported affected relatives [72–74], and despite the high prevalence of the disease, families that are informative for genetic linkage studies have been difficult to locate. Intra-familial differences in age of onset and severity of tremor [22,45] also suggest that environmental (or perhaps other genetic) factors may serve as modifiers of an underlying susceptibility genotype. Temporal trends in disease incidence or prevalence would also support the notion that environmental factors may contribute to the etiology of ET. A temporal trend in the annual incidence of ET was reported in Rochester, Minnesota [24], were the annual age-adjusted incidence per 100,000 rose from 5.8 in the period from 1935–1949, to 15.8 in the period from 1950–1964, and 23.5 in the period from 1965–1975. Increased recognition and diagnosis of the disorder may have contributed to this temporal trend.

Investigators suggested several potential environmental toxicants, including lead and β-carboline alkaloids [67], based on the observations that (1) acute or chronic exposure in humans results in action tremor and this action tremor shares clinical features with ET, (2) the underlying pathogenesis for the tremor is similar to that of ET because both involve cerebellar or cerebellar outflow pathway abnormalities, (3) the toxicant is highly ubiquitous, like ET, which is highly prevalent and geographically widespread, and (4) the slow accumulation of the toxicant in human tissue positively correlates with age, as ET is a disease of aging.

In a study of 100 ET patients and 143 controls, researchers analyzed blood lead concentrations using graphite furnace atomic absorption spectrophotometry and an industrial hygienist reviewed a lifetime occupational history [75]. Blood lead concentration was higher in ET patients than in controls (means = 3.3 ± 2.4 and $2.6 \pm 1.6\mu g/dl$; medians =

2.7 vs. 2.3 μg/dl, $p = 0.038$). After adjusting for confounding variables in a logistic regression model, blood lead concentration was associated with ET (OR per unit increase = 1.19, 95% CI = 1.03–1.37, $p = 0.02$). The prevalence of lifetime occupational lead exposure was similar in ET patients and controls, suggesting that the higher blood lead concentration in ET cases was not due to occupational lead exposure. Whether the association is due to increased exposure to lead or to a difference in lead kinetics in ET patients remains unknown and requires further investigation.

The β-carboline alkaloids, including harmane and harmine, are a group of highly tremorogenic chemicals. Laboratory animals injected with large doses of these chemicals acutely exhibit an action tremor that resembles ET [76]. Human volunteers acutely exposed to large doses display a reversible coarse tremor but the effect of low level, chronic exposure to β-carboline alkaloids is unknown. Sources both exogenous and endogenous to the body exist. β-carboline alkaloids are naturally present in small concentrations in the food chain, in commonly eaten plant-derived foods (wheat, rice, corn, barley) and in cooked meats. Also, these chemicals are normal body constituents and are produced *in vivo* by the cyclization of indole-alkylamines with aldehydes, occurring in most tissues in animals and humans. In a study of one hundred ET cases and one hundred controls [76], the median blood harmane concentration in ET cases ($5.21\,g^{-10}$/ml) was higher than that of controls ($2.28\,g^{-10}$/ml in controls, $p = 0.005$) and in a logistic regression model, the harmane concentration was associated with a diagnosis of ET (OR = 1.80, 95% CI = 1.10–2.93, $p = 0.02$), suggesting that these toxicants could play a role in the etiopathogenesis of ET.

V. DIAGNOSIS OF ESSENTIAL TREMOR

The diagnostic approach to patients with ET includes the following steps: a history, a physical examination, and, in some instances, selected laboratory tests [77]. Because a gene for ET has not yet been identified, there is no diagnostic genetic test for ET. Moreover, the utility of such a test would be limited for a variety of reasons. First, it is unknown what proportion of ET cases have an important genetic contribution, but this proportion may be much lower than 50% [13,22]. Second, in those individuals with a major genetic effect, multiple genes may be involved, either interacting within individuals, or as alternative etiologies in different patients. Finally, even in those individuals with a major genetic effect, environmental factors (e.g., toxicants) may be required to trigger onset of symptoms.

The following outline shows the diagnostic approach to a patient who is suspected of having ET. The first step is to obtain a history. During the history, information on the age of onset, localization of tremor, and evolution of tremor over time, along with family history information should be collected. Caffeine, cigarettes, and several medications, including lithium, prednisone, thyroxine, asthma inhalers, valproate, and selective serotonin re-uptake inhibitors, can exacerbate enhanced physiological tremor, which can resemble ET. Therefore, a complete inventory of all current medications (including inhalers), as well as caffeine and smoking habits, is important in order to exclude these as the cause of tremor or as contributors to tremor. Patients with tremor may also have disorders other than ET. These patients may have symptoms of these disorders at presentation. Thus, patients with hyperthyroidism may complain of diarrhea, weight loss, and heat intolerance and patients with PD may note a loss of normal facial expression, a change in normal arm swing, and slowness or stiffness, and patients with dystonia may notice pain or spasms in affected limbs.

During a physical examination, the clinician should carefully assess the characteristics of the tremor. Although many patients with PD manifest a postural or kinetic tremor [65], rest tremor is also present and affects approximately 85% [78] of patients with autopsy-proven PD. While rest tremor can accompany ET, it usually occurs in the setting of severe kinetic tremor of long duration. By contrast, patients with PD often have a rest tremor that occurs along with only mild or moderate postural or kinetic tremor of uncertain duration. Approximately 20–30% of patients with dystonia have a postural tremor that resembles ET, but on closer inspection, the tremor differs from that of ET (e.g., the tremor is often irregular and jerky rather than regularly oscillatory, and there may be a null point, which is a hand or arm position that they can find that will temporarily resolve the tremor). One must be careful here, because most tremors, especially the action tremor of ET and the rest tremor of PD, depend much upon the position of the limb, and patients can suppress or bring on these types of tremors with subtle changes in posture or limb positioning.

Two common clinical situations are the differentiation between ET and PD and ET and dystonic tremor. Some of the features of PD that generally do not occur in patients with ET are hemibody involvement (e.g., ipsilateral arm and leg) and bradykinesia and rigidity. The postural tremor of ET also tends to involve wrist flexion and extension whereas in PD, wrist rotation (esp., internal) often occurs. Features of dystonic tremor that do not occur in patients with pure ET are dystonic movements or postures, muscle hypertrophy, complaints of pain or pulling in the affected body region, a null point, and a nonrhythmic quality to the tremor.

The final step in evaluating the patient who is suspected of having ET is the laboratory work-up. If symptoms or signs of hyperthyroidism are present, then thyroid function tests should be performed. In any patient with action tremor who is under the age of forty, the possibility of Wilson disease should be explored with a serum ceruloplasmin. The ceruloplasmin is low (<20 mg/dl) in 95% of patients with Wilson disease [79]. If other clinical features suggestive of Wilson disease are present (e.g., dysarthria, dystonia, parkinsonism), then a careful slit lamp examination of the eye by an experienced ophthalmologist should be performed. Kayser-Fleischer rings on Descemet membrane are detectible in 99.3% of Wilson patients with neurological abnormalities [80].

Although PET has revealed a relative increase in cerebellar and red nuclear blood flow in some patients with ET [81–84], the diagnostic validity of this test has not been established. Some tertiary care centers provide quantitative computerized tremor analysis, with accelerometers attached to the arms, and that analysis may guide the clinician in distinguishing ET from other tremors, but its diagnostic validity has not been established. At present, the diagnosis of ET is clinical; there are no serological, radiological, or pathological markers for this disease. Because of the absence of these types of gold standards, one cannot assess the validity of the clinical diagnoses. However, one can assess the agreement between clinicians using the same clinical diagnostic criteria. To date, high reliability has been established for the use of one set of clinical criteria [85].

VI. NEUROIMAGING

Standard MRI has not demonstrated structural radiological abnormalities in ET patients, although MRI is not used routinely in the initial diagnosis or subsequent management of ET patients. Most ET patients never have MRI studies. In one study, twelve ET patients and fifteen controls had an MRI study using high-resolution proton density- and T2-weighted images, which did not reveal structural abnormalities of the brain [86]. Volumetric analyses of the cerebellum and other pertinent structures, however, were not performed. Although the pathology of ET has been limited, several postmortem cases have shown extensive Purkinje cell loss [54–56], and at least one has shown a notable amount of cerebellar cortical atrophy. One functional MRI (fMRI) study demonstrated bilateral cerebellar activation [86], and PET imaging studies have documented increased regional blood flow in the cerebellar hemispheres and red nucleus of ET cases during certain activation procedures (arm extension), and also occasionally at rest [81–84]. These studies suggest that cerebellar circuitry is involved in the initiation of tremor, and hence, blood flow to these regions is enhanced. An unusual feature of this cerebellar activation is that it is both ipsilateral and contralateral to the tremulous arm. In normal individuals without ET, the cerebellar hemispheres modulate movement predominantly in the ipsilateral and, to a far smaller extent, the contralateral limbs [87]. This suggests that in ET, the tremor in each arm is due to an abnormal pattern of input from both cerebellar hemispheres. In contrast to fMRI or PET, which assesses cerebral blood flow, [^{1}H] magnetic resonance spectroscopic imaging (MRSI) measures the concentrations of several intracellular metabolites. Using [^{1}H] MRSI, we demonstrated a reduction in NAA/tCR within the cerebellar cortex in ET cases, suggesting that there is cell damage or cell death in this region of the brain in ET (table 1) [50].

VII. ANIMAL MODELS OF DISEASE

There are no cellular or transgenic or knockout models of the disease. There are, however, several chemically induced animal models for ET. Acute exposure to the tremorogenic β-carboline alkaloids, such as harmane and harmaline, results in a generalized and intense action tremor in a broad range of laboratory species including mice, cats, and monkeys [88]. In human volunteers exposed to intravenous doses of 150–200 mg of harmine, neurological effects, including an acute coarse tremor, become apparent [89,90]. In animals, the tremor shares many features with ET including clinical features [91–93]; pharmacological responsiveness to benzodiazepines, alcohol, and barbiturates, which facilitate gamma-aminobutyric acid (GABA)-mediated inhibitory neurotransmission [94–96]; and underlying pathogenesis in cerebellar and GABAergic systems. The tremor-producing property of the beta-carboline alkaloids is related to their ability to enhance rhythmic firing in olivo-cerebellar neurons with secondary Purkinje cell degeneration [88,95]. Penitrem A, which is produced by the fungus *Penicillium crustosum*, is one of a group of tremor-producing agents produced by several fungi species [19]. Within ten minutes of an intraperitoneal injection, laboratory animals develop severe generalized 6–8 Hz tremors and ataxia that peaks within six hours but can persist to some extent for as long as two days. Despite widespread loss of Purkinje cells, particularly in the vermis and paravermis, the animals become normal within one week of the injection [19]. Finally, investigators have developed a $GABA_A$ receptor α1 subunit knock-out mouse model in which the animals develop a 25-Hz tremor when handled [97].

VIII. TREATMENT

The treatment of ET includes pharmacotherapy and surgery. Pharmacotherapy may be used to improve functional disability or to reduce the embarrassment that may be associated with ET. In mild cases without dysfunction or embarrassment, medications are not indicated. Surgery is indicated for severe cases that are refractory to medications. The following discussion focuses primarily on results from double-blind placebo-controlled trials.

Several issues deserve highlighting. First, the ultimate evidence of efficacy is reduced functional impairment rather than reduced amplitude of the tremor. Second, a large proportion of patients, on the order of 25% to 55%, do not respond to multiple medications. The factors that predict response to particular medications have not been identified. This problem can lead to frustration among patients and loss of confidence in their treating physician. Several factors may account for this high nonresponse rate. There is evidence, as noted above, that ET is not a homogeneous condition. Different clinical subtypes may differ with regard to their underlying etiology and pathogenesis [98]. Genetic heterogeneity occurs [15–17], and some subtypes may respond to a particular medication while others may not. In addition, little is known about the underlying pathophysiology of ET. Most current medications were discovered due to serendipity [99,100] rather than an understanding of the disease mechanisms. The neurotransmitter systems that are involved in ET are not clear, although GABAergic and catecholamine systems are a possibility [101,102]. Further elucidation of these mechanisms is critical in devising more disease-specific therapeutic interventions. Finally, patients who do respond to medications often respond only partially, and the tremor is rarely reduced to asymptomatic levels. The treatments are outlined in table 2.

Propranolol and primidone are the two front-line agents in the treatment of ET [65]. Peripheral β-adrenergic receptors [103] most probably mediate the effects of β-adrenergic blocking agents like propranolol, although researchers have debated whether central mechanisms may be involved as well. Several studies have demonstrated that propranolol, given in doses of 120 mg/day or more, results in a significant reduction in tremor compared with placebo [104], and, subjectively, 45% to 75% of study patients report that propranolol is more effective than the placebo in reducing their tremor. Although propranolol is generally well tolerated, there are several relative contraindications, including asthma, congestive heart failure, diabetes mellitus, and atrioventricular block. Propranolol is a nonselective β-adrenergic receptor antagonist, and it is more effective than antagonists with relatively selective β1 activity [103]. Trials of β1-selective agents such as atenolol and metroprolol have shown mixed results [103,105]. One study demonstrated that propranolol-LA is as effective as conventional propranolol [106].

Primidone, which is an anti-convulsant medication, is metabolized to phenylethylmalonamide and phenobarbitone. Phenylethylmalonamide itself has no therapeutic effect. While the barbiturate metabolite may contribute to the sustained therapeutic effect, the parent compound itself (primidone) is thought to mediate most of the acute and sustained effect [107–109]. Primidone is superior to phenobarbital in reducing tremor [110]. In doses of up to 750 mg/day, primidone significantly reduced tremor compared with placebo effect [107–110], however, tolerability is a common problem. Even at starting doses as low as 62.5 mg/day, an acute toxic reaction, consisting of nausea, vomiting, or ataxia has been reported in 22.7% [107] to 72.7% [108] of patients, requiring discontinuation of primidone in approximately 20% of patients in some studies [107].

Investigators have compared the two front-line agents, propranolol and primidone, in several studies. Primidone, at a dose of 750 mg/day, was compared with propranolol, at a dose of 120 mg/day, and each was significantly better than placebo [109]. However, neither was conclusively shown to be superior to the other. The mean reduction in tremor amplitude was 75.6% while patients were taking primidone compared with 59.7% on propranolol, but given the modest sample size of fourteen cases, this difference was not significant [109]. When investigators asked the study patients which of the two medications they preferred, a larger proportion chose primidone [109]. In another study, a 60% mean improvement occurred in patients taking primidone (250 mg/day in nine patients) versus a 35% improvement in twenty-two patients on maximum effective dose of propranolol (p value not reported) [111]. While initial tolerability is a sizeable problem with primidone, one study provides tentative evidence that long-term tolerability of primidone is superior to that of propranolol. In a study of twenty-five ET patients, acute adverse reactions occurred in 8% with propranolol and 32% with primidone. However, after one

TABLE 2 Medications Used to Treat ET

Medications	Usual therapeutic dose	Side effects
Propranolol	160 to 320 mg per day	Fatigue, impotence, headache, breathlessness, bradycardia, depression
Primidone	62.5 to 1000 mg per day	Sedation, nausea, vomiting
Gabapentin	1200 to 3600 mg per day	Drowsiness, fatigue, slurred speech, imbalance, nausea, dizziness
Topiramate	75 to 400 mg per day	appetite suppression, weight loss, paresthesias
Alprazalom	0.75 to 2.75 mg per day	Sedation, fatigue
Nimodipine	120 mg per day	Orthostatic hypotension
Theophylline	150 to 300 mg per day	None reported

year the significant side effects that the authors cited occurred in 0% with primidone compared with 17% taking propranolol [112].

Several other agents have been used with variable efficacy in the treatment of patients with ET. Among these is gabapentin, an anticonvulsant medication that is structurally similar to the inhibitory neurotransmitter GABA. There is some evidence that a disturbance of the GABAergic system occurs in ET [101]. Researchers have conducted three gabapentin trials, enrolling, in combination, a total of fifty-four patients. In two of the three trials, gabapentin (doses ranging from 1200 to 3600 mg/day) significantly reduced tremor compared with placebo, and in one of the two, its effect was similar to that of propranolol [113–115]. Gabapentin is generally well tolerated.

In a double-blind placebo-controlled trial, topiramate was administered to twenty-four patients at a single center [116]. The imputed intent-to-treat analyses using baseline observations carried forward for discontinuations demonstrated a significant effect of topiramate in most but not all outcomes. These results will need to be reproduced at other centers.

Benzodiazepines potentiate the effect of GABA by binding to the $GABA_A$ receptor. Although a variety of benzodiazepines, including diazepam and clonazepam are used to treat ET, alprazolam is the only benzodiazepine shown to be effective in ET in controlled trials. In one trial [117], alprazolam (dose ranging from 0.75 to 2.75 mg/day) significantly reduced tremor compared with placebo, and 75% of patients demonstrated at least some improvement. However, drowsiness or sedation occurred in 50% of the patients. Another agent, clonazepam did not significantly reduce tremor severity compared with placebo [118]. One problem with the benzodiazepines in general as a treatment for ET is that their anti-tremor effect often comes at a dose that is associated with sedation and/or cognitive slowing.

Calcium channel blockers have had variable success in treating ET. Trials of flunarizine, given at a dose of 10 mg/day have reported mixed results. In one trial, flunarizine significantly reduced tremor compared with placebo; thirteen of fifteen patients improved; however, none of the patients improved in a second trial [119]. Moreover, flunarazine is not available in the United States. In one trial [120], nimodipine, at a daily dose of 30 mg, significantly reduced tremor compared with placebo; eight of fifteen patients improved. Some calcium channel blockers may actually worsen tremor. Tremor was acutely worsened by 71% on average in a study of eight patients [121] on a single oral dose of 10 mg of nifedipine.

Intramuscular botulinum toxin injections may reduce tremor by producing weakness or by blocking gamma motor efferents and muscle spindle efferents. Patients with ET received one to two injections of botulinum toxin or placebo into the intrinsic muscles of the dominant hand in one trial [122]. Although tremor amplitude was significantly reduced, no significant improvement in function was observed. Also, the complication of muscle weakness made a truly blinded study impossible [122].

Action tremor may be mediated by neuronal loops that pass from the cerebellum to the cortex by way of the ventral intermediate nucleus of the thalamus. Clinicians have used two surgical approaches for tremor reduction. These approaches involve continuous deep-brain stimulation through an electrode implanted in the ventral intermediate nucleus of the thalamus and surgical lesioning of the ventral intermediate nucleus of the thalamus (i.e., thalamotomy). The two methods were compared in a prospective randomized single-blinded study [123]. Both procedures were equally effective in reducing tremor [123]. All patients had moderate to severe tremor at baseline and a complete resolution of tremor six months after treatment [123]. Investigators reported greater improvement with thalamic stimulation based on patients' self-reported measures of function. Adverse events were significantly more common in the thalamotomy group. These events included cognitive deterioration, dysarthria, and gait or balance disturbances [123]. Thalamic stimulation is the surgery of choice because fewer adverse events occur and the clinician can adjust the stimulator settings during follow-up care [124].

Nonprescription agents such as ethanol have also traditionally played a role in the treatment of ET. The effect of ethanol on tremor has been demonstrated in several studies. Growden and colleagues [125] documented a 46%–83% decrease in tremor amplitude, measured by accelerometry, in five ET patients—ten to fifteen minutes after the oral ingestion of ethanol. In another study [126], intravenous infusion of ethanol, but not placebo, significantly reduced tremor amplitude in fifteen ET patients. Finally, in a PET study [127], ethanol ingestion led to suppression of tremor and bilateral decreases in cerebellar blood flow in ET patients. One-third of ET patients report that their tremor is ethanol-responsive [128], although many are reluctant to use ethanol for a variety of reasons. First, older patients take medications with which the concurrent use of ethanol is often contraindicated. Second, while some patients report that a glass of wine during an evening social event will reduce the amplitude of their tremor, they are reluctant to use ethanol during day time hours, particularly while working, because of cognitive and soporific effects. Third, there are concerns about dependence and the social stigma of ethanol use. These factors all limit the use of ethanol.

In summary, treatment of ET should be reserved for patients who experience functional disability or embarrassment. Both primidone and propranolol are superior to placebo, and there is some evidence that primidone may be more effective than propranolol. However, this needs to be studied further. The long term tolerability of primidone may be superior, and, therefore, primidone is a reasonable first choice, and, if not tolerated, then propranolol is the second choice. Gabapentin and benzodiazepines are alternatives, although the latter may result in sedation at the doses required to treat tremor. If the patient does not respond to medications and is significantly disabled, then unilateral implantation of a deep brain thalamic stimulator is reasonable. The stimulator should be implanted in the thalamus contralateral to the more functionally disabled arm.

Video Legends

SEGMENT 1 Essential tremor—arm extension.

SEGMENT 2 Essential tremor—water pouring.

SEGMENT 3 Essential tremor—drawing an Archimedes spiral.

References

1. Louis, E.D., L.F. Barnes, S.M. Albert, L. Cote, F. Schneier, S.L. Pullman, and Q. Yu. 2001. Correlates of functional disability in essential tremor. *Mov Disord* **16**:914–920.
2. Louis, E.D., and P. Greene. 2000. Essential tremor. In *Merritt Textbook of Neurology*, 10th Edition. Ed. L.P. Rowland. pp. 678–679. Philadelphia: Lea & Febiger.
3. Hubble, J.P., K.L. Busenbark, and W.C. Koller. 1989. Essential tremor. *Clin Neuropharm* **12**:453–482.
4. Findley, L.J., and W.C. Koller. 1987. Essential tremor: A review. *Neurology* **37**:1194–1197.
5. Critchley, M. 1949. Observations on essential tremor (heredofamilial tremor). *Brain* **72**:113–139.
6. Stolze, H., G. Petersen, J. Raethjen, R. Wenzelburger, and G. Deuschl. 2000. Gait analysis in essential tremor—further evidence for a cerebellar dysfunction. *Mov Disord* **15**(Suppl 3):87.
7. Deuschl, G., R. Wenzelburger, K. Loffler, J. Raethjen, and H. Stolze. 2000. Essential tremor and cerebellar dysfunction. Clinical and kinematic analysis of intention tremor. *Brain* **123**:1568–1580.
8. Singer, C., J. Sanchez-Ramos, and Weiner. 1994. Gait abnormality in essential tremor. *Mov Dis* **9**:193–196.
9. Rajput, A.H., B. Rozdilsky, L. Ang, and A. Rajput. 1993. Significance of Parkinsonian manifestations in essential tremor. *Can J Neurol Sci* **20**:114–117.
10. Cohen, O., S. Pullman, E. Jurewicz, D. Watner, and E.D. Louis. 2003. Rest tremor in essential tremor patients: Prevalence, clinical correlates, and electrophysiological characteristics. *Arch Neurol* **60**: 405–410.
11. Gasparini, M., V. Bonifati, E. Fabrizio, G. Fabbrini, L. Brusa, G.L. Lenzi, G. Meco. 2001. Frontal lobe dysfunction in essential tremor. A preliminary study. *J Neurol* **248**:399–402.
12. Lombardi, W.J., D.J. Woolston, W.J. Roberts, and R.E. Gross. 2001. Cognitive deficits in patients with essential tremor. *Neurology* **57**:785–790.
13. Louis, E.D., and R. Ottman. 1996. How familial is familial tremor? Genetic epidemiology of essential tremor. *Neurology* **46**:1200–1205.
14. Bain, P.G., L.J. Findley, P.D. Thompson, M.A. Gresty, J.C. Rothwell, A.E. Harding, and C.D. Marsden. 1994. A study of hereditary essential tremor. *Brain* **117**:805–824.
15. Gulcher, J.R., P. Jonsson, A. Kong, et al. 1997. Mapping of a familial essential tremor gene, FET1, to chromosome 3q13. *Nature Genetics* **17**:84–87.
16. Higgins, J.J., J.M. Loveless, J. Jankovic, and P.I. Patel. 1998. Evidence that a gene for essential tremor maps to chromosome 2p in four families. *Mov Disord* **13**:972–977.
17. Higgins, L.T., J.J. Pho, and Nee. 1997. A gene (ETM) for essential tremor maps to chromosome 2p22–p25. *Mov Disord* **12**:859–864.
18. Elble, R.J. 1998. Animal models of action tremor. *Mov Disord* **13**(Suppl 3):35–39.
19. Cavanagh, J.B., J.L. Holton, C.C. Nolan, C.C. Ray, D.E. Naik, and P.G. Mantle. 1998. The effects of the tremorogenic mycotoxin penitrem A on the rat cerebellum. *Vet Pathol* **35**:53–63.
20. Louis, E.D., R. Ottman, and W.A. Hauser. 1998. How common is the most common adult movement disorder? Estimates of the prevalence of essential tremor throughout the world **13**:5–10.
21. Rautakorpi, I., J. Takala, R.J. Martilla, K. Sievers, and U.K. Rinne. 1982. Essential tremor in a Finnish population. *Acta Neurol Scandinav* **66**:58–67.
22. Louis, E.D., B. Ford, B. Frucht, L.F. Barnes, M-X. Tang, and R. Ottman. 2001. Risk of tremor and impairment from tremor in relatives of patients with essential tremor: A community based family study. *Ann Neurol* **49**:761–769.
23. Dogu, O., S. Sevin, H. Camdeviren, T. Sasmaz, R. Bugdayci, M. Aral, H. Kaleagasi, and E.D. Louis. 2003. Prevalence of essential tremor: Door-to-door neurological exams in Mersin Province, Turkey. *Neurology* **61**:1804–1807.
24. Rajput, A.H., K.P. Offord, C.M. Beard, and L.T. Kurland. 1984. Essential tremor in Rochester, Minnesota: A 45-year study. *J Neurol Neurosurg Psychiatry* **47**:466–470.
25. Louis, E.D., K. Marder, L. Cote, S. Pullman, B. Ford, D. Wilder, M.-X. Tang, et al. 1995. Differences in the prevalence of essential tremor among elderly African-Americans, Whites and Hispanics in Northern Manhattan, NY. *Arch Neurol* **52**:1201–1205.
26. Haerer, A.F., D.W. Anderson, and B.S. Schoenberg. 1992. Prevalence of essential tremor. Results from the Copiah county study. *Arch Neurol* **39**:750–751.
27. Louis, E.D., L.P. Fried, A.L. Fitzpatrick, W.T. Longstreth, and A.B. Newman. 2003. Regional and racial differences in the prevalence of physician diagnosed essential tremor in the United States. *Mov Disord* **18**:1035–1040.
28. Brennan, K.C., E. Jurewicz, B. Ford, S.L. Pullman, and E.D. Louis. 2002. Is essential tremor predominantly a kinetic or a postural tremor? A clinical and electrophysiological study. *Mov Disord* **17**: 313–316.
29. Lou, J.S., and J. Jankovic. 1991. Essential tremor: Clinical correlates in 350 patients. *Neurology* **41**:234–238.
30. Hubble, J.P., K.L. Busenbark, R. Pahwa, K. Lyons, and W.C. Koller. 1997. Clinical expression of essential tremor: Effects of gender and age. *Mov Disord* **12**:969–972.
31. Ashenhurst, E.M. 1973. The nature of essential tremor. *CMAJ* **109**: 876–878.
32. Louis, E.D., B. Ford, and S. Frucht. 2003. Factors associated with increased risk of head tremor in essential tremor: A community-based study in northern Manhattan. *Mov Disord* **18**:432–436.
33. Koller, W.C., and F.A. Rubino. 1985. Combined resting postural tremors. *Arch Neurol* **42**:683–684.
34. Brooks, D.J., E.D. Playford, V. Ibanez, et al. 1992. Isolated tremor and disruption of the nigrostriatal dopaminergic system: An 18F-Dopa PET study. *Neurology* **42**:1554–1560.
35. Louis, E.D., and E.C. Jurewicz. 2003. Olfaction in essential tremor patients with and without isolated rest tremor. *Mov Disord* **18**:1387–1389.
36. Lacritz, L.H., R. Dewey, Jr., C. Giller, and C.M. Cullum. 2002. Cognitive functioning in individuals with "benign" essential tremor. *J Int Neuropsychol Soc* **8**:125–129.
37. Vermilion, K., A. Stone, and D. Duane. 2001. Cognition and affect in idiopathic essential tremor. *Mov Disord* **16**:S30.
38. Duane, D.D., and K.J. Vermilion. 2002. Cognitive deficits in patients with essential tremor. *Neurology* **58**:1706.

39. Chatterjee, A., E.C. Jurewicz, L.M. Applegate, and E.D. Louis. 2004 Personality in essential tremor. *Neurology Neurosurg Psychiatry* **75**:958–961.
40. Louis, E.D., S.M. Bromley, E.C. Jurewicz, and D. Watner. 2002. Olfactory dysfunction in essential tremor: A deficit unrelated to disease duration or severity. *Neurology* **59**:1631–1633.
41. Ondo, W., K.D. Vuong, L. Sutton, and J. Jankovic. 2002. Assessment of hearing loss in essential tremor. *Neurology* **58**(Suppl 3):A219–A220.
42. Shukla, G., M. Bhatia, R.M. Pandey, and M. Behari. 2002. Peripheral silent periods in essential tremor. *J Neurol Sci* **199**:55–58.
43. Louis, E.D., K. Marder, E.C. Jurewicz, D. Watner, G. Levy, and H. Mejia-Santana. 2002. Body mass index in essential tremor. *Arch Neurol* **59**:1273–1277.
44. Dogu, O., S. Sevin, E.D. Louis, H. Kaleagasi, and M. Aral. 2004 Reduced body mass index in essential tremor: A population-based study in Mersin Province, Turkey. *Arch Neurol* **61**:386–389.
45. Larsson, T., and T. Sjogren. 1960. Essential tremor: A clinical and genetic population study. *Acta Psychiatrica Et Neurologica Scandinavica* **36**(Suppl 144):1–176.
46. Louis, E.D., R.A. Ottman, B. Ford, S. Pullman, M. Martinez, S. Fahn, and W.A. Hauser. 1997. The Washington Heights Essential Tremor Study: Methodologic issues in essential-tremor research. *Neuroepidemiology* **16**:124–133.
47. Rautakorpi, I. 1978. Essential Tremor. An epidemiological, clinical and genetic study. *Research Reports from the Department of Neurology*, No. 12, University of Turku, Finland.
48. Koller, W.C., N. Biary, and S. Cone. 1986. Disability in essential tremor: Effect of treatment. *Neurology* **36**:1001–1004.
49. Elble, R.J. 2000. Essential tremor frequency decreases with time. *Neurology* **55**:1547–1551.
50. Louis, E.D., D. Shungu, S. Chan, X. Mao, E.C. Jurewicz, and D. Watner. 2002. Metabolic abnormality in essential tremor: A ^{1}H Magnetic Resonance Spectroscopic Imaging Study. *Neurosci Lett* **333**:17–20.
51. Tedeschi, G., A. Bertolini, G. Campbell, et al. 1996. Reproducibility of proton MR spectroscopic imaging findings. *Am J Neuroradiol* **17**: 1871–1879.
52. Constantinidis, I. 1998. Magnetic resonance spectroscopy and the practing neurologist. *The Neurologist* **4**:77–98.
53. Ross, B.D., and S. Bluml. 1999. Neurospectroscopy. In *Euroimaging*. Ed. J.O. Greenberg. New York: The McGraw-Hill Companies, Inc.
54. Mylle, G., and L. Van Bogaert. 1948. Du tremblement essentiel non familial. *Monatsschr Psychiatr Neurol* **115**:80–90.
55. Hassler, R. 1939. Zur pathologischen Anatomie des senilen und des parkinsonistischen Tremor. *J Psychol Neurol* **49**:193–230.
56. Mylle, G., and L. Van Bogaert. 1940. Etudes anatomo-cliniques de syndromes hypercinetiques complexes. I. Sur le tremblement familial. *Mschr Psychiatr Neurol* **103**:28–43.
57. Herskovitz, E., and W. Blackwood. 1969. Essential (familial, hereditary) tremor: A case report. *J Neurol Neurosurg Psychiatry* **32**:509–511.
58. Bergamasco, I. 1907. Intorno ad un caso di tremore essenziale simulant in parte il quadro della sclerosi multipla. *Riv Pat Nerv Ment* **115**: 80–90.
59. Lapresle, J., P. Rondot, and G. Said. 1974. Idiopathic rest, attitude and action tremor. Anato-clinical study of one case. *Rev Neurol* (Paris) **130**:343–348.
60. Rajput, A.H., B. Rozdilsky, L. Ang, and A. Rajput. 1991. Clinicopathological observations in essential tremor: Report of six cases. *Neurology* **41**:1422–1424.
61. Frankl-Hochwart. 1903. A degenerescence hepato-lenticulaire (maladie de Wilson, pseudo-sclerose). Paris: Masson et Cie.
62. Boockvar, J., A. Telfeian, and G.H. Baltuch. 2000. Long-term deep brain stimulation in a patient with essential tremor: Clinical response and postmortem correlation with stimulator termination sites in ventral thalamus. *J Neurosurg* **93**:140–144.
63. Ellis, R.S. 1920. Norms for some structural changes in the human cerebellum from birth to old age. *J Comp Neurol* **32**:1–33.
64. Hall, T.C., A.K.H. Miller, and J.A.N. Corsellis. 1975. Variations in the human Purkinje cell population according to age and sex. *Neuropathol Appl Neurobiol* **1**:267–292.
65. Koller, W.C., B. Vetere-Overfield, and R. Barter. 1989. Tremors in early Parkinson disease. *Clin Neuropharmacol* **12**:293–297.
66. Tanner, C.M., S.M. Goldman, K.E. Lyons, D.A. Aston, J.W. Tetrud, M.D. Welsh, J.W. Langston, and W.C. Koller. 2001. Essential tremor in twins: An assessment of genetic vs. environmental determinants of etiology. *Neurology* **57**:1389–1391.
67. Louis, E.D. 2001. Etiology of essential tremor: Should we be searching for environmental causes? *Mov Disord* **16**:822–829.
68. Louis, E.D., L.F. Barnes, B. Ford, and R. Ottman. 2001. Family history information on essential tremor: Potential biases related to the source of the cases. *Mov Disord* **16**:320–324.
69. Louis, E.D., B. Ford, R. Ottman, and K.J. Wendt. 1999. Validity of family history data in essential tremor. *Mov Disord* **14**:456–461.
70. Weiss, K.M., R. Chakraborty, and P.P. Majumder. 1982. Problems in the assessment of relative risk of chronic disease among biological relatives of affected individuals. *J Chron Dis* **35**:539–551.
71. Louis, E.D., B. Ford, S. Frucht, and R. Ottman. 2001. Mild tremor in relatives of patients with essential tremor: What does this tell us about the penetrance of the disease? *Arch Neurology* **58**:1584–1589.
72. Salemi, G., G. Savettieri, W.A. Rocca, et al. 1994. Prevalence of essential tremor: A door-to-door survey in Terrasini, Sicily. *Neurology* **44**:61–64.
73. Hornabrook, R.W., and J.T. Nagurney. 1976. Essential tremor in Papau New Guinea. *Brain* **99**:659–672.
74. Martinelli, P., A.S. Gabellini, M.R. Gulli, and E. Lugaresi. 1987. Different clinical features of essential tremor: a 200-patient study. *Acta Neurol Scand* **75**:106–111.
75. Louis, E.D., E.C. Jurewicz, L. Applegate, P. Factor-Litvak, M. Parides, L. Andrews, V. Slavkovich, et al. 2003. Association between essential tremor and blood lead concentration. *Environ Health Perspect* **111**:1707–1711.
76. Louis, E.D., W. Zheng, E.C. Jurewicz, D. Watner, J. Chen, P. Factor-Litvak, and M. Parides. 2002. Elevation of blood β-carboline alkaloids in essential tremor. *Neurology* **59**:1940–1944.
77. Louis, E.D. 2001. Essential tremor. *N Engl J Med* **345**:887–891.
78. Louis, E.D., L.A. Klatka, Y. Lui, and S. Fahn. 1997. Comparison of extrapyramidal features in 31 pathologically confirmed cases of diffuse Lewy body disease and 34 pathologically confirmed cases of Parkinson disease. *Neurology* **48**:376–380.
79. Scheinberg, I.H., and I. Sternlieb. 1984. *Wilson disease*. Philadelphia: W.B. Saunders.
80. Walshe, J.M., and M. Yealland. 1992. Wilson disease: The problem of delayed diagnosis. *J Neurology Neurosurg Psychiatry* **55**:692–696.
81. Colebatch, J.G., L.J. Findley, R.S.J. Frackowiak, C.D. Marsden, and D.J. Brooks. 1990. Preliminary report: Activation of the cerebellum in essential tremor. *Lancet* **336**:1028–1030.
82. Hallet, M., and R.M. Dubinsky. 1993. Glucose metabolism in the brain of patients with essential tremor. *J Neurol Sci* **114**:45–48.
83. Wills, A.J., I.H. Jenkins, P.D. Thompson, L.J. Findley, and D.J. Brooks. 1994. Red nuclear and cerebellar but no olivary activation associated with essential tremor: A positron emission tomographic study. *Ann Neurol* **36**:636–642.
84. Jenkins, I.H., P.G. Bain, J.G. Colebatch, et al. 1993. A positron emission tomography study of essential tremor: Evidence for overactivity of cerebellar connections. *Ann Neurol* **34**:82–90.
85. Louis, E.D., B. Ford, and B. Bismuth. 1998. Reliability between two observers using a protocol for diagnosing essential tremor. *Mov Disord* **13**:287–293.

86. Bucher, S.F., K.C. Seelos, R.C. Dodel, M. Reiser, and W.H. Oertel. 1997. Activation mapping in essential tremor with functional magnetic resonance imaging. *Ann Neurol* **41**:32–40.
87. Grodd, W.E., E. Hulsmann, M. Lotze, D. Wildgruber, and M. Erb. 2001. Sensorimotor mapping of human cerebellum: fMRI evidence of somatotopic organization. *Hum Brain Mapp* **13**:55–73.
88. Ohearn, E., and M.E. Molliver. 1997. The olivocerebellar projection mediates ibogaine-induced degeneration of Purkinje cells: A model of indirect, trans-synaptic excitotoxicity. *J Neurosci* **17**:8828–8841.
89. Pennes, H.H., and P.H. Hoch. 1957. Psychotomimetics, clinical and theoretical considerations: harmine, Win-2299 and Nalline. *Am J Psychiatry* **113**:885–892.
90. Lewin, L. 1928. Untersuchungen uber Banisteria caapi. *Sp Arch Exp Pathol Pharmacol* **129**:133–149.
91. Milner, T.E., G. Cadoret, L. Lessard, and A.M. Smith, 1995. EMG analysis of harmaline-induced tremor in normal and three strains of mutant mice with Purkinje cell degeneration and the role of the inferior olive. *J Neurophysiol* **73**:2568–2577.
92. Trouvin, J.H., P. Jacqmin, C. Rouch, M. Lesne, and C.C. Jacquot. 1987. Benzodiazepine receptors are involved in taberanthine-induced tremor: *in vitro* and *in vivo* evidence. *Eur J Pharmacol* **140**:303–309.
93. Fuentes, J.A., and V.G. Longo. 1971. An investigation on the central effects of harmine, harmaline and related B-carbolines. *Neuropharmacology* **10**:15–23.
94. Cross, A.J., A. Misra, A. Sandilands, M.J. Taylor, and A.R. Green. 1993. Effect of chlormethiazole, dizocilpine and pentobarbital on harmaline-induced increase of cerebellar cyclic GMP and tremor. *Psychopharmacology* **111**:96–98.
95. Sinton, C.M., B.I. Krosser, K.D. Walton, and R.R. Llinas. 1989. The effectiveness of different isomers of octanol as blockers of harmaline-induced tremor. *Pflugers Arch* **414**:31–36.
96. Rappaport, M.S., R.T. Gentry, D.R. Schneider, and V.P. Dole. 1984. Ethanol effects on harmaline-induced tremor and increase of cerebellar cyclic GMP. *Life Sci* **34**:49–56.
97. Kralic, J.E., E.R. Korpi, T.K. O'Buckley, G.E. Homanics, and A.L. Morrow. 2002. Molecular and pharmacological characterization of $GABA_A$ receptor α1 subunit knockout mice. *J Pharmacol Exp Therap* **302**:1037–1045.
98. Louis, E.D., B. Ford, and L.F. Barnes. 2000. Clinical subtypes of essential tremor. *Arch Neurol* **57**:1194–1198.
99. Winkler, G.F., and R.R. Young. 1971. The control of essential tremor by propranolol. *Trans Am Neurol Assoc* **96**:66–68.
100. Obrien, M.D., A.R. Upton, and P.A. Toseland. 1981. Benign familial tremor treated with primidone. *BMJ* **282**:178–180.
101. Louis, E.D. 1999. A new twist for stopping the shakes? Revisiting GABAergic therapy for essential tremor. *Arch Neurol* **56**:807–808.
102. Rajput, A.H., O. Hornykiewicz, Y. Deng, S. Birdi, H. Miyashita, and R. Macaulay. 2001. Increased noradrenaline levels in essential tremor. *Neurology* **56**(Suppl 3):A302.
103. Jefferson, D., P. Jenner, and C.D. Marsden. 1979. β-Adrenoreceptor antagonists in essential tremor. *J Neurology Neurosurg Psychiatry* **42**:904–909.
104. Tolosa, E.S., and R.B. Loewenson. 1975. Essential tremor: Treatment with propranolol. *Neurology* **25**:1041–1044.
105. Dietrischson, P., and E. Espen. 1981. Effects of timolol and atenolol on benign essential tremor: Placebo-controlled studies based on quantitative recording. *J Neurology Neurosurg Psychiatry* **44**:677–683.
106. Cleeves, L., and L.J. Findley. 1988. Propranolol and propranolol-LA in essential tremor: A double blind comparative study. *J Neurol Neurosurg Psychiatry* **51**:379–384.
107. Findley, L.H., L. Cleeves, and S. Calzetti. 1985. Primidone in essential tremor of the hands and head: A double blind controlled clinical study. *J Neurol Neurosurg Psychiatry* **48**:911–915.
108. Sasso, E., E. Perucca, R. Fava, and S. Calzetti. 1990. Primidone in the long-term treatment of essential tremor: A prospective study with computerized quantitative analysis. *Clin Neuropharm* **13**:67–76.
109. Gorman, W.P., R. Cooper, P. Pocock, and M.J. Campbell. 1986. A comparison of primidone, propranolol, and placebo in essential tremor, using quantitative analysis. *J Neurol Neurosurg Psychiatry* **49**:64–68.
110. Sasso, E., E. Perucca, and S. Calzetti. 1988. Double-blind comparison of primidone and phenobarbital in essential tremor. *Neurology* **38**:808–810.
111. Koller, W.C., and V.L. Royse. 1986. Efficacy of primidone in essential tremor. *Neurology* **36**:121–124.
112. Koller, W.C., and B. Vetere-Overfield. 1989. Acute and chronic effects of propranolol and primidone in essential tremor. *Neurology* **39**: 1587–1588.
113. Gironell, A., J. Kulisevsky, M. Barbanoj, D. Lopez-Villegas, G. Hernandez, and B. Pascual-Sedano. 1999. A randomized placebo-controlled comparative trial of gabapentin and propranolol in essential tremor. *Arch Neurol* **56**:475–480.
114. Pahwa, R., K. Lyons, J.P. Hubble, et al. 1998. Double-blind controlled trial of gabapentin in essential tremor. *Mov Disord* **13**:465–467.
115. Ondo, W., C. Hunter, K. Dat Vuong, K. Schwartz, and J. Jankovic. 2000. Gabapentin for essential tremor: A multiple-dose, double-blind, placebo-controlled trial. *Mov Disord* **15**:678–682.
116. Connor, G.S. 2000. Efficacy of topiramate in treatment of essential tremor: A randomized, double-blind, placebo-controlled, cross-over study. *Ann Neurol* **48**:486.
117. Huber, S.J., and G.W. Paulson. 1988. Efficacy of alprazolam for essential tremor. *Neurology* **38**:241–243.
118. Thompson, C., A. Lang, J.D. Parkes, and C.D. Marsden. 1984. A double-blind trial of clonazepam in benign essential tremor. *Clin Neuropharm* **7**:83–88.
119. Curran, T., and A.E. Lang. 1993. Flunarizine in essential tremor. *Clin Neuropharm* **16**:460–463.
120. Biary, N., Y. Bahou, M.A. Sofi, W. Thomas, and S.M. Al Deeb. 1995. The effect of nimodipine on essential tremor. *Neurology* **45**:1523–1525.
121. Topaktas, S., R. Onur, and T. Dalkara. 1987. Calcium channel blockers and essential tremor. *Eur Neurol* **27**:114–119.
122. Jankovic, J., K. Schwartz, W. Clemence, A. Aswad, and J. Mordunt. 1996. A randomized, double-blind, placebo-controlled study to evaluate botulinum toxin type A in essential hand tremor. *Mov Disord* **11**:250–256.
123. Schuurman, P.R., D.A. Bosch, P.M.M. Bossuyt, et al. 2000. A comparison of continuous thalamic stimulation and thalamotomy for suppression of severe tremor. *N Engl J Med* **432**:461–468.
124. Hariz, G.M., M. Lindberg, and A.T. Bergenheim. 2002. Impact of thalamic deep brain stimulation on disability and health-related quality of life in patients with essential tremor. *J Neurol Neurosurg Psychiatry* **72**:47–52.
125. Growden, J.H., B.T. Shahani, and R.R. Young. 1975. The effect of alcohol on essential tremor. *Neurology* **25**:259–262.
126. Koller, W.C., and N. Biary. 1984. Effect of alcohol on tremors: comparison with propranolol. *Neurology* **34**:221–222.
127. Boecker, H., A.J. Wills, A. Ceballos-Baumann, et al. 1996. The effect of ethanol on alcohol-responsive essential tremor: A positron emission tomography study. *Ann Neurol* **39**:650–658.
128. Koller, W.C., K. Busenbark, and K. Miner. 1994. The relationship between essential tremor and other movement disorders. *Ann Neurol* **35**:717–723.

C H A P T E R

E3

Harmaline Tremor

MARK LeDOUX

Although tremor is a common sign of neurological disorders such as Parkinson disease, Wilson disease, and hereditary ataxia, most adults with clinically significant tremor have idiopathic or essential tremor (ET). Millions of Americans including at least four percent of adults over the age of fifty have ET, a bothersome and sometimes disabling movement disorder (Elble and Koller 1990; Louis et al. 1998). ET is a 4- to 12-Hz action tremor with a prominent postural and relatively milder kinetic component (Elble and Koller 1990). While ET mainly affects the arms, the head and voice are also often involved. Mechanical loads have little effect on the frequency of ET, which distinguishes ET from enhanced physiological tremor. The postural nature of ET often significantly interferes with activities of daily living such as eating and writing. For some patients, drinking from a glass without spilling becomes impossible. Persons with occupations dependent on manual dexterity such as secretaries with typing responsibilities, surgeons, and dentists may be forced into early retirement. The prevalence of ET increases with advancing age and men seem to be affected more frequently than women (Elble and Koller 1990; Hubble et al. 1997). In many patients, ET improves, sometimes dramatically, after the consumption of alcoholic beverages (Growdon et al. 1975). Medical treatments for ET include the drugs primidone and propranolol. Thalamic deep brain stimulation is employed in patients with incapacitating ET that does not respond well to medications. In many ET patients, the response to medical and surgical treatments may be inadequate, associated with significant side effects, or both.

The pathophysiology and etiology of ET are poorly understood. The drug harmaline has been shown to produce a generalized tremor at frequencies of 5–14 Hz in rodents, rabbits, cats, and primates by producing oscillatory firing of neurons within the inferior olive (IO). Harmaline-induced tremor has been proposed as a model for ET (Poirier et al. 1966; Llinás and Volkind 1973; Lamarre 1975, 1984; Batini et al. 1981; Bernard et al. 1984b). ET and harmaline tremor share numerous similarities and, as such, the latter may be a useful tool for understanding and treating the former.

I. PATHOPHYSIOLOGY OF ESSENTIAL TREMOR

ET is caused by a rhythmic 4- to 12-Hz entrainment of motor unit activity that forces the affected body part into oscillation of the same frequency. Characteristically, mechanical (mass) loads applied to the affected body part, such as a 500-gram weight applied to the dorsum of an ET patient's hand, have no significant effect on the frequency of ET, which remains in-phase with electromyographic (EMG) activity (Elble 1986; Homberg et al. 1987). Evidence from human studies suggests that ET is produced by a central nonlinear oscillator (Elble and Koller 1990). The IO is one such oscillator and has been proposed as a site of likely pathophysiological significance to ET.

Clinical-pathological correlations, positron emission tomography (PET), and functional magnetic resonance imaging (fMRI) point to the cerebellum and IO as sites possibly critical to the pathophysiology of ET. For instance, ET has been eliminated ipsilateral to cerebellar infarcts and contralateral to pontine lacunar infarcts. Moreover, ET patients tend to exhibit mild cerebellar gait ataxia (Hubble et al. 1997). PET and fMRI studies in ET patients have shown abnormal bilateral over-activity of cerebellar and red nuclear connections but found no evidence of intrinsic over-activity of the IO (Wills et al. 1994; Bucher et al. 1997). Another PET study suggested that circuits involving the IO are involved in the generation of ET because of glucose hypermetabolism in the medulla, although the IO was not definitively identified as the source of the increased medullary signal (Hallet and Dubinsky 1993).

Depending on study criteria and geographic location, 17% to 70% of patients have a positive family history of ET (Elble and Koller 1990; Louis et al. 1998). In families with ET, the inheritance pattern is autosomal dominant. Loci for ET were identified on chromosomes 3q13 (ETM1; Gulcher et al. 1997) and 2p24 (ETM2; Higgins et al. 1997). The ETM2 locus was reported in an American family of Czech descent and the EMT1 locus was found in Icelandic families. The ETM1 and EMT2 loci were excluded in other families with ET by pairwise and multipoint linkage analysis (Kovach et al. 2001). Therefore, studies to date indicate that ET is genetically heterogeneous.

Despite the apparent genetic heterogeneity of ET, certain clinical features of this disorder are common to most families with ET and to individuals with sporadic ET (Elble and Koller 1990). ET is predominantly a postural tremor with a mild to moderate kinetic component. A resting component can be seen in severe cases. Reduction of tremor with alcoholic beverages supports the diagnosis. Tremor does not affect the eyes and is usually asymptomatic in the lower extremities. In addition to the typical involvement of the upper extremities, the head, neck, and voice are commonly affected in ET. The frequency of ET (4–12 Hz) overlaps with the frequencies of most other tremors such that definitive identification of ET cannot be made by frequency alone. There is a strong negative correlation between tremor frequency and amplitude and a negative correlation between tremor frequency and patient age (Elble et al. 1994). The full range of tremor frequencies can be seen in the same family.

The physiological properties of ET indicate a central origin. The low-amplitude mechanical-reflex (MR) oscillation seen in both ET patients and normal subjects is produced by a combination of underdamped limb mechanics and the stretch reflex. The frequency of this component is determined in large part by the stiffness and mass of the limb. Mechanical (mass) loads have little effect on the frequency of ET but reduce the frequency of MR oscillations. In patients with ET, MR oscillation and ET can exhibit resonance when their frequencies are similar. However, when a mechanical (mass) load separates MR and essential tremors, resonance is abolished resulting in reduced tremor amplitude. With a mass load applied to the hand of ET patients and EMG electrodes over the extensor digitorum brevis muscle, spectral analysis of accelerometry recordings will produce two tremor peaks (MR and ET) while spectral analysis of the EMG will yield a single peak at the ET frequency (Elble 1986; Homberg et al. 1987).

II. ANIMAL MODELS OF ACTION TREMOR

Because the geometry and biomechanical properties of their limbs differ from humans, animal models *cannot* entirely mimic the kinematics of ET or, for that matter, any other human tremor. Furthermore, even skilled clinicians occasionally have difficulty distinguishing classic "tremor" disorders such as ET and Parkinson disease from one another. For instance, diagnostic confusion can arise because some patients with severe ET may exhibit a rest tremor and most patients with Parkinson disease have an action tremor. Thus, finding consensus on the face validity of animal models of human tremor disorders is often problematic.

Many animal models of action tremor are currently available to the research community. Action tremors are a prominent phenotypic feature of many rodents with spontaneous mutations; examples include trembler, vibrator, shiverer, and jumpy mice and zitter rats. Unlike humans with ET, however, these mutant rodents show severe pathological changes such as demyelination or spongiform degeneration of the peripheral and/or central nervous systems. In contrast, $GABA_A$ receptor α-1 subunit knock-out mice are pathologically normal and show an action tremor with both postural and kinetic components (Kralic et al. 2002).

Numerous pharmacological agents can induce action tremors. Unfortunately, only the tremors induced by harmaline and closely related compounds may have both face and predictive validity as models of ET. For example, the muscarinic-agonist tremorogenic agent, oxotremorine, produces a generalized tremor in a variety of mammalian species that does not require an intact olivocerebellar system. The oxotremorine tremor frequency (>12 Hz) is outside the range of human ET. Moreover, unlike ET, the tremor induced by oxotremorine does not improve significantly with moderate doses of ethanol (Rappaport et al. 1984).

In primates, the neurotoxin MPTP consistently produces three cardinal features of Parkinson disease: rigidity, bradykinesia, and postural instability. The characteristics and even the presence of tremor after exposure to MPTP are highly dependent on route of toxin administration, dosage, species, and the age of treated animals. In most reports, MPTP is actually associated with an action tremor with both postural and kinetic components rather than a resting tremor. In this regard, the tremorogenic effects of MPTP may depend, in part, on damage to the locus ceruleus. Although not commonly considered as a model of ET, the action tremor produced by MPTP is important because it may point to neural pathways involved in ET.

III. HARMALINE: ORIGINS AND CLINICAL EFFECTS

Harmaline, a β-carboline, is widely distributed in the plant kingdom (Figure 1). Plants within over eight botanical families manufacture harmaline, harmine, harmalol, harman, and related hallucinogenic alkaloids. Harmaline was first isolated from the seeds of Syrian rue (*Peganum harmala*), a wild desert shrub of Central Asia, Syria, and the Middle East. In Amazonia, harmaline, harmine and related alkaloids are derived from the bark and stems of ayahuasca (*Banisteriopsis caapi*). Ayahuasca and Syrian rue have been used in folk medicine for millennia. In some regions of the Middle East and North Africa, *Peganum harmala* is still used as an abortifacient and emmenagogue.

Few detailed accounts exist of human harmaline intoxication in the medical literature. For illustration, as described in a recent report from Iran, a thirty-five-year-old male patient consumed around 150 grams of *Peganum harmala* seeds and shortly thereafter, he experienced gastrointestinal distress, hematemesis, and visual hallucinations (Mahmoudian et al. 2002). His physicians noted tremors of the limbs and face. He was also tachycardic and hypotensive. Unfortunately, the reporting physicians did not provide a more detailed description of motor abnormalities in their patient. After a few hours, the signs and symptoms of toxicity resolved.

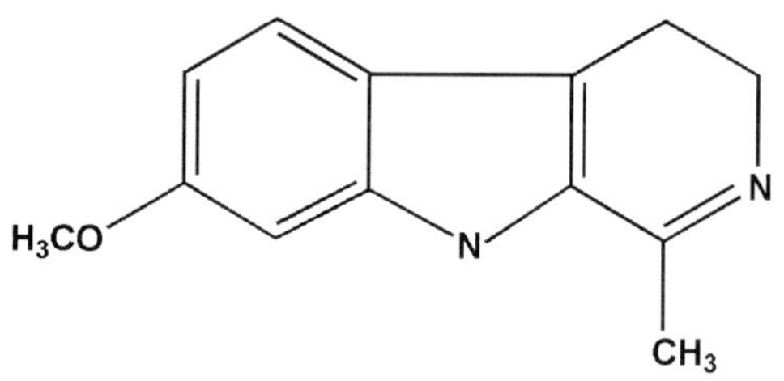

FIGURE 1 Two-dimensional structure of harmaline.

IV. CHARACTERISTICS OF HARMALINE TREMOR IN THE LABORATORY

A. Pharmacodynamics

Although harmaline is readily absorbed from the gut, most studies have employed intraperitoneal, subcutaneous, or intravenous administration. Different investigators have used a wide harmaline dosing range (0.5–100 mg/kg) to examine various aspects of olivocerebellar function. All mammals (e.g., mice, rats, rabbits, cats, monkeys) exhibit a readily perceptible tremor after receiving harmaline. In rodents and cats, a visible tremor is typically seen with dosages of 5 mg/kg and greater. After intravenous administration of harmaline, latency to tremor onset is one to two minutes. After subcutaneous and intraperitoneal administration, latency is three to ten minutes. Tremor amplitude typically plateaus within ten minutes of onset. Tremor duration depends on route of administration and dosage and ranges from thirty minutes to three hours.

Striking tolerance to repeated administration is a largely unexplained but critically important feature of harmaline pharmacology (Lutes et al. 1988; Wang and Fowler 2001). In some respects, the development of tolerance limits the utility of the harmaline model for testing drugs to treat tremor. Tolerance to harmaline tremor probably takes place within olivocerebellar pathways rather than at downstream motor sites (Lutes et al. 1988). More specifically, tolerance may be due to an altered Purkinje cell postsynaptic response to climbing fiber input (Lorden et al. 1988). In contrast, there appears to be much less tolerance to other neurological effects of harmaline (Stanford and Fowler 1998).

B. Frequency and Distribution of Harmaline Tremor

Harmaline tremor frequency has been reported as 5–14 Hz: 11–14 Hz (mice; Milner et al. 1995), 8–12 Hz (cats; Lamarre and Mercier 1971), 4.7–7.6 Hz (rhesus macaque; Ohye et al. 1970), and 10–12 Hz (rats; Yamazaki et al. 1979). Tremor frequency is seemingly independent of harmaline dosage. In contrast, tremor amplitude does depend, in large part, on harmaline dosage. Harmaline-induced tremor is an action tremor with both postural and kinetic components. At lower dosages, tremor may be present only intermittently. Tremor is accentuated by movement and it is most noticeable in the neck, trunk, and proximal muscles. Tremor can also be detected in the forelimbs (Stanford and Fowler 1998), whiskers, and facial muscles, however (Yang and Iadecola 1998). In one report, harmaline tremor disappeared from normal mice during swimming (Milner et al. 1995); one possible interpretation of this finding is that postural maintenance activates harmaline tremor.

Based on electromyographic (EMG) recordings, harmaline tremor is synchronous in agonist-antagonist muscle pairs such as the quadriceps and hamstrings (Lamarre and Mercier 1971; Milner et al. 1995). Moreover, EMG activity is synchronous in all muscles. For instance, EMG activity in the right deltoid and left hamstring muscles occurs simultaneously after administration of harmaline (Lamarre and Mercier 1971).

C. Additional Behavioral Effects

Besides tremor, a variety of neural and non-neural signs are seen after administration of harmaline to experimental animals. Even at relatively low dosages (5–10 mg/kg), most rodents exhibit decreased locomotor activity, mild ataxia, and hindlimb abduction (see video). With higher dosages, rodents may show hunched back, piloerection, and autonomic disturbances such as tachycardia and sialorrhea. In rodents, seizures may occur at dosages above 40 mg/kg.

D. Response of Harmaline Tremor to Drugs Used for ET

Most neurologists choose primidone as initial therapy for ET. Primidone is metabolized to phenobarbital and phenylmethylmalonamide. Pentobarbital, a commonly used anesthetic closely related to phenobarbital, inhibits harmaline tremor at comparatively low dosages (Cross et al. 1993). In contrast, a variety of β-blockers including propranolol have no significant effect on harmaline tremor (Iwata et al. 1993). Benzodiazepines are occasionally beneficial in some patients with ET. In one study, the benzodiazepine diazepam markedly reduced the power spectral density of harmaline tremor (Shinozaki et al. 1985).

V. NEURAL ORIGIN OF HARMALINE TREMOR

By creating neural lesions in stepwise fashion, Lamarre and colleagues localized the origin of harmaline tremor to the olivocerebellar pathways (Lamarre and Mercier 1971). Neither mid-collicular midbrain nor mid-thoracic spinal cord transactions eliminated harmaline-induced forelimb tremor. Furthermore, dorsal rhizotomy and lesions of the dorsal columns reduced only tremor amplitude. However, either bilateral lesions of the fastigial nuclei or sectioning of the inferior cerebellar peduncles eliminated harmaline (Lamarre and Mercier 1971). Because the fastigial nuclei send bilateral projections to the brainstem, unilateral lesions of the fastigial nucleus do not abolish harmaline tremor.

Harmaline produces rhythmic firing of neurons in the IO (de Montigny and Lamarre 1973; Llinás and Volkind 1973). The IO is the source of climbing fibers that synapse on the somas and proximal dendrites of Purkinje cells. IO neurons are electronically coupled through gap junctions and, under the influence of harmaline, they fire synchronously at 8–12 Hz. Despite a substantial body of work suggesting otherwise, experiments in connexin36 knock-out mice indicate that synchrony mediated by IO gap junctions does not play an essential role in the genesis of harmaline tremor (Long et al. 2002).

Perhaps independent of IO gap junctions, harmaline has been shown to increase both the auto- and cross-correlation of complex spike activity in the cerebellar cortex (Sasaki et al. 1989). Synchronous IO/climbing fiber activity entrains Purkinje cells in the vermal portions of the cerebellar cortex and neurons in the cerebellar nuclei, red nucleus, and brainstem reticular formation resulting in an 8- to 12-Hz postural tremor (Lamarre and Mercier 1971; Llinás and Volkind 1973; Lamarre 1975; Lamarre 1984). After injection of harmaline into cats, selected portions of the IO complex, the medial accessory olive (MAO), and caudolateral parts of the dorsal accessory olive (DAO) increase their metabolic activity (Batini et al. 1981). In rats injected with harmaline, increased metabolic activity is seen only in the MAO (Bernard et al. 1984b). Because the MAO and DAO make up only a small percentage of IO volume, the limited resolution of human PET studies may explain some of the discrepancies between metabolic studies of ET and harmaline-induced tremor.

The cerebellum receives climbing fibers from the IO and mossy fibers from several sites such the pons and spinal cord. The climbing fiber input to Purkinje cells is all-or-none with the excitatory post-synaptic potentials (EPSPs) producing a complex spike. Complex spikes exert an important influence on the responsiveness of Purkinje cells to subsequent synaptic inputs. After administration of harmaline, single-unit extracellular recordings from Purkinje cells show rhythmic complex spike activity and a marked suppression of simple spikes (Figure 2). IO afferents arise from multiple sites including the spinal cord, brainstem (including raphe nuclei and locus ceruleus), cerebellar nuclei, and frontal cortex. Afferents from the cerebellar nuclei are thought to be exclusively GABAergic. IO neurons are intrinsically rhythmic and electrotonically coupled through gap junctions (Benardo and Foster 1986; Llinás and Yarom 1986). Oscillations of IO neurons are mediated by a low threshold calcium conductance and reflect the properties of an ensemble of coupled neurons (Llinás and Yarom 1986). IO ensemble oscillation is heavily modulated by serotonin (5HT) and norepinephrine and can be induced by harmaline (Llinás and Yarom 1986).

Several additional lines of evidence support an essential role for the IO and climbing fiber innervation of Purkinje cells in the pathogenesis of harmaline tremor. First, climbing fibers begin to synapse on Purkinje cells in developing rat cerebellar cortex on Postnatal Days 10–12. For that reason, harmaline-induced tremor does not reliably appear in rats until Postnatal Day 13 (Henderson and Woolley et al.

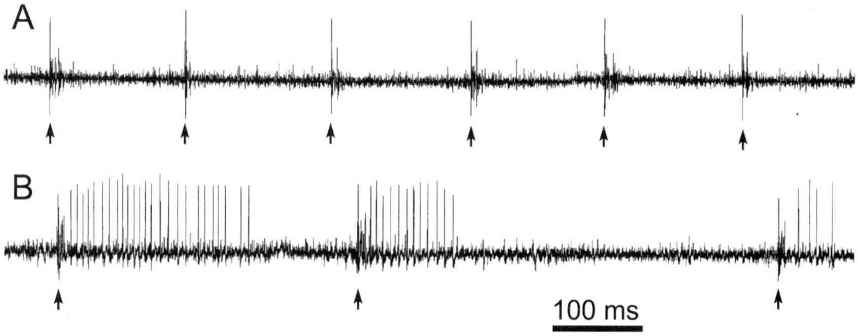

FIGURE 2 Harmaline-stimulated Purkinje cell spike trains from Postnatal Day 22 normal (**A**) and dystonic (**B**) rats. Complex spikes are marked with arrows. Reproduced with permission from Springer-Verlag (LeDoux, M.S., and J.F. Lorden. 2002. *Exp Brain Res* 145:457–467).

1970). Second, the IO is selectively and completely destroyed by the neurotoxin, 3-acetylpyridine (3-AP). After 3-AP IO elimination, rats do not produce tremor in response to harmaline (Bernard et al. 1984a). Third, mutant mice with Purkinje cell degeneration show either absent or reduced responses to harmaline (Milner et al. 1995).

Multiple experimental approaches have indicated that serotonergic systems, particularly the serotonergic innervation of the IO, may play a role in the expression of harmaline-induced tremor. 5HT increases the coherence and decreases the frequency of IO neuronal oscillations (Sugihara et al. 1995). The effects of pretreatment with the serotonin precursor, 5-hydroxytryptophan (5HTP), on harmaline tremor are dose-dependent (Kelly and Naylor 1974). When used at low dosages, 5HTP reduces harmaline tremor. In contrast, the intensity and duration of harmaline tremor are enhanced by high dosages of 5HTP. In rats, intraventricular administration of either 5,6-dihydroxytryptamine or 5,7-dihydroxytryptamine with desipramine pretreatment produces selective destruction of serotonergic synapses and axons. New axon sprouts appear five to seven days after injection and reinnervation of target neurons occurs in the IO. Harmaline tremor is attenuated in rats that have undergone serotonergic denervation and the reappearance of harmaline tremor parallels the time course of serotonergic reinnervation (Sjölund et al. 1977). In cats, harmaline tremor appears to originate in those parts of the IO (i.e., caudal medial accessory nucleus, caudolateral dorsal accessory nucleus) that receive a dense serotonergic innervation. In contrast, parts of the IO most sensitive to harmaline in rats do not correlate with the density of serotonergic innervation (Bernard et al. 1984a). One plausible interpretation of these various reports is that the effects of 5HT on harmaline tremor emerge at sites efferent to olivocerebellar pathways.

No specific sites of concentration were detected in a limited autoradiographic binding study with radiolabeled harmaline (Ho et al. 1970). Moreover, no mention was made of the IO in the report by Ho and co-workers (1970). Harmaline radioactivity was diffusely distributed in cortical and subcortical regions, and levels were high in the thalamus, hippocampus, and cerebellum. In another study, Deecher and colleagues (1992) used radioligand assays to prove that harmaline does not bind to a variety of receptor types (i.e., adrenergic, cannabinoid, dopamine, GABA, muscarinic, nicotinic, opiate, serotonin). In the same study, it was shown that harmaline binds to voltage-dependent sodium channels in the μM range. More recent work, however, indicates that harmaline may act as an inverse agonist at the NMDA receptor MK-801 binding site and open the cationic channel (Du et al. 1997). Relative concentration of NMDA receptors in the IO (Monaghan and Cotman 1985) and blockade of harmaline-induced tremor by the noncompetitive NMDA channel blocker dizocilpine are two pieces of evidence supporting this hypothesis (Du and Harvey 1997).

VI. USE OF HARMALINE TO STUDY OLIVOCEREBELLAR PATHWAYS AND MOTOR CONTROL

Harmaline is a powerful experimental method of activating the climbing fiber pathway. Harmaline has been used to show that rhythmic climbing fiber activation is associated with striking cGMP increases in cerebellar cortex (Biggio and Guidotti 1976). As another example, NADPH-diaphorase histochemistry and immunocytochemistry were used to demonstrate upregulation of nitric oxide synthase levels in cerebellar Purkinje cells days after the administration of harmaline. Thus, harmaline can be used to study the non-invasive induction of nitric oxide synthase and its relationship to excitotoxic events (Saxon and Beitz 1996).

In several mutant rodents with dystonia and/or ataxia, harmaline has been employed as a tool to examine the integrity of olivocerebellar structures. The dystonic rat, for instance, is insensitive to harmaline (see video; Lorden et al. 1985). Single-unit extracellular recordings have shown that harmaline-stimulated complex spike activity is faster and more rhythmic in normal than dystonic rats (LeDoux and Lorden 2002). In addition, there is much less harmaline-induced suppression of simple spike activity in dystonic rats in comparison with normal littermates (Figure 2).

The cerebellum is central to the processes of motor learning and motor coordination. By disrupting normal IO/climbing fiber physiology, harmaline can be utilized in behavioral paradigms to explore the roles of olivocerebellar pathways, particularly climbing fibers, in Pavlovian conditioning, fine motor control, and motor learning (Harvey and Romano 1993; Welsh 1998; Stanford and Fowler 1998). For example, low-dose harmaline (5 mg/kg) retards Pavlovian conditioning of the rabbit's nictitating membrane response without altering baseline levels of response, the level of non-associative responding to the conditioned stimulus or habituation to the conditioned stimulus (Harvey and Romano 1993).

VII. USE OF THE HARMALINE TREMOR MODEL AS A THERAPEUTIC SCREENING TOOL

The physiology and neurochemical anatomy of the IO provide a rich milieu for the development of drugs to treat ET. However, the relevance of harmaline-induced tremor to ET has not been completely established. For a case in point, previous physiological studies of harmaline-induced tremor in primates did not employ metabolic mapping or accelerometry thereby limiting comparisons to human ET. Moreover, the effects of alcohol and mechanical loads on harmaline-induced tremor have not been evaluated in primates (Poirier et al. 1966; Lamarre 1975). In addition, experiments are needed to clarify possible incongruities between human PET studies of ET and 2DG animal studies (e.g., cat, rat) of harmaline-induced tremor. Despite these concerns, harmaline tremor is similar to ET in terms of frequency, kinematics, response to ethyl alcohol, and cerebellar activation. Accordingly, harmaline tremor models have been used as tools to explore therapeutic options for ET.

A. Octanol

The marked reduction in the amplitude of ET seen with ethanol prompted a search for closely related small molecules to treat this movement disorder. Octanol isomers are structurally similar to ethanol and 1-octanol has been approved by the Food and Drug Administration for human use as a food additive. In the guinea pig brainstem slice preparation, 1-octanol acted as a potent antagonist of the low threshold calcium channel in IO neurons (Llinás and Yarom 1989). In a follow-up study using rats, all octanol isomers (i.e., 1-octanol, 2-octanol, 3-octanol, and 4-octanol) potently reduced harmaline tremor (Sinton et al. 1989). Quite recently, small doses of 1-octanol (1 mg/kg) were associated with significant reductions in ET tremor amplitude in six patients enrolled in a pilot study at the National Institutes of Health (Bushara et al. 2004). Thus, the harmaline tremor model successfully predicted the efficacy of 1-octanol in ET.

B. Vagus Nerve Stimulation

Vagus nerve stimulation (VNS) is one therapeutic option available for the management of patients with medically intractable epilepsy. Over the past decade, there has been substantial interest in applying VNS to a variety of additional psychiatric and neurological conditions, including ET. In a single study that utilized seven adult rats, investigators placed helical electrode leads around the left vagus nerve and recorded harmaline-induced tremor with a polygraph before, during, and after five minutes of VNS (Handforth and Krahl 2001). VNS suppressed harmaline tremor acutely. However, the effects of VNS lasted for only a few minutes stimulation ceased. Furthermore, there was no significant benefit of VNS in a pilot study of human ET (Handforth et al. 2000).

Acknowledgments

MSL has been supported by grants from the National Institutes of Health (K08 NS 01593 & R01 EY12232), Dystonia Medical Research Foundation, and Center of Genomics and Bioinformatics at the University of Tennessee Health Science Center.

Video Legends

SEGMENT 1 Open field behavior of a normal rat pup (1 bar on tail) at Postnatal Day 20 prior to the injection of Harmaline.

SEGMENT 2 Open field behavior of a normal rat pup (1 bar on tail) at Postnatal Day 20 after the injection of Harmaline (10 mg/kg). A generalized tremor is clearly apparent. Additionally, the rat exhibits abducted hind limbs, ataxia and decreased locomotor activity.

SEGMENT 3 Open field behavior of a dystonic rat pup (2 bars on tail) at Postnatal Day 20 prior to the injection of Harmaline.

SEGMENT 4 Open field behavior of a dystonic rat pup (2 bars on tail) at Postnatal Day 20 after the injection of Harmaline (10 mg/kg). No tremor is apparent.

SEGMENT 5 Open field behavior of the normal (1 bar on tail) and dystonic (2 bars on tail) rat pups at Postnatal Day 21. Rats are back to baseline on the day following injection of Harmaline.

SEGMENT 6 Open field behavior of a normal adult rat prior to the injection of Harmaline.

SEGMENT 7 Open field behavior of the normal adult rat after the injection of Harmaline (10 mg/kg). A generalized tremor is clearly apparent and spontaneous locomotor activity is markedly reduced.

SEGMENT 8 Open field behavior of the normal adult rat on the day following injection of Harmaline. The rat is back to its locomotor baseline.

References

Batini, C., C. Buisseret-Delmas, and M. Conrath-Verrier. 1981. Harmaline-induced tremor. I. Regional metabolic activity as revealed by [^{14}C]2-deoxyglucose in cat. *Exp Brain Res* **42**:371–382.

Bernard, J.F., C. Buisseret-Delmas, and S. Laplante. 1984a. Inferior olivary neurons: 3-acetylpyridine effects on glucose consumption, axonal transport, electrical activity and harmaline-induced tremor. *Brain Res* **322**: 382–387.

Bernard, J.F., C. Buisseret-Delmas, C. Compoint, and S. Laplante. 1984b. Harmaline induced tremor. III. A combined simple units, horseradish peroxidase, and 2-deoxyglucose study of the olivocerebellar system in the rat. *Exp Brain Res* **57**:128–137.

Benardo, L.S., and R.E. Foster. 1986. Oscillatory behavior in inferior olive neurons: mechanism, modulation, and aggregates. *Brain Res Bull* **17**: 773–784.

Biggio, G., and A. Guidotti. 1976. Climbing fiber activation and 3′,5′-cyclic guanosine monophosphate (cGMP) content in cortex and deep nuclei of cerebellum. *Brain Res* **107**:365–373.

Bucher, S.F., K.C. Seelos, R.C. Dodel, M. Reiser, and W.H. Oertel. 1997. Activation mapping in essential tremor with functional magnetic resonance imaging. *Ann Neurol* **41**:32–40.

Bushara, K.O., S.R. Goldstein, G.J. Grimes, Jr., A.H. Burstein, and M. Hallett. 2004. Pilot trial of 1-octanol in essential tremor. *Neurology* **62**:122–124.

Cross, A.J., A. Misra, A. Sandilands, M.J. Taylor, and A.R. Green. 1993. Effect of chlormethiazole, dizocilpine and pentobarbital on harmaline-induced increase in cerebellar cyclic GMP and tremor. *Psychopharm (Berl)* **111**:96–98.

Deecher, D.C., M. Teitler, D.M. Soderlund, W.G. Bornmann, M.E. Kuehne, and S.D. Glick. 1992. Mechanisms of action of ibogaine and harmaline congeners based on radioligand binding studies. *Brain Res* **571**: 242–247.

de Montigny, C., and Y. Lamarre. 1973. Rhythmic activity induced by harmaline in the olivo-cerebello-bulbar system of the cat. *Brain Res* **53**:81–95.

Du, W., and J.A. Harvey. 1997. Harmaline-induced tremor and impairment of learning are both blocked by dizocilpine in the rabbit. *Brain Res* **745**:183–188.

Du, W., V.J. Aloyo, and J.A. Harvey. 1997. Harmaline competitively inhibits [3H]MK-801 binding to the NMDA receptor in rabbit brain. *Brain Res* **770**:26–29.

Elble, R.J. 1986. Physiologic and essential tremor. *Neurology* **36**:225–231.

Elble, R.J., C. Higgins, K. Leffler, and L. Hughes. 1994. Factors influencing the amplitude and frequency of essential tremor. *Mov Disord* **9**: 589–596.

Elble, R.J., and W.C. Koller. 1990. *Tremor*. Baltimore: Johns Hopkins University Press.

Growdon, J.H., B.T. Shahani, and R.R. Young. 1975. The effect of alcohol on essential tremor. *Neurology* **25**:259–262.

Gulcher, J.R., P. Jonsson, A. Kong, K. Kristjansson, M.L. Frigge, A. Karason, I.E. Einarsdottir, et al. 1997. Mapping of a familial essential tremor gene, FET1, to chromosome 3q13. *Nat Genet* **17**:84–87.

Hallett, M., and R.M. Dubinsky. 1993. Glucose metabolism in the brain of patients with essential tremor. *J Neurol Sci* **114**:45–48.

Handforth, A., and S.E. Krahl. 2001. Suppression of harmaline-induced tremor in rats by vagus nerve stimulation. *Mov Disord* **16**:84–88.

Handforth, A., W.G. Ondo, S. Tatter, G.W. Mathern, R.K. Simpson, F. Walker, J.P. Sutton, et al. 2000. Effect of vagus nerve stimulation on essential tremor. *Neurology* **54**(Suppl 3):238.

Harvey, J.A., and A.G. Romano. 1993. Harmaline-induced impairment of Pavlovian conditioning in the rabbit. *J Neurosci* **13**:1616–1623.

Henderson, G.L., and D.E. Woolley. 1970. Ontogenesis of drug-induced tremor in the rat. *J Pharmacol Exp Ther* **175**:113–120.

Higgins, J.J., L.T. Pho, and L.E. Nee. 1997. A gene (ETM) for essential tremor maps to chromosome 2p22–p25. *Mov Disord* **12**:859–864.

Ho, B.T., G.E. Fritchie, J.E. Idänpään-Heikkilä, L.W. Tansey, and W.M. McIsaac. 1970. [^{3}H]Harmaline distribution in monkey brain; pharmacological and autoradiographic study. *Brain Res* **22**:397–401.

Homberg, V., H. Hefter, K. Reiners, and H.-J. Freund. 1987. Differential effects of changes in mechanical limb properties on physiological and pathological tremor. *J Neurol Neurosurg Psych* **50**:568–579.

Hubble, J.P., K.L. Busenbark, R. Pahwa, K. Lyons, and W.C. Koller. 1997. Clinical expression of essential tremor: effects of gender and age. *Mov Disord* **12**:969–972.

Iwata, S., M. Nomoto, and T. Fukuda. 1993. Effects of beta-adrenergic blockers on drug-induced tremors. *Pharmacol Biochem Behav* **44**: 611–613.

Kelly, D.M., and R.J. Naylor. 1974. Mechanisms of tremor induction by harmine. *Eur J Pharm* **27**:14–24.

Kovach, M.J., J. Ruiz, K. Kimonis, S. Mueed, S. Sinha, C. Higgins, S. Elble, et al. 2001. Genetic heterogeneity in autosomal dominant essential tremor. *Genet Med* **3**:197–199.

Kralic, J.E., E.R. Korpi, T.K. O'Buckley, G.E. Homanics, and A.L. Morrow. 2002. Molecular and pharmacological characterization of GABA(A) receptor alpha1 subunit knockout mice. *J Pharmacol Exp Ther* **302**: 1037–1045.

Lamarre, Y., and L.-A. Mercier. 1971. Neurophysiological studies of harmaline-induced tremor in the cat. *Can J Physiol Pharmacol* **49**:1049–1058.

Lamarre, Y. 1975. Tremorogenic mechanisms in primates. In *Advances in Neurology, Volume 10*. Edited by B.S. Meldrum and C.D. Marsden. New York: Raven Press. pp. 23–34.

Lamarre, Y. 1984. Animal models of physiological, essential and parkinsonian-like tremors. In *Movement Disorders: Tremors*. Edited by L.J. Findley and R. Capildeo. New York: Oxford University Press. pp. 183–194.

LeDoux, M.S., and J.F. Lorden. 2002. Abnormal spontaneous and harmaline-stimulated Purkinje cell activity in the awake genetically dystonic rat. *Exp Brain Res* **145**:457–467.

Llinás, R., and R.A. Volkind. 1973. The olivo-cerebellar system: functional properties as revealed by harmaline-induced tremor. *Exp Brain Res* **18**:69–87.

Llinás, R., and Y. Yarom. 1986. Oscillatory properties of guinea-pig inferior olivary neurones and their pharmacological modulation: an *in vitro* study. *J Physiol* **376**:163–182.

Long, M.A., M.R. Deans, D.L. Paul, and B.W. Connors. 2002. Rhythmicity without synchrony in the electrically uncoupled inferior olive. *J Neurosci* **22**:10898–10905.

Lorden, J.F., G.A. Oltmans, T.W. McKeon, J. Lutes, and M. Beales. 1985. Decreased cerebellar 3′,5′-cyclic guanosine monophosphate levels and insensitivity to harmaline in the genetically dystonic rat (dt). *J Neurosci* **5**:2618–2625.

Lorden, J.F., S.E. Stratton, L.E. Mays, and G.A. Oltmans. 1988. Purkinje cell activity in rats following chronic treatment with harmaline. *Neuroscience* **27**:465–472.

Louis, E.D., R. Ottman, and W.A. Hauser. 1998. How common is the most common movement disorder? Estimates of the prevalence of essential tremor throughout the world. *Mov Disord* **13**:5–10.

Lutes, J., J.F. Lorden, M. Beales, and G.A. Oltmans. 1988. Tolerance to the tremorogenic effects of harmaline: evidence for altered olivo-cerebellar function. *Neuropharmacology* **27**:849–855.

Mahmoudian, M., H. Jalilpour, and P. Salehian. 2002. Toxicity of *Peganum harmala*: review and a case report. *Iran J Pharm Ther* **1**:1–4.

Milner, T.E., G. Cadoret, L. Lessard, and A.M. Smith. 1995. EMG analysis of harmaline-induced tremor in normal and three strains of mutant mice with Purkinje cell degeneration and the role of the inferior olive. *J Neurophysiol* **73**:2568–2577.

Monaghan, D.T., and C.W. Cotman. 1985. Distribution of N-methyl-D-aspartate-sensitive L-[3H]glutamate binding sites in rat brain. *J Neurosci* **5**:2909–2919.

Ohye, C., R. Bouchard, L. Larochelle, P. Bédard, R. Boucher, B. Raphy, and L.J. Poirier. 1970. Effect of dorsal rhizotomy on postural tremor in the monkey. *Exp Brain Res* **10**:140–150.

Poirier, L.J., T.L. Sourkes, G. Bouvier, R. Boucher, and S. Carabin. 1966. Striatal amines, experimental tremor and the effect of harmaline in the monkey. *Brain* **89**:37–52.

Rappaport, M.S., R.T. Gentry, D.R. Schneider, and V.P. Dole. 1984. Ethanol effects on harmaline-induced tremor and increase of cerebellar cyclic GMP. *Life Sci* **34**:49–56.

Sasaki, K., J.M. Bower, and R. Llinás. 1989. Multiple Purkinje cell recording in rodent cerebellar cortex. *Eur J Neurosci* **1**:572–586.

Saxon, D.W., and A.J. Beitz. 1996. An experimental model for the non-invasive trans-synaptic induction of nitric oxide synthase in Purkinje cells of the rat cerebellum. *Neuroscience* **72**:157–165.

Shinozaki, H., K. Hirate, and M. Ishida. 1985. Further studies on quantification of drug-induced tremor in mice: effects of antitremorogenic agents on tremor frequency. *Exp Neurol* **88**:303–315.

Sinton, C.M., B.I. Krosser, K.D. Walton, and R.R. Llinás. 1989. The effectiveness of different isomers of octanol as blockers of harmaline-induced tremor. *Pflugers Arch* **414**:31–36.

Sjölund, B., A. Björklund, and L. Wiklund. 1977. The indolaminergic innervation of the inferior olive: 2. Relation to harmaline induced tremor. *Brain Res* **131**:23–37.

Stanford, J.A., and S.C. Fowler. 1998. At low doses, harmaline increases forelimb tremor in the rat. *Neurosci Lett* **241**:41–44.

Sugihara, I., E.J. Lang, and R. Llinás. 1995. Serotonin modulation of inferior olivary oscillations and synchronicity: a multiple-electrode study in the rat cerebellum. *Eur J Neurosci* **7**:521–534.

Wang, G., and S.C. Fowler. 2001. Concurrent quantification of tremor and depression of locomotor activity induced in rats by harmaline and physostigmine. *Psychopharmacology (Berl)* **158**:273–80.

Welsh, J.P. 1998. Systemic harmaline blocks associative and motor learning by the actions of the inferior olive. *Eur J Neurosci* **10**:3307–3320.

Wills, A.J., I.H. Jenkins, P.D. Thompson, L.J. Findley, and D.J. Brooks. 1994. Red nuclear and cerebellar but no olivary activation associated with essential tremor: a positron emission tomographic study. *Ann Neurol* **36**:637–642.

Yamazaki, M., C. Tanaka, and S. Takaori. 1979. Significance of central noradrenergic system on harmaline induced tremor. *Pharmacol Biochem Behav* **10**:421–427.

Yang, G., and C. Iadecola. 1998. Activation of cerebellar climbing fibers increases cerebellar blood flow. *Stroke* **29**:499–508.

C H A P T E R

E4

GABA$_A$ Receptor $\alpha 1$ Subunit Knockout Mice: A Novel Model of Essential Tremor

JESSICA L. OSTERMAN, JASON E. KRALIC, TODD K. O' BUCKLEY, GREGG E. HOMANICS and A. LESLIE MORROW

Deletion of GABA$_A$ receptor $\alpha 1$ subunits in mice results in a phenotype of kinetic tremor that mimics certain features of essential tremor disease. Knockout mice exhibit a tremor of approximately 16 to 22 Hz, whereas wild-type and heterozygous mice exhibit a physiological tremor in the range of 25 to 40 Hz. The tremor is observed early in life, and the power or amplitude of the oscillation is increased in 8-month-old mice compared to 4-month-old mice. The GABA$_A$ benzodiazepine receptor agonist diazepam and the GABAergic neuroactive steroid allopregnanolone exacerbate the tremor, whereas ethanol completely inhibits the tremor. Since the etiology of essential tremor is unknown, this animal model of genetic essential tremor may lead to an understanding of the pathophysiology of the disease and provide a valuable model system to develop therapeutic interventions.

I. BACKGROUND

Tremor is the most common movement disorder affecting the world's population, with a prevalence of 1% to 2% (McAuley, 2001; Goetz, 2001). The clinical ramifications of tremor can often be debilitating, rendering patients unable to write or even feed themselves (Goetz, 2001). Although tremor is often associated with neurological conditions, such as Parkinson disease, it is capable of manifesting itself in many other ways. Essential tremor, the most common of the tremor disorders, is a primary condition independent of any overlying disorder (Deuschl et al., 2000). Tremor is also commonly associated with substance withdrawal, and it is often a side effect of various drug treatments.

Whereas tremor can arise from a variety of external and internal means, all tremorogenic behavior falls under three main classifications, each defined by the conditions under which they occur (Cooper and Rodnitzky, 2000). Rest tremor is an involuntary oscillation of a body part that is completely supported against gravity (Smaga, 2003). The Parkinsonian tremor is a prime example of a resting tremor (Cooper, 2002). A kinetic tremor involves the same oscillatory pattern, but it takes place during movement or attempts at movement (Elble and Koller, 1990). An example of kinetic tremor is the oscillatory behavior associated with cerebellar disorders that arises from the demyelination of central nervous system axons (Goetz, 2001). The final classification is the postural tremor, which occurs when a posture is maintained against gravity (Elble and Koller, 1990). Essential tremor is characterized primarily by postural components, although the tremor tends to worsen upon movement, adding a kinetic component to the disease

(Goetz, 2001). Tremor occurring during alcohol or drug withdrawal is usually of a postural character (Goetz, 2001).

Whereas research on this common movement disorder continues, a pathway or regulatory mechanism for essential tremor has yet to be elucidated. Several brain regions, including the cerebellum, inferior olive, cerebral cortex, and thalamus, have all been implicated in the production of tremor behavior; however, the neurological origin of essential tremor remains elusive (Hellwig et al., 2001; McAuley, 2001). Similarly, the neurotransmitter systems involved in the production of essential tremor are unknown (Wilms et al., 1999). Current systems that are under investigation include the γ-aminobutyric acid (GABA), serotonin, and dopamine systems.

One of the major obstacles in the search for a tremor mechanism is the lack of an adequate animal model for essential tremor. Current models utilize drug-induced tremors, lesion-induced tremors, and models arising from mutant strains. The most common model system used today utilizes the drug harmaline to induce a temporary essential tremor in the animals. Harmaline is thought to act at the inferior olivary neurons, via blockade of GABA receptor junctions, allowing the neurons to fire synchronously (Wilms et al., 1999). Treatment with harmaline induces an 8- to 12-Hz tremor, which is apparent both at rest and during movement (Wilms et al., 1999). This drug-induced tremor, however, may be limited as a model system because of potential interactions between the tremor-inducing drug and experimental treatment drugs.

We have recently discovered a novel genetic animal model of tremor (Kralic, 2002a; Kralic et al., 2002b). This tremor has both postural and kinetic components, mimicking the pathology of essential tremor, and arises from the global deletion of GABA$_A$ receptor alpha-1 subunits. Tremor can be observed by the naked eye as the mice move freely about their cages; however, the tremor becomes significantly more pronounced upon suspension of the mice by their tails. In these knockouts, the tremor occurs primarily in the forelimbs and hindlimbs of the animal; however, it may also manifest itself in other areas that are more difficult to observe, such as the larynx and tongue. On average, the knockout mice ($\alpha 1^{-/-}$) exhibit a high amplitude tremor of approximately 16 to 22 Hz, whereas wild-type ($\alpha 1^{+/+}$) and heterozygous mice exhibit a low-amplitude physiological tremor in the range of 25 to 40 Hz (Kralic, 2002a).

II. GABA AND GABA$_A$ RECEPTORS

The amino acid GABA is the major inhibitory neurotransmitter in the human brain. GABA acts in opposition to excitatory neurotransmitters, such as glutamate and aspartate, and is essential for proper central nervous system (CNS) functioning (Kralic, 2002a). Failure of the GABA system to function properly can cause CNS hyperexcitability, leading to seizures and even death. Additionally, deficiencies in the GABA system can be linked to a variety of anxiety, sleep, and addiction disorders (Rudolph et al., 2001).

GABA actions are mediated via binding to one of three different types of GABA receptors—GABA$_A$, GABA$_B$, or GABA$_C$ receptors. GABA$_A$ and GABA$_C$ receptors are ligand-gated ion channel receptors, whereas GABA$_B$ receptors are metabotropic receptors (Purves et al., 2001). When activated by GABA, muscimol, isoguvacine, or a variety of other synthetic and endogenous substances, GABA$_A$ receptors gate chloride ion conductance through an integral channel, allowing for fast inhibitory action. GABA$_A$ receptors have multiple distinct drug recognition sites distributed both in the extracellular domain of the receptor as well as within the central pore (Morrow, 1995). Among others, benzodiazepines, barbiturates, neuroactive steroids, and ethanol all produce at least some of their actions via GABA$_A$ receptors (Morrow, 1995). GABA$_A$ receptors are pentameric, with varying combinations of subunits that form an integral ion channel (Sieghart and Sperk, 2002; Morrow, 1995). To date, twenty subunits have been identified, including six α subunits, four β, three γ, one δ, one ε, one π, and one θ subunit, although the most common combinations found within human brain are two α, two β, and one γ subunit or two α, two γ, and one β subunit (Sieghart and Sperk, 2002).

Of the alpha subunits available, the α1 subunit is the most abundant alpha subunit throughout the brain, so the global deletion of the α1 subunit in the knockout mice has major implications for distribution and composition of GABA receptors throughout the brain (Sieghart and Sperk, 2002). Interestingly, the appearance of tremor is the primary phenotype in these mice. The deletion of the α1 subunit in the knockout mice results in a decreased expression of β2/3 and γ2 subunits in the cerebral cortex and the cerebellum (Kralic, 2002a). The knockouts also exhibit an increased expression of α2 and α3 subunits in the cerebral cortex (Kralic, 2002a). Additionally, [^{3}H]muscimol, [^{35}S]TBPS, and [^{3}H] Ro-15-4513 binding assays have demonstrated the overall loss of 50% of GABA$_A$ receptors in the knockout mice (Kralic et al., 2002b). The deletion of the α1 subunit and the compensatory subunit alterations in the knockout brain also affect the properties of the remaining GABA$_A$ receptors. The ability of benzodiazepines such as diazepam to potentiate chloride ion flux was altered in the knockouts (Kralic et al., 2002c). In muscimol-stimulated chloride ion flux experiments, diazepam, a nonselective benzodiazepine for Type I and II benzodiazepine binding sites, was more capable of potentiating chloride ion flux, compared to the wild-type mice (Kralic et al., 2002c). Whereas numerous alterations are present in the knockouts at a molecular level, behavioral deficits are also observed in these deficient mice. The ability of diazepam to prevent bicuculline-induced seizures is completely lost in the knockout mice, and muscimol-stimulated $^{36}Cl^-$ uptake assays show a dramatic reduction in GABAergic tone, leading to increased seizure susceptibility in the knockout mice (Kralic et al., 2002b). This increased seizure susceptibility and loss of GABAergic tone may play a role in the pathology of the tremor. Decreased GABA inhibition leads to hyperexcitability in the knockout mice, which could manifest itself in the production of the tremor. In fact, individuals suffering from tremor have reported that self-administration of alcohol is effective in reducing tremor activity (Elble and Koller, 1990), indicating that increased inhibitory regulation of brain activity may play a role in tremor reduction. Controlled studies in patients with essential tremor have demonstrated that small amounts of alcohol suppress tremor symptoms (Growdon et al., 1975; Koller and Biary, 1984).

III. CHARACTERIZATION OF PATHOLOGICAL TREMOR GABA$_A$ RECEPTOR $\alpha 1$ SUBUNIT KNOCKOUT MICE

Whereas all animals exhibit a physiological tremor, the deletion of the $\alpha 1$ subunit in the $\alpha 1^{-/-}$ mice results in the expression of a pathological tremor with kinetic and postural components. Tremor measurements for the mice were obtained through the use of a tremor monitor developed within the Bowles Center for Alcohol Studies at the University of North Carolina at Chapel Hill. Each mouse was suspended by its tail from a cord attached to the center of a stereo speaker (Archer 3″ 8 Ωmax2 W). The vibrations from the surface of the speaker were transported to an amplifier (Realistic), where the signal from the speaker was augmented and then passed through an analog to digital converter. The a/d converter assigned voltage equivalents to the speaker vibrations. These voltage measurements were then transferred to a computer (Dell PC), where the voltage changes were recorded via a Pascal program developed in-house. Voltage recordings were made over a 22-sec period at a rate of 454 recordings per second. The data obtained from the program were analyzed in MatLab by Fourier transformation to determine the peak amplitude and average frequency of the tremor for each animal.

In addition to physiological tremor, the $\alpha 1^{-/-}$ mice exhibited a pathological tremor with increased mean amplitude and decreased mean frequency compared to the physiological tremor. The mean amplitude of the $\alpha 1^{-/-}$ mice was calculated to be 2.43×10^{12} N $\pm$ 4.15×10^{11} N ($n = 13$), and the mean frequency was calculated to be 19.30 Hz $\pm$ 0.95 Hz ($n = 13$) (Figure 1a). The physiological tremor of the $\alpha 1^{+/+}$ mice had an average amplitude of 0.26×10^{12} N $\pm$ 3.29×10^{11} N ($n = 16$), where N is an arbitrary unit of amplitude as dictated by the Fourier transform. The mean frequency of the physiological tremor in the $\alpha 1^{+/+}$ mice was 32.14 Hz $\pm$ 0.58 Hz ($n = 16$) (Figure 1b).

The effects of age on the amplitude of both the pathological and physiological tremor were examined. Whereas increasing age may affect the mechanics of neurotransmission and neuronal control in the central nervous system, the mean amplitude of the physiological tremor of the wild-type mice appeared to remain unaffected. The pathological tremor of the knockout mice, however, was significantly affected by age. Over a period of 4 months the mean tremor amplitude of the knockout mice was significantly increased. The 4-month-old $\alpha 1^{-/-}$ mice exhibited a pathological tremor with a mean amplitude of 2.43×10^{12} N $\pm$ 4.15×10^{11} N ($n = 13$), whereas the 8-month-old $\alpha 1^{-/-}$ mice exhibited a significantly more pronounced pathological tremor with a mean amplitude of 7.68×10^{12} N $\pm$ 2.68×10^{12} N ($n = 5$) ($p < 0.001$, one-way ANOVA, Newman-Keuls post hoc test) (Figure 2a). However, the physiological tremor exhibited by the $\alpha 1^{+/+}$ mice was unaffected over time. This increase in tremor behavior may indicate a further loss of GABAergic control in the knockout mice. As the knockout mice age, the weakening of neuronal circuitry in the tremorogenic regions of the brain may contribute to the increased amplitude of the pathological tremor.

IV. GABAERGIC DRUGS HAVE DIFFERING EFFECTS ON THE AMPLITUDE AND FREQUENCY OF THE PATHOLOGICAL TREMOR

The $\alpha 1^{-/-}$ mice were injected intraperitoneally with three different GABAergic drugs, and the effect of the drugs upon tremor was recorded. The saline-injected $\alpha 1^{-/-}$ mice exhibited a pathological tremor with a mean amplitude of 2.43×10^{12} N $\pm$ 4.15×10^{11} N ($n = 13$) and a mean frequency of 19.30 Hz $\pm$ 0.95 Hz ($n = 13$) (Figure 3a). The GABA agonist neurosteroid allopregnanolone (16 mg/kg) caused an increase in the mean amplitude and the mean frequency of the pathological tremor (Figure 3b). Diazepam (10 mg/kg) also resulted in elevated amplitude and frequency of the pathological tremor (Figure 3c). Ethanol (2.5 g/kg) dramatically reduced the mean amplitude of the pathological tremor while increasing the mean frequency (Figure 3d). Allopregnanolone is an endogenous neurosteroid that acts at GABA$_A$ receptors to enhance chloride ion flux (Morrow et al., 1989). It was expected that the ability of allopregnanolone to potentiate chloride ion flux would produce an increase in GABA-mediated inhibition and, consequently, a decrease in the severity of the pathological tremor. However, allopregnanolone exacerbated the mean amplitude of the tremor, completely debilitating the animals' attempts at movement. Likewise, diazepam is a benzodiazepine that acts at the benzodiazepine-binding sites of GABA$_A$ receptors to produce enhanced chloride ion flux (Kralic, 2002a). Since diazepam

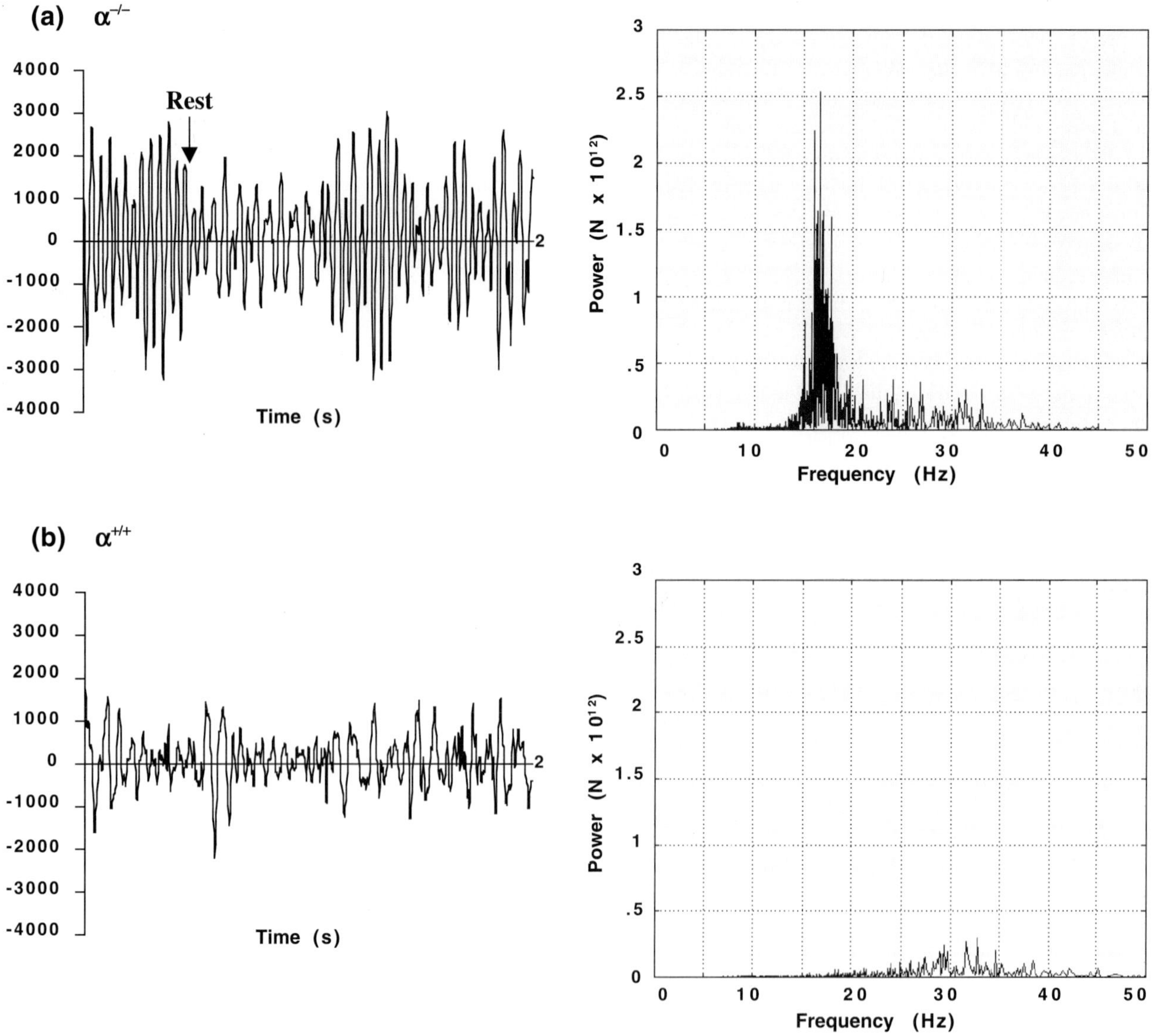

FIGURE 1 **Knockout mice exhibit a pronounced essential tremor.** Tremor measurements record the changes in voltage as a function of time to produce a tracing of the oscillatory movement of the animal. Fourier transforms produced in MatLab (frequency (Hz) on x-axis, amplitude (N) on y-axis) analyzed the average frequency of the tremor and the maximum amplitude achieved at that frequency. (a) Representative displacement tracing of $\alpha1^{-/-}$ animal over a period of 2 sec and a representative Fourier transform for the $\alpha1^{-/-}$ mice that exhibit a pathological tremor with a frequency ranging from 16 to 22 Hz and an average amplitude of 2.43×10^{12} N ($n = 13$, std. err. $= 4.15 \times 10^{11}$ N). (b) Representative displacement tracing of $\alpha1^{+/+}$ over a period of 2 sec and a representative Fourier transform for the $\alpha1^{+/+}$ mice that exhibit a physiological tremor with a frequency ranging from 25 to 40 Hz and an average amplitude of 0.26×10^{12} N ($n = 16$, std. err. $= 3.29 \times 10^{10}$ N).

is a nonselective benzodiazepine for Type I (α1-containing) and Type II (α2-, α3-, and α5-containing) binding sites and the ability of diazepam to potentiate chloride ion flux was enhanced in $\alpha1^{-/-}$ mice (Kralic, 2002a), diazepam should still mediate GABAergic inhibition in these mice. It was found that diazepam, much like allopregnanolone, exacerbated the mean amplitude and severity of the pathological tremor. These data suggest that loss of GABA$_A$ receptors in α1 subunit knockout mice may be complete in tremorogenic regions of brain, rendering GABAergic drugs ineffective as inhibitors of neuronal function at these sites.

Whereas this classical benzodiazepine and neurosteroid was ineffective in the reduction of the pathological tremor, ethanol, another drug that acts at GABA$_A$ receptors, was effective in reducing the mean amplitude of the tremor. The ability of ethanol to reduce the amplitude of the tremor may stem from ethanol's actions at other sites, including NMDA-type glutamate receptors, an excitatory class of receptors

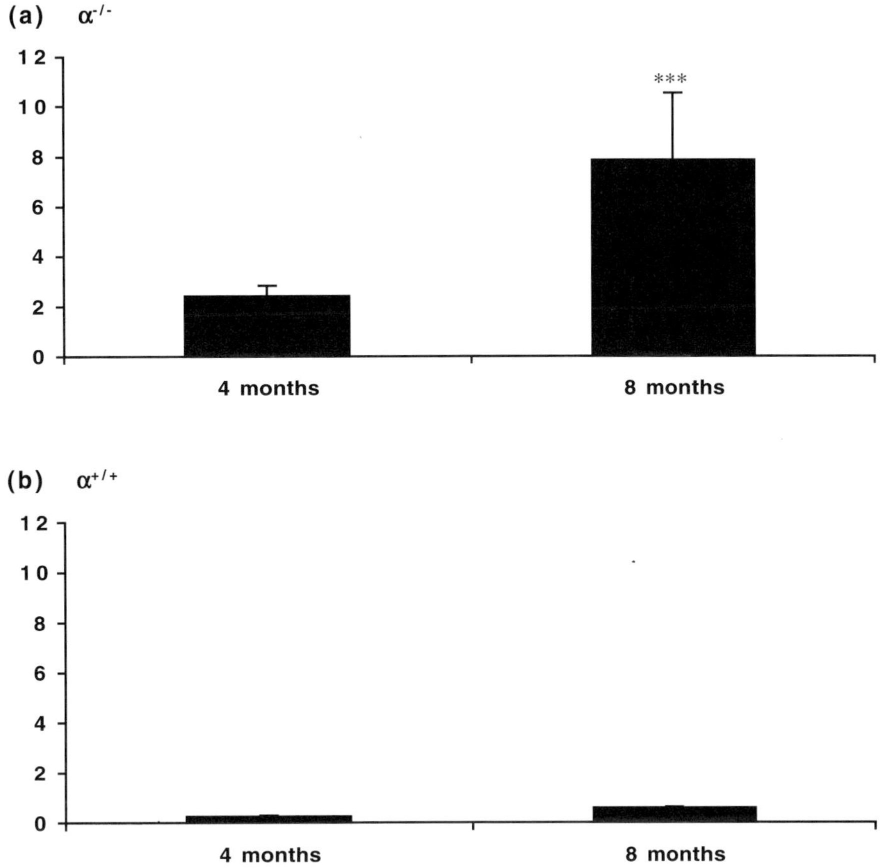

FIGURE 2 **Effect of age on amplitude of tremor in $\alpha 1^{-/-}$ and $\alpha 1^{+/+}$ mice.** Measurements of pathological tremor (16 to 22 Hz) in $\alpha 1^{-/-}$ and physiological tremor (30 to 35 Hz) in $\alpha 1^{+/+}$ mice of varying age. (a) The effect of age on the amplitude of pathological tremor in $\alpha 1^{-/-}$ mice. The average amplitude of the pathological tremor for the 4-month-old mice was determined to be 2.43×10^{12} N ($n = 13$, std. err = 4.15×10^{11} N), whereas the average amplitude of the 8-month-old mice was 7.68×10^{12} N ($n = 5$, std. err. = 2.68×10^{11} N). Age significantly affected the amplitude of the tremor in the $\alpha 1^{-/-}$ mice ($p < 0.001$). (b) The effect of age on the amplitude of the physiological tremor in $\alpha 1^{+/+}$ mice. The average tremor amplitude for the 4-month-old mice was determined to be 2.56×10^{11} N ($n = 16$, std. err. = 3.29×10^{10} N), whereas the average amplitude of the 8-month-old mice was 5.70×10^{11} N ($n = 4$, std. err. = 4.74×10^{10} N). Age did not significantly affect the amplitude of the tremor in the $\alpha 1^{+/+}$ mice ($p > 0.05$). Data represent the mean ±S.E.M. and were analyzed using a one-way ANOVA with Newman-Keuls post hoc test. ***, $p < 0.001$ statistical significance with respect to $\alpha 1^{+/+}$ mice.

thought to be involved in mediating the initial intoxicating and activating effects of ethanol at low doses (Hardman et al., 1995). At NMDA–type glutamate receptors, ethanol inhibits Ca^{2+} flux and NMDA–activated cyclic GMP, which in effect blocks excitatory neurotransmission (Crews et al., 1996). This evidence suggests that inhibition of the glutamate receptors may be primarily responsible for the ethanol-induced reduction of the pathological tremor. Furthermore, a central oscillator has been implicated in the effectiveness of alcohol in patients with essential tremor (Zeuner et al., 2003). The inferior olivary nucleus, a classic central oscillator, contains a high concentration of NMDA receptors (Monaghan and Cotman, 1985; Shaw et al., 1992). Ethanol could also modulate tremor via interactions with other glutamate receptors, voltage–gated Ca^{++} channels, and inhibition of adenosine transport, which increases adenosine-mediated inhibition in brain (Diamond et al., 2003). These possibilities are presently under investigation.

Although there is a global deletion of αl subunits, the loss of GABAergic inhibition in selected regions may account for the tremor activity. For example, harmaline is believed to act at the inferior olive, blocking $GABA_A$ receptor activity. Similarly, electronic coupling between inferior olivary neurons is reduced by cerebellar GABAergic input, lesioning of which leads to rhythmic oscillations of olivary neurons (Wilms et al., 1999). Therefore, loss of $GABA_A$ receptors at the inferior olive may enhance electronic coupling and lead to the observed tremor. It will be important

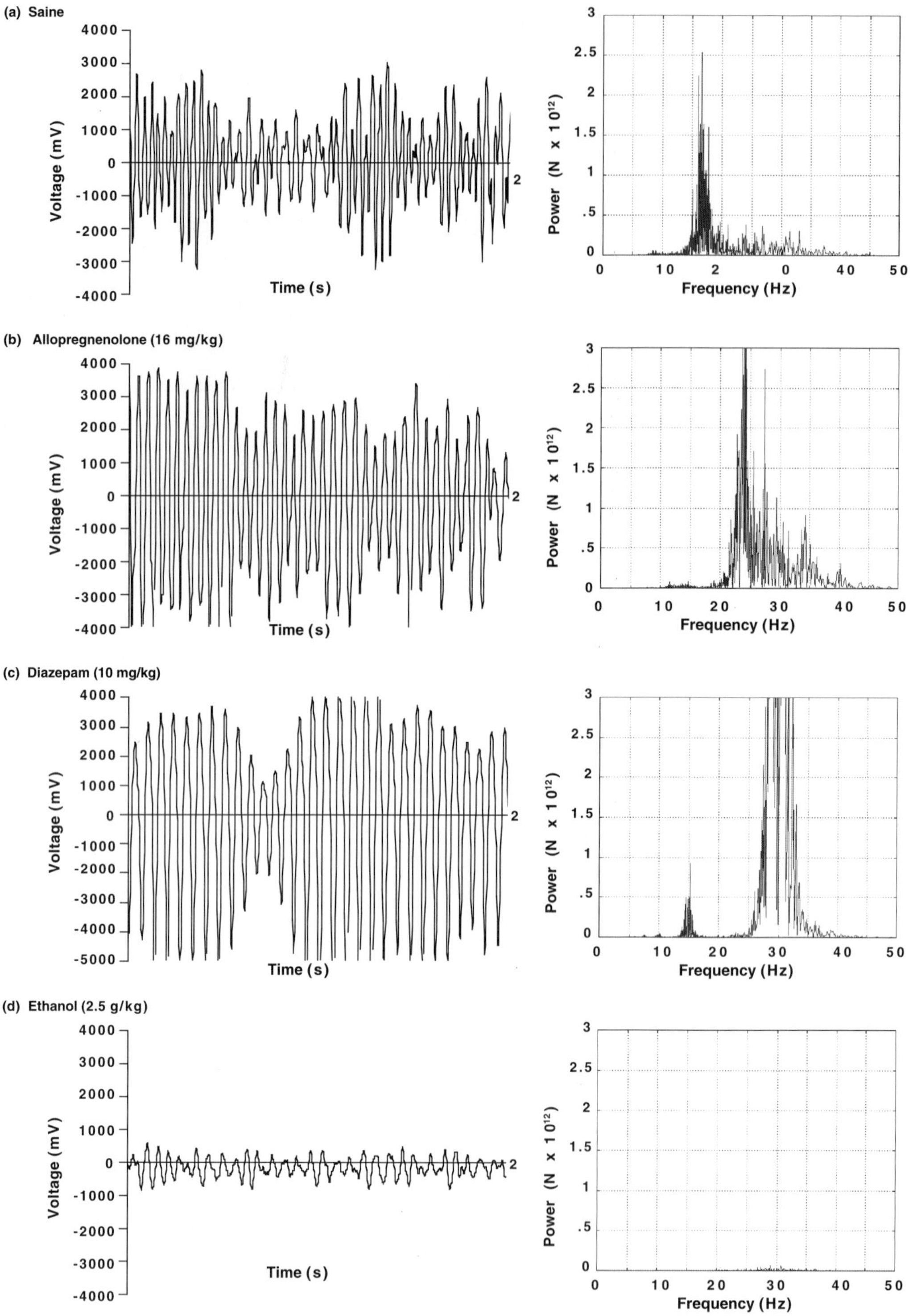

FIGURE 3 **Allopregnanolone and diazepam exacerbate the pathological tremor in $\alpha1^{-/-}$ mice, whereas ethanol ameliorates the tremor.** (a) Representative displacement tracing for the $\alpha1^{-/-}$ mice and a representative Fourier transform (frequency (Hz) on x-axis and amplitude (N) on y-axis) for the $\alpha1^{-/-}$ mice. The $\alpha1^{-/-}$ mice exhibit a tremor with an average amplitude of 2.43×10^{12} N (n = 13, std. err. = 4.15×10^{11} N) and an average frequency of 19.30 Hz (n = 13, std. err. = 0.95 Hz). (b) Representative displacement tracing for the allopregnanolone-injected (16 mg/kg) $\alpha1^{-/-}$ mice and a representative Fourier transform for these mice. Administration of allopregnanolone results in a tremor with an average amplitude of 6.32×10^{12} N (n = 6, std. err. = 1.99×10^{12} N) and an average frequency of 23.97 Hz (n = 6, std. err. = 1.32 Hz). (c) Representative displacement tracing for the diazepam-injected (10 mg/kg) $\alpha^{-/-}$ mice and a representative Fourier transform for these mice. Administration of diazepam results in a tremor with an average amplitude of 28.44×10^{12} N (n = 6, std. err. = 6.99×10^{12} N) and an average frequency of 27.51 Hz (n = 6, std. err. = 0.89 Hz). (d) Representative displacement tracing for the ethanol-injected (2.5 g/kg) $\alpha^{-/-}$ mice and a representative Fourier transform for these mice. Administration of ethanol resulted in a tremor with an average amplitude of 0.076×10^{12} N (n = 11, std. err. = 1.25×10^{10} N) and an average frequency of 29.72 Hz (n = 11, std. err. = 0.90 Hz).

to determine the role of a central oscillator, such as the olivary nucleus or thalamus, in the genesis of the tremor in $\alpha 1^{-/-}$ mice.

The production of $GABA_A$ $\alpha 1$ subunit–deficient mice represents a novel animal model of essential tremor. This model mimics the clinical manifestations of postural and intention tremor as well as sensitivity of the tremor to ethanol as well as the lack of sensitivity of the tremor to other GABAergic compounds such as diazepam. These mice exhibit a genetically encoded tremor that has provided a model system unencumbered with the complications from drug interactions or lesioning processes. The pathological tremor exhibited by the knockout mice has distinct frequency and amplitude components that were altered by age and the administration of various GABAergic drugs.

Whereas ethanol appears to have significant beneficial effects upon the tremor behavior exhibited by the mice in this model system, the addictive nature of ethanol poses complications for the clinical use of ethanol in the treatment of tremor. Ethanol is an extremely addictive substance, and dependence upon alcohol can be difficult to overcome. In fact, self-medication with ethanol has resulted in a 64% alcoholism rate in some populations of tremor patients (Schroeder and Nasrallah, 1982). The current studies investigating the ability of GABAergic drugs to modulate pathological tremor have provided direction for future experimental procedures investigating the pathology of the knockout tremor. Future studies may include drugs that mediate their actions through other sites of ethanol action, including the NMDA–type glutamate receptors (Deutsch et al., 1995). With continuing research on the mechanisms for genetic essential tremor and possible experimental treatments, a cure for essential tremor and other tremor behaviors may be realized in the foreseeable future.

References

Cooper, G., and R. Rodnitzky. 2000. The many forms of tremor: precise classification guides selection of therapy. *Postgraduate Medicine* **108**(1):57–70.

Crews, F.T., A.L. Morrow, H. Criswell, and G. Breese. 1996. Effects of Ethanol on Ion Channels. *International Review of Neurobiology Vol. 39.* pp. 283–367, Academic Press, New York.

Deuschl, G., R. Wenzelburger, K. Löffler, J. Raethjen, and H. Stolze. 2000. "Essential tremor and cerebellar dysfunction clinical and kinematic analysis of intention tremor." *Brain* **123**(8):1568–1580.

Deutsch, S.I., C.H. Park, L.G. Lukacs, C. Morn, L. Koetzner, and J. Mastropaolo. 1995. MK-801 alters the $GABA_A$ receptor complex and potentiates flurazepam's antiseizure efficacy. *Pharmacology Biochemistry and Behavior* **51**(4).909–915.

Elble, R.J., and W.C. Koller. 1990. *Tremor*. The Johns Hopkins University Press, Baltimore, Maryland.

Goetz, C., and S.S. Horn. 2001. Treatment of tremor and dystonia. *Neurologic Clinics* **19**(1):129–144, vi–vii.

Growdon, J.H., B.T. Shahani, and R.R. Young. 1975 The effect of alcohol on tremor. *Neurology* **25**:259–262.

Hardman, J.G., L. Limbird, P. Molinoff, R. Ruddon, and A. Gilman, eds. 1996. *The Pharmacological Basis of Therapeutics* Ninth Edition. McGraw-Hill, New York.

Hellwig, B., S. Haubler, B. Schelter, M. Lauk, B. Guschlbauer, J. Timmer, and C.H. Lucking. 2001. Tremor-correlated cortical activity in essential tremor. *The Lancet* **357**:519–523.

Koller, W.C., and N. Biary. 1984. Effect of alcohol on tremors: comparison with propranolol. *Neurology* **34**:221–222.

Kralic, J.E. 2002a. $GABA_A$ receptor $\alpha 1$ subunit knockout mice exhibit plasticity of GABAergic function and behavior. Ph.D. diss., University of North Carolina at Chapel Hill.

Kralic, J.E., E.R. Korpi, T.K. O'Buckley, G.E. Homanics, and A.L. Morrow. 2002b. Molecular and pharmacological characterization of $GABA_A$ receptor $\alpha 1$ subunit knockout mice. *The Journal of Pharmacology and Experimental Therapeutics* **302**(3):1037–1045.

Kralic, J.E., T.K. O'Buckley, R.T. Khisti, C.W. Hodge, G.E. Homanics, and A.L. Morrow. 2002c. $GABA_A$ Receptor alpha-1 subunit deletion alters receptor subtype assembly, pharmacological and behavioral responses to benzodiazepines and zolpidem. *Neuropharmacology* **43**:685–694.

McAuley, J.H. 2001. Does essential tremor originate in the cerebral cortex? *The Lancet* **357**:492–494.

Mehta, A.K., and M.K. Ticku. 1999. An update on $GABA_A$ receptors. *Brain Research Reviews* **29**:196–217.

Monaghan, D.T., and C.W. Cotman. 1985. Distribution of N-methyl-D-aspartate-sensitive L-[3H]glutamate-binding sites in rat brain. *Journal of Neuroscience* **5**, 2909–2919.

Morrow, A.L. 1995. Regulation of $GABA_A$ receptor function and gene expression in the central nervous system. *International Review of Neurobiology* **38**:1–41.

Morrow, A.L., J.R. Pace, R.H. Purdy, and S.M. Paul. 1989. Characterization of steroid interactions with γ-aminobutyric acid receptor-gated chloride ion channels: Evidence for multiple steroid recognition sites. *Molecular Pharmacology* **37**:263–270.

Purves, D., G.J. Augustine, D. Fitzpatrick, L.C. Katz, A.-S. LaMantia, J.O. McNamara, and S.M. Williams, eds. 2001. *Neuroscience* Sinauer Associates, Sunderland, Massachusetts.

Rudolph, U., F. Crestani, and H. Möhler. 2001. $GABA_A$ receptor subtypes: dissecting their pharmacological functions. *Trends in Pharmacological Sciences* **22**(4):188–194.

Schroeder, D., and H.A. Nasrallah. 1982. High alcoholism rate in patients with essential tremor. *American Journal of Psychiatry* **139**:1471–1473.

Shaw, P.J., P.G. Ince, M. Johnson, E.K. Perry, and J.M. Candy. 1992. The quantitative autoradiographic distribution of [3H]MK-801 binding sites in the normal human brainstem in relation to motor neuron diseases. *Brain Research* **572**:276–280.

Sieghart, W., and G. Sperk. 2002. Subunit composition, distribution and function of $GABA_A$ receptor subtypes. *Current Topics in Medical Chemistry* **2**:795–816.

Smaga, S. 2003. Tremor. *American Family Physician* **68**(8):1545–1552.

Wilms, H., J. Sievers, and G. Deuschl. 1999. Animal models of tremor [review]. *Movement Disorders* **14**(4):557–571.

Zeuner, K.E., F.M. Molloy, R.O. Shoge, S.R. Goldstein, R. Wesley, and M. Hallett. 2003. Effect of ethanol on the central oscillator in essential tremor. *Movement Disorders* **18**:1280–1285.

C H A P T E R

E5

Production and Physiological Study of Holmes Tremor in Monkeys

CHIHIRO OHYE

In this chapter, experimental production of a combined postural and resting tremor (*i.e.*, Holmes tremor) in monkeys is described. Following clinical studies on cases with tremor performed mainly in the nineteenth century, the production of Holmes tremor in monkeys has been attempted in many laboratories throughout the world. Based on these studies, it was revealed that the mesencephalic ventromedial tegmental (MVMT) area, including the red nucleus (mainly the parvocellular part), cell loss in the substantial nigra, and the cerebellothalamic tract were the essential neural elements necessary for the production of a combined postural and resting tremor compatible with the Holmes tremor seen in patients. Using stereotactic techniques with depth recording and ventriculography, an MVMT lesion between the red nucleus and substantia nigra was shown to be most successful for production of this type of tremor.

To elucidate the neural mechanism of this tremor, a series of physiological studies were conducted. Accordingly, rhythmic discharge time-locked with the tremor was searched by performing dorsal rhizotomies and microrecording along the neuraxis from the spinal cord, brain stem, and cerebellum to the thalamus. The results obtained led us to build a neural circuit mediating Holmes tremor.

Because tremor is a kind of distinct involuntary movement in humans, it has been known since the era of Galen (cited by Molina-Negro and Hardy, 1975), who described two types of tremor: resting type tremor and intentional type tremor. The systematic study of tremor, which was started in the clinical field by neurologists of the nineteenth century and then continued with the development of animal experiments in the early twentieth century, resulted in resting and/or ataxic tremor being produced in monkeys. It should be emphasized here that the true sense of tremor, either clinical or experimental, has been investigated in detail only in the higher primates, including humans. The definition of tremor is an involuntary rhythmic regular oscillation (of arm or leg) in one plane around one joint, according to the definition of French neurology. In this chapter the historical aspects of Holmes tremor and the author's own method of tremor production in animal models will be described, along with discussion of relevant physiological and clinical features of Holmes tremor.

I. HISTORICAL BACKGROUND

A. Clinical Analysis

In the history of study of tremor, clinical analyses have also seemed to be ahead of experimental studies. Probably the most important study on tremor was that by James Parkinson, who wrote "Essay on shaking palsy" in 1817. Since then, the resting type of tremor has been widely recognized as Parkinsonian tremor. Since the discovery of nigral degeneration by Tretiakoff (1919) and later by Hassler (1938), and its relation to dopamine deficiency by Hornykiewicz (1963), understanding of Parkinson disease has progressed dramatically. Curiously, however, despite accumulating studies on the nigrostriatal dopamine deficiency, origin and neural mechanism of tremor has still been under debate, as will be described in this chapter.

In the history of neurology another important study related to the tremor was the "Red Nucleus Syndrome," which includes ataxic tremor, sometimes also with resting tremor. Probably the first clinical report discussing the clinical pathology of this type of tremor was provided by Benedikt (1889), a neurologist in Vienna. He found three cases with a relatively unique tremor that included three common symptoms (*i.e.*, oculomotor palsy, hemiparesis, and Parkinsonian tremor) with some involuntary movement, on the side of the body contralateral to midbrain damage. In one of his cases, which was examined further at autopsy, he discussed the possibility that a tuberculoma located between the red nucleus and the cerebral peduncle might be responsible for the tremor production. (This midbrain lesion is now considered to involve substantia nigra pars compacta directly or indirectly.) Later, the great French neurologist Charcot (1903) appreciated this discovery and proposed naming similar cases the Benedikt syndrome. This syndrome is well known to practicing neurologists as a classic syndrome of focal midbrain damage. The findings of Benedikt were further confirmed by Holmes (1904) and Souques et al. (1930), who reported similar cases with tremor and midbrain lesion invading the red nucleus. However, now the clinical term of "Holmes tremor" is commonly used to describe the syndrome that consists of a low-frequency tremor that is present during both rest and intentional movements (Deuschl et al., 1989). Frequently a postural component is also present. The rhythm of Holmes tremor may be less regular than that of some other tremors and of large amplitude, giving it a "jerky" appearance. Frequently there is a delay of weeks to months between the causal cerebral insult and tremor onset.

B. Animal Experimental Tremor

Based on these clinical observations on the one hand and the interests of many research groups on primate anatomical-physiological correlative research on the other hand, many investigators were quite interested in the production of primate tremor models. Intentional, resting, and postural tremors were produced by making restricted lesions in the midbrain near the red nucleus. However, it was not easy to define the exact anatomical structures responsible for production of Parkinsonian resting tremor.

In years past, neuroscientists were interested in the Benedikt syndrome and other brainstem/midbrain syndromes as a portal toward understanding motor networks and the pathophysiology of movement disorders. Ogawa and Sano (1942) reported in Japanese an extensive experimental study in monkeys related to lesions of the mesencephalic tegmentum. The attention of this group was mainly focused on the various clinical symptoms seen after tegmental lesions. They described tremor in two monkeys (one tremor was spontaneous resting and the other was intentional) among ten monkeys. The authors discussed their findings in relation to Benedikt syndrome and suggested that damage to the red nucleus and the brachium conjunctivum might play a role in the production of tremor.

Around the same time that studies were going on in Japan, several laboratories in the United States were pursuing similar aims. Two different areas responsible for the production of tremor in monkey were described by separate groups. One was the study by Mettler's group in New York, which emphasized the cerebellar efferent fiber system (Carrea and Mettler, 1955; Mettler, 1966). Using either direct operative attack or stereotactic methods, they destroyed the superior cerebellar peduncle, decussation of superior cerebellar peduncles, superior peduncle and red nucleus, superior peduncle and basal ganglia, and interpeduncular nucleus, respectively. Thus, they produced among these monkeys, ataxia (eight cases), ataxia with static tremor (one case), ataxia with ataxic tremor and tremor (nine cases), and isolated tremor (three cases). They observed that, if the lesion was located caudal to the decussation, tremor appeared on the same side of the lesion, but, if the lesion was more rostral, tremor appeared on the contralateral side. They emphasized that rest tremors were produced by lesions along the cerebellar efferent fibers from the cerebellar nucleus through the superior cerebellar peduncles, as well as the decussation toward the thalamus, especially its ventral part. These findings are important but often neglected. They showed that the substantial nigra and tremor were not directly related and that a lesion in midbrain tegmentum is able to produce resting tremor.

The other U.S. group, represented by Ward in Chicago (Ward et al., 1948; Peterson et al., 1949; Jenker and Ward, 1953), claimed that the midbrain-pontine reticular formation was responsible for the production of postural tremor. Ward tried making different stereotactic lesions in the midbrain-pons-medulla to produce tremor in monkeys. The lesions destroyed the subthalamic nucleus, rostral part of midbrain tegmentum, decussation of cerebellar peduncles, medial part of midbrain-pontine-tegmentum, dorsomedial or dorsolateral part of pontine tegmentum, cerebral peduncle, and basal pons, respectively, and postural tremor appeared (in five monkeys among 24) only, with lesions destroying the midbrain ventromedial tegmentum. More correctly, the causal lesions were located just dorsal to the substantia nigra. The tremor (about 8 Hz) appeared from the day after operation to 8 days later and continued for up to 2.5 months.

Further study was reported by Carpenter and Stevens (1957), who made lesions in the cerebellar nuclei and/or superior cerebellar peduncle and observed resting tremor in five cases among 16, lasting for 100 days at maximum. Pathological examination revealed that, in the majority of the cases with tremor, the lesion was located in the dorsolateral part of the dentate nucleus and interpositus nucleus, with concomitant degeneration of the mid one-third of the superior cerebellar peduncle also. Lesions in the fastigial nucleus did not produce tremor. The resting tremor was also accompanied by an ataxic tremor. Later these investigators made a stereotactic lesion in the superior cerebellar peduncle and found marked resting tremor in three cases among eight, all on the ipsilateral side of the lesions, persisting for 100 days. Interestingly, ataxic tremor further continued after cessation of the resting tremor. Carpenter (1961) described that, for production of tremor, damage to the ascending cerebellar efferent fibers at the level of midbrain caudal to the red nucleus is necessary.

Aronson et al. (1962) tried to produce tremor in monkeys by electrical stimulation, by making a lesion in the brainstem or using reserpine. After lesioning the midbrain tegmentum, a resting tremor appeared along with an ataxic tremor but persisted for only a few days. Because the responsible lesion was found in the superior cerebellar peduncle *and* the nearby reticular formation, more pathophysiological emphasis was placed on the latter structure.

Stern (1966) attempted to clarify the core symptoms seen after destruction of the substantia nigra. He made nigral lesions in eight *Macaca* monkeys (five by a stereotactic method and three by direct incisions) and observed static tremor in two cases (one on the day of operation and one after a latency period of 1 week). The nigral lesion extended into the ventral portions of the superior cerebellar peduncle. It is noteworthy that he concluded that the central sign of nigral lesions was hypokinesia.

Velasco et al. (1979) used *Macaca* monkeys to study the tremor associated with midbrain ventromedial tegmental lesions. Their experimental method was unique in that they made lesions after recording electrical activity in the vicinity of the red nucleus with a concentric bipolar needle. They found rhythmic grouped discharges of 4 to 8 Hz in the red nucleus and substantia nigra pars compacta and made a lesion at the locations that included such grouped rhythmic discharges. Holmes tremor (4 to 8 Hz) appeared 1 to 20 days after lesion creation. Interestingly, an additional lesion dorsolateral to the first lesion arrested the tremor. Thus, they suggested that there exists both a tremor-producing and a tremor-suppressing system side by side in the midbrain tegmentum, although these investigators did not definitively define such systems. Importantly, these and earlier investigators were under the similar impression that, if the lesion was either too small or too large, Holmes tremor would not be manifested.

II. MIDBRAIN VENTROMEDIAL TEGMENTAL (MVMT) LESION

As described in the previous section, clinical and experimental studies strongly suggested that the midbrain ventromedial tegmental area is the most plausible candidate for production of Holmes tremor. It was Poirier's group in Quebec that helped to clarify this situation. According to one of their initial studies (Poirier, 1960), MVMT lesions induced postural or resting tremor in eight of 20 monkeys. In two cases contralateral tremor developed after unilateral lesions, and in two cases bilateral tremor was shown after bilateral lesions. In other cases tremor developed after repeated operations. Tremor was observed with short delay after operation in most of the cases. Tremor was often manifested by an elbow-flexed posture, which was exaggerated by excitation. In this sense it was described as a postural tremor. Mydriasis on the operated side, torticollis toward the operated side, contralateral hypotonia, hypokinesia, and ataxia were also observed in these monkeys. This type of tremor is exactly like our own model, as will be described. Pathological study revealed that the cell loss in the substantia nigra was due to damage to nigrostrial fibers, damage to the rubrospinal tract due to destruction of the magnocellular red nucleus, and damage to the superior cerebellar outflow tract.

The Canadian group clarified the neuronal elements involved in the ventrolateral tegmental lesion in 34 tremor monkeys with precise histopathological analyses (Poirier et al., 1969): the rubrospinal tract (crossed) from the magnocellular red nucleus, rubroolivary tract (uncrossed) from the parvocellular red nucleus, nucleus parabrachialis, ascending serotoninergic fibers from the pontine and mesencephalic reticular formations, and retrograde degeneration of nucleus dorsalis and nucleus centralis superior. In summary, they emphasized the involvement of ascending dopaminergic fibers and the rubro(parvocellular)-olivo-cerebello-rubral loop (Larochelle et al., 1970). Parallel to their studies of tremor, Poirier and co-workers contributed to the understanding of the neural mechanisms in Parkinson disease with the same animal models by showing decreased striatal dopamine levels that paralleled cell loss in the substantia nigra pars compacta (Poirier et al., 1969).

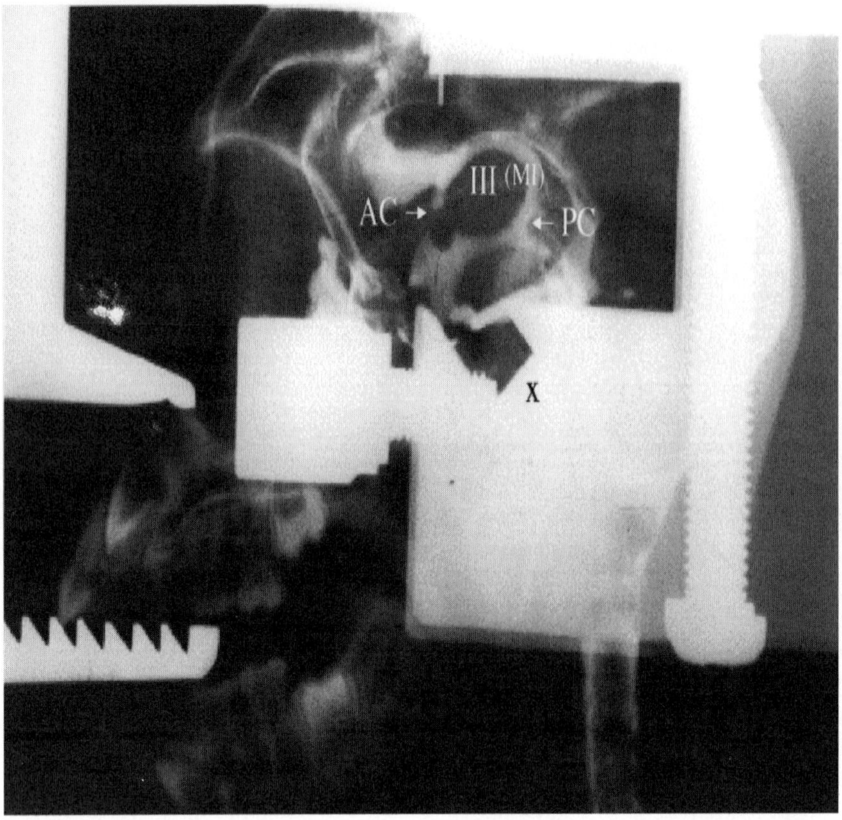

FIGURE 1 Ventriculography of a monkey sitting on a chair with stereotactic apparatus in place. AC, Anterior commissure; PC, posterior commissure; III, third ventricle; MI, massa intermedia; x, position of ear bar.

III. OUR OWN SERIES

A. Production of Tremor

Based on the work of other investigators, we knew the approximate location of neural structures critical to the pathophysiology of resting, postural, and kinetic tremors in primates. Our next step was to generate more exacting MVMT lesions using improved technical approaches. Following the principles and techniques laid out by Poirier's group, we subsequently applied human stereotactic methods in primates to create specific MVMT lesions. More specifically, we used ventriculography to visualize the third ventricle of monkeys and depth microrecording to identify the red nucleus zone (Ohye, 1979, 1988; Ohye et al., 1979).

A total of about 50 small monkeys (Java monkeys, *Macaca irus*) weighing less than 5 kg were used for our experiments. After fixing the head on animal stereotactic apparatus in sitting position under light Nembutal anesthesia (20 mg/Kg), two directional craniogams (lateral and frontal) were taken. For target planning, radiological and electrophysiological methods were used, as in human stereotactic surgery (Ohye, 1997). To perform ventriculography, a stereotactic needle puncture of the anterior horn of the lateral ventricle was per-formed, referring to the midline (4 mm lateral) and limbus sphenoidalis (about 10 mm above) on radiographic film (Percheron, 1975). Toward this tentative ventricular point, through a small hole by twist drill, a needle was slowly inserted. About 0.3 ml of radiopaque substance (Conray) was injected into the ventricular system to visualize the third ventricle on radiographic film. Usually it was not difficult to define the anterior commissure, posterior commissure, and intercommissural line (Figure 1). Our target area (MVMT) was found between the parvocellular red nucleus and substantia nigra (based on primate atlases, MVMT is located approximately a few millimeters anterior to the posterior commissure, several millimeters below the posterior commissure, and 1 to 2 mm lateral to the midline). Therefore, the parvocellular red nucleus is a good landmark to arrive at this optimal target for the production of tremor. To get to this critical point, depth microrecording was made to identify the red nucleus. This was not particularly difficult because the red nucleus showed very active spontaneous discharge, in contrast to the surrounding tegmental area, which showed only slight spontaneous activity (Figure 2).

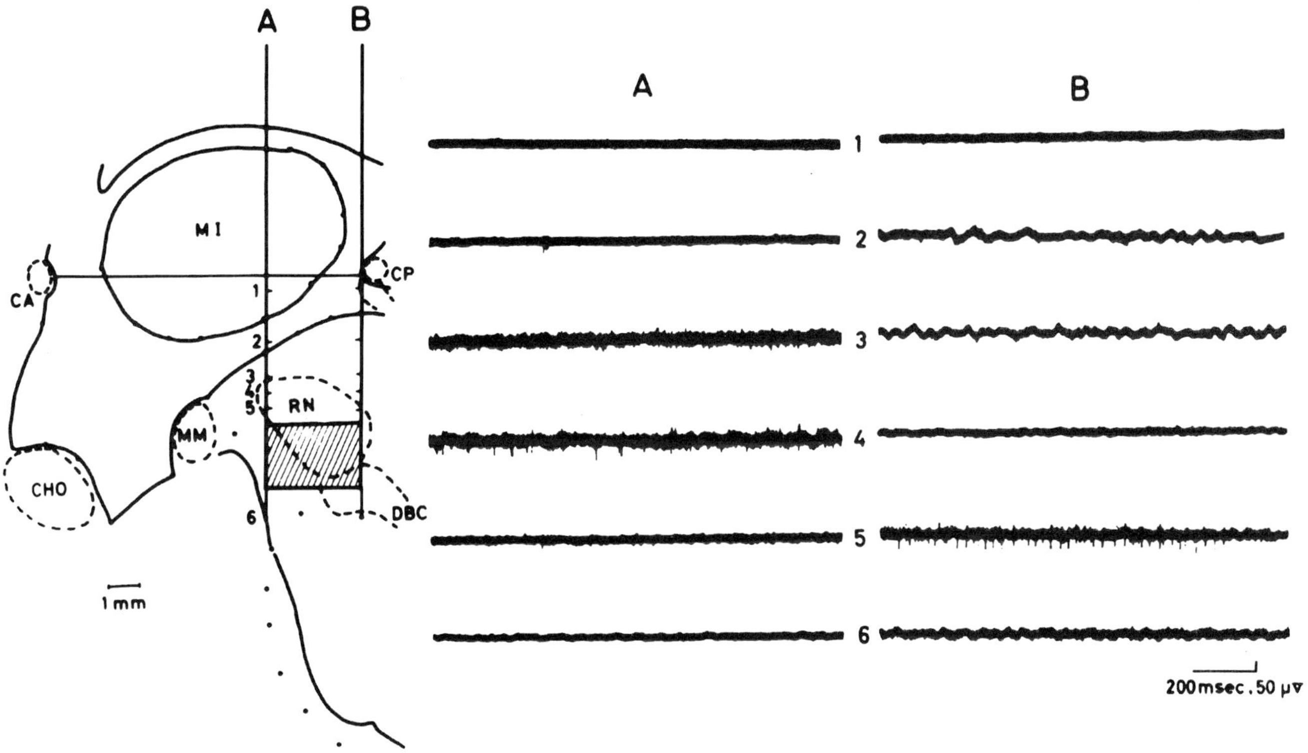

FIGURE 2 Microrecording in and around the red nucleus in a monkey. Vertical trajectory (A and B) by a pair of microelectrodes is shown on the left side, with the third ventricle traced from radiographic film. Examples of recorded depth activity at six different depths from each electrode (1 to 6) are shown on the right side. In this case, a hatched area was coagulated. Note that spontaneous activity increased in the red nucleus. CA, Anterior commissure; CP, posterior commissure; MI, massa intermedia; CHO, optic chiasma; MM, mammillary body; RN, red nucleus; DBC, decussation of brachium conjunctivum.

The recording electrode was a concentric bipolar needle type (outer diameter: 0.6 mm, interpolar distance: 200–300 µm, tip: 10 µm) that used a small tip size (effective tip length was 2 mm). We mainly used a vertical approach, although oblique anterior or posterior approaches were occasionally employed to avoid overlying cortical and thalamic damage. When microrecording indicated that the tip of the electrode was in or around the red nucleus, electrical stimulation (100 Hz, 5V, for 1–2 sec) was attempted in order to determine if responses consistent with third cranial nerve stimulation (pupillary constriction, various types of ocular movement, and palpebral opening) were observed.

After confirming the location of our electrode tip, radiofrequency coagulation lesions were made that included a part of the parvocellular red nucleus and MVMT area between the red nucleus and substantia niagra. A restricted coagulation was made with a pair of coagulation needles from Leksell's apparatus with an interval of 2 mm, using the radiofrequency thermocoagulator set at 65°C for 10 to 20 sec. The theoretical lesion volume was about 6 mm^3 (2 mm × 2 mm × 1.5 mm).

Immediately after coagulation, monkeys showed pupil dilatation, loss of light reaction, and ptosis on the operated side. These oculomotor signs lasted for about 1 month and then gradually improved to some extent. On the day following operations, torticollis toward the operated side, flexed posture of the contralateral limb at the elbow joint, and, often, forced circling toward the contralateral side were observed in most of the cases (Figure 3). The degree of head rotation was variable, almost 90 degrees in some cases. The flexed posture of the upper limb was rather constant, keeping the forearm flexed at 90 degrees at the elbow joint; fingers were extended naturally. The monkey was reluctant to use the affected limb; also, general movement became more or less hypokinetic. The leg did not show a particular posture but was also paretic and hypokinetic. These immediate changes improved to some extent within 1 month or so, but the flexed posture was maintained throughout. Among these three symptoms, mydriasis and torticollis did not directly relate to the later development of tremor.

The tremor appeared superimposing on the flexed upper limb gradually, but with some delay, usually of a few weeks (2 to 8 weeks, with a mean of 4 weeks). Exceptionally, there were cases in which the tremor appeared within a few days after the operation. The lower limb was also involved in

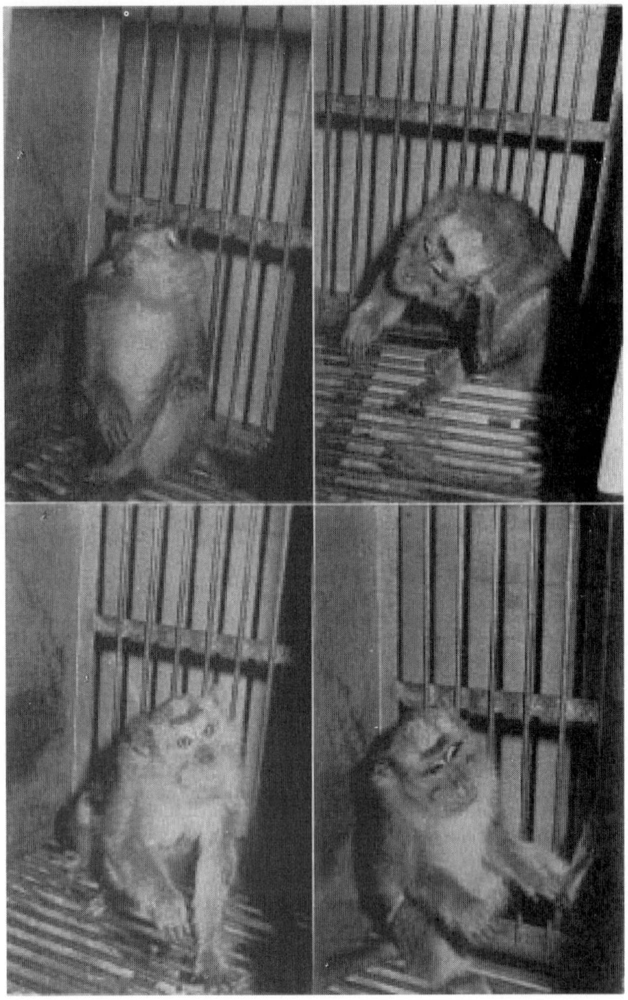

FIGURE 3 Four different postures of a left-sided MVMT lesioned monkey with spontaneous tremor. Note the flexed posture on the right upper limb and slight torticollis to the left. Mydriasis is not marked in this case.

one-third of the cases, but not so marked as the upper limb. It was not easy to determine the exact time of onset of tremor because it appeared first in the distal part of the contralateral limb and then spread to proximal parts. Once tremor appeared, it was continuous in the awake state, with reciprocal action between antagonistic muscles and appearing exaggerated in amplitude when the monkeys were excited. In a given monkey, tremor frequency was fairly constant. Frequency was mainly around 5 to 7 Hz, but variably up to 9 or even 10 Hz in some cases. Since the tremor was always accompanied by a flexed posture, we believed that it was better to define it as a postural tremor, although, at times, a marked hand-finger tremor with pill-rolling characteristics, as seen in Parkinson disease, was observed in the lesioned monkeys. Also, in some cases intentional tremor was manifest during certain movements as, for example, when reaching for food. The tremor tended to decrease gradually over the course of several months or years. In one case a postural tremor persisted for 7 years.

It is noteworthy that tremor was facilitated by administration of harmaline, a monoamine oxidase inhibitor. For example, when tremor decreased over time, harmaline enhanced tremor to its previous active state. Furthermore, during the latency period before appearance of tremor after lesion creation, harmaline permitted the tremor to become manifest. In this sense our success rate of tremor production was increased from about one-third to two-thirds of cases with harmaline.

Other pharmacological studies were undertaken to examine the effects of L-dopa on tremor (see Video). We found that a "proper" dose of L-dopa (for example, 100 mg) was able to reduce tremor amplitude but that larger dosages (e.g., 250 mg) temporarily induced choreiform movements in the affected limb(s), effectively converting tremor into dopa-induced dyskinesias. In this regard the effects of L-dopa on tremor were very similar to what is commonly seen in patients with Parkinson disease. It was also interesting to observe that frequent administration of L-dopa permanently changed the tremor into choreiform movements in one monkey.

Reserpine reversed the effects of L-dopa. Namely, when L-dopa converted tremor into choreiform movements, administration of reserpine (3 mg) arrested chorea acutely and subacutely suppressed general behavior, gradually resulting in a complete akinetic state that lasted for a couple of days prior to recovery to the baseline tremulous state. These studies clearly demonstrated the powerful effects of pharmacological agents on monkeys "primed" with focal lesions of central motor pathways.

B. Histological Analysis of MVMT Lesions

In the context of histopathological analysis, the precise work by Poirier's group provided a valuable framework for our own study. Keeping the proposed responsible neural elements involved in effective MVMT lesions in mind, we histologically examined the following elements in relation to the tremor: substantia nigra, parvocellular red nucleus, magnocellular red nucleus, and cerebellothalamic tract. In each case, areas of damage were estimated from examination of histological sections and plotted as circle graphs, as shown in Figures 4 and 5. Figure 5 summarizes the results in 14 cases, listed in the order of tremor severity. It seems likely that, as far as these neural elements were concerned, cell loss in the substantia nigra and parvocellular red nucleus is closely related to the production of Holmes tremor, confirming the previous conclusion of Poirier's group. Based on our results, we defined our optimum area (0-zone) for the production of tremor with a single destructive lesion. The ideal lesion should include the parvocellular red nucleus, with its ventral extend in the tegmental area almost

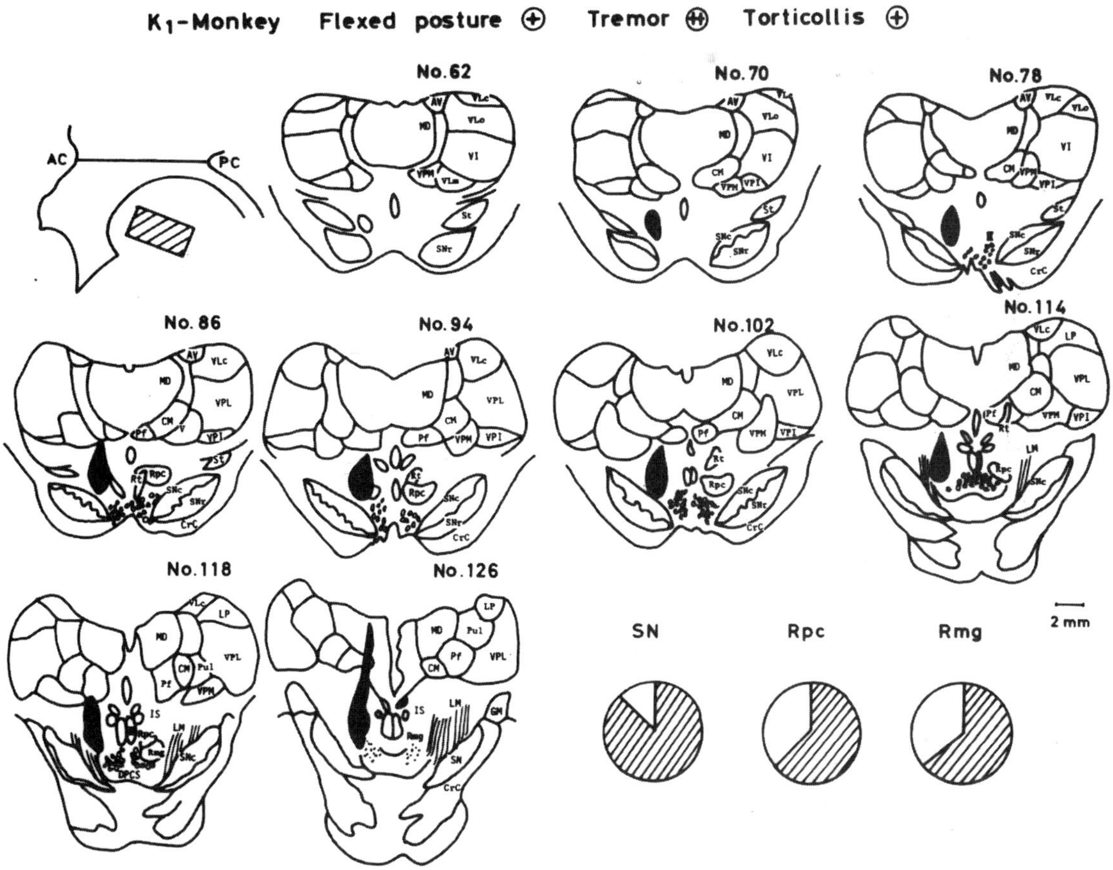

FIGURE 4 Drawings of a serial histological section of an MVMT lesioned monkey with typical flexed posture, spontaneous tremor, and torticollis. Extent of cell loss in the substantia nigra (SN), parvocellular red nucleus (RNpc), and magnocellular red nucleus (RNmg) was shown after counting several sampling areas on both sides, using a circle graph.

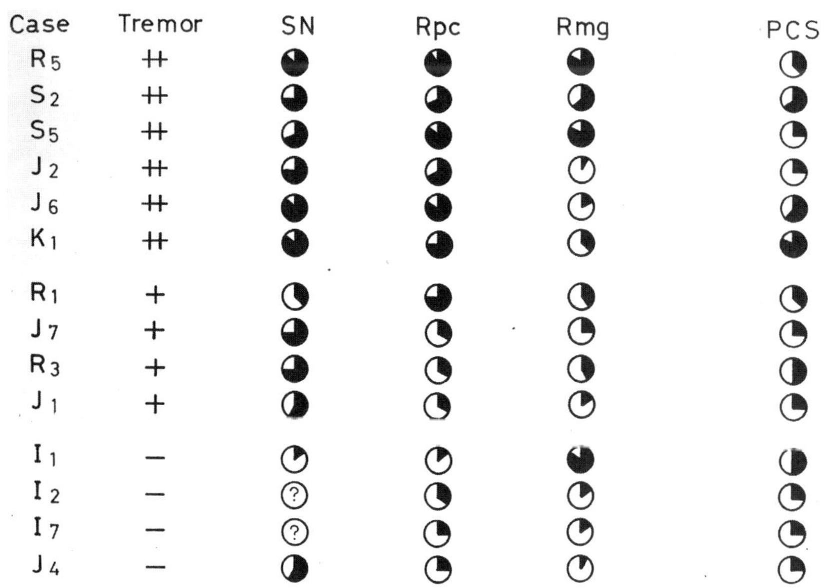

FIGURE 5 Damage to main mesencephalic structures shown for 14 MVMT lesioned monkeys with continuous spontaneous tremor (6 cases, ++), with temporary tremor (4 cases, +), and without tremor (4 cases, −). The extent of cell loss in SN, RNpc, RNmg, and superior cerebellar peduncle (PCS) is shown with circle graphs.

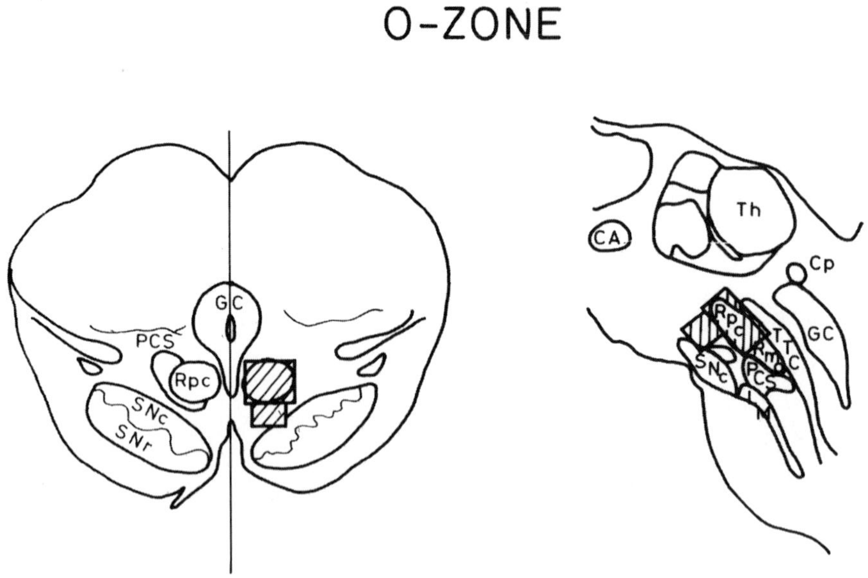

FIGURE 6 Optimal area (*hatched*) for MVMT lesions associated with Holmes tremor. *Left*, Coronal section; *right*, sagittal section; GC, central gray; Th, thalamus; TTC, central tegmental tract; LM, medial lemniscus.

touching the mediodorsal edge of the substantia nigra (Figure 6).

In order to verify that the previously mentioned elements are really necessary to produce Holmes tremor, we tried to destroy each element separately one by one, in random order (Ohye et al., 1988). This is schematically illustrated in Figure 7. So, in four monkeys, selective lesions were made (1) within the parvocellular red nucleus (either by radiofrequency coagulation or by injecting a small amount of kainic acid to destroy cellular elements), (2) at the level of decussation of the superior cerebellar peduncle to destroy the cerebellothalamic tract, and (3) at the mediodorsal part of the substantia nigra to interrupt the nigrostriatal fiber at its exit without invading the red nucleus, respectively. Operations were conducted always with the aid of radiological and electrophysiological control, as mentioned previously. Each lesion was made with an interval of several weeks or several months, with observation of whether or not the tremor appeared. Both spontaneous and harmaline-induced tremors were tested. The results obtained in four monkeys and, for comparison, one monkey with a standard MVMT lesion and another monkey with a red nucleus lesion are summarized in Figure 8. It was clearly revealed that only when all three elements were sufficiently (more than 50%) lesioned, irrespective of the order of destruction, a Holmes tremor appeared. Moreover, harmaline-induced tremor was easily manifest in those animals with lesions of all three neural elements, except in a single case with an inadequate lesion of the superior cerebellar peduncle. In this regard and as noted previously, the degree of response to harmaline tremor is a good indicator of damage to the cerebellar peduncle.

C. Physiological Study of Tremor in Monkeys

In order to elucidate the neuronal mechanism of tremor thus produced by MVMT lesion, several physiological studies were conducted.

1. Dorsal Root Section

In three monkeys with postural tremor, the ipsilateral cervical dorsal roots were cut (rhizotomy), to clarify the possible role of spinal reflex loops in tremor maintenance. In the study cited here, monkeys with cerebellar lesions were used (Ohye et al., 1970). Under general anesthesia, the spinal cord was exposed by laminectomy and the cervical dorsal roots from C2 to T2 were cut under direct visual control. The effect of the rhizotomy on the postural tremor was examined frequently by clinical observation, by EMG examination, and, finally, at autopsy. To facilitate the tremor, harmaline (3 mg/kg) was also utilized. After rhizotomy, monkeys showed sensory deficits and temporary monoparesis. Importantly, both spontaneous and harmaline-induced tremor persisted after deafferentation. Only a slight increase in the irregularity of tremor amplitude and rate was detected by EMG study. From this experiment the authors concluded that tremor rhythm originates centrally and is transferred to the spinal motor neuron pool via some descending tract. Moreover, the peripheral reflex loop serves to stabilize tremor amplitude and rhythm. Similar conclusions with respect to resting tremors were already made by the pioneering works of Foerster (1911) and Pollock and Davis (1930) in Parkinsonian patients.

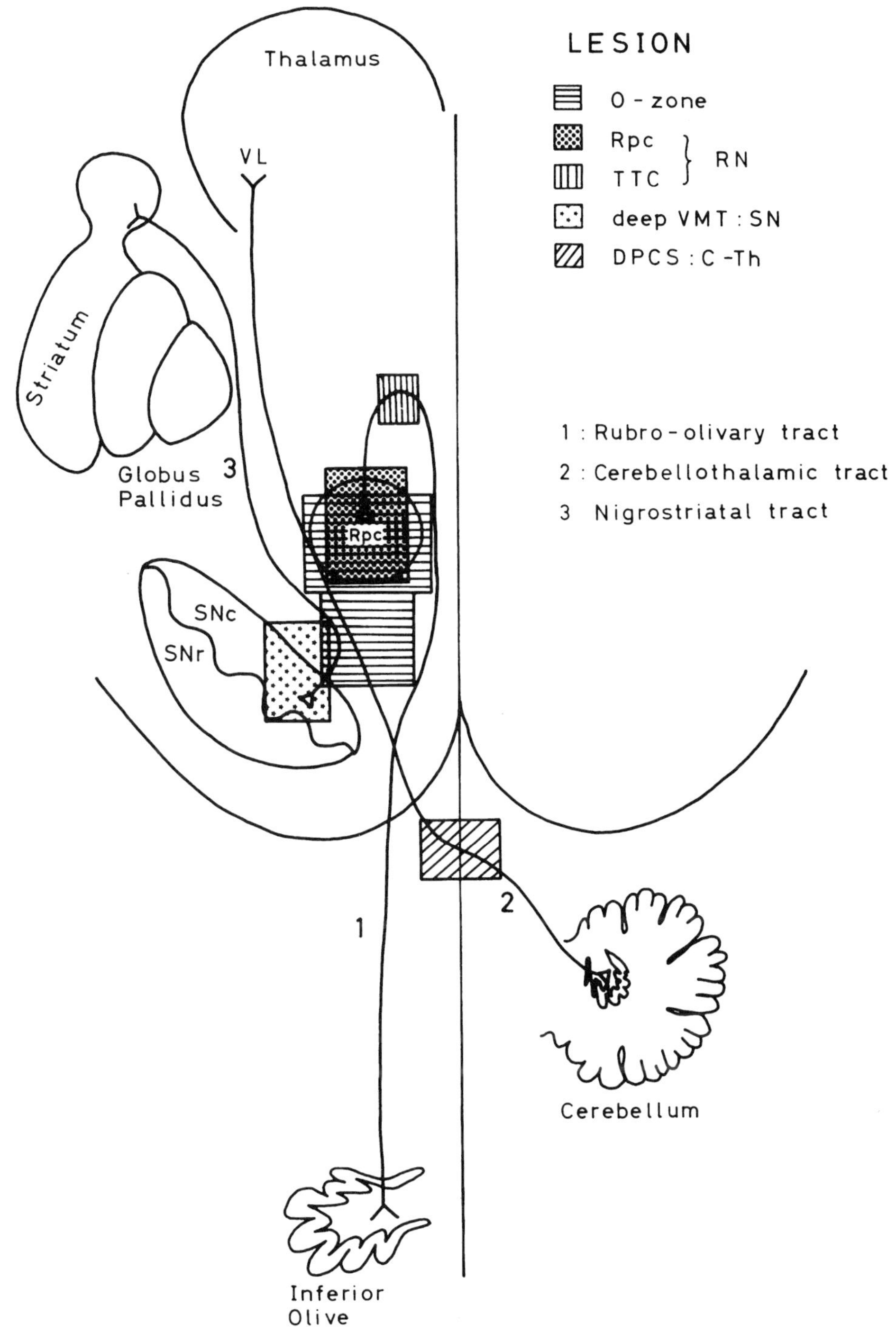

FIGURE 7 Schematic illustration of stepwise mesencephalic lesions in relation to the standard MVMT lesion (in the center). The main three tracts essential for Holmes tremor production are shown with numerals.

Autopsy studies in the deafferented monkeys revealed clear-cut degeneration of ascending tracts in the corresponding part of the ipsilateral cuneate fasciculus. Interestingly, in one monkey, rhizotomy induced concomitant degeneration of the dorsal spinocerebellar and lateral corticospinal tracts by the incidental interruption of the blood supply to the corresponding lateral column of the cervical cord. The findings in this case supported an important proposal that postural tremor can persist after complete interruption of the corticospinal tracts at the peduncular level (Poirier et al., 1969).

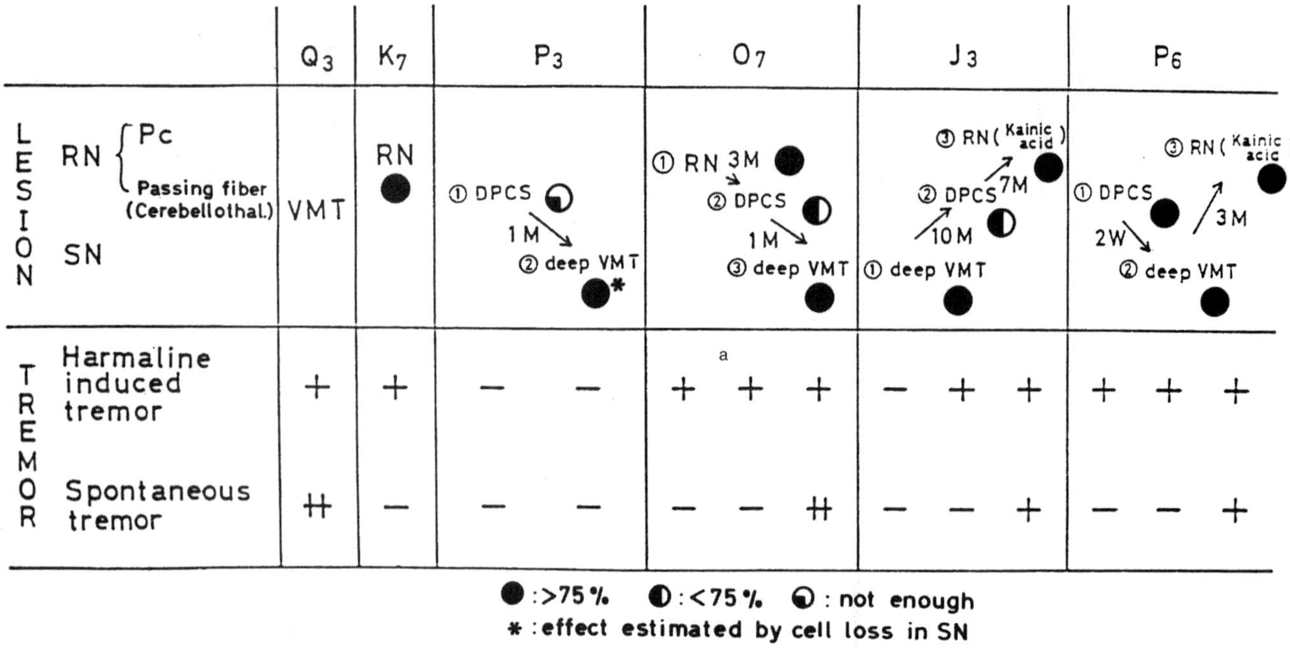

FIGURE 8 Sequential changes in the clinical manifestations of tremor (spontaneous and harmaline- induced) after stepwise sequential lesions (either electrolytic or kainic acid) in and around the MVMT region (red nucleus, substantia nigra, cerebellothalamic tract), as illustrated in Figure 7. Lesions were made separately, and consequent clinical states are described. Four monkeys were used for multiple lesions and two others (controls) for single lesions. (Reproduced from Ohye et al., 1988, with permission.)

2. Microrecording

a. Tremor Rhythm in the Spinal Cord

In the spinal cord of monkeys with Holmes tremor, microrecording was used to understand the descending and ascending pathways mediating the tremor rhythm (Ohye et al., 1984). For this purpose, a special metal plate (duralumine 5.5 × 5.5 × 4 mm) is fixed on the skull and by intermediate of this metal plate, monkey head is fixed to the stereotactic apparatus without giving pain (Percheron et al., 1973; Feger et al., 1978). For this study, a total of 30 small Java monkeys (*Macaca irus*) were used. After MVMT lesions, in most of the cases, postural tremor developed in the contralateral limb(s) with a delay of a couple of weeks. Once the tremor became stable and constant, microrecording from the spinal cord started. Systematic recordings were made to find rhythmic discharges time-locked with the tremor monitored by EMG. Several rhythmic discharges were found in the superficial portions of the ipsilateral dorsal column. These discharges were recognized as ascending tremor impulses in the lemniscal system, since they responded to light touch on certain areas of the corresponding arm. During cutaneous input, the rhythmic burst changed into tonic discharge. In addition, rhythmic discharges were detected in the spinocerebellar tracts of the lateral funiculus.

Searching for activity of descending nature, the following characteristics were adopted: (1) the spinal rhythmic burst preceded the EMG grouped discharge of tremor, and (2) burst discharge persisted after injection of curare with temporary artificial respiration to inhibit muscle contraction for a short period. Thus we found two distinct areas deep in the ventral quadrant of ipsilateral spinal cord. One was found around the dorsolateral corner of the ventral horn about 2 mm from the midline, ipsilateral to the tremulous upper limb. This kind of burst activity was found along rostrocaudal extent at almost the same distance from the midline and the same depth from the surface. Histological examination of one of the recorded points marked by ferrocyanide revealed that the point was located at the lateral edge of the ventral horn around Rexed's lamina VII at the C2 level. Because it was a positive spike (upward deflection in our recording), it was interpreted as electrical activity of fibers in a descending path. It was also interesting to note that, during the curarized state, tremor rate was slightly accelerated (Figure 9), probably due to unloading of the muscle contraction.

The other region showing characteristics of a descending tract was found about 0.5 mm lateral to the midline in the area of the anterior funiculus. In all monkeys it was located within 1 mm from the midline, deep in the ventral part of the spinal cord ipsilateral to the tremulous limb. In one case we attempted to electrolytically destroy the anterior funiculus and medial part of the ventral horn, as shown in Figure 10. It was concluded that the tremor rhythm was traversing downward through an ipsilateral midline structure, probably the reticulospinal tract in the anterior funiculus. Subsequently, tremor rhythm was transmitted to the motoneuron

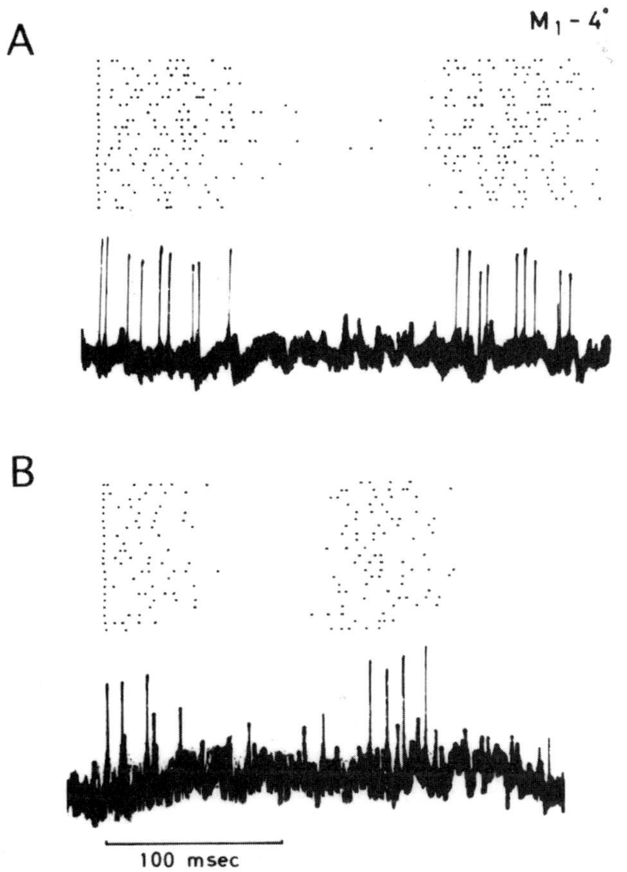

FIGURE 9 Raster display of the rhythmic grouped discharge time-locked with tremor recorded at two different states from the same point of the spinal cord in a monkey with spontaneous tremor. Recording site was the dorsolateral corner of the ventral horn, in this example. **A**, Usual state with spontaneous tremor. **B**, After immobilization with curare (0.2 mg). Note that the tremor rhythm was accelerated after curare.

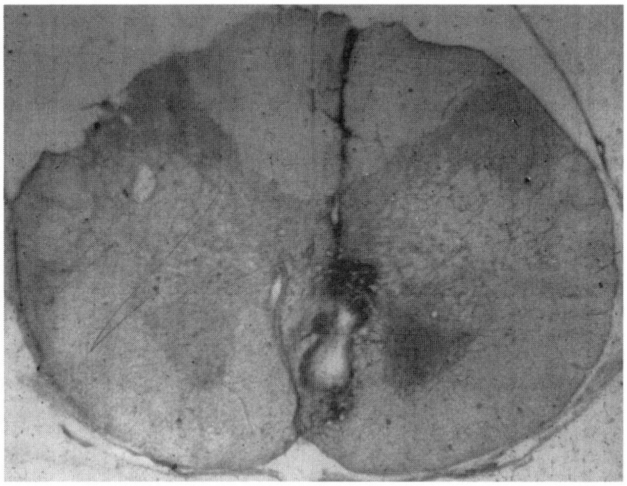

FIGURE 10 Histological section of the cervical cord showing a selective lesion in the anterior funiculus, where rhythmic grouped discharges time-locked with tremor were recorded. The spontaneous tremor was abolished after creation of the lesion.

pool via the dorsolateral corner of the ventral horn. It is well known that the reticulospinal tract is located in the anterior funiculus. This study showed that the descending tremor pathway does not necessarily utilize the pyramidal tract, as is commonly believed, but instead courses through the reticulospinal tract ipsilateral to tremor.

b. Tremor Rhythm in the Cerebellum

Although systematic recording was not conducted, rhythmic discharge related to tremor was surveyed in two cases. For this experiment, after fixing the monkey head to the stereotactic apparatus, an occipital craniectomy was performed to allow for access to the cerebellum. Up to twelve recording sessions were completed in each monkey. Recording sessions were separated by 3 to 7 days. Using inion as a surface landmark and considering spinocerebellar connections mentioned in the previous section, a 10-mm bilateral range and 10-mm rostrocaudal extent of cerebellum was explored. This area covered vermis and lobulus paramedianus. Rhythmic bursts related to the tremor were found only in the ipsilateral side, at two different depths, one of which was likely the Purkinje cell layer, less than 10 mm from the cortical surface; the other deeper one, at the level of the fourth ventricle, was one of the cerebellar nuclei, according to the sagittal view of the radiographic image. The former rhythmic discharge was time-locked with the tremor in the lower limb (ipsilateral rectus femoris muscle) and, when the tremor stopped as the tremulous muscle was held, the rhythmic discharge was desynchronized. Therefore, this tremor pathway was believed to belong to the ascending side, probably receiving spinocerebellar projections as expected, based on anatomical considerations.

c. Tremor Rhythm in the Brainstem

To monitor tremor-related rhythmic discharges at the level of the pons, light anesthesia with pentobarbital was necessary. Systematic microrecordings from the pontine level via a vertical approach through the cerebral cortex were performed in 18 experiments, utilizing a total of six monkeys. These experiments revealed rhythmic group discharges time-locked with tremor at the level of the mediodorsal pontine reticular formation, ipsilateral to the peripheral tremor, 2 mm from the midline, extending rostrocaudally about 10 mm along the aqueduct and the fourth ventricle in the sagittal view on radiographic film. It should be emphasized that this structure was assumed to be the origin of the pontine reticulospinal tract.

Considering that several rhythmic activities such as respiration, gait, and mastication originate at the level of the pontine reticular formation, the effects of low-frequency (3 to 10 Hz) stimulation were examined. When the rhythmic tremor-related discharge was isolated, the recording electrode was subsequently used for stimulation. Interestingly, low-frequency stimulation of 6 to 7 Hz was specifically effective to activate the tremor of the monkey whose

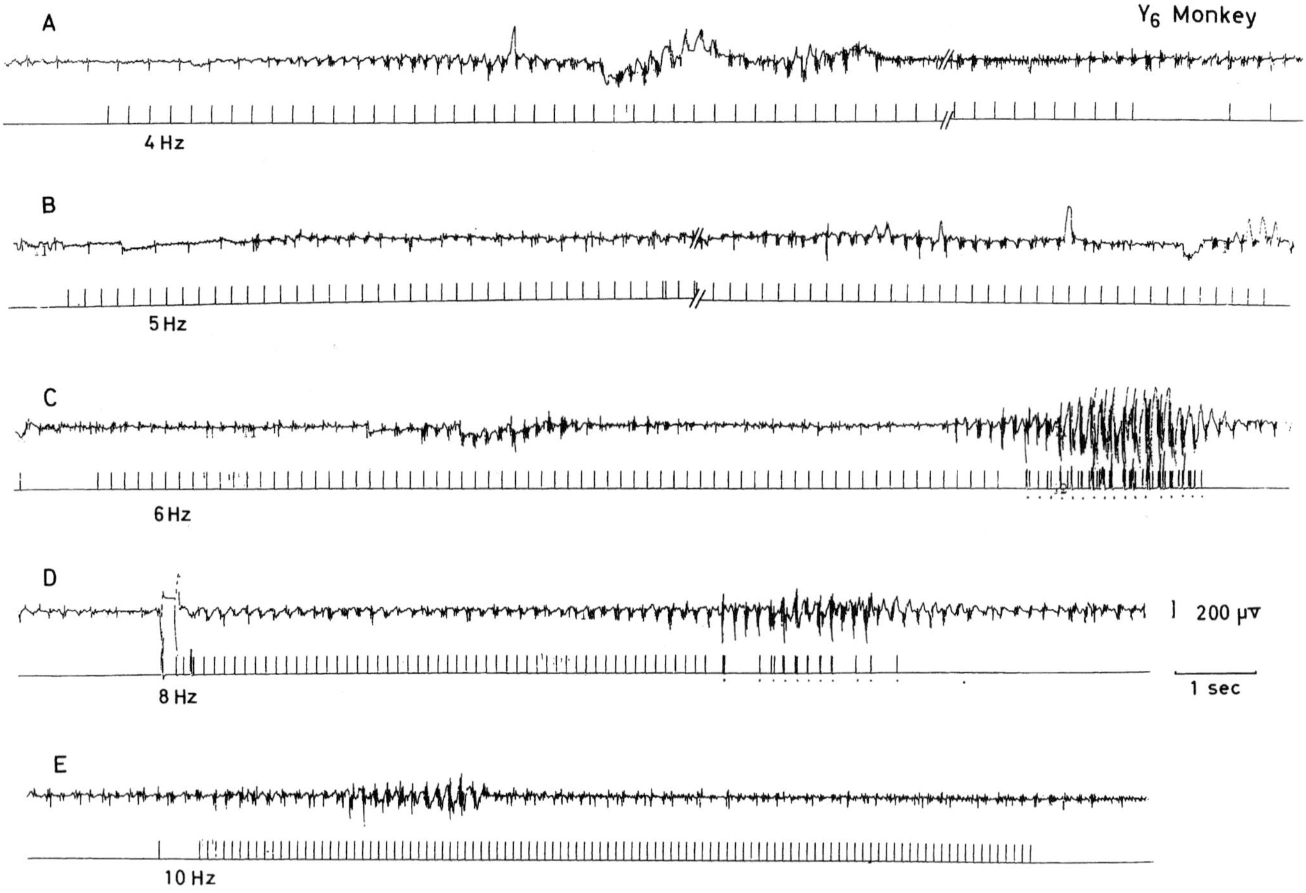

FIGURE 11 Electrical stimulation of the pontine medial tegmental point where tremor time-locked rhythmic discharges were recorded. Stimulation at different frequencies (4, 5, 6, 8, and 10 Hz) was delivered at about 0.1 mA. Notice that the pre-existing tremor was specifically exaggerated by the stimulation at 6 Hz, which coincided with that of the spontaneous tremor in this monkey. Upper trace: EMG from the right triceps muscle. Lower trace: signal of electrical stimulation.

recordings are shown in Figure 11. Also, the same stimulation paradigm at 7 Hz induced the original tremor with a latency of 10 to 20 sec when it was delivered during a tremor pause. It was confirmed that only stimulation ipsilateral to the original tremor was responsive to this activation procedure. Furthermore, when a type of feedback stimulation was given (*i.e.,* whenever the natural tremor began and amplitude was increasing to its plateau, electrical stimulation was delivered), it markedly accelerated the tremor.

The stimulation experiment in the pontine reticular formation strongly suggested that the reticulospinal tract–anterior funiculus of the spinal cord could be the descending pathway mediating the tremor rhythm. It is important to note that a recent study by Nandi et al. (2002) reported a similar result: that low-frequency stimulation of the pedunculopontine region produced tremor in the normal monkey.

d. Tremor Rhythm and Kinesthetic Response in the Thalamus

In the thalamus of five monkeys with tremor, we looked for the tremor rhythm in the ventralis posterior lateralis oralis (VPLo) nucleus, which is considered to be equivalent to the human ventralis intermedius (Vim) nucleus (Macchi and Jones, 1997). Similar to the tremor rhythm encountered in Parkinson disease, VPLo neurons in the monkeys with tremors showed almost the same characteristics as Vim neurons, namely time-locked rhythmic grouped discharges and kinesthetic responses to passive limb movement (Lamarre and Joffroy, 1979; Ohye and Albe-Fessard, 1978; Ohye et al., 1989, 1993). Furthermore, to clarify the possible ascending pathway to the kinesthetic zone, the dorsal columns were sectioned at a high cervical level bilaterally in one monkey. It was subsequently observed that the kines-

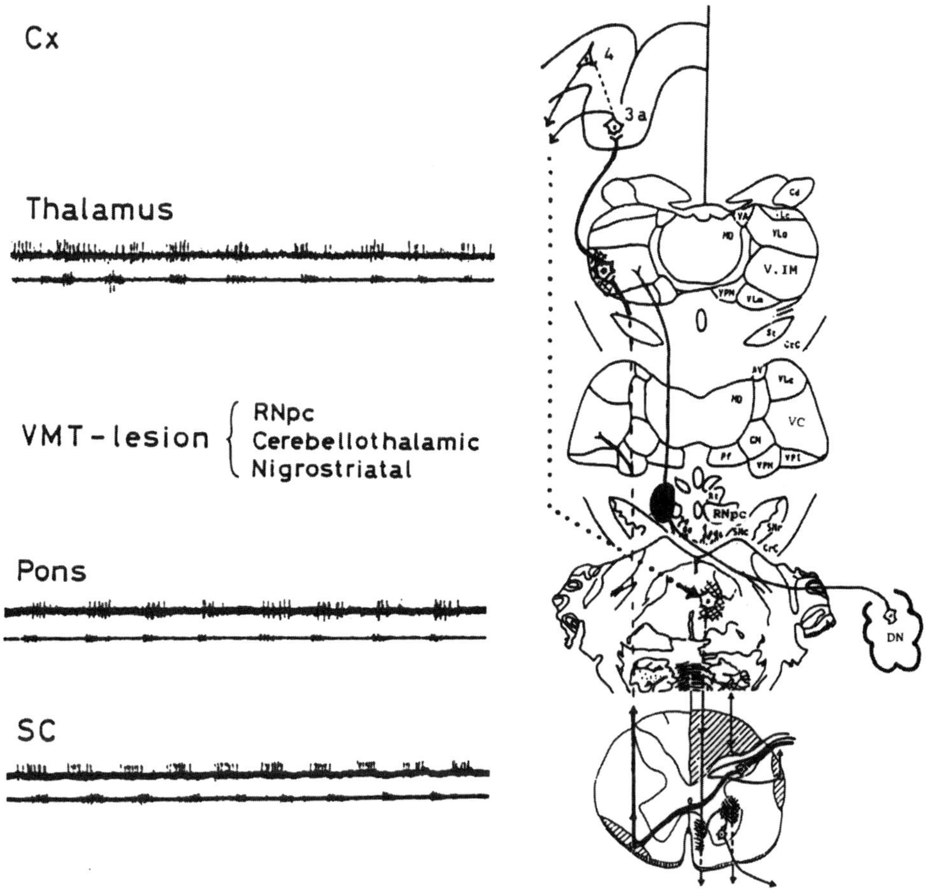

FIGURE 12 A hypothetical tremor mediating long-loop circuit, which integrates all of our experimental results in monkeys with our clinical experiences. (Modified from Ohye, 1987, with permission.)

thetic response in VPLo to electrical stimulation of a contralateral peripheral nerve (radial nerve in this case) was not affected. In another case, after spinal cord hemisection contralateral to the thalamus, the kinesthetic response in VPLo to the same electrical stimulation remained as before. This fact strongly suggested that an ascending route mediating the kinesthetic response and tremor rhythm may use a crossed pathway in the spinal cord, probably the spinothalamic tract (Ohye et al., 1993).

Although we did not try to destroy Vim as in human thalamotomy cases for Parkinson disease, Battista et al. (1969) reported abolition of experimentally produced tremor in monkeys with thalamotomy. In this sense, at the level of the thalamus, clinical data and primate experiments coincided with regard to tremor phenomena (Ohye and Albe-Fessard, 1978; Ohye et al., 1993).

IV. TREMOR-MEDIATING CIRCUIT

Taking into account both the experimental results on Holmes tremor in monkeys and observations in patients with Parkinson disease, we have proposed a hypothetical circuit mediating the tremor (Ohye, 1987): signals arising from the tremulous muscle (from the muscle spindles) go to the spinal cord, cross to take the spinothalamic tract of the contralateral side, ascend directly to the thalamic ventralis intermedius nucleus, go up to cortical area 3a deep in the central sulcus, descend to the contralateral pontine reticular formation probably by way of the pyramidal tract, come down through the spinal cord taking the reticulospinal tract in the anterior funiculus, and finally return to the tremulous muscle (Figure 12). To this main route many other accessory loops, for example, the spinal reflex loop, cerebello-thalamic-cortico-cerebellar loop, thalamo-cortico-basal ganglia-thalamic loop, and thalamo-cortico-reticular nucleus-thalamic loop, are joined to modify (e.g., amplify, synchronize, stabilize, recruit, suppress) the main stream. Since there are still missing or uncertain links such as thalamus to cortical area 3a and area 3a to the contralateral pontine reticular formation, we are still looking for data to complete the Holmes tremor circuit.

Video Legends

SEGMENT 1 Spontaneous tremor four months after left MVMT lesion (02:31:01 to 02:32:15).

SEGMENT 2 L-dopa test dose ten months after left MVMT lesion (02:32:16 to 02:32:43).

SEGMENT 3 Choreiform movements occurring 15 minutes after administration of L-dopa (02:32:43 to 02:34:06).

SEGMENT 4 Chorea and other hyperkinetic dyskinesias occurring 40 minutes after administration of L-dopa (02:34:06 to 02:35:04).

SEGMENT 5 Three hours after administration of L-dopa, tremor is once again present (02:35:04 to end).

Acknowledgments

This work was done in the Department of Neurosurgery, Gunma University. The author expresses sincere thanks to the collaboration of the following colleagues: Drs A. Fukamachi, S. Imai, I. Isobe, M. Miyazaki, H. Nakajima, T. Shibazaki, T. Hirai, H. Wada, Y. Nagaseki, Y. Kawashima, M. Hirato, and M. Matsumura.

References

Aronson, N.I., B.E. Becker, and W.A. McGovern. (1962). A study in experimental tremor. *Conf Neurol* **22**:397–429.

Battista, A.F., M. Goldstein, S. Nakatani, and M. Anagboste. (1969). The effect of ventrolateral thalamic lesions on tremor and the biosynthesis of dopamine in monkeys with lesions in the ventromedial tegmentum. *J Neurosurg* **31**:164–171.

Benedikt, M. (1889). Tremor with crossed oculomotor paralysis. In *The classical brain stem syndromes.* (Ed. J.K. Wolf), Charles C Thomas, Springfield, IL, pp. 101–109.

Carpenter, M.B. (1961). Brain stem and infratentorial neuraxis in experimental dyskinesia. *Arch Neurol* **5**:504–524.

Carpenter, M.B., and G.H. Stevens. (1957). Structural and functional relationship between the deep cerebellar nuclei and the brachium conjunctivum in the rhesus monkey. *J Comp Neurol* **107**:109–163.

Carrea, R.M.E., and F.A. Mettler. (1955). Functions of the primate brachium conjunctivum and related structures. *J Comp Neurol* **102**: 151–322.

Charcot, J. (1903). Le syndrome de Benedikt, Medecine moderne, p. 194.

Deuschl, G., P. Bain, and M. Brin. (1989). Consensus statement of the Movement Disorder Society on Tremor, Ad Hoc Scientific Committee. *Mov Disord* **13**(suppl 3):2–23.

Feger, J., C. Ohye, F. Gallouin, and D. Albe-Fessard. (1975). A stereotaxic technique for stimulation and recording in non-anesthetized monkeys: application to the determination of connection between caudate nucleus and substantia nigra. In *Advances in Neurology*. Vol.10 (B.S. Meldrum and C.D. Marsden, Eds.), pp. 35–45. Raven Press, New York.

Foerster, O. (1911). Resection of the posterior roots of spinal cord. *Lancet* **2**:76–79.

Hassler, R. (1938). Zur Pathologie der Paralysis agitans und des postenzephalitischen Parkinsonismus. *J Psychol Neurol* (Leipzig), **48**:387–476.

Holmes, G. (1904). On certain tremors in organic cerebral lesion. *Brain* **27**:327–375.

Hornykiewicz, O. (1963). Die topische lokalisation und das verhalten von noradrenalin und dopamin in der substantia nigra des normalen und parkinsonkranken menschen. *Wien klin Wschr* **75**:309–312.

Jenker, F.I., and A.A. Ward, Jr. (1953). Bulber reticular formation and tremor. *Arch Neurol Psychiatr* **79**:489–502.

Lamarre, Y., and A.J. Joffroy. (1979). Experimental tremor in monkey: Activity of thalamic and precentral cortical neurons in the absence of peripheral feedback. In *Advances in Neurology.* Vol. 24 (L.J. Poirier, T.I. Sourkes, and P. Bedard, Eds.) Raven Press, New York.

Larochelle, L., P. Bedard, R. Boucher, and L.J. Poirier. (1970). The rubro-olivo-cerebello-rubral loop and postural tremor in the monkey. *J Neurol Sci* **11**:53–64.

Macchi, G., and E.G. Jones. (1997). Toward an agreement on terminology of nuclear and subnuclear divisions of the motor thalamus. *J Neurosurg* **86**:670–685.

Mettler, F.A. (1966). Experimentally produced tremor. *Arch Neurol* **15**: 251–246.

Molina-Negro, P., and J. Hardy. (1975). Semiology of tremors. *Can J Neurol Sci* **2**:23–29.

Nandi, D., X. Liu, J. Winter, T.Z. Aziz, and J.F. Stein. (2002). Deep brain stimulation of the pedunculopontine region in the normal non-human primate. *J Clin Neurosci* **9**:170–174.

Ogawa, T., and Sano F. (1942). Zerstorungs versuche an die Mittelhirnhaube beim Affen mittels des Clarkeschen Apparates (in Japanese), *Z Anatomie* **20**:437–472.

Ohye, C. (1979). Primate model of Parkinsonian motor symptoms (in Japanese). *Adv Neurol Sci* **23**:949–955.

Ohye, C. (1987). Neural circuits involved in Parkinsonian motor disturbance studied in monkeys. *Eur Neurol* **26**(suppl 1):41–46.

Ohye, C. (1988). Experimental study on tremor (in Japanese). In *Modern Series of Physiological Sciences.* Vol. 10. *Physiology of Movement* (K. Sasaki and T. Hongo, Eds) pp. 243–258, Igaku-shoin, Tokyo.

Ohye, C. (1997). Functional organization of the human thalamus. In *Thalamus*, Vol. 2. (M. Steriade, E.G. Jones, D.A. McCormick, Eds.). pp. 517–542. Pergamon Press, Oxford.

Ohye, C. (1997). Thalamotomy for Parkinson's disease and other types of tremor. In *Textbook of Stereotactic and Functional Neurosurgery* (P.L. Gildenberg, R.R. Tasker, Eds.), pp. 1167–1178, McGraw-Hill, New York.

Ohye, C., and D. Albe-Fessard. (1978). Rhythmic discharges related to tremor in humans and monkeys. In *Abnormal Neuronal Discharges.* (N. Chalazonitis and M. Boisson, Eds.), pp. 37–48, Raven Press, New York.

Ohye, C., R. Bouchard, L. Larochelle, P. Bedard, R. Boucher, B. Raphy, and L.J. Poirer. (1970). Effect of dorsal rhizotomy on postural tremor in the monkey. *Exp Brain Res* **10**:140–150.

Ohye, C., S. Imai, H. Nakajima, T. Shibazaki, and T. Hirai. (1979). Experimental study of spontaneous postural tremor induced by a more successful tremor-producing procedure in the monkey. In *Advances in Neurology.* Vol. 24. (L.J. Poirier, T.I. Sourkes, and P. Bedard, Eds.), pp. 83–91, Raven Press, New York.

Ohye, C., T. Shibazaki, T. Hirai, Y. Kawashima, M. Hirato, M. Matsumura. (1993). Tremor mediating thalamic zone studied in humans and in monkeys. *Stereotact Func Neurosurg* **60**:136–145.

Ohye, C., T. Shibazaki, T. Hirai, Y. Nagaseki, H. Wada, Y. Kawashima, and M. Hirato. (1984). Possible descending pathways mediating spontaneous tremor in monkeys. In *Advances in Neurology.* Vol. 40. (R.G. Hassler and J.F. Christ, Eds.), pp. 181–188, Raven Press, New York.

Ohye, C., T. Shibazaki, T. Hirai, H. Wada, M. Hirato, Y. Kawashima. (1989). Further physiological observations on the ventralis intermedius neurons in the human thalamus. *J Neurophysiol* **61**:488–500.

Ohye, C., T. Shibazaki, T. Hirai, H. Wada, Y. Kawashima, M. Hirato, and M. Matsumura. (1988). A special role of the parvocellular red nucleus in lesion-induced spontaneous tremor in monkeys. *Behav Brain Res* **28**:241–243.

Percheron, G. (1975). Ventricular landmarks for the thalamic stereotaxy in macacs. *J Med Primatol* **4**:217–244.

Percheron. G., and N. Lacourly. (1973). L'imprecision de la stereotaxie thalamique utilisant les coordonnees de Horsley-Clarke chez le macaque. *Exp Brain Res* **18**:355–373.

Peterson, E.W., H.W. Magoun, W.S. McCulloch, and D.B. Lindsley. (1949). Production of postural tremor. *J Neurophysiol* **12**:371–384.

Poirier, L.J. (1960). Experimental and histological study of midbrain dyskinesias. *J Neurophysiol* **23**:534–551.

Poirier, L.J., G. Bouvier, P. Bedard, R. Boucher, L. Larochelle, A. Olivier, and P. Singh. (1969). Essai sur les circuits neuronaux impliques dans le tremblement postural et l'hypokinesie. *Rev Neurol* **120**:12–40.

Poirier, L.J., T.I. Sourkes, G. Bouvier, R. Boucher, and S. Carabin. (1966). Striatal amines, experimental tremor and the effect of harmaline in the monkey. *Brain* **89**:37–52.

Pollock, L.J., and L. Davis. (1930). Muscle tone in parkinsonian states. *Arch Neurol Psychiatr* (Chic). **23**:303–319.

Souques, A., O. Crouzon, and I. Bertrand. (1930). Revision du syndromes de Benedikt: A propos de l'autopsie d'un cas de ce syndrome. Forme tremochoreoathetoide et hypertonique de syndrome du noyau rouge. *Rev Neurol* **11**:377–417.

Stern, G. (1966). The effect of lesions in the substantia nigra. *Brain* **89**:449–478.

Tretiakoff, C. (1919). Contributions a l'etude de l'anatomie pathologique du locus niger de Sommering avec quelques deductions relatives a la pathogenie des troubles du tonus musculaire de la maladie de Parkinson. These, Paris.

Velasco, F., M. Velasco, R. Rome, and H. Maldonado. (1979). Production and suppression of tremor by mesencephalic tegmental lesion in monkeys. *Exp Neurol* **64**:516–527.

Ward, Jr., A.A., W.S. McCulloch, and H.W. Magoun. (1948). Production of an alternative tremor at rest in monkeys. *J Neurophysiol* **11**:317–330.

CHAPTER

E6

The Campus Syndrome in Pietrain Pigs

ANGELIKA RICHTER

Several inherited movement disorders in pigs, such as different types of congenital tremor, have been reported (Bradley and Wells, 1980; Bradley and Done, 1992; O'Toole et al., 1994; Bickardt, 1998; Beissner et al., 2003). Clinical interest in veterinary medicine is limited concerning hereditary neurological diseases in swine, because affected animals are usually omitted from breeding. However, well-defined animal models of tremor disorders in pigs can provide tools for the mapping and cloning of causative genes. The etiopathogenesis of tremor disorders in humans, a heterogeneous disease, is not well understood. Tremor models, such as the Campus syndrome in Pietrain pigs, may be helpful in giving insights into pathogenesis and in developing new effective treatments (Richter et al., 1995; Wissel et al., 1997; Tammen et al., 1999).

Apart from the Campus syndrome, four inherited tremor syndromes have been described in swine. A congenital sex-linked recessive type in Landrace pigs and an autosomal recessive form in Saddlebacks are both related to a type of hypomyelinogenesis (Done, 1976; Harding et al., 1973). The so-called "creeper syndrome" is an autosomal recessive primary myopathy in Pietrain pigs (Bradley and Wells, 1980). Finally, another type of tremor in Pietrain pigs is based on progressive neurodegeneration (O'Toole et al., 1994).

The Campus syndrome in the Pietrain breed, first observed in 1988 at the School of Veterinary Medicine Hannover (Hannover, Germany), represents a properly investigated tremor syndrome, as described in the following paragraphs. The syndrome shows several similarities to the human condition of orthostatic tremor (Richter et al., 1995; Wissel et al., 1997).

I. ORIGIN AND PHENOTYPE OF THE CAMPUS SYNDROME

A phenotypically unaffected boar of the Pietrain breed, named "Campus," was found to produce piglets with a severe movement disorder. By mating the boar Campus with healthy sows of different breeds, approximately 9% of the piglets were found to be affected (Richter et al., 1995).

In affected animals, the mean age of onset of the movement disorder was 27 days (range: 5 to 61 days). The affected pigs exhibited a high-frequency tremor when standing and during locomotion but not during rest in a lying position. Directly at the beginning of standing, an intensive tremor occurs first in the hindlimbs and a few seconds later in the forelimbs. During walking, the tremor persists and the gait is disturbed. The animals show muscle weakness after

30 to 90 sec of standing or walking and sink into a sternal position, at which point the tremor ceases immediately. No other neurological abnormalities occur. The intensity of tremor and muscle weakness worsens with age. Thereby, the recumbency becomes almost permanent. The affected pigs continue to drink and grow normally, while feed consumption is increased. The body weight gain in affected animals does not differ from that in unaffected siblings (Richter et al., 1995; Tammen et al., 1999).

The palpable consistency of the muscles in affected pigs was found to be comparable to that of unaffected animals. Furthermore, unaltered plasma concentrations of creatine kinase and aspartate aminotransferase suggested that the Campus syndrome was not a primary myopathy. The immediate disappearance of tremor when the pigs lay down may also argue against a role of a primary myopathy in the Campus syndrome (Richter et al., 1995). As shown by genotyping at the ryanodine receptor locus, an increased susceptibility to stress, an elevated body temperature of 40 to 41°C, and enhanced plasma lactate levels found in affected animals are not related to malignant hyperthermia, a common metabolic disorder of the skeletal muscle in swine (Fujii et al., 1991; Richter et al., 1995; Tammen et al., 1999). The expectancy of life is reduced to 3 to 18 months in pigs with the Campus syndrome. Most animals die before sexual maturity (Tammen et al., 1999).

II. PATHOLOGICAL EXAMINATIONS

Histopathological investigations of the brain and peripheral nerves did not disclose any pathological alterations (Schulze et al., 1996). Light and electron microscopic histopathological and morphometrical examinations of the skeletal muscles have shown angular atrophic muscle fibers (disseminated or in groups in the centers of muscle fascicles) of affected pigs. These changes are consistent with a secondary myopathy (Schulze et al., 1996).

III. INHERITANCE AND GENETIC MAPPING OF THE CPS

Extensive breeding studies excluded a recessive mode of inheritance and indicated that the Campus syndrome is an autosomal dominant disorder with a germline mutation in the healthy founder boar Campus (Tammen et al., 1999). This explains the unusual segregation rate of 8.7% among the offspring and an increased frequency of affected piglets among the offspring of affected sows. In view of the short life expectancy discussed above, breeding with the affected animals was limited and efforts to raise male affected animals for the collection of sperm failed. The expression of the tremor is obviously independent from the genetic background, because affected offspring were produced by mating Campus to sows from five different breeds (Tammen et al., 1999).

Tammen et al. (1999) found by a linkage analysis of 57 animals that the Campus syndrome gene maps to a region on porcine chromosome 7, which is flanked by the markers SW1418 and SW352, according to the map of Rohrer et al. (1997). Within this region the porcine genome maps are sparse for putative candidate genes. Bidirectional chromosome painting of the porcine and human genome shows that the porcine chromosome 7 is homologous to human chromosomes 6, 14, and 15 (HAS14) (Goureau et al., 1996). For example, the inhibitor of the transcription factor nuclear factor kappa B and the T-cell receptor alpha chain map to the region in which the Campus syndrome gene is located. Since the human dominant distal myopathy type 1 (MPD1) has been mapped to the homologous region of HSA14, Tammen et al. (1999) suggested that the Campus syndrome might serve as an animal model of MPD1. However, the phenotype of MPD1 is different from that of the Campus syndrome; e.g., tremor is absent in patients with MPD1 (Laing et al., 1995).

IV. NEUROPHYSIOLOGICAL EXAMINATIONS IN PIGS WITH THE CAMPUS SYNDROME

Neurophysiological studies demonstrated that the ulnar nerve motor conduction velocity was unaltered in pigs affected with the Campus syndrome in comparison to non-affected littermates (Wissel et al., 1997). At rest, quantitative electromyographic recordings (EMG) of the semitendinosus muscle did not disclose fibrillation potentials or positive sharp waves. The mean duration, amplitude, and shape of the single motor action potential did not reveal any myopathic changes.

When the Campus syndrome pigs were standing and exhibited a severe tremor, needle EMG showed a 14- to 15-Hz rhythmic EMG burst pattern in the semitendinosus muscle. An accelerometer was placed on the backs directly above the hindquarters of affected and non-affected pigs. The recordings showed a very low–amplitude 3.4-Hz tremor when the affected pigs were resting in a sternal position, whereas a high-amplitude 14-Hz tremor was detected when the pigs were standing (Richter et al., 1995; Wissel et al., 1997).

V. NEUROPHARMACOLOGICAL CHARACTERISTICS OF THE CAMPUS SYNDROME

In order to evaluate the pharmacology of the movement disorder, various drugs were administered via chronically implanted venous catheters (Richter et al., 1995). In contrast to human orthostatic tremor, which is known to respond to clonazepam and primidone (Deuschl et al., 1987; FitzGerald and Jankovic, 1991), the intensity of the tremor was not reduced by either clonazepam (0.1 to 0.2 mg/kg) or primidone (10 to 20 mg/kg) in affected pigs. Furthermore, phenobarbital (10 and 20 mg/kg), biperiden (0.4 to 1.4 mg/kg), and the atypical neuroleptic clozapine (5 and 10 mg/kg) failed to exert any beneficial effects in affected pigs (Richter et al., 1995).

VI. CONCLUSION

The Campus syndrome shares several common features with the human condition of orthostatic tremor. The neurophysiology of orthostatic tremor in humans is characterized by a highly typical 14- to 16-Hz tremor frequency (Thompson et al., 1986). Thus, the neurophysiological data in affected pigs showed a clear parallel to the human condition, whereas other described congenital tremor syndromes in swine show a frequency of 2 to 8 Hz (Bradley and Done, 1992). On the other hand, there are also differences between the Campus syndrome and orthostatic tremor. In contrast to the persistence of tremor during walking in affected pigs, orthostatic tremor is present during standing but usually disappears during walking. Only in severe cases does primary orthostatic tremor persist during gait (Deuschl et al., 1987; Deuschl and Krack, 1998). Furthermore, clonazepam has been reported to exert beneficial effects in patients with orthostatic tremor (Charles et al., 1999; Deuschl and Krack, 1998), whereas this benzodiazepine was not effective in Campus syndrome pigs. No animal model is yet available that exactly shares all features of any of the known tremor disorders in humans. Nevertheless, Campus syndrome pigs might be a useful model of human orthostatic tremor (Richter et al., 1995; Wilms et al., 1999; Wissel et al., 1997).

Video Legend

Pigs exhibit a moderately high amplitude 14–15 Hz generalized tremor.

References

Beissner, B., H. Hamann, and O. Distl. 2003. Prevalence of congenital anomalies of the pig breeds German Landrace and Pietrain in Bavaria. *Züchtungskunde* **75**:101–114.

Bickardt, K. 1998. Exertional myopathy and osteochondrosis of pigs as a result of breeding for growth rate. *Tierärztliche Umschau* **53**:129–134.

Bradley, R., and J.T. Done. 1992. Nervous and muscular systems. In *Diseases of Swine*. (A.D. Leman, B.E. Straw, W.L. Mengeling, S. D'Allaire, and D.J. Taylor, Eds.), pp. 62–87. Iowa State Univ. Press, Ames.

Bradley, R., and G.A.H. Wells. 1980. The pietrain "creeper" pig: A primary myopathy. In *Animal Models of Neurological Disease*. (F.C. Rose, and P.O. Behan, Eds.), pp. 34–64. Pitman, Tunbridge Wells.

Charles, P.D., G.J. Esper, T.L. Davis, R.J. Maciunas, and D. Robertson. 1999. Classification of tremor and update on treatment. *Am Fam Physician* **59**:1565–1572.

Deuschl, G., and P. Krack. 1998. Tremors: Differential diagnosis, neurophysiology, and pharmacology. In *Parkinson's Disease and Movement Disorders*. (J. Jankovic, and E. Tolosa, Eds.), pp. 419–452. Lippincott, Philadelphia.

Deuschl, G., C.H. Lücking, and I. Quintern. 1987. Orthostatischer Tremor: Klinik, Pathophysiologie und Therapie. *Z EEG-EMG* **18**:13–19.

Done, J.T. 1976. The congenital tremor syndrome in pigs. *Vet Annu* **16**:98–102.

FitzGerald, P.M., and J. Jankovic. 1991. Orthostatic tremor: an essential tremor variant. *Mov Disord* **6**:60–64.

Fujii, J., K. Otsu, F. Zorzato, S. De Leon, V.K. Khanna, J.E. Weiler, P.J. O'Brien, and D. MacLennan. 1991. Identification of a mutation in porcine ryanodine receptor associated with malignant hyperthermia. *Science* **253**:448–451.

Goureau, A., M. Yerle, A. Schmitz, J. Riquet, D. Milan, P. Pinton, G. Frelat, and J. Geljin. 1996. Human and porcine correspondance of chromosome segments using bidirectional chromosome painting. *Genomics* **36**:252–262.

Harding, J.D.J., J.T. Done, J.F. Harbourne, and J.F. Gilbert. 1973. Congenital tremor type A III in pigs: an inherited sex-linked cerebrospinal hypomyelinogenesis. *Vet Rec* **92**:527–529.

Laing, N.G., B.A. Laing, C. Meredith, S.D. Wilton, P. Robbine, K. Honeyman, S. Dorosz, H. Kozman, F.L. Mastaglia, and B.A. Kukulas. 1995. Autosomal dominant distal myopathy: linkage to chromosome 14. *Am J Hum Genet* **56**:422–427.

O'Toole, D., J. Ingram, V. Welch, K. Bardsley, C. Nunamaker, and G. Wells. 1994. An inherited lower motor disease of pigs: Clinical signs in two litters and pathology of an affected pig. *J Vet Diagn Invest* **6**:62–71.

Richter, A., J. Wissel, B. Harlizius, D. Simon, L. Schelosky, U. Scholz, W. Poewe, and W. Löscher. 1995. The "Campus syndrome": Neurological, neurophysiological and pharmacological characterization of a new hereditary movement disorder in pigs. *Exp Neurol* **134**:205–213.

Rohrer, G.A., L.J. Alexander, C.W. Beattie, P. Wilkie, G.H. Flickinger, L.H. Schook, A.A. Paszek, I. Andersson, P. Mariani, L. Marklund, M. Fredholm, B. Hayhelm, A.L. Archibald, V.H. Nielsen, D. Milan, and M.A.M. Groenen. 1997. A consensus linkage map for swine chromosome 7. *Anim Genet* **28**:223–229.

Schulze, L., C. Chavez, B. Harlizius, and J. Polenz. 1996. Hereditary progressive postural tremor in the pig: morphologic and morphometric study of the muscle alterations. *Eur J Vet Pathol* **2**:5–12.

Tammen, I., O. Schulze, J. Chavez-Moreno, D. Waberski, D. Simon, and B. Harlizius. 1999. Inheritance and genetic mapping of the Campus syndrome (CPS): A high-frequency tremor disease in pigs. *J Hered* **90**:472–476.

Thompson, P.D., J.C. Rothwell, and B.L. Day. 1986. The physiology of orthostatic tremor. *Arch Neurol* **43**:584–587.

Wilms, H., J. Sievers, and G. Deuschl. 1999. Animal models of tremor. *Mov Disord* **14**:557–571.

Wissel, J., B. Schwenger, A. Richter, W. Löscher, L. Schelosky, U. Scholz, and W. Poewe. 1997. A new tremor mutant in the Pietrain pig: An animal model of orthostatic tremor? A clinical and neurophysiological observation. *Mov Disord* **12**:743–746.

CHAPTER

F1

Pathophysiology, Neurophysiology, and Pharmacology of Human Myoclonus

MICHAEL R. PRANZATELLI

Myoclonus is a unique dyskinesia. It occurs physiologically as a muscle jerk on drowsiness or falling to sleep, during rapid eye movement (REM) sleep, and as hiccups. Myoclonus is also a developmental feature of the human nervous system, comprising the earliest fetal movements. In pathologic settings, myoclonus may be the only neurological abnormality, as in essential myoclonus, but more commonly it is a symptom of a larger neurological problem. The etiologic spectrum of symptomatic myoclonus is vast, but defining the underlying problem may provide the only opportunity for specific therapies. The approach to the patient should be to establish a specific etiologic diagnosis, using a battery of neurophysiologic, neuroradiologic, and other laboratory studies to localize the origin of the myoclonus and identify causative lesions. Drug treatment, which is largely empiric, must be systematic and aimed at restoring activities of everyday living. Multiple drug combinations are usually necessary for functional improvement. Recognition of quality-of-life issues should not be overshadowed by the often complex medical issues.

I. DEFINITION

Myoclonus is a brief involuntary muscle jerk originating in the central nervous system (Marsden et al., 1982), an isolated paroxysmal event or a symptom of many diseases. It affects all age groups and ranges in severity from trivial to severely disabling. Developmental and physiologic forms of myoclonus contribute to its uniqueness as a dyskinesia (Pranzatelli, 1993). Physiologic myoclonus occurs episodically throughout life as hiccups (singultus) and hypnic (sleep) jerks. Myoclonus is also distinguished from other movement disorders by its unusual association with epilepsy and ataxia and by the distinctive panels of drugs used in its treatment.

II. DIFFERENTIAL DIAGNOSIS

The shock-like abruptness and brevity of myoclonus help to differentiate it from superficially similar dyskinesias. Although it is sometimes confused with tics, which are commonly myoclonic in nature, tics are usually more complex in pattern and confined to the head and shoulders. Choreiform finger movements when a patient's hands are held outstretched may also appear myoclonic, but myoclonus is not typically confined to the fingers. When multiple dyskinesias are present, ancillary tests may be helpful in sorting them out. Periodic movements of sleep have sometimes been confused with "nocturnal myoclonus," which instead should be used to refer to myoclonic jerks during different

TABLE 1 Classification of Myoclonus[a]

Clinical	Etiologic	Neurophysiologic
Activation	Essential	Localization
Spontaneous		Cortical
Sensory-evoked	Symptomatic	Cortical reflex
Action-evoked	Genetic disorders	Spontaneous cortical
	Acquired disorders	Epilepsy partialis continua
		Cortico-reticular
Distribution		
Focal	Developmental	
Multifocal		Subcortical
Generalized	Physiologic	Reticular reflex
	Hiccups	Spontaneous reticular
Regularity	Hypnic jerks	Ballistic overflow
Rhythmic	Fragmentary nocturnal myoclonus	Oscillatory
Arrhythmic		Cortico-subcortical
Oscillatory		Spinal
Direction of joint displacement		Relation to muscle tone
		Positive
Upward		Negative
Downward		
		Relation to epilepsy
Synchrony		Epileptic
Synchronous		Cortical reflex
Asynchronous		Reticular reflex
		Primary generalized epileptic
		Non-epileptic
		Exaggerated startle
		Periodic movements of sleep
		Myoclonic tics
		Segmental myoclonus
		Physiologic myoclonus

[a]No one classification schema is sufficient, given all the aspects of myoclonus, and it is a useful exercise to apply each one to a new patient with myoclonus.

phases of sleep, such as fragmentary myoclonus (Anstead, 2000). The movements of restless legs are not truly myoclonic and are distinguished by the associated sensations. Although startle is a component of brainstem myoclonus, startle disorders such as hyperekplexia are discrete syndromes. It also has been suggested recently that essential myoclonus and myoclonic dystonia, both of which are sensitive to alcohol, are the same disorder. "Cortical tremor" implies a non-myoclonic disorder, but it is a form of cortical reflex myoclonus that looks similar clinically to essential tremor but is found in patients with myoclonus (Toro et al., 1993). The term "palatal myoclonus" has been used for many years to describe the rapid, rhythmic fluttering of the soft palate, but newer studies indicate that "palatal tremor" would be more appropriate.

III. CLASSIFICATION

A. Clinical

There are several types of myoclonus (Table 1). Spontaneous, reflex-induced, and movement-induced myoclonus can be differentiated clinically by the pattern of activation (Marsden et al., 1982). The most common of these is action myoclonus. Movement-induced myoclonus may be activated by the intention of an action or the action itself. Reflex myoclonus is activated by sound, light, touch, or passive movement of the limb. Myoclonus is also classified clinically by its body distribution, regularity, direction of limb or trunk displacement, and synchrony.

TABLE 2 Clinical Localization of Myoclonus[a]

Cortical	Subcortical	Spinal (segmental)
Focal	Generalized	Segmental
Distal musculature	Proximal and distal	Abdomen and lower limbs especially
One synergist muscle group	Agonist-antagonist co-contraction	Flexor groups predominantly
Rostrocaudal activation order	May propagate up brainstem	—
EMG event time-locked with EEG	Not time-locked	—
"Giant" (enhanced) SSEPs	Normal amplitude SSEPs	—

[a]Based on classification scheme by Marsden et al., 1982. Careful evaluation of the muscle groups affected by myoclonus in combination with electrophysiologic tests aids the clinician in localizing the origin of myoclonus.

B. Etiologic

The etiologic classification of myoclonus draws attention to the fact that myoclonus may occur as part of normal human development, under various physiological situations throughout life, and under abnormal circumstances, both in individuals who are otherwise well and in those who are not. The search for the underlying etiology of myoclonus is covered under Diagnostic Testing (Section VIII).

C. Neurophysiologic

1. Relation to Site of Origin

Cortical, subcortical, and spinal myoclonus are defined neurophysiologically, but there are also clinical clues (Table 2). Cortical myoclonus is focal and distal and found typically in the arm. Cortical reflex myoclonus may be activated by photic stimulation. Patients with subcortical myoclonus have both proximal and distal generalized myoclonus, which involves agonist and antagonist muscle groups. Spinal myoclonus may be limited to muscles innervated by a few or by multiple spinal segments and predominantly affects flexor muscles (Marsden et al., 1982). The contractions of diaphragmatic myoclonus often suppress normal breathing but can maintain adequate ventilation, possibly due to a generator source related to respiratory centers in the rostral medullar (Chen et al., 1995).

2. Relation to Muscle Tone

Patients with myoclonus may exhibit postural lapses that correspond with a silent period on electromyography (EMG). This brief lack of muscle activity that sometimes follows a muscle discharge has been called "negative myoclonus" or asterixis, in contradistinction to the muscle discharges denoted as "positive myoclonus" (Tassinari et al., 1995). Sudden loss of anti-gravitational muscle tone can be disabling and refractory to treatment (Toro et al., 1995). Many patients with severe myoclonus have a mixture of positive and negative myoclonus.

3. Relation to Epilepsy

These myoclonic categories can also be reshuffled as epileptic or non-epileptic myoclonus by the duration of EMG bursts (Hallett, 1985). Epileptic myoclonic jerks are briefer than non-epileptic myoclonic jerks, whether they are positive or negative (Shibasaki, 2000; Tassinari et al., 1995). Epileptic myoclonus EMG bursts last <50 msec when positive and ≤400 msec when negative. Non-epileptic myoclonus EMG bursts last 50 to 200 msec when positive and 200 to 500 msec when negative.

D. Rating Scales

Myoclonus can also be appraised through the use of rating scales. Most are designed for adults, focusing either on semi-quantitation of jerks or their impact on activities of daily living (Frucht et al., 2002). Pediatric rating scales for the evaluation of myoclonus are also available (Pranzatelli et al., 2001; Tate et al., 1995).

IV. CLINICAL SYNDROMES

The context in which myoclonus occurs aids diagnosis and helps organize the otherwise unruly heterogeneity of etiologies associated with myoclonus (Pranzatelli, 2003). It is routine to designate "dyskinesia-plus" syndromes in the etiologic classification of other movement disorders, and myoclonus is amenable to the same approach (Figure 1).

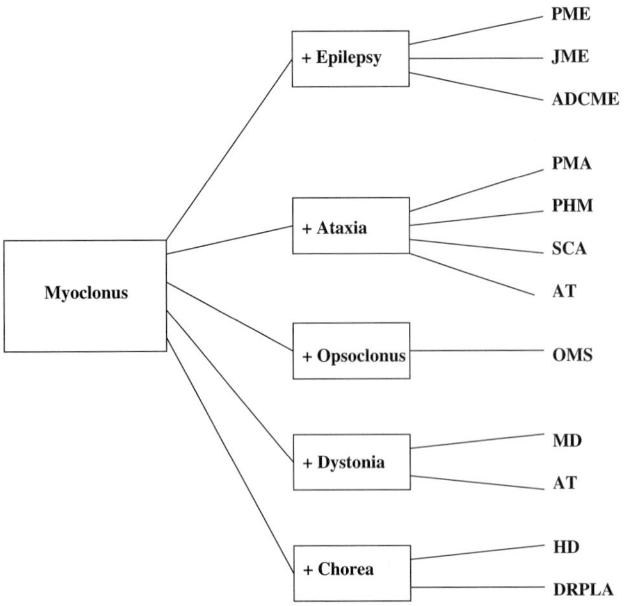

FIGURE 1 Myoclonus–plus syndromes describe the relation of myoclonus to epilepsy and other movement disorders. Abbreviations: ADCME, autosomal dominant cortical myoclonus and epilepsy; AT, ataxia-telangiectasia; DRPLA, dentatorubral-pallidolysian atrophy; OMS, opsoclonus-myoclonus syndrome; JME, juvenile myoclonus epilepsy; MD, myoclonus-dystonia; PHM, post-hypoxic myoclonus; PMA, progressive myoclonus ataxia; PME, progressive myoclonus epilepsy.

A. Physiologic Myoclonus, Otherwise Normal Individuals

Myoclonus is intrinsic to normal sleep physiology, occurring as paradoxical excitation in REM sleep. Beginning in fetal life, it is most abundant during the first 6 to 8 months postnatally and persists throughout life as fragmentary nocturnal myoclonus. Hypnic jerks, or myoclonus on sleep initiation, are associated with the sense of falling.

B. Non-physiologic Myoclonus, Otherwise Normal Individuals

1. Neonatal Sleep Myoclonus

The term benign neonatal sleep myoclonus specifies all the component features of this context-specific myoclonus. The diagnosis can be confirmed by waking the infant, which stops the myoclonus, or through proprioceptive input, by tapping on the limbs, which increases or elicits the jerks (Daoust-Roy and Seshia, 1992). When the myoclonus is rhythmic, the onset is late, or the syndrome persists, the diagnosis may be missed. The EEG is normal (Bye et al., 2000).

2. Essential Myoclonus

Essential myoclonus occurs in otherwise normal individuals and has an upper body distribution similar to myoclonic tics, with which it is most often confused. It is permanent, though nonprogressive.

3. Other Transient Syndromes

Benign myoclonus of early infancy is a term coined to designate non-epileptic spasms that otherwise resemble West syndrome (Maydell et al., 2001). Development and neurological examinations are normal, no treatment is required, and the prognosis is excellent. Self-limited myoclonus also occurs in normal children in the setting of fever (Rajakumar and Bodensteiner, 1996).

C. Myoclonus in Abnormal Individuals

1. Myoclonus and Epilepsy

a. Progressive Myoclonus Epilepsy (PME). PME presents in childhood or adolescence. Common to all the etiologies of PME is the presence of myoclonus and epilepsy and a progressive course, with a variable rate of progression (Uthman and Reichl, 2002). Ataxia and dementia are associated features in some types. The myoclonus affects speech and gait, is action-sensitive and stimulus-sensitive, and also occurs spontaneously (Pranzatelli et al., 1995). Although epileptic seizures may be the initial presentation, they gradually subside on treatment, but the myoclonus becomes relentless. The major types of PMEs are Unverricht-Lündborg disease (EPM1), mitochondrial encephalomyopathy (MERRF, MELAS, PEO), and Lafora disease (Berkovic et al., 1989). EPM1 is compatible with a normal life span, whereas the other two types are typically fatal in the second decade of life. Both may occur sporadically or by autosomal recessive inheritance. Patients with EPM1 tend to have absence or tonic-clonic seizures, whereas those with Lafora disease may have clonic-tonic-clonic seizures or partial epilepsy (Yoshimura et al., 2001). Many clinical features differentiate other types of PME, such as the funduscopic cherry red spot of sialidosis type I and the lactic acidosis and stroke-like episodes (MELAS) and progressive external ophthalmoplegia (PEO) of mitochondrial disorders (Minassian et al., 1995; Tobimatsu et al., 1985; Tomoda et al., 1991).

b. Juvenile Myoclonus Epilepsy (JME). JME represents primary generalized epilepsy in which myoclonic jerks occur independently of seizures, particularly on awakening. (Delgado-Escueta et al., 1999). It is sometimes combined with PME. Referring to it as "myoclonic epilepsy" is a misnomer.

c. Myoclonic Seizures. Because myoclonic seizures are a type of epilepsy and they have not been well characterized, this author does not include them in discussions of myoclonus as a movement disorder (Pranzatelli, 2002); however, some authors do (Fejerman, 1997; Minassian et al., 1995; Oguni et al., 2001).

2. Myoclonus and Ataxia

Myoclonus in the context of cerebellar ataxia is often part of a progressive disorder, such as ataxia-telangiectasia (AT), in which case other dyskinesias may be present, or spinocerebellar ataxia (SCA). Progressive myoclonus ataxia (PMA) can be associated with celiac disease (Bhatia et al., 1995), but in many instances a more specific diagnosis cannot be made (Marsden et al., 1990).

3. Myoclonus and Dystonia

The combination of myoclonus and dystonia without other abnormalities should suggest myoclonus-dystonia, a genetic entity. Alcohol-responsiveness and autosomal dominant inheritance have been described. The two dyskinesias also occur in many neurodegenerative disorders.

4. Myoclonus and Chorea

When chorea occurs with myoclonus, there are usually other neurological abnormalities as well. In dentatorubral-pallidoluysian atrophy (DRPLA), ataxia is also present (Ohizumi et al., 2002). In Huntington disease, cortical reflex myoclonus is a rare but disabling component (Thompson et al., 1994a).

5. Myoclonus and Opsoclonus

The opsoclonus-myoclonus syndrome (OMS) is a paraneoplastic disorder of all ages. Its presence signals the need for a thorough investigation for an occult neoplasm (Dalmau and Posner, 1997; Pranzatelli, 2000; Rojas-Marcos et al., 2003). Opsoclonus, also called "dancing eyes," refers to conjugate, darting eye movements. The myoclonus occurs principally with action, but also spontaneously and reflexly. Other features are gait ataxia, dysarthria, behavior problems, sleep disturbance, and cognitive impairment. The brain is caught in the "crossfire" of the immune system's attack on the tumor, which involves both B-cells and T-cells (Pranzatelli, 2000).

6. Myoclonus and Encephalopathy

a. Serotonin-Induced. The "serotonin syndrome" is an uncommon but potentially lethal drug reaction primarily in patients with psychiatric illness during treatment with serotonin reuptake inhibitors and other serotonin-potentiating agents (Pranzatelli, 1997). The serotonin syndrome is the prototype of drug-induced myoclonus. Patients also exhibit fever, confusion, restlessness, ataxia, hyperreflexia, and tremor.

b. Lance-Adams Syndrome. Postanoxic myoclonus follows coma most often due to myocardial infarction and anesthetic accidents. Stimulus-sensitive myoclonic jerks first appear in the intensive care setting. The majority of patients also have seizures. Later in the course, ataxia, dysarthria, and associated problems surface and the action myoclonus may be disabling (Fahn, 1979).

V. PATHOPHYSIOLOGY

Myoclonus is often one feature of a diffuse neurological disorder, so a gamut of neuropathologic lesions has obscured what might be an anatomic common denominator to myoclonus. MRI or CT scans of the head or spinal cord are normal in essential myoclonus and in some types of symptomatic myoclonus. MR spectroscopy is useful in evaluating subcortical structures and may be positive when other studies are negative.

A. Cortex

In cortical myoclonus, lack of inhibition facilitates the transcallosal and cortical spread of myoclonus (Hallett, 1985). Abnormal activation of sensorimotor cortex gives rise to cortical myoclonus, but whether abnormalities of both cortices are requisite remains controversial (Oguro et al., 2003). Both cortical and reticular reflex myoclonus occurs stimultaneously when the CNS is hyperexcitable at multiple levels (Table 3). In epileptic negative myoclonus, EEG–single photon emission CT (SPECT) indicates involvement of premotor cortex (Baumgartner et al., 1996). SPECT may demonstrate hypoperfusion associated with myoclonus (Berkovic et al., 1989; Oguro et al., 1997; Tanaka et al., 1997).

B. Brainstem

The most common forms of brainstem myoclonus appear to utilize the same circuitry as the normal startle reflex (Shibasaki, 2000). Brainstem myoclonus (Hallett, 2002) can be induced in experimental animals by injection of various drugs into the brainstem reticular formation at the nucleus gigantocellularis reticularis or anatomically related structures, such as the interior olives. This medullary reticular region has also been implicated in the paradoxically excitatory manifestation of myoclonus during REM sleep. In hereditary essential myoclonus, cerebral blood flow studies revealed reduction of cortical cerebral blood flow contralateral to the myoclonus, which suggests a brainstem or basal ganglia lesion.

C. Spinal Cord

Some forms of spinal myoclonus involve the propriospinal system (Rothwell, 2002). Release of a spinal stepping generator from supraspinal control has been proposed. Focal axial myoclonus and propriospinal myoclonus may coexist (Vertrugno et al., 2000). Spinal pathology, involving focal or multifocal lesions, is often found in segmental myoclonus at or above the level of the myoclonus.

D. Cerebellum

The role of the cerebellum in myoclonus has been debated, but the increased association of ataxia with myoclonus compared to other dyskinesias is inescapable. The cerebellar dentate nucleus was found to be abnormal in Alzheimer disease with myoclonus, due to an increase in the mean volume of large over small neurons in the dentate (Fukutani et al., 1999). Selective degeneration of the dentate nucleus and dentatorubrothalamic pathway was found in Gaucher type 3 with myoclonus (Verghese et al., 2000). In progressive myoclonus ataxia associated with celiac disease, the myoclonus is of cortical origin but the pathology is in the cerebellum, with Purkinje cell loss and Bergmann astrocytosis (Bhatia et al., 1995). Purkinje cell loss also occurs in post-anoxic myoclonus and could lead to myoclonus by causing thalamo-cortical and reticular hyperexcitability (Welsh et al., 2002).

VI. PHARMACOLOGY

More than one neurotransmitter system has been implicated in human myoclonic disorders through experiences with myoclonus-evoking drugs and intoxications in humans, the therapeutic use of many pharmacologically diverse categories of drugs, and cerebrospinal fluid studies of neurotransmitters or their metabolites in humans (Pranzatelli and Nadi, 1995).

A. Neurotransmitters

Without yet being able to identify which neurotransmitter is most proximal to the myoclonus induction mechanism, it is possible to say that GABA, glycine, serotonin, and glutamate seem to be primary (Snodgrass, 1990). Various types of myoclonus may involve different neurotransmitters locally and through projections, as they involve different anatomic pathways, but very few data are available in humans. Distinctive pharmacologic responses in diverse types of myoclonus may be based on unique circuitry of cortical, brainstem, and spinal myoclonus "generators' as well as the functional impact of specific human myoclonic disorders on the anatomy and physiology of that circuitry. In spinal cord of experimental animals, local circuitry includes GABA- and glycine-mediated inhibition of the Renshaw cell on spinal motor neurons. Neurotransmitter receptor subunit and ion channel disorders may be involved in some forms of hereditary myoclonus.

B. Animal Models

Gene knock-out animal models of myoclonus facilitate the study of links between gene defects and brain neuropharmacology. Of note are recent models of EPM1 (Pennacchio et al., 1996), neuronal ceroid lipofuscinosis (Gupta et al., 2001), and mitochondrial disorders (Wallace, 2002). Profound loss of GABAergic interneurons and an autoantibody inhibitory to glutamic acid decarboxylase are new findings in neuronal ceroid lipofuscinosis (Chattopadhyay et al., 2002; Cooper et al., 2002). Mice lacking potassium channels Kv3.1 and Kv3.3 display myoclonus (Espinosa et al., 2001). Pharmacologic animal models of myoclonus have been reviewed previously (Pranzatelli and Snodgrass, 1985; Rhyu et al., 1999).

VII. NEUROPHYSIOLOGY

A. Localization

Backaveraging, a computer-facilitated correlation of EEG and EMG activity, together with somatosensory-evoked responses, differentiate cortical, subcortical, and spinal myoclonus. A cortical electrical potential occurs just prior to the myoclonic jerk in cortical, but not subcortical, myoclonus (Shibasaki et al., 1994). Besides this time-locked EEG event, patients with cortical myoclonus have enlarged somatosensory-evoked potentials (SSEPs) and enhanced long loop reflexes (LLRs) (Toro et al., 1993). "Giant" SSEPs occur in the epilepsies (Figure 2), including myoclonic generalized seizures (Shibasaki, 2000). Cortical myoclonus is typical of PME, Angelman syndrome, and autosomal dominant cortical myoclonus and epilepsy (Guerrini et al., 1996; Guerrini et al., 2001; Tobimatsu et al., 1985). Advanced magnetograms (MEGs), which have three-dimensional resolution, have aided in the localization of the premyoclonus spike in cortical myoclonus, resolving the giant somatosensory evoked magnetic field (SEF) to sensory or motor cortex (Shibasaki, 2000).

In subcortical myoclonus, SSEPs are normal, and the muscle group activation indicates that discharges may actually propagate up the brainstem. A common type of subcortical myoclonus is reticular reflex myoclonus (Hallett, 1985). Physiologic myoclonus occurs without an enhanced evoked potential, such as during sleep or startle.

In spinal segmental myoclonus, there is segmental involvement of muscles with consistent rhythmicity and a rate of contraction ranging from 40 to 130 per minute. Flexor muscles are involved primarily. In propriospinal myoclonus, an uncommon form of spinal myoclonus, muscle involvement is not segmental. Myoclonic activity

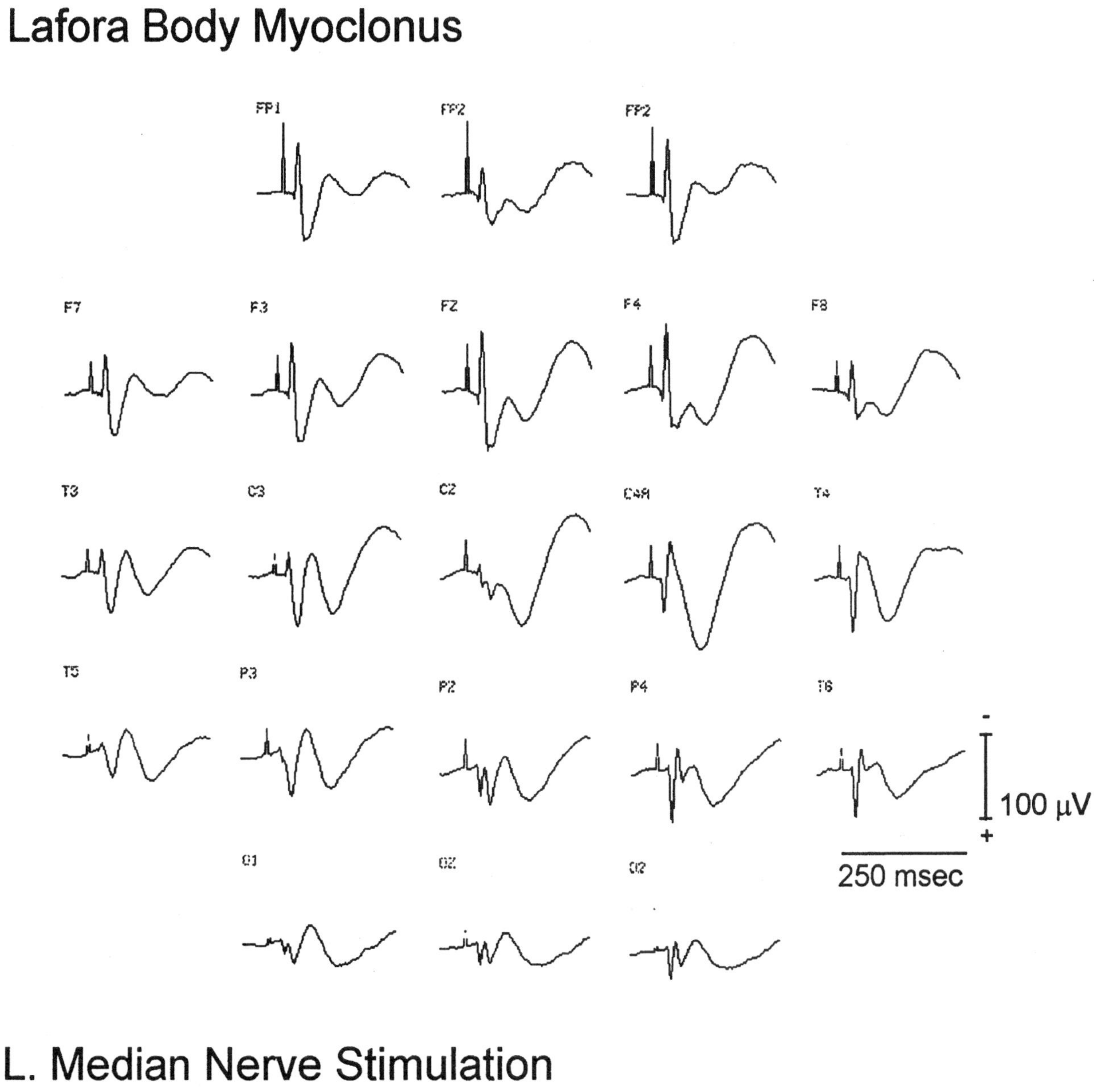

FIGURE 2 Enhanced contralateral somatosensory–evoked cortical potentials in Lafora disease following left median nerve stimulation, courtesy of Dr. Camillo Toro and Dr. Mark Hallett, Human Motor Control Section, National Institute of Neurological Disorders and Stroke, NIH, Bethesda, MD.

begins in spinally innervated muscles, propagating at low speed to rostral and caudal muscular segments (Montagna et al., 1997).

B. Relation to Epilepsy

Epileptic and non-epileptic myoclonus can be differentiated on EEG and EMG testing. The EMG burst in epileptic myoclonus is very short, and there is an EEG correlate. The innervation of muscles involved in jerking is synchronous, and the muscle groups affected may be activated either in a rostrocaudal or ascending fashion (Hallett, 1985). In contrast, non-epileptic myoclonus is associated with longer EMG discharges and asynchronous muscle group jerking. Muscles are activated in a segmental fashion without an EEG correlate (Marsden et al., 1982).

VIII. DIAGNOSTIC TESTING

The diagnostic evaluation of myoclonus (Figure 3) encompasses all of the efforts to classify myoclonus,

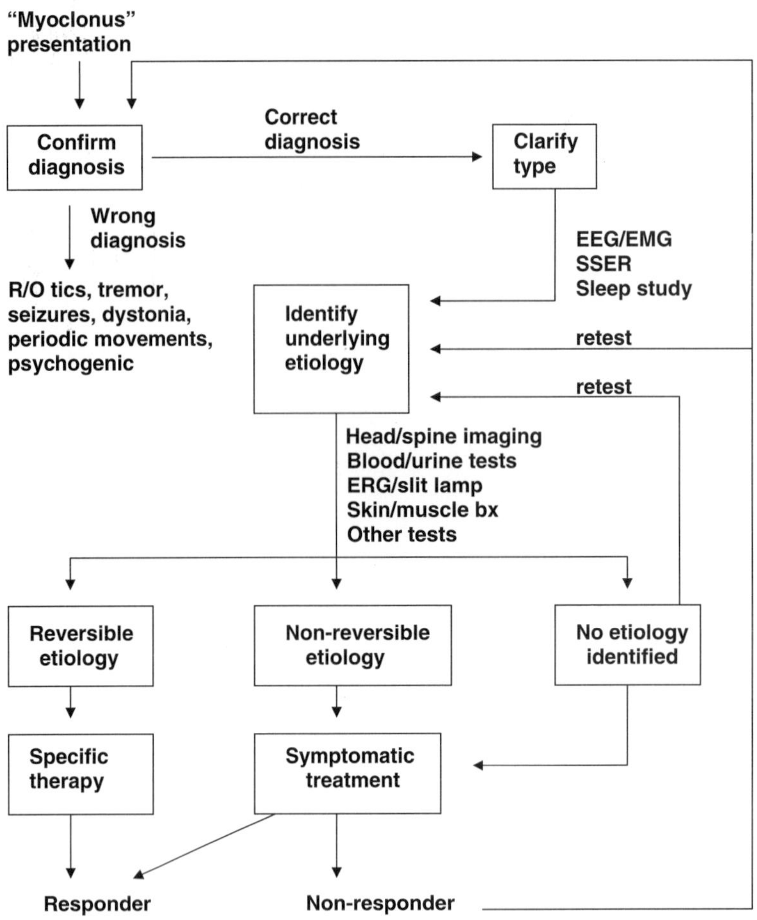

FIGURE 3 Schema for evaluation and treatment of a patient with myoclonus. Once the differential diagnosis of myoclonus has been considered and the diagnosis is confirmed, the most essential aspect is to identify the underlying etiology. The extent and type of diagnostic testing are often guided by associated features and presence of other organ system involvement. When myoclonus is part of a larger neurological syndrome and no etiology is found, it may be necessary to retest the patient at a later time. Symptomatic therapy is never a replacement for specific therapy when a reversible etiology has been uncovered.

differentiate it from non-myoclonic movements, and determine its specific context. Various neurophysiologic tests will have been employed. The next step is to use neuroimaging studies and laboratory tests to establish an etiology of myoclonus. Strong clues provided by the history may delimit the testing; otherwise, many studies may be necessary, requiring a systematic and staged approach.

A. Treatable or Reversible Etiologies

Recognizing treatable or reversible etiologies of myoclonus is crucial (Table 4) (Bhatia et al., 1992; Bhatia et al., 1995; Dale, 2003; DiFazio et al., 1998; Grech et al., 2001; Ozer et al., 2001; Pranzatelli, 1993). Many have been known for centuries, but new metabolic disorders are being discovered and novel microbial mechanisms surface regularly.

Drugs and intoxicants are important, and common causes of myoclonus (Ghaziuddin et al., 2001; Gordon, 2002; Maiteh and Daoud, 2001; McClain et al., 2001; Mercadante et al., 2001; Zaw et al., 2001). The pharmacologic diversity of agents, which span a multitude of clinical indications from antidepressants to narcotic analgesics, alerts the clinician to search for myoclonus-evoking drugs in every new case. Stopping the offending agent may be sufficient, but symptomatic therapy can be provided if necessary. Although propofol, used as an anesthetic, may occasionally induce myoclonus, for most patients with myoclonic disorders it is an effective agent for procedures (Tate et al., 1994). Intoxi-

TABLE 3 Pathophysiology of Epileptic Myoclonus[a]

Neurophysiologic feature	Cortical reflex	Reticular reflex	Primary generalized epileptic[b]
Hyperexcitability	Cortex	Caudal brainstem RF	cortex
Brain area involved	Small, focal contralateral SM cortex	Medullary NGR	? subcortical structures
Muscle involvement	Few, continuous focal/multifocal	Multiple, bilateral, with "jitter"[c] proximal > distal flexors > extensors	Small finger jerks or multiple, synchronous bilateral
Type of myoclonus	Action, reflex, spontaneous	Action, reflex, spontaneous	Minipolymyoclonus, spontaneous
Impulse propagation (activation)	Down brainstem	Up brainstem	Synchronous Ascending subcortical, then down brainstem
Timing of EEG event	Precedes jerk	Follows jerk	"Jitters" for small jerks
Distribution of EEG event	Focal	Generalized	Generalized
Clinical examples	EPC, Alzheimer?	Uremia	Absence; other primary generalized
Animal model	Focal PCN or alumina cream to motor cortex	Systemic PTZ, catechol, chloralose	Cortex bathed in dilated PCN

[a]Based on classification scheme by Hallett (1985). From Pranzatelli, 2002.
[b]Ascending subcortical impulses may arise in the reticular formation and nonspecific thalamic nuclei.
[c]"Jitter" refers to the EEG correlate fluctuating in time with respect to the jerk.
Abbreviations: SM, sensorimotor; RF, reticular formation; NGR, nucleus gigantocellularis reticularis; PCN, penicillin; PTZ, pentylenetetrazol; EPC, epilepsy partialis continua.

TABLE 4 Potentially Reversible Causes of Myoclonus[a]

Autoimmune disorders	Co-factor deficiency	Drugs/intoxications
Paraneoplastic syndromes, post-infectious and post-vaccinal disorders, celiac disease	Biotin, pyridoxine, cobalamin (congenital or infantile)	Psychotropic medications, antibiotics, insecticides, phenytoin, carbamazepine, anesthetics, narcotics, dopaminergic drugs; antineoplastic drugs, cardiovascular drugs, toxins (strychnine, lead)
Infections	**Metabolic disorders**	**Tumors**
Meningitis, encephalitis (EBV, Coxsackie B), HIV, group A beta-hemolytic streptococcal pharyngitis	Uremia, post-dialysis syndrome, hepatic failure, hyponatremia, hypoglycemia, aminoacidurias (maple syrup urine disease), urea cycle disorders, organic acidurias (medium-chain acyl-CoA dehydrogenase deficiency), Wilson disease	Brain or spinal cord tumors

[a]Not all conditions within a category of myoclonic disorders may be fully reversible, but etiology-specific treatments are preferable to non-specific treatments, as they may prevent further brain injury.

cants include industrial agents, pesticides, heavy metals, and substances of abuse. Specialized toxicology studies may be necessary.

Biochemical and histochemical tests allow specific etiologic diagnosis in many cases. They may include biotinidase, biotin, organic and amino acids, and urinary oligosaccharides, as well as evoked potentials, skin biopsies, slit lamp examination, muscle biopsy, and electroretinograms (Gascon et al., 1994). Antineuronal antibodies and antibodies to neurotransmitter pathway enzymes, such as glutamic acid decarboxylase (GAD), can be measured. Many molecular genetics tests for movement disorders are

TABLE 5 Some Genetic Disorders Associated with Myoclonus[a]

Disorder	Chromosome	Gene/Gene product
ADCME	2p11.1–q12.2	—
Angelman syndrome	15q11–q13	UBE3A, GABRB3(?)
Ataxia-telangiectasia	11q	ATM
Biotinidase deficiency	3p25	BTD gene/biotinidase
DRPLA	12p	DRPLA gene/atrophin-1
JME	6p, 15q	—
Mitochondrial		
MELAS		mt RNA (Leu (UUR))
MERRF		mt RNA (Lys)
PEO		Multiple point mutations and large deletions
Myoclonus-dystonia syndrome (DYT11)	7q21–q31 11q23	SGCE (gene for epsilon-sarcoglycan) D_2 dopamine receptor gene (?)
PME		
GM1-gangliosidosis	5p1.13	Beta-galactosidase gene
Juvenile Gaucher (type III)	1.q21	Glucocerebrosidase gene
Lafora (EPM2)	6q23–q25	EPM2A/laforin
NCL	16p12	CLN1, CLN2, CLN3/lysosomal enzymes and transmembrane proteins
Sialidosis, type 1	20	Sialidase gene
U-L disease (EPM1)	21q22.3	CSTB/cystatin B
SCA 2	12	SCA2 gene/ataxin-2

[a]From Pranzatelli, 2003.
ADCME, autosomal dominant cortical myoclonus and epilepsy.
DRPLA, dentatorubral-pallidoluysian atrophy.
JME, juvenile myoclonic epilepsy.
MERRF, mitochondrial encephalopathy with ragged red fibers.
MELAS, mitochondrial encephalopathy with lactic acidosis and stroke-like episodes.
NCL, neuronal ceroid lipofuscinosis.
PME, progressive myoclonus epilepsy.
SCA, spinocerebellar ataxia.

now available (Table 5) (Bespalova et al., 1997; Bonten et al., 2000; Borner et al., 2000; Delgado-Escueta et al., 1999; Guerrini et al., 2001; Klein et al., 2000; Larson et al., 1999; Minassian et al., 2001; Pagani et al., 2002; Pennacchio et al., 1996; Pshezhetsky and Ashmarina, 2001; Schols et al., 1997; Serratosa et al., 1999; Tomoda et al., 1991; Wisniewski et al., 2000; Wood et al., 2000; Zimprich et al., 2001). Determination of catecholamine precursors and metabolites in CSF may be helpful in diagnostically challenging cases (Hyland et al., 1998).

Factitious or psychogenic myoclonus may occur in adults and teenagers as one of the most common types of psychogenic movement disorders (Miyasaki et al., 2003). It is challenging to diagnose and treat. Clinical clues include incongruous findings, evidence of underlying psychopathology, suggestibility, and improvement with distraction or placebo (Monday and Jankovic, 1993). Poor outcome is associated with long duration of symptoms, insidious onset of movements, inability to accept the psychological nature of the movements, and psychiatric co-morbidity on Axis I diagnoses (Feinstein et al., 2001).

B. Non-reversible Etiologies

Non-reversible diseases associated with myoclonus constitute an extensive list of disorders without apparent connection (Table 6) (Blindauer, 2001; Caviness, 2002; Krauss et al., 1996; Rivest, 2003; Sejvar et al., 2003; Thompson et al., 1994a; Thompson, 1994b). These include genetic and acquired disorders, some resulting in a variety of structural lesions. Myoclonus is usually one of many neurologic abnormalities in these situations, and the other features help establish the diagnosis.

TABLE 6 Non-Reversible Myoclonic Disorders

Degenerative disorders	Brain anomalies	
Alper disease	Agenesis of corpus collosum	
Alzheimer disease	Dorsal and ventral defects	
Corticobasal degeneration	Hydranencephaly	
Hallervorden-Spatz disease	Migrational and proliferation disorders	
Leukodystrophies (Krabbe disease)		
Progressive myoclonus epilepsies	Porencephaly	
Spinocerebellar ataxias	Rett syndrome	
Metabolic disorders	**Neurocutaneous disorders**	**Acquired focal lesions**
Certain aminoacidurias	Incontinentia pigmenti	Head trauma
Leigh syndrome	Linear nevus sebaceum	Post-thalamotomy
Lysosomal storage diseases/trauma lipidoses	Sturge-Weber	Spinal cord
	Tuberous sclerosis	Stroke
		Tumor
Infections	**Toxins**	
Encephalitis (West Nile virus)	Bismuth	
Prion diseases (Creutzfeldt-Jakob)	DDT	

IX. TREATMENT

Treatment of the underlying etiology of myoclonus is preferable to symptomatic treatment. In drug-induced myoclonus, the offending agent should be stopped and symptomatic support given. The approach to myoclonus due to infections is directed to the source of the infection. When myoclonus occurs as the remote immunological effect of cancers, the therapy is aimed at the cancer and also against the autoimmune process (Pranzatelli, 2000). Not all types of myoclonus are equally remediable by drug therapy; spinal myoclonus may be especially difficult to treat (Hoehn and Cherington, 1977).

A. Drug Therapy

1. Antiepileptic Drugs

The principal treatment for myoclonus, whether epileptic or non-epileptic, is antiepileptic drugs (Table 7) (Capovilla et al., 1999; Mercadonte et al., 2001; Moretti et al., 2000; Wallace, 2001; Yoshimura et al., 2001). Anticonvulsants may have synergistic effects in myoclonus. The 1,3-substituted benzodiazepines clonazepam, nitrazepam, and lorazepam are particularly useful due to a combination of their anxiolytic, sedative, muscle relaxant, and anticonvulsant properties, but tolerance is limiting (Pranzatelli and Nadi, 1995). Valproate is the drug of choice for EPM1, but some patients are unusually sensitive to it and require low doses. However, not all are antimyoclonic; in epileptic patients, carbamazepine, gabapentin, lamotrigine, pregabalin, and vigabatrin may induce myoclonus, and lorazepam may evoke myoclonus in infants (Asconape et al., 2000; Eldridge et al., 1983; Genton et al., 1998; Guerrini et al., 1999; Huppertz et al., 2001; Janszky et al., 2000; Marciani et al., 1995; Nanba and Maegaki, 1999). Phenytoin worsens EPM1.

2. Other Neuroactive Drugs

a. Amino Acid Receptor–Active Drugs. Besides benzodiazepines, several other antimyoclonic drugs are thought to modulate GABA or excitatory amino acid receptors. Chloral hydrate may be used acutely or chronically in the treatment of refractory myoclonus in PME and, paradoxically, does not cause sedation (Pranzatelli and Tate, 2001). Baclofen, a GABA agonist, has been used in difficult or refractory cases of myoclonus such as spinal myoclonus or the EPM1 type of PME. Gamma-hydroxybutyric acid (sodium oxybate) is

TABLE 7 Pharmacotherapy of Specific Myoclonic Disorders

EPM1	PHM	OMS	Myoclonus-dystonia
Valproate	Clonazepam	ACTH	Trihexyphenidyl
Clonazepam	Valproate	Steroids	Sodium oxybate
Zonisamide	Piracetam	IVIG	
Piracetam	Levetiracetam	Chemotherapy	
Levetiracetam	L-5-HTP		
Chloral hydrate	Felbamate		
L-dopa induced/Parkinson		**PMA**	**Cortical reflex**
Methysergide		Acetazolamide	Lisuride
			Apomorphine
Diaphragmatic		**Spinal**	**Essential**
Phenytoin		Tetrabenazine	Primidone
Valproate		Baclofen	Propranolol
Epileptic negative		**Status myoclonus**	**Opioid-induced**
Ethosuximide		Phenobarbital	Clonazepam
		Chloral hydrate	Gabapentin
			Midazolam

advocated for alcohol-sensitive myoclonus but is a Schedule I drug (Agarwal and Frucht, 2003). Midazolam infusion may allow the continuation of long-term high-dose morphine for pain control in cancer patients, even in the presence of morphine-induced myoclonus. Dextromethorphan, a weak noncompetitive inhibitor at the dissociative anesthetic site within the ion channel associated with the NMDA glutamate receptor, has been used for non-ketotic hyperglycinemia.

b. Racetams. Piracetam is a first-generation prototype nootropic drug found by serendipity to be antimyoclonic only in cortical myoclonus (Brown et al., 1993; Gouliaev and Senning, 1994). Despite the high doses required (Ikeda et al., 1996), the safety index is excellent in children (Pranzatelli et al., 2001). Compared to levetiracetam, it has more antimyoclonic effect but little antiepileptic activity (Genton and Van Vleymen, 2000). Both have a place in the treatment of PME (Fedi et al., 2001) and post-hypoxic myoclonus (Krauss et al., 2001).

c. Serotonergic Drugs. The serotonin precursor 5-hydroxy-L-tryptophan (L-5-HTP), may be useful when conventional drugs have failed in posthypoxic myoclonus and photic cortical reflex myoclonus (Chadwick et al., 1977). L-5-HTP is not anti-myoclonic in all types of myoclonus, having a rather limited role in PME (Pranzatelli et al., 1995) and in OMS. It may induce the eosinophilia-myalgia syndrome. L-5-HTP is administered with a peripheral decarboxylase inhibitor such as carbidopa to limit the side effects, such as cramping and diarrhea. There is a rational basis for the use of serotonin receptor agonists and antagonists in myoclonic disorders (Pranzatelli, 1994), but this area is largely unexplored. Methysergide can offset L-dopa-induced myoclonus in Parkinson disease.

d. Dopaminergic Drugs. Lisuride and apomorphine have been used in the treatment of cortical reflex myoclonus (Obeso et al., 1986). Although apomorphine acts as a dopamine agonist, lisuride has serotonergic as well as dopaminergic properties. Tetrabenazine is a dopamine antagonist and dopamine storage depleter used occasionally to treat spinal myoclonus. Dopamine also can be modulated by estrogen (Kompoliti, 1999). When menstrual periods exacerbate myoclonus, use of oral contraceptives may improve the situation.

e. Other Drugs. Anticholinergic drugs such as trihexyphenidyl are an option in myoclonus-dystonia but have a limited role in the therapy of other myoclonic disorders. In progressive myoclonus ataxia, acetazolamide may be useful as an adjunctive therapy. One treatment for essential myoclonus is propranolol, or the selective beta-blockers metoprolol or nadolol, which lack intrinsic sympathomimetic activity.

3. Immunotherapy

B-cell and T-cell abnormalities have been described in autoimmune post-infectious or paraneoplastic myoclonus (Pranzatelli, 2000). Immunomodulation with intravenous immunoglobulins (IVIG) is one approach. Immunosuppressants, such as azathioprine, cyclophosphamide, and methotrexate, also may have a role. ACTH (corticotropin) is the gold standard for pediatric OMS, whereas corticosteroids are more often used in adults. Case reports suggest plasmapheresis may be effective (Yiu et al., 2001).

B. Metabolic Therapies

Co-factors and vitamins are vital to proper functioning of metabolic pathways. Coenzyme Q_{10}, L-carnitine, and creatine monohydrate may be combined in mitochondrial myopathies. Supplemental L-carnitine and a low-fat diet is the treatment of choice for medium-chain acyl-CoA dehydrogenase deficiency (MCAD), a disorder of fatty acid oxidation. Although biotin's mechanism of action in myoclonus remains uncertain, replacement therapy may be therapeutic in deficiencies of biotinidase, multiple carboxylases, or other biotin-dependent enzymes (Gascon et al., 1994). Response to biotin can occur infrequently in the absence of biotin or biotinidase deficiency. Response to thiamine was described in a case report of opsoclonic cerebellopathy.

C. Botulinum Toxin

Botulinum toxin injection prevents the release of acetylcholine at the neuromuscular junction, blocking involuntary movement but preserving strength. It temporarily alleviates painful myoclonus (Awaad et al., 1999). Both botulinum toxin A and B are commercially available. The current trend is to use low doses to reduce the chances of antibody formation. Effects last from weeks to months, and the injections must be repeated.

D. Transcranial Magnetic Stimulation (TMS)

A noninvasive, safe, and painless way to stimulate the human motor cortex in humans is TMS (Chen, 2000). Types include single-pulse, paired-pulse, and repetitive TMS (rTMS) (Amassian et al., 1995). Modulation of cortical excitability by rTMS has therapeutic potential in neurological and psychiatric disorders, as high-frequency rTMS (5 Hz) increases cortical excitability, whereas low-frequency stimulation (1 Hz) reduces cortical excitability (Triggs and Kirshner, 2001). Whereas only cortical structures are currently accessible, TMS seems capable of affecting activity in cortically linked deep brain structures (McDonald and Greenberg, 2000). The only serious side effect is a possible induction of seizures (Lisanby et al., 2001). Currently TMS is regarded largely as a research tool.

E. Quality of Life Issues

Whereas this discussion has focused on medical aspects of myoclonus, psychosocial issues should not be neglected. In severe cases, premature relegation to the wheelchair or bed may result from lack of exercise, obesity, depression, poor self-esteem, and lack of socialization. Companionship, rigorous efforts to increase independence, psychological counseling, and life-style changes can result in surprising functional gains. Taking the time to listen and helping to set practical and realistic expectations is an especially important aspect of the successful patient-physician relationship in myoclonic disorders.

Acknowledgements

Supported in part by grants from the American Medical Association Research and Education Foundation, the Children's Miracle Network, and the Southern Illinois University School of Medicine.

Video Legends

SEGMENT 1 **EPM1** (Unverricht-Lündborg Disease, Baltic or Mediterranean Myoclonus)

A. A 22-year-old man with cortical myoclonus. Despite taking several anti-epileptic drugs, his myoclonus periodically intensifies, like a seizure fragment. When asked to stand, he must first concentrate for several seconds to steady himself.

B. A 21-year-old woman with cortical tremor, a manifestation of cortical myoclonus. Her obesity is valproate-induced, but valproate has been her best drug.

SEGMENT 2 **Mitochondrial Myopathy**

A. Progressive External Ophthalmoplegia (PEO)
A 30-year-old man with severe action myoclonus and limb dysmetria. He also has a history of status epilepticus, peripheral neuropathy, and dementia. Neurophysiologic studies revealed his myoclonus to be subcortical in origin and he responded poorly to medication.

B. Mitochondrial Encephalopathy with Lactic Acidosis and Stroke-Like Episodes (MELAS)

1. A 25-year-old man with action myoclonus, ataxia, and a prominent seizure disorder despite taking several anti-epileptic drugs.
2. A 20-year-old female sibling with later onset and less severe symptoms. Having the patient drink from a cup is one of the best ways of eliciting the myoclonus.

SEGMENT 3 **EPM2** (Lafora Disease)
A 19-year-old man with multiple types of myoclonus, including sensory-evoked, action, and spontaneous myoclonus. He also manifests facial involvement, external ophthalmoplegia, and dementia. He was on several anti-epileptic drugs at the time of videotaping.

SEGMENT 4 **Sialidosis, Type 1** (Cherry Red Spot Myoclonus)
A non-ambulatory 20-year-old male with action myoclonus, ataxia, dysarthria, dystonia, cognitive impairment, and joint contractures. He has a brief seizure during the session.

SEGMENT 5 **Gaucher Disease, Type III** (Neuronopathic Form)

A. A 9-year-old boy with cortical myoclonus, infrequent seizures, behavior problems, dysarthria, ataxia, mental retardation, and tremor.

B. A non-ambulatory 31-year-old woman with cortical myoclonus and frequent complex partial seizures despite multiple anti-epileptic drugs.

SEGMENT 6 **Sleep Myoclonus**
A 5-year-old girl with episodic limb myoclonus only during sleep. A prolonged video-EEG recording revealed multiple myoclonic jerks, often occurring in clusters, without an EEG correlate—subcortical myoclonus.

SEGMENT 7 **Myoclonus-Dystonia**
A 4-year-old girl with myoclonus and action dystonia that emerge during tasks involving the hands, such as drawing and drinking from a cup. Neurological examination is otherwise normal. Anchoring of the elbow against the chest is a maneuver such patients use to steady their arms.

SEGMENT 8 **Ataxia-Telangiectasia**
A 12-year-old girl with enough spontaneous myoclonus to require her to use a seatbelt in her wheelchair. She also has significant dystonia.

SEGMENT 9 **Opsoclonus-Myoclonus-Ataxia**
A 4-year-old girl evaluated several years after resection of neuroblastoma and chemotherapy. She has marked gait ataxia, action myoclonus, and opsoclonus. The clinical course is one of neurological relapses with illness or tapering of immunotherapy.

SEGMENT 10 **Progressive Myoclonus Ataxia**
A 25-year-old woman with subcortical myoclonus and a pan-cerebellar syndrome. She has never had seizures.

References

Agarwal, P., and S.J. Frucht. 2003. Myoclonus. *Curr Opin Neurol* **16**: 515–521.

Amassian, V.E., R.Q. Cracco, P.S. Maccabee, J.B. Cracco, and K. Henry. 1995. Some positive effects of transcranial magnetic stimulation. *Adv Neurol* **67**:79–104.

Anstead, M. 2000. Pediatric sleep disorders: new developments and evolving understanding. *Curr Opin Pulm Med* **6**(6):501–506.

Asconape, J., A. Diedrich, and J. DellaBadia. 2000. Myoclonus associated with the use of gabapentin. *Epilepsia* **41**(4):479–481.

Awaad, Y., H. Tayem, A. Elgamal, and M.F. Coyne. 1999. Treatment of childhood myoclonus with botulinum toxin type A. *J Child Neurol* **14**(12):781–786.

Baumgartner, C., I. Podreka, A. Olbrich, K. Novak, W. Serles, S. Aull, G. Almer, S. Lurger, U. Pietrzyk, D. Prayer, and G. Lindinger. 1996. Epileptic negative myoclonus: An EEG-single-photon emission CT study indicating involvement of premotor cortex. *Neurology* **46**(3): 753–758.

Berkovic, S.F., S. Carpenter, A. Evans, G. Karpati, E.A. Shoubridge, F. Andermann, E. Meyer, J.L. Tyler, M. Diksic, and D. Arnold. 1989. Myoclonus epilepsy and ragged-red fibres (MERRF). 1. A clinical, pathological, biochemical, magnetic resonance spectrographic and positron emission tomographic study. *Brain* **112**(Pt 5):1231–1260.

Bespalova, I.N., S. Adkins, M. Pranzatelli, and M. Burmeister. 1997. Novel cystatin B mutation and diagnostic PCR assay in Unverricht-Lundborg (Baltic) progressive myoclonus epilepsy patient. *Am J Med Genet (Neuropsych Gen)* **74**(5):467–471.

Bhatia, K.P., P. Brown, R. Gregory, G.G. Lennox, H. Manji, P.D. Thompson, D.W. Ellison, and C.D. Marsden. 1995. Progressive myoclonic ataxia associated with coeliac disease. The myoclonus is of cortical origin, but the pathology is in the cerebellum. *Brain* **118**:1087–1093.

Bhatia, K., P.D. Thompson, and C.D. Marsden, 1992. "Isolated" postinfectious myoclonus. *J Neurol Neurosurg Psychiatry* **55**(11):1089–1091.

Blindauer, K. 2001. Myoclonus and its disorders. *Neurol Clin* **19**:723–734.

Bonten, E.J., W.F. Arts, M. Beck, A. Covanis, M.A. Donati, R. Parini, E. Zammarchi, and A. d'Azzo. 2000. Novel mutations in lysosomal neuraminidase identify functional domains and determine clinical severity in sialidosis. *Hum Mol Genet* **9**(18):2715–2725.

Borner, G.V., M. Zeviani, V. Tiranti, F. Carrara, S. Hoffmann, K.D. Gerbitz, H. Lochmuller, D. Pongratz, T. Klopstock, A. Melberg, E. Holme, and S. Paabo. 2000. Decreased aminoacylation of mutant tRNAs in MELAS but not in MERRF patients. *Hum Mol Genet* **9**(4):467–475.

Brown, P., M.J. Steiger, P.D. Thompson, J.C. Rothwell, B.L. Day, M. Salama, T. Waegemans, and C.D. Marsden. 1993. Effectiveness of piracetam in cortical myoclonus. *Mov Disord* **8**(1):63–68.

Bye, A.M., D.J. Kok, F.T. Ferenschild, and J.S. Vles. 2000. Paroxysmal non-epileptic events in children: a retrospective study over a period of 10 years. *J Paediatr Child Health* **36**(3):244–248.

Capovilla, G., F. Beccaria, P. Veggiotti, G. Rubboli, S. Meletti, and C.A. Tassinari. 1999. Ethosuximide is effective in the treatment of epileptic negative myoclonus in childhood partial epilepsy. *J Child Neurol* **14**(6):395–400.

Caviness, J.N. 2002. Epidemiology of myoclonus. *Adv Neurol* **89**:19–22.

Chadwick, D., M. Hallett, R. Harris, P. Jenner, E.T. Reynolds, and C.D. Marsden. 1977. Clinical, biochemical and physiological features distinguishing myoclonus responsive to 5-hydroxy-tryptophan, tryptophan with a monoamine oxidase inhibitor and clonazepam. *Brain* **100**: 455–487.

Chattopadhyay, S., M. Ito, J.D. Cooper, A.I. Brooks, T.M. Curran, J.M. Powers, and D.A. Pearce. 2002. An autoantibody inhibitory to glutamic acid decarboxylase in the neurodegenerative disorder Batten Disease. *Hum Mol Genet* **11**(12):1421–1431.

Chen, R. 2000. Studies of human motor physiology with transcranial magnetic stimulation. *Muscle Nerve Suppl* **9**:S26–S32.

Chen, R., H. Remtulla, and C.F. Bolton. 1995. Electrophysiological study of diaphragmatic myoclonus. *J Neurol Neurosurg Psychiatry* **58**(4): 480–483.

Cooper, J.D., P. Gupta, and E. Bihle. 2002. Profound loss of GABAergic interneurons in the PPT1 knockout mouse model of infantile neuronal ceroid lipofuscinosis. *Neuropathol Appl Neurobiol* **28**(2):158–159.

Dale, R.C. 2003. Autoimmunity and the basal ganglia: new insights into old diseases. *QJM* **96**:183–191.

Dalmau, J.O., and J.B. Posner. 1997. Paraneoplastic syndromes affecting the nervous system. *Semin Oncol* **24**:318–328.

Daoust-Roy, J., and S.S. Seshia. 1992. Benign neonatal sleep myoclonus: A differential diagnosis of neonatal seizures. *AJDC* **146**:1236–1241.

Delgado-Escueta, A.V., M.T. Medine, J.M. Serratosa, I.P. Castroviejo, M.N. Gee, K. Weissbecker, B.W. Westling, C.Y. Fong, M.E. Alonso, S. Cordova, P. Shah, S. Khan, J. Sainz, F. Rubio-Donnadieu, and R.S. Sparkes. 1999. Mapping and positional cloning of common idiopathic generalized epilepsies: juvenile myoclonus epilepsy and childhood absence epilepsy. *Adv Neurol* **79**:351–374.

DiFazio, M.P., J. Morales, and R. Davis. 1998. Acute myoclonus secondary to group A beta-hemolytic streptococcus infection: a PANDAS variant. *J Child Neurol* **13**(10):516–518.

Eldridge, R., M. Iivanainen, R. Stern, T. Koerber, and B.J. Wilder. 1983. "Baltic" myoclonus epilepsy: hereditary disorder of childhood made worse by phenytoin. *Lancet* **9**(8354):838–842.

Espinosa, F., A. McMahon, E. Chan, S. Wang, C.S. Ho, N. Heintz, and R.H. Joho. 2001. Alcohol hypersensitivity, increased locomotion, and spontaneous myoclonus in mice lacking the potassium channels Kv3.1 and Kv3.3. *J Neuro Sci* **21**(17):6657–6665.

Fahn, S. 1979. Posthypoxic action myoclonus: Review of the literature and report of two new cases with response to valproate and estrogen. *Adv Neurol* **26**:49–84.

Fedi, M., D. Reutens, F. Dubeau, E. Andermann, D. D'Agostino, and F. Andermann. 2001. Long-term efficacy and safety of piracetam in the treatment of progressive myoclonus epilepsy. *Arch Neurol* **58**(5): 781–786.

Feinstein, A., V. Stergiopoulos, J. Fine, and A.E. Lang. 2001. Psychiatric outcome in patients with a psychogenic movement disorder: a prospective study. *Neuropsychiatry Neuropsychol Behav Neurol* **14**(3):169–176.

Fejerman, N. 1997. Myoclonus and epilepsies. *Indian J Pediatr* **64**(5): 583–602.

Frucht, S.J., S.E. Leurgans, M. Hallett, and S. Fahn. 2002. The Unified Myoclonus Rating Scale. *Adv Neurol* **89**:361–376.

Fukutani, Y., N.J. Cairns, I.P. Everall, A. Chadwick, K. Isaki, and P.L. Lantos. 1999. Cerebellar dentate nucleus in Alzheimer's disease with myoclonus. *Dement Geriatr Cogn Disord* **10**:81–88.

Gascon, G.G., P.T. Ozand, and J. Brismar. 1994. Movement disorders in childhood organic acidurias. Clinical, neuroimaging, and biochemical correlations. *Brain Dev* **16** Suppl, 94–103.

Genton, P., V.H. Nguyen, and E. Mesdjian. 1998. Carbamazepine intoxication with negative myoclonus after the addition of clobazam. *Epilepsia* **39**:1115–1118.

Genton, P., and B. Van Vleymen. 2000. Piracetam and levetiracetam: close structural similarities but different pharmacological and clinical profiles. *Epileptic Disord* **2**(2):99–105.

Ghaziuddin, N., A. Iqbal, and S. Khetarpal. 2001. Myoclonus during prolonged treatment with sertraline in an adolescent patient. *J Child Adolesc Psychopharmacol* **11**(2):199–202.

Gordon, M.F. 2002. Toxin and drug-induced myoclonus. *Adv Neurol* **89**:49–76.

Gouliaev, A.H., and A. Senning. 1994. Piracetam and other structurally related nootropics. *Brain Res Rev* **19**:180–222.

Grech, V., C. Vella, and V. Mercieca. 2001. Temporary myoclonus with treatment of congenital transcobalamin 2 deficiency. *Pediatr Neurol* **24**(1):75–76.

Guerrini, R., A. Belmonte, L. Parmeggiani, and E. Perucca. 1999. Myoclonic status epilepticus following high-dosage lamotrigine therapy. *Brain Dev* **21**(6):420–424.

Guerrini, R., P. Bonanni, A. Patrignani, P. Brown, L. Parmeggiani, P. Grosse, P. Brovedani, F. Moro, P. Aridon, R. Carrozzo, and G. Casari. 2001. Autosomal dominant cortical myoclonus and epilepsy (ADCME) with complex partial and generalized seizures: A newly recognized epilepsy syndrome with linkage to chromosome 2p11.1-q12.2. *Brain* **124** (Pt 12):2459–2475.

Guerrini, R., T.M. De Lorey, P. Bonanni, A. Moncla, C. Dravet, G. Suisse, M.O. Livet, M. Bureau, P. Malzac, P. Genton, P. Thomas, F. Sartucci, P. Simi, and J.M. Serratosa. 1996. Cortical myoclonus in Angelman syndrome. *Ann Neurol* **40**(1):39–48.

Gupta, P., A.A. Sajombo, A. Atashband, K.E. Wisniewski, J.M. Shelton, J.A. Richardson, R.E. Hammer, and S.L. Hofmann. 2001. Disruption of PPT1 or PPT2 causes neuronal ceroid lipofuscinosis in knockout mice. *Proc Natl Acad Sci USA* **98**(24):13566–13571.

Hallett, M. 1985. Myoclonus: Relation to epilepsy. *Epilepsia* **26**:567–577.

Hallett, M. 2002. Neurophysiology of brainstem myoclonus. *Adv Neurol* **89**:99–102.

Hoehn, M.M., and M. Cherington. 1977. Spinal myoclonus. *Neurology* **27**:942–946.

Huppertz, H.J., T.J. Feuerstein, and A. Schulze-Bonhage. 2001. Myoclonus in epilepsy patients with anticonvulsive add-on therapy with pregabalin. *Epilepsia* **42**(6):790–792.

Hyland, K., L.A. Arnold, and J.M. Trugman. 1998. Defects of biopterin metabolism and biogenic amine biosynthesis: clinical, diagnostic, and therapeutic aspects. In: Fahn S, Marsden CD, DeLong M (eds), *Dystonia* **3**: Advances in Neurology, Vol 78. Philadelphia, Lippincott-Raven Publishers, 301–308.

Ikeda, A., H. Shibasaki, K. Tashiro, Y. Mizuno, and J. Kimura. 1996. Clinical trial of piracetam in patients with myoclonus: Nationwide multiinstitution study in Japan. *Mov Disord* **11**:691–700.

Janszky, J., G. Rasonyi, P. Halasz, S. Olajos, J. Perenyi, A. Szucs, T. Debreczeni. 2000. Disabling erratic myoclonus during lamotrigine therapy with high serum level—report of two cases. *Clin Neuropharmacol* **23**(2):86–89.

Klein, C., K. Schilling, R.J. Saunders-Pullman, J. Garrels, X.O. Breakefield, M.F. Brin, D. deLeon, D. Doheny, S. Fahn, J.S. Fink, L. Forsgren, J. Friedman, S. Frucht, J. Harris, G. Holmgren, B. Kis, R. Kurlan, M. Kyllerman, A.E. Lang, J. Leung, D. Raymond, J.D. Robishaw, G. Sanner, E. Schwinger, R.E. Tabamo, and M. Tagliati. 2000. A major locus for myoclonus-dystonia maps to chromosome 7q in eight families. *Am J Hum Genet* **67**(5),1314–1319.

Kompoliti, K. 1999. Estrogen and movement disorders. *Clin Neuropharmacol* **22**(6):318–326.

Krauss, G.L., A. Bergin, R.E. Kramer, et al. 2001. Suppression of post-hypoxic and post-encephalitic myoclonus with levetiracetam. *Neurology* **56**(3):411–412.

Krauss, J.K., R. Trankle, K.H. Kopp, Y.W. Cho, and S.G. Reich. 1996. Post-traumatic movement disorders in survivors of severe head injury. *Neurology* **47**,1488–1492.

Larson, G.P., S. Ding, R.G. Lafrenier, G.A. Rouleau, and T.G. Krotiris. 1999. Instability of the EPM1 minisatellite. *Hum Mol Genet* **8**(11): 1985–1988.

Lisanby, S.H., B. Luber, H.A. Sackeim, C. Schroeder, and H.A. Sackeim. 2001. Deliberate seizure induction with negative transcranial magnetic stimulation in nonhuman primates. *Arch Gen Psychiatry* **58**:199–200.

Maiteh, M., and A.S. Daoud. 2001. Myoclonic seizure following intravenous verapamil injection: case report and review of the literature. *Ann Trop Paediatr* **21**(3):271–272.

Marciani, M.G., M. Maschio, F. Spanedda, C. Iani, G.L. Gigli, and G. Bernardi. 1995. Development of myoclonus in patients with partial epilepsy during treatment with vigabatrin: an electro-encephalographic study. *Acta Neurol Scand* **91**(1):1–5.

Marsden, C.D., M. Hallett, and S. Fahn. 1982. The nosology and pathophysiology of myoclonus. In: Marsden CD, Fahn S (eds), *Movement Disorders*. London, Butterworths, 196–248.

Marsden, C.D., A.E. Harding, J.A. Obeso, and C.S. Lu. 1990. Progressive myoclonic ataxia (the Ramsay Hunt Syndrome). *Arch Neurol* **47**(10): 1121–1125.

Maydell, B.V., F. Berenson, A.D. Rothern, E. Wyllie, and P. Kotagal. 2001. Benign myoclonus of early infancy: an imitator of West's syndrome. *J Child Neurol* **16**(2):109–112.

McClain, B.C., L.A. Probst, and E. Pinter. 2001. Intravenous clonidine use in a neonate experiencing opioid-induced myoclonus. *Anesthesiology* **95**(2):549–550.

McDonald, W.M., and B.D. Greenberg. 2000. Electroconvulsive therapy in the treatment of neuropsychiatric conditions and transcranial magnetic stimulation as a pathophysiological probe in neuropsychiatry. *Depress Anxiety* **12**:135–143.

Mercadante, S., P. Villari, and F. Fulfaro. 2001. Gabapentin for opioid-related myoclonus in cancer patients. *Support Care Center* **9**(3): 205–206.

Minassian, B.A. 2001. Lafora's disease: towards a clinical, pathologic, and molecular synthesis. *Pediatr Neurol* **25**(1):21–29.

Minassian, B.A., J. Sainz, and A.V. Delgado-Escueta. 1995. Genetics of myoclonus and myoclonus epilepsies. *Clin Neurosci* **3**(4):223–235.

Miyasaki, J.M., D.S. Sa, N. Galvez-Jiminez, and A.E. Lang. 2003. Psychogenic movement disorders. *Can J Neurol Sci* **30** (Suppl 1), S94–100.

Monday, K., and J. Jankovic. 1993. Psychogenic myoclonus. *Neurol* **43**(2): 349–352.

Montagna, P., F. Provini, G. Plazzi, R. Luguori, and E. Lugaresi. 1997. Propriospinal myoclonus upon relaxation and drowsiness: a cause of severe insomnia. *Mov Disord* **12**(1):66–72.

Moretti, R., P. Torre, and R.M. Antonello. 2000. Opsoclonus-myoclonus syndrome: gabapentin as a new therapeutic proposal. *Eur J Neurol* **7**(4): 455–456.

Nanba, Y., and Y. Maegaki. 1999. Epileptic negative myoclonus induced by carbamazepine in a child with BECTS. Benign childhood epilepsy with centrotemporal spikes. *Pediatr Neurol* **21**(3):664–667.

Obeso, J.A., J.C. Rothwell, N.P. Quinn, A.E. Lang, J. Artieda, and C.D. Marsden. 1986. Lisuride in the treatment of myoclonus. *Adv Neurol* **43**:191–196.

Oguni, H., Y. Fukuyama, T. Tanaka, K. Kayashi, K. Hayashi, M. Funatsuka, M. Sakauchi, S. Shirakawa, and M. Osawa. 2001. Myoclonic-astatic epilepsy of early childhood—clinical and EEG analysis of myoclonic-astatic seizures, and discussions on the nosology of the syndrome. *Brain Dev* **23**(7):757–764.

Oguro, K., J. Kobayashi, H. Aiba, and J. Hojo. 1997. Opsoclonus-myoclonus syndrome with abnormal single photon emission computed tomography imaging. *Pediatr Neurol* **16**(4):334–336.

Oguro, K., K. Oya, C. Natori, H. Aiba, and H. Hojo. 2003. Cortical myoclonus in children. *Brain Dev* **25**:173–179.

Ohizumi, H., Y. Okuma, J. Fukae, K. Fujishima, K. Goto, and Y. Mizuno. 2002. Head tremor in dentatorubral-pallidoluysian atrophy. *Acta Neurol Scand* **106**:319–321.

Ozer, E.A., M. Turker, A.R. Bakiler, I. Yaprak, and C. Ozturk. 2001. Involuntary movements in infantile cobalamin deficiency appearing after treatment. *Pediatr Neurol* **25**(1):81–83.

Pagani, F., E. Buratti, C. Stuani, R. Bendix, T. Dork, and F.E. Baralle. 2002. A new type of mutation carries a splicing defect in ATM. *Nat Genet* **30**(4):426–429.

Pennacchio, L.A., A.E. Lehesjoki, N.E. Stone, V.L. Willour, K. Virtaneva, J. Miao, E. D'Amato, L. Ramirez, M. Faham, M. Koskiniemi, J.A. Warrington, R. Norio, A. de la Chapelle, D.R. Cox, and R.M. Myers. 1996. Mutations in the gene encoding cystatin B in progressive myoclonus epilepsy (EPM1). *Science* **271**(5256):1731–1734.

Pranzatelli, M.R. 1993. Myoclonic disorders. *Ped Ann* **22**(1):33–37.

Pranzatelli, M.R. 1994. Serotonin and human myoclonus: rationale for the use of serotonin receptor agonists and antagonists. *Arch Neurol* **51**: 605–617.

Pranzatelli, M.R. 1997. Serotonergic drugs and movement disorders in humans. *Drugs Today* **33**:379–392.

Pranzatelli, M.R. 2000. Paraneoplastic syndromes: an unsolved murder. *Sem Pediatr Neurol* **7**(2):118–130.

Pranzatelli, M.R. 2002. Infantile spasms vs. myoclonus: Is there a connection? In: Epilepsy, infantile spasms, and developmental encephalopathy. *Int Rev Neurobiol* **49**:285–314.

Pranzatelli, M.R. 2003. Myoclonus in childhood. *Sem Pediatr Neurol* **10**(1):41–51.

Pranzatelli, M.R., and N.S. Nadi. 1995. Mechanism of action of antiepileptic and antimyoclonic drugs. *Adv Neurol* **67**:329–360.

Pranzatelli, M.R., and S.R. Snodgrass. 1985. The pharmacology of myoclonus. *Clin Neuropharmacol* **8**:99–130.

Pranzatelli, M.R., and E.D. Tate. 2001. Chloral hydrate for progressive myoclonus epilepsy: a new look at an old drug. *Pediatr Neurol* **25**(5): 385–389.

Pranzatelli, M.R., E.D. Tate, I. Galvan, and A. Wheeler. 2001. Controlled pilot study of piracetam for pediatric opsoclonus-myoclonus. *Clin Neuropharmacol* **24**(6):352–357.

Pranzatelli, M.R., E. Tate, Y. Huang, R.H. Haas, J. Bodensteiner, S. Ashwal, and D. Franz. 1995. The neuropharmacology of progressive myoclonus epilepsy: response to 5-hydroxy-L-tryptophan. *Epilepsia* **36**:783–791.

Pranzatelli, M.R., A.L. Travelstead, E.D. Tate, T.J. Allison, E.J. Moticka, D.N. Franz, M.A. Nigro, J.T. Parke, D.A. Stumpf, and S.J. Verhulst. 2004. B- and T-cell markers in opsoclonus-myoclonus syndrome: Immunophenotyping of CSF lymphocytes. *Neurology* **62**:1526–1532.

Pshezhetsky, A.V., and M. Ashmarina. 2001. Lysosomal multienzyme complex: biochemistry, genetics and molecular pathophysiology. *Prog Nucleic Acid Res Mol Biol* **69**:81–114.

Rajakumar, K., and J.B. Bodensteiner. 1996. Febrile myoclonus: a survey of pediatric neurologists. *Clin Pediatr* (Phila) **35**(6):331–332.

Rhyu, I.J., L.C. Abbott, D.B. Walker, and C. Sotelo. 1999. An ultrastructural study of granule cell/Purkinje cell synapses in tottering (tg/tg), leaner (tg(la)/tg(la)) and compound heterozygous tottering/leaner (tg/tg(la)) mice. *Neurosci* **90**:717–728.

Rivest, J. 2003. Myoclonus. *Can J Neurol Sci* **30** Suppl 1, S53–58.

Rojas-Marcos, I., A. Rousseau, F. Keime-Guibert, R. Rene, S. Cartalat-Carel, J.Y. Delattre, and F. Graus. 2003. Spectrum of paraneoplastic neurologic disorders in women with breast and gynecologic cancer. *Medicine* **82**:216–223.

Rothwell, J.C. 2002. Pathophysiology of spinal myoclonus. *Adv Neurol* **89**:137–144.

Schols, L., S. Gispert, M. Vorgerd, A.M. Menezes Vieira-Saecker, P. Blanke, G. Auburger, G. Amoiridis, S. Meves, J.T. Epplen, H. Przuntek, S.M. Pulst, and O. Riess. 1997. Spinocerebellar ataxia type 2. Genotype and phenotype in German kindreds. *Arch Neurol* **54**(9):1073–1080.

Sejvar, J.J., M.B. Haddad, B.C. Tierney, G.L. Campbell, A.A. Marfin, J.A. Van Gerpen, A. Fleischauer, A.A. Leis, D.S. Stokic, and L.R. Petersen. 2003. Neurologic manifestations and outcome of West Nile virus infection. *JAMA* **290**:511–515.

Serratosa, J.M., P. Gomez-Garre, M.E. Gallaredo, B. Anta, D.B. de Bernabe, D. Lindhout, P.B. Augustijn, C.A. Tassinari, R.M. Malafosse, M. Topcu, D. Grid, C. Dravet, S.F. Berkovic, and S.R. de Cordoba. 1999. A novel protein tyrosine phosphatase gene is mutated in progressive myoclonus epilepsy of the Lafora type (EPM2). *Hum Mol Genet* **8**(2):345–352.

Shibasaki, H. 2000. Electrophysiological studies of myoclonus. *Muscle Nerve* **23**(3):321–335.

Shibasaki, H., A. Ikeda, T. Nagamino, T. Mima, K. Terada, N. Nishitani, M. Kanda, S. Takano, T. Hanazono, N. Kohara, et al. 1994. Cortical reflex negative myoclonus. *Brain* **117**:477–486.

Snodgrass, S.R. 1990. Myoclonus: analysis of monoamine, GABA, and other systems. *FASEB J* **4**:2775–2788.

Tanaka, S., S. Osari, M. Ozawa, H. Yamanouchi, Y. Goto, H. Matsuda, and I. Nonaka. 1997. Recurrent pain attacks in a 3-year-old patient with myoclonus epilepsy associated with ragged-red fibers (MERRF): a single-photon emission computed tomographic (SPECT) and electrophysiological study. *Brain Dev* **19**(3):205–208.

Tassinari, C.A., G. Rubboli, L. Parmeggiani, F. Valzania, R. Plasmati, P. Riguzzi, R. Michelucci, L. Volpi, D. Passarelli, S. Meletti, et al. 1995. Epileptic negative myoclonus. *Adv Neurol* **67**:181–197.

Tate, E., M.R. Pranzatelli, H. Ho, and A. Kim. 1995. A sensitive and semi-quantitative pediatric myoclonus evaluation scale. *Neurosci Nurs* **27**:287–291.

Tate, E.D., M.R. Pranzatelli, Yy. Huang, and R. Kaplan. 1994. An innovative approach to the problem of sedating children with opsoclonus-myoclonus syndrome: Effects on myoclonus and CSF monoamine metabolites. *Ann Neurol* **36**:543–544.

Thompson, P.D. 2002. Neurodegenerative causes of myoclonus. *Adv Neurol* **89**:31–34.

Thompson, P.D., K.P. Bhatia, P. Brown, M.B. Davis, M. Pires, N.P. Quinn, P. Luthert, M. Honovar, M.D. O'Brien, C.D. Marsden, et al. 1994a. Cortical myoclonus in Huntington's disease. *Mov Disord* **9**:633–641.

Thompson, P.D., B.L. Day, J.C. Rothwell, P. Brown, T.C. Britton, and C.D. Marsden. 1994b. The myoclonus in corticobasal degeneration. Evidence for two forms of cortical reflex myoclonus. *Brain* **117**:1197–1207.

Tobimatsu, S., R. Fukui, H. Shibasaki, M. Kato, and Y. Kuroiwa. 1985. Electrophysiological studies of myoclonus in sialidosis type 2. *Electroencephalogr Clin Neurophysiol* **60**(1):16–22.

Tomoda, A., M. Ikezawa, Y. Ohtani, T. Miike, and T. Kumamoto. 1991. Progressive myoclonus epilepsy: dentato-rubro-pallido-luysian atrophy (DRPLA) in childhood. *Brain Dev* **13**(4):266–269.

Toro, C., M. Hallett, J.C. Rothwell, P.T. Asselman, and C.D. Marsden. 1995. Physiology of negative myoclonus. *Adv Neurol* **67**:211–217.

Toro, C., A. Pascual-Leone, G. Deuschl, E. Tate, M.R. Pranzatelli, and M. Hallett. 1993. Cortical tremor: A common manifestation of cortical myoclonus. *Neurology* **43**:2346–2352.

Triggs, W.J., and H.S. Kirshner. 2001. Improving brain function with transcranial magnetic stimulation. *Neurology* **56**:429–430.

Uthman, B.M., and A. Reichl. 2002. Progressive myoclonic epilepsies. *Curr Treat Options Neurol* **4**:3–17.

Verghese, J., R.F. Goldberg, R.J. Desnick, M.E. Grace, J.E. Goldman, S.C. Lee, D.W. Dickson, and I. Rapin. 2000. Myoclonus from selective dentate nucleus degeneration in type 3 Gaucher disease. *Arch Neurol* **57**:389–395.

Vetrugno, R., F. Provini, G. Plazzi, M.L. Valentino, R. Liguori, E. Lugaresi, and P. Montagna. 2000. Focal myoclonus and propriospinal propagation. *Clin Neurophysiol* **111**:2175–2179.

Wallace, D.C. 2002. Animal models for mitochondrial disease. *Methods Mol Biol* **197**:3–54.

Wallace, S.J. 2001. Newer antiepileptic drugs: advantages and disadvantages. *Brain Dev* **23**(5):277–283.

Welsh, J.P., G. Yuen, D.G. Placantonakis, T.Q. Vu, F. Haiss, E. O'Hearn, M.E. Molliver, and S.A. Aicher. 2002. Why do Purkinje cells die so easily after global brain ischemia? Aldolase C, EAAT4, and the cerebellar contribution to posthypoxic myoclonus. *Adv Neurol* **89**:331–359.

Wisniewski, K.E., E. Kida, F. Connell, and N. Zhong. 2000. Neuronal ceroid lipofuscinoses: research update. *Neurol Sci* **21**(3 Suppl): 549–556.

Wood, J.D., F.C. Nucifara, K. Duan, C. Zhang, J. Wang, Y. Kim, G. Schilling, N. Sacchi, J.M. Liu, and C.A. Ross. 2000. Atrophin-1, the dentato-rubral and pallido-luysian atrophy gene product, interacts with ETO/MTG8 in the nuclear matrix and represses transcription. *J Cell Biol* **150**(5):939–948.

Yiu, V.W., T. Kovithavongs, L.F. McGonigle, and P. Ferreira. 2001. Plasmapheresis as an effective treatment for opsoclonus-myoclonus syndrome. *Pediatr Neurol* **24**(1):72–74.

Yoshimura, I., S. Kaneko, N. Yoshimura, and T. Murakami. 2001. Long-term observations of two siblings with Lafora disease treated with zonisamide. *Epilepsy Res* **46**(3):283–287.

Zaw, W., D.C. Knoppert, and O. da Silva. 2001. Flumazenil's reversal of myoclonic-like movements associated with midazolam in term newborns. *Pharmacotherapy* **21**(5):642–646.

Zimprich, A., M. Grabowski, F. Asmus, M. Naumann, D. Berg, M. Bertram, K. Scheidtmann, P. Kern, J. Winkelmann, B. Muller-Myhsok, L. Riedel, M. Bauer, T. Muller, M. Castro, T. Meitinger, T.M. Strom, and T. Gasser. 2001. Mutations in the gene encoding epsilon-sarcoglycan cause myoclonus-dystonia syndrome. *Nat Genet* **29**(1):66–69.

CHAPTER

F2

Post-Hypoxic Myoclonus in Rodents

KWOK-KEUNG TAI and DANIEL D. TRUONG

Myoclonus is a medical term used to describe brief, very rapid, sudden, shock-like involuntary jerking movements that involve small muscles or the whole body (Fahn, 1986). Myoclonus is manifested in a wide variety of neuropathological conditions affecting the central nervous system. Myoclonus can be classified based on anatomic distribution, pattern of contractions, pathophysiology, or etiology. One of the most disabling forms of myoclonus is known as post-hypoxic myoclonus, which is caused by brain damage resulting from a prolonged oxygen deprivation during cardiac arrest or anesthesia accidents during surgical operations. In addition, asthmatic attacks, airway obstruction, and drug intoxication can also trigger post-hypoxic myoclonus.

I. HISTORICAL BACKGROUND

Post-hypoxic myoclonus was originally reported by Lance and Adams in 1963, in which they described jerking movements exhibited by four patients in chronic post-hypoxic states. Since then, more than 100 cases have been reported in the literature, although the actual number of cases probably far exceeds this number, since many cases likely go unreported due to the subtlety of the symptoms. Patients suffering from post-hypoxic myoclonus are severely disabled, since their normally initiated movements can be interrupted by myoclonic jerks and pauses. Although patients with post-hypoxic myoclonus show signs of central nervous system dysfunction, the neuroanatomical substrate underlying this disorder remains largely unknown. In this regard, animal models may be useful in elucidating the mechanism of post-hypoxic myoclonus.

Early attempts at developing a rodent model of post-hypoxic myoclonus employed chemicals such as KCl (Truong et al., 1994), urea (Muscatt et al., 1986), or the pesticide p,p′-DDT (Chung and Van Woert, 1984). These models were complicated by the low survival rate of the animals, as well as other problems associated with the use of the chemicals, such as renal failure and cardiac injury. We have developed a rat model of post-hypoxic myoclonus, originally reported by Truong and colleagues (1994), in which rats are subjected to mechanical-induced cardiac arrest for a short duration of time. Cerebral hypoxic insults are induced during the cardiac arrest. These animals show jerking movements in response to auditory stimuli and other features of myoclonus that are similar to those observed in human myoclonus. This chapter provides an overall view of this rat model of post-hypoxic myoclonus, highlighting the behavioral, pharmacological, and neuroanatomical features that parallel those of human post-hypoxic myoclonus.

II. PROCEDURES FOR INDUCTION OF POST-HYPOXIC MYOCLONUS IN RATS

In this model, cardiac arrest is initiated by a mechanical obstruction of major cardiac vessels using an L-shaped loop, as described by Kawai et al. (1995), with some modifications. The procedures for the induction of post-hypoxic myoclonus are as follows: adult male, Sprague-Dawley rats weighing 220 to 240 g are anesthetized with intraperitoneal injections (i.p.) of ketamine (85 mg/kg) and xylazine (15 mg/kg, i.p.). Atropine (0.04 mg/kg, i.p.) is also administered to reduce respiratory secretions. The trachea is intubated with an 18 gauge catheter, which is then attached to a ventilator with settings of 175 ml/min of oxygen, 60 strokes per min. The rat is placed on a heating pad to maintain its body temperature at 37°C. In order to monitor the cardiac electrical activity and its function, electrocardiogram electrodes are attached to both arms and right leg of the rat to obtain an electrocardiogram. The left femoral artery and vein are catheterized to monitor arterial blood pressure and administer drugs that facilitate resuscitation.

Cardiac arrest is initiated and maintained by mechanically obstructing all of the major cardiac blood vessels, including the aorta, by hooking up the vessels with an L-shaped loop inserted into the rat body cavity. Chest compression is applied when the aorta is located between the hook and the fingers above the rat body cavity. The arterial blood pressure is maintained at 0 to 10 mm Hg. Under such low systemic arterial blood pressure, cerebral perfusion comes to a halt. In general, the mortality rate as a result of the operation procedures increases with a longer duration of cardiac arrest. Based on our experience, myoclonus develops only after a critical duration of cerebral hypoxia. A cardiac arrest for a duration of 8 minutes is a compromise at which myoclonus reliably develops following recovery, the survival rate is acceptable, and the severity of other neurological conditions is manageable.

Resuscitation begins at 8 minutes following cardiac arrest by resuming manual thoracic compression and by intravenous injection of 10 μg/kg epinephrine and 4 mEq/kg sodium bicarbonate. Following resuscitation, rats are weaned from the ventilator, the catheters are removed, and wounds are sutured. The animals are placed in an oxygen tent on a heating pad until completely recovered from the surgical coma.

III. BEHAVIOR AND EVALUATION OF POST-HYPOXIC MYOCLONUS IN RAT

One of the clinical features of post-hypoxic myoclonus is the trigger of myoclonic jerks in response to exogenous stimuli such as sound. The rat model of post-hypoxic myoclonus generated with the preceding procedures displays a behavioral profile similar to the myoclonus in humans. Patients who develop post-hypoxic jerks as a result of severe cerebral hypoxia usually are in a comatose state for a few days prior to the development of myoclonus. In this animal model, rats are also in a comatose state for 2 to 3 hours following cardiac arrest. Rats gradually regain consciousness but are non-ambulatory for the next 6 to 8 hours postsurgery. In the first 2 days after cardiac arrest, rats tend to develop spontaneous seizures. The types of seizures generated include tonic, partial seizures with wild running, and generalized clonic-tonic. In general, partial seizures are preceded by a short period of running, which is in turn preceded by myoclonic jerks. Running seizures can also be triggered in response to auditory stimuli as a result of environmental noise. Because the effects of running seizures are overwhelmingly intense in the first 2 days after cardiac arrest, they can mask the myoclonic jerks. Myoclonic jerks in response to auditory stimuli can occur while the rat is experiencing a seizure. Two days after the cardiac arrest, seizures decline gradually, whereas the myoclonic jerks persist.

Jerking movements in response to auditory stimuli can be ranked according to their intensity. The intensity of myoclonic jerks peaks on day 4 after cardiac arrest and then gradually declines to basal levels 34 days after surgery (Truong et al., 1994). For the purpose of evaluating myoclonic jerks in response to auditory stimuli, the rat is placed in a clear, Plexiglas cage for 10 min to let it habituate to the new environment prior to evaluation. The rat is then presented with 45 clicks of a metronome as the auditory stimulus. Each stimulus has a sound intensity of 96 dB with a duration of 40 ms at a frequency of 0.75 Hz. The involuntary muscle jerks in response to each stimulus are scored with the following criteria: 0 = no jerks; 1 = ear twitch; 2 = ear and head jerk; 3 = ear, head, and shoulder jerk; 4 = whole body jerk; and 5 = whole body jerk with jumping.

We examined whether the characteristics of this animal model are similar to those of post-hypoxic myoclonus syndrome in humans. In this rat model, hypoxic myoclonic jerks can last for more than 30 days, although the severity decreases over time (Figure 1). Evidence indicates that post-hypoxic myoclonus in humans lasts an average of 3 to 4 years (Werhahn et al., 1997). Considering that the rat has an average life span of 2½ years, the duration of 34 days may be approximately equivalent to 3 years in humans, assuming an average human life span of 80 years. Thus, the duration of myoclonus in our model approximates that observed in humans when calculated as a percentage of life span. Several additional factors that affect the severity of myoclonus in humans have also been examined in this rat model (Truong et al., 2000). Age is one of the factors in determining the severity of post-hypoxic myolconus in humans (Fahn, 1986), with severity of myoclonus increasing with age. In our model, cardiac arrest induces more

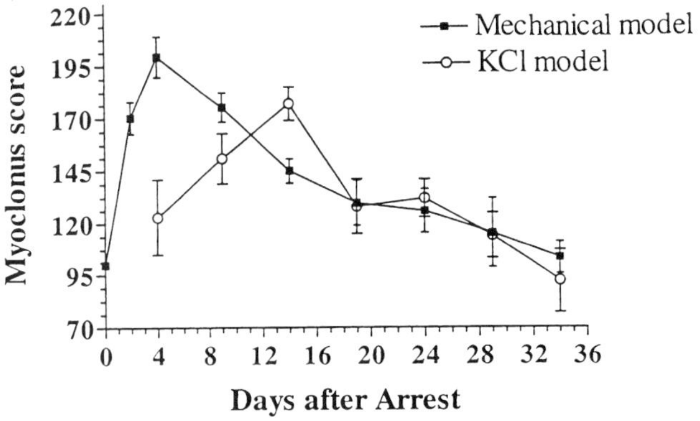

FIGURE 1 Time course of cardiac arrest-induced post-hypoxic myoclonus in rats using two different procedures. The myoclonus scores reach their peaks at 4 and 14 days for the mechanical- and potassium chloride (KCl)-induced models, respectively. Each point represents the mean ± SEM of six to ten animals. (Reprinted from *Clinical Neuroscience*, 96, Kanthasamy et al., Animal Models of Myoclonus, 236–245, Copyright (1995–1996), with permission from Association for Research in Nervous and Mental Disease.)

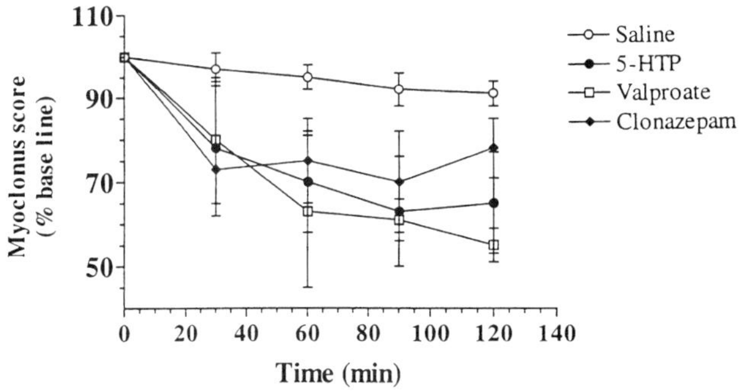

FIGURE 2 The antimyoclonic activity of clonazepam (0.5 mg/kg, i.p.), valporate (50 mg/kg, i.p.), and 5-HTP (100 mg/kg, i.p.) on cardiac arrest-induced post-hypoxic myoclonus. All three compounds significantly reduced the myoclonus scores of the rats when compared with saline-treated controls. Myoclonus scores are presented as a percentage of the initial response at time 0. (Reprinted from *Clinical Neuroscience*, 96, Kanthasamy et al., Animal Models of Myoclonus, 236–245, Copyright (1995–1996), with permission from Association for Research in Nervous and Mental Disease.)

severe myoclonus in adult rats than in the younger ones (Truong et al., 2000). We have also observed a relationship between cardiac arrest-induced mortality and increasing age of the animal.

IV. PHARMACOLOGICAL STUDIES FOR VALIDATION OF THE ANIMAL MODEL

Because myoclonus is often considered a component of an epileptic syndrome, antiepileptic drugs may be potentially useful for the treatment of this condition. Indeed, patients with myoclonus do respond to an array of antiepileptic agents. For example, clonazepam and valproate, two classical antiepileptic agents, can help reduce symptoms of post-hypoxic myoclonus in at least 50% of patients (Fahn, 1978; Fahn, 1986). In order to examine the validity of our model, we examined whether the rats with myoclonus also responded to antiepileptic agents. Results showed that both clonazepam and valproate significantly reduced myoclonus, as indicated by decreased myoclonus scores (Figure 2). The therapeutic effects of these two agents on myoclonus in this model occurred in a dose-related manner (Truong et al., 1994). Piracetam (2-oxo-1-pyrrolidine acetamide), a nootropic agent with an unknown mechanism of action, has also been shown to be effective in human myoclonus. Piracetam is found to be effective in reducing myoclonus in our animal model (Nguyen et al., 1999). More recently, levetiracetam, an analog of piracetam with remarkable effectiveness in human myoclonus (Genton and Gelisse 2000; Frucht et al., 2001), has also been shown to reduce myoclonus in our animal model (Truong, unpublished data). Based on these results, it appears that the pharmacological profile of our rat model of myoclonus is similar to that of human post-hypoxic myoclonus.

V. UNDERLYING DEFICITS IN GABAERGIC AND SEROTONERGIC ACTIVITY IN POST-HYPOXIC MYOCLONUS

The pharmacological studies may provide some insight into the cause of myoclonus following cerebral hypoxia insults. The mechanism of action of clonazepam is to enhance the activity of γ-aminobutyric acid (GABA), the major inhibitory neurotransmitter in the central nervous system, by increasing the frequency of opening of the $GABA_A$ receptor complex (Puia et al., 1991). Valproate enhances GABA activity by increasing the synthesis and decreasing the catabolism of GABA by inhibiting the enzyme GABA transaminase, which is responsible for intracellular GABA catabolism (Perucca, 2002). Because the mechanism of action of clonazepam and valproate is, in principle, to reduce neuronal activity by enhancing GABA channel activity, these observations suggest that hyperactivity of neuronal circuitry may be the underlying cause of myoclonus.

The neuronal substrate underlying post-hypoxic myoclonus is not currently known. Previous studies showed that the reticular thalamic nuclei (RTN) are a component of the pathway that triggers post-hypoxic myoclonus. In general, the thalamus is a neuronal structure of great importance in both sensory and motor systems. It is a crucial structure for organizing and integrating sensory information. It processes and channels the information to the key cortical areas, where further processing and integration take place.

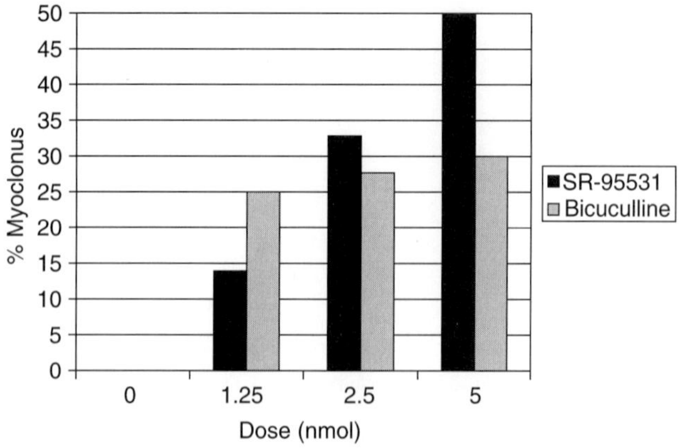

FIGURE 3 $GABA_A$ antagonist bicuculline or SR-95531 dose-dependently elicits spontaneous myoclonus following its microinjection into the lateral ventricles of the rats. (Reprinted from Wiley-Liss, Inc., a subsidiary of John Wiley & Sons, Inc., with permission.) (Matsumoto et al., 2000.)

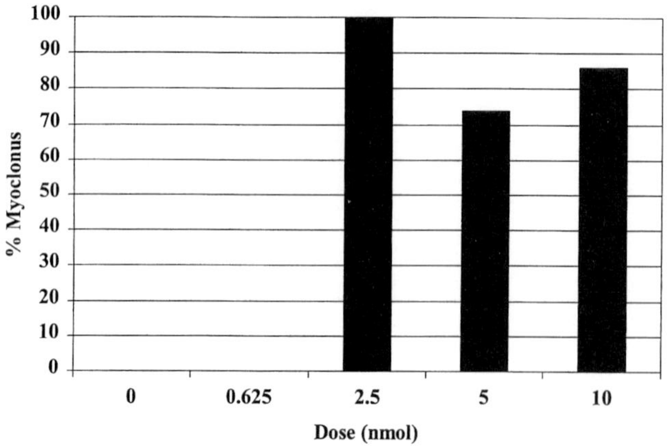

FIGURE 4 Bicuculline induces spontaneous myoclonus in rats following its microinjection into the reticular thalamic nucleus of the rats. (Reprinted from Wiley-Liss, Inc., a subsidiary of John Wiley & Sons, Inc., with permission.) (Matsumoto et al., 2000.)

With the exception of olfactory neuronal signal transmission, no sensory information reaches the cerebral cortex without prior processing in the thalamic nuclei.

Significantly, thalamic nuclei are generally involved in the complex neuroanatomical loops characteristic of motor systems that are associated with the pathways between the cerebellum and cerebral cortex and between the basal ganglia and cerebral cortex. Previous studies have shown that intracerebroventricular administration of the $GABA_A$ antagonists bicuculline or SR-95531 dose-dependently induce spontaneous myoclonus a few minutes following their administration (Figure 3) (Matsumoto et al., 2000). Microinjection of bicuculline into the RTN also elicits spontaneous, rhythmic myoclonus in rats in an apparent all-or-none effect, as bicuculline action on RTN does not occur in a dose-related manner (Figure 4) (Matsumoto et al., 2000). In addition, it has been shown that an increase in the availability of GABA by tiagabine, a GABA uptake inhibitor, can reduce myoclonus (Suzdak and Jansen, 1995; Jaw et al., 1996). Both $GABA_A$ and $GABA_B$ receptors are found in the RTN. Microinjection of phaclofen, a $GABA_B$ antagonist, into the RTN, does not induce spontaneous myoclonus, whereas topical cortical application (Robin et al., 1980a) as well as intracerebral injection of picrotoxin, a $GABA_A$ channel blocker, can elicit myoclonus (Robin et al., 1980b). As a result, it appears that $GABA_A$ but not $GABA_B$ receptors probably play a more pivotal role in the genesis of myoclonus. Taken together, these results indicate that pharmacological interventions that enhance GABAergic transmission at multiple levels along the neural axis of the central nervous system can attenuate post-hypoxic myoclonus, whereas manipulations that decrease GABAergic transmission trigger myoclonus.

It is believed that post-hypoxic myoclonus is a result of hyperactivity of neuronal circuitry in the cortex, cerebellum, and thalamus. More recently, excessive activity of the inferior olive has been shown to trigger myoclonus in the epilepsy-prone rat (Welsh et al., 1998) with a genetic form of myoclonic epilepsy. In an attempt to test this hypothesis in our model, we found that ablation of inferior olive does not attenuate post-hypoxic myoclonus in this rat model of post-hypoxic myoclonus. This suggests that the inferior olive may not be the trigger center for post-hypoxic myoclonus. The results also suggest that the substrate underlying myoclonic epilepsy and post-hypoxic myoclonus may be different and may possibly involve dysfunctions of different neuronal circuitries in the brain.

Using immediate early gene expression as a functional marker for neuronal activity to identify brain nuclei that exhibit hyperactivity, we found Fos immunoreactivity in the RTN in cardiac arrested rats that display myoclonic jerk in response to auditory stimuli (Figure 5). These results further support the notion that RTN plays an important role in the manifestation of post-hypoxic myoclonus. The findings have two possible implications. First, the observed RTN activity could simply signify a natural defense mechanism in response to auditory stimuli, the end result of which is to mitigate the muscle jerks as a result of stimuli. Most RTN neurons are GABAergic, and the Fos expressing neurons are likely to be GABAergic, although this has yet to be demonstrated experimentally. As a result, activation of the presumed GABAergic neurons leads to myoclonic jerks, which are regarded as an excitatory response, implying that the Fos-expressing GABAergic neurons in RTN may relay with another inhibitory center that in turn modulates the excitatory outputs triggering myoclonus. Although the RTN has no direct projections to the cortex, activation of RTN may indicate the involvement of cerebral cortex in the development of myoclonus in this animal model, as it is well documented that evoked cortical activity can still be achieved

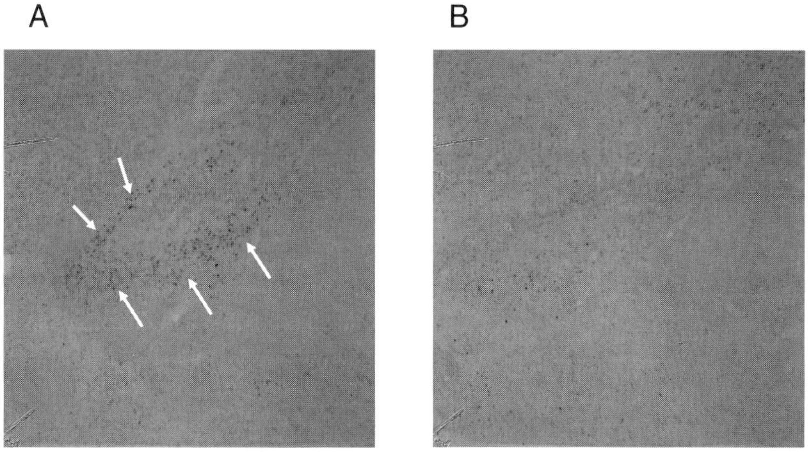

FIGURE 5 Coronal rat brain sections showing Fos immuoreactivity in the reticular thalamic nucleus in (A) rats manifesting myoclonic jerks in response to auditory stimuli following cardiac arrest–induced cerebral hypoxia for 8 minutes but not in control rats (B) which were also exposed to auditory stimuli but did not display myoclonic jerk reaction. The sections for immunohistochemical staining for Fos were visualized using the avidin-biotin peroxidase complex (ABC) method. The sections were incubated with anti-Fos protein antibody (1 : 10,000, Santa Cruz Biotechnology) for 48 hours at 4°C followed by biotinylated goat anti rabbit IgG (1 : 1000, Vector Labs) for 2 hours at room temperature. Then the sections were processed with the DAB nickel method (Vector Labs); the reactions lasted 8 minutes at room temperature.

indirectly with RTN inhibitory projections to some relay nuclei. Further studies are needed to substantiate these postulations.

Another neurotransmitter system of the central nervous system whose dysfunction has been implicated in the pathophysiology of post-hypoxic myoclonus is serotonin or 5-HT (Chadwick et al., 1977). Previous clinical study showed that 5-hydroxytryptophan (5-HTP), a precursor of 5-HT, shows therapeutic effectiveness in some myoclonus patients (De Lean et al., 1976). Concomitantly, the level of 5-HIAA, a 5-HT metabolite, in the cerebrospinal fluid of patients with post-hypoxic myoclonus, is lower than that of controls (De Lean et al., 1976). The improvement in myoclonus symptoms following 5-hydroxytryptophan treatment is associated with a significant elevation in the cerebrospinal fluid of 5-HIAA. These observations led to the hypothesis that functional deficiencies in the serotonergic transmission contribute to the manifestation of post-hypoxic myoclonus (Chadwick et al., 1977)

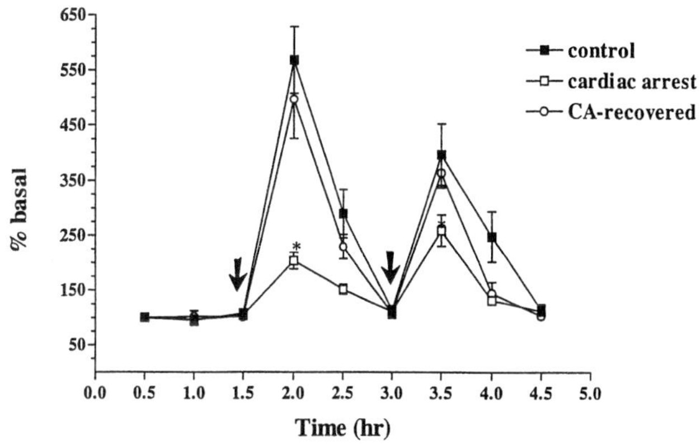

FIGURE 6 The dynamics of serotonin release in the rat model of post-hypoxic myoclonus. Microdialysis sampling performed in the frontal cortex. Both the basal and the stimulated levels of serotonin were collected at 30-min intervals. The arrows indicate KCl (100 mM) and NMDA (500 μM) stimulation. Values are mean ± SEM of 5 animals, *represents $p \leq 0.05$. (Reprinted from Wiley-Liss, Inc., a subsidiary of John Wiley & Sons, Inc., with permission.) (Kanthasamy et al., 2000.)

Myoclonus in our model can also be attenuated following the administration of 5-HTP (Figure 2) (Matsumoto et al., 1995a; Kanthasamy et al., 1995–1996). To evaluate the neurochemical dynamics of the serotonergic system in this animal model, extracellular release of serotonin and its metabolites was determined using *in vivo* microdialysis. Both basal and stimulated release of 5-HT and 5-HIAA were evaluated in the prefrontal cortex of the animal. The basal levels of 5-HT release among the control, post-hypoxic, and post-hypoxic recovered rats are similar. However, a significant reduction in KCl- and NMDA-stimulated release of 5-HT was observed between the control and the post-hypoxic animals (Figure 6). In addition, there exists an inverse relationship between the severity audiogenic myoclonus and the evoked striatal 5-HT release (Figure 7) as well as cortical 5-HIAA levels (Matsumoto et al., 1995b). These results indicate that a significant reduction in serotonergic neuronal

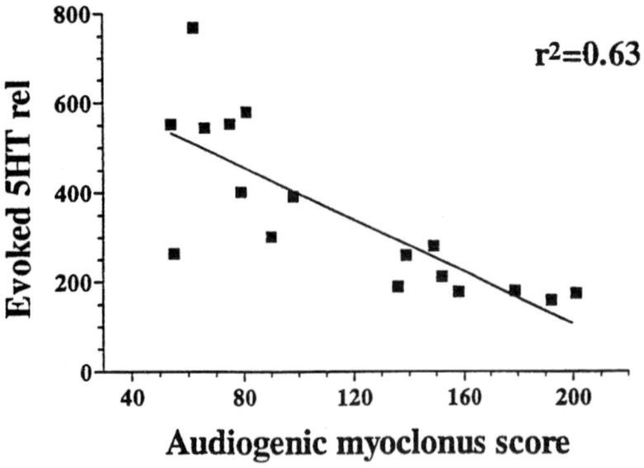

FIGURE 7 The relationship between 5-HT release and the audiogenic myoclonus activity. An inverse correlation was obtained when evoked 5-HT levels were plotted as a function of myoclonus score. (Reprinted from Wiley-Liss, Inc., a subsidiary of John Wiley & Sons, Inc., with permission.) (Kanthasamy et al., 2000.)

activity as a result of cardiac arrest-induced cerebral hypoxic insults.

Additional evidence to support the role of 5-HT in this rat model of post-hypoxic myoclonus comes from study with the use of serotonergic ligands. If serotonergic hypofunction is one of the underlying causes of myoclonus, the severity of myoclonus should be relieved by activating 5-HT receptors with 5-HT agonists. Previous study from our laboratory also showed that the audiogenic post-hypoxic myoclonus in this model can be attenuated with the administration of 5-HT-2 agonists and 5-HT-3 agonists, but not 5-HT-1A agonists (Matsumoto et al., 1995a), indicating that 5-HT-2 and 5-HT-3 but not 5-HT-1 receptors are involved in the development of post-hypoxic myoclonus. However, dysfunction of the 5-HT system underlying post-hypoxic myoclonus is still contradictory. Studies by others have shown that mesulergine, a 5-HT-2 receptor blocker, and methiothepin, a 5-HT-1 and 5-HT-2 receptor blocker, dose-dependently reduced post-hypoxic myoclonus in the rat (Pappert et al., 1999). In addition, immunostaining to evaluate the level of serotonin in brain sections from normal and post-hypoxic rats reveals no significant difference between them (Welsh et al., 2002). Results from these studies argue against the role of 5-HT in the pathophysiology of post-hypoxic myoclonus. Further studies are needed to resolve the discrepancies.

VI. NEURODEGENERATION REVEALED BY HISTOLOGY STUDIES

Autopsy in post-hypoxic myoclonus patients does not reveal significant lesions in the midline structure of the brain stem, where most serotonergic structures are located. This, together with the fact that myoclonic symptoms show improvement over time, suggests that post-hypoxic myoclonus is unlikely a progressive neurological condition that involves permanent structural damage of the brain. Instead, it is more likely associated with dysfunctions of certain neuroanatomical structures. Because the malfunctions of these circuitries result from hypoxia-induced injury, if this animal faithfully mimics cerebral hypoxia in humans, there should be some similarities in the brain structures that show injuries in this model compared with human cases. Studies using computerized tomography imaging showed both diffuse cortical and subcortical damage as well as myoclonic jerking movements in patients who had suffered severe cerebral hypoxia.

Histological studies have been performed in this animal model. Using Nissl staining and Fluoro-Jade histochemistry, a profound neuronal degeneration in the motor cortex and the primary and secondary somatosensory cortices of both hemispheres was found. Extensive neurodegeneration was also found in the thalamic reticular nucleus and in the hippocampus, including the CA1, CA2, and CA3 regions in rats with 8-minute, but not 4-minute, cardiac arrest. In addition, a severe loss of the Purkinje neurons in the cerebellum was also observed. Using monoclonal antibody targeting EAAC-1, the presynaptic neuronal glutamate transporter, in rat cerebellar brain sections, revealed a profound loss of the EAAC-1 expression in Purkinje cell layer of the cerebellum in 8-minute hypoxic rats (Truong et al., 2002). This indicates an impairment of function in the regions involved in motor coordination in this animal model of movement disorder.

VII. CONCLUSIONS

The rat model of post-hypoxic myoclonus presented in this chapter recapitulates a number of behavioral, pharmacological, and neuroanatomical features in patients who develop post-hypoxic myoclonus. As a result, this animal model will be of great value in identifying the neuroanatomical substrate underlying the manifestation of this syndrome in humans. In addition, the model is an invaluable tool for the evaluation of therapeutic efficacies of novel agents for the treatment of post-hypoxic myoclonus.

Acknowledgment

We thank Mary Ann Chapman for editorial assistance.

Video Legends

SEGMENT 1 Early period after cardiac arrest. In the first two days after cardiac arrest, rats exhibit seizure activity that may include both generalized and partial seizures. Partial seizures are typically preceded by a short period of running. "Running seizures" can be intense in the first two days after cardiac arrest. Myoclonic jerks in response to auditory stimuli can occur while the rat is experiencing a partial seizure. Two days after the cardiac arrest, seizures decline gradually whereas the myoclonic jerks persist.

SEGMENT 2 Late period after cardiac arrest. Myoclonic jerks in response to auditory stimuli.

References

Chadwick, D., M. Hallett, R. Harris, P. Jenner, E.H. Reynolds, and C.D. Marsden. 1977. Clinical, biochemical, and physiological features distinguishing myoclonus responsive to 5-hydroxytryptophan, tryptophan with a monoamine oxidase inhibitor, and clonazepam. *Brain* **100(3)**: 455–487.

Chung, E., and M.H. Van Woert. 1984. DDT myoclonus: sites and mechanism of action. *Exp Neurol* **85(2)**:273–282.

De Lean, J., J.C. Richardson, and O. Hornykiewicz. 1976. Beneficial effects of serotonin precursors in postanoxic action myoclonus. *Neurology* **26(9)**:863–868.

Fahn, S. 1978. Post-anoxic action myoclonus: improvement with valproic acid. *N Engl J Med* **299(6)**:313–314.

Fahn, S. 1986. Posthypoxic action myoclonus: literature review update. *Adv Neurol* **43**:157–169.

Frucht, S.J., E.D. Louis, C. Chuang, and S. Fahn. 2001. A pilot tolerability and efficacy study of levetiracetam in patients with chronic myoclonus. *Neurology* **57(6)**:1112–1114.

Genton, P, and P. Gelisse, 2000. Antimyoclonic effect of levetiracetam. *Epileptic Disord* **2(4)**:209–212.

Jaw, S.P., B. Nguyen, Q.T. Vuong, T.A. Trinh, M. Nguyen, and D.D. Truong. 1996. Effects of GABA uptake inhibitors on posthypoxic myoclonus in rats. Brain *Res Bull* **39(3)**:189–192.

Kanthasamy, A.G., R.R. Matsumoto, and D.D. Truong. 1995–96. Animal models of myoclonus. *Clin Neurosci* **3(4)**:236–245.

Kanthasamy, A.G., B.Q. Nguyen, and D.D. Truong. 2000. Animal model of posthypoxic myoclonus: II. Neurochemical, pathologic, and pharmacologic characterization. *Mov Disord* 15 Suppl **1**:31–38.

Kawai, K., L.P. Penix, N. Kawahara, C.A. Ruetzler, and I. Klatzo. 1995. Development of susceptibility to audiogenic seizures following cardiac arrest cerebral ischemia in rats. *J Cereb Blood Flow Metab* **15(2)**: 248–258.

Lance, J.W., and R.D. Adams. 1963. The syndrome of intention or action myoclonus as a sequel to hypoxic encephalopathy. *Brain* **86**:111–136.

Matsumoto, R.R., M.J. Hussong, and D.D. Truong. 1995a. Effects of selective serotonergic ligands on posthypoxic audiogenic myoclonus. *Mov Disord* **10(5)**:615–621.

Matsumoto, R.R., N. Aziz, and D.D. Truong. 1995b. Association between brain indole levels and severity of posthypoxic myoclonus in rats. *Pharmacol Biochem Behav* **50(4)**:533–538.

Matsumoto, R.R., D.D. Truong, K.D. Nguyen, A.T. Dang, T.T. Hoang, P.Q. Vo, and P. Sandroni. 2000. Involvement of GABA(A) receptors in myoclonus. *Mov Disord* 15(Suppl **1**):47–52.

Muscatt, S., J. Rothwell, J. Obeso, N. Leigh, P. Jenner, and C.D. Marsden. 1986. Urea-induced stimulus-sensitive myoclonus in the rat. *Adv Neurol* **43**:553–563.

Nguyen, B.Q., A.G. Kanthasamy, and D.D. Truong. 1999. Antimyoclonic effect of piracetam animal model of posthypoxic myoclonus. [Abstract] *Soc Neurosci* **25**:2052.

Pappert, E.J., C.G. Goetz, T.Q. Vu, Z.D. Ling, S. Leurgans, R. Raman, and P.M. Carvey. 1999. Animal model of post-hypoxic myoclonus: effects of serotonergic antagonists. *Neurology* **52**:16–21.

Perucca, E. 2002. Pharmacological and therapeutic properties of valproate: a summary after 35 years of clinical experience. *CNS Drugs* **16(10)**: 695–714.

Puia, G., S. Vicini, P.H. Seeburg, and E. Costa. 1991. Influence of recombinant gamma-aminobutyric acid-A receptor subunit composition on the action of allosteric modulators of gamma-aminobutyric acid-gated Cl-currents. *Mol Pharmacol* **39(6)**:691–696.

Robin, M.M., M.G. Palfreyman, M.M. Zraika, and P.J. Schechter. 1980a. Mapping of dyskinetic movements induced by local application of picrotoxin or (+)-gamma-acetylenic GABA on the rat motor cortex. *Eur J Pharmacol* **65(4)**:411–415.

Robin, M.M., M.G. Palfreyman, M.M. Zraika, and P.J. Schechter. 1980b. An analysis of the cortical and striatal involvement in dyskinesia induced in rats by intracerebral injection of GABA-transaminase inhibitors and picrotoxin. *Eur J Pharmacol* **62(4)**:319–327.

Suzdak, P.D., and J.A. Jansen. 1995. A review of the preclinical pharmacology of tiagabine: a potent and selective anticonvulsant GABA uptake inhibitor. *Epilepsia* **36(6)**:612–626.

Truong, D.D., A. Kanthasamy, B. Nguyen, R. Matsumoto, and P. Schwartz. 2000. Animal models of posthypoxic myoclonus: I. Development and validation. *Mov Disord* 15 Suppl **1**:26–30.

Truong, D.D., M. Kirby, A. Kanthasamy, and R.R. Matsumoto. 2002. Posthypoxic myoclonus animal models. *Adv Neurol* **89**:295–306.

Truong, D.D., R.R. Matsumoto, P.H. Schwartz, M.J. Hussong, and C.G. Wasterlain. 1994. Novel rat cardiac arrest model of posthypoxic myoclonus. *Mov Disord* **9(2)**:201–206.

Welsh, J.P., B. Chang, M.E. Menaker, and S.A. Aicher. 1998. Removal of the inferior olive abolishes myoclonic seizures associated with a loss of olivary serotonin. *Neuroscience* **82(3)**:879–897.

Welsh, J.P., D.G. Placantonakis, S.I. Warsetsky, R.G. Marquez, L. Bernstein, and S.A. Aicher. 2002. The serotonin hypothesis of myoclonus from the perspective of neuronal rhythmicity. *Adv Neurol* **89**:307–329.

Werhahn, K.J., P. Brown, P.D. Thompson, and C.D. Marsden. 1997. The clinical features and prognosis of chronic posthypoxic myoclonus. *Mov Disord* **12(2)**:216–220.

CHAPTER

F3

Baboon Model of Myoclonus

CARMEN SILVA-BARRAT and ROBERT NAQUET

Some predisposed *Papio papio* baboons may naturally present the following different types of myoclonia: myoclonia induced by movement and myoclonia induced by intermittent light stimulation.

Myoclonia induced by movement (MIM) is symmetrical and synchronous; its appearance is facilitated by active movements of the animals or by proprioceptive stimulations such as those caused by pressure on the sternum or by tension applied to a limb. Resembling a startle response, it is considered "non-epileptic" because of the absence of any abnormal electrocorticographic discharge.

Myoclonia induced by intermittent light stimulation (ILSM) is also symmetrical and synchronous; this myoclonia is always associated with electrocorticographic paroxysmal discharges, therefore it is considered "epileptic."

Pharmacological and electrophysiological data in animals and humans suggest that MIM has a brain stem origin. MIM is an important model with which to study *Papio papio* "movement disorders" and their relationship with "epilepsy."

I. BACKGROUND

Myoclonia induced by intermittent light stimulation (ILSM) in *Papio papio* baboons was discovered by Killam et al. (1966). It starts in the eyelids; it is followed by generalized myoclonus and eventually by a grand mal seizure. It is preceded by EEG paroxysmal discharges starting in fronto-rolandic areas (Fig. 1). The symptoms are analogous to those described in human photosensitive epilepsy, which is considered an "epileptic myoclonus." For this reason *Papio papio* was considered a good model with which to study ILS reflex epilepsy (Killam et al., 1967).

Myoclonia induced by movement or agitation (movement-induced myoclonus: MIM) never involves the face and predominates in the trunk. It is never preceded nor accompanied by EEG paroxysmal discharges (Fig. 1), and it never evolves into seizures. MIM was considered "non-epileptic" since it was not accompanied by EEG paroxysmal discharges. The structure generating them was not exactly determined, but numerous indirect arguments indicated that their most probable origin was in the lower brain stem. Such MIM symptoms resemble the one observed in human "movement disorders" (Guerrini et al., 2002) and appear as an exaggerated startle response corresponding to that named myoclonic jerks ("secousses myocloniques") (Gastaut, 1968). They also resemble "action myoclonus" (Lance and Adams, 1963) and "reticular reflex myoclonus" (Hallett et al., 1977).

Both ILSM and MIM are independent of each other and, on the basis of their symptomatology, are considered

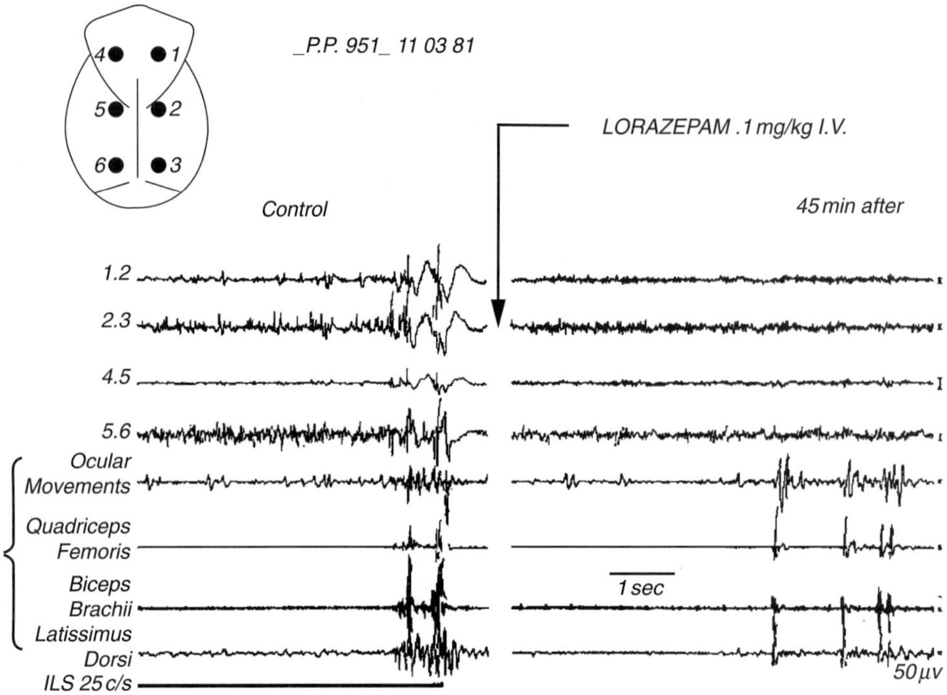

FIGURE 1 Effects of lorazepam on a photosensitive *Papio papio*. Before the injection of lorazepam (*left*), ILS induces epileptic myoclonus preceded by a paroxysmal discharge. The injection of lorazepam blocks epileptic myoclonus but induces the appearance of spontaneous myoclonus (*right*); this myoclonus may persist for 2 hr and is not accompanied by any EEG paroxysmal discharge.

different in their physiopathological origin. However, they may appear associated in the same wild animal or independently in other animals. Interestingly, all *Papio papio* show, at rest, in fronto-rolandic areas some isolated symmetrical or asymmetrical spike and waves frequently low in amplitude, considered in humans a sign of predisposition to "generalized epilepsy." The MIM characteristics of the *Papio papio* baboon will now be discussed.

II. CHARACTERSTICS OF MYOCLONUS INDUCED BY MOVEMENT

MIM may be present in baboons in the following three different situations.

1. Spontaneous MIM was first mentioned in a young non-photosensitive *Papio papio* captured during a mission in Senegal (Brailowsky et al., 1978). In fact, MIM exists in several *Papio papio* baboons, photosensitive or not, belonging to a group in which in general there exists a high predisposition to epilepsy.

2. Spontaneous MIM was also observed in animals in which the cerebellar vermis had been ablated to explore the possible effects of such lesions in photosensitive *Papio papio* (Brailowsky et al., 1978). The vermis ablation does not modify the degree of photosensitivity of the animals, but induced atonia and postural disturbances last for 2 to 3 weeks and then disappear. The MIM appeared from days to weeks after surgery and persisted throughout the survival time of the animal. It was violent, frequent, isolated, and induced by minimal movement or contact. Jerks were symmetrical and synchronous, mainly involving the truncular musculature and resembling a startle response. They were facilitated by active movements of the animals or by proprioceptive stimulations such as those caused by pressure on the sternum or by tension applied to a limb. After some proprioceptive stimulations, they appeared in long bursts similar to those described in hyperexplexia in children (Dalla Bernardina et al., 1989). In contrast, they disappeared completely when the animal was motionless or in the first stages of sleep.

3. MIM appearance is also favored by a benzodiazepine (BZ) injection (Fig. 2), which blocks ILSM (Cepeda et al., 1982; Valin et al., 1981, 1983; Naquet et al., 1985, Meldrum, 1986). Thus, during the first 10 to 20 min after the injection of diazepam or lorazepam, ILSM or movements do not induce myoclonus. Progressively ILSM comes back to its preexisting level; at the same time, MIM appears (Fig. 2). BZ-induced myoclonia increases in frequency and reaches

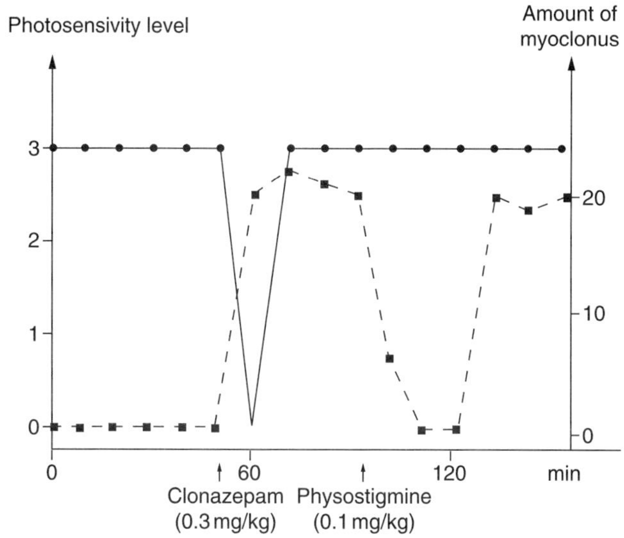

FIGURE 2 Differential reactivity of the epileptic, photic stimulation–induced myoclonus and the non-epileptic, movement-induced myoclonus in a photosensitive baboon. Ordinate (*left*): photosensitivity level: 1 = myoclonus of the eyelids; 2 = facial myoclonus; 3 = generalized myoclonus. Ordinate (*right*), amount of movement-induced myoclonus counted by 10-min. epochs (abscissa), from the EEG records. Clonazepam temporarily blocks the photic stimulation–induced myoclonus (*dots*) and facilitates the appearance of the non-epileptic myoclonus (*squares*), the two phenomena having different timings. Later, physostigmine makes the non-epileptic myoclonus disappear temporarily but has no action on the epileptic myoclonus.

a maximum, generally 5 hr later. Reaching this maximum, its frequency diminishes progressively during the following hours. BZ-induced myoclonus is never preceded or accompanied by any signs of EEG paroxysmal discharges and never evolves into seizures.

The facility to produce MIM (spontaneous or secondarily induced by cerebellectomy or BZ) seems to be the sign of a naturally greater or lesser predisposition of the *Papio papio* (Menini and Naquet, 1986; Rektor et al., 1986).

Electromyographic recordings have shown that MIM corresponds to brief contractions of the concerned muscles, lasting 30 ms on average, and occurring bilaterally and symmetrically. The trapezius is one of the first muscles involved in MIM. MIM was never preceded nor accompanied by any sign of EEG paroxysmal activity in all the recorded cortical structures. By using the back-averaging technique, any low-voltage signal preceding the jerk was detected, and only a somatic-evoked potential occurring in the fronto-parietal cortex 10 to 15 ms after the beginning of the myoclonic jerk was detected. Numerous subcortical structures from the thalamus to the brain stem were also recorded without any success (Rektor et al., 1993).

When comparing ILSM and MIM, it seems that the two types of myoclonus do not involve the same circuits. ILSM could involve cortical "epileptic" circuits, whereas MIM could involve "hyperexcitable" brainstem circuits. Based on these data, in the 1980s the first was called "epileptic myoclonus" and the second "non-epileptic myoclonus" (Menini and Naquet, 1986). However, differences between them need to be analyzed again.

ILSM and MIM may coexist in the same wild animal, presenting EEG paroxysmal discharges. In man, the presence of such discharges is considered a predisposition to epilepsy.

ILSM was considered the consequence of only hyperexcitable cortical circuits. It starts by myoclonus of the eyelids and progresses from there to the face, neck, and arms and may become generalized. If fronto-rolandic paroxysmal discharges precede any ILSM apparition, electrical stimulation of such cortical area never induces, at first, any eyelid myoclonus. In addition, ILSM progression evokes the possibility that the visual brainstem circuits, under control of cortical areas, play a role in their induction and progression (Naquet and Batini, 2002).

ILSM localized in the neck may be obtained in the chimera chicken after the graft of the mesencephalon of an embryonic photosensitive Fayoumi chicken (Fépi). Such mesencephalic ILSM never evolves into seizures. After a graft of the prosencephalon associated with mesencephalon, the animal presents the full spectrum of Fépi seizure. It has to be noted that audiogenic and photosensitive Fépi generalized seizures as well as rodent audiogenic seizures are never accompanied by EEG paroxysmal discharge during the fit (Batini et al., 1996; Avoli et al., 1990).

MIM induced after vermisectomy may be compared to the myoclonus induced by movement in human patients who present degenerative cerebellar syndromes generally associated with photosensitive epilepsy (Bradshaw, 1954).

III. PHARMACOLOGICAL REACTIVITY OF THE *PAPIO PAPIO* BABOON MYOCLONUS

Pharmacological study of the MIM raises the following interesting questions, which are not resolved at this time.

It was already noticed that BZ favored the apparition of MIM with a certain time lapse after its injection (10 to 20 min) and that it is durable and increases progressively during 3 to 5 hr (Valin et al., 1981). This effect was considered a BZ direct effect on MIM, as opposed to the antiepileptic effect on ILSM, which was brief and immediate. Moreover, an injection of Ro15-1788 (Valin et al., 1983), a specific antagonist of BZ receptors, progressively abolished BZ-induced MIM, but not spontaneous MIM.

Concerning the involvement of the GABAergic system on MIM, it was demonstrated that an epileptic GABA withdrawal syndrome appearing as rhythmic spikes appears in photosensitive or non-photosensitive baboons after withdrawal of chronic GABA infusion in the motor cortex

(Brailowsky et al., 1989). With this observation in mind, one is tempted to suggest that BZ-induced MIM is the expression of a rebound of brainstem hyperexcitability following cessation of BZ action. Nevertheless, even though BZ acts on GABA receptors, MIM is not fully GABA-mediated, since drugs acting directly on GABA receptors have no effect on them (Rektor et al., 1991). Therefore, results obtained with Ro-15-1788 may contradict the hypothesis of such a rebound effect in MIM induction.

The cholinergic system is involved in MIM generation. BZ-facilitating action was interpreted as the result of its indirect action on the cholinergic system (Rektor et al., 1986), given that BZ-induced MIM is blocked by physostigmine (Fig. 2), a substance that blocks acetylcholine esterase and increases the cerebral level of acetylcholine, but is potentiated by atropine (Rektor et al., 1984), an anticholinergic drug.

In addition, in most baboons, atropine alone (1 to 3 min after the injection) facilitates the appearance of MIM, which lasts several hours. Atropine-induced MIM, like BZ-induced MIM, is suppressed by physostigmine and is similar to that observed in *Papio papio* that have been vermisectomized or have had BZ administered to them. Whereas quinuclidinyl benzylate, a specific antagonist of central muscarinic receptors, induced MIM, this was not the case for methylquinuclidinyl benzylate, a methylated derivative that does not cross the blood-brain barrier and acts only on peripheral receptors. Interestingly, physostigmine blocks atropine-induced MIM, but at doses four times higher than those necessary to block BZ-induced MIM. These observations are in accordance with data in the literature, suggesting an interaction between BZ and the cholinergic system. Physostigmine is utilized for the treatment of BZ intoxications (Vogel, 1977), and BZ is part of the therapy against intoxication by organophosphates (Rump and Faff, 1976). Finally, other neurotransmitter systems such as noradrenergic and dopaminergic systems may influence MIM, although inconsistently (Rektor et al., 1989, 1991).

The complementary role played by drugs acting on acetylcholine or BZ receptors revealed by pharmacological studies confirms their importance to MIM production. However, they do not yet fully explain their mechanism of action on MIM induction or facilitation. Recently, it was observed that an epileptic midazolam withdrawal syndrome similar to the GABA withdrawal syndrome described in baboons could be provoked in rats after the interruption of a chronic midazolam treatment. This withdrawal syndrome was not blocked by cholinergic drugs, so it seems that the rhythmic spikes in the withdrawal syndrome provoked by GABAergic drugs are not under control of the cholinergic system. These results are in accordance with the involvement of different neuronal circuits for MIM and ILSM.

IV. ORIGIN OF MOVEMENT-INDUCED MYOCLONIA

The origin of *Papio papio* MIM remains unknown, but a cortical origin is unlikely for several reasons. First, MIM is never accompanied by any cortical EEG paroxysmal discharge. Second, in predisposed *Papio papio* baboons, no correlation exists between MIM and spontaneous or ILS-induced paroxysmal fronto-rolandic discharges (Menini and Naquet, 1986). Third, BZ action on ILSM and MIM is not time-locked. MIM starts almost at the same moment that ILSM stops, one facilitated by BZ and the other not (Fig. 1). Fourth, subcortical recordings suggest a brainstem origin although the precise locus has not been identified. Fifth, MIM facilitation after vermis ablation favors the hypothesis that this myoclonia originates in the low brain stem, and more probably in networks including the reticular formation (Rektor et al., 1993), as also suggested for the myoclonus observed in macaque monkeys after bilateral hemispherectomy (Denny-Brown, 1968).

The brainstem hypothesis is in accordance with MIM clinical characteristics, which concern the proximal musculature: the proximal musculature is mainly involved during activation of the reticulo-spinal motor system, whereas distal musculature is mainly involved during activation of the pyramidal system. Moreover, this hypothesis is in accordance with the presence, in the lower brain stem, of reflex centers responsible for the spino-bulbo-spinal reflexes observed in cats and monkeys under chloralose (Shimamura and Livingston, 1963; Shimamura et al., 1964), which can constitute the functional substrate responsible for MIM. Finally, this hypothesis is not in contradiction with the involvement of the different locations of receptors and networks involved in *Papio papio* MIM.

BZ receptors predominate in the *Papio papio* neocortex and are very important in the cerebellum (Mohler and Okada, 1977; Squires and Braestrup, 1977; Squires et al., 1979; Comar et al., 1979).

Several cholinergic neuronal populations have been described in the brain stem of *Papio papio* by using immunocytochemical techniques (Riche et al., 1987), implying the importance of the cholinergic system in this region.

In other species, it has been demonstrated that muscarinic receptors at this level present a very high affinity for ligands such as atropine or quinuclidinyl benzylate (Dawson and Poretski, 1983). In rodents, a myoclonus not associated with cortical paroxysmal discharges can be induced by 5HTP, a serotonin precursor, and transitorily blocked by methysergide, a serotonergic antagonist (Luscombe et al., 1982). The origin of this myoclonus is probably in the brain stem, where most of the serotonergic neurons are located. In the *Papio papio* the serotonergic system does not play an important role in MIM since it is neither suppressed nor facilitated by methysergide (Valin et al., 1983).

V. POSSIBLE MECHANISMS INVOLVED IN *PAPIO PAPIO* MYOCLONUS

The question as to whether or not *Papio papio* ILSM and MIM are linked remains open. Of 106 baboons tested for this purpose, 41 (39%) presented with ILSM, of which six also displayed MIM. Of the remaining 65 baboons, four had MIM (our unpublished observations). Statistical analysis of these data indicated that the two types of myoclonus are independent of each other. It is thus probable that brainstem dysfunction, even if it may be suspected in both cases, could implicate different circuits responsible for the two different types of myoclonus.

Hypotheses regarding the mechanisms involved in ILSM and MIM can be summarized as follows.

ILSM close to human photosensitive epilepsy has a cortical origin. Paroxysmal discharges that generate ILSM are located in the deep layers of the fronto-rolandic cortex (Silva-Barrat et al., 1988), where the pyramidal efferents originate. The neurochemical mechanisms at their origin involve GABAergic neurotransmission. Lloyd et al. (1986) have shown an inverse correlation between GABA levels in CSF and photosensitivity, and Brailowsky et al. (1989) showed that increasing GABA levels at the visual or fronto-rolandic cortices blocks ILS-induced EEG paroxysmal discharge and ILSM.

However, under the ILS effects, the following has been found.

In humans, induced myoclonus of the eyelids without any EEG paroxysmal discharge has been observed in some non-epileptic subjects. This myoclonia was considered as originating in the brain stem (Gastaut, 1973; Naquet and Poncet-Ramade, 1982).

In the chicken, neck myoclonia was induced in mesencephalic chimera with only an "epileptic" brain stem (Batini et al., 1996).

In photosensitive *Papio papio*, the start of myoclonus does not correspond to the region where the maximal amplitude and frequency of EEG paroxysmal discharges are observed (Menini and Naquet, 1986). An explanation would be that there is a circuit going from the fronto-rolandic cortex to the nuclei of the brainstem eyelid region (Naquet and Batini, 1996).

In the *Papio papio* baboon, electrical stimulation of this region of the fronto-rolandic area never induces eyelid myoclonus. Thus, it was proposed that, through EEG paroxysmal discharges, circuits starting in the fronto-rolandic area permit the start of ILSM in the high brain stem.

Papio papio MIM seems, as discussed above, to be different from *Papio papio* ILSM. Precisely, MIM is generated subcortically without cortical induction, and it occurs in the absence of any cortical or deep paroxysmal electrical phenomena. Denny-Brown (1968) proposed that the critical area for the generation of myoclonus is localized in the lower brain stem, but under control of the cortex and the thalamus. Regarding the role of the cerebellum in *Papio papio* MIM, vermis ablation has a facilitatory effect (Brailowsky et al., 1978), with no effects of such lesions on natural photosensitivity (Brailowsky et al., 1975). In humans, a cerebellar syndrome often includes ataxia, tremor, and intention myoclonus. From this evidence it can be suggested that the cerebellum has an inhibitory action on brainstem myoclonus.

In summary, after analysis of the symptoms and mechanisms at the origin of the different types of myoclonus presented by the *Papio papio*, the following conclusions can be suggested: MIM appears as a consequence of an inherited functional abnormality of the cholinergic system, given that a brainstem muscarinic dysfunction renders them extremely sensitive to muscarinic blockade, whereas ILSM appears as a consequence of an inherited functional abnormality of the GABAergic system (but not the cholinergic system) (Meldrum et al., 1970), which renders them very sensitive to any alteration. Nevertheless, both MIM and ILSM are very sensitive to dysfunction of BZ receptors and appear in animals predisposed to epilepsy.

These data raised many questions: MIM and ILSM—are they or are they not so different? Is one epileptic and the other not? Is one dependent on dysfunction of one neurotransmitter system and the other on another neurotransmitter system? We do not know yet, but their expression seems to predominate at the cortical or brainstem level. So, genetic research is needed for further comprehension of both pathologies.

VI. CONCLUSIONS

The *Papio papio* movement-induced myoclonus may result from a natural abnormality of some muscarinic receptors on neurons situated in a cerebral region until now undetermined but most probably situated in the lower brain stem. The exact nature of these myoclonia can be questioned. Even if they were named "non-epileptic" because they are never accompanied by EEG paroxysmal discharges and because the cerebral neocortex seems to play only a secondary role in their mechanisms, their characteristics are also observed in other well-known experimental models, from the chicken to rodents, presenting seizures without EEG paroxysmal discharges (Avoli et al., 1990; Malafosse et al., 1994). It is known that the ability to develop epileptiform discharges in the absence of convulsant drugs results from the intrinsic organization of the neuronal network in some structures, such as the neocortex or hippocampus. In these models, the absence of paroxysmal discharges could result from neuronal networks of the structures, involving particularly the reticular formation, but different from cortical neuronal networks.

References

Avoli, M., P. Gloor, K. Kostopoulos, and R. Naquet. 1990. In: *Generalized Epilepsy, Neurological Approaches.* Birkhäuser Eds. 481pp.

Batini, C., M.A. Teillet, R. Naquet, and N.M. Le Douarin. 1996. Brain chimeras in birds: application to the study of a genetic form of reflex epilepsy. *TINS* **19**:246–252.

Bradshaw, J. 1954. A study of myoclonus. *Brain* **77**:138–157.

Brailowsky, S., C. Menini, and R. Naquet. 1978. Myoclonus developing after vermisectomy in photosensitive Papio papio. *Electroenceph Clin Neurophysiol* **45**:82–89.

Brailowsky, S., C. Silva-Barrat, C. Menini, D. Riche, and R. Naquet. 1989. Effects of localized, chronic GABA infusions into different cortical areas of the photosensitive baboon Papio papio. *Electroenceph clin Neurophysiol* **72**:147–156.

Brailowsky, S., S. Walter, L. Larochelle, and R. Naquet. 1975. Cervelet et épilepsie photosensible chez le Papio papio: effets des lésions cérébelleuses sur la photosensibilité et les potentiels évoqués visuels. *Rev EEG Neurophysiol* **5**:247–251.

Cepeda, C., A. Valin, L. Calderazzo, J.M. Stutzmann, and R. Naquet. 1982. Myoclonies induites par certaines benzodiazépines chez le Papio papio. Comparaison avec les myoclonies induites par la stimulation lumineuse intermittente. *Rev EEG Neurophysiol* **12**:32–37.

Comar, D., M. Mazière, J.M. Godot, G. Berger, F. Soussaline, G. Menini, C. Arfel, and R. Naquet. 1979. Visualization of 11C-Flunitazepam displacement in the brain of the live baboon. *Nature (London)* **280**: 329–331.

Dalla Bernardina, B., E. Fontana, V. Colamaria, L. La Selva, D. Merlin, V. Sgro, and P. Scarpa. 1989. Neonatal Hyperexplexia. In: *Reflex seizures and reflex epilepsies.* A. Beaumanoir, H. Gastaut, and R. Naquet, eds. pp. 408–418.

Dawson, R.M., and M.A. Poretski. 1983. Comparision of the muscarinic cholinoreceptors and benzodiazepine receptors of guinea-pig brain and rat brain. *Neurochem Internat* **5**:369–374.

Denny-Brown, D. 1968. Quelques aspects physiologiques des myoclonies. *Rev Neurol (Paris)* **119**:121–129.

Gastaut, H. 1968. Séméiologie des myoclonies et nosologie analytique des syndromes myocloniques. *Rev Neurol* **119**:1–30

Gastaut, H. 1973. *Dictionnaire de l'Epilepsie. OMS.* Genève, 80p.

Guerrini, R., J. Aicardi, F. Andermann, and M. Hallett, eds. 2002. *Epilepsy and Movement Disorders.* Cambridge University Press.

Hallett, M., D. Chadwick, J. Adam, and C.D. Marsden. 1977. Reticular myoclonus: a physiological type of human post-hypoxic myoclonus. *J Neurol Neurosurg Psychiatr* **40**:253–264.

Killam, K.F., E.K. Killam, and R. Naquet. 1966. Mise en évidence chez certains singes d'un syndrome myoclonique, C.R. *Acad Sci (Paris)* **262**:1010–1012.

Killam, K.F., E.K. Killam, and R. Naquet. 1967. An animal model of light sensitive epilepsy. *Electroenceph clin Neurophysiol* **22**:497–513.

Lance, J.W., and R.D. Adams. 1963. The syndrome of intention or action myoclonus as a sequel to hypoxic encephalopathy. *Brain* **86**:11–136.

Lloyd, K.G., B. Scatton, C. Voltz, P. Bryere, A. Valin, and R. Naquet. 1986. Cerebrospinal fluid amino acid and monoamine metabolite levels of Papio papio: Correlation with photosensitivity. *Brain Res* **363**:390–394.

Luscombe, G., P. Jenner, and C.D. Marsden. 1982. Myoclonus in guinea pigs is induced by indole-containing but not piperazine-containing 5HT agonists. *Life Sci* **30**:1487–1494.

Malafosse, A., P. Genton, E. Hirsch, C. Marescaux, D. Broglin, and R. Bernasconi. 1994. In: *Idiopathic Generalized Epilepsies: Clinical, Experimental and Genetic Aspects.* John Libbey and Company Ltd.

Meldrum, B.S. 1986. Drugs Acting on Amino Acid Neurotransmitters. In *Advances in Neurology. Myoclonus.* Fahn, S., Marsden, C.D., and Van Woert, M. (Eds). Raven Press **43**:730pp.

Meldrum, B.S., R. Naquet, and E. Balzamo. 1970. Effects of atropine and eserine on the electroencephalogram, on behaviour and on light-induced epilepsy in the adolescent baboon *Papio-Papio. Electroenceph Clin Neurophysiol* **28**:449–458.

Menini, C., and R. Naquet. 1986. Les myoclonies. Des myoclonies du Papio papio à certaines myoclonies humaines. *Rev Neurol (Paris)*, **142**:3–28.

Möhler, H., and T. Okada. 1977. Benzodiazepine receptor: demonstration in the central nervous system. *Science* **198**:849–851.

Naquet, R., and C. Batini. 1996. Myoclonies et crises épileptiques réflexes du tronc cérébral. *Epilepsies* **8**:125–137.

Naquet, R., and C. Batini. 2002. Genetic Reflex Epilepsy from Chicken to Man: Relations between Genetic Reflex Epilepsy and Movement Disorders. In: R. Guerrini, J. Aicardi, F. Andermann, and M. Hallett, eds. In: *Epilepsy and Movement Disorders* Cambridge University Press. 29–46.

Naquet, R., and M. Poncet-Ramade. 1982. Paroxysmal Discharges Induced by Intermittent Light Stimulation. In: *Henri Gastaut and the Marseilles School's Contribution to the Neurosciences*) Broughton, R.J. (ed.). Elsevier Biomedical Press. Amsterdam. (EEG Suppl. No.35).

Naquet, R., A. Valin, and P. Bryère. 1985. Progabide, Benzodiazepines and Myoclonus in the Papio Papio. In: Bartholini, G. et al. (Eds). *Epilepsies et Agonists des Récepteurs du GABA: Recherche de Base et Thérapeutique.* Raven Press, New York. 159–171.

Rektor, I., P. Bryere, C. Silva-Barrat, and C. Menini. 1986. Stimulus-sensitive myoclonus of the baboon Papio papio: Pharmacological studies reveal interactions between benzodiazepines and the central cholinergic system. *Exper Neurol* **91**:13–22.

Rektor, I., P. Bryere, A. Valin, C. Silva-Barrat, R. Naquet, and C. Menini. 1984. Physostigmine antagonizes the benzodiazepine-induced myoclonus in the Papio papio baboon. *Neurosci Lett* **52**:91–96.

Rektor, I., C. Silva-Barrat, P. Barthuel, and C. Menini. 1991. Drugs influencing the GABAergic neurotransmission have no effect on the non-epileptic myoclonus of baboons. *Electroenceph clin Neurophysiol* **79**:148–152.

Rektor, I., M. Svejdova, C. Silva-Barrat, and C. Menini. 1989. Cholinergic system in the pathophysiology of some types of myoclonus. *Neurol in Europe* 582–586.

Rektor, I., M. Svejdova, C. Silva-Barrat, and C. Menini. 1993. The cholinergic system-dependent myoclonus of the baboon Papio Papio is a reticular reflex myoclonus. *Mov Disorders* **8**:28–32.

Riche, D., F. Conde, C. Silva-Barrat, and C. Menini. 1987. Morphology of different cholinergic groups of neurons in the hindbrain of the baboon. *Neurosci suppl* **22**:S784.

Rump, F., and J. Faff. 1976. Limitations of Pharmacotherapy in Organophosphate Intoxications. In: *Medical Protection against Chemical Warfare Agents. SIPRI and Almquist Wicksell International. Stockolm* Ch. 10.

Shimamura, M., and R.B. Livingston. 1963. Longitudinal conduction systems serving spinal and brainstem coordination. *J Neurophysiol* **26**: 258–272.

Shimamura, M., S. Mori, S. Matsushima, and B. Fujimori. 1964. On the spino-bulbo-spinal reflex in dogs, monkeys and man. *Jap J Physiol* **14**: 411–421.

Silva-Barrat, C., S. Brailowsky, G. Levesque, and C. Menini. 1988. Epileptic discharges induced by intermittent light stimulation in photosensitive baboons: A current source density study. *Epilepsy Res* **2**:1–8.

Squires, R.F., and C. Braestrup. 1977. Benzodiazepine receptors in rat brain, Nature (London), **266**:732–734.

Squires, R.F., R. Naquet, D. Riche, and C. Braestrup. 1979. Increased thermolability of benzodiazepine receptors in cerebral cortex of a baboon with spontaneous seizures. *Epilepsia* **20**:215–221.

Valin, A., C. Cepeda, E. Rey, and R. Naquet. 1981. Opposite effects of lorazepam on two kinds of myoclonus in the photosensitive Papio papio. *Electroenceph Clin Neurophysiol* **52**:647–651.

Valin, A., M. Kaijima, P. Bryere, and R. Naquet. 1983. Differential effect of the benzodiazepine antagonist Ro15-1788 on two types of myoclonus in baboon Papio papio. *Neurosci Lett* **38**:79–84.

Vogel, H.L. 1977. Intravenous use of physostigmine in the management of acute diazepam intoxication. *J Amer Osteopath Ass* **76**:349–351.

C H A P T E R

G1

Tourette Syndrome

HARVEY S. SINGER, CONSTANCE SMITH-HICKS, and DAVID LIEBERMAN

Establishing an animal model that mimics the Gilles de la Tourette syndrome is a major challenge to investigators of movement disorders wishing to decipher the mechanisms of this uniquely human disease. Tourette syndrome (TS) is a common, inherited neuropsychiatric disorder, characterized by the presence of chronic involuntary motor and vocal tics that wax and wane. In addition to tics, individuals with this syndrome often have a variety of concomitant psychopathologies, including obsessive-compulsive disorder (OCD), attention deficit hyperactivity disorder (ADHD), learning difficulties, and sleep abnormalities. TS is an inherited disorder, but the genetic abnormality and precise mode of transmission remain undetermined. Understanding of a role for nongenetic environmental influences is also evolving. The precise neuroanatomical localization remains unknown, but data suggest involvement of cortico-striato-thalamo-cortical (CSTC) circuits. At a cellular level, the distribution of classical neurotransmitters within CSTC circuits raises the possibility that a variety of transmitters could be involved in the pathobiology of TS.

I. TICS

Tics, the hallmark component of tic disorders, are involuntary, sudden, rapid, repetitive, nonrhythmic, stereotyped movements or vocalizations. They appear in a variety of forms, but are typically divided into simple and complex categories. Simple motor tics are brief rapid movements that often involve only one muscle group, *e.g.*, eye blink, head jerk, or shoulder shrug. Complex motor tics are abrupt movements that involve either a cluster of simple movements or a more coordinated sequence of movements. Complex motor tics may be non-purposeful (facial or body contortions), or appear to be more purposeful but actually serve no purpose (touching, hitting, smelling, jumping, obscene gestures), or have a dystonic character. Simple vocal tics include such sounds as grunting, barking, yelping, and throat clearing. Complex vocalizations include syllables, phrases, echolalia (repeating other people's words), palilalia (repeating one's own words), or coprolalia (obscene words). Coprolalia, one of the most distressing and recognizable symptoms, occurs in only about 10% of patients.[1]

Common characteristics of tics include: brief voluntary suppression; exacerbation by anxiety, excitement, anger, or fatigue; reduction during absorbing activities or sleep; and fluctuation over time. Premonitory urges or experiences (tickle, itch, discomfort, strange feelings) are reported in some TS patients before they make a tic movement or vocalization,[2] but tend to be noted less frequently in children. Misdiagnoses are common, *e.g.*, eye blinking tics may be thought to stem from ophthalmologic problems, ocular tics are confused with opsoclonus, throat-clearing tics are thought to be due to sinusitis or allergic conditions, involuntary sniffing frequently results in referral to an allergist, and a chronic persistent cough-like bark is diagnosed as asthma.

II. TOURETTE SYNDROME

A. Criteria

The formal criteria for Tourette syndrome, based on the Tourette Syndrome Classification Study Group,[3] include the presence of multiple motor tics and at least one vocal tic, a waxing and waning course, the presence of symptoms for at least 12 months, onset of symptoms occurring before the age of 21 years, absence of a precipitating illness (encephalitis, stroke, or degenerative disease) or medications, and the observation of tics by a knowledgeable observer.

B. Epidemiology and Outcome

Tourette syndrome occurs worldwide with common features in all cultures and races. Once considered a rare disorder, the estimated prevalence is now about 1% to 3% in regular school populations and higher in special education classes.[4–6] Tics are more common in males than in females (3 : 1), and the mean age of onset is between 6 and 7 years. There is no diagnostic laboratory test, nor is there a requirement for the presence of co-morbid disorders. Patients with TS often have normal neurological examinations and neuroradiographic studies. "Soft" signs, including abnormalities of coordination, fine motor performance, synkinesis, and motor restlessness, are often seen in affected children, especially if they have attention deficit hyperactivity disorder. The course of TS can be quite variable, but most studies suggest that tics improve in late adolescence or early adulthood.[7,8] Leckman and colleagues,[9] using a mathematical model to assess the time course of tic severity over the first 2 decades, have suggested that maximum tic severity occurs between the ages of 8 and 12 years and is then followed by a steady decline in symptoms. Early tic severity is not a good predictor of later tic severity.[10]

C. Genetics and Environmental Factors

Although Georges Gilles de la Tourette suggested an inherited nature for TS, the precise pattern of transmission and the identification of the gene remain elusive. Strong support for a genetic disorder is provided by studies of monozygotic twins that show an 86% concordance rate with TS, as compared to 20% in dizygotic twins.[11,12] Earlier proposals suggesting a sex-influenced autosomal dominant role of inheritance with variable expressivity as TS, chronic tic disorder, or OCD[13] have been seriously questioned. Other investigators have hypothesized that there is a single major locus in combination with a multifactorial background, *i.e.*, either additional genes or environmental factors.[14] The search for a genetic site is being actively pursued, but, despite several studies, to date no reproducible locus has been identified. In a systematic genome scan of 76 affected sib-pair families with a total of 110 sib-pairs, two regions (4q and 8p) showed a trend but did not reach statistical significance.[15] Genetic linkage studies on individuals with TS from an Afrikaner population in South Africa showed evidence for linkage or association for several markers,[16,17] one of which (D11S1377 on chromosome 11q23) is similar to that in a large French Canadian kindred.[18] Linkage studies to a large variety of candidate genes associated with specific synaptic markers have yielded no positive results.

A variety of environmental factors have been proposed as etiologic or modifying agents. Classical tics can be exacerbated by external factors (stress, anxiety, and fatigue), elevations of temperature, infections, and the use of other medications.[9,10,25] Postulated predisposing factors include low birth weight, conditions influencing intra-uterine growth,[26] exposure to medications or illicit drugs,[27,28] hyperthermia,[29,30] and infections.[31–34] A hypothesized role for infections, especially streptococcal infections, as a primary etiology for tics has been suggested for many years.[31,35–38] Proposals of relationships between tics and infectious agents are not, however, limited to Group A β-hemolytic streptococcal (GABHS) infection. Typical symptoms of TS have also been reported in isolated cases following acute infections with *Streptococcus pyogenes*, lyme borreliosis, and *Mycoplasma pneumoniae*,[33,34,39] and exacerbations have followed common colds.[40] Individuals may also have multiple motor and vocal tics that are associated with other medical conditions. This entity, designated "Tourettism," was first observed after an epidemic of encephalitis lethargica about 1920. Tics have also been reported in association with a variety of other acute and chronic neurologic disorders such as after head injury, stroke, cardiac surgery with bypass and hypothermia,[41] or infectious disease,[42] as well as in degenerative disorders including neuroacanthocytosis, Huntington disease, and Creutzfeldt-Jakob disease.[43,44]

D. Co-Morbid Problems

In his early descriptions, Georges Gilles de la Tourette noted the presence of a variety of co-morbid neurobehavioral problems, including obsessive-compulsive symptoms, anxieties, and phobias.[45] Recently, the list of associated problems has lengthened, and it has become clear that the psychopathology is more pervasive than was previously thought, *e.g.*, more than one-half of a large sample of TS patients sought counseling for neurobehavioral problems.[46] Although the presence of neurobehavioral problems is not required for the diagnosis of TS, their clinical impact on the affected patient is often more significant than are the tics themselves. Hence, in developing animal models it is essential that the investigator be aware of the potential psychopathologies that occur in TS.

1. ADHD

ADHD (inattention, hyperactivity, impulsivity) typically begins about age 4 to 5 years and, in TS patients, usually precedes the onset of tics by 2 to 3 years. The disorder is common in TS probands and is reported to affect about 50% (range: 21% to 90%) of referred cases. Its appearance is not associated with the concurrent severity of tics, although ADHD is common in those with more severe tic symptomatology.[47] Whether a genetic relationship exists between TS and ADHD remains controversial. Associated ADHD appears to be the most important contributing factor to poor school performance in a child with TS.[48,49] Comparisons between children with ADHD-only and TS plus ADHD have suggested that mood and anxiety problems were associated with ADHD rather than the presence of tics.[50] Investigators have also suggested that some of the increases in TS adult personality disorders are associated with the presence of childhood ADHD.[51]

2. OCD

The incidence of OCD in TS is typically reported to be in the range of 40% to 50%, although some studies report up to 60% to 89%. Obsessive behaviors generally emerge several years after the onset of tics, usually during early adolescence. Studies that compared obsessive-compulsive behaviors in persons with and without TS have suggested clinical differences. In patients with TS, symptoms usually include a need for order or routine and a requirement for things to be symmetrical or "just right." Hence, compulsions typically involve arranging, ordering, hoarding, touching, tapping, rubbing, counting, checking for errors, and "evening-up" rituals (performing activities until things are symmetrical or feel/look just right). Complex tics and compulsions represent a clinical spectrum of symptoms in TS, with many overlapping features. For example, it may be difficult to distinguish whether actions such as touching or picking represent complex tics or compulsions, and the two may be interwoven. There is evidence for a genetic association between obsessive-compulsive disorder and TS; however, OCD is etiologically heterogeneous and not all cases are associated with a chronic tic disorder.

3. Anxiety and Depression

Several studies have found an increased incidence of anxiety and depression in patients with TS.[47,52,53] In one report evaluating 100 children and adolescents, 76% met the criteria for mood disorder and 67% the criteria for non–obsessive-compulsive anxiety disorder.[53] Depressive symptoms are thought to be more severe in older female patients with TS who have echo phenomena. Some investigators believe that early onset and longer duration of tics correlates positively with depression, whereas others find no correlation between the two. Genetic studies show that major depressive disorder (MDD) is genetic but that TS and MDD are unrelated.[54]

4. Rage Attacks and Self-Injurious Behavior

Episodic outbursts (rage) and self-injurious behavior have been described in patients with TS.[55–57] It is unclear, however, whether these problems are related in etiology to TS or whether they represent other co-morbid conditions. In a study comparing 37 children who had TS and rage attacks to 31 children who did not have this symptom, those with rage were more likely to have ADHD, OCD, and oppositional defiant disorder.[56] In the case of self-injurious behavior, it is unclear whether these behaviors are due to the presence of other disruptive psychopathology, such as OCD or affective disorders.[55]

5. Other Psychopathologies

A variety of other behavioral/emotional problems have been identified in patients with TS. For example, in studies based on the Child Behavior Checklist (CBCL), up to two-thirds of TS subjects had abnormal scores, with clinical problems including obsessive-compulsive behaviors, aggressiveness, hyperactivity, immaturity, withdrawal, and somatic complaints.[58,59] The association of social withdrawal, somatic complaints, and immaturity with TS remains controversial.

6. Academic Difficulties

A variety of factors, including severe tics, psychosocial problems, ADHD, OCD, learning disabilities, and medications, can result in poor school performance in children with tics. Individuals with TS typically have normal levels of intellectual functioning, although there may be a discrepancy between performance and verbal IQ, an impairment of visual perceptual achievement, or a decrease in visual-motor skills.[60–62] Learning difficulties are most common in children who have both TS and ADHD.[63,64] Testing of executive function in children with TS with and without ADHD has indicated that those without ADHD perform significantly better in areas of executive function and perceptual organization.[63,65]

III. NEUROBIOLOGY OF TOURETTE SYNDROME

Despite a preponderance of evidence suggesting an organic rather than psychogenic origin for Tourette syndrome, the precise neurobiological abnormality remains speculative.

Neuroanatomically, there is increasing evidence confirming that cortico-striato-thalamo-cortical (CSTC) pathways represent the site of origin not only for tics but also for accompanying neuropsychiatric problems. Pathophysiological hypotheses are generally based on either *A,* excess thalamic excitation or impaired intracortical inhibition, or *B,* involvement of a specific neurotransmitter or synaptic component. Therefore, an animal model that displays altered synaptic circuitry or an altered neurotransmitter system may lead to the development of behavioral problems similar to those seen in TS.

There has been great difficulty in generating an animal model for TS, in part because the etiology of the underlying abnormalities is unclear. An animal model of TS should demonstrate dysfunction in brain regions causally affected by the disorder, should reflect the type of immune response thought to be active in the diseased brain, and should show abnormalities in neurotransmitter systems or second messengers or both that are inferred from human studies.

One unifying hypothesis for the pathogenesis of TS suggests that it is a developmental disorder resulting in dopaminergic hyperinnervation of the ventral striatum and the associated limbic system. The association between basal ganglia and limbic system structures may help explain the link between tics and complex behavioral problems. An abnormality in developmentally regulated, presumably genetically programmed, apoptosis may underlie the persistence of these dopaminergic projections, although the genetic basis for this is unknown.

Until such time that a genetic model for the disease can be generated, animal models will need to be developed through alterations of synaptic circuitry through microlesions, electrical stimulation, pharmacologic manipulation, or molecular biological alterations of neurotransmitter systems. These *in vitro* models will need to replicate the alterations expressed in TS patients if the animals are to express the phenotype themselves.

A. Neuroanatomic Localization

1. Circuitry

A series of parallel cortico-striato-thalamo-cortical (CSTC) circuits that link specific regions of the frontal cortex to subcortical structures[66–68] provide a unifying framework for understanding the interconnected neurobiological relationships that exist in TS. Five distinct parallel circuits have been described in primates, with each subserving a different function. Although presented as distinct pathways, there is evidence to suggest that these circuits may be more integrated than was previously thought.[69] This multiple convergent and divergent organization provides the capacity for integration and transformation of cortical information.[70]

The *motor* circuit, a potential site for generation of tics, originates primarily from the supplementary motor cortex and projects to the putamen in a somatotopic distribution. The *oculomotor* circuit, a potential site of origin for ocular tics, begins principally in the frontal eye fields and connects to the central region of the caudate. The *dorsolateral prefrontal* circuit links Brodmann's areas 9 and 10 with the dorsolateral head of the caudate and appears to be involved with executive function and motor planning. Dysfunction of this pathway could lead to attentional difficulties and poor results on Letter Word Fluency Testing.[71] The *lateral orbitofrontal* circuit originates in the inferolateral prefrontal cortex and projects to the ventromedial caudate. Orbitofrontal injury is associated with OCD, personality changes, disinhibition, irritability, and mania. Lastly, the *anterior cingulate* circuit arises in the anterior cingulate gyrus and projects to the ventral striatum (olfactory tubercle, nucleus accumbens, and ventral medial aspect of the caudate and putamen), which receives additional input from the amygdala, hippocampus, and entorhinal and perirhinal cortex. Mutism, apathy, and OCD are associated with this circuit. Dysfunction of the CSTC circuit may explain the loss of impulse control and apparent global disinhibition typically expressed by TS patients.

Abnormal activation of motor cortex via basal ganglia-thalamocortical circuits would be expected to cause relatively simple motor patterns, such as those observed in simple tics. Abnormal activation of premotor, supplementary motor, and cingulate motor areas would be expected to cause more elaborate motor patterns, similar to those observed in complex tics. Abnormal activation of the orbitofrontal cortex would be expected to cause even more elaborate motor patterns observed as compulsions. The premonitory symptoms would likewise be associated with abnormal activity of these areas. Thus, abnormal activation of motor areas may be associated with specific or nonspecific sensations, and activation of orbitofrontal areas may be associated with obsessions. Finally, abnormal disinhibition of dorsolateral prefrontal mechanisms may be associated with attention deficits. Although these proposed mechanisms for dysfunctional basal ganglia circuits and the consequent TS symptomatology are hypothetical, newer techniques of biochemistry, pharmacology, electrophysiology, molecular biology, and functional neuroimaging may stimulate formulation of more specific hypotheses to be tested, both in individuals with TS and in animal models of this disease.

2. Evidence Supporting A CSTC Anatomical Localization

Initial studies in TS focused primarily on the basal ganglia. Functional imaging studies identified abnormalities in glucose metabolism and perfusion of the basal ganglia, especially on the left.[72–74] In the HMPAO SPECT study of Moriarty et al.,[75] tic severity correlated with changes in the left lenticular nuclei. Volumetric MRI studies in TS showed significant differences in the symmetry of the putamen and lenticular region in children[76] and a reduction in the size of these structures in adults.[77] On the basis of a quantitative MRI study of monozygotic twins, other investigators have suggested that, rather than an abnormality of the lenticular region, the caudate may be the important site.[78] Transcranial magnetic stimulation (TMS) in children with tic disorders identified a shortened cortical silent period,[79] suggesting a deficiency of motor inhibition believed to be at the level of the basal ganglia. Lastly, in preliminary functional MRI studies, Peterson *et al.*[80] compared images acquired during periods of voluntary tic suppression with those acquired when subjects were allowed spontaneous expression of their tics. Significant changes in signal intensity were seen in the basal ganglia and thalamus as well as in connected cortical regions.

Complementing these TMS experiments, stimulation of the putamen by electrical or chemical means can provoke motor movements and tic-like vocal responses. Alexander and DeLong [81] showed that microstimulation of discrete striatal sites in the putamen of awake monkeys results in stereotyped movements of specific body parts, with increasing stimulation resulting in enhanced, but still stereotyped, muscle contraction. These data suggest that repeated activation of discrete sets of striatal matrisomes can produce repeated stereotyped movements. In contrast, microstimulation of the STN, GPi, or SNpr does not evoke movement. If a discrete population of striatal neurons becomes active due to excessive cortical or thalamic input to the striatum, or insufficient inhibition within the striatum, a stereotyped tic may result. Voluntary movement would be facilitated in a normal fashion but might be accompanied by unwanted facilitation of other motor patterns, resulting in tics accompanying the desired motor pattern (Mink, 2003). Interestingly, high-frequency stimulation of the median and rostral intralaminar thalamic nuclei produced a decrease in tics, implicating a role of these nuclei in the output of tonically active neurons in the striatum.

Large lesions of GPi or SNpr can disinhibit both desired and unwanted motor patterns, allowing not only normal initiation of the desired movement, but also inappropriate activation of competing motor patterns, resulting in involuntary movements. Thus, voluntary as well as involuntary movements are generated. Although smaller lesions of putamen, GPi, SNpr, or STN can produce unwanted motor output patterns, these patterns are not stereotyped and differ from tics. More work is needed in these areas to distinguish what features of the cortical and subcortical circuits give rise specifically to tic-like involuntary movements that can be modeled and examined more closely in the laboratory setting. In addition, further anatomical explanation of OCD and ADHD are required for the development of animal models.

More recent studies have emphasized and provided evidence for significant cortical dysfunction. Volumetric MRI studies have shown larger volumes of the dorsolateral prefrontal region in children with TS, but significantly smaller volumes in adults with the disorder.[82] Cortical white matter in children with TS is increased in the right frontal lobe[83] and decreased in the deep left frontal region.[84] Midsagittal measurements of the corpus callosum, which interconnect homologous cortical areas, have identified variable alterations in the size of this structure.[85,86] Functional MR imaging, in which images acquired during periods of voluntary tic suppression were compared with those during spontaneous expression of tics, suggests that tic suppression involves activation of the prefrontal cortex.[80] Event-related [^{15}O]H_2O PET combined with time-synchronized audio and videotaping identified aberrant activity in interrelated sensorimotor, language, executive, and paralimbic circuits.[87] Lastly, transcranial magnetic stimulation studies have suggested that tics may originate from impaired inhibition directly at the level of the motor cortex.[88,89]

B. Excess Striato-Thalamic Excitation or Abnormal Intracortical Inhibition?

1. Pathways

The striato-thalamic circuit is commonly subdivided into two pathways from the striatum to globus pallidus interna (GPi) and substantia nigra pars reticulata (SNpr) ("direct" and "indirect") and one extending from these neurons to the thalamus (Figure 1). The direct pathway transmits striatal information monosynaptically to the GPi and SNpr, whereas the indirect system conveys information to these same regions via a disynaptic relay from globus pallidus externa (GPe) to the subthalamic nucleus (STN). These parallel pathways have opposing effects on GABAergic GPi/SNpr output neurons (*i.e.,* the direct pathway inhibits and the indirect pathway stimulates) and, in turn, a reverse effect on thalamocortical (VA-VL) neurons. Both the GPi and SNpr receive innervation in a somatotopic organization: head and eyes represented in SNpr, and the rest of the body in the GPi. The thalamic targets of GPi/SNpr project to the frontal lobe, with the VA-VL thalamic complex providing excitatory innervation to motor-related cortical areas. Topographic representation noted in the striatum and globus pallidus are maintained within the thalamus and subsequent projections to the premotor and motor cortex.

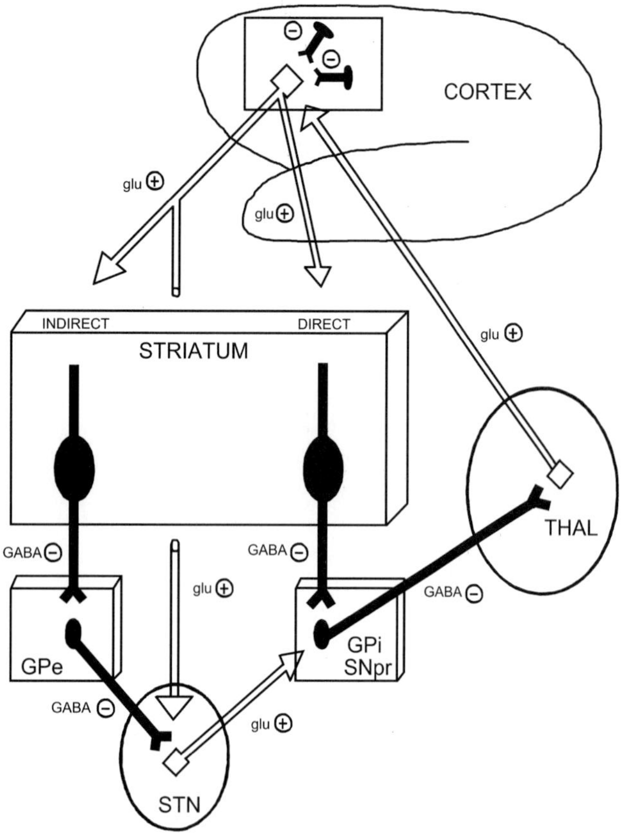

FIGURE 1 **Diagram of C-S-T-C pathways.** Proposed physiological mechanisms for tic symptoms include: a) disruption of the tonically active inhibitory GPi/SNpr output on excitatory thalamic nuclei, leading to excess excitement of cortical neurons, and b) excess excitement of frontal cortical neurons due to other causes, such as impaired inhibition or excessive dopaminergic innervation.

Abbreviations: GABA, gamma-aminobutyric acid; glu, glutamate; GPe, globus pallidus externa; GPi, globus pallidus interna; SNpr, substantia nigra pars reticulate; STN, subthalamic nucleus; THAL, thalamus.

A second model, known as the "center-surround" system, has also been proposed as a pathway that could disrupt striato-thalamic signals.[90] In this latter system, rapid direct and diffuse excitatory cortical inputs to subthalamic nucleus (STN) and slower more focused cortico-striatal pathways have a differential effect on the GPi/SNpr. As proposed, cortical initiation of a movement generates an excitatory signal to the STN, which then diffusely excites the GPi/SNpr, causing inhibition of the thalamocortical/brainstem motor mechanism (*i.e.,* stimulates the brake). In parallel, inputs from cortical areas projecting to the striatum are transferred to a focused, slower, more powerful, context-dependent direct output pathway that inhibits specific neurons in the GPi/SNpr. The effect of this inhibition is to disinhibit selectively the desired motor pattern (*i.e.,* selectively releasing the brake). Lastly, the indirect pathway acts to further focus the activity. In summary, the braking/acceleration of motor patterns enables the desired specific action while simultaneously inhibiting any competing movements.

2. Site of Abnormality

The basic pathobiological principle in all of the proposed pathways (direct-indirect, center-surround system, and striatal striosome–matrix compartment model, which was not discussed)[91] is a disruption of the tonically active inhibitory GPi/SNpr output on excitatory thalamic nuclei that, in turn, influences generation of motor patterns in the cortex or brain stem. Nevertheless, despite proposals of a primary subcortical abnormality, it is also possible that impaired inhibition occurs directly at the level of the motor cortex, or both.

Evidence supporting intracortical inhibitory pathways includes results from neurophysiological and transcranial magnetic stimulation (TMS) studies. Prepulse inhibition of the startle reflex, a measure of inhibitory sensorimotor gating, is deficient in TS.[92] Event-related brain potentials (ERPs), time-locked small voltage fluctuations recorded from the scalp that vary in amplitude as a function of stimulus perception or cognitive processes, have supported hypotheses of altered inhibitory processes or difficulties sustaining the process.[93–97] Results from studies of two response-locked ERPs, Bereitschaft and motor potentials, suggest that the inhibitory impairment involves abnormal modulation of motor excitation/inhibition circuits.[98] In TMS, the two most common measures are *pre-pulse inhibition* (PPI), also known as intracortical inhibition (ratio of amplitude of motor action potential generated by a suprathreshold stimulus to that after a conditioning paradigm that uses a subthreshold stimulus followed by a standard suprathreshold stimulus) and *cortical silent period* (period of electrical silence after the TMS–evoked motor excitation potential in a voluntarily contracted muscle). Although the results are somewhat variable among TS studies, all showed either reduced PPI and/or shortened cortical silent period.[79,89,99]

C. Abnormality of Synaptic Neurotransmission

The distribution of classical neurotransmitters within CSTC circuits raises the possibility that a variety of transmitters are involved in the pathobiology of TS. In general, current hypotheses are based on extrapolations from clinical trials evaluating the response to specific medications; from studies of CSF, blood, and urine in relatively small numbers of patients; from SPECT and PET investigations; and from neurochemical assays on a limited number of postmortem brain tissues. Genetic linkage has also been analyzed in an attempt to identify specific candidate genes that relate to components of neurotransmission.

The dopaminergic, GABAergic, cholinergic, serotonergic, noradrenergic, and opioid systems have all been investigated to varied degrees.[100–102] Which, if any, of these proposals represents the primary pathologic factor remains to be determined. Since many transmitter systems are interrelated in the production of complex actions, it is indeed possible, if not probable, that imbalances exist among several transmitter systems. Moreover, investigators must vigorously pursue mechanisms that could unify findings of alterations within multiple transmitter systems, *i.e.*, such possibilities as second-messenger pathways, vesicle release proteins, channelopathies, or synaptic membrane dysfunction. Furthermore, any hypotheses about specific neurotransmitter deficiencies must account for variability in tic manifestations, fluctuating symptoms, and potential resolution in adulthood.

The possibility of a dopaminergic abnormality in TS continues to receive strong consideration, because of the therapeutic response to neuroleptics, data from postmortem studies, and a variety of nuclear imaging protocols. If TS is associated with excess nigrostriatal dopaminergic activity, whether via postulated supersensitive dopamine receptors, dopamine hyperinnervation, abnormal presynaptic terminal function, increased vesicular dopamine release, or increased responsiveness to dopamine receptor activation, the result would be the disinhibition of excitatory neurons in the thalamus (see[102] for review).

On the basis of finding increased densities of prefrontal D2 receptor protein in postmortem tissue from three individuals with TS (two typical and one adult onset), we have recently proposed a prefrontal-dopaminergic model for this disorder.[103] That is, excess activation of postsynaptic pyramidal dopamine receptors would permit these neurons to fire more easily, leading to overstimulation of the striatal target. An excess inhibitory dopaminergic influence on cortical GABAergic interneurons would further increase excitatory pyramidal output. Since the dopamine transporter was also increased in the two typical cases of TS, a second possibility is an increased phasic dopamine release. Specifically, a reduction in tonic (basal) dopamine, postulated to be due to an overactive dopamine transporter system, could result in a system with elevated DA receptors and an excessive phasic release of dopamine. A similar proposal has been used to explain several neurochemical changes in TS, including elevated intrasynaptic dopamine release after a pharmacologic challenge with amphetamine.[104] In support of the aforementioned hypothesis, tics can be exacerbated by stimulants that increase DA release and block reuptake and by environmental stimuli (stress, anxiety) that increase phasic DA release. Despite the aforementioned proposals, some investigators have emphasized that abnormalities of dopamine fail to explain many clinical and laboratory observations, including the description of unchanged tics in four adults who developed parkinsonism and received treatment with L-dopa[105] and the coexistence of tics and dopa-responsive dystonia.[106]

D. Neuroimmunological Disorder?

Pathophysiologically, based on a Sydenham chorea (SC) model, an immune-mediated mechanism involving molecular mimicry (*i.e.*, antibodies produced against GABHS cross-react with neuronal tissue in specific brain regions) has been proposed for a subset of children with TS. Labeled as *p*ediatric *a*utoimmune *n*europsychiatric *d*isorders *a*ssociated with *s*treptococcal infection (PANDAS), this entity has attained widespread notoriety in both scientific and lay publications. First formally proposed in 1998,[31] diagnostic criteria include the presence of OCD and/or tic disorder; prepubertal age at onset; sudden, "explosive" onset of symptoms and/or a course of sudden exacerbations and remissions; a temporal relationship between symptoms and GABHS; and the presence of neurological abnormalities, including hyperactivity and choreiform movements. The existence of this entity has been supported by several clinical, neuroradiographic, and laboratory studies. More specifically, additional cohorts have been described;[107] familial studies have shown that first-degree relatives of children with PANDAS have higher rates of tic disorders and OCD than do those in the general population.[108] Furthermore, volumetric analyses in children with PANDAS show that the average size of the caudate, putamen, and globus pallidus is significantly larger in those with PANDAS than in healthy children.[109] There are reports of improvement of tics/OCD after plasma exchange or the use of intravenous immunoglobulin,[110] and the finding that a trait marker for susceptibility in rheumatic fever (the monoclonal antibody D8/17) has an enhanced expression in individuals with PANDAS.[111] Nevertheless, despite these findings, concerns have been raised about the existing clinical criteria used to define this disorder,[112,113] the failure to identify abnormal antineuronal antibodies,[114] and the inability of PANDAS sera to induce stereotypes after infusion into rodent striatum.[115,116] Taken together, these findings suggest that, although PANDAS is an intriguing hypothesis, convincing evidence supporting an immune-mediated process is not yet available.

IV. CONCLUSIONS

Tourette syndrome is a common disorder characterized by chronic motor and vocal tics and frequent psychiatric comorbidities. Evidence supports a genetic inheritance, but environmental factors may have a significant role. The disorder arises from abnormalities within CSTC circuits, with likely disruption of tonically active inhibitory GPi/SNpr output on excitatory thalamic nuclei or changes of cortical inhibition. Although abnormalities occur within dopaminergic systems, the precise cellular mechanism has not been identified. An immune-mediated mechanism remains an unproven hypothesis. Active research continues, and the availability of animal models would be of major benefit.

References

1. Goldenberg, J.N., S.B. Brown, and W.J. Weiner. 1994. Coprolalia in younger patients with Gilles de la Tourette syndrome. *Mov Disord* **9**:622–625.
2. Leckman, J.F., and B.S. Peterson. 1993. The pathogenesis of Tourette's syndrome: epigenetic factors active in early CNS development. *Biol Psychiatry* **34**:425–427.
3. The Tourette Syndrome Classification Study Group. 1993. Definitions and classification of tic disorders. *Arch Neurol* **50**:1013–1016.
4. Kurlan, R., M.P. McDermott, C. Deeley, P.G. Como, C. Brower, S. Eapen, E.M. Andresen, et al. 2001. Prevalence of tics in schoolchildren and association with placement in special education. *Neurology* **57**:1383–1388.
5. Mason, A., S. Banerjee, V. Eapen, H. Zeitlin, and M.M. Robertson. 1998. The prevalence of Tourette syndrome in a mainstream school population. *Dev Med Child Neurol* **40**:292–296.
6. Robertson, M.M. 2003. Diagnosing Tourette syndrome: is it a common disorder? *J Psychosom Res* **55**:3–6.
7. Erenberg, G., R.P. Cruse, and A.D. Rothner. 1987. The natural history of Tourette syndrome: a follow-up study. *Ann Neurol* **22**:383–385.
8. Pappert, E.J., C.G. Goetz, E.D. Louis, L. Blasucci, and Leurgans, S. 2003. Objective assessments of longitudinal outcome in Gilles de la Tourette's syndrome. *Neurology* **61**:936–940.
9. Leckman, J.F., H. Zhang, A. Vitale, F. Lahnin, K. Lynch, C. Bondi, Y.S. Kim, et al. 1998. Course of tic severity in Tourette syndrome: the first two decades. *Pediatrics* **102**:14–19.
10. Goetz, C.G., C.M. Tanner, G.T. Stebbins, G. Leipzig, and W.C. Carr. 1992. Adult tics in Gilles de la Tourette's syndrome: description and risk factors. *Neurology* **42**:784–788.
11. Price, R.A., K.K. Kidd, D.J. Cohen, D.L. Pauls, and J.F. Leckman. 1985. A twin study of Tourette syndrome. *Arch Gen Psychiatry* **42**: 815–820.
12. Hyde, T.M., B.A. Aaronson, C. Randolph, K.C. Rickler, and D.R. Weinberger. 1992. Relationship of birth weight to the phenotypic expression of Gilles de la Tourette's syndrome in monozygotic twins. *Neurology* **42**:652–658.
13. Pauls, D.L., and J.F. Leckman. 1986. The inheritance of Gilles de la Tourette's syndrome and associated behaviors. Evidence for autosomal dominant transmission. *N Engl J Med* **315**:993–997.
14. Walkup, J.T., M.C. LaBuda, H.S. Singer, J. Brown, M.A. Riddle, and O. Hurko. 1996. Family study and segregation analysis of Tourette syndrome: evidence for a mixed model of inheritance. *Am J Hum Genet* **59**:684–693.
15. Genetics TTSAICf. 1999. A complete genome screen in sib pairs affected by Gilles de la Tourette syndrome. *Am J Hum Genet* **65**: 1428–1436.
16. Simonic, I., G.S. Gericke, J. Ott, and J.L. Weber. 1998. Identification of genetic markers associated with Gilles de la Tourette syndrome in an Afrikaner population. *Am J Hum Genet* **63**:839–846.
17. Simonic, I., D.R. Nyholt, G.S. Gericke, D. Gordon, N. Matsumoto, D.H. Ledbetter, J. Ott, et al. 2001. Further evidence for linkage of Gilles de la Tourette syndrome (GTS) susceptibility loci on chromosomes 2p11, 8q22 and 11q23–24 in South African Afrikaners. *Am J Med Genet* **105**:163–167.
18. Merette, C., A. Brassard, A. Potvin, H. Bouvier, F. Rousseau, C. Emond, L. Bissonnette, et al. 2000. Significant linkage for Tourette syndrome in a large French Canadian family. *Am J Hum Genet* **67**:1008–1013.
19. Hebebrand, J., M.M. Nothen, A. Ziegler, B. Klug, H. Neidt, K. Eggermann, G. Lehmkuhl, et al. 1997. Nonreplication of linkage disequilibrium between the dopamine D4 receptor locus and Tourette syndrome. *Am J Hum Genet* **61**:238–239.
20. Barr, C.L., K.G. Wigg, E. Zovko, P. Sandor, and L.C. Tsui. 1997. Linkage study of the dopamine D5 receptor gene and Gilles de la Tourette syndrome. *Am J Med Genet* **74**:58–61.
21. Barr, C.L., K.G. Wigg, A.J. Pakstis, R. Kurlan, D. Pauls, K.K. Kidd, L.C. Tsui, et al. 1999. Genome scan for linkage to Gilles de la Tourette syndrome. *Am J Med Genet* **88**:437–445.
22. Devor, E.J., R.M. Dill-Devor, and H.J. Magee. 1998. The Bal I and Msp I polymorphisms in the dopamine D3 receptor gene display, linkage disequilibrium with each other but no association with Tourette syndrome. *Psychiatr Genet* **8**:49–52.
23. Thompson, M., D.E. Comings, L. Feder, S.R. George, and B.F. O'Dowd. 1998. Mutation screening of the dopamine D1 receptor gene in Tourette's syndrome and alcohol dependent patients. *Am J Med Genet* **81**:241–244.
24. Stober, G., J. Hebebrand, S. Cichon, M. Bruss, H. Bonisch, G. Lehmkuhl, F. Poustka, et al. 1999. Tourette syndrome and the norepinephrine transporter gene: results of a systematic mutation screening. *Am J Med Genet* **88**:158–163.
25. Erenberg, G., and S. Fahn. 1996. Tourette syndrome. *Arch Neurol* **53**:588.
26. Burd, L., R. Severud, M.G. Klug, and J. Kerbeshian. 1999. Prenatal and perinatal risk factors for Tourette disorder. *J Perinat Med* **27**: 295–302.
27. Klawans, H.L., D.K. Falk, P.A. Nausieda, and W.J. Weiner. 1978. Gilles de la Tourette syndrome after long-term chlorpromazine therapy. *Neurology* **28**:1064–1066.
28. Singer, W.D. 1981. Transient Gilles de la Tourette syndrome after chronic neuroleptic withdrawal. *Dev Med Child Neurol* **23**:518–521.
29. Kessler, A.R. 2002. Tourette syndrome associated with body temperature dysregulation: possible involvement of an idiopathic hypothalamic disorder. *J Child Neurol* **17**:738–744.
30. Scahill, L., P.J. Lombroso, G. Mack, P.J. Van Wattum, H. Zhang, A. Vitale, and J.F. Leckman. 2001. Thermal sensitivity in Tourette syndrome: preliminary report. *Percept Mot Skills* **92**:419–432.
31. Swedo, S.E., H.L. Leonard, M. Garvey, B. Mittleman, A.J. Allen, S. Perlmutter, L. Lougee, et al. 1998. Pediatric autoimmune neuropsychiatric disorders associated with streptococcal infections: clinical description of the first 50 cases. *Am J Psychiatry* **155**:264–271.
32. Muller, N., M. Riedel, S. Forderreuther, C. Blendinger, and M. Abele-Horn. 2000. Tourette's syndrome and mycoplasma pneumoniae infection. *Am J Psychiatry* **157**:481–482.
33. Riedel, M., A. Straube, M.J. Schwarz, B. Wilske, and N. Muller. 1998. Lyme disease presenting as Tourette's syndrome. *Lancet* **351**:418–419.
34. Greenberg, B.D., D.L. Murphy, and S.E. Swedo. 1998. Symptom exacerbation of vocal tics and other symptoms associated with streptococcal pharyngitis in a patient with obsessive-compulsive disorder and tics. *Am J Psychiatry* **155**:1459–1460.
35. Selling, L. 1929. The role of infection in the etiology of tics. *Arch Neurol Psychiatry* **22**:1163–1171.
36. Brown, E.E. 1957. Tics (habit spasms) secondary to sinusitis. *Arch Pediatr* **74**:39–46.
37. Matarazzo, E.B. 1992. Tourette's syndrome treated with ACTH and prednisone: Report of two cases. *J Child Adolesc Psychopharmacol* **2**:215–226.
38. Kiessling, L.S. 1989. Tic disorders associated with evidence of invasive group A beta hemolytic streptococcal disease, abstracted. *Dev Med Child Neurol* **31**:48.
39. Muller, N., M. Riedel, A. Straube, W. Gunther, and B. Wilske. 2000. Increased anti-streptococcal antibodies in patients with Tourette's syndrome. *Psychiatry Res* **94**:43–49.

40. Hoekstra, P.J., C.G. Kallenberg, J. Korf, and R.B. Minderaa. 2002. Is Tourette's syndrome an autoimmune disease? *Mol Psychiatry* **7**: 437–445.
41. Singer, H.S., P.S. Dela Cruz, M.T. Abrams, S.C. Bean, and A.L. Reiss. 1997. A Tourette-like syndrome following cardiopulmonary bypass and hypothermia: MRI volumetric measurements. *Mov Disord* **12**:588–592.
42. Northam, R.S., and H.S. Singer. 1991. Postencephalitic acquired Tourette-like syndrome in a child. *Neurology* **41**:592–593.
43. Sacks, O.W. 1982. Acquired Tourettism in adult life. *Adv Neurol* **35**:89–92.
44. Jankovic, J., and T. Ashizawa. 1995. Tourettism associated with Huntington's disease. *Mov Disord* **10**:103–105.
45. Tourette, Gdl. 1885. Étude sur une affection nerveuse caractérisée par l'incoordination motrice accompagnée d'écholalie et de copralalie. *Arch Neurol Vol* **9**:19–42, 158–200.
46. Stefl, M.E. 1984. Mental health needs associated with Tourette syndrome. *Am J Public Health* **74**:1310–1313.
47. Robertson, M.M., M.R. Trimble, and A.J. Lees. 1988. The psychopathology of the Gilles de la Tourette syndrome. A phenomenological analysis. *Br J Psychiatry* **152**:383–390.
48. Park, S., P.G. Como, L. Cui, and R. Kurlan. 1993. The early course of the Tourette's syndrome clinical spectrum. *Neurology* **43**:1712–1715.
49. Abwender, D.A., P.G. Como, R. Kurlan, K. Parry, K.A. Fett, L. Cui, S. Plumb, et al. 1996. School problems in Tourette's syndrome. *Arch Neurol* **53**:509–511.
50. Spencer, T., J. Biederman, M. Harding, D. O'Donnell, T. Wilens, S. Faraone, B. Coffey, et al. 1998. Disentangling the overlap between Tourette's disorder and ADHD. *J Child Psychol Psychiatry* **39**: 1037–1044.
51. Robertson, M.M. 2000. Tourette syndrome, associated conditions and the complexities of treatment. *Brain* 123 Pt **3**:425–462.
52. Comings, B.G., and D.E. Comings. 1987. A controlled study of Tourette syndrome. V. Depression and mania. *Am J Hum Genet* **41**:804–821.
53. Coffey, B.J., and K.S. Park. 1997. Behavioral and emotional aspects of Tourette syndrome. *Neurol Clin* **15**:277–289.
54. Pauls, D.L., J.F. Leckman, and D.J. Cohen. 1994. Evidence against a genetic relationship between Tourette's syndrome and anxiety, depression, panic and phobic disorders. *Br J Psychiatry* **164**:215–221.
55. Robertson, M.M. 1992. Self-injurious behavior and Tourette syndrome. *Adv Neurol* **58**:105–114.
56. Budman, C.L., R.D. Bruun, K.S. Park, M. Lesser, and M. Olson. 2000. Explosive outbursts in children with Tourette's disorder. *J Am Acad Child Adolesc Psychiatry* **39**:1270–1276.
57. Budman, C.L., L. Rockmore, J. Stokes, and M. Sossin. 2003. Clinical phenomenology of episodic rage in children with Tourette syndrome. *J Psychosom Res* **55**:59–65.
58. Singer, H.S., and L.A. Rosenberg. 1989. Development of behavioral and emotional problems in Tourette syndrome. *Pediatr Neurol* **5**:41–44.
59. Walkup, J.T., L.A. Rosenberg, J. Brown, and H.S. Singer. 1992. The validity of instruments measuring tic severity in Tourette's syndrome. *J Am Acad Child Adolesc Psychiatry* **31**:472–477.
60. Golden, G.S. 1984. Psychologic and neuropsychologic aspects of Tourette's syndrome. *Neurol Clin* **2**:91–102.
61. Bornstein, R.A. 1990. Neuropsychological performance in children with Tourette's syndrome. *Psychiatry Res* **33**:73–81.
62. Brookshire, B.L., I.J. Butler, L. Ewing-Cobbs, and J.M. Fletcher. 1994. Neuropsychological characteristics of children with Tourette syndrome: evidence for a nonverbal learning disability? *J Clin Exp Neuropsychol* **16**:289–302.
63. Schuerholz, L.J., T.L. Baumgardner, H.S. Singer, A.L. Reiss, and M.B. Denckla. 1996. Neuropsychological status of children with Tourette's syndrome with and without attention deficit hyperactivity disorder. *Neurology* **46**:958–965.
64. Faraone, S.V., J. Biederman, B.K. Lehman, T. Spencer, D. Norman, L.J. Seidman, I. Kraus, et al. 1993. Intellectual performance and school failure in children with attention deficit hyperactivity disorder and in their siblings. *J Abnorm Psychol* **102**:616–623.
65. Harris, E.L., L.J. Schuerholz, H.S. Singer, M.J. Reader, J.E. Brown, C. Cox, J. Mohr, et al. 1995. Executive function in children with Tourette syndrome and/or attention deficit hyperactivity disorder. *J Int Neuropsychol Soc* **1**:511–516.
66. Alexander, G.E., M.R. DeLong, and P.L. Strick. 1986. Parallel organization of functionally segregated circuits linking basal ganglia and cortex. *Annu Rev Neurosci* **9**:357–381.
67. Alexander, G.E., and M.D. Crutcher. 1990. Functional architecture of basal ganglia circuits: neural substrates of parallel processing. *Trends Neurosci* **13**:266–271.
68. Cummings, J.L. 1993. Frontal-subcortical circuits and human behavior. *Arch Neurol* **50**:873–880.
69. Gerfen, C.R., and C.J. Wilson. 1996. The basal ganglia. Handbook of chemical neuroanatomy. Amsterdam: Elsevier.
70. Graybiel, A.M., T. Aosaki, A.W. Flaherty, and M. Kimura. 1994. The basal ganglia and adaptive motor control. *Science* **265**:1826–1831.
71. Schuerholz, L.J., H.S. Singer, and M.B. Denckla. 1998. Gender study of neuropsychological and neuromotor function in children with Tourette syndrome with and without attention-deficit hyperactivity disorder. *J Child Neurol* **13**:277–282.
72. Riddle, M.A., A.M. Rasmusson, S.W. Woods, and P.B. Hoffer. 1992. SPECT imaging of cerebral blood flow in Tourette syndrome. *Adv Neurol* **58**:207–211.
73. Stoetter, B., A.R. Braun, C. Randolph, J. Gernert, R.E. Carson, P. Herscovitch, and T.N. Chase. 1992. Functional neuroanatomy of Tourette syndrome. Limbic-motor interactions studied with FDG PET. *Adv Neurol* **58**:213–226.
74. Baxter, L.R., and B.J. Guze. 1993. Neuroimaging. In: Kurlan, R., ed. Handbook of Tourette's and related tic and behavioral disorders. New York: Marcel Dekker, 289.
75. Moriarty, J., D.C. Costa, B. Schmitz, M.R. Trimble, P.J. Ell, and M.M. Robertson. 1995. Brain perfusion abnormalities in Gilles de la Tourette's syndrome. *Br J Psychiatry* **167**:249–254.
76. Singer, H.S., A.L. Reiss, J.E. Brown, E.H. Aylward, B. Shih, E. Chee, E.L. Harris, et al. 1993. Volumetric MRI changes in basal ganglia of children with Tourette's syndrome. *Neurology* **43**:950–956.
77. Peterson, B., M.A. Riddle, D.J. Cohen, L.D. Katz, J.C. Smith, M.T. Hardin, and J.F. Leckman. 1993. Reduced basal ganglia volumes in Tourette's syndrome using three-dimensional reconstruction techniques from magnetic resonance images. *Neurology* **43**:941–949.
78. Hyde, T.M., M.E. Stacey, R. Coppola, S.F. Handel, K.C. Rickler, and D.R. Weinberger. 1995. Cerebral morphometric abnormalities in Tourette's syndrome: a quantitative MRI study of monozygotic twins. *Neurology* **45**:1176–1182.
79. Ziemann, U., F. Tergau, J. Netz, and V. Homberg. 1997. Delay in simple reaction time after focal transcranial magnetic stimulation of the human brain occurs at the final motor output stage. *Brain Res* **744**:32–40.
80. Peterson, B.S., P. Skudlarski, A.W. Anderson, H. Zhang, J.C. Gatenby, C.M. Lacadie, J.F. Leckman, et al. 1998. A functional magnetic resonance imaging study of tic suppression in Tourette syndrome. *Arch Gen Psychiatry* **55**:326–333.
81. Alexander, G.E., and M.R. DeLong. 1985. Microstimulation of the primate neostriatum. II. Somatotopic organization of striatal microexcitable zones and their relation to neuronal response properties. *J Neurophysiol* **53**:1417–1430.
82. Peterson, B.S., L. Staib, L. Scahill, H. Zhang, C. Anderson, J.F. Leckman, D.J. Cohen, et al. 2001. Regional brain and ventricular volumes in Tourette syndrome. *Arch Gen Psychiatry* **58**:427–440.

83. Fredericksen, K.A., L.E. Cutting, W.R. Kates, S.H. Mostofsky, H.S. Singer, K.L. Cooper, D.C. Lanham, et al. 2002. Disproportionate increases of white matter in right frontal lobe in Tourette syndrome. *Neurology* **58**:85–89.
84. Kates, W.R., M. Frederikse, S.H. Mostofsky, B.S. Folley, K. Cooper, P. Mazur-Hopkins, O. Kofman, et al. 2002. MRI parcellation of the frontal lobe in boys with attention deficit hyperactivity disorder or Tourette syndrome. *Psychiatry Res* **116**:63–81.
85. Baumgardner, T.L., H.S. Singer, M.B. Denckla, M.A. Rubin, M.T. Abrams, M.J. Colli, and A.L. Reiss. 1996. Corpus callosum morphology in children with Tourette syndrome and attention deficit hyperactivity disorder. *Neurology* **47**:477–482.
86. Peterson, B.S., J.F. Leckman, J.S. Duncan, R. Wetzles, M.A. Riddle, M.T. Hardin, and D.J. Cohen. 1994. Corpus callosum morphology from magnetic resonance images in Tourette's syndrome. *Psychiatry Res* **55**:85–99.
87. Stern, E., D.A. Silbersweig, K.Y. Chee, A. Holmes, M.M. Robertson, M. Trimble, C.D. Frith, et al. 2000. A functional neuroanatomy of tics in Tourette syndrome. *Arch Gen Psychiatry* **57**:741–748.
88. Ziemann, U., W. Paulus, and A. Rothenberger. 1997. Decreased motor inhibition in Tourette's disorder: evidence from transcranial magnetic stimulation. *Am J Psychiatry* **154**:1277–1284.
89. Moll, G.H., H. Heinrich, G.E. Trott, S. Wirth, N. Bock, and A. Rothenberger. 2001. Children with comorbid attention-deficit-hyperactivity disorder and tic disorder: evidence for additive inhibitory deficits within the motor system. *Ann Neurol* **49**:393–396.
90. Mink, J.W. 2001. Basal ganglia dysfunction in Tourette's syndrome: a new hypothesis. *Pediatr Neurol* **25**:190–198.
91. Graybiel, A.M., J.J. Canales, and C. Capper-Loup. 2000. Levodopa-induced dyskinesias and dopamine-dependent stereotypies: a new hypothesis. *Trends Neurosci* **23**:S71–S77.
92. Swerdlow, N.R., B. Karban, Y. Ploum, R. Sharp, M.A. Geyer, and A. Eastvold. 2001. Tactile prepuff inhibition of startle in children with Tourette's syndrome: in search of an "fMRI-friendly" startle paradigm. *Biol Psychiatry* **50**:578–585.
93. Johannes, S., C. Kube, B.M. Wieringa, M. Matzke, and T.F. Munte. 1997. Brain potentials and time estimation in humans. *Neurosci Lett* **231**:63–66.
94. Johannes, S., B.M. Wieringa, W. Nager, K.R. Muller-Vahl, R. Dengler, and T.F. Munte. 2001. Electrophysiological measures and dual-task performance in Tourette syndrome indicate deficient divided attention mechanisms. *Eur J Neurol* **8**:253–260.
95. Johannes, S., B.M. Wieringa, W. Nager, K.R. Muller-Vahl, R. Dengler, and T.F. Munte. 2002. Excessive action monitoring in Tourette syndrome. *J Neurol* **249**:961–966.
96. Oades, R.D., A. Dittmann-Balcar, R. Schepker, C. Eggers, and D. Zerbin. 1996. Auditory event-related potentials (ERPs) and mismatch negativity (MMN) in healthy children and those with attention-deficit or tourette/tic symptoms. *Biol Psychol* **43**:163–185.
97. van Woerkom, T.C., R.A. Roos, and J.G. van Dijk. 1994. Altered attentional processing of background stimuli in Gilles de la Tourette syndrome: a study in auditory event-related potentials evoked in an oddball paradigm. *Acta Neurol Scand* **90**:116–123.
98. O'Connor, K., M.E. Lavoie, and M. Robert. 2001. Preparation and motor potentials in chronic tic and Tourette syndromes. *Brain Cogn* **46**:224–226.
99. Moll, G.H., S. Wischer, H. Heinrich, F. Tergau, W. Paulus, and A. Rothenberger. 1999. Deficient motor control in children with tic disorder: evidence from transcranial magnetic stimulation. *Neurosci Lett* **272**:37–40.
100. Singer, H.S. 1997. Neurobiology of Tourette syndrome. *Neurol Clin* **15**:357–379.
101. Singer, H.S. 2000. Current issues in Tourette syndrome. *Mov Disord* **15**:1051–1063.
102. Singer, H.S., and K. Minzer. 2004. Neurobiology of Tourette syndrome: concepts of neuroanatomical localization and neurochemical abnormalities. Brain and Development, in press.
103. Minzer, K., O. Lee, J.J. Hong, and H.S. Singer. 2004. Increased prefrontal D2 protein in Tourette syndrome: a postmortem analysis of frontal cortex and striatum. *J Neurol Sci* in press.
104. Singer, H.S., S. Szymanski, J. Giuliano, F. Yokoi, A.S. Dogan, J.R. Brasic, Y. Zhou, et al. 2002. Elevated intrasynaptic dopamine release in Tourette's syndrome measured by PET. *Am J Psychiatry* **159**:1329–1336.
105. Kumar, R., and A.E. Lang. 1997. Coexistence of tics and parkinsonism: evidence for non-dopaminergic mechanisms in tic pathogenesis. *Neurology* **49**:1699–1701.
106. Romstad, A., E. Dupont, B. Krag-Olsen, K. Ostergaard, P. Guldberg, and F. Guttler. 2003. Dopa-responsive dystonia and Tourette syndrome in a large Danish family. *Arch Neurol* **60**:618–622.
107. Murphy, M.L., and M.E. Pichichero. 2002. Prospective identification and treatment of children with pediatric autoimmune neuropsychiatric disorder associated with group A streptococcal infection (PANDAS). *Arch Pediatr Adolesc Med* **156**:356–361.
108. Lougee, L., S.J. Perlmutter, R. Nicolson, M.A. Garvey, and S.E. Swedo. 2000. Psychiatric disorders in first-degree relatives of children with pediatric autoimmune neuropsychiatric disorders associated with streptococcal infections (PANDAS). *J Am Acad Child Adolesc Psychiatry* **39**:1120–1126.
109. Giedd, J.N., J.L. Rapoport, M.A. Garvey, S. Perlmutter, and S.E. Swedo. 2000. MRI assessment of children with obsessive-compulsive disorder or tics associated with streptococcal infection. *Am J Psychiatry* **157**:281–283.
110. Perlmutter, S.J., S.F. Leitman, M.A. Garvey, S. Hamburger, E. Feldman, H.L. Leonard, and S.E. Swedo. 1999. Therapeutic plasma exchange and intravenous immunoglobulin for obsessive-compulsive disorder and tic disorders in childhood. *Lancet* **354**: 1153–1158.
111. Swedo, S.E., H.L. Leonard, B.B. Mittleman, A.J. Allen, J.L. Rapoport, S.P. Dow, M.E. Kanter, et al. 1997. Identification of children with pediatric autoimmune neuropsychiatric disorders associated with streptococcal infections by a marker associated with rheumatic fever. *Am J Psychiatry* **154**:110–112.
112. Kurlan, R. 1998. Tourette's syndrome and "PANDAS": will the relation bear out? Pediatric autoimmune neuropsychiatric disorders associated with streptococcal infection. *Neurology* **50**:1530–1534.
113. Singer, H.S., and C. Loiselle. 2003. PANDAS: a commentary. *J Psychosom Res* **55**:31–39.
114. Singer, H.S., C.R. Loiselle, O. Lee, K. Minzer, S.E. Swedo, and F.H. Grus. 2004. Anti-basal ganglia antibody abnormalities in PANDAS. in press.
115. Loiselle, C.R., O. Lee, T.H. Moran, and H.S. Singer. 2003. Striatal microinfusion of Tourette syndrome and PANDAS sera: failure to induce behavioral changes. *Mov Disord* In press.
116. Singer, H.S., J.W. Mink, J. Hallett, and P. Lombroso, Unpublished data.
117. Mink, J.W. 2003. The basal ganglia and involuntary movements: impaired inhibition of competing motor patterns. *Arch Neurol* **60**: 1365–1368.

CHAPTER

G2

Animal Models of Tourette Syndrome

KATHLEEN BURKE and PAUL J. LOMBROSO

Animal models advance medical research by providing investigators with a means to test hypotheses about disease mechanisms and treatments. The value of an animal model is based on the extent to which that model is homologous with the causes and symptoms of a specific human disease (Willner, 1986; McKinney, 2001; Overall, 2000). In many instances a somatic disease can be fully reproduced in an animal because the etiology is clearly defined (for example, a bacterial infection), the symptoms are obvious and quantifiable (fever, swelling, pain) and relieved by treatments known to be effective in humans (antibiotics). In contrast, psychiatric syndromes emerge from complex and largely unknown genetic, developmental, and social interactions that give rise to changes in mood, cognition, and behavior that seem to be uniquely human (McKinney, 1998). Nevertheless, although an entire syndrome cannot be modeled, selected components of a syndrome can be studied in animal preparations, and these "partial models" of psychiatric disorders have proven to be heuristically valuable (McKinney, 2001).

Tourette syndrome is a phenotypically complex disorder involving disturbances in movement, cognition, and behavior. The disorder is inherited and also associated with a number of environmental risk factors present during development (reviewed in Leckman, 2002). In this chapter we present three "partial animal models" of Tourette syndrome that represent distinct approaches to investigating pathological mechanisms associated with this disorder.

I. TOURETTE SYNDROME

Tourette syndrome (TS) is a neuropsychiatric disorder characterized by abrupt, repeated motor movements and vocalizations, or tics. The disorder typically begins in early childhood (mean age of seven), with motor tics appearing first, followed by vocal tics one to two years later. Boys are affected four to eight times more frequently than girls. The tics occur in bouts, which can vary in frequency, intensity, and anatomical location. Stress, anxiety, and fatigue may exacerbate tic expression. For most individuals, symptoms decrease or even disappear during adolescence and early adulthood; however, 25% of individuals with clinically diagnosed TS become chronically disabled in adulthood by severe motor and vocal tics (Shapiro et al., 1988).

Patients with TS often display symptoms of other psychopathies such as hyperactivity, aggressiveness, obsessive-compulsive disorder (OCD), depression, and anxiety. Other commonly noted difficulties include sleep disturbances, learning disabilities, and speech problems. About 50% of TS patients referred to clinics have sufficient attentional, impulsive, and hyperactive symptoms to warrant the diagnosis of attention deficit with hyperactivity disorder (ADHD) (Cohen et al., 1992; Bruun and Budman, 1992; Comings and Comings, 1987). In many children, the attentional and disruptive behaviors produce greater impairment than the tics themselves. Over 60% of patients with TS also report obsessive and compulsive symptoms during the course of their illness (Pauls et al., 1986, 1991). Typically, these symptoms begin in early adolescence (mean age of eleven years) (Jagger et al., 1982). The obsessional thoughts and compulsive behaviors often become more prominent during later adolescence and, in some cases, the full-blown OCD symptom picture becomes even more burdensome than the original tic symptomatology. The OCD symptoms are more likely to have aggressive or sexual content than OCD patients without tics (George et al., 1993), although a significant number of patients have contamination and contagion concerns, as well as checking and cleaning compulsions. Distinctive features of tic-related forms of OCD are the need to "even things up," or repeat actions until they feel "just right" (Leckman et al., 1993, 1994).

A. Characteristics of Tics

Tics are classified as either simple or complex. Simple motor tics involve repetitive contractions of one or a few muscle groups, most often the facial muscles. The most common simple tic, blinking, is usually the first tic to appear with disease onset. Other facial tics include squinting, grimacing, nose twitching, and oral movements such as licking the lips or biting the lips or tongue. Jerking of the head or extremities, shoulder shrugging, and pulling at clothing are also common simple tics (reviewed in Comings, 1990; Leckman, 2002). Throat clearing is the most frequently observed vocal tic, but vocalizations can be as diverse as sniffing, barking, spitting, humming, screaming, coughing, and grunting. Complex motor tics involve coordinated patterns of movement such as jumping, touching, smelling or kissing oneself, or others. Complex vocal tics occur in less than 25% of cases and include echolalia, coprolalia, or uttering nonsense syllables. Complex tics can involve combinations of motor and vocal tics, such as jumping and humming (Comings, 1990).

Most individuals with TS report that uncomfortable physical sensations or mental states, "premonitory urges," precede or accompany tics. These sensations are described as itching, pressure, or "crawling feelings," and are often localized to specific body parts such as the hands and shoulders (Leckman et al., 1993; Swerdlow and Leckman, 2002). Performance of the tic relieves these sensations. Interestingly, many patients experience these premonitory urges as involuntary, and tic performance as intentional (Leckman et al., 1993). Tics can be suppressed temporarily, but premonitory sensations continue to increase until the tic is performed (Leckman et al., 1993).

B. Involvement of the Basal Ganglia

While the neural mechanisms responsible for tic production are largely unknown, abnormalities in basal ganglia function have been consistently demonstrated in TS. The basal ganglia consist of interconnected subcortical structures in the forebrain, diencephalon, and midbrain that are involved in movement, learning, motivation, and reward. The basal ganglia include the striatum (caudate, nucleus accumbens, and putamen) the subthalamic nucleus, the globus pallidus (pars interna and externa), and the substantia nigra (pars reticulata and compacta). The striatum and subthalamic nucleus (STN) are the input structures of the basal ganglia, receiving excitatory, somatotopically organized glutamatergic afferents from the frontal cortex (STN and striatum) and from the parietal temporal and occipital cortex (striatum) (Alexander et al., 1994; Mink, 2001). In addition, the striatum receives dopaminergic projections from the substantia nigra pars compacta (SNpc) and ventral tegmental area. The basal ganglia output structures, the substantia nigra pars reticulata (SNpr) and the globus pallidus pars interna (GPi), are tonically active GABAergic neurons that project to the VA and VL thalamus. These thalamic nuclei, in turn, send excitatory projections back to the cortex.

Signals from different cortical areas enter the striatum through parallel, segregated loops that direct signals through specific areas of the basal ganglia and thalamus (Alexander, 1994). Cortical afferents make excitatory glutamatergic synaptic connections with striatal medium spiny projection neurons (MSNs). MSNs are distributed between two striatal compartments, the striosomes and the matrix, and can be distinguished by differences in neuropeptide content and level of dopamine receptor subtype expression (Graybiel et al., 2000). Sensorimotor cortical afferents project to MSNs in the matrix, and corticolimbic afferents project to striosomal MSNs. Within the matrix, MSNs are organized into matrisomes, groups of neurons that receive input from the same cortical areas (Graybiel et al., 2000). MSNs inhibit their target neurons by releasing GABA.

MSNs in the matrix give rise to two opposing signaling pathways: the direct and indirect pathways (Albin et al., 1989; Graybiel et al., 2000). MSNs of the direct pathway express D1 receptors and project to the SNpr and GPi. Neurons of these output nuclei are GABAergic and tonically active, so excitation of the direct pathway inhibits SNpr and GPi neurons, with release of excitatory thalamic neurons. Thus the net effect of direct pathway stimulation is increased excitation of cortical neurons. MSNs of the indirect pathway express D2 receptors and project to the GPe, which projects, in turn, to the SNpr. Stimulation of the indirect pathway thus inhibits GPe neurons, releasing glutamatergic STN neurons from inhibition. Excitatory STN neurons in turn, activate GABAergic SNpr neurons, leading to decreased thalamic drive to the cortex. Striosomal MSNs are not part of the CSTC loops, but project to the SNpc; striosomal activation leads to decreased nigrostriatal dopamine release.

Investigators believe that executing normal movement depends, in part, on a balance between the direct pathway, which facilitates movement release, and the indirect pathway, which inhibits movement release. Some investigators have suggested that increased striatal dopamine activity in TS may cause tic expression either by stimulating direct pathway activity via D1 receptors or by suppressing indirect pathway activity via D2 receptors (Hallett, 1993; Black, 1997).

Alternatively, Mink (2001) has proposed a scheme in which the net inhibitory output of the basal ganglia tonically suppresses the activity of motor pattern generators in the cortex and brainstem. Execution of a voluntary movement requires that projection neurons of the selected motor pattern generator simultaneously increase basal ganglia inhibitory input to competing pattern generators while reducing basal ganglia inhibitory input to themselves (Mink, 2001). Mink has proposed that abnormalities in specific matrisomes cause them to be active at inappropriate times, leading to the release of unwanted movements such as tics (Mink, 2001).

II. MODELING TOURETTE SYNDROME IN RODENTS

Because the genetic and pathophysiological etiologies of TS are unknown, no animal models of the disorder exist that have true construct validity (McKinney, 1998). However, investigators have a variety of methods that can induce abnormal repetitive movements in rodents that mimic elements of tic behavior. Stereotypies are simple or complex movement sequences that are repeated excessively, invariantly, and purposelessly (Ridley, 1994; Mason, 1991). These behaviors are species specific and emerge when an animal is subjected to stress or confinement in a low stimulus environment such as a zoo or laboratory animal colony (Ridley, 1994; Mason, 1991). For example, laboratory mice housed in propylene bins frequently engage in "cage stereotypies" such as mouthing the bars of the wire cage top (Wurbel, 2001; Garner and Mason, 2002). It is generally accepted that stereotypies develop from functional, motivated behaviors such as foraging or defense that are normally terminated when the goals (food, escape) are achieved (Dantzer, 1991; Wurbel, 2001). In captive situations, these goals are repeatedly frustrated, and sensory feedback from the motor behaviors serves to trigger further execution of the behaviors in the absence of motivation or environmental stimulus (Dantzer, 1991).

Garner and Mason (2002) provided compelling evidence that stereotypical behaviors reflect disorders of basal ganglia dysfunction. These investigators hypothesized that if stereotypies emerge as a result of disinhibition of behavioral selection, other behaviors mediated by the basal ganglia should also show evidence of disinhibition. Garner and Mason (2002) reported that caged voles expressing stereotypies also had enhanced rates of behavioral initiation, increased impulsivity, impaired extinction learning, and increased "knowledge-action" dissociation—the inability to suppress a previous incorrect response despite knowledge of the correct response. These results are consistent with behavioral findings of impulsivity and inattention in individuals with TS (Leckman, 2002).

A. Measuring Stereotypies in Rodents

Stereotypic behavior in rodents can be elicited by a variety of methods, including isolation rearing, lesioning of specific brain structures, administration of drugs that affect CSTC neurotransmission, and, more recently, genetic manipulations (Ridley, 1994; Campbell et al., 1999). Despite the diversity of induction procedures, methods used to evaluate stereotypical behaviors are essentially similar. Observers who are blind to the experimental conditions test the animal either in its home cage or in a special test chamber. Behavior ratings can be categorical, recording the presence or absence of a specific behavior, or quantitative, measuring the frequency and duration of each behavior. Most behavior rating scales are based on the Creese-Iverson stereotypy scale (Creese and Iverson, 1973). This scale consists of six categories of behavior: 0) asleep or motionless; 1) active, moving about the cage; 2) predominantly active with bursts of stereotyped activity; 3) stereotyped activity occurring along a fixed path; 4) stereotyped behaviors occurring in one location of the cage with sniffing or rearing in one location; 5) stereotyped behavior in one location, with bursts of gnawing or licking; and 6) continual gnawing or licking of the cage. This scale was developed from behavioral observations of rats exposed to increasing doses of amphetamine, and behaviors such as sniffing, licking, and gnawing are species specific and selectively promoted by amphetamine. Substitution of other repetitive behaviors is necessary in evaluating other species.

Behavioral scoring is often done in real time, using at least two observers blind to treatment conditions. However, because some orofacial movements may be subtle and easily missed, videotaping the observation sessions is preferred. The most common method of scoring uses time sampling procedures, in which investigators record behavior over a specified time at predetermined intervals in the testing session. For example, in our laboratory, we record animal behaviors over a one-minute period, at five-minute intervals in a thirty-minute test session.

In addition to the traditional observation methods described here, automated methods of stereotypy detection and analysis are now available that appear to offer greater sensitivity and ease of use (Campbell et al., 1998; Fowler, 2001).

B. Psychostimulant Model

The "dopamine hypothesis" of TS holds that excessive dopaminergic transmission in corticostriatothalamic (CSTC) circuits is responsible for the pathophysiology of TS. This hypothesis developed largely from clinical observations that drugs that block dopamine D2 receptors relieve tic symptoms in the majority of TS patients (Challas, 1967; Shapiro and Shapiro, 1988; Shapiro et al., 1989). Drugs that block dopamine synthesis or vesicular uptake were also reported to be helpful (Sweet et al., 1974; Jankovic et al., 1984), while drugs that increased synaptic dopamine concentrations often worsened tic symptoms (Erenberg et al., 1985). However, aside from these pharmacologic studies, little evidence supports the presence of dopaminergic abnormalities in TS patients. Early reports of decreased concentrations of homovanillic acid (HVA), the major dopamine metabolite in the cerebrospinal fluid of TS patients (Butler et al., 1979; Cohen et al., 1978; Singer et al., 1982) have been contradicted by more recent findings in a comprehensive study of TS, OCD, and control populations (Leckman et al., 1995). Postmortem examinations of brain dopamine and HVA concentrations, as well as tyrosine hydroxylase activity, have also failed to identify differences between TS and control populations (Anderson et al., 1992a,b). However, recent PET and SPECT imaging studies examining dopamine release have provided intriguing but inconclusive evidence of changes in dopamine receptor densities and phasic dopamine release in TS patients (reviewed in Singer and Wendlandt, 2001).

1. Description of the Model

Since the first report that amphetamine induces oral stereotypies in rodents, investigators have intensively studied psychostimulant effects on behavior and neurochemistry (Randrup et al., 1963). The ability of these drugs to reliably induce a set of characteristic behaviors in rodents provides an opportunity to examine the neural circuits and molecular mechanisms underlying behavioral disinhibition. The indirect dopamine receptor agonist amphetamine has been particularly well studied in this regard. Amphetamine increases synaptic dopamine concentrations through multiple mechanisms, including reversal of the synaptic and vesicular monamine transporters and inhibition of monoamine oxidase (Florin et al., 1994).

The behavioral profiles elicited by acute systemic amphetamine administration have been well described (for reviews see Randrup and Munkvad, 1974; Robinson and Becker, 1986; and Florin et al. 1994). In low doses (0.3–1.5 mg/kg), amphetamine stimulates increased locomotor behavior, primarily vertical- (rearing) and forward-directed movements. At intermediate doses (1.5–2.5 mg/kg) these movements increase in frequency, but are interrupted by brief periods of decreased locomotion accompanied by repetitive head and limb movements and sniffing. Amphetamine doses greater than 2.5 mg/kg induce a behavior pattern characterized by an early and late phase of increased locomotor behavior separated by a prolonged period of stereotypy. During the stereotypy phase, the animal remains in a particular area of the cage and engages in repeated movements of the head and forelimbs, and may continuously sniff, lick, or bite the cage or bedding. Repeated daily injections of amphetamine increase in the magnitude and duration of the locomotor and stereotypy responses. In addition, at high doses, the interval to onset of the stereotypy phase is decreased.

2. Relevance to Tourette Syndrome

Although the psychostimulant model is not unique to TS, it has provided a wealth of information about the role of the basal ganglia in the release of normal and repetitive behaviors that has advanced understanding of this disorder. Thus this model continues to have considerable heuristic value in TS research. One significant recent finding is the discovery of a potential role for striosomes in the activation of stereotypic behavior.

The relationship between stereotypies and striosomal activation may be the single most important *recent* discovery relevant to TS (Canales and Graybiel, 2000). Expression of immediate early genes such as *fos* and *jun* is a marker of neuronal activation in the striatum (Graybiel, 2000). Graybiel and colleagues had previously discovered that repeated administration of the psychostimulants amphetamine and cocaine increased the number of neurons expressing these markers (Graybiel et al., 1990). In an elegant series of studies, Graybiel and colleagues compared the amount of striatal immediate early gene expression with the intensity of stereotypy expression induced by repeated administration of amphetamine and cocaine (Canales and Graybiel, 2000). Results of this study showed that the ratio of striosomal to matrix activation was tightly correlated with the intensity of stereotypy expression (Canales and Graybiel, 2000). These findings suggested that in addition to the indirect-direct pathways regulating movement inhibition and release, another pathway exists that regulates movement frequency and selection (Canales and Graybiel, 2000). Striosomes receive cortical input from the limbic orbitofrontal and anterior cingulate cortex and project to the substantia nigra, thus regulating the availability of dopamine to the striatum

(Graybiel, 2000). Enhanced activation of striosomal neurons may promote stereotypy expression by altering normal patterns of reward and saliency signaling by corticostriatal and nigrostriatal pathways, decreasing the range of behaviors selected and increasing the repetition of those behaviors (Canales and Graybiel, 2000).

C. The Transgenic Model

While Graybiel's findings clearly established a role for the basal ganglia in the expression of stereotypies, they also emphasized the need to investigate cortical contributions to this behavior. Hyperactivation of glutamatergic cortical projection neurons has been proposed as a causative mechanism in TS and several lines of evidence support this hypothesis (Weeks, 1996). Seizures of the cingulate cortex, a secondary motor area associated with integration of motor and affective information give rise to involuntary vocalizations and orofacial movements (Levin and Duchowny, 1991; Mazars, 1970). PET scans show decreased perfusion in this area in TS patients, and fMRI showed increased signal intensity in this region during tic suppression. (Chase et al., 1986). The ability of most TS patients to voluntarily suppress their tics suggests involvement of the medial prefrontal cortex, and imaging studies have shown an increase in basal glucose metabolism in the medial prefrontal and orbitofrontal cortices (Chase et al., 1986; Cunningham and Jones, 1993). Two studies using transcranial magnetic stimulation (TMS) have found evidence of abnormalities in the primary motor cortex of TS patients (Zieman et al., 1997; Greenberg et al., 2000).

1. Description of the Model

The D1CT-7 transgenic mouse is currently the best animal model for investigating the effects of cortical hyperactivity on stereotypy expression. This animal line, developed by Dr. Frank Burton at the University of Minnesota, expresses a transgene made by fusing the promoter region for the human D1 receptor with the enzymatic portion of cholera toxin subunit alpha 1 (A1) gene (Burton et al., 1991; Campbell et al., 1999). The A1 subunit catalyzes the transfer of an ADP-ribose moiety from NADH to the alpha subunit of activated heterotrimeric Gs proteins (Burton et al., 1991). Because ribosylation of Gs inhibits its intrinsic GTPase ability, the molecule remains in an irreversibly active state. The net cellular effect is hyperresponsiveness to all afferent stimuli and enhanced neurotransmitter release due to chronic activation of adenylate cyclase with elevation of cAMP levels and its associated downstream targets (Campbell, 1999).

Interestingly, despite the fact that D1 expression is highest in the basal ganglia, expression of the D1CT transgene is restricted to the piriform cortex layer II, and somatosensory cortex layers II–III, and the amygdalar intercalated nucleus (ICN) (Campbell, 1999). Neurons in these layers of the somatosensory and piriform cortex project laterally and also to deeper layer output neurons that innervate the dorsal and ventral striatum, respectively (Campbell, 1999). The ICN regulates excitatory output from the basolateral and central amygdaloid nuclei, which project to the prefrontal cortex and ventral striatum (Campbell, 1999).

The behaviors of D1CT-7 mice are consistent with heightened activity of the anatomical regions expressing the transgene. The mice are generally hyperactive and exhibit perseveration in all behaviors; however, in contrast to psychostimulant-induced stereotypies, D1CT-7 mice can be easily distracted during these behaviors (Campbell, 1999). Initial studies indicated that these mice exhibited behaviors that appeared to be primarily compulsive. For example, D1CT-7 mice of both sexes were observed to engage in persistent biting of themselves and their cage mates. However, "resident-intruder" behavioral assays revealed that D1CT-7 mice are actually less aggressive than control littermates; moreover, the biting behavior emerged prepubertally, and occurred during social grooming but not fighting (Campbell, 1999). Taken together, these findings indicated that biting behavior was likely to be analogous to trichotillomania, a hair-pulling compulsion related to TS and obsessive compulsive disorder (Van Ameringen et al., 1999; Campbell, 1999).

Recent behavioral studies indicate that in addition to compulsive behaviors, D1CT-7 mice exhibit repetitive jerking movements, or "twitches," of the head, trunk, and limbs that have several characteristics of tics (Nordstrom and Burton, 2002; McGrath et al., 2000). The twitches are simple or complex combinations of jerking movements, and occurred in flurries (defined as twitches that occurred at intervals of five seconds or less). Interestingly, males exhibited more "tic flurries" than females. Like TS, the onset of twitching occurred developmentally, appearing as early as postnatal day 16 (Nordstrum and Burton, 2002). Finally, administration of clonidine, an alpha2 adrenergic agonist used for tic suppression in TS, significantly reduced the number of twitches in D1CT-7 mice (Nordstrum and Burton, 2002).

2. Relevance to Tourette Syndrome

Based on the above information, D1CT-7 mice appear to have the greatest behavioral homology to TS of any animal model reported so far. Further studies examining the neural substrates of the compulsive and tic-like behaviors of these mice may provide valuable insights into normal and abnormal mechanisms by corticostriatal loops that regulate behavioral selection and release. Moreover, the similarity of the D1CT-7 behaviors to tic behaviors suggests that this model may have good predictive validity in developing therapeutic drugs for the treatment of tics.

D. The Autoimmune Model

The hypothesis that infections may trigger tic disorders is not new. In 1929, Selling proposed that the majority of tics arise from "... toxic encephalitis due to absorption from an extracerebral focus" and presciently suggested treatment directed toward "early recognition and proper handling of infection" (Selling, 1929). However, research into the relationship between infections and tic disorders really began in the last decade, spurred in large part by a renewed interest in Sydenham chorea (SC) as a neuropsychiatric manifestation of poststreptococcal rheumatic fever.

SC is the most common acquired choreiform movement disorder of childhood, affecting females more often than males. Characteristic symptoms include rapid, involuntary contractions of facial, trunk, and limb muscles, but children with SC often display tics, emotional lability, and symptoms of obsessive compulsive and attention deficit disorders (Swedo, 1994; Mercadante, 2000). A finding key to understanding how streptococcal infection could produce motor and psychiatric symptoms was the discovery of antibodies in the serum of SC patients that reacted with basal ganglia nuclei and streptococcal antigens (Husby, 1976). Kiessling and colleagues (1993) hypothesized that a similar "molecular mimicry" could be the pathogenic mechanism in some cases of TS and OCD. Antineuronal antibodies were present in the sera from a cohort of children with recent onset of tics following streptococcal infections. In 1998, National Institute of Mental Health (NIMH) defined a new diagnostic subgroup of individuals with childhood onset tics and OCD: pediatric autoimmune neuropsychiatric disorders associated with streptococcal infection (PANDAS) (Swedo et al., 1998). Criteria for diagnosis included the presence of tics or OCD symptoms with a prepubertal onset, evidence of streptococcal infection, episodic symptom severity, and neurological abnormalities (Swedo et al., 1998).

Molecular mimicry, or binding of streptococcal antibodies to human basal ganglia epitopes, remains the proposed mechanism for post streptococcal tic expression in PANDAS patients. One hypothesis suggests that children expressing high levels of the B-cell surface receptor D8/17 are more vulnerable to developing rheumatic fever and neuropsychiatric disorders following Group A beta-hemolytic streptococci (GABHS) infection (Bessen, 2001).

1. Description of the Model

To establish a causal role for autoantibodies in the pathogenesis of TS, it was necessary to demonstrate that passive transfer of serum from TS patients would induce ticlike behaviors in animal models (Archelos, 2000). Hallett and colleagues (2000) were the first to report the induction of stereotypy expression following infusion of sera into the striatum of adult male rats. In this procedure, cannulae were stereotaxically implanted into the striatum of anesthetized rats. After a one-week recovery period to allow reestablishment of the blood brain barrier, the animal was again anesthetized and the cannulae were connected to polyethylene tubing filled with serum from TS patients or normal controls. The serum was driven through the cannulae by an osmotic pump implanted subcutaneously in the animal's back. Behavior was scored every day for the three days of serum infusion, and for three days after the infusion was stopped. Results of behavior scoring showed that during the period of infusion, animals that received TS sera exhibited significant increases in licking and ultrasonic vocalizations as compared to controls (Hallett et al., 2000). During the post infusion period, licking and head shaking were significantly increased in this group as compared to controls (Hallett et al., 2000).

A subsequent study by Taylor and colleagues (2002) compared induction of oral stereotypies in rats infused with TS sera containing high levels of autoantibodies, TS sera with low levels of autoantibodies, and sera from normal controls. In this study, the cannulae were implanted in the ventrolateral striatum, a region associated with the expression of oral behaviors (Kelley et al., 1988). Results of this study also showed significant increases in oral stereotypy expression in rats receiving TS serum containing high levels of antineuronal and antinuclear antibodies. However, a third laboratory was unable to replicate these findings (Loiselle et al., 2003).

2. Relevance to Tourette Syndrome

In light of the contradictory findings obtained with the autoimmune model, investigators cannot draw any conclusions yet regarding its value as an animal model of TS. However, it has been shown that therapies directed toward reducing circulating autoantibody levels in PANDAS patients provide symptom relief (Perlmutter et al., 1999). These clinical findings emphasize the need to develop experimental models in order to identify the components of the immune response that are responsible for generating tic behavior in susceptible children.

Acknowledgments

This work was supported by the National Association of Research on Schizophrenia and Depression (NARSAD), and the National Institutes of Health grants MH049351, MH01527, MH52711 (PJL). We thank Dr. Surojit Paul for helpful comments on the manuscript.

Video Legends

PSYCHOSTIMULANT MODEL OF TOURETTE SYNDROME

SEGMENT 1 Baseline.

SEGMENT 2 5 minutes after amphetamine injection.

SEGMENT 3 11 minutes after amphetamine injection.

SEGMENT 4 15 minutes after amphetamine injection.

SEGMENT 5 25 minutes after amphetamine injection.

Typical oral stereotypes associated with the psychostimulant model

SEGMENT 6 Head up sniffing.

SEGMENT 7 Head down sniffing.

SEGMENT 8 Nose poking.

SEGMENT 9 Nose poking with biting.

SEGMENT 10 Licking.

Another feature of the psychostimulant model

SEGMENT 11 Rat ignores novel object.

References

Albin, R.L., A.B. Young, and J.B. Penney. 1989. The functional anatomy of basal ganglia disorders. *Trends Neurosci* **12**:366–375.

Alexander, G.E. 1994. Basal ganglia-thalamocortical circuits: Their role in control of movements. *J Clin Neurophysiol* **11**:420–431.

Anderson, G.M., E.S. Pollak, D. Chatterjee, J.F. Leckman, M.A. Riddle, and D.J. Cohen. 1992a. Postmortem analysis of subcortical monoamines and amino acids in Tourette syndrome. *Adv Neurol* **58**:123–133.

Anderson, G.M., E.S. Pollak, D. Chatterjee, J.F. Leckman, M.A. Riddle, and D.J. Cohen. 1992b. Brain monoamines and amino acids in Gilles de la Tourette's syndrome: a preliminary study of subcortical regions. *Arch Gen Psychiatry* **49**:584–586.

Archelos, J.J., and H.P. Hartung. 2000. Pathogenetic role of autoantibodies in neurological diseases. *Trends Neurosci* **23**:317–327.

Bessen, D.E. 2001. Genetics of childhood disorders: XXXII. Autoimmune disorders, part 5: streptococcal infection and autoimmunity, an epidemiological perspective. *J Am Acad Child Adolesc Psychiatry* **40**: 1346–1348.

Black, K.J., M.H. Gado, and J.S. Perlmutter. 1997. PET measurement of dopamine D2 receptor-mediated changes in striatopallidal function. *J Neurosci* **17**:3168–3177.

Bruun, R.D., and C.L. Budman. 1992. The natural history of Tourette syndrome. *Adv Neurol* **58**:1–6.

Burton, F.H., K.W. Hasel, F.E. Bloom, and J.G. Sutcliffe. 1991. Pituitary hyperplasia and gigantism in mice caused by a cholera toxin transgene. *Nature* **350**:74–77.

Butler, I.J., S.H. Koslow, W.E. Seifert, Jr., R.M. Caprioli, and H.S. Singer. 1979. Biogenic amine metabolism in Tourette syndrome. *Ann Neurol* **6**:37–39.

Campbell, K.M., L. de Lecea, D.M. Severynse, M.G. Caron, M.J. McGrath, S.B. Sparber, L.Y. Sun, and F.H. Burton. 1999. OCD-like behaviors caused by a neuropotentiating transgene targeted to cortical and limbic D1+ neurons. *J Neurosci* **19**:5044–5053.

Campbell, K.M., R.M. Rohland, M.J. McGrath, S.D. Satoskar, and F.H. Burton. 1998. Detecting subtle differences in behavior using waveform display analysis. *Physiol Behav* **64**:83–91.

Canales, J.J., and A.M. Graybiel. 2000. A measure of striatal function predicts motor stereotypy. *Nat Neurosci* **3**:377–383.

Challas, G., J.L. Chapel, and R.L. Jenkins. 1967. Tourette's disease: Control of symptoms and its clinical course. *Int J Neuropsychiatry* **3**:Suppl. 1:95–109.

Chase, T.N., V. Geoffrey, M. Gillespie, and G.H. Burrows. 1986. Structural and functional studies of Gilles de la Tourette syndrome. *Rev Neurol (Paris)* **142**:851–855.

Cohen, D.J., A.J. Friedhoff, J.F. Leckman, and T.N. Chase. 1992. Tourette syndrome: Extending basic research to clinical care, the clinical phenotype, and natural history. *Adv Neurol* **58**:341–362.

Cohen, D.J., B.A. Shaywitz, B. Caparulo, J.G. Young, and M.B. Bowers, Jr. 1978. Chronic, multiple tics of Gilles de la Tourette's disease. CSF acid monoamine metabolites after probenecid administration. *Arch Gen Psychiatry* **35**:245–250.

Comings, D.E. 1990. *Tourette's Syndrome and Human Behavior*. Duarte, California: Hope Press.

Comings, D.E., and B.G. Comings. 1987. A controlled study of Tourette syndrome. I-VI. *Am J Hum Genet* **41**:701–838.

Creese, I., and S.D. Iversen. 1973. Blockage of amphetamine induced motor stimulation and stereotypy in the adult rat following neonatal treatment with 6-hydroxydopamine. *Brain Res* **55**:369–382.

Cunningham, V.J., and T. Jones. 1993. Spectral analysis of dynamic PET studies. *J Cereb Blood Flow Metab* **13**:15–23.

Dantzer, R. 1991. Stress, stereotypies and welfare. *Behavioural Processes* **25**:95–102.

Erenberg G., R.P. Cruse, and A.D. Rothner. 1985. Gilles de la Tourette's syndrome: effects of stimulant drugs. *Neurology* **35**:1346–1348.

Florin, S.M., R. Kuczenski, and D.S. Segal. 1994. Regional extracellular norepinephrine responses to amphetamine and cocaine and effects of clonidine pretreatment. *Brain Res* **654**:53–62.

Fowler, S.C., B.R. Birkestrand, R. Chen, S.J. Moss, E. Vorontsova, G. Wang, and T.J. Zarcone. 2001. A force-plate actometer for quantitating rodent behaviors: Illustrative data on locomotion, rotation, spatial patterning, stereotypies, and tremor. *J Neurosci Methods* **107**:107–124.

Garner, J.P., and G.J. Mason. 2002. Evidence for a relationship between cage stereotypies and behavioural disinhibition in laboratory rodents. *Behav Brain Res* **136**:83–92.

Graybiel, A.M., R. Moratalla, and H.A. Robertson. 1990. Amphetamine and cocaine induce drug-specific activation of the c-fos gene in striosome matrix compartments and limbic subdivisions of the striatum. *Proc Natl Acad Sci USA* **87**:6912–6916.

Graybiel, A.M., T. Aosaki, A.W. Flaherty, M. Kimura. 1994. The basal ganglia and adaptive motor control. *Science* **265**:1826–1831.

Graybiel, A.M., J.J. Canales, and C. Capper-Loup. 2000. Levodopa-induced dyskinesias and dopamine-dependent stereotypies: A new hypothesis. *Trends Neurosci* **23**:S71–77.

Greenberg, B.D., U. Ziemann, G. Cora-Locatelli, A. Harmon, D.L. Murphy, J.C. Keel, and E.M. Wassermann. 2000. Altered cortical excitability in obsessive-compulsive disorder. *Neurology* **54**:142–147.

Hallett, J.J., C.J. Harling-Berg, P.M. Knopf, E.G. Stopa, and L.S. Kiessling. 2000. Anti-striatal antibodies in Tourette syndrome cause neuronal dysfunction. *J Neuroimmunol* **111**:195–202.

Hallett, M. 1993. Physiology of basal ganglia disorders: An overview. *Can J Neurol Sci* **20**:177–183.

Husby, G., I. van de Rijn, J.B. Zabriskie, Z.H. Abdin, and R.C. Williams, Jr. 1976. Antibodies reacting with cytoplasm of subthalamic and caudate nuclei neurons in chorea and acute rheumatic fever. *J Exp Med* **144**:1094–1110.

Jagger, J., B.A. Prusoff, D.J. Cohen, K.K. Kidd, C.M. Carbonari, and K. John. 1982. The epidemiology of Tourette syndrome: A pilot study. *Schizophr Bull* **8**:267–278.

Jankovic, J., D.G. Glaze, J.D. Frost, Jr. 1984. Effect of tetrabenazine on tics and sleep of Gilles de la Tourette's syndrome. *Neurology* **34**:688–692.

Kelley, A.E., C.G. Lang, and A.M. Gauthier. 1988. Induction of oral stereotypy following amphetamine microinjection into a discrete subregion of the striatum. *Psychopharmacology (Berl)* **95**:556–569.

Kiessling, L.S., A.C. Marcotte, and L. Culpepper. 1993. Antineuronal antibodies in movement disorders. *Pediatrics* **92**:39–43.

Leckman, J.F. 2002. Tourette's syndrome. *The Lancet* **360**:1577–1586.

Leckman, J.F., D.E. Walker, and D.J. Cohen. 1993. Premonitory urges in Tourette's syndrome. *Am J Psychiatry* **150**:98–102.

Leckman, J.F., D.E. Walker, W.K. Goodman, D.L. Pauls, and D.J. Cohen. 1994. "Just right" perceptions associated with compulsive behaviors in Tourette's syndrome. *Am J Psychiatry* **151**:675–680.

Leckman J.F., W.K. Goodman, G.M. Anderson, M.A. Riddle, P.B. Chappell, M.T. McSwiggan-Hardin, C.J. McDougle, et al. 1995. Cerebrospinal fluid biogenic amines in obsessive compulsive disorder, Tourette's syndrome, and healthy controls. *Neuropsychopharmacology* **12**:73–86.

Levin, B., and M. Duchowny. 1991. Childhood obsessive-compulsive disorder and cingulate epilepsy. *Biol Psychiatry* **30**:1049–1055.

Loiselle, C.R., O. Lee, T.H. Moran, and H.S. Singer. 2003. Striatal microinfusion of Tourette syndrome and PANDAS sera: Failure to induce behavioral changes. *Movement Disorders* **19**:406–415.

Loiselle, C.R., O. Lee, T.H. Moran, and H.S. Singer. 2004. Striatal microinfusion of Tourette syndrome and PANDAS sera: failure to induce behavioral changes. *Mov Disord* **19**:390–396.

Mason, G.J. 1991. Stereotypies and suffering. *Behavioral Processes* **25**: 103–115.

Mazars, G. 1970. Criteria for identifying cingulate epilepsy. *Epilepsia* **11**:41–47.

McGrath, M.J., K.M. Campbell, C.R. Parks, and F.H. Burton. 2000. Glutamatergic drugs exacerbate symptomatic behavior in a transgenic model of comorbid Tourette's syndrome and obsessive-compulsive disorder. *Brain Res* **877**:23–30.

McKinney, W.T. 2001. Overview of the past contributions of animal models and their changing place in psychiatry. *Semin Clin Neuropsychiatry* **6**(1):68–78.

McKinney, W.T., R. Gardner, G.W. Barlow, and M.T. McGuire. 1994. Conceptual basis of animal models in psychiatry: a conference summary. *Ethology and Sociobiology* **15**:369–382.

Mercadante, M.T., G.F. Busatto, P.J. Lombroso, L. Prado, M.C. Rosario-Campos, R. do Valle, M.J. Marques-Dias, et al. 2000. The psychiatric symptoms of rheumatic fever. *Am J Psychiatry* **157**:2036–2038.

Mink, J.W. 2001. Basal ganglia dysfunction in Tourette's syndrome: A new hypothesis. *Pediatr Neurol* **25**:190–198.

Nordstrom, E.J., and F.H. Burton. 2002. A transgenic model of comorbid Tourette's syndrome and obsessive-compulsive disorder circuitry. *Mol Psychiatry* **7**:617–625, 524.

Overall, K.L. 2000. Natural animal models of human psychiatric conditions: Assessment of mechanism and validity. *Prog Neuropsychopharmacol Biol Psychiatry* **24**:727–776.

Pauls, D.L., C. Raymond, J. Stevenson, and J.F. Leckman. 1991. A family study of Gilles de la Tourette syndrome. *Am J Hum Genet* **48**:154–163.

Pauls, D.L., K.E. Towbin, J.F. Leckman, G. Zahner, and D.J. Cohen. 1986. Gilles de la Tourette's syndrome and obsessive-compulsive disorder: Evidence supporting a genetic relationship. *Arch Gen Psychiatry* **43**: 1180–1182.

Perlmutter, S.J., S.F. Leitman, M.A. Garvey, S. Hamburger, E. Feldman, H.L. Leonard, and S.E. Swedo. 1999. Therapeutic plasma exchange and intravenous immunoglobulin for obsessive-compulsive disorder and tic disorders in childhood. *The Lancet* **354**:1153–1158.

Randrup, A., and I. Munkvad. 1974. Pharmacology and physiology of stereotyped behavior. *J Psychiatr Res* **11**:1–10.

Randrup A., I. Munkvad, and P. Udsen. 1963. Adrenergic Mechanisms and Amphetamine Induced Abnormal Behaviour. *Acta pharmacol Toxicol (Copenh)* **20**:145–157.

Rebec, G.V. 1984. Auto- and postsynaptic dopamine receptors in the central nervous system. *Monogr Neural Sci* **10**:207–223.

Ridley, R.M. 1994. The psychology of perseverative and stereotyped behaviour. *Progress in Neurobiology* **44**:221–231.

Robinson, T.E., and J.B. Becker. 1986. Enduring changes in brain and behavior produced by chronic amphetamine administration: a review and evaluation of animal models of amphetamine psychosis. *Brain Res* **396**:157–198.

Selling, L. 1929. The role of infection in the etiology of tics. *Arch Neurol Psychiatry* **22**:1163–1171.

Shapiro, A.K., E.S. Shapiro, J.G. Young, and T.E. Feinberg. 1988. History of Tourette and tic disorders. In *Gilles de la Tourette Syndrome*. Ed. A.K. Shapiro, J.G. Young, T.E. Feinberg. pp. 1–27. New York: Raven Press.

Shapiro, E., A.K. Shapiro, G. Fulop, M. Hubbard, J. Mandeli, J. Nordlie, and R.A. Phillips. 1989. Controlled study of haloperidol, pimozide and placebo for the treatment of Gilles de la Tourette's syndrome. *Arch Gen Psychiatry* **46**:722–730.

Singer H.S., and J.T. Wendlandt. 2001. Neurochemistry and synaptic neurotransmission in Tourette syndrome. *Adv Neurol* **85**:163–178.

Singer H.S., L.E. Tune, I.J. Butler, R. Zaczek, and J.T. Coyle. 1982. Clinical symptomatology, CSF neurotransmitter metabolites, and serum haloperidol levels in Tourette syndrome. *Adv Neurol* **35**:177–183.

Sweet, R.D., R. Bruun, E. Shapiro, and A.K. Shapiro. 1974. Presynaptic catecholamine antagonists as treatment for Tourette syndrome. Effects of alpha methyl para tyrosine and tetrabenazine. *Arch Gen Psychiatry* **31**:857–861.

Swedo, S.E., and H.L. Leonard. 1994. Childhood movement disorders and obsessive compulsive disorder. *J Clin Psychiatry* **55 Suppl**:32–37.

Swedo, S.E., H.L. Leonard, M. Garvey, B. Mittleman, A.J. Allen, S. Perlmutter, S. Dow, et al. 1998. Pediatric autoimmune neuropsychiatric disorders associated with streptococcal infections: Clinical description of the first 50 cases. *Am J Psychiatry* **155**:264–271.

Swerdlow, N.R., and J.F. Leckman. 2002. Tourette Syndrome and Related Tic Disorders, In *Neuropsychopharmacology: The Fifth Generation of Progress*. Ed. Kenneth L. Davis, Dennis Charney, Joseph T. Coyle, and C. Nemeroff. Lippincott, Philadelphia, PA: Williams & Wilkins.

Taylor, J.R., S.A. Morshed, S. Parveen, M.T. Mercadante, L. Scahill, B.S. Peterson, R.A. King, et al. 2002. An animal model of Tourette's syndrome. *Am J Psychiatry* **159**:657–660.

Van Ameringen, M., C. Mancini, J.M. Oakman, and P. Farvolden. 1999. The potential role of haloperidol in the treatment of trichotillomania. *J Affect Disord* **56**:219–226.

Weeks, R.A., N. Turjanski, and D.J. Brooks. 1996. Tourette's syndrome: A disorder of cingulate and orbitofrontal function? *Q J M* **89**:401–408.

Wilner, P. 1986. Validation criteria for animal models of human mental disorders: learned helplessness as a paradigm case. *Prog Neuropsychopharmacol Biol Psychiat* **10**:677–690.

Wurbel, H. 2001. Ideal homes? Housing effects on rodent brain and behavior. *Trends Neurosci* **24**:207–211.

Ziemann, U., W. Paulus, and A. Rothenberger. 1997. Decreased motor inhibition in Tourette's disorder: Evidence from transcranial magnetic stimulation. *Am J Psychiatry* **154**:1277–1284.

CHAPTER

H1

Paroxysmal Dyskinesias in Humans

KAILASH P. BHATIA

I. HISTORICAL ASPECTS, CLASSIFICATION, AND DEFINITION OF PAROXYSMAL MOVEMENT DISORDERS

Mount and Reback (1940) first used the term "paroxysmal dystonic choreoathetosis" (PDC) when reporting a 23-year-old man with attacks of choreo dystonia lasting many hours [1]. He was from a family with many others similarly affected [1]. In 1941, Smith and Heersema reported what they called "periodic dystonia" [2]; their cases were probably similar to those of Kertesz (1967), who introduced the new term paroxysmal *kinesigenic* choreo athetosis (PKC) [3], noting that attacks in their cases were induced by a sudden movement, hence, kinesigenic. Kertesz, however, felt that this condition probably represented a *forme fruste* of the disorder described by Mount and Reback, and not a separate entity. Between attacks the patients in both disorders appeared to be entirely normal. As more cases of these two conditions were reported in the literature, certain clinical characteristics of the two conditions became clear. For instance, it became apparent that episodes in PDC could last several hours and were often precipitated by drinking alcohol, coffee, or tea, and by fatigue and smoking [4,5]. In this regard, Lance (1977), when describing a four-generation family, observed that "the (dystonic) attacks lasted up to 4 hours, were precipitated by alcohol, emotion, or fatigue." This family appears to have the same condition as that described by Mount and Reback termed "paroxysmal dystonic choreoathetosis" [6]. Lance tried to differentiate this from paroxysmal kinesigenic choreoathetosis, mentioning that an analysis of 100 cases of PKC showed that the attacks were brief, lasting less than 5 minutes, were precipitated by sudden movement or startle, and usually responded well to phenytoin or barbiturates. He divided the kinesigenic form into a familial group (72% of cases) and a sporadic group (28% of cases). In the same paper, a family was reported that Lance called the *intermediate form*, in which episodes of dystonia (choreoathetosis) were provoked by continued exertion and lasted for up to 30 minutes or so. Lance thus classified the paroxysmal dyskinesias based primarily on duration of attacks into three types: [1] PKC, in which there were brief attacks up to 5 minutes induced by sudden movement; [2] PDC, in which attacks were not induced by sudden movement and were of long duration up to 4 hours; and [3] paroxysmal exercise-induced dystonia (PED), the intermediate type, in which attacks were induced by prolonged exercise but the duration was more than 5 minutes but less than what was seen in typical PDC [6]. Demerkiran and Jankovic [7] more recently proposed a modification of the earlier classification of Lance [6]. They

TABLE 1 Causes of Secondary Paroxysmal Dyskinesias

Multiple sclerosis
Vascular lesions
Metabolic disorders/endocrine
Hypoparathyroidism
Thyroid dysfunction
Hypoglycemia
Hyperglycemia
Trauma
Central-head injuries
Peripheral trauma
CNS infections
HIV
Other
Post encephalitis
Post kernicterus
Brain tumors
Other causes

suggested replacing the term choreoathetosis with dyskinesias, as a variety of different movements can be seen in these disorders. They also suggested two broad groupings of these disorders, namely "paroxysmal kinesigenic dyskinesia" (PKD) if the disorder was induced by sudden movement, and "paroxysmal non-kinesigenic dyskinesia" (PNKD) if it was not. Those cases in which exercise was the precipitating cause were described as paroxysmal exercise-induced dyskinesia (PED). These terms broadly correlate to PKC, PDC, and the intermediate variety of the old classification. It had also become clear over the years that, apart from idiopathic familial cases, secondary or symptomatic cases due to a variety of etiologies could cause similar paroxysmal dyskinesias.

Paroxysmal dyskinesias are a rare group of conditions manifesting as abnormal involuntary movements that recur episodically and last for only a brief duration [8]. The abnormal movements may be choreic, dystonic, ballistic, or a mixture of these. Between episodes the patient is generally normal. The condition may be inherited or acquired. This chapter will focus on the idiopathic (primary) group of paroxysmal movement disorders, providing an update with regard to the clinical and genetic aspects and the pathophysiology of these conditions [9]. Table 1 shows the common causes of secondary (symptomatic) dyskinesias; readers are referred to a recent review article [10] about this group of disorders, which will not be covered here further.

II. PAROXYSMAL KINESIGENIC DYSKINESIA (PKD/PKC)

As first mentioned by Kertesz (1967), in this condition brief dyskinetic episodes are precipitated by *sudden* movement [3]. Typically this involves getting up suddenly from a chair when sitting, quickly responding to a telephone call, or breaking into a sudden run when spotting a bus. Rarely, episodes occur at rest and even during sleep. An "aura-like" sensation in the affected limb occurs in about 60% of cases with PKD [11]. Dystonia is the common manifestation sometimes associated with chorea or ballism; attacks commonly involve the hemi-body, in some almost always on the same side or alternating sides [11]. Rarely the episodes become generalized. Speech can be affected, but consciousness is not lost. Typically PKD attacks are very brief and frequent, and an attack will last from seconds to 1 to 2 minutes, occasionally up to 5 minutes. There can be dozens of attacks per day. After an attack there is usually a short refractory period before another attack can be triggered. The kinesigenic form usually occurs from early childhood; in a recently reported series of 26 idiopathic cases, the mean age of onset was 13 years (range, 1 to 39 years) [11]. Males are more commonly affected (8,11); in this series by Houser and associates, the male to female ratio was 7 : 1 [11]. Most cases are idiopathic and apparently sporadic. Family history is present in about 23% of cases and usually follows an autosomal dominant pattern of inheritance [11]. An association with epilepsy has been recognized in some familial cases with PKD. This was first reported in two papers describing families with the affected person having infantile convulsions with later onset of episodes of paroxysmal choreoathetosis (called *i*nfantile *c*onvulsions and *c*horeo*a*thetosis (ICCA) syndrome [12,13]. These families were linked to the pericentromic region of chromosome 16p12–q12 [12,13]. In both these reports, attacks of paroxysmal choreoathetosis in the affected person resembled PKD in being very brief, frequent, and induced by sudden exertion. Thereafter, reports of families with typical PKD with or without epilepsy have appeared to show linkage to the same region of chromosome 16 [14–16].

PKD patients respond dramatically to low doses of antiepileptics, with a particular sensitivity to carbamazepine, which is the drug of choice (11); response to phenytoin is also good. The attack frequency of PKD wanes over time, decreasing considerably or abating in adulthood.

III. PAROXYSMAL NON-KINESIGENIC DYSKINESIA (PNKD)/PDC

PNKD attacks can be spontaneous but often are precipitated by alcohol or coffee, as mentioned in the earliest descriptions of the disorder (1). The episode, once started, usually lasts many hours; however, unlike PKD, the episodes are infrequent, with long attack-free intervals. Idiopathic PNKD also has its onset in childhood or teenage years with intermittent episodes, which tend to be a mixture of dystonia and chorea [17]. As with PKD, more males than females are affected (1.4 : 1) [17], and after onset in childhood there is a tendency for the attacks to wane with age.

The initial report by Mount and Reback was of a family with a clear autosomal dominant pattern of inheritance; other families reported also showed a similar pattern [1,18–21]. Generally typical PNKD/PDC cases have no detectable abnormalities between attacks, although there was one report of a patient with PDC who also had some interictal dystonia [17] and another of a family with PDC with interictal myokymia [22]. There was also a report of a large German family in whom affected members had PNKD along with spasticity as well as other symptoms, including perioral paresthesias, double vision, headache, and generalized myoclonic jerks often culminating in a seizure with unconsciousness [23]. Because some affected persons also had marked spastic paraparesis, this condition is referred to as *CSE* (choreoathetosis/spasticity, episodic movement disorder) [23], making this condition quite different from typical PNKD. Two groups have linked families with typical autosomal dominant PNKD to chromosome 2q, although the gene has not yet been identified [19,20]. In the family with CSE mentioned above with PNKD and spasticity, it has been linked to a different locus on chromosome 1p; again, the gene remains unknown [23].

PNKD is quite difficult to treat compared with PKD, as these cases do not usually benefit from antiepileptics. Some patients may respond to levodopa [24]; other drugs, including anticholinergics, acetazolamide, and benzodiazepines such as clonazepam, have been tried with limited success.

IV. PAROXYSMAL EXERCISE-INDUCED DYSKINESIA (PED)

In this disorder the attacks begin after 10 or 15 min of continuing exercise, rather than at the initiation of movement [25]. The attacks are usually dystonic and appear in the body part involved in the exercise, most commonly the legs after prolonged walking or running; even focal dystonia of the jaw after chewing gum has been reported [26]. Exposure to cold [27], passive movements and vibration [28], as well as transcranial magnetic stimulation of the motor cortex [29] have been reported to induce attacks apart from exercise in persons affected with this disorder. The dystonic episodes usually wane 10 to 15 minutes after the provoking activity or exercise is stopped, and the patient is usually normal between episodes. PED is a rare disorder; apart from a handful of sporadic cases, only a few families have been described, mostly with an autosomal dominant pattern of inheritance [25]. Initially it was believed that familial PED might be a forme fruste of PNKD [30]. However, linkage to the PNKD locus on chromosome 2q has been excluded in at least one family with typical PED [26]. Also, it is becoming clear that there may be some overlap clinically between PKD and PED with regard to triggering factors. For example, the dyskinetic attacks in patients with the so-called ICCA syndrome mentioned earlier could be triggered both by sudden movements and by ongoing exercise. Interestingly, in this regard a recessive family with rolandic epilepsy, episodes of exercise-induced dystonia, and writer's cramp (RE-PED-WC syndrome) has been linked to chromosome 16p 12–11.2 [31] in the same region as the families with the ICCA syndrome [12,13], again suggesting a possible overlap between these disorders.

However, unlike typical PKD, anticonvulsants are only occasionally useful for PED; in this regard clonazepam but not carbamazepine may be helpful [25]. Levodopa, acetazolamide, and anticholinergics can sometimes be beneficial, but drug treatment is usually disappointing [25].

V. PAROXYSMAL HYPNOGENIC DYSKINESIA (PHD)

This disorder has been added to the three classic forms of paroxysmal dyskinesias described above. In this condition episodes of paroxysmal dyskinesia occur in sleep, hence the term "hypnogenic." Lugaresi and Cirignotta (1981) described five patients who had attacks almost every night [32]. Further similar sporadic and familial cases were described [33–36]. In a typical episode the patient awakens with a cry and has involuntary dystonic and ballistic thrashing movements, mainly of the legs (but can spread to the arm and neck), lasting up to 45 seconds, with no detectable concurrent EEG abnormalities. Several attacks can occur each night. This disorder was often misdiagnosed and thought to represent night terrors or some other type of sleep disorder [36]. It has recently become clear that in most of these cases, especially the familial variety, these nocturnal dyskinesias are due to mesial frontal lobe seizures (which are often difficult to pick up on surface EEG recordings) [34,35]. ADNFLE (*a*utosomal *d*ominant *n*octurnal *f*rontal *l*obe *e*pilepsy) was the eponym given to describe this condition in six families in whom affected members had typical PHD attacks [35]. The gene responsible for ADNFLE has been discovered in a few families and is usually due to an abnormality in the family of nicotinic acetylcholine receptor genes (see section below).

VI. OTHER EXAMPLES OF PAROXYSMAL DYSKINESIAS

A. Paroxysmal Benign Torticollis of Infancy

This is a relatively rare disorder with onset in infancy with episodes of torticollis with or without tortipellvis [37]. The duration is hours rarely up to a few days. The episodes are infrequent, with one to two occurring in a day at times.

There have been some suggestions of a relationship to migraine (basilar variety) and kinestosis [37]. This is because, with time, episodes of head tilt become less prominent, replaced by vertigo, vomiting, lassitude, and migraine-like headaches. Recently, two cases with BPT were described from families with familial hemiplegic migraine linked with calcium channel gene (CACLNA1) [38]. This is interesting, given the hypothesis (see below) that the paroxysmal dyskinesias may be to due to ion channel abnormalities.

B. Familial Hyperekplexia (Startle Disease)

Hyperekplexia, also known as hereditary startle disease, is a rare neurogenetic disorder characterized by exaggerated startle response and neonatal hypertonia [39,40]. This is predominantly an autosomal dominant disease, with many fewer autosomal recessive and sporadic cases reported. The disease is rare, and the prevalence remains unknown. It mainly affects northern European descendants. Suhren and associates, describing kindred in 1966, called it "hyperexplexia" (Greek) [40], which was subsequently changed to "hyperekplexia." Clinically there is a difference between newborns and adults. Newborns with hyperekplexia manifest diffuse hypertonia, hyperreflexia, and exaggerated startle response to noise and handling shortly after birth [39,40]. The startle attack can be easily elicited by tapping on the nose and consists of sudden head retraction and body tonic flexion. The hypertonicity and hyperreflexia are transient and usually diminish spontaneously after the first year of life, although early motor milestones may be delayed due to hypertonicity. Those affected may refuse to ambulate in their early childhood because of the fear of frequent falls due to exaggerated startle reflex, which usually persists into adult life. The abnormal startle response is usually triggered by loud or unexpected noises and constitutes sudden stiffness and fall to the ground with arms by both sides and without loss of consciousness. Patients can suffer severe injuries, including facial laceration and skull or limb fractures, from the attacks. They often have an uncertain gait, with the fear of falling. Untreated adults with hyperekplexia can be severely debilitated and eventually wheelchair-bound to avoid severe injury from frequent falls with excessive startle response. Routine investigations, including imaging, are normal in primary hyperekplexia, as there is no gross or microscopic pathology in the nervous system. Specialized electromyographic (EMG) reflex studies, recording the response of head and limb muscles to acoustic and tactile stimuli, have demonstrated higher sensitivity, shorter latency, higher muscle response amplitude, and much less habituation in hyperekplexia, as compared to normal controls [41–43]. The earliest responder to the stimuli is the sternocleidomastoid muscle, suggesting a brainstem origin of the reflex. Hyperekplexia is a highly treatable disease, with clonazepam the drug of choice, which dramatically diminishes exaggerated startle response [44]. However, it does not reduce infantile hypertonicity to the same degree. Patients usually require high doses (0.1 to 0.2 mg/kg/day) of clonazepam and tolerate it very well without loss of effectiveness over time [44]. With regard to genetics, the hyperekplexia gene was initially linked to the long arm of chromosome 5 (5q33–35) by a linkage study in a large kindred study; subsequently, the alpha 1 subunit of the inhibitory glycine receptor (GLRA1) gene was found to be the defective gene in hyperekplexia [45–49]. The inhibitory glycine receptor is a member of the neurotransmitter–gated ion channel superfamily that includes GABA, glutamate, and nicotinic acetylcholine receptors. It is a ligand–gated chloride channel provoking postsynaptic hyperpolarization, which mediates synaptic inhibition in brainstem and spinal cord, where it is primarily expressed. Several missense mutations of GLRA1 gene have been identified in families with autosomal dominant hyperekplexia [46–49]. Most cases of the sporadic hyperekplexia do not carry mutations in GLRA1 gene, although compound heterozygous mutations in GLRA1 gene have been described.

C. Familial Dyskinesia and Facial Myokymia (FDFM)

Recently a novel autosomal dominant disorder characterized by adventitious movements that sometimes appear choreiform and that are associated with perioral and periorbital myokymia has been described, called familial dyskinesia and facial myokymia (FDFM) [50]. It was reported in a single five-generation family, with 18 affected members (ten males and eight females). The disorder is said to have an early childhood or adolescent onset; the involuntary movements are *paroxysmal* at early ages, but increase in frequency and severity, and may become constant in the third decade. Thereafter, there is no further deterioration, and there may even be improvement in old age. The adventitious movements are worsened by anxiety but not by voluntary movement, startle, caffeine, or alcohol. All known paroxysmal dyskinesia loci were excluded in this family, which may suggest that a novel gene underlies this condition.

VII. PATHOPHYSIOLOGY

Since the very first descriptions of the paroxysmal movement disorders, there has been much controversy regarding their pathophysiology. Many authors regard these to be a form of reflex epilepsy, perhaps involving the thalamus or the basal ganglia, particularly with reference to PKD/PKC as an example [51,52]. Their main arguments are the paroxysmal nature of the attacks, the aura at onset, the nonprogressive (often remitting) character of the disorder, and the excellent response to anticonvulsants [51]. The absence of seizure discharges on EEG in the majority of cases, the absence of evolution of the attacks into generalized or focal convulsions, and the lack of an associated loss of consciousness or amnesia is said to fit in with the possibility of a subcortical, rather than cortical, focus. Also in support of this are cases in which both epilepsy and paroxysmal dyskinesia are present, both aspects responding to antiepileptics [12,13,53].

On the other hand, a basal ganglia disorder is a view favored by some authors based on the clinical characteristics of the involuntary movements, the absence of EEG abnormalities during attacks, the occurrence of symptomatic PKC due to lesions, or conditions known to affect basal ganglia [10]. There has been support for this extrapyramidal theory based on special electrophysiological studies known to be abnormal in basal ganglia disorders. Abnormalities of contingent negative variation (CNV), which, normalized with phenytoin therapy in PKC, have been reported [54], as well as abnormalities of the premotor (*Bereitschafts*) potential in the same disorder [11]. Abnormally decreased choline/creatine ratios in the basal ganglia were found on magnetic resonance spectroscopy in PKC [55], and increased perfusion of the thalamus was noted on SPECT scans [56]. Furthermore, increased CSF dopamine metabolites have been noted following an attack in both PNKD and PED [21,57], and decreased presynaptic dopamine decarboxylase activity with increased D2 postsynaptic receptors has been suggested by 18 fluorodopa and raclopride scan changes, respectively, in PNKD [58].

Although this debate is still inconclusive, what is clear is that the paroxysmal dyskinesias have many similarities to other episodic disorders of the nervous system, such as episodic ataxias and periodic paralysis, thus suggesting a common pathophysiological mechanism [9]. More and more paroxysmal neurological disorders are now being discovered to be caused by gene mutations regulating ion channels [59–64] called channelopathies. The periodic paralyses were found to be caused by mutations in voltage-gated sodium [61] and calcium [62] channels. Subsequently, the two forms of episodic ataxias (EA1 and EA2) were shown to be caused by mutations of voltage-gated potassium [59] and calcium channels [64]. It is interesting to observe the similarities between PKD and episodic ataxia type 1 (EA1). EA1 is characterized by periodic ataxia, frequently provoked by kinesigenic stimuli similar to the attacks of PKC; the episodes are brief, lasting from seconds to a few minutes, and they can occur several times a day [65]. Both PKC and EA1 have an early age of onset, and both have the tendency to abate in adulthood. Although EA1 typically responds to acetazolamide like PKD does, anticonvulsants may reduce EA1 attacks in some patients and also help the interictal myokymia seen in this disorder [65,66]. Like the paroxysmal dyskinesias, many of these other paroxysmal disorders have similar precipitating factors such as stress, fatigue, and diet. There is also an overlap for many of these disorders with regard to drug treatment. For example, acetazolamide is helpful not only for periodic paralysis, but also for myotonia, episodic ataxias [63], and some paroxysmal dyskinesias [25]. Carbamazepine, an antiepileptic, is also very effective in patients with paroxysmal kinesigenic dyskinesia. There are also reports of families with multiple episodic disorders, for example, paroxysmal dyskinesia in a family with episodic ataxia and association of episodic problems such as migraine and epilepsy in families with paroxysmal dyskinesias [16,26]. Thus, like periodic paralysis and episodic ataxias, the familial paroxysmal dyskinesias may also be caused by defects in genes regulating ion channels [2].

VIII. GENES/GENETIC LOCI

A. Paroxysmal Kinesigenic Dyskinesia (PKC/PKD)

Szepetowski and colleagues linked four French families with what was described as the "ICCA syndrome" (infantile convulsions and paroxysmal choreoathetosis) to the pericentromeric region of chromosome 16 [12]. Linkage to the same locus was further confirmed in a Chinese family said to have a similar disorder [13]. Although description of the paroxysmal dyskinetic episodes in these reports was rather limited, they did seem similar to PKD. Not surprisingly, eight Japanese families [14] and an African-American kindred [15], both with typical PKC, were also linked to the pericentromeric region of chromosome 16. In these Japanese families there was an increased prevalence of afebrile infantile convulsions; therefore, it was suggested that one gene may be responsible for both PKC and ICCA [14]. However, the PKC interval identified in the African-American family in which individuals had PKC alone (and no infantile seizures) overlaps by 3.4 cM with the ICCA region and by 9.8 cM with the PKC region identified in Japanese families. Thus at the moment it is unclear whether there are two genes or a single gene in this interval that could give rise to both ICCA and PKC in these families. Furthermore, an autosomal recessive family with rolandic epilepsy, paroxysmal exercise-induced dyskinesia, and writer's cramp (RE-PED-WC) syndrome (see above in the section on Clinical Features) has also been linked to chromosome 16 within the ICCA region but outside the 3.4 cM overlap between ICCA and PKC [31]. Thus, RE-PED-WC is probably allelic to ICCA but not PKC. Furthermore, an Indian family with PKC has been linked to a second locus on chromosome 16q, distinct from the locus of the Japanese families with PKC [16], thus suggesting that there may be a family of genes causing paroxysmal disorders on the pericentromeric region of chromosome 16 [16]. Since the gene is likely to be an ion channel gene, different candidate genes, including the sodium/hydrogen exchanger and other ion channel genes, have been considered and excluded [67] and the gene remains unknown. There are also families with PKC that do not link to chromosome 16 at all [68], thus suggesting at least one more locus and confirming that PKD is genetically heterogeneous.

B. Paroxysmal Non-Kinesigenic Dyskinesia (PNKD)

Two separate groups reported linkage to microsatellite markers on distal 2q (2q31–q36) [20–21]. This was further confirmed in a British family (69) and also other families with typical PNKD and autosomal dominant inhertitance [70–72]. It appears therefore that there is *genetic homogeneity* for typical familial PNKD/PDC. A variety of candidate genes (mostly ion channels), including the acid-sensing ion channels (ASICs) and others, have been excluded in the area of linkage [70,73–74], but the gene has not been found.

C. Autosomal Dominant Nocturnal Frontal Lobe Epilepsy (ADNFLE)

In an Australian family, Phillips et al. (1995) mapped an ADNFLE locus on chromosome 20q13.2; the obvious candidate was the alpha 4 subunit of the neuronal acetylcholine receptor (*CHRNA4*) gene [75]. Two different mutations—a missense mutation and a 3-bp insertion—were then identified in the CHRNA4 gene in the Australian family and in a Norwegian family, respectively [76,77]. However, another family with ADNFLE was linked not to *CHRNA4* on chromosome 20q but to a novel locus on chromosome 15q24 close to a *CHRNA3/CNRNA5/CHRNB4* nicotinic acetylcholine receptor gene cluster [78]. Also, in seven other families with ADNFLE and in seven sporadic cases, linkage to the ADNFLE loci on chromosome 20q13.2 and 15q24 was excluded, thereby suggesting the existence of at least a third ADNFLE locus and supporting the fact that ADNFLE is a genetically heterogeneous disease [78].

D. Other Paroxysmal Dyskinesias

Benign positional torticollis (BPT) of infancy has been reported in four cases from families with familial hemiplegic migraine, which is linked to a calcium channel gene (CACLNA1) [38]. It is not clear whether there were any functional mutations of the CACLNA1 in these cases and whether this applies to all cases with BPT. Further reports are awaited.

With regard to the startle syndrome, hyperekplexia, as mentioned above, this is due to the defective alpha 1 subunit of the inhibitory glycine receptor (GLRA1) gene [45–46]. The inhibitory glycine receptor is a member of the neurotransmitter–gated ion channel superfamily that includes GABA, glutamate, and nicotinic acetylcholine receptors. It is a ligand–gated chloride channel, provoking postsynaptic hyperpolarization, which mediates synaptic inhibition in brain stem and spinal cord, where it is primarily expressed. Several missense mutations of GLRA1 gene have been identified in families with autosomal dominant hyperekplexia [47–49]. These missense mutations result in amino acid

TABLE 2 Mapped Loci/Genes for Familial Paroxysmal Dyskinesia Conditions

Condition	Chromosome	Gene	Ion channel
PNKD			
Familial paroxysmal non-kinesigenic dyskinesia (PNKD)	2q33–35	not known	not known
Paroxysmal choreoathetosis/spasticity	1p	not known	not known
PKD/ICCA			
Infantile convulsions & paroxysmal choreoathetosis (ICCA)	16p12–q12	not known	not known
Familial paroxysmal kinesigenic dyskinesias (PKD)	16p11.2–q12.1	not known	not known
PED			
Autosomal recessive RE-WC-PED syndrome	16p12–11.2	not known	not known
HPD			
Autosomal dominant nocturnal frontal lobe epilepsy (ADNFLE)	20q13	*CHRNA4*	Ach receptor
Autosomal dominant nocturnal frontal lobe epilepsy (ADNFLE)	15q24	*CHRNA3*	Ach receptor
Familial Hyperekplexia (Startle disease)	5q	*GLRA1*	Glycine receptor
BPT			
Benign positional torticollis of infancy	19p	CACNA1	Calcium channel
FDFM			
Familial dyskinesia and facial myokymia	not known	not known	not known

Ach = Nicotinic acetylcholine receptor, GLRA1 = alpha 1 subunit of the glycine receptor gene.

changes; the most common mutations are G1192T and G1192A in exon 6 that result in the substitution of uncharged amino acids (leucine and glutamine, respectively) for Arg271, a highly conserved amino acid among different species. The Arg271 mutations have been reported in at least 12 independent families from the Netherlands, the United States, the United Kingdom, and Switzerland. Three reported autosomal recessive hyperekplexia cases were also caused by mutations in the GLRA1 gene [48].

IX. CONCLUSIONS

The paroxysmal dyskinesias are a heterogeneous group of disorders that share the feature of an episodic hyperkinetic movement disorder. There are many similarities between the paroxysmal dyskinesias and other intermittent neurological disorders such as periodic paralysis, episodic ataxias, epilepsy, and migraine, suggesting a common pathophysiology. The list of linked gene loci causing the paroxysmal dyskinesia phenotypes is growing rapidly (Table 2), although the genes for most of these conditions are still to be identified. It is, however, likely that the paroxysmal dyskinesias (such as the episodic ataxias and other such conditions) are also caused by defective ion channel genes.

Video Legends

SEGMENT 1 Paroxysmal non-kinesigenic dyskinesia (PNKD).

SEGMENT 2 Paroxysmal kinesigenic dyskinesia (PKD)

SEGMENT 3 Paroxysmal exercise-induced dyskinesia (PED).

References

1. Mount, L.A., and S. Reback. 1940. Familial paroxysmal choreoathetosis: preliminary report of a hitherto undescribed clinical syndrome. *Arch Neurol Psychiatry* **44**:841–847.
2. Smith, L.A., and P.H. Heersema. 1941. Periodic dystonia. *Mayo Clin Proc* **16**:842–846.
3. Kertesz, A. 1967. Paroxysmal kinesigenic choreoathetosis. An entity within the paroxysmal choreoathetosis syndrome. Description of 10 cases, including 1 autopsied. *Neurology* **17**:680–690.
4. Forssman, H. 1961. Hereditary disorder characterized by attacks of muscular contractions, induced by alcohol amongst other factors. *Acta Med Scand* **170**:517–533.
5. Lance, J.W. 1963. Sporadic and familial varieties of tonic seizures. *J Neurol Neurosurg Psychiatry* **26**:51–59.
6. Lance, J.W. 1977. Familial paroxysmal dystonic choreoathetosis and its differentiation from related syndromes. *Ann Neurol* **2**:285–293.
7. Demirkirin, M., and J. Jankovic. 1995. Paroxysmal dyskinesias: clinical features and classification. *Ann Neurol* **38**:571–579.
8. Fahn, S. 1994. The paroxysmal dyskinesias. In: Marsden C.D., and S. Fahn. Movement Disorders 3, Butterworth-Heinmann Ltd, Oxford 310–345.
9. Bhatia, K.P., R.C. Griggs, and L.J. Ptacek. 2000. Episodic movement disorders as channelopaties. *Mov Disord* **15**:429–433.
10. Blakeley, J., and J. Jankovic. 2002. *Mov Disord* **17**:726–734.
11. Houser, M.K., V.L. Soland, K.P. Quinn, N.P. Bhatia, and C.D. Marsden. 1999. Paroxysmal kinesigenic choreoathetosis: a report of 26 cases. *J Neurol* **246**:120–126.
12. Szepetowski, P., J. Rochette, P. Berquin, C. Piussan, G.M. Lathrop, and A.P. Monaco. 1997. Familial infantile convulsions and paroxysmal choreoathetosis: a new neurological syndrome linked to the pericentromic region of human chromosome 16. *Am J Hum Genet* **61**:889–898.
13. Lee, W.L., A. Tay, H.T. Ong, L.M. Goh, A.P. Monaco, and P. Szepetowski. 1998. Association of infantile convulsions with paroxysmal dyskinesias (ICCA syndrome): confirmation of linkage to human chromosome 16p12–q12 in a Chinese family. *Hum Genet* **103**:608–612.
14. Tomita. H., S. Nagamitsu, K. Wakui, Y. Fukushima, K. Yamada, M. Sadamatsu, A. Masui, et al. 1999. Paroxysmal kinesigenic choreoathetosis locus maps to chromosome 16p11.2–q12.1. *Am J Hum Genet* **65**:1688–1697.
15. Bennett, L.B., E.S. Roach, and A.M. Bowcock. 2000. A locus for paroxysmal kinesigenic dyskinesia maps to human chromosome 16. *Neurology* **54**:125–130.
16. Valente, E.M., S.D. Spacey, G.M. Wali, K.P. Bhatia, P.H. Dixon, N.W. Wood, and M.B. Davis. 2000. A second paroxysmal kinesigenic choreoathetosis locus (EKD2) mapping on 16q13–q22.1 indicates a family of genes which give rise to paroxysmal disorders on human chromosome 16. *Brain* **123**:2040–2045.
17. Bressman, S.B., S. Fahn, and R.E. Burke. 1988. Paroxysmal nonkinesigenic dystonia. *Adv Neurol* **50**:403–413.
18. Richards, R.N., and H.J. Barnett. 1968. Paroxysmal dystonic choreoathetosis. A family study and review of the literature. *Neurology* **18**:461–469.
19. Fink, J.K., S. Rainer, J. Wilkowski, S.M. Jones, A. Kume, P. Hedera, R. Albin, et al. 1996. Paroxysmal dystonic choreoathetosis: tight linkage to chromosome 2q. *Am J Hum Genet* **59**:140–145.
20. Fouad, G.T., S. Servidei, S. Durcan, E. Bertini, and L.J. Ptacek. 1996. A gene for familial dyskinesia (FPD1) maps to chromosome 2q. *Am J Hum Genet* **59**:135–139.
21. Jarman, P.R., K.P. Bhatia, C. Davie, S.J. Heales, N. Turjanski, S.D. Taylor-Robinson, C.D. Marsden, and N.W. Wood. 2000. Paroxysmal dystonic choreoathetosis: clinical features and investigation of pathophysiology in a large family. *Mov Disord* **15**:648–657.
22. Byrne, E., O. White, and M. Cook. 1991. Familial dystonic choreoathetosis with myokimia; a sleep responsive disorder. *J Neurol Neurosurg Psychiatry* **54**:1090–1092.
23. Auburger, G., T. Ratzlaff, A. Lunkes, H.W. Nelles, B. Leube, F. Binkofski, H. Kugel, et al. 1996. A gene for autosomal dominant paroxysmal choreoathetosis/spasticity (CSE) maps to the vicinity of a potassium channel gene cluster on chromososme 1p, probably within 2cM between D1S443 and D1S197. *Genomics* **31**:90–94.
24. Fink, J.K., P. Hedera, J.G. Mathay, and R. Albin. 1997. Paroxysmal dystonic choreoathetosis linked to chromosome 2q: clinical analysis and proposed pathophysiology. *Neurology* **49**:177–183.
25. Bhatia, K.P., V.L. Soland, M.H. Bhatt, N.P. Quinn, and C.D. Marsden. 1997. Paroxysmal exercise-induced dystonia: eight new sporadic cases and a review of the literature. *Mov Disord* **12**:1007–1012.
26. Munchau, A., E.M. Valente, G.A. Shahidi, L.H. Eunson, M.G. Hanna, N.P. Quinn, A.H.V. Schapira, N.W. Wood, and K.P. Bhatia. 2000. A new family with paroxysmal exercise-induced dystonia and migraine: a clinical and genetic study. *J Neurol Neurosurg Psychiatry* 68 :609–614.
27. Wali, G.M. 1992. Paroxysmal hemidystonia induced by prolonged exercise and cold. *J Neurol Neurosurg Psychiatry* **55**:236–237.
28. Plant, G.T., A.C. Williams, C.J. Early, and C.D. Marsden. 1984. Familial paroxysmal dystonia induced by exercise. *J Neurol Neurosurg Psychiatry* **47**:275–279.

29. Meyer, B.-U., K. Irlbacher, and H. Meierkord. 2001. Analysis of stimuli triggering attacks of paroxysmal dystonia induced by exertion. *J Neurol Neurosurg Psychiatry* **70**:247–251.
30. Kurlan, R., J. Behr, L. Medved, and I. Shoulson. 1987. Familial paroxysmal dystonic choreoathetosis: a family study. *Mov Disord* **2**:187–192.
31. Guerrini, R., P. Bonanni, N. Nardocci, L. Parmeggiani, M. Piccirilli, M. De Fusco, P. Aridon, et al. 1999. Autosomal recessive rolandic epilepsy with paroxysmal exercise-induced dystonia and writers cramp: delineation of the syndrome and gene mapping to chromosome 16p12–11.2. *Ann Neurol* **45**:344–352.
32. Lugaresi, E., and F. Cirignotta. 1981. Hypnogenic paroxysmal dystonia: epileptic seizure or a new syndrome? *Sleep* **4**:129–138.
33. Lee, B.I., R.P. Lesser, C.E. Pippenger, H.H. Morris, H. Luders, D.S. Dinner, W.S. Corrie, et al. 1985. Familial paroxysmal hypnogenic dystonia. *Neurology* **35**:1357–1360.
34. Tinuper, P., A. Cerullo, F. Cirignotta, P. Cortelli, E. Lugaresi, and P. Montagna. 1990. Nocturnal paroxysmal dystonia with short lasting attacks: three cases with evidence for an epileptic frontal lobe origin of seizures. *Epilepsia* **31**:549–556.
35. Scheffer, I.E., K.P. Bhatia, I. Lopes-Cendes, D.R. Fish, C.D. Marsden, E. Andermann, F. Andermann, et al. 1995. Autosomal dominant nocturnal frontal lobe epilepsy. A distinctive clinical disorder. *Brain* **118**:61–73.
36. Scheffer, I.E., K.P. Bhatia, I. Lopes-Cendes, D.R. Fish, C.D. Marsden, F. Andermann, E. Andermann, et al. 1994. Autosomal dominant frontal lobe epilepsy misdiagnosed as a sleep disorder. *Lancet* **43**:515–517.
37. Drigo, P., G. Carli, and A.M. Laverda. 2000. Benign paroxysmal torticollis of infancy. *Brain Dev* **22**(3):169–172.
38. Giffin, N.J., S. Benton, and P.J. Goadsby. 2002. Benign paroxysmal torticollis of infancy: four new cases and linkage to CACNA1A mutation. *Dev Med Child Neurol* **44**(7):490–493.
39. Andermann, F., D.L. Keene, E. Andermann, and L.F. Quesney. 1980. Startle disease or hyperekplexia: future delineation of the syndrome. *Brain* **103**:985–997.
40. Suhren, O., G.W. Bruyn, and A. Tuynman. 1966. Hyperexplexia. A hereditary startle syndrome. *J Neurol Sci* **3**:577–605.
41. Brown, P., J.C. Rothwell, P.D. Thompson, T.C. Britton, B.L. Day, and C.D. Marsden. 1991. The hyperekplexias and their relationship to the normal startle reflex. *Brain* **114**:1903–1928.
42. Tijssen, M.A., L.M. Voorkamp, G.W. Padberg, and J.G. van Dijk. 1997. Startle responses in hereditary hyperekplexia. *Arch Neurol* **54**:388–393.
43. Matsumoto, J., P. Fuhr, M. Nigro, and M. Hallett. 1992. Physiological abnormalities in hereditary hyperekplexia. *Ann Neurol* **32**:41–50.
44. Tijssen, M.A., H.C. Schoemaker, P.J. Edelbroek, R.A. Roos, A.F. Cohen, and J.G. van Dijk. 1997. The effects of clonazepam and vigabatrin in hyperekplexia. *J Neurol Sci* **149**(1):63–67.
45. Shiang, R., S.G. Ryan, Y.Z. Zhu, T.J. Fielder, R.J. Allen, A. Fryer, S. Yamashita, P. O'Connell, and J.J. Wasmuth. 1995. Mutational analysis of familial and sporadic hyperekplexia. *Ann Neurol* **38**(1):85–91.
46. Shiang, R., S.G. Ryan, Y.Z. Zhu, A.F. Hahn, P. O'Connell, and J.J. Wasmuth. 1993. Mutations in the alpha 1 subunit of the inhibitory glycine receptor cause the dominant neurologic disorder, hyperekplexia. *Nat Genet* **5**(4):351–358.
47. Milani, N., L. Dalpra, A. del Prete, R. Zanini, and L. Larizza. 1996. A novel mutation (Gln266>His) in the alpha 1 subunit of the inhibitory glycine-receptor gene (GLRA1) in hereditary hyperekplexia. *Am J Hum Genet* **58**:420–422.
48. Rees, M.I., M. Andrew, S. Jawad, and M.J. Owen. 1994. Evidence for recessive as well as dominant forms of startle disease (hyperekplexia) caused by mutations in the alpha 1 subunit of the inhibitory glycine receptor. *Hum Mol Genet* **3**(12):2175–2179.
49. Tijssen, M.A., R. Shiang, J. van Deutekom, R.H. Boerman, J.J. Wasmuth, L.A. Sandkuijl, R.R. Frants, and G.W. Padberg. 1995. Molecular genetic reevaluation of the Dutch hyperekplexia family. *Arch Neurol* **52**(6):578–582.
50. Fernandez, M., W. Raskind, J. Wolff, M. Matsushita, E. Yuen, W. Graf, H. Lipe, and T. Bird. 2001. Familial dyskinesia and facial myokymia (FDFM): a novel movement disorder. *Ann Neurol* **49**:486–492.
51. Lishman, W.A., C.D. Symonds, C.W. Whitty, and R.G. Wilson. 1962. Seizures induced by movement. *Brain* **85**:93–108.
52. Kinast, M., G. Erenberg, and A.D. Rothner. 1980. Paroxysmal choreoathetosis, report of five cases and review of the literature. *Pediatrics* **65**:74–77.
53. Guerrini, R., R. Sanchez-Carpintero, T. Deonna, M. Santucci, K.P. Bhatia, T. Moreno, L. Parmeggiani, and B.D. Bernardina. 2002. Early-onset absence epilepsy and paroxysmal dyskinesia. *Epilepsia* **43**(10): 1224–1229.
54. Franssen, H., C. Fortgens, A.E. Wattendorff, and T.C.A.M. Van Woerom. 1983. Paroxysmal kinesigenic choreoathetosis and abnormal contingent negative variation. A case report. *Arch Neurol* **40**:381–385.
55. Kim, M.O., J.H. Im, C.G. Choi, M.C. Lee, and M.R. Proton. 1998. Spectroscopic findings in paroxysmal kinesigenic dyskinesia. *Mov Disord* **13**:570–575.
56. Shirane, S., M. Sasaki, D. Kogure, H. Matsuda, and T. Hashimoto. 2001. Increased ictal perfusion of the thalamus in paroxysmal kinesigenic dyskinesia. *J Neurol Neurosurg Psychiatry* **71**:408–410.
57. Barnett, M.H., P.R. Jarman, S.J. Heales, and K.P. Bhatia. 2002. Further case of paroxysmal exercise-induced dystonia and some insights into pathogenesis. *Mov Disord* **17**:1386–1387.
58. Lombroso, C.T., and A. Fischman. 1999. Paroxysmal non-kinesigenic dyskinesia: pathophysiological investigations. *Epileptic Disord* **1**:187–193.
59. Browne, D.L., S.T. Gancher, J.G. Nutt, E.R. Brunt, E.A. Smith, P. Kramer, and M. Litt. 1994. Episodic ataxia myokimia syndrome is associated with point mutations in the human potassium channel gene, KCNA1. *Nature Genet* **8**:136–140.
60. Vahedi, K., A. Joutel, P. Van Bogaert, A. Ducros, J. Maciazeck, J.F. Bach, M.G. Bousser, et al. 1995. A gene for hereditary paroxysmal cerebellar ataxia maps to chromosome 19. *Ann Neurol* **37**:289–293.
61. Ptacek, L.J., R. Tawil, R.C. Griggs, G. Meola, P. McManis, R.J. Barohn, J.R. Mendell, et al. 1994. Sodium channel mutations in acetazolamide-responsive myotonia congenita, paramyotonia congenita, and hyperkalemic periodic paralysis. *Neurology* **44**:1500–1503.
62. Jurkat-Rott, K., F. Lehmann-Horn, A. Elbaz, R. Heine, R.G. Gregg, K. Hogan, P.A. Powers, et al. 1994. A calcium-channel mutation causing hypokalemic periodic paralysis. *Hum Mol Genet* **3**:1415–1419.
63. Kramer, P.L., Q. Yue, S.T. Gancher, J.G. Nutt, R. Baloh, E. Smith, D. Browne, et al. 1995. A locus for the nystagmus-associated form of episodic ataxia maps to an 11-cm region on chromosome 19p. *Am J Hum Genet* **57**:182–185.
64. Ophoff, R.A., G.M. Terwindt, M.N. Vergouwe, R. van Eijk, P.J. Oefner, S.M. Hoffman, J.E. Lamerdin, et al. 1996. Familial hemiplegic migraine and episodic ataxia type-2 are caused by mutations in the Ca^{2+} channel gene CACNLIA4. *Cell* **87**:543–552.
65. Brunt, E.R.P., and T.W. Van Weerden. 1990. Familial paroxysmal kinesigenic ataxia and continuous myokimia. *Brain* **113**:1361–1382.
66. Griggs, R.C., R.T. Moxley III, R.A. Lafralane, and J. McQuillen. 1978. Hereditary paroxysmal ataxia, response to acetazolamide. *Neurology* **28**:1259–1264.
67. Spacey, S.D., B.I. Szczygielski, J.E. McRory, G.M. Wali, N.W. Wood, and T.P. Snutch. 2002. Mutation analysis of the sodium/hydrogen exchanger gene (NHE5) in familial paroxysmal kinesigenic dyskinesia. *J Neural Transm* **109**:1189–1194.
68. Spacey, S.D., E.M. Valente, G.M. Wali, T.T. Warner, P.R. Jarman, A.H. Schapira, P.H. Dixon, M.B. Davis, K.P. Bhatia, and N.W. Wood. 2002. Genetic and clinical heterogeneity in paroxysmal kinesigenic dyskinesia: evidence for a third EKD gene. *Mov Disord* **17**:717–725.

69. Jarman, P.R., M.B. Davis, S.V. Hodgson, C.D. Marsden, and N.W. Wood. 1997. Paroxysmal dystonic choreoathetosis. Genetic linkage studies in a British family. *Brain* **120**:2125–2130.
70. Raskin, W.H., T. Bolin, J. Wolff, J. Fink, M. Matsushita, M. Litt, H. Lipe, et al. 1998. Further localization of a gene for paroxysmal dystonic choreoathetosis to a 5-cM region on chromosome 2q34. *Hum Genet* **102**:93–97.
71. Hofele. K., R. Benecke, and G. Auburger. 1997. Gene locus FPD1 of the dystonic Mount-Reback type of autosomal-dominant paroxysmal choreoathetosis. *Neurology* **49**:1252–1257.
72. Matsuo, H., K. Kamakura, M. Saito, M. Oakano, T. Nagase, Y. Tadano, K. Kaida, et al. 1999. Familial paroxysmal dystonic choreoathetosis: clinical findings in a large Japanese family and genetic linkage to 2q. *Arch Neurol* **56**:721–726.
73. Matsuo, H., K. Kamakura, S. Matsushita, T. Ohmori, M. Okano, Y. Tadano, S. Tsuji, and S. Higuchi. 1999. Mutational analysis of the anion exchanger 3 gene in familial paroxysmal dystonic choreoathetosis linked to chromosome 2q. *Am J Med Genet* **88**:733–737.
74. Grunder, S., H.S. Geisler, S. Rainier, and J.K. Fink. 2001. Acid-sensing ion channel (ASIC) 4 gene: physical mapping, genomic organisation, and evaluation as a candidate for paroxysmal dystonia. *Eur J Hum Genet* **9**:672–676.
75. Phillips, H.A., I.E. Scheffer, S.F. Berkovic, V.E. Holloway, G.R. Sutherland, and J.C. Mulley. 1995. Localization of a gene for autosomal dominant nocturnal frontal lobe epilepsy to chromosome 20q 13.2. *Nat Genet* **10**:117–118.
76. Steinlein, O.K., J.C. Mulley, P. Propping, R.H. Wallace, H.A. Phillips, G.R. Sutherland, I.E. Scheffer, et al. 1995. A missense mutation in the neuronal nicotinic acetylcholine receptor alpha4 subunit is associated with autosomal dominant nocturnal frontal lobe epilepsy. *Nat Genet* **11**:201–202.
77. Steinlein, O.K., A. Magnusson, J. Stoodt, S. Bertrand, S. Weiland, S.F. Berkovic, K.O. Nakken, et al. 1997. An insertion mutation of the CHRNA4 gene in a family with autosomal dominant nocturnal frontal lobe epilepsy. *Hum Mol Genet* **6**:943–947.
78. Phillips, H.A., I.E. Scheffer, K.M. Crossland, K.P. Bhatia, D.R. Fish, C.D. Marsden, S.J. Howell, et al. 1998. Autosomal dominant nocturnal frontal-lobe epilepsy: genetic heterogeneity and evidence for a second locus at 15q24. *Am J Hum Genet* **63**:1108–1116.

C H A P T E R

H2

The Genetically Dystonic Hamster: An Animal Model of Paroxysmal Dystonia

ANGELIKA RICHTER

The genetically dystonic hamster (gene symbol: dt^{sz}) shows the phenotypic characteristics of paroxysmal non-kinesigenic dyskinesia in which episodes of dystonia and choreoathetosis occur spontaneously or can be provoked by stress, excitement, and intake of methylxanthines (Löscher et al., 1989; Richter and Löscher, 1998, 2002). Paroxysmal dyskinesias in humans can be divided into several subtypes, such as paroxysmal non-kinesigenic dyskinesia (paroxysmal dystonic choreoathetosis; brief: paroxysmal dystonia), paroxysmal kinesigenic dyskinesia (paroxysmal kinesigenic choreoathetosis), the exertion-induced and hypnogenic paroxysmal dyskinesias (Demirkiran and Jankovic, 1995; Nardocci et al., 2002; see also Chapter H1). The underlying defects in human paroxysmal dyskinesias remain unknown (Fahn, 1994). The dt^{sz} mutant hamster is one of the most extensively examined genetic animal models of movement disorders. The genetically dystonic hamsters represent an excellent model that can be helpful (1) to give new insights into the pathogenesis of this movement disorder and (2) to identify new strategies for the treatment of paroxysmal dystonia (Nardocci et al., 2002).

I. CLINICAL SIGNS IN GENETICALLY DYSTONIC HAMSTERS

The dt^{sz} mutant hamster, an inbred line of Syrian hamsters, exhibits attacks of generalized dystonic and choreoathetotic movements in response to mild stress and sometimes also spontaneously (Richter and Löscher, 1998). These motor impairments are transmitted by an autosomal recessive gene (Löscher et al., 1989). Since the genome of Syrian hamsters is not well characterized, the gene defect in mutant hamsters has not yet been identified. Initially, the symptoms were misdiagnosed as reflex epilepsy (Yoon et al., 1976). Therefore, the original gene symbol was *sz* (for seizures).

More detailed investigations demonstrated that the attacks are not epileptic seizures but show several features in common with paroxysmal non-kinesigenic dystonic choreoathetosis (PDC) in humans (Löscher et al., 1989). In brief, episodes of twisting movements and abnormal postures last several hours in mutant hamsters and can be precipitated by stress and methylxanthines (caffeine, theophylline), whereas the progression of dystonic symptoms is often aborted by sleep (Nardocci et al., 2002; Richter and Hamann, 2001; Richter and Löscher, 1998, 2002). The consciousness is obviously not altered during attacks because the animals react to different external stimuli. Altered EMG patterns, *i.e.*, cocontractions of opposing muscles, found in dt^{sz} hamsters are comparable to those determined in patients with dystonia (Löscher et al., 1989; Richter and Löscher, 1998). EEG recordings failed to disclose any ictal or interictal epileptogenic activities in cortical areas, hippocampus, basal ganglia nuclei (striatum, globus pallidus), or nucleus ruber (Gernert et al., 1997; 1998; Löscher et al., 1989). The mutant hamster was, therefore, renamed by the gene symbol dt^{sz} (*dt* for dystonic).

Effects of drug treatment in the dt^{sz} mutant are similar to those reported in patients with paroxysmal dystonia (Fahn, 1994). Benzodiazepines and neuroleptics exerted beneficial effects, whereas classical antiepileptics such as phenytoin were not effective or even worsened dyskinesia in mutant hamsters. In view of the comparable drug response, the dt^{sz} hamster is suitable for preclinical drug testing (Richter and Löscher, 1998).

By using histological standard techniques, no morphological abnormalities could be detected within the CNS of mutant hamsters. Neither signs of neurodegeneration nor a general retardation of brain development seems to be involved in the syndrome of mutant hamsters (Burgunder et al., 1999; Nobrega et al., 1999; Wahnschaffe et al., 1990).

The vitality is normal in mutant hamsters. The paroxysmal nature of the dystonic syndrome allows an undisturbed food and water intake. The age-dependent time-course of dystonia contributes to an unaltered fertility, although the onset of puberty was found to be retarded in male and female dt^{sz} hamsters (Löscher et al., 1995).

Together, the genetically dystonic hamster can be considered as a valid animal model of idiopathic paroxysmal dystonia (Nardocci et al., 2002; Richter and Löscher, 2002).

II. RATING THE SEVERITY OF DYSTONIA AND AGE-DEPENDENCE OF DYSKINESIA

In mutant hamsters, dystonic attacks can be reproducibly induced by stress, such as handling (Löscher et al., 1989). After the stressful stimuli, dt^{sz} hamsters develop a sequence of abnormal movements and postures. In addition to the predominant dystonic postures, twisting movements in these animals are similar to choreoathetosis in humans. The severity of dystonic episodes can be rated by the following score-system (Richter and Löscher, 1998): *stage 1*, flat body posture; *stage 2*, facial contortions, rearing with forelimbs crossing, and disturbed gait with hyperextended forepaws (see Figure 1, *A*); *stage 3*, hyperextended hindlimbs so that the animals appear to walk on tiptoes; *stage 4*, twisting

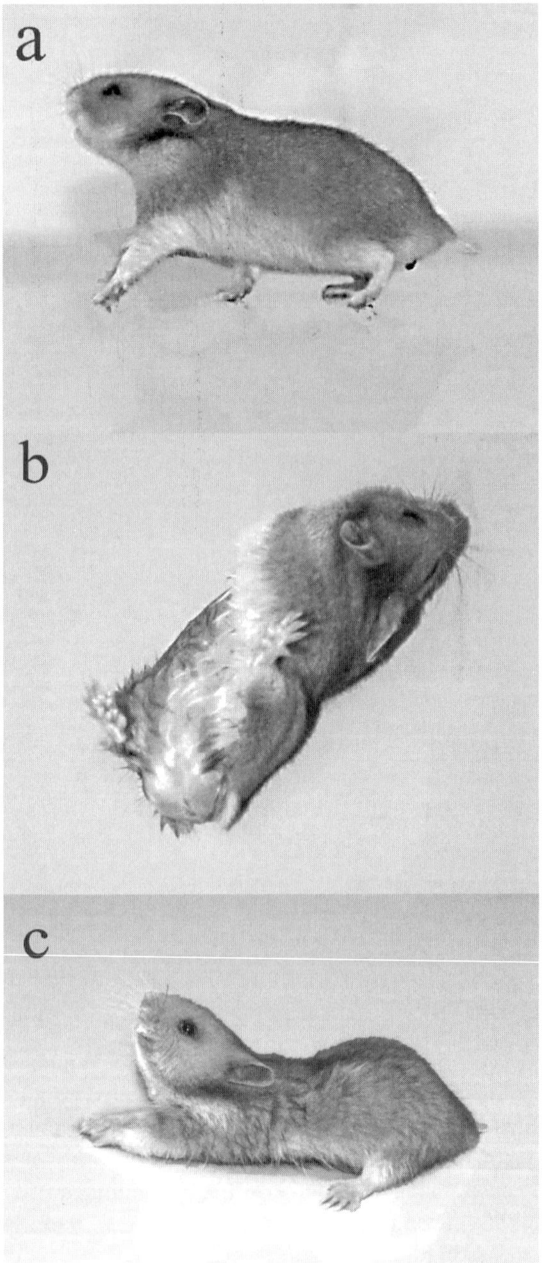

FIGURE 1 Dystonic movements and postures in dt^{sz} hamsters. The dyskinetic syndrome in mutant hamsters consists of a sequence of motor disturbances. Therefore, the severity of dystonia can be rated according to a six-point score system. Not all animals reach all the six stages, which are described in section II. The individual stage is usually reached within 3 hr. Thereafter the hamster completely recovers. The pictures show some of the most often occurring symptoms in mutant hamsters, *e.g.*, (a) hyperextension of the forepaws (*stage 2*), (b) abnormal tonus in the back muscles and twisting movements of the trunk, which cause falling (*stage 4*), (c) immobilization in a twisted, hunched posture; opisthotonus, hind- and forelimbs tonically extended forward (*stage 6*).

movements and loss of balance (Figure 1, *B*); *stage 5*, hindlimbs hyperextended caudally; and *stage 6*, immobilization in a twisted, hunched posture with hindlimbs and forelimbs tonically extended forward (Figure 1, *C*). The individual maximum stage of dystonia is usually reached within 3 hr after the hamsters are placed in the new cage. Thereafter, the hamsters completely recover.

The severity of dyskinetic symptoms shows an age-dependent time-course, with first occurrence of dystonic attacks on about day 16 of life. The severity reaches a maximum at an age of 30 to 40 days of life. Then the severity continuously reduces until a complete remission of the stress-inducible disorder is observed at an age of about 10 wk (*e.g.*, Löscher et al., 1995; Richter and Löscher, 1998, 2000). Nevertheless, paroxysmal dystonia in mutant hamsters is obviously not really transient because relapses of dystonia occur in females during late pregnancy (Löscher et al., 1995) and because lamotrigine and riluzole can provoke an exacerbation of dystonic attacks in male and female hamsters over 10 wk of age (Richter et al., 1994, 1997).

III. EFFECTS OF SYSTEMIC DRUG TREATMENTS IN MUTANT HAMSTERS

The score-system for rating severity of dystonic attacks, as described above, is suitable to examine drug effects on the severity of dyskinesia in mutant hamsters (Löscher et al., 1989; Richter and Löscher, 2002). Among drugs tested in dt^{sz} hamsters during the last years, most marked beneficial effects were observed after acute treatments with various GABA-potentiating drugs, antidopaminergic compounds, and adenosine receptor agonists, whereas drugs that disturb GABAergic inhibition or compounds known to cause an increase of the dopaminergic activity worsened the dystonic syndrome (Nardocci et al., 2002; Richter and Hamann, 2001; Richter and Löscher, 1998, 1999, 2002). Methylxanthines (caffeine, theophylline) and sodium channel blockers caused an aggravation of dystonia in mutant hamsters (Richter et al., 1997; Richter and Hamann, 2001). Chronic administration of phenobarbital also worsened dystonia in the dt^{sz} mutant (possibly related to a GABA-mediated depolarization), whereas acute treatment with this drug exerted antidystonic efficacy (Richter and Löscher, 2000). Apart from NMDA receptor NR2B subtype selective antagonists, various NMDA and AMPA receptor antagonists exerted beneficial effects in the hamster model (Richter and Löscher, 1998; Richter, 2003). Further examples of compounds that reduced the severity to dystonia were cannabinoids and a kappa-opioid receptor agonist (Richter and Löscher, 1998, 2002b).

The pharmacological data were in part helpful for interpretations of neurochemical findings in mutant hamsters. Particularly, microinjections of compounds into brain regions in which neurochemical changes were detected can contribute to the understanding of the pathophysiology.

IV. PATHOPHYSIOLOGICAL FINDINGS IN THE GENETICALLY DYSTONIC HAMSTER

In order to identify the underlying mechanism of the dystonic syndrome, the dt^{sz} mutant has been extensively examined by neurochemical, immunohistological, and electrophysiological investigations (in comparison to nondystonic control hamsters). The paroxysmal nature of dyskinesias in dt^{sz} hamsters provides the possibility for a separation of changes that are secondary to abnormal motor patterns (examinations in the absence *versus* in the presence of dystonic attacks). In addition, the age-dependence of paroxysmal dystonia gives insights into the importance of changes for the occurrence of dystonia by ontogenetic studies, *i.e.*, alterations detected at an age of maximum severity should disappear or at least be reduced in older animals after spontaneous remission of stress-inducible attacks. Over the last decade, various neurotransmitter systems (monoamines, inhibitory and excitatory amino acids) and neuropeptides (Friedman et al., 2002; Nobrega et al., unpublished observations) were investigated. The main findings of neurochemical, immunohistochemical, and electrophysiological studies are summarized in the following paragraphs.

A. Neurochemical Changes in the dt^{sz} Mutant

Neurochemical examinations included 14 to more than 100 brain regions and subregions. Most changes were detected in the striatum and ventral thalamic nuclei of dt^{sz} hamsters (Richter and Löscher, 1998, 2002). There is strong evidence that disturbed GABAergic inhibition and enhanced dopaminergic and glutamatergic activity are critically involved in the dystonic syndrome of dt^{sz} hamsters.

1. Changes in the Dopaminergic System

Determinations of the levels of dopamine and its metabolites in tissue homogenates of different brain regions, examinations of tyrosine hydroxylase by immunohistochemistry and by *in-situ* hybridization as well as analyses of dopamine transporter binding did not show any abnormalities in brains of dystonic hamsters (Burgunder et al., 1999; Löscher et al., 1994; Nobrega et al., 1999). In view of an unaltered density of dopaminergic neurons and of their terminals, the dopaminergic system appears to be intact in this animal model. Autoradiographic analyses of dopamine receptor density, however, revealed a reduced dopamine D_1 and D_2 receptor binding in the dorsal striatum (Nobrega et al., 1996). With regard to pharmacological observations in mutant hamsters, this could be due to a receptor down-regulation as a consequence of an enhanced dopamine release. Dopamine receptor antagonists, *e.g.*, haloperidol and clozapine, exerted beneficial effects, whereas compounds that increase dopaminergic activity aggravated dystonia after systemic administrations in mutant hamsters (Nobrega et al., 1999; Richter and Löscher, 1993, 1998). Striatal injections of the dopamine D_2 receptor agonist quinpirole significantly worsened the dystonic syndrome, whereas combined microinjections of D_1 and D_2 receptor antagonists exerted striking beneficial effects (Rehders et al., 2000). Recently, determinations of extracellular monoamine levels by microdialysis revealed that the striatal concentrations are normal in the absence of dyskinesia, but the extracellular dopamine levels were significantly increased during the manifestation of a dystonic episode in the striatum of dt^{sz} hamsters in comparison to control animals (Hamann and Richter, 2004).

These data indicate that striatal dopaminergic overactivity is critically involved in the occurrence of dyskinetic episodes in mutant hamsters. With regard to the recent findings by microdialysis, an enhanced release of dopamine in the striatum of mutant hamsters is not a persistent abnormality but occurs temporarily during a stress-induced dystonic attack. The dopaminergic dysfunctions are possibly secondary to impaired GABAergic inhibition.

2. Examinations of the GABAergic System and of Excitatory Amino Acids

In the striatum of dt^{sz} hamsters the GABA levels were found to be reduced at an age of maximum severity but not after remission of paroxysmal dystonia (Löscher and Hörstermann, 1992). The striatal expression of the GABA-synthesizing enzyme glutamic acid decarboxylase was also reduced in dystonic hamsters (Burgunder et al., 1999). An increased affinity and density of benzodiazepine binding sites on the $GABA_A$ receptor in the striatum, determined in mutant hamsters at the age of most marked severity of paroxysmal dystonia, but not in older animals after the remission of stress-inducible dyskinesia, could reflect an up-regulation of these sites (Pratt et al., 1995). This interpretation referred to previous pharmacological observations that demonstrated that GABAmimetic drugs exerted marked antidystonic efficacy after systemic administrations (Richter and Löscher, 1998). Indeed, the neurochemical changes of GABA can be explained by a significant deficit of striatal parvalbumin-immunoreactive GABAergic interneurons in dt^{sz} hamsters at the most sensitive age (Gernert et al., 2000). These interneurons constitute only 3% to 5% of the cells in the rodent striatum but are the main inhibitory source in the striatum (Kawaguchi et al., 1995; Koos and Tepper, 1999). Striatal microinjections of agonists at the GABA and benzodiazepine binding sites of the $GABA_A$ receptor were found to exert beneficial effects in mutant hamsters, supporting the functional relevance of the reduction of striatal GABAergic interneurons (Hamann and Richter, 2002).

Hence, a retarded development of striatal parvalbumin-reactive GABAergic interneurons probably plays a critical role in the pathogenesis of paroxysmal dystonia in the hamster model. This persistent structural defect can explain several previous pharmacological, neurochemical, and electrophysiological findings in dt^{sz} hamsters (Richter and Löscher, 2002). The paroxysmal nature of the movement disorder, however, indicates that additional changes are essential for the manifestation of dystonia, such as a temporary increase of dopamine release in the striatum.

There is also evidence that glutamatergic overactivity contributes to the manifestation of severe dystonic attacks in dt^{sz} hamsters (Richter and Löscher, 1998, 2002). In the dt^{sz} mutant, NMDA and AMPA receptor antagonists exerted beneficial effects (Richter and Löscher, 1998). Recently, the basal levels of the polyamine spermine were found to be increased in the forebrain of dystonic hamster (Richter and Morrison, 2003). Decreases of NMDA receptors in the ventrolateral thalamus and reductions of AMPA receptors, *e.g.*, in the striatum, were detected during the expression of a dystonic attack, but not in the absence of dystonic symptoms (Nobrega et al., 1997, 2002). Examinations in cortico-striatal slice preparations suggested that an increased excitability of cortico-striatal communication appears to be mediated, at least in part, by an enhanced presynaptic release probability at glutamatergic synapses (Köhling et al., 2003). This could also be related to a deficit of GABAergic interneurons.

B. Studies on the Neuronal Activity in dt^{sz} Hamsters

2-Deoxyglucose (2-DG)-uptake studies, undertaken in mutant hamsters during the manifestation of a dystonic attack, have reflected increased (synaptic and axonal) activity in the dorsomedial striatum, in the ventromedial, ventrolateral, and ventral anterior nuclei of the thalamus, in the medial vestibular nucleus, and in the nucleus ruber, whereas a reduced uptake was found in the reticular thalamic nucleus and in the deep cerebellar nuclei (Richter et al., 1998). This study was helpful to decide which nuclei could be involved in the manifestation of this movement disorder and should be therefore investigated in more detail, but the strength of the 2-DG method is limited. Therefore, single unit recordings were carried out in anesthetized (fentanyl/gallamine) hamsters when dystonic attacks were absent.

With regard to several neurochemical changes and an enhanced 2-DG-uptake in the dorsal striatum, single unit recordings were at first done from striatal GABAergic projection neurons. These recordings revealed an increased basal activity (+58%) of striatal projection neurons in dt^{sz} hamsters (Gernert et al., 1999b). This is not related to sodium channel dysfunctions, as shown by *in vitro* electrophysiological investigations (Siep et al., 2002). Probably, the enhanced activity of striatal projection neurons is based on the deficiency of striatal GABAergic interneurons (Gernert et al., 2000).

A significantly reduced discharge pattern of GABAergic neurons (−69%) was found in the entopeduncular nucleus (the homologue of the internal segment of the globus pallidus, GPi, in primates) of mutant hamsters (Gernert et al., 2000). Furthermore, the firing patterns were found to be more irregular in the entopeduncular nucleus of dyskinetic animals (Gernert et al., 2002). The age-dependent spontaneous remission of dystonia coincided with a normalization of the discharge rate and discharge pattern in the entopeduncular nucleus (Bennay et al., 2001; Gernert et al., 2002). Supporting the relevance of an abnormal basal ganglia output in the pathophysiology of dystonia, recent high-frequency stimulation of the entopoduncular nucleus has been shown to improve the dyskinetic syndrome in mutant hamsters (Harnack et al., 2004).

In the globus pallidus (globus pallidus externus in primates), the neuronal activity only tended to be increased (+40%) with a wide range, and no significant changes of the discharge rates could be detected in the substantia nigra pars reticulata of mutant hamsters at the most sensitive age of dystonia (Gernert et al., 1999b). Thus, in contrast to the (direct) striato-entopeduncular pathway, the neuronal activity is obviously not significantly disturbed within the striatonigral and (indirect) striato-pallidal pathway, at least in the

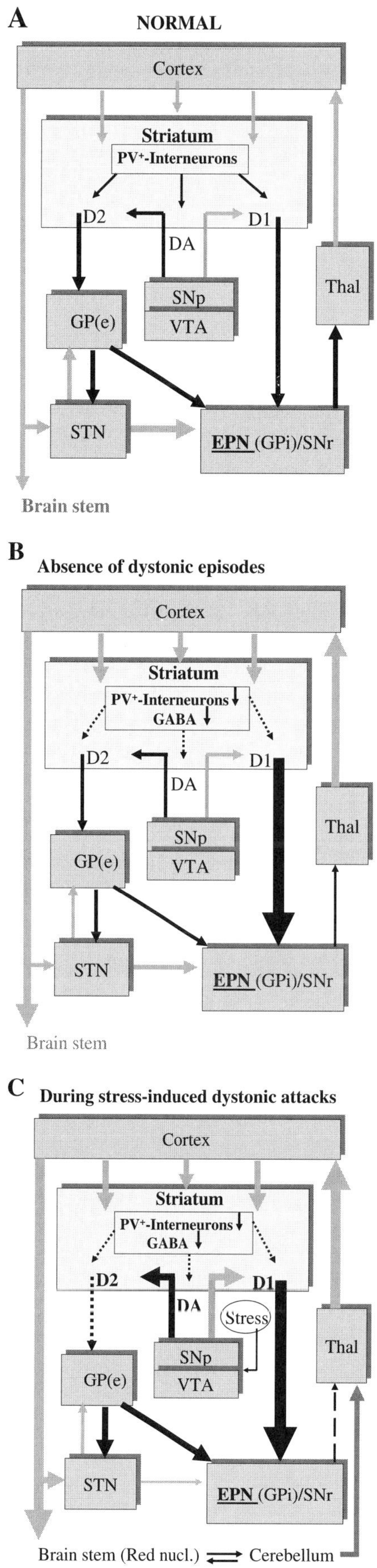

FIGURE 2 Schematic diagram of the basal ganglia motor circuit in normal (A), dt^{sz} mutant hamsters in the absence of dystonic attacks (B), and during a dystonic attack (C). Inhibitory connections are represented by black arrows, and excitatory projections by gray arrows. Changes in neuronal activities are indicated by the thickness of the arrows. As shown by single unit recordings in anaesthetized hamsters (fentanyl, gallamine), *i.e.*, in the absence of dystonia (B), the activity of striatal GABAergic projection neurons was significantly increased, which is probably related to the deficit of striatal parvalbumin-reactive (PV+) inhibitory interneurons. The consequence is a dramatic decrease of the entopeduncular activity (EPN, globus pallidus internus (GPi) in primates), whereas no significant changes were found in the globus pallidus (GP, in primates the external (e) segment) or in the substantia nigra pars reticulata (SNr). As shown by microinjections and microdialysis, enhanced extracellular dopaminergic levels during stress-induced dystonic episodes seem to be an important factor for the manifestation of dyskinesia in mutant hamsters (C). A temporary enhanced stimulation of dopamine D2 receptors, which are thought to be predominantly located on the striatopallidal neurons, should result in a further decrease of the entopeduncular activity. There is evidence that an increased activity of glutamatergic corticostriatal neurons may also contribute to the manifestation of dyskinetic symptoms in mutant hamsters.

absence of dystonic attacks (Richter and Löscher, 2002). Recent findings of changes in the striatal extracellular dopamine levels (Hamann and Richter, 2004) and also in the expression of opioid peptide precursors (Nobrega et al., unpublished observations), however, let us assume that an abnormal dopaminergic activation of the indirect pathway is involved during the occurrence of dystonic episodes. The current concept of basal ganglia dysfunctions in the hamster model, as shown in Figure 2, has to be examined by further single unit recordings from different basal ganglia nuclei in *freely moving* dt^{sz} hamsters.

In cortico-striatal slice preparations, field responses were larger, paired-pulse accentuation was more pronounced, and LTP was stronger in the dt^{sz} mutant than in control hamsters. An increased excitability of cortico-striatal communication mediated by an enhanced presynaptic release probability at glutamatergic synapses (Köhling et al., 2003) could be related to the deficit of striatal inhibitory interneurons (see above) or to reduced cortical inhibition.

V. SUMMARY AND CONCLUSIONS

In summary, striatal dysfunctions resulting in an abnormal basal ganglia output are critically involved in paroxysmal dyskinesia in the hamster model, as illustrated in Figure 2. The finding of a reduced discharge rate and an irregular firing pattern of entopeduncular neurons in mutant hamsters substantiates the hypothesis of the pathophysiology of dyskinesias in humans (Vitek and Giroux, 2000; Wichmann and DeLong, 1996). The suggestion that paroxysmal dyskinesias are due to sodium channel defects is not supported by the investigations in the hamster model (Siep et al., 2002). Changes in the dopaminergic system have been hypothesized to be responsible for dystonia (Todd and Perlmutter, 1998). In the hamster model, the trigger of dystonic episodes (stress) probably leads to a temporary increased dopaminergic and glutamatergic activation of striatal projection neurons as a consequence of a disinhibition because of a deficit of striatal GABAergic interneurons (Figure 2, *C*). In patients, dyskinesias are often associated with striatal lesions (Bhatia and Marsden, 1994; Craver et al., 1996). The inborn deficit of striatal GABAergic interneurons in dt^{sz} hamsters indicates that the GABAergic system deserves attention in human dyskinesias, particularly in types in which GABA-potentiating drugs exert beneficial effects, such as in paroxysmal dystonia (Fahn, 1994). Interestingly, recent examinations in patients with focal dystonia supported this view. By using two-dimensional J-resolved magnet resonance spectroscopy, the GABA levels were found to be reduced in the striatum and in the sensorimotor cortex of dystonian patients (Levy and Hallett, 2002).

Although most changes were found in the basal ganglia–thalamocortical circuit, it should be emphasized that abnormalities were also detected in the cerebellum, red nucleus, vestibular nuclei, and limbic structures of dystonic hamsters. These changes are possibly also relevant for the induction of dyskinesia by stress, anxiety, and excitement (limbic structures, such as the hippocampus) and for the occurrence of specific clinical features, *e.g.*, opisthotonus and torticollis mediated by vestibular and rubrospinal abnormalities.

The genetically dystonic hamster represents a unique animal model of inherited paroxysmal dystonia. This animal model shows high face, predictive, and constructive validity. The primary defect probably differs dependent of the type of dystonia or paroxysmal dyskinesia in humans, but these defects may finally result in common alterations of the neuronal activity with the consequence to provoke similar symptoms. Animal models that allow invasive examinations can be useful to enhance our knowledge about the underlying mechanisms.

Acknowledgment

The examinations of genetically dystonic hamsters were funded by the Deutsche Forschungsgemeinschaft and in part by the Dystonia Medical Research Foundation.

Video Legends

STAGE 1 Flat body posture.

STAGE 2 Facial contortions, rearing with forelimbs crossing, disturbed gait with hyperextended forepaws.

STAGE 3 Hyperextended hindlimbs so that the animals appear to walk on tiptoes.

STAGE 4 Twisting movements and loss of balance.

STAGE 5 Hindlimbs hyperextended caudally.

STAGE 6 Immobilization in a twisted, hunched posture with hind- and forelimbs tonically extended forward.

References

Bennay, M., M. Gernert, and A. Richter. 2001. Spontaneous remission of paroxysmal dystonia coincides with normalization of entopeduncular activity in dt^{sz} mutants. *J Neurosci* **21**:RC153(1–4).

Bhatia, K.P., and C.D. Marsden. 1994. The behavioural and motor consequences of focal lesions of the basal ganglia in man. *Brain* **117**: 859–876.

Burgunder, J.-M., A. Richter, and W. Löscher. 1999. Expression of cholecystokinin, somatostatin, thyrotropin-releasing hormone, glutamic acid decarboxylase and tyrosine hydroxylase genes in the central nervous motor systems of the genetically dystonic hamster. *Exp Brain Res* **129**:114–120.

Craver, R.D., M.C. Duncan, and J.S. Nelson. 1996. Familial dystonia and choreoathetosis in three generations associated with bilateral striatal necrosis. *J Child Neurol* **11**:185–188.

Demirkiran, M., and J. Jankovic. 1995. Paroxysmal dyskinesias: clinical features and classification. *Ann Neurol* **38**:571–579.

Fahn, S. 1994. The paroxysmal dyskinesias. In *Movement Disorders 3* (Marsden, C.D., and Fahn, S., Eds.), pp. 311–345. Butterworth-Heinemann, Oxford.

Friedman, Y., A. Richter, R. Raymond, W. Löscher, and J.N. Nobrega. 2002. Regional decreases in NK-3, but not NK-1 tachykinin receptor binding in dystonic hamster (dt^{sz}) brains. *Neuroscience* **112**:639–645.

Gernert, M., M. Bennay, M. Fedrowitz, J.H. Rehders, and A. Richter. 2002. Altered discharge pattern of basal ganglia output neurons in an animal model of idiopathic dystonia. *J Neurosci* **22**:7244–7253.

Gernert, M., M. Hamann, M. Bennay, W. Löscher, and A. Richter. 2000. Deficit of striatal parvalbumin-reactive GABAergic interneurons and decreased basal ganglia output in a genetic rodent model of idiopathic paroxysmal dystonia. *J Neurosci* **20**:7052–7058.

Gernert, M., A. Richter, and W. Löscher. 1997. The electrical activity is impaired in the red nucleus of dt^{sz} hamsters with paroxysmal dystonia: an EEG power spectrum analysis of depth electrode recordings. *Brain Res* **760**:102–108.

Gernert, M., A. Richter, and W. Löscher. 1999a. Alterations in spontaneous single unit activity of striatal subdivisions during ontogenesis in mutant dystonic hamsters. *Brain Res* **821**:277–285.

Gernert M., A. Richter, and W. Löscher. 1999b. In vivo extracellular electrophysiology of pallidal neurons in dystonic and nondystonic hamsters. *J Neurosi Res* **57**:894–905.

Gernert, M., A. Richter, and W. Löscher. 1999c. A subconvulsive dose of pentylenetetrazole increases the firing rate of substantia nigra pars reticulata neurons in dystonic but not in non-dystonic hamsters. *Synapse* **33**:259–267.

Gernert, M., A. Richter, C. Rundfeldt, and W. Löscher. 1998. Quantitative EEG analysis of depth electrode recordings from several brain regions of mutant hamsters with paroxysmal dystonia discloses frequency changes in the basal ganglia. *Mov Disord* **13**:509–521.

Hamann, M., and A. Richter. 2002. Effects of striatal injections of $GABA_A$ receptor agonists and antagonists in a genetic animal model of paroxysmal dystonia. *Eur J Pharmacol* **443**:59–70.

Hamann, M., and A. Richter. 2004. Striatal increase of extracellular dopamine levels during dystonic episodes in a genetic model of paroxysmal dyskinesia. *Neurobiol Dis* **16**:78–84.

Harnack, D., M. Hamann, W. Meissner, R. Morgenstern, A. Kupsch, and A. Richter. 2004. High-frequency stimulation of the entopeduncular nucleus improves dystonia in dt^{SZ} hamsters. *Neuroreport* **15**:1391–1393.

Kawaguchi, Y., C.J. Wilson, S.J. Augood, and P.C. Emson. 1995. Striatal interneurons: chemical, physiological and morphological characterization. *Trends Neurosci* **18**:527–535.

Köhling, R., U. Koch, A. Richter, M. Hamann, and E.-J. Speckmann. 2003. Cortico-striatal communication in dystonic dt^{sz} hamster brain slices. *Eur J Physiol* **445**:S27.

Koos, T., and J.M. Tepper. 1999. Inhibitory control of neostriatal projection neurons by GABAergic interneurons. *Nature Neurosci* **2**:467–472.

Levy, L.M., and M. Hallett. 2002. Impaired brain GABA in focal dystonia. *Ann Neurol* **51**:93–101.

Löscher, W., R. Annies, and A. Richter. 1994. Marked regional disturbances in brain metabolism of monoaminergic neurotransmitters in the genetically dystonic hamster. *Brain Res* **658**:199–208.

Löscher, W., T. Blanke, A. Richter, and H.-O. Hoppen. 1995. Gonadal sex hormones and dystonia: experimental studies in genetically dystonic hamsters. *Mov Disord* **10**:92–102.

Löscher, W., J.E. Jr. Fisher, D. Schmidt, G. Fredow, D. Hönack, and W.B. Iturrian. 1989. The *sz* mutant hamster: a genetic model of epilepsy or of paroxysmal dystonia? *Mov Disord* **4**:219–232.

Löscher, W., and D. Hörstermann. 1992. Abnormalities in amino acid neurotransmitters in discrete brain regions of genetically dystonic hamsters. *J Neurochem* **59**:689–694.

Nardocci, N., E. Fernandez-Alvarez, N.W. Wood, S.D. Spacy, and A. Richter. 2002. The paroxysmal dyskinesias. In *Epilepsy and Movement Disorders.* (Guerrini, R., Aicardi, J., Andermann, F., Hallett, M., Eds.), pp. 125–139. Cambridge University Press, Cambridge.

Nobrega, J.N., M. Gernert, W. Löscher, R. Raymond, T. Belej, and A. Richter. 1999. Tyrosine hydroxylase immunreactivity and [3H]WIN 35,428 binding to the dopamine transporter in a hamster model of idiopathic paroxysmal dystonia. *Neuroscience* **92**:211–217.

Nobrega, J.N., J.H. Parkes, P. Wong, R. Raymond, and A. Richter. Altered expression of preproenkephalin and prodynorphin mRNA in a genetic model of paroxysmal dystonia, Unpublished observations.

Nobrega, J.N., R. Raymond, K. Barlow, M. Hamann, and A. Richter. 2002. Changes in AMPA receptor binding in an animal model of inborn paroxysmal dystonia. *Exp Neurol* **176**:371–376.

Nobrega, J.N., A. Richter, D. Jiwa, R. Raymond, and W. Löscher. 1997. Autoradiographic analysis of NMDA receptor binding in dystonic hamster brains. *Brain Res* **744**:161–165.

Nobrega, J.N., A. Richter, N. Tozman, D. Jiwa, and W. Löscher. 1996. Quantitative autoradiography reveals regionally selective changes in dopamine D_1 and D_2 receptor binding in the genetically dystonic hamster. *Neuroscience* **71**:927–936.

Pratt, D.G., H. Möhler, A. Richter, and W. Löscher. 1995. Regionally selective and age-dependent alterations in benzodiazepine receptor binding in the genetically dystonic hamsters. *J Neurochem* **64**:2153–2158.

Rehders, J.H., W. Löscher, and A. Richter. 2000. Evidence for striatal dopaminergic overactivity in paroxysmal dystonia indicated by microinjections in a genetic rodent model. *Neuroscience* **97**:267–277.

Richter, A. 2003. The NMDA receptor NR2B subtype selective antagonist Ro 25-6981 aggravates paroxysmal dyskinesia in the dt(s2) mutant. Eur J Pharmacol **458**:107–110.

Richter, A., J.M. Brotchie, A.R. Crossman, and W. Löscher. 1998. [^{3}H]-2-Deoxyglucose uptake study in mutant dystonic hamsters: Abnormalities in discrete brain regions of the motor system. *Mov Disord* **13**:718–725.

Richter, A., M. Gernert, and W. Löscher. 1997. Prodystonic effects of riluzole in an animal model of idiopathic dystonia related to decreased total power in the red nucleus? *Eur J Pharmacol* **332**:133–142.

Richter, A., and M. Hamann. 2001. Effects of adenosine receptor agonists and antagonists in a genetic animal model of primary dystonia. *Br J Pharmacol* **134**:343–352.

Richter, A., and W. Löscher. 1993. The atypical neuroleptic clozapine exerts antidystonic activity in a mutant hamster model. Comparison with haloperidol. *Eur J Pharmacol* **242**:309–312.

Richter, A., and W. Löscher. 1998. Pathophysiology of idiopathic dystonia: findings from genetic animal models. *Prog Neurobiol* **54**:633–677

Richter, A., and W. Löscher. 1999. Gabapentin decreases the severity of dystonia at low doses in a genetic animal model of paroxysmal dystonic choreoathetosis. *Eur J Pharmacol* **369**:335–338.

Richter, A., and W. Löscher. 2000. Paradoxical aggravation of paroxysmal dystonia during chronic treatment with phenobarbital in a genetic rodent model. *Eur J Pharmacol* **397**:343–350.

Richter, A., and W. Löscher. 2002a. Animal models of paroxysmal dyskinesia. *Adv Neurol* **89**:443–451.

Richter, A., and W. Löscher. 2002b. Effects of pharmacological manipulations of cannabinoid receptors on severity of dystonia in a genetic model of paroxysmal dyskinesia. *Eur J Pharmacol* **454**:145–151.

Richter, A., P.-A. Löschmann, and W. Löscher. 1994. The novel antiepileptic drug lamotrigine exerts prodystonic effects in a mutant hamster model of generalized dystonia. *Eur J Pharmacol* **264**:345–351.

Richter, A., and L.D. Morrison. 2003. Polyamines in a genetic animal model of paroxysmal dyskinesia. *Brain Res* **981**:168–173.

Siep, E., A. Richter, W. Löscher, E.-J. Speckmann, and R. Köhling. 2002. Sodium currents in striatal neurons from dystonic dt^{sz} hamsters: altered response to lamotrigine. *Neurobiol Dis* **9**:258–268.

Todd, R.D., and J.S. Perlmutter. 1998. Mutational and biochemical analysis of dopamine in dystonia. *Molec Neurobiol* **16**:135–147.

Vitek, J.L., and M. Giroux. 2000. Physiology of hypokinetic and hyperkinetic movement disorders: Model for dyskinesia. *Ann Neurol* **47**: 131–140.

Wahnschaffe, U., G. Fredow, P. Heintz, and W. Löscher. 1990. Neuropathological studies in a mutant hamster model of paroxysmal dystonia. *Mov. Disord.* **5**, 286–293.

Wichmann, T., and M.R. DeLong. 1996. Functional and pathophysiological models of the basal ganglia. *Curr Opin Neurobiol* **6**:751–758.

Yoon, C.H., J.S. Peterson, and D. Corrow. 1976. Spontaneous seizures: a new mutation in Syrian golden hamsters. *J Heredity* **67**:115–116.

CHAPTER

H3

Mouse Models of Hyperekplexia

LORE BECKER and HANS WEIHER

Hyperekplexia is a rare hereditary human disease caused by deficiencies of the inhibitory glycine receptor (GlyR) system. Patients develop startle-induced, transient, generalized muscle contractions, which are often accompanied with hypertonia. Dominant and recessive mutations in the $\alpha1$ and β subunit of the GlyR have been found associated with the disease. Several animal models of this neurological disease exist. Spontaneous mouse mutants carrying mutations in the evolutionary strongly conserved $\alpha1$ and β subunit of the murine receptor have been analyzed in some detail. These mutants display characteristic phenotypes resembling the motor deficits in hyperekplexia patients. Depending upon the amount of remaining GlyR activity or expression, the mutant mice show the phenotype, to different extents. It is characterized by an exaggerated startle reflex, inducible tremor and rigidity, and an impaired righting response. In addition to the spontaneous mouse mutants, transgenic models have been generated. In order to mimic the conditions of human hyperekplexia as closely as possible, a human hyperekplexia-associated, dominant negative mutation in the GlyRα1 subunit with altered agonist affinity (R271Q) was introduced as a transgene into mice. Analysis of the motor abilities of these mice revealed that the expression of this mutant subunit in tg271Q-300 mice caused a specific dominant disease phenotype similar to the ones displayed by the GlyR deficient mutants. Electrophysiological studies on spinal cord neurons revealed strong reduction in both, the glycinergic as well as the GABAergic, inhibitory systems pointing towards physiological interactions between the two inhibitory systems. This may be relevant for the development of pharmacological intervention in diseases involving impaired inhibitory synaptic transmission. Therefore, pharmacological studies on tg271Q-300 animals have been initiated.

I. HYPEREKPLEXIA—GENETICS AND THERAPY

Hereditary hyperekplexia, or startle disease, is a genetic neuromotor disease occurring at low frequency (Andrew and Owen, 1997; Schofield, 2002; Zhou et al., 2002). The condition is characterized by severe neonatal hypertonia and an exaggerated startle reflex in response to unexpected tactile or auditory stimulation (Brown, 2002; Morley et al., 1982). Due to the early appearance of the symptoms, it is also called stiff-baby syndrome, and life-threatening apnea can occur (Lingam et al., 1981; Praveen et al., 2001). The symptoms generally improve with age and the hypertonia diminishes, but adult patients still display an exaggerated startle response when stimulated by a sudden noise or touch. Therefore, patients may suffer serious injuries from falling during

TABLE 1 Genotype and Phenotype of Spontaneous GlyR Mutations in Mammals

Species	Subunit residue(s)	Disease/Phenotype	Functional effect	Reference
human	α_1 S231P	Hyperekplexia	recessive inheritance	(Humeny et al., 2002)
human	α_1 I244Q	Hyperekplexia	recessive inheritance	(Rees et al., 1994)
human	α_1 P250T	Hyperekplexia	reduced ligand affinity, low conductance, rapid desensitization	(Breitinger et al., 2001) (Saul et al., 1999)
human	α_1 R252Q/H	Hyperekplexia	membrane insertion	(Vergouwe et al., 1999)
human	α_1 R252H/R392H	Hyperekplexia	compound heterozygous, membrane insertion	(Vergouwe et al., 1999)
human	α_1 V260M	Hyperekplexia		(del Giudice et al., 2001)
human	α_1 Q266H	Hyperekplexia	channel gating	(Moorhouse et al., 1999)
human	α_1 S271T	Hyperekplexia		(Lapunzina et al., 2003)
human	α_1 R271L/Q	Hyperekplexia	altered ligand affinity, altered conductance	(Shiang et al., 1993) (Rajendra et al., 1994) (Langosch et al., 1994)
human	α_1 K276E	Hyperekplexia	channel gating	(Lewis et al., 1998) (Elmslie et al., 1996)
human	α_1 Y279C	Hyperekplexia		(Shiang et al., 1995) (Kwok et al., 2001)
human	deletion of GlyRα_1	Hyperekplexia		(Brune et al., 1996)
human	βG229D/exon5 loss	Hyperekplexia	compund heterozygous, ligand binding	(Rees et al., 2002)
mouse	deletion in GlyRα_1	*oscillator(spd^{ot})*	recessive inheritance, lethal at 3 wks postnatal	(Buckwalter et al., 1994) (Kling et al., 1997)
mouse	insertion in GlyRβ	*spastic (spa)*	β subunit expression decreased by 90%, GlyR levels 10–20%	(Kingsmore et al., 1994) (Mulhardt et al., 1994)
mouse	α_1 A52S	*spasmodic (spd)*	altered ligand affinity	(Ryan et al., 1994) (Saul et al., 1994)
cattle	deletion of GlyRα_1	myoclonus	loss of GlyRα_1	(Pierce et al., 2001)

startle-induced seizures. Genetic analyses by Shiang and associates first identified mutations in the GlyRα_1 subunit of the strychnine-sensitive inhibitory glycine receptor (GlyR) (Shiang et al., 1993). Since this original finding, several further mutations in this GlyRα_1 and in the β-subunit genes of this receptor have been found associated with genetically dominant as well as recessive inheritance (Breitinger and Becker, 2002; Breitinger et al., 2001; Brune et al., 1996; del Giudice et al., 2001; Elmslie et al., 1996; Lapunzina et al., 2003; Lewis et al., 1998; Moorhouse et al., 1999; Rees et al., 1994; Rees et al., 2001; Rees et al., 2002; Saul et al., 1999; Schofield, 2002; Shiang et al., 1995; Vergouwe et al., 1999) (Table 1).

Originally benzodiazepines have been introduced for the treatment of this condition with some success (Becker, 1992; Ryan et al., 1992), as in the autoimmune disease "stiff-man syndrome", which is associated with autoantibodies against the GABA$_A$-receptor system (Stayer and Meinck, 1998). Therefore, an involvement of the receptor for the neurotransmitter γ-aminobutyric acid (GABA) was hypothesized, but no association of the disease with mutations of GABA$_A$ receptor subunits was found. Although genetic diagnosis is possible, today the options for treatment of the disease are still limited. Thus, the benzodiazepine treatment has remained the only therapy so far, and it is thought that it acts through compensatory mechanisms between the two major systems of synaptic inhibition—GABA$_A$ and glycine (Zhou et al., 2002). However, pharmacological approaches addressing the glycine receptor directly are likely to improve the therapeutic situation.

II. THE INHIBITORY GLYCINE RECEPTOR

The inhibitory glycine receptor (GlyR) mediates fast synaptic inhibition mainly in the brainstem and spinal cord (Betz, 1992). In higher areas of the central nervous system, this function is carried out by GABA$_A$ receptors, but both receptor systems overlap in their sites of action. They both belong to a superfamily of membrane–bound neurotransmitter receptors constituting ligand–gated ion channels. This family includes excitatory, acetylcholine– and serotonin–activated sodium–conducting ion channels, as well as inhibitory chloride–conducting ion channels activated by GABA and glycine (Breitinger and Becker, 2002; Grenningloh et al., 1987; Rajendra et al., 1997; Schofield, 2002; Vannier and Triller, 1997).

The members of this receptor family generally represent pentameric complexes of different subunit proteins. The subunits within this family are relatively homologous to

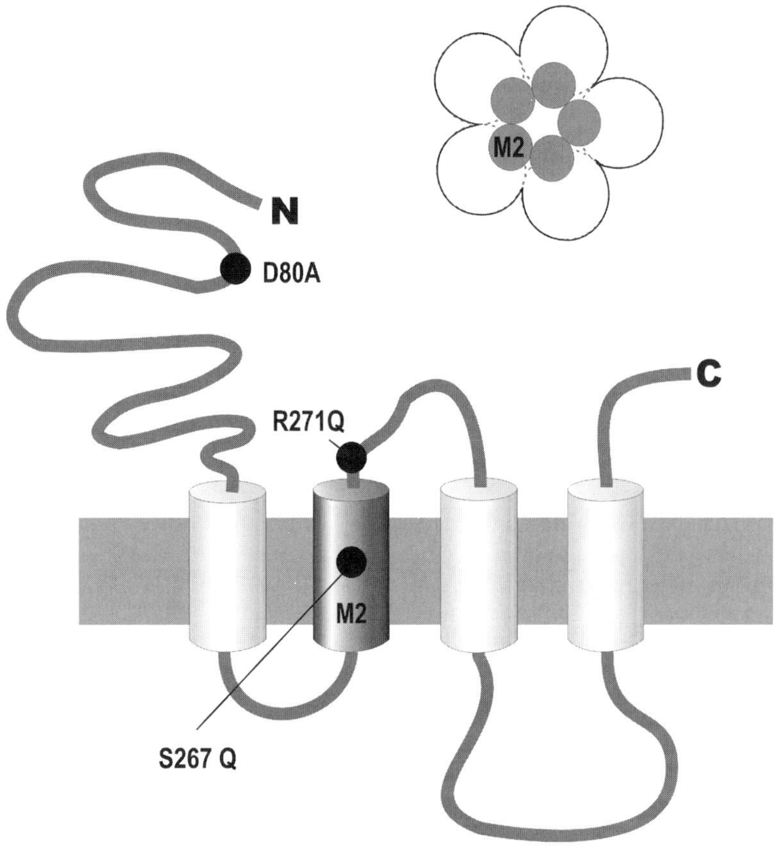

FIGURE 1 Schematic drawing of the human glycine receptor α_1 subunit. M2 depicts the transmembrane region that forms the inside of the channel as indicated in the small scheme.

each other, and all consist of five hydrophilic regions of variable size interrupted by four transmembrane domains. Figure 1 depicts a schematic drawing of a typical subunit of this kind, the α_1 subunit of the strychnine-sensitive glycine receptor (GlyRα_1), as it is found in adult humans.

The adult GlyR in rodents as well as in humans consists of three ligand-binding α_1 subunits and two structural β subunits (Kuhse et al., 1993; Langosch et al., 1988). The respective M2 transmembrane regions form the ion channel (Bormann et al., 1993) (Figure 1). Binding of the natural ligand glycine leads to gating of the channel and subsequent influx of chloride ions. Thereby hyperpolarization occurs, inhibiting neuronal firing. In addition to the natural ligand glycine, the GlyR binds and responds to several other ligands, such as the amino acids taurine and β-alanine. The alkaloid strychnine binds specifically and with high affinity to the glycine receptor as a competitive antagonist *in vitro* and *in vivo* (Pfeiffer and Betz, 1981). Acute poisoning results in severe generalized hypotonia and convulsions (Becker, 1992; Dittrich et al., 1984; Smith, 1990). Subconvulsive doses lead to hyperresponsiveness to sensory stimuli due to the reduction of inhibition, thereby disturbing the balance between excitatory and inhibitory signalling. These symptoms are similar to those observed in hereditary hyperekplexia or startle disease. Analogous syndromes have been identified in other mammals, including horse (Gundlach et al., 1993), cattle (Gundlach, 1990; Pierce et al., 2001), and mouse (White and Heller, 1982). Analyses of the underlying mechanisms revealed mutations in genes of the GlyR in humans (Breitinger and Becker, 2002; Shiang et al., 1993), as well as mice (Buckwalter et al., 1994; Kingsmore et al., 1994; Mulhardt et al., 1994; Ryan et al., 1994; Saul et al., 1994), and cattle (Pierce et al., 2001). The glycine receptor structure and function is highly conserved between mammalian species, emphasizing the importance of this system in evolution.

The subunit composition of the GlyR underlies developmental and spatial variation. Early in development, a homopentamer of the neonatal α_2 subunit forms the receptor complex (Becker et al., 1992), whereas a switch to the α_1/β subunit complex occurs in humans around birth (Ryan et al., 1994), and in mice 2 weeks postnatally (Becker et al., 1988; Ryan et al., 1994). In addition to α_1 and α_2, two more α-subunits with so far unknown function, α_3 (Kuhse et al., 1990) and α_4 (Matzenbach et al., 1994) exist. However, the different isoforms of the GlyRα subunit are expressed in different temporal and spatial limits (Malosio et al., 1991). Further variability is introduced by the existence of several α subunit splice variants of unknown function (Vannier and Triller, 1997). In contrast, the GlyRβ-subunit, which is responsible for positioning the adult GlyR complex to the synapse through binding the cytoplasmatic anchoring protein gephyrin (Kirsch et al., 1996), does not display isoform variation. It is widely expressed in the nervous system, and the role of β subunit expression in regions without α subunit co-expression is unclear. Thus it is not known if it forms complexes with any other neurotransmitter subunit than GlyRα_1. As demonstrated by work on mouse mutants, however, GlyRα_1 requires the expression of the β subunit to form the adult GlyR in animals (Kingsmore et al., 1994; Mulhardt et al., 1994).

The GlyR activity can be regulated on several levels. In addition to the ligand binding, its function can be modulated by intracellular phosphorylation of the α_1 and the β subunit (Ruiz-Gomez et al., 1991; Vaello et al., 1994). Furthermore, Zn^{2+} ions affect receptor activity in a concentration-dependent manner (Laube et al., 2000), and several alcohols and anesthetics have been reported to modify the activity of reconstituted receptors in tissue culture and in *Xenopus* oocytes, whereby the potentiating effect of ethanol on GlyR function should be emphasized (Belelli et al., 1999; Mascia et al., 1998; Mascia et al., 2000; Mihic, 1999; Miller, 2002).

The molecular functions of the GlyR subunits have been investigated in many studies by mutational analyses in tissue culture or other heterologous systems. To investigate the complex interactions with other transmitter systems relevant *in vivo*, in hyperekplexia as well as in other diseases, mutant and transgenic animal models were analyzed.

III. GLYCINE RECEPTOR DEFICIENCIES IN SPONTANEOUS AND TRANSGENIC MUTANT MICE

A. Spontaneous Mutants

In mice, spontaneous mutations affecting GlyR subunits have been described. In contrast to the human mutations, only recessive inheritance was observed. A summary of the spontaneous mouse mutations is given in Table 1.

1. Oscillator (spd^{ot})

The recessive mouse mutant *oscillator* carries a microdeletion of eight base pairs in the GlyRα_1 gene leading to a premature stop codon (Buckwalter et al., 1994). The consequence is a complete loss of GlyR in adult homozygous animals due to lack of the α_1 subunit (Kling et al., 1997). The absence of adult GlyR function in homozygous *oscillator* mice manifests itself with the development of progressively worsening neurological symptoms at about day 15 of life. Initially, a startle-induced fine motor tremor and a delayed righting reflex are observed. When brought into a supine position, the mice are not able to right themselves instantly. Within several days the tremor becomes permanent and disables the animals completely, leading to death before the age of about 21 days (Buckwalter et al., 1994). The phenotype onset occurs at the age when the isoform-switch between the neonatal α_2 and the adult α_1/β isoform of the receptor takes place due to expression changes in the animal (Becker et al., 1992). It should be noted that this onset is later than the perinatal appearance of the symptoms in hyperekplexia patients and, it is supposed that the isotype switch in humans happens earlier. A partial loss of GlyR expression in heterozygous animals causes only a very mild phenotype detectable as an enhanced acoustic startle (Kling et al., 1997).

2. Spasmodic (spd)

Another GlyRα_1 subunit mutation, in the recessive mutant *spasmodic*, represents a missense mutation changing an alanine to serine (A52S). This was shown to reduce the agonist affinity of the mutant receptor (Ryan et al., 1994; Saul et al., 1994). The mutation reduces the ethanol potentiation in recombinant GlyR (Mascia et al., 1996) but does not alter the sensitivity towards certain anesthetics (Quinlan et al., 2002). Homozygous *spasmodic* mice therefore display reduced GlyR function but are viable. Their phenotype includes an exaggerated startle reflex (Plappert et al., 2001), *i.e.*, a physical overreaction to unexpected noise or touch (Brown, 2002), and startle-induced tremor episodes. The impaired righting response (Lane et al., 1987) in these mutants is less pronounced, than in homozygous *oscillator* animals. In addition, these animals display a clenching of the hind feet when held suspended by the tail, instead of the outward movement of the limbs in *wildtype* mice (Simon, 1997).

3. Spastic (spa)

A very similar phenotype is shown by homozygous *spastic* animals, the first GlyR mutant described (White and Heller, 1982), in which the GlyRβ gene is expressed to only 10% to 20% due to an LINE1-insertion into intron 6 compromising mRNA splicing of this gene (Kingsmore et al., 1994; Mulhardt et al., 1994). Because the β-subunit is essential for adult GlyR assembly and function, in these animals the number of membrane-bound GlyRs is strongly reduced (Becker et al., 1986; Becker et al., 1992; White and Heller, 1982). An even greater loss of [^{3}H]strychnine binding was found in a meanwhile extinct mutant, *spastic albany* (*spa*^{alb}) displaying a lethal phenotype resembling the functional null mutant *oscillator*. The phenotype of *spastic* is not that

TABLE 2 Transgene Expression and Phenotype in Different GlyRα_1 Transgenic Mice

Transgene	tg271Q-				tg271R-		
mouse line	300	382	331	354	783	791	803
genotype	+/+ +/–	+/+ +/–	+/+ +/–	+/+ +/–	+/+ +/–	+/+ +/–	+/+ +/–
expression level	+++++	+++	+	+	+++++	++	+
"hyperekplectic"	n.a. ++	+ –	(+) –	– –	– –	– –	– –
hind limb dysfunction	– –	– –	– –	– –	n.a. ++	+ –	(+) –

n.a.: not analyzed.

strong and may vary dependent upon genetic background (Becker, 1990; von Wegerer et al., 2003). Gradually increasing GlyR expression by introduction of β-subunit–expressing transgenes generated mice with weakened phenotypes, depending upon the levels of GlyR activity. Even temporal changes in phenotype strength, that is, symptomatic weakening with age, as observed in human hyperekplexia, could be reproduced in a mouse model constructed in this way (Becker et al., 2000). Thus, from the data reviewed so far, it revealed that, depending upon the levels of remnant GlyR activity, mice show motor deficiencies with different severity closely resembling the human disease symptoms. The high structural homology between human and mouse GlyRα_1 genes further encouraged activities to test a human hyperekplexia disease gene in mice directly.

B. Transgenic Mouse Models

1. A Mouse Model of Human Hyperekplexia

a. Generation of Transgenic Mice Expressing a Hyperekplexia-specific Human Glyrα_1 Subunit

The most frequent, genetically dominant form of human startle disease is associated with a mutation in pos. 271 on the outside of the membrane-spanning region M2, in which a glutamine substitutes for an arginine (R271Q) (Breitinger and Becker, 2002; Shiang et al., 1993) (Figure 1, Table 1). Also changes to leucine have been found in patients at this position (R271L) (Shiang et al., 1993). Recombinant expression of the respective disease genes resulted in glycine receptors with impaired glycine as well as taurine and β-alanine responses in tissue culture and in *Xenopus* oocytes (Langosch et al., 1994; Rajendra et al., 1994). Binding of the natural ligand glycine to the mutant receptor is diminished, whereas the competitive antagonist strychnine binds to the mutant receptor with unchanged affinity in these heterologous systems (Langosch et al., 1994; Rajendra et al., 1994).

An animal model of this genetically dominant form of the disease was generated by introducing the human R271Q mutant cDNA under the control of a neuron-specific promoter as a transgene in mice (Becker et al., 2002). Several lines with different expression levels were derived (Table 2). It revealed that, dependent upon expression levels, the mutant transgenics (tg271Q) displayed a phenotype very similar to the spontaneous mutant *spastic* and *spasmodic*. The results obtained with these animals are discussed in detail below.

As a control, the nonmutant human GlyRα_1 gene was expressed in transgenic lines as well. Mice expressing the human wt GlyRα_1 transgene showed additional ligand binding, documenting the formation of receptors composed of transgenic human GlyRα_1 and endogenous murine GlyRβ subunits. Such chimeric receptors are functional, since the lethal phenotype of the null mutation *oscillator* is rescued, when the transgene is bred into this genetic background (Becker et al., 2002). This functional interspecies rescue is important for the evaluation of the data obtained with the mutant GlyRα_1 transgene.

b. Phenotypic Analysis of tg271Q-300 Mice

Using several mouse models of differential GlyR function, qualitative and quantitative assays have been developed to measure GlyR function (Becker et al., 2000; Simon, 1997). These were used to characterize the disease phenotype in the tg271Q transgenic hyperekplexia model strains. As depicted schematically in Table 2, it was found that the strongest expressing strain, tg271Q-300, showed a phenotype when the transgene was present heterozygously, while two other strains showed gene dosage effects, whereby a phenotype was seen only in homozygotes. One weakly expressing strain did not show a phenotype at all. Further characterization of the phenotype was restricted to tg271Q-300 mice. Transgenic overexpression of the unmutated human GlyRα_1 subunit, although rescuing a GlyRα_1 null mutation *oscillator*, evokes a phenotype very different from the one of the *spastic* or *spasmodic* mice described above. Also dependent upon expression level of the additional α_1 subunit, the mice showed a slowly progressing hind limb disorder, characterized by malcoordination and muscle wasting. Degeneration of motoneurons was found in the spinal cord of these animals (Becker et al., manuscript in preparation).

tg271Q-300 animals display an exaggerated startle reflex inducible by acoustic and especially tactile stimuli, as well

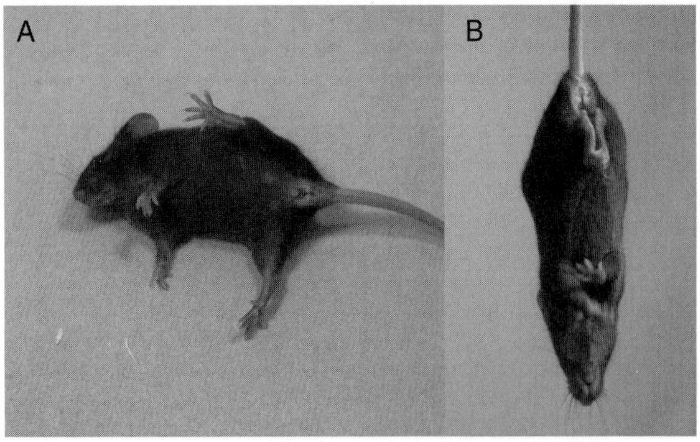

FIGURE 2 Tg271Q-300 mice show an impaired righting reflex (A) and hind feet clenching when picked up by the tail (B).

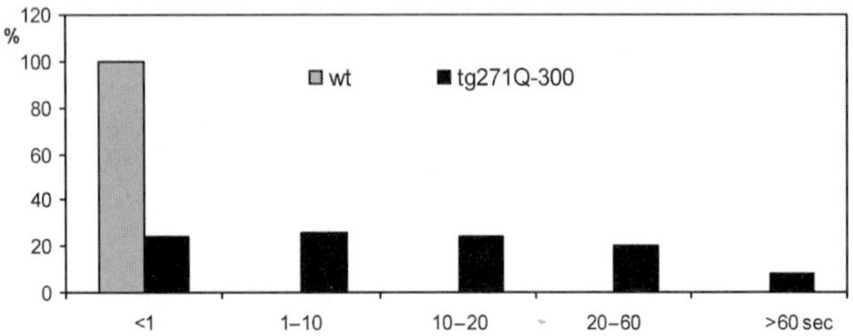

FIGURE 3 Phenotypic analysis of tg271Q-300 animals. Time required to right after being turned to the back.

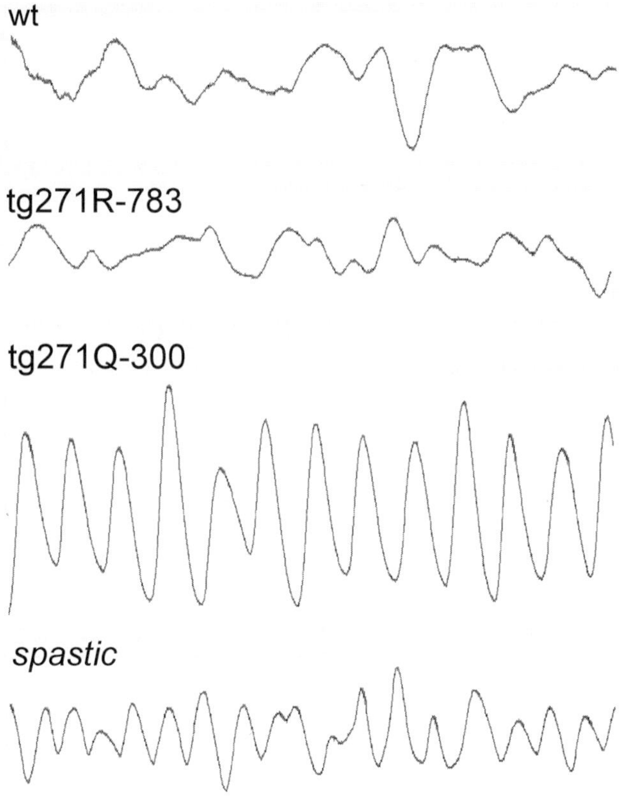

FIGURE 4 Tremor recordings of different mouse strains. Each trace represents the recording of 0.5 sec.

as an impaired righting response. Mice with reduced GlyR function stay on their backs when turned around (Figure 2, *A*) and, depending upon the remnant GlyR function, get back onto their feet faster or slower. Thus, the righting time is a measure of phenotype strength and inversely correlated to GlyR function. This measurement has indeed shown to be a reliable and easily quantifiable marker for this behavior (Becker et al., 2000; Becker et al., 2002; Hartenstein et al., 1996). As shown in Figures 2, *A* and 3, tg271Q-300 animals were severely impaired with respect to this ability. Also, very much like *spastic* and *spasmodic* animals, tg271Q-300 mice showed tremors inducible by sudden noise or handling stress. The vibrations caused by this tremor can be measured using an electromechanical transducer developed for this purpose. The traces obtained from an experiment of this kind are shown in Figure 4. tg271-Q300 animals showed tremor frequencies of about 25 to 30 Hz, similar to those recorded from *spastic* mice, which also are in accord with the frequencies appearing in human hyperekplexia (Stayer and Meinck, 1998). The amplitude of the recordings appeared to be stronger in tg271Q-300 animals than in *spastic* animals and, unlike in preterminal *oscillator* mice, the tremor was not permanent but inducible (Becker et al., 2002). tg271R mice expressing the human wt GlyRα1 subunit did not display tremor (Figure 4). Finally, the tg271Q-300 animals showed a hind feet clenching behavior when picked up by the tail (Figure 2, *B*).

c. Modification of Inhibitory Transmission in the Spinal Cord of tg271Q-300 Mice

To investigate whether the GlyR dependent neuromotor inhibition was impaired in this hyperekplexia model, patch clamp analyses on α-motoneurons in the ventral horn of spinal cord slices of postnatal days 14–19 transgenic mice were performed (Becker et al., 2002). The postsynaptic currents (PSC) can be blocked completely by inhibiting the glutamate, glycine, and $GABA_A$ receptors altogether. Selective blocking of the glutamatergic and GABAergic components with kynurenic acid and bicuculline revealed that the glycinergic component was reduced in the tg271Q-300 transgenics by 69.8% (Figure 5, *B*). In addition to the restricted GlyR function, these animals showed an almost complete loss of GABAergic inhibition as well (90.9% reduction), evident after blocking with kynurenic acid and strychnine (Figure 5, *B*). This result is evidence for an interaction between the two inhibitory transmitter systems, the glycinergic and the GABAergic one. No involvement of diminished $GABA_A$ receptor binding has been found so far in these mice, which suggests that the interaction is regulated more likely at a physiological level than by regulation of the amount of $GABA_A$ receptors. These data demonstrate non-compensatory interactions between the different inhibitory signalling

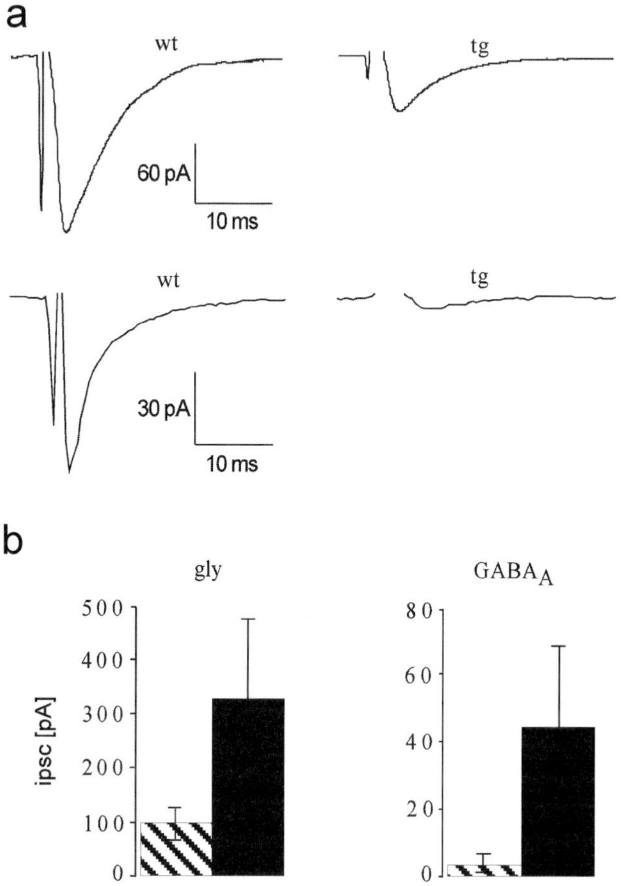

FIGURE 5 Electrically evoked ipscs from spinal cord neurons. (a): representative tracings from individual measurements on spinal cord neurons of nontransgenic (*left*) and tg271Q-300 (*right*) mice. *Top*: Glycinergic component of the ipsc. *Bottom*: $GABA_A$ receptor-mediated ipsc. (b): summary of the electrophysiolgical data: Mean amplitudes of the glycine receptor-mediated (*left*) and $GABA_A$ receptor-mediated ipscs for tg271Q-300 animals (*striped bars*) and nontransgenic controls (*filled bars*). In tg271Q-300 the glycinergic component was reduced from −331.2 ± 124.8 pA to −100.1 ± 23.8 pA. The GABA-Rb_A receptor-mediated component was −4.1 ± 3.0 pA for tg271Q-300 mice, in comparison to −45.0 ± 25.4 pA in the controls (figure taken from Becker et al., 2002).

pathways in the animal model. Such interactions may have been suggested by earlier findings: Glycine and $GABA_A$ receptors have been found to be co-expressed (Bohlhalter et al., 1994) and co-released (Jonas et al., 1998) and are clustered in the synapse due to binding to the accessory protein gephyrin (Dumoulin et al., 2000; Essrich et al., 1998; Feng et al., 1998; Kneussel et al., 1999). In gephyrin-deficient mice the GlyR and the $GABA_A$ receptor clustering was reduced (Essrich et al., 1998; Feng et al., 1998; Kneussel et al., 1999). Furthermore, these results may provide a rationale for the success of benzodiazepine treatment of genetic GlyR defects (Ryan et al., 1992; Zhou et al., 2002). The symptomatic similarity between *stiff-man syndrome*, an autoimmune disease affecting the GABAergic system, and genetic GlyR defects with respect to electromyographic data (Stayer and Meinck, 1998) is due to the partially parallel and overlapping function of the two inhibitory transmitter systems. In tg271Q-300 animals an interaction of these two systems was clearly demonstrated. Targeted mutation of certain $GABA_A$ receptor subunits does also lead to neuromotor modifications, *e.g.*, an intention tremor in $GABA_A\alpha_1$ negative mice (Kralic et al., 2002; Sur et al., 2001).

The results obtained from tg271Q-300 mice are in contrast with early studies on *spastic* mice, in which a compensatory increase of GABAergic signalling has been postulated (White and Heller, 1982). This raised the question of whether these data might be due to the dominant nature of the hyperekplexia transgene producing a gene product physically cross-reacting with the $GABA_A$ receptor. However, von Wegerer and associates corroborated the results obtained with the 271Q-300 transgene with *spastic* mice displaying a loss of wt GlyR expression to about 20% (von Wegerer et al., 2003). Thus, all recent data argue against compensation in motoneurons.

It should be noted, however, that these data only concern motoneuron regulation. Yet GABA and glycine modulate sensory pathways as well, and electrophysiological studies on superficial dorsal horn (SFDH) neurons, important for nociceptive processing, indeed revealed such a compensatory increase of GABAergic signalling (Graham et al., 2003). Interestingly, compensation was only seen in *spastic* mice that still have some GlyR expression, but not in the *oscillator* mutant, completely lacking adult GlyR. Future studies will reveal if compensation occurs in tg271Q-300 animals, as these, by displaying reduced agonist affinity instead of reduced GlyR expression, feature a different mechanism of signal interruption. The tg271Q-300 animals resemble human hyperekplexia closely; therefore, the results from this model should be relevant to the human disease.

More recently, von Wegerer and associates have shown that not only the inhibitory, but also the excitatory, transmission in these animals is modified; whereas no change is observed with AMPA/kainate receptor transmission, the NMDA-mediated EPSC is significantly enhanced (von Wegerer et al., manuscript in preparation). These data show that the imbalance between excitatory and inhibitory signalling due to the $GlyR\alpha_1$ mutation causes complex physiological dysregulations.

2. Other $GlyR\alpha_1$ Mutations Introduced in Mice

To elucidate the molecular function of the $GlyR\alpha_1$ subunit, numerous mutations have been produced and analyzed for their electrophysiological and pharmacological properties in heterologous systems, such as transfected tissue culture cells and *Xenopus* oocytes. Ultimately, the properties of mutated molecules and, specifically, disease mechanisms are preferably studied in animal models *in vivo*. Along these lines, several other mutations were introduced into the genome and studied in mice, in addition to the one associated with human startle disease described above. Mutating the serine 267 to a glutamine (S267Q) in heterologous systems leads to a decreased efficacy of the GlyR rather than to reduced agonist binding (Figure 1) (Findlay et al., 2003). In "knock in" mice, this mutation produced homozygous lethality, phenotypically resembling the full loss-of-function phenotype of homozygous *oscillator* mice. In heterozygotes, this mutation produced a stronger startle phenotype than that of heterozygous oscillator mice, indicating the dominant negative nature of the mutation (Findlay et al., 2003). The same mutation abolishes the possibility to potentiate GlyR activity by ethanol *in vitro*. Transgenic mice, overexpressing a GlyRα_1 (S267Q) mutant subunit, exhibit decreased ethanol sensitivity (Findlay et al., 2002).

In order to study the role of Zn^{2+} ions in the function of GlyR *in vivo,* "knock in" mice have been produced carrying a substitution of an aspartic acid by an alanine residue in their GlyRα_1 subunit at position 80 (D80A) in the N-terminal extracellular portion of GlyRα_1 (Figure 1). This position is not involved in agonist binding but rather is critical for Zn^{2+} regulation of the GlyR activity (Laube et al., 2000). Consistent with previous data on transfected cells or injected *Xenopus* oozytes, the modification of the glycine response by Zn^{2+} ions in spinal cord neurons from homozygous mutant (D80A) mice was affected. These mice produced a characteristic hyperekplexia phenotype, although milder than tg271Q-300 or even *spastic* and *spasmodic* animals. Thus, the Zn^{2+} regulation of GlyR activity (Laube et al., 2000) is important for its function *in vivo* (Hirzel et al., manuscript in preparation).

IV. HYPEREKPLEXIA MODELS TO DEVELOP AND TEST THERAPEUTIC INTERVENTION

In order to understand the pathological mechanisms acting in GlyR disease, pharmacological treatments have been applied to some of the animal models described above. For example, it has been shown in transgenic animals overexpressing the glycine receptor mutation (S267Q) that this mutant GlyR renders mice more resistant to ethanol (Findlay et al., 2002); these results provide *in vivo* evidence for the hypothesis that the GlyR is an important target for motor incoordination and anesthetic properties of ethanol action (Mihic, 1999; Mihic et al., 1997; Sebe et al., 2003). Quinlan and associates have found modified ethanol responses in mice with mutant GlyR (Quinlan et al., 2002). Application of cannabinoids to GlyR mutant mice have so far not produced evidence for a potential benefit of such agents in GlyR disease (D. Baker, unpublished observation). The use of such models to develop and test therapeutic intervention has just begun. Thus, we have recently shown that the anesthetic propofol, which potentiates glycinergic inhibition (Bansinath et al., 1995; Dong and Xu, 2002), transiently rescues completely the phenotype of tg271Q-300 mice in subhypnotic and subanesthetic doses and may therefore be suited for intervention with acute seizures (O'Shea et al., 2004). However, this may only be the starting point for a search for better medications. The complex interactions of the glycinergic system with other neurotransmitter systems are not yet fully understood. Further studies in the described animal models provide the possibilities to explore the underlying mechanisms in the mammalian organism.

Acknowledgments

We thank Bodo Laube, David Baker, and Jörg von Wegerer and their co-workers for communication of unpublished results. The support of this work through grants from the Bundesministerium für Bildung und Forschung and the Thyssen Foundation are gratefully acknowledged.

Video Legends

SEGMENT 1 Hyperekplectic mice (transgenic 271Q-300). Postnatal Day 15.

SEGMENT 2 Oscillator mice. Postnatal Day 15.

SEGMENT 3 Two hyperekplectic (transgenic 271Q-300) mice and one wild-type mouse. Startle induced by clapping hands.

SEGMENT 4 Two hyperekplectic (transgenic 271Q-300) mice and one wild-type mouse. Startle induced with noise.

SEGMENT 5 Hyperekplectic mice (transgenic 271Q-300). Impaired righting reflex.

SEGMENT 6 Non-transgenic mice. Tail suspension test.

SEGMENT 7 Hyperekplectic mice (transgenic 271Q-300). Tail suspension test.

The following segments relate to human wild-type transgenic (271R-783) control mice. Neurodegeneration phenotype.

SEGMENT 8 Tail suspension test.

SEGMENT 9 Open field behavior.

References

Andrew, M., and M.J. Owen. 1997. Hyperekplexia: abnormal startle response due to glycine receptor mutations. *Br J Psychiatry*, **170**:106–108.

Bansinath, M., V.K. Shukla, and H. Turndorf. 1995. Propofol modulates the effects of chemoconvulsants acting at GABAergic, glycinergic, and glutamate receptor subtypes. *Anesthesiology*, **83**:809–815.

Becker, C.M. 1990. Disorders of the inhibitory glycine receptor: the spastic mouse. *Faseb J*, **4**:2767–2774.

Becker, C.-M. 1992. Convulsants Acting at the Inhibitory Glycine Receptor. In H. Herken, F.F.H. (ed.), *Handbook of Experimental Pharmacology*. Springer-Verlag, Vol. 102, pp. 539–575.

Becker, C.M., I. Hermans-Borgmeyer, B. Schmitt, and H. Betz. 1986. The glycine receptor deficiency of the mutant mouse spastic: evidence for normal glycine receptor structure and localization. *J Neurosci*, **6**:1358–1364.

Becker, C.M., W. Hoch, and H. Betz. 1988. Glycine receptor heterogeneity in rat spinal cord during postnatal development. *Embo J*, **7**:3717–3726.

Becker, C.M., V. Schmieden, P. Tarroni, U. Strasser, and H. Betz. 1992. Isoform-selective deficit of glycine receptors in the mouse mutant spastic. *Neuron*, **8**:283–289.

Becker, L., B. Hartenstein, J. Schenkel, J. Kuhse, H. Betz, and H. Weiher. 2000. Transient neuromotor phenotype in transgenic spastic mice expressing low levels of glycine receptor beta-subunit: an animal model of startle disease. *Eur J Neurosci*, **12**:27–32.

Becker, L., J. von Wegerer, J. Schenkel, H.U. Zeilhofer, D. Swandulla, and H. Weiher. 2002. Disease-specific human glycine receptor alpha1 subunit causes hyperekplexia phenotype and impaired glycine- and GABA(A)-receptor transmission in transgenic mice. *J Neurosci*, **22**:2505–2512.

Belelli, I., I. Pistis, J.A. Peters, and J.J. Lambert. 1999. General anaesthetic action at transmitter-gated inhibitory amino acid receptors. *Trends Pharmacol Sci*, **20**:496–502.

Betz, H. 1992. Structure and function of inhibitory glycine receptors. *Q Rev Biophys*, **25**:381–394.

Bohlhalter, S., H. Mohler, and J.M. Fritschy. 1994. Inhibitory neurotransmission in rat spinal cord: co-localization of glycine- and GABAA-receptors at GABAergic synaptic contacts demonstrated by triple immunofluorescence staining. *Brain Res*, **642**:59–69.

Bormann, J., N. Rundstrom, H. Betz, and D. Langosch. 1993. Residues within transmembrane segment M2 determine chloride conductance of glycine receptor homo- and hetero-oligomers. *Embo J*, **12**:3729–3737.

Breitinger, H.G., and C.M. Becker. 2002. The inhibitory glycine receptor-simple views of a complicated channel. *Chembiochem*, **3**:1042–1052.

Breitinger, H.G., C. Villmann, K. Becker, and C.M. Becker. 2001. Opposing effects of molecular volume and charge at the hyperekplexia site alpha 1(P250) govern glycine receptor activation and desensitization. *J Biol Chem*, **276**:29657–29663.

Brown, P. 2002. The startle syndrome. *Mov Disord*, **17 Suppl 2**:S79–82.

Brune, W., R.G. Weber, B. Saul, M. von Knebel Doeberitz, C. Grond-Ginsbach, K. Kellerman, H.M. Meinck, and C.M. Becker. 1996. A GLRA1 null mutation in recessive hyperekplexia challenges the functional role of glycine receptors. *Am J Hum Genet*, **58**:989–997.

Buckwalter, M.S., S.A. Cook, M.T. Davisson, W.F. White, and S.A. Camper. 1994. A frameshift mutation in the mouse alpha 1 glycine receptor gene (Glra1) results in progressive neurological symptoms and juvenile death. *Hum Mol Genet*, **3**:2025–2030.

del Giudice, E.M., G. Coppola, G. Bellini, G. Cirillo, G. Scuccimarra, and A. Pascotto. 2001. A mutation (V260M) in the middle of the M2 pore-lining domain of the glycine receptor causes hereditary hyperekplexia. *Eur J Hum Genet*, **9**:873–876.

Dittrich, K., M.J. Bayer, and L.A. Wanke. 1984. A case of fatal strychnine poisoning. *J Emerg Med*, **1**:327–330.

Dong, X.P., and T.L. Xu. 2002. The actions of propofol on gamma-aminobutyric acid-A and glycine receptors in acutely dissociated spinal dorsal horn neurons of the rat. *Anesth Analg*, **95**:907–914.

Dumoulin, A., S. Levi, B. Riveau, B. Gasnier, and A. Triller. 2000. Formation of mixed glycine and GABAergic synapses in cultured spinal cord neurons. *Eur J Neurosci*, **12**:3883–3892.

Elmslie, F.V., S.M. Hutchings, V. Spencer, A. Curtis, T. Covanis, R.M. Gardiner, and M. Rees. 1996. Analysis of GLRA1 in hereditary and sporadic hyperekplexia: a novel mutation in a family cosegregating for hyperekplexia and spastic paraparesis. *J Med Genet*, **33**:435–436.

Essrich, C., M. Lorez, J.A. Benson, J.M. Fritschy, and B. Luscher. 1998. Postsynaptic clustering of major GABAA receptor subtypes requires the gamma 2 subunit and gephyrin. *Nat Neurosci*, **1**:563–571.

Feng, G., H. Tintrup, J. Kirsch, M.C. Nichol, J. Kuhse, H. Betz, and J.R. Sanes. 1998. Dual requirement for gephyrin in glycine receptor clustering and molybdoenzyme activity [see comments]. *Science*, **282**:1321–1324.

Findlay, G.S., R. Phelan, M.T. Roberts, G.E. Homanics, S.E. Bergeson, G.F. Lopreato, S.J. Mihic, Y.A. Blednov, and R.A. Harris. 2003. Glycine receptor knock-in mice and hyperekplexia-like phenotypes: comparisons with the null mutant. *J Neurosci*, **23**:8051–8059.

Findlay, G.S., M.J. Wick, M.P. Mascia, D. Wallace, G.W. Miller, R.A. Harris, and Y.A. Blednov. 2002. Transgenic expression of a mutant glycine receptor decreases alcohol sensitivity of mice. *J Pharmacol Exp Ther*, **300**:526–534.

Graham, B.A., P.R. Schofield, P. Sah, and R.J. Callister. 2003. Altered inhibitory synaptic transmission in superficial dorsal horn neurones in spastic and oscillator mice. *J Physiol*, **551**:905–916.

Grenningloh, G., A. Rienitz, B. Schmitt, C. Methfessel, M. Zensen, K. Beyreuther, E.D. Gundelfinger, and H. Betz. 1987. The strychnine-binding subunit of the glycine receptor shows homology with nicotinic acetylcholine receptors. *Nature*, **328**:215–220.

Gundlach, A.L. 1990. Disorder of the inhibitory glycine receptor: inherited myoclonus in Poll Hereford calves. *Faseb J*, **4**:2761–2766.

Gundlach, A.L., G. Kortz, T.C. Burazin, J. Madigan, and R.J. Higgins. 1993. Deficit of inhibitory glycine receptors in spinal cord from Peruvian Pasos: evidence for an equine form of inherited myoclonus. *Brain Res*, **628**:263–270.

Hartenstein, B., J. Schenkel, J. Kuhse, B. Besenbeck, C. Kling, C.M. Becker, H. Betz, and H. Weiher. 1996. Low level expression of glycine receptor beta subunit transgene is sufficient for phenotype correction in spastic mice. *Embo J*, **15**:1275–1282.

Humeny, A., T. Bonk, K. Becker, M. Jafovi-Boroujerdi, U. Stephani, K. Reuter and C.M. Becker. 2002. A novel recessive hyperekplexia allele GLRA1 (S231R): genotying by MACDI-TOF mass spectrometry and functional characterisation as a determinant of cellular glycine trafficking. *Eur J Human Genet* **10**:188–196.

Jonas, P., J. Bischofberger, and J. Sandkuhler. 1998. Corelease of two fast neurotransmitters at a central synapse [see comments]. *Science*, **281**: 419–424.

Kingsmore, S.F., B. Giros, D. Suh, M. Bieniarz, M.G. Caron, and M.F. Seldin. 1994. Glycine receptor beta-subunit gene mutation in spastic mouse associated with LINE-1 element insertion. *Nat Genet*, **7**:136–141.

Kirsch, J., G. Meyer, and H. Betz. 1996. Synaptic targeting of ionotropic neurotransmitter receptors. *Mol Cell Neurosci*, **8**:93–98.

Kling, C., M. Koch, B. Saul, and C.M. Becker. 1997. The frameshift mutation oscillator (Glra1(spd-ot)) produces a complete loss of glycine receptor alpha1-polypeptide in mouse central nervous system. *Neuroscience*, **78**:411–417.

Kneussel, M., J.H. Brandstatter, B. Laube, S. Stahl, U. Muller, and H. Betz. 1999. Loss of postsynaptic GABA(A) receptor clustering in gephyrin-deficient mice. *J Neurosci*, **19**:9289–9297.

Kralic, J.E., E.R. Korpi, T.K. O'Buckley, G.E. Homanics, and A.L. Morrow. 2002. Molecular and pharmacological characterization of GABA(A) receptor alpha1 subunit knockout mice. *J Pharmacol Exp Ther*, **302**: 1037–1045.

Kuhse, J., B. Laube, D. Magalei, and H. Betz. 1993. Assembly of the inhibitory glycine receptor: identification of amino acid sequence motifs governing subunit stoichiometry. *Neuron*, **11**:1049–1056.

Kuhse, J., V. Schmieden, and H. Betz. 1990. Identification and functional expression of a novel ligand binding subunit of the inhibitory glycine receptor. *J Biol Chem*, **265**:22317–22320.

Kwok, J.B., S. Raskin, G. Morgan, S.A. Antoniuk, I. Bruk, and P.R. Schofield. 2001. Mutations in the glycine receptor alpha 1 subunit

(GLRA1) gene in hereditary hyperekplexia pedigrees: evidence for non-penetrance of mutation Y279C. *J Med Genet*, 38:E17.

Lane, P.W., A.L. Ganser, A.L. Kerner, and W.F. White. 1987. Spasmodic, a mutation on chromosome 11 in the mouse. *J Hered*, **78**:353–356.

Langosch, D., B. Laube, N. Rundstrom, V. Schmieden, J. Bormann, and H. Betz. 1994. Decreased agonist affinity and chloride conductance of mutant glycine receptors associated with human hereditary hyperekplexia. *Embo J*, **13**:4223–4228.

Langosch, D., L. Thomas, and H. Betz. 1988. Conserved quaternary structure of ligand-gated ion channels: the postsynaptic glycine receptor is a pentamer. *Proc Natl Acad Sci U S A*, **85**:7394–7398.

Lapunzina, P., J.M. Sanchez, M. Cabrera, A. Moreno, A. Delicado, M.L. De Torres, A.M. Mori, J. Quero, and I. Lopez Pajares. 2003. Hyperekplexia (startle disease): A novel mutation (S270T) in the M2 domain of the GLRA1 gene and a molecular review of the disorder. *Mol Diagn*, **7**:125–128.

Laube, B., J. Kuhse, and H. Betz. 2000. Kinetic and mutational analysis of Zn2+ modulation of recombinant human inhibitory glycine receptors. *J Physiol*, **522 Pt 2**:215–230.

Lewis, T.M., L.G. Sivilotti, D. Colquhoun, R.M. Gardiner, R. Schoepfer, and M. Rees. 1998. Properties of human glycine receptors containing the hyperekplexia mutation alpha1(K276E), expressed in Xenopus oocytes. *J Physiol*, **507 (Pt 1)**:25–40.

Lingam, S., J. Wilson, and E.W. Hart. 1981. Hereditary stiff-baby syndrome. *Am J Dis Child*, **135**:909–911.

Malosio, M.L., B. Marqueze-Pouey, J. Kuhse, and H. Betz. 1991. Widespread expression of glycine receptor subunit mRNAs in the adult and developing rat brain. *Embo J*, **10**:2401–2409.

Mascia, M.P., S.J. Mihic, C.F. Valenzuela, P.R. Schofield, and R.A. Harris. 1996. A single amino acid determines differences in ethanol actions on strychnine-sensitive glycine receptors. *Mol Pharmacol*, **50**:402–406.

Mascia, M.P., J.R. Trudell, and R.A. Harris. 2000. Specific binding sites for alcohols and anesthetics on ligand-gated ion channels. *Proc Natl Acad Sci USA*, **97**:9305–9310.

Mascia, M.P., M.J. Wick, L.D. Martinez, and R.A. Harris. 1998. Enhancement of glycine receptor function by ethanol: role of phosphorylation. *Br J Pharmacol*, **125**:263–270.

Matzenbach, B., Y. Maulet, L. Sefton, B. Courtier, P. Avner, J.L. Guenet, and H. Betz. 1994. Structural analysis of mouse glycine receptor alpha subunit genes. Identification and chromosomal localization of a novel variant. *J Biol Chem*, **269**:2607–2612.

Mihic, S.J. 1999. Acute effects of ethanol on GABAA and glycine receptor function. *Neurochem Int*, **35**:115–123.

Mihic, S.J., Q. Ye, M.J. Wick, V.V. Koltchine, M.D. Krasowski, S.E. Finn, M.P. Mascia, C.F. Valenzuela, K.K. Hanson, E.P. Greenblatt, R.A. Harris, and N.L. Harrison. 1997. Sites of alcohol and volatile anaesthetic action on GABA(A) and glycine receptors. *Nature*, **389**:385–389.

Miller, K.W. 2002. The nature of sites of general anaesthetic action. *Br J Anaesth*, **89**:17–31.

Moorhouse, A.J., P. Jacques, P.H. Barry, and P.R. Schofield. 1999. The startle disease mutation Q266H, in the second transmembrane domain of the human glycine receptor, impairs channel gating. *Mol Pharmacol*, **55**:386–395.

Morley, D.J., D.D. Weaver, B.P. Garg, and O. Markand. 1982. Hyperexplexia: an inherited disorder of the startle response. *Clin Genet*, **21**:388–396.

Mulhardt, C., M. Fischer, P. Gass, D. Simon-Chazottes, J.L. Guenet, J. Kuhse, H. Betz, and C.M. Becker. 1994. The spastic mouse: aberrant splicing of glycine receptor beta subunit mRNA caused by intronic insertion of L1 element. *Neuron*, **13**:1003–1015.

O'Shea, S.M., L. Becker, H. Weiher, H. Betz, and B. Laube. 2004. Propofol Restores the Function of "Hyperekplexic" Mutant Glycine Receptors in Xenopus Oocytes and Mice. *J Neurosci*, **24**:2322–2327.

Pfeiffer, F., and H. Betz. 1981. Solubilization of the glycine receptor from rat spinal cord. *Brain Res*, **226**:273–279.

Pierce, K.D., C.A. Handford, R. Morris, B. Vafa, J.A. Dennis, P.J. Healy, and P.R. Schofield. 2001. A nonsense mutation in the alpha1 subunit of the inhibitory glycine receptor associated with bovine myoclonus. *Mol Cell Neurosci*, **17**:354–363.

Plappert, C.F., P.K. Pilz, K. Becker, C.M. Becker, and H.U. Schnitzler. 2001. Increased sensitization of acoustic startle response in spasmodic mice with a mutation of the glycine receptor alpha1-subunit gene. *Behav Brain Res*, **121**:57–67.

Praveen, V., S.K. Patole, and J.S. Whitehall. 2001. Hyperekplexia in neonates. *Postgrad Med J*, **77**:570–572.

Quinlan, J.J., C. Ferguson, K. Jester, L.L. Firestone, and G.E. Homanics. 2002. Mice with glycine receptor subunit mutations are both sensitive and resistant to volatile anesthetics. *Anesth Analg*, **95**:578–582.

Rajendra, S., J.W. Lynch, K.D. Pierce, C.R. French, P.H. Barry, and P.R. Schofield. 1994. Startle disease mutations reduce the agonist sensitivity of the human inhibitory glycine receptor. *J Biol Chem*, **269**:18739–18742.

Rajendra, S., J.W. Lynch, and P.R. Schofield. 1997. The glycine receptor. *Pharmacol Ther*, **73**:121–146.

Rees, M.I., M. Andrew, S. Jawad, and M.J. Owen. 1994. Evidence for recessive as well as dominant forms of startle disease (hyperekplexia) caused by mutations in the alpha 1 subunit of the inhibitory glycine receptor. *Hum Mol Genet*, **3**:2175–2179.

Rees, M.I., T.M. Lewis, J.B. Kwok, G.R. Mortier, P. Govaert, R.G. Snell, P.R. Schofield, and M.J. Owen. 2002. Hyperekplexia associated with compound heterozygote mutations in the beta-subunit of the human inhibitory glycine receptor (GLRB). *Hum Mol Genet*, **11**:853–860.

Rees, M.I., T.M. Lewis, B. Vafa, C. Ferrie, P. Corry, F. Muntoni, H. Jungbluth, J.B. Stephenson, M. Kerr, R.G. Snell, P.R. Schofield, and M.J. Owen. 2001. Compound heterozygosity and nonsense mutations in the alpha(1)-subunit of the inhibitory glycine receptor in hyperekplexia. *Hum Genet*, **109**:267–270.

Ruiz-Gomez, A., M.L. Vaello, F. Valdivieso, and F., Mayor. Jr. 1991. Phosphorylation of the 48-kDa subunit of the glycine receptor by protein kinase C. *J Biol Chem*, **266**:559–566.

Ryan, S.G., M.S. Buckwalter, J.W. Lynch, C.A. Handford, L. Segura, R. Shiang, J.J. Wasmuth, S.A. Camper, P. Schofield, and P. O'Connell, 1994. A missense mutation in the gene encoding the alpha 1 subunit of the inhibitory glycine receptor in the spasmodic mouse. *Nat Genet*, **7**:131–135.

Ryan, S.G., S.L. Sherman, J.C. Terry, R.S. Sparkes, M.C. Torres, and R.W. Mackey. 1992. Startle disease, or hyperekplexia: response to clonazepam and assignment of the gene (STHE) to chromosome 5q by linkage analysis. *Ann Neurol*, **31**:663–668.

Saul, B., T. Kuner, D. Sobetzko, W. Brune, F. Hanefeld, H.M. Meinck, and C.M. Becker. 1999. Novel GLRA1 missense mutation (P250T) in dominant hyperekplexia defines an intracellular determinant of glycine receptor channel gating. *J Neurosci*, **19**:869–877.

Saul, B., V. Schmieden, C. Kling, C. Mulhardt, P. Gass, J. Kuhse, and C.M. Becker. 1994. Point mutation of glycine receptor alpha 1 subunit in the spasmodic mouse affects agonist responses. *FEBS Lett*, **350**:71–76.

Schofield, P.R. 2002. The role of glycine and glycine receptors in myoclonus and startle syndromes. *Adv Neurol*, **89**:263–274.

Sebe, J.Y., E.D. Eggers, and A.J. Berger. 2003. Differential effects of ethanol on GABA(A) and glycine receptor-mediated synaptic currents in brain stem motoneurons. *J Neurophysiol*, **90**:870–875.

Shiang, R., S.G. Ryan, Y.Z. Zhu, T.J. Fielder, R.J. Allen, A. Fryer, S. Yamashita, P. O'Connell, and J.J. Wasmuth. 1995. Mutational analysis of familial and sporadic hyperekplexia. *Ann Neurol*, **38**:85–91.

Shiang, R., S.G. Ryan, Y.Z. Zhu, A.F. Hahn, P. O'Connell, and J.J. Wasmuth. 1993. Mutations in the alpha 1 subunit of the inhibitory glycine receptor cause the dominant neurologic disorder, hyperekplexia. *Nat Genet*, **5**:351–358.

Simon, E.S. 1997. Phenotypic heterogeneity and disease course in three murine strains with mutations in genes encoding for alpha 1 and beta glycine receptor subunits. *Mov Disord*, **12**:221–228.

Smith, B.A. 1990. Strychnine poisoning. *J Emerg Med*, **8**:321–325.

Stayer, C., and H.M. Meinck. 1998. Stiff-man syndrome: an overview. *Neurologia*, **13**:83–88.

Sur, C., K.A. Wafford, D.S. Reynolds, K.L. Hadingham, F. Bromidge, A. Macaulay, N. Collinson, G. O'Meara, O. Howell, R. Newman, J. Myers, J.R. Atack, G.R. Dawson, R.M. McKernan, P.J. Whiting, and T.W. Rosahl. 2001. Loss of the major GABA(A) receptor subtype in the brain is not lethal in mice. *J Neurosci*, **21**:3409–3418.

Vaello, M.L., A. Ruiz-Gomez, J. Lerma, and F. Mayor. Jr. 1994. Modulation of inhibitory glycine receptors by phosphorylation by protein kinase C and cAMP-dependent protein kinase. *J Biol Chem*, **269**: 2002–2008.

Vannier, C., and A. Triller. 1997. Biology of the postsynaptic glycine receptor. *Int Rev Cytol*, **176**:201–244.

Vergouwe, M.N., M.A. Tijssen, A.C. Peters, R. Wielaard, and R.R. Frants. 1999. Hyperekplexia phenotype due to compound heterozygosity for GLRA1 gene mutations. *Ann Neurol*, **46**:634–638.

von Wegerer, J., K. Becker, D. Glockenhammer, C.M. Becker, H.U. Zeilhofer, and D. Swandulla. 2003. Spinal inhibitory synaptic transmission in the glycine receptor mouse mutant spastic. *Neurosci Lett*, **345**:45–48.

White, W.F., and A.H. Heller. 1982. Glycine receptor alteration in the mutant mouse spastic. *Nature*, **298**:655–657.

Zhou, L., K.L. Chillag, and M.A. Nigro. 2002. Hyperekplexia: a treatable neurogenetic disease. *Brain Dev*, **24**:669–674.

CHAPTER

H4

Bovine Hyperekplexia

JULIE A. DENNIS, PETER A. WINDSOR, PETER R. SCHOFIELD, and PETER J. HEALY

Inherited congenital myoclonus is an autosomal recessive disease in Poll Hereford cattle and a model of human hyperekplexia or startle disease. It is characterized by spontaneous and stimulus-responsive myoclonic spasms that resemble tetany. A ten-day reduction in the mean gestation length for affected calves may be a consequence of fetal spasms, their skeletal sequelae, or both. High velocity muscle tremors can occasionally be detected as an audible hum. Cranial nerve functions are unimpaired. Macro and microscopic abnormalities are considered the result of severe spasms of the dominant adductor musculature of the pelvic limbs and are limited to skeletal lesions in the coxae. The lesions most commonly involve fracture of the acetabular cartilage and erosion of the femoral head, though fractures of the femoral head can occur. Strychnine binding studies reveal a severe deficiency of functional glycine receptor sites. Results of immunohistochemistry indicate a loss of cell surface immunoreactivity with monoclonal antibody to α and β subunits of the glycine receptor. The causative mutation is C → A transversion at position 156 in exon 2 of the α1 subunit of the glycine receptor, resulting in the substitution of tyrosine with a termination codon (Tyr24Ter). The result is an absence of the glycine receptor α1 subunit and a marked reduction in the number of functional glycine receptors in the spinal cord. Reduction in glycine receptor expression levels explains the ICM phenotype, which provides additional information on the consequences of glycine receptor dysfunction.

I. HISTORY

Hyperekplexia in newborn Hereford calves was first identified in the United States of America and published as Hereditary Neuraxial Oedema (HNO) (Cordy et al., 1969). Subsequently, a similar clinical syndrome was observed in newborn polled Hereford calves in Australia (Blood and Gay, 1971) and England (Weaver, 1974), and in polled Hereford crossbred calves in New Zealand (Davis et al., 1975). Breeding records of the American herds were considered consistent with autosomal recessive inheritance of the condition. No data were presented with the Australian and English cases to corroborate this conclusion, though the New Zealand cases were born to Poll Hereford cross Holstein cows mated with a Poll Hereford bull. Subsequent investigations confirmed that the hyperekplexic component of the HNO syndrome was inherited in an autosomal recessive manner (Healy et al., 1985) and resolved disparities in the association between hyperekplexia and edema of the neuraxis in some reports of HNO syndrome (Healy et al., 1986; Harper et al., 1986a).

In the initial American report (Cordy et al., 1969) three of twelve affected calves examined had severe spongy vacuolation of the white matter of the central nervous system (CNS). The degree of vacuolation in the remaining nine cases was minor and recorded as microvacuolation. Clinicians recorded that one calf had fractures of the epiphyseal plates of both femurs. Blood and Gay (1971) did not observe significant microscopic lesions in the CNS of nine cases they studied. Studies on thirteen HNO affected calves born in Tasmania (Donaldson and Mason, 1984) revealed five with significant lesions in the hips, and ten with histological lesions consistent with HNO as described by Cordy and colleagues (1969).

By examining the records of the laboratory component of the veterinary diagnostic service in New South Wales Agriculture, investigators established that during the late 1970s and early 1980s HNO was the most common diagnosis offered to field veterinarians investigating suspected inherited diseases in newborn calves. In response, investigators established an experimental breeding herd by purchasing cows and bulls reputed to be parents of calves that displayed stimulus responsive myoclonic spasms and were unable to stand. During 1981, 1982, and 1983, fourteen of fifty-six calves born in the herd displayed, from birth, myoclonic whole body spasms with stimulus response similar to those described by Cordy and colleagues (1969), Blood and Gay (1971), Davis and colleagues (1974), and Donaldson and Mason (1984). None of the fourteen calves born in this experimental breeding herd could rise from birth unassisted, yet all displayed normal mentation, with absence of severe spongy vacuolation of the CNS. Thirteen of the fourteen calves had lesions in the hip joints, the most common being flattening of the acetabular fossa and eburnation of the femoral head. Investigators proposed that a separate disorder was most likely to be present in the polled Hereford population to account for cases of calves with edema of the neuraxis (Harper et al., 1986a; Healy et al., 1986).

Investigators established a smaller breeding herd comprising parents of calves that had severe spongy vacuolation of the CNS. All twenty-one calves born in this herd could rise unassisted following birth, but six developed clinical signs of progressive CNS dysfunction within thirty-six hours of birth. These six calves were euthanazed between three and five days of age because of progressive higher central nervous dysfunction, and all had severe spongy vacuolation of the CNS. Estimates of amino and ketoacid concentrations in body fluids and tissues indicated extreme elevations of the branched chain amino acids, valine, leucine, and isoleucine, and their derived ketoacids. This finding was consistent with the calves being affected with branched chain ketoacid dehydrogenase deficiency, or maple syrup urine disease (MSUD) (Healy et al., 1986).

The two breeding experiments, and results of clinical, biochemical, and pathological examinations, clearly confirmed that the syndrome previously known as HNO comprised two distinct entities, both of which are inherited as autosomal recessives. The condition, characterized by spontaneous and stimulus-responsive myoclonic spasms that were evident from birth, was given the descriptive title, inherited congenital myoclonus (ICM) (Harper et al., 1986a). The disease characterized by progressive CNS dysfunction, with elevated concentrations of branched chain keto and amino acids, is clearly bovine MSUD (Harper et al., 1986b).

II. CLINICAL FEATURES

Major clinical features of bovine hyperekplexia (ICM) are shown in the accompanying visual presentation. The segments demonstrate stimulus-responsive and occasional spontaneous myoclonic spasms that are characteristic of this defect and present at birth. Though the calves display normal mentation and suckling reflexes, they cannot gain sternal recumbency or stand unassisted. Assisting the affected calf to stand results in extreme muscular rigidity and severe adduction of the pelvic limbs, consistent with profound release of lower motor neuron inhibition.

Observations based on matings of obligate heterozygotes in the experimental herd provided evidence of the prenatal expression of the bovine disease. Myoclonic responses to tactile stimulation of the lumbosacral region of a 254-day fetus (normal bovine gestation is 282 days), recovered from a cow euthanazed due to metastasizing squamous cell carcinoma, provided evidence of the prenatal occurrence of myoclonic spasms. This evidence was supported by the existence of chronic tissue reaction adjacent to the fractured femoral head in the hip joint of a stillborn hydranencephaly-affected calf. The calf was rendered decerebrate as a consequence of inadvertent intra-uterine infection towards the end of the first trimester of gestation with the insect-borne Akabane virus. Whole body spasms were observed in a newborn calf when the lumbosacral region of the calf was licked by its dam approximately twenty seconds after birth (see video). In addition, the average gestation length for ICM-affected calves is approximately ten days shorter than that of unaffected half-siblings, suggesting a disturbance in the normal fetal/maternal relationship, possibly generated by steroid responses in the fetus to the hip joint lesions (Healy et al., 1985).

Affected calves are usually observed to be bright and alert and are found lying in lateral recumbency, though Blood and Gay (1971) recorded that some could gain sternal recumbency. In contrast, only one of the fourteen affected calves born in the ICM experimental herd attained sternal recumbency with the limbs drawn under the body, and that

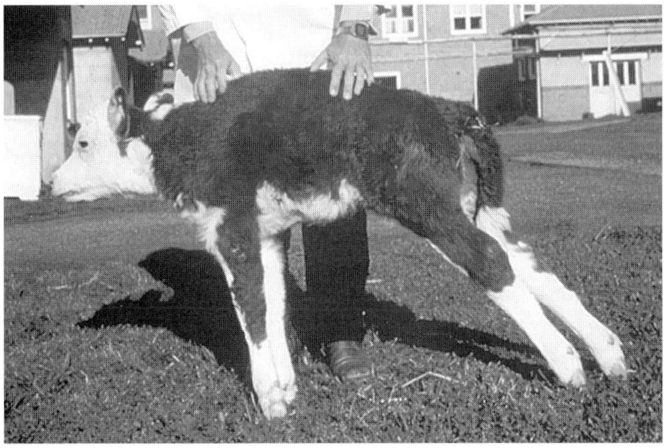

FIGURE 1 Poll Hereford calf affected with ICM and supported in standing position. Note the typical "sawhorse" stance.

TABLE 1 Lesions in the Coxae of Fifty Hyperekplexic Calves

Lesion	Number of cases
Unilateral acetabular fracture	5
Bilateral acetabular fracture	5
Unilateral acetabular fracture, erosion of femoral head	7
Bilateral acetabular fracture, erosion of femoral head	16
Unilateral femoral head fracture	7
Bilateral femoral head fracture	7
Unilateral femoral head luxation	2
Bilateral femoral head luxation	1
Pelvis limb atrophy	1
No lesion	1

was only possible with human assistance. All of the fourteen calves could raise their heads, flex their necks laterally, and elevate the anterior thorax to approximately 45 degrees to the vertical for extended periods of time. As the calves could not gain even sternal recumbency, none could stand without assistance (Healy et al., 1985).

When investigators attempted to stand affected calves by lifting them under the thorax, the calves displayed severe muscular rigidity, resembling tetany, accompanied by apnea and a high velocity muscular tremor that was occasionally detected as an audible hum. The calves could be held in this "sawhorse" posture with minor lateral support (Figure 1). Upon removal of the support, the calves fell to the ground and the rigidity was sustained for up to five seconds (see video). Hyperpnoea followed cessation of the muscle rigidity, and occasionally calves bellowed upon recovery, suggesting they had experienced pain. When investigators shifted support of the standing calf to the posterior abdomen, the whole body rigidity and apnea ceased. By holding affected calves vertically in this manner, investigators could demonstrate the calves responding to postural changes with compensatory lateral movement of the forelimbs, although the movements were "clumsy" and interrupted by occasional myoclonic jerks (Harper et al., 1986a).

The severity of the myoclonic response diminished with repeated tactile stimuli, suggesting calves could voluntarily override the immediate myoclonic responses to, at least, tactile stimuli. Affected calves were "trained" to stand with the assistance of a sling supporting the thorax and abdomen. Following an extended period in the sling, two calves could walk forward, without support, for up to 1.5 meters. However, as is clearly demonstrated in the video, when the calf places a hoof on concrete, a myoclonic jerk and upward motion occurs just before the generalized startle and muscular rigidity. The animal then loses its precarious balance and falls laterally to the ground.

Affected calves were maintained for up to eight weeks of age with adequate feeding and nursing. Their mentation, sucking reflex, and other cranial nerve function tests were normal (Harper et al., 1986a), and they learned to recognize the approach of a feeding bottle, supporting the observation that cranial functions were unimpaired.

III. PATHOLOGY

In fifty ICM-affected calves examined in an expanded study that included referred cases, investigators found spongy change in the cerebellar white matter in only one subject. The cause of this lesion was not established. However, given its uncommon appearance in ICM-affected calves, the lesion was most likely associated with another unrecognized insult to the individual.

The contents of Table 1 show that lesions in the coxae were a common finding in hyperekplexic calves. They include deep linear contusions in the cranial portion of the acetabular fossa, and erosions of the corresponding articular surface of the head of the femur. Some erosions were so deep that the hyperemic subendochondral bone was exposed. Fragments of bone were encapsulated in close proximity to fractures of the femoral neck. Investigators also frequently observed hemorrhage and fibrosis in the joint capsule and surrounding tissue (Harper et al., 1986a). The severity of the hip joint lesions is evident on the X-ray images depicted in the video. No other pathology has been associated with ICM.

IV. PHARMACOLOGY

Investigators assessed the clinical effects of orally administering various drugs that affect CNS function in affected calves. Daily treatment (total doses bracketed) with levodopa (6 g), carbidopa (0.6 g), carbamazepine (17.6 g), phenytoin sodium (5.4 g), sodium valproate (7 g), and baclofen (0.75 g) had no detectable effect on clinical outcome. Treatment with thiopentone sodium (0.5 g) and diazepam (0.01 g) alleviated muscle spasms, but this was probably a secondary effect to generalized CNS depression at these dose rates. Treatment with xylazine (0.01 g) and acetyl promazine maleate (0.02 g) led to increased frequency and severity of myoclonic spasms, with some calves developing severe tetany and apnea lasting almost sixty seconds. Administration of a calcium preparation had no clinical effect. In summary, administration of antiepileptic and anticonvulsant drugs at therapeutic doses did not alleviate the clinical signs of bovine ICM (Harper et al., 1986a).

V. BIOCHEMISTRY

A. Clinical Chemistry

Biochemical findings were unremarkable in calves affected with ICM. Plasma and CSF concentrations of calcium, magnesium, phosphate, glucose, urea, protein, and albumin (plasma only) were similar to concentrations in clinically normal calves. In addition, investigators observed no differences between normal and affected calves in plasma activities of alkaline phosphatase, creatine kinase, aspartate aminotransferase, gamma glutamyl transferase, or ornithine carbamoyltransferase. Creatine kinase and aspartate aminotransferase activities in CSF were also unremarkable (Dennis, 1987).

B. Neurotransmitters

The apparent failure of ICM-affected calves to moderate motor responses, and some clinical similarities to tetanus and strychnine poisoning, led investigators to hypothesize that the disease could be caused by an abnormality in an inhibitory feedback mechanism in the brainstem or spinal cord, most probably involving failure of lower motor neuron inhibition. This hypothesis prompted a detailed investigation into amino acid, organic acid, and catecholamine concentrations in various tissues and body fluids, with particular emphasis on the inhibitory neurotransmitters, glycine, taurine, and gamma-aminobutyric acid (GABA) (Dennis, 1987).

Although glycine has an inhibitory effect on the spinal cord when applied iontophoretically and is the most potent of the known inhibitory neurotransmitters (Curtis et al., 1968), investigators observed no differences between normal and affected calves in free glycine concentrations in plasma, serum, CSF, spinal cord, and thirteen physio-anatomically distinct regions within the cerebellum and cerebral cortex. The other free amino acid neurotransmitters analyzed in plasma and CSF—GABA, taurine, aspartate, glutamate, and noradrenalin—were also similar between the two phenotypes. Taurine concentrations were significantly higher in some regions of the brain of ICM-affected calves (medulla oblongata, pons, white matter of the cerebellum, and substantia nigra), but the significance, if any, of this observation remains unknown. GABA concentrations were not significantly different between the phenotypes for any of the thirteen brain sites analyzed (Dennis, 1987).

C. Strychnine Receptor Studies

Bovine ICM shares some similarity to the clinical signs of subconvulsive strychnine poisoning. Strychnine acts to block the inhibitory amino acid transmitter, glycine (Curtis and Johnston, 1974), by interacting with the postsynaptic glycine receptor (Young and Snyder, 1973). Researchers conducted a series of experiments to investigate the uptake and release of glycine in spinal cord extracts from ICM-affected calves using radiolabelled strychnine. Receptor site function studies in synaptosome preparations demonstrated that only 5% strychnine binding occurred in ICM-affected calves compared with controls, indicating a severe deficiency of functional glycine receptor sites. $GABA_A$ receptor binding sites were not significantly different between ICM calves and controls, confirming the results were selective for the glycine receptor. Investigators also demonstrated a 240% increase in the rate of glycine uptake by spinal cord synaptosomes in affected calves, and they postulated that this increase might be a compensatory mechanism for the lack of functional post synaptic receptors (Gundlach et al., 1988).

VI. IMMUNOHISTOCHEMISTRY

Researchers used immunohistochemistry to investigate the cellular expression of the glycine receptor in cattle. A monoclonal antibody (Mab-4a) raised against an epitope common to all subunits in the glycine receptor (Schroder et al., 1991) revealed a marked difference in staining patterns between control and affected animals. The immunoreaction in the control group was obvious in the cytoplasm and the cell surface membrane of the spinal neurons, but confined to just the cytoplasm in spinal neurons of affected calves. The absence of staining on the cell surface membrane in spinal cord from ICM-affected individuals was consistent with a failure of glycine receptor assembly at the cell surface (Pierce et al., 2001).

VII. MOLECULAR GENETICS

A. Characterization of the Bovine Glra1 and Glrb Genes

The [^{3}H] strychnine binding studies in spinal cord implicated the inhibitory glycine receptor subunit genes as the most likely group of candidate genes responsible for myoclonus in Poll Hereford calves. The adult spinal cord glycine receptor is a pentameric complex, being composed of three ligand binding α1 subunits and two structural β subunits (Langosch et al., 1988). The $\alpha 1/\beta$ glycine receptor is clustered in the synaptic membrane via the cytoplasmic anchoring protein, gephyrin (Kuhse et al., 1995). The bovine Glra1 and Glrb genes were isolated from bovine λ phage and bacterial artificial chromosome (BAC) genomic DNA libraries using radiolabelled probes based on the corresponding human cDNA sequences. The genomic organization between Glra1 and Glrb was similar, with both genes comprising nine exons ranging in size from 68 bp to over 470 bp, and splice junctions consistent with consensus splice sequences (Mount, 1982). An alternative splice acceptor site was identified in the Glra1 gene upstream of exon 9. Investigators predict that the subsequent insertion of twenty-four nucleotides into the cDNA will encode a further eight amino acids. Both splice variants were utilized in cattle (Pierce et al., 2001) and have been observed in rat (Malosio et al., 1991), mouse (Ryan et al., 1994), and probably human (Shiang et al., 1993) Glra1 genes. The bovine Glra1 coding region consists of 1,374 nucleotides, encoding a 457-amino acid protein, while the Glrb coding region is 1,494 nucleotides and encodes a 475-amino acid protein. The protein sequence in the bovine Glra1 gene shares 99% and 99.8% identity with the mouse and human sequence, respectively (Pierce et al., 2001).

B. Identification of the Disease-Causing Mutation

Amplification and sequencing of both strands of genomic DNA from affected calves revealed a substitution of adenine for cytidine at position 156 of the Glra1 gene (156C $\rightarrow$ A) when compared with normal controls. The transversion is predicted to substitute a termination codon in place of a tyrosine codon at position 24 in exon 2, resulting in a truncated, nonfunctional Glra1 subunit of the glycine receptor complex. Results of amplification and sequencing of genomic DNA from a further twelve affected calves and seven obligate heterozygotes (animals known to have produced ICM-affected offspring) confirmed the expectation that the 156A allele cosegregated with the disease. The twelve affected calves were homozygous for the 156A allele, and the seven obligate heterozygotes were heterozygous at the 156 site (156C/A) (Pierce et al., 2001).

The 156A mutation deletes a *Bci*VI restriction endonuclease cleavage site. Amplification of a 375 bp region flanking the 156 site, gel purification of the product, and incubation with *Bci*VI followed by gel electrophoresis, yielded 201 bp and 174 bp fragments with homozygous wild-type sequence. A single band corresponding to the uncut 375 bp product was observed in homozygous mutant sequence, and heterozygous sequence revealed all three fragments of 375, 201, and 174 bp (Pierce et al., 2001). The *Bci*VI genotyping assay results were consistent with the sequencing data on animals representing the three ICM genotypes. However, the assay worked reliably only on gel purified PCR product, necessitating development of a robust genotyping procedure that could be applied commercially.

C. Genotyping for Bovine ICM

A robust genotyping assay was developed for routine use on crude hair root extracts, using a double mismatch amplification procedure to incorporate at least one *Acc*I restriction site into the 273 bp amplicon (Healy et al., 2002). A single nucleotide mismatch near the 3′ end of the sense primer enabled discrimination between the alleles by creating an *Acc*I recognition site in the wild-type amplicon, but not the mutant amplicon. In addition, a dinucleotide mismatch was engineered near the 3′ end of the antisense primer to create an *Acc*I site in the amplicon that was independent of the ICM alleles. This latter mismatch acted as an internal control by providing confirmation of activity of *Acc*I regardless of the ICM genotype. Figure 2 depicts the restriction fragment pattern visualized in an ethidium bromide-stained agarose gel in calves representing the three possible genotypes. Complete digestion by *Acc*I is obvious by comparing the shorter (252 bp and/or 232 bp) fragments in lanes 3 to 8 with the longer undigested fragment in lane 2 (273 bp).

VIII. PREVALENCE

In an extensive management system with infrequent supervision of breeding herds, the numbers of cases of ICM reported to veterinarians are unlikely to reflect the true incidence of the disease. Before the molecular basis of the disease was identified, some Poll Hereford breeders chose the expensive and time-consuming option of breeding experiments using obligate heterozygote cows to predict the ICM genotype of elite bulls (Healy et al., 1987). This procedure required the cows to be superovulated, inseminated with the test semen, and the resulting embryos flushed and transferred to recipient cows. Fifteen live, unaffected calves

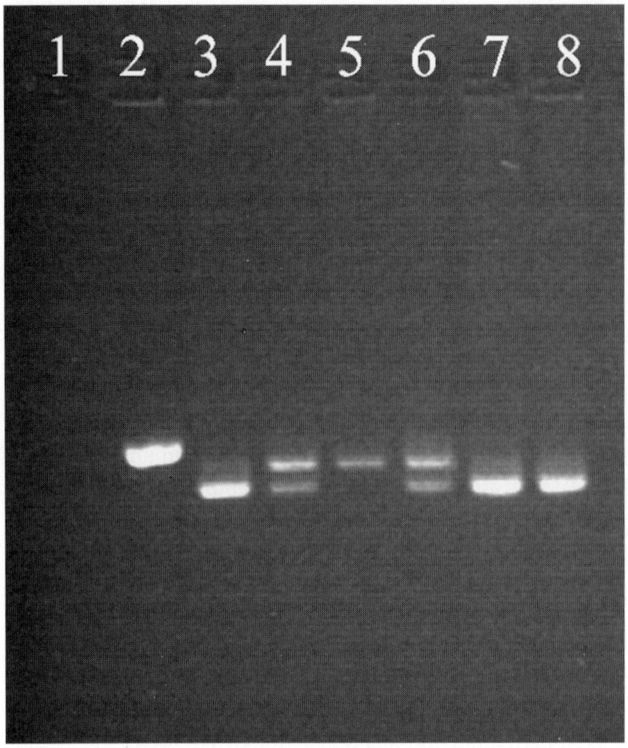

FIGURE 2 Agarose gel electrophoresis of PCR products digested with *Acc*I. Lane 1 = DNA blank, lanes 2 to 5 = purified control DNA samples of undigested amplicon (2), and amplicon digested with *Acc*I from homozygous wild-type (3), heterozygote (4) and homozygous mutant (5) cattle, and lanes 6 to 8 = crude DNA extracts from tail hair roots from a heterozygote (6) and two homozygous wild-type subjects (7 and 8)

were required for a 98.7% probability that the bull would be homozygous wild-type for ICM. Of the four bulls "genotyped" by this procedure in 1985, two produced affected calves. Development of a PCR-based method for genotyping individuals at the Glra1 156 site has provided a relatively inexpensive alternative to breeding experiments, and made it possible to obtain an estimate of the prevalence of heterozygotes in the breeding population, and thence deduce probable incidence of the disease.

Genotyping results on 218 saleyard bull samples collected in 1992, 163 sale bull samples collected in 1993, and 74 slaughter bull samples collected between 2000 and 2001 revealed a heterozygote frequency of 3.1% (Healy et al., 2002). In light of this information, the Australian Poll Hereford Society implemented a mandatory genotyping program in 2002 for bulls entering artificial insemination centers. In the ensuing eighteen-month period, 149 samples were genotyped at the Glra 156 site, with one heterozygote identified (unpublished data). If the observed reduction in heterozygotes in the last two years accurately reflects expected statistics in the Australian Poll Hereford herd, then science has provided the means to minimize the economic and animal welfare implications of bovine hyperekplexia.

IX. RELATIONSHIP TO OTHER INHERITED STARTLE SYNDROMES

Mutations in the α1 subunit of the glycine receptor gene are responsible for hereditary hyperekplexia or startle disease in humans (Shiang et al., 1993; reviewed in Vafa and Schofield, 1998). Similarly, α1 subunit mutations are responsible for the mouse mutants *spasmodic* (Ryan et al., 1994; Saul et al., 1994) and *oscillator* (Buckwalter et al., 1994). Mutations in the β subunit of the glycine receptor have been defined in the mutant mouse *spastic* (Kingsmore et al., 1994; Mulhardt et al., 1994) and recently in humans (Rees et al., 2002).

The disease phenotypes of the various inherited startle syndromes all result from either a loss of glycine receptor responsiveness to neurotransmitter or from a reduction in glycine receptor expression levels (Rajendra and Schofield, 1995). For example, the Ala52Ser mutation in the extracellular signal transduction domain of the *spasmodic* mouse causes a reduced decay time of synaptic miniature inhibitory postsynaptic currents (mIPSCs) via impaired receptor function (Callister et al., 1999). This results in a reduction in the total hyperpolarizing charge carried by this receptor. Likewise, the *spastic* mutation results in a reduction of glycine β subunits and a marked reduction in functional glycine receptors. Thus the *spastic* mutation exerts its effect by reducing the amplitude of the mIPSC (Callister et al., 1999). The bovine ICM mutation results in the absence of glycine receptor α1 subunit and thus a marked reduction in functional glycine receptors. This result fits within the conceptual framework that explains the phenotypic effects of the various startle syndrome mutations (see Figure 3). Missense mutations in the genes encoding the glycine receptor result in reduced receptor sensitivity and are responsible for startle syndromes in humans (hyperekplexia) and mice (*spasmodic*). Mutations that reduce the levels of receptor expression or result in truncated receptor proteins are responsible for startle syndromes in mice (*spastic* and *oscillator*) and cattle (myoclonus). In both cases, the consequences of the mutations converge physiologically leading to reduced glycinergic inhibition in the spinal cord and brainstem, resulting in hypertonia and an excessive startle response.

X. CONCLUSIONS

ICM, a bovine model of human hyperekplexia, first emerged as HNO in the 1960s in polled Hereford cattle on several continents. Ten years later, ICM was considered the most common inherited disease of newborn calves in Australia. Studies confirmed that the initial reports of HNO confused two separate autosomal recessive diseases with differing clinical, pathological, and biochemical features—ICM and MSUD. Clinical findings of prenatal stimulus-

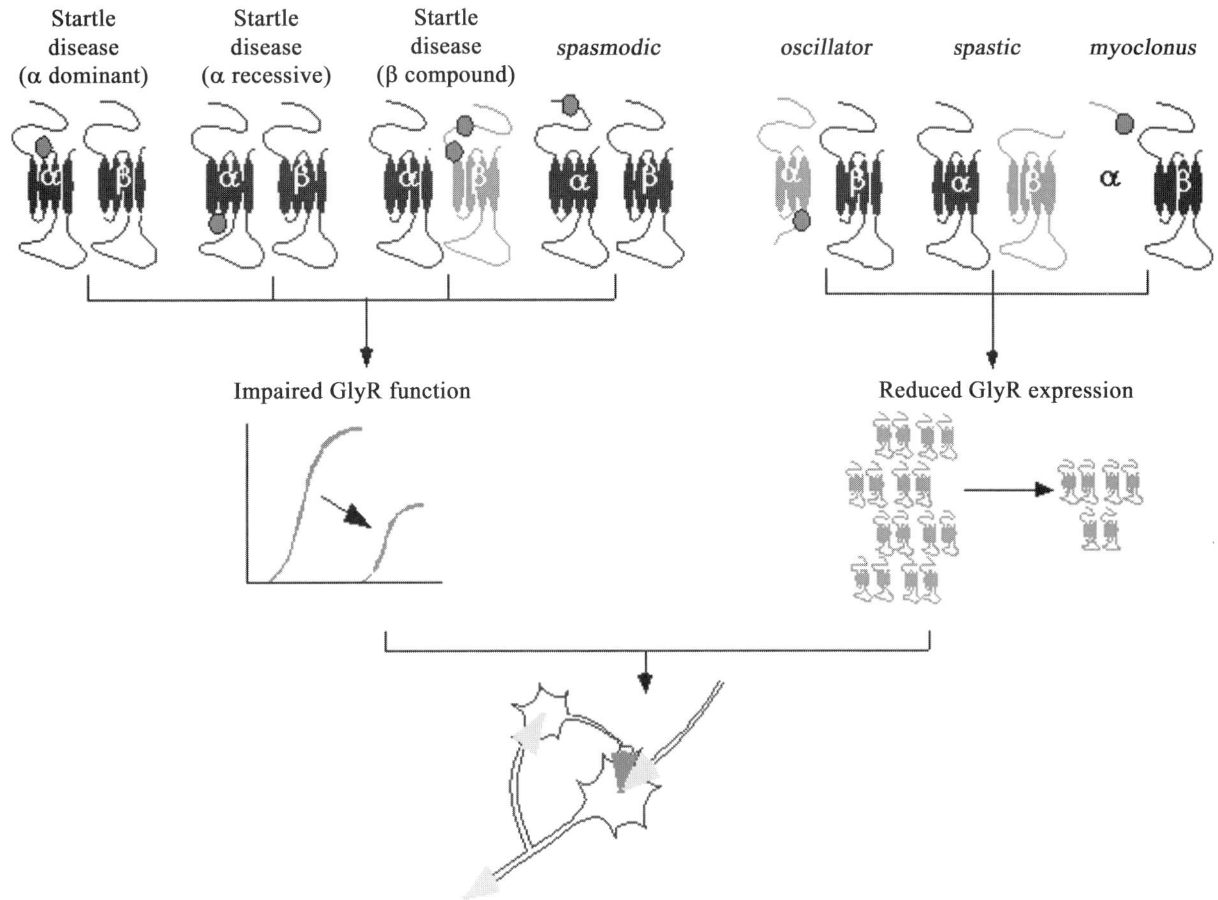

FIGURE 3 Convergent physiology of startle disorders. Mutations in the glycine receptor (GlyR) exert their effect by either impairing GlyR responsiveness to the neurotransmitter (startle disease (humans) and *spasmodic* (mice)), or by reducing GlyR expression levels (*oscillator*, *spastic* (mice) and *myoclonus* (cattle). The phenotypic expression is excessive startle response and hypertonia.

responsive myoclonic jerks and severe tetanic spasms characteristic of ICM were the result of a failure of glycine-mediated inhibitory neurotransmission, as demonstrated by the loss of [^{3}H] strychnine binding sites from brainstem and spinal cord extracts in affected calves. The disease-causing mutation replaces a tyrosine codon at position 24 with a termination codon (Tyr24Ter) in the α1 subunit of the glycine receptor, resulting in the synthesis of a truncated polypeptide that lacks function. Identification of the mutation (156C → A) has facilitated development of an efficient heterozygote detection test that will be pivotal in ensuring the current prevalence of the disease in Poll Herefords remains low. Definition of the clinical, pathological, biochemical, and molecular aspects of ICM is the result of breeding experiments and laboratory studies involving many disciplines. The result is the characterization of a recessive inherited neurological disorder in cattle that provides a model for investigating the role of neurotransmitter receptors.

Acknowledgments

The authors are indebted to Tom Braz for compilation of the video from various archived sources and Lowan Turton for final preparation of the figures. The birth sequence and calf walking segments have been reproduced with permission from Wiley-Liss, Inc., a subsidiary of John Wiley & Sons, Inc., in *Movement Disorders* Vol. 17, No. 4, 2002, pp. 743–744 entitled "Bovine myoclonus: model of human hyperekplexia (Startle Disease)" by P.J. Healy, K.D. Pierce, J.A. Dennis, P.A. Windsor, and P.R. Schofield.

Video Legends

SEGMENT 1 Whole body spasms were observed in a newborn calf when the lumbosacral region of the calf was licked by its dam approximately 20 seconds after birth.

SEGMENT 2 Attempts to stand affected calves results in severe muscular rigidity. Calves can be held in this "sawhorse" posture with minor lateral support. Upon removal of support, calves fall to the ground and rigidity is sustained for up to five seconds

SEGMENT 3 When the calf places a hoof on concrete, a myoclonic jerk and upward motion is elicited just prior to the generalized startle and muscular rigidity, resulting in the animal losing its precarious balance and falling laterally to the ground.

SEGMENT 4 Lesions in the coxae were a common finding in hyperekplexic calves. These include deep linear contusions in the cranial portion of the acetabular fossa and erosions of the corresponding articular surface of the femoral head. The severity of the hip joint lesions is evident on the radiographic images.

References

Blood, D.C., and C.C. Gay. 1971. Hereditary neuraxial oedema of calves. *Aust Vet J* **47**:520.

Buckwalter, M.S., S.A. Cook, M.T. Davisson, and W. White. 1994. A frameshift mutation in the mouse α1 glycine receptor gene (Glra1) results in progressive neurological symptoms and juvenile death. *Hum Mol Genet* **3**:2025–2030.

Callister, R.J., P.R. Schofield, and P. Sah. 1999. The use of murine mutants to study glycine receptor function. *Clin Exp Pharmacol Physiol* **26**: 929–931.

Cordy, D.R., W.P.C. Richards, and C. Stormont. 1969. Hereditary neuraxial oedema in Hereford calves. *Pathol Vet* **6**:487–501.

Curtis, D.R., L. Hosli, G.A.R. Johnston, and I.H. Johnston. 1968. The hyperpolarisation of spinal mononeurones by glycine and related amino acids. *Exp Brain Res* **5**:235–258.

Curtis, D.R., and G.A.R. Johnston. 1974. Amino acid transmitters in the mammalian central nervous system. *Rev Physiol Biochem Pharmacol* **69**:97–188.

Davis, G.B., E.J. Thompson, and R.J. Kyle. 1975. Hereditary neuraxial oedema of calves. *N Z Vet J* **23**:181.

Dennis, J.A. 1987. Amino acid composition of body fluids and nervous tissue of normal calves and those affected with neuraxial oedema. *Masters Thesis*, School of Biological Sciences, Macquarie University, Sydney.

Donaldson, C., and R.W. Mason. 1984. Hereditary neuraxial oedema in a Poll Hereford herd. *Aust Vet J* **61**:188–189.

Gundlach, A.L., P.R. Dodd, C.S.G. Grabara, W.E.I. Watson, G.A.R. Johnston, P.A.W. Harper, J.A. Dennis, and P.J. Healy. 1988. Deficit of spinal cord glycine/strychnine receptor in inherited myoclonus of Poll Hereford calves. *Science* **241**:1807–1809.

Harper, P.A.W., P.J. Healy, and J.A. Dennis. 1986a. Inherited congenital myoclonus of Polled Hereford calves (so called neuraxial oedema): A clinical, pathological and biochemical study. *Vet Rec* **119**:59–62.

Harper, P.A.W., P.J. Healy, and J.A. Dennis. 1986b. Maple syrup urine disease as a cause of spongiform encephalopathy in calves. *Vet Rec* **119**:62–65.

Healy, P.J., P.A.W. Harper, and J.K. Bowler. 1985. Prenatal occurrence and mode of inheritance of neuraxial oedema in Poll Hereford calves. *Res Vet Sci* **38**:96–98.

Healy, P.J., P.A.W. Harper, and J.A. Dennis. 1986. Diagnosis of neuraxial oedema in calves. *Aust Vet J* **63**:95.

Healy, P.J., J.A. Dennis, P.A.W. Harper, and T.D. Heath. 1987. Determination of the congenital myoclonus genotype of bulls by multiple ovulation-embryo transfer. *Aust Vet J* **64**:224–225.

Healy, P.J., J.A. Dennis, P.A. Windsor, K.D. Pierce, and P.R. Schofield. 2002. Genotyping cattle for inherited congenital myoclonus and maple syrup urine disease alleles. *Aust Vet J* **80**:695–697.

Kingsmore, S.F., B. Giros, D. Suh, M. Bieniarz, M.G. Caron, and M.F. Seldin. 1994. Glycine receptor β-subunit gene mutation in *spastic* mouse associated with LINE-1 element insertion. *Nat Genet* **7**:136–141.

Kuhse, J., H. Betz, and J. Kirsch. 1995. The inhibitory glycine receptor: Architecture, synaptic localization and molecular pathology of a postsynaptic ion-channel complex. *Curr Opin Neurobiol* **5**:318–323.

Langosch, D., L. Thomas, and H. Betz. 1988. Conserved quaternary structure of ligand-gated ion channels: The postsynaptic glycine receptor is a pentamer. *Proc Natl Acad Sci USA* **85**:7394–7398.

Malosio, M.-L., G. Grenningloh, J. Kuhse, V. Schmieden, B. Schmitt, P. Prior, and H. Betz. 1991. Alternative splicing generates two variants of the α1 subunit of the inhibitory glycine receptor. *J Biol Chem* **266**: 2048–2053.

Mount, S.M. 1982. A catalogue of splice junction sequences. *Nucl Acid Res* **10**:459–472.

Mulhardt, C., M. Fischer, P. Gass, D. Simon-Chazottes, J.L. Guenet, J. Kuhse, H. Betz, and C.M. Becker. 1994. The spastic mouse: Aberrant splicing of glycine receptor beta subunit mRNA caused by intronic insertion of L1 element. *Neuron* **13**:1003–1015.

Pierce, K.D., C.A. Handford, R. Morris, B. Vafa, J.A. Dennis, P.J. Healy, and P.R. Schofield. 2001. A nonsense mutation in the α1 subunit of the inhibitory glycine receptor associated with bovine myoclonus. *Mol Cell Neurosci* **17**:354–363.

Rajendra, S., and P.R. Schofield. 1995. Molecular mechanisms of inherited startle syndromes. *Trends Neurosci* **18**:80–82.

Rees, M.I., T.M. Lewis, J.B.J. Kwok, G. Mortier, P. Govaert, R.G. Snell, P.R. Schofield, and M.J. Owen. 2002. Hyperekplexia associated with compound heterozygote mutations in the β-subunit of the human inhibitory glycine receptor (*GLRB*). *Hum Mol Genet* **11**:853–860.

Ryan S.G., M.S. Buckwalter, J.W. Lynch, C.A. Handford, L. Segura, R. Shiang, J.J. Wasmuth, et al. 1994. A missense mutation in the gene encoding the α1 subunit of the inhibitory glycine receptor in the spasmodic mouse. *Nat Genet* **7**:131–135.

Saul, B., V. Schmieden, C. Kling, C. Mulhardt, P. Gass, J. Kuhse, and C.M. Becker. 1994. Point mutation of glycine receptor alpha 1 subunit in the spasmodic mouse affects agonist responses. *FEBS Lett* **350**:71–76.

Schroder, S., W. Hoch, C.M. Becker, G. Grenningloh, and H. Betz. 1991. Mapping of antigenic epitopes on the alpha 1 subunit of the inhibitory glycine receptor. *Biochem* **30**:42–47.

Shiang, R., S.G. Ryan, Y.-Z. Zhu, A.F. Hahn, P. O'Connell, and J.J. Wasmuth. 1993. Mutations in the α1 subunit of the inhibitory glycine receptor cause the dominant neurologic disorder, hyperekplexia. *Nat Genet* **5**:351–357.

Vafa, B., and P.R. Schofield. 1998. Heritable mutations in the glycine, $GABA_A$ and nicotinic acetylcholine receptors provide new insights into the ligand-gated ion channel receptor superfamily. *Int Rev Neurobiol* **42**:285–332.

Weaver, A.D. 1974. Erbliches neuraxiales odem bei hornlosen Hereford-Kalbern. *Deutsche Tieraerztl Wochenschr* **81**:549–604.

Young, A.B., and S.H. Snyder. 1973. Strychnine binding associated with glycine receptors of the central nervous system. *Proc Natl Acad Sci USA* **70**:2832–2836.

C H A P T E R

H5

Movement Disorders in *Drosophila* Mutants of Potassium Channels and Biogenic Amine Pathways

LYLE FOX, ATSUSHI UEDA, BRETT BERKE, I-FENG PENG and CHUN-FANG WU

The ease of isolating mutations affecting locomotion control in *Drosophila melanogaster* has facilitated genetic analysis of movement disorders. Screening for mutations that cause leg shaking in adult flies, for example, has led to the cloning and subunit identification of *Shaker* and related channels, delineating the diversity of the K^+ channel family. Rhythmic components of several behaviors, such as larval locomotion, have been well studied by morphometric quantitative analysis. Mutations affecting K^+ channels and biogenic amine systems with defined molecular lesions provide useful entry points to reveal components of the genetic network controlling patterned activity underlying locomotion control. The regulation of membrane excitability and its behavioral consequences through ion channel interactions have been revealed by double mutant studies of identified K^+ channels with their interacting Na^+ and Ca^{2+} channels. Altered membrane excitability affects the developmental plasticity of activity-dependent neuronal growth. Studies at the larval neuromuscular junction and in cultured neurons indicate the Ca^{2+}- and cAMP-mediated activity-dependent processes are affected by hyperexcitability. As demonstrated in double-mutant studies, systematic enhancer and suppressor screens can uncover interacting components in the gene network controlling a given phenotype. Many genes described here have homologous counterparts and conserved mutant phenotypes across phyla, including humans. In the post-genomic era, established experimental paradigms in *Drosophila* can help provide a comprehensive understanding of how mutations of a candidate gene exert effects at all levels, from molecules and cells to circuits and behaviors.

I. INTRODUCTION

A large collection of mutants in the fruit fly, *Drosophila melanogaster*, has provided abundant genetic information for improving our understanding of locomotion control and movement disorders. In particular, investigators are extensively studying behavioral consequences of mutations in ion channels and transmitter systems in *Drosophila*. Here we focus on K^+ channel mutations, first identified and cloned in *Drosophila* (Table 1), leading to the elucidation of the function and structure of the various K^+ channels that are conserved in different species, including humans (Coetzee et al., 1999). We also review mutations of biogenic amine pathways that modulate motor output of central pattern generators involved in locomotion control. A number of genes encoding components in these pathways are now well-characterized in *Drosophila* at the molecular and biochemical levels (Table 1).

TABLE 1 *Drosophila* Mutants of Ion Channels, Biogenic Amines, and Second Messenger Pathways

Mutant	Gene product	Cellular role	Phenotype	Reference[a]
		Ion channels		
Sh (Shaker)	Voltage-activated K^+ channel α subunit	I_A	Leg shaking, wing scissoring, NMJ transmission and growth	Kaplan and Trout 1969; Jan et al. 1977; Salkoff and Wyman 1981; Tanouye et al. 1981; Ganetzky and Wu 1982a; Wu and Haugland 1985; Kamb et al. 1987; Papazian et al. 1987; Solc et al. 1987; Baumann et al. 1988; Schwartz et al. 1988; Baker and Salkoff 1990; Haugland and Wu 1990
Shab	Voltage-activated K^+ channel α subunit	I_K	Heat-induced paralysis and wings up	Butler et al. 1989; Hegde et al. 1999; Singh and Singh 1999; Chopra et al. 2000
Hk (Hyperkinetic)	Voltage-activated K^+ channel β subunit	I_A modulation	Leg shaking, enhanced startle reflex, slower habituation rate	Kaplan and Trout 1969; Ikeda and Kaplan 1970a,b; Stern and Ganetzky 1989; Wang and Wu 1996; Chouinard et al. 1995; Engel and Wu 1998; Yao and Wu 1999a
eag (ether a go-go)	Voltage-activated K^+ channel, modulatory α subunit	Multiple K^+ channel modulation	Leg shaking, NMJ transmission and growth, courtship conditioning, larval locomotion deficit	Kaplan and Trout 1969; Ganetzky and Wu 1983; Wu et al. 1983b; Burg and Wu 1989; Budnik et al. 1990; Warmke et al. 1991; Griffith et al. 1994; Wang et al. 2002
slo (slowpoke)	Ca^{2+}-activated K^+ channel α subunit	I_{CF} (BK)	Heat-induced "sticky feet," poor flight, courtship defect, slower habituation rate	Elkins et al. 1986; Atkinson et al. 1991; Singh and Wu 1989, 1990; Saito and Wu 1991; Gho and Ganetzky 1992; Warbington et al. 1996; Engel and Wu 1998
para^ts^ (paralytic, temperature-sensitive)	Voltage-activated Na^+ channel	I_{Na}	Temperature-sensitive action potential block and paralysis, larval locomotion deficit	Suzuki et al. 1971; Siddiqi and Benzer 1976; Wu and Ganetzky 1980; Suzuki and Wu 1984; Loughney et al. 1989; O'Dowd et al. 1989; Wang et al. 1997a, 2002
nap^ts^ (no-action potential, temperature-sensitive)	A unique allele of *mle* RNA helicase	Reduced expression of *para* Na^+ channels	Temperature-sensitive action potential block and paralysis	Wu et al. 1978; Ganetzky and Wu 1982b; Wu et al. 1983a; Burg and Wu 1986; Kernan et al. 1991
cac (cacophony)	Voltage-activated Ca^{2+} channel	I_{Ca} (?)	Courtship song defect	Von Schilcher 1976, 1977; Smith et al. 1996; Kawasaki et al. 2000
sei^ts^ (seizure, temperature-sensitive)	K^+ channel, an *eag*-related gene (*erg*)	Inward rectifier K^+ current (?)	Temperature-sensitive paralysis	Jackson et al. 1985; Elkins and Ganetzky 1990; Warmke and Ganetzky 1994; Titus et al. 1997; Wang et al. 1997b
qvr (quiver)	Unknown	I_A modulation	Leg shaking, reactive oxygen species (ROS) sensitive, larval locomotion deficit	Humphreys et al. 1996; Wang et al. 2000, 2002
		Biogenic Amines		
Mutant	**Gene product**	**Cellular role**	**Phenotype**	**Reference[a]**
Tβh (tyramine β-hydroxylase)	tyramine β-hydroxylase	Synthesis of octopamine from tyramine	Egg laying, courtship, and larval locomotion deficits	Monastirioti et al. 1996; McClung and Hirsh 1999; Saraswati et al. 2004
iav (inactive)	Unknown	Reduced tyramine and octopamine levels	Inactive flies, cocaine sensitization, courtship and larval locomotion deficits	Kaplan 1977; Homyk and Sheppard 1977; O'Dell et al. 1987; O'Dell 1994; McClung and Hirsh 1999; Saraswati et al. 2004
Ddc (DOPA decarboxylase)	DOPA decarboxylase	Dopamine and serotonin synthesis	Odor conditioning and larval locomotion deficits	Hirsh and Davidson 1981; Wright et al. 1981; Tempel et al. 1984

(continued)

TABLE 1 (*continued*)

Second Messenger Pathways				
Mutant	**Gene product**	**Cellular role**	**Phenotype**	**Reference**[a]
dnc (dunce)	cAMP-specific phosphodiesterase	cAMP hydrolysis	NMJ transmission and growth, odor and courtship conditioning, aberrant spike firing, faster habituation rate, growth cone motility and Ca^{2+} dynamics	Dudai et al. 1976; Byers et al. 1981; Tully and Quinn 1985; Gailey et al. 1985; Zhong and Wu 1991b; Zhong et al. 1992; Engel and Wu 1996; Kim and Wu 1996; Zhao and Wu 1997; Berke and Wu 2002
rut (rutabaga)	Ca^{2+}/calmodulin-responsive adenylyl cyclase	cAMP synthesis	NMJ transmission and growth, odor and courtship conditioning, aberrant spike firing, slower habituation rate, growth cone motility and Ca^{2+} dynamics	Acevez-Pina et al. 1983; Livingstone et al. 1984; Gailey et al. 1985; Tully and Quinn 1985; Zhong and Wu 1991b; Levin et al. 1992; Zhong et al. 1992; Engel and Wu 1996; Kim and Wu 1996; Berke and Wu 2002
for (foraging)	cGMP-dependent protein kinase	Phosphorylation of serine and threonine in proteins	Food gathering, NMJ transmission and growth, habituation rate, hyperexcitability	Osborne et al. 1997; Renger et al. 1999; Engel et al. 2000

[a]Selected references for behavior, *in situ* physiology, and cloning.

Many genes introduced here have orthologs or homologs across phyla. Some physiological and behavioral consequences of their mutations are also conserved in both invertebrates and vertebrates. Therefore, *Drosophila* mutant phenotypes may provide useful insights into mechanisms of human diseases and promising therapeutic strategies. In *Drosophila*, researchers can use mutant alleles of different severity, ranging from mild, extreme, or lethal, to investigate the full impact of a mutant gene. Mutant individuals carrying lethal alleles can still be propagated in genetic stocks. Defects in cellular and molecular mechanisms can be elucidated in cultured cells or at the embryonic, larval, or adult stage to provide a comprehensive understanding of phenotype expression. Furthermore, *Drosophila* neurogenetics facilitates the study of genetic interactions to explore mechanistic links among molecules and between biochemical pathways. Novel phenotypes not present in each single mutant may emerge in double mutants to help reveal unexpected functional relationships among gene products.

In the same vein, investigators can design experiments to screen for genes involved in complex traits. It is well known that in vertebrate mutants and human patients, many alleles of a diseased gene do not manifest identical syndromes among individual carriers because of differences in environmental and genetic factors, including variation at other genetic loci in the background. Such genetic complexity can be analyzed and interacting genes uncovered in a systematic manner by identifying enhancers or suppressors of a given phenotype. As we will highlight in the following sections, studies of three K^+ channel genes, *Sh, eag*, and *Hk*, first discovered in *Drosophila* (Kaplan and Trout, 1969), have culminated in the elucidation of K^+ channel structure-function relationships, including those for the auxiliary subunits. For example, studies of *Hk* and *Sh* mutations have revealed the identity and modulatory function of the *Hk* β subunit for the *Sh* K^+ channel through a stereotypic interaction between the two genes (Table 1). Another strong phenotypic enhancement in double-mutant studies has demonstrated the functional specialization of the two K^+ channel α subunits separately encoded by the *eag* and *Sh* genes (Table 1). Alternatively, phenotypic suppression can result from counterbalancing effects of two different genes. *Sh* mutant flies display characteristic motor disorders associated with nerve hyperexcitability and enhanced synaptic transmission that are suppressed by reducing Na^+ channel expression with the nap^{ts} mutation (Figure 1, Table 1). The above observations suggest a strategy for using a sensitized genetic background to uncover genes with only mild or modifying effects on a particular phenotype. These approaches of preserving extreme alleles, making double-mutant combinations, and conducting systematic enhancer and suppressor screens are conceptually and technically well established in *Drosophila*.

II. LOCOMOTION CONTROL: ROLES OF ION CHANNELS AND BIOGENIC AMINES

Investigators have implicated a number of *Drosophila* genes in behavioral repertoires, such as aggression, courtship, learning, flying, and walking (Tully and Quinn, 1985; Gailey and Hall, 1989; Buchner, 1991; Baier et al., 2002; Ueda and Kidokoro, 2002). Components of these behaviors are generated and controlled by networks of

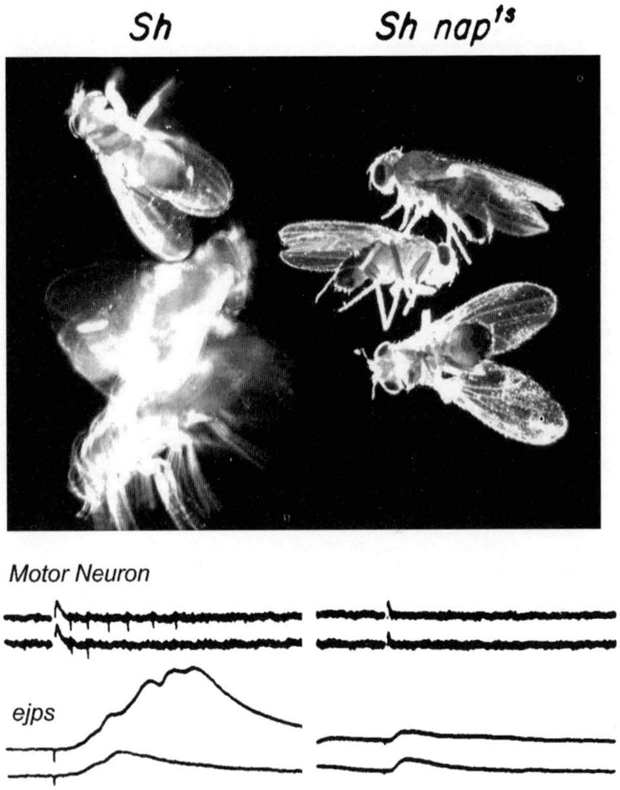

FIGURE 1 Suppression of *Shaker* (*Sh*) hyperexcitability by *no-action potential* (nap^{ts}). *Sh* mutant flies display vigorous leg shaking under ether anesthesia and hyperexcitability at the larval neuromuscular junction, manifesting increased excitatory junctional potentials (EJPs) correlated with supernumerary spikes of the motor axon. The leg-shaking behavior and enhanced neuromuscular transmission are suppressed in *Sh* nap^{ts} double mutants, demonstrating the counterbalancing effects of reducing a K$^+$ current by *Sh* mutations and decreased Na$^+$ channel expression by the nap^{ts} mutation. 23°C. Low Ca^{2+} saline (0.2 mM).

neurons termed central pattern generators (Marder and Calabrese, 1996; Marder, 2000; MacKay-Lyons, 2002). The activity of these networks depends on the K$^+$ channels expressed in neurons and can be modulated by biogenic amines like dopamine, octopamine, and serotonin (Harris-Warrick and Marder, 1991; Calabrese, 1998; Kiehn et al., 2000; Harris-Warrick, 2002; Grillner, 2003).

Octopamine and tyramine affect locomotor activity in adult flies (Kaplan, 1977; Homyk and Sheppard, 1977; O'Dell and Burnet, 1988). Quantitative analysis of stereotypic rhythmic behaviors in flies, including walking and flying, is particularly well suited for localizing the central networks and identifying some cellular components involved in locomotion control (Strauss and Heisenberg, 1990; Wolf and Heisenberg, 1990; Martin et al., 1998, 1999; Frye and Dickenson, 2001).

Larval crawling is a rhythmic, stereotyped behavior that has been highlighted in foraging and phototaxis studies (Sokolowski, 1980; Sawin-McCormack et al., 1995). Using video recordings and software like the Dynamic Image Analysis System (DIAS), researchers can analyze larval crawling morphometrically and dissect it into discrete, quantifiable parameters. This approach has demonstrated the distinct roles of different ion channels or biogenic amines in locomotion control (Wang et al., 1997a, 2002; Suster and Bate, 2002; Saraswati et al., 2004). The outlines of crawling larvae from successive video frames are stacked in Figure 2 to show that wild-type (WT) larvae crawl in a stereotypic pattern composed of periods of forward locomotion interspersed with periods of pausing. The pausing or "searching" episodes consist of periods of lateral head movements without forward locomotion (Wang et al., 1997a, 2002). Ion channel mutants display crawling patterns different from that of wild-type larvae (Figure 2). Larvae with mutations in the gene encoding a Na$^+$ channel, $para^{ts}$ (Table 1), or a K$^+$ channel α subunit, *eag* (Table 1), exhibit shorter periods of forward locomotion and more frequent searching episodes than WT (CS and OR) larvae. By contrast, mutations in the genes encoding the α subunit (*Sh*) or β subunit (*Hk*) of a transient K$^+$ channel (Table 1) lengthen the periods of forward locomotion and reduce the frequency of searching episodes. In addition, locomotion of *qvr* mutants (Table 1) resembles that of *Sh* and *Hk* larvae, consistent with specific defects in the *Sh* transient K$^+$ current in the three mutants (Wang et al., 2002).

Morphometric analysis of the video recordings has revealed defective crawling parameters that are not readily detectable by eye. For example, forward locomotion involves alternating extension of the anterior body segments and contraction of the posterior segments (Green et al., 1983; Berrigan and Pepin, 1995; Wang et al., 1997a). Difference pictures produced by overlapping the outlines of crawling larvae from successive video frames (Figure 3A; Wang et al., 1997a) help determine the temporal relationship between head extension and tail retraction during locomotion. Figure 3B shows abnormal phase relationships of head extension and tail retraction for $para^{ts}$ and *Hk* mutants, suggesting poor coordination of contraction cycles.

Investigators have also studied larval locomotion in mutants with altered levels of the biogenic amines, *Tβh*, *iav*, and *Ddc* (Table 1). In *Tβh* mutants, the enzyme tyramine β-hydroxylase, for octopamine synthesis, is disrupted, which increases tyramine and reduces octopamine levels. In *iav* mutants, the activity of tyrosine decarboxylase, which converts tyrosine to tyramine, is reduced. In *Ddc* mutants, DOPA decarboxylase, necessary for the synthesis of dopamine and serotonin, is defective. Each of these mutants with altered amine levels exhibits characteristic defects in locomotion (Figure 2C). Both *Tβh* and *iav* travel less distance than wild-type larvae. In *Tβh* larvae, the decrease is due to increased searching episodes and especially inefficient translocation whereas in *iav* larvae, it is primarily due to reduced stride frequency (Saraswati et al., 2004). By contrast, *Ddc* mutants have longer periods of forward locomo-

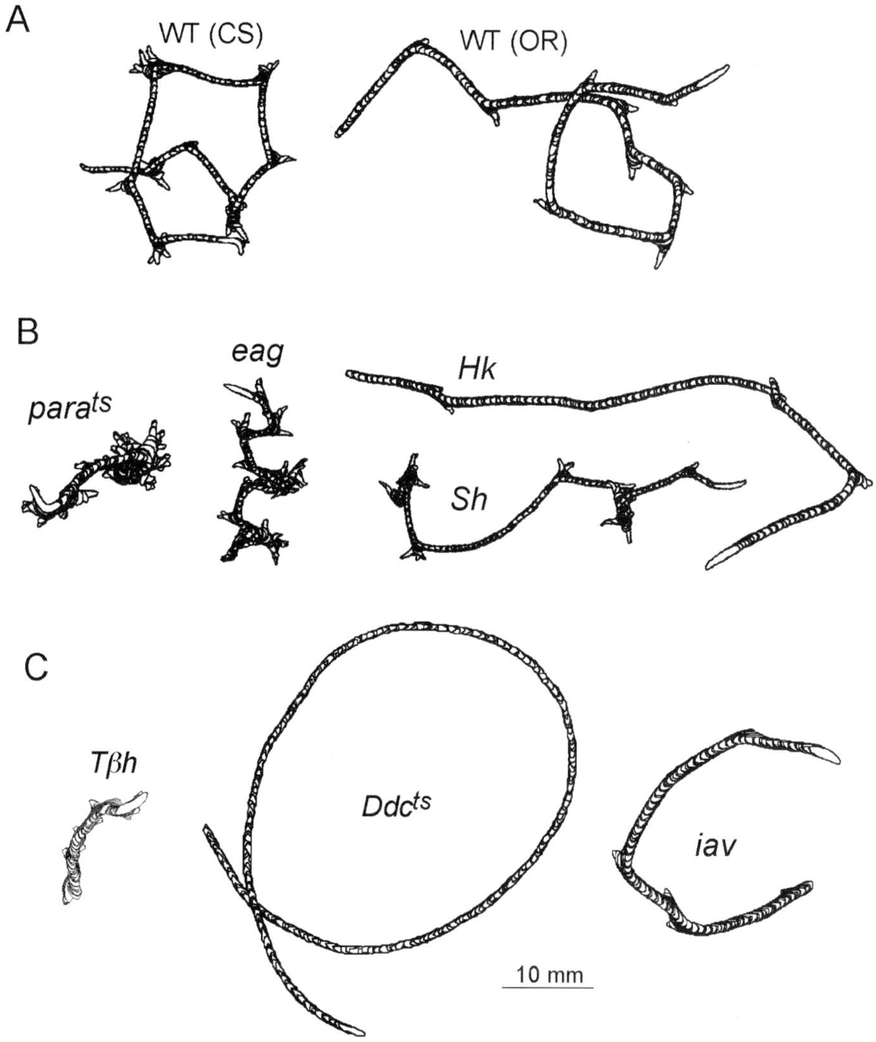

FIGURE 2 Representative crawling patterns of mutant larvae defective in ion channels and biogenic amine systems. The body outlines of third instar larvae crawling on an agarose substrate were captured by video recording at two frames per second for two minutes. Larval locomotion is composed of periods of forward translocation interspersed with periods of "searching." Crawling patterns of wild-type (WT) larvae of the Canton-S (CS) and Oregon-R (OR) strains are compared with those of mutants defective in Na^+ (*para^{ts}*) and K^+ (*eag*, *Hk* and *Sh*) channels and in biogenic amine systems (*Tβh*, *Ddc* and *iav*). (Modified from Wang et al. 1997a, 2002; Saraswati et al. 2004.)

tion. Some *Ddc* mutants exhibit a circular crawling pattern related to a maintained direction change over time (Figure 2C). Investigators have used targeted transgene expression to inhibit neurotransmitter release in the neural networks involved in locomotion control. Transgenic larvae that express tetanus toxin in a small population of neurons, including both dopaminergic and peptidergic neurons, also crawled in a circular pattern (Suster et al., 2003). It should be noted that a dopamine deficiency in the mouse model for Parkinson disease often produces circling (Kaakkola and Teravainen, 1990).

Modulating the excitability of the central neurons that generate motor programs or modulating the properties of peripheral synapses and muscles that produce the movements can change animal behavior. In *Drosophila* larvae, investigators can readily study changes in the coordination of neuronal activity or muscle responses because the body-wall muscle fibers and the related motor neurons have been identified (Crossley, 1978; Johansen et al., 1989; Atwood et al., 1993; Jia et al., 1993; Landgraf et al., 1997; Hoang and Chiba, 2001) and are accessible for electrophysiological recording (Jan and Jan, 1976a,b; Wu et al., 1978; Broadie and Bate, 1993; Kidokoro and Nishikawa, 1994). Researchers can record the output of the motor neurons *en passant* from segmental nerves with a suction electrode, and they can monitor the synaptic potentials simultaneously at the neuromuscular junction using either an intracellular electrode (Figure 1) or extracellular focal patch electrode

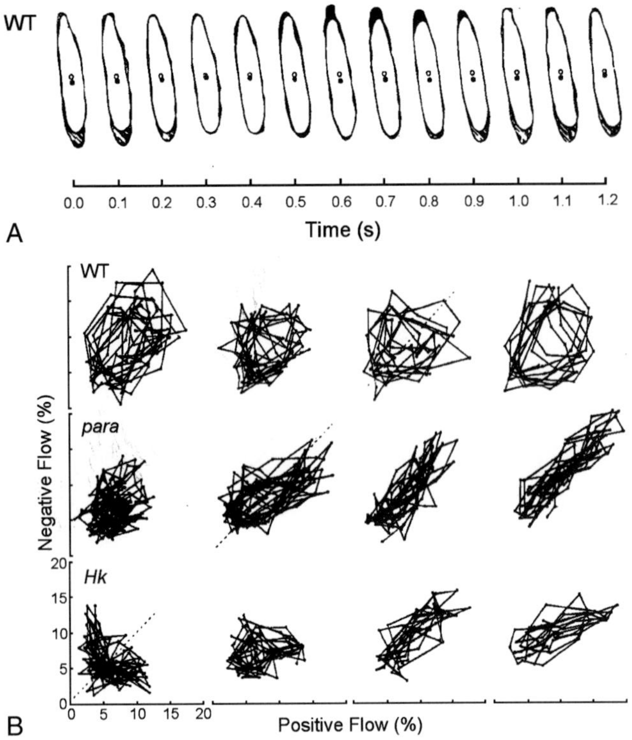

FIGURE 3 Morphometric analysis of larval locomotion. **A.** Displacement of the body perimeter during a peristaltic contraction cycle during forward locomotion. Filled and shaded areas in the pictures represent head extension (positive flow) and tail retraction (negative flow), respectively. For each picture, two frames at 0.4 s apart are overlaid to accentuate the body flow. The "centroids" are indicated with circles. **B.** The relationship between positive and negative flows of the body perimeter is revealed by a phase plot composed of superimposed frames acquired at 0.2 s apart. For a complete contraction cycle, a phase lag for the tail retraction generates circular loops around the 45° diagonal (dashed line). The phase lag is altered in *para^{ts}* and *Hk* larvae, resulting in more compact or irregular trajectories. (Adapted from Wang et al. 1997a.)

(Figure 4). Using these techniques, rhythmic bursting patterns of spike activities have been found in the motor neurons that innervate the segmental body-wall muscles (Budnik et al., 1990; Cooper and Neckameyer, 1999; Cattaert and Birman, 2001; Barclay et al., 2002) as well as pharyngeal muscles that help produce mouth hook movements during larval locomotion (Gorczyca et al., 1991). Mutations altering K^+ channel function or biogenic amine levels change motor patterns (Figure 4). For example, *eag Sh* double mutants exhibit abnormal sustained activity that is partially restored in *eag Sh nap^{ts}* triple-mutant larvae (Budnik et al., 1990). Manipulating biogenic amine levels in *Tβh* and *Ddc^{ts}* mutants alters the bursting duration and interburst interval (Saraswati, Fox, and Wu, unpublished), consistent with results from pharmacological manipulations of the dopaminergic system (Cooper and Neckameyer, 1999). Immunocytology of the *Drosophila* brain also suggests an important role for dopamine, octopamine, and serotonin in motor control, showing that these transmitters are expressed in discrete nonoverlapping populations of neurons with a profuse innervation of the central nervous system (Monastirioti, 1999).

In addition to the central effects of the biogenic amines, they also affect body-wall muscles innervated by neurons immunoreactive for octopamine or tyramine (Keshishian et al., 1993; Monastirioti et al., 1995; Nagaya et al., 2002). Exogenous application of octopamine, tyramine, and dopamine modifies the strength of synaptic transmission at the larval neuromuscular junction (Cooper and Neckameyer, 1999; Nishikawa and Kidokoro, 1999; Kutsukake et al., 2000; Nagaya et al., 2002).

III. MOVEMENT DISORDERS IN *DROSOPHILA*: NEURONAL EXCITABILITY, SYNAPTIC TRANSMISSION, AND INTERACTIONS AMONG ION CHANNEL GENES

Investigators have discovered many ion channel genes by mutational analysis of movement disorders. For example, early attempts to isolate mutant flies that exhibit leg shaking during ether anesthesia (Kaplan and Trout, 1969) have led to the identification of three major K^+ channel genes: *Sh*, *eag*, and *Hk* (Table 1). Screening for flies that become paralyzed at high temperatures (Suzuki, 1970; Wu et al., 1978; Elkins et al., 1986) has yielded "temperature-sensitive" mutants of the *para^{ts}* and *nap^{ts}* genes, encoding a Na^+ channel and a helicase regulating its expression, and the *slo* gene encoding a Ca^{2+}-activated K^+ channel (Table 1).

To reveal the functional interactions among these K^+ and Na^+ channel genes within neural circuits of interest, investigators can compare double-mutant phenotypes with those of the corresponding single mutants. For instance, the leg-shaking behavior of *Sh* mutant flies is enhanced in *eag Sh* double mutants, whereas the shaking of *Sh* and *Hk* is suppressed by adding the *nap^{ts}* mutation in *Sh nap^{ts}* and *Hk nap^{ts}* double mutants, indicating functional interactions in neurons expressing these two K^+ channel subunits and the Na^+ channel regulated by *nap^{ts}* (Figure 1; Ganetzky and Wu, 1982a). The *eag Sh* double mutants also exhibit qualitatively different phenotypes, including altered wing posture and impaired flight (Ganetzky and Wu, 1985; Stern et al., 1990; Engel and Wu, 1992), whereas *para^{ts} nap^{ts}* double mutations are completely lethal (Wu and Ganetzky, 1980). Many other double-mutant combinations exhibit unexpected interactions among channel genes. *Hk* mutations increase the readiness of a jump-and-flight escape reflex. The enhanced escape reflex in *Hk* is, however, suppressed in *Hk Sh* double mutants by *Sh* mutations (Kaplan and Trout, 1974), which also increase the reflex response, although to a lesser extent than *Hk* (Kaplan and Trout, 1969). This suppression can be explained by the fact that *Hk* encodes a β-subunit that mod-

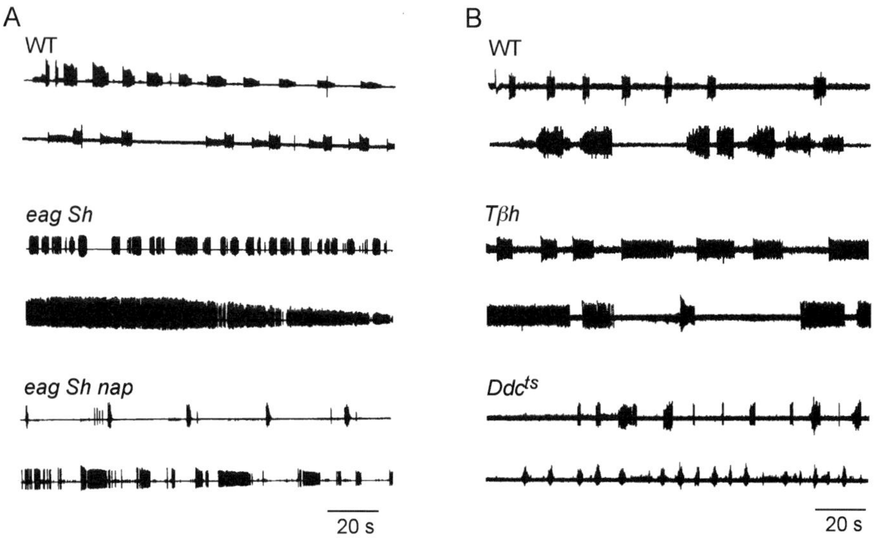

FIGURE 4 Patterns of neuronal activity recorded from a neuromuscular preparation of WT and mutant larvae. **A.** Spontaneous activity focally recorded from motor nerve entry points of body-wall muscles 6 and 7. Spikes are primarily grouped in short bursts for WT larvae, whereas *eag Sh* double mutants exhibit sustained abnormal activity. Wild type-like bursting activity is partially restored in *eag Sh nap* triple mutants. **B.** Spontaneous spike activity recorded from segmental nerves innervating body-wall muscles of WT, *Tβh*, and Ddc^{ts} larvae. Bursting activity is altered in *Tβh*, and Ddc^{ts} mutants. (**A.** Adapted from Budnik et al. 1990.)

ulates the *Sh* K^+-channel α subunit (Table 1). Thus expression of *Hk* phenotypes depends on functionally intact *Sh* subunits (Yao and Wu, 1999a). Another example involves an interaction between mutations in the *cac* Ca^{2+} channel and *slo* Ca^{2+}-activated K^+ channel genes (Table 1), both producing abnormal courtship songs generated by aberrant wing beats (Figure 5). The *cac slo* double mutant exhibits striking nonadditive defects in courtship song patterning (Figure 5), whereas *cac* song defects are partially rescued by either nap^{ts} or $para^{ts}$ in the corresponding double mutants (Peixoto and Hall, 1998). This indicates functional links between *slo* Ca^{2+}-activated K^+ channels and *cac* Ca^{2+} channels, and between *cac* Ca^{2+} channels and *para* Na^+ channels in a central pattern generator and its associated neural circuits for courtship song production.

In 1970 Ikeda and Kaplan first reported the electrophysiological phenotypes of movement disorders in *Drosophila* mutants. Recordings from the thoracic ganglia and motor nerve bundles (Ikeda and Kaplan, 1970a,b, 1974) have demonstrated that the ether-induced leg-shaking behavior in *Hk* flies is correlated with rhythmic bursting activity of motor neurons (Figure 6). The rhythmic bursts are generated independently in left and right halves of the thoracic ganglia. In gynandromorph mosaics of *Hk*, the *Hk* mutant tissue in the thorax, but not the brain, determines the ipsilateral leg shaking (Figure 6B,C). Investigators have also documented well the enhanced excitability in the jump-and-flight reflex circuits in K^+ channel mutant flies. Action potential broad-

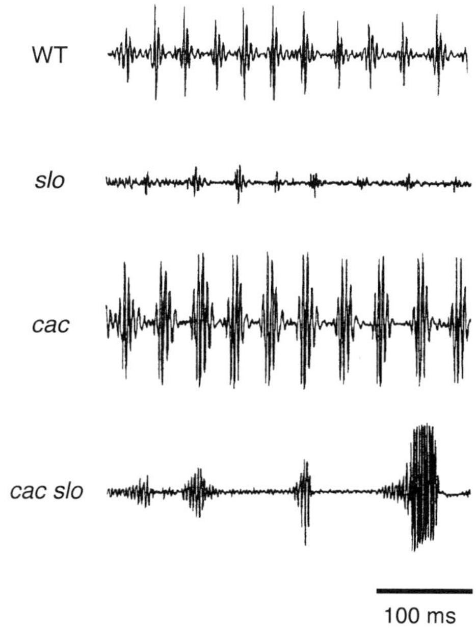

FIGURE 5 Courtship song generated by wing beats in WT, *slo*, *cac*, and *cac slo* mutant male flies. Audio recordings demonstrate the role of Ca^{2+}-dependent currents in courtship song generation using *slo* (Ca^{2+}-activated K^+ channel) and *cac* (Ca^{2+} channel) mutations. Courtship songs of *slo* flies have lower amplitude and longer interpulse intervals, whereas abnormal large-amplitude polycyclic songs are emitted by *cac* mutant flies. Note that synergistic interactions between *cac* and *slo* in the *cac slo* double mutant produce strikingly different song patterns. (Modified from Peixoto and Hall 1998.)

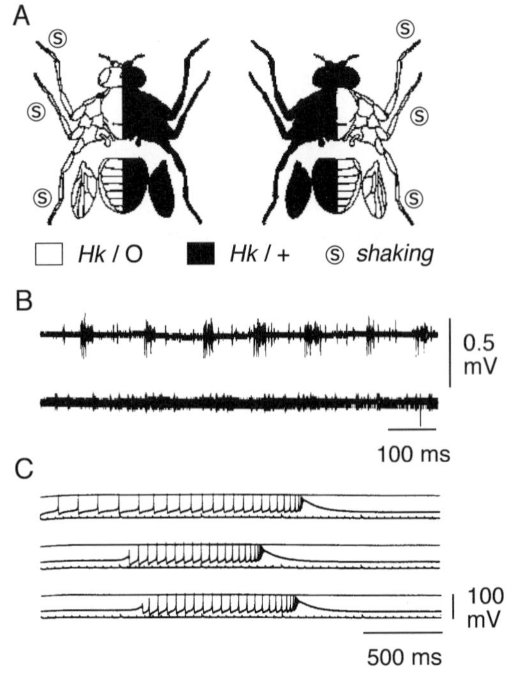

FIGURE 6 Mosaic and electrophysiological analyses of ether-induced leg-shaking behavior in *Hk* flies. **A.** Leg shaking in *Hk* gynandromorph mosaics composed of *Hk*/O male (white) and *Hk*/+ female tissue (black). Heterozygous *Hk*/+ female tissue is phenotypically normal. Loss of the X chromosome during development produces patches of X/O male tissue and reveals recessive *Hk* phenotypes in the mosaic flies. (left) A bilateral mosaic. (right) A thorax-abdomen bilateral mosaic, with a heterozygous head. Shaking is observed at the legs marked s. Note that leg shaking is associated with the ipsilateral thoracic *Hk*/O tissue and is independent of the genotype of the head tissue. **B.** and **C.** Electrical activities in the thoracic ganglia during ether anesthesia. **B.** A simultaneous extracellular recording from a bilateral pair of motor regions shows periodic bursting activity on the male side (*Hk*/O, upper trace) but not on the female side (*Hk*/+, lower trace). **C.** A consecutive intracellular recording from a pacemaker-like neuron of a homozygous *Hk*/*Hk* female shows rhythmic activity and bursting discharges. (Modified from Ikeda and Kaplan 1970b, 1974.)

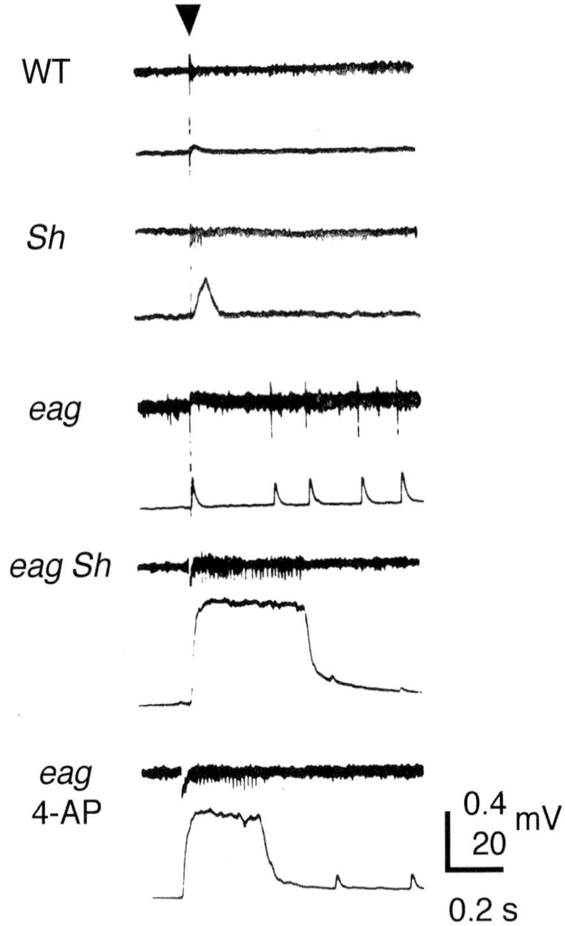

FIGURE 7 Simultaneous nerve and muscle recordings from WT and *Sh*, *eag*, and *eag Sh* larvae. Upper and lower traces indicate motor-axon activities recorded extracellularly from the segmental nerve, and EJPs recorded intracellularly from the body-wall muscle fibers, respectively. At low external Ca^{2+} concentrations (0.1–0.2 mM), nerve stimulation (arrowhead) evokes enhanced neuromuscular transmission in mutant larvae. In *Sh*, a single stimulus causes multiple firing of the motor axons (cf. Figure 1), resulting in enhanced transmitter release. In *eag*, slow but repetitive firing of motor axons, correlated with EJPs, occurs spontaneously. Combining *eag* and *Sh* in double mutants produces striking synergistic effects, resulting in greatly prolonged EJPs correlated with bursts of motor axon spikes, a phenotype mimicked by treating *eag* with a *Sh* channel blocker, 4-AP. (Adapted from Ganetzky and Wu 1985.)

ening and repetitive firing have been reported in the giant fiber axons of these circuits in *Sh* mutants (Tanouye et al., 1981; Tanouye and Ferrus, 1985). The motor output of the giant fiber circuits is increased to different degrees in *Hk*, *Sh*, *eag*, and *eag Sh* double mutants (Engel and Wu, 1992), consistent with the enhanced jump-and-flight escape reflex (Kaplan and Trout, 1969).

Investigators have extensively analyzed defects from membrane excitability in the larval neuromuscular preparation, in which pre- and postsynaptic elements are readily accessible for physiological and morphological studies. As shown in Figure 7, *Sh* mutants manifest extra spikes in the presynaptic motor axon, correlating with larger postsynaptic excitatory junctional potentials (EJPs) upon nerve stimulation, whereas *eag* mutants exhibit spontaneous nerve firing and concomitant EJPs (Jan et al., 1977; Ganetzky and Wu, 1982b, 1983). As in the adult double mutant, *eag Sh* larvae also manifest qualitatively new phenotypes. Large, prolonged EJPs appear in *eag Sh* larvae and are driven by repetitive firing of the motor neuron (Figure 7). Pharmacological studies support the idea that *Sh* and *eag* preferentially affect distinct K^+ currents mediated by separate K^+ channel subunits at the neuromuscular junction (Jan et al., 1977; Ganetzky and Wu, 1983, 1985). The effects of *Sh* mutations can be mimicked in WT by applying 4-aminopyridine (4-AP), a blocker of the transient I_A, and the striking phenotype of *eag Sh* double mutants can be mimicked by applying 4-AP to *eag* larvae (Figure 7). Finally, a nonspecific K^+ channel blocker, tetraethylammonium (TEA), can phenocopy *eag Sh* defects in WT. Subsequently, voltage-clamp analysis of K^+ currents in larval muscles demonstrated that *Sh* affects I_A and *eag* affects several identified K^+ currents (Zhong and Wu, 1991a, 1993).

The above experiments demonstrate the interactions among the various K^+, Na^+, and Ca^{2+} channel genes, that lead to striking physiological consequences. Similar interactions have revealed morphological alterations, indicating the roles of ion channels in activity-dependent neuronal development.

IV. ACTIVITY-DEPENDENT NEURONAL GROWTH IN HYPEREXCITABLE K+ CHANNEL MUTANTS

A number of studies demonstrate that neuronal spikes and synaptic activity regulate the final projection pattern of terminal arbors (Hubel et al., 1977; Harris, 1981; Meyer, 1982; Cline and Constantine-Paton, 1989). In *Drosophila*, activity-dependent neuronal growth has been well-demonstrated in several hyperexcitable K^+ channel mutants (Table 1). In addition to the striking electrophysiological defects (Figures 4A and 7), the number of synaptic boutons and terminal branches at the larval neuromuscular junction increase in *eag Sh* (Figure 8A) and *Hk eag* double mutants, in contrast to no obvious defects in the single mutants (Budnik et al., 1990). Overgrowth is due to the effects of hyperexcitability. In addition to the genetic manipulation of K^+ channels, enhancing Na^+ channel expression (duplication of the para gene) achieves similar effects. Reducing para Na^+ channel expression (in nap mutants) suppresses the effects (Budnik et al., 1990).

Numerous signaling pathways are implicated in the neuronal plasticity manifested in activity-dependent growth (Bailey and Kandel, 1993; Kennedy, 1994). It is important to ask which signaling pathways mediate the K^+ channel-dependent growth of axonal arbors in *Drosophila*. The cAMP (Zhong et al., 1992), PKG (Renger et al., 1999), and CaMK (Griffith et al., 1994) pathways all regulate aspects of terminal arborization at the larval neuromuscular junction in an activity-dependent manner. We focus here on the cAMP system, and its well-characterized interaction with K^+ channels. The *dnc* mutations, which increase cAMP levels by reducing cAMP-specific phosphodiesterase activity (Byers et al., 1981), increase the growth of larval motor terminals (Figure 8B). Branch and bouton numbers are further increased when excitability is enhanced by *Sh* mutations in *dnc Sh* double mutants (Figure 8B). However, this effect is reversed in *dnc rut Sh* triple mutants (Zhong et al., 1992; Zhong and Wu, 2004), in which defects in the *rut* adenylyl cyclase decrease cAMP levels (Livingstone et al., 1984). Electrical activity can increase Ca^{2+} accumulation (Cohan et al., 1987) and in turn enhance cAMP production via Ca^{2+}/calmodulin (CaM) stimulation of the *rut* adenylyl cyclase, which is blocked by the *rut* mutation. In many systems, cAMP-induced gene transcription, mediated by the cAMP response element binding protein (CREB), can lead to activity-dependent changes in synaptic efficacy (Bailey and Kandel, 1993; Yin and Tully, 1996). At *Drosophila* neuromuscular junctions, activation of CREB and expression of the fasII adhesion molecule may mediate the effects of *eag Sh* and *dnc* mutations in the activity-dependent development of motor terminal arbors (Davis et al., 1996; Schuster et al., 1996).

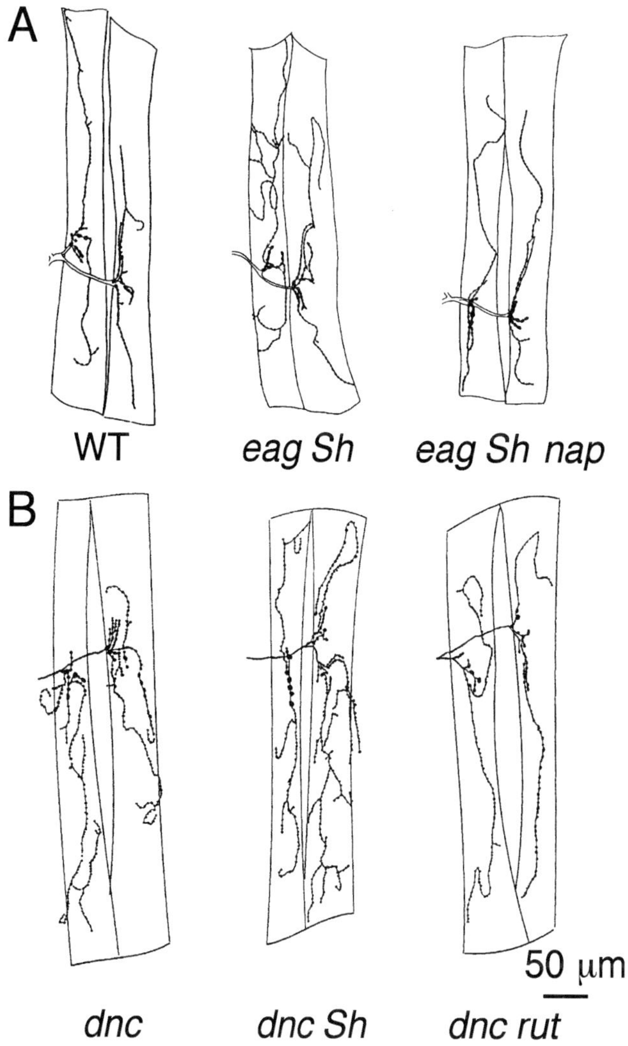

FIGURE 8 Altered motor axon terminal arbors in ion channel and cAMP cascade mutants. **A.** Camera lucida drawings of immunohistochemically stained axon terminals on muscles 12 and 13 of third instar larvae reveal extreme ramification in *eag Sh* double mutants. This alteration is suppressed by nap^{ts}. **B.** In *dnc*, the extent of ramification is increased and can be further enhanced when combined with the hyperexcitability mutation *Sh*, even though *Sh* alone does not significantly affect axonal terminal growth. The overgrowth in *dnc* is suppressed by a reduction in cAMP synthesis due to the *rut* mutation. (Modified from Budnik et al. 1990 and Zhong et al. 1992.)

The morphology of axonal arbors at the neuromuscular junction of third instar larvae is the cumulative result of several developmental processes including axon elongation, guidance, and branching, as well as synapse formation and stabilization. Axon elongation and guidance in *Drosophila*, as in other species (Meyer et al., 1982; Shatz, 1990), appears to be independent of action potential generation. Abnormal branching of identified sensory axons has not been detected in *eag Sh* or *para nap* double-mutant mechanosensory neurons in adult flies (Burg and Wu, 1986, 1989) and suppression of motor neuron activity by tetrodotoxin (TTX) or *para* and *nap* mutations does not prevent embryonic muscle innervation (Broadie and Bate, 1993). In aspects of growth that are activity-dependent, investigators have focused on a prominent structural specialization at the end of growing axons, the neuronal growth cone. Nerve terminal branching involves the transition from the axonal growth cone into a mature presynaptic terminal, a process well documented at the *Drosophila* larval neuromuscular junction (Halpern et al., 1991; Yoshihara et al., 1997). In other species, neuronal activity affects growth cone morphology (Cohan and Kater, 1986) and may underlie transient increases in growth cone Ca^{2+} levels observed at choice points along the projection pathway (Gomez and Spitzer, 1999).

Growth cone behavior and the underlying Ca^{2+} dynamics during nerve terminal arborization may be altered in hyperexcitable K^+ channel mutants. "Giant" neuron cultures made from cytokinesis-arrested neuroblasts (Wu et al., 1989) can facilitate analysis of the contributions made by individual K^+ channel subunits in growth cones and other cellular regions in activity-dependent growth. For example, K^+ channel mutations including *Sh* indeed alter the size of growth cones in culture (Figure 10A). In addition, *Sh* and *slo* mutations lead to excessive spontaneous Ca^{2+} increases in the growth cone (Figure 10B). A role for action potentials is suggested in triggering spontaneous Ca^{2+} transients and in the enlarged growth cones because both can be suppressed by TTX (Berke and Wu, unpublished observations).

High K^+ depolarization-induced Ca^{2+} transients are larger and more dynamic in the growth cone than in the cell body in WT cultures (Figure 9; Berke and Wu, 2002). Similarly, *slo* mutations produce larger spontaneous Ca^{2+} transients (Figure 10C) and broaden action potentials more in axon terminals than near the soma of cultured neurons (Saito and Wu, 1991). These phenotypes indicate roles for voltage- and Ca^{2+}-activated K^+ currents in regulating Ca^{2+} dependent growth cone behaviors.

Localized Ca^{2+} increases in the growth cone periphery may be important for stimulating local growth *in vivo* (Lau et al., 1999) and for growth cone turning induced by guidance molecules in culture (Song and Poo, 1999; Zheng, 2000). The large growth cones in "giant" neuron cultures facilitate local optical measurements and reveal larger high K^+-induced Ca^{2+} transients at the leading edge of motile

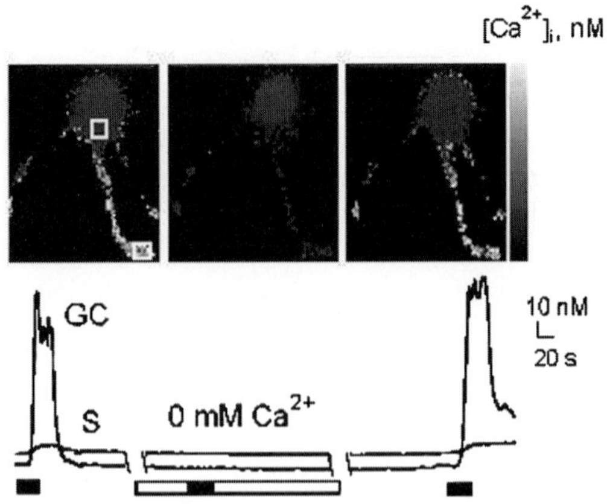

FIGURE 9 Differences in depolarization-induced Ca^{2+} signaling between the growth cone and soma in cultured neurons. Intracellular Ca^{2+} increases in response to depolarization induced by high K^+ saline (60 mM, black bars) are shown by fluorescence absorption by the Ca^{2+} indicator fura-2 (Grynkiewicz et al. 1985). Ca^{2+} levels in selected regions (boxes) are shown in the traces, and grayscale images show representative Ca^{2+} levels at the peak of the response (scale bar shown at right). The dynamic range of the Ca^{2+} increase over time is larger within the growth cone (GC) than soma (S). The response is reversibly eliminated in 0 mM Ca^{2+} saline (white bar). (Adapted from Berke and Wu 2002.)

growth cones compared to their central domain (Berke and Wu, 2002). cAMP may be important in sub-cellular Ca^{2+} dynamics because both *dnc* and *rut* mutations disrupt this local pattern (Berke and Wu, 2002) and suppress lamellipodial expansion and contraction during growth cone motility (Kim and Wu, 1996). Further analysis with *Drosophila* mutations can identify the K^+ and Ca^{2+} channel types (Table 1) contributing to the electrical activities of growth cones and local Ca^{2+} dynamics.

Several second-messenger cascades are implicated in growth cone behaviors cued by guidance molecules, including the signaling pathways of cAMP, cGMP-dependent protein kinase (PKG), and the Ca^{2+}/CaM-dependent protein kinase (CaMK). Using Drosophila mutants defective in second messenger systems, investigators can examine aspects of growth cone physiology and behavior related to the actions of known guidance molecules (Dickson, 2002). Flies with defects in the PKG and CaMK pathways exhibit enhanced synaptic transmission and motor terminal growth at larval neuromuscular junctions (de Belle et al., 1989; Griffith et al., 1994; Wang et al., 1994; Renger et al., 1999). Interestingly, application of growth factors and biogenic amines increases growth cone Ca^{2+} dynamics and regulates its motility in culture (Haydon et al., 1984; Cohan et al., 1987; McCobb et al., 1988; Song and Poo, 1999). Furthermore, biogenic amines such as dopamine and serotonin modulate neuronal activity by stimulating the cAMP pathway (Svenningsson et al., 2003), which in *Drosophila* controls K^+ channel-mediated changes in membrane excitability (Renger et al. 1999; Yao and Wu, 1999b). PKG mutants (*for*, Table 1) have altered foraging behavior

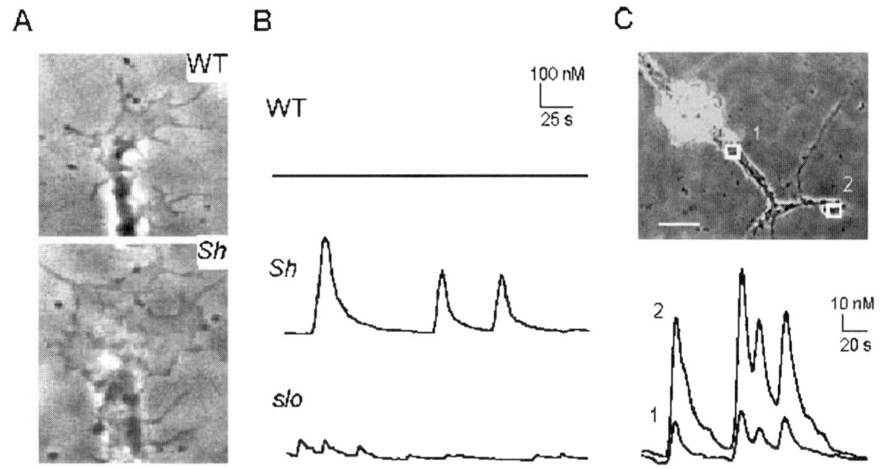

FIGURE 10 Hyperexcitability mutations enhance spontaneous Ca^{2+} transients and increase growth cone size in neuronal cultures. **A.** Representative phase-contrast images of growth cones demonstrating increased growth cone size in *Sh*. Scale bar, 4 µm. **B.** In contrast to WT growth cones, *Sh* and *slo* growth cones exhibit robust Ca^{2+} transients in the absence of stimulation. **C.** Spontaneous Ca^{2+} transients are larger in growth cones than near the soma of cultured *slo* neurons. Ca^{2+} is estimated in the squares labeled 1 and 2. Scale bar, 10 µm.

(Osborne et al., 1997) and conditional CaMK inhibition in *ala* transformants disrupts courtship conditioning (Griffith et al., 1993). Further analysis of second messenger-dependent growth and excitability will undoubtedly help reveal how K^+ channels participate in the activity-dependent formation of neural circuits subserving these different behavioral tasks.

V. ALTERATIONS OF NERVE AND MUSCLE EXCITABILITY IN K^+ CHANNEL MUTANTS

A. K^+ Current Defects

Membrane excitability is determined by ion fluxes across the cell membrane driven by electrochemical gradients. Na^+ and Ca^{2+} influxes control membrane depolarization whereas ensuing outward K^+ currents are the major repolarizing force. Disrupting the balance between inward and outward currents by mutations or pharmacological agents affecting specific K^+ channels can alter membrane excitability and neuronal activity in different manners.

K^+ channels constitute the most diverse ion channel family (Coetzee et al., 1999). *Drosophila* mutants have provided the necessary entry points for the molecular studies of a variety of K^+ channels in different species. As mentioned above, *Drosophila slo* and *Hk* mutations were instrumental in the discovery of the α subunits of Ca^{2+}-activated K^+ channels and the β subunit for *Sh* channels, respectively (Table 1). Based on sequence homology to the *Sh* gene that encodes I_A channel α subunits, the *Shab*, *Shaw*, and *Shal* genes were later identified to encode other types of voltage-activated K^+ channel α subunits in *Drosophila* (Table 1). This finding has led to subsequent identification of mammalian *Sh* family homologs, the K^+ channel subunits Kv1, 2, 3, and 4, associated with different transient and delayed K^+ currents (Coetzee et al., 1999). Similar homologue searches using *eag* have identified additional members of the EAG family (Table 1): *erg* (*eag-related gene*, also known as *seizure* (*sei*)), and *elk* (*eag-like channel*). Their homologs have been subsequently implicated in human diseases, for example, Human *erg* (*Herg*) in the long-QT syndrome (Sanguinetti, 1999).

Mutants of the *Sh and erg* genes have revealed differential defects in K^+ currents, reflecting the *in vivo* function of individual K^+ currents. Investigators have identified four K^+ current components with distinct kinetics and gating mechanisms in *Drosophila* larval body-wall muscle fibers: the transient and delayed voltage-activated I_A and I_K, and the fast and slow Ca^{2+}-activated I_{CF} and I_{CS} (Singh and Wu 1989). Null mutations of *Sh* eliminate I_A in muscle cells (Figure 11A; Wu and Haugland, 1985), but only partially remove the transient K^+ current in neurons (Baker and Salkoff, 1990; Tsunoda and Salkoff, 1995b; Peng and Wu, unpublished). In addition to *Sh*, another subunit, *Shal*, may also contribute to the transient K^+ current in neurons as both *Sh* and *Shal* currents exhibit fast inactivation in the *Xenopus* oocyte expression system (Wei et al., 1990). A null mutation of *Shab* only partially removes I_K in both muscle cells (Singh and Singh, 1999) and neurons (Peng and Wu, unpublished), consistent with the idea that *Shaw* as well as *Shab* contribute to the sustained I_K (Wei et al., 1990; Tsunoda and Salkoff, 1995a,b). The gene *slo* encodes channels responsible for a

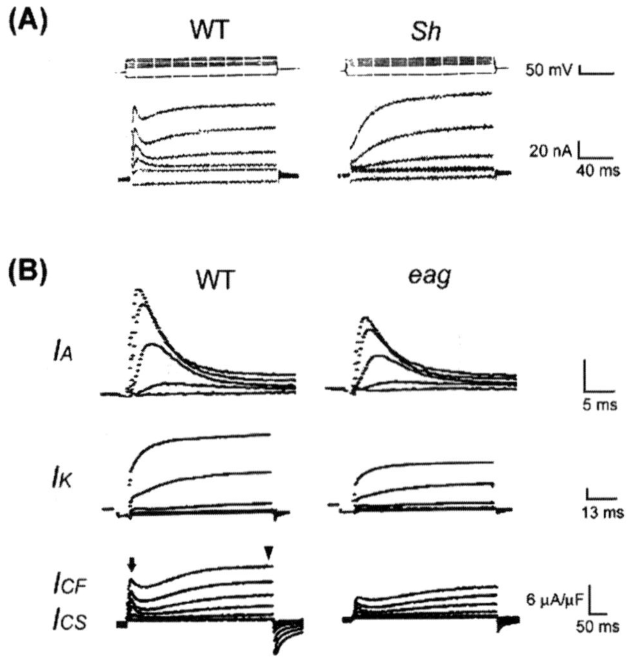

FIGURE 11 Differential effects of *Sh* and *eag* mutations on four K^+ currents. Four outward K^+ currents can be recorded in larval muscle fibers using two-electrode voltage clamp. **A.** Voltage-activated I_A and I_K in Ca^{2+}-free saline. Total outward currents in a *Sh* null mutant demonstrate a lack of the early transient I_A without changing the delayed I_K. **B.** Pre-pulse depolarization inactivates I_A, enabling measurement of I_K. The difference between the responses without and with pre-pulse conditioning is I_A. Furthermore, Ca^{2+}-activated I_{CF} (arrow) and I_{CS} (arrowhead) can be isolated in saline containing Ca^{2+} as well as 4-AP and quinidine that block voltage-activated I_A and I_K. Note that the eag^{X6} mutation reduces all four K^+ currents. (Modified from Wu and Haugland 1985; Zhong and Wu 1991a.)

Ca^{2+}-activated K^+ current in neurons (Saito and Wu, 1991) and I_{CF} in muscle (Elkins et al., 1986; Singh and Wu, 1989; Komatsu et al., 1990). The gene encoding I_{CS} channel subunits responsible for the slow Ca^{2+}-activated K^+ current has yet to be identified. Mutational studies in larval muscles have also demonstrated that the *Hk* β subunit modulates *Sh* channels affecting a wide range of I_A properties, including its amplitude, activation, and inactivation (Wang and Wu, 1996). Mutations of another gene, *qvr*, specifically disrupt *Sh* I_A without altering other K^+ currents (Wang et al., 2000).

In contrast to the effects of *Sh*, *Shab*, *slo*, *Hk*, and *qvr* mutations on specific currents, *eag* mutations affect multiple K^+ currents. In *eag* larval muscle, all four K^+ currents (I_A, I_K, I_{CF}, and I_{CS}) are reduced (Figure 11B; Zhong and Wu, 1991a). Physical interaction between *Sh* and *eag* subunits is suggested by allele-specific interactions between *Sh* and *eag* in double-mutant combinations (Zhong and Wu, 1993) and by co-expression studies in *Xenopus* oocytes (Chen et al., 1996, 2000). Thus, the *eag* subunit may be able to interact with multiple K^+ channel subunits and provides a convergent point for cyclic nucleotide modulation of K^+ currents (Zhong and Wu, 1993). A putative cyclic nucleotide-binding domain has been found in the C-terminal region of the *eag* subunit (Guy et al., 1991) and a cGMP analog strongly enhances I_K in muscle, which is blocked by *eag* mutations (Zhong and Wu, 1993).

B. Enhanced Spontaneous Spike Activities and Altered Firing Patterns

Several physiological preparations have revealed the consequences of K^+ current defects in *Drosophila* mutants. Spontaneous spike activities are markedly enhanced in the motor neurons of larval body-wall muscle (Figure 4A), in adult thoracic ganglion neurons (Figure 6C), and in the motor output of the adult giant fiber escape pathway (Engel and Wu, 1998).

Neuronal activities are controlled by intrinsic membrane properties and interactions among neurons in a circuit. *Drosophila* neuronal cultures are particularly suitable for studying endogenous ion currents in isolated neurons in relation to spontaneous firing patterns (Saito and Wu, 1991; Zhao and Wu, 1997; Yao and Wu, 1999a). In particular, analysis of *Hk* and *Sh* mutants has provided insights into the regulation of the neuronal quiescent state. In dissociated embryonic giant neuron cultures, the majority of WT cells (>85%) are quiescent and the remaining cells show three types of spontaneous spiking activities (Figure 12). Irregular activities (sporadic and plateau spiking patterns) occur in a small population (~8%) and rhythmic activity (persistent spiking pattern) is generated in an even smaller population (~4%). Both *Sh* and *Hk* mutations increase the percentage of neurons firing spontaneously (Figure 12B). *Sh* mutations increase the population with irregular activities (~25%), while *Hk* neurons exhibit excessive persistent pacemaker-like firing (~20%). Significantly, the enhancement of spontaneous firing is not additive in *Hk Sh* double mutants, as *Hk Sh* neurons do not show increased rhythmic activity but express a phenotype indistinguishable from that of *Sh* (Figure 12B). This finding is consistent with the fact that the *Hk* β subunit modulates *Sh* I_A channels (Wang and Wu, 1996) and implies that the pacemaker-like activity of *Hk* mutants rely on the function of intact *Sh* α subunits (Figure 6; Ikeda and Kaplan, 1974; Yao and Wu, 1999a). Therefore, misregulation of *Hk-Sh* subunit interaction leads to excessive spontaneous rhythmic spiking in certain types of neurons.

In addition to firing patterns, the properties of individual action potentials are relevant to motor control. *Drosophila* mutations have helped delineate the role of K^+ channel subunits in shaping action potentials as well as firing patterns. Intracellular recordings from the cervical giant fiber show delayed repolarization and increased action potential duration for several *Sh* alleles (Tanouye and Ferrus, 1985), establishing a role for *Sh* I_A in axons and in motor axon terminals

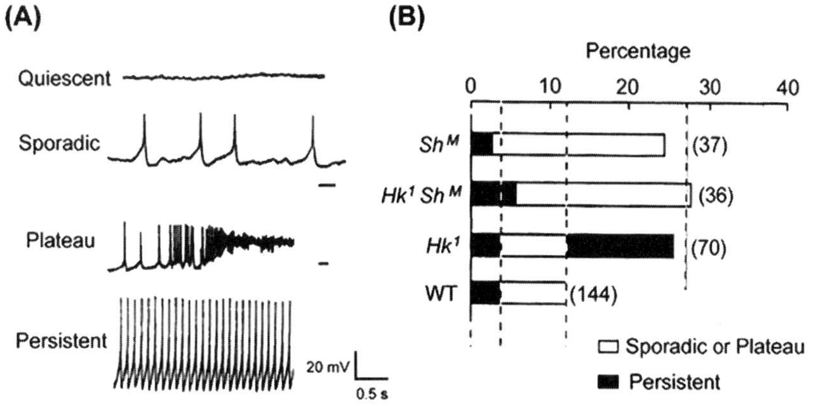

FIGURE 12 Spontaneous firing patterns in WT and *Sh* and *Hk* neurons. **A.** Four types of spontaneous activities are seen in isolated cultured neurons. Quiescent—no spontaneous spike activity; sporadic—occasional single or clusters of spikes; plateau—bursts of spike activities that turn into sustained depolarization; persistent—sustained rhythmic spike activity. **B.** The percentage of neurons exhibiting different spontaneous firing patterns among genotypes suggests possible roles for *Sh* and *Hk* in the maintenance of the quiescent state. Note that *Sh* and *Hk* mutants have a similar reduction in the number of quiescent neurons. Persistent pacemaker-like activities are increased in *Hk* cultures, whereas irregular activities (sporadic or plateau) are increased in *Sh* cultures. Significantly, only the *Sh*, but not *Hk*, phenotype is expressed in the *Hk Sh* double mutant. (Modified from Yao and Wu 1999a.)

(Figure 1). In some cultured *Hk* neurons, the action potential duration is broadened up to tenfold (Yao and Wu, 1999a), suggesting another consequence of mutations in the *Hk* β subunit. In contrast to I_A mutants (*Sh* and *Hk*), *Shab* mutants with defects in I_K fail to maintain membrane repolarization during sustained depolarizing currents and cannot support several common firing patterns (Peng and Wu, unpublished).

The *slo* mutant phenotypes have demonstrated a role for Ca^{2+}-activated K^+ channels in regulating Na^+ and Ca^{2+} in action potentials in functionally specialized cell types and subcellular regions. In *Drosophila* muscle, Na^+ channels are absent and Ca^{2+} influx supports the membrane depolarization (Singh and Wu, 1999). In adult and larval muscles (Elkins et al., 1986; Singh and Wu, 1990), *slo* mutations severely prolong the depolarization phase of action potentials by at least an order of magnitude, especially upon I_A inactivation after the initial spikes (Figure 13B). In neurons, Na^+ influx dominates axonal and somatic depolarization whereas Ca^{2+} channels are abundant in nerve terminals and growth cones. In some cultured neurons, *slo* mutants exhibit action potential-broadening (Figure 13), which is most striking in the nerve terminals (Saito and Wu, 1991), consistent with a role of *slo* channels in controlling Ca^{2+} spike shape. Regulation of Ca^{2+} influx through Ca^{2+} spike shaping by *slo* channels thus plays a central role for neurotransmitter release in mature nerve terminals (Gho and Ganetzky, 1992; Warbinton et al., 1996) and are implicated in growth cone motility, neurite elongation, and axonal pathfinding as mentioned above.

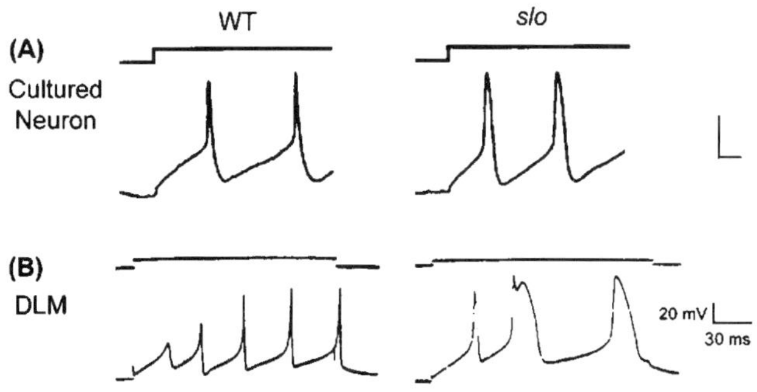

FIGURE 13 Alterations in action potential shape and firing patterns in *slo* mutants. **A.** Action potentials elicited by current injection from cultured WT and *slo* neurons. Duration of action potentials is increased in *slo* neurons. **B.** Regenerative voltage responses to constant current injection from WT and *slo* adult flight muscles (DLMs). The action potentials from *slo* muscles exhibit broadening, which becomes more pronounced after the first spike due to inactivation of transient I_A. (Modified from Saito and Wu 1991; Elkins et al. 1985.)

VI. CONCLUSIONS

We have seen that mutational analysis in conjunction with molecular studies of genes in *Drosophila* has provided a gold mine of information about movement disorders. Many genes described here have homologous counterparts in vertebrates and their mutant phenotypes are often conserved across phyla. *Drosophila* mutant studies at the different levels of analyses have a broad implication since many cellular functions and even some motor patterns are also conserved in different species. Uncovering phenotypes at all levels, from molecules and cells to networks and behavior, provides a means to fill the conceptual gaps between the defective molecular mechanisms and the manifestation of altered higher functions. For instance, further functional analyses of the *Shaker* (*Sh*) gene and its interacting partners may yield useful clues for exploring possible mechanisms and new treatments for ataxia and related disorders derived from mutations of the *Sh* homologs in humans (Coetzee et al., 1999). Similarly, mutants of the *seizure* (*sei^{ts}*) gene are defective in the *erg* K^+ channel and are characterized by high temperature-induced seizure and paralysis (Table 1). Comparative studies of *sei^{ts}* and functionally related genes may help uncover a range of physiological and behavioral alterations beyond the long QT syndrome associated with mutations in a human homolog, the *Herg* K^+ channel (Sanguinetti, 1999). This information is relevant because the *Herg* channel is expressed outside of cardiac tissue (Saganich et al., 2001).

In the post-genomic era, the rate of discovery of new candidate genes involved in movement disorders will likely accelerate. Considering the function of many candidate genes is still unknown, it becomes increasingly important to understand the *in vivo* role of the putative genes and the interacting gene network. In addition to delineating the molecular diversity of ion channels and biogenic amine pathways, the biological control of their cell type-dependent synthesis, subcellular targeting, and functional modulation calls for *in vivo* studies in a genetically tractable system. *Drosophila* will be a higher organism of choice for examining alleles of different extremities, for constructing double mutants, and for screening systematically for interacting genes because such approaches are technically and financially more feasible in *Drosophila* than vertebrate model systems.

In addition to the studies based on classical point mutations and chromosomal aberrations as described above, P-element insertion lines are available for transposon-induced mutagenesis, transgene introduction, and enhancer detection (Lindsley and Zimm, 1992; www.flybase.org). These genetic tools offer an unprecedented flexibility and precision for functional and developmental analyses of the nervous system. Investigators can achieve temporal and spatial control of transgene expression. Exogenous promoters (e.g., heat-shock promoter) introduced together with the transgene can be used for conditional expression, enabling an assessment of gene action in different developmental time windows.

The GAL4-UAS binary system, originated from yeast and later introduced into *Drosophila* by P-element-mediated transformation (Brand and Perrimon, 1993), has made it possible to genetically alter targeted cell populations. An insertion of a GAL4 construct that occurs in close proximity to an endogenous enhancer element in the host genome (enhancer trap) causes the cargo transgene in a UAS construct to be expressed in a particular cell type or lineage in a pattern reflecting the enhancer's expression during development. For example, through genetic crosses, different GAL4-enhancer trap drivers can be combined with a UAS-GFP (green fluorescent protein) construct to selectively mark subsets of cells. This expression has enabled an examination of different K^+ currents in defined neuronal populations in culture (Peng and Wu, unpublished). In principle, a proper collection of GAL4 drivers should allow identification of neuronal cell types that are particularly susceptible to *Sh*, *Hk* and *eag* mutations. Such information may reveal how differential expression of distinct K^+ channel subunits generates different patterns of neuronal spiking activities associated with specific cell types. In larval neuromuscular junction development, the GAL4-UAS system has also demonstrated a presynaptic role of cAMP for nerve terminal arborization through targeted expression of the *dnc* phosphodiesterase (Cheung et al., 1999). As the structure and development of the various sensory and motor systems have been characterized, a large array of GAL4-UAS combinations will allow researchers to investigate the action of a given gene at critical anatomical sites and developmental stages in generating higher functions.

With the different genetic tools now available, investigators can conduct a broad-based analysis of motor control and movement disorders by well-developed molecular, cellular, physiological, and behavioral paradigms in *Drosophila*. Mechanistic analyses and functional characterizations of candidate genes in different cell types and neuronal circuits will elucidate a full range of phenotypes at different levels, from molecules, cells, and networks, to behavior.

References

Aceves-Pina, E.O., R. Booker, J.S. Duerr, M.S. Livingstone, W.G. Quinn, R.F. Smith, P.P. Sziber, et al. 1983. Learning and memory in *Drosophila*, studied with mutants. *Cold Spring Harb Symp Quant Biol* **48**:831–839.

Atkinson, N.S., G.A. Robertson, and B. Ganetzky. 1991. A component of calcium-activated potassium channels encoded by the *Drosophila slo* locus. *Science* **253**:551–555.

Atwood, H.L., C.K. Govind, and C.-F. Wu. 1993. Differential ultrastructure of synaptic terminals on ventral longitudinal abdominal muscles in *Drosophila* larvae. *J Neurobiol* **24**:1008–1024.

Baier, A., B. Wittek, and B. Brembs. 2002. *Drosophila* as a new model organism for the neurobiology of aggression? *J Exp Biol* **205**: 1233–1240.

Bailey, C.H., and E.R. Kandel. 1993. Structural change accompanying memory storage. *Ann Rev Physiol* **55**:397–426.

Baker, K., and L. Salkoff. 1990. The *Drosophila Shaker* gene codes for a distinctive K^+ current in a subset of neurons. *Neuron* **4**:129–140.

Barclay, J.W., H.L. Atwood, and R.M. Robertson. 2002. Impairment of central pattern generation in *Drosophila* cysteine string protein mutants. *J Comp Physiol A* **188**:71–78.

Baumann, A., A. Grupe, A. Ackermann, and O. Pongs. 1988. Structure of the voltage-dependent potassium channel is highly conserved from

Drosophila to vertebrate central nervous systems. *EMBO J* **7**: 2457–2463.

Berke, B.A., and C.-F. Wu. 2002. Regional calcium regulation within cultured *Drosophila* neurons: Effects of altered cAMP metabolism by the learning mutations *dunce* and *rutabaga*. *J Neurosci* **22**:4437–4447.

Berrigan, D., and D.J. Pepin. 1995. How maggots move: Allometry and kinematics of crawling in larval diptera. *J Insect Physiol* **41**:329–337.

Brand, A.H., and N. Perrimon. 1993. Targeted gene expression as a means of altering cell fates and generating dominant phenotypes. *Development* **118**:401–415.

Broadie, K.S., and M. Bate. 1993. Development of the embryonic neuromuscular synapse of *Drosophila melanogaster*. *J Neurosci* **13**:144–166.

Buchner, E. 1991. Genes expressed in the adult brain of *Drosophila* and effects of their mutations on behavior: A survey of transmitter- and second messenger-related genes. *J Neurogenet* **7**:153–192.

Budnik, V., Y. Zhong, and C.-F. Wu. 1990. Morphological plasticity of motor axons in *Drosophila* mutants with altered excitability. *J Neurosci* **10**:3754–3768.

Bulter, A., A. Wei, K. Baker, and L. Salkoff. 1989. A family of putative potassium channel genes in *Drosophila*. *Science* **243**:943–947.

Burg, M., and C.-F. Wu. 1986. Differentiation and central projections of peripheral sensory cells with action-potential block in *Drosophila* mosaics. *J Neurosci* **6**:2968–2976.

Burg, M., and C.-F. Wu. 1989. Central projections of peripheral mechanosensory cells with increased excitability in *Drosophila* mosaics. *Dev Biol* **131**:505–514.

Byers, D., R.L. Davis, and J.A. Kiger. 1981. Defect in cAMP phosphodiesterase due to the *dunce* mutation of learning in *Drosophila melanogaster*. *Nature* **289**:79–81.

Calabrese, R.L. 1998. Cellular, synaptic, network, and modulatory mechanisms involved in rhythm generation. *Curr Opin Neurobiol* **8**:710–717.

Cattaert, D., and S. Birman. 2001. Blockade of the central generator of locomotor rhythm by noncompetitive NMDA receptor antagonists in *Drosophila* larvae. *J Neurobiol* **48**:58–73.

Chen, M.L., T. Hoshi, and C.-F. Wu. 1996. Heteromultimeric interactions among K^+ channel subunits from *Shaker* and *eag* families in *Xenopus* oocytes. *Neuron* **17**:535–542.

Chen, M.-L., T. Hoshi, and C.-F. Wu. 2000. *Sh* and *Eag* K^+ channel subunit interaction in frog oocytes depends on level and time of expression. *Biophys J* **79**:1358–1368.

Chopra, M., G.G. Gu, and S. Singh. 2000. Mutations affecting the delayed rectifier potassium current in *Drosophila*. *J Neurogenet* **14**:107–123.

Chouinard, S.W., G.F. Wilson, A.K. Schlimgen, and B. Ganetzky. 1995. A potassium channel β subunit related to the aldo-keto reductase superfamily is encoded by the *Drosophila* hyperkinetic locus. *Proc Natl Acad Sci USA* **92**:6763–6767.

Cheung, U.S., A.J. Shayan, G.L. Boulianne, and H.L. Atwood. 1999. *Drosophila* larval neuromuscular junction's responses to reduction in cAMP in the nervous system. *J Neurobiol* **40**:1–13.

Cline, H.T., and M. Constantine-Paton. 1989. NMDA receptor antagonists disrupt the retinotectal topographic map. *Neuron* **3**:413–426.

Coetzee, W.A., Y. Amarillo, J. Chiu, A. Chow, D. Lau, T. McCormack, H. Moreno, et al. 1999. Molecular diversity of K^+ channels. *Ann NY Acad Sci* **868**:233–285.

Cohan, C., and S. Kater. 1986. Suppression of neurite elongation and growth cone motility by electrical activity. *Science* **232**:1638–1640.

Cohan, C.S., J.A. Connor, and S.B. Kater. 1987. Electrically and chemically mediated increases in intracellular calcium in neuronal growth cones. *J Neurosci* **7**:3588–3599.

Cooper, R.L., and W.S. Neckameyer. 1999. Dopaminergic modulation of motor neuron activity and neuromuscular function in *Drosophila melanogaster*. *Comp Biochem Physiol B* **122**:199–210.

Crossley, C.A. 1978. The morphology and development of the *Drosophila* muscular system. In *The genetics and biology of* Drosophila. Ed. Ashburner and Wright. Vol. **2b**, pp. 449–559. New York: Academic Press.

Davis, G.W., C.M. Schuster, and C.S. Goodman. 1996. Genetic dissection of structural and functional components of synaptic plasticity. III. CREB is necessary for presynaptic functional plasticity. *Neuron* **17**: 669–679.

Dickson, B.J. 2002. Molecular mechanisms of axon guidance. *Science* **298**:1959–1964.

de Belle, J.S., A.J. Hilliker, and M.B. Sokolowski. 1989. Genetic localization of *foraging* (*for*): A major gene for larval behavior in *Drosophila melanogaster*. *Genetics* **123**:157–163.

Dudai, Y., Y.N. Jan, D. Byers, W.G. Quinn, and S. Benzer. 1976. *dunce*, a mutant of *Drosophila* deficient in learning. *Proc Natl Acad Sci USA* **73**: 1684–1688.

Elkins, T., B. Ganetzky, and C.-F. Wu. 1986. A *Drosophila* mutation that eliminates a calcium-dependent potassium current. *Proc Natl Acad Sci USA* **83**:8415–8419.

Elkins, T., and B. Ganetzky. 1990. Conduction in the giant nerve fiber pathway in temperature-sensitive paralytic mutants of *Drosophila*. *J Neurogenet* **6**:207–219.

Engel, J.E., and C.-F. Wu. 1992. Interactions of membrane excitability mutations affecting potassium and sodium currents in the flight and giant fiber escape systems of *Drosophila*. *J Comp Physiol A* **171**: 93–104.

Engel, J., and C.-F. Wu. 1996. Altered habituation of an identified escape circuit in *Drosophila* memory mutants. *J Neurosci* **16**:3486–3499.

Engel, J.E., and C.-F. Wu. 1998. Genetic dissection of functional contributions of specific potassium and sodium currents in the flight and giant fiber escape systems of *Drosophila*. *J Comp Physiol A* **171**:93–104.

Engel, J.E., X.-J. Xie, M.B. Sokolowski, and C.-F. Wu. 2000. A cGMP-dependent protein kinase gene, *foraging*, modifies habituation-like response decrement of the giant fiber escape circuit in *Drosophila*. *Learn and Mem* **7**:341–352.

Frye, M.A., and M.H. Dickinson. 2001. Fly flight: A model for the neural control of complex behavior. *Neuron* **32**:385–388.

Gailey, D.A., and J.C. Hall. 1989. Behavior and cytogenetics of *fruitless* in *Drosophila melanogaster*: Different courtship defects caused by separate, closely linked lesions. *Genetics* **121**:773–785.

Gailey, D.A., J.C. Hall, and R.W. Siegel. 1985. Reduced reproductive success for a conditioning mutant in experimental populations of *Drosophila melanogaster*. *Genetics* **111**:795–804.

Ganetzky, B., and C.-F. Wu. 1982a. Indirect suppression involving behavioral mutants with altered nerve excitability in *Drosophila melanogaster*. *Genetics* **100**:597–614.

Ganetzky, B., and C.-F. Wu. 1982b. *Drosophila* mutants with opposing effects on nerve excitability: Genetic and spatial interactions in repetitive firing. *J Neurophysiol* **47**:501–514.

Ganetzky, B., and C.-F. Wu. 1983. Neurogenetic analysis of potassium currents in *Drosophila*: Synergistic effects on neuromuscular transmission in double mutants. *J Neurogenet* **1**:17–28.

Ganetzky, B., and C.-F. Wu. 1985. Genes and membrane excitability in *Drosophila*. *Trends in Neurosci* **8**:322–326.

Gho, M., and B. Ganetzky. 1992. Analysis of repolarization of presynaptic motor terminals in *Drosophila* larvae using potassium-channel-blocking drugs and mutations. *J Exp Biol* **170**:93–111.

Gomez, T., and N. Spitzer. 1999. *In vivo* regulation of axon extension and pathfinding by growth-cone calcium transients. *Nature* **397**:350–355.

Gorczyca, M.G., V. Budnik, K. White, and C.-F. Wu. 1991. Dual muscarinic and nicotinic action on a motor program in *Drosophila*. *J Neurobiol* **22**:391–404.

Green, C.H., B. Burnet, and K.J. Connolly. 1983. Organization and patterns of interspecific and intraspecific variation in the behavior of *Drosophila* larvae. *Anim Behav* **31**:282–291.

Griffith, L.C., L.M. Verselis, K.M. Aitken, C.P. Kyriacou, W. Danho, and R.J. Greenspan. 1993. Inhibition of calcium/calmodulin-dependent protein kinase in *Drosophila* disrupts behavioral plasticity. *Neuron* **10**:501–509.

Griffith, L.C., J. Wang, Y. Zhong, C.-F. Wu, and R.J. Greenspan. 1994. Calcium/calmodulin-dependent protein kinase II and potassium channel subunit Eag similarly affect plasticity in *Drosophila*. *Proc Natl Acad Sci USA* **91**:10044–10048.

Grillner, S. 2003. The motor infrastructure: From ion channels to neuronal networks. *Nat Rev Neurosci* **4**:573–586.

Grynkiewicz, G., M. Poenie, and R. Tsien. 1985. A new generation of Ca^{2+} indicators with greatly improved fluorescence properties. *J Bio Chem* **260**:3440–3450.

Guy, H.R., S.R. Durell, J. Warmke, R. Drysdale, and B. Ganetzky. 1991. Similarities in amino acid sequences of *Drosophila* Eag and cyclic nucleotide-gated channels. *Science* **254**:730.

Halpern, M.E., A. Chiba, J. Johansen, and H. Keshishian. 1991. Growth cone behavior underlying the development of stereotypic synaptic connections in *Drosophila* embryos. *J Neurosci* **11**:3227–3238.

Harris, W.A. 1981. Neural activity and development. *Ann Rev Phys* **43**:689–710.

Harris-Warrick, R.M., and E. Marder. 1991. Modulation of neural networks for behavior. *Annu Rev Neurosci* **14**:39–57.

Harris-Warrick, R.M. 2002. Voltage-sensitive ion channels in rhythmic motor systems. *Curr Opin Neurobiol* **12**:646–651.

Haugland, F.N., and C.F. Wu. 1990. A voltage-clamp analysis of gene-dosage effects of the *Shaker* locus on larval muscle potassium currents in *Drosophila*. *J Neurosci* **10**:1357–1371.

Haydon, P.G., D.P. McCobb, and S.B. Kater. 1984. Serotonin selectively inhibits growth cone motility and synaptogenesis of specific identified neurons. *Science* **236**:561–564.

Hegde, P., G.G. Gu, D. Chen, S.J. Free, and S. Singh. 1999. Mutational analysis of the *Shab*-encoded delayed rectifier K^+ channels in *Drosophila*. *J Biol Chem* **274**:22109–22113.

Hirsh, J., and N. Davidson. 1981. Isolation and characterization of the dopa decarboxylase gene of *Drosophila melanogaster*. *Mol Cell Biol* **1**:475–85.

Hoang, B., and A. Chiba. 2001. Single-cell analysis of *Drosophila* larval neuromuscular synapses. *Dev Biol* **229**:55–70.

Homyk, T., and D.E. Sheppard. 1977. Behavioral mutants of *Drosophila melanogaster*. I. Isolation and mapping of mutations which decrease flight ability. *Genetics* **87**:95–104.

Hubel, D.H., T.N. Wiesel, and S. LeVay. 1977. Plasticity of ocular dominance columns in monkey striate cortex. *Philos Trans R Soc Lond B Biol Sci* **278**:377–409.

Humphreys, J.M., B. Duyf, M.L. Joiner, J.P. Phillips, and A.J. Hilliker. 1996. Genetic analysis of oxygen defense mechanisms in *Drosophila melanogaster* and identification of a novel behavioural mutant with a *Shaker* phenotype. *Genome* **3**:749–757.

Ikeda, K., and W.D. Kaplan. 1970a. Patterned neural activity of a mutant *Drosophila melanogaster*. *Proc Natl Acad Sci USA* **66**:765–772.

Ikeda, K., and W.D. Kaplan. 1970b. Unilaterally patterned neural activity of gynandromorphs, mosaic for a neurological mutant of *Drosophila melanogaster*. *Proc Natl Acad Sci USA* **67**:1480–1487.

Ikeda, K., and W.D. Kaplan. 1974. Neurophysiological genetics in *Drosophila melanogaster*. *Am Zool* **14**:1055–1066.

Jackson, F.R., J. Gitschier, G.R. Strichartz, and L.M. Hall. 1985. Genetic modifications of voltage-sensitive sodium channels in *Drosophila*: Gene dosage studies of the *seizure* locus. *J Neurosci* **5**:1144–1151.

Jan, L.Y., and Y.N. Jan. 1976a. Properties of the larval neuromuscular junction in *Drosophila melanogaster*. *J Physiol* **262**:189–214.

Jan, L.Y., and Y.N. Jan. 1976b. L-glutamate as an excitatory transmitter at the *Drosophila* larval neuromuscular junction. *J Physiol* **262**:215–236.

Jan, Y.N., L.Y. Jan, and M.J. Dennis. 1977. Two mutations of synaptic transmission in *Drosophila*. *Proc R Soc Lond B* **198**:87–108.

Jia, X.X., M. Gorczyca, and V. Budnik. 1993. Ultrastructure of neuromuscular junctions in *Drosophila*: Comparison of wild type and mutants with increased excitability. *J Neurobiol* 24:1025–1044.

Johansen, J., M.E. Halpern, K.M. Johansen, and H. Keshishian. 1989. Stereotypic morphology of glutamatergic synapses on identified muscle cells of *Drosophila* larvae. *J Neurosci* **9**:710–725.

Kaakkola, S., and H. Teravainen. 1990. Animal models of parkinsonism. *Pharmacol Toxicol* **67**:95–100.

Kamb, A., L.E. Iverson, and M.A. Tanouye. 1987. Molecular characterization of *Shaker*, a *Drosophila* gene that encodes a potassium channel. *Cell* **50**:405–413.

Kaplan, W.D. 1977. *iav: inactive. Drosophila Inf Serv* **52**:1.

Kaplan, W.D., and W.E. Trout III. 1969. The behavior of four neurological mutants of *Drosophila*. *Genetics* **61**:339–409.

Kaplan, W.D., and W.E. Trout. 1974. Genetic manipulation of an abnormal jump response in *Drosophila*. *Genetics* **77**:721–739.

Kawasaki, F., R. Felling, and R.W. Ordway. 2000. A temperature-sensitive paralytic mutant defines a primary synaptic calcium channel in *Drosophila*. *J Neurosci* **20**:4885–4889.

Kennedy, M.B. 1994. The biochemistry of synaptic regulation in the central nervous system. *Ann Rev Biochem* **63**:571–600.

Kernan, M.J., M.I. Kuroda, R. Kreber, B.S. Baker, and B. Ganetzky. 1991. *nap^{ts}*, a mutation affecting sodium channel activity in *Drosophila*, is an allele of *mle*, a regulator of X chromosome transcription. *Cell* **66**:949–959.

Keshishian, H., A. Chiba, T.N. Chang, M.S. Halfon, E.W. Harkins, J. Jarecki, L. Wang, et al. 1993. Cellular mechanisms governing synaptic development in *Drosophila melanogaster*. *J Neurobiol* **24**:757–787.

Kidokoro, Y., and K. Nishikawa. 1994. Miniature endplate currents at the newly formed neuromuscular junction in *Drosophila* embryo and larvae. *Neurosci Res* **19**:143–154.

Kiehn, O., O. Kjaerulff, M.C. Tresch, and R.M. Harris-Warrick. 2000. Contributions of intrinsic motor neuron properties to the production of rhythmic motor output in the mammalian spinal cord. *Brain Res Bull* **53**:649–659.

Kim, Y., and C.-F. Wu. 1996. Reduced growth cone motility in cultured neurons from *Drosophila* memory mutants with a defective cAMP cascade. *J Neurosci* **16**:5593–5602.

Komatsu, A., S. Singh, P. Rathe, and C.-F. Wu. 1990. Mutational and gene dosage analysis of calcium-activated potassium channels in *Drosophila*: Correlation of micro- and macroscopic currents. *Neuron* **4**:313–321.

Kutsukake, M., A. Komatsu, D. Yamamoto, and S. Ishiwa-Chigusa. 2000. A tyramine receptor gene mutation causes a defective olfactory behavior in *Drosophila melanogaster*. *Gene* **245**:31–42.

Landgraf, M., T. Bossing, G.M. Technau, and M. Bate. 1997. The origin, location, and projections of the embryonic abdominal motoneurons of *Drosophila*. *J Neurosci* **17**:9642–9655.

Lau, P., R. Zucker, and D. Bentley. 1999. Induction of filopodia by direct local elevation of intracellular calcium ion concentration. *J Cell Bio* **145**:1265–1275.

Levin, L.R., P.L. Han, P.M. Hwang, P.G. Feinstein, R.L. Davis, and R.R. Reed. 1992. The *Drosophila* learning and memory gene *rutabaga* encodes a Ca^{2+}/Calmodulin-responsive adenylyl cyclase. *Cell* **68**: 479–489.

Lindsley, D.L., and G.G. Zimm. 1992. *The Genome of* Drosophila melanogaster. San Diego: Academic Press.

Livingstone, M.S., P.P. Sziber, and W.G. Quinn. 1984. Loss of Ca/CaM responsiveness in AC of *rutabaga*, a *Drosophila* learning mutant. *Cell* **37**:205–215.

Loughney, K., R. Kreber, and B. Ganetzky. 1989. Molecular analysis of the *para* locus, a sodium channel gene in *Drosophila*. *Cell* **58**:1143–1154.

MacKay-Lyons, M. 2002. Central pattern generation of locomotion: A review of the evidence. *Phys Ther* **82**:69–83.

Marder, E. 2000. Motor pattern generation. *Curr Opin Neurobiol* **10**: 691–698.

Marder, E., and R.L. Calabrese. 1996. Principles of rhythmic motor pattern generation. *Physiol Rev* **76**:687–717.

Martin, J.R., R. Ernst, and M. Heisenberg. 1998. Mushroom bodies suppress locomotor activity in *Drosophila melanogaster. Learn and Mem* **5**:179–191.

Martin, J.R., T. Raabe, and M. Heisenberg. 1999. Central complex substructures are required for the maintenance of locomotor activity in *Drosophila melanogaster. J Comp Physiol A* **185**:277–288.

McClung, C., and J. Hirsh. 1999. The trace amine tyramine is essential for sensitization to cocaine in *Drosophila. Curr Biol* **9**:853–860.

McCobb, D.P., P.G. Haydon, and S.B. Kater. 1988. Dopamine and serotonin inhibition of neurite elongation of different identified neurons. *J Neurosci Res* **19**:19–26.

Meyer, R.L. 1982. Tetrodotoxin blocks the formation of ocular dominance columns in goldfish. *Science* **18**:589–591.

Monastirioti, M., M. Gorczyca, J. Rapus, M. Eckert, K. White, and V. Budnik. 1995. Octopamine immunoreactivity in the fruit fly *Drosophila melanogaster. J Comp Neurol* **356**:275–287.

Monastirioti, M., C.E. Linn, and K. White. 1996. Characterization of *Drosophila tyramine-hydroxylase* gene and isolation of mutant flies lacking octopamine. *J Neurosci* **16**:3900–3911.

Monastirioti, M. 1999. Biogenic amine systems in the fruit fly *Drosophila melanogaster. Microscop Res Tech* **45**:106–121.

Nagaya, Y., M. Kutsukake, S.I. Chigusa, and A. Komatsu. 2002. A trace amine, tyramine, functions as a neuromodulator in *Drosophila melanogaster. Neurosci Lett* **329**:324–328.

Nishikawa, K., and Y. Kidokoro. 1999. Octopamine inhibits synaptic transmission at the larval neuromuscular junction in *Drosophila melanogaster. Brain Res* **837**:67–74.

O'Dell, K., J.F. Coulon, J.C. David, C. Papin, S. Fuzeau-Braesch, and J.M. Jallon. 1987. La mutation *inactive* produit une marquée d'octopamine dans le cerveau des *Drosophiles. CR Acad Sci Série III* **305**:199–202.

O'Dell, K., and B. Burnet. 1988. The effects on locomotor activity and reactivity of the hypoactive and inactive mutations of *Drosophila melanogaster. Heredity* **61**:199–207.

O'Dell, K.M. 1994. The *inactive* mutation leads to abnormal experience-dependent courtship modification in male *Drosophila melanogaster. Behav Genet* **24**:381–388.

O'Dowd, D.K., S.E. Germeraad, and R.W. Aldrich. 1989. Alterations in the expression and gating of *Drosophila* sodium channels by mutations in the *para* gene. *Neuron* **2**:1301–1311.

Osborne, K.A., A. Robichon, E. Burgess, S. Butland, R.A. Shaw, A. Coulthard, H.S. Pereira, et al. 1997. Natural behavior polymorphism due to a cGMP-dependent protein kinase of *Drosophila. Science* **277**:834–836.

Papazian, D.M., T.L. Schwarz, B.L. Tempel, Y.N. Jan, and L.Y. Jan. 1987. Cloning of genomic and complementary DNA from *Shaker. Science* **237**:749–753.

Peixoto, A.A., and J.C. Hall. 1998. Analysis of temperature sensitive mutants reveals new genes involved in the courtship song of *Drosophila. Genetics* **148**:827–838.

Renger, J.J., W.D. Yao, M.B. Sokolowski, and C.-F. Wu. 1999. Neuronal polymorphism among natural alleles of a cGMP-dependent kinase gene, *foraging*, in *Drosophila. J Neurosci* **19**:RC28 (1–8).

Saito, M., and C.-F. Wu. 1991. Expression of ion channels and mutational effects in giant *Drosophila* neurons differentiated from cell division-arrested embryonic neuroblasts. *J Neurosci* **11**:2135–2150.

Salkoff, L., and R. Wyman. 1981. Genetic modification of potassium channels in *Drosophila Shaker* mutants. *Nature* **293**:228–230.

Saganich, M.J., E. Machado, and B. Rudy. 2001. Differential expression of genes encoding subthreshold-operating voltage-gated K^+ channels in brain. *J Neurosci* **21**:4609–4624.

Sanguinetti, M.C. 1999. Dysfunction of delayed rectifier potassium channels in an inherited cardiac arrhythmia. *Ann NY Acad Sci* **868**:406–413.

Saraswati, S., L.E. Fox, D.R. Soll, and C.-F. Wu. 2004. Tyramine and octopamine have opposite effects on the locomotion of *Drosophila* larvae. *J Neurobiol* **58**:425–441.

Sawin-McCormack, E.P., M.B. Sokolowski, and A.R. Campos. 1995. Characterization and genetic analysis of *Drosophila melanogaster* photobehavior during larval development. *J Neurogenet* **10**:119–135.

Schuster, C.M., G.W. Davis, R.D. Fetter, and C.S. Goodman. 1996. Genetic dissection of structural and functional components of synaptic plasticity. I. Fasciclin II controls synaptic stabilization and growth. *Neuron* **17**:641–654.

Schwarz, T.L., D.L. Tempel, D.M. Papazian, Y.N. Jan, and L.Y. Jan. 1988. Multiple potassium-channel components are produced by alternative splicing at the *Shaker* locus of *Drosophila. Nature* **331**:137–142.

Shatz, C.F. 1990. Impulse activity and the patterning of connections during CNS development. *Neuron* **5**:745–756.

Siddiqi, O., and S. Benzer. 1976. Neurophysiological defects in temperature-sensitive paralytic mutants of *Drosophila melanogaster. Proc Natl Acad Sci USA* **73**:3253–3257.

Singh, A., and S. Singh. 1999. Unmasking of a novel potassium current in *Drosophila* by a mutation and drugs. *J Neurosci* **19**:6838–6843.

Singh, S., and C.-F. Wu. 1989. Complete separation of four potassium currents in *Drosophila. Neuron* **2**:1325–1329.

Singh, S., and C.-F. Wu. 1990. Properties of potassium currents and their role in membrane excitability in *Drosophila* larval muscle fibers. *J Exp Biol* **152**:59–76.

Singh, S., and C.-F. Wu. 1999. Ionic currents in larval muscles of *Drosophila. Intern Rev Neurobiol* **43**:191–220.

Smith, L.A., X. Wang, A.A. Peixoto, E.K. Neumann, L.M. Hall, and J.C. Hall. 1996. A *Drosophila* calcium channel α1 subunit gene maps to a genetic locus associated with behavioral and visual defects. *J Neurosci* **16**:7868–7879.

Sokolowski, M.B. 1980. Foraging strategies of *Drosophila melanogaster*: A chromosomal analysis. *Behav. Genet.* **10**:291–302.

Solc, C.K., Zagotta, W.N., and Aldrich, R.W. 1987. Single-channel and genetic analyses reveal two distinct A-type potassium channels in *Drosophila. Science* **236**:1094–1098.

Song, H.-J., and M.-M. Poo. 1999. Signal transduction underlying growth cone guidance by diffusible factors. *Curr Opin Neurobiol* **9**:355–363.

Stern, M., and B. Ganetzky. 1989. Altered synaptic transmission in *Drosophila Hyperkinetic* mutants. *J Neurogenet* **5**:215–228.

Stern, M., R. Kreber, and B. Ganetzky. 1990. Dosage effects of a *Drosophila* sodium channel gene on behavior and axon excitability. *Genetics* **124**:133–143.

Strauss, R., and M. Heisenberg. 1990. Coordination of legs during straight walking and turning in *Drosophila melanogaster. J Comp Physiol A* **167**:403–412.

Suster, M.L., and M. Bate. 2002. Embryonic assembly of a central pattern generator without sensory input. *Nature* **416**:174–178.

Suster, M.L., J.R. Martin, C. Sung, and S. Robinow. 2003. Targeted expression of tetanus toxin reveals sets of neurons involved in larval locomotion in *Drosophila. J Neurobiol* **55**:233–246.

Suzuki, D.T. 1970. Temperature-sensitive mutations in *Drosophila melanogaster. Science* **170**:695–706.

Suzuki, D.T., T. Grigliatti, and R. Williamson. 1971. Temperature-sensitive mutations in *Drosophila melanogaster.* VII. A mutation (*para^{ts}*) causing reversible adult paralysis. *Proc Natl Acad Sci USA* **68**:890–893.

Suzuki, N., and C.-F. Wu. 1984. Altered sensitivity to sodium channel-specific neurotoxins in cultured neurons from temperature-sensitive paralytic mutants of *Drosophila. J Neurogenet* **1**:255–238.

Svenningsson, P., E.T. Tzavara, R. Carruthers, I. Rachleff, W. Sigrid, M. Nehls, D.L. McKinzie, et al. 2003. Diverse psychomimetics act through a common signaling pathway. *Science* **302**:1412–1415.

Tanouye, M.A., and A. Ferrus. 1985. Action potentials in normal and *Shaker* mutant of *Drosophila. J Neurogenet* **2**:253–271.

Tanouye, M.A., A. Ferrus, and S.C. Fujita. 1981. Abnormal action potentials associated with the *Shaker* complex locus of *Drosophila*. *Proc Natl Acad Sci USA* **78**:6548–6552.

Tempel, B.L., M.S. Livingstone, and W.G. Quinn. 1984. Mutations in the dopa decarboxylase gene affect learning in *Drosophila*. *Proc Natl Acad Sci USA* **81**:3577–3581.

Titus, S.A., J.W. Warmke, and B. Ganetzky. 1997. The *Drosophila erg* K^+ channel polypeptide is encoded by the seizure locus. *J Neurosci* **17**: 875–881.

Tsunoda, S., and L. Salkoff. 1995a. Genetic analysis of *Drosophila* neurons: *Shal*, *Shaw*, and *Shab* encode most embryonic potassium currents. *J Neurosci* **15**:1741–1754.

Tsunoda, S., and L. Salkoff. 1995b. The major delayed rectifier in both *Drosophila* neurons and muscle is encoded by *Shab*. *J Neurosci* **15**: 5209–5221.

Tully, T., and W.G. Quinn. 1985. Classical conditioning and retention in normal and mutant *Drosophila melanogaster*. *J Comp Physiol A* **157**: 263–277.

Ueda, A., and Y. Kidokoro. 2002. Aggressive behaviors of female *Drosophila melanogaster* are influenced by their social experience and food resources. *Physiol Entomol* **27**:21–28.

von Schilcher, F. 1976. The behavior of *cacophony*, a courtship song mutant in *Drosophila melanogaster*. *Behav Biol* **17**:187–196.

von Schilcher, F. 1977. A mutation which changes courtship song in *Drosophila melanogaster*. *Behav Genet* **7**:251–259.

Wang, J., J. Renger, L. Griffith, R. Greenspan, and C.-F. Wu. 1994. Concomitant alterations of physiological and developmental plasticity in *Drosophila* CaMKII-inhibited synapses. *Neuron* **13**: 1373–1384.

Wang, J.W., and C.-F. Wu. 1996. *In vivo* functional role of the *Drosophila Hyperkinetic* β subunit in gating and inactivation of *Shaker* K^+ channels. *Biophys J* **71**:3167–3176.

Wang, J.W., A.W. Sylwester, D. Reed, D.A. Wu, D.R. Soll, and C.-F. Wu. 1997a. Morphometric description of the wandering behavior in *Drosophila* larvae: aberrant locomotion in Na^+ and K^+ channel mutants revealed by computer-assisted motion analysis. *J Neurogenet* **11**: 231–254.

Wang, X.J., E.R. Reynolds, P. Deak, and L.M. Hall. 1997b. The *seizure* locus encodes the *Drosophila* homolog of the HERG potassium channel. *J Neurosci* **17**:882–890.

Wang, J.W., J.M. Humphreys, J.P. Phillips, A.J. Hilliker, and C.F. Wu. 2000. A novel leg-shaking *Drosophila* mutant defective in a voltage-gated K^+ current and hypersensitive to reactive oxygen species. *J Neurosci* **20**: 5958–5964.

Wang, J.W., D.R. Soll, and C.-F. Wu. 2002. Morphometric description of the wandering behavior in *Drosophila* larvae: A phenotypic analysis of K^+ channel mutants. *J Neurogenet* **16**:45–63.

Warbington, L., T. Hillman, C. Adams, and M. Stern. 1996. Reduced transmitter release conferred by mutations in the slowpoke-encoded Ca^{2+}-activated K^+ channel gene of *Drosophila*. *Invert Neurosci* **2**:51–60.

Warmke, J., R. Drysdale, and B. Ganetzky. 1991. A distinct potassium channel peptide encoded by the *Drosophila eag* locus. *Science* **252**: 1560–1562.

Warmke, J.W., and B. Ganetzky. 1994. A family of potassium channel genes related to *eag* in *Drosophila* and mammals. *Proc Natl Acad Sci USA* **91**:3438–3442.

Wei, A., M. Covarrubias, A. Butler, K. Baker, M. Pak, and L. Salkoff. 1990. K^+ current diversity is produced by an extended gene family conserved in *Drosophila* and mouse. *Science* **248**:599–603.

Wolf, R., and M. Heisenberg. 1990. Visual control of straight flight in *Drosophila melanogaster*. *J Comp Physiol A* **167**:269–283.

Wright, T.R.F., R. Steward, K.W. Bentley, and P.N. Adler. 1981. The genetics of dopa decarboxylase in *Drosophila melanogaster*. III. Effects of a temperature sensitive dopa decarboxylase deficient mutation on female fertility. *Dev Genet* **2**:223–235.

Wu, C.-F., B. Ganetzky, L.Y. Jan, Y.-N. Jan, and S. Benzer. 1978. A *Drosophila* mutant with a temperature-sensitive block in nerve conduction. *Proc Natl Acad Sci USA* **8**:4047–4051.

Wu, C.-F., and B. Ganetzky. 1980. Genetic alteration of nerve membrane excitability in temperature-sensitive paralytic mutants of *Drosophila melanogaster*. *Nature* **286**:814–816.

Wu, C.-F., N. Suzuki, and M.-M. Poo. 1983a. Dissociated neurons from normal and mutant *Drosophila* larval central nervous systems in cell culture. *J Neurosci* **3**:1888–1899.

Wu, C.-F., B. Ganetzky, F. Haugland, and A.-X. Liu. 1983b. Potassium currents in *Drosophila*: Different components affected by mutations of two genes. *Science* **220**:1076–1078.

Wu, C.-F., and F.N. Haugland. 1985. Voltage clamp analysis of membrane currents in larval muscle fibers of *Drosophila*: Alteration of potassium currents in *Shaker* mutants. *J Neurosci* **5**:2626–2640.

Wu, C.-F., K. Sakai, M, Saito, and Y. Hotta. 1989. Giant *Drosophila* neurons differentiated from cytokinesis-arrested embryonic neuroblasts. *J Neurobiol* **21**:499–507.

Yao, W., and C.-F. Wu. 1999a. Auxiliary *Hyperkinetic* β subunit of K^+ channels: Regulation of firing properties and K^+ currents in *Drosophila* neurons. *J Neurophysiol* **81**:2472–2484.

Yao, W., and C.-F. Wu. 1999b. Regulation of firing patterns through modulation of non-Sh K^+ currents by calcium/calmodulin-dependent kinase II in *Drosophila* embryonic neurons. *Ann NY Acad Sci* **868**:450–453.

Yin, J.C., and T. Tully. 1996. CREB and the formation of long-term memory. *Curr Opin Neurobiol* **6**:264–268.

Yoshihara, M., M.B. Rueben, and Y. Kidokoro. 1997. Transition from growth cone to functional motor nerve terminal in *Drosophila* embryos. *J Neurosci* **17**:8408–8426.

Zhao, M., and C.-F. Wu. 1997. Alterations in frequency coding and activity dependence of excitability in cultured neurons of *Drosophila* memory mutants. *J Neurosci* **17**:2187–2199.

Zheng, J.Q. 2000. Turning of nerve growth cones induced by localized increases in intracellular calcium ions. *Nature* **403**:89–93.

Zhong, Y., and C.-F. Wu. 1991a. Alteration of four identified K^+ currents in *Drosophila* muscle by mutations in *eag*. *Science* **252**:1562–1564.

Zhong, Y., and C.-F. Wu. 1991b. Altered synaptic plasticity in *Drosophila* memory mutants with a defective cyclic AMP cascade. *Science* **251**: 198–201.

Zhong, Y., V. Budnik, and C.-F. Wu. 1992. Synaptic plasticity in *Drosophila* memory and hyperexcitable mutants: Role of cAMP cascade. *J Neurosci* **12**:644–651.

Zhong, Y., and C.-F. Wu. 1993. Modulation of different K^+ currents in *Drosophila*: A hypothetical role for the Eag subunit in multimeric K^+ channels. *J Neurosci* **13**:4669–4679.

Zhong, Y., and C.-F. Wu. 2004. Neuronal activity and adenylyl cyclase in environment-dependent plasticity of axonal outgrowth in *Drosophila*. *J Neurosci* **24**:1439–1445.

CHAPTER

11

Progressive Supranuclear Palsy and Corticobasal Degeneration

IRENE LITVAN

Over the past few years, investigators have made major progress in understanding the tauopathies: progressive supranuclear palsy (PSP) and corticobasal degeneration (CBD). These disorders share biological and clinical commonalities that question their existence as separate nosological entities. In 1964 Steele and colleagues [1] first described PSP as a distinct clinicopathological entity, and Rebeiz, Kolodny, and Richardson first described CBD in 1967 as "corticodentatonigral degeneration with neuronal achromasia" [2]. Considered largely to be motor disorders until recently, PSP and CBD also exhibit cognitive and psychiatric disturbances [3–4] and both are four-repeat tauopathies [5].

Although patients with frontotemporal dementia and Parkinsonism associated with chromosome 17 abnormalities (FTDP-17) may present with PSP, CBD, or both phenotypes, to date investigators have found no mutations in sporadic PSP or CBD. Patients with sporadic PSP and CBD exhibit several polymorphisms in tau, constituting an extended tau haplotype (H1), which is much more frequently present in these patients than in the general population [6]. Whether PSP and CBD are different phenotypes of the same disorder, or different nosologic disorders, is debatable. It is likely that other risk factors, such as oxidative injury, inflammation, or nerve growth factor deficiency, in addition to the H1 tau haplotype, are required for patients to manifest PSP or CBD (Figure 1). The relation between PSP/CBD and the atypical Parkinsonism in the West Indies [7–8], which seems associated with neurotoxins found in tropical fruits, also needs further investigation.

No biological markers exist for the diagnosis of these disorders. Pathology constitutes the gold standard diagnosis [9] and the proposed neuropathologic criteria for both disorders are accurate and reliable [5,10]. While the clinical criteria to diagnose PSP have been operationalized and highly specific [11–12], clinical criteria to diagnose CBD has not undergone such a process [13–14] and its diagnosis remains challenging [9]. Because misdiagnosis in CBD is frequent, patients with a lateralized CBD phenotype are labeled with CB syndrome, whereas the term "CBD" is reserved for those with a neuropathologically confirmed diagnosis [9]. On the other hand, because both possible and probable criteria from the National Institute of Neurologic Disorders and Stroke (NINDS)-SPSP had high specificity and positive predictive value and were highly reliable [12], the probable NINDS-SPSP criteria was renamed as *clinically definite* and the possible NINDS-SPSP criteria as *clinically probable* [4]. In this chapter, epidemiologic, clinical, nosologic, pathologic, laboratory, and management aspects of these disorders will be discussed.

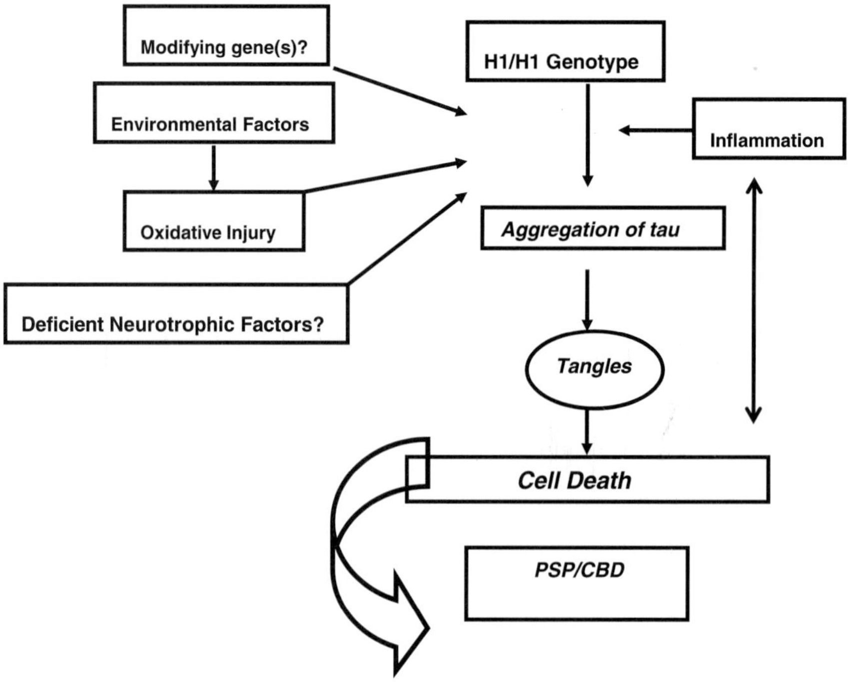

FIGURE 1 Pathways to neurodegeneration and phenotypic presentations as PSP and CBD.

I. EPIDEMIOLOGIC ASPECTS

PSP and CBD are better recognized but still underdiagnosed. PSP is currently considered the most common atypical neurodegenerative parkinsonian disorder [15–17]. The estimated prevalence of PSP is 6.0–6.4/100,000 in two population-based prevalence studies conducted in the United Kingdom and a general population-based survey in Olmsted County, Minnesota, using currently accepted diagnostic criteria for PSP [15–17].

The incidence of PSP increases with age. The crude incidence rate for PSP in Olmsted County, Minnesota, is 1.1 per 100,000 per year, which increased from 1.7 cases per 100,000 per year at ages fifty to fifty-nine years to 14.7 per 100,000 per year at ages eighty to ninety-nine years [15,18]. Investigators believe that increased recognition of PSP by neurologists and non-neurologists, and better study designs and case-definitions have led to higher incidence and prevalence estimates.

No data exists on the incidence or prevalence of CBD, but like PSP, CBD is clearly underdiagnosed [19]. One large movement disorder clinic reported that subjects with a CB syndrome constitute 0.9% of the patients with Parkinsonism [20]. Based on those findings, Togasaki and Tanner [21] estimated that the number of people who develop the CB syndrome in the population would be 4–6% of those with Parkinsonism. Based on the incidence of PD, they estimated that the incidence rate of patients with a CB syndrome would be 0.62–0.92/100.000 each year and based on the incidence and survival of CBD of 7.9 yrs, they estimated that the prevalence rate would be 4.9–7.3/100.000. However, this estimate overestimates the patients with a CB syndrome since subjects were evaluated in a tertiary center that specialized in differentiating these disorders. On the other hand, this estimate does not include the patients with CBD presenting with a dementia phenotype.

In PSP, clinicians estimate median survival time from symptom onset to be five to six years. Early falls, speech and swallowing problems, diplopia, and early need for a percutaneous gastrostomy (PEG) predict reduced survival [22]. To evaluate disease progression in PSP, Goetz and colleagues [23] recently analyzed fifty PSP patients: twenty-one were followed until death (mean duration of surveillance 53.6 months) and twenty-nine were followed in an ongoing fashion (mean duration of surveillance 46.2 months). They found that the first target sign in 48% of the sample was inability to walk (median disease duration 58 months); in 55% it was unintelligible speech (median disease duration 71 months); and as a composite end point, speech and gait accounted for 98% of the sample's first target point. The need for a nasogastric tube was only rarely the first target sign (8%). Despite individual patient patterns, the distinct temporal separation between gait, speech, and swallowing endpoints suggests that interventions that alter the progression of all or only one area of dysfunction can be reliably tested in PSP. Hence, survival analyses for neuroprotective studies in PSP can now use a composite outcome defined as the time to the first of either unintelligible speech or gait dysfunction.

II. CLINICAL ASPECTS

A. Progressive Supranuclear Palsy

Typically, PSP presents in the seventh decade with early postural instability, vertical supranuclear gaze palsy, pseudobulbar palsy, frontal subcortical dementia, and Parkinsonism characterized by bradykinesia and axial rigidity, not benefiting from levodopa therapy. Initial presentation is most frequently one of postural instability (manifested as unexplained or unexpected falls), followed by speech, gait, swallowing, and oculomotor disturbances [11,22,24–30]. Falls usually occur backwards, but they can occur in any direction [24,27]. When postural instability and falls are the only features of the disease, an abnormal response to the postural reflex may be the only abnormality in the patient's examination. PSP patients usually exhibit axial more than limb muscle involvement [27,31] (see video segment 1). Sitting "en bloc" is also a characteristic feature, as is an absent, poor, or waning response to levodopa. A few PSP patients do show a moderate transient response from dopaminergic agents, but most do not; indeed, this may be because many PSP patients have little or no limb Parkinsonism. PSP patients rarely develop levodopa-induced involuntary movements, and if they do, they usually develop dystonia. Clinicians infrequently observe the disproportionate retrocollis that was once thought of as characteristic of, but may observe other types of dystonia, such as blepharospasm (and more rarely limb dystonia) [32]. In those cases dopaminergic medication should be cautiously reduced or discontinued, to rule out the possibility of treatment-induced symptoms.

While mobility problems are the most common early feature in PSP, visual symptoms are often functionally disabling [22]. Marked slowing of vertical saccades, or rapid eye movement between two stimuli (see video segment 2), usually precedes the development of vertical supranuclear gaze palsy, which takes about three years to manifest (see video segment 3). Supranuclear vertical gaze palsy after the age of forty and severe postural instability and falls within the first year of symptom onset are the main features that allow clinicians to make a definite clinical diagnosis of PSP. Blink rate usually becomes profoundly sparse in PSP. The combination of rare blinking, facial dystonia, and gaze abnormalities leads to the development of particular "staring and non-blinking faces."

Patients with PSP may also present with either prominent or early-onset severe speech or swallowing difficulties. PSP patients classically have a hypokinetic-spastic dysarthria. Clinicians may also observe speech preservation and anomia, but not true aphasia. Severe sialorrhea may be observed in PSP, even at early stages of the disease. In addition, PSP patients may have difficulty judging the amount of food they can swallow and tend to take oversized mouthfuls or overstuff their mouths when eating.

Florid frontal lobe symptomatology (impaired abstract thought, decreased verbal fluency) including motor perseveration and frontal behavioral disturbances (primarily apathy, but also disinhibition and anxiety) usually manifest at early stages in PSP [33–39]. Executive dysfunction (difficulty with planning, problem-solving, concept-formation, and social cognition) may be the presenting symptom in some PSP patients and is a frequent feature throughout the disease.

In general, symptoms progress steadily for an average of five to six years. Clinicians have infrequently reported neuropathologically confirmed PSP cases without ophthalmoplegia, dementia, or those that present only with dementia or akinesia. PSP patients only rarely present with asymmetric Parkinsonism, akinesia, dementia, unilateral dystonia, or ideomotor apraxia.

Several features should make one suspect that a patient may suffer from PSP. The following list outlines those common features:

(1) *Early instability and falls, particularly during the first year of symptom onset.* However, early instability and falls may also develop in patients with CBD when asymmetric symptoms develop in the lower extremities, although it is rare [40]. Instability and falls may also develop early in Multiple System Atrophy (MSA), although these symptoms are usually present when patients already exhibit autonomic disturbances.

(2) *Marked slowing of vertical saccades.* The saccades in CBD may have an increased latency, but normal speed, and are similarly affected in the vertical and horizontal plane, whereas in MSA, the saccades have normal speed and latency. Although *supranuclear gaze palsy* is key in diagnosing PSP, it may occasionally be present in patients with dementia with Lewy bodies, arteriosclerotic pseudo-Parkinsonism, MSA, Creutzfeldt-Jakob disease, Whipple disease, or CBD [41].

(3) *Early prominent or severe speech and swallowing difficulties.* The patient may exhibit overstuffing the mouth (squirrel sign) when eating, but the pseudobulbar palsy features may also be present in CBD.

(4) *Florid frontal lobe symptomatology.* This symptom usually manifests at early stages in PSP, whereas it is typically less evident or manifests later in the other parkinsonian disorders. On the other hand, pyramidal signs (usually bilateral) present later in PSP, whereas

asymmetric pyramidal signs may present earlier and more frequently in CBD.

B. Corticobasal Degeneration and Corticobasal Syndrome

CBD usually has a combination of features including neurobehavioral, cognitive, and movement dysfunction. It usually presents in the sixth or seventh decade with either a CB syndrome (characterized by slowly progressive unilaterally jerky, tremulous, akinetic, rigid, and apraxic extremity held in a fixed dystonic posture and displaying cortical lateralized features such as an alien limb syndrome, a progressive aphasia, or visuospatial disturbances), or with dementia syndrome characterized by a frontal dementia phenotype followed by bilateral Parkinsonism. The main CBD phenotypes reflect its diverse anatomic involvement [9,40, 42–44]. The most known presentation of CBD is its CB syndrome, occurring in at least 40% of autopsy-confirmed patients [43,45,46]. Depending on the hemisphere affected, the CB syndrome includes, in addition to a unilateral akinetic-rigid syndrome unresponsive to L-dopa and associated with dystonic postures and myoclonus, an ideomotor apraxia, language disturbances, alien limb syndrome, or sensory or visual neglect syndrome [44, 47–48]. Speech, but not swallowing, disturbances may also occur early. Early falls are unusual unless the symptoms manifest in the lower limbs.

On the other hand, CBD patients presenting with the dementia phenotype typically exhibit severe cognitive deficits, particularly, frontal lobe disturbances characterized by severe executive dysfunction and attention deficit (with or without expressive aphasia), and later, development of bilateral motor (e.g., non-L-dopa responsive Parkinsonism, pyramidal signs) and urinary disturbances (incontinence) [49,51–52]. Differentiating patients with the CB syndrome (lateralized) from those with a dementia phenotype is important due to prognostic implications, since initial cognitive decline often leads to early placement in nursing home facilities and is associated with shorter survival [40].

While some studies show that patients with the CB syndrome usually exhibit CBD pathologically [13], other studies point to a significant number of cases in which this phenotype corresponds to other disorders, including PSP, Alzheimer disease (AD), basal ganglia infarctions, and dementia with Lewy bodies (DLB) [9,53–55]. The dementia phenotype is difficult to differentiate from Pick disease, FTDP-17, or dementia lacking distinctive histological features. Interestingly, FTDP-17 with a P301S mutation in exon 10 of the tau gene may present with either a frontotemporal dementia or a CB syndrome [56], suggesting that the same primary gene defect in tau can lead to two distinct clinical phenotypes.

III. NOSOLOGIC CONTROVERSIES

The cause or causes of CBD and PSP, as well as most neurodegenerative diseases, are unknown. CBD and PSP share clinical, anatomic, genetic, and pathologic features. Both may present with frontal cognitive disturbances, Parkinsonism not responding to levodopa therapy, and oculomotor, speech, and swallowing disturbances [55–56]. Both share the same abnormal aggregation of tau forming mainly four-repeat aggregates [59–60]. In PSP and CBD, no amyloid deposition occurs, and tau aggregates in neurons and glia mainly as four-repeat isoforms, altering the three-repeat:four-repeat ratio [61–64]. In addition, PSP and CBD are associated with the inheritance of an extended haplotype in the tau gene (H1) [6,65]. Investigators have observed that coding and splice-site mutations in the tau gene cause FTDP-17, which demonstrates that tau dysfunction is sufficient to induce neurodegeneration [61,66–68]. The parallels between FTDP-17 and PSP/CBD also include FTDP-17 patients with defined tau mutations (e.g., P-301, N279K) who share many clinical and pathological features with PSP and CBD [56,69–70] such as selective deposition of four-repeat tau. To date, none of the rarely reported familial cases of PSP [71,72] are due to FTDP-17 mutations or non-tau mutated genes.

The similarities between PSP and CBD have led investigators to question whether the two disorders are distinct nosologic entities or different phenotypes of the same disorder [9]. Recently validated neuropathologic diagnostic criteria [5] emphasize the presence of tau-immunoreactive lesions in neurons, glia, and cell processes in these disorders and also provide good differentiation between PSP and CBD. Moreover, protein sequencing and immunochemical analysis demonstrated differences between these disorders [72]. While in PSP brains (n = 8) a 33 kDa band predominated in the low molecular weight tau fragments, two closely related bands of approximately 37 kDa predominated in CBD brains (n = 6). Protein sequencing and immunochemical analyses showed that the 33 kDa band and the 37 kDa doublet consisted of the carboxyl half of tau with different amino termini. This study suggests that different proteolytic processing of abnormal tau may occur in PSP and CBD. Despite these findings, the controversy continues [9,50].

IV. NEUROPATHOLOGIC FINDINGS

Investigators have published and validated consensus criteria for the pathologic diagnosis of PSP and CBD [5,10, 64]. Macroscopically, midbrain and pontine tegmentum atrophy and pallor of the substantia nigra are the most relevant findings in PSP, whereas CBD is characterized by asymmetric parietofrontal or frontotemporal cortical atrophy.

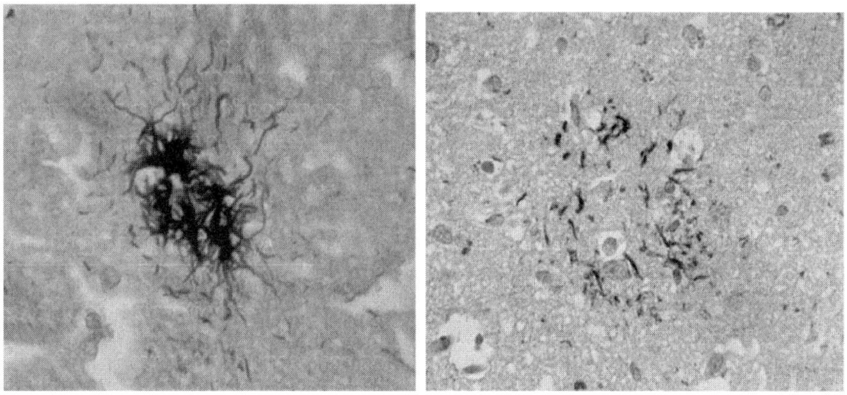

FIGURE 2 Morphological markers in CBD (astrocytic plaque) and PSP (tufted astrocyte). (Courtesy of Dr. Ian McKenzie.)

Microscopically, accumulation of phosphorylated tau protein in both neurons and glia is observed in both disorders. Immunocytochemistry with tau, as well as phosphorylated neurofilament or αB-crystallin tau positive threads, coiled bodies, and tangles are shared lesions of CBD and PSP. The characteristic lesions in PSP are neurofibrillary tangles, neuropil threads (fibrillar structures intensely reactive with tau antibody), and "tufted astrocytes" (tau fills the entire length of the cellular processes and equally distributes in all directions) (Figure 2). These lesions usually involve the substantia nigra, locus ceruleus, globus pallidus, subthalamic nucleus, midbrain tegmentum, cerebellar dentate nucleus, and pontine nuclei, but the precentral and premotor areas may also be affected. In CBD, neuronal loss, gliosis, tau-positive "astrocytic plaques" (accumulation of tau in the distal processes of the astrocyte, Figure 2), thread-like lesions, and oligodendroglial coiled bodies in gray and white matter, most often in the superior frontal gyrus, superior parietal gyrus, pre- and postcentral gyri, and striatum are characteristic. Superficial spongiosis may be prominent in the maximally affected cortical gyri, and achromatic, ballooned neurons immunoreactive to phosphorylated neurofilament or αB-crystallin are usually present in CBD, but their absence does not preclude this diagnosis.

Dysfunction in the microtubule-associated tau is present in both PSP and CBD. This feature is supported by the presence of tau positive inclusions, hyperphosphorylation of tau that disrupts binding to microtubules, and by transgenic mice with the P301L mutation exhibiting clinical and neuropathologic findings similar to those found in these disorders (see Chapter 3).

Investigators must further investigate whether, in addition to the H1 haplotype, inflammation, oxidative injury, or additional genetic factors lead to aggregation of tau that affects different neuronal populations (Figure 1) and manifests with different phenotypic presentations. Further characterization of the cascade of events in tau dysfunction and neurodegeneration will be critical to developing therapy.

V. LABORATORY INVESTIGATIONS

At present, it is unclear whether or not ancillary studies would improve the diagnostic accuracy of these disorders and, if so, which studies would have higher positive predictive value, be less invasive, and more economic. Thus far, studies evaluating the overall concentration of tau (phosphorylated and not phosphorylated) in cerebrospinal fluid (CSF) have not been useful in appropriately differentiating these disorders.

Electrooculographic recording may help distinguish PSP patients from CBD at an early stage [74–75], since PSP patients have decreased horizontal saccade amplitude and velocity but normal latency, while for CBD patients opposite results are observed. Investigators report that the antisaccade task (looking in the direction opposite to a visual stimulus), which correlates well with frontal lobe dysfunction, is markedly impaired in patients with PSP, although it may be impaired in patients with AD as well. Slight or no saccade impairment occurs in Parkinson disease patients (PD) and MSA patients with Parkinsonism (i.e., those with no cerebellar signs).

Brainstem auditory evoked potentials are normal in PSP. However, other neurophysiological measures of brainstem function are abnormal, reflecting the widespread pathological alteration in the pons and mesencephalon in these patients. While the blink reflex to an electrical stimulus is normal, the orbicularis oculi response is absent in patients with PSP exhibiting a mentalis response to electrical stimulation of the median nerve. This finding differentiates PSP patients from those with CBD, PD, and MSA, all of whom present simultaneous responses of the orbicularis oculi and

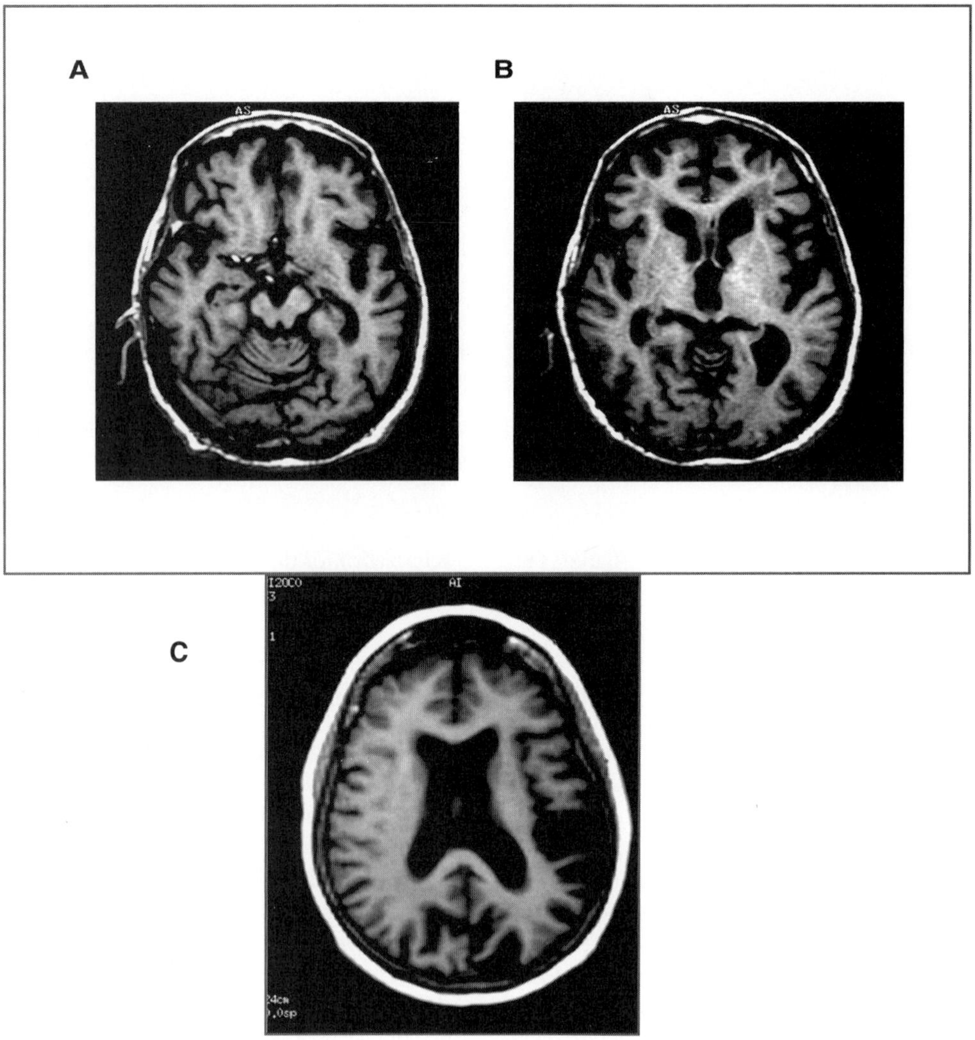

FIGURE 3 MRI abnormalities in PSP. (A) Midbrain atrophy; (B) dilation of third ventricle. Midbrain atrophy measured by an anteroposterior (AP) diameter equal or less than 13.4 mm [76] *or* an AP diameter equal or less than 17 mm in addition to dilation of third ventricle [96] have been proposed as radiologic features that help distinguish PSP from related Parkinsonian disorders, particularly Parkinson disease and MSA. (C) MRI of a patient with autopsy-confirmed CBD. Note the asymmetric cortical atrophy in CBD.

mentalis muscles after electrical stimulation of the median nerve [76].

A few studies suggest that evoked potentials [77] may help differentiate patients with PSP from those with CBD, but the small sample size of these studies precludes significant conclusions.

Magnetic resonance imaging (MRI) and positron emission tomography (PET) studies may contribute to the diagnosis of these disorders. Thinning of the quadrigeminal plate, particularly in its superior part, better seen in sagittal MRI sections, and dilation of the third ventricle support a diagnosis of PSP (Figures 3A, 3B) [78–79]. Minimal signal abnormalities in the periaqueductal region can also be seen in proton density MRI. CT or MRI of the brain showing asymmetric atrophy in the posterior frontal or parietal areas can also support the diagnosis of CBD [80] (Figure 3C). MSA should be suspected when there is atrophy of the pons, middle cerebellar peduncles and cerebellum, or altered signal intensity in the putamen. MRI may also rule out multi-infarct states, hydrocephalus, or tumors. However, investigators are still questioning whether or not the use of routine MRI could help differentiate PSP from CBD [81].

Another technique that may help distinguish PSP patients from those with CBD is three-dimensional MRI-based volumetry [82]. Using this technique, Groschel and colleagues found significant reduction in average brain, brainstem, midbrain, and frontal gray matter volumes in patients with probable, possible, or definite PSP (n = 33), whereas patients with CBD (n = 18) showed atrophy of parietal cortex and corpus callosum. With the exception of reduced midbrain volumes in PSP, the measured volumes of anatomical structures had an extensive overlap with the normal range. Using postmortem confirmed cases, the volumes of midbrain, parietal white matter, temporal gray matter, brainstem, frontal white matter, and pons were identified to best differentiate between PSP (n = 8), CBD (n = 7), and normal controls (n = 22). Investigators correctly predicted diagnosis for 76% of the PSP patients, 83% of CBD patients, and 95% of normal controls. Although asymmetries were not relevant in this study, they were in another study [83] that showed asymmetric parietal atrophy present in 93% of fifteen patients, frontal atrophy in 60%, and dilation of the lateral ventricles in 60%. In addition, at least two of these abnormalities were present in 80% of MRIs in patients with CBD. However, about half of CBD patients do not present with asymmetrical features (dementia phenotype).

Magnetic resonance spectroscopy imaging has detected different patterns of cortical and subcortical involvement in PSP, CBD, and PD patients as compared with controls [84]. PSP patients had reduced NA/Cre in the brainstem, centrum semiovale, frontal and precentral cortex, and reduced NA/Cho in the lentiform nucleus. On the other hand, when compared with control subjects, CBD patients had reduced NA/Cre in the centrum semiovale, and reduced NA/Cho in the lentiform nucleus and parietal cortex. Although magnetic resonance spectroscopy can find significant group differences, it seems that this technique does not help differentiate between individual patient groups.

Although PET studies have been used in research protocols to differentiate atypical Parkinsonian disorders from each other, and from PD, these investigations are not widely available in clinical practice and, except for asymmetries, hardly differentiate PSP from CBD [85]. Results of a recent study suggest that functional MRI can show parietal and motor cortex dysfunction in CBD before structural and even single-photon emission computed tomography changes become evident [85]. Furthermore, investigators have not yet established whether or not PET studies contribute to a definite diagnosis in patients with questionable disorders. ^{18}F-Fluorodeoxyglucose PET scans and ^{123}IMP-single photon emission computed tomography (SPECT) blood flow studies both show marked reduction in frontal and striatal metabolism in PSP. Frontal hypometabolism in PSP is secondary to deafferentation and cortical pathology. However, this finding is not specific to PSP. PET measures of striatal dopamine D_2 receptor density using ^{76}Br-bromospiperone, or ^{11}C-raclopride are also significantly reduced in most PSP patients, but again, these findings are not specific to PSP. Hypometabolism of glucose in the frontal cortex and decreased ^{18}F-fluorodopa uptake in the presynaptic nigrostriatal dopaminergic system (with similar reduction in both putamen and caudate) are also shown by PET in PSP patients. On the other hand, asymmetric PET findings are the main results in CBD [86–88].

VI. MANAGEMENT

No curative therapies exist for PSP and CBD [90–91]. Due to the widespread involvement of dopaminergic and nondopaminergic neurotransmitter systems, current neurotransmitter replacement therapies in PSP and CBD are not very helpful [92–93]; however, each symptom patients exhibit can be managed (Table 1). Future studies should systematically evaluate whether or not symptomatic palliative therapies (e.g., speech therapy, physical therapy) improve the quality of life or survival of PSP patients (e.g., by preventing aspiration).

Accurate diagnosis of these disorders is relevant for prognosis and management because complications vary. Development of biologic therapies for PSP and CBD require additional pathogenetic studies. Accurate diagnosis is also necessary to understand the etiopathogenesis of these disorders, which in turn, may allow for the development of biologic therapeutic strategies to stop or slow disease progression. Recently developed four-repeat tau-transgenic animal models resembling PSP [92–95] will likely accelerate efforts to discover more effective therapies. Given the recent progress made in understanding tau's significance in the development of neurodegeneration, the most promising approaches may be those that aim to prevent the abnormal aggregation of the microtubule-associated protein tau. In view of the proposed pathogenesis (Figure 1), additional biologic targets with therapeutic potential include free radical scavengers, cell metabolism enhancers, and anti-

TABLE 1 Palliative Therapies

Symptom	Therapy
Dysarthria	Speech therapy; communication aids
Dysphagia	Speech therapy; straws; food thickeners; soft, processed food; percutaneous endoscopic gastrostomy (PEG)
Decreased rate of eye blink	Artificial tears (avoid exposure keratitis)
Visual disturbances	Visual prisms; talking books
Gait instability	Weighted walkers; physiotherapy
Dystonia (blepharospasm)	Botulinum toxin (except antecollis)
Antecollis	Avoid botulinum toxin; prismatic spectacles and/or cervical collars sometimes helpful
Myoclonus	Clonazepam, piracetam, valproate
Depression	Antidepressants; support therapy
Emotional incontinence	Amitriptyline
Drooling	Anticholinergics (use cautiously)
Patient and family support	Social services; lay associations (e.g., Society for PSP, Inc.-SPSP, PSP Association)

inflammatory agents (non-steroidals) that cross the blood-brain barrier. Agents that could block microglial activation, such as minocyline, may prove to be of therapeutic value. Investigators hope the translation of successful therapeutic approaches in animal models will soon be translated into effective bench therapies.

Video Legends

SEGMENT 1 Progressive supranuclear palsy. Motor disturbances affect axial (gait, neck) more than limb muscles (tapping, alternating movements). There are impaired postural reflexes with the backward pull test. The patient would have fallen, unless aided by the examiner {2:55:32 to 2:56:05}.

SEGMENT 2 Progressive supranuclear palsy. Vertical saccades are much slower than horizontal saccades {2:54:06 to 2:54:20}.

SEGMENT 3 Progressive supranuclear palsy. Severe limitation in the vertical range of ocular motor movements affects voluntary gaze, saccades and optokinetic nystagmus. Vertical pursuit, convergence and Doll's head maneuver are shown on the video. Horizontal saccades are slow and hypometric {2:53:35 to 2:54:06}.

SEGMENT 4 Corticobasal degeneration. A 76-year-old female with a 3–4 year history of progressive loss of control of her right hand. In the year preceding this video, she had begun to fall occasionally. In addition, her speech had slowed. Ideomotor apraxia, focal myoclonus, and dystonia are described and/or shown in this brief history and examination {2:54:22 to 2:55:32}.

References

1. Steele, J.C., J.C. Richardson, and J. Olszewski. 1964. Progressive Supranuclear Palsy. *Arch Neurol* **10**:333–359.
2. Rebeiz, J.J., E.H. Kolodny, and E.P. Richardson, Jr. 1967. Corticodentatonigral degeneration with neuronal achromasia: a progressive disorder of late adult life. *Trans Am Neurol Assoc* **92**:23–26.
3. Graham, N.L., T.H. Bak, and J.R. Hodges. 2003. Corticobasal degeneration as a cognitive disorder. *Mov Disord* **18**:1224–1232.
4. Frattali, C., J.R. Duffy, I. Litvan, A.D. Patsalides, and J. Grafman. 2003. Yes/no reversals as neurobehavioral sequela: A disorder of language, praxis, or inhibitory control? *Eur J Neurol* **10**:103–106.
5. Dickson, D.W., C. Bergeron, S.S. Chin, C. Dvyckaerts, D. Horoupian, K. Ikeda, K. Jellinger, et al. 2002. Office of Rare Diseases neuropathologic criteria for corticobasal degeneration. *J Neuropathol Exp Neurol* **61**:935–946.
6. Houlden, H., M. Baker, H.R. Morris, N. MacDonald, S. Pickering-Brown, J. Adamson, A.J. Lees, et al. 2001. Corticobasal degeneration and progressive supranuclear palsy share a common tau haplotype. *Neurology* **56**:1702–1706.
7. Caparros-Lefebvre, D., and A. Elbaz. 1999. Possible relation of atypical parkinsonism in the French West Indies with consumption of tropical plants: A case-control study. Caribbean Parkinsonism Study Group. *Lancet* **354**:281–286.
8. Caparros-Lefebvre, D., N. Sergeant, A. Lees, A. Camuzat, S. Daniel, A. Lannuzel, A. Brice, et al. 2002. Guadeloupean parkinsonism: A cluster of progressive supranuclear palsy-like tauopathy. *Brain* **125**:801–811.
9. Boeve, B.F., A.E. Lang, and I. Litvan. 2003. Corticobasal degeneration and its relationship to progressive supranuclear palsy and frontotemporal dementia. *Ann Neurol* **54**:S15–S19.
10. Litvan, I., J.J. Hauw, J.J. Bartko, P.L. Lantos, S.E. Daniel, D.S. Horoupian, A. McKee, et al. 1996. Validity and reliability of the preliminary NINDS neuropathologic criteria for progressive supranuclear palsy and related disorders. *J Neuropathol Exp Neurol* **55**:97–105.
11. Litvan, I., Y. Agid, D. Calne, G. Campbell, B. Dubois, R.C. Duvoisin, C.G. Goetz, et al. 1996. Clinical research criteria for the diagnosis of progressive supranuclear palsy (Steele-Richardson-Olszewski syndrome): Report of the NINDS-SPSP international workshop. *Neurology* **47**:1–9.
12. Lopez, O.L., I. Litvan, K.E. Catt, R. Stowe, W. Klunk, D.I. Kaufer, J.T. Becker, et al. 1999. Accuracy of four clinical diagnostic criteria for the diagnosis of neurodegenerative dementias. *Neurology* **53**:1292–1299.
13. Litvan, I., Y. Agid, C. Goetz, J. Jankovic, G.K. Wenning, J.P. Brandel, E.C. Lai, et al. 1997. Accuracy of the clinical diagnosis of corticobasal degeneration: A clinicopathologic study. *Neurology* **48**:119–125.
14. Litvan, I., K.P. Bhatia, D.J. Burn, C.G. Goetz, A.E. Lang, I. McKeith, N. Quinn, et al. 2003. Movement Disorders Society Scientific Issues Committee report: SIC Task Force appraisal of clinical diagnostic criteria for Parkinsonian disorders. *Mov Disord* **18**:467–486.
15. Bower, J.H., D.M. Maraganore, S.K. McDonnell, and W.A. Rocca. 1997. Incidence of progressive supranuclear palsy and multiple system atrophy in Olmsted County, Minnesota, 1976 to 1990. *Neurology* **49**: 1284–1288.
16. Schrag, A., Y. Ben-Shlomo, and N.P. Quinn. 1999. Prevalence of progressive supranuclear palsy and multiple system atrophy: a cross-sectional study. *Lancet* **354**:1771–1775.
17. Nath, U., Y. Ben-Shlomo, R.G. Thomson, H.R. Morris, N.W. Wood, A.J. Lees, and D.J. Burn. 2001. The prevalence of progressive supranuclear palsy (Steele-Richardson- Olszewski syndrome) in the UK. *Brain* **124**:1438–1449.
18. Bower, J.H., D.M. Maraganore, S.K. McDonnell, and W.A. Rocca. 1999. Incidence and distribution of parkinsonism in Olmsted County, Minnesota, 1976 to 1990. *Neurology* **52**:1214–1220.
19. Litvan, I. 1997. Progressive supranuclear palsy and corticobasal degeneration. *Baillieres Clin Neurol* **6**:167–185.
20. Stacy, M., and J. Jankovic. 1992. Differential diagnosis of Parkinson's disease and the parkinsonism plus syndromes. *Neurol Clin* **10**:341–359.
21. Togasaki, D.M., and C.M. Tanner. 2000. Epidemiologic aspects. *Adv Neurol* **82**:53–59.
22. Nath, U., Y. Ben-Shlomo, R.G. Thomson, A.J. Lees, and D.J. Burn. 2003. Clinical features and natural history of progressive supranuclear palsy: A clinical cohort study. *Neurology* **60**:910–916.
23. Goetz, C.G., S. Leurgans, A.E. Lang, and I. Litvan. 2003. Progression of gait, speech and swallowing deficits in progressive supranuclear palsy. *Neurology* **60**:917–922.
24. Maher, E.R., and A.J. Lees. 1986. The clinical features and natural history of the Steele-Richardson-Olszewski syndrome (progressive supranuclear palsy). *Neurology* **36**:1005–1008.
25. Walsh, J.S., H.G. Welch, and E.B. Larson. 1990. Survival of outpatients with Alzheimer-type dementia. *Ann Intern Med* **113**:429–434.
26. Tolosa, E., F. Valldeoriola, and M.J. Marti. 1994. Clinical diagnosis and diagnostic criteria of progressive supranuclear palsy (Steele-Richardson-Olszewski syndrome). *J Neural Transm Suppl* **42**:15–31.
27. Litvan, I., C.A. Mangone, A. McKee, M. Verny, A. Parsa, K. Jellinger, L. D'Olhaberriague, et al. 1996. Natural history of progressive supranuclear palsy (Steele-Richardson-Olszewski syndrome) and clinical predictors of survival: A clinicopathological study. *J Neurol Neurosurg Psychiatry* **60**:615–620.
28. Verny, M., K.A. Jellinger, J.J. Hauw, C. Bancher, I. Litvan, and Y. Agid. 1996. Progressive supranuclear palsy: A clinicopathological study of 21 cases. *Acta Neuropathol* **91**:427–431.
29. Santacruz, P., B. Uttl, I. Litvan, and J. Grafman. 1998. Progressive supranuclear palsy: A survey of the disease course. *Neurology* **50**: 1637–1647.

30. Wenning, G.K., G. Ebersbach, M. Verny, K.R. Chavdhuri, K. Jellinger, A. McKee, W. Poewe, et al. 1999. Progression of falls in postmortem-confirmed parkinsonian disorders. *Mov Disord* **14**:947–950.
31. Verny, M., C. Duyckaerts, Y. Agid, and J.J. Hauw. 1996. The significance of cortical pathology in progressive supranuclear palsy. Clinico-pathological data in 10 cases. *Brain* **119**:1123–1136.
32. Barclay, C.L., and A.E. Lang. 1997. Dystonia in progressive supranuclear palsy. *J Neurol Neurosurg Psychiatry* **62**:352–356.
33. Pillon, B., B. Dubois, F. Lhermitte, and Y. Agid. 1986. Heterogeneity of cognitive impairment in progressive supranuclear palsy, Parkinson's disease, and Alzheimer's disease. *Neurology* **36**:1179–1185.
34. Grafman, J., I. Litvan, C. Gomez, and T.N. Chase. 1990. Frontal lobe function in progressive supranuclear palsy. *Arch Neurol* **47**:553–558.
35. Grafman, J., H. Weingartner, P.A. Newhouse, K. Thompson, F. Lalonde, I. Litvan, S. Molchan, et al. 1990. Implicit learning in patients with Alzheimer's disease. *Pharmacopsychiatry* **23**:94–101.
36. Pillon, B., B. Dubois, A. Ploska, and Y. Agid. 1991. Severity and specificity of cognitive impairment in Alzheimer's, Huntington's, and Parkinson's diseases and progressive supranuclear palsy. *Neurology* **41**:634–643.
37. Pillon, B., B. Deweer, A. Michon, C. Malapani, Y. Agid, and B. Dubois. 1994. Are explicit memory disorders of progressive supranuclear palsy related to damage to striatofrontal circuits? Comparison with Alzheimer's, Parkinson's, and Huntington's diseases. *Neurology* **44**: 1264–1270.
38. Litvan, I., M.S. Mega, J.L. Cummings, and L. Fairbanks. 1996. Neuropsychiatric aspects of progressive supranuclear palsy. *Neurology* **47**:1184–1189.
39. Litvan, I., J.S. Paulsen, M.S. Mega, and J.L. Cummings. 1998. Neuropsychiatric assessment of patients with hyperkinetic and hypokinetic movement disorders. *Arch Neurol* **55**:1313–1319.
40. Litvan, I., D.A. Grimes, and A.E. Lang. 2000. Phenotypes and Prognosis: Clinicopathologic Studies of Corticobasal Degeneration. In *Advances in Neurology*. Ed. I. Litvan, C.K. Goetz, and A.E. Lang. pp. 183–196. Philadelphia: Lippincott Williams and Wilkins.
41. Daniel, S.E., V.M. de Bruin, and A.J. Lees. 1995. The clinical and pathological spectrum of Steele-Richardson-Olszewski syndrome (progressive supranuclear palsy): A reappraisal. *Brain* **118**:759–770.
42. Bergeron, C., M.S. Pollanen, L. Weyer, S.E. Black, and A.E. Lang. 1996. Unusual clinical presentations of cortical-basal ganglionic degeneration. *Ann Neurol* **40**:893–900.
43. Grimes, D.A., A.E. Lang, and C. Bergeron. 1999. Dementia is the most common presentation of cortical-basal ganglionic degeneration. *Neurology* **53**:1969–1974.
44. Tang-Wai, D.F., K.A. Josephs, B.F. Boeve, D.W. Dickson, J.E. Parisi, and R.C. Petersen. 2003. Pathologically confirmed corticobasal degeneration presenting with visuospatial dysfunction. *Neurology* **61**:1134–1135.
45. Gibb, W.R., P.J. Luthert, and C.D. Marsden. 1989. Corticobasal degeneration. *Brain* **112**:1171–1192.
46. Riley, D.E., A.E. Lang, A. Lewis, L. Resch, P. Ashby, G. Horny Kiewicz, S. Black. 1990. Cortical-basal ganglionic degeneration. *Neurology* **40**:1203–1212.
47. Wenning, G.K., I. Litvan, J. Jankovic, R. Granata, C.A. Mangone, A. McKee, W. Poewe, et al. 1998. Natural history and survival of 14 patients with corticobasal degeneration confirmed at postmortem examination. *J Neurol Neurosurg Psychiatry* **64**:184–189.
48. Boeve, B., D. Dickson, J. Duffy, J. Bartleson, M. Trenerry, and R. Petersen. 2003. Progressive nonfluent aphasia and subsequent aphasic dementia associated with atypical progressive supranuclear palsy pathology. *Eur Neurol* **49**:72–78.
49. Grimes, D.A., C.B. Bergeron, and A.E. Lang. 1999. Motor neuron disease-inclusion dementia presenting as cortical-basal ganglionic degeneration. *Mov Disord* **14**:674–680.
50. Frattali, C.M., J. Grafman, N. Patronas, F. Makhlouf, and I. Litvan. 2000. Language disturbances in corticobasal degeneration. *Neurology* **54**:990–992.
51. Bergeron, C., A. Davis, and A.E. Lang. 1998. Corticobasal ganglionic degeneration and progressive supranuclear palsy presenting with cognitive decline. *Brain Pathol* **8**:355–365.
52. Boeve, B.F., D.M. Maraganore, J.E. Parisi, J.E. Ahlskog, N. Graff-Radford, R.J. Caselli, D.W. Dickson, et al. 1999. Pathologic heterogeneity in clinically diagnosed corticobasal degeneration. *Neurology* **53**:795–800.
53. Bhatia, K.P., M.S. Lee, J.O. Rinne, T. Revesz, F. Scavavalli, L. Davies, C.D. Marsden. 2000. Corticobasal degeneration look-alikes. *Adv Neurol* **82**:169–182.
54. Bugiani, O., J.R. Murrell, G. Giaccone, M. Hasegawa, G. Ghigo, M. Tabaton, M. Morbin, et al. 1999. Frontotemporal dementia and corticobasal degeneration in a family with a P301S mutation in tau. *J Neuropathol Exp Neurol* **58**:667–677.
55. Litvan, I., Y. Agid, J. Jankovic, C. Goetz, J.P. Brandel, E.C. Lai, G. Wenning, et al. 1996. Accuracy of clinical criteria for the diagnosis of progressive supranuclear palsy (Steele-Richardson-Olszewski syndrome). *Neurology* **46**:922–930.
56. Litvan, I., G. Campbell, C.A. Mangone, M. Verny, A. McKee, K.R. Chavdhuri, K. Jellinger, et al. 1997. Which clinical features differentiate progressive supranuclear palsy (Steele-Richardson-Olszewski syndrome) from related disorders? A clinicopathological study. *Brain* **120**:65–74.
57. Spillantini, M.G., and M. Goedert. 1998. Tau protein pathology in neurodegenerative diseases. *Trends Neurosci* **21**:428–433.
58. Buee, L., and A. Delacourte. 1999. Comparative biochemistry of tau in progressive supranuclear palsy, corticobasal degeneration, FTDP-17 and Pick's disease. *Brain Pathol* **9**:681–693.
59. Goedert, M., R.A. Crowther, and M.G. Spillantini. 1998. Tau mutations cause frontotemporal dementias. *Neuron* **21**:955–958.
60. Sergeant, N., A. Wattez, and A. Delacourte. 1999. Neurofibrillary degeneration in progressive supranuclear palsy and corticobasal degeneration: Tau pathologies with exclusively "exon 10" isoforms. *J Neurochem* **72**:1243–1249.
61. Chambers, C.B., J.M. Lee, J.C. Troncoso, S. Reich, and N.A. Muma. 1999. Overexpression of four-repeat tau mRNA isoforms in progressive supranuclear palsy but not in Alzheimer's disease. *Ann Neurol* **46**:325–332.
62. Hauw, J.J., S.E. Daniel, D. Dickson, D.S. Horoupian, K. Jellinger, P.L. Lantos, A. McKee, et al. 1994. Preliminary NINDS neuropathologic criteria for Steele-Richardson-Olszewski syndrome (progressive supranuclear palsy). *Neurology* **44**:2015–2019.
63. Di Maria, E., M. Tabaton, T. Vigo, G. Abbruzzese, E. Bellone, C. Donati, E. Frasson, et al. 2000. Corticobasal degeneration shares a common genetic background with progressive supranuclear palsy. *Ann Neurol* **47**:374–377.
64. D'Souza, I., P. Poorkaj, M. Hong, D. Nochlin, V.M. Lee, T.D. Bird, G.D. Schellenberg. 1999. Missense and silent tau gene mutations cause frontotemporal dementia with parkinsonism-chromosome 17 type, by affecting multiple alternative RNA splicing regulatory elements. *Proc Natl Acad Sci U S A* **96**:5598–5603.
65. Iijima, M., T. Tabira, P. Poorkaj, G.D. Schellenberg, J.Q. Trojanowsk, V.M. Lee, M.L. Schmidt, et al. 1999. A distinct familial presenile dementia with a novel missense mutation in the tau gene. *Neuroreport* **10**:497–501.
66. Grover, A., H. Houlden, M. Baker, J. Adamson, J. Lewis, G. Prihar, S. Pickering-Brown, et al. 1999. 5′ splice site mutations in tau associated with the inherited dementia FTDP-17 affect a stem-loop structure that regulates alternative splicing of exon 10. *J Biol Chem* **274**:15134–15143.
67. Bird, T.D., D. Nochlin, P. Poorkaj, M. Cherrier, J. Kaye, H. Payami, E. Peskind, et al. 1999. A clinical pathological comparison of three

families with frontotemporal dementia and identical mutations in the tau gene (P301L). *Brain* **122**:741–756.

68. van Swieten, J.C., M. Stevens, S.M. Rosso, P. Rizzu, M. Joosse, I. de Koning, W. Kamphorst, et al. 1999. Phenotypic variation in hereditary frontotemporal dementia with tau mutations. *Ann Neurol* **46**:617–626.
69. Rojo, A., R.S. Pernaute, A. Fontan, P.G. Ruiz, J. Honnorat, T. Lynch, S. Chin, et al. 1999. Clinical genetics of familial progressive supranuclear palsy. *Brain* 122 (Pt 7):1233–1245.
70. Morris, H.R., R. Katzenschlager, J.C. Janssen, J.M. Brown, M. Ozansoy, N. Quinn, T. Revesz, et al. 2002. Sequence analysis of tau in familial and sporadic progressive supranuclear palsy. *J Neurol Neurosurg Psychiatry* **72**:388–390.
71. Arai, T., K. Ikeda, H. Akiyama, T. Nonaka, M. Hasegawa, K. Ishiguro, S. Iritani, et al. 2004. Identification of amino-terminally cleaved tau fragments that distinguish progressive supranuclear palsy from corticobasal degeneration. *Ann Neurol* **55**:72–79.
72. Vidailhet, M., S. Rivaud, N. Gouider-Khouja, B. Pillon, A.M. Bonnet, B. Gaymard, Y. Agid, et al. 1994. Eye movements in parkinsonian syndromes. *Ann Neurol* **35**:420–426.
73. Rivaud-Pechoux, S., M. Vidailhet, G. Gallouedec, I. Litvan, B. Gaymard, and C. Pierrot-Deseilligny. 2000. Longitudinal ocular motor study in corticobasal degeneration and progressive supranuclear palsy. *Neurology* **54**:1029–1032.
74. Valls-Sole, J. 2000. Neurophysiological characterization of parkinsonian syndromes. *Neurophysiol Clin* **30**:352–367.
75. Okuda, B., H. Tachibana, M. Takeda, K. Kawabata, and M. Sugita. 1998. Asymmetric changes in somatosensory evoked potentials correlate with limb apraxia in corticobasal degeneration. *Acta Neurol Scand* **97**:409–412.
76. Warmuth-Metz, M., M. Naumann, I. Csoti, and L. Solymosi. 2001. Measurement of the midbrain diameter on routine magnetic resonance imaging: A simple and accurate method of differentiating between Parkinson disease and progressive supranuclear palsy. *Arch Neurol* **58**:1076–1079.
77. Morris, H.R., J.R. Vaughan, S.R. Datta, R. Bandopadhyay, H.A. Rohan De Silv, A. Schrag, et al. 2000. Multiple system atrophy/progressive supranuclear palsy: Alpha-synuclein, synphilin, tau, and APOE. *Neurology* **55**:1918–1920.
78. Savoiardo, M. 2003. Differential diagnosis of Parkinson's disease and atypical parkinsonian disorders by magnetic resonance imaging. *Neurol Sci* **24 Suppl 1**:S35–S37.
79. Yekhlef, F., G. Ballan, F. Macia, O. Delmer, C. Sourgen, and F. Tison. 2003. Routine MRI for the differential diagnosis of Parkinson's disease, MSA, PSP, and CBD. *J Neural Transm* **110**:151–169.
80. Groschel, K., T.K. Hauser, A. Luft, N. Patronas, J. Dichgans, I. Litvan, J.B. Schultz. 2004. Magnetic resonance imaging-based volumetry differentiates progressive supranuclear palsy from corticobasal degeneration. *NeuroImage* In Press.
81. Ballan, G., F. Tison, V. Dousset, M. Vidailhet, Y. Agid, and P. Henry. 1998. MRI in corticobasal degeneration. *Rev Neurol* **154**:224–227.
82. Tedeschi, G., I. Litvan, S. Bonavita, et al. 1997. Proton magnetic resonance spectroscopic imaging in progressive supranuclear palsy, Parkinson's disease and corticobasal degeneration. *Brain* **120**:1541–1552.
83. Ukmar, M., R. Moretti, P. Torre, R.M. Antonello, R. Longo, and A. Bava. 2003. Corticobasal degeneration: Structural and functional MRI and single-photon emission computed tomography. *Neuroradiology* **45**:708–712.
84. Pirker, W., S. Asenbaum, G. Bencsits, et al. 2000. [123I]beta-CIT SPECT in multiple system atrophy, progressive supranuclear palsy, and corticobasal degeneration. *Mov Disord* **15**:1158–1167.
85. Brooks, D.J. 2000. Functional imaging studies in corticobasal degeneration. *Adv Neurol* **82**:209–215.
86. Hossain, A.K., Y. Murata, L. Zhang, S. Taura, Y. Saitoh, H. Mizusawa, K. Oda, et al. 2003. Brain perfusion SPECT in patients with corticobasal degeneration: Analysis using statistical parametric mapping. *Mov Disord* **18**:697–703.
87. Litvan, I., D.W. Dickson, J.A. Buttner-Ennever, A. Delacourte, M. Hutton, B. Dubois, L.J. Golbe, et al. 2000. Research goals in progressive supranuclear palsy. First International Brainstorming Conference on PSP. *Mov Disord* **15**:446–458.
88. Kompoliti, K., C.G. Goetz, I. Litvan, K. Jellinger, and M. Verny. 1998. Pharmacological therapy in progressive supranuclear palsy. *Arch Neurol* **55**:1099–1102.
89. Kompoliti, K., C.G. Goetz, B.F. Boeve, D.M. Maraganore, J.E. Ahlskog, C.D. Marsden, K.P. Bhatin, et al. 1998. Clinical presentation and pharmacological therapy in corticobasal degeneration. *Arch Neurol* **55**:957–961.
90. Litvan, I., R. Blesa, K. Clark, P. Nichelli, J.R. Atack, M.M. Mouradian, J. Grafman, et al. 1994. Pharmacological evaluation of the cholinergic system in progressive supranuclear palsy. *Ann Neurol* **36**:55–61.
91. Litvan, I. 2001. Diagnosis and management of progressive supranuclear palsy. *Semin Neurol* **21**:41–48.
92. Lewis, J., E. McGowan, J. Rockwood, H. Melrose, P. Nacharaju, M. Van Slegtenhorst, K. Gwinn-Hordy, et al. 2000. Neurofibrillary tangles, amyotrophy and progressive motor disturbance in mice expressing mutant (P301L) tau protein. *Nat Genet* **25**:402–405.
93. Hutton, M., J. Lewis, D. Dickson, S.H. Yen, and E. McGowan. 2001. Analysis of tauopathies with transgenic mice. *Trends Mol Med* **7**: 467–470.
94. Wittmann, C.W., M.F. Wszolek, J.M. Shulman, P.M. Salvaterra, J. lewis, M. Hutton, M.B. Feany. 2001. Tauopathy in *Drosophila*: Neurodegeneration without neurofibrillary tangles. *Science* **293**:711–714.
95. Klein, R.L., W.L. Lin, D.W. Dickson, J. Lewis, M. Hutton, K. Duff, E.M. Meyer, et al. 2004. Rapid neurofibrillary tangle formation after localized gene transfer of mutated tau. *Am J Pathol* **164**:347–353.
96. Schrag, A., C.D. Good, K. Miszkiel, H.R. Morris, C.J. Mathias, A.J. Lees, N.P. Quinn. 2000. Differentiation of atypical parkinsonian syndromes with routine MRI. *Neurology* **54**:697–702.

CHAPTER

12

Genetic Susceptibility and Animal Modeling of PSP

PARVONEH POORKAJ NAVAS, IAN D'SOUZA, and GERARD D. SCHELLENBERG

Progressive supranuclear palsy (PSP) is a neurodegenerative disorder characterized by Parkinsonism, rigidity, pseudobulbar palsy, axial dystonia, postural instability, and supranuclear gaze palsy. PSP is generally a sporadic disorder; however, familial clustering has been reported, suggesting that heritable genetic components contribute to the onset or progression of the disease. PSP is pathologically characterized by neurodegeneration, gliosis, and intracellular inclusions that include neurofibrillary tangles composed of hyper-phosphorylated tau proteins. Discovery of an association between the microtubule associated protein tau (gene –[*MAPT*]) A0 allele and an extended tau H1 haplotype with PSP presents *MAPT* as a candidate gene for PSP; however, coding sequence *MAPT* mutations in PSP are rare and functional susceptibility alleles have not yet been identified or characterized. To date, seven different mutations in the *MAPT* gene have been identified in individuals with PSP or PSP-like phenotypes; however, phenotypic overlap with probands harboring the same tau mutation and atypical forms of frontotemporal dementia confound the ability to generate a *MAPT* transgenic mouse model of PSP. The role of tau in PSP and which *MAPT* mutations should be used to generate a transgenic mouse model of PSP are discussed. Rationales, with regard to the available experimental and pathological data relating to *MAPT* and PSP, are presented for mutation and expression construct selection, and a reliable method for generating mutant genomic *MAPT* transgenes is discussed in detail.

I. GENETIC CONTRIBUTIONS IN PSP

In PSP, the age of onset for initial symptoms ranges from fifty-five to past eighty years, with a five to six year duration of disease before death [11,95,116]. PSP is clinically characterized by Parkinsonism and prominent vertical gaze palsy [43,127]. Patients can also exhibit deficits in visual attention, information processing, long-term memory, conceptualization, and social cognition [70,84,86,102,106]. PSP is one of a number of Parkinsonian disorders that manifest as dementias, movement disorders, or both and share neuropathology that includes ubiquitinated neurofibrillary tangles (NFTs) comprised of hyperphosphorylated tau proteins and ubiquitinated α-synuclein proteins (found in the form of Lewy bodies [LBs]) [108]. These overlapping neurodegenerative diseases include Parkinson disease (PD), Parkinsonism-Dementia Complex of Guam (PDC-G) and Guamanian-ALS (ALS-G), frontotemporal dementia with Parkinsonism chromosome-17 type (FTDP), and progressive supranuclear palsy (PSP). Among these diseases, all but

TABLE 1 Insoluble Deposits of Tau and Other Proteins in Sporadic and Hereditary Tauopathies

Tauopathy and affected regions of the brain	Neuronal forms and isoforms of insoluble tau	Additional disease-defining protein deposits
Alzheimer disease (AD): entorhinal cortex hippocampus neocortex	NFTs (typically flame-shaped) neuropil threads Predominantly paired helical filaments composed of: 3R and 4R tau isoforms	β amyloid (plaques) α-synuclein (Lewy bodies)
Corticobasal degeneration (CBD): cerebral cortex deep cerebellar nuclei substantia nigra	PHF-like filaments and straight tubules Extensive neuropil threads (in both gray and white matter) predominantly 4R tau isoforms	Glial tau inclusions in: astrocytes oligodendrocytes (coiled bodies) Astrocytic plaques
Guam-ALS/PDC dementia complex: hippocampus neocortex spinal cord	NFTs: Isolated paired and unpaired straight and helical filaments 3R and 4R tau isoforms	
Frontotemporal dementia (FTDP): frontal and temporal cortex	NFTs composed of: 3R and 4R tau isoforms or 3R tau isoforms or 4R tau isoforms	Some glial tau inclusions
Pick disease (PiD): hippocampus neocortex	Pick bodies, a mixture of: wide, straight filaments wide, twisted filaments exclusively 3R tau isoforms	
Progressive supranuclear palsy (PSP): basal ganglia brainstem cerebellum subthalamus	NFTs (typically round or globose) Predominantly straight filaments, 4R tau isoforms	Glial tau inclusions in: astrocytes (tufted astrocytes) oligodendrocytes (coiled bodies)

PD are also classified as tauopathies (disorders in which tau pathology is a disease-defining characteristic). Other neurodegenerative disorders classified within this family of tauopathies include Pick disease (PiD), corticobasal degeneration (CBD), Alzheimer disease (AD), and Lewy body variants of AD. Each of these neurodegenerative disorders has a unique and characteristic combination of neuronal and/or glial cell depositions of insoluble tau proteins and intra/extra-cellular depositions of characteristic disease-related proteins (table 1).

The cellular and molecular pathology in PSP includes subcortical neuronal degeneration and gliosis, where NFTs are observed in the nigrostriatal pathway, the basal forebrain, the tegmental nuclei; and the *locus ceruleus*. Minor neocortical pathology is also seen in the hippocampus and anterior association cortex [48]. Positioning of these subcortical lesions within the frontal lobe significantly affects the cholinergic and dopaminergic neurotransmitter systems resulting in frontal lobe hypometabolism [8]. Amyloid β peptide deposition and neuritic plaques found in Alzheimer disease (AD) are absent in PSP [31,53,61]. The NFTs and related pathological filaments observed in PSP are composed primarily of the microtubule associated protein tau and are similar but not identical to those observed in AD and in some cases of FTDP [121,123,128]. Although PSP and AD tau filaments share the same phospho-tau epitopes, the abnormal tau-containing filaments in PSP are predominantly straight or a mixture of straight and paired helical filament (PHF) structures, while in AD, pathological filaments are predominantly PHFs [39,110,131].

PSP is generally a sporadic disorder [42,44]; however, investigators have reported familial clustering of PSP, suggesting that in some rare PSP families, heritable genetic components contribute to onset or progression of the disease [13,26,36,98]. Discovery of a genetic association between PSP and a short tandem repeat polymorphism (A0 allele, characterized by eleven TG repeats) within *MAPT* (the gene encoding tau) presents *MAPT* as a candidate gene for PSP [20,58]. Subsequent studies expanded this A0 allelic association to an extended H1 haplotype composed of the A0 allele and eight additional single nucleotide polymorphisms (SNPs) spanning *MAPT* (Figure 1A), where the H1 haplotype is overrepresented in sporadic PSP subjects when compared with normal control subjects [82,127]. An additional two missense mutations in exon 4a (an exon expressed only in the peripheral nervous system) are associated with the H1 haplotype and PSP. The genetic association between the H1 haplotype and PSP has been confirmed in multiple independent Caucasian PSP populations [6,85,99]; however, *MAPT* mutations in PSP are rare and investigators have identified no other candidate PSP susceptibility genes [4,99,100,104,105,126]. Because most PSP cases are spo-

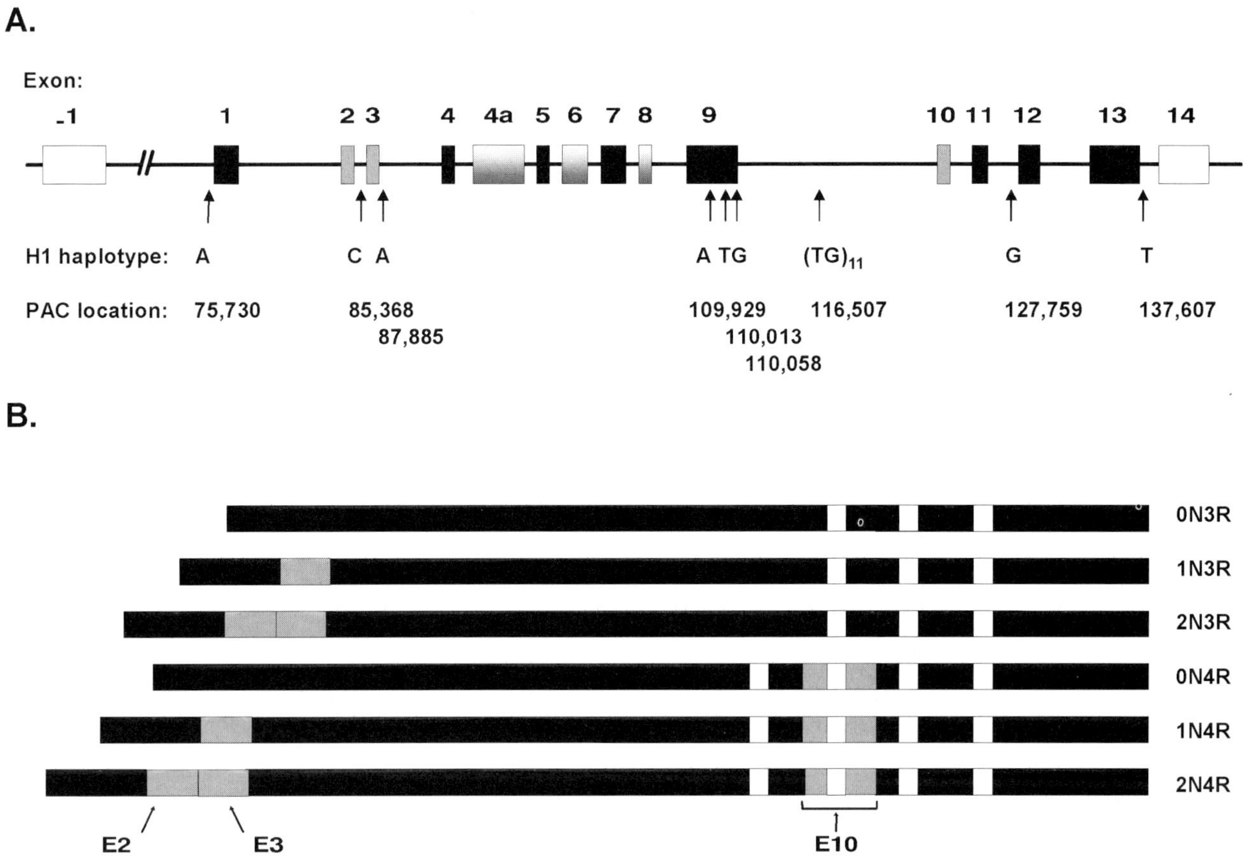

FIGURE 1 The tau H1 haplotype and alternative splicing of *MAPT*. (**A**) Genomic representation of *MAPT* spanning 133.9 Kb. Exon and intron sizes are not accurately represented. Noncoding exons are represented as white boxes, peripheral nervous system alternative spliced exons are represented with white-to-gray gradation, and central nervous system (CNS) alternatively spliced exons are represented in grey. Relative genomic locations of the single nucleotide polymorphisms (SNPs) and A0 dinucleotide repeat comprising the tau H1 haplotype are indicated by arrows. Nucleotides comprising the H1 haplotype are found on human *MAPT* PAC 61D6 (Genbank Accession # AC091628). SNP locations (nucleotide position) on PAC 61D6 are aligned below the corresponding nucleotides. (**B**) *MAPT* has fifteen exons, of which six coding exons undergo alternative splicing. In the adult human CNS, six splice variants are produced by alternative inclusion of amino terminal exons 2 and 3 (0N, 1N, or 2N inclusions), and carboxy terminus exon 10 (E10). Inclusion of E10 generates a four repeat isoform (4R tau with four microtubule binding domains) while exclusion of E10 generates 3R tau. Microtubule binding domains are represented in white.

radic and can vary both clinically and pathologically, investigators have suggested that low penetrance or nongenetic environmental interactions may contribute to the onset, progression, and phenotype of the disease [83].

Recently investigators have proposed that two subtypes of PSP may exist (clinically typical and atypical) with pathologically diagnosed PSP; typical PSP patients are more likely to have *MAPT* H1 haplotypes and deposits of straight hyperphosphorylated tau filaments and atypical patients are more likely to have highly varied clinical syndromes that often resemble idiopathic PD [91]. Atypical presentations of PSP may also represent co-occurrence of PD and PSP, in which α-synuclein and tau positive inclusions are concomitant [71]. Whether a genetic link exists between tau mutations and the manifestation of Parkinsonism remains to be more thoroughly examined, although recent studies may support this hypothesis with proposals that *MAPT* may be associated with some forms of PD [87,117]. Investigators have identified a single heterozygous mutation in the *parkin* gene (mutations in *parkin* are responsible for autosomal recessive juvenile-onset PD) in one sporadic PSP subject; however, heterozygous single mutations in *parkin* are not known to cause disease and *parkin* mutation carrier frequencies for unaffected control populations have not been published [90,114]. Thus, the role of *parkin* mutations in PSP is unclear. Currently *MAPT* is the only gene that has been conclusively and reproducibly linked to disease in sporadic PSP populations.

II. THE ROLE OF TAU IN NEURODEGENERATION

Tau is found primarily in neurons of the central nervous system (CNS), although it is also detected to a lesser degree in oligodendrocytes, astrocytes, and in some non-neuronal tissues [49,134]. Tau proteins play a fundamental role in neurite outgrowth and stabilization and regulates the assembly, dynamic behavior, and spatial organization of microtubules in neurons and possibly glia [15,16]. Normally, tau proteins are found as a family of six soluble cytoplasmic isoforms (resulting from alternative splicing of exons 2, 3, and 10) that are located in the axonal compartment of CNS neurons [16]. Inclusion of exon 10 (E10) generates a four-repeat isoform (4R tau containing four microtubule [MT] binding domains) while exclusion of E10 generates 3R tau (Figure 1B). In neurodegenerative tauopathies, hyperphosphorylated tau proteins are aberrantly deposited in varied filamentous forms (straight filaments, paired helical filaments –[PHFs], and neuropil threads) and as aggregated forms of PHFs called NFTs.

The role of tau in neurodegeneration is best understood in FTDP where missense and silent/intronic mutations in the gene for tau (*MAPT*) result in an autosomal dominant group of syndromes with overlapping behavioral, cognitive, and motor features, and neuropathologic features that include frontotemporal atrophy, neuronal cell loss, and gliosis [7,32,56]. At least two FTDP families have NFTs and all probably have some form of tau pathology. In the Seattle A family (tau $^{V}337^{M}$ mutation), the NFTs are microscopically indistinguishable from those in AD [121,122,128]. *MAPT* mutations act both at the biochemical level (by affecting the microtubule binding properties) and at the level of mRNA splicing [2,17,19,24,25,62]. Pathologic FTDP mutations within intron 10 (I10) splice donor sequences and within E10 enhancer and silencer sequences also alter normal 4R/3R tau isoform ratios [24,25]. These intronic FTDP mutations demonstrate that tau gene regulation and expression are involved in both neurodegeneration and tau pathology.

A. *MAPT* Gene Structure

The human tau gene (17q21) is flanked by two unrelated neuronally expressed genes: the receptor gene for the corticotropin releasing factor (CRFR, GenBank accession #L23332), located 55 Kb upstream of the tau promoter and a gene of unknown function, and KIAA1267 (GenBank accession #AB033093), located 1.6 Kb downstream of the terminal polyadenylation signal for *MAPT* [104]. Although Genscan, BLAST, and PowerBlast analyses of human and mouse tau genomic sequences identify only tau gene exons that are known, recent publication of *Saitohin*, an intronless gene located ~2.6 Kb downstream from tau E9 (within intron 9), provides evidence for an expressed, embedded gene within tau [21]. The *Saitohin* gene is not conserved across species (human vs. mouse comparison) [104]. A single polymorphic site within *Saitohin* ($^{Q}7^{R}$) is in disequilibrium with the tau H1 haplotype and in disequilibrium with PSP; however, investigators have not identified a role for this polymorphism in neurological disease [22,27,136].

Expression of the gene encoding tau is highly regulated both at the developmental and tissue-specific levels and particularly at the mRNA splicing stage. This regulation differs between rodents and humans. Human *MAPT* has fifteen exons spanning a genomic distance of 133.9 Kb (which includes 3′ and 5′ UTR sequences), and six of fourteen coding exons undergo alternative splicing [3,59,60]. In the fetal CNS, a single tau isoform lacking all alternatively spliced exons is produced. In the adult human CNS, six splice variants are produced by inclusion of alternative exons 2, 3, and 10 [40]. In the adult human brain, the 3R/4R ratio is approximately one [62,72]. In contrast, in the adult rodent brain, three isoforms are present where all forms contain E10 and only E2 and E3 are alternatively spliced [19,72]. Tau mRNA encodes microtubule-binding domains that are imperfect eighteen amino acid repeats separated by thirteen to fourteen amino acid inter-repeat regions that are dissimilar; E10 encodes one binding repeat and one inter-repeat. Depending on whether E10 is excluded or included, tau has either three (3R tau) or four (4R tau) microtubule binding repeats, respectively. The functional consequence of adding E10 is that 4R tau binds microtubules with a higher affinity compared to 3R tau [14,50]. In PSP, tau filaments in the neocortical regions are composed of only the two larger species of tau (4R tau only) [115,135]. In contrast, in AD and other related dementias, NFTs contain six tau protein isoforms (3R and 4R tau) [1]. For purposes of clinical diagnosis, while tau levels are often elevated in cerebrospinal fluid (CSF) from subjects with AD, FTDP, and CBD, CSF tau levels in PSP subjects are not different from nondemented subjects [74].

The use of other alternatively spliced exons (4a, 6, and 8) appears to be confined to the peripheral nervous system (PNS) in humans, although low levels of E4a- and E6-containing transcripts are found in human and rodent brain [12,37,38,88,89,137]. In addition, in some mouse transcripts, the intron between E13 and E14 is removed by RNA splicing, while in other mouse transcripts and in all described rat and human transcripts, the equivalent sequences are retained [76]. Polyadenylation site usage is also regulated and *MAPT* transcripts have either a short 200–250 nt 3′ untranslated region (3′ UTR) or a much longer ~4 kb 3′ UTR [41,111].

B. *MAPT* Mutations

MAPT mutations can be classified according to location (exonic or intronic) and according to disease-causing mechanism (biochemical or splicing) [18,64,124]. Mutations within the constitutively expressed exons (E1, E9, and E11–E13) alter the biochemical properties of tau and its ability to bind to MTs and to initiate MT bundling. Muta-

TABLE 2 PSP-Associated *MAPT* Mutations and Pathological Manifestations

MAPT mutation (reference)	Sarkosyl extracted filaments	Isoforms of insoluble tau	Cellular pathology	*In vitro* mutation effects
$^{R}5^{H}$, exon 1 [105]	straight	4R	mainly glia	↓ MT assembly ↑ filament formation
$^{R}5^{L}$, exon 1 [103]	mainly straight	4R	neurons and glia	↓ MT assembly
$^{N}279^{K}$, exon 10 [18,28]	twisted ribbons, some straight	4R	neurons and glia	↑ E10 splicing
del296N homo, exon 10 [100]	ND‡	ND	Not determined	↑ E10 splicing
$^{S}305^{S}$, exon 10 [126]	ND	ND	neurons and glia	↑ E10 splicing
E10+16, intron 10 [64,93]	wide twisted ribbons	4R	neurons and glia	↑ E10 splicing
$^{R}406^{W}$, exon 13 [64,112]	PHF and straight	3R/4R	mainly neurons	↓ MT assembly

‡ND = not determined.

tions within the alternatively spliced E10 can cause disease by multiple mechanisms: by altering the biochemical properties of tau (e.g., $^{P}301^{L}$) or by disrupting the normal regulation of E10 splicing (e.g., $^{N}279^{K}$, $^{L}284^{L}$, $^{S}305^{N}$) [24,25,62]. A single mutation within tau E12 ($^{E}342^{V}$) is associated with increased expression of E10 protein isoforms [81]. For some autosomal dominant FTDP families, genetic linkage analysis has clearly localized the disease-causing defect to the *MAPT* region of chromosome 17 and yet no mutations have been identified in the *MAPT* open-reading frame or in the intronic sequences immediately flanking exons [78]. Investigators presume that mutations in these families are within as yet unidentified intronic regulatory sequences or in flanking genomic sequences. Currently, no known mutations or functional polymorphisms occur within the PNS-expressed *MAPT* exons or within the *MAPT* untranslated regions.

MAPT mutations can result in a phenotype resembling PSP (table 2); however, the majority of these cases are classified as atypical FTDP [28,100,107,120,126]. The most common *MAPT* mutation ($^{P}301^{L}$) has been identified in one subject that has a PSP-like phenotype; however, other subjects with the same mutation present phenotypically with FTDP and CBD [64]. Recently, investigators identified a previously documented intronic E10 + 16 *MAPT* mutation in a subject presenting clinically with early-onset PSP [93]. This mutation and other intronic *MAPT* mutations previously were shown to alter tau mRNA splicing and cause overproduction of 4R tau protein isoforms [25]. Pathological examination of brain tissue from the E10 + 16 subject revealed diffuse and globular tau-positive inclusions, NFTs, neuropil threads, and coiled bodies. Senile plaques were absent [93].

Although, most *MAPT* mutations are within or flanking the microtubule binding domains, investigators identified two amino terminal tau mutations in subjects with tau pathology that is characteristic of PSP. Two different substitutions at the same amino acid site ($^{R}5^{H}$ and $^{R}5^{L}$) were identified in unrelated subjects with pathological documentation of abnormal accumulations of 4R tau and PSP-like straight filaments [54,105]. The $^{R}5^{H}$ mutation was identified in a subject with marked depigmentation of the substantia nigra, severe neuronal loss, and gliosis—although the subject lacked the characteristic supranuclear gaze palsy of PSP and had widespread plaque deposition in the cerebral cortex [54]. The $^{R}5^{L}$ point mutation was found in a sixty-two-year-old Caucasian female diagnosed with a gait disorder, postural instability, vertical supranuclear gaze palsy, and lid retraction [105]. Pathology included neuronal loss, depigmentation, and astrocytosis of the substantia nigra and locus ceruleus, and neuronal loss and astrocytosis of the cerebellar dentate nucleus. Globose NFTs, oligodendroglial tangles, and coiled bodies satisfied the criteria for PSP.

Biochemical and functional analyses of 5^{L} tau proteins show altered solubility when compared with wild-type tau proteins. Biochemical analysis of tau from the $^{R}5^{L}$ brain identified all six tau isoforms with equal amounts of 4R and 3R isoforms, suggesting that the amino terminal mutation does not significantly influence mRNA splicing. Insoluble tau from the cortical gray and white matter consisted of predominantly 4R tau isoforms (with and without both amino terminal insertions); however, in sub-cortical areas only two 4R tau isoforms were present (0N4R and 1N4R) [105]. Soluble tau in the frontal and temporal cortices was 1.5- to 2-fold higher for the $^{R}5^{L}$ case when compared to normal controls. Functional assays using recombinant mutant tau show that the 5^{L} mutation alters the ability of tau to promote MT assembly, delays the assembly initiation, and lowers the mass of MTs formed [105]. More recent *in vitro* studies of the $^{R}5^{L}$ mutation provide further evidence that mutation of the amino terminus enhances tau protein polymerization [33].

Although investigators have identified seven tau mutations in subjects with clinical presentations of PSP, tau mutations in PSP are rare [57,92,105]. The lack of tau coding sequence or intronic mutations in the majority of sporadic PSP cases suggests that mutations in a regulatory sequence predispose to PSP [104,105]. The fact that 4R tau is predominant in PSP tau aggregates suggests that the common PSP mutation may be in an unidentified regulatory site that controls E10 splicing.

III. ANIMAL MODELS OF TAUOPATHIES

Investigators have generated a number of AD and FTDP mouse models using transgenic (Tg), knock-out (KO), and knock-in methodologies, and by crossing these models to examine transgene synergism; however, no published mouse model completely recapitulates AD or FTDP disease phenotypes and pathology. Researchers have also generated presenilin (PS), amyloid precursor protein (APP), and tau KO mice in which they have observed a significant phenotype of embryonic lethality in homozygous PS KO mice [51,55,118]. Transgenic cDNA mice expressing wild-type (WT) or mutant PS, APP, or tau proteins develop some features of AD pathology. Mutant APP (Aβ) Tg mice exhibit significant amyloid deposition, but lack significant levels of associated neuronal loss, have no neurofibrillary tangles, and have minimal behavioral deficits [9,34,63,75]. Mutant PS1 cDNA Tg mice have increased levels of $A\beta_{1-42}$ and knock-in PS1 $^{P}264^{L}$ Tg mice exhibit accelerated amyloid deposition in a manner that depends on gene dosage, but similarly have minimal neuronal loss, behavioral deficits, or abnormal tau/NFT deposits [29,119].

Investigators have created neurofibrillary tangle mouse models using both mutant and WT cDNAs encoding various isoforms of the tau protein and genomic PACs (P1 artificial chromosomes) that express all six tau isoforms. Overexpressing WT tau cDNA mice have pretangle lesions or tangles (mouse dependent), but no associated plaques or neuronal loss. Mutant cDNA mice have tangles or tangle-like filaments in the hippocampus, cerebellum, and spinal cord [46,47,129]. The most significant tau phenotype is observed in the MoPRP-P301L tau cDNA mice, which exhibit motor dysfunction and neuronal loss in the spinal cord [80]. Genomic PAC mice exhibit appropriate tissue-specific and developmentally appropriate expression but have no tangles, abnormal behavior, or pathology [30]. Through crosses between the APP/PS/tau transgenic mice investigators have identified a synergism between these AD/FTDP genes, where plaque and tangle pathology is increased and occurs earlier in double Tg mice than in single Tg mice [10,79]. Researchers have also published a transgenic *C. elegans* model of tauopathy, where overexpression of FTDP tau mutations results in neurodegeneration, defective neurotransmission, accumulation of insoluble tau, and a quantifiable presynaptic defect [73].

Investigators have published no animal models for PSP; however, the tools for generating such a model now exist. Utilizing the current knowledge of PSP-associated *MAPT* mutations, the overrepresentation of the H1 haplotype in PSP, and the behavioral and pathological data ascertained from existing animal models of tauopathies, investigators can now generate a *MAPT* transgenic mouse model of PSP. The goal of generating an optimal animal model of PSP that recapitulates the movement disorders exhibited in PSP, the neuronal loss and gliosis, and the deposition of 4R tau as straight filaments and NFTs, relies on the successful and appropriate expression of a *MAPT* mutation that manifests in human subjects as clinical and pathological PSP.

IV. CONSIDERATIONS IN GENERATING A MOUSE MODEL OF PSP

A. Mutation Selection and Transgenic Expression Constructs

In order to generate a *MAPT* Tg mouse that pathologically and phenotypically models PSP and does not simply provide another mouse model of FTDP, one must evaluate which PSP-associated tau mutation should be introduced. Of the seven *MAPT* mutations identified in PSP-like cases, four of the mutations lie within or flanking alternatively spliced tau E10 ($^{N}279^{K}$, $^{S}305^{S}$, E10 + 16, and del296N-homozygous) and influence tau mRNA splicing mechanisms [24,25,52]. Investigators have also identified two of these mutations ($^{N}279^{K}$ and E10 + 16) in clinically diagnosed cases of atypical FTDP and thus, these mutations may be equally as likely to manifest as a PSP or FTDP phenotype in the transgenic mouse [18,103,132]. The remaining two PSP-associated splicing mutations may also represent atypical cases of FTDP, although researchers have identified them only in the single PSP-like probands/families [100,138]. Three of the PSP *MAPT* mutations are located in constitutively expressed tau exons. The $^{R}406^{W}$ mutation, identified in one PSP subject, has also been identified in additional probands with more typical FTDP presentations [109,112,133]. This mutation has been used to generate transgenic cDNA mice as a model for FTDP. Although aged $^{R}406^{W}$ Tg mice form straight tau filaments and have memory deficits suggestive of PSP, other pathological characteristics in $^{R}406^{W}$ transgenic mouse brains are more representative of FTDP, where the majority of tau deposits are flame-shaped rather than globose NFTs [130]. The remaining two amino terminal tau mutations, $^{R}5^{H}$ and $^{R}5^{L}$, are rare and unique to individuals who pathologically have tau deposits in the form of PSP-like straight filaments. Because the only amino terminal tau mutations identified thus far are associated with PSP pathology, and because the $^{R}5^{L}$ substitution is the sole *MAPT* mutation associated with an autopsy-documented case that met criteria for the diagnosis of PSP, the 5^L substitution presents as the most likely mutation to manifest as PSP in an animal model.

When creating a mouse model of PSP, investigators must also consider how the chosen mutation should be expressed in the transgenic animal. To date the majority of tau transgenic mouse models express single mutant isoforms with variable amino terminal inserts, where a heterologous promoter (most use the mouse prion- and Thy-1 promoters) drives expression of the tau transgene [45,65,77]. One disadvantage to this approach is that the heterologous promoter likely generates an expression pattern that differs from the normal promoter. Although these tauopathy models have significantly advanced the understanding of the role of abnormal tau in NFT formation, none reproduce the true disease state, in which all six tau isoforms are expressed in an appropriate developmentally regulated manner. Some of the pathological and behavioral deficits exhibited by these mice may be due in part to an imbalance in tau isoform expression or to inappropriate developmental and cellular regulation. Although the pathological end results of these expressed transgenes may represent a tauopathy disease state, they likely exemplify significantly different disease mechanisms than would cause human disease.

While investigators often use intronless cDNA expression constructs to evaluate the biochemical properties of mutant proteins *in vivo*, regulated splicing does not occur, and as such, *MAPT* splicing mutations cannot be evaluated. Splicing mutations can only be evaluated *in vivo* by using genomic constructs that contain the entire gene locus [5]. Whole gene constructs provide for mRNA expression that is controlled by native regulatory elements such as endogenous promoters, enhancers, potentially regulatory large intronic distances, and alternative polyadenylation signals. Investigators have documented appropriate regulation of human *MAPT* in a mouse neuronal environment in *MAPT* transgenic PAC mice, which express all six human tau isoforms in a tissue-specific and developmentally appropriate manner [30]. The basic regulatory mechanisms for human splicing that are to be characterized in transgenic models of tau splicing mutations are mimicked in mice, as evidenced by an appropriate developmental switch from 3R tau to 4R tau isoform expression in adult transgenic mice.

Because soluble tau levels in the $^R5^L$ brain frontal and temporal cortices are higher than those of normal controls, but are the same as normal controls in parietal and occipital cortices, the $^R5^L$ substitution potentially alters the biochemical properties of tau proteins and may also affect regional specific gene expression. The PSP-associated tau H1 haplotype may also interact with the mutation or other regulatory mechanisms to influence gene expression. Therefore, *in vivo* analysis of *MAPT* expression and splicing, and the influence of flanking regulatory sequences can only be evaluated if the expression of tau is driven by its endogenous promoter in the context of a whole gene construct. Based on the pathological data from the $^R5^L$ brain, the association of the tau H1 haplotype with PSP, and the clinical and pathological manifestations associated with PSP *MAPT* mutations, a mutagenized *MAPT* genomic clone, where the 5^L tau mutation is embedded within the tau H1 haplotype, is the most likely transgene to manifest as PSP (and not FTDP) in an animal model. Investigators have published a fully characterized *MAPT* PAC clone (with a background H1 haplotype, Figure 1A) that is available for site-directed mutagenesis [104].

B. Genomic Clone Mutagenesis

Yeast artificial chromosomes (YACs) were among the first large insert genomic clones used for gene expression in transgenic animals; however, YACs are often unstable, exhibiting chimerism, deletions, and rearrangements [101]. In contrast to YAC clones, P1 artificial chromosomes (PACs) and bacterial artificial chromosomes (BACs) are generally stable and not typically chimeric. Because average insert sizes range from 90 to 300 Kb, a typical gene and its flanking regulatory sequences are often encompassed within a single clone [67]. With growing numbers of commercially available human and mouse genomic clones and readily accessible sequences from the Human Genome Project, readily available technologies have met the need for new methods of BAC/PAC genetic engineering, allowing bacterial mediated site-directed mutagenesis [23,66,68,69,94,97, 125]. Most methods use homologous recombination between the genomic target clone and a mutagenized gene target fragment. Investigators use antibiotic counterselection and temperature-sensitive replication to isolate mutagenized clones away from wild-type clones and recombination vectors. Of the published recombination systems, these authors have found great success in their efforts of mutagenizing a human *MAPT* PAC using the pDF-25 recombination vector published by Imam and colleagues (2000) [66].

Mutagenesis using the *E. coli* integrating plasmid pDF-25 is a reproducible methodology that allows the introduction of point mutations, deletions, or insertions via homologous recombination within PAC-containing host *DH10B* cells. The pDF-25 vector encodes the following genes: (1) the rec A gene, allowing homologous recombination in the *E. coli* host; (2) the rep A gene (temperature-sensitive-TS1), allowing replication of the pDF-25 plasmid as a circular cytoplasmic molecule only at a 30°C permissive temperature; (3) a WT rpsL1 gene (rpsL+), allowing host cell resistance to only low concentrations of Str (streptomycin); and (4) the chloramphenicol resistance gene (Cm). The host *DH10B* cells are rec A mutant (disallowing homologous recombination in the absence of the pDF-25 vector), have a mutated rpsL gene (causing high Str resistance), and are Kanamycin (Kan) resistant due to the presence of the Kan gene on the PAC arms. Mutations in the

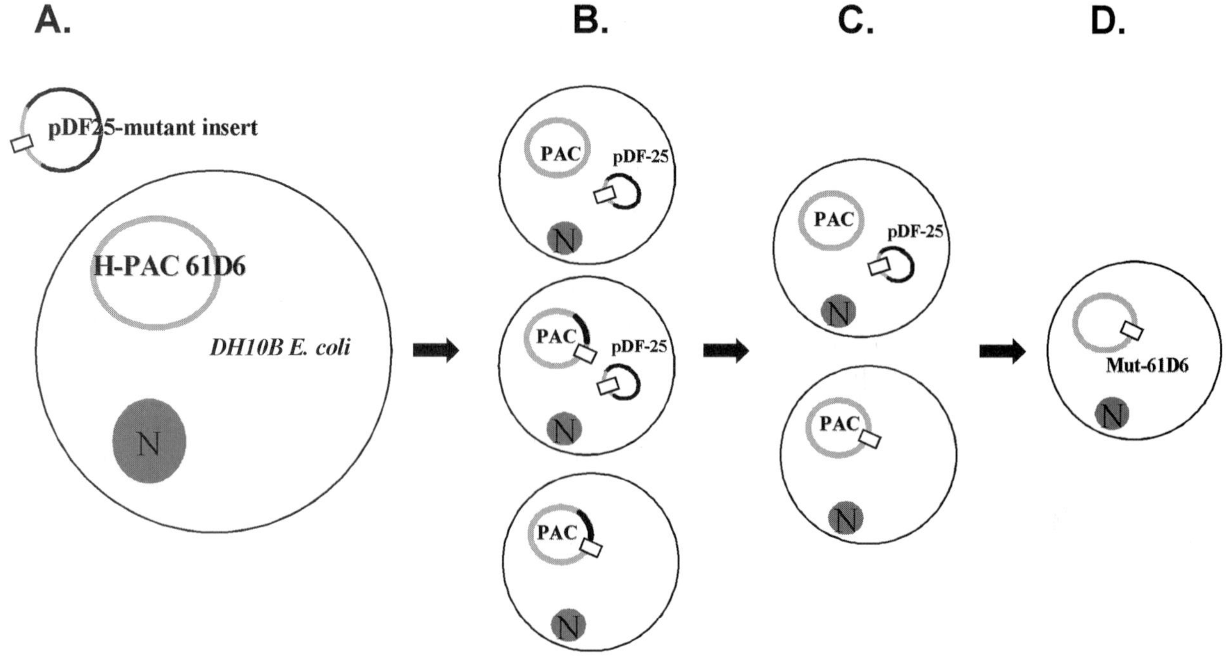

Step:	A.	B.	C.	D.
Procedure:	Electroporation	Integration	Excision	Segregation
Selection temperature:	30 °C	42 °C	42 °C	37 °C
Selection antibiotic:	Kan/Cm	Kan/Cm	Kan	Kan/Str
Characterization:		colony PCR restriction enzyme digest	colony PCR restriction enzyme digest	PCR, PFGE sequencing

FIGURE 2 PAC site-directed mutagenesis in *DH10B E. coli* cells using the pDF-25 vector and homologous recombination [66]. H-PAC 61D6 (represented as a light grey plasmid) host cells are represented with dark grey nuclei (N); homologous 61D6 PAC sequences within the pDF-25 vector are represented in light grey with the inserted mutation indicated by a white rectangle; relative plasmid sizes are not accurately represented. **(A)** PAC containing *DH10B* cells are electroporated with mutant pDF-25 and plated under selection for at least twenty hours; transformed cells grow slowly under temperature and double antibiotic selection. **(B)** Colonies are re-plated at a nonpermissive temperature disallowing nonintegrated plasmid replication. Integration of the homologous PAC sequences into H-PAC61D6 results in duplication of the target sequence (one wild type and one mutant) separated by pDF-25 vector sequences. **(C)** The recombination vector is excised from the integrated clones using antibiotic selection for the PAC arms only. Excision randomly removes either wild-type or mutant sequences. **(D)** Bacterial colonies that harbor either or both the wild-type and mutant PACs (but have lost the recombination vector) are selected for by growth under high concentrations of Str (200 μg/ml). Wild-type and mutant PACs within the same bacterial host cell can be segregated to individual daughter cells by restreaking and Kan selection. Kan, kanamycin; Cm, chloramphenical; Str, streptomycin; PFGE, pulse field gel electrophoreses.

rpsL gene (found in the host *DH10B* cells) alter the binding affinity of 30S ribosomal proteins for Str (Str binds to the 30S subunit causing misreading and bacterial cell death), leading to resistance at high concentrations of streptomycin. Gene products that modify Str (rpsL+ on pDF-25) confer only low concentration Str resistance.

The published human *MAPT* PAC (201 Kb, H-PAC 61D6 Genbank # AC091628) encodes the PSP-associated tau H1 haplotype and is easily mutagenized using the pDF-25 vector (Figure 2). The complete mutagenesis process, from transformation of the pDF-25 vector into the H-PAC 61D6 containing *DH10B* cells to isolation of a characterized clone for micro-injection, takes approximately six weeks. Multiple clones can be mutagenized simultaneously. Homologous sequence inserts harboring the mutation to be introduced, with a minimum of 50–300 nt flanking the mutation site (allowing efficient recombination), are blunt-end ligated into the *Nae* I site of pDF-25 (attempts to subclone recombination fragments into other polycloning site sequences in pDF-25 have been unsuccessful) and sequenced to confirm cloning fidelity.

To generate a mouse model of PSP, H-PAC 61D6 can be used to create a mutant 5^L *MAPT* PAC with a single G→T transversion in tau exon 1, recapitulating the *MAPT* coding sequences in the $^R5^L$ PSP subject. An overnight culture of H-PAC 61D6 containing *DH10B* cells is used to inoculate a 20 ml liquid culture (Kan selection). After 1.5 hours of shaking, the cells are induced with 0.5 mM IPTG (isopropyl-beta-D-thiogalactopyranoside) to increase plasmid copy numbers. Induced bacteria are harvested five hours later and used to prepare electro-competent cells by standard protocols [113]. H-PAC 61D6-*DH10B* cells are electroporated with purified 5^L mutant pDF-25 DNA [113]. Transformed H-PAC 61D6-*DH10B* cells are grown under Kan + Cm selection (25 µg/ml each) at 30°C overnight, allowing recombination between homologous sequences where the target sequence is now duplicated (one mutant and one wild type) with the pDF-25 vector in between. Transformed clones harboring the PAC (Kan resistance) and pDF-25 vector (Cm resistance) are arrayed on fresh Kan + Cm selection plates and placed at 43°C overnight, disallowing nonintegrated plasmid replication. Positive clones, with the integrated pDF25-mutant vector can be screened for sequence-specific integration using long-range PCR primers located outside of the recombined sequence. Correctly integrated clones with accurate long-range PCR fragment sizes (pDF25 vector length + mutant insert length + wild type sequence length), are regridded and selected using Kan (25 µg/ml) at 43°C overnight, allowing random excision of the recombination vector, such that a single copy of the target sequence remains as either WT-61D6 (5^R) or mutant 5^L-61D6. Growth at 43°C overnight disallows replication of pDF-25. Selected colonies are screened directly using colony PCR and diagnostic restriction enzyme digests that identify an altered enzyme recognition sequence introduced by the 5^L encoding point mutation. Colonies containing 5^L-61D6 sequences are reselected using Kan + high Str. Growth on high Str assures the loss of the rpsL + allele and thus the pDF-25 vector. Because the electro-competent host cells were induced and contained several copies of H-PAC 61D6, a small percentage of the selected clones will harbor both WT and mutant PACs; these colonies can be restreaked under Kan selection, allowing segregation of the WT and mutant clones into separate daughter cells.

E. coli clones harboring the introduced 5^L mutation and the WT 61D6 clone are then used for direct DNA isolation or to make preparative agarose plugs containing high molecular weight bacterial genomic and super-coiled PAC DNA [35]. Pulsed field gel electrophoresis resolves the high molecular weight bacterial genomic DNA away from unmodified WT 61D6 or modified 5^L PAC DNAs allowing direct comparison of WT and mutated PAC sizes [96]. DNA from 5^L-61D6 PACs that are the same size as the unmodified PAC (201 kb) can be isolated directly from the agarose plugs and characterized by PCR amplification of coding exons and long-range PCR of introns (WT and mut-61D6 PAC DNAs are amplified simultaneously allowing a direct comparison of exon content and intron size). Final confirmation of the introduced mutation and the flanking recombined sequences is performed by direct sequencing of mutant PAC DNAs.

Bacterial site-directed mutagenesis of the *MAPT* PAC provides significant advantages for studying the $^R5^L$ PSP mutation in a mouse model. It allows the characterization of transgene expression in the context of coding and flanking sequence regulatory elements and in the context of the PSP-associated H1 haplotype. To date, investigators have introduced three different tau mutations ($^V337^M$, $^N279^K$, and $^R5^L$) into H-PAC 61D6 using site-directed mutagenesis and the verified constructs used to generate transgenic mice that express mutant tau isoforms (P. Poorkaj and G. Shellenberg, unpublished results). Investigators are currently pathologically and phenotypically characterizing these transgenic lines and hopefully the lines will recapitulate the PSP and PSP-like disease states ($^N279^K$ and $^R5^L$) by more accurately representing the disease mechanisms that occur in humans.

References

1. Anderton, B., and G. Gibb. 1997. Cytoskeletal probes in neurodegenerative disease and the characteristics of tau in progressive supranuclear palsy (PSP). In *Abstracts: Progressive supranuclear palsy (PSP Europe International Workshop). Mov Disord* **236**:262–264.
2. Andreadis, A., J.A. Broderick, and K.S. Kosik. 1995. Relative exon affinities and suboptimal splice site signals lead to non-equivalence of two cassette exons. *Nucleic Acids Res* **23**:3585–3593.
3. Andreadis, A., W.M. Brown, and K.S. Kosik. 1992. Structure and novel exons of the human-tau gene. *Biochemistry* **31**:10626–10633.
4. Baker, M., I. Litvan, H. Houlden, J. Adamson, D. Dickson, J. Pereztur, J. Hardy, et al. 1999. Association of an extended haplotype in the tau gene with progressive supranuclear palsy. *Hum Molec Genet* **8**:711–715.
5. Barghorn, S., Q. Zheng-Fischhofer, M. Ackmann, J. Biernat, M. von Bergen, E.-M. Mandelkow, and E. Mandelkow. 2000. Structure, microtubule interactions, and paired helical filament aggregation by tau mutants of frontotemporal dementias. *Biochemistry* **39**:11714–11721.
6. Bennett, P., V. Bonifati, U. Bonuccelli, C. Colosimo, M. De Mari, G. Fabbrini, R. Marconi, et al. 1998. Direct genetic evidence for involvement of tau in progressive supranuclear palsy. European Study Group on Atypical Parkinsonism Consortium. *Neurology* **51**:982–5.
7. Bird, T.D., E.M. Wijsman, D. Nochlin, M. Leehey, S.M. Sumi, H. Payami, P. Poorkaj, et al. 1997. Chromosome 17 and hereditary dementia: Linkage studies in three non-Alzheimer families and kindreds with late onset FAD. *Neurology* **48**:949–954.
8. Blin, J., M. Ruberg, and J.C. Baron. 1992. Positron emission tomography studies. In *Progressive supranuclear palsy: clinical and research approaches*. pp. 155–168. New York: Oxford University Press.

9. Bondolfi, L., M. Calhoun, F. Ermini, H. G. Kuhn, K. H. Wiederhold, L. Walker, M. Staufenbiel, and M. Jucker. 2002. Amyloid-associated neuron loss and gliogenesis in the neocortex of amyloid precursor protein transgenic mice. *J Neuroscience* **22**:515–522.
10. Boutajangout, A., K. Leroy, N. Touchet, M. Authelet, V. Blanchard, G. Tremp, L. Pradier, and J. P. Brion. 2002. Increased tau phosphorylation but absence of formation of neurofibrillary tangles in mice double transgenic for human tau and Alzheimer mutant (M146L) presenilin-1. *Neurosci Lett* **318**:29–33.
11. Bowen, J.H., D.M. Maraganore, S.K. McDonnell, and W.A. Rocca. 1997. Incidence of progressive supranuclear palsy and multiple system atrophy in Olmsted County, Minnesota, 1976–1990. *Neurology* **49**:1284–1288.
12. Boyne, L.J., A. Tessler, M. Murray, and I. Fischer. 1995. Distribution of big tau in the central nervous system of the adult and the developing rat. *J Comp Neurol* **358**:279–293.
13. Brown, J., P. Lantos, M. Stratton, P. Roques, and M. Rossor. 1993. Familial progressive supranuclear palsy. *J Neurol Neurosurg Psych* **56**:473–476.
14. Butner, K.A., and M.W. Kirschner. 1991. Tau protein binding to microtubules through a flexible array of distributed weak sites. *J Cell Biol* **115**:717–730.
15. Caceres, A., and K.S. Kosik. 1990. Inhibition or neurite polarity by tau antisense oligonucleotides in primary cerebellar neurons. *Nature* **343**:461–463.
16. Caceres, A., S. Potrebic, and K.S. Kosik. 1991. The effect of tau antisense oligonucleotides on neurite formation of cultured cerebellar macroneurons. *J Neurosci* **11**:1515–1523.
17. Chen, W.T., W.K. Liu, and S.H. Yen. 1994. Expression of tau exon 8 in different species. *Neurosci Lett* **172**:167–170.
18. Clark, L.N., P. Poorkaj, Z. Wszolek, D.H. Geschwind, Z.S. Nasreddine, B. Miller, D. Li, et al. 1998. Pathogenic implications of mutations in the tau gene in pallido-ponto-nigral degeneration and related neurodegenerative disorders linked to chromosome 17. *Proc Natl Acad Sci U S A* **95**:13103–13107.
19. Collet, J., L. Fehrat, H. Pollard, L.R. Depouplana, G. Charton, A. Bernard, J. Moreau, et al. 1997. Developmentally regulated alternative splicing of mRNAs encoding N-terminal tau variants in the rat hippocampus: Structural and functional implications. *Eur J Neurosci* **9**:2723–2733.
20. Conrad, C., A. Andreadis, J. Trojanowski, D. Dickson, D. Kang, X. Chen, W. Wiederholt, et al. 1997. Genetic evidence for the involvement of Tau in progressive supranuclear palsy. *Ann Neurol* **47**:277–281.
21. Conrad, C., C. Vianna, M. Freeman, and P. Davies. 2002. A polymorphic gene nested within an intron of the tau gene: Implications for Alzheimer's disease. *Proc Natl Acad Sci U S A* **99**:7751–7756.
22. Cook, L., C.E. Brayne, D. Easton, J.G. Evans, J. Xuereb, N.J. Cairns, and D.C. Rubinsztein. 2002. No evidence for an association between Saitohin Q7R polymorphism and Alzheimer's disease. *Ann Neurol* **52**:690–691.
23. Court, D.L., S. Swaminathan, D. Yu, H. Wilson, T. Baker, M. Bubunenko, J. Sawitzke, and S.K. Sharan. 2003. Mini-lambda: a tractable system for chromosome and BAC engineering. *Gene* **315**: 63–69.
24. D'Souza, I., P. Poorkaj, M. Hong, D. Nochlin, V.M.Y. Lee, T.D. Bird, and G.D. Schellenberg. 1999. Missense and silent tau gene mutations cause front temporal dementia with parkinsonism—chromosome 17 type by affecting multiple alternative RNA splicing regulatory elements. *Proc Natl Acad Sci U S A* **96**:5598–5603.
25. D'Souza, I., and G.D. Schellenberg. 2000. Determinants of 4 repeat tau expression: Coordination between enhancing and inhibitory splicing sequences for exon 10 inclusion. *J Biol Chem* **275**:17700–17709.
26. David, N.J., E.A. Mackey, and J.L. Smith. 1968. Further observations in progressive supranuclear palsy. *Neurology* **18**:349–356.
27. De Silva, R., A. Hope, A. Pittman, M.E. Weale, H.R. Morris, N.W. Wood, and A.J. Lees. 2003. Strong association of the Saitohin gene Q7 variant with progressive supranuclear palsy. *Neurology* **61**:407–409.
28. Delisle, M.B., J.R. Murrell, R. Richardson, J.A. Trofatter, O. Rascol, X. Soulages, M. Mohr, et al. 1999. A mutation at codon 279 (N279K) in exon 10 of the Tau gene causes a tauopathy with dementia and supranuclear palsy. *Acta Neuropathol* **98**:62–77.
29. Duff, K., C. Eckman, C. Zehr, X. Yu, C.M. Prada, J. Pereztur, M. Hutton, et al. 1996. Increased amyloid-beta 42(43) in brains of mice expressing mutant presenilin 1. *Nature* **383**:710–713.
30. Duff, K., H. Knight, L.M. Refolo, S. Sanders, X. Yu, M. Picciano, B. Malester, et al. 2000. Characterization of pathology in transgenic mice over-expressing human genomic and cDNA tau transgenes. *Neurobiol Dis* **7**:87–98.
31. Flament, S., A. Delacourte, M. Verny, J. Hauw, and F. Javoy-Agid. 1991. Abnormal tau proteins in progressive supranuclear palsy. Similarities and differences with the neurofibrillary degeneration of the Alzheimer type. *Acta Neuropathol* **81**:591–596.
32. Foster, N.L., K. Wilhelmsen, A.A.F. Sima, M.Z. Jones, C.J. D'Amato, S. Gilman, and conference participants. 1997. Frontotemporal dementia and Parkinsonism linked to chromosome 17: A consensus conference. *Ann Neurol* **41**:706–715.
33. Gamblin, T.C., R.W. Berry, and L.I. Binder. 2003. Tau polymerization: Role of the amino terminus. *Biochemistry* **42**:2252–2257.
34. Games, D., D. Adams, R. Alessandrini, R. Barbour, P. Berthelette, C. Blackwell, T. Carr, et al. 1995. Alzheimer-type neuropathology in transgenic mice overexpressing V717F beta-amyloid precursor protein. *Nature* **373**:523–527.
35. Gautom, R.K. 1997. Rapid pulsed-field gel electrophoresis protocol for typing of Escherichia coli O157:H7 and other gram-negative organisms in 1 day. *J Clin Microbiol* **35**:2977–80.
36. Gazeley, S., and J.A. Maguire. 1996. Familial progressive supranuclear palsy. *Clin Neuropathol* 15:215–220.
37. Georgieff, I., R.K.H. Liem, W. Mellado, J. Nunez, and M.L. Shelanski. 1991. High molecular weight tau: Preferential localization in the peripheral nervous system. *J Cell Sci* **100**:55–60.
38. Georgieff, I., R.K.M. Liem, D. Couchie, C. Mavilia, J. Nunez, and M.L. Shelanski. 1993. Expression of high molecular weight tau in the central and peripheral nervous system. *J Cell Sci* **105**:729–737.
39. Ghatak, N.R., D. Nochlin, and M.G. Hadfield. 1980. Neurofibrillary pathology in progressive supranuclear palsy. *Acta Neuropathol* **52**: 73–76.
40. Goedert, M., M.G. Spillantini, R. Jakes, D. Rutherford, and R.A. Crowther. 1989. Multiple isoforms of human microtubule-associated protein tau: Sequences and localization in neurofibrillary tangles of Alzheimer's disease. *Neuron* **3**:519–526.
41. Goedert, M., C.M. Wischik, R.A. Crowther, J.E. Walker, and A. Klug. 1988. Cloning and sequencing of the cDNA encoding a core protein of the paired helical filament of Alzheimer disease: Identification as the microtubule-associated protein tau. *Proc Natl Acad Sci U S A* **85**: 4051–4055.
42. Golbe, L.I. 1996. The epidemiology of progressive supranuclear palsy. *Adv Neurol* **69**:25–31.
43. Golbe, L.I., P.H. Davis, B.S. Schoenberg, and R.C. Duvoisin. 1988. Prevalence and natural history of progressive supranuclear palsy. *Neurology* **38**:1031–1034.
44. Golbe, L.I., R.S. Rubin, R.P. Cody, J.M. Belsh, R.C. Duvoisin, C. Grosmann, F.E. Lepore, et al. 1996. Follow-up study of risk factors in progressive supranuclear palsy. *Neurology* **47**:148–154.
45. Gotz, J. 2001. Tau and transgenic animal models. *Brain Research Reviews* **35**:266–286.
46. Gotz, J., F. Chen, J. Vandorpe, and R.M. Nitsch. 2001. Formation of neurofibrillary tangles in P301L tau transgenic mice induced by A beta 42 fibrils. *Science* **293**:1491–1495.

47. Gotz, J., M. Tolnay, R. Barmettler, F. Chen, A. Probst, and R.M. Nitsch. 2001. Oligodendroglial tau filament formation in transgenic mice expressing G272V tau. *Eur J Neuroscience* **13**:2131–2140.
48. Grafman, J., I. Litvan, and M. Stark. 1995. Neuropsychological features of progressive supranuclear palsy. *Brain Cognit* **28**:311–320.
49. Gu, Y.J., F. Oyama, and Y. Ihara. 1996. Tau is widely expressed in rat tissues. *J. Neurochem* **67**:1235–1244.
50. Gustke, N., B. Trinczek, J. Biernat, E.M. Mandelkow, and E. Mandelkow. 1994. Domains of tau protein and interactions with microtubules. *Biochemistry* **33**:9511–9522.
51. Harada, A., K. Oguchi, S. Okabe, J. Kuno, S. Terada, T. Ohshima, R. Sato-Yoshitake, et al. 1994. Altered microtubule organization in small-caliber axons of mice lacking tau protein. *Nature* **36**:488–491.
52. Hasegawa, M., M.J. Smith, M. Iijima, T. Tabira, and M. Goedert. 1999. FTDP-17 mutations N279K and S305N in tau produce increased splicing of exon 10. *FEBS Lett* **443**:93–96.
53. Hauw, J.J., S.E. Daniel, D. Dickson, D.S.J.K. Horoupian, P.L. Lantos, A. McKee, M. Tabaton, and I. Litvan. 1994. Preliminary NINDS neuropathologic critical for Steele-Richardson-Olszewski syndrome (progressive supranuclear palsy). *Neurology* **44**:2015–2019.
54. Hayashi, S., Y. Toyoshima, M. Hasegawa, Y. Umeda, K. Wakabayashi, S. Tokiguchi, T. Iwatsubo, and H. Takahashi. 2002. Late-onset frontotemporal dementia with a novel exon 1 (Arg5His) tau gene mutation. *Ann Neurol* **51**:525–530.
55. Herreman, A., D. Hartmann, W. Annaert, P. Saftig, K. Craessaerts, L. Serneels, L. Umans, et al. 1999. Presenilin 2 deficiency causes a mild pulmonary phenotype and no changes in amyloid precursor protein processing but enhances the embryonic lethal phenotype of presenilin 1 deficiency. *Proc Natl Acad Sci U S A* **96**:11872–7.
56. Heutink, P., M. Stevens, P. Rizzu, E. Bakker, J.M. Kros, A. Tibben, M.F. Niermeijer, et al. 1997. Hereditary frontotemporal dementia is linked to chromosome 17q21–q22: A genetic and clinicopathological study of three Dutch families. *Ann Neurol* **41**:150–159.
57. Higgins, J.J., R.L. Adler, and J.M. Loveless. 1999. Mutational analysis of the tau gene in progressive supranuclear palsy. *Neurology* **53**:1421–1424.
58. Higgins, J.J., I. Litvan, L.T. Pho, W. Li, and L.E. Nee. 1998. Progressive supranuclear gaze palsy is in linkage disequilibrium with the tau and not the alpha-synuclein gene. *Neurology* **50**:270–273.
59. Himmler, A. 1989. Structure of the bovine tau gene: Alternatively spliced transcripts generate a protein family. *Mol Cell Biol* **9**:1389–1396.
60. Himmler, A., D. Drechsel, M.W. Kirschner, and D.W. Martin. 1989. Tau consists of a set of proteins with repeated C-terminal microtubule-binding domains and variable N-terminal domains. *Mol Cell Biol* **9**:1381–1388.
61. Hof, P.R., A. Delacourte, and C. Bouras. 1992. Distribution of cortical neurofibrillary tangels in progressive supranuclear palsy: A quantitative analysis of six cases. *Acta Neuropathol* **84**:45–51.
62. Hong, M., V. Zhukareva, V. Vogelsberg-Ragaglia, Z. Wszolek, L. Reed, B.I. Miller, D.H. Geschwind, T.D. Bird, et al. 1998. Mutation-specific functional impairments in distinct tau isoforms of hereditary FTDP-17. *Science* **282**:1914–1917.
63. Hsiao, K. K., D.R. Borchelt, K. Olson, R. Johannsdottir, C. Kitt, W. Yunis, S. Xu, et al. 1995. Age related CNS disorder and early death in transgenic FVB/N mice overexpressing Alzheimer amyloid precursor proteins. *Neuron* **15**:1203–1218.
64. Hutton, M., C.L. Lendon, P. Rizzu, M. Baker, S. Froelich, H. Houlden, S. Pickering-Brown, et al. 1998. Association of missense and 5′-splice-site mutations in tau with the inherited dementia FTDP-17. *Nature* **393**:702–705.
65. Hutton, M., J. Lewis, D. Dickson, S.H. Yen, and E. McGowan. 2001. Analysis of tauopathies with transgenic mice. *Trends Mol Med* **7**:467–470.
66. Imam, A.M., G.P. Patrinos, M. de Krom, S. Bottardi, R.J. Janssens, E. Katsantoni, A.W. Wai, et al. 2000. Modification of human beta-globin locus PAC clones by homologous recombination in *Escherichia coli. Nucleic Acids Res* **28**:E65.
67. Ioannou, P.A., C.T. Amemiya, J. Garnes, P.M. Kroisel, H. Shizuya, C. Chen, M.A. Batzer, and P.J. de Jong. 1994. A new bacteriophage P1-derived vector for the propagation of large human DNA fragments. *Nat Genet* **6**:84–89.
68. Jamsai, D., M. Nefedov, K. Narayanan, M. Orford, S. Fucharoen, R. Williamson, and P.A. Ioannou. 2003. Insertion of common mutations into the human beta-globin locus using GET Recombination and an EcoRI endonuclease counterselection cassette. *J Biotechnol* **101**:1–9.
69. Jamsai, D., M. Orford, M. Nefedov, S. Fucharoen, R. Williamson, and P.A. Ioannou. 2003. Targeted modification of a human beta-globin locus BAC clone using GET Recombination and an I-Scei counter-selection cassette. *Genomics* **82**:68–77.
70. Johnson, R., I. Litvan, and J. Grafman. 1991. Progressive supranuclear palsy: Altered sensory processing leads to degraded cognition. *Neurology* **41**:1257–1262.
71. Judkins, A.R., M.S. Forman, K. Uryu, D.A. Hinkle, A.K. Asbury, V.M.Y. Lee, and J.Q. Trojanowski. 2002. Co-occurrence of Parkinson's disease with progressive supranuclear palsy. *Acta Neuropathologica* **103**:526–530.
72. Kosik, K.S., L.D. Orecchio, S. Bakalis, and R.L. Neve. 1989. Developmentally regulated expression of specific tau sequences. *Neuron* **2**:1389–1397.
73. Kraemer, B.C., B. Zhang, J.B. Leverenz, J.H. Thomas, J.Q. Trojanowski, and G.D. Schellenberg. 2003. Neurodegeneration and defective neurotransmission in a *Caenorhabditis elegans* model of tauopathy. *Proc Natl Acad Sci U S A* **100**:9980–9985
74. Kuda, T., M. Shoji, H. Arai, S. Kawashima, and T.C. Saido. 1997. Reduction of plasma glutamyl aminopeptidase activity in sporadic Alzheimer's disease. *Biochem Biophys Res Comm* **231**:526–530.
75. Kulnane, L.S., and B.T. Lamb. 2001. Neuropathological characterization of mutant amyloid precursor protein yeast artificial chromosome transgenic mice. *Neurobiol Dis* **8**:982–992.
76. Lee, G., N. Cowan, and M. Kirschner. 1988. The primary structure and heterogeneity of tau protein from mouse brain. *Science* **239**:285–288.
77. Lee, V.M.Y., M. Goedert, and J.Q. Trojanowski. 2001. Neurodegenerative tauopathies. *Ann Rev Neurosci* **24**:1121–1159.
78. Lendon, C.L., T. Lynch, J. Norton, D.W. Mckeel, F. Busfield, N. Craddock, S. Chakraverty, et al. 1998. Hereditary dysphasic disinhibition dementia: A frontotemporal dementia linked to 17q21–22. *Neurology* **50**:1546–1555.
79. Lewis, J., D.W. Dickson, W.L. Lin, L. Chisholm, A. Corral, G. Jones, S.H. Yen, N. Sahara, et al. 2001. Enhanced neurofibrillary degeneration in transgenic mice expressing mutant tau and APP. *Science* **293**: 1487–1491.
80. Lewis, J., E. McGowan, J. Rockwood, H. Melrose, P. Nacharaju, M. Van Slegtenhorst, et al. (2000). Neurofibrillary tangles, amyotrophy and progressive motor disturbance in mice expressing mutant (P301L) tau protein. *Nat Genet* **25**:402–405.
81. Lippa, C.F., V. Zhukareva, T. Kawarai, K. Uryu, M. Shafiq, L.E. Nee, J. Grafman, et al. 2000. Frontotemporal dementia with novel tau pathology and a Glu342Val tau mutation. *Ann Neurol* **48**.850–858.
82. Litvan, I. 1998. Progressive supranuclear palsy revisited. *Acta Neurologica Scandinavica* **98**:73–84.
83. Litvan, I., D.W. Dickson, J.A. Buttner-Ennever, A. Delacourte, M. Hutton, B. Dubois, L.I. Golbe, et al., and participants in the First International Brainstorming Conference on PSP. 2000. Research goals in progressive supranuclear palsy. First International Brainstorming Conference on PSP. *Move Disord* **15**:446–458.

84. Litvan I., J. Grafman, C. Gomez, and T.N. Chase. 1989. Memory impairment in patients with progressive supranuclear palsy. *Arch Neurol* **46**:765–767.

85. Liu, W.K., T.V. Le, J. Adamson, M. Baker, N. Cookson, J. Hardy, M. Hutton, et al. 2001. Relationship of the extended tau haplotype to tau biochemistry and neuropathology in progressive supranuclear palsy. *Ann Neurol* **50**:494–502.

86. Maher, E.R., E.M. Smith, and A.J. Lees. 1985. Cognitive deficits in the Steele-Richardson-Olszewski syndrome (progressive supranuclear palsy). *J Neurol Neurosurg Psych* **48**:1234–1239.

87. Martin, E.R., W.K. Scott, M.A. Nance, R.L. Watts, J.P. Hubble, W.C. Koller, K. Lyons, et al. 2001. Association of single-nucleotide polymorphisms of the tau gene with late-onset Parkinson disease. *JAMA* **286**:2245–2250.

88. Mavilia, C., D. Couchie, M.G. Mattei, M.P. Nivez, and J. Nunez. 1993. High and low molecular weight tau proteins are differentially expressed from a single gene. *J Neurochem* **61**:1073–1081.

89. Mavilia, C., D. Couchie, and J. Nunez. 1994. Diversity of high-molecular weight tau proteins in different regions of the central nervous system. *J Neurochem* **63**:2300–2306.

90. Morales, B., A. Martinez, I. Gonzalo, L. Vidal, R. Ros, E. Gomez-Tortosa, A. Rabano, et al. 2002. Steele-Richardson-Olszewski syndrome in a patient with a single C212Y mutation in the parkin protein. *Mov Disord* **17**:1374–1380.

91. Morris, H.R., G. Gibb, R. Katzenschlager, N.W. Wood, D.P. Hanger, C. Strand, T. Lashley, et al. 2002. Pathological, clinical and genetic heterogeneity in progressive supranuclear palsy. *Brain* **125**:969–975.

92. Morris, H.R., R. Katzenschlager, J.C. Janssen, J.M. Brown, M. Ozansoy, N. Quinn, T. Revesz, et al. 2002. Sequence analysis of tau in familial and sporadic progressive supranuclear palsy. *J Neurol Neurosurg Psych* **72**:388–390.

93. Morris, H.R., Y. Osaki, J. Holton, A.J. Lees, N.W. Wood, T. Revesz, and N. Quinn. 2003. Tau exon 10 + 16 mutation FTDP-17 presenting clinically as sporadic young onset PSP. *Neurology* **61**:102–104.

94. Narayanan, K., R. Williamson, Y. Zhang, A.F. Stewart, and P.A. Ioannou. 1999. Efficient and precise engineering of a 200 kb beta-globin human/bacterial artificial chromosome in E. coli DH10B using an inducible homologous recombination system. *Gene Ther* **6**:442–447.

95. Nath, U., Y. Benshlomo, R.G. Thomson, H.R. Morris, N.W. Wood, A.J. Lees, and D.J. Burn. 2001. The prevalence of progressive supranuclear palsy (Steele-Richardson-Olszewski syndrome) in the UK. *Brain* **124**:1438–1449.

96. Navas, P.A., Q. Li, K.R. Peterson, R.A. Swank, A. Rohde, J. Roy, and G. Stamatoyannopoulos. 2002. Activation of the beta-like globin genes in transgenic mice is dependent on the presence of the beta-locus control region. *Hum Mol Genet* **11**:893–903.

97. Nefedov, M., R. Williamson, and P.A. Ioannou. 2000. Insertion of disease-causing mutations in BACs by homologous recombination in Escherichia coli. *Nucleic Acids Res* **28**:E79

98. Ohara, S., K. Kondo, H. Morita, K. Maruyama, S. Ikeda, and N. Yanagisawa. 1992. Progressive supranuclear palsy-like syndrome in two siblings of a consanguineous marriage. *Neurology* **42**:1009–1014.

99. Pastor, P., M. Ezquerra, E. Tolosa, E. Munoz, M.J. Marti, F. Valldeoriola, J.L. Molinuevo, et al. 2002. Further extension of the H1 haplotype associated with progressive supranuclear palsy. *Move Disord* **17**:550–556.

100. Pastor, P., E. Pastor, C. Carnero, R. Vela, T. Garcia, G. Amer, E. Tolosa, and R. Oliva. 2001. Familial atypical progressive supranuclear palsy associated with homozygosity for the delN296 mutation in the tau gene. *Ann Neurol* **49**:263–267.

101. Peterson, K.R., P.A. Navas, Q. Li, and G. Stamatoyannopoulos. 1998. LCR-dependent gene expression in beta-globin YAC transgenics: detailed structural studies validate functional analysis even in the presence of fragmented YACs. *Hum Mol Genet* **7**:2079–2088.

102. Pillon, B., B. Dubois, F. Lhermitte, and Y. Agid. 1986. Heterogeneity of cognitive impairment in progressive supranuclear palsy, Parkinson's disease and Alzheimer's disease. *Neurology* **36**:1179–1185.

103. Poorkaj, P., M. Grossman, E. Steinbart, H. Payami, A. Sadovnick, D. Nochlin, T. Tabira, et al. 2001. Frequency of tau gene mutations in familial and sporadic cases of non-Alzheimer dementia. *Arch Neurol* **58**(3):383–387.

104. Poorkaj, P., A. Kas, I. D'Souza, Y. Zhou, O. Pham, M.V. Olson, and G.D. Schellenberg. 2001. A genomic sequence analysis of the mouse and human microtubule-associated protein tau. *Mamm Genome* **12**:700–712.

105. Poorkaj, P., N.A. Muma, V. Zhukareva, E.J. Cochran, K.M. Shannon, H. Hurtig, W.C. Koller, et al. 2002. A $^{R}5^{L}$ tau mutation in a subject with a progressive supranuclear palsy phenotype. *Ann Neurol* **52**: 511–516.

106. Rafal, R. 1992. Visually guided behavior. In *Progressive supranuclear palsy: clinical and research approaches*. pp. 204–222. New York: Oxford Univ. Press.

107. Reed, L.A., T.J. Grabowski, M.L. Schmidt, J.C. Morris, A. Goate, A. Solodkin, G.W. Vanhoesen, et al. 1997. Autosomal dominant dementia with widespread neurofibrillary tangles. *Ann Neurol* **42**: 564–572.

108. Riess, O., and R. Kruger. (1999). Parkinson's disease—a multifactorial neurodegenerative disorder. *J Neural Trans* Supplement **56**: 113–125.

109. Rosso, S.M., L. Donker Kaat, T. Baks, M. Joosse, I. de Koning, Y. Pijnenburg, D. de Jong, et al. 2003. Frontotemporal dementia in the Netherlands: Patient characteristics and prevalence estimates from a population-based study. *Brain* **126**:2016–22.

110. Roy, S., C.K. Datta, A. Hirano, N.R. Ghatak, and H.M. Zimmerman. 1974. Electron microscopic study of neurofibrillary tangles in Steele-Richardson-Olszewski syndrome. *Acta Neuropathol* **29**:175–179.

111. Sadot, E., R. Marx, J. Barg, L. Behar, and I. Ginzburg. 1994. Complete sequence of 3′-untranslated region of tau from rat central nervous system. *J Mol Biol* **241**:325–331.

112. Saito, Y., A. Geyer, R. Sasaki, S. Kuzuhara, E. Nanba, T. Miyasaka, K. Suzuki, and S. Murayama. 2002. Early-onset, rapidly progressive familial tauopathy with R406W mutation. *Neurology* **58**:811–813.

113. Sambrook, J., E.F, Fritsch, and T. Maniatis. 1989. In *Molecular cloning: A laboratory manual*, 2nd edition. New York: Cold Spring Harbor Laboratory Press.

114. Sanchez, M.P., I. Gonzalo, J. Avila, and J.G. De Yebenes. 2002. Progressive supranuclear palsy and tau hyperphosphorylation in a patient with a C212Y parkin mutation. *J Alzheimers Dis* **4**:399–404.

115. Schmidt, M.L., R. Huang, J.A. Martin, J. Henley, M. Mawaldewan, H.I. Hurtig, V.M.Y. Lee, and J.Q. Trojanowski. 1996. Neurofibrillary tangles in progressive supranuclear palsy contain the same tau epitopes identified in Alzheimer's disease PHF tau. *J Neuropath Exp Neurol* **55**:534–539.

116. Schrag, A., Y. Benshlomo, and N. P. Quinn. 1999. Prevalence of progressive supranuclear palsy and multiple system atrophy: A cross-sectional study. *Lancet* **354**:1771–1775.

117. Scott, W.K., M.A. Nance, R.L. Watts, J.P. Hubble, W.C. Koller, K. Lyons, R. Pahwa, et al. 2001. Complete genomic screen in Parkinson disease: Evidence for multiple genes. *JAMA* **286**:2239–44.

118. Shen, J., R.T. Bronson, D.F. Chen, W.M. Xia, D.J. Selkoe, and S. Tonegawa. 1997. Skeletal and CNS defects in presenilin-1-deficient mice. *Cell* **89**:629–639.

119. Siman, R., A.G. Reaume, M.J. Savage, S. Trusko, Y.G. Lin, R.W. Scott, and D.G. Flood. 2000. Presenilin-1 P264L knock-in mutation: Differential effects on A beta production, amyloid deposition, and neuronal vulnerability. *J Neurosci* **20**:8717–8726.

120. Soliveri, P., G. Rossi, D. Monza, F. Tagliavini, S. Piacentini, A. Albanese, O. Bugiani, and F. Girotti. 2003. A case of dementia

Parkinsonism resembling progressive supranuclear palsy due to mutation in the tau protein gene. *Arch Neurol* **60**:1454–6.

121. Spillantini, M.G., T.D. Bird, and B. Ghetti. 1998. Frontotemporal dementia and Parkinsonism linked to chromosome 17: A new group of tauopathies. *Brain Pathol* **8**:387–402.
122. Spillantini, M.G., R.A. Crowther, and M. Goedert. 1996. Comparison of the neurofibrillary pathology in Alzheimer's disease and familial presenile dementia with tangles. *Acta Neuropathol* **92**:42–48.
123. Spillantini, M.G., M. Goedert, R.A. Crowther, J.R. Murrell, M.R. Farlow, and B. Ghetti. 1997. Familial multiple system tauopathy with presenile dementia: A disease with abundant neuronal and glial tau filaments. *Proc Natl Acad Sci U S A* **94**:4113–4118.
124. Spillantini, M.G., J.R. Murrell, M. Goedert, M.R. Farlow, A. Klug, and B. Ghetti. 1998. Mutation in the tau gene in familial multiple system tauopathy with presenile dementia. *Proc Natl Acad Sci U S A* **95**:7737–7741.
125. Stamm, S., T.G. Zhang, D.M. Marr, and D. M. Helfman. 1994. A sequence compilation and comparison of exons that are alternatively spliced in neurons. *Nucleic Acids Res* **22**:1515–1526.
126. Stanford, P.M., G.M. Halliday, W.S. Brooks, B.J. Kwok, C.E. Storet, H. Creasey, J.G.L. Morris, et al. 2000. Progressive supranuclear palsy caused by a novel silent mutation in exon 10 of the tau gene. *Brain* **123**:880–893.
127. Steele, J.C., J.C. Richardson, and J. Olszewski. 1964. Progressive supranuclear palsy. *Arch Neurol* **10**:333–359.
128. Sumi, S.M., T.D. Bird, D. Nochlin, and M.A. Raskind. 1992. Familial presenile dementia with psychosis associated with cortical neurofibrillary tangles and neurodegeneration of the amygdala. *Neurology* **42**:120–127.
129. Tanemura, K., T. Akagi, M. Murayama, N. Kikuchi, O. Murayama, T. Hashikawa, Y. Yoshiike, et al. 2001. Formation of filamentous tau aggregations in transgenic mice expressing V337M human tau. *Neurobiol Dis* **8**:1036–1045.
130. Tatebayashi, Y., T. Miyasaka, D.H. Chui, T. Akagi, K. Mishima, K. Iwasaki, M. Fujiwara, et al. 2002. Tau filament formation and associative memory deficit in aged mice expressing mutant (R406W) human tau. *Proc Natl Acad Sci U S A* **99**:13896–901.
131. Tomonaga, M. 1977. Ultrastructure of neurofibrillary tangles in progressive supranuclear palsy. *Acta Neuropathol* **37**:177–181.
132. Tsuboi, Y., M. Baker, M.L. Hutton, R.J. Uitti, O. Rascol, M.B. Delisle, X. Soulages, et al. 2002. Clinical and genetic studies of families with the tau N279K mutation (FTDP-17). *Neurology* **59**:1791–1793.
133. van Swieten, J. C., M. Stevens, S.M. Rosso, P. Rizzu, M. Joosse, I. Dekoning, W. Kamphorst, et al. 1999. Phenotypic variation in hereditary frontotemporal dementia with tau mutations. *Ann Neurol* **46**: 617–626.
134. Vanier, M.T., P. Neuville, L. Michalik, and J.F. Launay. 1998. Expression of specific tau exons in normal and tumoral pancreatic acinar cells. *J Cell Sci* **111**:1419–1432.
135. Vermersch, P., Y. Robitaille, L. Bernier, A. Wattez, D. Gauvreau, and A. Delacourte. 1994. Biochemical mapping of neurofibrillary degeneration in a case of progressive supranuclear palsy: Evidence for general cortical involvement. *Acta Neuropathol* **87**:572–577.
136. Verpillat, P., S. Ricard, D. Hannequin, B. Dubois, J. Bou, A. Camuzat, L. Pradier, et al. 2002. Is the Saitohin gene involved in neurodegenerative diseases? *Ann Neurol* **52**:829–832.
137. Wei, M.-L., and A. Andreadis. 1998. Splicing of a regulated exon reveals additional complexity in the axonal microtubule-associated protein tau. *J Neurochem* **70**:1346–1356.
138. Wszolek, Z. K., Y. Tsuboi, R.J. Uitti, L. Reed, M.L. Hutton, and D.W. Dickson. 2001. Progressive supranuclear palsy as a disease phenotype caused by the S305S tau gene mutation. *Brain* **124**:1666–1668.

C H A P T E R

13

Rodent Models of Tauopathies

JADA LEWIS and EILEEN McGOWAN

I. TAUOPATHIES

The term "tauopathies" refers to a family of neurodegenerative diseases that includes frontotemporal dementia and Parkinsonism linked to chromosome 17 (FTDP-17), progressive supranuclear palsy (PSP), corticobasal degeneration (CBD), and Pick disease. Tauopathies are neuropathologically characterized by fibrillar lesions composed of aggregated tau protein (Spillantini and Goedert, 1998). These tau inclusions are primarily composed of filaments of hyperphosphorylated tau protein with paired helical, twisted ribbon, or straight morphologies (Kidd, 1964; Yagishita et al., 1981; Flament et al., 1991; Spillantini and Goedert, 1998). Despite the common tau pathology, tauopathies represent a diverse group of disorders with multiple and highly varied clinical manifestations.

FTDP-17 is an autosomal dominant condition caused by mutations in the microtubule-associated protein tau; the most commonly identified mutation is P301L, which resides within exon 10 encoding one of four microtubule-binding domains (Hutton et al., 1998; Poorkaj et al., 1998; Spillantini et al., 1998). To date, more than thirty mutations in approximately 100 families have been reported [for a current listing of tau mutations, see the Alzheimer Disease & Frontotemporal Dementia Mutation Database (web address: molgen-www.uia.ac.be) maintained by Marc Cruts and Roos Rademakers]. FTDP-17 patients display a highly diverse set of clinical and pathological features that are likely determined, at least in part, by the nature of the mutation in each family. Nonetheless, investigators used a general set of clinical and pathological features to define FTDP-17 (Foster et al., 1997), including behavioral, cognitive, and motor disturbances. Neuropathology generally includes degeneration of the frontal and temporal lobes with prominent neuronal loss and gliosis. Most families display prominent neuronal loss in the substantia nigra; however, the involvement of other subcortical regions and the hippocampus is variable. Spongioform change is observed in the superficial layers of the cortex with balloon neurons present in some families. Although investigators have observed tau inclusion pathology in all families with defined tau mutations, the nature of the tau inclusions varies in distribution, morphology, filament type, and isoform content. For example, a report on three families with the P301L mutation demonstrated some common phenotypic and neuropathological characteristics; however, age of onset (49.0 to 64.3 years), disease duration (5.4 to 8.0 years), presence of Parkinsonism, and the distribution of neuropathology (including within the brain stem) were highly variable (Bird et al., 1999).

PSP is an uncommon Parkinsonian movement disorder that is associated with early postural instability and supranuclear vertical gaze palsy (Litvan and Hutton, 1998). The brains of PSP patients have neurofibrillary tangles that are primarily localized to the basal ganglia, diencephalon, and the brainstem (Dickson, 1999; Ishizawa and Dickson, 2001). Brainstem regions that are usually affected in PSP include the locus ceruleus, pontine nuclei, and pontine tegmentum. Additionally, the cerebellar dentate nuclei and spinal cord are frequently affected in PSP patients; however, the spinal cord is not commonly studied (Dickson, 1999; Ishizawa and Dickson, 2001).

CBD is generally a sporadic disorder characterized by neurofibrillary lesions and ballooned neurons (Dickson, 1999). Tau pathology in CBD is located in the substantia nigra, locus ceruleus, and the raphe nuclei. The fibrillar tau lesions that are observed in both PSP and CBD contain predominantly four-repeat tau-isoforms; however, PSP lesions generally consist of straight filaments whereas CBD lesions contain twisted ribbon filaments (Spillantini and Goedert, 1998; Dickson, 1999).

Classic Pick disease, like CBD, is characterized by ballooned neurons plus tau positive, argyrophilic inclusions termed "Pick bodies." Pick bodies are frequently observed in the limbic and paralimbic cortices and the ventral temporal lobe and are composed of both straight and twisted filaments (Dickson, 2001). Yet another tauopathy, amyotrophic lateral sclerosis-Parkinsonism-dementia of Guam is largely characterized by neurofibrillary lesions in the subcortical brain regions as well in the spinal cord. Although this condition is essentially restricted to the island of Guam, it is currently uncertain to what degree genetic and environmental factors contribute to the development of this disease.

Alzheimer disease can also be considered a tauopathy due to the neurofibrillary pathology that is a hallmark of the disease. The other major pathological lesion in AD is the senile plaque composed of amyloid β. Therefore, AD can be considered to straddle two major disease classifications—the tauopathies and the amyloidoses.

II. THE TAU GENE

In 1998 investigators identified the first mutations in the tau gene (MAPt) in patients with FTDP-17 (Hutton et al., 1998; Spillantini et al., 1998; Poorkaj et al., 1998). The tau gene, located on human chromosome 17q21 (Neve et al., 1986), encodes the tau protein that binds tubulin, stabilizing microtubules through microtubule-binding domains. In addition to its maintenance role in the cytoarchitecture of neurons, and sometimes glia, tau also plays a role in axonal transport (LoPresti et al., 1995; Ebneth et al., 1998).

The function of the tau protein is regulated, in part, by both alternative splicing and phosphorylation. Alternative splicing of exons 2, 3, and 10 in tau mRNA produces six major tau isoforms (termed 0N3R, 1N3R, 2N3R, 0N4R, 1N4R, and 2N4R) (Goedert et al., 1989a, 1989b). Exons 2 and 3 encode N terminal domains, while exon 10 encodes one of four microtubule-binding domains. Exons 9, 11, and 12 encode the other three microtubule-binding domains. Tau proteins encoded from mRNA lacking exons 2 and 3 are referred to as 0N isoforms, whereas the presence of exon 2 alone or exons 2 and 3 together results in 1N or 2N isoforms, respectively. Similarly, tau mRNA containing exon 10 results in the tau isoforms with four microtubule-binding domains (4R); however, when exon 10 is absent, 3R tau is produced.

III. RODENT MODELS OF TAUOPATHY

The variable clinical, biochemical, and neuropathological features of each disease show the diversity of the human tauopathies. PSP and CBD as well as some cases of FTDP-17 appear to involve mainly four-repeat tau isoforms, whereas the tauopathy found in Alzheimer disease involves all six tau isoforms (Spillantini and Goedert, 1998). PSP, CBD, and ALS-FTD often have significant motor components, unlike AD and FTDP-17 where cognitive dysfunction is often the primary manifestation. Over the past five years, the advances in the genetics and biochemistry of the tauopathies have given researchers great tools to develop rodent models exhibiting a wide variety of tau neuropathological, biochemical, and behavioral features that represent the spectrum of human tauopathies. Some of these models express wild-type human tau while others express transgenic tau with mutations linked to the human tauopathy FTDP-17. In some cases, the resultant tauopathy occurs in the context of other pathological manipulations (i.e., kinase activation or amyloid plaque formation). As investigators publish additional studies and produce new models, the choice of mouse strain, tau isoform, and promoter clearly play a significant role in the ability of a transgenic line to model human tauopathy. This review will focus on the tau transgenic mouse models generated over the last five years, with emphasis on detailing the motor phenotypes present in each line.

A. Models Expressing Human Tau Alone

1. Tau Transgenics without Motor Phenotype

A number of tau transgenic mouse models lack any defined motor dysfunction. The absence of a motor phenotype in these tau transgenic mouse models may be influenced largely by the pattern of tau expression and the degree of tau pathology; however, the background strain and the choice of tau isoform may also affect disease development. In general, tau mice that lack motor dysfunction develop only early tau pathological changes such as pretangles. The promoters that drive the expression in these models vary, as do the levels of expression and the background mouse strains. Most of these models do not have high transgene expression in regions likely to affect motor function (i.e., the spinal cord). In all but one model lacking a motor phenotype, the tau transgene was the human 2N4R tau isoform (see table 1).

Duff and colleagues (2000) created a transgenic line, termed 8c, that expressed all six human tau isoforms from a wild-type human P1-derived artificial chromosome (PAC) containing the human tau promoter. Although all six human tau isoforms were expressed in this model, there was a significant bias toward three-repeat tau production. This model, generated in the hybrid background strain of Swiss Webster/DBA2/C57BL6 mice, lacked any profound characteristics of human tauopathy despite an almost fourfold overexpression of the human tau transgene. Although these mice exhibited little tau pathology alone, this group of researchers created a double transgenic line that has substantial tau pathology (Andorfer et al., 2003—see "Models expressing tau in combination with other proteins").

In an attempt to produce an aggressive mouse model of human tauopathy, Lim and colleagues (2001) utilized the

TABLE 1
A. Wild-type Tau Transgenic Models

Transgenic line	Transgene	Pathology	Behavior/Phenotype	Ref.
T44 line 7	MoPrP 0N3R tau	Tau immunoreactive axonal spheroids, rare NFT in old mice	Progressive motor weakness	Ishihara et al. 1999; Ishihara et al. 2001
8c	PAC (human tau)	Tau positive pretangles and dendritic processes	None	Duff et al. 2000
Tα1-3RT tau (line14)	Tα1-tubulin 0N, 1N, 2N3R tau	Tau fibrillary glial inclusions, loss of oligodendrocytes with aging	Progressive motor weakness, olfactory dysfunction	Higuchi et al. 2002; Macknin et al. 2004
htau40-1	Mo Thy-1.2 2N4R tau	Axonopathy, dystrophic neurites	Mild motor impairment	Spittaels et al. 1999; Tilleman et al. 2002
ALZ17	Mo Thy-1.2 2N4R tau	Pretangles, axonopathy, dystrophic neurites	Hindlimb clasping in aged mice	Probst et al. 2000

B. Mutant Tau Transgenic Models

Transgenic line	Transgene	Pathology	Behavior/Phenotype	Ref.
JNPL3	MoPrP P301L (0N4R) tau	Neuronal loss, pretangles and NFT, tau positive glial inclusions, axonopathy; apoptotic oligodendrocytes	Hindlimb weakness progressing to dystonia, loss of righting, reduced lifespan	Lewis et al. 2000; Zehr et al. 2004
pR5	Mo Thy-1.2 P301L (2N4R) tau	Pretangles and occasional NFT in cortes, brain stem and spinal cord	None	Götz et al. 2001
Line 2541	Mo Thy-1 P301S (0N4R) tau	Neuronal loss, NFT in limbic cortex, brain stem and spinal cord	general muscle weakness, tremor, leading to severe paraparesis	Allen et al. 2002
VLW	Mo Thy-1 G272V, P301L, R406W (2N4R) tau	Dystrophic neurites, pretangles, increased lysosomal bodies	None	Lim et al. 2001
G272V tau	MoPrP/tTA/tetOp G272V (2N4R) tau	Pretangles; tau filamentous inclusions in oligodendroglia	None	Götz et al. 2001
214	PDGFβ V337M (2N4R) tau	Tau immunoreactive pretangles	Abnormal performance in the elevated plus maze; hyperactivity	Tanemura et al. 2002
Tg748, Tg502, Tg492, Tg483	CamKII R406W (2N4R) tau	Pretangles, occasional NFT in aged mice	Impaired contextual and cued fear responses	Tatebayashi et al. 2002
RW	MoPrP R406W (2N4R) tau	Tau inclusions in the spinal cord, cerebellum, cortex, and hippocampus; impaired slow axonal transport of mutant tau	Progressive motor impairment (dystonia)	Zhang et al. 2004

(continues)

TABLE 1 *(continued)*
C. Multigenic/Modified Models

Transgenic line	Transgene/ Modification	Pathology	Behavior/Phenotype	Ref.
TAPP	Tg2576 × JNPL3 [HaPrP APP695$_{swe}$ × MoPrP P301L (0N4R) tau]	Amyloid pathology, neuronal loss, increased limbic neurofibrillary pathology	Similar to JNPL3	Lewis et al. 2001
3xTg-AD	PS1$_{M146V}$knockin/ Thy1.2 APP(695)$_{SWE}$/ Thy1.2 P301L (4R0N) tau	Amyloid pathology, precedes neurofibrillary pathology	None	Oddo et al. 2003; Oddo et al. 2004
P25/T	human p25 × JNPL3 [human p25 × MoPrP P301L (0N4R) tau]	Increased tau accumulation and pathology in brainstem compared to JNPL3	Similar to JNPL3	Noble et al. 2003
Htau	PAC (human tau)/ mouse × tau knock-out [8c × tau k.o.]	Progressive tau pathology in neocortex, hippocampus and hypothalamus; aggregated tau and PHFs present from nine months.	None	Andorfer et al. 2003
CNP tau-P301L/α-syn	M2 × Line 6 [BGH A53T human α-synuclein × CNP P301L (1N4R) tau*]	Filamentous tau and α-syn inclusions in oligodendroglia	Limb-twitch phenotype	Giasson et al. 2003
pR5	Tau P301L plus Aβ brain infusion	Cortical/hippocampal infusion of Aβ fibrils leads to fivefold increase in NFTs in the amygdala	As described for pR5	Götz et al. 2001
**Rat model	AAV2 (4R2N) P301L-tau	NFT in basal forebrain, AAV2-mutant tau injected into medial septum	None	Klein et al. 2004

*BGH: bovine growth hormone promoter, CNP: 2′-3′-cyclic nucleotide 3′-phosphodiesterase promoter.
**Direct infusion of AAV2-mutant tau into rat brain tissue.

mouse Thy-1 promoter to drive expression of the human 4R2N isoform containing three different FTDP-17 associated mutations (G272V, P301L, and R406W). This model, termed VLW, was generated on a C57BL6/CBA background. The researchers observed dystrophic neurites and hyperphosphorylated tau in the cortex and the hippocampus; however, tau phosphorylation at tangle-defining epitopes was absent (Ser396/404). This absence of phosphorylation at this epitope may be due to its close proximity to the R406W mutation included in the transgene. Although sarkosyl-insoluble tau filaments were isolated from the VLW mice, immunogold analysis of tau phosphorylation was not assessed in either the extracts or in tissue. Lim and colleagues (2001) reported increased lysosomal bodies in conjunction with tau immunostaining, which suggests that lysosomal abnormalities may result even from early tau dysfunction.

Tanemura and colleagues (2001, 2002) generated transgenic mice on a C57BL6/SJL background that expressed the 2N4R isoform of tau containing the FTDP-17-associated V337M mutation under the control of the PDGFβ promoter. These animals developed early markers of tau dysfunction (pretangles) in the hippocampus that reportedly resulted in behavioral deficits. The deficits included hyperactivity and impaired performance on the elevated plus maze test often used as a test for anxiety. No motor dysfunction was observed.

Tatebayashi and colleagues (2002) used the CamKII promoter to express the 2N4R tau isoform containing the R406W mutation. The researchers generated this model on the C57BL6/SJL background. Despite the significant transgenic tau overexpression (nearly eighteen-fold) that was primarily distributed in forebrain neurons, the researchers observed mainly pretangles with only occasional tangles in mice up to eighteen months of age. Interestingly, impaired contextual and cued fear responses were reported in conjunction with this tauopathy. No motor dysfunction was noted.

Götz and colleagues (2001a) used a bigenic system to drive expression of the 2N4R tau isoform containing the FTDP-17-associated G272V mutation. This model expressed the tetracycline transactivator protein directed by the mouse prion promoter, allowing activation of the tau transgene, which was under control of the tetOp promoter sequence. These G272V tau transgenic mice were created on the C57BL6/DBA2 background. The researchers identified Thioflavin-S positive tau inclusions in the oligodendrocytes of the spinal cord; however, these aggregates were not silver positive. Pretangles were identified in the neurons of the G272V mice.

Götz and colleagues (2001b) also created transgenic mice expressing the 2N4R human tau isoform containing the P301L mutation under control of the mouse Thy-1 promoter. This model, termed pR5, was generated on a C57BL6/DBA2 background. Investigators observed pretangles and occasional neurofibrillary tangles in the brainstem, spinal cord, amygdala, and cortex of these animals (Götz et al., 2001b; Pennanen et al., 2004). Despite tau pathology within regions that control motor function and significant neuronal apoptosis, no motor abnormalities were observed in this model. The pR5 mice had greater levels of apoptosis than that reported for other P301L/S models (Zehr et al., 2004; Allen et al., 2002), which will be discussed in great detail below. Investigators reported increased exploratory behavior and loss of conditioned taste aversion in association with the tau aggregates identified in the amygdala of these P301L animals (Pennanen et al., 2004).

2. Tau Transgenics with a Motor Phenotype

Researchers made several attempts to model tauopathies using the wild-type human 2N4R tau isoform driven by the mouse Thy-1 promoter in FVB/N and C57BL6/DBA2 strain backgrounds (Spittaels et al., 1999; Probst et al., 2000). Despite transgenic overexpression up to tenfold over endogenous mouse tau levels, expression of human wild-type four-repeat tau on its own has resulted in models that develop only early markers of tauopathy characterized by pretangles, dystrophic neurites, and axonopathy; mature neurofibrillary lesions are absent from these models. Gliosis was generally associated with the tau pathology in the cortex and spinal cords of these animals. Additionally, mild motor impairments have been reported in conjunction with the limited tau pathologies.

Adult mouse tau is almost exclusively composed of four-repeat isoforms; however, adult humans express both three- and four-repeat tau (Goedert et al., 1989b; Kosik et al., 1989). In order to more closely model the context in which human tauopathies occur, two groups have attempted to express human three-repeat tau in transgenic mice. Ishihara and colleagues (1999, 2001) expressed the 0N3R wild-type human isoform under the murine prion promoter using the C57BL6/DBA2 background mouse strain. The tauopathy in these animals progressed from pretangles and axonal spheroids to occasional neurofibrillary tangles in older animals (one to two neurofibrillary tangles per section in two-year-old animals), and therefore, these mice represent a good model of tau dysfunction as it relates to aging. Investigators reported progressive motor weakness in these animals that likely reflected the tau immunopositive axonal spheroids and tau inclusions observed in the spinal cord.

Higuchi and colleagues (2002) overexpressed all three-repeat human tau isoforms (0N3R, 1N3R, and 2N3R) under the control of the T1α-tubulin promoter in the C57BL6/SJL background strain. Formic acid-insoluble tau accumulated in the spinal cord and cerebellum of twelve-month-old animals. By twenty-four months of age, fibrillar tau inclusions were evident in oligodendrocytes, but not in neurons, with a concomitant reduction in oligodendrocytes with age. The tau pathology was reminiscent of oligodendroglial-coiled bodies similar to those found in CBD and PSP. Researchers reported motor impairment in this model, manifesting as an impaired ability to stand on a slanted surface and hindlimb dystonia, and decreased olfactory function (Higuchi et al., 2002; Macknin et al., 2004).

In 2000 Lewis and colleagues generated transgenic mice that expressed the human 0N4R tau isoform containing the FTDP-17-associated P301L mutation. These P301L tau mice, termed JNPL3, developed a tauopathy characterized by neurofibrillary tangles and pretangles (Figure 1), reactive gliosis, neuronal loss, amyotrophy, and motor and behavioral dysfunction. The motor phenotype in these animals resembles aspects of human PSP, FTD-ALS, and some cases of FTDP-17 that have been attributed to the tau P301L mutation. Neurofibrillary tangles, both Thioflavin-S and Gallyas positive, were frequent in the neurons of the spinal cord and the brain, particularly in the basal telencephalon. Pretangles had a wider distribution throughout the brain. Neuronal loss was extensive in regions of concentrated tau pathology (e.g., the spinal cord and some brainstem nuclei). Pathological tau initially accumulated in axons, then only subsequently were the formation of the pretangle and filamentous tangles structures in neuronal cell bodies evident (Figure 2).

The presence of mainly straight filaments in the tau lesions likely reflects the transgenic expression of only a single tau isoform as opposed to twisted ribbon or paired helical filaments observed in the context of the expression of multiple tau isoforms in human tauopathies. Additionally, silver positive, neurofibrillary tau lesions were also identified in oligodendrocytes of the JNPL3 mice (Lin et al., 2003). In contrast to data from Götz and colleagues (2001b), oligodendrocytes, but not neurons, underwent apoptosis in this JNPL3 tau transgenic line (Zehr et al., 2004). Biochemically, transgenic tau, but not mouse tau, became progressively detergent insoluble with age. Notably, a 64kD species of tau accumulated in the detergent-insoluble fraction with age and disease progression, which represented an abnormal hyperphosphorylated species of 0N4R tau (Sahara et al., 2002). Investigators have observed this same species of 64kD insoluble tau in all human tauopathies in which the 0N4R isoform plays a role in the disease (Spillantini and

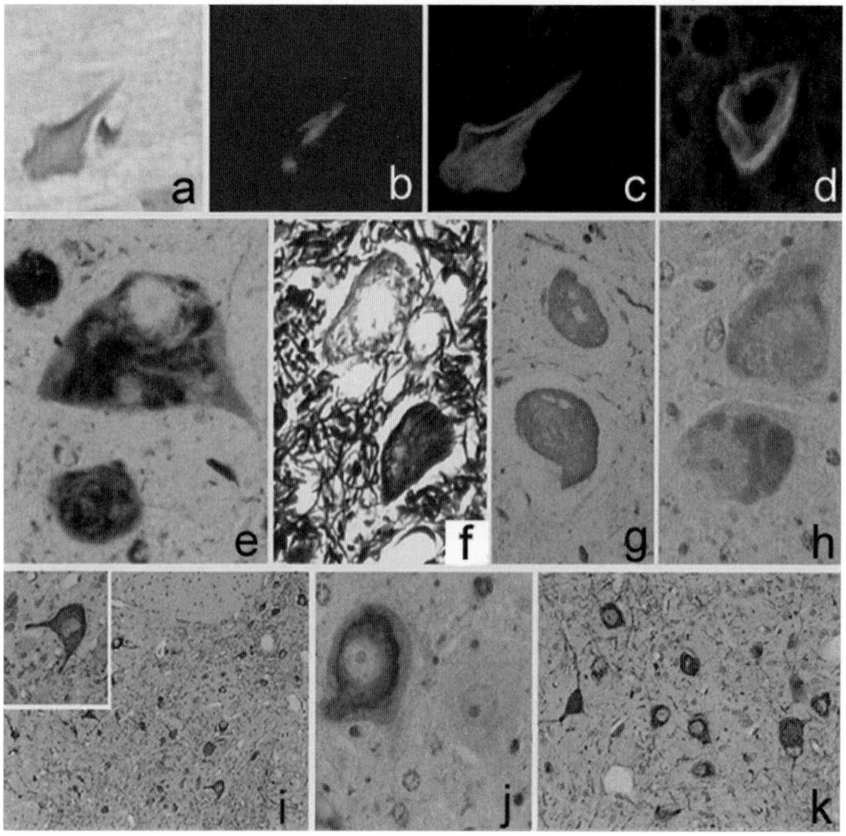

FIGURE 1 (See color version on DVD) Neurofibrillary tangles in the JNPL3 mice contain fibrillar, hyperphosphorylated tau. (a) Congo red staining under light microscope, (b) with polarization, and (c) with confocal microscopy demonstrates the fibrillary nature of the neurofibrillary tangles in the JNPL3 animals. These lesions are also positive for Thioflavin-S (d) as well as a variety of silver stains: Gallyas (e), Bielschowsky (f), and Bodian (g). Some of the neurofibrillary tangles were also immunopositive for ubiquitin (h). Both neurofibrillary tangles from the JNPL3 animals contained hyperphosphorylated tau-AT8 (i), AT180 (j), and CP13 (k).

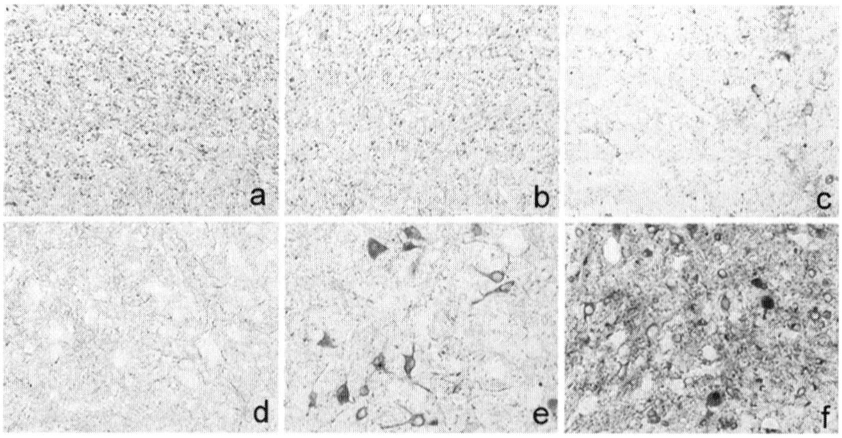

FIGURE 2 (See color version on DVD) Tau pathology in the white and gray matter of the spinal cord of JNPL3 mice. White matter (a–c) and gray matter (d–f) from 2M, 8M, and 12M JNPL3 female mice respectively are shown immunostained with MC-1, which detects an abnormal conformation of tau associated with human tauopathy. Abnormal tau accumulates first within the axons before accumulating within the neuronal cell bodies.

Goedert, 1998). Transgenic tau expression was equivalent to endogenous levels in the male mice and twofold endogenous tau levels in the female mice. This expression difference was reflected in the age of onset for the tauopathy in female versus male transgenic mice—females develop the disease approximately six months earlier than males.

Although the motor phenotype in the JNPL3 animals does not represent all human tauopathies, it can be a reliable marker for tau pathology and neuronal loss in the spinal cord, thereby allowing easy screening of therapeutic measures against tau dysfunction. Progressive behavioral symptoms include abnormal escape extension following tail elevation, progressive dystonia of hind limbs and tail, hunched posture, inability to right or slowed righting, poor performance or inability to complete the rope hand test, and weight loss. Onset of the initial motor dysfunction is often accompanied by docility and reduced vocalization and grooming. Based on the performance on rope hang, righting, and tail hang tests, we devised a simple scale to rate motor dysfunction in the JNPL3 mice (table 2). In the accompanying video, a JNPL3 mouse that would be classified at "severe stage" exhibits general ambulation difficulty, tail hang abnormalities, and inability to perform the rope hang test. Additionally, the gait test in which the paws of mice are colored with non-toxic ink to track gait abnormalities helps in following the progression of the motor phenotype, and thus the tauopathy, in the JNPL3 model. These behavioral tests are simple and do not require any specialized equipment. The motor dysfunction scale can be applied to any mouse model, not only tau models that exhibit a motor phenotype. This profound motor dysfunction has complicated the use of more complex behavioral tests, such as the Morris Water Maze, to track the progression of the tauopathy; however, recent data indicate that the extent of tau lesions in the hippocampus and neocortex results in impaired cognition as measured by water maze tasks (Arendash et al., 2004).

These JNPL3 mice were originally generated on a Swiss Webster/DBA2/C57BL6 hybrid background strain (Lewis et al., 2000), and the majority of the published data is from JNPL3 mice maintained on the outbred Swiss Webster background. However, recent evidence from our lab and others indicates that strain may influence the development and manifestation of tauopathy in this and other tau models (e.g., increasing C57BL6 strain in the background of JNPL3 animals delays the onset of tauopathy by as much as twofold over the normal age). Detailed analysis of these and other tau mouse models may reveal one or more modulators of tauopathy that do not affect the expression of the tau transgene but may affect key processes in the onset and progression of the disease.

Neurofibrillary tangles, neuronal loss, and motor dysfunction also characterize the transgenic model, Line 2541, which expresses the same human tau isoform, 0N4R, as in the JNPL3 animals but with the P301S mutation (Allen et al., 2002). Transgene expression was driven by the murine Thy-1 promoter in the C57BL6/CBA background mouse strain. Neurofibrillary tangles and pretangles develop in the spinal cord, brain stem, and in the limbic cortex and significant neuronal loss occurs in the spinal cord [at levels approaching 50%, similar to that observed in the JNPL3 animals (Lewis et al., 2000)]. No evidence of neuronal

TABLE 2 Motor Impairment Scale for JNPL3 Mice

Tests
Tail Hang (Score 0–2)
0—When lifted by tail, animal displays escape response
1—Animal does not exhibit full escape response, inward trend is evident
2—Animal maintains legs in scissored, clasped, or dystonic position
Righting Reflex (Score 0–2)
0—Mouse can right when placed supine
1—Mouse righting slowed
2—Mouse unable to right within 10 seconds
Rope Hang (Score 0–2) performed twice
0—Can complete test with at least three paws and tail within 2 minutes
1—Can hold on to rope without falling until 2 min. limit; does not complete
2—Falls before 2 minutes without completion
3—Unable to perform test

Motor Impairment Score:
1) Calculate S1 and S2 individually using the motor task tables:

S1		**Righting reflex**		
Tail Hang		**0**	**1**	**2**
	0	0	2	4
	1	10	12	14
	2	14	16	22

S2		**Rope 2**			
Rope 1		**0**	**1**	**2**	**3**
	0	0	1	3	5
	1	1	2	4	6
	2	3	4	5	7
	3	5	6	7	8

2) Add S1 and S2 scores from Motor task tables to determine stage of disease:

Total score (S1 + S2)	**Disease stage**
0–12	Normal
13–20	Mild/Early
21–23	Moderate/Mid
24–30	Severe/End

apoptosis was observed. The "half twisted" ribbon filaments observed in this P301S model were composed of human, not murine, tau. Biochemically, the insoluble, hyperphosphorylated tau isolated from this P301S model was similar to that obtained from cases of human tauopathy. Line 2541 mice (Allen et al., 2002) developed motor abnormalities similar to the JNPL3 mouse model reported by Lewis and colleagues (2000), including muscle weakness and paraparesis. Researchers achieved these phenotypic, pathological, and biochemical similarities between the JNPL3 and Line 2541 models using the same tau isoform and human tau with a mutation within the same codon; however, mouse strain and promoter were different.

Most recently, Zhang and colleagues generated transgenic mice, termed RW, that expressed the 2N4R human tau isoform containing the R406W mutation under the murine prion promoter. The RW transgenic mice were generated on the C57BL6/C3H background strain. Biochemically, the transgenic RW tau protein had reduced solubility and its ability to bind microtubules decreased with age. Somatodendritic accumulation of tau occurred in the spinal cord, neocortex, hippocampus, and cerebellum. Some of these aggregates were positive for Thioflavin-S, but silver staining was not reported. Ultrastructural analysis confirmed straight tau filaments within the inclusions. Reactive astrocytosis was also observed. Interestingly, the expression of the mutant tau protein in the RW mice impaired slow axonal transport of the mutant tau protein, likely leading to the somatodendritic accumulation of the tau protein. The RW mice developed motor impairment characterized by progressive hindlimb dystonia, which investigators assessed by the tail elevation test; approximately one-third of the RW mice developed motor impairments by twelve months of age. Additionally, the RW mice had a reduced lifespan, resulting in 90% mortality by two years of age compared to the nontransgenic mice and transgenic mice expressing wild-type 2N4R tau.

B. Models Expressing Tau in Combination with Other Protein(s)

Expression of wild-type human tau alone in transgenic mice has not resulted in a model of mature tauopathy; however, this appears to be due in part to the presence of murine tau in these transgenic mice. Andorfer and colleagues (2003) bred the wild-type human tau PAC mice (8c, Duff et al., 2000) to mice that lack the murine tau gene. Neither the 8c mice (Duff et al., 2000) nor the tau knockout mice (Tucker et al., 2001) developed tau pathology alone. The resulting offspring, termed Htau, expressed only human tau. These mice developed a progressive tauopathy that was characterized by the accumulation of insoluble, hyperphosphorylated tau protein in neurons of the neocortex and hippocampus. Ultrastructural analysis of the sarkosyl insoluble tau from these Htau mice showed paired helical filaments with a similar periodicity to PHFs isolated from human AD brain. Although these mice modeled many aspects of human tauopathies through wild-type tau expression, future studies that detail the degree of neurodegeneration and cognitive deficits present in these mice would be useful. This study was the first to demonstrate that abundant neurofibrillary pathology can be generated in a wild-type tau transgenic model.

The generation of tau transgenic mouse models has allowed the field to examine the interaction of tau protein with other proteins such as the amyloid precursor protein and alpha-synuclein. Lewis and colleagues (2001) bred the Tg2576 mouse model, which expresses mutant APP with the Swedish double mutation and develops significant amyloid plaque pathology (Hsiao et al., 1996), to the JNPL3 model (Lewis et al., 2000), which develops tau neurofibrillary tangles. Similar timing and distribution of amyloid plaque formation occurred between the parental Tg2576 line and the bigenic TAPP offspring. Neurofibrillary tau pathology occurred in the spinal cord, brain stem, and deep cerebellar nuclei as observed in the JNPL3 parental line; however, tangle pathology was significantly increased in the limbic system and the olfactory cortex of the TAPP animals, supporting an interaction between Aβ or APP and tau. Götz and colleagues (2001c) observed similar enhancement of neurofibrillary tau pathology following direct injection of Aβ42 fibrils into the brains (cortex and hippocampus) of P301L mice (pR5 line) (Götz et al., 2001b). These two studies, taken together, strongly support a pathogenic interaction between tau and amyloid beta in both our mouse models, but also in human Alzheimer disease.

Giasson and colleagues (2003) created a tau transgenic mouse model expressing the 1N4R tau isoform under the direction of the 2′,3′-cyclic nucleotide 3′-phosphodiesterase promoter named Line 6. To determine if an interaction existed between alpha-synuclein and tau, these P301L mice were bred to mice expressing wild-type alpha-synuclein (table 1). The tau and synuclein lines lacked inclusions of either protein up to eighteen months of age; however, bigenic synuclein/tau animals developed both Thioflavin-S positive tau and synuclein inclusions in oligodendrocytes from twelve months of age, suggesting that these two proteins may interact in the fibrillization of the other. These bigenic mice developed a limb-twitch phenotype that coincided with the detection of the Thioflavin positive inclusions. The results of these mouse models suggest that both tau and synuclein could potentially play a role in human synucleinopathies and tauopathies.

Oddo and colleagues (2003a, 2003b) attempted to develop a triple transgenic mouse model of Alzheimer disease, called 3xTg AD, by expressing the P301L 0N4R tau and APP (695)Swe genes on a gene-targeted mutant (M146V) presenilin 1 "knock-in" background. Intracellular accumulation of amyloid beta in this triple transgenic model occurred before the extracellular Aβ deposits, and the accumulated intracellular Aβ caused synaptic dysfunction. Later, investigators first observed extracellular amyloid deposits in the cortex and then in the hippocampus. These deposits preceded detectable tau pathology, which first developed in the hippocampus and then in the cortex. No motor phenotype has been reported for this model. These animals should prove useful for the study of amyloid and tau pathologies and for studies of how both intracellular and extracellular amyloid beta contribute to the disease process.

The role of specific kinases in the hyperphosphorylation of tau remains controversial. In an effort to determine the impact of enhanced cdk5 activity on tau pathology, Noble and colleagues (2003) bred the mutant P301L mice, JNPL3 (Lewis et al., 2000) with transgenic mice that express p25, the constitutive activator of the cdk5 (Ahlijanian et al., 2000). Tau hyperphosphorylation and tau neurofibrillary lesions were increased in the double transgenic mice, suggesting that either cdk5 on its own, or perhaps in conjunction with another kinase such as GSK3β, can influence the development of tauopathy. These data suggest that strategies aimed at reducing the activity of specific tau kinases have potential therapeutic value against human tauopathy.

In another approach, Klein and colleagues (2004) infused adeno-associated virus (serotype 2) incorporating 2N4R P301L human tau DNA into the medial septal region of rats to create the first rat model of tauopathy. Argyrophilic tau neurofibrillary tangles, pretangles, and neuropil threads were evident in the basal forebrain as early as one month post-transfection. The demonstration that tau neurofibrillary pathology can be rapidly induced in rats through gene transfer should make this a useful model to study tau-induced neurodegeneration.

IV. CONCLUSIONS

With pathology ranging from initial tau hyperphosphorylation to mature neurofibrillary tangles, a wide range of rodent models of tauopathy are now available. These models facilitate testing of potential tau therapeutics, determining the interaction of related proteins, observing disease-related gene expression, mapping disease progression, and determining environmental or molecular factors that may influence the impact of tau dysfunction. Despite these major advances over the past five years, our understanding of tauopathies would benefit from the development of gene-targeted mouse models with specific tau mutations or alterations. Gene-targeted tau mouse models would allow us to examine the effects of mutations in the context of endogenous isoform production and levels of expression, as well as proper spatial and temporal distribution of the tau protein. Negating these complicating factors that occur in all the current overexpressing wild-type and mutant tau models may allow us to fully understand the impact of tau dysfunction on the neurodegenerative process.

By generating transgenic mouse models that employ inducible systems of gene expression (i.e., tetracycline-off conditional system), we could explore which disease stages may be reversible. These studies would help us understand the degradation process for both normal and abnormal tau protein. Additionally, by creating an inducible tau transgenic mouse that does not express the transgene until aging has occurred, we can explore the exact role that aging plays in the disease process.

Although several mouse lines exist that model mature tauopathy, including the Htau mice created by Andorfer and colleagues (2003), none currently combine wild-type tau expression to form paired helical, filamentous tau inclusions distributed only in regions directly relevant to human tauopathies, neuronal loss, and cognitive dysfunction. Detailed studies of the currently available models should help guide the future generations of tau modeling so that the goal of the perfect rodent model of tauopathy can be met.

Video Legends

SEGMENT 1 Line test. JNPL3 tau transgenic mice show hind limb clasping and marked difficulty grasping onto a horizontal line.

SEGMENT 2 Walking test. JNPL3 tau transgenic mice show marked locomotor difficulty due to a combination of bradykinesia and quadriparesis.

References

Ahlijanian, M.K., N.X. Barrezueta, R.D. Williams, A. Jakowski, K.P. Kowsz, S. McCarthy, T. Coskran, et al., 2000. Hyperphosphorylated tau and neurofilament and cytoskeletal disruptions in mice overexpressing human p25, an activator of Cdk5. *Proc Natl Acad Sci U S A* **97**:2910–2915.

Andorfer, C., Y. Kress, M. Espinoza, R. de Silva K.L. Tucker, Y.-A. Barde, K. Duff, and P. Davies. 2003. Hyperphosphorylation and aggregation of tau in mice expressing normal human tau isoforms. *J Neurochem* **86**: 582–590.

Allen, B., E. Ingram, M. Takao, M.J. Smith, R. Jakes, K. Virdee, H, Yoshida, et al. 2002. Abundant tau filaments and nonapoptotic neurodegeneration in transgenic mice expressing human P301S tau protein. *J Neurosci* **22**:9340–9351.

Arendash, G.W., J. Lewis, R.E. Leighty, E. McGowan, J.R. Cracchiolo, M. Hutton, and M.F. Garcia. 2004. Multi-metric behavioral comparison of APPsw and P301L models of Alzheimer's disease: Linkage of poorer cognitive performance to tau pathology in the forebrain. *Brain Res* **1–2**: 29–41.

Bird, T.D., D. Nochlin, P. Poorkaj, M. Cherrier, J. Kaye, H. Payami, E. Peskind, et al. 1999. A clinical pathological comparison of three families with frontotemporal dementia and identical mutations in the tau gene (P301L). *Brain* **122**:741–756.

Dickson, D.W. 1999. Neuropathologic differentiation of progressive supranuclear palsy and corticobasal degeneration. *J Neurol* **246 (Suppl 2)**:6–15.

Dickson, D.W. 2001. Neuropathology of Pick's Disease. *Neurology* **56 (Suppl 4)**:S16–S20.

Duff, K., H. Knight, L.M. Refolo, S. Sanders, X. Yu, M. Picciano, B. Malester, et al. 2000. Characterization of pathology in transgenic mice over-expressing human genomic and cDNA tau transgenes. *Neurobiol Dis* **7**:87–98.

Ebneth, A., R. Godemann, K. Stamer, S. Illenberger, B. Trinczek, and E. Mandelkow. 1998. Overexpression of tau protein inhibits kinesin-dependent trafficking of vesicles, mitochondria, and endoplasmic reticulum: Implications for Alzheimer's disease. *J Cell Biol* **143**:777–794.

Flament, S., A. Delacourte, M. Verny, J.J. Hauw, and F. Javoy-Agid. 1991. Abnormal tau proteins in progressive supranuclear palsy. Similarities and differences with the neurofibrillary degeneration of the Alzheimer type. *Acta Neuropathol (Berl)* **81**:591–596.

Foster, N.L., K. Wilhelmsen, A.A. Sima, M.Z. Jones, C.J. D'Amato, and S. Gilman. 1997. Frontotemporal dementia and Parkinsonism linked to chromosome 17: A consensus conference. Conference Participants. *Ann Neurol* **41**:706–715.

Giasson, B.I., M.S. Forman, M. Higuchi, L.I. Golbe, C.L. Graves, P.T. Kotzbauer, J.Q. Trojanowski, and V.M.-Y. Lee. 2003. Initiation and synergistic fibrillization of tau and alpha-synuclein. *Science* **300**:636–640.

Goedert, M., M.G. Spillantini, M.C. Potier, J. Ulrich, and R.A. Crowther. 1989a. Cloning and sequencing of the cDNA encoding an isoform of microtubule-associated protein tau containing four tandem repeats: Differential expression of tau protein mRNAs in human brain. *EMBO J* **8**:393–399.

Goedert, M., M.G. Spillantini, R. Jakes, D. Rutherford, and R.A. Crowther. 1989b. Multiple isoforms of human microtubule-associated protein tau: Sequences and localization in neurofibrillary tangles of Alzheimer's disease. *Neuron* **3**:519–526.

Götz, J., M. Tolnay, R. Barmettler, F. Chen, A. Probst, and R.M. Nitsch. 2001a. Oligodendroglial tau filament formation in transgenic mice expressing G272V tau. *Eur J Neurosci* **13**:2131–2140.

Götz, J., F. Chen, R. Barmettler, and R.M. Nitsch. 2001b. Tau filament formation in transgenic mice expressing P301L tau. *J Biol Chem* **276**:529–534.

Götz, J., F. Chen, J. van Dorpe, and R.M. Nitsch. 2001c. Formation of neurofibrillary tangles in P301L tau transgenic mice induced by Abeta fibrils. *Science* **293**:1491–1495.

Higuchi, M., T. Ishihara, B. Zhang, M. Hong, A, Andreadis, J.Q. Trojanowski, and V.M.-Y. Lee. 2002. Transgenic mouse model of tauopathies with glial pathology and nervous system degeneration. *Neuron* **35**:433–446.

Hsiao, K., P. Chapman, S. Nilsen, C. Eckman, Y. Harigaya, S. Younkin, F. Yang, and G. Cole. 1996. Correlative memory deficits, Abeta elevation, and amyloid plaques in transgenic mice. *Science* **274**:99–102.

Hutton, M., C.L. Lendon, P. Rizzu, M. Baker, S. Froelich, H. Houlden, S. Pickering-Brown, et al. 1998. Association of missense and 5′-splice site mutations in tau with the inherited dementia FTDP-17. *Nature* **393**: 702–705.

Ishihara, T., M. Hong, B. Zhang, Y. Nakagawa, M.K. Lee, J.Q. Trojanowski, and V.M.-Y. Lee. 1999. Age-dependent emergence and progression of a tauopathy in transgenic mice overexpressing the shortest human tau isoform. *Neuron* **24**:751–762.

Ishihara, T., B. Zhang, M. Higuchi, Y. Yoshiyama, J.Q. Trojanowski, and V.M. Lee. 2001. Age-dependent induction of congophilic neurofibrillary tau inclusions in tau transgenic mice. *Am J Pathol* **158**:555–562.

Ishizawa, K., and D.W. Dickson. 2001. Microglial activation parallels system degeneration in progressive supranuclear palsy and corticobasal degeneration. *J Neuropathol Exp Neurol* **60**:647–657.

Ishizawa, T., N. Sahara, K. Ishiguro, J. Kersh, E. McGowan, J. Lewis, M. Hutton, D.W. Dickson, and S.-H. Yen. 2003. Co-localization of glycogen synthase kinase-3 with neurofibrillary tangles and granulovacular degeneration in transgenic mice. *Am J Pathol* **163**:1057–1067.

Kidd, M. 1964. Alzheimer's Disease—an electron microscopical study. *Brain* **87**:307–320.

Klein, R.L., W.L. Lin, D.W. Dickson, J. Lewis, M. Hutton, K. Duff, E.M. Meyer, and M.A. King. 2004. Rapid neurofibrillary tangle formation after localized gene transfer of mutated tau. *Am J Pathol* **1**:347–353.

Kins, S., A. Crameri, D.R.H. Evans, B.A. Hemmings, R. Nitsch, J. Götz. 2001. Reduced PP2A activity induces tau hyperphosphorylation and altered compartmentalization of tau in transgenic mice. *J Biol Chem* **276**:38193–38200.

Kosik, K.S., L.D. Orecchio, S. Bakalis, and R.L. Neve. 1989. Developmentally regulated expression of specific tau sequences. *Neuron* **2**: 1389–1397.

Lewis, J., E. McGowan, J. Rockwood, H. Melrose, P. Nacharaju, M. Van Slegtenhorst, K. Gwinn-Hardy, et al. 2000. Neurofibrillary tangles, amyotrophy and progressive motor disturbance in mice expressing mutant (P301L) tau protein. *Nat Genet* **25**:402–405.

Lewis, J., D.W. Dickson, W.L. Lin, L. Chisholm, A. Corral, G. Jones, S.H. Yen, et al. (2001) Enhanced neurofibrillary degeneration in transgenic mice expressing mutant tau and APP. *Science* **293**:1487–1491.

Lim, F., F. Hernandez, J.J. Lucas, P. Gomez-Ramos, M.A. Moran, and J. Avila. 2001. FTDP-17 Mutations in tau transgenic mice provoke lysosomal abnormalities and tau filaments in forebrain. *Mol Cell Neurosci* **18**:702–714.

Lin, W.-L., J. Lewis, S.-H. Yen, M. Hutton, and D.W. Dickson, 2003. Filamentous tau in oligodendrocytes and astrocytes of transgenic mice expressing the human tau isoform with the P301L mutation. *Am J Pathol* **162**:213–218.

Litvan, I., and M. Hutton. 1998. Clinical and genetic aspects of progressive supranuclear palsy. *J Geriatr Psychiatry Neurol* **11**:107–114.

LoPresti, P., S. Szvehet, S.C. Papasozomenos, R.P. Zinkowski, and L.I. Binder. (1995) Functional implications for the microtubule-associated protein tau: Localization in oligodendrocytes. *Proc Natl Acad Sci U S A* **92**:10369–10373.

Macknin, J.B., M. Higuchi, V.M. Lee, J.Q. Trojanowski, and R.L. Doty. 2004. Olfactory dysfunction occurs in transgenic mice overexpressing human tau protein. *Brain Res* **1000**:174–178.

Neve, R.L., P. Harris, K.S. Kosik, D.M. Kurnit, and T.A. Donlon. 1986. Identification of cDNA clones for the human microtubule-associated protein tau and chromosomal localization of the genes for tau and microtubule-associated protein 2. *Brain Res* **387**:271–280.

Noble, W., V. Olm, K. Takata, E.O.M Casey, J. Meyerson, K. Gaynor, J. LaFrancois, et al. 2003. Cdk5 is a key factor in tau aggregation and tangle formation in vivo. *Neuron* **38**:555–565.

Oddo, S., A. Caccamo, J.D. Shepherd, M.P. Murphy, T.E. Golde, R. Kayed, R. Metherate, et al. 2003a. Triple-transgenic model of Alzheimer's disease with plaques and tangles: Intracellular Ab and synaptic dysfunction. *Neuron* **39**:409–421.

Oddo, S., A. Caccamo, M. Kitazawa, B.P. Tseng, and F.M. LaFerla. 2003b. Amyloid deposition precedes tangle formation in a triple transgenic model of Alzheimer's Disease. *Neurobiol Aging* **24**:1063–1070.

Pennanen, L., H. Welzl, P. D'Adamo, R.M. Nitsch, and J. Götz. 2004. Accelerated extinction of conditioned taste aversion in P301L tau transgenic mice. *Neurobiol Dis* **3**:500–509.

Poorkaj, P., T.D. Bird, E. Wijsman, E. Nemens, R.M. Garruto, L. Anderson, A. Andreadis, et al. 1998. Tau is a candidate gene for chromosome 17 frontotemporal dementia. *Ann Neurol.* **43**:815–825.

Probst, A., J. Götz, K.H. Wiederhold, M. Tolnay, C. Misti, A.L. Jaton, M. Hong, et al. 2000. Axonopathy and amyotrophy in mice transgenic for human four-repeat tau protein. *Acta Neuropathol* **99**:469–481.

Sahara, N., J. Lewis, M. DeTure, E. McGowan, D.W. Dickson, M. Hutton, and S.-H. Yen. 2002. Assembly of tau in transgenic animals expressing P301L tau: alterations of phosphorylation and solubility. *J Neurochem* **83**:1498–1508.

Spillantini, M.G., J.R. Murrell, M. Goedert, M.R. Farlow, A. Klug, and B. Ghetti. 1998. Mutation in the tau gene in familial multiple system tauopathy with presenile dementia. *Proc Natl Acad Sci USA* **95**:7737–7741.

Spillantini, M.G., and M. Goedert. 1998. Tau protein pathology in neurodegenerative diseases. *Trends Neurosci* **21**:428–433.

Spittaels, K., C. Van den Haute, J. Van Dorpe, K. Bruynseels, K. Vandezande, I. Laenen, H. Geerts, et al. 1999. Prominent axonopathy in the brain and spinal cord of transgenic mice overexpressing four-repeat human tau protein. *Am J Pathol* **155**:2153–2165.

Tanemura, K., T. Akagi, M. Murayama, N. Kikuchi, O. Murayama, Y. Hashikama, Y. Yoshiike, et al. 2001. Formation of filamentous tau aggregates in transgenic mice expressing V337M human tau. *Neurobiol Disease* **8**:1036–1045.

Tanemura, K., M. Murayama, T. Akagi, T. Hashikawa, T. Tominaga, M. Ichikawa, H. Yamaguchi, and A. Takashima. 2002. Neurodegeneration with tau accumulation in a transgenic mouse expressing V337M human tau. *J Neurosci* **22**:133–141.

Tatebayashi, Y., T. Miyasaka, D.-H. Chui, T. Akagi, K.-I. Mishima, K. Iwasaki, M. Fujiwara, et al. 2002. Tau filament formation and associative memory deficit in aged mice expressing mutant (R406W) human tau. *Proc Natl Acad Sci U S A* **99**:13896–13901.

Tucker, K.L., M. Meyer, and Y.A. Barde. 2001. Neurotrophins are required for nerve growth during development. *Nat Neurosci* **4**:29–37.

Yagashita, S., Y. Itoh, W. Nan, and N. Amano. 1981. Reappraisal of the fine structure of Alzheimer's neurofibrillary tangles. *Acta Neuropathol (Berl)* **54**:239–246.

Zehr, C., J. Lewis, E. McGowan, J. Crook, W.L. Lin, K. Godwin, J. Knight, et al. 2004. Apoptosis in oligodendrocytes is associated with axonal degeneration in P301L tau mice. *Neurobiol Dis* **3**:553–562.

Zhang, B., M. Higuchi, Y. Yoshiyama, T. Ishihara, M.S. Forman, D. Martinez, S. Joyce, et al. 2004. Retarded axonal transport of R406W mutant tau in transgenic mice with a neurodegenerative tauopathy. *J Neurosci* **24**:4657–4667.

C H A P T E R

J1

Clinical Spectrum and Pathological Features of Multiple System Atrophy

CARLO COLOSIMO, FELIX GESER, and GREGOR K. WENNING

I. HISTORICAL REVIEW

The term multiple system atrophy (MSA) was introduced by Graham and Oppenheimer in 1969 to denote a neurodegenerative disease characterized clinically by any combination of autonomic, parkinsonian, cerebellar, or pyramidal symptoms and signs and pathologically by cell loss and gliosis in the basal ganglia and olivopontocerebellar system. Previously, cases of MSA were reported under the rubrics of olivopontocerebellar atrophy (OPCA), idiopathic orthostatic hypotension (IOH) or progressive autonomic failure (PAF), Shy-Drager syndrome (SDS), and striatonigral degeneration (SND). Although Dejerine and Thomas were the first to introduce the term OPCA in 1900, reporting two sporadic cases of late-onset ataxia, the case of Stauffenberg in 1918, diagnosed in life as OPCA, was the first to associate cerebellar, parkinsonian, and autonomic features with identified pathological lesions not only of olives, pons, and cerebellum, but also of basal ganglia (Quinn, 1994).

Name and Address for Correspondence, Carlo Colosimo, M.D., Dipartimento di Scienze Neurologiche, Università La Sapienza, viale dell'Università 30, I-00185 Rome, Italy, phone +39 06 4991-4711; fax +39 06 4457-705, e-mail: carlo.colosimo@uniroma1.it

The term SND was introduced in 1960 by van der Eecken, Adams, and van Bogaert (van der Eecken et al., 1960; Adams et al., 1961; Adams et al., 1964), who noted pronounced shrinkage and brownish discoloration of the putamen and pallidum as well as depigmentation of the substantia nigra in three patients with progressive and severe parkinsonism associated with cerebellar, pyramidal, and autonomic features. Earlier reports of SND probably include those of Fleischhacker (1924) and Scherer (1933a; 1933b) (Berciano et al., 1998; Wenning et al., 2000b). In 1960 Shy and Drager reported two cases with marked autonomic failure, slurred speech, ataxia, Parkinsonian features, pyramidal signs, and distal muscle wasting. Postmortem examination of Case 2 demonstrated pathological lesions consistent with MSA, including involvement of the intermediolateral cell column. Subsequently, the term SDS was erroneously widened to include cases of Parkinson disease (PD) and autonomic failure. Its further use has therefore been discouraged (Quinn et al., 1995). In 1989, Papp and colleagues reported the presence of glial cytoplasmic inclusions (GCIs) in the brains of patients with MSA regardless of presentation (SND, OPCA, and SDS). GCIs were not present in a large series of patients with other neurodegenerative disorders. The abundant presence of GCIs in all clinical subtypes of MSA introduced grounds for considering SDS, SND, and sporadic OPCA as one disease entity characterized by neuronal multisystem degeneration based on unique oligodendroglial inclusion pathology. Subsequently, neuronal and axonal inclusions were also identified in MSA brains; however, they were less numerous compared to GCIs (Papp and Lantos, 1992; Papp and Lantos, 1994). In the late nineties, α-synuclein immunostaining was recognized as the most sensitive marker of inclusion pathology in MSA, being superior to ubiquitin immunostaining which had previously been used (Wakabayashi et al., 1998c; Spillantini et al., 1998). Due to these advances in molecular pathogenesis, MSA has been firmly established as α-synucleinopathy along with PD and dementia with Lewy bodies (DLB) (Dickson et al., 1999). In parallel, the clinical recognition greatly improved following the introduction of diagnostic criteria. In 1989, Quinn first proposed a list of diagnostic criteria for MSA (Quinn, 1989b). Cases were classified as definite only when neuropathological confirmation was obtained. In the late nineties, a number of pitfalls associated with the Quinn criteria were identified and Consensus diagnostic criteria were therefore developed in 1998 (Gilman et al., 1998; Gilman et al., 1999). The Consensus (or Gilman) criteria have since been widely established in the research community and in movement disorders clinics. However, both Quinn and Consensus criteria remain to be validated prospectively.

II. MORPHOLOGICAL PATTERN OF VULNERABILITY

A. Gross Neuropathology of MSA

External examination of the brain is usually normal in MSA. However, when there is a significant involvement of the olivopontocerebellar system the appearances are characteristic. The cerebellum is small, with the hemispheres far from covering the occipital poles. The white matter of the cerebellum appears grey and the folia atrophic. The basis pontis and middle cerebellar peduncles are reduced. In the medulla, the protuberance of the inferior olives may be reduced. Occasionally, macroscopic abnormality is confined to the brainstem pigmented nuclei, and in these instances it is impossible to make a distinction from PD on naked-eye appearance alone (Daniel, 1999). In SND, the putamen is shrunken with grey-green discoloration. When pathology is severe, there may be a cribriform appearance. Atrophy and discoloration of the caudate nucleus and pallidum are less common. The substantia nigra invariably shows decreased pigmentation and the locus coeruleus may also appear pale.

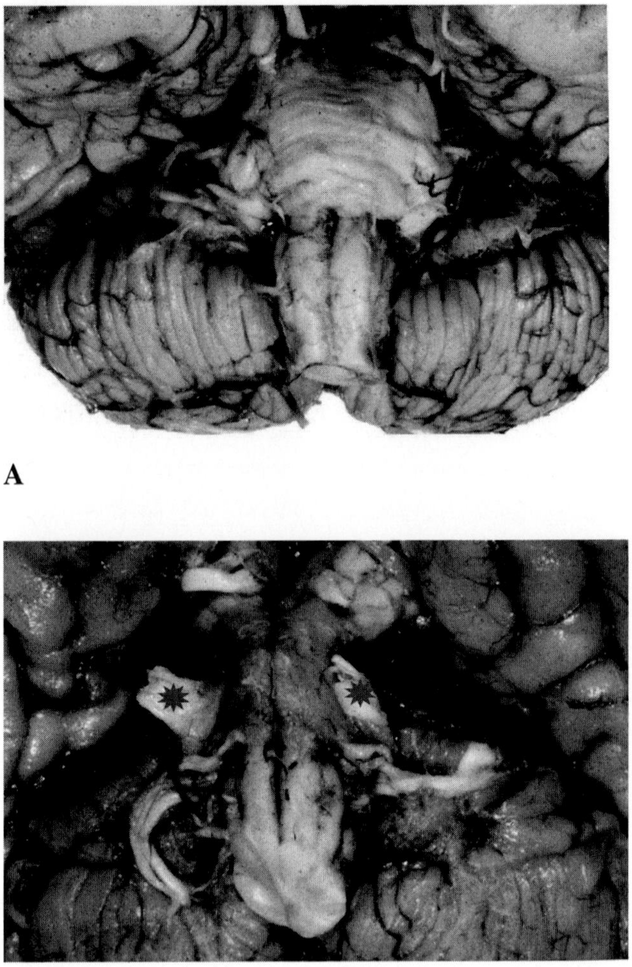

A

B

FIGURE 1 Macroscopic appearance of the brainstem. When compared with normal (A) in MSA (B) the pons and middle cerebellar peduncles are atrophic and the trigeminal nerves (*) are prominent (Daniel, 1999).

B. Microscopic Neuropathology of MSA

1. Cellular Inclusions

Glial inclusion formation is a prominent feature of MSA pathology (Quinn, 1994). Although inclusions have been described in five cellular sites, i.e., in oligodendroglial and neuronal cytoplasm and nuclei as well as in axons (Papp and Lantos, 1992), glial cytoplasmic inclusions (GCIs) (Papp et al., 1989) are most ubiquitous and appear to represent the subcellular hallmark lesion of MSA (Lantos, 1998). Their distribution selectively involves basal ganglia, supplementary and primary motor cortex, the reticular formation, basis pontis, the middle cerebellar peduncles, and the cerebellar white matter (Lantos, 1998; Papp and Lantos, 1994). Staining with antibodies against ubiquitin, α- and β-tubulin, and tau indicates an origin from cytoskeletal proteins. More recently, MSA has been recognized as an α-synucleinopathy with prominent glial cytoplasmic inclusion pathology (Wakabayashi et al., 1998a) (Figure 3). There also may be rod-like nuclear inclusions accompanying cytoplasmic inclusions in oligodendrocytes (Papp and Lantos, 1992).

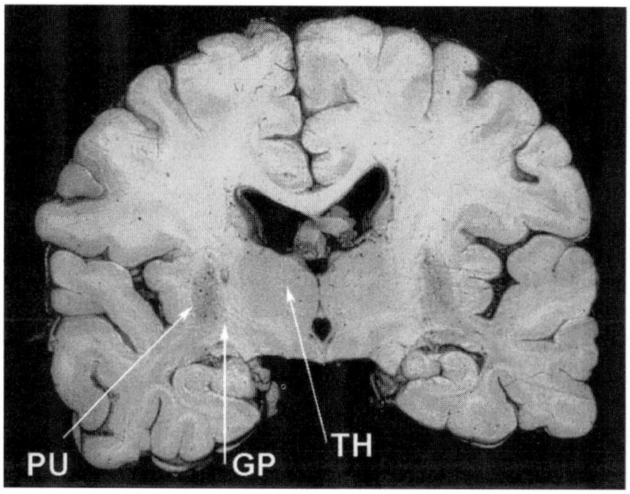

FIGURE 2 Coronal slice of cerebrum. The putamena are symmetrically shrunken. Pallida are atrophic. PU: Putamen, GP: Globus Pallidus, TH: Thalamus. (Reprinted with permission from Elsevier; *The Lancet Neurology* 2004. **3**:93–103.)

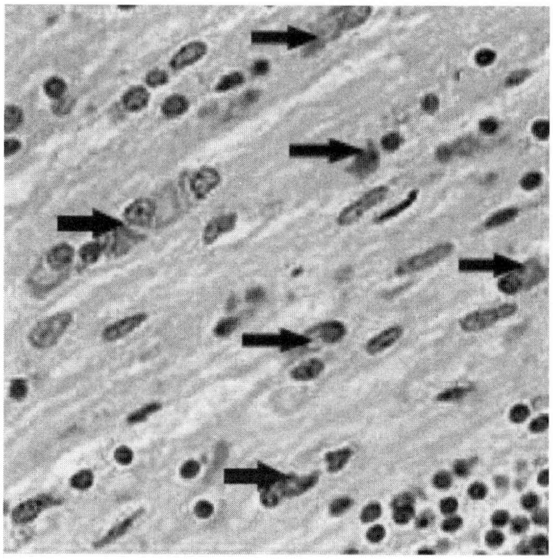

FIGURE 3 (See color version on DVD) α-synuclein immunostaining reveals GCIs in subcortical white matter. (Reprinted with permission from Whitehouse Publishing; ACNR 2004. **3**:5–10.)

Nuclear and cytoplasmic inclusions also occur in neurones and are ubiquitinated but distinguishable from those in oligodendrocytes by a lack of immunoreactivity for cytoskeletal proteins. Despite the different immunohistochemical reactions of the various inclusions described, electron microscopy invariably shows irregular filaments composed of 20–30 μm tubules (Papp and Lantos, 1992).

2. Striatonigral Degeneration (SND)

The striatonigral system is the main site of pathology, but less severe degeneration can be widespread (Figures 1 and 2) and usually includes the olivopontocerebellar system (Wenning et al., 1996b). In early stages, the putaminal lesion shows a distinct topographical distribution with a predilection for the caudal and dorsolateral regions (Kume et al., 1993). GCIs predominate, while nerve cell loss and gliosis can be difficult to identify without the aid of glial fibrillary acidic protein (GFAP) immunostaining. The majority of reports indicate that the small neurones, which normally outnumber the large by about 170 to 1, are preferentially affected (Papp and Lantos, 1992; Kume et al., 1993). As the disease progresses, the entire putamen is usually affected with the result that bundles of striatopallidal fibers are narrowed and poorly stained for myelin. When atrophy is severe, the neuropil becomes rarefied with very few remaining nerve cells lying among hypertrophic astrocytes. Brown pigment granules accumulate in astrocytes, macrophages, and around blood vessel walls; these granules have been identified as containing lipofuscin, neuromelanin, and iron (Daniel, 1999).

Nerve cell loss and gliosis occurs in the caudate nucleus, but rarely to the extent found in putamen; the dorsomedial region is usually most affected with gliosis extending through the striatal bridges. The globus pallidus may appear uninvolved or show a reduction of myelinated fibers with gliosis and variable neuronal depletion. Pallidal atrophy is generally considered to be secondary to loss of putaminal efferents (Ito et al., 1996); however, in occasional cases where there is definite neuronal degeneration, this may represent a trans-synaptic effect or primary involvement.

Degeneration of pigmented nerve cells occurs in the substantia nigra pars compacta (SNC), while non-pigmented cells of the pars reticulata are reported as normal. The caudolateral region is most severely affected with neuronal depletion, glial hyperplasia, and granules of neuromelanin lying free in the neuropil and within macrophages. The appearances are usually of a more active type of degeneration when compared with that of PD; the neuropil is often vacuolated and occasionally there are microglial nodules and evidence of neuronophagia in addition to a diffuse increase of microglia. The topographical patterns of neurodegeneration involving the motor neostriatum, efferent pathways, and nigral neurones reflect their anatomical relationship and suggest a common denominator or "linked" degeneration (Kume et al., 1993).

3. Olivopontocerebellar Atrophy (OPCA)

The brunt of pathology is in the olivopontocerebellar system, while the involvement of striatum and substantia nigra is less severe. The basis pontis is atrophic, with loss of pontine neurones and transverse pontocerebellar fibers. In sections stained for myelin, the intact descending corticospinal tracts stand out against the degenerate transverse fibers and the middle cerebellar peduncles. Many authors report a disproportionate depletion of fibers from the middle

TABLE 1 Frequency (%) of Individual Clinical Features in Three Series of MSA

	Series 1 (n = 168)	Series 2 (n = 100)	Series 3 (n = 35)
Sex ratio (Male : Female)	1.4 : 1	1.9 : 1	1.2 : 1
Mean age at onset (yrs)	54.1	52.5	55
Median survival (yrs)	6.0	9.3	7.3
Autonomic symptoms	71	97	97
Postural faintness (incl. syncope)	na	53	31
Syncope	24	15	20
Urinary incontinence	56	71	51
Urinary retention	18	27	34
Fecal incontinence	12	2	3
Impotence	43	90	62
Parkinsonism	84	91	100
Tremor	64	66	80
present at rest	40	29	34
pill-rolling	7	9	11
Cerebellar signs	59	52	34
Gait ataxia	54	37	29
Limb ataxia	51	47	31
Pyramidal signs	48	61	54
Stridor	9	34	34
Dysarthria	79	96	89
Antecollis	4	15	9
Myoclonus	na	31	29

Legend: Series 1 refers to the series of well-documented pathologically proven MSA cases reported in the literature (Wenning et al., 1997b) excluding the 35 confirmed cases from the UK Parkinson's Disease Society Brain Bank that constitute Series 3 (Wenning et al., 1995). Series 2 refers to the clinical series of 100 cases with probable MSA (Wenning et al., 1994a) (Wenning and Quinn, 1997). na: not available.

cerebellar peduncles compared with the loss of pontine neurones, an observation which led to the suggestion of a "dying back" process (Oppenheimer, 1984).

In MSA, cerebellar atrophy is often stated to be greatest in the neocerebellum, whereas the palaeocerebellum is involved in primary cerebellar cortical degenerations. However, in several examples of MSA, pathology is most severe in the vermis (Takei and Mirra, 1973; Wenning et al., 1996b) or, alternatively, vermis and hemispheres may be equally affected. There is loss of Purkinje nerve cells and accompanying astrocytosis, resulting in isomorphic gliosis in the molecular layer. Both the folial and central hemispheric white matter is reduced in amount while that around the dentate nucleus and within the hilus is well preserved. Due to the loss of Purkinje cell axon terminals, increased gliosis occurs in the dentate nucleus but there is usually no neuronal depletion at this site (Daniel, 1999). In medulla there is loss of neurones in the inferior and accessory olivary nuclei with increased gliosis. A lack of topographic relationship between neuronal cell loss in inferior olives and cerebellar cortex suggests that these may be primary unrelated degenerations (Wenning et al., 1996b).

4. Autonomic Failure

Autonomic failure in MSA is caused by dysfunction of:

1. central and preganglionic efferent autonomic activity,
2. neuronal networks in the brainstem controlling cardiovascular and respiratory function, and
3. the neuroendocrine component of the autonomic regulation via the hypothalamopituitary axis.

A supraspinal contribution to the autonomic failure of MSA is now well established (Daniel, 1999). Cell loss is reported in dorsal motor nucleus of the vagus (Sung et al., 1979) and involves catecholaminergic neurons of ventrolateral medulla (Benarroch et al., 1998). Cell loss has also been described for the Edinger-Westphal nucleus and posterior hypothalamus (Shy and Drager, 1960), including the tuberomamillary nucleus (Nakamura et al., 1996). Papp and Lantos

TABLE 2 "Red Flags": Warning Features of MSA

Motor red flags	Definition
Poorly levodopa responsive parkinsonism	As defined by the Consensus diagnostic criteria[12]
Cerebellar ataxia	As defined by the Consensus diagnostic criteria[12]
Pyramidal signs	As defined by the Consensus diagnostic criteria[12]
Early instability and falls	H&Y III within 3 years of disease onset
Rapid progression (wheelchair sign) despite dopaminergic treatment	H&Y V within 5 years of disease onset
Orofacial dystonia/dyskinesias	Atypical spontaneous or levodopa induced dystonia/dyskinesia predominantly affecting orofacial muscles, occasionally resembling risus sardonicus of cephalic tetanus.
Axial dystonia	Pisa syndrome (subacute axial dystonia with a severe tonic lateral flexion of the trunk, head, and neck) or early severe camptocormia
Disproportionate antecollis	Chin-on-chest, neck can only with difficulty be passively and forcibly extended to its normal position. Despite severe chronic neck flexion, flexion elsewhere is minor.
Jerky tremor	Irregular myoclonic (jerky) postural or action tremor of the hands and/or fingers.
Dysarthria	Atypical quivering, irregular, severely hypophonic or slurring high-pitched dysarthria, which tends to develop earlier, be more severe and be associated with more marked dysphagia compared to PD.
Non-motor red flags	
Severe dysautonomia	As defined by the Consensus diagnostic criteria[12]
Abnormal respiration	Nocturnal (harsh or strained, high pitched inspiratory sounds) or diurnal inspiratory stridor, involuntary deep inspiratory sighs/gasps, sleep apnea (arrest of breathing for ≥10 secs), and excessive snoring (increase from premorbid level, or newly arising).
REM sleep behavior disorder	Intermittent loss of muscle atonia and appearance of elaborate motor activity (striking out with arms in sleep often with talking/shouting) associated with dream mentation.
Cold hands/feet	Coldness and color change (purple/blue) of extremities not due to drugs with blanching on pressure and poor circulatory return.
Raynaud's phenomenon	Painful "white finger," which may be provoked by ergot drugs.
Emotional incontinence	Crying inappropriately without sadness or laughing inappropriately without mirth.

H&Y, Hoehn and Yahr Staging. (Reprinted with permission from Elsevier; *The Lancet Neurology* 2004. **3**:93–103).

(1994) have shown marked involvement of brainstem pontomedullary reticular formation with GCIs, providing a supraspinal histological counterpart for impaired visceral function. Autonomic neuronal degeneration also affects the locus coeruleus (Wenning et al., 1997b). Degeneration of sympathetic preganglionic neurones in the intermediolateral column of the thoracolumbar spinal cord is considered contributory to orthostatic hypotension (Daniel, 1999). It is noteworthy that there is not always a strong correlation between nerve cell depletion or gliosis and the clinical degree of autonomic failure. It is estimated that more than 50% of cells within the intermediolateral column need to decay before symptoms become evident (Oppenheimer, 1980).

Disordered bladder, rectal, and sexual function in SND and OPCA have been associated with cell loss in parasympathetic preganglionic nuclei of the spinal cord. These neurons are localized rostrally in Onuf's nucleus between sacral segments S2 and S3, and more caudally in the inferior intermediolateral nucleus, chiefly in the S3 to S4 segments (Konno et al., 1986).

In the peripheral component of the autonomic nervous system, Bannister and Oppenheimer (1972) have described atrophy of the glossopharyngeal and vagus nerves. No pathology has been reported in the visceral enteric plexuses or in the innervation of glands, blood vessels, or smooth muscles. Sympathetic ganglia have not often been examined in pathological studies of autonomic failure, and have seldom been described quantitatively. In a few cases there were either no obvious or mild abnormalities in sympathetic ganglia. Any morphological changes reported in sympathetic ganglionic neurons in MSA have tended to be nonspecific (Spokes et al., 1979), falling within the normal age-related range of appearances (Matthews, 1999).

5. Additional Sites of Pathology

A variety of other neuronal populations are noted to show cell depletion and gliosis with considerable differences in vulnerability from case to case. Various degrees of abnormality in the cerebral hemisphere, including Betz cell loss, were detected in pathologically proven MSA cases (Tsuchiya et al., 2000; Wakabayashi et al., 1998b; Konagaya et al., 1999; Konagaya et al., 2002). Fujita et al. (1993) demonstrated a distinct laminar astrocytosis of the motor cortices in the fifth layer in four of six sporadic OPCA cases and in none of five control cases by immunohistochemistry for glial fibrillary acidic protein. In three autopsy cases of MSA, cerebellar cortical lesions were more conspicuous in the vermis than in the hemisphere (Tsuchiya et al., 1998). These neuropathological findings differ from the established theory that cerebellar lesions of MSA are more pronounced in the hemisphere than in the vermis. The degree of cerebellar cortical lesions in these cases increased in relation to the duration of the disease. Furthermore, anterior horn cells may show some depletion but rarely to the same extent as that occurring in motor neuron disease (Konno et al., 1986; Sima et al., 1993). Laryngeal stridor is a common feature of MSA and may occur as a presenting sign (Wu et al., 1996) or, more often, in later stages of the disease. Depletion of large myelinated nerve fibers in the recurrent laryngeal nerve which innervates intrinsic laryngeal muscles has been demonstrated in MSA patients with vocal cord palsy (Hayashi et al., 1997).

6. Differential Diagnosis

From a neuropathological viewpoint, there is little cause for confusion of MSA with other neurodegenerative conditions. The GCI is the hallmark that accompanies signs of degeneration involving striatonigral and olivopontocerebellar systems. Similar inclusions have been described in several other diseases, including progressive supranuclear palsy (PSP), corticobasal degeneration (CBD) (Daniel et al., 1995), and familial OPCA (Berciano and Ferrer, 1996); however, they are infrequent and require careful search. GCI are distinctly different from filamentous oligodendroglial inclusions, called coiled bodies, found in other neurodegenerative diseases, including PSP, CBD, and argyrophilic grain disease (Braak and Braak, 1989; Yamada and McGeer, 1990; Chin and Goldman, 1996).

Rarely MSA may be combined with additional pathologies. Lewy bodies (LBs) have been reported in 8–10 percent of MSA cases and show a distribution comparable with that of PD (Wenning and Quinn, 1994). This frequency is similar to that of controls and suggests an incidental finding related to aging and/or presymptomatic PD. Isolated reports of unusual clinicopathological cases occur and include overlap of MSA with PSP and CBD (Ansorge et al., 1997a, Takanashi et al., 2002), MSA with Alzheimer disease and PD (Ansorge et al., 1997b), and MSA with atypical Pick disease (Horoupian and Dickson, 1991).

III. BIOCHEMICAL/ NEUROPHARMACOLOGICAL FINDINGS

A. Biochemical Findings

Neurochemical studies have shown alterations consistent with sites of major pathology. Calcineurin, a marker for medium-sized spiny neurons, is decreased in striosomes of the putamen and in the efferent pathway of the globus pallidus and substantia nigra (Goto et al., 1989b). Ito et al. (1996) also reported that regardless of clinical presentation, there is reduced immunoreactivity for additional markers of the striatal efferent system, including metenkephalin, substance P, and calbindin. In the SNC, tyrosine hydroxylase (TH) containing dopaminergic neurons are depleted. Similar neurones in the C1 and A2 regions of the medulla also showed reduced TH activity, which has been associated with orthostatic hypotension (Kato et al., 1995).

Biochemical analyses have found only minor differences in reduced striatal and nigral dopamine content in MSA when compared with PD (Brucke et al., 1997). However, unlike PD, mitochondrial respiratory chain function in the substantia nigra is normal in MSA (Gu et al., 1997). An increase in total iron content appears to reflect sites of primary damage and occurs in both PD and MSA substantia nigra, as well as in MSA striatum (Dexter et al., 1991). Decreased noradrenaline levels are reported in septal nuclei, nucleus accumbens, hypothalamus, and locus ceruleus, while a consistent deficit of choline acetyltransferase is found in red nucleus, dentate, pontine, and inferior olivary nuclei, with variable involvement of the striatum and additional areas (Spokes et al., 1979). Cerebellar and, in particular, Purkinje cell damage has been indicated by reduced levels of glutamate dehydrogenase (Plaitakis et al., 1993), amino acid binding sites (Price et al., 1993), and cerebrospinal fluid (CSF) calbindin-D (Kiyosawa et al., 1993). Holmberg et al. (1998) showed that the content of neurofilament (NFL) in CSF was significantly higher in both PSP and MSA compared to PD patients, reflecting the degree of ongoing neuronal degeneration affecting mainly the axonal compartment.

Several studies have measured CSF content of biogenic amine metabolites/derivates, thiamine, neuropeptide Y, substance P, or corticotropin-releasing hormone in MSA patients (Gonzalez-Quevedo et al., 1993; Botez et al., 2001; Orozco et al., 1989; Martignoni et al., 1992; Nutt et al., 1980; Suemaru et al., 1995). Botez et al. (2001) measured levels of the dopamine metabolite homovanillic acid (HVA), the serotonin metabolite 5-hydroxindoleacetic acid (5HIAA) and precursor tryptophan, as well as the noradrenaline metabolite 3-methoxy-4-hydroxyphenylethylene glycol (MHPG), and thiamine in the CSF of patients with OPCA (among others), as compared with sex- and age-matched control subjects. CSF HVA, MHPG, and thiamine values were markedly lower than those in control patients, whereas CSF 5HIAA values showed only a trend towards lower levels than control subjects.

B. Neuropharmacological Findings

The combination of nigral and striatal degeneration is the core pathology underlying parkinsonism in MSA. The degenerative process affects nigrostriatal dopaminergic transmission at both pre- and post-synaptic sites (Fearnley and Lees, 1991; Kume et al., 1993). Pathologically, the loss of dopaminergic neurons in MSA-P is comparable to that found in PD (Tison et al., 1995a). Only a few patients with MSA exhibit a presynaptic pattern with minimal putaminal changes (Tison et al., 1995a; Wenning et al., 1994c; Berciano et al., 2002). There is a close anatomical relationship between nigral and striatal degeneration in MSA-P. Degeneration of pigmented dopaminergic neurons begins and predominantly involves the ventrolateral tier of SNC, which in turn projects to the dorsolateral posterior putamen. The latter is the predominant site of striatal degeneration in MSA. Several post-mortem immunohistochemical and autoradiographical, as well as in vivo neuroimaging studies, suggest that both striatal outflow pathways are affected: encephalin-containing striatal neurons projecting to the external globus pallidus that carry dopamine D_2 receptors (indirect pathway) and substance P (SP)-containing cells projecting to internal globus pallidus and substantia nigra pars reticulata (SNR) that carry D_1 receptors (direct pathway) (Quik et al., 1979; Cortes et al., 1989; Brooks et al., 1992; Churchyard et al., 1993; Vogels et al., 2000; Goto et al., 1989a; Goto et al., 1989c; Goto et al., 1990; Goto et al., 1996; Schelosky et al., 1993; van Royen et al., 1993; Ito et al., 1996).

In accordance with the topographical projection of the putamen onto pallidal segments, the posterolateral portions of the external and internal globus pallidus, and the ventrolateral portion of the substantia nigra are deafferented from striatal projections (Brooks et al., 1992).

Progressive loss of striatal dopamine receptors and striatal output systems might explain levodopa unresponsiveness in most MSA-P patients (Tison et al., 1995a; Ito et al., 1996; Parati et al., 1993; Rajput et al., 1990). Those patients with a good initial response to levodopa would thus have less striatal damage than those with absent or poor initial response. However, there is evidence suggesting that the response to levodopa does not always depend solely on the degree of striatal cell loss (Wenning et al., 1994c). In vivo PET studies by Brooks et al. (1992) have also failed to clearly correlate therapeutic response with striatal D_2 receptor status. Additional loss of D_1 and opiate receptors could also be an important factor underlying dopaminergic unresponsiveness in MSA-P (Burn et al., 1995), as well as other changes downstream of striatum itself.

IV. MOLECULAR BIOLOGY

The discovery of GCIs in MSA brains firmly established glial pathology as a biological hallmark of this disorder, akin to the LB of PD. GCIs are argyrophilic and half moon, oval, or conical in shape (Lantos, 1998; Papp et al., 1989). They consist of 20 to 30 nm diameter filaments and contain the classical cytoskeletal antigens, ubiquitin and tau (Lantos, 1998; Cairns et al., 1997a). Furthermore, α-synuclein, a presynaptic protein which is affected by point mutations in some families with autosomal dominant PD (Goedert and Spillantini, 1998) and which is present in LBs (Spillantini et al., 1997), has also been observed in both neuronal and glial cytoplasmic inclusions (Wakabayashi et al., 1998c; Arima et al., 1998; Tu et al., 1998) in brains of patients with MSA. The accumulation of α-synuclein into filamentous inclusions appears to play a mechanistic role in the pathogenesis of several α-synucleinopathies including PD, dementia with LBs, Down syndrome, familial AD, sporadic AD, MSA, and other synucleinopathies (Trojanowski et al., 2002). The α-synuclein accumulation in these inclusions appears to precede their ubiquitination, because α-synuclein antibodies detect a greater number of inclusions than ubiquitin antibodies (Gai et al., 1998). Importantly, α-synuclein, but not ubiquitin, antibodies also reveal numerous degenerating neurites in the white matter of MSA cases (Gai et al., 1998). This suggests that an as yet unrecognized degree of pathology may be present in the axons of MSA cases, although whether neuronal/axonal α-synuclein pathology precedes glial α-synuclein pathology has not been examined.

V. PATHOGENESIS/MECHANISM OF DISEASE

The α-synuclein pathway appears to be the key pathway to selective loss of glia and neurons in MSA. The differential distribution of α-synuclein deposits and associated neuronal pathology (SND, OPCA, and spinal cord) suggests variability of pathogenetic mechanisms underlying the multifaceted disease process of MSA.

MSA, as reflected in its current definition, is regarded as a sporadic disease (Wenning et al., 1993) and no confirmed familial cases of MSA have yet been described. Even so, it is conceivable that genetic factors may play a role in the etiology of the disease. However, initial screening studies for candidate genes revealed no risk factors (Bandmann et al.,

1997; Nicholl et al., 1999). Other recent studies have further looked for polymorphisms or mutations in candidate genes, which may predispose an individual toward developing MSA. The apolipoprotein ε4 allele is not over-represented in MSA when compared with controls, and there have been conflicting reports of the association of a cytochrome P-450-2D6 polymorphism with MSA (Iwahashi et al., 1995; Bandmann et al., 1995; Cairns et al., 1997b).

The pathogenetic role of α-synuclein is still unclear. Inactivation of the α-synuclein gene by homologous recombination did not lead to a severe neurological phenotype (Abeliovich et al., 2000). Therefore, loss of function of the α-synuclein protein is unlikely to account for its role in neurodegeneration. Mice lacking α-synuclein were found to show increased release of striatal dopamine, indicating that this protein could function as an activity-dependent, negative regulator of neurotransmission in the striatum. While there is strong evidence that α-synuclein participates in the pathogenesis of some types of familial PD (Polymeropoulos et al., 1997; Kruger et al., 1998), no mutations have been found in the entire coding region of the α-synuclein gene in MSA (Ozawa et al., 1999) or in sporadic forms of PD (El-Agnaf et al., 1998). However, polymorphisms in the α-synuclein gene have been identified in PD (Kruger et al., 1999). They may also increase the risk of developing MSA by promoting α-synuclein protein aggregation. Polymorphisms in codons 1 to 39 of the α-synuclein gene, a domain related to interaction with synphilin-1, or indeed polymorphisms in the synphilin-1 gene itself, or in the genes of other protein-interacting partners of α-synuclein, may also need to be considered in the pathogenesis of MSA (Engelender et al., 1999). The number of α-synuclein protein-interacting partners has expanded to include 14-3-3 protein chaperones, protein kinase C, extracellular regulated kinase, and BAD, a molecule that regulates cell death (Ostrerova et al., 1999). Nevertheless, association studies with genetic polymorphisms for α-synuclein have so far been negative in MSA (Bandmann, 1997; Morris et al., 2000).

Gilman et al. (1996) have reported an MSA-like phenotype including GCI like (α-synuclein negative) inclusions in one SCA1 (spinocerebellar ataxia type 1) family. Other SCA mutations (except for SCA-2 [Bösch et al., 2002a]) have not been reported to present with MSA-like features (Schöls et al., 2000; Ranum et al., 1995; Silveira et al., 1996; Leggo et al., 1997; Futamura et al., 1998; Moseley et al., 1998). Conversely, the majority of MSA-C patients do not appear to have expanded SCA1 and SCA3 alleles (Bandmann et al., 1997). Indeed, MSA-C appears to be a frequent form of sporadic cerebellar ataxia of late onset. Nearly thirty percent of sporadic adult-onset ataxia patients suffer from MSA (Abele et al., 2002). This finding corresponds well to data of a study of sporadic OPCA patients who were followed up for ten years (Gilman et al., 2000). Within this period, seventeen out of fifty-one patients developed autonomic failure or Parkinsonism, indicating a diagnosis of MSA.

To summarize, the up-to-date knowledge about the role of α-synuclein and its aggregation in neurodegenerative disorders remains unclear. It is not yet elucidated how the expression and aggregation of α-synuclein in glial cells affects their biology as well as the glia-neuron interactions, which might be a critical step in the pathogenesis of α-synucleinopathies. Whether environmental factors influence α-synuclein aggregation and the survival of glial and neuronal cells remains unknown as well.

VI. CLINICAL PICTURE

A. Introduction

In a series of one hundred cases of clinically probable MSA (Wenning et al., 1994a; Wenning and Quinn, 1997), at the last evaluation, 97% of patients with MSA had autonomic failure, 91% had parkinsonism, 52% had cerebellar features and 61% had pyramidal features. Autonomic failure may be associated with either levodopa unresponsive parkinsonism in 80% of cases (MSA-P subtype) or with cerebellar ataxia in 20% of cases (MSA-C subtype). There is commonly clinical and subclinical evidence of autonomic failure in both MSA variants.

B. Presenting Features

MSA patients may present with parkinsonism that usually responds poorly to levodopa. This has been identified as the most important early clinical discriminator of MSA and PD (Quinn, 1989b; Schwarz et al., 1992; Schelosky et al., 1993; Wenning et al., 2000a), although a subgroup of MSA patients may show a good or, rarely, excellent, but usually short-lived, response to levodopa (Hughes et al., 1992; Parati et al., 1993; Bösch et al., 2002b). Progressive ataxia may also be the presenting feature of MSA (Schulz et al., 1994; Wenning et al., 1997a). In Japan, cerebellar presentation of MSA appears to be more common than the parkinsonian variant compared to Western countries (Watanabe et al., 2002). Autonomic failure with symptomatic orthostatic hypotension and/or urogenital disturbance may accompany the motor disorder in up to 50 percent of patients at disease onset.

Unusual presentations in pathologically proven cases have included stroke-like episodes evolving into parkinsonism (Lambie et al., 1947), REM sleep disorder (Tison et al., 1995b), pseudo-TIAs in the anterior or posterior circulation (Bannister and Oppenheimer, 1972; Klein et al., 1995) as well as limb shaking attacks (Litvan, personal communication).

C. Features of Established Disease

1. Parkinsonism

Bradykinesia, rigidity, postural tremor, as well as dysequilibrium and gait unsteadiness characterize parkinsonism associated with MSA. Jerky postural tremor and, less commonly, tremor at rest may be superimposed. Frequently, patients exhibit orofacial dystonia associated with a characteristic quivering high-pitched dysarthria. Postural stability is compromised early on; however, recurrent falls at disease onset are unusual in contrast to PSP. The clinical data in table 1 are derived from three MSA series (Wenning and Quinn, 1997): one hundred sixty-eight well-documented clinicopathological cases of MSA reported in the literature (Wenning et al., 1997b), one hundred cases of clinically probable MSA (Wenning et al., 1994a), and thirty-five cases of pathologically confirmed MSA from the United Kingdom Parkinson's Disease Society Brain Bank (UKPDSBB) (Wenning et al., 1995). The vast majority of patients in the three series (84 to 100%) developed parkinsonism. Pure MSA-P (parkinsonism without cerebellar signs) represented the single most common motor subtype ranging from 40% (literature) through 48% (clinical series) to 66% (UKPDSBB series). In contrast, pure MSA-C (cerebellar ataxia without parkinsonism) was absent in the UKPDSBB series, and present in 9% of patients in the clinical series, and in 16% in the literature series. It has been suggested that a symmetrical atremulous picture might distinguish MSA-P from PD (Fearnley and Lees, 1990; Albanese et al., 1995; Colosimo et al., 1995; Gouider-Khouja et al., 1995). However, motor disturbance was asymmetrical in 74% of patients in the clinical series, and unilateral at onset in 47% of literature cases, and in many of the UKPDSBB cases. Also, some sort of tremor was present in 64 to 80% of cases, and tremor present at rest was observed in 29 to 40% of cases. Even so, a classical pill-rolling resting tremor was reported in only 7 to 9% of subjects. Therefore, the differential diagnosis of MSA-P and PD may be quite difficult in the early stages due to a number of overlapping features such as rest tremor or asymmetrical akinesia and rigidity. Furthermore, levodopa-induced improvement of parkinsonism may be seen in 30% of MSA-P patients; however, the benefit is transient in most of them. Levodopa-induced dyskinesia affecting orofacial and neck muscles occurs in 50% of MSA-P patients, sometimes in the absence of motor benefit (Bösch et al., 2002b; Hughes et al., 1992). In most instances, a fully developed clinical picture of MSA-P evolves within five years of disease onset, allowing a clinical diagnosis during follow-up (Wenning et al., 2000a).

2. Dysautonomia

Dysautonomia is characteristic of both MSA subtypes, primarily comprising urogenital and orthostatic dysfunction.

a. Urogenital Dysfunction

Urinary incontinence (71%) or retention (27%) are frequent, often early in the course or as presenting symptoms, (Wenning et al., 1994a/1999c; Beck et al., 1994; Sakakibara et al., 2000a). Disorders of micturition generally occur more commonly, earlier, and to a more severe degree in MSA than in PD (Beck et al., 1994). Urinary retention can be caused or exacerbated by benign prostatic hypertrophy or, in women, by perineal laxity secondary to difficult childbirth or uterine descent. In men, the urological symptoms of pollakiuria, urgency, nocturia, and incontinence, together with hesitancy and incomplete emptying or chronic retention, may simulate those of prostatic outflow obstruction. In a series of patients with probable MSA, 43% of males had undergone futile prostatic or bladder neck surgery before the correct diagnosis was made, although more than half had neurological symptoms or signs at the time of the procedure (Beck et al., 1994). Stress incontinence occurred in 57% of the women and half of these had undergone surgery. The results of surgery were also poor (Beck et al., 1994; Chandiramani et al., 1997). Fecal incontinence was much rarer (2–12%) (Wenning and Quinn, 1997), despite frequent severe denervation of the external anal sphincter, suggesting that the mechanisms of urinary and fecal continence are distinct in MSA.

Early impotence is virtually universal in men with MSA. In a series of sixty-two MSA patients, impotence occurred in 96% of the men and was the first symptom alone in 37% (Beck et al., 1994). Reduced genital sensitivity with or without impaired libido has recently been reported in the majority of female MSA patients (Oertel et al., 2003). In addition, MSA patients may note increased constipation and hypo- or anhydrosis.

b. Orthostatic Dysfunction

Based on Shy and Drager's description (1960), recurrent syncopal attacks are commonly regarded as a typical feature of MSA. However, severe orthostatic hypotension with recurrent (more than three) syncopes was reported in only 15% of subjects, whereas postural faintness was present, but only to a mild or moderate degree, in up to 53% of cases (Wenning et al., 1994a/1999c). Analysis of a detailed questionnaire and autonomic function tests in a series of 121 patients with clinically diagnosed MSA showed that urinary symptoms (96%) were more common than orthostatic symptoms (43%) (Sakakibara et al., 2000a) (see IX.A.). Orthostatic hypotension is frequently associated with impaired or absent reflex tachycardia upon standing. Dopaminergic drugs may provoke or worsen orthostatic hypotension. Recumbent arterial hypertension, mainly due to loss of baroreflexes, may be seen in a few patients with severe cardiovascular autonomic failure (Bannister and Mathias, 1999a).

3. Cerebellar Disorder

The cerebellar disorder comprises gait ataxia, limb kinetic ataxia, and scanning dysarthria as well as cerebellar oculomotor disturbances. Cerebellar signs, most commonly manifesting as a wide-based ataxic gait developed in 34 to 59% of patients (Wenning and Quinn, 1997; Schulz et al., 1994) (see table 3). However, a subgroup of patients presented with narrow-based unsteady gait due to more marked impairment of postural reflexes (Wenning et al., 1997a). Spontaneous and/or gaze-evoked nystagmus, often subtle, was detected in 23 to 25% of patients (Wenning et al., 1997a or Wenning et al., 1994a), and cerebellar scanning dysarthria may occur. The finding of a mixed dysarthria with combinations of hypokinetic, ataxic, and spastic components is consistent with both the overall clinical and the neuropathologic changes in MSA (Kluin et al., 1996; Garratt et al., 1994).

Patients with MSA-C usually develop additional noncerebellar symptoms and signs, but before doing so may be indistinguishable from other patients with idiopathic late-onset cerebellar ataxia, many of whom have a disease clinically restricted to cerebellar signs and pathologically to degeneration of the cerebellum and olives (Abele et al., 2002; Wenning et al., 2004).

TABLE 3 Consensus Statement: Clinical Domains, Features, and Criteria Used in the Diagnosis of MSA

I. Autonomic and urinary dysfunction

A. Autonomic and urinary features

1. Orthostatic hypotension (by 20 mmHg systolic or 10 mmHg diastolic)
2. Urinary incontinence or incomplete bladder emptying

B. Criterion for autonomic failure or urinary dysfunction in MSA

Orthostatic fall in blood pressure (by 30 mmHg systolic or 15 mmHg diastolic) or urinary incontinence (persistent, involuntary partial, or total bladder emptying, accompanied by erectile dysfunction in men) or both

II. Parkinsonism

A. Parkinsonian features

1. Bradykinesia (slowness of voluntary movement with progressive reduction in speed and amplitude during repetitive actions)
2. Rigidity
3. Postural instability (not caused by primary visual, vestibular, cerebellar, or proprioceptive dysfunction)
4. Tremor (postural, resting, or both)

B. Criterion for Parkinsonism in MSA

Bradykinesia plus at least one of items 2 to 4

III. Cerebellar dysfunction

A. Cerebellar features

1. Gait ataxia (wide-based stance with steps of irregular length and direction)
2. Ataxic dysarthria
3. Limb ataxia
4. Sustained gaze-evoked nystagmus

B. Criterion for cerebellar dysfunction in MSA

Gait ataxia plus at least one of items 2 to 4

IV. Corticospinal tract dysfunction

A. Corticospinal tract features

1. Extensor plantar responses with hyperreflexia

B. Corticospinal tract dysfunction in MSA: no corticospinal tract features are used in defining the diagnosis of MSA

*A feature (A) is a characteristic of the disease and a criterion (B) is a defining feature or composite of features required for diagnosis.

Reproduced with kind permission from Gilman et al., *J Neurol Sci* 1999;163:94–98.

4. Pyramidal Signs

Although pyramidal signs may be elicited in up to 61% of MSA patients (Wenning and Quinn, 1997), obvious spastic paraparetic gait or significant pyramidal weakness should cast doubt upon the clinical diagnosis of MSA.

D. Other Clinical Features

Besides the poor response to levodopa, and the additional presence of pyramidal or cerebellar signs or autonomic failure as major diagnostic clues, certain other features may either raise suspicion of MSA, or at least suggest that one might not be dealing with PD (Quinn, 1989b). These early warning signs of MSA, so-called "red flags," are listed in table 2.

Camptocormia (bent spine) has been associated with PD for a long time. It is characterized by severe forward flexion of the thoracolumbar spine, which increases while walking and disappears in the recumbent position (Djaldetti et al., 1999). In contrast with other skeletal disorders of the spine such as kyphosis, the deformity in camptocormia is not fixed and is corrected by passive extension or lying in the supine position. Evaluation of this disorder can indeed be challenging, and often no definite diagnosis is made (Umapathi et al., 2002).

Subacute *Pisa's syndrome*, a form of severe axial dystonia, has also been reported in MSA (Colosimo, 1998). However, Pisa's syndrome is a non-specific feature of Parkinsonism and it may also emerge in patients with other neurodegenerative conditions.

Tremulous myoclonic jerks, usually affecting the fingers, of small amplitude, and often stretch-sensitive, occur in a number of patients with MSA, but are otherwise rare in non-demented PD patients (Quinn, 1989b; Salazar et al., 2000).

A more frequent and characteristic feature suggesting MSA is the development of a disproportionate *antecollis* (Langston, 1936; Neumann, 1977; Caplan, 1984; Quinn, 1989a; Rivest et al., 1990; Bösch et al., 2002b) hampering feeding, communication, and vision. The pathophysiological basis remains uncertain (myopathy, focal dystonia?). Botulinum toxin injections into sternocleidomastoid muscles are usually unrewarding and worsen dysphagia (Thobois et al., 2001). Other manifestations of focal dystonia are less common, but may include *axial, facial and hand dystonia, torticollis*, and *dystonic toe movements*. Levodopa exposure may worsen dystonic movements in the absence of anti-Parkinsonian benefit (Bösch et al., 2002b).

Nighttime respiratory stridor, commonly attributed to vocal cord paralysis (Williams et al., 1979; Hughes et al., 1998), but perhaps reflecting dystonia of the vocal cords (Merlo et al., 2002) is also a helpful diagnostic pointer. Nocturnal stridor has been considered a poor prognostic feature. Analysis of survival curves of 30 patients with follow-up information showed a significantly shorter survival from the sleep evaluation, but not from disease onset, for patients with stridor compared with those without (Silber et al., 2000). Inspiratory stridor was documented in 9 to 34% (Wenning and Quinn, 1997) of patients and occurred at any time point in the disease process. In fact, several cases have presented acutely with laryngeal palsy requiring tracheostomy (Kew et al., 1990) or nasotracheal intubation (Flügel et al., 1984). Tracheostomy in later disease stages may be more controversial. In contrast, stridor is very uncommon in PD.

Speech impairment develops in virtually all MSA patients and is probably largely related to laryngeal dysfunction (Garratt et al., 1994). It tends to be dominated by hypophonic monotony or a scanning quality according to clinical subtype (Kluin et al., 1996). In addition to the low volume monotony of parkinsonism, a quivering, irregular, severely hypophonic or slurring *dysarthria* is often so characteristic that the diagnosis can be suggested by listening to the patient on the telephone (Caplan, 1984). Dysarthria tends to develop earlier, be more severe, and be associated with more marked dysphagia in MSA compared to PD (Muller et al., 2001).

MSA patients are prone to sleep-related breathing disorders, often resulting in nighttime oxygen desaturation (Wenning and Quinn, 1997). They also often show disrupted sleep with rapid eye movement (REM) phase alterations and may present with isolated *REM behavior disorder* (*RBD*) (Tison et al., 1995b; Plazzi et al., 1997). Sleep disorders are more common in patients with MSA than in those with PD after the same duration of the disease, reflecting the more diffuse underlying pathological process in MSA (Ghorayeb et al., 2002).

Abnormal sudomotor function, sympathetic skin response, impaired heat tolerance, and skin temperature regulation have been described in MSA (Cohen et al., 1987; Sandroni et al., 1991; Kihara et al., 1991). Furthermore, patients with MSA often have cold, dusky, violaceous hands, with poor circulatory return after blanching by pressure. Changes in skin color or temperature were easily detected by Klein et al. (1997), and suggest a defect in neurovascular control of distal extremities.

VII. CORE CHARACTERISTICS OF THE DISEASE

The extrapyramidal features appear similar to those in PD, including bradykinesia with rigidity, postural instability, hypokinetic speech, and occasionally tremor, usually with a poor or unsustained response to chronic levodopa therapy. The signs of cerebellar dysfunction include disorders of extraocular movements, ataxic speech, and ataxia of limb movements and gait resulting in postural instability and frequent falls. Autonomic insufficiency results in orthostatic hypotension, urinary retention or incontinence, and impotence, often accompanied by constipation and decreased sweating. Parkinsonian, cerebellar, and autonomic features often occur in combination in MSA, but one or, in some patients, two features may predominate.

VIII. CLINICAL DIAGNOSTIC CRITERIA

The clinical diagnosis of MSA is fraught with difficulty and there are no pathognomonic features to discriminate the common (80% of cases) parkinsonian variant (MSA-P) from PD. In a clinicopathologic study conducted by Litvan et al. (1997), primary neurologists (who followed up the patients clinically) identified only 25% of MSA patients at the first visit (42 months after disease onset). Even at last neurological follow-up (74 months after disease onset), half of the patients were misdiagnosed and the correct diagnosis in the other half was established on average four years after disease onset. Mean rater sensitivity for movement disorder specialists was higher but still suboptimal at the first (56%) and last (69%) visit.

Consistent with this observation, most of the MSA patients identified in the epidemiological survey by Schrag et al. (1999) were only diagnosed during the study, suggesting that MSA is poorly recognized in clinical practice and is commonly mistaken for PD due to a number of overlapping features (Wenning et al., 2000a). Osaki et al. (2002) assessed the accuracy of clinical diagnosis of MSA in the United Kingdom. This study demonstrated that clinical diagnosis maintained until death by neurologists was incorrect in eight of fifty-nine (14%) cases and application of either Quinn or Consensus criteria improved the clinical diagnosis of MSA at first, but not at last visit. In an earlier clinicopathological study, twelve of thirty-five MSA cases remained misdiagnosed as PD until death (Wenning et al., 1995). MSA may be also confused with PSP or other atypical Parkinsonian disorders (Wenning et al., 2000a; Litvan et al., 1996).

Clinical diagnostic criteria for MSA were proposed by Quinn in 1989. These criteria were slightly modified in 1994 to include an investigation (sphincter EMG); furthermore, the category possible MSA-OPCA was defined for the first time (Quinn, 1994). According to this schema, patients are

TABLE 4 Consensus Statement: Diagnostic Categories of MSA

I. Possible MSA
One criterion plus two features from separate other domains. When the criterion is Parkinsonism, a poor levodopa response qualifies as one feature (hence only one additional feature is required).

II. Probable MSA
Criterion for autonomic failure/urinary dysfunction plus poorly levodopa-responsive Parkinsonism or cerebellar dysfunction.

III. Definite MSA
Pathologically confirmed by the presence of a high density of glial cytoplasmic inclusions in association with a combination of degenerative changes in the nigrostriatal and olivopontocerebellar pathways.

*The features and criteria for each clinical domain are shown in table 3.

Reproduced with kind permission from Gilman et al., *J Neurol Sci* 1999;163:94–98.

TABLE 5 Consensus Statement: Exclusion Criteria for the Diagnosis of MSA

I. History
Symptomatic onset under 30 years of age

Family history of a similar disorder

Systemic disease or other identifiable causes for features listed in Table 6

Hallucinations unrelated to medication

II. Physical examination
DSM-IV criteria for dementia

Prominent slowing of vertical saccades or vertical supranuclear gaze palsy[a]

Evidence of focal cortical dysfunction such as aphasia, alien limb syndrome, and parietal dysfunction

III. Laboratory investigation
Metabolic, molecular genetic, and imaging evidence of an alternative cause of features listed in Table 6

[a]In practice, MSA is most frequently confused with PD or PSP. Mild limitation of upward gaze alone is nonspecific, whereas a prominent (>50%) limitation of upward gaze or any limitation of downward gaze suggests PSP. Before the onset of vertical gaze limitation, a clinically obvious slowing of voluntary vertical saccades is usually easily detectable in PSP and assists in the early differentiation of these two disorders. (Reproduced with kind permission from Gilman et al., *J Neurol Sci* 1999;163:94–98.)

classified as either SND or OPCA type MSA depending on the predominance of parkinsonism or cerebellar ataxia. These criteria define two levels of clinical diagnostic certainty (possible, probable) and reserve a definite diagnosis to neuropathological confirmation. So far, sensitivity and specificity of the Quinn criteria have never been prospectively determined. Two retrospective validation studies have shown good specificity, but poor sensitivity of these criteria (Litvan et al., 1998; Osaki et al., 2002).

In April 1998 an International Consensus Conference was convened to develop optimized criteria for a clinical diagnosis of MSA (Gilman et al., 1998; Gilman et al., 1999). The Consensus criteria have since been widely established in the research community as well as at movement disorders clinics. They define three diagnostic categories of increasing certainty: possible, probable, and definite. The diagnoses of possible and probable MSA are based on the presence of specific clinical features (tables 3 and 4). In addition, exclusion criteria must be considered (table 5). A definite diagnosis requires a typical neuropathological lesion pattern with α-synuclein-positive GCIs (Dickson et al., 1999). The main differences between Quinn and Consensus criteria are reported in table 6.

A retrospective evaluation of the Consensus criteria on pathologically proven cases showed excellent positive predictive values (PPV) for both possible and probable MSA; however, sensitivity for probable MSA was poor (Osaki et al., 2002). Interestingly, the Consensus criteria and Quinn's criteria had similar PPVs. While such formal diagnostic criteria are important for certain types of clinical research, they add little to the problem of detecting early cases, and improved screening instruments are certainly needed.

TABLE 6 Comparative Synopsis of Quinn's vs. Consensus Criteria for the Diagnosis of MSA

	Quinn's	Consensus
Categories	Possible, probable and definite	Possible, probable and definite
Items included	Clinical features and sphincter EMG	Clinical features only
Definition of clinical features	++	+ ++
Ease of application	+++	++
Sensitivity	++	+/++
Specificity	+++	+++
Retrospective validation	yes	yes
Prospective validation	no	no

IX. TIME COURSE OF THE DISEASE

MSA usually manifests in middle age, affects both sexes, and progresses relentlessly with a mean survival significantly shorter than PD (Ben-Shlomo et al., 1997; Wenning et al., 1994a; Wenning et al., 1997b).

A. Onset

MSA is a disease that commonly causes clinical symptoms beginning in the sixth decade, although occasionally symptoms commence as early as the fourth decade (Sima et al., 1993). In a series of one hundred cases of MSA reported by Wenning et al. (1994a), the median age of onset was 53 and the range was 33 to 76 years. In a meta-analysis of 433 cases, mean age of onset was 54.2 years (range 31 to 78) (Ben Shlomo et al., 1997). Latency to onset, but not duration, of symptomatic orthostatic hypotension or urinary incontinence differentiates PD from other parkinsonian syndromes, particularly MSA. Wenning et al. (1999c) found significant group differences for latency, but not duration, of symptomatic orthostatic hypotension and urinary incontinence: Latencies to onset of either feature were short in patients with MSA, intermediate in patients with DLB, CBD, and PSP, and long in those with PD. Symptomatic orthostatic hypotension occurring within the first year after disease onset predicted MSA in 75% of cases; early urinary incontinence was less predictive for MSA (56%). It is likely that urinary dysfunction is more common and often an earlier manifestation than orthostatic hypotension in patients with MSA, although subclinical cardiovascular abnormalities appear in the early stage of the disease (Sakakibara et al., 2000a). The responsible sites seem to be central and peripheral for both dysfunctions.

Latencies to onset of falls were short in PSP patients, intermediate in MSA, DLB, and CBD, and long in PD (Wenning et al., 1999a). Recurrent falls occurring within the first year after disease onset predicted PSP in 68% of the patients. Conversely, latency to onset, but not duration, of recurrent falls differentiates PD from other parkinsonian disorders.

B. Progression

MSA is a chronically progressive disease characterized by the gradual onset of neurological symptoms and accumulation of disability reflecting involvement of the systems initially unaffected. Thus, patients who present initially with extrapyramidal features commonly progress to develop autonomic disturbances, cerebellar disorders, or both. Conversely, patients who begin with symptoms of cerebellar dysfunction often progress to develop extrapyramidal or autonomic disorders, or both. Patients whose symptoms initially are autonomic may later develop other neurological disorders.

Progression to different Hoehn and Yahr (HY) stages was evaluated in eighty-one pathologically confirmed patients with parkinsonism. Patients with PD showed significantly longer latencies to each HY stage than patients with atypical parkinsonian disorders (APD). In fact, development of a HY-III within one year of motor onset accurately predicted an APD. However, the progression to each HY stage was unhelpful in distinguishing the APD from each other. Once patients with PD and APD became wheelchair-bound, both had equally short survival times (Müller et al., 2000). In a more recent study (Watanabe et al., 2002), median intervals from onset to aid-requiring walking, confinement to a wheelchair, a bedridden state, and death were three, five, eight, and nine years, respectively.

C. Prognosis

MSA is a progressive disorder associated with a shortened life span, with death occurring on average within about 10 years of symptom onset. In one clinical study, the median survival from onset of symptoms was 9.5 years (Wenning et al., 1994a), and in another 7.5 years (Testa et al., 1996), whereas more recently, Tison et al. (2000b) showed a mean disease duration of 6.8 years. Similar average survivals were reported in two autopsy-verified series of MSA patients, 8.7 years in one (Wenning et al., 1995), and 8.0 years in another (Hughes et al., 1992). Schulz et al. (1994) found among 32 cases a median survival time after onset of motor symptoms of 4 years in SND and 9.1 years in OPCA. In a meta-analysis of 433 cases of pathologically proven MSA over a 100-year period survival showed a secular trend from a median duration of 4.9 years for publications between 1887 and 1970 to 6.8 years between 1991 and 1994 (Ben-Shlomo et al., 1997). Older age of onset was associated with shorter survival; the hazard ratio for patients with onset after 60 years was 1.8 compared with patients between 31 and 49 years. Cerebellar features were associated with marginally increased survival. These results demonstrate the poor prognosis for patients with MSA but may be biased toward the worst cases.

X. EPIDEMIOLOGY

Determining the incidence and prevalence of MSA is difficult, as only a few epidemiologic studies have been reported. Estimates of the prevalence of MSA (per 100,000 in the population) in different studies ranged from 1.9 to 4.9 (Tison et al., 2000b; Wermuth et al., 1997; Schrag et al., 1999; Chio et al., 1998). The annual incidence of MSA was estimated to be about 0.6 cases per 100,000 persons or 3.0/100,000 people over the age of fifty years (Bower et al., 1997). These figures are similar to those of other well-known neurodegenerative disorders such as Huntington disease or motor neuron disease. Analytical epidemiology of MSA is even poorer: A case-control study in North America showed an increased risk of MSA associated with occupational exposure to organic solvents, plastic monomers and additives, pesticides, and metals (Nee et al., 1991). Smoking habits seem to be less frequent in MSA cases (as in PD cases) than in healthy controls. The fact that the inverse association with smoking found previously in PD is shared by MSA but not by PSP lends epidemiologic support to the notion that different smoking habits are associated with different groups of neurodegenerative disease (Vanacore et al., 2000).

XI. INVESTIGATIONS

A. Introduction

The clinical diagnosis of MSA rests largely on history and physical examination. Additional investigations are particularly helpful in excluding differential diagnoses; however, they may also support a presumptive clinical diagnosis. MSA-P patients are usually misdiagnosed as PD early in their disease. Regular follow-up is therefore required to detect development of atypical features suggestive of MSA.

B. Autonomic Function Tests

Autonomic function tests are a mandatory part of the diagnostic process and clinical follow-up in patients with MSA. Findings of severe autonomic failure early in the course of the disease make the diagnosis of MSA more likely, although the specificity in comparison to other neurodegenerative disorders is unknown in a single patient. Pathological results of autonomic function tests may account for a considerable number of symptoms in MSA patients and should prompt specific therapeutic steps to improve quality of life and prevent secondary complications like ascending urinary infections or injuries due to hypotension-induced falls.

1. Cardiovascular Function

A history of postural faintness or other evidence of orthostatic hypotension, e.g., neck ache on rising in the morning or posturally related changes of visual perception, should be sought in all patients in whom MSA is suspected. After taking a comprehensive history, testing of cardiovascular function should be performed according to Consensus recommendations (Consensus statement on the definition of orthostatic hypotension, pure autonomic failure, and multiple system atrophy, 1996; Braune et al., 1999a). A drop in systolic blood pressure (BP) of 20 mm Hg or more, or in diastolic BP of 10 mm Hg or more, compared with baseline within a standing time of three minutes is defined as orthostatic hypotension (Consensus statement on the definition of orthostatic hypotension, pure autonomic failure, and multiple system atrophy, 1996), and must lead to more specific assessment. This is based on continuous non-invasive measurement of blood pressure and heart rate during tilt table testing (Bannister and Mathias, 1999b; Braune et al., 1996a, Braune et al., 1996b). Although abnormal cardiovascular test results may provide evidence of sympathetic and/or parasympathetic failure, they do not differentiate autonomic failure associated with PD versus MSA (Riley and Chelimsky, 2003).

In MSA, cardiovascular dysregulation appears to be caused by central rather than peripheral autonomic failure. During supine rest noradrenaline levels (representing postganglionic sympathethic efferent activity) are normal (Ziegler et al., 1977; Polinsky et al., 1981), and there is no denervation hypersensitivity, which indicates a lack of increased expression of adrenergic receptors on peripheral neurons (Polinsky et al., 1981). Uptake of the noradrenaline analogue metaiodobenzylguanidine is normal in postganglionic cardiac neurons (Braune et al., 1999b; Orimo et al., 1999; Takatsu et al., 2000; Taki et al., 2000) (see XII.F) and the response to tilt is impaired with little increase in noradrenaline. In contrast, mainly postganglionic sympathetic dysfunction is thought to account for autonomic failure associated with PD. In keeping with this assumption, both basal and tilted noradrenaline levels are low.

2. Neuroendocrine Testing

In vivo studies in MSA, which involved testing of the endocrine component of the central autonomic nervous systems (the hypothalamic-pituitary axis) with a variety of challenge procedures, provided evidence of impaired humoral responses of the anterior and the posterior parts of the pituitary gland with impaired secretion of adrenocorticotropic hormone (ACTH) (Polinsky et al., 1987), growth hormone (Kimber et al., 1997), and vasopressin/ADH (Kaufmann et al., 1992), respectively. Although these observations can be made in virtually all patients in an advanced stage of the disease, their prevalence during the early course of MSA is unknown.

There is an ongoing debate about the diagnostic value of the growth-hormone response to clonidine (CGH-test), a neuropharmacological assessment of central adrenergic function, in PD and MSA. Clonidine is a centrally active alpha 2-adrenergic agonist which lowers blood pressure predominantly by reducing CNS sympathetic outflow. Kimber et al. (1997) showed that a normal serum GH increase in response to clonidine infusion was present in fourteen PD patients (without autonomic deficit) and in nineteen patients with PAF, but was absent in thirty-one patients with MSA. In a further study (Tranchant et al., 2000), GH levels remained stable after clonidine infusion in all seven of MSA patients but increased in only twelve of the nineteen PD patients, while remaining stable in the other seven. No correlation was found with the presence of orthostatic hypotension. The authors conclude that the GH response to clonidine infusion has a very high sensitivity for the diagnosis of

MSA, but it cannot be used as a diagnostic test because of its poor specificity.

3. Bladder Function

Assessment of bladder function is mandatory in MSA and usually provides evidence of involvement of the autonomic nervous system at an early stage of the disease. Following a careful history regarding frequency of voiding, difficulties in initiating or suppressing voiding, and the presence and degree of urinary incontinence, standard urinalysis should exclude infection. Post-void residual volume needs to be determined sonographically or via catheterization to initiate intermittent self-catheterization (ISC) in due course. In some patients only cystometry can discriminate between hypocontractile detrusor function and a hyperreflexic sphincter-detrusor dyssynergy.

The nature of bladder dysfunction is different in MSA and PD. Although pollakiuria and urgency are common in both disorders, marked urge or stress incontinence with continuous leakage is not a feature of PD. Urodynamic studies show a characteristic pattern of abnormality in MSA patients (Kirby et al., 1986). In the early stages there is often detrusor hyperreflexia, often with bladder neck incompetence due to abnormal urethral sphincter function, which result in early pollakiuria and urgency followed by urge incontinence. Later on, the ability to initiate a voluntary micturition reflex and the strength of the hyperreflexic detrusor contractions diminish, and the bladder may become atonic, accounting for increasing postmicturition residual urine volumes.

The detrusor hyperreflexia may result from a disturbance of the pontine micturition center (Beck et al., 1994; Wenning et al., 1996b). Alternatively, degeneration of the substantia nigra and other regions of the basal ganglia that are important in the control of micturition may contribute to urological symptoms. The atonic bladder in advanced MSA has been related to the progressive degeneration of the intermediolateral columns of the thoracolumbar spinal cord (Beck et al., 1994); however, this remains speculative.

4. Sexual Function

Sexual dysfunction is a frequent and early symptom of MSA, particularly in male patients. Since male MSA patients frequently develop erectile failure in their forties, and therefore experience substantial impairment of their sexual performance, expert uroneurological advice should be sought for further investigation and implementation of appropriate therapeutic intervention. The pathophysiology of impotence in MSA is unclear; however, it is likely to include central autonomic disturbance and, more rarely, peripheral factors such as venous leakage.

5. Thermoregulation

Abnormalities on tests of sudomotor function, sympathetic skin response, heat tolerance, and skin temperature regulation have been reported in MSA patients (Cohen et al., 1987; Sandroni et al., 1991; Kihara et al., 1991; Santens et al., 1996; Klein et al., 1997). The thermoregulatory sweat test (TST) as a test of preganglionic sympathetic function detects sweating by a color change of an indicator after thermal stimulation, whereas the quantitative sudomotor axon reflex test (QSART) measures an axon reflex mediated by the postganglionic sympathetic sudomotor axon following stimulation of sweat glands with acetylcholine. In MSA, using TST and QSART, both pre- and postganglionic sympathetic failure has been reported (Kihara et al., 1991). However, the sensitivity and specificity of these tests in MSA are unknown and they require specialist experience and equipment.

The pathogenesis of anhidrosis associated with MSA remains unclear. This symptom may be entirely the result of central autonomic dysfunction, or due to (additional) postganglionic sympathetic dysfunction. The latter proposal is supported by tests using direct cholinergic stimulation of peripheral parasympathetic nerves (Baser et al., 1991; Cohen et al., 1987; Sandroni et al., 1991).

6. Gastrointestinal Function

Gastrointestinal motility in MSA has not been investigated in detail, and a single study comparing anorectal function in MSA and PD demonstrated that most patients in both groups showed an abnormal straining pattern, decreased anal tone, or both dysfunctions (Stocchi et al., 2000). The authors suggested that although bowel and anorectal dysfunctions do not differentiate MSA from PD, both abnormalities occur earlier and develop faster in MSA than in PD.

XII. IMAGING

A. Computerized Tomography (CT)

CT scan abnormalities including cerebellar or brainstem atrophy have been reported in patients with a variety of clinical labels such as OPCA, MSA, idiopathic cerebellar ataxia and non-familial degenerative disease (Huang and Plaitakis, 1984; Uematsu et al., 1987; Staal et al., 1990; Klockgether et al., 1990a; Wessel et al., 1993). All of these studies have been biased towards the OPCA type of MSA and in some of them familial and sporadic OPCA were lumped together (Uematsu et al., 1987; Wessel et al., 1993). However, in patients presenting with idiopathic late-onset cerebellar ataxia subclinical brainstem atrophy preceding other clinical symptoms of OPCA by months to years has been reported (Klockgether et al., 1990a). In another CT study focusing on MSA-P (Wenning et al., 1994b), subclinical cerebellar atrophy was detected in 25% of "pure" MSA-P cases. However, all of them had additional autonomic and pyramidal signs that allowed a diagnosis of MSA to be made on clinical grounds alone, suggesting some limitations of this diagnostic tool in routine clinical practice (Wenning et al., 1994b).

B. Routine Magnetic Resonance Imaging (MRI)

MRI scanning of patients with MSA often, but not always, reveals atrophy of cerebellar vermis and, less marked, of cerebellar hemispheres (Schrag et al., 2000). There is also evidence of shrinkage of pons as well as middle cerebellar peduncles (Schulz et al., 1994), differentiating MSA-C from cortical cerebellar atrophy (CCA). The pattern of infratentorial atrophy visible on MRI correlates with the pathological process of OPCA affecting cerebellar vermis and hemispheres, middle cerebellar peduncles, pons, and lower brainstem (Klockgether et al., 1990b). The MRI changes may be indistinguishable from those of patients with autosomal dominant cerebellar ataxias (Wüllner et al., 1993). On the other hand, MRI measures of basal ganglia pathology in MSA are less well established and naked eye assessments are often unreliable. Only in advanced cases may putaminal atrophy be detectable and may correlate with severity of extrapyramidal symptoms (Wakai et al., 1994).

Common abnormalities on MRI may include not only infratentorial atrophy, but also signal abnormalities on T2-weighted images within the pontocerebellar system and putamen. Signal hyperintensities sometimes seen within the pons and middle cerebellar peduncles are thought to reflect degeneration of pontocerebellar fibers and therefore, together with marked atrophy in these areas, indicate a major site of pathology in OPCA type MSA (Savoiardo et al., 1990; Schulz et al., 1994). The characteristic infratentorial signal change on T2-weighted 1.5 Tesla MRI ("hot cross bun" sign) may also corroborate the clinical diagnosis of MSA (Schrag et al., 2000). Putaminal hypointensities in supposedly APD were first reported in 1986 by two groups using a 1.5 Tesla magnet and T2-weighted images (Pastakia et al., 1986; Drayer et al., 1986). This change has subsequently been observed by others in cases clinically thought to have MSA (O'Brien et al., 1990; Olanow, 1992; Wakai et al., 1994; Schulz et al., 1994), and in cases with pathological confirmation (Lang et al., 1994; Schwarz et al., 1996). A lateral to medial as well as posterior to anterior gradient is also well established with the most prominent changes in the posterolateral putamen (Pastakia et al., 1986; Wakai et al., 1994; Lang et al., 1994). This putaminal hypointensity has been proposed as a sensitive and specific abnormality in patients with MSA, and to reflect increased iron deposition. However, similar abnormalities may occur in patients with classical PD (Stern et al., 1989; Schrag et al., 1998) or may represent incidental findings in patients without basal ganglia disorders. The notion of increased iron deposition has been challenged by Brooks and colleagues (1989) and later by Schwarz and colleagues (1996). It was recently shown that hypointense putaminal signal changes were more often observed in MSA than in PD patients using T2*-weighted gradient echo (GE) but not T2-weighted fast spin echo images, indicating that T2*-weighted GE sequences are of diagnostic value for patients with Parkinsonism (Kraft et al., 2002).

Increased putaminal relative to pallidal hypointensities may be seen, as well as a slit-like hyperintense band lateral to the putamen (Schwarz et al., 1996; Konagaya et al., 1993; Konagaya et al., 1994). These changes are consistent with a clinical diagnosis of MSA. However, they also appear to be nonspecific and have also been noted in clinically diagnosed PD and PSP (Schrag et al., 1998; Schrag et al., 2000). But it is the pattern consisting of hypointense and hyperintense T2 changes within the putamen which is a highly specific MRI sign of MSA, while hypointensity alone remains a sensitive, but nonspecific sign of MSA (Kraft et al., 1999). The hyperintense signal correlated with the most pronounced reactive microgliosis and astrogliosis as well as highest iron content in one MRI-postmortem study (Schwarz et al., 1996). Others have reported that the slit hyperintensity in the putaminal margin may represent widened intertissue space due to a severe shrinkage and rarefaction of this nucleus (Konagaya et al., 1998). However, in spite of these speculations the nature of this abnormal signal intensity has remained uncertain.

C. Diffusion-Weighted Imaging (DWI)

Diffusion-weighted imaging (DWI) may represent a useful diagnostic tool that can provide additional support for a diagnosis of MSA-P. It was demonstrated by Schocke et al. (2002), that DWI, even if measured in the slice direction only, is able to discriminate MSA-P and both patients with PD and healthy volunteers on the basis of putaminal rADC (regional apparent diffusion coefficients) values. The increased putaminal rADC values in MSA-P are likely to reflect ongoing striatal degeneration, whereas most neuropathologic studies reveal intact striatum in PD. But since in PSP compared to PD patients rADCs were also significantly increased in both putamen and globus pallidus (Seppi et al., 2003), increased putaminal rADC values do not discriminate MSA-P from PSP.

D. Magnetic Resonance Volumetry

Whether magnetic resonance volumetry will contribute to the differential diagnosis of MSA from other parkinsonian disorders remains to be confirmed. Schulz et al. (1999) found significant reductions in mean striatal and brainstem volumes in patients with MSA-P, MSA-C, and PSP, whereas patients with MSA-C and MSA-P also showed a reduction in cerebellar volume. Total intracranial volume-normalized magnetic resonance imaging-based volumetric measurements provide a sensitive marker to discriminate typical and atypical parkinsonism. Voxel-based morphometry (VBM) confirmed previous region of interest (ROI)-based volumetric studies (Schulz et al., 1999) showing basal ganglia and infratentorial volume loss in MSA-P patients (Brenneis et al., 2003). These data revealed prominent cortical volume loss in MSA-P mainly comprising the cortical targets of striatal projections, consistent with the established frontal lobe impairment of MSA patients (Robbins et al., 1992).

E. Magnetic Resonance Spectroscopy (MRS)

In general, MRS studies have generated conflicting observations of limited relevance to differential diagnosis. Proton magnetic resonance spectroscopy (MRS) is a noninvasive method that provides information about the chemical pathology of disorders affecting the central nervous system. The largest peak visible with MRS is derived from N-acetylaspartate (NAA), an amino acid contained almost exclusively within neurons and their processes in the adult brain (Urenjak et al., 1993). Debate has surrounded MRS findings in MSA. Davie et al. (1995) showed reduced NAA/Cr in the putamen in MSA compared with PD and controls. Federico et al. (1999) have also shown reduced NAA/Cr and NAA/Cho in MSA compared with controls and reduced NAA/Cr in MSA compared with PD. More recently, others have failed to confirm this finding (Hu et al., 1998; Clarke and Lowry, 2000).

F. Functional Imaging

Functional imaging methods for the differential diagnosis of parkinsonian disorders can be divided into investigations of receptor binding and glucose metabolism. Studies of receptor binding in disorders with parkinsonism examine the presynaptic nigrostriatal neurons by evaluating the dopa decarboxylase activity and the dopamine transporter (DAT), and the postsynaptic dopaminergic function evaluating the dopamine D2 receptor. More recently, SPECT and PET ligands have become available to study cardiac sympathetic innervation as well. Acknowledging the lack of comparative studies, iodobenzamide (IBZM) and metaiodobenzylguanidine (MIBG) SPECT as well as fluorodeoxyglucose (FDG) PET (when available) appear to be helpful functional imaging tools that may support an early clinical diagnosis of MSA.

The Hammersmith Cyclotron Unit, using PET, found that putaminal uptake of the presynaptic dopaminergic markers [^{18}F]fluorodopa and S-[^{11}C]nomifensine (Brooks et al., 1990a/b) was similarly reduced in MSA and PD; in approximately half the MSA subjects, caudate uptake was also markedly reduced, as opposed to only moderate reduction in PD. However, discriminant function analysis of striatal [^{18}F]fluorodopa uptake performed poorly in separating MSA and PD patients (Burn et al., 1994). Measurements of striatal dopamine D_2 receptor densities using raclopride and PET failed to differentiate between PD and APD, demonstrating a similar loss of densities in patients with advanced PD, MSA, and PSP (Brooks et al., 1992).

PET studies using other ligands such as [^{11}C]diprenorphine (non-selective opioid receptor antagonist) (Burn et al., 1995) and [^{18}F] FDG (de Volder, 1989; Eidelberg et al., 1993; Perani et al., 1995) have proved more consistent in detecting striatal degeneration and in distinguishing patients with MSA-P from those with PD, particularly when combined with a dopamine D2 receptor scan. Widespread functional abnormalities in MSA-C have been demonstrated using [^{18}F] FDG and PET (Gilman et al., 1994). Reduced metabolism was most marked in the brainstem and cerebellum, but other areas such as the basal ganglia and cerebral cortex were also involved, supporting its nosological status as the cerebellar subtype of MSA.

SPECT evaluation of DAT using [^{123}I]beta-CIT may be useful in differentiating true parkinsonism from patients with essential tremor and patients with "lower body parkinsonism" due to a subcortical vascular encephalopathy. MSA and PSP cannot be separated from PD by this method alone (Brucke et al., 2000). However, MSA patients may show a more symmetric DAT loss, consistent with the more symmetric clinical motor dysfunction observed in this condition. SPECT imaging studies of patients with dopa naive parkinsonism have used [^{123}I] IBZM as a D2 receptor ligand (Schwarz et al., 1992; Schelosky et al., 1993). A good response to apomorphine and subsequent benefit from chronic dopaminergic therapy was observed in subjects with normal IBZM binding, whereas subjects with reduced binding failed to respond. Some of these patients developed other atypical clinical features suggestive of MSA during follow-up (Schwarz et al., 1993). Other SPECT studies have also revealed significant reductions of striatal IBZM binding in clinically probable MSA subjects compared to PD patients (Brücke et al., 1993; Schulz et al., 1994) or controls (Brücke et al., 1993; van Royen et al., 1993). An example is shown in Figure 4. There has been much debate about the mechanisms of levodopa-unresponsiveness in MSA; in addition to loss of striatal dopamine binding sites, alterations further downstream probably also contribute to this clinical finding (Tison et al., 1995a). However, striatal IBZM binding is also reduced in other APD such as PSP (van Royen et al., 1993) limiting its predictive value for an early diagnosis of MSA.

Scintigraphic visualization of postganglionic sympathetic cardiac neurons was found to differentiate patients with

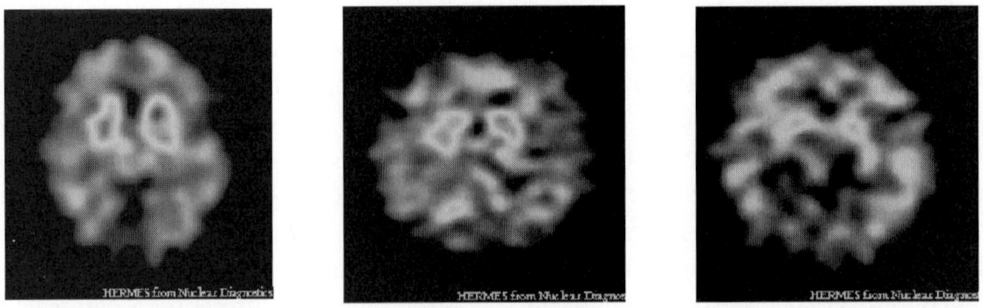

FIGURE 4 (See color version on DVD) Examples of IBZM SPECT images at the level of the striatum in patients with untreated (A) and treated (B) PD compared to a patient with early MSA-P (C). There is normal (A) or only mildly reduced (B) loss of striatal dopamine D2 receptors in the PD patients compared to almost complete loss in early MSA-P. (Innsbruck MSA Study Group, unpublished data).

MSA from patients with PD (Braune et al., 1999b; Orimo et al., 1999; Takatsu et al., 2000; Taki et al., 2000). Considering all reports published so far, standard scintigraphy with [^{123}I] MIBG, which has been used to detect pheochromocytoma cells for years, was able to correctly allocate each of about seventy patients with MSA versus more than 200 patients with PD, because all patients in the latter group showed a severely reduced cardiac uptake of the radioactive ligand. This method appears to be a highly sensitive and specific tool to discriminate between MSA and PD within two years of onset of symptoms; however, the test cannot distinguish MSA from other APD such as PSP (Yoshita, 1998).

XIII. NEUROPHYSIOLOGY

A. External Anal and Urethral Sphincter Electromyography (EMG)

The external anal or urethral sphincter EMG is a common investigation in patients with suspected MSA. Due to degeneration of Onuf's nucleus, both anal and urethral external sphincter muscles undergo denervation and re-innervation. Abnormality of the striated urethral sphincter EMG in MSA was first shown by Martinelli and Coccagna (1978). Subsequently, Kirby et al. (1986) confirmed the presence of polyphasia and abnormal prolongation of individual motor units in MSA, and also examined the potential diagnostic role of sphincter EMG in patients with MSA and PD (Eardley et al., 1989). Sixteen (62%) of tweny-six patients with probable MSA, and only one (8%) of thirteen with probable PD had a pathological EMG result. Anal sphincter EMGs are generally better tolerated, and yield identical results (Beck et al., 1994). In at least 80% of patients with MSA, EMG of the external anal sphincter reveals signs of neuronal degeneration in Onuf's nucleus with spontaneous activity and increased polyphasia (Pramstaller et al., 1995; Ravits et al., 1996; Schwarz et al., 1997; Palace et al., 1997; Tison et al., 2000a). However, these findings do not reliably differentiate between MSA and other forms of APD. An abnormal anal sphincter examination was present in five of twelve (41.6%) PSP patients (Valldeoriola et al., 1995). Furthermore, several investigators have also demonstrated neurogenic changes of external anal sphincter muscle in advanced stages of PD (Libelius and Johansson, 2000; Giladi et al., 2000; Jost and Schimrigk 1996). Also, chronic constipation, previous pelvic surgery, or vaginal deliveries can be confounding factors which may induce non-specific abnormalities (Colosimo et al., 2000). In summary, in patients with probable MSA, abnormal sphincter EMG, as compared to control subjects, has been found in the vast majority of patients, including those who, as yet, have no urological or anorectal problems. The prevalence of abnormalities in the early stages of MSA is as yet unclear. Patients with PD as a rule do not show severe sphincter EMG abnormalities in the early stage of the disease, unless other causes for sphincter denervation are present. With such criteria, the sensitivity of the method is, however, relatively low (Vodusek, 2001).

B. Evoked Potentials

In general, the value of evoked potential studies in the diagnosis of MSA is limited. Prasher and Bannister (1986) compared BAEPs in twenty patients with PD, fourteen patients with MSA and autonomic failure and six patients with pure autonomic failure (PAF). Abnormal latencies or amplitude ratios (wave V/I) were identified in MSA, one PD and none of the PAF patients. The authors proposed that these changes might be due to disruption of the auditory pathway in the superior olivary complex. However, in a subsequent study in twenty patients with probable MSA, routine BAEPS were found to be completely normal in almost 50% of the cases, with only minimal alterations in the rest (Smith, personal communication). Magnetic evoked potentials (MEP) are often, but not always, normal in MSA (Sobue et al., 1992; Wenning and Smith, 1997; Abbruzzese et al., 1997). Somatosensory, visual, and acoustic evoked potentials may show prolonged latencies in up to 40% of patients

(Abele et al., 2000a; Kodama et al., 1999), but many patients show no abnormalities of central efferent and afferent neuronal pathways (Abele et al., 2000a; Abbruzzese et al., 1997).

C. Electroneurography

To study the frequency and severity of peripheral neuropathy in MSA, Abele et al. (2000b) performed nerve conduction studies (NCS) in 42 MSA patients suffering from either MSA-C or MSA-P. Overall, abnormal nerve conduction was present in 24% of the patients. Abnormalities were significantly more frequent in MSA-P (43%) compared to MSA-C (14%). The data provide evidence that the peripheral nervous system is differentially affected in MSA-P and MSA-C.

Some investigators (Montagna et al., 1983; Cohen et al., 1987; Sobue et al., 1992; Terao et al., 1994) have suggested that both somatic anterior horn cells and peripheral nerves are commonly affected in MSA, and their involvement has therefore been regarded as part of the clinical spectrum of MSA. Indeed, muscle wasting was reported in the original description by Shy and Drager (1960). However, despite the occasional presence of pathological changes in anterior horn cells (Terao et al., 1994), somatic nerves (Tohgi et al., 1982; Galassi et al., 1982), and muscle (Bannister et al., 1999), clinical symptomatology is usually mild or absent. Furthermore, in the clinical series of Wenning et al. (1994a) of 100 MSA patients only 4 had focal wasting, and only 1 had fasciculations.

D. Startle Response

Excessive auditory startle responses (ASR) may also help differentiate MSA both from PD and other forms of APD (Kofler et al., 2001). The auditory startle reaction to an unexpected loud stimulus is mediated by a brainstem reflex originating in the nucleus reticularis pontis caudalis, being distributed up the brainstem and down the spinal cord along slowly conducting pathways. Exaggerated ASR is a characteristic feature of MSA patients and may reflect disinhibition of lower brainstem nuclei due to the degenerative disorder.

XIV. OTHER INVESTIGATIONS

CSF-NFL and levodopa tests combined with discriminant analysis may contribute to the differential diagnosis of Parkinsonian syndromes (Holmberg et al., 2001). Whereas the CSF-NFL and levodopa tests predicted 79% and 85% correct diagnoses (PD or non-PD [MSA and PSP]), respectively, the combined test predicted 90% correct diagnoses. The authors conclude that the CSF-NFL and levodopa tests provide detailed information of clinical variables on which the clinical diagnostic criteria are based. As they are pathologically unrelated, the diagnostic precision increases compared to clinical diagnoses when they are combined.

Patients with MSA usually retain normal intelligence levels, but abnormalities of neuropsychological function have been described (Meco et al., 1996). In a few studies, a distinctive pattern of cognitive defects was found, suggesting normal intelligence but disorders of frontal lobe function (Robbins et al., 1992; Brown et al., 2002). These included difficulties with attentional set shifting when extradimensional shifting was required, impairment in subject-ordered tests of spatial working memory, and deficits in speed of thinking (rather than of accuracy) in the Tower of London task. Another study in patients with MSA-P demonstrated impairment on category and phonemic fluency, frontal behaviors, trail making tests A and B, and free recall in the Grober and Buschke test (Pillon et al., 1995). These patients were normal on all other tests, including the revised Wechsler Adult Intelligence Scale verbal and memory scales.

XV. TREATMENT

Because of the small number of randomized controlled trials, the practical management of MSA is largely based on empirical evidence, except for a few controlled studies on midodrine.

A. Autonomic Failure

Unfortunately there is no causal therapy for autonomic dysfunction currently available to clinicians. Therefore, the therapeutic strategy is defined by clinical symptoms and impairment of quality of life in these patients. Due to the progressive course of MSA, a regular review of the treatment is mandatory to adjust measures according to clinical needs. The concept of treating symptoms of orthostatic hypotension is based on the increase of intravasculature volume and the reduction of volume shift to lower body parts when changing into an upright position. The selection and combination of the following options depends on the severity of symptoms and their practicability in the individual patient, but not on the extent of blood pressure drop during tilt test. Nonpharmacological options include sufficient fluid intake, high salt diet, more frequent but smaller meals per day to reduce postprandial hypotension by spreading the total carbohydrate intake, and custom-made elastic body garments. During the night, head-up tilt increases intravasculature volume up to 1 L within a week, which is particularly helpful in improving hypotension early in the morning. This approach is particularly successful in combination with fludrocortisone, which further supports sodium retention.

The next group of drugs to use is the sympathomimetics. These include ephedrine (with both direct and indirect effects) which is often valuable in central autonomic disorders such as MSA. With higher doses, side effects include tremulousness, loss of appetite, and urinary retention in men.

Among the large number of vasoactive agents that have been evaluated in MSA, only one, the directly acting α-agonist midodrine, meets the criteria of evidence-based medicine (Jankovic et al., 1993; Low et al., 1997; Wright et al., 1998). Side effects are usually mild and only rarely lead to discontinuation of treatment because of urinary retention or pruritus predominantly on the scalp. Another promising drug appears to be the noradrenaline precursor L-threo-dihydroxy-phenylserine (L-threo-DOPS), which has been used in this indication in Japan for years and whose efficacy has now been shown by a recent open, dose-finding trial (Mathias et al., 2001). If the preceding drugs do not produce the desired effect, then selective targeting is needed. The somatostatin analogue, octreotide, often is beneficial in postprandial hypotension (Alam et al., 1995), presumably because it inhibits release of vasodilatory gastrointestinal peptides (Raimbach et al., 1989); importantly, it does not enhance nocturnal hypertension (Alam et al., 1995). The vasopressin analogue desmopressin, which acts on renal tubular vasopressin-2 receptors, reduces nocturnal polyuria and improves morning postural hypotension (Mathias et al., 1986). The peptide erythropoietin may be beneficial in some patients by raising red cell mass, secondarily improving cerebral oxygenation (Perera et al., 1995; Winkler et al., 2001). A broad range of drugs have been used in the treatment of postural hypotension (Mathias and Kimber, 1999). Unfortunately, the value and side effects of many of these drugs have not been adequately determined in MSA patients using appropriate endpoints.

In neurogenic bladder dysfunction including residual urine clean intermittent catheterization three to four times per day is a widely accepted approach to prevent secondary consequences from failure to micturate. It can become necessary to provide the patient with a permanent transcutaneous suprapubic catheter if mechanical obstruction in the urethra or motor symptoms of MSA prevent uncomplicated catheterization. Pharmacological options with anti- or procholinergic or -adrenergic substances are usually not successful to adequately reduce post-void residual volume in MSA, but anticholinergic agents like oxybutynin can improve symptoms of detrusor hyperreflexia or sphincter-detrusor dyssynergy in the early course of the disease (Beck et al., 1994). Recently, α-adrenergic receptor antagonists (prazosin and moxisylyte) have been shown to improve voiding with reduction of residual volumes in MSA patients (Sakakibara et al., 2000b). Urological surgery must be avoided in these patients because worsening of bladder control post-operatively is most likely (Beck et al., 1994).

The necessity of a specific treatment of sexual dysfunction must be evaluated individually in each MSA patient. Male impotence can be partially circumvented by the use of intracavernosal papaverine, prostaglandin E1, or penile implants (Colosimo and Pezzella, 2002). Preliminary evidence in PD patients (Zesiewicz et al., 2000) had suggested that sildenafil may also be successful in treating erectile failure in MSA: A recent trial confirmed the efficacy of this compound in MSA, but also suggested caution because of the frequent cardiovascular side-effects (Hussain et al., 2001).

Constipation is relieved by an increase in intraluminal fluid which may be achieved by a macrogol-water solution (Eichhorn and Oertel, 2001). Inspiratory stridor develops in about 30% of patients, occasionally from the disease onset. Continuous positive airway pressure (CPAP) may be helpful in some of these patients (Iranzo et al., 2000). In only about 4% is a tracheostomy needed and performed.

B. Motor Disorder

1. General Approach

Because the results of drug treatment for the motor disorder of MSA are generally poor, other therapies are all the more important. Physiotherapy helps maintain mobility and prevent contractures, and speech therapy can improve speech and swallowing and provide communication aids. Dysphagia may require feeding via a nasogastric tube or even percutaneous endoscopic gastrostomy (PEG). These management decisions should be based on careful clinical judgment, taking into account the expectations of both patient and caregivers. Occupational therapy helps to limit the handicap resulting from the patient's disabilities and should include a home visit. Provision of a wheelchair is usually dictated by the liability to fall because of postural instability and gait ataxia but not by akinesia and rigidity per se. Psychological support for patients and partners should be stressed.

2. Parkinsonism

Parkinsonism is the predominating motor disorder of MSA and therefore represents a major target for therapeutic intervention. Although less effective than in PD and despite the lack of controlled trials, levodopa replacement represents the mainstay of anti-parkinsonian therapy in MSA. Open-label studies suggest that up to 30 to 40% of MSA patients may derive benefit from levodopa at least transiently (Parati et al., 1993; Wenning et al., 1994a). Occasionally, a beneficial effect is evident only when seemingly unresponsive patients deteriorate after levodopa withdrawal (Hughes et al., 1992). Pre-existing orthostatic hypotension is often unmasked or exacerbated in levodopa-treated MSA

TABLE 7 Therapeutic Studies in MSA since 1993

Agent/Reference	Target	Number of patients	Design	Dose	Outcome measures	Results	Side effects
Amantadine (Botez et al., 1996)	Ataxia	30 (OPCA)	randomized, controlled, double-blind	200 mg/day	reaction and movement times	improvement on seven out of eight variables	
Amantadine (Colosimo et al., 1996)	Parkinsonism	5	open label	400–600 mg/day	UPDRS III	no benefit	
Levodopa (Parati et al., 1993)	Parkinsonism	8	single challenge, open label	250 mg	UPDRS III	moderate improvement in four patients	
Levodopa and apomorphine (Rossi et al., 2000)	Parkinsonism	28	single challenge, open label	levodopa: 250 mg; apomorphine 1.5–4.5 mg	UPDRS III	mean motor score improvement up to 14.3%	frequent nausea with apomorphine
Metoclopramide (Magnifico et al., 2001)	OH	6	acute challenge, controlled	20 mg over 20 min	BP	no benefit	supine hypotension with lack of heart rate increase
Midodrine (Jankovic et al., 1993)	OH	97	randomized, controlled, double-blind	7.5–30 mg/day	BP, symptoms of OH	effective	scalp pruritus, supine hypertension, urgency
Midodrine (Low et al., 1997)	OH	40	randomized, controlled, parallel	30 mg/day	BP, symptoms of OH, global relief score	effective, well tolerated	pilomotor reaction, supine hypertension, urinary retention
Midodrine (Wright et al., 1998)	OH	25	acute challenge, controlled, crossover	2.5–20 mg	BP, global assessment	effective	
Octreotide (Bordet et al., 1994)	OH	5	open label	300 μg/day	BP	functional improvement	
Octreotide (Bordet et al., 1995)	OH	9	acute challenge, randomized, controlled, double-blind	100 μg	BP, norepinephrine level	partial improvement, well tolerated	
Threo-DOPS (Freeman et al., 1999)	OH	10	acute challenge, randomized, controlled, crossover	1 g/day	BP, norepinephrine level, quality of life questionnaire	effective, well tolerated	no major side effects
Threo-DOPS (Mathias et al., 2001)	OH	26	open, dose ranging	200–600 mg/day	BP, symptoms related to OH	effective and well tolerated	no supine hypertension
Sildenafil (Hussain et al., 2001)	Impotence	12	controlled, double-blind	50 mg/day	erectile function questionnaire	effective	significant OH in three patients

UPDRS, Unified PD Rating Scale.
OH, Orthostatic hypotension.

associated with autonomic failure. In contrast, psychiatric or toxic confusional states appear to be less common than in PD (Wenning et al., 1994a). Results with dopamine agonists have been even more disappointing (Lees, 1999). Severe psychiatric side-effects occurred in a double-blind trial of six patients on lisuride, with nightmares, visual hallucinations, and confusional states (Lees and Bannister, 1981). Wenning et al. (1994a) reported a response to oral dopamine agonists only in four of forty-one patients. None of thirty patients receiving bromocriptine improved, but three of ten who received pergolide had some benefit. Twenty-two percent of the levodopa responders had good or excellent response to at least one orally active dopamine agonist in addition. Anti-Parkinsonian effects were noted in four of twenty-six MSA patients treated with amantadine (Wenning et al., 1994a); however, there was no significant improvement in an open study of nine patients with APD, including five subjects with MSA (Colosimo et al., 1996).

Blepharospasm and limb dystonia, but not antecollis, may respond well to local injections of botulinum toxin A.

3. Cerebellar Ataxia

There is no effective therapy for the progressive ataxia of MSA-C. Occasional successes have been reported with cholinergic drugs, amantadine, 5-hydroxytryptophan, isoniazid, baclofen, and propanolol; however, for the large majority of patients these drugs proved to be ineffective.

C. Future Therapeutic Approaches

Two European research initiatives (EMSA-SG, NNIPPS) are presently conducting multi-center intervention trials in MSA. These trials will radically change our approach to MSA. For the first time, prospective data concerning disease progression will become available, enabling us to reliably identify predictors of survival. Secondly, a specific rating instrument (Unified MSA Rating Scale, UMSARS) including a video teaching tape has been developed by EMSA-SG (Wenning et al., 2002) to standardize severity assessments in specialized clinics and research programs worldwide. Furthermore, surrogate markers of the disease process will be identified by the EMSA-SG and NIPPS trials using structural and functional neuroimaging. These markers will allow planning for future Phase III intervention trials more effectively. Research into the etiopathogenesis and neuropathology of MSA is being conducted by several groups thanks to a number of animal models which have become available as testbeds for preclinical intervention studies (Wenning et al., 1996a; Scherfler et al., 2000; Wenning et al., 1999b; Waldner et al., 2001). This work will hopefully lead to a multitude of neuroprotective candidate agents ready for evaluation during the next decade.

D. Conclusion

During the last fifteen years, major advances have been made in our understanding of the cellular pathology of MSA. At the same time, the first multi-center intervention trials have been launched in Europe. Although therapeutic options are limited at present, there is a real hope for a radical change of our approach to this devastating illness.

Acknowledgments

GKW received grants from the Fonds zur Förderung der wissenschaftlichen Forschung (FWF, Vienna), Nationalbank (Vienna), Bundesministerium für Bildung, Wissenschaft und Kultur (BMWK, Vienna), and the EC (Fifth framework programme).

References

Abbruzzese, G., R. Marchese, and C. Trompetto. 1997. Sensory and motor evoked potentials in multiple system atrophy: comparative study with Parkinson's disease. *Mov Disord* **12**:315–321.

Abele, M., K. Burk, L. Schols, S. Schwartz, I. Besenthal, J. Dichgans, C. Zuhlke, O. Riess, and T. Klockgether. 2002. The aetiology of sporadic adult-onset ataxia. *Brain* **125**:961–968.

Abele, M., J.B. Schulz, K. Burk, H. Topka, J. Dichgans, and T. Klockgether. 2000a. Evoked potentials in multiple system atrophy (MSA). *Acta Neurol Scand* **101**:111–115.

Abele, M., J.B. Schulz, K. Burk, H. Topka, J. Dichgans, and T. Klockgether. 2000b. Nerve conduction studies in multiple system atrophy. *Eur Neurol* **43**:221–223.

Abeliovich, A., Y. Schmitz, I. Farinas, D. Lundberg, W.H. Ho, P.E. Castillo et al. 2000. Mice lacking alpha-synuclein display functional deficits in the nigrostriatal dopamine system. *Neuron* **25**:239–252.

Adams, R.D., L. van Bogaert, and H. van der Eecken. 1961. Dégénérescences nigro-striées et cérébello-nigro-striees. *Psychiatria et Neurologia* **142**:219–259.

Adams, R.D., L. van Bogaert, and H. van der Eecken. 1964. Striato-nigral degeneration. *J Neuropath Exp Neurol* **23**:584–608.

Alam, M., G. Smith, K. Bleasdal-Barr, D.V. Pavitt, and C.J. Mathias. 1995. Effects of the peptide release inhibitor, octreotide, on daytime hypotension and on nocturnal hypertension in primary autonomic failure. *J Hypertens* **13**:1664–1669.

Albanese, A., C. Colosimo, A.R. Bentivoglio, R. Fenici, G. Melillo, C. Colosimo et al. 1995. Multiple system atrophy presenting as parkinsonism: clinical features and diagnostic criteria. *J Neurol Neurosurg Psychiatry* **59**:144–151.

Ansorge, O., A.J. Lees, D.J. Brooks, and S.E. Daniel. 1997a. Multiple system atrophy presenting as progressive supranuclear palsy and vice-versa: two unusual cases. *Mov Disord* **12(suppl.1)**:96.

Ansorge, O., A.J. Lees, and S.E. Daniel. 1997b. Pathological overlap of Alzheimer's disease, Parkinson's disease and multiple system atrophy. *Neuropathol Appl Neurobiol* **23**:179.

Arima K., K. Ueda, N. Sunohara, K. Arakawa, S. Hirai, M. Nakamura, H. Tonozuka-Uehara, and M. Kawai. 1998. NACP/alpha-synuclein immunoreactivity in fibrillary components of neuronal and oligodendroglial cytoplasmic inclusions in the pontine nuclei in multiple system atrophy. *Acta Neuropathol* (Berl) **96**:439–444.

Bandmann, O., G.K. Wenning, N.P. Quinn, and A.E. Harding. 1995. Arg296 to Cys296 polymorphism in exon 6 of cytochrome P-450-2D6 (CYP2D6) is not associated with multiple system atrophy. *J Neurol Neurosurg Psychiatry* **59**:557.

Bandmann, O., M.G. Sweeney, S.E. Daniel, G.K. Wenning, N. Quinn, C.D. Marsden, and N.W. Wood. 1997. Multiple-system atrophy is genetically distinct from identified inherited causes of spinocerebellar degeneration. *Neurology* **49**:1598–1604.

Bannister, R., M. Ellison, and J. Morgan-Hughes. 1999. Histological studies of skeletal and smooth muscles in autonomic failure. In: Mathias C.J., Bannister R., eds. Autonomic Failure. A Textbook of Clinical Disorders of the Autonomic Nervous System. *Oxford: University Press* 340–341.

Bannister, R., and C.J. Mathias. 1999a. Clinical features and evaluation of the primary chronic autonomic failure syndromes. In: Mathias C.J., Bannister R., eds. Autonomic Failure. A Textbook of Clinical Disorders of the Autonomic Nervous System. *Oxford: University Press* 307–316.

Bannister, R., and C.J. Mathias. 1999b. Investigation of autonomic disorders. In: Mathias C.J., Bannister R., eds. Autonomic failure. A Textbook of Clinical Disorders of the Autonomic Nervous System. *Oxford: University Press* 169–195.

Bannister, R., and D.R. Oppenheimer. 1972. Degenerative diseases of the nervous system associated with autonomic failure. *Brain* **95**:457–474.

Baser, S.M., J. Meer, R.J. Polinsky, and M. Hallett. 1991. Sudomotor function in autonomic failure. *Neurology* **41**:1564–1566.

Beck, R.O., C.D. Betts, and C.J. Fowler. 1994. Genitourinary dysfunction in multiple system atrophy: clinical features and treatment in 62 cases. *J Urol* **151**:1336–1341.

Benarroch, E.E., I.L. Smithson, P.A. Low, and J.E. Parisi. 1998. Depletion of catecholaminergic neurons of the rostral ventrolateral medulla in multiple systems atrophy with autonomic failure. *Ann Neurol* **43**:156–163.

Ben-Shlomo, Y., G.K. Wenning, F. Tison, and N.P. Quinn. 1997. Survival of patients with pathologically proven multiple system atrophy: a meta-analysis. *Neurology* **48**:384–393.

Berciano, J., O. Combarros, J.M. Polo, J. Pascual, and A. Oterino. 1998. Who first described striatonigral degeneration? *Neurology* **50(suppl 4)**: 120.

Berciano, J., and I. Ferrer. 1996. Glial and neuronal cytoplasmic inclusions in familial olivopontocerebellar atrophy. *Ann Neurol* **40**:819–820.

Berciano, J., F. Valldeoriola, I. Ferrer, J. Rumia, J. Pascual, C. Marin, M.J. Rey, and E. Tolosa. 2002. Presynaptic parkinsonism in multiple system atrophy mimicking Parkinson's disease: a clinicopathological case study. *Mov Disord* **17**:812–816.

Bordet, R., J. Benhadjali, C. Libersa, and A. Desteè. 1994. Octreotide in the managment of orthostatic hypotension in multiple system atrophy: pilot trial of chronic administration. *Clin Neuropharmacol* **17**:380–383.

Bordet, R., J. Benhadjali, A. Desteè, A. Belabbas, and C. Libersa. 1995. Octreotide effects on orthostatic hypotension in patients with multiple system atrophy: a controlled study of acute administration. *Clin Neuropharmacol* **18**:83–89.

Bösch, S.M., M. Schocke, K. Seppi, P. Hollosi, W. Poewe, and G.K. Wenning. 2002a. Abnormal striatal dopaminergic function in SCA2 revealed by beta-CIT and IBZM SPECT. *Mov Disord* **17(Suppl 5)**:311.

Bösch, S.M., G.K. Wenning, G. Ransmayr, and W. Poewe. 2002b. Dystonia in multiple system atrophy. *J Neurol Neurosurg Psychiatry* **72**:300–303.

Botez, M.I., T. Botez-Marquard, R. Elie, O.L. Pedraza, K. Goyette, and R. Lalonde. 1996. Amantadine hydrochloride treatment in heredodegenerative ataxias: a double blind study. *J Neurol Neurosurg Psychiatry* **61**:259–264.

Botez, M.I., and S.N. Young. 2001. Biogenic amine metabolites and thiamine in cerebrospinal fluid in heredodegenerative ataxias. *Can J Neurol Sci* **28**:134–140.

Bower, J.H., D.M. Maraganore, S.K. McDonnell, and W.A. Rocca. 1997. Incidence of progressive supranuclear palsy and multiple system atrophy in Olmsted County, Minnesota, 1976 to 1990. *Neurology* **49**: 1284–1288.

Braak, H., and E. Braak. 1989. Cortical and subcortical argyrophilic grains characterize a disease associated with adult onset dementia. *Neuropathol Appl Neurobiol* **15**:13–26.

Braune, S., A. Auer, J. Schulte-Mönting, S. Schwerbrock, and C.H. Lücking. 1996a. Cardiovascular parameters: sensitivity to detect autonomic dysfunction and influence of age and sex in normal subjects. *Clinical Autonomic Research* **6**:3–15.

Braune, S., J. Schulte-Monting, S. Schwerbrock, and C.H. Lucking. 1996b. Retest variation of cardiovascular parameters in autonomic testing. *J Auton Nerv Syst* **60**:103–107.

Braune, S., M. Elam, R. Baron, and P.A. Low. 1999a. Assessment of blood pressure regulation. The International Federation of Clinical Neurophysiology. *Electroencephalogr Clin Neurophysiol Suppl* **52**: 287–291.

Braune, S., M. Reinhardt, R. Schnitzer, A. Riedel, and C.H. Lücking. 1999b. Cardiac uptake of (123I)MIBG separates Parkinson's disease from multiple system atrophy. *Neurology* **53**:1020–1025.

Brenneis, C., K. Seppi, M.F. Schocke, J. Müller, E. Luginger, S. Bösch, W. Löscher, C. Büchel, W. Poewe, and G.K. Wenning. 2003. Voxel-based morphometry detects cortical atrophy in the parkinson variant of multiple system atrophy. *Mov Disord* **18**:1132–1138.

Brooks, D.J., P. Luthert, D. Gadian, and C.D. Marsden. 1989. Does signal-attenuation on high-field T2-weighted MRI of the brain reflect regional cerebral iron deposition? Observations on the relationship between regional cerebral water proton T2-values and iron levels. *J Neurol Neurosurg Psychiatry* **52**:108–111.

Brooks, D.J., V. Ibanez, G.V. Sawle et al. 1990a. Differing patterns of striatal 18-F-Dopa uptake in Parkinson's disease, multiple system atrophy and progressive supranuclear palsy. *Ann Neurol* **28**:547–555.

Brooks, D.J., E.P. Salmon, C.J. Mathias et al. 1990b. The relationhip between locomotor disability, autonomic dysfunction, and the integrity of the striatal dopaminergic system in patients with multiple system atrophy, pure autonomic failure, and Parkinson's disease, studied with PET. *Brain* **113**:1539–1552.

Brooks, D.J., V. Ibanez, G.V. Sawle, E.D. Playford, N. Quinn, C.J. Mathias, A.J. Lees, C.D. Marsden, R. Bannister, and R.S. Frackowiak. 1992. Striatal D2 receptor status in patients with Parkinson's disease, striatonigral degeneration, and progressive supranuclear palsy, measured with 11C-raclopride and positron emission tomography. *Ann Neurol* **31**: 184–192.

Brown, R.G., B. Pillon, I. Uttner, C. Payan, L. Lacomblez, Members of the Neuropsychology Working Group and NNIPPS Consortium. 2002. Cognitive function in patients with Progressive Supranuclear Palsy (PSP) and Multiple System Atrophy (MSA). *Mov Disord* **17(Suppl 5)**: 221.

Brücke, T., S. Wenger, and S. Asenbaum. 1993. Dopamine D2 receptor imaging and measurement with SPECT. *Adv Neurol* **60**:494–500.

Brücke, T., S. Asenbaum, W. Pirker, S. Djamshidian, S. Wenger, C. Wober, C. Muller, and I. Podreka. 1997. Measurement of the dopaminergic degeneration in Parkinson's disease with [123I] beta-CIT and SPECT. Correlation with clinical findings and comparison with multiple system atrophy and progressive supranuclear palsy. *J Neural Transm Suppl* **50**:9–24.

Brücke, T., S. Djamshidian, G. Bencsits, W. Pirker, S. Asenbaum, and I. Podreka. 2000. SPECT and PET imaging of the dopaminergic system in Parkinson's disease. *J Neurol* **247**:IV/2–7.

Burn, D.J., G.V. Sawle, and D.J. Brooks. 1994. Differential diagnosis of Parkinson's disease, multiple system atrophy, and Steele-Richardson-Olszewski syndrome: discriminant analysis of striatal 18F-dopa PET data. *J Neurol Neurosurg Psychiatry* **57**:278–284.

Burn, D.J., J.O. Rinne, N.P. Quinn, A.J. Lees, C.D. Marsden, and D.J. Brooks. 1995. Striatal opioid receptor binding in Parkinson's disease, striatonigral degeneration and Steele-Richardson-Olszewski syndrome. A [11C]diprenorphine PET study. *Brain* **118**:951–958.

Cairns, N.J., P.F. Atkinson, D.P. Hanger, B.H. Anderton, S.E. Daniel, and P.L. Lantos. 1997a. Tau protein in the glial cytoplasmatic inclusions of multiple system atrophy can be distinguished from abnormal tau in Alzheimer's disease. *Neurosci Lett* **230**:49–52.

Cairns, N.J., P.F. Atkinson, T. Kovacs, A.J. Lees, S.E. Daniel, and P.L. Lantos. 1997b. Apolipoprotein E ε4 allele frequency in patients with multiple system atrophy. *Neurosci Lett* **221(2–3)**:161–164.

Caplan, L.R. 1984. Clinical features of sporadic (Dejerine-Thomas) olivopontocerebellar atrophy. *Adv Neurol* **41**:217–224.

Chandiramani, V.A., J. Palace, and C.J. Fowler. 1997. How to recognize patients with parkinsonism who should not have urological surgery. *Br J Urol* **80**:100–104.

Chin, S.S., and J.E. Goldman. 1996. Glial inclusions in CNS degenerative diseases. *J Neuropathol Exp Neurol* **55**:499–508.

Chio, A., C. Magnani, and D. Schiffer. 1998. Prevalence of Parkinson's disease in northwestern Italy: comparison of tracer methodology and clinical ascertainment of cases. *Mov Disord* **13**:400–405.

Churchyard, A., G.A. Donnan, A. Hughes, D.W. Howells, D. Woodhouse, J.Y. Wong, R.M. Kalnins, F.A. Mendelsohn, and G. Paxinos. 1993. Dopa resistance in multiple-system atrophy: loss of postsynaptic D2 receptors. *Ann Neurol* **34**:219–226.

Clarke, C.E., and M. Lowry. 2000. Basal ganglia metabolite concentrations in idiopathic Parkinson's disease and multiple system atrophy measured by proton magnetic resonance spectroscopy. *Eur J Neurol* **7**:661–665.

Cohen, J., P. Low, R. Fealey, S. Sheps, and N.S. Jiang. 1987. Somatic and autonomic function in progressive autonomic failure and multiple system atrophy. *Ann Neurol* **22**:692–699.

Colosimo, C. 1998. Pisa syndrome in a patient with multiple system atrophy. *Mov Disord* **13**:607–609.

Colosimo, C., A. Albanese, A.J. Hughes, V.M. de Bruin, and A.J. Lees. 1995. Some specific clinical features differentiate multiple system atrophy (striatonigral variety) from Parkinson's disease. *Arch Neurol* **52(3)**:294–298.

Colosimo, C., M. Inghilleri, and K.R. Chaudhuri. 2000. Parkinson's disease misdiagnosed as multiple system atrophy by sphincter electromyography. *J Neurol* **247**:559–561.

Colosimo, C., M. Merello, and F.E. Pontieri. 1996. Amantadine in parkinsonian patients unresponsive to levodopa: a pilot study. *J Neurol* **243**: 422–425.

Colosimo, C., and F.R. Pezzella. 2002. The symptomatic treatment of multiple system atrophy. *Eur J Neurol* **9**:195–199.

Consensus statement on the definition of orthostatic hypotension, pure autonomic failure, and multiple system atrophy. 1996. *J Neurol Sci* **144**: 218–219.

Cortes, R., M. Camps, B. Gueye, A. Probst, and J.M. Palacios. 1989. Dopamine receptors in human brain: autoradiographic distribution of D1 and D2 sites in Parkinson syndrome of different etiology. *Brain Res* **483(1)**:30–38.

Daniel, S.E. 1999. The neuropathology and neurochemistry of multiple system atrophy. In: Mathias C.J., Bannister R., eds. Autonomic Failure. A Textbook of Clinical Disorders of the Autonomic Nervous System. *Oxford: Oxford University Press* 321–328.

Daniel, S.E., J.F. Geddes, and T. Revesz. 1995. Glial cytoplasmic inclusions are not exclusive to multiple system atrophy. *J Neurol Neurosurg Psychiatry* **58**:262.

Davie, C.A., G.K. Wenning, G.J. Barker, P.S. Tofts, B.E. Kendall, N. Quinn et al. 1995. Differentiation of multiple system atrophy from idiopathic Parkinson's disease using proton magnetic resonance spectroscopy. *Ann Neurol* **37**:204–210.

Dejerine, J., and A.A. Thomas. 1900. L'atrophie olivo-ponto-cérébelleuse. *Nouvelle Iconographie de le Salpêtrière* **13**:330–370.

De Volder, A.G., J. Francart, C. Laterre, G. Dooms, A. Bol, C. Michel et al. 1989. Decreased glucose utilization in the striatum and frontal lobe in probable striatonigral degeneration. *Ann Neurol* **26**:239–247.

Dexter, D.T., A. Carayon, F. Javoy-Agid, Y. Agid, F.R. Wells, S.E. Daniel, A.J. Lees, P. Jenner, and C.D. Marsden. 1991. Alterations in the levels of iron, ferritin and other trace metals in Parkinson's disease and other neurodegenerative diseases affecting the basal ganglia. *Brain* **114**: 1953–1975.

Dickson, D.W., W. Lin, W.K. Liu, and S.H. Yen. 1999. Multiple system atrophy: a sporadic synucleinopathy. *Brain Pathol* **9**:721–732.

Djaldetti, R., R. Mosberg-Galili, H. Sroka, D. Merims, and E. Melamed. 1999. Camptocormia (bent spine) in patients with Parkinson's disease—characterization and possible pathogenesis of an unusual phenomenon. *Mov Disord* **14**:443–447.

Drayer, B.P., W. Olanow, P. Burger, G.A. Johnson, R. Herfkens, and S. Riederer. 1986. Parkinson Plus Syndrome: diagnosis using high field MR imaging of brain iron. *Radiology* **159**:493–498.

Eardley, I., N.P. Quinn, C.J. Fowler, R.S. Kirby, H.F. Parkhouse, C.D. Marsden et al. 1989. The value of urethral sphincter electromyography in the differential diagnosis of parkinsonism. *British Journal of Urology* **64**:360–362.

Eichhorn, T.E., and W.H. Oertel. 2001. Macrogol 3350/electrolyte improves constipation in Parkinson's disease and multiple system atrophy. *Mov Disord* **16**:1176–1177.

Eidelberg, D., S. Takikawa, J.R. Moeller, V. Dhawan, K. Redington, T. Chaly et al. 1993. Striatal hypometabolism distinguishes striatonigral degeneration from Parkinson's disease. *Ann Neurol* **33**:518–527.

El-Agnaf, O.M., M.D. Curran, A. Wallace, D. Middleton, C. Murgatroyd, A. Curtis, R. Perry, and E. Jaros. 1998. Mutation screening in exons 3 and 4 of alpha-synuclein in sporadic Parkinson's and sporadic and familial dementia with Lewy bodies cases. *Neuroreport* **9**:3925–3927.

Engelender, S., Z. Kaminsky, X. Guo, A.H. Sharp, R.K. Amaravi, J.J. Kleiderlein, R.L. Margolis, J.C. Troncoso, A.A. Lanahan, P.F. Worley, V.L. Dawson, T.M. Dawson, and C.A. Ross. 1999. Synphilin-I associates with alpha-synuclein and promotes the formation of cytosolic inclusions. *Nat Genet* **22**:110–114.

Fearnley, J.M., and A.J. Lees. 1991. Ageing and Parkinson's disease: substantia nigra regional selectivity. *Brain* **114**:2283–2301.

Fearnley, J.M., and A.J. Lees. 1990. Striatonigral degeneration. A clinicopathological study. *Brain* **113**:1823–1842.

Federico, F., I.L. Simone, V. Lucivero, D.M. Mezzapesa, M. de Mari, P. Lamberti et al. 1999. Usefulness of proton magnetic resonance spectroscopy in differentiating parkinsonian syndromes. *Ital J Neurol Sci* **20(4)**:223–229.

Fleischhacker, H. 1924. Afamiliäre chronisch progressive Erkrankung des mittleren Lebensalters vom Pseudosklerosetyp. *Z Gesamte Neurol Psychiatrie* **91**:1–22.

Freeman, R., L. Landsberg, and J. Young. 1999. The treatment of neurogenic orthostatic hypotension with 3,4-DL-threodihydroxyphenylserine: a randomized, placebo-controlled, crossover trial. *Neurology* **53**:2151–2157.

Flugel, K.A., T.A. Mosler, and R.H. Wild. 1984. Bulbar paralytic symptoms including acute vocal cord paralysis in Shy-Drager syndrome. *Nervenarzt* **55(6)**:293–298.

Fujita, T., M. Doi, T. Ogata, I. Kanazawa, and H. Mizusawa. 1993. Cerebral cortical pathology of sporadic olivopontocerebellar atrophy. *J Neurol Sci* **116(1)**:41–46.

Futamura, N., R. Matsumura, Y. Fujimoto, H. Horikawa, A. Suzumura, and T. Takayanagi. 1998. CAG repeat expansions in patients with sporadic cerebellar ataxia. *Acta Neurol Scand* **98**:55–59.

Gai, W.P., J.H. Power, P.C. Blumbergs, and W.W. Blessing. 1998. Multiple-system atrophy: a new alpha-synuclein disease? *Lancet* **352(9127)**:547–548.

Galassi, G., R. Nemni, A. Baraldi, M. Gibertoni, and A. Colombo. 1982. Peripheral neuropathy in multiple system atrophy with autonomic failure. *Neurology* **32**:1116–1121.

Garratt, H., G.K. Wenning, C. Barnes, R. Howard, and N.P. Quinn. 1994. Speech dysfunction and levodopa response in multiple system atrophy. *New Trends in Clinical Neuropharmacology* 207–208.

Ghorayeb, I., F. Yekhlef, V. Chrysostome, E. Balestre, B. Bioulac, and F. Tison. 2002. Sleep disorders and their determinants in multiple system atrophy. *J Neurol Neurosurg Psychiatry* **72**:798–800.

Giladi, N., E.S. Simon, A.D. Korczyn, G.B. Groozman, Y. Orlov, H. Shabtai, and V.E. Drory. 2000. Anal sphincter EMG does not distinguish between multiple system atrophy and Parkinson's disease. *Muscle Nerve* **23**:731–734.

Gilman, S., R.A. Koeppe, L. Junck, K.J. Kluin, M. Lohman, and R.T. St. Laurent. 1994. Patterns of cerebral glucose metabolism detected with positron emission tomography differ in multiple system atrophy and olivopontocerebellar atrophy. *Ann Neurol* **36**:166–175.

Gilman, S., A.A. Sima, L. Junck, K.J. Kluin, R.A. Koeppe, M.E. Lohman, and R. Little. 1996. Spinocerebellar ataxia type 1 with multiple system degeneration and glial cytoplasmic inclusions. *Ann Neurol* **39(2)**:241–255.

Gilman, S., P. Low, N. Quinn, A. Albanese, Y. Ben-Shlomo, C. Fowler, H. Kaufmann, T. Klockgether, A. Lang, P. Lantos, I. Litvan, C. Mathias, E. Oliver, D. Robertson, I. Schatz, and G. Wenning. 1998. Consensus statement on the diagnosis of multiple system atrophy. American Autonomic Society and American Academy of Neurology. *Clin Auton Res* **8**:359–362.

Gilman, S., P.A. Low, N. Quinn, A. Albanese, Y. Ben-Shlomo, C.J. Fowler, H. Kaufmann, T. Klockgether, A.E. Lang, P.L. Lantos, I. Litvan, C.J. Mathias, E. Oliver, D. Robertson, I. Schatz, and G.K. Wenning. 1999. Consensus statement on the diagnosis of multiple system atrophy. *J Neurol Sci* **163**:94–98.

Gilman, S., R. Little, J. Johanns, M. Heumann, K.J. Kluin, L. Junck, and R.A. Koeppe, 2000. Evolution of sporadic olivopontocerebellar atrophy into multiple system atrophy. *Neurology* **55**:527–532.

Goedert, M., and M.G. Spillantini. 1998. Lewy body diseases and multiple system atrophy as alpha-synucleinopathies. *Mol Psychiatry* **3**:462–465.

Gonzalez-Quevedo, A., J.C. Garcia, R. Fernandez, and L. Fernandez Cartaya. 1993. Monoamine metabolites in normal human cerebrospinal fluid and in degenerative diseases of the central nervous system. *Bol Estud Med Biol* **41**:13–19.

Goto, S., A. Hirano, and S. Matsumoto. 1989a. Subdivisional involvement of nigrostriatal loop in idiopathic Parkinson's disease and striatonigral degeneration. *Ann Neurol* **26**:766–770.

Goto, S., A. Hirano, and R.R. Rojas-Corona. 1989b. Calcineurin immunoreactivity in striatonigral degeneration. *Acta Neuropathol (Berl)* **78**:65–71.

Goto, S., A. Hirano, and R.R. Rojas-Corona. 1989c. Immunohistochemical visualization of afferent nerve terminals in human globus pallidus and its alteration in neostriatal neurodegenerative disorders. *Acta Neuropathol (Berl)* **78**:543–550.

Goto, S., A. Hirano, and S. Matsumoto. 1990. Met-enkephalin immunoreactivity in the basal ganglia in Parkinson's disease and striatonigral degeneration. *Neurology* **40**:1051–1056.

Goto, S., S. Matsumoto, Y. Ushio, and A. Hirano. 1996. Subregional loss of putaminal efferents to the basal ganglia output nuclei may cause parkinsonism in striatonigral degeneration. *Neurology* **47**:1032–1036.

Gouider-Khouja, N., M. Vidailhet, A.M. Bonnet, J. Pichon, and Y. Agid. 1995. "Pure" striatonigral degeneration and Parkinson's disease: a comparative clinical study. *Mov Disord* **10**:288–294.

Graham, J.G., and D.R. Oppenheimer. 1969. Orthostatic hypotension and nicotine sensitivity in a case of multiple system atrophy. *J Neurol Neurosurg Psychiatry* **32**:28–34.

Gu, M., M.T. Gash, J.M. Cooper, G.K. Wenning, S.E. Daniel, N.P. Quinn, C.D. Marsden, and A.H. Schapira. 1997. Mitochondrial respiratory chain function in multiple system atrophy. *Mov Disord* **12**:418–422.

Hayashi, M., E. Isozaki, M. Oda, H. Tanabe, and J. Kimura. 1997. Loss of large myelinated nerve fibers of the recurrent laryngeal nerve in patients with multiple system atrophy and vocal cord palsy. *J Neurol Neurosurg Psychiatry* **62**:234–238.

Holmberg, B., B. Johnels, P. Ingvarsson, B. Eriksson, and L. Rosengren. 2001. CSF-neurofilament and levodopa tests combined with discriminant analysis may contribute to the differential diagnosis of parkinsonian syndromes. *Park Relat Disord* **8**:23–31.

Holmberg, B., L. Rosengren, J.E. Karlsson, and B. Johnels. 1998. Increased cerebrospinal fluid levels of neurofilament protein in progressive supranuclear palsy and multiple-system atrophy compared with Parkinson's disease. *Mov Disord* **13**:70–77.

Horoupian, D.S., and D.W Dickson. 1991. Striatonigral degeneration, olivopontocerebellar atrophy and "atypical" Pick disease. *Acta Neuropathol (Berl)* **81(3)**:287–295.

Hu, M.T.M., A. Simmons, A. Glover et al. 1998. Proton magnetic resonance spectroscopy of the putamen in Parkinson's disease and multiple system atrophy. *Mov Disord* **13**:182.

Huang, Y.P., and A. Plaitakis. 1984. Morphological changes of olivopontocerebellar atrophy in computed tomography and comments on its pathogenesis. *Adv Neurol* **41**:39–85.

Hughes, A.J., C. Colosimo, B. Kleedorfer, S.E. Daniel, and A.J. Lees. 1992. The dopaminergic response in multiple system atrophy. *J Neurol Neurosurg Psychiatry* **55**:1009–1013.

Hughes, R.G., K.P. Gibbin, and J. Lowe. 1998. Vocal fold abductor paralysis as a solitary and fatal manifestation of multiple system atrophy. *J Laryngeol Otol* **112(2)**:177–178.

Hussain, I.F., C.M. Brady, M.J. Swinn, C.J. Mathias, and C.J. Fowler. 2001. Treatment of erectile dysfunction with sildenafil citrate (Viagra) in parkinsonism due to Parkinson's disease or multiple system atrophy with observations on orthostatic hypotension. *J Neurol Neurosurg Psychiatry* **71**:371–374.

Iranzo, A., J. Santamaria, and E. Tolosa. 2000. Continuous positive air pressure eliminates nocturnal stridor in multiple system atrophy. Barcelona Multiple System Atrophy Study Group. *Lancet* **356**:1329–1330.

Ito, H., H. Kusaka, S. Matsumoto, and T. Imai. 1996. Striatal efferent involvement and its correlation to levodopa efficacy in patients with multiple system atrophy. *Neurology* **47**:1291–1299.

Iwahashi, K., R. Miyatake, Y. Tsuneoka, Y. Matsuo, Y. Ichikawa, K. Hosokawa, K. Sato, and T. Hayabara. 1995. A novel cytochrome P-450IID6 (CYPIID6) mutant gene associated with multiple system atrophy. *J Neurol Neurosurg Psychiatry* **58**:263–264.

Jankovic, J., J.L. Gilden, B.C. Hiner, H. Kaufmann, D.C. Brown, C.H. Coghlan, M. Rubin, and F.M. Fouad-Tarazi. 1993. Neurogenic orthostatic hypotension: a double-blind, placebo-controlled study with midodrine. *Am J Med* **95**:38–48.

Jost, W.H., and K. Schimrigk. 1996. Urinary incontinence in patients with Parkinson syndrome. *Wien Klin Wochenschr* **108**:296–302.

Kato, S., M. Oda, H. Hayashi, T. Shimizu, M. Hayashi, A. Kawata, and H. Tanabe. 1995. Decrease of medullary catecholaminergic neurons in multiple system atrophy and Parkinson's disease and their preservation in amyotrophic lateral sclerosis. *J Neurol Sci* **132**:216–221.

Kaufmann, H., E. Oribe, M. Miller, P. Knott, M. Wiltshire-Clement, and M.D. Yahr. 1992. Hypotension-induced vasopressin release distinguishes between pure autonomic failure and multiple system atrophy with autonomic failure. *Neurology* **42**:590–593.

Kew, J., M. Gross, and P. Chapman. 1990. Shy-Drager syndrome presenting as isolated paralysis of vocal cord abductors. *BMJ* **300**.1441.

Kihara, M., J. Suganoya, and A. Takahashi. 1991. The assessment of sudomotor dysfunction in multiple system atrophy. *Clin Auton Res* **1**:297–302.

Kimber, J.R., L. Watson, and C.J. Mathias. 1997. Distinction of idiopathic Parkinson's disease from multiple system atrophy by stimulation of growth-hormone release with clonidine. *Lancet* **349**:1877–1881.

Kirby, R., C.J. Fowler, J. Gosling, and R. Bannister. 1986. Urethro-vesical dysfunction in progressive autonomic failure with multiple system atrophy. *J Neurol Neurosurg Psychiatry* **49**:554–562.

Kiyosawa, K., K. Mokuno, N. Murakami, T. Yasuda, A. Kume, Y. Hashizume, A. Takahashi, and K. Kato. 1993. Cerebrospinal fluid 28-kDa calbindin-D as a possible marker for Purkinje cell damage. *J Neurol Sci* **118**:29–33.

Klein, C., G.K. Wenning, and N.P. Quinn. 1995. Pseudotransitory ischemic attacks as the initial symptom of multiple system atrophy. *Nervenarzt* **66**:133–135.

Klein, C., R. Brown, G. Wenning, and N. Quinn. 1997. The "cold hand sign" in multiple system atrophy. *Mov Disord* **12**:514–518.

Klockgether, T., J. Faiss, M. Poremba, and J. Dichgans. 1990a. The development of infratentorial atrophy in patients with idiopathic cerebellar ataxia of late onset: a CT study. *J Neurol* **237**:420–423.

Klockgether, T., G. Schroth, H.C. Diener, and J. Dichgans. 1990b. Idiopathic cerebellar ataxia of late onset: natural history and MRI morphology. *J Neurol Neurosurg Psychiatry* **53**:297–305.

Kluin, K.J., S. Gilman, M. Lohmann, and L. Junck. 1996. Characteristics of the dysarthria of multiple system atrophy. *Arch Neurol* **53**:545–548.

Kodama, Y., T. Ieda, M. Hirayama, Y. Koike, H. Ito, and G. Sobue. 1999. Auditory brainstem responses in patients with autonomic failure with Parkinson's disease and multiple system atrophy. *J Auton Nerv Syst* **77**: 184–189.

Kofler, M., J. Müller, G.K. Wenning, L. Reggiani, P. Hollosi, S. Bösch et al. 2001. The auditory startle reaction in parkinsonian disorders. *Mov Disord* **16**:62–71.

Konagaya, M., Y. Konagaya, H. Honda, and M. Iida. 1993. A clinico-MRI study of extrapyramidal symptoms in multiple system atrophy—linear hyperintensity in the outer margin of the putamen. *No To Shinkei* **45**: 509–513.

Konagaya, M., Y. Konagaya, and M. Iida. 1994. Clinical and magnetic resonance imaging study of extrapyramidal symptoms in multiple system atrophy. *J Neurol Neurosurg Psychiatry* **57**:1528–1531.

Konagaya, M., M. Sakai, Y. Matsuoka, Y. Goto, M. Yoshida, and Y. Hashizume. 1998. Patho-MR imaging study in the putaminal margin in multiple system atrophy. *No To Shinkei* **50**:383–385.

Konagaya, M., M. Sakai, Y. Matsuoka, Y. Konagaya, and Y. Hashizume. 1999. Multiple system atrophy with remarkable frontal lobe atrophy. *Acta Neuropathol (Berl)* **97**:423–428.

Konagaya, M., Y. Konagaya, M. Sakai, Y. Matsuoka, and Y. Hashizume. 2002. Progressive cerebral atrophy in multiple system atrophy. *J Neurol Sci* **195**:123–127.

Konno, H., T. Yamamoto, Y. Iwasaki, and H. Iizuka. 1986. Shy-Drager syndrome and amyotrophic lateral sclerosis. Cytoarchitectonic and morphometric studies of sacral autonomic neurons. *J Neurol Sci* **73**: 193–204.

Kraft, E., C. Trenkwalder, and D.P. Auer. 2002. T2-weighted MRI differentiates multiple system atrophy from Parkinson's disease. *Neurology* **59**:1265–1267.

Kraft, E., J. Schwarz, C. Trenkwalder, T. Vogl, T. Pfluger, and W.H. Oertel. 1999. The combination of hypointense and hyperintense signal changes on T2-weighted magnetic resonance imaging sequences: a specific marker of multiple system atrophy? *Arch Neurol* **56**:225–228.

Kruger, R., W. Kuhn, T. Muller, D. Woitalla, M. Graeber, S. Kosel, H. Przuntek, J.T. Epplen, L. Schols, and O. Riess. 1998. Ala30Pro mutation in the gene encoding alpha-synuclein in Parkinson's disease. *Nat Genet* **18**:106–108.

Kruger, R., A.M. Vieira-Saecker, W. Kuhn, D. Berg, T. Muller, N. Kuhnl, G.A. Fuchs, A. Storch, M. Hungs, D. Woitalla, H. Przuntek, J.T. Epplen, L. Schols, and O. Riess. 1999. Increased susceptibility to sporadic Parkinson's disease by a certain combined alpha-synuclein/apolipoprotein E genotype. *Ann Neurol* **45**:611–617.

Kume, A., A. Takahashi, and Y. Hashizume. 1993. Neuronal cell loss of the striatonigral system in multiple system atrophy. *J Neurol Sci* **117**:33–40.

Lambie, C.G., O. Latham, and G.L. MacDonald. 1947. Olivo-ponto-cerebellar atrophy (Marie's ataxia). *Medical Journal of Australia* **2**: 626–632.

Lang, A.E., T. Curran, J. Provias, and C. Bergeron. 1994. Striatonigral degeneration: iron deposition in putamen correlated with the slit-like void signal of magnetic resonance imaging. *Can J Neurol Sci* **21**:311–318.

Langston, W. 1936. Orthostatic hypotension: report of a case. *Ann Int Med* **10**:688–695.

Lantos, P.L. 1998. The definition of multiple system atrophy: a review of recent developments. *J Neuropathol Exp Neurol* **57**:1099–1111.

Lees, A.J., and R. Bannister. 1981. The use of lisuride in the treatment of multiple system atrophy with autonomic failure (Shy Drager syndrome). *J Neurol Neurosurg Psychiatry* **44**:347–351.

Lees, A.J. 1999. The treatment of the motor disorders of multiple system atrophy. In: C.J. Mathias, R. Bannister, Eds. Autonomic Failure. *Oxford: University Press* 357–363.

Leggo, J., A. Dalton, P.J. Morrison, A. Dudge, M. Connarty, M.J. Kotze, et al. 1997. Analysis of spinocerebellar ataxia types 1, 2, 3, and 6, dentatorubral-pallidoluysian atrophy, and Friedreich's ataxia genes in spinocerebellar ataxia patients in the UK. *J Med Genet* **34**:982–985.

Libelius, R., and F. Johannson. 2000. Quantitative electromyography of the external anal sphincter in Parkinson's disease and multiple system atrophy. *Muscle & Nerve* **23**:1250–1256.

Litvan, I., Y. Agid, D. Calne, G. Campbell, B. Dubois, R.C. Duvoisin, C.G. Goetz, L.I. Golbe, J. Grafman, J.H. Growdon, M. Hallett, J. Jankovic, N.P. Quinn, E. Tolosa, and D.S. Zee. 1996. Clinical research criteria for the diagnosis of progressive supranuclear palsy (Steele-Richardson-Olszewski syndrome): report of the NINDS-SPSP international workshop. *Neurology* **47**:1–9.

Litvan, I., C.G. Goetz, J. Jankovic, G.K. Wenning, V. Booth, J.J. Bartko, A. McKee, K. Jellinger, E.C. Lai, J.P. Brandel, M. Verny, K.R. Chaudhuri, R.K. Pearce, and Y. Agid. 1997. What is the accuracy of the clinical diagnosis of multiple system atrophy? A clinicopathologic study. *Arch Neurol* **54**:937–944.

Litvan, I., V. Booth, G.K. Wenning, J.J. Bartko, C.G. Goetz, A. McKee, J. Jankovic, K. Jellinger, E.C. Lai, J.P. Brandel, M. Verny, K.R. Chaudhuri, R.K. Pearce, and Y. Agid. 1998. Retrospective application of a set of clinical diagnostic criteria for the diagnosis of multiple system atrophy. *J Neural Transm* **105**:217–227.

Low, P.A., J.L. Gilden, R. Freeman, K.N. Sheng, and M.A. McElligott. 1997. Efficacy of midodrine vs placebo in neurogenic orthostatic hypotension. A randomized, double-blind multicenter study. Midodrine Study Group. *JAMA* **277**:1046–1051.

Magnifico, F., G. Pierangeli, G. Barletta, et al. 2001. The cardiovascular effects of metoclopramide in multiple system atrophy and pure autonomic failure. *Clin Auton Res* **11**:163–168.

Martignoni, E., F. Blandini, F. Petraglia, C. Pacchetti, G. Bono, and G. Nappi. 1992. Cerebrospinal fluid norepinephrine, 3-methoxy-4-hydroxyphenylglycol and neuropeptide Y levels in Parkinson's disease, multiple system atrophy and dementia of the Alzheimer type. *J Neural Transm [Park Dis Dement Sect]* **4**(3):191–205.

Martinelli, P., and G. Coccagna. 1978. Etude electromyographique du sphincter strie de l'anus dans trois cas de syndrome de Shy-Drager. In: L. Arbus, J. Cadilhac, Eds. Electromyographie. *Toulouse: Premieres Journees Languedociennes d'Electromyographie* 321–326.

Mathias, C.J., P. Fosbraey, D.F. da Costa, A. Thornley, and R. Bannister. 1986. The effect of desmopressin on nocturnal polyuria, overnight weight loss, and morning postural hypotension in patients with autonomic failure. *BMJ (Clin Res Ed)* **293**:353–354.

Mathias, C.J., and J.R. Kimber. 1999. Postural hypotension: causes, clinical features, investigation, and management. *Annu Rev Med* **50**:317–336.

Mathias, C.J., J.M. Senard, S. Braune, L. Watson, A. Aragishi, J.E. Keeling, et al. 2001. L-threo-dihydroxyphenylserine (L-threo-DOPS; droxidopa) in the management of neurogenic orthostatic hypotension: a multinational, multi-center, dose-ranging study in multiple system atrophy and pure autonomic failure. *Clin Auton Res* **11**:235–242.

Matthews, M.R. 1999. Autonomic ganglia and preganglionic neurones in autonomic failure. In: Mathias CJ, Bannister R, eds. Autonomic Failure. A Textbook of Clinical Disorders of the Autonomic Nervous System. *Oxford: University Press* 329–339.

Meco, G., M. Gasparini, and F. Doricchi. 1996. Attentional functions in multiple system atrophy and Parkinson's disease. *J Neurol Neurosurg Psychiatry* **60**:393–398.

Merlo, I.M., A. Occhini, C. Pacchetti, and E. Alfonsi. 2002. Not paralysis, but dystonia causes stridor in multiple system atrophy. *Neurology* **58**: 649–652.

Montagna, P., P. Martinelli, N. Rizzuto, A. Salviati, F. Rasi, and E. Lugaresi. 1983. Amyotrophy in Shy-Drager syndrome. *Acta Neurol Belg* **83**:142–157.

Morris, H.R., J.R. Vaughan, S.R. Datta, R. Bandopadhyay, H.A. Rohan De Silva, A. Schrag, et al. 2000. Multiple system atrophy/progressive supranuclear palsy: alpha-synuclein, synphilin, tau, and APOE. *Neurology* **55**:1918–1920.

Moseley, M.L., K.A. Benzow, L.J. Schut, T.D. Bird, C.M. Gomez, P.E. Barkhaus, K.A. Blindauer, M. Labuda, M. Pandolfo, M.D. Koob, and L.P. Ranum. 1998. Incidence of dominant spinocerebellar and Friedreich triplet repeats among 361 ataxia families. *Neurology* **51**:1666–1671.

Muller, J., G.K. Wenning, M. Verny, A. McKee, K.R. Chaudhuri, K. Jellinger, W. Poewe, and I. Litvan. 2001. Progression of dysarthria and dysphagia in postmortem-confirmed parkinsonian disorders. *Arch Neurol* **58**:259–264.

Müller, J., G.K. Wenning, K. Jellinger, A. McKee, W. Poewe, and I. Litvan. 2000. Progression of Hoehn and Yahr stages in parkinsonian disorders: a clinicopathologic study. *Neurology* **55**:888–891.

Nakamura, S., K. Ohnishi, M. Nishimura, T. Suenaga, I. Akiguchi, J. Kimura, and T. Kimura. 1996. Large neurons in the tuberomammillary nucleus in patients with Parkinson's disease and multiple system atrophy. *Neurology* **46**:1693–1696.

Nee, L.E., M.R. Gomez, J. Dambrosia, S. Bale, R. Eldridge, and R.J. Polinsky. 1991. Environmental—occupational risk factors and familial associations in multiple system atrophy: a preliminary investigation. I **1**:9–13.

Neumann, M.A. 1977. Pontocerebellar atrophy combined with vestibular-reticular degeneration. *J Neuropathol Exp Neurol* **36**:321–337.

Nicholl, D.J., P. Bennett, L. Hiller, V. Bonifati, N. Vanacore, G. Fabbrini, et al. 1999. A study of five candidate genes in Parkinson's disease and related neurodegenerative disorders. European Study Group on Atypical Parkinsonism. *Neurology* **53**:1415–1421.

Nutt, J.G., E.A. Mrox, S.E. Leeman, A.C. Williams, W.K. Engel, and T.N. Chase. 1980. Substance P in human cerebrospinal fluid: reductions in peripheral neuropathy and autonomic dysfunction. *Neurology* **30**:1280–1285.

O'Brien, C., J.H. Sung, R.E. McGeachie, and M.C. Lee. 1990. Striatonigral degeneration: clinical, MRI, and pathologic correlation. *Neurology* **40**:710–711.

Oertel, W.H., T. Wachter, N. Quinn, G. Ulm, and D. Brandstädter. 2003. Reduced genital sensitivity in female patients with multiple system atrophy of parkinsonian type (MSA-P). *Mov Disord* **18**:430–432.

Olanow, C.W. 1992. Magnetic resonance imaging in parkinsonism. *Neurol Clin* **10**:405–420.

Oppenheimer, D. 1984. Diseases of the basal ganglia, cerebellum and motor neurons. In: J.H. Adams, J.A.N. Corsellis, L.W. Duchen, eds. Greenfield's Neuropathology. *New York: Wiley* 699–747.

Oppenheimer, D.R. 1980. Lateral horn cells in progressive autonomic failure. *J Neurol Sci* **46**:393–404.

Orimo, S., E. Ozawa, S. Nakade, T. Sugimoto, and H. Mizusawa. 1999. (123)I-metaiodobenzylguanidine myocardial scintigraphy in Parkinson's disease. *J Neurol Neurosurg Psychiatry* **67**:189–194.

Orozco, G., R. Estrada, T.L. Perry, J. Arana, R. Fernandez, A. Gonzalez-Quevedo, J. Galarraga, and S. Hansen. 1989. Dominantly inherited olivopontocerebellar atrophy from eastern Cuba. Clinical, neuropathological, and biochemical findings. *J Neurol Sci* **93**:37–50.

Osaki, Y., G.K. Wenning, S.E. Daniel, A. Hughes, A.J. Lees, C.J. Mathias, and N. Quinn. 2002. Do published criteria improve clinical diagnostic accuracy in multiple system atrophy? *Neurology* **59**:1486–1491.

Ostrerova, N., L. Petrucelli, M. Farrer, N. Mehta, P. Choi, J. Hardy, and B. Wolozin. 1999. alpha-synuclein shares physical and functional homology with 14-3-3 proteins. *J Neurosci* **19**:5782–5791.

Ozawa, T., H. Takano, O. Onodera, H. Kobayashi, T. Ikeuchi, and R. KoideI. 1999. No mutation in the entire coding region of the alpha-synuclein gene in pathologically confirmed cases of multiple system atrophy. *Neurosci Lett* **270**:110–112.

Palace, J., V.A. Chandiramani, and C.J. Fowler. 1997. Value of sphincter electromyography in the diagnosis of multiple system atrophy. *Muscle & Nerve* **20**:1396–1403.

Papp, M.I., J.E. Kahn, and P.L. Lantos. 1989. Glial cytoplasmic inclusions in the CNS of patients with multiple system atrophy (striatonigral degeneration, olivopontocerebellar atrophy and Shy-Drager syndrome). *J Neurol Sci* **94**:79–100.

Papp, M.I., and P.L. Lantos. 1992. Accumulation of tubular structures in oligodendroglial and neuronal cells as the basic alteration in multiple system atrophy. *J Neurol Sci* **107**:172–182.

Papp, M.I., and P.L. Lantos. 1994. The distribution of oligodendroglial inclusions in multiple system atrophy and its relevance to clinical symptomatology. *Brain* **117**:235–243.

Parati, E.A., V. Fetoni, G.C. Geminiani, P. Soliveri, P. Giovannini, D. Testa, S. Genitrini, T. Caraceni, and F. Girotti. 1993. Response to L-dopa in multiple system atrophy. *Clin Neuropharmacol* **16**:139–144.

Pastakia, B., R. Polinsky, G. Di Chiro, J.T. Simmon, R. Brown, and L. Wener. 1986. Multiple system atrophy (Shy-Drager syndrome): MR imaging. *Radiology* **159**:499–502.

Perani, D., S. Bressi, D. Testa, F. Grassi, P. Cortelli, S. Genitrini, et al. 1995. Clinical/metabolic correlations in multiple system atrophy. A fludeoxyglucose F18 positron emission tomography study. *Arch Neurol* **52**:179–185.

Perera, R., L. Isola, and H. Kaufmann. 1995. Effect of recombinant erythropoietin on anemia and orthostatic hypotension in primary autonomic failure. *Clin Auton Res* **5**:211–213.

Pillon, B., N. Gouider-Khouja, B. Deweer, M. Vidailhet, C. Malapani, B. Dubois, et al. 1995. Neuropsychological pattern of striatonigral degeneration: comparison with Parkinson's disease and progressive supranuclear palsy. *J Neurol Neurosurg Psychiatry* **58**:174–179.

Plaitakis, A., P. Flessas, A.B. Natsiou, and P. Shashidharan. 1993. Glutamate dehydrogenase deficiency in cerebellar degenerations: clinical, biochemical and molecular genetic aspects. *Can J Neurol Sci* **20** Suppl **3**:S109–116.

Plazzi, G., R. Corsini, and F. Provini. 1997. REM sleep behavior disorders in multiple system atrophy. *Neurology* **48**:1094–1097.

Polinsky, R.J., R.T. Brown, G.K. Lee, K. Timmers, J. Culman, O. Foldes, I.J. Kopin, and L. Recant. 1987. Beta-endorphin, ACTH, and catecholamine responses in chronic autonomic failure. *Ann Neurol* **21**:573–577.

Polinsky, R.J., I.J. Kopin, M.H. Ebert, and V. Weise. 1981. Pharmacologic distinction of different orthostatic hypotension syndromes. *Neurology* **31**:1–7.

Polymeropoulos, M.H., C. Lavedan, E. Leroy, S.E. Ide, A. Dehejia, A. Dutra, et al. 1997. Mutation in the alpha-synuclein gene identified in families with Parkinson's disease. *Science* **276**:2045–2047.

Pramstaller, P., G.K. Wenning, S.J.M. Smith, R.O. Beck, N.P. Quinn, and C.J. Fowler. 1995. Nerve conduction studies, skeletal muscle EMG, and sphincter EMG in multiple system atrophy. *J Neurol Neurosurg Psychiatry* **58**:618–621.

Prasher, D., and R. Bannister. 1986. Brain stem auditory evoked potentials in patients with multiple system atrophy with progressive autonomic failure (Shy-Drager syndrome). *J Neurol Neurosurg Psychiatry* **49**:278–289.

Price, R.H., R.L. Albin, S.Y. Sakurai, R.J. Polinsky, J.B. Penney, and A.B. Young. 1993. Cerebellar excitatory and inhibitory amino acid receptors in multiple system atrophy. *Neurology* **43**:1323–1328.

Quik, M., E.G. Spokes, A.V. Mackay, and R. Bannister. 1979. Alterations in [3H]spiperone binding in human caudate nucleus, substantia nigra and frontal cortex in the Shy-Drager syndrome and Parkinson's disease. *J Neurol Sci* **43**:429–437.

Quinn, N. 1989a. Disproportionate antecollis in multiple system atrophy. *Lancet* **1**:844.

Quinn, N. 1989b. Multiple system atrophy—the nature of the beast. *J Neurol Neurosurg Psychiatry* **52 (suppl)**:78–89.

Quinn, N. 1994. Multiple system atrophy. In: Marsden C.D., Fahn S., eds. Mov Disord 3. *London: Butterworth-Heinemann* 262–281.

Quinn, N.P., G. Wenning, and C.D. Marsden. 1995. The Shy-Drager syndrome. What did Shy and Drager really describe? *Arch Neurol* **52**: 656–657.

Raimbach, S.J., P. Cortelli, J.S. Kooner, R. Bannister, S.R. Bloom, and C.J. Mathias. 1989. Prevention of glucose-induced hypotension by the somatostatin analogue octreotide (SMS 201–995) in chronic autonomic failure: haemodynamic and hormonal changes. *Clin Sci (Lond)* **77**: 623–628.

Rajput, A.H., B. Rozdilsky, A. Rajput, and L. Ang. 1990. Levodopa efficacy and pathological basis of Parkinson syndrome. *Clin Neuropharmacol* **13**:553–558.

Ranum, L.P., J.K. Lundgren, L.J. Schut, M.J. Ahrens, S. Perlman, J. Aita, et al. 1995. Spinocerebellar ataxia type 1 and Machado-Joseph-disease: incidence of CAG expansions among adult-onset ataxia patients from 311 families with dominant, recessive, or sporadic ataxia. *Am J Hum Genet* **57**:603–608.

Ravits, J., M. Hallett, J. Nilsson, R. Polinsky, and J. Dambrosia. 1996. Electrophysiological tests of autonomic function in patients with idiopathic autonomic failure syndromes. *Muscle & Nerve* **19**:758–763.

Riley, D.E., and T.C. Chelimsky. 2003. Autonomic nervous system testing may not distinguish multiple system atrophy from Parkinson's disease. *J Neurol Neurosurg Psychiatry* **74**:56–60.

Rivest, J., N. Quinn, and C.D. Marsden. 1990. Dystonia in Parkinson's disease, multiple system atrophy, and progressive supranuclear palsy. *Neurology* **40**:1571–1578.

Robbins, T.W., M. James, K.W. Lange, A.M. Owen, N.P. Quinn, and C.D. Marsden. 1992. Cognitive performance in multiple system atrophy. *Brain* **115**:271–291.

Rossi, P., C. Colosimo, E. Moro, P. Tonali, and A. Albanese. 2000. Acute challenge with apomorphine and levodopa in parkinsonism. *Eur Neurol* **43**:95–101.

Sakakibara, R., T. Hattori, T. Uchiyama, K. Kita, M. Asahina, A. Suzuki, and T. Yamanishi. 2000a. Urinary dysfunction and orthostatic hypotension in multiple system atrophy: which is the more common and earlier manifestation? *J Neurol Neurosurg Psychiatry* **68**:65–69.

Sakakibara, R., T. Hattori, T. Uchiyama, T. Suenaga, H. Takahashi, T. Yamanishi, K. Egoshi, and N. Sekita. 2000b. Are alpha-blockers involved in lower urinary tract dysfunction in multiple system atrophy? A comparison of prazosin and moxisylyte. *J Auton Nerv Syst* **79**:191–195.

Salazar, G., J. Valls-Sole, M.J. Marti, H. Chang, and E.S. Tolosa. 2000. Postural and action myoclonus in patients with parkinsonian type of multiple system atrophy. *Mov Disord* **15**:77–83.

Sandroni, P., J.E. Ahlskog, R.D. Fealy, and P.A. Low. 1991. Autonomic involvement in extrapyramidal and cerebellar disorders. *Clin Auton Res* **1**:147–155.

Santens, P., L. Crevits, and C. van der Linden. 1996. Raynaud's phenomenon in a case of multiple system atrophy. *Movement Disorders* **11**:586–588.

Savoiardo, M., L. Strada, and F. Girotti F. 1990. Olivopontocerebellar atrophy: MR diagnosis and relationship to multisystem atrophy. *Radiology* **174**:693–696.

Schelosky, L., J. Hierholzer, L. Wissel, M. Cordes, and W. Poewe. 1993. Correlation of clinical response in apomorphine test with D2-receptor status as demonstrated by 123I IBZM-SPECT. *Mov Disord* **8(4)**:453–458.

Scherer, H.J. 1933a. Beiträge zur pathologischen Anatomie des Kleinhirns. III. Mitteilung: Genuine Kleinhirnatrophien. *Z Gesamte Neurol Psychiatrie* **145**:335–405.

Scherer, H.J. 1933b. Extrapyramidale Störungen bei der olivopontocerebellären Atrophie. *Z Gesamte Neurol Psychiatrie* **145**:406–419.

Scherfler, C., Z. Puschban, I. Ghorayeb, G.P. Goebel, F. Tison, K. Jellinger, et al. 2000. Complex motor disturbances in a sequential double lesion rat model of striatonigral degeneration (multiple system atrophy). *Neuroscience* **99**:43–54.

Schocke, M., K. Seppi, R. Esterhammer, C. Kremser, W. Jaschke, W. Poewe, et al. 2002. Diffusion-weighted MRI differentiates the Parkinson variant of multiple system atrophy from PD. *Neurology* **58**:575–580.

Schöls, L., S. Szymanski, S. Peters, H. Przuntek, J.T. Epplen, C. Hardt, et al. 2000. Genetic background of apparently idiopathic sporadic cerebellar ataxia. *Hum Genet* **107**:132–137.

Schrag, A., D. Kingsley, C. Phatouros, C.J. Mathias, A.J. Lees, S.E. Daniel, et al. 1998. Clinical usefulness of magnetic resonance imaging in multiple system atrophy. *J Neurol Neurosurg Psychiatry* **65**:65–71.

Schrag, A., Y. Ben-Shlomo, and N.P. Quinn. 1999. Prevalence of progressive supranuclear palsy and multiple system atrophy: a cross-sectional study. *Lancet* **354**:1771–1775.

Schrag, A., C.D. Good, K. Miszkiel, H.R. Morris, C.J. Mathias, A.J. Lees, et al. 2000. Differentiation of atypical parkinsonian syndromes with routine MRI. *Neurology* **54**:697–702.

Schulz, J.B., T. Klockgether, D. Petersen, M. Jauch, W. Muller-Schauenburg, S. Spieker, et al. 1994. Multiple system atrophy: natural history, MRI morphology, and dopamine receptor imaging with 123IBZM-SPECT. *J Neurol Neurosurg Psychiatry* **57**:1047–1056.

Schulz, J.B., M. Skalej, D. Wedekind, A.R. Luft, M. Abele, K. Voigt, et al. 1999. Magnetic resonance imaging-based volumetry differentiates idiopathic Parkinson's syndrome from multiple system atrophy and progressive supranuclear palsy. *Ann Neurol* **45**:65–74.

Schwarz, J., K. Tatsch, G. Arnold, T. Gasser, C. Trenkwalder, C.M. Kirsch, et al. 1992. 123I-iodobenzamide-SPECT predicts dopaminergic responsiveness in patients with de novo parkinsonism. *Neurology* **42**:556–561.

Schwarz, J., K. Tatsch, G. Arnold, M. Ott, C. Trenkwalder, C.M. Kirsch, and W.H. Oertel. 1993. 123I-iodobenzamide-SPECT in 83 patients with de novo parkinsonism. *Neurology* **43**:17–20.

Schwarz, J., S. Weis, and E. Kraft. 1996. Signal changes on MRI and increases in reactive microgliosis, astrogliosis, and iron in the putamen of two patients with multiple system atrophy. *J Neurol Neurosurg Psychiatry* **60**:98–101.

Schwarz, J., M. Kornhuber, C. Bischoff, and A. Straube. 1997. Electromyography of the external anal sphincter in patients with Parkinson's disease and multiple system atrophy: frequency of abnormal spontaneous activity and polyphasic motor unit potentials. *Muscle & Nerve* **20(9)**:1167–1172.

Seppi, K., M.F.H. Schocke, R. Esterhammer, C. Kremser, C. Brenneis, J. Mueller, S. Boesch, W. Jaschke, W. Poewe, and G.K. Wenning. 2003. DWI discriminates PSP from PD, but not from the parkinson variant of multiple system atrophy. *Neurology* **60**:922–927.

Shy, G.M., and G.A. Drager. 1960. A neurological syndrome associated with orthostatic hypotension. A clinicopathological study. *Arch Neurol* **2**:511–527.

Silber, M.H., and S. Levine. 2000. Stridor and death in multiple system atrophy. *Mov Disord* **15(4)**:699–704.

Silveira, I., I. Lopes-Cendes, S. Kish, P. Maciel, C. Gaspar, P. Coutinho, et al. 1996. Frequency of spinocerebellar ataxia type 1, dentatorubro-pallidoluysian atrophy, and Machado-Joseph disease mutations in a large group of spinocerebellar ataxia patients. *Neurology* **46**:214–218.

Sima, A.A.F., M. Caplan, C.J. D'Amato, M. Pevzner, and J.W. Furlong. 1993. Fulminant multiple system atrophy in a young adult presenting as motor neuron disease. *Neurology* **43**:2031–2035.

Sobue, G., S. Terao, T. Kachi, E. Ken, Y. Hashizume, T. Mitsuma, et al. 1992. Somatic motor efferents in multiple system atrophy with autonomic failure: a clinico-pathological study. *J Neurol Sci* **112**:113–125.

Spillantini, M.G., R.A. Crowther, R. Jakes, N.J. Cairns, P.L. Lantos, and M. Goedert. 1998. Filamentous alpha-synuclein inclusions link multiple system atrophy with Parkinson's disease and dementia with Lewy bodies. *Neurosci Lett* **251**:205–208.

Spillantini, M.G., M.L. Schmidt, V.M. Lee, J.Q. Trojanowski, R. Jakes, and M. Goedert. 1997. Alpha-synuclein in Lewy bodies. *Nature* **388**:839–840.

Spokes, E.G., R. Bannister, and D.R. Oppenheimer. 1979. Multiple system atrophy with autonomic failure: clinical, histological and neurochemical observations on four cases. *J Neurol Sci* **43**:59–82.

Staal, A., J.D. Meerwaldt, K.K. van Dongen, P.G.H. Mulder, and H.F.M. Busch. 1990. Non-familial degenerative disease and atrophy of brainstem and cerebellum. Clinical and CT data in 47 patients. *J Neurol Sci* **95**: 259–269.

Stauffenberg. 1918. Zur Kenntnis des extrapyramidalen motorischen Systems und Mitteilung eines Falles von sog. "Atrophie olivo-pontocérébelleuse." *Z Gesamte Neurol Psychiatrie* **39**:1–55.

Stern, M.B., B.H. Braffman, B.E. Skolnick, H.I. Hurtig, and R.I. Grossman. 1989. Magnetic resonance imaging in Parkinson's disease and parkinsonian syndromes. *Neurology* **39**:1524–1526.

Stocchi, F., D. Badiali, L. Vacca, L. D'Alba, F. Bracci, S. Ruggieri, M. Torti, A. Berardelli, and E. Corazziari. 2000. Anorectal function in multiple system atrophy and Parkinson's disease. *Mov Disord* **15**:71–76.

Suemaru, S., K. Suemaru, K. Kawai, S. Miyata, K. Nobukuni, Y. Ihara, R. Namba, K. Urakami, and K. Hashimoto. 1995. Cerebrospinal fluid corticotrophin-releasing hormone in neurodegenerative diseases: reduction in spinocerebellar degeneration. *Life Sci* **57**:2231–2235.

Sung, J.H., A.R. Mastri, and E. Segal. 1979. Pathology of Shy-Drager syndrome. *J Neuropathol Exp Neurol* **38**:353–368.

Takanashi, M., S. Ohta, S. Matsuoka, H. Mori, and Y. Mizuno. 2002. Mixed multiple system atrophy and progressive supranuclear palsy: a clinical and pathological report of one case. *Acta Neuropathol (Berl)* **103(1)**: 82–87.

Takatsu, H., K. Nagashima, M. Murase, H. Fujiwara, H. Nishida, and H. Matsuo. 2000. Differentiating Parkinson disease from multiple-system atrophy by measuring cardiac iodine-123 metaiodobenzylguanidine accumulation. *JAMA* **284(1)**:44–45.

Takei, Y., and S. Mirra. 1973. Striatonigral degeneration: a form of multiple system atrophy with clinical parkinsonism. In: Zimmermann H.M., ed. Progress in Neuropathology, Vol. 2. *New York: Grune & Stratton* 217–251.

Taki, J., K. Nakajima, E.H. Hwang, I. Matsunari, K. Komai, and M. Yoshita. 2000. Peripheral sympathetic dysfunction in patients with Parkinson's disease without autonomic failure is heart selective and disease specific. *Eur J Nucl Med* **27**:566–573.

Terao, S., G. Sobue, Y. Hashizume, T. Mitsuma, and A. Takahashi. 1994. Disease-specific patterns of neuronal loss in the spinal ventral horn in amyotrophic lateral sclerosis, multiple system atrophy and X-linked recessive bulbospinal neuronopathy, with special reference to the loss of small neurons in the intermediate zone. *J Neurol* **241**:196–203.

Testa, D., G. Filippini, M. Farinotti, E. Palazzini, and T. Caraceni. 1996. Survival in multiple system atrophy: a study of prognostic factors in 59 cases. *J Neurol* **243**:401–404.

Thobois, S., E. Broussolle, L. Toureille, and C. Vial. 2001. Severe dysphagia after botulinum toxin injection for cervical dystonia in multiple system atrophy. *Mov Disord* **16**:764–765.

Tison, F., G.K. Wenning, S.E. Daniel, and N. Quinn. 1995a. The pathophysiology of parkinsonism in multiple system atrophy. *Eur J Neurol* **2**:435–444.

Tison, F., G.K. Wenning, N.P. Quinn, and S.J. Smith. 1995b. REM sleep behaviour disorder as the presenting symptom of multiple system atrophy. *J Neurol Neurosurg Psychiatry* **58**:379–380.

Tison, F., P. Arne, C. Sourgen, V. Chrysostome, and F. Yeklef. 2000a. The value of external anal sphincter electromyography for the diagnosis of multiple system atrophy. *Mov Disord* **15**:1148–1157.

Tison, F., F. Yekhlef, V. Chrysostome, and C. Sourgen. 2000b. Prevalence of multiple system atrophy. *Lancet* **355**:495–496.

Tohgi, H., M. Tabuchi, M. Tomonaga, and N. Izumiyama. 1982. Selective loss of small myelinated and unmyelinated fibers in Shy-Drager syndrome. *Acta Neuropathologica (Berlin)* **57**:282–286.

Tranchant, C., C. Guiraud-Chaumeil, A. Echaniz-Laguna, and J.M. Warter. 2000. Is clonidine growth hormone stimulation a good test to differentiate multiple system atrophy from idiopathic Parkinson's disease? *J Neurol* **247(11)**:853–856.

Trojanowski, J.Q. 2002. Tauists, baptists, syners, apostates, and new data. *Ann Neurol* **52(3)**:263–265.

Tsuchiya, K., E. Ozawa, C. Haga, S. Watabiki, M. Ikeda, M. Sano, K. Ooe, K. Taki, and K. Ikeda. 2000. Constant involvement of the Betz cells and pyramidal tract in multiple system atrophy: a clinicopathological study of seven autopsy cases. *Acta Neuropathol (Berl)* **99(6)**:628–636.

Tsuchiya, K., S. Watabiki, M. Sano, H. Iobe, H. Shiotsu, K. Taki, and K. Hashimoto. 1998. Distribution of cerebellar cortical lesions in multiple system atrophy: a topographic neuropathological study of three autopsy cases in Japan. *J Neurol Sci* **155(1)**:80–85.

Tu, P.H., J.E. Galvin, M. Baba, B. Giasson, T. Tomita, S. Leight, S. Nakajo, T. Iwatsubo, J.Q. Trojanowski, and V.M. Lee. 1998. Glial cytoplasmatic inclusions in white matter oligodendrocytes of multiple system atrophy brains contain insoluble alpha-synuclein. *Ann Neurol* **44**:415–422.

Uematsu, D., J. Hamada, and F. Gotoh. 1987. Brainstem auditory evoked responses and CT findings in multiple system atrophy. *J Neurol Sci* **77**:161–171.

Umapathi, T., V. Chaudhry, D. Cornblath, D. Drachman, J. Griffin, and R. Kuncl. 2002. Head drop and camptocormia. *J Neurol Neurosurg Psychiatry* **73**:1–7.

Urenjak, J., S.R. Williams, D.G. Gadian, and M. Noble. 1993. Proton nuclear magnetic resonance spectroscopy unambiguously identifies different neuronal cell types. *J Neurosci* **13**:981–989.

Valldeoriola, F., J. Valls-Sole, E.S. Tolosa, and M.J. Marti. 1995. Striated anal sphincter denervation in patients with progressive supranuclear palsy. *Mov Disord* **10(5)**:550–555.

Vanacore, N., V. Bonifati, G. Fabbrini, C. Colosimo, R. Marconi, D. Nicholl, et al. 2000. Smoking habits in multiple system atrophy and progressive supranuclear palsy. *Neurology* **54**:114–119.

van der Eecken, H., R.D. Adams, and L. van Bogaert. 1960. Striopallidal-nigral degeneration. A hitherto undescribed lesion in paralysis agitans. *J Neuropathol Exp Neurol* **19**:159–161.

van Royen, E., N.F. Verhoeff, J.D. Speelman, E.C. Wolters, M.A. Kuiper, and A.G. Janssen. 1993. Multiple system atrophy and progressive supranuclear palsy. Diminished striatal D2 dopamine receptor activity demonstrated by 123I-IBZM single photon emission computed tomography. *Arch Neurol* **50**:513–516.

Vodusek, B. 2001. Sphincter EMG and differential diagnosis of multiple system atrophy. *Mov Disord* **16**:600–607.

Vogels, O.J., J. Veltman, W.J. Oyen, and M.W. Horstink. 2000. Decreased striatal dopamine D2 receptor binding in amyotrophic lateral sclerosis (ALS) and multiple system atrophy (MSA): D2 receptor down-regulation versus striatal cell degeneration. *J Neurol Sci* **180**:62–65.

Wakabayashi, K., S. Hayashi, A. Kakita, M. Yamada, Y. Toyoshima, M. Yoshimoto, and H. Takahashi. 1998a. Accumulation of alpha-synuclein/NACP is a cytopathological feature common to Lewy body disease and multiple system atrophy. *Acta Neuropathol (Berl)* **96(5)**:445–452.

Wakabayashi, K., T. Ikeuchi, A. Ishikawa, and H. Takahashi. 1998b. Multiple system atrophy with severe involvement of the motor cortical areas and cerebral white matter. *J Neurol Sci* **156**:114–117.

Wakabayashi, K., M. Yoshimoto, S. Tsuji, and H. Takahashi. 1998c. Alpha-synuclein immunoreactivity in glial cytoplasmic inclusions in multiple system atrophy. *Neurosci Lett* **249**:180–182.

Wakai, M., A. Kume, A. Takahashi, T. Ando, and Y. Hashizume. 1994. A study of parkinsonism in multiple system atrophy: clinical and MRI correlation. *Acta Neurologica Scandinavica* **90**:225–231.

Waldner, R., Z. Puschban, C. Scherfler, K. Seppi, K. Jellinger, and W. Poewe. 2001. No functional effects of embryonic neuronal grafts on motor deficits in a 3-nitropropionic acid rat model of advanced striatonigral degeneration (multiple system atrophy). *Neuroscience* **102**: 581–592.

Watanabe, H., Y. Saito, S. Terao, T. Ando, T. Kachi, E. Mukai, et al. 2002. Progression and prognosis in multiple system atrophy: an analysis of 230 Japanese patients. *Brain* **125**:1070–1083.

Wenning, G.K., S. Wagner, S.E. Daniel, and N.P. Quinn. 1993. Multiple system atrophy: sporadic or familial? *Lancet* **342**:681.

Wenning, G.K., Y. Ben-Shlomo, M. Magalhaes, S.E. Daniel, and N.P. Quinn. 1994a. Clinical features and natural history of multiple system atrophy. An analysis of 100 cases. *Brain* **117**:835–845.

Wenning, G.K., R. Jäger, B. Kendall, et al. 1994b. Is cranial computerized tomography (CT) useful in the diagnosis of multiple system atrophy? *Mov Disord* **9**:333–336.

Wenning, G.K., N. Quinn, M. Magalhaes, C. Mathias, and S.E. Daniel. 1994c. "Minimal change" multiple system atrophy. *Mov Disord* **9**:161–166.

Wenning, G.K., and N. Quinn. 1994. Are Lewy bodies non-specific epiphenomena of nigral damage? *Mov Disord* **9**:378–379.

Wenning, G.K., Y. Ben-Shlomo, M. Magalhaes, S.E. Daniel, and N.P. Quinn. 1995. Clinicopathological study of 35 cases of multiple system atrophy. *J Neurol Neurosurg Psychiatry* **58**:160–166.

Wenning, G.K., R. Granata, P.M. Laboyrie, N.P. Quinn, P. Jenner, and C.D. Marsden. 1996a. Reversal of behavioural abnormalities by fetal allografts in a novel rat model of striatonigral degeneration. *Mov Disord* **11**:522–532.

Wenning, G.K., F. Tison, L. Elliott, N.P. Quinn, and S.E. Daniel. 1996b. Olivopontocerebellar pathology in multiple system atrophy. *Mov Disord* **11**:157–162.

Wenning, G.K., E. Kraft, R. Beck, C.J. Fowler, C.J. Mathias, N.P. Quinn, and A.E. Harding. 1997a. Cerebellar presentation of multiple system atrophy. *Mov Disord* **12**:115–117.

Wenning, G.K., F. Tison, Y. Ben-Shlomo, S.E. Daniel, and N.P. Quinn. 1997b. Multiple system atrophy: a review of 203 pathologically proven cases. *Mov Disord* **12**:133–147.

Wenning, G.K., and N.P. Quinn. 1997. Multiple system atrophy. In: Quinn N.P. ed. Parkinsonism. *Bailliere's Clin Neurol* **6**:187–204.

Wenning, G.K., and S.J.M. Smith. 1997. Magnetic brain stimulation in multiple system atrophy. *Mov Disord* **12**:452–453.

Wenning, G.K., G. Ebersbach, M. Verny, K.R. Chaudhuri, K. Jellinger, A. McKee, et al. 1999a. Progression of falls in postmortem-confirmed parkinsonian disorders. *Mov Disord* **14**:947–950.

Wenning, G.K., R. Granata, Z. Puschban, C. Scherfler, and W. Poewe. 1999b. Neural transplantation in animal models of multiple system atrophy: a review. *J Neural Transm* **55**:103–113.

Wenning, G.K., C. Scherfler, R. Granata, S. Bösch, M. Verny, and K.R. Chaudhuri. 1999c. Time course of symptomatic orthostatic hypotension and urinary incontinence in patients with postmortem confirmed parkinsonian syndromes: a clinicopathological study. *J Neurol Neurosurg Psychiatry* **67**:620–623.

Wenning, G.K., Y. Ben-Shlomo, A. Hughes, S.E. Daniel, A.J. Lees, and N.P. Quinn. 2000a. What clinical features are most useful to distinguish definite multiple system atrophy from Parkinson's disease? *J Neurol Neurosurg Psychiatry* **68**:434–440.

Wenning, G.K., K.J. Jellinger, N.P. Quinn, and W.H. Poewe. 2000b. An early report of striatonigral degeneration. *Mov Disord* **15**:159–162.

Wenning, G.K., K. Seppi, C. Sampaio, N.P. Quinn, W. Poewe, and F. Tison. 2002. European Multiple System Atrophy Study Group (EMSA-SG): Validation of the Unified MSA Rating Scale (UMSARS). *Mov Disord* **17 (suppl 5)**:252.

Wenning, G.K., C. Colosimo, F. Geser, and W. Poewe. 2004. Multiple system atrophy. *Lancet Neurol* **3**:93–103

Wenning, G.K., and F. Geser. 2004. Diagnosis and treatment of multiple system atrophy: an update. *Advances in Clinical Neuroscience & Rehabilitation* **3**:5–10.

Wermuth, L., P. Joensen, N. Bunger, and B. Jeune. 1997. High prevalence of Parkinson's disease in the Faroe Islands. *Neurology* **49**:426–432.

Wessel, K., G.P. Huss, H. Brückmann, and D. Kömpf. 1993. Follow-up of neurophysiological tests and CT in late-onset cerebellar ataxia and multiple system atrophy. *J Neurol* **240**:168–176.

Williams, A., D. Hanson, and D.B. Calne. 1979. Vocal cord paralysis in the Shy-Drager syndrome. *J Neurol Neurosurg Psychiatry* **42**:151–153.

Winkler, A.S., J. Marsden, M. Parton, P.J. Watkins, and K.R. Chaudhuri. 2001. Erythropoietin deficiency and anaemia in multiple system atrophy. *Mov Disord* **16**:233–239.

Wright, R.A., H.C. Kaufmann, R. Perera, T.L. Opfer-Gehrking, M.A. McElligott, and K.N. Sheng. 1998. A double-blind, dose-response study of midodrine in neurogenic orthostatic hypotension. *Neurology* **51**:120–124.

Wu, Y.R., C.M. Chen, L.S. Ro, S.T. Chen, and L.M. Tang. 1996. Vocal cord paralysis as an initial sign of multiple system atrophy in the central nervous system. *J Formos Med Assoc* **95**:804–806.

Wüllner, U., T. Klockgether, D. Petersen, T. Naegele, and J. Dichgans. 1993. Magnetic resonance imaging in hereditary and idiopathic ataxia. *Neurology* **43**:318–325.

Yamada, T., and P.L. McGeer. 1990. Oligodendroglial microtubular masses: an abnormality observed in some human neurodegenerative diseases. *Neurosci Lett* **120**:163–166.

Yoshita, M. 1998. Differentiation of idiopathic Parkinson's disease from striatonigral degeneration and progressive supranuclear palsy using iodine-123 meta-iodobenzylguanidine myocardial scintigraphy. *J Neurol Sci* **155**:60–67.

Zesiewicz, T.A., M. Helal, and R.A. Hauser. 2000. RA Sildenafil citrate (Viagra) for the treatment of erectile dysfunction in men with Parkinson's disease. *Mov Disord* **15**:305–308.

Ziegler, M.G., C.R. Lake, and I.J. Kopin. 1977. The sympathetic-nervous-system defect in primary orthostatic hypotension. *N Engl J Med* **296**: 293–297.

CHAPTER

J2

Double-Lesion Animal Models of Multiple System Atrophy

IMAD GHORAYEB, NADIA STEFANOVA, PIERRE-OLIVIER FERNAGUT, GREGOR KARL WENNING, and FRANÇOIS TISON

Multiple system atrophy is a neurodegenerative disease of undetermined etiology that occurs sporadically and manifests itself as a combination of Parkinsonian, autonomic, cerebellar, and pyramidal signs. There is at present no effective therapy to reverse this condition. Levodopa-unresponsive Parkinsonism dominates the clinical syndrome of multiple system atrophy of the striatonigral degeneration subtype, a condition that is characterized by a dual pathology affecting nigral dopaminergic neurons and their striatal output neurons. Experimental models reproducing salient pathological and clinical features are needed to better understand the underlying pathophysiology of Parkinsonian motor signs and levodopa-unresponsiveness. In the following chapter, we demonstrate the feasibility of such models in rodents and in non-human primates. In rodents, a "double toxin-double lesion" unilateral stereotaxic approach using intrastriatal sequential or combined quinolinic acid (QA) + 6-hydroxydopamine (6-OHDA), and a "single toxin-double lesion" using either intrastriatal 3-nitropropionic acid (3NP) or 1-methyl-4-phenylpyridinium ion (MPP^+) were explored. In mice and non-human primates, systemic combined and sequential chronic 1-methyl-4-phenyl-1,2,3,6-tetrahydropyridine (MPTP) + 3NP injections were used. In rodents, complex motor symptoms were induced by the combined striatal and nigral lesions that were different from those induced by a single striatal or nigral lesion. In primates, the most relevant clinical aspects were the occurrence of asymmetrical hindlimb dystonia predicting the striatal lesion and the subsequent emergence of a levodopa-unresponsive Parkinsonism. The latter was associated with a decreased density of dopaminoceptive medium spiny neurons of both the indirect and direct striatal outflow pathways as observed in striatonigral degeneration. Altogether, our results clearly demonstrate that clinical and pathological features associated with striatonigral degeneration can be reproduced by neurotoxic treatments in both rodents and non-human primates. These models will be helpful to understand the degenerative process in multiple system atrophy and to explore new therapeutic strategies prior to clinical applications in humans.

I. INTRODUCTION

The use of animal models represents an essential part of basic neuroscience research efforts to improve the understanding, prevention, and treatment of neurological conditions. Without such models, it would be impossible to investigate such topics as the underlying mechanisms of neuronal cell damage and death, or to screen new compounds for possible neuroprotective or neurorestorative strategies. The relevance of information gained during experimental conditions will determine the adequacy of any one particular model. In line with this, the development of rodent and primate models of Parkinson (PD) and Huntington (HD) disease, replicating either nigral ("PD-like") or striatal ("HD-like") pathology, has yielded major advances in the understanding of the pathogenesis of these diseases (Jenner, 2003; Brouillet et al., 1999) and provided the opportunity to identify and assess new therapeutic strategies for rational clinical trials (Gross et al., 1999; Benabid et al., 2000; Rosas et al., 1999). Here, we review contributions demonstrating the feasibility of animal models to investigate multiple system atrophy (MSA). We conclude that the integration of phenotypic rodent and non-human primate models into programs seeking to identify novel treatment strategies for neurodegenerative disease can significantly speed progress toward finding cures for this devastating disease.

II. MULTIPLE SYSTEM ATROPHY

A. Clinical Features

MSA is a sporadic, progressive adult onset degenerative disease of the nervous system of unknown cause. The disease manifests clinically with any combination of Parkinsonian, pyramidal, cerebellar, urinary, and autonomic symptoms (Lantos, 1998). Recent Consensus criteria have recommended that patients with predominantly Parkinsonian features should be classified as MSA-P, formerly striatonigral degeneration (SND), whereas those with predominantly cerebellar features are designated MSA-C, formerly olivopontocerebellar atrophy (OPCA) (Gilman et al., 1999). Parkinsonism is the principal motor feature in MSA, developing in 80% of cases (Tison et al., 1995). Unlike in PD, Parkinsonism in the majority of MSA patients responds poorly and temporarily to levodopa treatment (Tison et al., 1995). The prognosis of MSA is therefore depressingly poor, with a rapidly progressive course, leading to dramatically reduced life expectancy (Ben-Shlomo et al., 1996).

B. Neuropathological Findings

Pathologically, MSA is characterized by a neuronal multisystem degeneration (striatonigral, olivopontocerebellar and autonomic) with neuronal loss and abnormal insoluble glial cytoplasmic inclusions (GCIs) containing fibrillar aggregates of α-synuclein (Lantos, 1998). This molecular form of α-synuclein contrasts sharply with normal α-synuclein, which is an abundant soluble presynaptic protein in brain neurons (Dev et al., 2003).

Degenerative changes in somatotopically related areas of the substantia nigra pars compacta (SNc) and of the striatum represent the neuropathological substrate of MSA-P/SND (Tison et al., 1995; Goto et al., 1989; Fearnley et Lees, 1990; Wenning et al., 1997). It is characterized by the combined loss of dopaminergic neurons of the ventrolateral part of the SNc, such as in PD, and of their striatal target cells in the caudal and dorsolateral putamen (Fearnley and Lees, 1990; Kume et al., 1993; Tison et al., 1995; Goto, 1996). This striatal degeneration, which is broadly similar to that found in HD, results in a decreased density of dopaminoceptive medium spiny neurons containing either GABA and pre-pro-enkephalin A (PPA) ("indirect pathway", bearing dopamine D2 receptors) or substance P (SP) ("direct pathway," bearing dopamine D1 receptors) (Churchyard et al., 1993; Kume et al., 1993; Goto et al., 1996; Goto et al., 1990; Goto et al., 1989; Tison et al., 1995), accounting for the levodopa unresponsiveness observed in most patients (Fearnley and Lees, 1990; Tison et al., 1995; Wenning et al., 1997). However, the relative contribution of nigral and striatal degeneration in producing Parkinsonian motor impairment and the functional changes occurring downstream these degenerating structures remains poorly known (Fearnley and Lees, 1990; Tison et al., 1995; Goto et al., 1996). GCIs are observed throughout the cortico-striato-pallido-cortical loops and may also contribute to basal ganglia dysfunction (Lantos, 1998). However, the degree to which either the neuronal loss or the GCI accumulation contributes to the Parkinsonism observed in MSA remains, at present, entirely speculative (Tison et al., 1995).

C. MSA Pathogenesis: Current Hypothesis

The etiology of MSA has yet to be delineated (Wenning et al., 2003). A genetic component seems unlikely. Familial clustering has never been reported (Wenning et al., 1993), and screening studies for candidate genes revealed no risk factors (Bandmann et al., 1997; Nicholl et al., 1999). Environmental factors, including cigarette smoking, have not been clearly linked to MSA but are likely to play a role given the absence of genetic contributions (Klockgether et al., 1998; Vanacore et al., 2000). The detection of α-synuclein in GCIs has yielded an attractive, albeit poorly understood, link with the other α-synucleinopathies such as PD and dementia with Lewy bodies (Jaros and Burn, 2000). Unlike rare forms of familial PD caused by mutations in α-synuclein, disease mechanisms in most α-synucleinopathies implicate wild-type α-synuclein and seem to converge around oxidative damage and impairments in protein catabolism (Dev et al., 2003). It is not known whether these causalities involve α-synuclein from the beginning, but defects in the handling of this protein seem to contribute to disease progression because accumulation of toxic α-synuclein leads to neuron damage (Dev et al., 2003). Further clues to the pathogenesis of MSA may be found through exploration of mediators of apoptosis, trophic factor, and other influences that may disrupt the oligodendroglia-neuron-axon functional unit (Wenning et al., 2003).

III. ANIMAL MODELS OF MSA

A. General Considerations

Although the etiology of this devastating illness has not yet been found, phenotypic animal models of MSA-P/SND (i.e., nigral plus striatal degeneration) are required to sort out main issues concerning its underlying pathogenesis, and as a test-bed for the evaluation of yet lacking new therapeutic proposals. Such models are thought to mimic the salient pathological and motor behavioral features of MSA-P/SND rather than aiming to replicate the still unknown primary pathological process. Hence, the combined destruction of the nigrostriatal pathway and of the striatum by specific neurotoxins constitutes the basic premise to model the core neuropathological hallmark of Parkinsonism associated with MSA-P/SND in animals. In our work, we used well-established neurotoxins that produce nigral and striatal lesions in animal models that had been developed to mimic the core pathological features of PD and HD.

B. Contribution of Experimental Neurotoxins to Animal Models of MSA-P/SND

1. 6-Hydroxydopamine

6-Hydroxydopamine (6-OHDA), a hydroxylated analogue of the natural dopamine neurotransmitter, is one of the most common neurotoxins used experimentally to model nigral degeneration (Sachs and Jonsson, 1975). Given that 6-OHDA is unable to cross the blood-brain barrier, specific central neuronal lesions can be generated only after direct intracerebral administration. Thus, in experimental rodent models of PD, 6-OHDA is preferentially injected stereotaxically into the striatum, the SNc, or the ascending medial forebrain bundle (MFB), to destroy the nigral dopaminergic neurons and thus to reproduce the pathological features responsible for motor impairments in PD (Ungerstedt, 1968; Ichitani et al., 1991; Sauer and Oertel, 1994). Once injected, 6-OHDA is taken up into the dopaminergic terminals via high-affinity dopamine uptake. It then accumulates into dopaminergic neurons to exert its deleterious effects through complex but interacting mechanisms involving oxidative stress (Kumar et al., 1995) and mitochondrial defects through respiratory chain enzyme complex I and IV inhibition (Glinka and Youdim, 1995; Blum et al., 2001). In our rodent models 6-OHDA was injected either into the striatum or in the MFB.

2. Quinolinic Acid

Quinolinic acid (QA) is a well-known endogenous tryptophan metabolite at the kynurenine level, and a potent neurotoxin exhibiting glutamate agonist properties with relative selectivity for the *N*-methyl-D-aspartate (NMDA) receptor (Stone, 1993). It exerts its neurotoxic actions through mechanisms involving excitotoxicity, reactive oxygen species formation and oxidative stress (Foster et al., 1983; Behan et al., 1999; Santamaria et al., 2001). When injected into the striatum, QA produces a selective pattern of striatal neuronal degeneration with loss of GABAergic projecting medium spiny neurons and relative sparing of somatostatin/neuropeptide Y/NADPH-diaphorase containing interneurons depending on animal age and QA injection speed (Figueredo-Cardenas et al., 1997 and 1998). This particular pattern of QA-induced striatal lesion shows prominent similarities to the striatal pathology seen in HD (Ferrante et al., 1985), and thus was used to provide experimental rat and monkey models of HD (Beal et al., 1986; Ferrante et al., 1993). In our rodent models QA was injected into the striatum.

3. 3-Nitropropionic Acid

3-Nitropropionic acid (3NP) is another neurotoxic compound that causes neuronal degeneration within the basal ganglia when injected systematically or directly into the striatum. 3NP is a mitochondrial toxin that inhibits both complex II-III of the respiratory chain and the tricarboxylic acid through inactivation of the succinate dehydrogenase (SDH) enzyme (Alston et al., 1977). Acute and chronic inhibition of SDH by systematic injection of 3NP has been used to produce animal models for HD in both rats and monkeys (Brouillet et al., 1999). 3NP neurotoxicity involves three interacting processes, namely energy impairment, excitotoxicity, and oxidative stress (Alexi et al., 1998). However, the mechanisms by which 3NP produces lesions in the striatum are not fully characterized. While impairment of energy metabolism occurs throughout all cells of the body and brain, it is the striatum that is most severely affected (Gould and Gustine, 1982; Gould et al., 1985), partly because of a preferential vulnerability of the GABAergic neurons, which make up the bulk of the neurons in the striatum, to tricarboxylic acid cycle inhibition (Hassel and Sonnewald, 1995).

4. 1-Methyl-4-phenyl 1,2,3,6 tetrahydropyridine and 1-methyl-4-phenylpyridinium ion

1-methyl-4-phenyl-1,2,3,6-tetrahydropyridine (MPTP) is considered a powerful drug which induces nigral degeneration in animals and was shown to induce PD-like symptoms in several species including mouse, dog, cat, and monkey

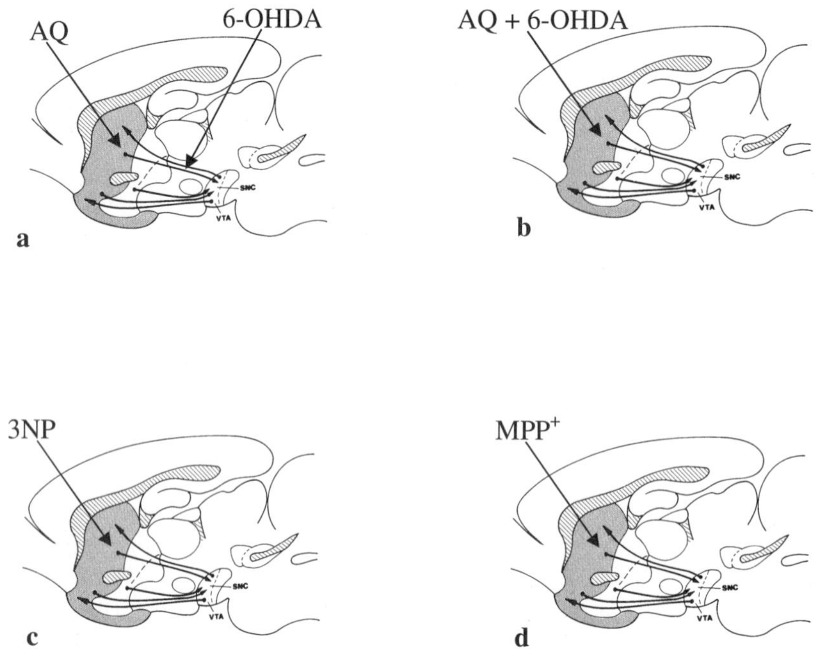

FIGURE 1 In vivo models of MSA-P/SND in rats using different unilateral stereotaxic approaches.
a, b: The "double toxin-double lesion" approach (**a**: Wenning et al., 1996; Scherfler et al., 2000. **b**: Ghorayeb et al., 2001).
c, d: The "single toxin-double lesion" approach (**c**: Waldner et al., 2001. **d**: Ghorayeb et al., 2002).

(Burns et al., 1983; Heikkila et al., 1984; Langston et al., 1984; Schneider and Markham, 1986; Wilson et al., 1987; Gerlach and Riederer, 1996). When systematically administered to animals, MPTP crosses the blood-brain barrier and is converted, mainly in glial cells, into its effective form, 1-methyl-4-phenylpyridinium ion (MPP^+), by monoamine oxidase B. MPP^+ then accumulates in dopaminergic cells after selective uptake by dopamine transporter (Chiba et al., 1985; Pifl et al., 1993; Santiago et al., 1996). Once inside the cells, MPP^+ leads to a major inhibition of complex I of the mitochondrial respiratory chain but also to oxidative stress, both triggering cell death (Blum et al., 2001). Interestingly, it has also been demonstrated that MPP^+ toxicity is not restricted to dopaminergic neurons. In rats, MPP^+ can induce a dose-dependent loss of striatal GABAergic neurons (Heikkila et al., 1985; Altar et al., 1986) likely through an NMDA-dependent excitotoxic mechanism (Storey et al., 1992).

C. The Unilateral Stereotaxic Approach in Rats

1. Double Toxin-Double Lesion Paradigm

In rodents, several attempts have been undertaken to reproduce the core pathological features of SND underlying levodopa-unresponsive Parkinsonism in MSA-P/SND. A unilateral "double toxin-double lesion" approach using sequential dopaminergic denervation by injection of 6-OHDA into the MFB, followed by ipsilateral excitotoxic striatal lesioning by QA, was developed first (Wenning et al., 1996) (Figure 1a). Subsequently, different experimental paradigms with primary nigral or striatal lesions followed by complementary secondary striatal or nigral lesions were tested to explore the relative contribution of the nigral and the striatal lesion to the Parkinsonian symptoms (Schefler et al., 2000).

It is well established that unilateral striatal or SNc degeneration produces an asymmetric and quantifiable motor behavior. This allows easy and reliable control of the extent of the lesion and the potential benefits of therapeutic treatments. However, the motor consequences of a combined striatal and nigral lesion were never before reported in detail. In our experiments, the motor symptoms of the unilateral striatonigral double lesion were characterized and quantified by using behavioral tests that are known to reflect motor function impairment after striatal or nigral lesioning such as the spontaneous and drug-induced rotational behavior (Ungerstedt and Arbuthnott, 1970; Fuxe and Ungerstedt, 1976; Dunnett and Iversen, 1982a,b; Fornaguera et al., 1994; Hudson et al., 1993; Kafetzopoulos et al., 1988; Schwarting and Huston, 1996), the "stepping test" (Olsson et al., 1995), the "balance test" (Scherfler et al., 2000), and the "staircase test" (paw reaching) (Montoya et al., 1991).

This rodent experimental model showed that a sequential unilateral lesioning of MFB and striatum results in complex behavioral changes with mainly bilateral paw reaching impairment more marked contralateral to the lesion (Scherfler et al., 2000), and in a characteristic drug-induced rotational response with the abolition of the apomorphine-induced contralateral rotation secondary to the QA striatal lesioning in the 6-OHDA rats (Wenning et al., 1996; Puschban et al., 2000a,b). These results suggest that both nigral and striatal pathology contribute to Parkinsonism in MSA-P/SND, and the lack of circling in response to apomorphine appears to be analogous to the lack of therapeutic benefit seen in MSA-P/SND patients. Indeed, histopathological evaluation of the striatal lesion indicated marked loss of dopamine and cyclic adenosine 3′:5′-monophosphate-regulated phosphoprotein 32 (DARPP-32) expression in the dorsolateral striatum accounting for the reduction in contralateral apomorphine-induced rotation (Wenning et al., 1996). However, in a separate experiment, the reduction of apomorphine rotation in double-lesioned rats did not correlate with residual surface areas and specific dopamine D1 and D2 receptor binding on the lesioned relative to the intact side (Puschban et al., 2000). Inter-individual variations in striatal degeneration occasionally extending to ventral striatal pathways known to augment circling behavior (Pycock and Marsden, 1978) may account for the lack of correlations in our double-lesioned rats. Histological studies also revealed extensive unilateral nigral and striatal lesions with evidence of an intriguing and complex interaction between the two lesions, producing distinct histological changes depending on the lesion sequence (nigrostriatal versus striatonigral lesion sequence) (Wenning et al., 1996; Scherfler et al., 2000).

This initial 6-OHDA/QA model served to evaluate neurotransplantation approaches with evidence indicating that embryonic mesencephalic grafts alone or combined with striatal grafts partially reverse drug-induced rotation asymmetries without improving deficits of complex motor function (Wenning et al., 1996; Puschban et al., 2000a,b). These preliminary results are in accordance with anecdotal clinical evidence of incomplete motor benefit produced by embryonic mesencephalic grafts in one MSA-P/SND patient misdiagnosed as PD (Spencer et al., 1992).

Thus, although the relevance of this sequential model is indisputable, a number of drawbacks limited its usefulness. Firstly, and as previously noted by Buisson et al. (1991), primary dopaminergic denervation by 6-OHDA modified subsequent sensitivity to striatal QA. Secondly, the complete nigral degeneration did not account for the anatomical relationship between the loss of the ventrolateral nigral dopaminergic neurons and dorsolateral striatal target neurons typically observed in the human disease (Fearnley and Lees, 1990; Kume et al., 1993; Tison et al., 1995). Hence, the severity of the induced lesions may have limited the effectiveness of neurorestorative intervention (Wenning et al., 1996; Puschban et al., 2000a,b).

By using this "double toxin-double lesion" approach, we subsequently established a modified partial unilateral model of early-stage SND based on simultaneous low dose QA and 6-OHDA injections into the lateral sector of the rat striatum, the putaminal equivalent of the rat striatum (Ghorayeb et al., 2001) (Figure 1b). This strategy was designed to induce simultaneous and anatomically related striatal and nigral degeneration closely reflecting the human disease process (Tison et al., 1995) and to avoid reduction of QA striatal toxicity by prior dopamine depletion. As for the aforementioned experiments, behavioral analysis comprised spontaneous and dopaminergic drug-induced rotations, the "stepping test" and the "staircase test" (Olsson et al., 1995; Montoya et al., 1991). The open-field "thigmotactic scanning" behavior, which explores sensorimotor integration, was also analyzed (Schwarting et al., 1991; Schwarting et al., 1993; Schwarting and Huston, 1996). Behavioral deficits and histopathological changes were compared in four rat groups including a control group, a striatal/QA-lesioned group, an SNc/6-OHDA-lesioned group, and a striatonigral/QA + 6-OHDA-lesioned group. Interestingly, this double toxin striatal administration again resulted in a unique motor behavior characterized mainly by reduction of the spontaneous amphetamine- and apomorphine-induced rotational bias observed in the SNc-lesioned and in the striatum-lesioned groups and bilateral impairment of the skilled paw use. This ipsilateral effect was also observed by Scherfler et al. (2000) and may account for the severity of Parkinsonism in MSA-P/SND. Simultaneous QA and 6-OHDA also reduced the thigmotactic bias observed in the 6-OHDA rats indicating that functional asymmetry in dopaminergic-depleted rats requires the integrity of striatal projection neurons.

Histopathology revealed a more marked striatal cell loss, increased astrogliosis, and severe reduction of the lesioned striatal surface after simultaneous QA and 6-OHDA injections than was noted after QA alone, consistent with an exacerbation of QA striatal toxicity by additional 6-OHDA. By contrast, at the presynaptic level, the mean loss of tyrosine hydroxylase (TH)-positive neurons in the ipsilateral SNc of the double-toxin group was less marked than in the 6-OHDA group, reflecting a possible protective action of intrastriatal QA upon 6-OHDA retrograde SNc degeneration. Although this intrastriatal combined intoxication paradigm did not prevent previously described complex interactions between QA and 6-OHDA (Venero et al., 1995; Scherfler et al., 2000), it clearly improves the clinical and pathological phenotype of the previously proposed model and produces a rodent model of early stage MSA-P/SND more suitable for early therapeutic interventions.

2. Single Toxin-Double Lesion Paradigm

The simplified "single toxin-double lesion" strategy serves to avoid neurotoxin interactions encountered in our first experiments (Wenning et al., 1996; Ghorayeb et al., 2001; Scherfler et al., 2000). It is based on the use of a single toxin to elicit degeneration in both the striatum and the SNc, producing MSA-P/SND-like pathology. A number of mitochondrial respiratory chain inhibitors are helpful candidates for this approach, including 3NP and MPP^+. In line with this, we first tested intrastriatal 3NP injection in order to create a rat model of advanced MSA-P/SND and to assess the effects of embryonic allografts upon drug-induced rotation asymmetries and complex-motor behavioral deficits measured by paw reaching tests (Waldner et al., 2001) (Figure 1c). Unfortunately, significant dopamine depletion (–45%) was reached only when almost complete destruction of the injected striatum was achieved such that the severity of the striatal lesion precluded the functional effect of the embryonic neuronal co-grafts upon the recovery of the amphetamine- and apomorphine-induced rotations and skilled forelimb use. To avoid 3NP-induced massive destruction, MPP^+, the active metabolite of the MPTP, was used as an alternative candidate. Although the rat is poorly sensitive to the neurotoxic effects of systematically administered MPTP (Chiueh et al., 1984), intrastriatal administration of MPP^+ does cause retrograde and irreversible damage to the dopaminergic system (Heikkila et al., 1985; Bradbury et al., 1986), and also produces marked excitotoxic lesions of the striatum (Storey et al., 1992; Espejo et al., 1998) thereby providing an alternative "single toxin-double lesion" approach for modeling MSA-P/SND (Figure 1d).

As for our combined QA/6-OHDA "double toxin-double lesion" approach, we explored the motor behavior effects of a single stereotaxic intrastriatal injection of MPP^+, compared to a "pure" retrograde dopaminergic lesion with 6-OHDA, and a "pure" striatal lesion with QA and controls. We hypothesized that intrastriatal MPP^+ will replicate the combined nigral and striatal motor deficit pattern with its histopathological correlates, comparable to that found in our previously described "double toxin-double lesion" MSA-P/SND rat models (Ghorayeb et al., 2001).

Interestingly, MPP^+ administration resulted in loss of the amphetamine-induced ipsilateral bias observed in the 6-OHDA group and of the apomorphine-induced ipsilateral bias observed in the QA group. This is a relatively constant and specific pattern that we and others observed with the combination of dopaminergic nigral and lateral striatal lesions relative to the apomorphine-induced rotations (Friehs et al., 1991; Barker and Dunnett, 1994; Ghorayeb et al., 2001). By contrast, changes in amphetamine-induced rotations are less consistent and depend greatly upon the size and location of the striatal lesion (Barker and Dunnett, 1994; Schwarting and Huston, 1996; Wenning et al., 1996; Fricker et al., 1996). Globally, this MPP^+ rotational pattern was similar to that observed in either the sequential or the simultaneous QA + 6-OHDA double-lesioned model (Wenning et al., 1996; Puschban et al., 2000a,b; Ghorayeb et al., 2001) and was also consistent with a combined striatal and nigral lesion, although a possible role of extra-striatal lesions such as the retrograde degeneration of the thalamic parafascicular nucleus in the MPP^+ rats cannot be ruled out (Ahlenius et al., 1982; Ghorayeb et al., 2002). However, it seems that the effects of both striatal and nigral lesions cancel each other out because lesions induce rotations in opposite directions and, as mentioned in our "double toxin-double lesion" paradigm, this lack of dopaminergic drugs circling can also be viewed as a "dopaminergic resistance" due to the striatonigral lesion similar to the levodopa-unresponsive Parkinsonism seen in human patients (Tison et al., 1995).

No thigmotactic scanning asymmetry was observed in the MPP^+ rats compared to the QA and the 6-OHDA rats, whereas MPP^+ elicited a bilateral stepping adjustment deficit similar to that found in the QA group when compared to controls. Also, a more severe and significant contralateral deficit in paw reaching was present when compared to controls, 6-OHDA, and QA groups. This unique pattern of thigmotactic bias may be due to a complex effect of the combined striatal and nigral lesions upon sensorimotor integration and exploratory behavior (Ghorayeb et al., 2001), although one would expect a more pronounced (additive effect), as for the paw reaching, or similar bias as in the 6-OHDA or QA rats, as for the stepping test. Again, the retrograde degeneration in the thalamic parafascicular nucleus may have played a role (Ghorayeb et al., 2002). Altogether, and as it has previously been demonstrated, our results suggest that combining a striatal and a nigral lesion does not simply add up, nor does it attenuate behavioral deficits arising from single striatal and nigral lesion, but rather generates novel types of behavioral disturbances, such as ipsilateral motor deficits and postural adjustment impairments (Scherfler et al., 2000; Ghorayeb et al., 2001; Waldner et al., 2001).

Histopathology revealed a significant reduction of the striatal surface (–48%) with neuronal loss and astrogliosis in the MPP^+ group grossly similar to that found in the QA group. Contrary to the latter group, however, loss of intrastriatal and striatal-crossing fiber bundles was observed in the MPP^+ group as there was also some retrograde degeneration in the ipsilateral thalamic parafascicular nucleus. The mean loss of dopaminergic cells in the ipsilateral SNc in MPP^+ rats was less marked (–49%) than in the 6-OHDA rats (–64%) and was not significant in QA rats (–5%). Thus, the present experiment shows that a single unilateral intrastri-

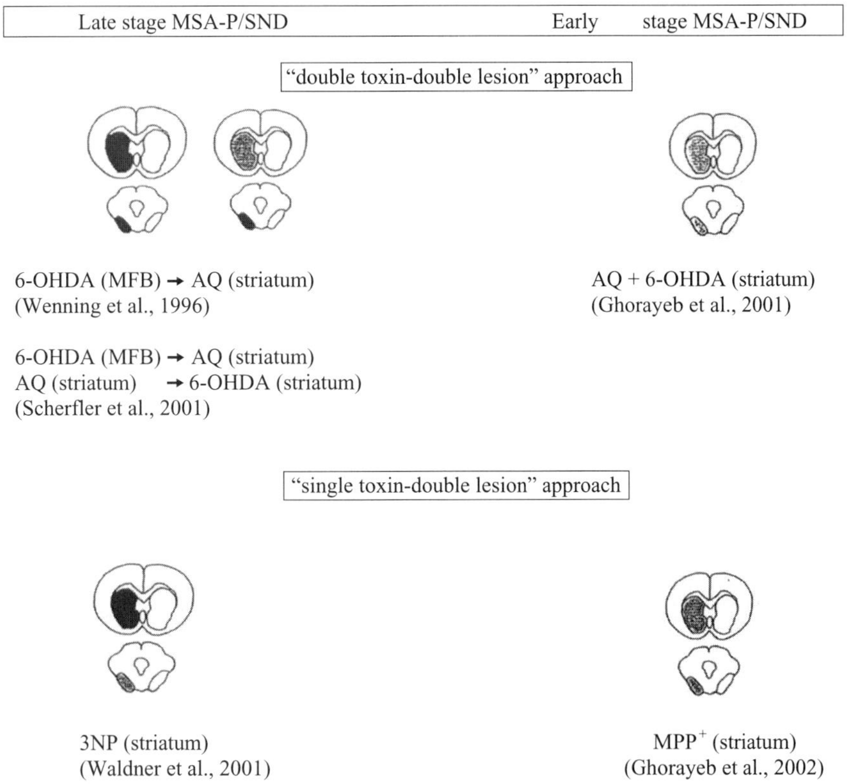

FIGURE 2 Different shades of grey showing variable degree of striatal and nigral lesion severity produced by the different unilateral stereotaxic approaches in rats, with the black standing for severe lesions, grey for mild, and white for absence of lesion.
MFB: medial forebrain bundle.

atal administration of MPP^+ induces a unique motor behavior closely resembling that which is observed in our previously established "double toxin-double lesion" models and resulting from almost equal nigral and striatal degeneration. This "single toxin-double lesion" paradigm may thus advantageously replace or complement these later models, particularly in regards to the better lesion volume control obtained with a single toxin, and serve as a rat model of early stage SND.

3. Rat Models Conclusion

Behavioral and histological analysis of our unilateral double-lesion rat models relevant to a striatonigral lesion is in accordance with expected results. However, these experiments produced several rat models mimicking various degrees of disease severity due principally to interaction between the nigral and the striatal lesions (Figure 2). This complex interaction was overcome by using a single toxin intrastriatal injection such as 3NP or MPP^+. Regarding MPP^+, we were able to produce more "balanced" nigral and striatal lesions to achieve a rat model of early stage MSA-P/SND.

D. The Systemic Toxic Approach in Mice and Non-Human Primates

Even if it constitutes a relevant approach for initial exploratory studies, the stereotaxic unilateral rat model still has limitations. Firstly, the stereotaxic unilateral lesioning approach is an invasive and time-consuming procedure that poorly mimics the natural history and time course of a disease with a diffuse progressive degenerative process. This aspect can be partly circumvented by switching to a systemic MPTP + 3NP subacute/chronic intoxication approach in species sensitive to the toxic effects of these compounds, namely mice and monkeys. Secondly, even if it can reveal unexpected behavioral abnormalities like ipsilateral impairments, the rat model lacks clinical pertinence. In fact, the repertoire of clinical symptoms in the non-human primate is closer to that seen in humans than is that seen in rats (Langston et al., 1984; Hantraye et al., 1993; Bezard et al., 1997). Thirdly, the anatomical and functional organization of the basal ganglia in humans is closer to that of monkeys than to that of rodents (Hedreen et al., 1991; Aubert et al., 2000). Finally, even if the rat model remains an interesting starting point for new pathophysiological hypothesis and new therapeutic strategies testing, non-human primate studies are necessary to yield results with therapeutic relevance and possible therapeutic implications in humans (Benazzouz et al., 1993; Guyot et al., 1997; Kendall et al., 1998; Palfi et al., 1998).

1. The MPTP + 3NP Mouse Model of MSA

The systemic administration of MPTP + 3NP in mouse models allows a dynamic approach of the neurodegenerative process and its behavioral consequences. While being closer to the human situation, this strategy applied to the mouse is also better suited to explore the dopaminergic modulation of striatal damage by allowing the use of a greater number of animals and the study of transgenic mice with modified α-synuclein or key regulatory actor expression in dopaminergic neurons. Using multiple sequential paradigms of MPTP and 3NP administration, a first mouse model was developed (Stefanova et al., 2003). Prior lesioning with MPTP reduced 3NP-induced striatal damage while prior 3NP administration reduced MPTP-induced nigral degeneration.

We subsequently developed a combined MPTP + 3NP mouse model in order to reproduce the co-occurrence of nigral and striatal degeneration as is thought to be the case in the human disease. Contrary to all previous sequential double lesion attempts which showed a "protective" effect of a first nigral deafferentation, this combined model showed that MPTP can potentiate 3NP-induced striatal damage (neuronal loss and astroglial activation) provided the nigral and striatal compromise coexists (Fernagut et al., 2004). Behaviorally, MPTP + 3NP-treated mice had a more severe and long-lasting motor disorder (clinical scale, rotarod, pole test, beam traversing) consistent with the increased severity of Parkinsonism in MSA-P. These results are consistent with previous reports indicating that elevated striatal dopaminergic levels increase the sensitivity to 3NP (Reynolds et al., 1998; Fernagut et al., 2002). The mechanisms involved (dopamine-induced oxidative stress, stimulation of D1 and D2 receptors, etc.) remain to be determined. Since rat, and more recently, mouse models underlined the importance of dopaminergic neurotransmission homeostasis upon the neural degeneration process in the nigrostriatal system, our results plead toward an assessment of the possible role of dopaminergic therapy on striatal degeneration natural history.

2. The MPTP + 3NP Non-Human Primate Model of MSA

For the first time, we explored the feasibility of a non-human primate model of MSA-P/SND. For this, candidate neurotoxins included MPTP, which produces a highly selective loss of dopaminergic neurons of the SNc through acute/subacute or chronic systemic administration (Bezard et al., 1998) and 3NP, which produces striatal excitotoxic lesions exhibiting "HD-like" pathology (Brouillet and Hantraye, 1995). Our intoxication paradigm used sequential systemic administration of MPTP and 3NP in *Macaca fascicularis* monkeys (Ghorayeb et al., 2000), and this intoxication paradigm was further validated in a subsequent experiment using additional monkeys and a more chronic intoxication approach (Ghorayeb et al., 2002).

Motor status was monitored every day by direct observation using a semi-quantitative scale for primate Parkinsonism (Bezard et al., 1997), and after emergence of stable MPTP-induced Parkinsonism, general motor activity was assessed at baseline and one hour after levodopa challenge tests with a dose that was determined to constantly produce a ≥50% motor improvement. Following this experimental setting, we clearly demonstrated that sequential systemic administration of MPTP and 3NP in non-human primates replicates the neuropathological substrate of levodopa-unresponsive Parkinsonism associated with MSA-P/SND with however marked inter-individual susceptibility that was not gender-related (Ghorayeb et al., 2002). In fact, levodopa reversed the Parkinsonian motor features that appeared following MPTP administration, consistent with the integrity of dopaminoceptive striatal outflow pathways. Subsequent 3NP intoxication increased the severity of Parkinsonism and almost abolished the beneficial anti-Parkinsonian effect of levodopa, while occasionally producing facial dyskinesia without motor benefit, as it is occasionally observed in MSA-P/SND (Hughes et al., 1992). This loss of efficacy of levodopa occurred concomitantly with the appearance of an asymmetrical hindlimb dystonia indicating striatal damage as demonstrated by in vivo MRI in our first experiment (Ghorayeb et al., 2000). Histopathologically, there was a bilateral pre- and post-synaptic lesion of the nigrostriatal system, with almost complete loss of dopaminergic neurons and with circumscribed lesions of the dorsolateral putamen and the ventral head of the caudate nucleus surrounded by a more diffuse metabolic failure as evidenced by cytochrome oxidase histochemistry. In contrast to that seen in the human disease where the caudatus nucleus is relatively spared compared to the putamen, our first model displayed roughly equal damage affecting the caudate nucleus and putamen (Figure 3). In the second experiment, tissue damage predominated within the putamen and to a lesser degree in the caudate nucleus. In our monkey model, and as also demonstrated in our rodent models (Schefler et

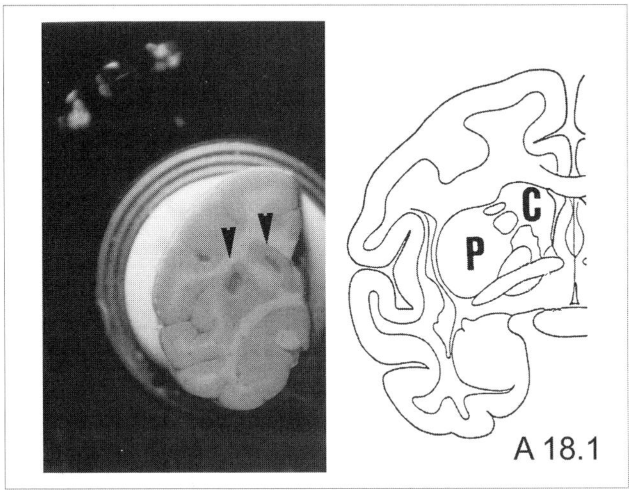

FIGURE 3 Macroscopic photograph of the monkey striatum at the commissural level and its corresponding drawing at the same anatomical level. Arrowheads show both putaminal and caudate nucleus lesions. **P**: putamen; **C**: caudate nucleus.

al., 2000; Ghorayeb et al., 2001 and 2002), additional striatal lesions aggravated the motor symptoms, suggesting that both nigral and striatal damage play a role in the severity of Parkinsonism in MSA-P/SND. The complementary striatal lesion also abolished the levodopa response, in agreement with previous clinicopathological observations by Fearnley and Lees (1990), suggesting a correlation of putaminal cell loss and levodopa-unresponsiveness. The core striatal lesion in our model was devoid of PPA and SP neurons, whereas the somatostatin interneurons (NADPH-, diaphorase-, and neuropeptide Y-containing neurons) were preserved, consistent with findings in 3NP-primate models and in QA-rodent models of HD (Beal et al., 1993; Roberts et al., 1993). It is not clear, however, whether or not such interneurons or cholinergic interneurons are preserved in MSA (Tison et al., 1995; Fearnley and Lees, 1990; Goto et al., 1996).

Our model displaying circumscribed lesions does not, however, replicate the diffuse pathological process seen in MSA with numerous GCIs in subcortical motor regions. Moreover, the absence of α-synuclein-positive GCIs in our model, despite severe neuronal pathology reminiscent of SND, may limit its impact since it has been suggested, but yet not demonstrated, that glial pathology may represent a primary pathogenic event in the human disease (Lantos, 1998). Alternatively, GCIs formation may be secondary to the chronic process of the human disease, as well as aging-related factors, both of which may be taken into account in future experiments using modifications of the double lesion protocol reported here. As in our "double toxin-double lesion" rat models, complex interactions between the two degenerating sites was revealed. In the SNc, 3NP may have potentiated the toxic effect of MPTP, accounting for the rather severe dopaminergic denervation reminiscent of that found in MSA-P (Tison et al., 1995; Fearnley and Lees, 1990; Goto et al., 1996). On the other hand, primary dopaminergic denervation may have reduced the subsequent striatal sensitivity to 3NP, explaining the need for relatively high doses to obtain striatal damage in our animal (Maragos et al., 1998).

3. Systemic Models Conclusion

We provide evidence that the levodopa-unresponsive Parkinsonism and "SND-like" pathologic changes characteristic of MSA-P/SND may be modeled in mice and non-human primates by either combined or acute/sub-acute sequential systemic administration of MPTP and 3NP. Ethical considerations, time-consuming experiments, and the need for a great number of animals due to marked individual susceptibility to neurotoxins are, however, limiting factors for the use of monkeys in routine experiment settings. Therefore, systemic mouse models may be used preferentially for drug pre-screening requiring a high number of animals before testing in monkeys. However, and although the motor disorders elicited in MPTP + 3NP mice have been now well delineated, the phenotypic model of MSA in non-human primates will still provide a unique mean for final experimental efficacy testing of new therapeutic strategies in laboratory animals with cerebral anatomy and behavioral repertoire close to that of humans. This is particularly important when considering the potential use of new therapeutic approaches such as deep brain stimulation that must be assessed for its efficiency and safety in a situation that mimics as far as possible the clinical situation before trials in human patients.

IV. CONCLUDING REMARKS AND FUTURE DIRECTIONS

There is a large body of evidence indicating that the neuropathological substrate of Parkinsonism associated with MSA-P comprises degenerative changes in the SNc and striatum. Both the etiology and pathogenesis of the disease process underlying MSA, however, remain elusive. Bringing together observations coming from our improved phenotypic double-lesion rodent and non-human primate models, it is therefore possible to formulate new pathophysiological hypotheses for MSA-P/SND, which would help to propose new therapeutic strategies. Ultimately, animal models reflecting both neuronal and glial lesions need to be developed. Specific alterations of oligodendroglial and microglial function may be replicated using transgenic mice. These novel MSA models may shed light on the poorly understood interaction between glial and neuronal dysfunction (Stefanova et al., 2001).

Acknowledgments

Centre Hospitalier de Bordeaux and CNRS.

Abbreviations

3NP: 3-nitropropionic acid
6-OHDA: 6-hydroxydopamine
GCIs: glial cytoplasmic inclusions
HD: Huntington disease
MFB: medial forebrain bundle
MSA: multiple system atrophy
MPTP: 1-methyl-4-phenyl-1,2,3,6-tetrahydropyridine
MPP^+: 1-methyl-4-phenylpyridinium ion
PD: Parkinson disease
PPA: pre-pro-enkephalin A
QA: quinolinic acid
SNc: substantia nigra pars compacta
SND: striatonigral degeneration
SP: substance P
TH: tyrosine hydroxylase

References

Ahlenius, S., N.E. Anden, and M. Grabowska-Anden. 1982. Apomorphine-induced ipsilateral turning in rats with unilateral lesions of the parafascicular nucleus. *Exp Brain Res* **47**:270–276.

Alexi, T., P.E. Hughes, R.L. Faull, and C.E. Williams. 1998. 3-Nitropropionic acid's lethal triplet: cooperative pathways of neurodegeneration. *Neuroreport* **9**:R57–64.

Alston, T.A., L. Mela, and H.J. Bright. 1977. 3-Nitropropionate, the toxic substance of Indigofera, is a suicide inactivator of succinate dehydrogenase. *Proc Natl Acad Sci U S A* **74**:3767–3771.

Altar, C.A., R.E. Heikkila, L. Manzino, and M.R. Marien. 1986. 1-Methyl-4-phenylpyridine (MPP+): regional dopamine neuron uptake, toxicity, and novel rotational behavior following dopamine receptor proliferation. *Eur J Pharmacol* **131**:199–209.

Aubert, I., I. Ghorayeb, E. Normand, and B. Bloch. 2000. Phenotypical characterization of the neurons expressing the D1 and D2 dopamine receptors in the monkey striatum. *J Comp Neurol* **418**:23–32.

Bandmann, O., M.G. Sweeney, S.E. Daniel, G.K. Wenning, N. Quinn, C.D. Marsden, and N.W. Wood. 1997. Multiple-system atrophy is genetically distinct from identified inherited causes of spinocerebellar degeneration. *Neurology* **49**:1598–1604.

Barker, R., and S.B. Dunnett. 1994. Ibotenic acid lesions of the striatum reduce drug-induced rotation in the 6-hydroxydopamine-lesioned rat. *Exp Brain Res* **101**:365–374.

Beal, M.F., E. Brouillet, B.G. Jenkins, R.J. Ferrante, N.W. Kowall, J.M. Miller, R. Storey, R. Srivastava, B.R. Rosen, and B.Y. Hyman. 1993. Neurochemical and histologic characterization of striatal excitotoxic lesions produced by the mitochondrial toxin 3-nitropropionic acid. *J Neurosci* **13**:4181–4192.

Beal, M.F., N.W. Kowall, D.W. Ellison, M.F. Mazurek, K.J. Swartz, and J.B. Martin. 1986. Replication of the neurochemical characteristics of Huntington's disease by quinolinic acid. *Nature* **321**:168–171.

Behan, W.M., M. McDonald, L.G. Darlington, and T.W. Stone. 1999. Oxidative stress as a mechanism for quinolinic acid-induced hippocampal damage: protection by melatonin and deprenyl. *Br J Pharmacol* **128**:1754–1760.

Benabid, A.L., P.P. Krack, A. Benazzouz, P. Limousin, A. Koudsie, and P. Pollak. 2000. Deep brain stimulation of the subthalamic nucleus for Parkinson's disease: methodologic aspects and clinical criteria. *Neurology* **55(12 Suppl 6)**:S40–44.

Benazzouz, A., C. Gross, J. Feger, T. Boraud, and B. Bioulac. 1993. Reversal of rigidity and improvement in motor performance by subthalamic high-frequency stimulation in MPTP-treated monkeys. *Eur J Neurosci* **5**:382–389.

Ben-Shlomo, Y., G.K. Wenning, F. Tison, and N.P. Quinn. 1996. Survival of patients with pathologically-proven multiple system atrophy: a meta-analysis. *Neurology* **48**:384–393.

Bezard, E., C. Imbert, and C.E. Gross. 1998. Experimental models of Parkinson's disease: from the static to the dynamic. *Rev Neurosci* **9**:71–90.

Bezard, E., C. Imbert, X. Deloire, B. Bioulac, and C.E. Gross. 1997. A chronic MPTP model reproducing the slow evolution of Parkinson's disease: evolution of motor symptoms in monkey. *Brain Res* **766**:107–112.

Blum, D., S. Torch, N. Lambeng, M. Nissou, A. Benabid, R. Sadoul, and J. Verna. 2001. Molecular pathways involved in the neurotoxicity of 6-OHDA, dopamine and MPTP: contribution to the apoptotic theory in Parkinson's disease. *Prog Neurobiol* **65**:135–172.

Bradbury, A.J., B. Costall, A.M. Domeney, P. Jenner, M.E. Kelly, C.D. Marsden, and R.J. Naylor. 1986. 1-methyl-4-phenylpyridine is neurotoxic to the nigrostriatal dopamine pathway. *Nature* **319**:56–57.

Brouillet, E., and P. Hantraye. 1995. Effects of chronic MPTP and 3-nitropropionic acid in nonhuman primates. *Curr Opin Neurol* **8**:469–473.

Brouillet, E., F. Conde, M.F. Beal, and P. Hantraye. 1999. Replicating Huntington's disease phenotype in experimental animals. *Prog Neurobiol* **59**:427–468.

Buisson, A., V. Plateau, M. Plotkine, and R.G. Boulu. 1991. Nigrostriatal pathway modulates striatum vulnerability to quinolinic acid. *Neurosci Lett* **131**:257–259.

Burns, R.S., C.C. Chiueh, S.P. Markey, M.H. Ebert, D.M. Jacobowitz, and I.J. Kopin. 1983. A primate model of parkinsonism: selective destruction of dopaminergic neurons in the pars compacta of the substantia nigra by N-methyl-4-phenyl-1,2,3,6-tetrahydropyridine. *Proc Natl Acad Sci U S A* **80**:4546–4550.

Chiba, K., A.J. Trevor, and N. Castagnoli, Jr. 1985. Active uptake of MPP+, a metabolite of MPTP, by brain synaptosomes. *Biochem Biophys Res Commun* **128**:1228–1232.

Chiueh, C.C., S.P. Markey, R.S. Burns, J.N. Johannessen, A. Pert, and I.J. Kopin. 1984. Neurochemical and behavioral effects of systemic and intranigral administration of N-methyl-4-phenyl-1,2,3,6-tetrahydropyridine in the rat. *Eur J Pharmacol* **100**:189–194.

Churchyard, A., G.A. Donnan, A. Hughes, D.W. Howells, D. Woodhouse, J.Y. Wong, R.M. Kalnins, F.A. Mendelsohn, and G. Paxinos. 1993. Dopa resistance in multiple-system atrophy: loss of postsynaptic D2 receptors. *Ann Neurol* **34**:219–226.

Dev, K.K., K. Hofele, S. Barbieri, V.L. Buchman, and H. van der Putten. 2003. Part II: alpha-synuclein and its molecular pathophysiological role in neurodegenerative disease. *Neuropharmacology* **45**:14–44.

Dunnett, S.B., and S.D. Iversen. 1982a. Sensorimotor impairments following localized kainic acid and 6-hydroxydopamine lesions of the neostriatum. *Brain Res* **248**:121–127.

Dunnett, S.B., and S.D. Iversen. 1982b. Spontaneous and drug-induced rotation following localized 6-hydroxydopamine and kainic acid-induced lesions of the neostriatum. *Neuropharmacology* **21**:899–908.

Espejo, M., S. Ambrosio, J. Llorens, and B. Cutillas. 1998. Intrastriatal grafts of fetal mesencephalic cell suspensions in MPP+-lesioned rats: a microdialysis study in vivo. *Neurochem Res* **23**:1217–1223.

Fearnley, J.M., and A.J. Lees. 1990. Striatonigral degeneration. A clinicopathological study. *Brain* **113**:1823–1842.

Fernagut, P.O., E. Diguet, B. Bioulac, and F. Tison. 2004. MPTP potentiates 3-nitropropionic acid-induced striatal damage in mice: reference to striatonigral degeneration. *Exp Neurol* **185**:47–62.

Fernagut, P.O., E. Diguet, N. Stefanova, M. Biran, G.K. Wenning, P. Canioni, B. Bioulac, and F. Tison. 2002. Subacute systemic 3-nitropropionic acid intoxication induces a distinct motor disorder in adult C57Bl/6 mice: behavioral and histopathological characterisation. *Neuroscience* **114**:1005–1017.

Ferrante, R.J., N.W. Kowall, M.F. Beal, E.P. Richardson Jr., E.D. Bird, and J.B. Martin. 1985. Selective sparing of a class of striatal neurons in Huntington's disease. *Science* **230**:561–563.

Ferrante, R.J., N.W. Kowall, P.B. Cipolloni, E. Storey, and M.F. Beal. 1993. Excitotoxin lesions in primates as a model for Huntington's disease: histopathologic and neurochemical characterization. *Exp Neurol* **119**:46–71.

Figueredo-Cardenas, G., C.L. Harris, K.D. Anderson, and A. Reiner. 1998. Relative resistance of striatal neurons containing calbindin or parvalbumin to quinolinic acid-mediated excitotoxicity compared to other striatal neuron types. *Exp Neurol* **149**:356–372.

Figueredo-Cardenas, G., Q. Chen, and A. Reiner. 1997. Age-dependent differences in survival of striatal somatostatin-NPY-NADPH-diaphorase-containing interneurons versus striatal projection neurons after intrastriatal injection of quinolinic acid in rats. *Exp Neurol* **146**: 444–457.

Fornaguera, J., R.J. Carey, J.P. Huston, and R.K.W. Schwarting. 1994. Behavioral asymmetries and recovery in rats with different degrees of unilateral striatal dopamine depletion. *Brain Res* **664**:178–188.

Foster, A.C., J.F. Collins, and R. Schwarcz. 1983. On the excitotoxic properties of quinolinic acid, 2,3-piperidine dicarboxylic acids and structurally related compounds. *Neuropharmacology* **22**:1331–1342.

Fricker, R.A., L.E. Annett, E.M. Torres, and S.B. Dunnett. 1996. The placement of a striatal ibotenic acid lesion affects skilled forelimb use and the direction of drug-induced rotation. *Brain Res Bull* **41**:409–416.

Friehs, G.M., R.G. Parker, L.S. He, S.J. Haines, D.A. Turner, and T.J. Ebner. 1991. Lesioning of the striatum reverses motor asymmetry in the 6-hydroxydopamine rodent model of parkinsonism. *J Neural Transplant Plast* **2**:141–156.

Fuxe, K., and U. Ungerstedt. 1976. Antiparkinsonian drugs and dopaminergic neostriatal mechanisms: studies in rats with unilateral 6-hydroxydopamine (=6-OH-DA)-induced degeneration of the nigro-neostriatal DA pathway and quantitative recording of rotational behavior. *Pharmacol Ther [B]* **2**:41–47.

Gerlach, M., and P. Riederer. 1996. Animal models of Parkinson's disease: an empirical comparison with the phenomenology of the disease in man. *J Neural Transm* **103**:987–1041.

Ghorayeb, I., P.O. Fernagut, I. Aubert, E. Bezard, W. Poewe, G.K. Wenning, and F. Tison. 2000. Toward a primate model of L-dopa-unresponsive parkinsonism mimicking striatonigral degeneration. *Mov Disord* **15**:531–536.

Ghorayeb, I., P.O. Fernagut, N. Stefanova, G.K. Wenning, B. Bioulac, and F. Tison. 2002. Dystonia is predictive of subsequent altered dopaminergic responsiveness in a chronic 1-methyl-4-phenyl-1,2,3,6-tetrahydropyridine+3-nitropropionic acid model of striatonigral degeneration in monkeys. *Neurosci Lett* **335**:34–38.

Ghorayeb, I., Z. Puschban, P.O. Fernagut, C. Scherfler, R. Rouland, G.K. Wenning, and F. Tison. 2001. Simultaneous intrastriatal 6-hydroxydopamine and quinolinic acid injection: a model of early-stage striatonigral degeneration. *Exp Neurol* **167**.133–147.

Gilman, S., P. Low, N. Quinn, A. Albanese, Y. Ben-Shlomo, C. Fowler, H. Kaufmann, T. Klockgether, A. Lang, P. Lantos, I. Litvan, C. Mathias, E. Oliver, D. Robertson, I. Schatz, and G. Wenning. 1998. Consensus statement on the diagnosis of multiple system atrophy. American Autonomic Society and American Academy of Neurology. *Clin Auton Res* **8**:359–362.

Glinka, Y.Y., and M.B. Youdim. 1995. Inhibition of mitochondrial complexes I and IV by 6-hydroxydopamine. *Eur J Pharmacol* **292**:329–332.

Goto, S., A. Hirano, and S. Matsumoto. 1989. Subdivisional involvement of nigrostriatal loop in idiopathic Parkinson's disease and striatonigral degeneration. *Ann Neurol* **26**:766–770.

Goto, S., A. Hirano, and S. Matsumoto. 1990. Met-enkephalin immunoreactivity in the basal ganglia in Parkinson's disease and striatonigral degeneration. *Neurology* **40**:1051–1056.

Goto, S., S. Matsumoto, Y. Ushio, and A. Hirano. 1996. Subregional loss of putaminal efferents to the basal ganglia output nuclei may cause parkinsonism in striatonigral degeneration. *Neurology* **47**:1032–1036.

Gould, D.H., and D.L. Gustine. 1982. Basal ganglia degeneration, myelin alterations, and enzyme inhibition induced in mice by the plant toxin 3-nitropropanoic acid. *Neuropathol Appl Neurobiol* **8**:377–393.

Gould, D.H., M.P. Wilson, and D.W. Hamar. 1985. Brain enzyme and clinical alterations induced in rats and mice by nitroaliphatic toxicants. *Toxicol Lett* **27**:83–89.

Gross, C.E., T. Boraud, D. Guehl, B. Bioulac, and F. Bezard. 1999. From experimentation to the surgical treatment of Parkinson's disease: prelude or suite in basal ganglia research? *Prog Neurobiol* **59**:509–532.

Guyot, M.C., S. Palfi, J.M. Stutzmann, M. Maziere, P. Hantraye, and E. Brouillet. 1997. Riluzole protects from motor deficits and striatal degeneration produced by systemic 3-nitropropionic acid intoxication in rats. *Neuroscience* **81**:141–149.

Hantraye, P., M. Varastet, M. Peschanski, D. Riche, P. Cesaro, J.C. Willer, and M. Maziere. 1993. Stable parkinsonian syndrome and uneven loss of striatal dopamine fibres following chronic MPTP administration in baboons. *Neuroscience* **53**:169–178.

Hassel, B., and U. Sonnewald. 1995. Selective inhibition of the tricarboxylic acid cycle of GABAergic neurons with 3-nitropropionic acid in vivo. *J Neurochem* **65**:1184–1191.

Hedreen, J.C., and M.R. DeLong. 1991. Organization of striatopallidal, striatonigral, and nigrostriatal projections in the macaque. *J Comp Neurol* **304**:569–595.

Heikkila, R.E., A. Hess, and R.C. Duvoisin. 1984. Dopaminergic neurotoxicity of 1-methyl-4-phenyl-1,2,5,6-tetrahydropyridine in mice. *Science* **224**:1451–1453.

Heikkila, R.E., W.J. Nicklas, and R.C. Duvoisin. 1985. Dopaminergic toxicity after the stereotaxic administration of the 1-methyl-4-phenylpyridinium ion (MPP+) to rats. *Neurosci Lett* **59**:135–140.

Heikkila, R.E., W.J. Nicklas, and R.C. Duvoisin. 1985. Dopaminergic toxicity after the stereotaxic administration of the 1-methyl-4-phenylpyridinium ion (MPP+) to rats. *Neurosci Lett* **59**:135–140.

Hudson, J.L., C.G. van Horne, I. Strömberg, S. Brock, J. Clayton, J. Masserano, B.J. Hoffer, and G.A. Gerhardt. 1993. Correlation of apomorphine-induced turning with nigrostriatal dopamine content in unilateral 6-hydroxydopamine lesioned rats. *Brain Res* **626**:167–174.

Ichitani, Y., H. Okamura, Y. Matsumoto, I. Nagatsu, and Y. Ibata. 1991. Degeneration of the nigral dopamine neurons after 6-hydroxydopamine injection into the rat striatum. *Brain Res* **549**:350–353.

Jaros, E., and D.J. Burn. 2000. The pathogenesis of multiple system atrophy: past, present, and future. *Mov Disord* **15**:784–788.

Jenner, P. 2003. The contribution of the MPTP-treated primate model to the development of new treatment strategies for Parkinson's disease. *Parkinsonism Relat Disord* **9**:131–137.

Kafetzopoulos, E., V. Vlaha, and S. Konitsiotis. 1988. Different patterns of rotational behavior in rats after dorsal or ventral striatal lesions with ibotenic acid. *Pharmacol Biochem Behav* **29**:403–406.

Kendall, A.L., F.D. Rayment, E.M. Torres, H.F. Baker, R.M. Ridley, and S.B. Dunnett. 1998. Functional integration of striatal allografts in a primate model of Huntington's disease. *Nat Med* **4**:727–729.

Klockgether, T., K. Burk, U. Wullner, G. Wenning, J.B. Schulz, G. Doller, K. Wessel, P. Huss, A. Kramer, and R. Ludtke. 1998. Risk factors for idiopathic cerebellar ataxia of late onset. *J Neurol Sci* **160**:171–174.

Kumar, R., A.K. Agarwal, and P.K. Seth. 1995. Free radical-generated neurotoxicity of 6-hydroxydopamine. *J Neurochem* **64**:1703–1707. Erratum in: *J Neurochem* 1995;65:1906.

Kume, A., A. Takahashi, and Y. Hashizume. 1993. Neuronal cell loss of the striatonigral system in multiple system atrophy. *J Neurol Sci* **117**:33–40.

Langston, J.W., L.S. Forno, C.S. Rebert, and I. Irwin. 1984. Selective nigral toxicity after systemic administration of 1-methyl-4-phenyl-1,2,5,6-tetrahydropyrine (MPTP) in the squirrel monkey. *Brain Res* **292**: 390–394.

Lantos, P.L. 1998. The definition of multiple system atrophy: a review of recent developments. *J Neuropath Exp Neurol* **57**:1099–1111.

Maragos, W.F., R.S. Jakel, Z. Pang, and J.W. Geddes. 1998. 6-hydroxydopamine injections into the nigrostriatal pathway attenuate striatal malonate and 3-nitropropionic acid lesions. *Exp Neurol* **154**:637–644.

Montoya, C.P., H.L. Campbell, K.D. Pemberton, and S.B. Dunnett. 1991. The "staircase test": a measure of independent forelimb reaching and grasping abilities in rats. *J Neurosci Methods* **36**:219–228.

Nicholl, D.J., P. Bennett, L. Hiller, V. Bonifati, N. Vanacore, G. Fabbrini, R. Marconi, C. Colosimo, P. Lamberti, F. Stocchi, U. Bonuccelli, P. Vieregge, D.B. Ramsden, G. Meco, and A.C. Williams. 1999. A study of five candidate genes in Parkinson's disease and related neurodegenerative disorders. European Study Group on Atypical Parkinsonism. *Neurology* **53**:1415–1421.

Olsson, M., G. Nikkhah, C. Bentlage, and A. Björklund. 1995. Forelimb akinesia in the rat Parkinson model: differential effects of dopamine agonists and nigral transplants as assessed by a new stepping test. *J Neurosci* **15**:3863–3875.

Palfi, S., F. Conde, D. Riche, E. Brouillet, C. Dautry, V. Mittoux, A. Chibois, M. Peschanski, and P. Hantraye. 1998. Fetal striatal allografts reverse cognitive deficits in a primate model of Huntington disease. *Nat Med* **4**:963–966.

Pifl, C., B. Giros, and M.G. Caron. 1993. Dopamine transporter expression confers cytotoxicity to low doses of the parkinsonism-inducing neurotoxin 1-methyl-4-phenylpyridinium. *J Neurosci* **13**: 4246–4253.

Puschban, Z., C. Scherfler, R. Granata, P. Laboyrie, N.P. Quinn, P. Jenner, W. Poewe, and G.K. Wenning. 2000b. Autoradiographic study of striatal dopamine re-uptake sites and dopamine D1 and D2 receptors in a 6-hydroxydopamine and quinolinic acid double-lesion rat model of striatonigral degeneration (multiple system atrophy) and effects of embryonic ventral mesencephalic, striatal or co-grafts. *Neuroscience* **95**:377–388.

Puschban, Z., R. Waldner, K. Seppi, N. Stefanova, C. Humpel, C. Scherfler, M. Levivier, W. Poewe, and G.K. Wenning. 2000a. Failure of neuroprotection by embryonic striatal grafts in a double lesion rat model of striatonigral degeneration (multiple system atrophy). *Exp Neurol* **164**:166–175.

Pycock, C.J., and C.D. Marsden. 1978. The rotating rodent: a two component system? *Eur J Pharmacol* **47**:167–175.

Reynolds, D.S., R.J. Carter, and A.J. Morton. 1998. Dopamine modulates the susceptibility of striatal neurons to 3-nitropropionic acid in the rat model of Huntington's disease. *J Neurosci* 18:10116–10127.

Roberts, R.C., A. Ahn, K.J. Swartz, M.F. Beal, and M. DiFiglia. 1993. Intrastriatal injection of quinolinic acid or kainic acid: differential patterns of cell survival and the effects of data analysis on outcome. *Exp Neurol* **124**:274–282.

Rosas, H.D., W.J. Koroshetz, B.J. Jenkins, Y.I. Chen, D.L. Hayden, M.F. Beal, and M.E. Cudkowicz. 1999. Riluzole therapy in Huntington's disease (HD). *Mov Disord* **14**:326–330.

Sachs, C., and G. Jonsson. 1975. Mechanisms of action of 6-hydroxydopamine. *Biochem Pharmacol* **24**:1–8.

Santamaria, A., M.E. Jimenez-Capdeville, A. Camacho, E. Rodriguez-Martinez, A. Flores, and S. Galvan-Arzate. 2001. In vivo hydroxyl radical formation after quinolinic acid infusion into rat corpus striatum. *Neuroreport* **12**:2693–2696.

Santiago, M., A. Machado, and J. Cano. 1996. Nigral and striatal comparative study of the neurotoxic action of 1-methyl-4-phenylpyridinium ion: involvement of dopamine uptake system. *J Neurochem* **66**:1182–1190.

Sauer, H., and W.H. Oertel. 1994. Progressive degeneration of nigrostriatal dopamine neurons following intrastriatal terminal lesions with 6-hydroxydopamine: a combined retrograde tracing and immunocytochemical study in the rat. *Neuroscience* **59**:401–415.

Scherfler, C., Z. Puschban, I. Ghorayeb, G.P. Goebel, F. Tison, K. Jellinger, W. Poewe, and G.K. Wenning. 2000. Complex motor disturbances in a sequential double lesion rat model of striatonigral degeneration (multiple system atrophy). *Neuroscience* **99**:43–54.

Schneider, J.S., and C.H. Markham. 1986. Neurotoxic effects of N-methyl-4-phenyl-1,2,3,6-tetrahydropyridine (MPTP) in the cat. Tyrosine hydroxylase immunohistochemistry. *Brain Res* **373**:258–267.

Schwarting, R.K., H. Steiner, and J.P. Huston. 1991. Asymmetries in thigmotactic scanning: evidence for a role of dopaminergic mechanisms. *Psychopharmacology (Berl)* **103**:19–27.

Schwarting, R.K.W., and J.P. Huston. 1996. The unilateral 6-hydroxydopamine lesion model in behavioral brain research. Analysis of functional deficits, recovery and treatments. *Prog Neurobiol* **50**:275–331.

Schwarting, R.K.W., R. Goldenberg, H. Steiner, J. Fornaguera, and J.P. Huston. 1993. A video image analyzing system for open-field behavior in the rat focusing on behavioral asymmetries. *J Neurosci Methods* **49**:199–210.

Spencer, D.D., R.J. Robbins, F. Naftolin, K.L. Marek, T. Vollmer, C. Leranth, R.H. Roth, L.H. Price, A. Gjedde, and B.S. Bunney, et al. 1992. Unilateral transplantation of human fetal mesencephalic tissue into the caudate nucleus of patients with Parkinson's disease. *N Engl J Med* **327**:1541–1548.

Stefanova, N., L. Klimaschewski, W. Poewe, G.K. Wenning, and M. Reindl. 2001. Glial cell death induced by overexpression of alpha-synuclein. *J Neurosci Res* **65**:432–438.

Stefanova, N., Z. Puschban, P.O. Fernagut, E. Brouillet, F. Tison, M. Reindl, K.A. Jellinger, W. Poewe, and G.K. Wenning. 2003. Neuropathological and behavioral changes induced by various treatment paradigms with MPTP and 3-nitropropionic acid in mice: towards a model of striatonigral degeneration (multiple system atrophy). *Acta Neuropathol* **106**:157–166.

Stone, T.W. 1993. Neuropharmacology of quinolinic and kynurenic acids. *Pharmacol Rev* **45**:309–379.

Storey, E., B.T. Hyman, B. Jenkins, E. Brouillet, J.M. Miller, B.R. Rosen, and M.F. Beal. 1992. 1-Methyl-4-phenylpyridinium produces excitotoxic lesions in rat striatum as a result of impairment of oxidative metabolism. *J Neurochem* **58**:1975–1978.

Storey, E., B.Y. Hyman, B. Jenkins, E. Brouillet, J.M. Miller, B.R. Rosen, and M.F. Beal. 1992. 1-Methyl-4-phenylpyridinium produces excitotoxic lesions in rat striatum as a result of impairment of oxidative metabolism. *J Neurochem* **58**:1975–1978.

Tison, F., G.K. Wenning, S.E. Daniel, and N.P. Quinn. 1995. The pathophysiology of parkinsonism in multiple system atrophy. *Eur J Neurol* **2**:435–444.

Ungerstedt, U. 1968. 6-Hydroxy-dopamine induced degeneration of central monoamine neurons. *Eur J Pharmacol* **5**:107–110.

Ungerstedt, U., and G.W. Arbuthnott. 1970. Quantitative recording of rotational behavior in rats after 6-hydroxy-dopamine lesions of the nigrostriatal dopamine system. *Brain Res* **24**:485–493.

Vanacore, N., V. Bonifati, G. Fabbrini, C. Colosimo, R. Marconi, D. Nicholl, U. Bonuccelli, F. Stocchi, P. Lamberti, G. Volpe, G. De Michele, I. Iavarone, P. Bennett, P. Vieregge, and G. Meco. 2000. Smoking habits in multiple system atrophy and progressive supranuclear palsy. European Study Group on Atypical Parkinsonisms. *Neurology* **54**:114–119.

Venero, J.L., M. Romero-Ramos, M. Revuelta, A. Machado, and J. Cano. 1995. Intrastriatal quinolinic acid injections protect against 6-hydroxydopamine-induced lesions of the dopaminergic nigrostriatal pathway. *Brain Res* **672**:153–158.

Waldner, R., Z. Puschban, C. Scherfler, K. Seppi, K. Jellinger, W. Poewe, and G.K. Wenning. 2001. No functional effects of embryonic neuronal grafts on motor deficits in a 3-nitropropionic acid rat model of advanced striatonigral degeneration (multiple system atrophy). *Neuroscience* **102**:581–592.

Wenning, G.K., F. Geser, M. Stampfer-Kountchev, and F. Tison. 2003. Multiple system atrophy: an update. *Mov Disord* **18** Suppl 6:S34–42.

Wenning, G.K., F. Tison, Y. Ben-Shlomo, S.E. Daniel, and N.P. Quinn. 1997. Multiple system atrophy: a review of 203 pathologically proven cases. *Mov Disord* **12**:133–147.

Wenning, G.K., R. Granata, P.M. Laboyrie, N.P. Quinn, P. Jenner, and C.D. Marsden. 1996. Reversal of behavioral abnormalities by fetal allografts in a novel rat model of striatonigral degeneration. *Mov Disord* **11**:522–532.

Wenning, G.K., S. Wagner, S. Daniel, and N.P. Quinn. 1993. Multiple system atrophy: sporadic or familial? *Lancet* **342**:681.

Wilson, J.S., B.H. Turner, G.D. Morrow, and P.J. Hartman. 1987. MPTP produces a mosaic-like pattern of terminal degeneration in the caudate nucleus of dog. *Brain Res* **423**:329–332.

C H A P T E R

13

A Mouse Model for Multiple System Atrophy

DIANNE M. PEREZ

Multiple system atrophy (MSA) is an adult-onset sporadic progressive neurodegenerative disorder of unknown etiology that is clinically characterized by the variable combination of signs of autonomic failure (urinary incontinence, postural faintness, impotence, urinary retention, fecal incontinence), Parkinsonism (akinesia, bradykinesia, tremor, rigidity, and dyskinesia), cerebellar ataxia (gait ataxia, limb ataxia, intention tremor, and nystagmus), and pyramidal signs (hyperreflexia, spasticity, extensor plantar response). Parkinsonian features predominate in 80% of patients (MSA-P subtype), and cerebellar ataxia is the major motor feature in 20% of patients (MSA-C subtype). MSA affects both men and women in their sixth decade and progresses relentlessly until death after an average of nine years' survival from onset of symptoms. Currently available therapeutic strategies for MSA are to keep the patient comfortable and to provide some respite for the patient's symptoms. To date, there are no treatment strategies that arrest or delay the progression of MSA. The symptoms that are frequently targeted for symptomatic treatment include Parkinsonism, orthostatic hypotension, bladder urgency/incontinence, myoclonus, dystonia, depression, dysphagia, dysarthria, sialorrhea, and gait disorder. In more than 90% of the MSA patients, these therapeutic interventions provide no meaningful symptomatic relief. For example, in >90% of MSA-P patients Parkinsonian features fail to respond to L-dopa, the best available anti-Parkinsonian medicine.

We have generated a transgenic mouse model that systemically overexpresses the α_{1B}-adrenergic receptor (AR) (Zuscik et al., 2000). Adrenergic receptors mediate the sympathetic nervous system by binding epinephrine and norepinephrine. The role of this receptor in the central nervous system (CNS) is unknown but is thought to be stimulatory in nature, to affect the release of other neurotransmitters, and to be involved in locomotion. Our transgenic mouse model develops a neurodegenerative disease that is similar to MSA. This was unexpected. We do not yet understand why α_{1B}-AR overexpression would lead to traits similar to MSA. We are not suggesting that the cause of MSA is due to a defect in this gene. Since the same cell types (neurons and oligodendrocytes) in key areas of the brain are degenerating, this is likely the reason for the similarity to the symptoms of MSA. Nevertheless, this mouse model should be useful in deciphering the neurotransmission pathways involved with MSA and may lead to some therapeutic recourse for patients.

I. BACKGROUND

A. Adrenergic Receptors

Adrenergic receptors (ARs) are glycosylated integral membrane proteins that are activated by selectively binding the catecholamines norepinephrine and epinephrine (Graham and Lanier, 1986). ARs, as determined by their different pharmacological specificities, physiological effects, and primary structure, are classified as α_1, α_2, β_1, β_2, and β_3. By transducing the external chemical stimulus into an intracellular signal, these receptors regulate the sympathetic nervous system and, thus, play a crucial role in a variety of tissue-specific responses, including those involved in cardiovascular function. ARs belong to the superfamily of at least 1,000 distinct G-protein-coupled receptors sharing a common structural motif (Strader et al., 1989). This motif consists of seven transmembrane (TM) domains of 20 to 28 hydrophobic amino acids, which interestingly, form the ligand-binding site in an analogous manner to the visual transducing protein rhodopsin, where the ligand ll-*cis* retinal, sits in the binding pocket formed within the membrane bilayer (Oprian et al., 1987). Over 80% of all hormones signal through these types of receptors, making them applicable for study from drug targeting perspectives.

B. α_1-Adrenergic Receptor Subtypes

α_1ARs are a group of heterogeneous but related proteins. The cDNAs are separate gene products and have been isolated for three subtypes (α_{1A}, α_{1B}, α_{1D}), all three of which we have cloned and characterized. We remain a major contributor to the study of their pharmacology, structure-function, and physiological effects (Perez et al., 1991; Ramarao et al., 1992; Perez et al., 1994). α_1ARs are delineated according to their primary sequence and their affinity for subtype-selective antagonists, such as WB4101 and 5-methylurapidil (Hanft et al., 1989). α_{1A}ARs have a high affinity for these competitive antagonists. Conversely, α_{1B}- and α_{1D}-ARs have a low affinity for these same ligands. However, there are no selective drugs available with at least 1,000-fold affinity difference between the subtypes. This is needed to prevent cross-talk between the subtypes. Even more problematic are the endogenous agonists, norepinephrine and epinephrine, which have similar affinities among all adrenergic receptors (α_1, α_2, β_1, β_2, and β_3).

C. Adrenergic Receptor Subtypes and the CNS

The effects of norepinephrine in the CNS are often considered as preparatory for the processing of information (i.e., "clearing the decks") (Holets, 1990). This is generally achieved in the forebrain by depression of inhibitory responses and by potentiating the effects of excitatory signals. As mentioned earlier, since there are no truly subtype-specific agonists and antagonists, it is hard to allocate a particular CNS effect to any one of the subtypes. α_2ARs are the most widely studied because their sedative effects via activation are mediated through the brain (presynaptic release) (Macdonald and Scheinin, 1995). The β-ARs in the CNS have been implicated in modulation of arousal as well as neuronal and behavioral plasticity (Hopkins and Johnston, 1988). The α_1ARs are the least understood of the central ARs. This is surprising in that the overall density of the α_1ARs matches that of the α_2ARs and far exceeds that of the βARs. The activation of α_1ARs can have a facilitatory effect on neuronal transmission in the neocortex. In the somatosensory areas of the cortex, α_1AR activation has been found to increase the excitation seen after administration of glutamate or acetylcholine (Mouradian et al., 1991). α_1ARs also cause excitatory responses in subcortical areas such as the medial and lateral geniculate nuclei, the reticular thalamic nucleus, dorsal raphe, and spinal motor neurons. It appears that this activation is largely due to a decrease in resting potassium conductance and not to a robust increase in calcium conductance (McCormick et al., 1991). α_1ARs may modulate both weak and strong activation of the pyramidal neurons in the neocortex and may play a role in long-term potentiation. α_1ARs may affect many brain functions via non-neuronal mechanisms since they are also localized to glial cells (Lerea & McCarthy, 1989). The activation of α_1ARs has been found to increase calcium transients in hippocampal astrocytes. α_1AR activation could modulate the buffering of potassium ions, uptake of neurotransmitters, gene expression, or glycogenolysis by astrocytes and, therefore, could secondarily affect synaptic transmission.

D. Adrenergic Receptors in Movement Control

1. α_1AR Subtypes and Dopaminergic Inter-relationships

There is anatomical and functional evidence for interactions between ascending systems such as the noradrenergic and dopaminergic (DA) systems. Electrophysiological studies have shown that prazosin, a specific-α_1-antagonist administered systemically, can decrease the burst firing and can regularize the firing pattern of dopaminergic neurons located in the ventral tegmental area innervating the limbic striatum and neocortex (Andersson et al., 1994; Grenhoff & Svensson, 2003). In another study, the activation of the mesocortical dopaminergic neurons by stimulation of the ventral tegmental area induced a marked inhibition of the spontaneous activity of prefrontal cortical cells, suggesting that complex interactions between cortical dopamine receptors (D2, D1) and α_1ARs are involved in the regulation of cortical cells by the ventral tegmentum. They confirm that stimulation of cortical α_1ARs hampers the functional activity of cortical D1 and D2 receptors (Gioanni et al., 1998). Biochemical and behavioral studies have also evidenced functional antagonism between cortical DA and NA systems mediated by D1 and α_1-ARs. In cultured embryonic cortical neurons, following the DA-mediated desensitization of D1 transmission, the application of methoxamine, an α_1-agonist, accelerated the re-sensitization of the D1 receptor-mediated response, indicating that the corresponding receptors were located on the same cells and suggesting that stimulation of the α_1AR could block D1 transmission (Trovero et al., 1994). Norepinephrine and dopamine concentrations throughout the cerebral cortex of Parkinsonian subjects are 50% those of controls (Scatton et al., 1983). This decrease probably results from degeneration of noradrenergic neurons in the locus coeruleus which projects to the cortex, demonstrated histologically and biochemically in subjects with PD. The contribution of this lesion to the symptoms of PD is unknown. It may relate to the dementia in these patients since the lesion is also found in subjects with Alzheimer disease (Bondareff et al., 1981). α_1ARs are increased in the pre-frontal cortex of patients with demented PD. The modification of the receptor number seems to be related to the lesion of the noradrenergic pathway from the locus coeruleus to the cortex (Cash et al., 1984).

In animal studies, locomotor activity can be assessed in an open-field model, which determines a forced ambulation since there is no option for hiding. Eventually the mice reduce their ambulation, which is considered to be partially dependent on memory as the mouse recognizes the familiarity of its surroundings. Enhanced horizontal locomotion in an open-field is thought to be linked to increased activity of the dopaminergic system in the ventral striatum. Therefore, the modulation of locomotor activity is usually considered in the context of activation of the mesolimbic-dopaminergic pathway. Activation of central α_1ARs can enhance locomotor activity as assessed in an open-field. Intraventricular injection of phenylephrine or methoxamine enhances horizontal ambulation (Heal, 1990). Prazosin administered systemically or directly into the cortex was able to diminish hyperlocomotion induced by *d*-amphetamine, presumably due to the reduced release of the functional part of the subcortical DA (Darracq et al., 1998). In a recent study (Berretta et al., 2000), perfusion of an α_1AR agonist, phenylephrine, increased the spontaneous firing of reticulata cells of the substantia nigra.

The only information that has been published from the recent α_1AR knockout (KO) models is that α_{1B}AR is thought to be involved in the interactions between noradrenergic and dopaminergic neurons, specifically in the nucleus accumbens which controls the actions of psychostimulants, such as D-amphetamine.

Here, the α_{1B}AR was shown to control the locomotor and rewarding effects of opiates and amphetamine by controlling the release, by amphetamine, of extracellular dopamine (Drouin et al., 2002). α_{1B}AR KO decreased the release of dopamine, confirming a role of this subtype in controlling dopamine release. Therefore, in our overexpression model, the α_{1B}AR could cause excessive release of dopamine, possibly leading to an excitotoxic condition and then to neurodegeneration, a popular etiological hypothesis for Parkinson disease (Graham et al., 1978). The KO studies are also confirmatory with our transgenic Parkinsonian MSA model, which suggests a link between the α_{1B}AR and dopamine regulation.

2. Direct Interactions of α_{1B}ARs and Locomotion Control

Recent studies have suggested that α_1ARs, and perhaps specifically, the α_{1B}AR subtype, are involved in movement control (Stone et al., 1999; Stone et al., 2001). A series of studies using intraventicular injection of terazosin produced a dose-dependent and complete inhibition of active behavior and movement (catalepsy) without sedation in mice. This inhibition could be reversed by co-administration of the α_1AR specific agonist, phenylephrine, but not with dopaminergic agonists. The α_1AR subtype involved was believed to be the α_{1B}AR due to the use of chloroethylclonidine, a mildly selective alkylating agent for the α_{1B}AR, and mRNA localization arguments.

II. CONSTRUCTION OF THE TRANSGENE

The mice were generated by first isolating the murine promoter for the α_{1B}AR. We had also characterized this promoter in various cell lines to demonstrate α_{1B}AR specificity *in vitro* (Zuscik et al., 1999). The murine promoter for the α_{1B}AR (4 kb in length) was cloned in front of either a wild-type (W) cDNA or two different constitutively active forms of the α_{1B}AR, which we term S (single mutant) or T (triple mutant) (Figure 1). Therefore, these mutants are always signaling even though an agonist is not present. We have previously characterized these mutants *in vitro* (Hwa et al., 1997; Perez et al., 1996). We have also recently generated another transgenic mouse that overexpresses .the α_{1B}AR wild-type receptor with enhanced green fluorescent protein (EGFP) attached at its C-terminus. Since there are no good antibodies against adrenergic receptors for localization studies, we generated this animal to show the cell types and areas in the brain that contain the α_{1B}AR. Thus, our transgenic system is designed to achieve systemic overexpression but only in tissues that naturally express the α_{1B}AR. This is vastly different but more physiologically relevant than most other transgenic animals that use tissue-specific promoters

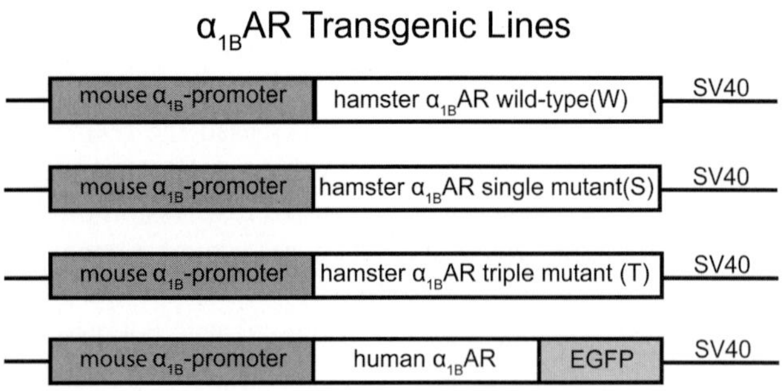

FIGURE 1 α_{1B}AR transgenic lines. EGFP, enhanced green fluorescent protein.

which might not endogenously express the protein in question. The animals also develop naturally postnatally with the over-stimulated receptor and would mimic an animal with an inborn error.

To confirm overexpression of the transgene at the protein level, we performed ligand binding on whole tissues using an α_1-specific antagonist as the radiolabel (I^{125}-HEAT). We measured anywhere from 2–5-fold overexpression in all α_{1B}AR-containing tissues (i.e., liver, heart, brain, kidney, spleen) whereas we found very little if any specific binding in α_{1B}AR-negative tissues such as skeletal muscle (Zuscik et al., 2000). In whole brain, overexpression was 2–3-fold overall and may have been even higher in discrete regions.

To confirm constitutive signaling, we examined inositol phosphate release (the second messenger of the α_1AR) in the livers and kidneys of each of the transgenic lines. All lines displayed elevated levels of basal signal transduction over non-transgenic controls. Wild-type (W) levels were also elevated, but were not as robust as the S and T lines. To further verify promoter fidelity and confirm localization of the α_{1B}AR in the brain, we performed *in situ* mRNA hybridization in areas of the brain previously thought to express this receptor (Zuscik et al., 2000). Transcript was localized to areas of the cortex, thalamus, and hypothalamus, which is consistent in both the rat and the mouse with previously published reports.

III. PHENOTYPE

A. General Characteristics

At birth, the mice appear normal, but homozygous mice breed poorly. We believe that poor breeding is not an artifact of transgenics since only S and T lines (which demonstrate constitutive signaling) have the breeding problems. Therefore, all analyses of phenotype are performed on heterozygous mice. The transgenic lines do experience a reduced body weight (20–30%) at twelve months of age, but not before. We believe the reduced body weight and breeding difficulties are due to the beginning of neurological problems and autonomic failure, which manifests at about one year of age. Also, the mice have a reduced longevity, which begins its significance at one year. About 75% of the mice survive to eighteen months, compared to 97% for normals.

In general, the phenotype follows the rank order of severity in symptoms: W < S < T. We do see some aspects of degeneration in the WT line, but this usually appears at a much older age. The phenotype is much more apparent in biochemical assays (autonomic dysfunction, see below) which are more sensitive in detecting abnormalities. The rank order of severity is consistent with the constitutive activity of the receptor mutants and the measured amount of basal signal transduction differences measured (Zuscik et al., 2000).

B. Locomotion Deficits

Beginning at three months of age, the transgenics display a locomotion deficit (see Video). All transgenic lines show reduced horizontal movement as well as total distance traveled, and the phenotype is age progressive. Hindlimb dysfunction was even more apparent when one measured the rearing behavior or the ability of the mice to get up on their hindlimbs. In the video, the long-tailed mouse is a normal non-transgenic, while the clipped-tailed mice are transgenic. The most severely affected mice have an elongated body stride because of hindlimb distention, dragging, and abnormal gait. In the video, the transgenic mice never get up on their hindpaws, in contrast to normal mice, in which this is part of their behavior movement pattern.

In initial experiments, both the horizontal activity as well as rearings can be rescued/improved with the four-week administration of an α_1-antagonist (terazosin) as well as the dopamine precursor, L-Dopa, to the drinking water. L-Dopa was administered along with carbidopa. Since both an α_1-antagonist and a dopamine agonist can alleviate the symptoms, it is also suggested that these two pathways are linked (adrenergic and dopaminergic), as well as the phenotype mimicking a Parkinsonian syndrome. Although the majority of MSA patents are typically unresponsive to L-dopa, a significant minority (i.e., 25%) do respond positively. It is thought that varying extents of putaminal damage could be responsible for the differing motor response to L-dopa in MSA patients (Parati et al., 1993). In our mouse model, there is substantial apoptosis in the caudate/putamen region (see section on apoptosis).

C. Neurodegeneration

Neurodegeneration was prominent in the cerebellum and medulla. Other areas affected were in the basal ganglia, periaqueductal gray, spinal cord, thalamus, hypothalamus, and cerebral cortex (Zuscik et al., 2000; Papay et al., 2002). In the cerebellum, vacuoles were prominent in the molecular areas. These vacuoles had highly chromagenic nuclei with a sickle-cell shape, suggesting apoptosis. The molecular areas of the cerebellum also expressed the α_{1B}AR EGFP tagged receptor in the transgenic mouse model (Papay et al., 2004). Another highly degenerative area was the medulla, especially in the inferior olives and pons, suggesting the mice had more of the OPCA form of MSA. Expression of the α_{1B}AR EGFP-tagged receptor (Papay et al., 2004) was also demonstrated here. There was also Purkinje cell degeneration, indicative of the phenotype in MSA, called "the baskets are empty." We previously showed an H&E stain of Purkinje cell loss as well as granular and molecular cell loss in Papay et al. (2002). Based on data from the transgenic mouse line expressing α_{1B}AR-EGFP, the receptor is located in Purkinje cells, as well as the granular cell layer and the overexpression of even the wild-type receptor is sufficient to cause Purkinje cell degeneration. As demonstrated in the apoptosis section, the degeneration of the Purkinje cell is likely due to the nuclear degradation, followed by the cytoplasmic deterioration, again suggestive of an apoptotic mechanism.

In previous publications, we showed degeneration in the periaqueductal grey (Zuscik et al., 2000) and the intermediolateral grey columns of the spinal cord (Papay et al., 2002), an area of degeneration in MSA. We can also demonstrate α_{1B}AR expression of the EGFP protein in these same areas of the spinal cord (Papay et al., 2004). Degeneration of the basal ganglia was previously demonstrated by showing loss of dopaminergic neurons as assessed by tyrosine hydroxylase immunohistochemistry and a response to L-dopa (Zuscik et al., 2002).

In general, the expression of the α_{1B}AR EGFP-tagged receptor co-localized with areas undergoing degeneration, suggesting a direct effect by the over-stimulation of the receptor. This is also verified by the use of prazosin, an α_{1B}AR antagonist, which can improve the symptoms of locomotion and later is shown to protect against neuronal loss (Papay et al., 2002). Recently, we have demonstrated by NEUN, GFAP, CC1, and NG2 antibody co-localization that the α_{1B}AR is expressed in neurons and not astrocytes. Although at lower levels, α_{1B}AR is also expressed in the developing oligodendrocyte (NG2-positive cells). Weaker expression is noted in mature oligodendrocytes (CC1-positive cell).

D. Autonomic Dysfunction

Since the mice were showing similarities to a Parkinsonian syndrome, we thought to test the hypothesis that the mice were also undergoing autonomic failure, which is seen to varying degrees in MSA. We first tested the plasma levels for various stress hormones and the catecholamines epinephrine and norepinephrine. Epinephrine is released from the adrenal under sympathetic nervous regulation and norepinephrine can be measured in the blood as leakage from nerve ending discharges. Both are considered ways of measuring sympathetic output. We found that the transgenic mice had 40% reduced levels of ACTH and CRF as well as cortisol (Zuscik et al., 2001). In measuring catecholamine release, transgenic mice had a 50% reduction, followed by a 20–25% reduction by the W transgenic line. In additional studies, we determined that the transgenic mice had lower blood pressure, both basally and when stimulated by phenylephrine, compared to non-transgenics (Zuscik et al., 2001). This reduction in blood pressure was not due to changes in vasoconstriction; isolated vessel preparations demonstrated no changes from normals. In fact, the reduction in blood pressure is opposite to an expected phenotype of increasing blood pressure since α_1AR is the major vasoconstrictor force in blood vessels. We also measured lower heart rate (Zuscik et al., 2001) via echocardiography, but the lower heart rate disappears when the hearts are examined *ex vivo* (Ross et al., 2003). Since the *ex vivo* heart no longer has autonomic influences, the lower heart rate is likely due to decreased sympathetic control. Since the mice have reproduction problems, reductions in body weight later in life, lower blood pressure, and lower stress hormones and catecholamine, together with the neurodegeneration, we believe that the phenotype most resembles autonomic dysfunction, which is seen in various degrees in MSA.

E. α-Synuclein Inclusion Bodies

Cytoplasmic and/or neuronal inclusion bodies are also typically seen in neurodegenerative diseases. In Parkinson disease, there are Lewy bodies; in multiple system atrophy, there are α-synuclein and ubiquitin inclusions in oligodendrocytes (Papp et al., 1989). Most neurodegenerative diseases have inclusion bodies and the types of proteins found in these bodies, as well as their localization, may be different depending upon the disease. It is not known whether these bodies are a contributing factor or a consequence in the generation of the disease. Overexpression of alpha-synuclein in a transgenic mouse under a PDGF receptor promoter resulted in a Parkinsonian-like phenotype (Masliah et al., 2000). Other proteins that have been found in these inclusions include tau, RAb5, Rabaptin-5, alpha B-crystallin, and α- and β-tubulins.

We showed that the transgenic mice are positive for two different proteins typically found in inclusion bodies, ubiquitin and α-synuclein, present in the caudate and cerebellum (Papay et al., 2002). The staining is in both the white and grey matter. To identify the cell types in the brain contained in these inclusions, cells were identified by FITC-labeled antibodies against oligodendrocytes, neurons, or astrocytes and fluorescently determined if they co-localized with the α-synuclein inclusion bodies, labeled with rhodamine-labeled antibodies. The α-synuclein-positive inclusion

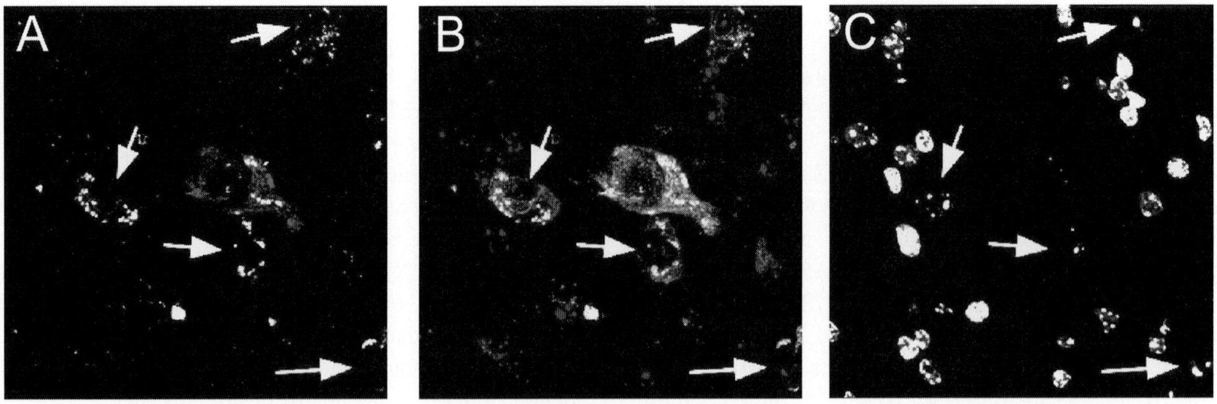

FIGURE 2 Confocal microscopy of neuronal inclusion bodies. Numerous punctate α-synuclein inclusion bodies (**A**) localize to the cytoplasm of neurons (**B**). Neurons have large vacuoles that originate from fragmented nuclei (arrows). Normal nuclei are stained with DAPI (**C**).

bodies co-localized to oligodendrocytes and neurons, but not to astrocytes. Upon higher magnification (Figure 2), neurons showed several α-synuclein-positive inclusions (yellow upon colocalization, white arrows) and cell death was apparent with vacuolization of the nucleus containing fragmented DAPI-stained nuclei. Neuronal nuclei in transgenic mice appeared apoptotic as measured by the number of hyperchromatic and/or amorphic nuclei (yellow arrows).

α_{1B}AR transgenic mice showed an increase in abnormal aggregated forms of α-synuclein, which also increased its nitrated content with age (Papay et al., 2002). It has also been shown that α-synuclein is the major protein modified by nitration in MSA and found in the signature inclusions of neurons and oligodendrocytes (Giasson et al., 2000). The α-synuclein in our transgenic mouse model does not increase its content compared to normals, but only its aggregational properties. Of note, the vast majority of synucleinopathies occurs despite the normal expression levels of α-synuclein.

F. Apoptosis

In the transgenic mice, we have shown increased TUNEL staining in the substantia nigra and caudate/putamen (Zuscik et al., 2000). Using an antibody that recognizes only the activated form of caspase 3, we can also demonstrate caspase 3 activation in the white matter tracts of the caudate/putamen and cerebellum (Yun et al., 2003). However, caspase 3 activation also occurred in the grey matter, particularly in the medulla and cerebral cortex (Yun et al., 2003).

To further characterize the neurodegeneration and to explore potential mechanisms of α_{1B}AR-induced neurodegeneration, we performed gene chip studies on the brains of 3–4, 8–10, and 12–16 month old T mice compared with age-matched normals (Yun et al., 2003). We performed this analysis as a snapshot of gene expression changes through disease progression. Of particular note are the many genes involved in apoptosis, synaptic vesicle function, neurodegenerative disorders (especially inclusion bodies), and glial function. An abbreviated list of genes showing altered expression is shown in table 1.

IV. THE POTENTIAL USE OF α_1AR ANTAGONISTS TO TREAT MSA

In the mouse model, we have shown that oral administration of the α_1AR antagonist (terazosin) can reverse some of the symptoms associated with MSA (i.e., locomotion) and can delay or protect the brain from the neurodegeneration and formation of the α-synuclein inclusion bodies (Papay et al., 2002). A previous clinical study (Sakakibara et al., 2000) used prazosin and moxisylyte (both α_1-adrenergic receptor antagonists, like terazosin) in MSA patients. After a 4-week treatment, 38% of the patients had reductions in residual urine volume and lessening of urinary symptoms. Side effects due to orthostatic hypotension were seen in 23% of the patients and were common in patients with postural hypotension of more than −30 mmHg at trial entry. No other adverse side effects were reported. Terazosin is approved by the FDA for treatment of hypertension and benign prostatic hyperplasia. This drug works by relieving the contractile tone of smooth muscle, providing vasodilation of the vasculature or dilation of the prostatic smooth muscle for urinary relief. α_1AR antagonists have not been tested for their ability to improve locomotion deficits or other symptoms of autonomic failure. However, since we have shown in our mouse model that terazosin improves locomotion and can reverse the neurodegeneration and there is good evidence in the literature that terazosin is safely tolerated in MSA patients when given for urinary tract symptoms, we propose to test the hypothesis that administration of

TABLE 1 Gene Expression Profiles (Oligonucleotide Arrays) of Transgenic Mice vs. Normal Controls

Apoptotic genes	**3–4 Month**	**8–10 Month**	**12–18 Month**
BIK-like killer protein (death agonist) (pro-apop)	+6.1 ± 2	NC	NC
Met proto-oncogene (Anti-apop, PI3, Akt pathway)	+5.6 ± 2	NC	NC
Tumor necrosis factor ligand (CD40) (pro-apop)	+4.2 ± 0.2	NC	NC
Transforming growth factor β (pro-apop)	+5 ± 0	NC	−2.5 ± 0.5
Interferons β and γ or receptors (pro-apop)	NC	−3.3 ± 0.4	−1.8 ± 0.3
Cytochrome c-synthetase (pro-apop)	NC	NC	−2.8 ± 0.5
Insulin-like growth factor 2 receptor (anti-apop)	−9.3 ± 1.4	NC	+7.7 ± 0.3
Summary: Pro-apop upregulated and anti-apop downregulated in 3–4M mice; opposite true in older mice.			
Synaptic proteins			
Interleukin 7 receptor (neuronal growth)	+4.3 ± 0.5	NC	NC
Synaptobrevin-like protein (neurotransmitter release)	+3.4 ± 0.7	NC	NC
NIPSNAP1 (transmitter release)	+1.6 ± 0.05	NC	NC
Synaptophysin (synaptic vesicle recycling)	−1.8 ± 0.05	NC	NC
Synaptotagmin (SNARE; neurotransmitter release)	NC	−2.3 ± 0.2	−1.9 ± 0.1
RAB7 (transport vesicles)	NC	NC	−1.7 ± 0.1
Summary: Neurotransmission increased in 2–3M mice; neurotransmitter and vesicle transport down-regulated in old mice.			
Glutamate and calcium regulation			
NMDA receptor R1	NC	+2.3 ± 0.2	+2.8 ± 0.2
AMPA receptor α1	NC	+1.9 ± 0.1	+2.1 ± 0.1
GABA-A receptor	NC	NC	−1.9 ± 0.1
CAM PKII (plasticity; Phosphor. α-synuclein)	−10.5 ± 3	+4.5 ± 0.9	+3.85 ± 0.5
Plasma membrane Ca+2-ATPase (pump Ca out)	NC	+5.2 ± 1	+6.1 ± 0.9
Na HCO_3 Cotransport (active with increased Ca)	NC	+1.9 ± 0.1	+2.4 ± 0.1
Glutamate decarboxylase (breakdown of Glu)	NC	NC	+2.7 ± 0.3
Glutamate-ammonia ligase (converts Glu to Gln)	NC	NC	+1.5 ± 0.3
Summary: Glutamate and calcium dysregulation (excessive stimulation) appears in older not younger mice.			
Neurodegenerative-associated proteins			
Mitochondrial-specific NADH5 (oxidative stress)	+4.7 ± 1.5	NC	NC
α-tubulin (inclusions)	+1.65 ± 0.1	NC	NC
Microtubule-associated Tau (inclusions)	+1.6 ± 0.02	NC	NC
Summary: Inclusion proteins upregulate in young not older mice.			
Glia cell-associated proteins			
Myelin-associated oligodendrocyte basic protein	−3.4 ± 0.4	NC	NC
Glia cell adhesion	NC	NC	+2.2 ± 0.3

(Age matched). Genes reported are fold changes. Summation of each class of genes appears in bold.

NC, no change. Data taken from (Yun et al., 2003).

terazosin to MSA patients will improve locomotion and autonomic symptoms. We are currently enrolling MSA patients in a double-blind, placebo-controlled, two-phased study to determine the efficacy of terazosin to improve the symptoms commonly associated with MSA.

V. DIFFERENCES IN HUMAN MSA VERSUS MOUSE MSA MODEL

In summary, transgenic mice showed evidence of neurodegeneration that was noticeable when the mice approached midlife by histology in the spinal cord, medulla, and cerebellum as well as in other areas of the brain. Immunohistochemistry of the substantia nigra with an antibody against tyrosine hydroxylase indicated that transgenic mice had a loss of dopaminergic neurons and were partially responsive to L-dopa treatment, suggesting a Parkinsonian syndrome. The mice had a locomotion deficit that included a reduced ability to walk because of hindlimb distention and gait problems. Transgenic mice also had certain aspects of autonomic dysfunction (Zuscik et al., 2001). Taking these results together, we suggest that the mice resemble the human form of MSA. In a recently published study from our lab (Papay et al., 2002), we found α-synuclein inclusions in the white matter and striatum but also in grey matter. We have found that these inclusion bodies co-localize with oligodendrocytes and neurons, which is a criterion for the MSA diagnosis. We report TUNEL staining with caspase 3-activation, consistent with suggestions in the literature that MSA brains undergo a significant amount of apoptosis (Probst-Cousin et al., 1998). Our mouse model also had excessive tyrosine-nitration of abnormal forms of α-synuclein, the major protein modified by nitration in MSA, and found in the signature inclusions of oligodendrocytes. We have also shown Purkinje cell loss in the cerebellum and degeneration of the intermediolateral columns of the spinal cord (Papay et al., 2002), areas affected in the OPCA form of MSA. However, the transgenic mice display seizures (Kunieda et al., 2002) and have degeneration in areas not typically seen in MSA, such as the cerebral cortex. Therefore, the two models are similar but indeed different.

There is another report of a transgenic mouse model of oligodendrocyte-targeted α-synuclein overexpression, which is thought to mimic the MSA model (Kahle et al., 2002). However, while this model did produce hyperphosphorylation of serine 129, just as in PD and MSA, there are no locomotion defects or neurodegeneration present in this mouse model even when the mice are eighteen months old. These results suggest that pathology of the oligodendrocyte alone or the expression of α-synuclein alone is not sufficient to produce the symptoms of MSA and suggests that our mouse model, which displays both the appropriate inclusion bodies (in oligodendrocytes as well as neurons) and has clinical presentation of locomotion/gait/neurodegeneration consistent with human MSA, may be an appropriate mouse model to study mechanisms of pathology associated with MSA.

Video Legends

SEGMENT 1 Two α_{1B}-adrenergic receptor (AR) transgenic mice (snipped tails) and one normal mouse are shown during open field behavior. The α_{1B}AR transgenic mice are smaller and show decreased rearing activity.

SEGMENT 2 An α_{1B}-adrenergic receptor (AR) transgenic mouse from another line. Note the presence of a "wobbly" gait.

References

Graham, R.M., and S.M. Lanier. 1986. In: The Heart and Cardiovascular System (ed. HA Fozzard et al.), pp. 1059–1095, Chapter 50, Raven Press, NY.

Strader, C.D., I.S. Sigal, R.A. Dixon. 1987. Structural basis of β-adrenergic receptor function. *FASEB J* **3**:1825–1832.

Oprian, D., T. Sakmar, T. Nakayama, H.B. Chen, B. Knox, S. Karnik, R. Franke, H.G. Khorana. 1987. Discussions in Neurosciences. *FENS* **3**:20–28.

Perez, D.M., M.T. Piascik, and R.M. Graham. 1991. RM: Solution-phase library screening for the identification of rare clones: Isolation of an α1d-adrenergic receptor cDNA. *Mol Pharmacol* **40**:876–883.

Ramarao, C.S., J.M.K. Denker, D.M. Perez, R.P. Riek, R.M. Graham. 1992. Genomic organization of the human α1b-adrenergic receptor. *J Biol Chem* **267**:21936–21945.

Perez, D.M., M.T. Piascik, N. Malik, R.J. Gaivin, R.M. Graham. 1994. Cloning, expression and tissue distribution of the rat homolog of the bovine α1c-adrenergic receptor provide evidence for its classification as the α1a-subtype. *Mol Pharmacol* **46**:823–831.

Hanft, G., G. Gross, J.J. Beckeringh, and C. Korstanjc. 1989. α1-Adrenoceptors: the ability of various agonists and antagonists to discriminate between two distinct [3H] prazosin binding sites. *J Pharm Pharmacol* **41**:714–716.

Holets, V.R. (1990) The anatomy and function of noradrenaline in the mammalian brain. In D.J. Heal & C.A. Marsden (Eds.), *The Pharmacology of Noradrenaline in the Central Nervous System* (pp. 1–40). New York: Oxford University Press.

Macdonald, E., and M. Scheinin. 1995. Distribution and pharmacology of α2-adrenoceptors in the central nervous system. *J Physiol Pharmacol* **46**:241–258.

Hopkins, W.F., and D. Johnston. 1988. Noradrenergic enhancement of long term potentiation at mossy fiber synapses in the hippocampus. *J Neurophysiol* **59**:667–687.

Mouradian, R.D., F.M. Sessler, and B.D. Waterhouse. 1991. Noradrenergic potentiation of excitatory transmitter action in cerebrocortical slices: evidence for mediation by an α1-receptor-lined second messenger pathway. *Brain Res* **546**:83–95.

McCormick, D.A., H.C. Pape, and A. Williamson. 1991. Actions of norepinephrine in the cerebral cortex and thalamus: implications for function of the central noradrenergic system. *Prog Brain Res* **88**:293–305.

Lerea, L.S., and K.D. McCarthy. 1989. Astroglial cells are heterogeneous with respect to expression of the α1-adrenergic receptor. *Glia* **2**:135–147.

Andersson, J.L., M. Marcus, G.G. Nomikos, and T.H. Svensson. 1994. Prazosin modulates the changes in firing pattern and transmitter release induced by raclopride in the mesolimbic, but not in the nigrostriatal dopaminergic system. *Naunyn Schmiedebergs Arch Pharmacol* **349**: 236–243.

Grenhoff, J., and T.H. Svensson. 2003. Prazosin modulates the firing pattern of dopamine neurons in rat ventral tegmental area. *Eur J Pharmacol* **233**:79–84.

Gioanni, Y., A.M. Thierry, J. Glowinski, and J.P. Tassin. 1998. α1-Adrenergic, D1 and D2 receptors interactions in the prefrontal cortex: implications for the modality of action of different types of neuroleptics. *Synapse* **30**:362–370.

Trovero, F., P. Marin, J.P. Tassin, J. Premont, and J. Glowinski. 1994. Accelerated resensitization of the D1 dopamine receptor-mediated response in cultured cortical and striatal neurons from the rat: respective role of α1-adrenergic and N-methyl-D-aspartate receptors. *J Neurosci* **14**: 6280–6288.

Scatton, B., F. Javoy-Agid, L. Rouquier, B. Dubois, and Y. Agid. 1983. Reduction of cortical dopamine, noradrenaline, serotonin and their metabolites in Parkinson's disease. *Brain Res* **275**:321–328.

Bondareff, W., C.Q. Mountjoy, and M. Roth. 1981. Selective loss of neurons of origin of adrenergic projection to cerebral cortex (nucleus locus coeruleus) in senile dementia. *Lancet* **1**:783–784.

Cash, R., M. Ruberg, R. Raisman, and Y. Agid. 1984. Adrenergic receptors in Parkinson's disease. *Brain Res* **322**:269–275.

Heal, D.J. 1990. The effects of drugs on behavioural models of central noradrenergic function. In D.J. Heal & D.A. Marsden (Eds.), *The Pharmacology of Noradrenaline in the Central Nervous System* (pp. 266–315). New York: Oxford University Press.

Darracq, L., G. Blanc, J. Glowinski, and J.P. Tassin. 1998. Importance of the noradrenergic-dopamine coupling in the locomotor activating effects of d-amphetamine. *J Neurosci* **18**:2729–2739.

Zuscik, M.J., M.T. Piascik, and D.M. Perez. 1999. Cloning, cell-type specificity and regulatory function of the murine α1b-adrenergic receptor promoter. *Mol Pharmacol* **56**:1288–1297.

Hwa, J., R. Gaivin, J. Porter, and D.M. Perez. 1997. Synergism of constitutive activity in α1-adrenergic receptor activation. *Biochemistry* **36**:633–639.

Perez, D.M., J. Hwa, R. Gaivin, M. Mathur, F. Brown, and R.M. Graham. 1996. Constitutive activation of a single effector pathway: evidence for multiple activation states of a G-protein-coupled receptor. *Mol Pharmacol* **49**:112–122.

Masliah, E., E. Rockenstein, I. Veinbergs, M. Mallory, M. Hashimoto, A. Takeda, Y. Sagara, A. Sisk, L. Mucke. 2000. Dopaminergic loss and inclusion body formation in alpha-synuclein mice: implications for neurodegenerative disorders. *Science* **287**:1265–1269.

Drouin, C., L. Darracq, F. Trovero, G. Blanc, J. Glowinski, S. Cotecchia, and J.P. Tassin. 2002. α1B-Adrenergic receptors control locomotor and rewarding effects of psychostimulants and opiates. *J Neuroscience* **22**: 2873–2884.

Graham, D.G., S.M. Tiffany, W.R. Bell, and W.F. Gutknecht. 1978. Autooxidation versus covalent binding of quinones as the mechanism of toxicity of dopamine, 6-hydroxydopamine and related compounds toward C1300 neuroblastoma cells in vitro. *Mol Pharmacol* **14**:644–653.

Stone, E.A., Y. Zhang, H. Rosengarten, J. Yeretsian, D. Quartermain. 1999. Brain alpha1-adrenergic neurotransmission is necessary for behavioral activation to environmental change in mice. *Neuroscience* **94**:1245–1252.

Stone, E.A, Y. Lin, A. Itteera, D. Quarterman. 2001. Pharmacological evidence for the role of central alpha1Badrenoceptors in the motor activity and spontaneous movement of mice. *Neuropharmacology* **40**:254–261.

Kahle, P.J., M. Neumann, L. Ozmen, V. Muler, H. Jacobsen, W. Spooren, B. Fuss, B. Mallon, W.B. Macklin, H. Fujiwara, M. Hasegawa, T. Iwatsubo, H.A. Kretzschmar, and C. Haass. 2002. Hyperphosphorylation and insolubility of α-synuclein in transgenic mouse oligodendrocytes. *EMBO Reports* **3**:583–588.

Kunieda, T., M.J. Zuscik, A. Boongird, D.M. Perez, H.O. Lüders, I.M. Najm. 2002. Systemic overexpression of the α1B-adrenergic receptor in mice: An animal model of epilepsy. *Epilepsia* **43**:1324–1329.

Zuscik, M.J., D. Chalothorn, D. Hellard, C. Deighan, A. McGee, C. Daly, D.J.J. Waugh, S.A. Ross, R.J. Gaivin, A. Moorehead, J. Thomas, E.F. Plow, J.C. McGrath, M.T. Piascik, and D.M. Perez. 2001. Hypotension, autonomic failure and cardiac hypertrophy in transgenic mice overexpressing the α1b-adrenergic receptor. *J Biol Chem* **276**:13738–13743.

Papay, R., R. Gaivin, D.F. McCune, B.R. Ronabaugh, W.B. MacKlin, J.C. McGrath, and D.M. Perez. 2004. The mouse α_{1B}-adrenergic receptor is expressed in neurons and NG2 oligodendrocytes. *J Comp Neurol* (in press).

Papay, R., M.T. Zuscik, S.A. Ross, J. Yun, D.F. McCune, P. Gonzalez-Cabrera, R. Gaivin, W.B. Macklin, J. Drazba, and D.M. Perez. 2002. Mice expressing the α1b-adrenergic receptor induces a synucleinopathy with excessive tyrosine nitration but decreased phosphorylation. *J Neurochem* **83**:1–12.

Probst-Cousin, S., C.H. Rickert, K.W. Schmid, F. Gullotta. 1998. Cell death mechanisms in multiple system atrophy. *J Neuropathol Exp Neurol* **57**:814–821.

Zuscik, M.J., S. Sand, S.A. Ross, D.J.J. Waugh, R.J. Gaivin, D. Morilak, and D.M. Perez. 2000. Overexpression of the α_{1B} adrenergic receptor causes apoptotic neurodegeneration: a multiple system atrophy. *Nature Medicine* **6**:1388–1394, 2000.

Sakakibara, R., T. Hattori, T. Uchiyama, T. Suenaga, H. Takahashi, T. Yamanishi, K. Egoshi, N. Sekita. 2000. Are alpha-blockers involved in lower urinary tract dysfunction in multiple system atrophy? A comparison of prazosin and moxisylyte. *J Auton Nerv Syst* **79(2–3)**:191–195.

Berretta, N., G. Bernardi, and N.B. Mercuri. 2000. Alpha(1)-adrenoceptor-mediated excitation of substantia nigra pars reticulata neurons. *Neuroscience* **98**:599–604.

Parati, E.A., V. Fetoni, G.C. Geminiani, P. Soliveri, P. Giovannini, D. Testa, S. Genitrini, T. Caraceni, F. Girotti. 1993. Response to L-DOPA in multiple system atrophy. *Clin Neuropharmacol* **Apr;16(2)**:139–144.

Ross, S.A., D. Chalothorn, J. Yun, P.J. Gonzalez-Cabrera, D.F. McCune, B. Rorabaugh, M.T. Piascik, and D.M. Perez. 2003. The alpha(1B)-adrenergic receptor decreases the inotropic response in the mouse Langendorff heart model. *Cardiovasc Res* **60**:598–607.

Papp, M.I., J.E. Kahn, P.L. Lantos. 1989. Glial cytoplasmic inclusions in the CNS of patients with multiple system atrophy (striatonigral degeneration, olivopontocerebellar atrophy and Shy-Drager syndrome). *J Neurol Sci* **94**:79–100.

Giasson, B.I., J.E. Duda, I.V. Murray, Q. Chen, J.M. Souza, H.I. Hurtig, H. Ischiropoulos, J.Q. Trojanowski, and V.M. Lee. 2000. Oxidative damage linked to neurodegeneration by selective alpha-synuclein nitration in synucleinopathy. *Science* **290**:985–989.

Yun, J., R.J. Gaivin, D.F. McCune, B. Atthaporn, R.S. Papay, Z. Ying, P.J. Gonzalez-Cabrera, I. Najm, and D.M. Perez. 2003. Gene expression profiles of neurodegeneration induced by the α1b-adrenergic receptor: NMDA/GABAA dysregulation and apoptosis. *Brain* **126**: 2667–2681.

Clinical and Pathological Features of Hereditary Ataxias

TETSUO ASHIZAWA and S.H. SUBRAMONY

Hereditary ataxias have been recognized as a heterogeneous group of diseases based on their clinical and histopathological features (Greenfield, 1963; Harding, 1981b). Diagnosis of specific disorders is complicated by the considerable phenotypic variability and marked overlap of clinical features among the hereditary ataxias. Recent progress in the field of molecular and human genetics allowed for identification of genetic loci or mutations responsible for many of these diseases and DNA testing now can identify the mutation in 60–70% of patients with hereditary ataxia.

An increasing number of genetic animal models of hereditary ataxias are becoming available. These genetically engineered animals provide a powerful means to study disease mechanisms, which is essential for development of rational treatment strategies. These animal models are also used to screen available drugs for their efficacy in treating the disease. Although the disease phenotypes of animal models may resemble the human diseases, there are almost always some differences. The differences may be attributable to the species-specific phenotypic expression of the disease, but they could also be due to the technological strategies used to create the animal models. Whether an animal model is a faithful model of human disease is an important question. Comparing the phenotype of an animal model with the clinical and pathological features of the disease in humans is a critical step in assessing the value of animal models in the research investigation of the disease.

In this chapter, we will review the clinical and histopathological features of inherited ataxias. For the most part, we will focus on the diseases for which the causative genetic mutation has been identified. Readers may also refer to recent reviews of hereditary ataxias (Rosa and Ashizawa, 2002; Evidente et al., 2000) and dominant hereditary ataxias (Subramony et al., 1999; Klockgether et al., 2000; Stevanin et al., 2000). Additional information on genetic ataxias can also be found at the following websites: the Neuromuscular Disease Center of Washington University (http://www.neuro.wustl.edu/neuromuscular/ataxia/aindex.html/) and the Online Mendelian Inheritance in Man (OMIM; http://www.ncbi.nlm.nih.gov/omim/).

Work in the laboratory of TA has been supported by NIH/NINDS grant #1 RO1 NS41547-01. Work in the laboratory of SHS has been supported by Grants from the Luckyday Foundation and the Stangle Ataxia Research Fund.

I. AUTOSOMAL DOMINANT ATAXIA

A. Spinocerebellar ataxias (SCAs)

Autosomal dominant spinocerebellar ataxias (ADCAs) are a group of heterogeneous disorders which have been clinically classified into three major classes, i.e., ADCA-I, II, and III (Harding, 1981b and 1993). Assignment of genetic loci and identification of pathogenic mutations have led to re-classification of these disorders under the nomenclature of "spinocerebellar ataxias (SCAs)." To date, 21 diseases including SCAs 1–8, 10–19, and 21–22, and dentatorubral pallidoluysian atrophy (DRPLA), have been assigned to genetic loci, and disease causing mutations have been found in 11: SCAs 1–3, 6–8, 10, 12, 14, 17, and DRPLA) (table 1) (reviewed in Rosa and Ashizawa, 2002). Clinical phenotypes of SCAs have been roughly correlated with Harding's classification. ADCA-I, which includes SCAs 1, 2, 3, 4, 12, 13, 17, 18 (GDB accession #:11507789), 19 (Verbeek et al., 2002), and 21 (Vuillaume et al., 2002), consists of a cerebellar syndrome variably accompanied by other nervous system dysfunctions, including ophthalmoplegia, pyramidal and extrapyramidal signs, dementia, dorsal column signs, motor neuron disease, and peripheral neuropathy. DRPLA, though not bearing the prefix of "SCA," also belongs to ADCA-I. ADCA-II is characterized by retinopathy that accompanies cerebellar ataxia and other neurological abnormalities. Currently, SCA7 is the sole disorder with known gene locus in this class. ADCA-III is a pure cerebellar syndrome, which includes SCAs 5, 6, 8, 10, 11, 14, 15, 16, and 22 (Chung et al., 2003). However, phenotypic variability and overlaps among different SCAs complicate the relationships between these two (ADCAs vs. SCAs) classifications. For example, diseases categorized as ADCA-I may present with pure cerebellar ataxia, especially at the onset of the diseases, while some disorders of the ADCA-III class, such as SCA6 and SCA8, may have "extra-cerebellar" neurological features. Conversely, Harding's classification has one-to-one correlation with SCA7, since retinopathy develops in virtually all patients with SCA7 and no other genetic loci have been identified for ADCA-II. Other characteristic clinical features may further differentiate SCAs in the same ADCA category and, accordingly, they will be described in this chapter under each SCA subtype.

The ADCA classes are roughly correlated with the regions of gross pathological abnormalities in these disorders. Brains of patients with ADCA-I show atrophy of the cerebellum and brainstem, similar to that seen in sporadic olivopontocerebellar atrophy. Other parts of the brain, as well as spinal cord and peripheral nerves, may show abnormalities corresponding to the clinical phenotype. Patients with ADCA-II show retinal degeneration in addition to widespread atrophy of the cerebellum, cerebrum and brainstem. ADCA-III patients show cerebellar atrophy with no or little atrophy of the brainstem or other parts of the nervous system. These gross pathological changes are recognizable *in vivo* on brain imaging studies, such as the magnetic resonance imaging (MRI) and computerized tomography (CT). Although histological changes in these disorders are most severe in the regions of atrophy, microscopic abnormalities may be much more widespread than atrophied areas in the central nervous system. In at least some SCAs, experimental data suggest that neuronal dysfunction without neuronal loss is sufficient to cause the clinical phenotype. However, the histological changes in patients at autopsy invariably involve neuronal loss, and some histological abnormalities are specific for the genotype of the diseases. A good example is an accumulation of proteins containing expanded polyglutamine tracts, which are seen in patients with ADCAs caused by an expansion of coding CAG repeats, such as SCAs 1, 2, 3, 6, 7, and 17, and DRPLA (Orr, 2001). The mutant protein aggregates are located mainly in the nucleus in SCAs 1, 3, 7, and 17, while they are seen in cytoplasm in SCA2 and in both nucleus and cytoplasm in SCA6. The neuronal inclusions contain the polyglutamine tracts, interacting proteins, and proteins from the ubiquitin-degradation pathway (see Orr, 2001). Whether these aggregates, or soluble oligomers and monomers, of the expanded polyglutamine tracts are responsible for the disease remains controversial (Klement et al., 1998). The pathogenicity of the mutant protein in these diseases appears to involve protein misfolding, sequestration of transcription co-activators and co-repressors, and/or other gain of function mechanisms (Zoghbi and Orr, 2000).

In SCA8, SCA10, and SCA12, the repeat expansion is located in the untranslated regions of their respective genes. The pathogenic mechanisms of these SCAs remain to be investigated. SCAs 4, 5, 11, 13, 15, 16, 18, 19, 21, and 22 have been mapped, but their mutations have not been identified. SCAs 1, 2, 3, 6, 7, 8, 10, and 17 appear to be more frequent ADCAs than others. According to large screenings from different populations around the world, known SCAs constitute about 60–80% of the ADCA families. The incidence of the different types of SCA around the world is variable and a few SCA types have been recognized only in a single family (table 1).

1. SCA1

The mutation responsible for SCA1 is an expanded CAG repeat encoding a polyglutamine tract in the *SCA1* gene (table 1) (Banfi et al., 1994). The clinical phenotype of SCA1 is classified as ADCA-1 (Zoghbi, 1995; Sasaki et al., 1996). Typical onset with cerebellar ataxia, usually in the order of broad-based gait, limb ataxia, and dysarthria is often followed by hand tremor and oculomotor signs, which include intermittent nystagmus, slowed saccadic velocity, and limitation of up-gaze. Patients with SCA1 may also exhibit bulbar and upper motor neuron signs including lingual fasciculations, non-cerebellar dysphagia and dysarthria, and brisk deep tendon reflexes and limb spasticity. Mild peripheral neuropathy may also be found. In an advanced stage, patients become wheelchair-bound with severe disability, necessitating total nursing care, and fre-

TABLE 1 Autosomal Dominant Cerebellar Ataxia (ADCA)

Disease	Locus	Type of mutation / Gene product	Normal alleles	Pathogenic alleles	Distribution (number of families)	% of total SCA
ADCA I						
SCA-1	6p22–p23	*CAG expansion / ataxin-1*	6–44	40–81	worldwide	5–15%
SCA-2	12q23–24.1	*CAG expansion / ataxin-2*	14–31	34–59	Cuba, worldwide	5–15%
SCA-3/MJD	14q24.3–q32.1	*CAG expansion / ataxin-3*	14–33	56–200	Portugal, worldwide	30–50%
SCA-4	16q22.1	*unknown*			USA, Japan (7 families)	?
SCA-12	5p31–p33	*CAG expansion / 5¢UTR of PPP2R2B*	17–28	55–78	USA, India (2 families)	rare
SCA-13	19q13.3–13.4	*unknown*			France (1 family)	rare
SCA-17	6q27	*Interrupted CAG expansion / TBP*[a]	27–44	47–63	Japan, Germany	rare
SCA-18	7q31–q32	*unknown*			USA	?
SCA-19	1p21–q21	*unknown*			Holland (1 family)	rare
SCA-21	7p21.3–p15.1	*unknown*			France (1 family)	rare
ADCA II						
SCA-7	3p12–p13	*CAG expansion / ataxin-7*	7–19	37–300	Worldwide	?
ADCA III						
SCA-5	11cen	*Unknown*			USA (1 family)	rare
SCA-6	19p13.1	*CAG expansion / CACNLA1A*[a]	4–17	19–30	Worldwide	5–10%
SCA-8	13q21	*CTG expansion / 3¢UTR region of SCA8*	15–91	107–127		?
SCA-10	22q13	*ATTCT expansion / intron 9 of SCA10*	10–22	800–4500	Mexico	rare
SCA-11	15q14–q21.3	*Unknown*			England (1 family)	rare
SCA-14	19q13.4–qter	*Point mutations / PRKCG*[a]			Japan, Europe (2 families)	rare
SCA-16	8q22.1–q24.1	*Unknown*			Japan	rare
SCA-22	1p21–q23	*Unknown*			China	?
Episodic Ataxia						
EA type 1	12p13	*Missense mutations/ KCNA1*[a]			Worldwide	
EA type 2	19p13	*Missense mutations/ CACNLA1A*[a]			Worldwide	
	12p12					
DRPLA		*CAG expansion / atrophin-1*	7–35	54–83	Japan	20% (Japan)

[a]TBP (TATA binding protein); KCNA1 (potassium voltage-gated channel 1); CACNLA1A (α1A-voltage-gated calcium channel subunit); PRKCG (protein kinase C gamma).

D: Diagnosis available = Commercially (C), Research (R), Non-available (N). *SCA9* was reported as a new ataxia locus based on the analysis of a family in which other SCA loci were excluded in 1997 (Higgins et al., Movement Disorders). The *SCA9* locus has not been mapped, and it is unknown whether this locus is distinct from newer SCA loci. SCA20 is apparently reserved but it does not appear on the Genome Database. SCA23 has been mapped (GDB accession #: 11510207) but the phenotype has not been described in the literature.

quent choking and aspiration pneumonia threaten their lives. The phenotype of the disease appears to be relatively homogeneous within and between families. Neuro-imaging studies typically show atrophy of cerebellar cortex, vermis, and brainstem.

SCA1 families show anticipation, i.e., progressively earlier onset with increasing severity of the disease in successive generations, especially when the disease is transmitted by an affected father (Matilla et al., 1993; Zoghbi, 1995). The length of the repeat expansion inversely correlates with the age of onset, and the length of the expanded repeat becomes progressively larger in successive generations (Ranum et al., 1994a; Genis et al., 1995).

Gross pathological changes of SCA1 brain consist of overall reduction in the size of the cerebellum, especially in the vermis, without consistent atrophy of the pons (Figure 1), which are compatible with findings on brain MRI (Burk et al., 1996). Genis et al., (1995) reported that brains from three patients with SCA1 showed primary damage to cerebellar Purkinje cells. However, neuronal loss is also found in

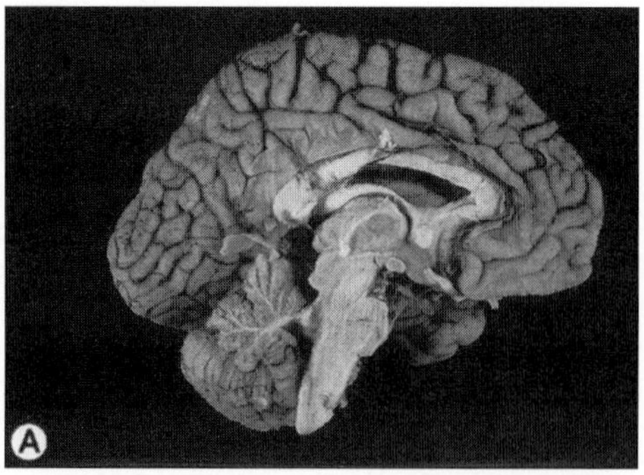

FIGURE 1 The midsagittal section of the brain of a patient with SCA1. Note atrophy of the cerebellar vermis and modest dilatation of the fourth ventricle resulting from the vermian atrophy. Gross pontine atrophy is absent in spite of microscopic neuronal loss in the basis pontis. (Obtained from Koeppen, 2002.)

the gray matter of basis pontis, inferior olivary nuclei, and dentate nucleus. These cell losses were associated with loss or bizarre morphological changes of dendrites and "empty baskets" (Figure 2). Furthermore, torpedoes in the granular layer of the cerebellum are abundant, although parallel fibers are well-preserved (Koeppen, 2002). The cerebellum of SCA1 patients and SCA1 transgenic animals shows neuronal degeneration with ubiquitinated nuclear inclusions including ataxin1 (Figure 3). There has been evidence to suggest that the inclusions may be the result of cells' effort to eliminate toxic mutant ataxin1 protein (Zoghbi and Orr, 2000).

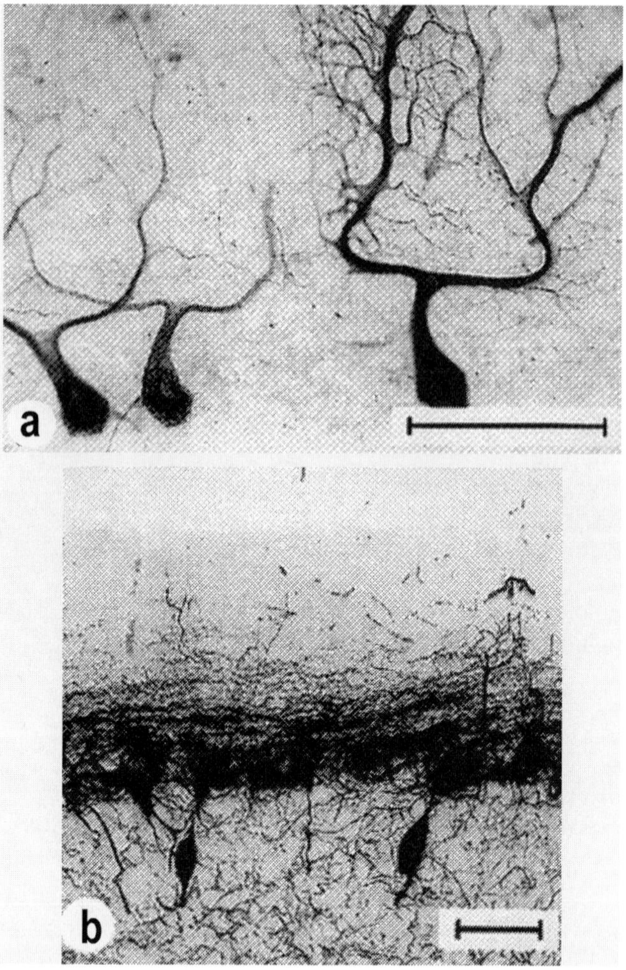

FIGURE 2 Microscopic findings of the cerebellum of an SCA1 patient. **a**, Although the number of Purkinje cells is decreased, dendritic arborization of the remaining Purkinje cells is simplified or lost. **b**, The internal third of cerebellar molecular layer shows abundant parallel fibers with empty baskets and axonal interruption. (Modified from Koeppen, 2002.)

2. SCA2

The polyglutamine repeat expansion in SCA2 is in the ataxin 2 protein encoded by the *SCA2* gene on chromosome 2q23–24.1 (table 1) (Pulst et al., 1996; Sanpei et al., 1996; Imbert et al., 1996). The CAG repeat lengths inversely correlate with the age of onset, and tend to expand further during paternal transmission with anticipation (Riess et al., 1997).

Patients with SCA2 show gait ataxia, which is characteristically accompanied by slow saccades, kinetic or postural tremor, and decrease of muscle tone and tendon reflexes. SCA2 patients may also have Parkinsonian features, dystonia, chorea, supranuclear ophthalmoplegia, and dementia. MRI of the brain shows non-specific cerebellar or pontocerebellar atrophy. Nerve conduction studies often show evidence of axonal sensory-motor neuropathy.

Macroscopic changes of SCA2 brains are characterized by dramatic cerebellar and pontine atrophy, similar to sporadic olivo-ponto-cerebellar atrophy (OPCA) (Figure 4). MRI of the brain of SCA2 patients clearly shows these dramatic changes (Figure 5). The most conspicuous microscopic findings are severe loss of Purkinje cells and cells in the pontine and olivary nuclei. Cells in the dentate nuclei and the substantia nigra are preserved. In advanced stages, neuronal losses are more extensive, involving regions such as substantia nigra, striatum, pallidum, and later even the neocortex. The spinal cord may also show severe atrophy of the dorsal columns and reduction in the number of neurons in the motor pool and Clarke's nuclei (Pang et al., 2000). This widespread degeneration pattern is clearly more extensive than most other spinocerebellar ataxias, and involves regions known to degenerate in Huntington disease and multi-system atrophy (Estrada et al., 1999). SCA2 has an intriguing pathophysiological difference from other polyglutamine diseases; ataxin-2, the protein product of the *SCA2* gene, is diffusely and densely distributed in the cytoplasm in cerebellar neurons of SCA2 patients (Figure 6). The ataxin-2 loaded neurons are particularly numerous in the pontine nuclei (Huynh et al., 2000), and have been shown to contain ubiquitin (Koyano et al., 1999). SCA2 patients show the most severe overall synaptic destruction in cerebellum and brain stem (Koeppen et al., 2002).

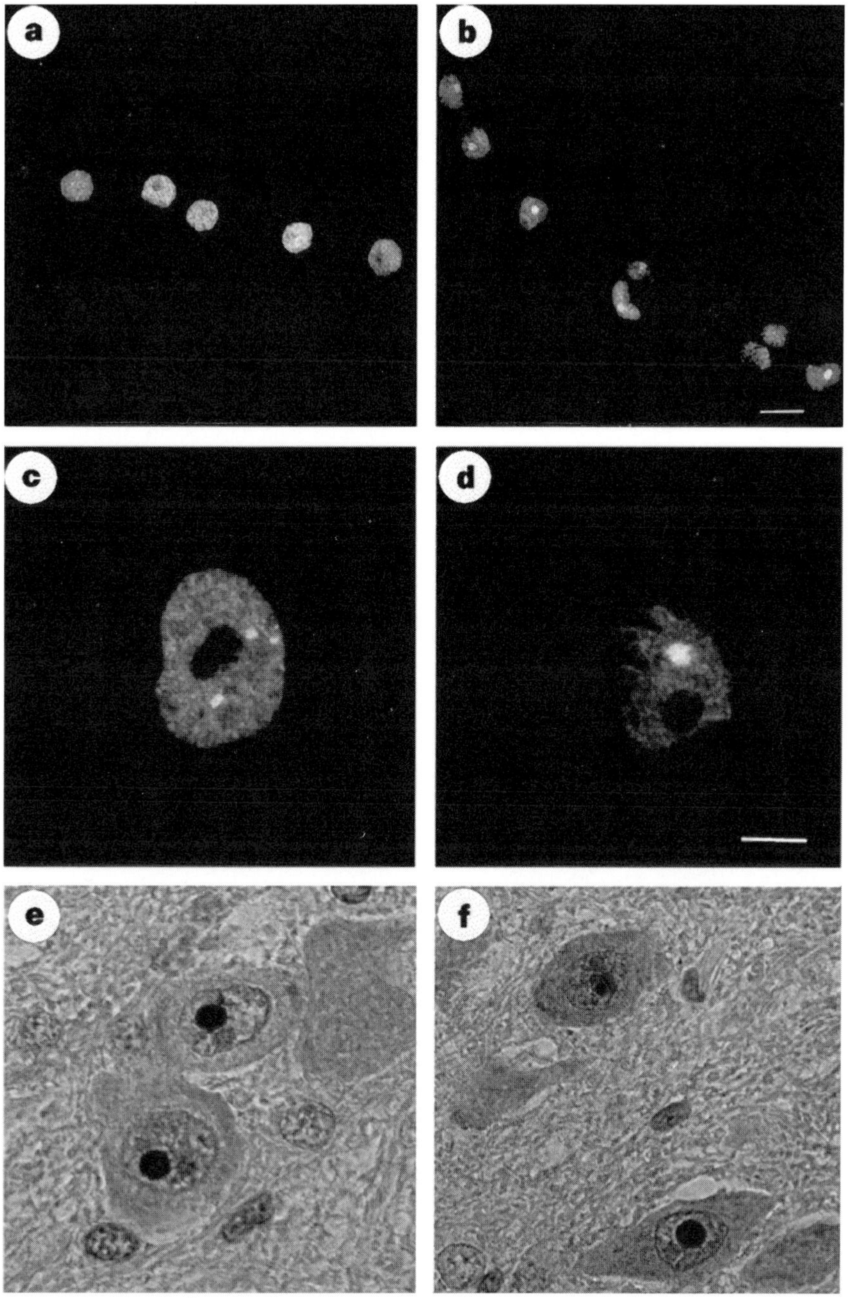

FIGURE 3 Immunofluorescence of ataxin-1 within the cerebellar Purkinje cell nuclei of an SCA1 transgenic mouse model and neurons of an SCA1 patient. **a**, **c**, Localization of wild-type ataxin-1 with 30 repeats; **b**, **d**, localization of mutant ataxin-1 with 82 repeats in the Purkinje cells of transgenic mice (**a**, **b**, a 10-μm series of confocal images; **c**, **d**, a single confocal Z scan). **e**, **f**, Ataxin-1 (**e**) and ubiquitin (**f**) immunostaining of neurons is shown in the nucleus pontis centralis from an SCA1 patient with an expanded allele of 82 repeats. (From Skinner et al., 1997.)

3. SCA3/MJD (Machado-Joseph disease)

SCA3, also known as Machado-Joseph disease (MJD), was originally described in Portuguese Azorean families (Romanul et al., 1977) and is now recognized with a worldwide distribution. In this disease, the *MJD* gene on 14q31.1 shows an expansion of a CAG repeat encoding a polyglutamine tract (Table 1) (Kawaguchi, 1994). Clinical manifestations are variable; in addition to cerebellar ataxia and ophthalmoplegia, the early-onset disease is manifested with spasticity, dystonia, and an akinetic syndrome, whereas the late-onset SCA3 is mainly presented with cerebellar ataxia

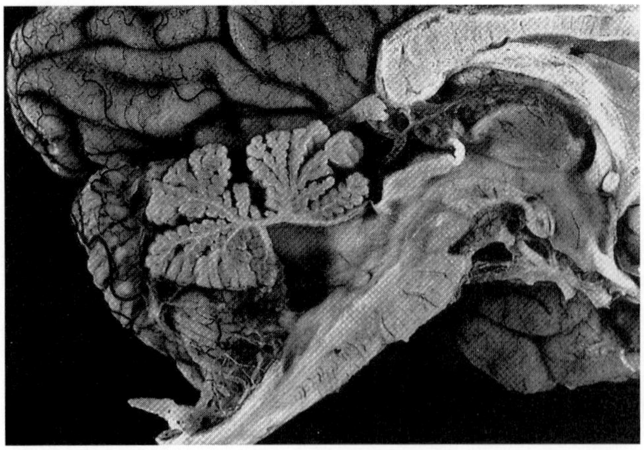

FIGURE 4 The midsagittal section of the brain from a patient with SCA2. Severe cerebellar and pontine atrophy, wide interfolial spaces, and dilatation of the fourth ventricle and aqueduct are shown. The uvula and nodulus of the vermis are not significantly atrophied. (Obtained from Koeppen, 2002.)

and ophthalmoparesis with minimal extrapyramidal symptomatology (Matilla et al., 1995; Cancel, 1995). The extrapyramidal signs are a characteristic, but not exclusive, feature of the SCA3 phenotype (Matilla et al., 1995). Patients with typical MJD show eyelid retraction and facial fasciculations. There is an inverse correlation between the age of onset and the expanded CAG repeat length. The severity of the disease as well as the presence of peripheral neuropathy appears to be dependent on the length of the expansion, with short and very large pathological alleles lacking neuropathy (Durr, 1996).

Macroscopically, brains of patients with SCA3/MJD show a small cerebellum due to severe atrophy of the dentate nucleus and its afferent fibers, but characteristically spare the cerebellar cortex and the inferior olivary nucleus (Koeppen, 2002) (Figure 7). Pontine atrophy may be absent in some cases but severe in others. Microscopically, there is a striking loss of neurons in the dentate nucleus, where

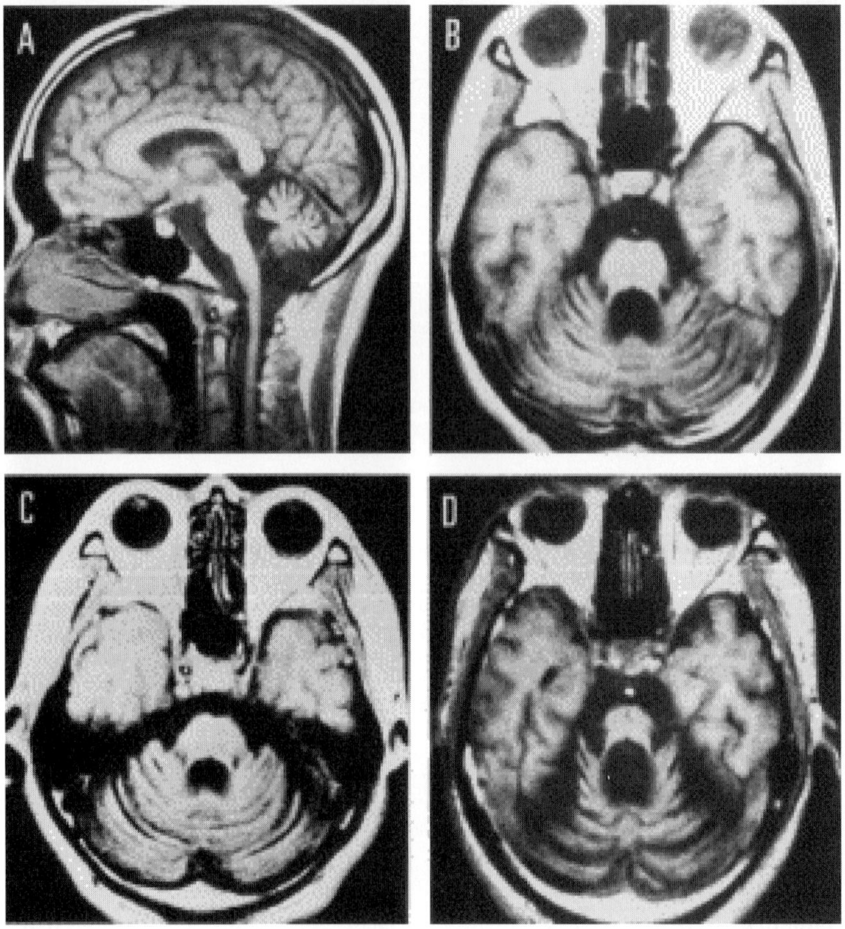

FIGURE 5 T1-weighted brain MRI of three SCA2 patients. Mediosagittal plane (A) and axial images at the level of the pons (B) show atrophy of the cerebellum and the brain stem in a 21 year-old-patient with the disease duration 5 years and 51 CAGs. Similar axial images show mild brain stem and cerebellar atrophy in a 61-year-old patient with 4 year duration and 36 CAGs (C), compared with more severe atrophy in a 39-year-old patient with a 14 year disease duration and 43 CAGs (D). (From Mizushima et al., 1998.)

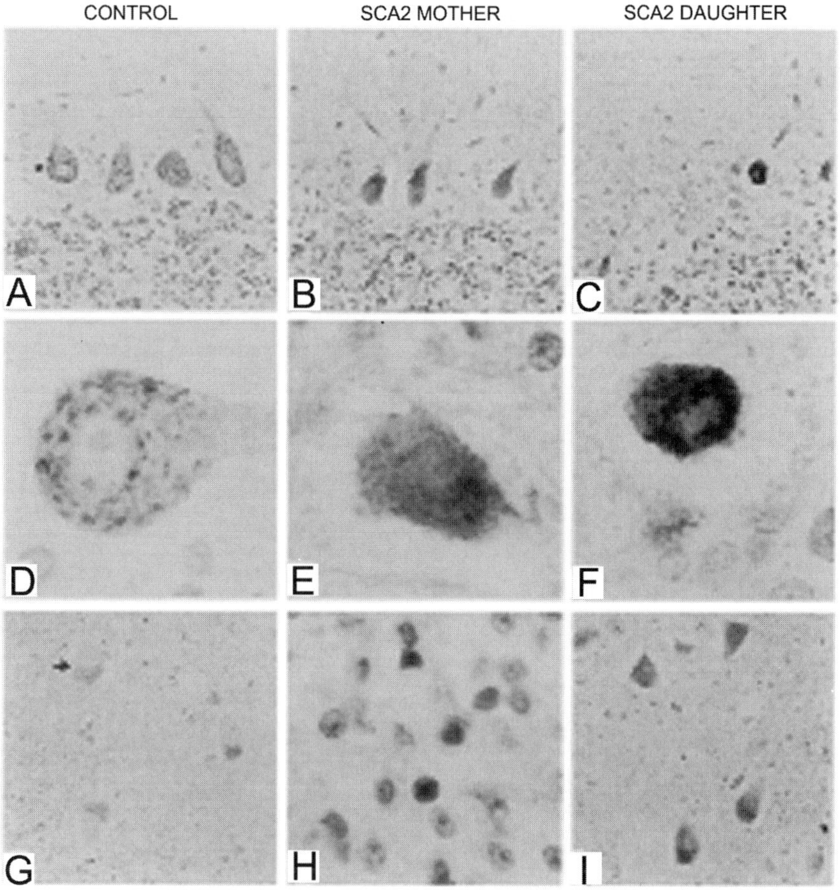

FIGURE 6 Ataxin-2 in the cerebellum of SCA2 patients. Levels of ataxin-2 immunoreactivity in the cerebellum from a 49-year-old female with SCA2 (B, E and H), and her 41-year-old daughter with SCA2 (C, F and I) are more diffuse and intense than in the cerebellum of a 49-year-old female control (A, D and G). A–C are cerebellar cortex, D–F are Purkinje cells, G and I are dentate neurons, and H is cerebellar granule neurons. Nuclear immunoreactivity was seen in some granular neurons (H). (From Huynh et al., 1998.)

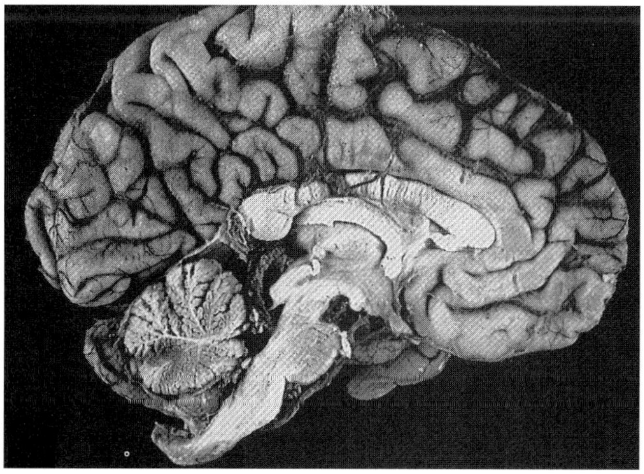

FIGURE 7 The midsagittal section of the brain from a patient with SCA3/MJD. The cerebellum is small although the cerebellar cortex is spared. (From Koeppen, 2002.)

the remaining neurons often show dendritic expansion and pathological abundance of synaptic terminals (grumose degeneration). In the spinal cord, the lesions may be similar to those in Friedreich ataxia. The dorsal nucleus shows severe neuronal loss. Atrophy of the dorsal and lateral funiculi is not as severe as Friedreich ataxia, corresponding to the relative preservation of dorsal root ganglia and corticospinal tracts. The ventral spinocerebellar tracts are severely affected. Motor neurons in the anterior horn are also depleted. Patients with SCA3/MJD often have peripheral polyneuropathy, which shows a variable loss of large myelinated fibers and distal axonopathy with relative hypomyelination (Lin and Soong, 2002).

Intranuclear and intracytoplasmic inclusions containing expanded polyglutamines and ubiquitin are found in the affected regions of the brain. Intranuclear aggregates have been seen in areas outside the most severely affected regions, including the cerebral cortex, thalamus, and autonomic ganglia (Yamada et al., 2001). Only cytoplasmic inclusions, but not intranuclear inclusions were found in the spinal motor neurons (Hayashi et al., 2003). Intranuclear inclusions have been shown to be immunopositive for several transcription factors such as TATA-binding protein (TBP), TBP-associated factor (TAF(II)130), Sp1, cAMP-responsive element-binding protein (CREB), and CREB-binding protein, suggesting that neuronal degeneration in polyglutamine diseases may result from nuclear depletion of transcription factors containing the glutamine-rich domain (Yamada et al., 2000). However, nuclear shrinkage and deformity in MJD brains were attenuated in neurons harboring nuclear aggregates, suggesting that nuclear inclusions are not necessarily toxic to neurons (Uchihara et al., 2002). Thus, the pathogenic role of nuclear inclusions requires further investigation.

4. SCA6

SCA6 belongs to ADCA-III, although patients in advanced stages of the disease may also show dystonia and other dyskinesias and abnormalities in tendon reflexes (Ikeuchi et al., 1997). Extraocular movement abnormalities are characterized by horizontal and oblique gaze nystagmus and an abnormal vestibulo-ocular reflex (Gomez et al., 1997; Sugawara et al., 2000). Some phenotypic overlap with the allelic disease, EA-2, has been noted (Geschwind et al., 1997; Jodice et al., 1997). MRI of the brain shows atrophy of the cerebellum, but some patients may show atrophy of the pons, middle cerebellar peduncles, and red nucleus (Murata et al., 1998; Nagai et al., 1998; Gomez et al., 1997). The SCA6 mutation is a small CAG repeat expansion within the α1A-voltage-dependent calcium channel subunit (*CACNLA1A*) gene (Zhuchenko et al., 1997). Expanded alleles in patients show 19–30 CAGs while normal alleles contain 4–17 CAGs (Table 1) (Zhuchenko et al., 1997; Matsuyama et al., 1997; Katayama et al., 2000). Although the age of onset inversely correlates with the expanded repeat size among different families, the expanded repeat is usually stably transmitted within each family (Matsuyama et al., 1997; Riess et al., 1997; Ishikawa et al., 1997). In rare cases, however, mild expansions have been reported during transmissions (Shimazaki et al., 2001; Shizuka et al., 1998). Cases with homozygous expansions suggested a gene dosage effect on the age of onset (Matsuura et al., 1997; Ikeuchi et al., 1997; Takiyama et al., 1998; Geschwind et al., 1997), but the relationship of the progression rate of the disease with the repeat size may not be as straightforward as the age of onset (Kato et al., 2000). Anticipation has been described in French (Stevanin et al., 1997), Japanese (Matsuyama et al., 1997), and Taiwanese (Soong et al., 2001) kindreds, in the absence of changes in the CAG repeat size. Some patients have no

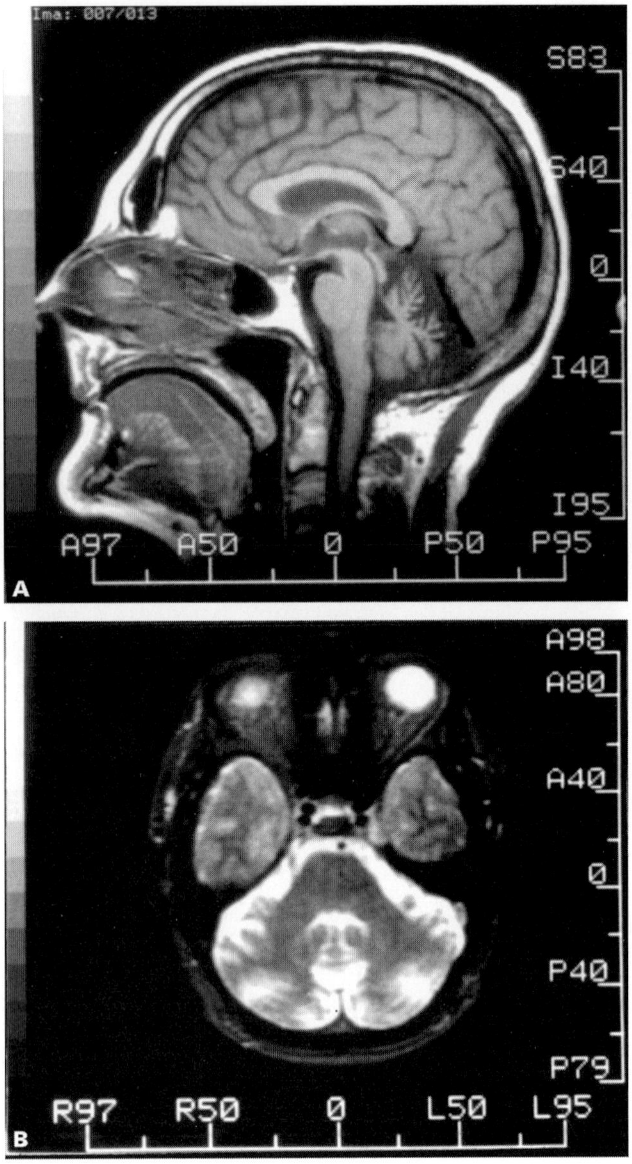

FIGURE 8 T1-weighted brain MRI in a 47-year-old patient with SCA6 after a disease duration of 12 years. Mediosagittal plane (A) and axial images at the level of the middle cerebellar peduncles (B). (From Schols et al., 1998.)

family history and their diagnosis would have been a sporadic ataxia if genetic testing were not done.

Gross pathological findings correlate with brain MRI (Figure 8), i.e., severe atrophy of cerebellum with sparing of the uvula and nodulus (Figure 9), which is also seen in other types of dominant ataxias. Microscopically, Purkinje cell loss with depleted dendritic arbors is the major feature, while loss of granular cells and parallel fibers is variable. Neurons of dentate nucleus are generally preserved although small cell gliosis is evident. The inferior olivary nucleus shows variable atrophy (Subramony et al., 1996; Gomez et al., 1997; Takahashi et al., 1998; Koeppen et al., 2002).

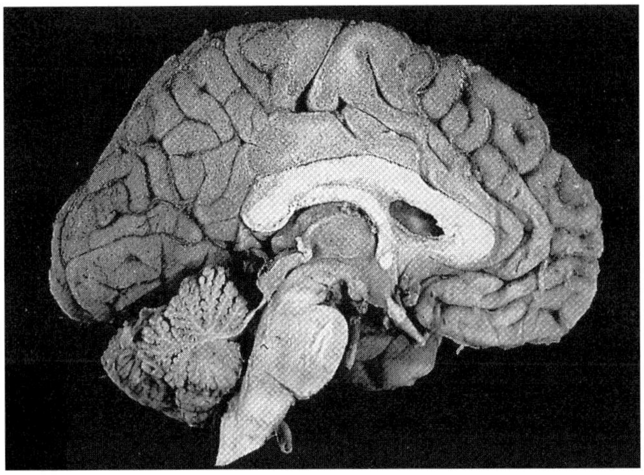

FIGURE 9 The midsagittal section of the brain from a patient with SCA6. The cerebellum is greatly reduced in size. The folia of the superior vermis are narrowed and reveal wide spaces between them, whereas the uvula and nodulus are better preserved. (From Koeppen, 2002.)

Although the expansion size of the CAG repeat is smaller than any other pathogenic CAG expansions, the polyglutamine tract in a densely packed membrane protein may allow small expansions to aggregate (Ishikawa et al., 1999; Ishikawa et al., 2001). A key question is whether the pathogenic mechanism of SCA6 involves a gain of toxic function by the expanded polyglutamine tract or perturbation of the gating of P/Q-type channels (Restituito et al., 2000). It has been postulated that protein interactions altered by the expanded polyglutamine tract might cause gating abnormalities (Gomez, 2001).

5. SCA7

SCA7 is characterized by cerebellar ataxia and progressive pigmentary maculopathy, which are accompanied by a wide spectrum of clinical features including pyramidal and extrapyramidal signs, ophthalmoplegia, dementia, hypoacusia, hypotonia, and auditory hallucinations (David et al., 1998). SCA7 belongs to ADCA-II. Slowing of voluntary and involuntary saccadic eye movements have been recognized as an early sign of SCA7 (Oh et al., 2001). Anticipation is well documented in families of SCA7, with cases of the juvenile and infantile SCA7 in the later generations. The infantile form occurs only on paternal transmission and shows severe hypotonia, cerebral and cerebellar atrophy, early visual loss, congestive heart failure, and patent ductus arteriosus (Benton et al., 1998).

SCA7 is caused by an expansion of a CAG repeat coding for a polyglutamine tract in the *SCA7* (*ataxin-7*) gene on chromosome 3p (Table 1) (David et al., 1997; Koob et al., 1998). The expansion size is the major determinant of both severity of the disease and age of onset (Del-Favero et al., 1998; Johansson et al., 1998). Intermediate alleles with 28–36 repeats are prone to expand further, accounting for *de novo* mutation cases (Stevanin et al., 1998; Giunti et al., 1999). Intergenerational expansion of the CAG repeat is particularly prominent with paternal transmission (Gouw et al., 1998). The expanded CAG repeat in sperm shows massive size increases, potentially causing putative embryonic lethality or dysfunctional sperm (Monckton et al., 1999).

Although autopsy reports have not been available for SCA7, brains of ADCA-II patients macroscopically show olivopontocerebellar atrophy (Koeppen, 2002). The optic nerves, chiasm, and the lateral geniculate nuclei also show atrophy. Microscopically, severe Purkinje cell loss and neuronal depletion in the inferior olivary nuclei and the basis pontis are accompanied by fiber loss in the spinocerebellar tracts and dorsal column of the spinal cord. The mutant ataxin-7 protein with the polyglutamine expansion is considered pathogenic via a gain of toxic function mechanism (Kaytor et al., 1999; Cancel et al., 2000; Yvert et al., 2000; Einum et al., 2001).

6. SCA8

Patients with SCA8 show primarily the ADCA-III phenotype, which is variably associated with pyramidal and cognitive dysfunction (Day et al., 2000; Juvonen et al., 2000). SCA8 patients have an expansion of a non-coding CTG repeat in the *SCA8* gene on chromosome 13q21 (Koob et al., 1999). The CTG repeat expands to the pathogenic range of 100 to 152 repeats in patients, while normal individuals have 15 to 91 CTGs (Table 1). Many SCA patients have expanded alleles with interruptions by CCG, CTA, CTC, CCA, or CTT, which may newly arise or change from generation to generation (Moseley et al., 2000). Affected individuals usually inherit an expanded allele from their mothers with an instability bias toward further expansion, whereas paternal transmissions mostly result in smaller alleles due to *en mass* contraction of the expanded alleles to the normal range (<100 CTGs) in the sperm (Day et al., 2000; Moseley et al., 2000; Silveira et al., 2000). However, expanded repeats in Japanese patients with the ADCA-III phenotype showed 89–155 CTGs with paternal anticipation (Ikeda et al., 2000). SCA8 pedigrees show variable penetrance (Day et al., 2000; Ikeda et al., 2000). There has been no evidence of correlation between the repeat size and the age of onset. Haplotype analyses showed multiple origins for the SCA8 expansions (Juvonen et al., 2000).

SCA8 contains no open reading frame, but the most 5′ exon is transcribed through the first exon of another gene, *KLHL1*, which is transcribed in the opposite orientation. This raises the possibility that the SCA8 transcript is an endogenous antisense RNA for *KLHL1*. Both *SCA8* and *KLHL1* are primarily expressed in specific brain tissues affected by SCA8 (Nemes et al., 2000). Other gain-of-function mechanisms involving the mutant SCA8 transcript have not been investigated, but are by no means excluded.

Alleles longer than 100 CTG repeats at the *SCA8* locus have been found in 1.2% (14 of 1,120) of major psychosis patients and 0.7% (5 of 710) of normal control subjects who had no family history of ataxia (Vincent et al., 2000). This lack of absolute specificity of the CTG repeat expansion for SCA8 has raised the possibility that CTG expansions at the *SCA8* locus are a rare polymorphism rather than the disease-causing mutation (Worth et al., 2000; Stevanin et al., 2000b).

7. SCA10

Patients with SCA10 show the ADCA-III phenotype. Additionally, however, SCA10 patients often have epilepsy with generalized motor seizures, complex partial seizures, or both. Some patients have variable combinations of mild cognitive dysfunction, sensory polyneuropathy, and soft corticospinal tract signs (Rasmussen et al., 2001). Anticipation is observed with considerable interfamilial variability. The disease has, so far, been confined to families of the Mexican (Matsuura et al., 2000; Rasmussen et al., 2001) and Brazilian (unpublished data) populations. The SCA10 mutation is an expansion of the ATTCT pentanucleotide repeat located in intron 9 of the *SCA10* (*E46L*) gene on chromosome 22q13 (Matsuura et al., 2000). The normal alleles have 10–21 ATTCTs while patients with SCA10 have 800–4500 repeats (Table 1). The expansion size correlates inversely with the age of onset. The mechanism of the disease remains unknown. Although there have been no autopsy reports of patients with SCA10, MRI of the brain of SCA10 patients shows cerebellar atrophy similar to that seen in other ADCA-III. In spite of epilepsy, there has been no evidence of cerebral cortical abnormalities on MRI.

8. SCA12

SCA12 is clinically characterized by ataxia, upper body tremor, corticospinal tract signs, hypokinesia, and dementia, which typically start in adulthood. In the late stage, some patients exhibit psychiatric manifestations, including depression, anxiety, or delusions. There has been no evidence of anticipation in SCA12. Brain MRI shows cerebellar and cerebral cortical atrophy. The mutation of SCA12 is a CAG repeat expansion in the 5′ untranslated region of the *PPP2R2B* gene on chromosome 5p31–p33 (Table 1) (Holmes et al., 1999). The disease is described in two populations, one from the United States and the other from India (Fujigasaki et al., 2001). It has been postulated that the expansion of the CAG repeat upregulates *PPP2R2B* expression.

9. SCA14

SCA14 is localized to 19q13.4 (Yamashita et al., 2000; Brkanac et al., 2002). In a Japanese family, the family members with a late onset (>39 years old) exhibited pure cerebellar ataxia, whereas those with an early onset (<27 years old) first showed intermittent axial myoclonus followed by ataxia. Other neurological signs were sparse, and neuroimaging studies revealed atrophy confined to the cerebellum. Another family of English and Dutch descent showed a mean age of onset in the third decade, presenting with gait ataxia, dysmetria, dysarthria, abnormal eye movements, and hyperreflexia without cognitive impairment, myoclonus, or sensory loss (Brkanac, 2002). Chen et al. (2003) identified three different non-conservative missense mutations in the C1 domain of the protein kinase C-gamma (*PRKCG*) gene. Immunohistochemical studies of cerebellar tissues from a patient demonstrated reduced staining for both PKC-gamma and ataxin-1 in Purkinje cells, whereas staining for calbindin was preserved.

10. SCA17

An expansion of CAG repeats of the TATA-binding protein (*TBP*) gene was initially reported in a Japanese patient with sporadic cerebellar ataxia and intellectual deterioration associated with *de novo* expansion (Koide et al., 1999). Subsequent reports of familial cases with this repeat expansion in Japanese and German families demonstrated that SCA17 is an ADCA-I (Nakamura et al., 2001; Zuhlke et al., 2001). Japanese families showed phenotypes resembling Huntington disease or DRPLA (Nakamura et al., 2001). The neuropathology of SCA17 has been classified as a "pure cerebellar" or "cerebello-olivary" degeneration. In the cerebellar cortex, the molecular layer is thinned with a striking Purkinje cell loss, empty baskets, axonal torpedoes, and unusual dendritic expansions. However, intranuclear neuronal inclusions with immunoreactivity to anti-TBP and antipolyglutamine were extensively distributed throughout the brain gray matter, including basis pontis; nucleus raphe; dorsomedian nucleus of the thalamus; midbrain tegmentum; tegmentum of the medulla oblongata; nucleus basalis of Meynert; stellate and basket neurons of the molecular layer; and the pyramidal neurons (including Betz cells) of the frontal cortex (Rolfs et al., 2003; Nakamura et al., 2001). Immunoreactivity was absent from Purkinje cells, the neurons of the dentate nucleus, putamen, globus pallidus, thalamic nuclei other than the dorsomedian nucleus, the medial accessory olivary nuclei, and the spinal cord. The nuclear inclusions are much larger than those seen in SCA2 and SCA3.

11. DRPLA

DRPLA is most frequent in Japan, although a few isolated families have been recognized worldwide (see Potter, 1995). The mutation is an expansion of a polyglutamine-coding CAG repeat in the *DRPLA* gene on chromosome 12p

(Koide et al., 1994; Nagafuchi et al., 1994). Early onset of the disease includes ataxia, myoclonus epilepsy, and progression to dementia, while adult-onset cases show cerebellar ataxia and psychiatric symptoms, which may accompany seizures (Potter, 1995; Nielsen et al., 1996) and choreoathetotic abnormal movements, resembling a "Huntington-like" phenotype (Warner et al., 1995). Families with DRPLA show conspicuous anticipation, and the age of onset and severity correlate with the length of the CAG expansion. The mutation in the *DRPLA* gene has also been found in the Haw River Syndrome, which has somewhat different clinical characteristics from DRPLA (Burke et al., 1994).

The hallmark of brain histopathology is atrophy of dentatorubral and pallidoluysian system as the name of the disorder implies, but occasional degenerative lesions are found in the cerebral white matter, putamen, Goll's nucleus of the medulla oblongata, and lateral corticospinal and Goll's tract of the spinal cord (Oyanagi, 2000). The neuropathological spectrum in Caucasian patients with DRPLA is essentially identical to those described in Japanese patients with DRPLA (Becher et al., 1997). Expanded polyglutamine stretches are diffusely accumulated in nucleoplasm of the wide variety of neurons in the central nervous system. Like Huntington disease and Machado-Joseph disease, the inclusions in DRPLA are immunopositive for several transcription factors such as TATA-binding protein (TBP), TBP-associated factor (TAF(II)130), Sp1, cAMP-responsive element-binding protein (CREB), and CREB-binding protein, suggesting that neuronal degeneration may result from nuclear depletion of transcription factors containing the glutamine-rich domain (Yamada et al., 2002).

B. Episodic Ataxia (EA)

Episodic ataxia (EA) is an autosomal dominant disease, which belongs to a class of diseases known as channelopathies. Intermittent ataxia is the hallmark of EA, but patients with EA usually exhibit disease-specific interictal neurological signs.

1. EA type 1 (EA1)

EA1 patients have missense mutations in *KCNA1* (a potassium channel gene) on chromosome 12p (Browne et al., 1994). Episodic ataxia and dysarthria lasting seconds to minutes are precipitated by exercise or startle with the onset in childhood to adolescence. During and between attacks, patients with EA1 show myokymia around the eyes, lips, or fingers (Litt et al., 1994).

2. EA type 2 (EA2)

Patients with EA2 show mild to severe intermittent cerebellar ataxia associated with interictal nystagmus, diplopia, and migraine. Attacks may last for minutes to a few days. Episodes are provoked by stress and exercise but not startle. The EA2 mutations are in the α-1A subunit of the calcium channel (*CACNA1*A) gene, which has also shown mutations in familial hemiplegic migraine 1 (FHM1) and spinocerebellar ataxia type 6 (SCA6) (Ophoff et al., 1996). Missense mutations tend to cause FHM1 while non-sense or splice site mutations usually cause EA2 (Tournier-Lasserve, 1999) although many exceptions to this rule have been documented (Denier et al., 2001). Overlaps in clinical manifestations have been found, suggesting that EA2, FHM1, and SCA6 represent a clinical continuum caused by distinct mutations in *CACNA1A* (Jen and Geschwind, 2001). An identical mutation could give various clinical expressions of these allelic disorders in the same EA2 family. Progressive permanent ataxia has been found in some cases of EA2, but the molecular mechanism of the neuronal degeneration in EA2 remains unknown (Jen and Geschwind, 2001). The disease may respond to the treatment with acetazolamide (Griggs et al., 1978; see Battistini et al., 1999).

II. AUTOSOMAL RECESSIVE ATAXIA WITH CHILDHOOD OR JUVENILE ONSET

A. Friedreich ataxia (FRDA)

Friedreich ataxia (FRDA) is the most frequent autosomal recessive ataxia, accounting for 30–40% of Caucasians with autosomal recessive ataxias (Cosee et al., 1997). Moreover, there has been no report of FRDA among Sub-Saharan Africans, Amerindians, and peoples from China, Japan, and Southeast Asia (Labuda et al., 2000). The disease presents as a progressive spinocerebellar degeneration with typical onset before the age of 25 years, especially around childhood or puberty (7–14 years) (Harding, 1981a). Unsteady gait with profound proprioceptive sensory loss is the presenting manifestation in most cases, with subsequent development of leg weakness, dysarthria, upper limb ataxia, distal sensory loss, and absence of reflexes. With increasing weakness of the arm and leg muscles, scoliosis and high-arched feet develop. Nerve conduction studies show evidence of sensory axonal peripheral neuropathy. The clinical boundary of FRDA was expanded to the "late onset" (after 25 years old) Friedreich ataxia (LOFA) and Friedreich ataxia with retained reflexes (FARR) as patients with these phenotypic variants do have the FRDA mutations (Klockgether et al., 1993; Ragno et al., 1997). Patients with FRDA often develop a hypertrophic cardiomyopathy (Harding and Hewer, 1983) and impaired glucose tolerance or diabetes mellitus (Finocchiaro et al., 1988).

Neuropathology of FRDA is characterized by degeneration of the dorsal root ganglia, Clarke's columns, dorsal columns, corticospinal/spinocerebellar tracts, spinocerebellar tracts, cerebellum, pons, and medulla (Oppenheimer, 1979). The small size of the spinal cord, especially at thoracic level, is seen in both early-onset and late–onset cases, suggesting developmental hypoplasia instead of acquired atrophy (Koeppen, 2002). Dorsal roots are thin, but anterior roots are normal in thickness. Anterior spinocerebellar tracts and anterior corticospinal tracts are relatively spared compared with posterior spinocerebellar tracts and lateral corticospinal tracts, respectively. Severe neuronal loss is found in the nucleus dorsalis of Clarke. Dorsal root ganglia also show severe neuronal loss and proliferation of satellite cells. Peripheral nerves in some patients with Friedreich ataxia show loss of large myelinated fibers, foreshortened internodes, and even some evidence of segmental demyelination and remyelination, but most of the cases exhibit only minor axonal changes (reviewed in Koeppen, 2002). In the cerebellum, the dentate nucleus is more severely involved than the cerebellar cortex. In severe cases, the superior cerebellar peduncles are thinned. These lesions have been interpreted as results of "dying back" neuropathy in sensory nerves, dorsal spinal roots, dorsal columns, and corticospinal tracts. The nucleus dorsalis may be affected by transneuronal degeneration. However, the lesion in the dentate nucleus is not explainable by the dying back phenomenon. Alternative hypothesis would be that these lesions are primary targets of frataxin deficiency. However, there has been no convincing evidence to support this hypothesis, unlike in the heart where hypertrophy with increased endomysial connective tissues results from oxidative damages to myocardium due to frataxin deficiency.

Most FRDA patients have an expansion of the trinucleotide GAA in intron 1 of the *FRDA* gene, which encodes a protein named frataxin (Campuzano et al., 1996; Puccio and Koenig, 2000; Pandolfo, 2001). The normal number of repeats is 6–28, while affected individuals have 60–1800. Compound heterozygotes in which one chromosome has a GAA expansion and the other chromosome has a point mutation account for 2–4% of the cases. Clinical manifestations of these compound heterozygotes may differ from those with homozygous GAA expansions (see Forrest et al., 1998). Patients who are homozygous for frataxin point mutations have not been reported to date, and it has been postulated that such mutations would cause a lethal phenotype (see discussion in Pandolfo, 2001). There is an inverse correlation between the size of the GAA expansion and the age of onset, severity of the disease, and the occurrence of cardiomyopathy and diabetes; small-expanded alleles (i.e. <400 repeats) are found in patients with FARR or LOFA (Puccio and Koenig, 2000). Genetic heterogeneity in FRDA has been proposed, and the second locus has recently been identified as FRDA2 (Christodoulou et al., 2001).

Frataxin is a mitochondrial protein that plays a role in iron homeostasis. Deficiency of frataxin results in mitochondrial iron accumulation, defects in specific mitochondrial enzymes, enhanced sensitivity to oxidative stress, and eventually free-radical mediated cell death (Alper and Narayanan, 2003; Bradley et al., 2000). Oral administrations of idebenone (a free-radical scavenger, analogue of coenzyme Q10) have improved the cardiac hypertrophy and, potentially, cardiac function (Buyse et al., 2003; Mariotti et al., 2003; Hausse et al., 2002; Rustin et al., 1999). A recently developed mouse model of FRDA (Puccio et al., 2001) raises a hope for providing a powerful means to explore many of these hypotheses and potential treatments.

B. Ataxia with Vitamin E Deficiency (AVED)

Vitamin E deficiency may be presented with a phenotype that closely resembles FRDA. Patients with a previous diagnosis of FRDA and a negative genetic test for FRDA should be tested for serum vitamin E levels, which are very low (<5 μg/ml) in this disease. Although several diseases are known to lead to secondary vitamin E deficiency, mutations in the *TTP1* gene (Ouahchi et al., 1995) on chromosome 8q13, encoding the α-tocopherol transfer protein, (Catignani et al., 1977) are the disease-causing mutations in autosomal recessive ataxia with primary vitamin E deficiency. Early onset and severe forms of the disease are caused by truncating or missense mutations in well-conserved amino acids (Cavalier et al., 1998). Early replacement therapy may prevent progression of the disease (Jackson et al., 1996; Schuelke et al., 1999).

C. Abetalipoproteinemia (Bassen-Kornzweig Disease-BKD)

This rare autosomal recessive disorder causes secondary Vitamin E deficiency, with a phenotype consisting of spinocerebellar degeneration, peripheral neuropathy, and retinitis pigmentosa (Triantafillidis et al., 1998), resembling AVED. Peripheral blood smear shows acanthocytosis ("thorny" red blood cells) in BKD patients (see Stevenson and Hardie, 2001). Symptoms of BKD begin in childhood, with steatorrhoea and fat malabsorption. Mutations in the microsomal trygliceride transfer protein (MTP) gene on 4q22–24 (Sharp et al., 1993; Narcisi et al., 1995) account for a part of the BKD patients. Vitamin E replacement therapy prevents further progression of the neurological symptoms. Hypobetalipoproteinemia is a genetically distinct disorder with a similar clinical presentation to BKD.

D. Cayman Ataxia

Cayman ataxia is a recessive congenital ataxia restricted to one area of Grand Cayman Island. Individuals with Cayman ataxia have hypotonia from birth, variable psychomotor retardation and cerebellar dysfunction, including nystagmus, intention tremor, dysarthria, ataxic gait, and truncal ataxia (Nystuen et al., 1996). Imaging studies show cerebellar hypoplasia. The pathogenic mutations are located in *ATCAY*, which encodes a neuron-restricted protein called caytaxin (Bomar et al., 2003). Caytaxin contains a CRAL-TRIO motif common to proteins that bind small lipophilic molecules. Interestingly, alpha-tocopherol transfer protein (TTPA) also contains CRAL-TRIO motif. However, three-dimensional protein structural modeling predicts that the caytaxin ligand is more polar than vitamin E.

E. Autosomal Recessive Spastic Ataxia of Charlevoix-Saguenay (ARSACS)

This autosomal recessive ataxia presents itself with early onset ataxia initially manifested with gait ataxia, which is followed by progressive axonal neuropathy, spastic paraplegia and variably associated hypermyelination of retinal-nerve fibers (Bouchard et al., 1998). Intelligence is usually normal, although lowered IQ has been recognized in some cases. MRI studies show cerebellar atrophy. The gene on chromosome 13q11 (Bouchard et al., 1998), was identified as *SACS*, which has a single giant exon (12,794 bp) encoding a protein named sacsin, a putative chaperone highly expressed in the granular cell layer of the cerebellum (Engert et al., 2000). Mutations in the *SACS* gene were also found in eighteen patients with ARSACS in Tunisia (El Euch-Fayache et al., 2003). The same *SACS* locus has been linked to the hereditary ataxia in two Turkish families (Gucuyener et al., 2001).

F. Disorders Associated With Defective DNA Repair

1. Ataxia telangiectasia (AT)

Ataxia telangiectasia (AT) presents with gait ataxia during infancy or childhood (Crawford, 1998), and is associated with ocular apraxia, slow horizontal saccades, cerebellar syndrome, dystonic postures, chorea, tics or jerks, dysphagia, and choking, as well as peripheral neuropathy, which develop with the progression of the disease. Patients with AT also show dermatological signs, such as telangiectasia, premature senile keratosis and graying of the hair, and immunological abnormalities including atrophy of thymus and lymphoid tissues, lymphopenia, low levels of immunoglobulins. Increased sensitivity to DNA damage is the basis of AT, and lymphomas, leukemia, and other cancers are found in about 20% of patients with AT. Elevated serum α-fetoprotein levels are observed in about 90–95% of AT patients. Non-random chromosomal aberrations (i.e., chromosomes 7 and 14) are observed in lymphocytes. Survival after the age of 30 is rare. The disease is caused by mutations in the gene *ATM* (ataxia telangiectasia, mutated) on 11q22–23 (Savitsky et al., 1995), encoding a protein with serine/threonine kinase activity from the family of the phosphatidyl inositol-3-kinases (Lavin and Shiloh, 1997). *ATM* mutations have not been found in other cerebellar syndromes without additional clinical phenotype recognized in AT (Hassin-Baer et al., 1999). Conversely, a mutation in the gene *hMRE11*, involved in double strand break repair, has been found in an ataxic patient with an AT-like phenotype (Stewart et al., 1999).

2. Early Onset Ataxia with Oculomotor Apraxia and Hypoalbuminemia (EAOH)

The clinical hallmark of EAOH is early onset cerebellar ataxia associated with oculomotor apraxia and hypoalbuminemia (Barbot et al., 2001; Dawson, 2001; Date et al., 2001). The disease locus is located on 9q13 (Moreira et al., 2001a) and point mutations have been found in the *APTX* gene which encodes aprataxin, a new HIT/Zn-finger protein involved in DNA single-strand break repair (Date et al., 2001; Moreira et al., 2001b). Severe motor neuropathy dominates the clinical picture in the advanced phases of the disease, in which ocular apraxia evolves into external ophthalmoplegia (Barbot et al., 2001). Chorea, mental deterioration, scoliosis, pes cavus, and hypercholesterolemia are also present (Shimazaki et al., 2002; Le Ber et al., 2003). Brain CT and MRI show marked cerebellar atrophy. Nerve biopsy revealed depletion of large myelinated fibers.

3. Spinocerebellar Ataxia with Axonal Neuropathy (SCAN1)

A Saudi Arabian family affected with autosomal recessive spinocerebellar ataxia with axonal neuropathy (SCAN1) showed a homozygous mutation in tyrosyl-DNA phosphodiesterase 1 (*TDP1*) (Takashima et al., 2002). *TDP1* is a DNA repair gene whose deficiency in humans does not predispose to neoplasia or dysfunctions in rapidly replicating tissues, but instead causes spinocerebellar ataxia with axonal neuropathy (SCAN1) by affecting large, terminally differentiated, non-dividing neuronal cells. TDP1 repairs covalently bound topoisomerase I-DNA complexes and is essential for preventing the formation of double-strand breaks that result when stalled topoisomerase I complexes interfere with DNA replication in yeast.

Xeroderma pigmentosum (XP), Cockayne's syndrome (CS), and Trichothiodystrophy (TTD) are also often associated with ataxia (Rapin et al., 2000).

Video Legends

SEGMENT 1 Ataxia, unknown genotype. Patient with episodes of ataxia, followed by permanent ataxia of unknown genotype. The video shows 1) cerebellar dysarthria, 2) nystagmus with downbeat components (the patient has oscillopsia and diplopia), 3) normal saccade velocity, 4) mild finger-to-nose ataxia, 5) dysdiadokokinesia, 6) normal deep tendon reflexes, 7) heel-to-shin ataxia, and 8) severe stance and gait ataxia.

SEGMENT 2 Advanced SCA3 (Machado-Joseph disease). The video shows 1) restricted eye movements, "ocular stare," and temoralis and facial muscle atrophy, 2) slow saccades, 3) gaze improves with horizontal, but not vertical oculocephalic reflex, 4) gaze palsy is supranuclear, 5) mild tongue atrophy with fasciculations, 6) severe dysarthria, 7) muscles generally wasted, but weakness is mild, 8) severe abnormality of rapid alternating movements, 9) finger-to-nose ataxia and slow movements, 10) left foot exhibits a dystonic posture, 11) left knee reflex is brisk, and ankle reflexes are absent, and 12) the patient cannot stand.

SEGMENT 3 Friedrich ataxia. Teenager with FA of five years' duration. The video shows 1) eye movements are normal, 2) mild ataxia on finger-to-nose testing, 3) absent reflexes in the arms, 4) vibration and position sense are normal in finger, 5) mild weakness in distal leg muscles, 6) absent reflexes in legs, 7) bilateral extensor plantar reflexes, 8) proprioception is defective in legs, 9) mild gait ataxia with a broad base, and 10) heel-to-shin ataxia.

References

Alper, G., and V. Narayanan. 2003. Friedreich's ataxia. *Pediatr Neurol* **28**:335–341.

Banfi, S., A. Servadio, M. Chung, et al., 1994. Identification and characterization of the gene causing type 1 spinocerebellar ataxia. *Nat Genet* **7**:513–520.

Barbot, C., P. Coutinho, R. Chorão, et al. 2001. Recessive ataxia with ocular apraxia: review of 22 Portuguese patients. *Arch Neurol* **58**:201–205.

Battistini, S., S. Stenirri, M. Piatti, et al. 1999. A new CACNA1A gene mutation in acetazolamide-responsive familial hemiplegic migraine and ataxia. *Neurology* **53**:38–43.

Becher, M.W., D.C. Rubinsztein, J. Leggo, M.V. Wagster, O.C. Stine, N.G. Ranen, M.L. Franz, M.H. Abbott, M. Sherr, J.C. MacMillan, L. Barron, M. Porteous, P.S. Harper, and C.A. Ross. 1997. Dentatorubral and pallidoluysian atrophy (DRPLA). Clinical and neuropathological findings in genetically confirmed North American and European pedigrees. *Mov Disord* **12**:519–530.

Benton, C., R. de Silva, S. Rutledge, et al. 1998. Molecular and clinical studies in SCA-7 define a broad clinical spectrum and the infantile phenotype. *Neurology* **51**:1081–1086.

Bomar, J.M., P.J. Benke, E.L. Slattery, R. Puttagunta, L.P. Taylor, E. Seong, A. Nystuen, W. Chen,R.L. Albin, P.D. Patel, R.A. Kittles, V.C. Sheffield, and M. Burmeister. 2003. Mutations in a novel gene encoding a CRAL-TRIO domain cause human Cayman ataxia and ataxia/dystonia in the jittery mouse. *Nat Genet* **35**:264–269.

Bouchard, J., A. Richter, J. Mathieu, et al. 1998. Autosomal recessive spastic ataxia of Charlevoix-Saguenay. *Neuromuscul Disord* **8**:474–479.

Bradley, J., J. Blake, S. Chamberlain, et al. 2000. Clinical, biochemical and molecular genetic correlations in Friedreich's ataxia. *Hum Mol Genet* **9**:275–282.

Brkanac, Z., L. Bylenok, M. Fernandez, M. Matsushita, H. Lipe, J. Wolff, D. Nochlin, W.H. Raskind, and T.D. Bird. 2002. A new dominant spinocerebellar ataxia linked to chromosome 19q13.4-qter. *Arch Neurol* **59**:1291–1295.

Browne, D., S. Gancher, J. Nutt, et al. 1994. Episodic ataxia/myokymia syndrome is associated with point mutations in the human potassium channel gene, KCNA1. *Nat Genet* **8**:136–140.

Burk, K., M. Abele, M. Fetter, et al. 1996. Autosomal dominant cerebellar ataxia type I clinical features and MRI in families with SCA1, SCA2 and SCA3. *Brain* **119**:1497–1505.

Burke, J., M. Wingfield, K. Lewis, et al. 1994. The Haw River syndrome: dentatorubropallidoluysian atrophy (DRPLA) in an African-American family. *Nat Genet* **7**:521–524.

Buyse, G., L. Mertens, G. Di Salvo, I. Matthijs, F. Weidemann, B. Eyskens, W. Goossens, N. Goemans, G.R. Sutherland, and J.L. Van Hove. 2003. Idebenone treatment in Friedreich's ataxia: Neurological, cardiac, and biochemical monitoring. *Neurology* **60**:1679–1681.

Campuzano, V., L. Montermini, M. Molto, et al. 1996. Friedreich's ataxia: autosomal recessive disease caused by an intronic GAA triplet repeat expansion. *Science* **271**:1423–1427.

Cancel, G., N. Abbas, G. Stevanin, et al. 1995. Marked phenotypic heterogeneity associated with expansion of a CAG repeat sequence at the spinocerebellar ataxia 3/Machado-Joseph disease locus. *Am J Hum Genet* **57**:809–816.

Cancel, G., C. Duyckaerts, M. Holmberg, et al. 2000. Distribution of ataxin-7 in normal human brain and retina. *Brain* **123**:2519–2530.

Catignani, G., and J. Bieri. 1977. Rat liver alpha-tocopherol binding protein. *Biochim Biophys Acta* **497**:349–357.

Cavalier, L., K. Ouahchi, H. Kayden, et al. 1998. Ataxia with isolated vitamin E deficiency: heterogeneity of mutations and phenotypic variability in a large number of families. *Am J Hum Genet* **62**:301–310.

Chen, D.H. , Brkanac, C.L. Verlinde, X.J. Tan, L. Bylenok, D. Nochlin, M. Matsushita, H. Lipe, J. Wolff, M. Fernandez, P.J. Cimino, T.D. Bird, and W.H. Raskind. 2003. Missense mutations in the regulatory domain of PKC gamma: a new mechanism for dominant nonepisodic cerebellar ataxia. *Am J Hum Genet* **72**:839–849.

Christodoulou, K., F. Deymeer, P. Serdaroglu, et al. 2001. Mapping of the second Friedreich's ataxia (FRDA2) locus to chromosome 9p23-p11: evidence for further locus heterogeneity. *Neurogenetics* **3**:127–132.

Chung, M.Y., Y.C. Lu, N.C. Cheng, and B.W. Soong. 2003. A novel autosomal dominant spinocerebellar ataxia (SCA22) linked to chromosome 1p21-q23. *Brain* **126**:1293–1299.

Cossee, M., M. Schmitt, V. Campuzano, et al. 1997. Evolution of the Friedreich's ataxia trinucleotide repeat expansion: founder effect and premutations. Proc. *Natl Acad Sci U S A* **94**:7452–7457.

Crawford, T. 1998. Ataxia telangiectasia. *Semin Pediatr Neurol* **5**:287–294.

Date, H., O. Onodera, H. Tanaka, et al. 2001. Early-onset ataxia with ocular motor apraxia and hypoalbuminemia is caused by mutations in a new HIT superfamily gene. *Nat Genet* **29**:184–188.

David, G., N. Abbas, G. Stevanin, et al. 1997. Cloning of the SCA7 gene reveals a highly unstable CAG repeat expansion. *Nat Genet* **17**:65–70.

David, G., A. Durr, G. Stevanin, et al. 1998. Molecular and clinical correlations in autosomal dominant cerebellar ataxia with progressive macular dystrophy (SCA7). *Hum Mol Genet* **7**:165–167.

Dawson, D. 2001. Recessive ataxia with ocular motor apraxia. *Arch Neurol* **58**:173–174.

Day, J., L. Schut, M. Moseley, et al. 2000. Spinocerebellar ataxia type 8: clinical features in a large family. *Neurology* **55**:649–657.

Del-Favero, J., L. Krols, A. Michalik, et al. 1998. Molecular genetic analysis of autosomal dominant cerebellar ataxia with retinal degeneration (ADCA type II) caused by CAG triplet repeat expansion. *Hum Mol Genet* **7**:177–186.

Denier, C., A. Ducros, A. Durr, et al. 2001. Missense CACNA1A mutation causing episodic ataxia type 2. *Arch Neurol* **58**:292–295.

Durr, A., G. Stevanin, G. Cancel, et al. 1996. Spinocerebellar ataxia 3 and Machado-Joseph disease: clinical, molecular, and neuropathological features. *Ann Neurol* **39**:490–499.

Einum, D., J. Townsend, L. Ptacek, et al. 2001. Ataxin-7 expression analysis in controls and spinocerebellar ataxia type 7 patients. *Neurogenetics* **3**:83–90.

El Euch-Fayache, G., I. Lalani, R. Amouri, I. Turki, K. Ouahchi, W.Y. Hung, S. Belal, T. Siddique, and F. Hentati. 2003. Phenotypic features and genetic findings in sacsin-related autosomal recessive ataxia in Tunisia. *Arch Neurol* **60**:982–988.

Engert, J., P. Berube, J. Mercier, et al. 2000. ARSACS, a spastic ataxia common in northeastern Quebec, is caused by mutations in a new gene encoding an 11.5-kb ORF. *Nat Genet* **24**:120–125.

Estrada, R., J. Galarraga, G. Orozco, A. Nodarse, and G. Auburger. 1999. Spinocerebellar ataxia 2 (SCA2): morphometric analyses in 11 autopsies. *Acta Neuropathol (Berl)* **97**:306–310.

Evidente, V., K. Gwinn-Hardy, L. Caviness, et al. 2000. Hereditary ataxias. *Mayo Clin Proc* **75**:475–490.

Finocchiaro, G., G. Baio, P. Micossi, et al. 1988. Glucose metabolism alterations in Friedreich's ataxia. *Neurology* **38**:1292–1296.

Forrest, S., M. Knight, M. Delatycki, et al. 1998. The correlation of clinical phenotype in Friedreich ataxia with the site of point mutations in the FRDA gene. *Neurogenetics* **1**:253–257.

Fujigasaki, H., I. Verma, A. Camuzat, et al. 2001. SCA12 is a rare locus for autosomal dominant cerebellar ataxia: a study of an Indian family. *Ann Neurol* **49**:117–121.

Fujigasaki, H., J.J. Martin, P.P. De Deyn, A. Camuzat, D. Deffond, G. Stevanin, B. Dermaut, C. Van Broeckhoven, A. Durr, and A. Brice. 2001. CAG repeat expansion in the TATA box-binding protein gene causes autosomal dominant cerebellar ataxia. *Brain* **124**:1939–1947.

Genis, D., T. Matilla, V. Volpini, et al. 1995. Clinical, neuropathologic, and genetic studies of a large spinocerebellar ataxia type 1 (SCA1) kindred: (CAG)n expansion and early premonitory signs and symptoms. *Neurology* **45**:24–30.

Geschwind, D., S. Perlman, K. Figueroa, et al. 1997. Spinocerebellar ataxia type 6. Frequency of the mutation and genotype-phenotype correlations. *Neurology* **49**:1247–1251.

Giunti, P., G. Stevanin, P. Worth, et al. 1999. Molecular and clinical study of 18 families with ADCA type II: evidence for genetic heterogeneity and de novo mutation. *Am J Hum Genet* **64**:1594–1603.

Gomez, C., R. Thompson, J. Gammack, et al. 1997. Spinocerebellar ataxia type 6: gaze-evoked and vertical nystagmus, Purkinje cell degeneration, and variable age of onset. *Ann Neurol* **42**:933–950.

Gomez, C. 2001. Polyglutamine aggregates in SCA6 Purkinje cells: a tale of two toxicities. *Neurology* **56**:1618–1619.

Gouw, L., M. Castaneda, C. McKenna, et al. 1998. Analysis of the dynamic mutation in the SCA7 gene shows marked parental effects on CAG repeat transmission. *Hum Mol Genet* **7**:525–532.

Greenfield, J.G., and W. Blackwood. 1963. "Greenfield's Neuropathology." Williams & Wilkins, Baltimore.

Griggs, R., R. Moxley 3rd, R. Lafrance, et al. 1978. Hereditary paroxysmal ataxia: response to acetazolamide. *Neurology* **28**:1259–1264.

Gucuyener, K., K. Ozgul, C. Paternotte, et al. 2001. Autosomal recessive spastic ataxia of Charlevoix-Saguenay in two unrelated Turkish families. *Neuropediatrics* **32**:142–146.

Harding, A., and R. Hewer. 1983. The heart disease of Friedreich's ataxia: a clinical and electrocardiographic study of 115 patients, with an analysis of serial electrocardiographic changes in 30 cases. *Q J Med* **52**:489–502.

Harding, A. 1981a. Friedreich's ataxia: a clinical and genetic study of 90 families with an analysis of early diagnostic criteria and intrafamilial clustering of clinical features. *Brain* **104**:589–620.

Harding, A. 1981b. Genetic aspects of autosomal dominant late onset cerebellar ataxia. *J Med Genet* **18**:436–441.

Harding, A.E. 1993. Clinical features and classification of inherited ataxias. *Adv Neurol* **61**:1–14.

Hassin-Baer, S., A. Bar-Shira, S. Gilad, et al. 1999. Absence of mutations in ATM, the gene responsible for ataxia telangiectasia in patients with cerebellar ataxia. *J Neurol* **246**:716–719.

Hayashi, M., K. Kobayashi, and H. Furuta. 2003. Immunohistochemical study of neuronal intranuclear and cytoplasmic inclusions in Machado-Joseph disease. *Psychiatry Clin Neurosci* **57**:205–213.

Hausse, A.O., Y. Aggoun, D. Bonnet, D. Sidi, A. Munnich, A. Rotig, and P. Rustin. 2002. Idebenone and reduced cardiac hypertrophy in Friedreich's ataxia. *Heart* **87**:346–349.

Higgins, J.J., D.H. Morton, N. Patronas et al. 1997. An autosomal recessive disorder with posterior column ataxia and retinitis pigmentosa. *Neurology* **49**:1717–1720.

Holmes, S., E. O'Hearn, M. McInnis, et al. 1999. Expansion of a novel CAG trinucleotide repeat in the 5′ region of PPP2R2B is associated with SCA12. *Nat Genet* **23**:391–392.

Huynh, D.P., M.R. Del Bigio, D.H. Ho, and S.M. Pulst. 1998. Expression of ataxin-2 in brains from normal individuals and patients with Alzheimer's disease and spinocerebellar ataxia 2. *Ann Neurol* **45**:232–241.

Huynh, D.P., K. Figueroa, N. Hoang, et al. 2000. Nuclear localization or inclusion body formation of ataxin-2 are not necessary for SCA2 pathogenesis in mouse or human. *Nat Genet* **26**:44–50.

Ikeda, Y., M. Shizuka-Ikeda, M. Watanabe, et al. 2000. Asymptomatic CTG expansion at the SCA8 locus is associated with cerebellar atrophy on MRI. *J Neurol Sci* **182**:76–79.

Ikeuchi, T., H. Takano, R. Koide, et al. 1997. Spinocerebellar ataxia type 6: CAG repeat expansion in alpha1A voltage-dependent calcium channel gene and clinical variations in Japanese population. *Ann Neurol* **42**:879–884.

Imbert, G., F. Saudou, G. Yvert, et al. 1996. Cloning of the gene for spinocerebellar ataxia 2 reveals a locus with high sensitivity to expanded CAG/glutamine repeats. *Nat Genet* **14**:285–291.

Ishikawa, K., H. Tanaka, M. Saito, et al. 1997. Japanese families with autosomal dominant pure cerebellar ataxia map to chromosome 19p13.1–p13.2 and are strongly associated with mild CAG expansions in the spinocerebellar ataxia type 6 gene in chromosome 19p13.1. *Am J Hum Genet* **61**:336–346.

Ishikawa, K., H. Fujigasaki, H. Saegusa, et al. 1999. Abundant expression and cytoplasmic aggregations of [alpha]1A voltage-dependent calcium channel protein associated with neurodegeneration in spinocerebellar ataxia type 6. *Hum Mol Genet* **8**:1185–1193.

Ishikawa, K., K. Owada, Ishida, et al. 2001. Cytoplasmic and nuclear polyglutamine aggregates in SCA6 Purkinje cells. *Neurology* **56**:1753–1756.

Jackson, C., A. Amato, and R. Barohn. 1996. Isolated vitamin E deficiency. *Muscle Nerve* **19**:1161–1165.

Jen, J., and D. Geschwind. 2001. Ataxia and calcium channels: what a headache! *Arch Neurol* **58**:179–180.

Jodice, C., E. Mantuano, L. Veneziano, et al. 1997. Episodic ataxia type 2 (EA2) and spinocerebellar ataxia type 6 (SCA6) due to CAG repeat expansion in the CACNA1A gene on chromosome 19p. *Hum Mol Genet* **6**:1973–1978.

Johansson, J., L. Forsgren, O. Sandgren, et al. 1998. Expanded CAG repeats in Swedish spinocerebellar ataxia type 7 (SCA7) patients: effect of CAG repeat length on the clinical manifestation. *Hum Mol Genet* **7**:171–176.

Juvonen, V., M. Hietala, M. Paivarinta, et al. 2000. Clinical and genetic findings in Finnish ataxia patients with the spinocerebellar ataxia 8 repeat expansion. *Ann Neurol* **48**:354–361.

Katayama, T., Y. Ogura, H. Aizawa, et al. 2000. Nineteen CAG repeats of the SCA6 gene in a Japanese patient presenting with ataxia. *J Neurol* **247**:711–712.

Kato, T., F. Tanaka, M. Yamamoto, et al. 2000. Sisters homozygous for the spinocerebellar ataxia type 6 (SCA6)/CACNA1A gene associated with different clinical phenotypes. *Clin Genet* **58**:69–73.

Kawaguchi, Y., T. Okamoto, M. Taniwaki, et al. 1994. CAG expansions in a novel gene for Machado-Joseph disease at chromosome 14q32.1. *Nat Genet* **8**:221–228.

Kaytor, M., L. Duvick, P. Skinner, et al. 1999. Nuclear localization of the spinocerebellar ataxia type 7 protein, ataxin-7. *Hum Mol Genet* **8**: 1657–1664.

Klement, I.A., P.J. Skinner, M.D. Kaytor, et al. 1998. Ataxin-1 nuclear localization and aggregation: role in polyglutamine-induced disease in SCA1 transgenic mice. *Cell* **95**:41–53.

Klockgether, T., S. Chamberlain, U. Wullner, et al. 1993. Late-onset Friedreich's ataxia. Molecular genetics, clinical neurophysiology, and magnetic resonance imaging. *Arch Neurol* **50**:803–806.

Klockgether, T., U. Wullner, A. Spauschus, et al. 2000. The molecular biology of the autosomal-dominant cerebellar ataxias. *Mov Disord* **15**: 604–612.

Koide, R., T. Ikeuchi, O. Onodera, et al. 1994. Unstable expansion of CAG repeat in hereditary dentatorubral-pallidoluysian atrophy (DRPLA). *Nat Genet* **6**:9–13.

Koide, R., S. Kobayashi, T. Shimohata, et al. 1999. A neurological disease caused by an expanded CAG trinucleotide repeat in the TATA-binding protein gene: a new polyglutamine disease? *Hum Mol Genet* **8**:2047–2053.

Koeppen, A.H. 2002. Neuropathology of the inherited ataxias. *In* "The cerebellum and its disorders" (M.U. Manto and M. Pandolfo, Eds). Cambridge University Press, New York, pp. 387–405.

Koob, M., K. Benzow, T. Bird, et al. 1998. Rapid cloning of expanded trinucleotide repeat sequences from genomic DNA. *Nat Genet* **18**:72–75.

Koob, M., M. Moseley, L. Schut, et al. 1998. An untranslated CTG expansion causes a novel form of spinocerebellar ataxia (SCA8) *Nat Genet* **21**:379–384.

Koutnikova, H., V. Campuzano, F. Foury, et al. 1997. Studies of human, mouse and yeast homologues indicate a mitochondrial function for frataxin. *Nat Genet* **16**:345–351.

Koyano, S., T. Uchihara, H. Fujigasaki, A. Nakamura, S. Yagishita, and K. Iwabuchi. 1999. Neuronal intranuclear inclusions in spinocerebellar ataxia type 2: triple-labeling immunofluorescent study. *Neurosci Lett* **273**:117–120.

Labuda, M., D. Labuda, C. Miranda, et al. 2000. Unique origin and specific ethnic distribution of the Friedreich ataxia GAA expansion. *Neurology* **54**:2322–2334.

Lavin, M., and Y. Shiloh. 1997. The genetic defect in ataxia-telangiectasia. *Annu Rev Immunol* **15**:177–202.

Le Ber, I., M.C. Moreira, S. Rivaud-Pechoux, C. Chamayou, F. Ochsner, T. Kuntzer, M. Tardieu, G. Said, M.O. Habert, G. Demarquay, C. Tannier, J.M. Beis, A. Brice, M. Koenig, and A. Durr. 2003. Cerebellar ataxia with oculomotor apraxia type 1: clinical and genetic studies. *Brain* **126**:2761–2772.

Lin, K.P., and B.W. Soong. 2002. Peripheral neuropathy of Machado-Joseph disease in Taiwan: a morphometric and genetic study. *Eur Neurol* **48**:210–217.

Litt, M., P. Kramer, D. Browne, S. Gancher, E.R. Brunt, D. Root, T. Phromchotikul, C.J. Dubay, and J. Nutt. 1994. A gene for episodic ataxia/myokymia maps to chromosome 12p13. *Am J Hum Genet* **55**:702–709.

Mariotti, C., A. Solari, D. Torta, L. Marano, C. Fiorentini, and S. Di Donato. 2003. Idebenone treatment in Friedreich patients: One-year-long randomized placebo-controlled trial. *Neurology* **60**:1676–1679.

Matilla, T., V. Volpini, D. Genis, J. Rosell, J. Corral, A. Davalos, A. Molins, and X. Estivill. 1993. Presymptomatic analysis of spinocerebellar ataxia type 1 (SCA1) via the expansion of the SCA1 CAG-repeat in a large pedigree displaying anticipation and parental male bias. *Hum Mol Genet* **2**:2123–2128.

Matilla, T., A. McCall, S. Subramony, et al. 1995. Molecular and clinical correlations in spinocerebellar ataxia type 3 and Machado-Joseph disease. *Ann Neurol* **38**:68–72.

Matsumura, R., N. Futamura, Y. Fujimoto, S. Yanagimoto, H. Horikawa, A. Suzumura, and T. Takayanagi. 1997. Spinocerebellar ataxia type 6. Molecular and clinical features of 35 Japanese patients including one homozygous for the CAG repeat expansion. *Neurology* **49**:1238–1243.

Matsuura, T., T. Yamagata, D. Burgess, et al. 2000. Large expansion of the ATTCT pentanucleotide repeat in spinocerebellar ataxia type 10. *Nat Genet* **26**:191–194.

Matsuyama, Z., H. Kawakami, H. Maruyama, et al. 1997. Molecular features of the CAG repeats of spinocerebellar ataxia 6 (SCA6). *Hum Mol Genet* **6**:1283–1287.

Mizushima, K., M. Watanabe, K. Abe, M. Aoki, Y. Itoyama, M. Shizuka, K. Okamoto, and M. Shoji. 1998. Analysis of spinocerebellar ataxia type 2 in Gunma Prefecture in Japan: CAG trinucleotide expansion and clinical characteristics. *J Neurol Sci* **156**:180–185.

Monckton, D., M. Cayuela, F. Gould, et al. 1999. Very large (CAG)(n) DNA repeat expansions in the sperm of two spinocerebellar ataxia type 7 males. *Hum Mol Genet* **8**:2473–2478.

Moreira, M.C., C. Barbot, N. Tachi, et al. 2001. Homozygosity mapping of Portuguese and Japanese forms of ataxia-oculomotor apraxia to 9p13, and evidence for genetic heterogeneity. *Am J Hum Genet* **68**:501–508.

Moreira, M.C., C. Barbot, N. Tachi, et al. 2001b. The gene mutated in ataxia-ocular apraxia 1 encodes the new HIT/Zn-finger protein aprataxin. *Nat Genet* **29**:189–193.

Moseley, M., L. Schut, T. Bird, et al. 2000. SCA8 CTG repeat: en masse contractions in sperm and intergenerational sequence changes may play a role in reduced penetrance. *Hum Mol Genet* **9**:2125–2130.

Murata, Y., H. Kawakami, S. Yamaguchi, et al. 1998. Characteristic magnetic resonance imaging findings in spinocerebellar ataxia 6. *Arch Neurol* **55**:1348–1352.

Nagafuchi, S., H. Yanagisawa, K. Sato, et al. 1994. Dentatorubral and pallidoluysian atrophy expansion of an unstable CAG trinucleotide on chromosome 12p. *Nat Genet* **6**:14–18.

Nagai, Y., T. Azuma, M. Funauchi, et al. 1998. Clinical and molecular genetic study in seven Japanese families with spinocerebellar ataxia type 6. *J Neurol Sci* **157**:52–59.

Nakamura, K., S. Jeong, T. Uchihara, et al. 2001. SCA17, a novel autosomal dominant cerebellar ataxia caused by an expanded polyglutamine in TATA-binding protein. *Hum Mol Genet* **10**:1441–1448.

Narcisi, T., C. Shoulders, S. Chester, et al. 1995. Mutations of the microsomal triglyceride-transfer-protein gene in abetalipoproteinemia. *Am J Hum Genet* **57**:1298–1310.

Nemes, J., K. Benzow, M. Moseley, et al. 2000. The SCA8 transcript is an antisense RNA to a brain-specific transcript encoding a novel actin-binding protein (KLHL1). *Hum Mol Genet* **9**:1543–1551.

Nielsen, J., S. Sorensen, L. Hasholt, et al. 1996. Dentatorubral-pallidoluysian atrophy. Clinical features of a five-generation Danish family. *Mov Disord* **11**:533–541.

Nystuen, A., P.J. Benke, J. Merren, E.M. Stone, and V.C. Sheffield. 1996. A cerebellar ataxia locus identified by DNA pooling to search for linkage disequilibrium in an isolated population from the Cayman Islands. *Hum Mol Genet* **5**:525–531.

Oh, A., K. Jacobson, J. Jen, et al. 2001. Slowing of voluntary and involuntary saccades: an early sign in spinocerebellar ataxia type 7. *Ann Neurol* **49**:801–804.

Ophoff, R., G. Terwindt, M. Vergouwe, et al. 1996. Familial hemiplegic migraine and episodic ataxia type-2 are caused by mutations in the Ca2+ channel gene CACNL1A4. *Cell* **87**:543–552.

Oppenheimer, D. 1979. Brain lesions in Friedreich's ataxia. *Can J Neurol Sci* **6**:173–176.

Orr, H.T. 2001. Beyond the Qs in the polyglutamine diseases. *Genes Dev* **15**:925–932.

Ouahchi, K., M. Arita, H. Kayden, et al. 1995. Ataxia with isolated vitamin E deficiency is caused by mutations in the alpha-tocopherol transfer protein. *Nat Genet* **9**:141–145.

Pandolfo, M. 2001. Molecular basis of Friedreich ataxia. *Mov Disord* **16**: 815–821.

Potter, N., M. Meyer, A. Zimmerman, et al. 1995. Molecular and clinical findings in a family with dentatorubral-pallidoluysian atrophy. *Ann Neurol* **37**:273–277.

Puccio, H., and M. Koenig. 2000. Recent advances in the molecular pathogenesis of Friedreich ataxia. *Hum Mol Genet* **9**:887–892.

Puccio, H., D. Simon, M. Cossee, et al. 2001. Mouse models for Friedreich ataxia exhibit cardiomyopathy, sensory nerve defect and Fe-S enzyme deficiency followed by intramitochondrial iron deposits. *Nat Genet* **27**:181–186.

Pulst, S., A. Nechiporuk, T. Nechiporuk, et al. 1996. Moderate expansion of a normally biallelic trinucleotide repeat in spinocerebellar ataxia type 2. *Nat Genet* **14**:269–276.

Ragno, M., G. De Michele, F. Cavalcanti, et al. 1997. Broadened Friedreich's ataxia phenotype after gene cloning. Minimal GAA expansion causes late-onset spastic ataxia. *Neurology* **49**:1617–1620.

Rapin, I., Y. Lindenbaum, D. Dickson, et al. 2000. Cockayne syndrome and xeroderma pigmentosum. *Neurology* **55**:1442–1449.

Rasmussen, A., T. Matsuura, L. Ruano, et al. 2001. Clinical and genetic analysis of four Mexican families with spinocerebellar ataxia type 10. *Ann Neurol* **50**:234–239.

Restituito, S., R. Thompson, J. Eliet, et al. 2000. The polyglutamine expansion in spinocerebellar ataxia type 6 causes a beta subunit-specific enhanced activation of P/Q-type calcium channels in Xenopus oocytes. *J Neurosci* **20**:6394–6403.

Riess, O., L. Schols, H. Bottger, et al. 1997. SCA6 is caused by moderate CAG expansion in the alpha1A-voltage-dependent calcium channel gene. *Hum Mol Genet* **6**:1289–1293.

Rolfs, A., A.H. Koeppen, I. Bauer, P. Bauer, S. Buhlmann, H. Topka, L. Schols, and O. Riess. 2003. Clinical features and neuropathology of autosomal dominant spinocerebellar ataxia (SCA17). *Ann Neurol* **54**: 367–375.

Romanul, F., H. Fowler, J. Radvany, et al. 1977. Azorean disease of the nervous system. *N Engl J Med* **296**:1505–1508.

Rosa, A.L., and T. Ashizawa. 2002. Genetic ataxia. *Neurol Clin* **20**: 727–757.

Rustin, P., J. von Kleist-Retzow, K. Chantrel-Groussard, et al. 1999. Effect of idebenone on cardiomyopathy in Friedreich's ataxia: a preliminary study. *Lancet* **354**:477–479.

Sanpei, K., H. Takano, S. Igarashi, et al. 1996. Identification of the spinocerebellar ataxia type 2 gene using a direct identification of repeat expansion and cloning technique, DIRECT. *Nat Genet* **14**:277–284.

Sasaki, H., T. Fukazawa, T. Yanagihara, et al. 1996. Clinical features and natural history of spinocerebellar ataxia type 1. *Acta Neurol Scand* **93**:64–71.

Savitsky, K., A. Bar-Shira, S. Gilad, et al. 1995. A single ataxia telangiectasia gene with a product similar to PI-3 kinase. *Science* **268**:1749–1753.

Schols, L., R. Kruger, G. Amoiridis, H. Przuntek, J.T. Epplen, and O. Riess. 1998. Spinocerebellar ataxia type 6: genotype and phenotype in German kindreds. *J Neurol Neurosurg Psychiatry* **64**:67–73.

Schuelke, M., E. Mayatepek, M. Inter, et al. 1999. Treatment of ataxia in isolated vitamin E deficiency caused by alpha-tocopherol transfer protein deficiency. *J Pediatr* **134**:240–244.

Sharp, D., L. Blinderman, K. Combs, et al. 1993. Cloning and gene defects in microsomal triglyceride transfer protein associated with abetalipoproteinaemia. *Nature* **365**:65–69.

Shimazaki, H., Y. Takiyama, K. Sakoe, et al. 2001. Meiotic instability of the CAG repeats in the SCA6/CACNA1A gene in two Japanese SCA6 families. *J Neurol Sci* **185**:101–107.

Shimazaki, H., Y. Takiyama, K. Sakoe, K. Ikeguchi, K. Niijima, J. Kaneko, M. Namekawa, T. Ogawa, H. Date, S. Tsuji, I. Nakano, and M. Nishizawa. 2002. Early-onset ataxia with ocular motor apraxia and hypoalbuminemia: the aprataxin gene mutations. *Neurology* **59**:590–595.

Shizuka, M., M. Watanabe, Y. Ikeda, et al. 1998. Molecular analysis of a de novo mutation for spinocerebellar ataxia type 6 and (CAG)n repeat units in normal elder controls. *J Neurol Sci* **161**:85–87.

Silveira, I., I. Alonso, L. Guimaraes, et al. 2000. High germinal instability of the (CTG)n at the SCA8 locus of both expanded and normal alleles. *Am J Hum Genet* **66**:830–840.

Skinner, P.J., B.T. Koshy, C.J. Cummings, I.A. Klement, K. Helin, A. Servadio, H.Y. Zoghbi, and H.T. Orr. 1997. Ataxin-1 with an expanded glutamine tract alters nuclear matrix-associated structures. *Nature* **389**: 971–974.

Stevanin, G., A. Durr, G. David, et al. 1997. Clinical and molecular features of spinocerebellar ataxia type 6. *Neurology* **49**:1243–1246.

Stevanin, G., P. Giunti, G. Belal, et al. 1998. De novo expansion of intermediate alleles in spinocerebellar ataxia 7. *Hum Mol Genet* **7**:1809–1813.

Stevanin, G., A. Durr, and A. Brice. 2000a. Clinical and molecular advances in autosomal dominant cerebellar ataxias, from genotype to phenotype and physiopathology. *Eur J Hum Genet* **8**:4–18.

Stevanin, G., A. Herman, A. Durr, et al. 2000b. Are (CTG)n expansions at the SCA8 locus rare polymorphisms? *Nat Genet* **24**:213- 215.

Stevenson, V., and R. Hardie. 2001. Acanthocytosis and neurological disorders. J. Neurol. **248**:87–94.

Stewart, G., R. Maser, T. Stankovic, et al. 1999. The DNA double-strand break repair gene hMRE11 is mutated in individuals with an ataxia-telangiectasia-like disorder. *Cell* **99**:577–587.

Subramony, S.H., J.D. Fratkin, B.V. Manyam, and R.D. Currier. 1996. Dominantly inherited cerebello-olivary atrophy is not due to a mutation at the spinocerebellar ataxia-I, Machado-Joseph disease, or Dentato-Rubro-Pallido-Luysian atrophy locus. *Mov Disord* **11**:174–180.

Subramony, S., P. Vig, and D. McDaniel. 1999. Dominantly inherited ataxias. *Semin Neurol* **19**:419–425.

Sugawara, M., I. Toyoshima, C.Wada, et al. 2000. Pontine atrophy in spinocerebellar ataxia type 6. *Eur Neurol* **43**:17–22.

Takahashi, H., T. Ikeuchi, Y. Honma, S. Hayashi, and S. Tsuji. 1998. Autosomal dominant cerebellar ataxia (SCA6): clinical, genetic and neuropathological study in a family. *Acta Neuropathol (Berl)* **95**:333–337.

Takashima, H., C.F. Boerkoel, J. John, G.M. Saifi, M.A. Salih, D. Armstrong, Y. Mao, F.A. Quiocho, B.B. Roa, M. Nakagawa, D.W. Stockton, and J.R. Lupski. 2002. Mutation of TDP1, encoding a topoisomerase I-dependent DNA damage repair enzyme, in spinocerebellar ataxia with axonal neuropathy. *Nat Genet* **32**:267–272.

Takiyama, Y., K. Sakoe, M. Namekawa, et al. 1998. A Japanese family with spinocerebellar ataxia type 6 which includes three individuals homozygous for an expanded CAG repeat in the SCA6/CACNL1A4 gene. *J Neurol Sci* **158**:141–147.

Tournier-Lasserve, E. 1999. CACNA1A mutations: hemiplegic migraine, episodic ataxia type 2, and the others. *Neurology* **53**:3–4.

Triantafillidis, J., G. Kottaras, S. Sgourous, et al. 1998. A-beta-lipoproteinemia: clinical and laboratory features, therapeutic manipulations, and follow-up study of three members of a Greek family. *J Clin Gastroenterol* **26**:207–211.

Uchihara, T., K. Iwabuchi, N. Funata, and S. Yagishita. 2002. Attenuated nuclear shrinkage in neurons with nuclear aggregates–a morphometric study on pontine neurons of Machado-Joseph disease brains. *Exp Neurol* **178**:124–128.

Verbeek, D.S., J.H. Schelhaas, E.F. Ippel, F.A. Beemer, P.L. Pearson, and R.J. Sinke. 2002. Identification of a novel SCA locus (SCA19) in a Dutch autosomal dominant cerebellar ataxia family on chromosome region 1p21-q21. *Hum Genet* **111**:388–393.

Vincent, J., M. Neves-Pereira, A. Paterson, et al. 2000. An unstable trinucleotide-repeat region on chromosome 13 implicated in spinocerebellar ataxia: a common expansion locus. *Am J Hum Genet* **66**:819–829.

Vuillaume, I., D. Devos, S. Schraen-Maschke, C. Dina, A. Lemainque, F. Vasseur, G. Bocquillon, P. Devos, C. Kocinski, C. Marzys, A. Destee, and B. Sablonniere. 2002. A new locus for spinocerebellar ataxia (SCA21) maps to chromosome 7p21.3–p15.1. *Ann Neurol* **52**:666–670.

Warner, T., L. Williams, R. Walker, et al. 1995. A clinical and molecular genetic study of dentatorubropallidoluysian atrophy in four European families. *Ann Neurol* **37**:452–459.

Worth, P.F., H. Houlden, P. Giunti, et al. 2000. Large, expanded repeats in SCA8 are not confined to patients with cerebellar ataxia. *Nat Genet* **24**:214.

Yamada, M., S. Tsuji, and H. Takahashi. 2000. Pathology of CAG repeat diseases. *Neuropathology* **20**:319–325.

Yamada, M., S. Hayashi, S. Tsuji, and H. Takahashi. 2001. Involvement of the cerebral cortex and autonomic ganglia in Machado-Joseph disease. *Acta Neuropathol (Berl)* **101**:140–144.

Yamada, M., S. Tsuji, and H. Takahashi. 2002. Genotype-phenotype correlation in CAG-repeat diseases. *Neuropathology* **22**:317–322.

Yamashita, I., H. Sasaki, I. Yabe, et al. 2000. A novel locus for dominant cerebellar ataxia (SCA14) maps to a 10.2-cM interval flanked by D19S206 and D19S605 on chromosome 19q13.4-qter. *Ann Neurol* **48**: 156–163.

Yvert, G., K.S. Lindenberg, S. Picaud, et al. 2000. Expanded polyglutamines induce neurodegeneration and transneuronal alterations in cerebellum and retina of SCA7 transgenic mice. *Hum Mol Genet* **9**: 2491–2506.

Zhuchenko, O., J. Bailey, P. Bonnen, et al. 1997. Autosomal dominant cerebellar ataxia (SCA6) associated with small polyglutamine expansions in the alpha 1A-voltage-dependent calcium channel. *Nat Genet* **15**:62–69.

Zoghbi, H.Y. 1995. Spinocerebellar ataxia type 1. *Clin Neurosci* **3**:5–11.

Zoghbi, H.Y., and H.T. Orr. 2000. Glutamine repeats and neurodegeneration. *Ann Rev Neurosc* **23**:217–247.

Zuhlke, C., Y. Hellenbroich, A. Dalski, et al. 2001. Different types of repeat expansion in the TATA-binding protein gene are associated with a new form of inherited ataxia. *Eur J Hum* ••

C H A P T E R

K2

Acquired Ataxias

SUSAN L. PERLMAN

Ataxia is incoordination or clumsiness of movement that is not the result of muscle weakness. It is caused by cerebellar, vestibular, or proprioceptive sensory (large fiber/posterior column) dysfunction. The focus of this chapter will be on acquired disorders causing cerebellar-mediated ataxic symptoms.

Cerebellar ataxia is produced by lesions of the cerebellum or its afferent or efferent connections in the cerebellar peduncles, red nucleus, pons, medulla, or spinal cord. Crossed connections between the frontal cerebral cortex and the cerebellum may allow unilateral frontal disease to mimic a contralateral cerebellar problem.

Cerebellar ataxia causes irregularities in the rate, rhythm, amplitude, and force of voluntary movements, especially at initiation and termination of motion, resulting in "jerky" trajectories (dysynergia), terminal tremor, and overshoot (dysmetria) in limbs. Speech can become dysrhythmic (scanning dysarthria) and articulation slurred, with irregular breath control. Difficulty swallowing or frank choking may also be present. Similar changes can be seen in control of eye movement, with jerky (saccadic) pursuit, gaze-evoked nystagmus, and overshoot. Muscle tone is decreased, resulting in defective posture maintenance and reduced ability to check excessive movement (rebound or sway). Truncal movement is unsteady, feet are held wider apart during standing and walking, and the ability to stand on one foot or with feet together or to walk a straight line is diminished. Altered cerebellar connections to brainstem oculomotor and vestibular nuclei may result in sensations of "dizziness" or environmental movement (oscillopsia). Vestibular ataxia has prominent vertigo (directional spinning sensations) and spares the limbs and speech. Sensory ataxia has no vertigo or dizziness, also spares speech, worsens when the eyes are closed (positive Romberg sign), and is accompanied by decreased vibration and joint position sense.

Cerebellar influence is ipsilateral (the right hemisphere controls the right side of the body), and within the cerebellum are regions responsible for particular functions (midline—gait, head and trunk control, eye movement control; superior vermis—gait; hemispheres—limb tone and control, eye movement control, speech). Cerebellar signs on the neurological exam can help determine whether a process is unilateral or involves the entire cerebellum and whether a particular region of the cerebellum has been targeted (vermis, outflow tracts, etc.). Certain etiologies may then become more likely.

I. DIAGNOSIS OF NON-GENETIC ATAXIA

The genetically-mediated ataxias typically have insidious onset and relatively slow (months to years), symmetrical progression—affecting both sides of the body and moving from the legs to the arms to speech or from midline (gait/trunk) to hemispheric (limb) structures to deep outflow pathways (increasing tremor). Acquired ataxias may have more sudden or subacute onset and progression (weeks to months) and be asymmetrical or frankly focal in presentation. Acute onset with no progression suggests a monophasic insult (injury, vascular event or hemorrhage, anoxia). Subacute onset with progression suggests infectious/inflammatory/immune processes, metabolic or toxic derangements, or neoplastic/mass effects.

The neurological history may provide clues to cause relating to associated illnesses, medication use, or lifestyle/environmental exposures. The neurological examination can be supplemented by neural imaging (brain or spine magnetic resonance scanning/MRI or computed tomography/CT) and electrophysiological studies (electromyogram and nerve conduction/EMG-NCV; evoked potential testing—visual/VER, brainstem/BAER, somatosensory/SSER; electronystagmography of oculomotor and vestibular pathways/ENG; electroencephalogram/EEG), to confirm the anatomic localization of the process and often the actual etiology (mass lesion of a specific type, stroke or hemorrhage, inflammation/infection or vasculitis, demyelination, characteristic regional atrophy). Additional laboratory studies can be ordered (blood; urine; spinal fluid; biopsy of muscle, nerve, or brain). The presence of a known genetic disorder does not rule out the presence of additional acquired insults that might alter the presentation and course of the symptoms of ataxia and warrant further investigation.

Similarly, the absence of a clear family history does not rule out the role of genetic factors in an apparently sporadic disorder. There may be no family history because the history wasn't taken, because the information is unavailable (adoption, loss of contact, non-cooperation, paternity issues), because of non-dominant inheritance patterns (recessive, X-linked, maternal), or because of specific genetic processes (anticipation, incomplete penetrance, mosaicism) that modify disease presentation in the pedigree. Genetic studies of large groups of patients with sporadic ataxia have shown an average of 4–29% with one of the triplet repeat disorders (SCA) and 2–11% with Friedreich ataxia (Futamura et al., 1998; Giuffrida et al., 1999; Hsieh et al., 2000; Jardim et al., 2001; Leggo et al., 1997; Maruyama et al., 2002; Moseley et al., 1998; Pujana et al., 1999; Ramesar et al., 1997; Schols et al., 1997; Schols et al., 1998; Schols et al., 2000; Soong et al., 2001; Storey et al., 2000). Research is also ongoing in the identification of genetic susceptibility factors or genes that may participate in multifactorial pathologic processes affecting the cerebellum (Chataway et al., 1999; Jardim et al., 2003; Li et al., 2003; Sun et al., 2003).

II. PATHOPHYSIOLOGY OF CEREBELLAR DYSFUNCTION

The anatomic, physiologic, and chemical complexity of the cerebellum provides multiple avenues for disruption of normal functioning by a variety of agents and insults. The intracerebellar neuronal network receives sensory input and feedback information from the rest of the neuraxis and projects from the deep cerebellar nuclei to all components of the voluntary and postural motor systems, except the basal ganglia.

Afferent fibers exceed efferent fibers by a ratio of about 40 : 1 and include the glutamatergic climbing fibers (from the contralateral inferior olive) and the faster conducting mossy fibers, as well as other cholinergic and monoaminergic fibers. The climbing fibers and mossy fibers (via the glutamatergic granule cells/parallel fibers) excite the cortex and deep cerebellar nuclei, while the cortex (primarily via the GABAergic Purkinje cells) inhibits the deep nuclei. There are an estimated 15 million Purkinje cells and 10–100 billion granule cells in the adult brain. These cells are the types most frequently lost in diseases of the cerebellum.

The intracerebellar neurons are arranged in three cortical layers—the surface molecular layer, the Purkinje cell layer, and the granular cell layer. Basket cells and stellate cells are the GABAergic inhibitory interneurons of the molecular layer; outnumbering their target Purkinje cells 10 : 1. All three of these cell types share the same parallel fiber input from the granular cell layer. Lugaro cells and Golgi cells are the predominantly GABAergic (possibly also glycine) inhibitory interneurons of the granular cell layer, both receiving input from the Purkinje cells and the latter also from the parallel fibers. The Lugaro cells target the basket and stellate cells, while the Golgi cells modulate mossy fiber/brush cell input to the granule cells. Nitric oxide (released from parallel fibers) and glial structures may also play modulatory roles in the cerebellum.

With the exception of some Purkinje cell projections to the lateral vestibular nuclei, all cerebellar output is from the deep cerebellar nuclei (fastigial nuclei bilaterally to the vestibular and reticular nuclei of the brainstem; interpositus nuclei to the thalamus, red nucleus, pontine nuclei, and superior colliculus; and dentate nuclei to thalamus and red nucleus). In the absence of movement, the output cells maintain a high firing rate, which is modulated during movement and also anticipates movement to aid in initiation.

Any process which interferes with neuronal cell membrane structure; dendrite/axon maintenance; synaptic stability; neurotransmitter production, storage, release, and recovery; energy production; apoptotic equilibrium; or the structure and function of associated glial cells can cause cerebellar dysfunction and disease.

III. CONGENITAL ETIOLOGIES

Congenital ataxic syndromes (without other features such as mental retardation and spasticity) are rare. They present with gross and fine motor delay, feeding problems, titubation of head and trunk when the child begins to try to sit, and nystagmus. Progressive early-onset cerebellar diseases are typically genetically determined (inborn errors of metabolism, X-linked or maternal disorders, early-onset dominant disorders). Congenital non-progressive syndromes are also frequently genetic and include cerebellar/vermian agenesis and hypoplasia (which may be minimally symptomatic); more complex cerebellar dysgenesis disorders (Joubert's syndrome; pontoneocerebellar hypoplasia; granule cell layer hypoplasia; Gillespie syndrome; Paine syndrome; disequilibrium syndrome); and the congenital malformations. The latter conditions, which may have contributory genetic factors or environmental causes of developmental disruption, include the Chiari malformations (types I–IV, of increasing severity of displacement of the cerebellar tonsils, inferior vermis, and associated brainstem regions below the foramen magnum) and the cystic posterior fossa malformations (Dandy-Walker and variants, megacisterna magna, Blake's pouch cyst). These may require surgical intervention to decompress the posterior fossa structures and treat associated dysraphism, meningomyelocele, and hydrocephalus.

The cerebellum has the longest period of embryological development of any major structure of the brain, beginning at 32 days post-fertilization and not completing neuronal migration until one year post-natally, remaining vulnerable to teratogenic insult throughout. The flocculonodular lobe (archicerebellum or vestibulocerebellum) forms at 8–9 weeks; the paleocerebellum or spinocerebellum (anterior vermis, followed in 30–60 days by its associated hemispheric tissue) forms at 10–11 weeks; and the neocerebellum (posterior vermis, followed by it associated hemisphere) forms at 13–14 weeks. Most malformation syndromes involve the paleocerebellum. Partial aplasia affects the caudal portion rather than the rostral, due to this craniocaudal pattern of formation.

Lhermitte-Duclos syndrome, a focal enlargement of the cerebellum, represents a failure of migration of the Purkinje cells, with reactive hypertrophy of the granule cells, forming a cerebellar gangliocytoma (Lhermitte & Duclos, 1920).

The most common acquired, non-progressive, congenital cerebellar syndromes are caused by peri-natal trauma and hypercoagulable or hemorrhagic vascular events ("ataxic cerebral palsy") (Mercuri et al., 1997; Nelson & Lynch, 2004; Ozduman et al., 2004). Fetal stroke is estimated to complicate 1 in 4000 full-term births.

IV. TRAUMATIC AND VASCULAR ETIOLOGIES

Open or closed head injury, with traumatic brain injury, is a leading cause of death in children and young adults (Goldstein, 1990). 100,000 survivors per year will have long-term disabling residua, and 2% will live in a persistent vegetative state. Head injury is most often a result of car or motorcycle accidents (49%), often complicated by alcohol intake (Kraus et al., 1989). Accidental falls in the elderly account for 29% of cases of head injury, and 90% of significant intracranial injury in infants is due to child abuse (Billmire & Myers, 1985). Major injuries within the posterior fossa are seen in 3.3% of all head trauma (Tsai et al., 1980), usually intra-axial brainstem (36%) or cerebellar (25%) parenchymal damage, and less commonly epidural (25%) or subdural (14%) hematomas and subarachnoid hemorrhage.

Cerebellar parenchymal injury can be via concussion, contusion, diffuse axonal injury from shearing forces, or delayed intracerebellar hematoma. Progressive post-traumatic events include free radical release and excitotoxicity, cell membrane and blood-brain barrier dysfunction, and release of inflammatory cytokines and vasoreactive substances, which can lead to edema and increased intracranial pressure (Miller, 1993). Traumatic dissection of vertebral arteries (especially following neck injury), direct vessel damage associated with skull fracture, or spasm of basal arteries due to subarachnoid hemorrhage may lead to embolic or ischemic cerebellar stroke. Vertebral artery dissection usually leads to occlusion of the posterior inferior cerebellar artery and features of the lateral medullary syndrome (Wallenberg's syndrome—unilateral Horner's syndrome with eyelid droop/ptosis and small pupil/miosis, as well as loss of pain and temperature sensation on the opposite side). In severe head trauma, localizing cerebellar symptoms and signs may be overshadowed by altered level of consciousness or associated brainstem or supratentorial damage.

Treatment centers on support of vital functions, control of increased intracranial pressure, surgical intervention for space-occupying lesions (evacuation of hematomas and decompression for diffuse brain swelling), and ultimately intensive rehabilitation to enhance plastic neuronal change and outcome. Long-term complications of cerebellar injury include delayed-onset tremor from reorganization of outflow pathways (Louis et al., 1996), segmental myoclonus (eg. palatal myoclonus) from disruption of the dentate-rubro-olivary pathway and olivary hypertrophy (Kawata et al., 1996), and superficial siderosis (deposition of hemosiderin from hemorrhage on the leptomeninges), which can lead to cerebellar signs and hearing loss (Bracchi et al., 1993).

Cerebellar stroke can be ischemic (arterial embolic or atherosclerotic thrombosis), hemorrhagic (10%), mixed (ischemia with secondary bleed, hemorrhage with vasospasm), or due to thrombosis of cerebellar venous structures and results in symptoms and signs in the vascular territory affected. The posterior inferior cerebellar artery arises from the vertebral artery and supplies the posterior and caudal cerebellum. Deficits in its distribution include the lateral medullary syndrome described above; ipsilateral impairment of facial sensation; ipsilateral limb incoordination and tremor; and ataxia of gait, trouble swallowing, vertigo, and eye movement abnormalities. The anterior inferior cerebellar artery arises from the first third of the basilar artery and supplies the pons, middle cerebellar peduncle, and the flocculus. Stroke in these areas causes ipsilateral impairment of facial sensation and strength; ipsilateral limb incoordination; altered speech and swallowing; vertigo and tinnitus; and some ataxia of gait and impaired sensation of the contralateral body. The superior cerebellar artery arises from the top of the basilar artery and supplies the superior cerebellum. Loss of its blood supply causes primarily ipsilateral limb incoordination and tremor; ataxia of gait; altered speech; and some eye movement abnormalities. Stroke in the distribution of the superior cerebellar artery is most likely to result in later onset of palatal or jaw myoclonus (Freeman & Jaffe, 1941). Thrombosis of the veins draining from the cerebellar surface into the transverse sinus or of the superior vermian vein into the vein of Galen causes bilateral cerebellar signs and is seen in hypercoagulable states, including pregnancy, oral contraceptive use, and diabetics with the hyperosmolar state; with infections near the base of the skull; and as a complication of intracranial surgery (Andeweg, 1999).

Cerebellar infarction may also lead to regional cerebellar edema with increased posterior fossa pressures, delayed loss of consciousness, and the risk in 20–25% of potentially lethal brainstem compression, tonsillar herniation, and acute hydrocephalus (Amarenco, 1991).

As with cerebellar trauma, treatment is supportive, with close monitoring for complications and the use of intensive rehabilitation to ensure optimal recovery. Thrombolytic therapy for acute ischemic stroke increases reperfusion and may improve the ability of patients to survive stroke without disability (Hacke et al., 1988). Risk factors for recurrent stroke (hypertension, hyperlipidemia, diabetes, hypercoagulable factors, cigarette smoking, vascular stenosis, embolic sites) need to be identified and addressed and the use of antiplatelet agents considered.

Risk factors for hemorrhage include complications of anticoagulation therapy, other coagulation disorders, trauma, brain metastases, and vascular defects (aneurysm, arteriovenous malformation, angioma, hemangioblastoma), some of which may be familial (eg. Von Hippel Lindau disease) and require genetic consultation and counseling, in addition to possible surgical intervention.

V. INFECTIOUS ETIOLOGIES

Infectious agents of all classes can target the central nervous system directly or via exotoxins (eg. pertussis (Askelof & Gillenius, 1982; Setta et al., 1999)), via delayed antigen-antibody reactions involving molecular mimicry (eg. antigens of infectious agents and epitopes in the cerebellum), via mechanisms not completely understood (eg. cerebellar degeneration associated with HIV infection (Tagliati et al., 1998)), and possibly from the deleterious effects of high fever on cerebellar neurons (Yaqub et al., 1987). Causative organisms can usually be identified by visualization or culture from spinal fluid samples. Antibodies specific for the infectious agent can also be detected. There may be evidence for increased synthesis of immunoglobulins in the central nervous system (elevated cerebrospinal fluid IgG synthesis rates), although this is also seen in some non-infectious CNS inflammatory conditions. Rarely brain biopsy will be necessary to establish an infectious etiology. Treatment utilizes appropriate anti-microbial regimens (broad coverage often being started before the culture results are ready, then modified for the specific agent found), as well as supportive measures, steroids for associated brain edema, and, when necessary, surgical intervention (decompression, shunting).

Bacteria may gain access to the brain by colonizing and locally invading the mucous membranes of the nasopharynx with direction extension to the meninges. Alternatively, bacteria can spread hematogenously to the subarachnoid space and meninges, where the resultant inflammatory reaction promotes blood-brain barrier permeability, vasogenic edema, altered blood flow/stroke, and possible direct neuronal toxicity. Typical early symptoms can be fever, confusion, headache, vomiting, and neck stiffness, followed by focal neurological signs. Bacteria may also enter the nervous system through anatomic defects in the skull or parameningeal sites, such as the paranasal sinuses or middle ear. Individuals with a history of head trauma, prior neurosurgery, alcoholism, tuberculosis, cancer, or immunodeficiency are at greater risk to develop infection (Garvey, 1983).

Children with complications of otologic infection or with cyanotic heart disease and patients with septic emboli related to other chronic systemic disease may develop cerebellar abscess, where the initial headache and ataxia may be quickly superceded by signs of altered consciousness, brainstem compression, obstructive hydrocephalus, and tonsillar herniation, necessitating urgent surgical intervention.

The most common bacterial pathogens are enteric Streptococcal species, *Escherichia coli*, and *Listeria monocytogenes* in infants; *Neisseria meningitides* (meningococcus), *Strep. pneumoniae* (pneumococcus), and *Haemophilus influenzae* in children and young adults; and *Strep. pneumoniae*, *Listeria monocytogenes*, and Gram-negative bacilli in older adults and in individuals with impaired cellular immunity. Immunization is available against *Haemophilus influenzae* for children; against *Neisseria meningitides* for military recruits, college students, and those in areas of ongoing epidemics; and against *Strep. pneumoniae* for older adults and splenectomized patients. Patients with head injury, neurosurgery, or a cerebrospinal fluid shunt are more likely to develop Staphylococcal and Gram-negative bacilli infections (Quagliarello & Scheld, 1997).

Tuberculous granulomas affecting the basal meninges and arteries (causing cranial neuropathies and stroke) usually result from reactivation of earlier latent infection that seeded the meninges and surface of the brain. Individuals with a history of pulmonary tuberculosis, alcoholism, steroid treatment, HIV infection, or other conditions that impair the immune response are at greatest risk for this.

Tropheryma whippelii, an actinomycete (filamentous bacterial class, which also includes *Nocardia*) and the causative bacterium of **Whipple's disease**, leads to granulomatous infection of the small intestine, regional lymph nodes, liver, heart, lungs, and central nervous system, preferentially the deep brain structures and cerebellum. Gastrointestinal and joint symptoms are prominent, with associated cerebellar ataxia, myoclonus/myorhythmia (classically affecting visual convergence, jaw, tongue, and neck muscles), dementia, seizures, insomnia, hyperphagia, and polydipsia (Perkin & Murray-Lyon, 1998). Accurate diagnosis may require duodenal or brain biopsy, with PCR assay for *T. whippelii*-specific DNA sequences (Lynch et al., 1997). Aggressive and lengthy antibiotic treatment (up to two years) may stop progression of neurological signs, but cerebellar deficits may remain disabling. Disease can recur in one third of cases (Singer, 1998).

Spirochetal infections (Lyme disease, syphilis) typically manifest neurologic signs weeks to years after the primary infection, in both central (meningitis, meningoencephalitis, cranial neuropathies) and peripheral (spinal radiculopathies, peripheral neuropathies) locations. The ataxia of syphilis (tabes dorsalis) is sensory in origin, due to involvement of dorsal root ganglia and posterior columns.

Systemic **fungal infections** may invade the central nervous system hematogenously from internal organ or skin sites or by direct extension from parameningeal sites (orbits, paranasal sinuses), causing meningitis, focal abscess, parenchymal granulomas, infarction due to vasculitis, or communicating hydrocephalus. Their clinical presentation can resemble that of tuberculosis. Diabetes, carcinoma, hematological malignancy, AIDS, organ transplantation, steroid or cytotoxic drug treatment, prolonged antibiotic therapy, and intravenous drug use predispose to these often opportunistic infections, which include cryptococcus, coccidioides, candida, aspergillus, mucor, histoplasma, and blastomyces. Anti-fungal therapy has frequent complications, may require long-term maintenance regimens, and may not prevent neurological residua.

Parasitic infections (protozoal—*malaria, toxoplasma, naegleria, acanthamoeba*; helminthic—*cysticercosis, angiostrongylus*; rickettsial—*Rocky Mountain spotted fever*) are also more common in immunocompromised patients and cause meningoencephalitic symptoms (altered mental status, seizures, myoclonus, ataxia) or focal mass lesions.

Viral and viral-associated cerebellar syndromes can present as a straightforward cerebellitis or a more complicated illness with extracerebellar features (dystonia, myoclonus, brainstem signs, seizures, altered mental status). They can occur within hours of the acute infection or develop slowly over a month, implying both direct infectious or toxic mechanisms and delayed, post-infectious, immune-mediated demyelination. Many infectious agents have been documented to precede an acute/subacute cerebellitis. In children the most common viruses are varicella (1 in 1000 cases of varicella infection will develop ataxia), measles, mumps, rubella, infectious mononucleosis, parvovirus B19, and hepatitis A. Rubella infection contracted in utero may also cause a chronic progressive panencephalitis with prominent ataxia, similar to subacute sclerosing panencephalitis that may follow measles infection. Cerebellitis has also been seen following vaccination for diphtheria-tetanus-pertussis, mumps-measles-rubella, varicella, influenza, and hepatitis B (Mancini et al., 1996; Sunaga et al., 1995).

In adults, Epstein-Barr virus, influenza, parainfluenza, the enteroviruses (polio, coxsackie, echo), herpes simplex virus, varicella zoster virus, cytomegalovirus, adenovirus, HIV-1, and mumps are reported, but the causative agent cannot be identified in up to 35% of cases (Klockgether et al., 1993).

Children and young adults with acute cerebellitis have an 80–90% chance for good functional recovery within seven to eight months, with minimal residua in 10–40% and rare cerebellar atrophy (Hayakawa & Katoh, 1995). Older patients may not recover as favorably as those less than 40 years of age, being more likely to be left with permanent cerebellar disability and cerebellar atrophy.

Anti-viral agents (eg. acyclovir) started within the first few days of a viral infection (eg. Varicella) can reduce the duration and severity of the acute illness, but may not interfere with the subsequent immunologic response (Dangond et al., 1993). The effect of steroids on modifying the outcome of viral-mediated cerebellitis is also not confirmed, although adrenocorticotrophic hormone (ACTH) reduces symptoms in up to 85% of children with post-viral opsoclonus-myoclonus syndrome ("dancing eyes-dancing feet"). Plasmapheresis and high-dose intravenous immunoglobulin therapy have been used to try to stop the progression of ataxia in the Miller-Fisher variant of Guillain-Barré syndrome, a post-infectious disorder which may include ataxia, ophthalmoplegia, and areflexia (Zifko et al., 1994) and has been associated with IgG antibodies directed against GQ1b or GT1b ganglioside (Nagashima et al., 2004).

Individuals with altered cell-mediated immunity (AIDS, lymphoma, inherited immunodeficiency syndromes) are at risk of developing **progressive multifocal leukoencephalopathy (PML)**, a severe demyelinating disease of the central nervous system. It begins focally, usually in the parieto-occipital white matter and progresses over weeks to months, causing altered mental status, visual deficits, and motor weakness. The cerebellum is affected in 13% (Jones et al., 1982). It is caused by a neurotropic papovavirus (JC virus), which is transported from the kidney by infected B-lymphocytes to the brain, where it may persist as a latent infection of oligodendroglia until it is reactivated during the immunosuppressed state (Brink & R.F., 1996).

Sporadic Creutzfeldt-Jakob disease (sCJD), the most common of the human prion disorders (transmissible spongiform encephalopathies/TSE), typically presents in the seventh decade as a rapidly progressive dementia with myoclonus, but may also have an ataxic form. There may be an incubation period of months to years after exposure (dietary, corneal transplantation or dura mater grafting of infected tissues, treatment with cadaveric human growth hormone). Variant Creutzfeldt-Jakob disease has earlier onset (third decade) and prominent psychiatric and ataxic features, and it may relate to human exposure to bovine spongiform encephalopathy ("mad-cow disease"). Diagnosis may be difficult clinically, but electroencephalography, brain magnetic resonance scanning with diffusion-weighted imaging, and specialized spinal fluid studies can be helpful. Brain biopsy may be necessary to confirm this diagnosis (Will, 2003).

VI. NEOPLASTIC AND PARANEOPLASTIC ETIOLOGIES

Primary or metastatic tumors, complications of antineoplastic therapy (surgery, radiation, and chemotherapy), delayed-onset superficial siderosis, secondary vascular and infectious lesions, and the remote effects of cancer (most often felt to be immune-mediated) can all affect the cerebellum.

Space-occupying lesions of the posterior fossa can directly damage regions of the cerebellum or cause mass effects (herniations, obstructive hydrocephalus, increased intracranial pressure) manifesting initially as headache, vomiting, and papilledema, and progressing to focal brainstem deficits, altered levels of consciousness, cardiorespiratory instability, and death.

Cerebellar medulloblastomas represent 20% of pediatric primary brain tumors and are also associated with certain inherited disorders (eg. ataxia-telangiectasia, basal cell nevus syndrome). Cerebellar astrocytomas (10–20%), as well as fourth ventricle ependymomas (10–20%) and brainstem gliomas (10–20%), are also more common in children (Ullrich & Pomeroy, 2003). Metastatic disease to the cerebellum, as well as extrinsic meningiomas and schwannomas are more common in adults (Zabek, 2003). Meningiomas and schwannomas may present before the age of twenty in patients with neurofibromatosis type 1 or 2 (von Recklinghausen's disease). Rarer tumors are the cerebellar hemagioblastomas (a common manifestation in the dominantly inherited von Hippel Lindau disease), the congenital ectodermally-derived epidermoid and dermoid cysts, primary central nervous system lymphomas, and the quasineoplasm syndromes—Lhermitte-Duclos disease (dysplastic cerebellar gangliocytoma) and Langerhans' cell histiocytosis (eosinophilic granuloma, causing ataxia with diabetes insipidus).

The paraneoplastic cerebellar syndromes evolve slowly over weeks to months, may present up to five years before an occult carcinoma manifests itself, and can be identified in approximately 50% of patients by antibodies in serum or cerebrospinal fluid. Anti-Yo antibodies are associated with ovarian and breast cancer and target certain Purkinje cell cytoplasmic 34 and 62 kD proteins (Drlicek et al., 1997; Furneaux et al., 1990). Anti-Ri antibodies are also associated with breast and gynecologic tumors, but target 55 and 80 kD proteins found in all neuronal nuclei and cause a specific syndrome of opsoclonus and myoclonus, distinct from the syndrome seen with small cell lung cancer and neuroblastoma. Anti-Hu (small cell lung cancer; targeting a 35–40 kD neuronal nuclear protein), anti-CV2 (small cell lung cancer, uterine sarcoma, malignant thymoma; targeting a 66 kD oligodentrocyte cytoplasmic protein), anti-Tr (Hodgkin's lymphoma; targeting Purkinje cell body and dendrites), and anti-Ma1 (parotid, breast, and colon cancer; targeting a 37 kD neuronal protein) cause cerebellar degeneration similar to the anti-Yo syndrome. Diagnostic evaluation should include a brain magnetic resonance imaging study, serum or cerebrospinal fluid studies for paraneoplastic antibodies, and an aggressive evaluation for occult neoplasm, if the source is not already known. Treatment consists of removal of the source of the antibody (the underlying tumor) and suppression of the immune response (plasmapheresis; intravenous immunoglobulin infusion; anti-T and B cell drugs, eg. tacrolimus, mycophenolate mofetil; or other immunosuppressant agents, eg. corticosteroids, cyclophosphamide) (Darnell & Posner, 2003). Recovery depends on stopping the cerebellar disease process before there is significant loss of Purkinje cells (Graus et al., 1992).

VII. OTHER IMMUNE-MEDIATED ETIOLOGIES

Antibodies directed against the cerebellum have been found in other cerebellar syndromes not related to prior viral infection or underlying carcinoma.

Gluten enteropathy (celiac sprue) is associated with immune-mediated neurologic disease, due to cross-reacting antibodies produced in response to the gluten sensitive small bowel disorder. Anti-gliadin antibodies target the Purkinje cell and can be seen in individuals without gastrointestinal symptoms or the tissue transglutaminase and endomysial antibodies associated with the gut disease. They are reported to occur in up to 27% of individuals with sporadic ataxia and 37% of patients with dominantly inherited ataxia, possibly as a result of Purkinje cell degeneration and antigen release. The pathologic role of these antibodies and the effect of the gluten-free diet or immunomodulating therapy is under investigation in this syndrome (Bushara et al., 2001; Hadjivassiliou et al., 2003a; Hadjivassiliou et al., 2003b).

In insulin-dependent diabetes, antibodies directed against glutamic acid decarboxylase in spinal cord are known to cause stiff-person syndrome and, in rare cases, cerebellar ataxia (Iwasaki et al., 2001; Kono et al., 2001). This is suspected to be due to a functional decline in GABA neurons in spinal cord and cerebellum, as a result of presynaptic impairment of inhibitory synapses (Mitoma et al., 2000). It may be steroid-responsive (Lauria et al., 2003).

VIII. METABOLIC AND TOXIC ETIOLOGIES

Several acquired **endocrine disorders** are associated with cerebellar ataxia, usually related to thyroid dysfunction or a disturbance of calcium/parathyroid metabolism. These conditions will typically show signs of endocrine as well as neurologic disease.

Hypothyroidism in adults manifests a slowly progressive superior vermian syndrome, with gait instability and truncal titubation and less common involvement of eye movement and arms. Cognitive dysfunction, seizures, myoclonus, deep tendon reflex changes, and myopathy may also be present (Harayama et al., 1983). Hyperthyroidism (eg. as seen in Hashimoto's thyroiditis) may cause postural tremor and episodic gait ataxia, as well as motor unit fasciculations, choreoathetosis, seizures, confusion, and psychiatric symptoms. While the deficits in Hashimoto's are felt to be immune-mediated and may respond to steroids, the hyperthyroid-related reduction of low density lipoproteins and associated reduction in vitamin E levels (as also seen in abeta/hypobetalipoproteinemia) may also contribute to the cerebellar dysfunction (Asayama et al., 1989). Amiodarone treatment can interfere with thyroid function and may contribute to ataxia on that basis.

Hypo- and hyperparathyroidism (primary, secondary, and pseudo) are associated with cerebellar dysfunction, but the mechanism is not fully understood.

Many **toxic exposures** can target the cerebellum, the most common being ethanol consumption, which has been found to affect the structure and function of both granule and Purkinje cells in animals. 27–47% of individuals with alcoholism will develop cerebellar degeneration (Torvik, 1987), primarily in the superior vermis, but frequently affecting other parts of the neuraxis (Fadda & Rossetti, 1998). Anti-convulsant medication (phenytoin, carbamazepine, barbiturates, gabapentin, lamotrigine, topiramate, vigabatrin), anti-neoplastics (cytosine arabinoside, 5-fluorouracil, methotrexate), and other agents (amiodarone, bismuth, bromides, cimetidine, cyclosporin, isoniazid, lindane, lithium, mefloquine, perhexiline maleate) can cause cerebellar dysfunction, either acutely or with chronic use. Heavy metal intoxication (germanium, lead, manganese, mercury, methylmercury, thallium), exposure to benzene or toluene derivatives, insecticide/herbicide poisoning (carbon disulfide, chlordecone, phosphin), and recreational drug use (cocaine, heroin, phencyclidine) can all cause irreversible cerebellar damage. Purkinje cells are extremely sensitive to hyperthermic damage, anoxia (including carbon monoxide poisoning), and any process that interferes with oxidative metabolism (acute and chronic B vitamin deficiencies—eg. thiamine, vitamin B12; cyanide poisoning; certain shellfish neurotoxins—eg. saxitoxin from *Mylilus*) (Manto & Jacquy, 2002).

IX. NON-GENETIC ATAXIAS OF UNKNOWN ETIOLOGY

In a study of 112 patients with sporadic ataxia (Abele et al., 2002), with onset after the age of 20 (median age 56) and with no identifiable family history or other cause, 29% met criteria for possible or probable multiple system atrophy, 13% had an unexpected genetically-mediated ataxia (6% SCA6, 3% SCA3, 1% SCA2, 4% Friedreich ataxia), and 58% remained with unknown etiology. 15% of these unknowns were positive for anti-gliadin antibodies (none had anti-GAD antibodies), but 9% of the inherited ataxias were also positive.

Currently, over half the adults presenting with late-onset, sporadic cerebellar ataxia will not be able to be given a specific diagnosis or prognosis. Some will progress rapidly, others indolently. All will suffer some disability. About one-third will develop multiple system atrophy, with its severe morbidity and mortality. Some will ultimately be found to suffer from as yet unknown processes related to the immune system or environmental factors or cerebellar homeostasis. Basic research with the animal models of cerebellar disease will shed much needed light on the etiology and pathophysiology of cerebellar ataxia and ultimately reveal pathways to treatment.

Video Legends

Congenital cerebellar hypoplasia in a 7-year-old male

SEGMENT 1 Primary position and gaze-evoked nystagmus

SEGMENT 2 Mild limb dysarthria

SEGMENT 3 Mild difficulty with tandem gait

Immune-mediated cerebellar ataxia of five years' duration in a 55-year-old male

SEGMENT 1 Moderate limb dysmetria

SEGMENT 2 Moderate gait ataxia with widened base and truncal instability requiring bilateral support

Idiopathic late-onset ataxia of two years' duration in a 68-year-old male

SEGMENT 1 Moderate dysarthria with scanning type speech

SEGMENT 2 Moderate arm dysmetria

SEGMENT 3 Moderate leg dysmetria with terminal tremor. This patient is unable to walk.

References

Abele, M., K. Burk, L. Schols, S. Schwartz, I. Besenthal, J. Dichgans, C. Zuhlke, O. Riess, and T. Klockgether. 2002. The aetiology of sporadic adult-onset ataxia. *Brain* **125**:961–968.

Amarenco, P. 1991. The spectrum of cerebellar infarctions. *Neurology* **41**: 973–979.

Andeweg, J. 1999. Consequences of the anatomy of deep venous outflow from the brain. *Neuroradiology* **41**:233–241.

Asayama, K., K. Dobashi, H. Hayashibe, and K. Kato. 1989. Vitamin E protects against thyroxine-induced acceleration of lipid peroxidation in cardiac and skeletal muscles in rats. *J Nutr Sci Vitaminol (Tokyo)* **35**:407–418.

Askelof, P., and P. Gillenius. 1982. Effect of lymphocytosis-promoting factor from Bordetella pertussis on cerebellar cyclic GMP levels. *Infect Immun* **36**:958–961.

Billmire, M.E., and P.A. Myers. 1985. Serious head injury in infants: accident or abuse? *Pediatrics* **75**:340–342.

Bracchi, M., M. Savoiardo, F. Triulzi, D. Daniele, M. Grisoli, G.B. Bradac, C. Agostinis, D. Pelucchetti, and G. Scotti. 1993. Superficial siderosis of the CNS: MR diagnosis and clinical findings. *AJNR Am J Neuroradiol* **14**:227–236.

Brink, N.S., and R.F.M. 1996. Clinical presentation, diagnosis, and therapy of progressive multifocal leukoencephalopathy. *J Infect* **32**:97–102.

Bushara, K.O., S.U. Goebel, H. Shill, L.G. Goldfarb, and M. Hallett. 2001. Gluten sensitivity in sporadic and hereditary cerebellar ataxia. *Ann Neurol* **49**:540–543.

Chataway, J., S. Sawcer, F. Coraddu, R. Feakes, S. Broadley, H.B. Jones, D. Clayton, J. Gray, P.N. Goodfellow, and A. Compston. 1999. Evidence that allelic variants of the spinocerebellar ataxia type 2 gene influence susceptibility to multiple sclerosis. *Neurogenetics* **2**:91–96.

Dangond, F., E. Engle, L. Yessayan, and M.H. Sawyer. 1993. Pre-eruptive varicella cerebellitis confirmed by PCR. *Pediatr Neurol* **9**:491–493.

Darnell, R.B., and J.B. Posner. 2003. Paraneoplastic syndromes involving the nervous system. *N Engl J Med* **349**:1543–1554.

Drlicek, M., G. Bianchi, G. Bogliun, B. Casati, W. Grisold, C. Kolig, U. Liszka-Setinek, L. Marzorati, E. Wondrusch, and G. Cavaletti. 1997. Antibodies of the anti-Yo and anti-Ri type in the absence of paraneoplastic neurological syndromes: a long-term survey of ovarian cancer patients. *J Neurol* **244**:85–89.

Fadda, F., and Z.L. Rossetti. 1998. Chronic ethanol consumption: from neuroadaptation to neurodegeneration. *Prog Neurobiol* **56**:385–431.

Freeman, W., and D. Jaffe. 1941. Occlusion of superior cerebellar artery: Report of a case with necropsy. *Arch. Neurol. Psychiatry* **46**:115–126.

Furneaux, H.M., M.K. Rosenblum, J. Dalmau, E. Wong, P. Woodruff, F. Graus, and J.B. Posner. 1990. Selective expression of Purkinje-cell antigens in tumor tissue from patients with paraneoplastic cerebellar degeneration. *N Engl J Med* **322**:1844–1851.

Futamura, N., R. Matsumura, Y. Fujimoto, H. Horikawa, A. Suzumura, and T. Takayanagi. 1998. CAG repeat expansions in patients with sporadic cerebellar ataxia. *Acta Neurol Scand* **98**:55–59.

Garvey, G. 1983. Current concepts of bacterial infections of the central nervous system. Bacterial meningitis and bacterial brain abscess. *J Neurosurg* **59**:735–744.

Giuffrida, S., R. Saponara, A. Trovato Salinaro, D.A. Restivo, E. Domina, M. Papotto, F. Le Pira, A. Nicoletti, A. Trovato, and D.F. Condorelli. 1999. Identification of SCA2 mutation in cases of spinocerebellar ataxia with no family history in mid-eastern Sicily. *Ital J Neurol Sci* **20**:217–221.

Goldstein, M. 1990. Traumatic brain injury: a silent epidemic. *Ann Neurol* **27**:327.

Graus, F., F. Vega, J.Y. Delattre, I. Bonaventura, R. Rene, D. Arbaiza, and E. Tolosa. 1992. Plasmapheresis and antineoplastic treatment in CNS paraneoplastic syndromes with antineuronal autoantibodies. *Neurology* **42**:536–540.

Hacke, W., H. Zeumer, A. Ferbert, H. Bruckmann, and G.J. del Zoppo. 1988. Intra-arterial thrombolytic therapy improves outcome in patients with acute vertebrobasilar occlusive disease. *Stroke* **19**:1216–1222.

Hadjivassiliou, M., G.A. Davies-Jones, D.S. Sanders, and R.A. Grunewald. 2003a. Dietary treatment of gluten ataxia. *J Neurol Neurosurg Psychiatry* **74**:1221–1224.

Hadjivassiliou, M., R. Grunewald, B. Sharrack, D. Sanders, A. Lobo, C. Williamson, N. Woodroofe, N. Wood, and A. Davies-Jones. 2003b. Gluten ataxia in perspective: epidemiology, genetic susceptibility and clinical characteristics. *Brain* **126**:685–691.

Harayama, H., T. Ohno, and T. Miyatake. 1983. Quantitative analysis of stance in ataxic myxoedema. *J Neurol Neurosurg Psychiatry* **46**:579–581.

Hayakawa, H., and T. Katoh. 1995. Severe cerebellar atrophy following acute cerebellitis. *Pediatr Neurol* **12**:159–161.

Hsieh, M., S.J. Lin, J.F. Chen, H.M. Lin, K.M. Hsiao, S.Y. Li, C. Li, and C.J. Tsai. 2000. Identification of the spinocerebellar ataxia type 7 mutation in Taiwan: application of PCR-based Southern blot. *J Neurol* **247**:623–629.

Iwasaki, H., R. Sato, M. Shichiri, and Y. Hirata. 2001. A patient with type 1 diabetes mellitus and cerebellar ataxia associated with high titer of circulating anti-glutamic acid decarboxylase antibodies. *Endocr J* **48**: 261–268.

Jardim, L., I. Silveira, M.L. Pereira, M. do Ceu Moreira, P. Mendonca, J. Sequeiros, and R. Giugliani. 2003. Searching for modulating effects of SCA2, SCA6 and DRPLA CAG tracts on the Machado-Joseph disease (SCA3) phenotype. *Acta Neurol Scand* **107**:211–214.

Jardim, L.B., I. Silveira, M.L. Pereira, A. Ferro, I. Alonso, M. do Ceu Moreira, P. Mendonca, F. Ferreirinha, J. Sequeiros, and R. Giugliani. 2001. A survey of spinocerebellar ataxia in South Brazil—66 new cases with Machado-Joseph disease, SCA7, SCA8, or unidentified disease-causing mutations. *J Neurol* **248**:870–876.

Jones, H.R., E.T. Hedley Whyte, S.R. Friedberg, J.E. Kelleher, and J. Krolikowski. 1982. Primary cerebellopontine mutlitfocal leucoencephalopathy diagnosed premortem by cerebellar biopsy. *Ann Neurol* **11**:199–202.

Kawata, Y., T. Suzuki, H. Kagaya, R. Omi, H. Shiroto, and K. Ebina. 1996. An MRI analysis of brain-stem and cerebellar lesions and olivary hypertrophy. *Neuroradiology* **38**:441–443.

Klockgether, T., G. Doller, U. Wullner, D. Petersen, and J. Dichgans. 1993. Cerebellar encephalitis in adults. *J Neurol* **240**:17–20.

Kono, S., H. Miyajima, M. Sugimoto, Y. Suzuki, Y. Takahashi, and A. Hishida. 2001. Stiff-person syndrome associated with cerebellar ataxia and high glutamic acid decarboxylase antibody titer. *Intern Med* **40**: 968–971.

Kraus, J.F., H. Morgenstern, D. Fife, C. Conroy, and P. Nourjah. 1989. Blood alcohol tests, prevalence of involvement, and outcomes following brain injury. *Am J Public Health* **79**:294–299.

Lauria, G., D. Pareyson, M.G. Pitzolu, and E. Bazzigaluppi. 2003. Excellent response to steroid treatment in anti-GAD cerebellar ataxia. *Lancet Neurol* **2**:634–635.

Leggo, J., A. Dalton, P.J. Morrison, A. Dodge, M. Connarty, M.J. Kotze, and D.C. Rubinsztein. 1997. Analysis of spinocerebellar ataxia types 1, 2, 3, and 6, dentatorubral-pallidoluysian atrophy, and Friedreich's ataxia genes in spinocerebellar ataxia patients in the UK. *J Med Genet* **34**: 982–985.

Lhermitte, J., and P. Duclos. 1920. Sur un ganlioneurome diffus du cortex du cervelet. *Bull Assoc Fancaise Etude Cancer* **9**:99M12.

Li, Y.J., S.A. Oliveira, P. Xu, E.R. Martin, J.E. Stenger, C.R. Scherzer, M.A. Hauser, W.K.Scott, G.W. Small, M.A. Nance, R.L. Watts, J.P. Hubble, W.C. Koller, R. Pahwa, M.B. Stern, B.C. Hiner, J. Jankovic, C.G. Goetz, F. Mastaglia, L.T. Middleton, A.D. Roses, A.M. Saunders, D.E. Schmechel, S.R. Gullans, J.L. Haines, J.R. Gilbert, J.M. Vance, and M.A. Pericak-Vance. 2003. Glutathione S-transferase omega-1 modifiesage-at-onset of Alzheimer disease and Parkinson disease. *Hum Mol Genet* **12**:3259–3267.

Louis, E.D., T. Lynch, B. Ford, P. Greene, S.B. Bressman, and S. Fahn. 1996. Delayed-onset cerebellar syndrome. *Arch Neurol* **53**:450–454.

Lynch, T., J. Odel, D.N. Fredericks, E.D. Louis, S. Forman, H. Rotterdam, S. Fahn, and D.A. Relman. 1997. Polymerase chain reaction-based detection of Tropheryma whippelii in central nervous system Whipple's disease. *Ann Neurol* **42**:120–124.

Mancini, J., B. Chabrol, E. Moulene, and N. Pinsard. 1996. Relapsing acute encephalopathy: a complication of diphtheria-tetanus-poliomyelitis immunization in a young boy. *Eur J Pediatr* **155**:136–138.

Manto, M.U., and J. Jacquy. 2002. Other cerebellotoxic agents. *In* "The Cerebellum and its Disorders" (M.U. Manto, and M. Pandolfo, Eds.), pp. 342–366, Cambridge University Press, Cambridge.

Maruyama, H., Y. Izumi, H. Morino, M. Oda, H. Toji, S. Nakamura, and H. Kawakami. 2002. Difference in disease-free survival curve and regional distribution according to subtype of spinocerebellar ataxia: a study of 1,286 Japanese patients. *Am J Med Genet* **114**:578–583.

Mercuri, E., J. He, W.L. Curati, L.M. Dubowitz, F.M. Cowan, and G.M. Bydder. 1997. Cerebellar infarction and atrophy in infants and children with a history of premature birth. *Pediatr Radiol* **27**:139–143.

Miller, J.D. 1993. Head injury. *J Neurol Neurosurg Psychiatry* **56**:440–447.

Mitoma, H., S.Y. Song, K. Ishida, T. Yamakuni, T. Kobayashi, and H. Mizusawa. 2000. Presynaptic impairment of cerebellar inhibitory synapses by an autoantibody to glutamate decarboxylase. *J Neurol Sci* **175**:40–44.

Moseley, M.L., K.A. Benzow, L.J. Schut, T.D. Bird, C.M. Gomez, P.E. Barkhaus, K.A. Blindauer, M. Labuda, M. Pandolfo, M.D. Koob, and L.P. Ranum. 1998. Incidence of dominant spinocerebellar and Friedreich triplet repeats among 361 ataxia families. *Neurology* **51**:1666–1671.

Nagashima, T., M. Koga, M. Odaka, K. Hirata, and N. Yuki. 2004. Clinical correlates of serum anti-GT1a IgG antibodies. *J Neurol Sci* **219**:139–145.

Nelson, K.B., and J.K. Lynch. 2004. Stroke in newborn infants. *Lancet Neurol* **3**:150–158.

Ozduman, K., B.R. Pober, P. Barnes, J.A. Copel, E.A. Ogle, C.C. Duncan, and L.R. Ment. 2004. Fetal stroke. *Pediatr Neurol* **30**:151–162.

Perkin, G.D., and I. Murray-Lyon. 1998. Neurology and the gastrointestinal system. *J Neurol Neurosurg Psychiatry* **65**:291–300.

Pujana, M.A., J. Corral, M. Gratacos, O. Combarros, J. Berciano, D. Genis, I. Banchs, X. Estivill, and V. Volpini. 1999. Spinocerebellar ataxias in Spanish patients: genetic analysis of familial and sporadic cases. The Ataxia Study Group. *Hum Genet* **104**:516–522.

Quagliarello, V.J., and W.M. Scheld. 1997. Treatment of bacterial meningitis. *N Engl J Med* **336**:708–716.

Ramesar, R.S., S. Bardien, P. Beighton, and A. Bryer. 1997. Expanded CAG repeats in spinocerebellar ataxia (SCA1) segregate with distinct haplotypes in South African families. *Hum Genet* **100**:131–137.

Schols, L., S. Gispert, M. Vorgerd, A.M. Menezes Vieira-Saecker, P. Blanke, G. Auburger, G. Amoiridis, S. Meves, J.T. Epplen, H. Przuntek, S.M. Pulst, and O. Riess. 1997. Spinocerebellar ataxia type 2. Genotype and phenotype in German kindreds. *Arch Neurol* **54**:1073–1080.

Schols, L., R. Kruger, G. Amoiridis, H. Przuntek, J.T. Epplen, and O. Riess. 1998. Spinocerebellar ataxia type 6: genotype and phenotype in German kindreds. *J Neurol Neurosurg Psychiatry* **64**:67–73.

Schols, L., S. Szymanski, S. Peters, H. Przuntek, J.T. Epplen, C. Hardt, and O. Riess. 2000. Genetic background of apparently idiopathic sporadic cerebellar ataxia. *Hum Genet* **107**:132–137.

Setta, F., M. Baecke, J. Jacquy, J. Hildebrand, G. Monseu, and M.U. Manto. 1999. Cerebellar ataxia following whooping cough. *Clin Neurol Neurosurg* **101**:56–61.

Singer, R. 1998. Diagnosis and treatment of Whipple's disease. *Drugs* **55**: 699–704.

Soong, B.W., Y.C. Lu, K.B. Choo, and H.Y. Lee. 2001. Frequency analysis of autosomal dominant cerebellar ataxias in Taiwanese patients and clinical and molecular characterization of spinocerebellar ataxia type 6. *Arch Neurol* **58**:1105–1109.

Storey, E., D. du Sart, J.H. Shaw, P. Lorentzos, L. Kelly, R.J. McKinley Gardner, S.M. Forrest, I. Biros, and G.A. Nicholson. 2000. Frequency of spinocerebellar ataxia types 1, 2, 3, 6, and 7 in Australian patients with spinocerebellar ataxia. *Am J Med Genet* **95**:351–357.

Sun, G., J.J. Gargus, D.T. Ta, and L.E. Vickery. 2003. Identification of a novel candidate gene in the iron-sulfur pathway implicated in ataxia-susceptibility: human gene encoding HscB, a J-type co-chaperone. *J Hum Genet* **48**:415–419.

Sunaga, Y., A. Hikima, T. Ostuka, and A. Morikawa. 1995. Acute cerebellar ataxia with abnormal MRI lesions after varicella vaccination. *Pediatr Neurol* **13**:340–342.

Tagliati, M., D. Simpson, S. Morgello, D. Clifford, R.L. Schwartz, and J.R. Berger. 1998. Cerebellar degeneration associated with human immunodeficiency virus infection. *Neurology* **50**:244–251.

Torvik, A. 1987. Brain lesions in alcoholics: neuropathological observations. *Acta Med Scand Suppl* **717**:47–54.

Tsai, F.Y., J.S. Teal, H.H. Itabashi, J.E. Huprich, G.B. Hieshima, and H.D. Segall. 1980. Computed tomography of posterior fossa trauma. *J Comput Assist Tomogr* **4**:291–305.

Ullrich, N.J., and S.L. Pomeroy. 2003. Pediatric brain tumors. *Neurol Clin* **21**:897–913.

Will, R.G. 2003. Acquired prion disease: iatrogenic CJD, variant CJD, kuru. *Br Med Bull.* **66**:255–265.

Yaqub, B.A., A.K. Daif, and C.P. Panayiotopoulos. 1987. Pancerebellar syndrome in heat stroke: clinical course and CT scan findings. *Neuroradiology* **29**:294–296.

Zabek, M. 2003. Primary posterior fossa tumours in adult patients. *Folia Neuropathol* **41**:231–236.

Zifko, U., M. Drlicek, G. Senautka, and W. Grisold. 1994. High dose immunoglobulin therapy is effective in the Miller Fisher syndrome. *J Neurol* **241**:178–179.

C H A P T E R

K3

Animal Models of Spinocerebellar Ataxia Type 1 (SCA1)

MICHAEL D. KAYTOR and HARRY T. ORR

Expansion of a polyglutamine repeat within the *SCA1*-encoded protein ataxin-1 causes the neurodegenerative disease spinocerebellar ataxia type 1 (SCA1). Numerous animal models have been generated that recapitulate many aspects of SCA1 pathogenesis. Studies using these animal models have led to numerous conclusions regarding the pathogenic potential of mutant ataxin-1. While protein folding and clearance pathways are important in the development of disease, ataxin-1 nuclear inclusion formation is not required for initiation of disease. In the case of SCA1, Purkinje cells are the last neurons to form nuclear inclusions but the most susceptible to the toxic effects of mutant ataxin-1, suggesting inclusion formation may be a protective event. Nuclear localization of mutant ataxin-1 is necessary but not sufficient to induce pathogenesis. A single amino acid, serine 776, within ataxin-1 was found to be important in disease progression. Serine 776 of both wild-type and mutant ataxin-1 is phosphorylated. Preventing phosphorylation of this residue by replacing it with alanine results in a mutant protein found in the nucleus that is not pathogenic. Other modifiers of ataxin-1 induced neurodegeneration include components of RNA processing and protein processing pathways. Importantly, as wild-type ataxin-1 is found in the nucleus and to be phosphorylated on serine 776, the disease pathway likely acts through ataxin-1's normal cellular pathway(s).

I. INTRODUCTION

Spinocerebellar ataxia type 1 (SCA1) is an autosomal dominant adult onset neurological disorder in which individuals typically survive only 10–15 years after the first appearance of symptoms (Zoghbi and Ballabio, 1995). Clinically, SCA1 patients exhibit ataxia, dysarthria, and bulbar dysfunction. Pathologically, there is Purkinje cell loss in the cerebellar cortex and loss of neurons in the inferior olivary nuclei, cerebellar dentate nuclei, and the red nuclei. SCA1 is caused by the expansion of a polyglutamine tract within the *SCA1* encoded protein ataxin-1 (Orr et al., 1993). An inverse relationship exists between the length of the repeat tract and the age of onset and severity of disease (Ranum et al., 1994). The longer the mutant CAG repeat, the earlier the age of onset and the more severe the clinical symptoms. In the general population the number of CAG repeats is highly variable, ranging from 6–44 triplet repeats. Alleles with repeat tracts longer than 20 typically have between 1 and 3 CAT interruptions (Chung et al., 1993). Mutant alleles have repeat tracts that contain 39–82 CAG repeats that lack CAT interruptions. Thus, the interruption might be an important factor in the intergenerational stability of the longer normal alleles.

SCA1 is a member of a group of neurodegenerative disorders known as the polyglutamine diseases. To date, this group includes spinobulbar muscular atrophy (SBMA), dentatorubropallidoluysian atrophy (DRPLA), Huntington disease (HD), and the spinocerebellar ataxias (SCA1, SCA2, SCA3/MJD, SCA6, SCA7, and SCA17) (Nakamura et al., 2001; Zoghbi and Orr, 2000). Other than the CAG repeat tract, the gene products associated with these disorders share no significant homology. A common feature among the polyglutamine diseases is the aberrant deposition of the mutant protein (Kaytor and Warren, 1999). Most often these accumulations are found within the nucleus of neurons. The role that nuclear inclusions play in disease pathogenesis remains controversial. Of particular interest is the cell-specificity of pathogenesis. Despite widespread expression of these proteins in the brain and other tissues only a certain subset of neurons is vulnerable to neurodegeneration in each of the disorders.

Ataxin-1 is a novel protein of unknown function, which has been shown to bind RNA and to interact with specific proteins (Orr and Zoghbi, 2001). The subcellular localization of ataxin-1 varies depending on cell type. For example, in lymphoblastoid cells ataxin-1 is found primarily in the cytoplasm, while in neurons ataxin-1 is mostly nuclear (Cummings et al., 1998; Servadio et al., 1995; Skinner et al., 1997). Ataxin-1 shares a region of homology, termed the AXH domain, with the transcription factor HBP1 (de Chiara et al., 2003). This region is postulated to be a protein–protein interaction and RNA binding motif. Not surprisingly, the region of ataxin-1 that is involved in RNA binding and in its interactions with other proteins maps within the AXH domain (Yue et al., 2001).

The use of animal models has been crucial in understanding cellular and molecular aspects of disease pathogenesis in SCA1 and the other polyglutamine disorders. Numerous SCA1 models have implicated the importance of the subcellular localization of the mutant protein, the role of the nuclear inclusions, protein folding, and clearance and post-translational modification in disease. In this chapter we will focus on the animal models used to investigate each of these aspects as they relate to SCA1 pathogenesis.

II. UNCOVERING SCA1 PATHOGENIC MECHANISMS VIA ANIMAL MODELS

A. Expanded Polyglutamine-Mediated Dominant Gain of Function

To gain insight into the function of wild-type ataxin-1 and to determine if SCA1 is due to a loss or gain of function mutation, *Sca1* null mice have been generated. Mice lacking ataxin-1 failed to show any overt signs of ataxia or evidence of Purkinje cell pathology (Matilla et al., 1998). The *Sca1* null mice displayed both motor and spatial learning deficits, suggesting that ataxin-1 has a role in both cerebellar and hippocampal-mediated learning. In humans, large deletions within 6p22–23 spanning the *SCA1* gene do not cause SCA1 (Davies et al., 1999). Together, these data indicate that SCA1 is not caused by loss of ataxin-1 function, supporting a toxic gain-of-function model.

In a further effort to test a gain-of-function hypothesis, *SCA1* transgenic mice have been made. These mice focused on developing a model to allow the examination of pathogenesis in a single cell type, the cerebellar Purkinje cells, a prominent site of pathology in patients. Studies on patient material have revealed reduced Purkinje cell dendritic arborization associated with a reduction in number of small spiny dendritic processes (Ferrer et al., 1994; Koeppen, 1991). In addition, axonal torpedo bodies have been observed in the Purkinje cells. To model Purkinje cell pathology seen in SCA1, the strong Purkinje cell-specific promoter (*Pcp2/L7*) was used to direct expression of a human *SCA1* cDNA to the cerebellar Purkinje cells (Burright et al., 1995). Two transgenic lines were extensively characterized (Figure 1). The first expressed a wild-type *SCA1* allele containing 30 glutamine repeats, ataxin-1[30Q], while the second expressed a mutant *SCA1* allele containing 82 repeats, ataxin-1[82Q]. The B05 mice expressing mutant ataxin-1 developed severe ataxia and progressive Purkinje cell

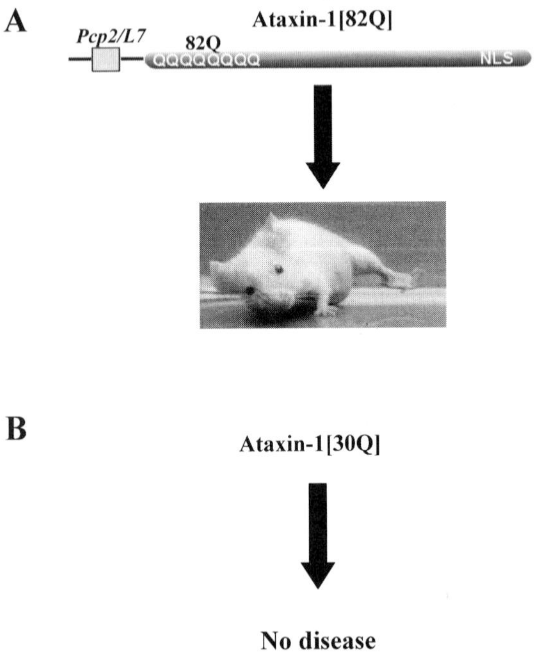

FIGURE 1 SCA1 is due to a dominant gain-of-function mutation. A) *SCA1* B05 transgenic mice expressing mutant ataxin-1 with 82 glutamine repeats develop severe ataxia. B) *SCA1* A02 transgenic mice expressing wild-type ataxin-1 with 30 glutamine repeats fail to develop any signs of disease.

pathology. In contrast, A02 transgenic mice expressing wild-type ataxin-1 failed to develop any signs of ataxia or neurodegeneration. These studies indicated that neurodegeneration of Purkinje cells results from the expression of mutant ataxin-1 and reinforced the toxic gain-of-function model for polyglutamine-induced pathogenesis.

In B05 mice, mutant ataxin-1 localized to a single nuclear inclusion similar to what has been seen in tissue samples from SCA1 patients (Skinner et al., 1997). The appearance of these inclusions, which were ubiquitinated, contained components of the 26S proteasome and molecular chaperones preceded the onset of ataxia by about six weeks (Cummings et al., 1998). The first sign of mild cerebellar impairment in the B05 mice occurred at five weeks of age, as evidenced by a slight deficit in rotarod performance (Clark et al., 1997). At this age there were no signs of gait abnormalities or balance problems. By twelve weeks, as assessed by home cage behavior, the motor impairment progressed to visible ataxia that worsened with age. The first pathological sign detected in the B05 mice was the appearance of cytoplasmic vacuoles in the Purkinje cells at postnatal day 25 (Clark et al., 1997; Skinner et al., 2001). By six weeks of age, a loss of proximal dendritic branches and a decrease in the number of dendritic spines became apparent. Thus, Purkinje cells that overexpress mutant ataxin-1 develop features that are seen in SCA1 patients.

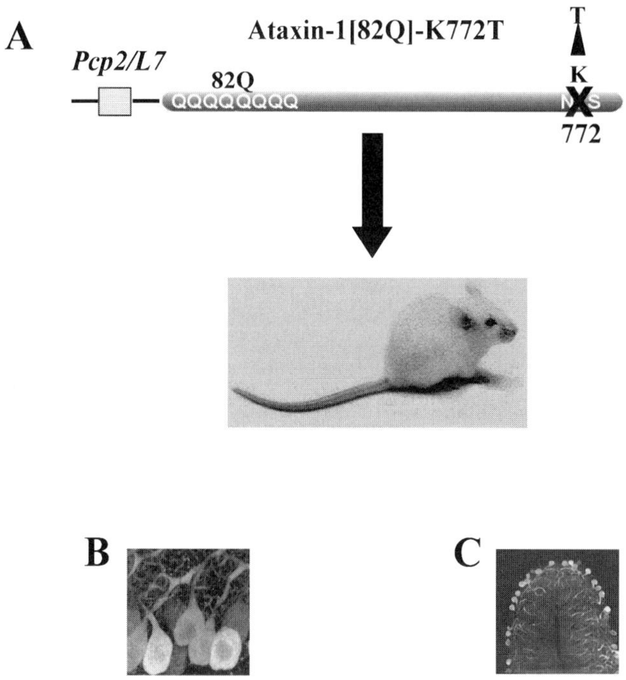

FIGURE 2 Nuclear localization of mutant ataxin-1 is required to induce pathogenesis. A) *SCA1* K772T transgenic mice expressing mutant ataxin-1 with a non-functional nuclear localization signal fail to develop any signs of disease. B) Ataxin-1[82Q]-K772T localizes to the cytoplasm of cerebellar Purkinje cells. C) *SCA1* K772T transgenic mice exhibit no signs of Purkinje cell degeneration.

B. Subcellular Localization

Ataxin-1 is widely expressed in the normal human brain and peripheral tissues. Within neurons, ataxin-1 is predominantly nuclear with some cytoplasmic ataxin-1 found in Purkinje cells and brain stem nuclei (Cummings et al., 1998; Servadio et al., 1995; Skinner et al., 1997). Cell culture studies found that mutant ataxin-1 confers nuclear alterations. Specifically, mutant ataxin-1 causes nuclear-matrix associated promyelocytic leukaemia protein (PML) containing bodies to be redistributed, altering its normal nuclear localization (Skinner et al., 1997). PML was often found sequestered with mutant ataxin-1 within the large nuclear inclusions. In both tissue culture cells and Purkinje cells of transgenic mice, ataxin-1 was found to be associated with the nuclear matrix. Taken together, these results suggest that the primary site of pathogenesis is nuclear. However, in Purkinje cells ataxin-1 is also found in the cytoplasm. Pathologically, the first sign of disease is cytoplasmic vacuoles (Clark et al., 1997). The possible role of nuclear-mediated pathogenesis and predominant nuclear localization of ataxin-1 stimulated the identification of a functional nuclear localization signal (NLS) in the C-terminus of the protein (Klement et al., 1998). To directly determine whether nuclear expression of mutant ataxin-1 is required to induce pathogenesis, transgenic mice expressing mutant ataxin-1 with a single point mutation, K772T, preventing nuclear localization of the protein were generated and characterized (Figure 2). Like previous *SCA1* mice, expression of this transgene was directed to the cerebellar Purkinje cells using the *Pcp2/L7* promoter. In these ataxin-1[82Q]-K772T mice, the mutant protein was found predominantly in the cytoplasm of Purkinje cells. Compared to the B05 transgenic mice, ataxin-1[82Q]-K772T mice express a comparable amount of protein, yet there was no indication of cytoplasmic inclusions in the ataxin-1[82Q]-K772T mice. Ataxin-1[82Q]-K772T mice do not develop ataxia or signs of Purkinje cell degeneration. Thus, the ataxin-1[82Q]-K772T mice do not develop the cerebellar dysfunction characteristic of the B05 *SCA1* transgenic mice, despite expressing comparable levels of mutant ataxin-1 in Purkinje cells. This indicates that nuclear expression of mutant ataxin-1 is necessary for pathogenesis and that polyglutamine-mediated nuclear alterations are critical for disease in transgenic mice.

C. Protein Folding, Clearance, and Solubility

A pathological hallmark in most of the polyglutamine disorders is the presence of nuclear inclusions containing the mutant protein (Zoghbi and Orr, 2000). The role that these inclusions have in disease pathogenesis remains controversial. In SCA1, ataxin-1 multimerization is mediated by intramolecular interactions via a self-association domain (SAD) (Burright et al., 1997). To test the role of ataxin-1 self-association in pathogenesis, *SCA1* transgenic mice were

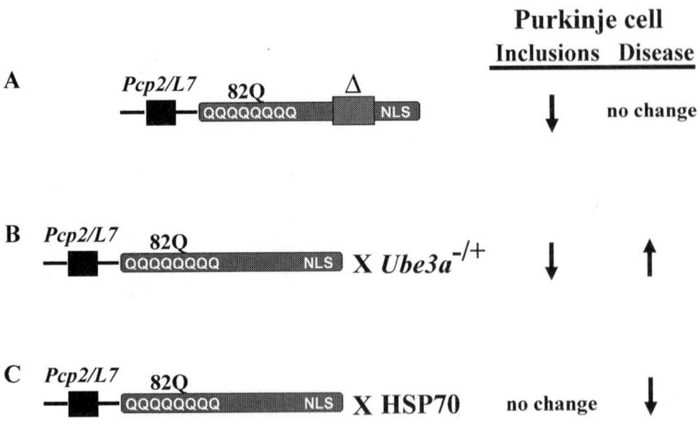

FIGURE 3 Intracellular protein processing pathways are involved in SCA1 pathogenesis. Changes in Purkinje cells are relative to *SCA1* B05 transgenic mice. A) Mutant ataxin-1 self-association is not required for SCA1 pathogenesis. Deletion of the ataxin-1 self-association domain results in fewer nuclear inclusions but no change in disease. B) Protein clearance pathways are involved in SCA1 pathogenesis. Deletion of the E3 ubiquitin ligase encoded by *Ube3a* results in fewer nuclear inclusions but a more severe disease. C) Protein folding pathways are involved in SCA1 pathogenesis. Overexpression of the molecular chaperone HSP70 does not affect nuclear inclusion formation but does mitigate disease.

generated in which the self-association region was deleted (Klement et al., 1998). Ataxin-1[77Q]-ΔSAD localized to the nucleus of Purkinje cells. However, in spite of nuclear localization ataxin-1[77Q]-ΔSAD transgenic mice did not have nuclear aggregates. Ataxin-1[77Q]-ΔSAD mice did develop ataxia and Purkinje cell pathology (Figure 3A). A progressive Purkinje cell pathology similar to that observed in the B05 mice was apparent in these mice. This included the appearance of cytoplasmic vacuoles at three weeks, shrinkage of the molecular layer by eight weeks and the appearance of heterotopic Purkinje cells at twelve weeks. The performance of the ataxin-1[77Q]-ΔSAD mice on the accelerating rotarod at twelve weeks of age is compromised compared to non-transgenic littermates. This deficit was similar to that observed for the B05 mice at twelve weeks of age. Hence, despite the absence of detectable nuclear inclusions, ataxin-1[77Q]-ΔSAD mice had histological and neurological alterations similar to B05 mice. Thus, ataxin-1 nuclear inclusion formation is not required for initiation of SCA1 pathogenesis. Further characterization of the ataxin-1[77Q]-ΔSAD mice found that the deleted protein–protein interaction region did not affect the initiation of disease, but did substantially suppress disease progression (Skinner et al., 2002). This suggests a role for the protein–protein interaction region in disease progression. Moreover, mutant ataxin-1 induced initiation of disease and disease progression likely involve distinct events.

Polyglutamine-containing nuclear inclusions contain ubiquitin and have been shown to redistribute chaperones and components of the ubiquitin proteasome pathway (Berke and Paulson, 2003; Cummings and Zoghbi, 2000). Inhibition of the proteasome pathway increased formation of ataxin-1 inclusions, which was accompanied by an increase in the amount of detergent-insoluble ataxin-1 (Cummings et al., 1999). Ubiquitin was conjugated similarly to both wild-type and mutant ataxin-1, suggesting that ubiquitination of ataxin-1 is not influenced by the length of the polyglutamine repeat. However, mutant ataxin-1 was more resistant to degradation *in vitro*, suggesting a role for the ubiquitin-proteasome pathway in SCA1 pathogenesis. To test this hypothesis, *SCA1* transgenic mice were crossed to mice deficient in a component of the ubiquitin-proteasome pathway (Cummings et al., 1999). *Ube3a* encodes an E3 ubiquitin ligase responsible for the addition of ubiquitin moiety to a substrate targeting it for 26S proteasome-mediated degradation. *Ube3a* has a unique expression pattern; the paternal allele is silenced in cerebellar Purkinje cells due to tissue-specific imprinting. Maternal deficiency of the *Ube3a* gene product (E6-AP) causes the human genetic disorder Angelman syndrome. Mental retardation, hyperactivity, seizures, ataxia, and inappropriate laughter characterize Angelman syndrome. *Ube3a* deficiency results in no histological abnormalities of the cerebellum. Offspring from *SCA1* B05 mice crossed to the *Ube3a* deficient mice that carried both a mutant *SCA1* allele and a targeted disruption of the maternal *Ube3a* allele were extensively characterized (Figure 3B). The Purkinje cells of these bi-transgenic animals contained significantly fewer nuclear inclusions. However, the Purkinje cell pathology in these mice was significantly worse than that observed in the mice with a functional copy of *Ube3a*. Thus, lack of this E3 ligase greatly accelerates polyglutamine-induced pathology in *SCA1* transgenic mice, indicating that nuclear inclusions are not necessary to induce pathogenesis.

Molecular chaperones work together with the ubiquitin-proteasome pathway to recognize and hydrolyze misfolded proteins. Nuclear inclusions from both SCA1 patient tissue and transgenic mice stained positive for the molecular chaperones Hsp70 and Hsp40 (Cummings et al., 1998). This suggests that expansion of the polyglutamine repeat within ataxin-1 leads to a misfolded protein that is inefficiently cleared by the ubiquitin-proteasome pathway. In support of this, overexpression of an Hsp40 chaperone (HDJ-2) reduced mutant ataxin-1 inclusion formation in tissue culture cells. Studies using Drosophila have also found that overexpression of molecular chaperones suppressed polyglutamine-induced cell toxicity (Fernandez-Funez et al., 2000; Kazemi-Esfarjani and Benzer, 2000; Warrick et al., 1998).

To further investigate whether altered protein folding and deficient protein clearance are involved in polyglutamine-induced pathogenesis *SCA1* B05 transgenic mice were crossed to mice overexpressing the molecular chaperone HSP70 (Cummings et al., 2001). Overexpression of HSP70 did mitigate the phenotype of the B05 mice (Figure 3C). *SCA1* B05 transgenic mice overexpressing HSP70 recovered

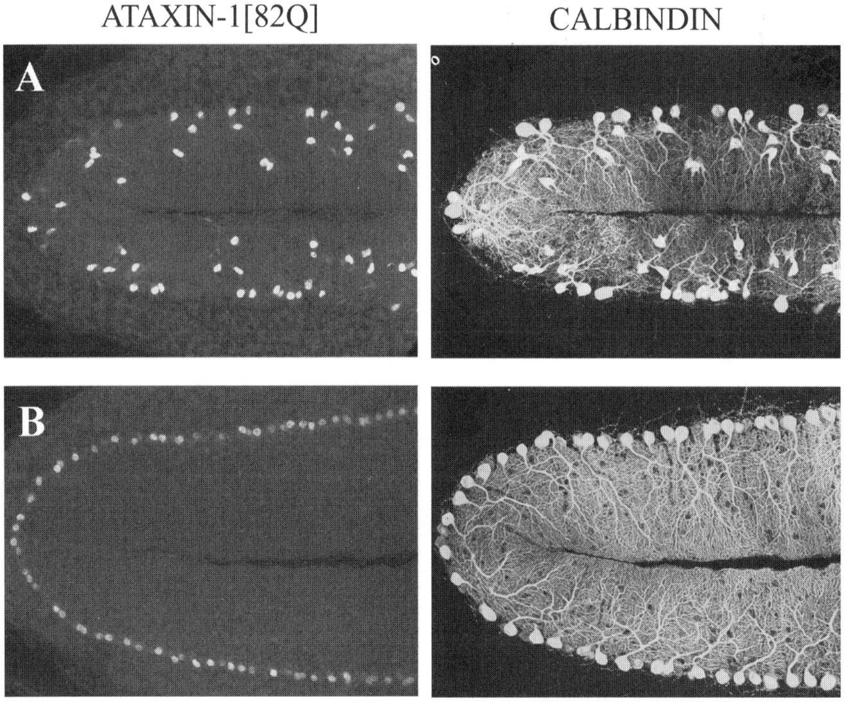

FIGURE 4 Ataxin-1[82Q]-A776 is substantially less pathogenic in *SCA1* transgenic mice. Purkinje cell morphology was assessed by calbindin immunofluorescence and mutant protein expression by ataxin-1 immunofluorescence. A) 27-week-old *SCA1* B05 transgenic mouse expressing ataxin-1[82Q]-S776. B) 27-week-old *SCA1* A776 transgenic mouse expressing ataxin-1[82Q]-A776. Reprinted with permission from Elsevier Science.

the ability to perform on the rotarod. This rescue was dose dependent as B05/HSP70$^{tg/tg}$ animals performed better than B05/HSP70$^{tg/-}$ animals on the rotarod. HSP70 also ameliorates Purkinje cell pathological changes. B05/HSP70$^{tg/tg}$ mice have Purkinje cells with thicker and more robust dendritic arborization and fewer heterotopic Purkinje cells compared to the neurons within B05 cerebella. Interestingly, overexpression of HSP70 did not alter the prevalence of nuclear inclusions. Suppression of the disease phenotype in the absence of any notable alterations in the properties of mutant ataxin-1 found in nuclear inclusions further indicates that inclusions are not a prominent aspect of disease pathogenesis. Molecular chaperones may modulate the folding and degradation of pathogenic non-sequestered mutant ataxin-1.

Purkinje cells are not the sole type of neuron affected in SCA1; neurons within the brain stem and spinal cord also degenerate. In an attempt to faithfully recapitulate the full spectrum of pathological changes observed in SCA1, an expanded polyglutamine tract was introduced via homologous recombination into the endogenous murine *Sca1* locus. The endogenous murine *Sca1* locus contains two glutamines. Two knockin lines have been generated; one with 78 CAG repeats the other with 154 repeats. In the first, murine *Sca1* with 78 repeats, mutant ataxin-1 was not pathogenic (Lorenzetti et al., 2000). These mice were not ataxic as observed by home cage behavior, nor did they have any of the neuropathological changes that are observed in other transgenic models of SCA1 out to eighteen months of age. Thus, mutant ataxin-1 with 78 repeats expressed at endogenous levels was not sufficient to induce any detectable pathological changes. In contrast, overexpression of mutant ataxin-1 with 82 repeats in the *SCA1* B05 transgenic mice is pathogenic (Figure 4). Together, these data suggest that, in mice, disease is a function of polyglutamine length, protein level, and time of exposure. To circumvent these variables, a second knockin that harbored 154 repeats within the murine *Sca1* locus was generated (Watase et al., 2002). These mice did develop a neurological disorder reminiscent of the human disease. The mice had motor coordination deficits and Purkinje cell pathology with cell loss that worsened progressively with increasing age. In addition, growth retardation, cognitive defects, and premature death were also observed. Of note, reduced Purkinje cell dendritic arborization was also observed early in the disease process, while cell loss was not evident until the end-stage of the disease. As surmised previously, this confirms that Purkinje cell dysfunction, and not cell loss, is responsible for the early stages of pathogenesis.

One of the prominent findings within the polyglutamine diseases is the appearance of neuronal intranuclear inclusions. In the adult mouse brain, ataxin-1 localizes primarily within the nucleus of neurons, and mutant ataxin-1 typically to a singular nuclear foci (Servadio et al., 1995; Skinner et al., 1997). In the *Sca1*$^{154Q/2Q}$ mice, intranuclear inclusions were found within numerous neuronal populations. Of importance, inclusions were less frequent in the most susceptible groups of neurons compared to cortical or hippocampal neurons, which are only mildly affected in SCA1. For example, by twenty weeks of age, less than 0.5% of the Purkinje cells contained inclusions, while more than 80% of the neurons in other regions had inclusions. This is consistent with previous reports that the nuclear inclusions do not initiate disease in *SCA1* transgenic animals. It suggests that the most susceptive neurons may be those unable to efficiently sequester mutant ataxin-1 into inclusions in a timely manner. Purkinje cells are the last cells in which mutant ataxin-1 containing aggregates are observed but are the most susceptible cells in SCA1. Selective neuronal vulnerability in SCA1 and the other polyglutamine disorders may result from a combination of protein solubility and factors involved in a pathway that results in formation of nuclear inclusions that contain the mutant protein. As discussed earlier, these factors may include components of the ubiquitin-proteasome pathway and molecular chaperones. Such factors may be rate-limiting in susceptible neurons resulting in their increased vulnerability to polyglutamine-mediated toxicity.

D. Genetic Modifiers and Mediators

Drosophila has proven to be a powerful model system that has been extremely useful in elucidating the genetic pathways that are involved in polyglutamine-induced neurodegeneration. Directed expression of mutant ataxin-1 to the retina produced a severe form of neurodegeneration (Fernandez-Funez et al., 2000). In addition to the observed retinal pathology nuclear inclusions were also observed. Interestingly, the wild-type form of the protein produced a mild form of neurodegeneration. Whether or not the intrinsic toxicity of normal ataxin-1 is relevant to the human disease is not known. The power of Drosophila genetics is evident in the ability to carry out genetic screens to identify genes that modify the initial phenotype. Toward this end, a genetic screen of modifiers of the polyglutamine-induced pathogenesis in these *SCA1* transgenic flies yielded several insightful genes. Modifier genes that suppress or enhance ataxin-1-induced neurodegeneration were identified. Mutations within numerous genes within ubiquitin-proteasome pathway enhanced ataxin-1-induced neurodegeneration. These include ubiquitin, a ubiquitin carboxy-terminal hydrolyase, as well as genes involved in ubiquitin conjugation. Another group of enhancers included numerous transcriptional cofactors. Enhancers and suppressors were found that contained an RNA-binding domain. A Drosophila protein (dDNAJ-1) which is homologous to the HSP40 chaperone suppressed neurodegeneration. The modifiers identified cemented the importance of protein folding and clearance pathways, RNA processing pathways, and transcriptional homeostasis in the development of disease.

In SCA1 the cerebellar Purkinje cells are affected, in HD the striatal neurons, while in SBMA the spinal motor neurons are most susceptible (Zoghbi and Orr, 2000). Although progress has been made in understanding the selective vulnerability of specific subsets of neurons in each of the polyglutamine disorders, the underlying mechanism remains a mystery. One hypothesized cellular response for mutant polyglutamine damage is the activation of apoptotic machinery, suggesting apoptotic cell loss as a central component of the disease (Paulson et al., 2000). However, in *SCA1* transgenic mice the ataxic phenotype is present well before any evidence of cell loss, arguing that neuronal dysfunction and not cell loss is central to SCA1 pathogenesis (Clark et al., 1997). In contrast, numerous studies have implicated the activation of an apoptotic pathway in polyglutamine-mediated neurodegeneration (Li et al., 2000; Ona et al., 1999; Sanchez et al., 1999; Warrick et al., 1998). In addition to being a central component of apoptotic pathways p53 has been linked to neuronal cell death, including ties to polyglutamine-mediated pathogenesis (Jana et al., 2001; Trettel et al., 2000). To further investigate the role of p53 in SCA1, B05 transgenic mice were crossed to mice lacking p53 (Shahbazian et al., 2001). In these mice a reduction in the severity of later features of the disease was observed. These included fewer heterotopic Purkinje cells, slowed dendritic thinning, and amelioration of the shrinkage of the molecular layer. Interestingly, no signs of apoptotic cell death were observed in the *SCA1* mice, suggesting that the mitigating effects of p53 are independent of neuronal cell death. Thus, p53 acts after the initiation of neuropathological alterations to promote the progression of SCA1 pathogenesis.

Neuronal susceptibility and disease progression are not solely dependent on the length of the mutant polyglutamine tract. Numerous reports have found that a mutant polyglutamine peptide isolated from the intact sequence is much more toxic than when it is imbedded within the entire protein (Wellington and Hayden, 2000; Zoghbi and Botas, 2002). This argues that the context of the protein surrounding the mutant tract may lessen the pathogenic consequences of a mutant polyglutamine tract. Sequences outside of the polyglutamine tract may also be involved in cell specific neurodegeneration. Animal models have been crucial in understanding the processes that modify SCA1 disease progression. Nuclear localization of mutant ataxin-1 is necessary for pathogenesis, as *SCA1* transgenic mice in which the nuclear localization signal was mutated (to prevent nuclear import) did not develop ataxia (Klement et al., 1998). In the

TABLE 1 Biological Properties of Ataxin-1 in *SCA1* Transgenic Mice

Transgenic	pQ length	Localization	Inclusions	P-S776[a]	Disease
A02	30Q	nuclear	–	+	no
B05	82Q	nuclear	++++	+	yes
K772T	82Q	cytoplasmic	–	+/–	no
ΔSAD	77Q	nuclear	–	+	yes
A776	82Q	nuclear	+	–	no

[a]Serine 776 phosphorylated ataxin-1 determined by immunohistochemical analysis (Emamian et al., 2003).

absence of the E3 ubiquitin ligase (*Ube3a*) inclusion formation and pathogenesis was accelerated (Cummings et al., 1999). These results implicated a role for protein folding, clearance, and subcellular localization in pathogenesis. Protein phosphorylation is a prominent mechanism to regulate protein degradation and subcellular localization (Hunter, 2000). To investigate this possibility further purified ataxin-1 was subjected to mass spectroscopy analysis to identify potential sites of phosphorylation. Towards this end, the serine at residue 776 of ataxin-1 was found to be phosphorylated (Emamian et al., 2003). To further investigate the role of this phosphorylation event in mutant ataxin-1 subcellular localization and neuronal dysfunction the serine residue was mutated to alanine, thus preventing its phosphorylation. Mutation of this residue to an alanine in transgenic mice (A776) resulted in a significant dampening of the pathogenic effects of mutant ataxin-1. By both behavioral analyses and by assessing Purkinje cell morphology, mutation of serine 776 to alanine rendered mutant ataxin-1 in effect innocuous. Mutation of this residue did not affect the subcellular localization of mutant ataxin-1, indicating that phosphorylation of this residue is not required for nuclear transport.

In tissue culture cells, mutation of serine 776 to alanine drastically reduced the ability of mutant ataxin-1 to form inclusions. In cells expressing ataxin-1[82Q]-A776, less than 1 in 1000 cells contained nuclear inclusions. In contrast, in cells expressing ataxin-1[82Q]-S776, at least 60% contained nuclear inclusions. As expected, this reduction in inclusion formation coincided with an increase in extractable soluble mutant ataxin-1. In ataxin-1[82Q]-A776 transgenic mice, the ability of the mutant protein to form nuclear inclusions was similarly diminished. The reduction of ataxin-1[82Q]-A776 nuclear inclusions suggests that the cell is able to more efficiently handle the mutant protein. Consistent with this is the increased solubility of the ataxin-1[82Q]-A776 protein. Polyglutamine tract expansion and nuclear localization of mutant ataxin-1 within Purkinje cells are not sufficient to induce disease SCA1 pathogenesis. A single amino acid within mutant ataxin-1, serine 776, also plays a critical role in pathogenesis.

III. CONCLUDING REMARKS

Animal models of the polyglutamine diseases have been extremely useful in gaining insights into the pathogenic mechanism(s) of these disorders. In the case of SCA1, numerous transgenic mouse and Drosophila models have been used to uncover many important aspects of the disease. At this time the data indicate that nuclear localization of the mutant protein is required for disease, nuclear inclusions are not necessary to initiate disease, and protein folding and clearance pathways are vital to the disease process. In fact, formation of inclusions may be a cellular defense mechanism against polyglutamine-mediated toxicity. Neurons that are the last to form inclusions are the most vulnerable to neurodegeneration. Hence, perhaps neuron-specific rate-limiting components of protein folding and clearance pathways are responsible for the cell-specific neurodegeneration observed in each of the polyglutamine disorders. Finally, events outside of the CAG repeat in *cis* can modulate pathogenesis. Mutation of serine 776 of ataxin-1 to alanine dampened the pathogenicity of mutant ataxin-1. Moreover, this mutation rendered the mutant ataxin-1 substantially more soluble, perhaps allowing for more prompt disposal of the mutant protein by the neuron.

An important and relevant conclusion has come out of the numerous *SCA1* transgenic mouse studies; the disease pathway appears to be acting through ataxin-1's normal cellular pathway(s) (table 1). Aspects involved in the normal cellular role of ataxin-1 appear to require nuclear localization and phosphorylation of the protein on serine 776. Both the wild-type and mutant ataxin-1 are primarily found in the nucleus of neurons. Preventing the mutant protein from entering the nucleus by mutating the NLS signal prevents disease. Second, both wild-type and mutant ataxin-1 are phosphorylated. Mutation of serine 776 in the mutant protein mitigates disease. Thus, defining the role of phosphorylated ataxin-1 in the nucleus may provide further insights into SCA1 pathogenesis.

The progress made to date in developing an understanding of the disease process in SCA1 has uncovered numerous potential sites for therapeutic intervention. These include upregulation of molecular chaperone or protein degradation pathways, regulation of subcellular localization and altering the solubility of the mutant protein. In addition, modulation of ataxin-1 phosphorylation and mutant-specific protein–protein interactions are promising avenues to further investigate.

References

Berke, S.J.S., and H.L. Paulson. 2003. Protein aggregation and the ubiquitin proteasome pathway: gaining the UPPer hand on neurodegeneration. *Curr Opin Genet Dev* **13**:253–261.

Burright, E.N., et al. 1995. SCA1 transgenic mice: A model for neurodegeneration caused by an expanded CAG trinucleotide repeat. *Cell* **82**: 937–948.

Burright, E.N., et al. 1997. Identification of a self-association region within the *SCA1* gene product, ataxin-1. *Hum Mol Genet* **6**:513–518.

Chung, M.Y., et al. 1993. Evidence for a mechanism predisposing to intergenerational CAG repeat instability in spinocerebellar ataxia type I. *Nat Genet* **5**:254–258.

Clark, H.B., et al. 1997. Purkinje cell expression of a mutant allele of *SCA1* in transgenic mice leads to disparate effects on motor behaviors, followed by a progressive cerebellar dysfunction and histological alterations. *J Neurosci* **17**:7385–7395.

Cummings, C.J., et al. 1998. Chaperone suppression of aggregation and altered subcellular proteasome localization imply protein misfolding in SCA1. *Nat Genet* **19**:148–154.

Cummings, C.J., et al. 1999. Mutation of the E6-AP ubiquitin ligase reduces nuclear inclusion frequency while accelerating polyglutamine-induced pathology in *Sca1* mice. *Neuron* **24**:879–892.

Cummings, C.J., et al. 2001. Over-expression of inducible HSP70 chaperone suppresses neuropathology and improves motor function in SCA1 mice. *Hum Mol Genet* **10**:1511–1518.

Cummings, C.J., and H.Y. Zoghbi. 2000. Fourteen and counting: unraveling trinucleotide repeat diseases. *Hum Mol Genet* **9**:909–916.

Davies, A.F., et al. 1999. Delineation of two distinct 6p deletion syndromes. *Hum Genet* **104**:64–72.

de Chiara, C., et al. 2003. The AXH module: an independently folded domain common to ataxin-1 and HBP1. *FEBS Lett* **551**:107–112.

Emamian, E.S., et al. 2003. Serine 776 of ataxin-1 is critical for polyglutamine-induced disease in SCA1 transgenic mice. *Neuron* **38**:375–387.

Fernandez-Funez, P., et al. 2000. Identification of genes that modify ataxin-1-induced neurodegeneration. *Nature* **408**:101–106.

Ferrer, I., et al. 1994. The Purkinje cell in olivopontocerebellar atrophy. A golgi and immunohistochemical study. *Neuropathol Appl Neurobiol* **20**:38–46.

Hunter, T. 2000. Signaling 2000 and beyond. *Cell* **100**:113–127.

Jana, N.R., et al. 2001. Altered proteasomal function due to the expression of polyglutamine-expanded truncated N-terminal huntingtin induces apoptosis by caspase activation through mitochondrial cytochrome c release. *Hum Mol Genet* **10**:1049–1059.

Kaytor, M.D., and S.T. Warren. 1999. Aberrant protein deposition and neurological disease. *J Biol Chem* **274**:37507–37510.

Kazemi-Esfarjani, P., and S. Benzer. 2000. Genetic suppression of polyglutamine toxicity in Drosophila. *Science* **287**:1837–1840.

Klement, I.A., et al. 1998. Ataxin-1 nuclear localization and aggregation: Role in polyglutamine-induced disease in *SCA1* transgenic mice. *Cell* **95**:41–53.

Koeppen, A.H. 1991. The Purkinje cell and its afferents in human hereditary ataxia. *J Neuropath Expt Neurol* **50**:505–514.

Li, S.-H., et al. 2000. Intranuclear huntington increases the expression of caspase-1 and induces apoptosis. *Hum Mol Genet* **9**:2859–2867.

Lorenzetti, D., et al. 2000. Repeat instability and motor incoordination in mice with a targeted expanded CAG repeat in the Sca1 locus. *Hum Mol Genet* **9**:779–785.

Matilla, A., et al. 1998. Mice lacking ataxin-1 display learning deficits and decreased hippocampal paired-pulse facilitation. *J Neurosci* **18**:5508–5516.

Nakamura, K., et al. 2001. SCA17, a novel autosomal dominant cerebellar ataxia caused by an expanded polyglutamine in TATA-binding protein. *Hum Mol Genet* **10**:1441–1448.

Ona, V.O., et al. 1999. Inhibition of caspase-1 slows disease progression in a mouse model of Huntington's disease. *Nature* **399**:263–267.

Orr, H.T., et al. 1993. Expansion of an unstable trinucleotide CAG repeat in spinocerebellar ataxia type 1. *Nat Genet* **4**:221–226.

Orr, H.T., and H.Y. Zoghbi. 2001. SCA1 molecular genetics: a history of a 13 year collaboration against glutamines. *Hum Mol Genet* **10**:2307–2311.

Paulson, H.L., et al. 2000. Polyglutamine disease and neuronal cell death. *Proc Natl Acad Sci U S A* **97**:12957–12958.

Ranum, L.P.W., et al. 1994. Molecular and clinical correlations in spinocerebellar ataxia type 1: evidence for familial effects on the age at onset. *Am J Hum Genet* **55**:244–252.

Sanchez, I., et al. 1999. Caspase-8 is required for cell death induced by expanded polyglutamine repeats. *Neuron* **22**:623–633.

Servadio, A., et al. 1995. Expression analysis of the ataxin-1 protein in tissues from normal and spinocerebellar ataxia type 1 individuals. *Nat Genet* **10**:94–98.

Shahbazian, M.D., et al. 2001. Reduction of Purkinje cell pathology in SCA1 transgenic mice by p53 deletion. *Neurobiol Dis* **8**:974–981.

Skinner, P.J., et al. 1997. Ataxin-1 with an expanded glutamine tract alters nuclear matrix-associated structures. *Nature* **389**:971–974.

Skinner, P.J., et al. 2001. Altered trafficking of membrane proteins in purkinje cells of SCA1 transgenic mice. *Am J Pathol* **159**:905–913.

Skinner, P.J., et al. 2002. Amino acids in a region of ataxin-1 outside of the polyglutamine tract influence the course of disease in SCA1 transgenic mice. *Neuromolecular Med* **1**:33–42.

Trettel, F., et al. 2000. Dominant phenotypes produced by the HD mutation in STHdh(Q111) striatal cells. *Hum Mol Genet* **9**:2799–2809.

Warrick, J.M., et al. 1998. Expanded polyglutamine protein forms nuclear inclusions and causes neural degeneration in *Drosophila*. *Cell* **93**: 939–949.

Watase, K., et al. 2002. A long CAG repeat in the mouse Sca1 locus replicates SCA1 features and reveals the impact of protein solubility on selective neurodegeneration. *Neuron* **34**:905–919.

Wellington, C.L., and M.R. Hayden. 2000. Caspases and neurodegeneration: on the cutting edge of new therapeutic approaches. *Clin Genet* **57**:1–10.

Yue, S., et al. 2001. The spinocerebellar ataxia type 1 protein, ataxin-1, has RNA-binding activity that is inversely affected by the length of its polyglutamine tract. *Hum Mol Genet* **10**:25–30.

Zoghbi, H.Y., and A. Ballabio. 1995. Spinocerebellar ataxia type 1. *In* "The metabolic and molecular basis of inherited disease" (C.R. Scriver, A.L. Beaudet, W.S. Sly, and D. Valle, Ed.), pp. 4559–4568. McGraw Hill, New York.

Zoghbi, H.Y., and J. Botas. 2002. Mouse and fly models of neurodegeneration. *Trends Genet* **18**:463–471.

Zoghbi, H.Y., and H.T. Orr. 2000. Glutamine repeats and neurodegeneration. *Annu Rev Neurosci* **23**:217–247.

C H A P T E R

K4

Spinocerebellar Ataxia Type 2 (SCA2)

STEFAN-M. PULST

SCA2 is a neurodegenerative disease caused by expansion of an unstable CAG repeat in the SCA2 or ataxin-2 gene on human chromosome 12. SCA2 typically shows a phenotype of progressive ataxia accompanied by slow saccadic eye movements, but a wide phenotypic spectrum is observed including L-dopa-responsive Parkinsonism. Ataxin-2 is a member of a novel protein family that is evolutionarily conserved. The wide separation between normal and pathological repeat ranges seen in other CAG repeat disorders is not present in SCA2; alleles with reduced penetrance exist. Transgenic mice expressing mutant ataxin-2[Q58] show progressive functional and morphologic deficits. Knockdown of the ataxin-2 ortholog in the worm and fly is an embryonic lethal. Ataxin-2 knockout in the mouse causes weight gain due to hyperphagia.

I. SCA2: THE HUMAN PHENOTYPE

In addition to ataxic gait and other cerebellar findings, many patients have slow saccadic eye movements. Tendon reflexes may be brisk during the first years of life, but absent several years later. Analysis of a large number of SCA2 pedigrees has indicated a wide range of phenotypic manifestations that make SCA2 indistinguishable from other SCAs in the individual patient. Some findings, however, are particularly common in SCA2. These are slow saccades, peripheral neuropathy, and dementia. Deficits of frontal executive function are also frequent in SCA2, even in early stages of the disease (reviewed in Pulst, 2003).

Movement disorders are common in SCA2. Geschwind et al. (1997) found a relatively high incidence of dystonia or chorea, and myoclonus is prominent in Cuban SCA2 patients, especially in those with early onset (Pulst, personal observation). Parkinsonism and even L-dopa-responsive Parkinsonism without significant ataxia has recently been recognized as a feature of SCA2 mutations (reviewed in Payami et al., 2003).

II. ATAXIN-2: NORMAL FUNCTION

The ataxin-2 cDNA sequence predicts a protein with 1,312 amino acids with the CAG repeat coding for polyglutamine (Pulst et al., 1996; Sanpei et al., 1996). The 5′-sequence of the SCA2 cDNA is extremely GC rich and two potential ATG initiation codons can be identified. The most 5′ ATG is located 78 bp downstream of an in-frame stop codon. Usage of this translation initiation site predicts a protein of 140.1 . The second ATG, which has a better Kozak consensus sequence, is located just 5′ to the CAG repeat and would result in a protein with relative M.W. of 125. Proteins observed by Western blot analysis and conservation of the 5′ ATG in the mouse (Nechiporuk et al., 1998) suggest that the 5′ ATG is the predominant site of translation initiation.

By Northern blot analysis, a 4.5 kb *SCA2* transcript is recognized in RNAs from brain, heart, placenta, liver, skeletal muscle, and pancreas with little expression in lung or kidney (Pulst et al., 1996; Sanpei et al., 1996; Imbert et al., 1996). Antibodies to ataxin-2 recognize a 145 kDa protein in mouse and human brains (Nechiporuk et al., 1998; Huynh et al., 1999). The protein expression is not restricted to those neuronal populations that show the most severe degeneration.

Homology searches using the cDNA and amino acid sequences have identified homologies with several proteins (Figure 1). Significant sequence homology was detected with a protein designated ataxin-2 related protein (A2RP) and the mouse SCA2 protein (Pulst et al., 1996; Figueroa et al., 2003). A2RP is also known under the name A2D for Ataxin-2 Domain protein (Meunier et al., 2002). A motif predicted to bind to poly(A)-binding protein is present in ataxin-2 and A2RP (Kozlov et al., 2001). The polyglutamine tract in human ataxin-2 is not present in A2RP or in mouse ataxin-2 suggesting that it may not be important for the normal function of ataxin-2. Ataxin-2 interacts with a protein (A2BP) that is the human homolog of the *C. elegans* protein fox-1 (Shibata et al., 2000).

III. EFFECTS OF REDUCED ATAXIN-2 EXPRESSION IN THE WORM, THE FLY, AND THE MOUSE

Animal models have begun to unravel the normal and pathologic function of ataxin-2. Human ataxin-2 has 44%

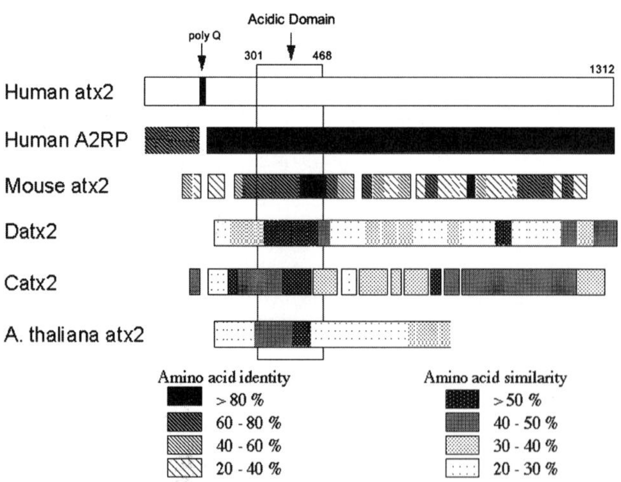

FIGURE 1 Ataxin-2 homologs and orthologs. Amino acid sequence identity (for vertebrate sequences) or similarity (for invertebrate and plant sequences) is indicated by degree of shading. Highly conserved domains are boxed.

amino acid similarity with its worm ortholog (Figure 1). Using the endogenous promoter coupled with a GFP expression vector, Kiehl et al. (2000) studied the expression of Catx-2. Strong expression in adult muscle and nervous system was seen. Catx-2 was also heavily expressed in the embryo. The use of RNA interference (RNAi) allowed knockdown of expression of the ataxin-2 ortholog in *C. elegans*. Injection of RNAi or addition to the media resulted in early embryonic lethality. Knockdown of the A2BP1 ortholog, known as fox-1, resulted in even more significant reduction in egg cell mass.

Similar observations have been made in the fly. Loss of Datx2 results in a recessive lethal phenotype. Datx2 is abundant in nurse cells and the oocyte and appears to be exclusively cytoplasmic. Hypomorphic Datx2 alleles cause egg chambers to arrest at a stage when nurse cells transport their cytoplasmic contents into the oocyte through intracytoplasmatic bridges.

Even in the absence of GAL4-induced expression, several Datx2 transgenes were able to rescue the Datx2 larval lethality. Although flies rescued with specific transgenes continued to show a motor and rough eye phenotype, bristle defects were common in all rescued flies as a consequence of reduced *Datx* function. Actin bundles in these bristles were shorter and thinner than in wild-types. Aberrant actin structures were also detected in the fly eye, when eye imaginal discs from wild-type flies, *Datx2* mutants, and flies overexpressing *Datx2* were compared. Increased or decreased Datx2 expression resulted in abnormal punctate actin aggregates. These results suggest that the normal cellular role for *Datx2* is dosage sensitive.

An ataxin-2 deficient mouse line has been generated by homologous recombination. These lines do not develop apparent neurodegeneration and have no gross tissue or developmental changes. These observations support the hypothesis that polyQ expansion does not lead to a loss of function in SCA2 (Figueroa et al., 2004).

Quite surprisingly, ataxin-2 deficient mice showed weight gain beginning at approximately three months (Figure 2). Heterozygous animals had an intermediate phenotype. Weight gain was caused by hyperphagia; food restriction to 4 g of rodent chow per day resulted in a weight similar to that of wild-type littermates.

IV. ATAXIN-2: ABNORMAL FUNCTION

In SCA2 brains, antibodies to ataxin-2 or to expanded polyglutamine repeats show intense cytoplasmic staining that appears significantly stronger than in simultaneously stained control brains. Instead of a finely granular staining pattern, the entire cytoplasm is strongly immunoreactive in SCA2 brains. Huynh et al. (1999) did not detect intranuclear inclusions in Purkinje and dentate neurons. Koyano

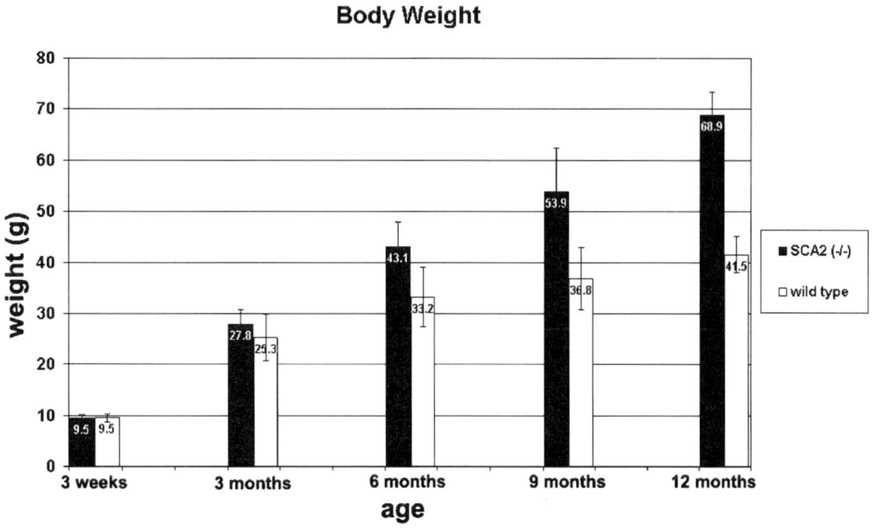

FIGURE 2 Body weight in ataxin-2 deficient mice (*Sca2*$^{-/-}$) and wild-type mice of the same background (C57BL/6J:129X1/SVJ). Ataxin-2 deficiency leads to significant obesity.

et al. (1999) reported ubiquitinated intranuclear inclusions in about 1 to 2% of neurons in affected areas except in Purkinje neurons. This suggested that the formation of intranuclear inclusions is a late event and not necessary for pathogenesis in SCA2. Pang et al. (2002), however, detected intranuclear inclusions in a larger number of neurons in the brainstem and the cortex in two brains from SCA2 patients. These authors also reported on the presence of intranuclear inclusions in glial cells, confirming the observations by Huynh et al. (1999) that ataxin-2 staining in glial cells was increased in SCA2 brains.

V. TRANSGENIC MOUSE LINES EXPRESSING MUTANT ATAXIN-2

Huynh et al. (2000) expressed full-length human ataxin-2 under the control of the Purkinje cell specific Pcp2 promoter in C57BL/6JxDBA/2J mice. Only mice expressing ataxin-2 with 58 glutamine repeats (ataxin-2[Q58]), but not those with ataxin-2[Q22] showed progressive motor deficits and morphologic alterations.

A. Functional Testing of Transgenic Lines

Three independent functional tests were performed to determine the effect of transgene expression on Purkinje cell function: clasping, footprinting, and rotarod analysis. Clasping is a non-specific phenotype seen in mice with motor deficits due to lesions in various neurologic systems. It describes a tendency to fold the hindlegs when held by the tail for at least one minute. Clasping was observed at four to five months in line Q58-19, and at eight to twelve months in the Q58-11 line. In Q58-5B animals, no clasping was observed up to twenty-six weeks of age. Q22-4 and Q22-5 animals did not show clasping up to twelve months.

Stride length was significantly altered in mice expressing mutant ataxin-2 compared with wild-type mice or mice expressing ataxin-2[Q22] (Figure 3A). In the Q58-19 line, stride length was significantly reduced by 19% at eight weeks. At sixteen weeks, all three ataxin-2[Q58] lines showed similar reductions in stride length. Mice expressing ataxin-2[Q22] showed no significant reduction in stride length compared to wild-type mice even at twelve months (Figure 3A). Thus, the functional deficits were specific to expression of mutant ataxin-2 and the deficits were progressive with time.

For rotarod testing, mice were placed on a rod that rotated at increasing speeds from 4 to 40 rotations per minute for a total of 10 minutes (Figure 3B). The time that mice were able to stay on the rod was measured and compared between groups of mice. Rotarod testing of lines Q58-11 and Q58-5B confirmed these functional deficits. Wild-type, heterozygous, and homozygous Q58-11 mice were tested at six, fourteen- to sixteen and twenty-six weeks. At six weeks, motor performance of transgenic animals was not different from wild-type mice. At sixteen weeks, homozygous Q58-11 mice already performed poorly on rotarod testing, whereas heterozygous Q58-11 animals performed as well as wild-type. Although mice from the Q58-5B line exhibited later stride-length deficits than those from the Q58-11 line, their rotarod performance matched that of the Q58-11 mice. The functional deficits were progressive. At twenty-six weeks, both heterozygous and homozygous Q58-11 animals showed severely impaired motor performance. The rotarod

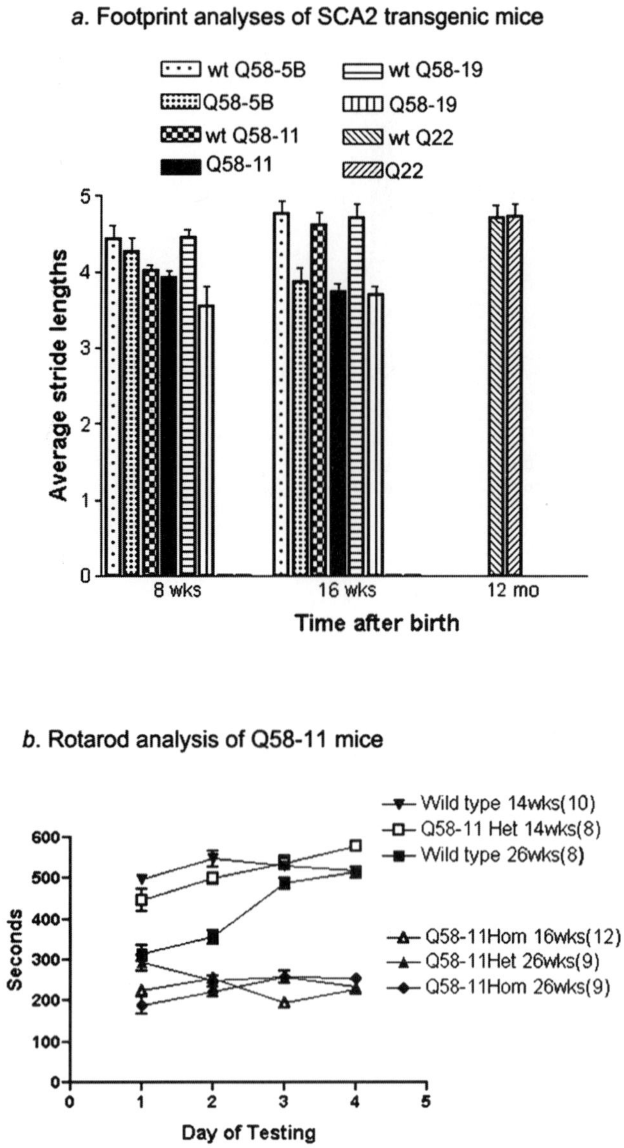

FIGURE 3 Functional analysis of ataxin-2 [Q58] transgenic mouse lines by footprint and rotarod analyses.

A) Progressive decline of stride length in three transgenic lines expressing mutant ataxin-2[Q58] compared with wild-type littermates designated wtQ58-5B, wt Q58-11, and wt Q58-19. Animals expressing the normal ataxin-2[Q22] have normal stride length even at twelve months of age.

B) Rotarod analysis of line Q58-11. Mice in line 58Q-11 show a progressive motor deficit. Four trials were conducted each day and the average time on the rotarod is shown for each day. This paradigm was repeated for days 2 to 4. Doubling of the gene dosage by breeding to homozygosity increases the motor deficit and results in abnormal performance that is already detectable at sixteen weeks. Note the variability in performance of two groups of wild-type animals at fourteen and twenty-six weeks, indicating the need for simultaneous evaluation of control groups in the rotarod testing paradigm. Numbers in parentheses denote number of animals per trial.

performance of animals expressing ataxin-2[Q22] was not significantly different from wild type animals.

B. Morphologic Changes in Transgenic Lines

Labeling with antibodies to either ataxin-2 or 1C2 antibody did not reveal intranuclear inclusions, although Purkinje cell cytoplasm labeled intensely with these antibodies in animals expressing ataxin-2[Q58]. Ubiquitin-labeling was undetectable in Purkinje cells of wild-type and transgenic animals. To characterize dendritic morphology of Purkinje cells an antibody to Calbindin28K was used (Figure 4). Calbindin28K is expressed in the cytoplasm and dendritic processes of cerebellar Purkinje cells. Calbindin immunoreactivity is significantly reduced in Purkinje cells of patients with SCAs. All three transgenic lines expressing ataxin-2[Q58] showed a reduction in Calbindin staining. This reduction was progressive. Loss of the dendritic arbor was closely followed by a loss in PC number. The percentage of surviving Purkinje cells showed a progressive decline. At twenty-four to twenty-seven weeks, Purkinje cell number was reduced by 50 to 53% in lines Q58-5B, Q58-11, and Q58-19. Compared with wild-type mice, mice expressing ataxin-2[Q22] showed no reduction in Purkinje cell number even at one year of age.

VI. COMPARISON OF THE SCA1 AND SCA2 MOUSE MODELS

The transgenic SCA1 and SCA2 mouse models share several crucial features that permit comparisons of the phenotype (Burright et al., 1995; Klement et al., 1998). In both models, the transgene is expressed under control of the PcP2 promoter that targets expression to Purkinje cells. In addition, both models express a full-length cDNA. Although the precise lengths of the polyQ tracts are different, 82 repeats in the SCA1 model and 58 glutamines in the SCA2 model, the polyQ tracts are similar with regard to polyQ repeat lengths in patients; both correspond to juvenile onset in the respective disease. The behavioral phenotype is similar in both models, although SCA1 mice (line B05) have an earlier disease onset and more severe progression, which may be related to greater gene copy number and higher expression levels. The most significant difference lies in the observation that in the SCA1 mouse model intranuclear localization of the gene product is necessary for pathogenesis (Klement et al., 1998, 1999). Cytoplasmic expression of ataxin-1 in Purkinje cells obtained by deletion of a nuclear localization signal in ataxin-1 results in mice with a normal behavioral phenotype without altered Purkinje cells. In contrast, in the SCA2 model cytoplasmic localization of ataxin-2 is sufficient. Intranuclear inclusion bodies or intranuclear aggregates are not observed at the light microscopic level in mice expressing ataxin-2[Q58].

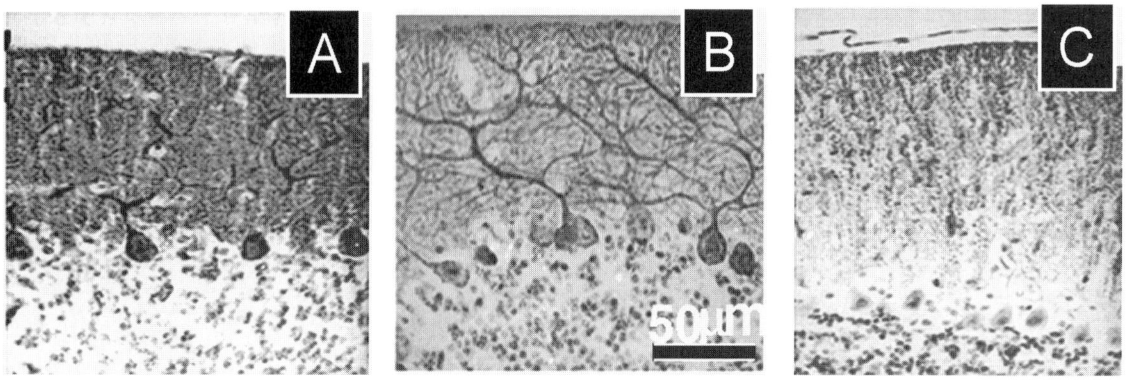

FIGURE 4 Decreased calbindin staining in cytoplasm and dendrites of cerebellar Purkinje cells in mice expressing mutant ataxin-2[Q58]. Calbinding 28K labeling of Purkinje cells of wild-type mice (A), mice expressing an ataxin-2[Q22] transgene (B), and mice expressing a mutant ataxin-2[Q58] transgene. Mice were between four and seven weeks of age. Bar: 50 μ.

Acknowledgments

This work was supported by the Carmen and Louis Warschaw Endowment for Neurology, F.R.I.E.N.D.s of Neurology, the National Ataxia Foundation, and grant RO1-NS33123 from the National Institutes of Health.

Video Legends

SEGMENT 1 Spontaneous tremor four months after left MVMT lesion (02:31:01 to 02:32:15).

SEGMENT 2 L-dopa test dose ten months after left MVMT lesion (02:32:16 to 02:32:43).

SEGMENT 3 Choreiform movements occurring 15 minutes after administration of L-dopa (02:32:43 to 02:34:06).

SEGMENT 4 Chorea and other hyperkinetic dyskinesias occurring 40 minutes after administration of L-dopa (02:34:06 to 02:35:04).

SEGMENT 5 Three hours after administration of L-dopa, tremor is once again present (02:35:04 to end).

References

Burright, E.N., H.B. Clark, A. Servadio, T. Matilla, R.M. Feddersen, W.S. Yunis, L.A. Duvick, H.Y. Zoghbi, and H.T. Orr. 1995. SCA1 transgenic mice: a model for neurodegeneration caused by an expanded CAG trinucleotide repeat. *Cell* **82**:937–948.

Figueroa, K.P., T.R. Kiehl, X. Xu, and S.M. Pulst. 2004. Knock-out of the ataxin-2 (SCA2) gene causes hyperphagia and marked obesity. *Neurology (Suppl.).*

Figueroa, K.P., and S.M. Pulst. 2003. Identification and expression of the gene for human ataxin-2 related protein (A2RP) on chromosome 16. *J Exp Neurol*

Geschwind, D.H., S. Perlman, C.P. Figueroa, L.J. Treiman, and S.M. Pulst. 1997. The prevalence and wide clinical spectrum of the spinocerebellar ataxia type 2 trinucleotide repeat in patients with autosomal dominant cerebellar ataxia. *Am J Hum Genet* **60**:842–850.

Huynh, D.P., M.R. Del Bigio, D.H. Ho, and S.M. Pulst. 1999. Expression of ataxin-2 in brains from normal individuals and patients with Alzheimer's disease and spinocerebellar ataxia 2. *Ann Neurol* **45**:232–241.

Huynh, D.P., K.P. Figueroa, N. Hoang, and S.M. Pulst. 2000. Nuclear localization or inclusion body formation are not necessary for SCA2 pathogenesis in man or mouse. *Nat Genet* **2**:44–50.

Imbert, G., F. Saudou, G. Yvert, D. Devys, Y. Trottier, J.M. Garnier, C. Webe, J.L. Mandel, G. Cancel, N. Abbas, A. Dürr, O. Didierjean, G. Stevanin, Y. Agid, and A. Brice. 1996. Cloning of the gene for spinocerebellar ataxia 2 reveals a locus with high sensitivity to expanded CAG/glutamine repeats. *Nat Genet* **14**:285–291.

Kiehl, T.R., H. Shibata, and S.M. Pulst. 2000. The ortholog of human ataxin-2 is essential for early embryonic patterning in *C. elegans*. *J Mol Neurosci* **15**:231–241.

Klement, I.A., P.J. Skinner, M.D. Kaytor, H. Yi, S.M. Hersch, H.B. Clark, H.Y. Zoghbi, and H.T. Orr. 1998. Ataxin-1 nuclear localization and aggregation: role in polyglutamine-induced disease in SCA1 transgenic mice. *Cell* **95**:41–53.

Klement, I.A., H.Y. Zoghbi, and H.T. Orr. 1999. Pathogenesis of polyglutamine-induced disease: a model for SCA1. *Mol Genet Metab* **66**:172–178.

Koyano, S., T. Uchihara, H. Fujigasaki, A. Nakamura, S. Yagishita, and K. Iwabuchi. 1999. Neuronal intranuclear inclusions in spinocerebellar ataxia type 2: triple-labeling immunofluorescent study. *Neurosci Lett* **273**:117–20.

Kozlov, G., J.F. Trempe, K. Khaleghpour, A. Kahvejian, I. Ekiel, and K. Gehring. 2001. Structure and function for the C-terminal structure and function of the C-terminal PABC domain of human poly(A)-binding protein. *Proc Natl Acad Sci U S A* **98**:4409–4413.

Meunier, C., D. Bordereaux, F. Porteu, S. Gisselbrecht, S. Chretien, and G. Courtois. 2002. Cloning and characterization of a family of proteins associated with Mpl. *J Biol Chem* **277**:9139–9147.

Nechiporuk, T., D.P. Huynh, K. Figueroa, S. Sahba, A. Nechiporuk, and S.M. Pulst. 1998. The mouse SCA2 gene: cDNA sequence, alternative splicing and protein expression. *Hum Mol Genet* **8**:1301–1309.

Pang, J.T., P. Giunti, S. Chamberlain, R. Vitaliani, T. Scaravilli, L. Martinian, N.W. Wood, F. Scaravilli, and O. Ansorge. 2002. Neuronal intranuclear inclusions in SCA2: a genetic morphological and immunohistochemical study of two cases. *Brain* **125**:656–663.

Payami, H., J. Nutt, S. Gancher, T. Bird, M.G. McNeal, W.K. Seltzer, J. Hussey, P. Lockhart, K. Gwinn-Hardy, A.A. Singleton, A.B. Singleton,

J. Hardy, and M. Farrer. 2003. SCA2 may present as levodopa-responsive Parkinsonism. *Mov Disord* **218**:425–429.

Pulst, S.M., A. Nechiporuk, T. Nechiporuk, S. Gispert, X.N. Chen, I. Lopes-Cendes, S. Pearlman, S. Starkman, G. Orozco-Diaz, A. Lunkes, P. DeJong, G.A. Rouleau, G. Auburger, J.R. Korenberg, C. Figueroa, and S. Sahba. 1996. Moderate expansion of a normally biallelic trinucleotide repeat in spinocerebellar ataxia type 2. *Nat Genetics* **14**: 269–276.

Pulst, S.M. 2003. Spinocerebellar ataxia 2 (SCA2). In *Genetics of Movement Disorders* (S.M. Pulst, Ed.), pp. 45–55. Academic Press, New York.

Sanpei, K., H. Takano, S. Igarashi, T. Sato, M. Oyake, H. Sasaki, A. Wakisaka, K. Tashiro, Y. Ishida, T. Ikeuchi, R. Koide, M. Saito, A. Sato, T. Tanaka, S. Hanyu, Y. Takiyama, M. Nishizawa, N. Shimizu, Y. Nomura, M. Segawa, K. Iwabuchi, I. Eguchi, H. Tanaka, H. Takahashi, and S. Tsuji. 1996. Identification of the spinocerebellar ataxia type 2 gene using a direct identification of repeat expansion and cloning technique, DIRECT. *Nat Genetics* **14**:277–284.

Shibata, H., D.P. Huynh, and S.M. Pulst. 2000. A novel protein with RNA binding motifs interacts with ataxin-2. *Hum Mol Genet* **9**:1303–1313.

CHAPTER

K5

SCA7 Mouse Models

DOMINIQUE HELMLINGER and DIDIER DEVYS*

Spinocerebellar ataxia type 7 (SCA7) is an adult-onset neurodegenerative disorder belonging to the clinically and genetically heterogeneous group of autosomal dominant cerebellar ataxias (ADCAs) (Konigsmark and Weiner, 1970; Harding, 1993). ADCA type I-III is characterized by progressive degeneration of the cerebellum, brainstem, and spinocerebellar tracts. In ADCA type II (SCA7), cerebellar ataxia is associated with progressive pigmentary macular degeneration and loss of visual acuity (Benomar et al., 1994; Enevoldson et al., 1994; Gouw et al., 1994; Martin et al., 1994). SCA7 patients typically present with gait and limb ataxia consistently associated with dysarthria and variably with additional symptoms, such as a pyramidal syndrome, dysphagia, and oculomotor abnormalities.

The onset of SCA7 is usually in the second to fourth decade (median, 30 years), but can vary from a few months to over 70 years ((Michalik et al., 2003) and refs. therein). Although cerebellar ataxia is usually the presenting symptom, patients with an earlier onset of the disease tend to develop visual impairment before ataxia (Johansson et al., 1998). SCA7 is characterized by a marked clinical anticipation as the age at onset is, on average, 20 years earlier in the offspring compared to the affected parents. SCA7 juvenile- or infantile-onset patients show a more rapid progression and a broader spectrum of phenotypes than adult-onset patients, with both neuronal and non-neuronal tissues being affected in infantile cases (Benton et al., 1998; David et al., 1998; Johansson et al., 1998).

Pathologically, SCA7 presents as an olivocerebellar atrophy with massive neuronal loss and gliosis in the cerebellum, mainly affecting Purkinje cells and the dentate nucleus, in inferior olive nuclei and mild loss of neurons in basis pontis and substantia nigra. Degenerative changes in the retina initially affect cone photoreceptors, but progress toward a cone-rod dystrophy (Enevoldson et al., 1994; Gouw et al., 1994; Martin et al., 1994). Importantly, several infantile SCA7 cases have been reported with limited cell loss throughout the central nervous system (CNS), which is probably due to the short duration of the disease (Carpenter and Schumacher, 1966; Ryan et al., 1975; de Jong et al., 1980; Traboulsi et al., 1988).

I. GENETICS OF SCA7

SCA7 is caused by the expansion of a CAG trinucleotide repeat within the coding region of the *SCA7* gene (David

*To whom correspondence should be addressed.
Email: devys@igbmc.u-strasbg.fr

et al., 1997; Del-Favero et al., 1998; Koob et al., 1998). Eight other neurodegenerative disorders, including Huntington disease (HD), spinal and bulbar muscular atrophy (SBMA), dentatorubral and pallidoluysian atrophy (DRPLA), and other spinocerebellar ataxias (SCA1, SCA2, SCA3, SCA6, and SCA17), are also caused by a CAG repeat expansion leading to an abnormally long polyglutamine (polyQ) tract in the respective proteins (Cummings and Zoghbi, 2000; Zoghbi and Orr, 2000).

Normal SCA7 alleles contain a pure CAG repeat which is polymorphic ranging from 4 to 35 repeats, although about 75% of normal alleles carry 10 CAG. Mutant SCA7 alleles contain between 38 and 70 repeats, but extreme expansions have been documented (up to 460) (Benton et al., 1998; Johansson et al., 1998; van de Warrenburg et al., 2001). As for other polyQ disorders, longer SCA7 CAG repeats are correlated with earlier onset and more rapid progression of the disease. In SCA7, repeats larger than 70 CAG typically lead to juvenile cases (onset below ten years, death within a few years) while those larger than 150 CAG result in infantile cases (onset below two years, death within a few months) (Michalik et al., 2003). Clinical anticipation has been described in all polyQ disorders and is explained by an intergenerational instability of expanded CAG repeats. The SCA7 mutation is the most unstable among polyQ disorders, as CAG repeats expand at almost every maternal or paternal transmission. Importantly, the largest CAG repeats found in juvenile and infantile cases are always transmitted by affected fathers carrying moderate expanded repeats (Benton et al., 1998; van de Warrenburg et al., 2001), in agreement with the extreme instability of the SCA7 CAG repeat in male germ line (Monckton et al., 1999). Importance of genomic context for SCA7 CAG repeat instability has been suggested based upon studies comparing transgenic mice carrying a SCA7 mutation either in a genomic fragment or in a cDNA construct. The CAG repeat was highly unstable specifically in its proper genomic context (Libby et al., 2003).

Genetic and molecular studies indicate that expanded polyQ tracts confer a toxic gain-of-function to the otherwise unrelated proteins (Cummings and Zoghbi, 2000; Zoghbi and Orr, 2000; Ross, 2002). Despite widespread expression of all these genes throughout the brain and other tissues, only a specific subset of neuronal populations is vulnerable in each of these diseases. However, severe juvenile-onset cases display significant overlap in phenotypes, indicating that neurons usually spared can be targets for mutant protein toxic effect.

SCA7 is unique among all polyQ disorders in that it is the only one affecting the retina, which is particularly suitable for phenotypic and molecular analysis. Furthermore, SCA7 is the only one in which infantile cases with extremely large expansions are found. This appeared favorable for generating a detectable neurological phenotype over the mouse life-span, using either very long CAG/polyQ tracts or cell-type specific overexpression of cDNA constructs with modest repeat lengths (Table 1). Many SCA7 mouse models have been generated and have provided significant new insights into SCA7 pathogenesis that advanced our understanding of the mechanisms potentially implicated in polyQ disorders.

II. ATAXIN-7, THE PROTEIN MUTATED IN SCA7

A. Normal Function

Ataxin-7 is an 892 amino acid protein of unknown function. Initial sequence analysis predicted a bipartite nuclear localization signal (NLS, position 378–393). We recently searched for ataxin-7 homologue genes in various vertebrate genomes and identified four ataxin-7 paralogues in *Homo sapiens*, *Mus musculus*, *Brachydanio rerio*, and *Fugu rubripes* (Helmlinger et al., 2004b). Notably, sequence comparison of ataxin-7 family members revealed three conserved blocks: block I (residues 126–176 in human ataxin-7), block II (residues 341–400) and block III (residues 508–565) (Figure 1). The expandable polyQ motif, located N-terminal to block I, is present in human ataxin-7 and in its vertebrate orthologues, but is absent in ataxin-7 paralogues. Using human ataxin-7 block, I and II as query sequences, we and others retrieved several ataxin-7 homologues in more distant species, such as *Anophele gambiae*, *Caenorhabditis briggsae*, and *Saccharomyces cerevisiae* (Mushegian et al., 2000; Scheel et al., 2003). In these genomes, a single ataxin-7 sequence was found and characterized by a weakly conserved block I (16% identity between *H. sapiens* and *S. cerevisiae*) located N-terminal to a highly conserved block II (42% identity between *H. sapiens* and *S. cerevisiae*) and by absence of block III. Two glutamine-rich regions (11 and 8 Qs) are found in the C-terminal part of ataxin-7 yeast orthologue (SGF73) (Figure 1).

SGF73 has been recently identified as a new component of the yeast SAGA (Spt/Ada/Gcn5 acetylase) multi-subunit complex (Gavin et al., 2002; Sanders et al., 2002), a co-activator required for transcription of a subset of RNA polymerase II-dependent genes (Grant et al., 1997; Grant et al., 1998). We showed that human ataxin-7 is an integral component of the TATA-binding protein-free TAF-containing transcriptional complexes (TFTC), which are mammalian homologues of yeast SAGA (Helmlinger et al., 2004b). These complexes contain GCN5 histone acetylase activity and were shown to preferentially acetylate histone H3 in both free and nucleosomal contexts and to activate

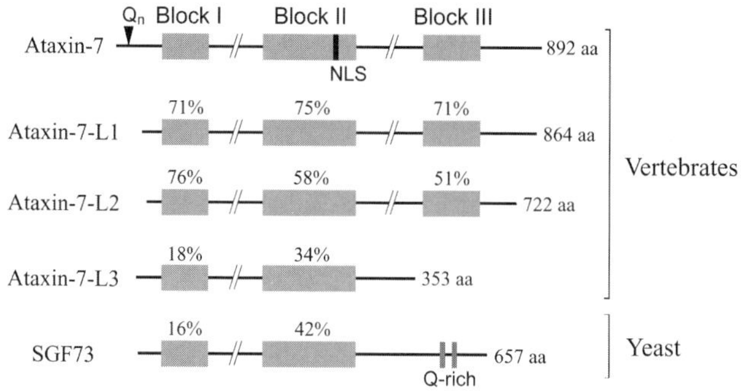

FIGURE 1 Identification of an ataxin-7 gene family and conserved domains in ataxin-7 homologues. Schematic representation of the four ataxin-7 paralogue genes that were found in vertebrates (human, mouse, and fish). A single ataxin-7 orthologue gene was found in yeast. For each conserved block (grey boxes), sequence identities of human ataxin-7 paralogues and yeast SGF73 are indicated relative to human ataxin-7. Only human ataxin-7 contains an expandable polyQ motif (shown as black triangle), located in the N-terminal part of the protein. Yeast SGF73 contain two glutamine-rich (Q-rich, represented as dark grey boxes) motifs in its C-terminal part. The nuclear localization signal (NLS, black block) is also indicated in human ataxin-7.

transcription on chromatin templates (Wieczorek et al., 1998; Brand et al., 1999; Martinez et al., 2001).

B. Expression Levels and Subcellular Localization

Northern blot analysis showed that *SCA7* expression is ubiquitous including different brain regions and non-neuronal tissues (David et al., 1997; Strom et al., 2002). In particular, Lindenberg et al. 2000 showed by *in situ* hybridization that *SCA7* mRNA is found in both affected and unaffected neurons (Lindenberg et al., 2000). In agreement, ataxin-7 protein levels vary between distinct brain regions, but are not markedly elevated in SCA7-vulnerable neurons.

Regional distribution of ataxin-7 immunoreactivity does not differ between patients and controls. Several studies using different antibodies suggest that endogenous ataxin-7 subcellular localization varies between neuronal types, being either nuclear, cytoplasmic, or even both (Cancel et al., 2000; Lindenberg et al., 2000; Einum et al., 2001; Jonasson et al., 2002; Strom et al., 2002). However, ataxin-7 is not preferentially nuclear in neurons affected in SCA7 pathology.

Finally, the ataxin-7 NLS has been shown to be functional in transfected mammalian cells (Kaytor et al., 1999; Zander et al., 2001). However, a recent study suggested that ataxin-7 NLS might be located in the C-terminal part of the protein (Chen et al., 2004). Recombinant normal ataxin-7 was found nuclear in all neuronal types from different transgenic mice (Garden et al., 2002; Helmlinger et al., 2004a) and Yoo et al. showed that endogenous mouse ataxin-7 is predominantly nuclear in the cerebellum using fractionation experiments (Yoo et al., 2003).

III. SCA7 PATHOGENESIS

A. Phenotypic Abnormalities of SCA7 Mouse Models

All generated SCA7 mouse models express full-length ataxin-7, but differ in the size of the polyQ expansion and in the neuronal types targeted (table 1). Four SCA7 transgenics models have been generated using heterologous promoters. Platelet-derived growth factor chain B (PDGF-B) and prion (Prp) promoters led to widespread overexpression of mutant ataxin-7 with 90 to 128 Qs, while rhodopsin (Rho) and Pcp2 promoters led to a restricted overexpression of the transgene product (Yvert et al., 2000; La Spada et al., 2001; Yvert et al., 2001; Garden et al., 2002). The P7E and R7E models show dysfunction of Purkinje cells and rod photoreceptors, respectively, two cell types affected in the human disease. Yoo et al. generated SCA7 knock-in mice by introducing a 266 CAG repeat into the *Sca7* locus by homologous recombination, leading to expression of the mutant protein at endogenous levels and in the proper spatio-temporal pattern (Yoo et al., 2003).

In knock-in and transgenic models, widespread expression of mutant ataxin-7 in the CNS causes adult-onset and progressive neurological phenotype leading to premature death. These mice typically present with gait ataxia and motor incoordination which is quantified by progressive impairment of rotarod performance. As disease progresses, symptoms become more complex and variable among the different models although tremors, weight loss, and hypoactivity are consistently observed. Phenotypic differences are likely brought out by variable expression patterns and by distinct genetic backgrounds used to generate these mice. Also, differences in mutant ataxin-7 expression levels and polyQ length likely account for specific severity reported in the different models. Despite expression in peripheral organs such as heart and kidney, Prp mice (6076 line) do not show pathology in these tissues. However, knock-in mice display muscle wasting with kyphosis, although muscle pathology was not assessed.

Knock-in mice have been generated using a 266 CAG repeat expansion found in an infantile SCA7 patient and present symptoms strikingly similar to those reported in this patient, with comparable disease onset (one month) and progression (death around five months). Interestingly, Yoo et al. showed that mice compound heterozygous for an expanded and a null *Sca7* allele (*Sca7* 266Q/-) display a phenotype comparable to *Sca7* 266Q/5Q mice, demonstrating that SCA7 pathology results from a gain of function

TABLE 1 SCA7 Mouse Models

Model design			Expression		Phenotype			
Promoter	Protein length	PolyQ length	Level	Cell type	Onset	Severity[a]	Death	Line Refs
TRANSGENIC SCA7 MICE								
Rhodopsin	full-length	90Q	High	Rods (retina)	1 mo[b] (ERG[c])	+++	No	R7E[d] (Yvert et al., 2000)
Pcp-2	full-length	90Q	Moderate	Purkinje	11 mo (rotarod)	+	No	P7E[d] (Yvert et al., 2000)
PDGF-B	full-length	128Q	Moderate	CNS	5 mo	+/++	8 mo/No	B7E2[d] (Yvert et al., 2001)
Prp	full-length	92Q	Moderate	CNS	3 mo (ERG; rotarod)	+++	5 mo	6076[d] (La Spada et al., 2001; Garden et al., 2002)
KNOCK-IN SCA7 MICE								
Endogenous	full-length	266Q	Endogenous		1 mo (ERG; rotarod)	+++	5 mo	H10[d] (Yoo et al., 2003)

[a] The number of plus signs denotes the severity of the phenotype, from + (mild) to +++ (severe).
[b] mo: months.
[c] ERG: electroretinograpy.
[d] Data summarized in this table were obtained from the most characterized lines in each study.

mutation and not from a partial loss of ataxin-7 normal function. Furthermore, enhanced toxicity reported in homozygous *Sca7* 266Q/266Q mice and in homozygous R7E mice indicates a gene dosage effect (Yoo et al., 2003; Helmlinger et al., 2004a).

As demonstrated for other polyQ disorders, prolonged exposure of neurons to mutant proteins is necessary for neuronal dysfunction. Thus, it was shown that either high overexpression of mutant ataxin-7 or very long polyQ tracts were required to produce a phenotype during the mouse's short life-span. Indeed, no ataxic phenotype was detected in one Prp line (line 6529) which expresses mutant ataxin-7 at 0.75-fold the endogenous level. Severe neurological phenotype and premature death are produced by overexpression of ataxin-7 with 92 Qs (2.5-fold the endogenous level) in another Prp line (line 6561) or by endogenous level of ataxin-7 with an extremely large polyQ expansion (266 Qs).

B. Neuropathological Features of SCA7 Mice

Reduced size of Purkinje cell bodies has been described in two transgenic models (P7E and Prp lines) and in the knock-in model (Yvert et al., 2000; Garden et al., 2002; Yoo et al., 2003). Purkinje cell pathology correlated with the onset of neurological signs and occurred without significant cell loss, as suggested by normal cell counts and by absence of apoptotic cells. Targeted overexpression of mutant ataxin-7 in Purkinje cells produced a mild and late-onset neurological phenotype associated with reduced dendritic arborization in 16 months-old P7E animals (Table 1). Interestingly, Garden et al. also observed reduced arborization of Purkinje cells in 5-month-old 6076 mice, in which transgene expression could be detected only in the granular and molecular cell layers, but not in the Purkinje cells (Garden et al., 2002). These findings suggest that mutant ataxin-7 could exert its toxic effect on Purkinje cells in a non-cell autonomous manner. At variance with observations made in the transgenic models, Purkinje neurons from the SCA7 knock-in mice exhibit normal dendritic arborization (Yoo et al., 2003). Interestingly, SCA1 knock-in mice present Purkinje cell pathology with marked reduction of dendritic arborization and significant cell loss (Watase et al., 2002). Although Purkinje cells are affected in both SCA1 and SCA7 knock-in mice, the dissimilar neuronal pathology highlights the importance of protein context in polyQ induced toxicity.

C. Retinal Pathology of SCA7 Mice

SCA7 is unique among all polyQ disorders as it is the only one commonly affecting the retina in addition to the brain. Using different SCA7 mouse models, numerous studies have attempted to decipher the specific mechanisms that underlie SCA7 restricted retinal involvement. Furthermore, mouse retina is a valuable tissue in which to study neurodegeneration as neuronal dysfunction and

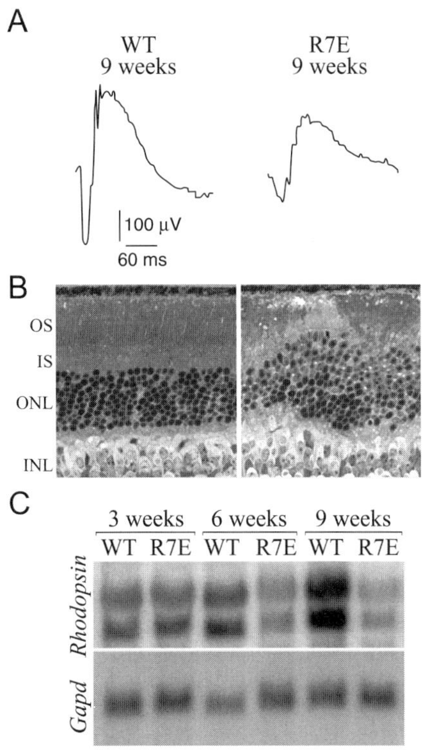

FIGURE 2 Electrophysiogical, histological, and transcriptional abnormalities in the retina from SCA7 transgenic mice (R7E mice). (**A**) Scotopic electroretinographic (ERG) responses from wild-type and R7E mice at 9 weeks of age. Each recording corresponds to the average response of one animal at maximal light intensities (from 0 to 1.4 log cd s m-2). Decrease of ERG response was concomitant to progressive thinning of the segment layer. (**B**) Histologically, the photoreceptor nuclear layer (ONL) is completely disrupted by numerous whorls that correspond to focal thinning of the outer segments (OS) layer. OS, outer segment; IS, inner segment; ONL, outer nuclear layer; INL, inner nuclear layer. (**C**) Rhodopsin mRNA levels are progressively and severely reduced in SCA7 mice. Northern blot of total RNA extracted from wild-type and R7E mice at 3, 6, and 9 weeks of age was hybridized with rhodopsin and Gapd probes, as an internal control. Constant expression of rhodopsin in aging wild-type mice contrasted with a progressive diminution of rhodopsin mRNA up to almost undetectable levels in nine-week-old R7E mice.

neuropathological features can be directly assessed on living animals using electroretinography (ERG) and fundus examination, respectively. Retinal dysfunction was quantified by recording electrophysiological responses from the different retinal neuronal types in two transgenic models (R7E and Prp lines) and in the knock-in model (Yvert et al., 2000; Garden et al., 2002; Yoo et al., 2003). Scotopic (dark-adapted) ERGs record both rod photoreceptors (a-wave) and rod-initiated post-synaptic responses (b-wave) while photopic (light-adapted) ERGs record cone photoreceptor-initiated responses. Early-onset decrease of ERG recordings was observed in all SCA7 models and eventually led to complete absence of photoreceptor responses (Figure 2A). In R7E mice, in which transgene expression is restricted to rod photoreceptors, scotopic a-wave amplitude progressively decreased up to flat recordings from one year of age. In mouse models expressing mutant ataxin-7 in the entire retina, scotopic a- and b-waves are severely affected. Scotopic b-wave decrease may have resulted from decreased input of the rod photoreceptors or from a defect in rod bipolar cells. In the latter models (knock-in and Prp lines), cone-mediated responses were shown to be affected before rod-mediated responses, raising the possibility that mouse cone photoreceptors may be more sensitive to mutant ataxin-7, similar to the human pathology. However, mouse cone photoreceptors may simply be particularly sensitive to any polyQ expansion, as suggested by occurrence of a cone-rod dystrophy in an HD mouse model (Helmlinger et al., 2002).

In R7E mice, fundoscopy revealed white retinal spots across the retina corresponding to areas of photoreceptor segment loss observed by histology (Helmlinger et al., 2004a). The most prominent pathological feature of the retina from all SCA7 mouse models is a progressive thinning of photoreceptors outer and inner segments, in which phototransduction takes place. Shortening of the segments is homogenous in knock-in mice whereas it is periodic in R7E transgenic mice, giving a wavy aspect to the photoreceptor nuclear layer (Figure 2B). This observation might be related to mosaic onset of rhodopsin promoter expression (Zack et al., 1991). In contrast to what was observed in the cerebellum from SCA7 mice, significant photoreceptor cell loss was consistently evidenced by cell counting and TUNEL staining in the retina from SCA7 mice. However, photoreceptor degeneration was limited, as knock-in and R7E mice retained 70–80% of photoreceptors until terminal stages of the disease. Furthermore, ERG abnormalities appeared prior to photoreceptor cell loss, which was detectable at fifteen weeks of age in knock-in mice and from one year of age in R7E mice. Finally, all three models showed Müller glial cells activation, which is an indicator of photoreceptor degeneration, as revealed by an increased GFAP staining (Rattner et al., 2001).

Using R7E transgenic mice, we recently reported that rhodopsin promoter activity was early and dramatically repressed, suggesting that downregulation of photoreceptor-specific genes plays a major role in polyQ-induced retinal dysfunction (Section III.H). Since the rhodopsin promoter drives mutant ataxin-7 expression in these SCA7 mice, we assessed whether downregulation of mutant SCA7 transgene would reverse retinopathy progression and aggregate formation. Although residual expression of mutant ataxin-7 was found negligible from nine weeks of age, SCA7 transgenic mice showed a progressive decline of photoreceptor activity leading to a complete loss of electroretinographic responses from one year of age (Helmlinger et al., 2004a). At this age, aggregates were cleared in only half of the photoreceptors, indicating that their formation is not fully reversible in this model (Section III.D). These results suggest that mutant ataxin-7-induced toxicity might not be reversible beyond a given pathological threshold. However, high and stable expression levels of mutant ataxin-7 may have more deleterious effects, suggesting that transgene silencing might have slowed retinopathy progression in R7E mice. Regardless, this observation contrasts with previous studies showing that phenotypic abnormalities were reversed after suppression of mutant Huntington expression in a conditional HD mouse model (HD94) (Yamamoto et al., 2000). In R7E mice, disease progression despite long-term extinction of mutant ataxin-7 expression, could be due to a combination of irreversible transcriptional abnormalities and of partial persistence of aggregates (Section III.D).

D. Aggregation of Mutant Ataxin-7 into Nuclear Inclusions

As for other polyglutamine disease-causing proteins, mutant ataxin-7 aggregates and forms nuclear inclusions (NIs), which were first detected by immunohistology performed on post-mortem brain. Several studies using different anti-ataxin-7 antibodies showed that NIs were not particularly enriched in SCA7-vulnerable neurons (Mauger et al., 1999; Cancel et al., 2000; Einum et al., 2001; Jonasson et al., 2002). However, regional distribution of NIs varied between these different studies.

All generated SCA7 mouse models display numerous NIs, both in regions that are affected in patients (*e.g.*, cerebellum, inferior olive nucleus or retina) and in non-affected areas (*e.g.*, cerebral cortex or hippocampus) (Yvert et al., 2001; Garden et al., 2002; Yoo et al., 2003). In all SCA7 transgenic mice, aggregates became detectable at the onset of neurological symptoms and gradually accumulated as disease progressed (Yvert et al., 2000; La Spada et al., 2001; Yvert et al., 2001; Garden et al., 2002). This observation was not reproduced in SCA7 knock-in mice, in which aggregates formed after the onset of neuronal dysfunction (Yoo et al., 2003). However, NIs developed earlier in cone than in rod photoreceptors from these mice, agreeing with an earlier onset of cone dysfunction as assessed by specific ERG recordings. In the early steps of SCA7 knock-in mice pathogenesis, mutant ataxin-7 could be detected only as insoluble material by Western blot analysis of cerebellar extracts, before apparition of visible NIs in Purkinje cells. Together with the observation that expanded polyQ impedes ataxin-7 turnover (Section III.F), these results strongly suggest that mutant ataxin-7 is accumulating faster in affected neurons. Insoluble microaggregates that cannot be detected by conventional microscopy, were recently identified in other polyQ models and could themselves be pathogenic (reviewed in (Michalik and Van Broeckhoven, 2003)). Taken together, the different studies performed in patients and animal models of different polyQ disorders provided challenging results that did not answer the question as to whether polyQ aggregation initiates pathogenesis *per se* or exacerbates the disease already progressing because of the presence of soluble mutant protein.

As described in section III.C, aggregate clearance was observed in about one half of photoreceptors from one-year-old R7E mice, whereas mutant ataxin-7 expression was lost starting at two months of age. Despite long-term loss of mutant ataxin-7 expression and normal proteasomal activity (D.H., unpublished results), a significant number of rods retained aggregates, even in two-year-old R7E mice. Our results suggest that, in this model, aggregate formation is rapid while their clearance is partial and much slower than previously reported in an inducible HD model (Martin-Aparicio et al., 2001). In addition, fluorescence imaging of living cells expressing polyQ expansions revealed the co-existence of stable and dynamic aggregates (Stenoien et al., 2002), which could explain the observation that aggregate formation was not fully reversible in R7E mice.

Many studies have reported abnormal accumulation of a variety of essential proteins into polyQ aggregates from patients and animal models. In SCA7 mice, NIs were consistently stained for ubiquitin, 19S and 20S proteasome subunits, and different chaperones (HSP70, HSC70, and HDJ2) (La Spada et al., 2001; Yvert et al., 2001; Yoo et al., 2003). It has been proposed that recruitment and sequestration of transcription factors, particularly those containing a glutamine-rich motif (*e.g.*, CREB-binding protein (CBP)), would interfere with their normal function, thereby contributing to pathogenesis. Different studies performed in various polyQ models provided challenging results regarding the involvement of a loss of CBP function in polyQ pathogenesis (McCampbell et al., 2000; Steffan et al., 2000; Nucifora et al., 2001; Yu et al., 2002; Taylor et al., 2003). In all SCA7 transgenic models, CBP was found associated with aggregates but without any evidence of depletion from its normal localization. Moreover, Yoo et al. reported that CBP was found associated with NIs late in pathogenesis (eighteen weeks of age, *i.e.*, just before death) while these knock-in mice displayed severe transcriptional defects as early as four weeks of age (Yvert et al., 2001; Yoo et al., 2003). Yvert et al. performed an extensive screen for transcription factors recruitment into NIs and found that none of them was depleted from the nucleoplasm. Furthermore, there was no correlation between the presence of a glutamine-rich motif in the respective transcription factors and their likelihood to be recruited into NIs. Finally, they characterized NI distribution and content in chaperones, proteasome components, and transcription factors in mice overexpressing mutant ataxin-7 throughout the CNS (B7E2 transgenic mice) and reported no obvious differences that would explain regional degeneration specificity observed in patients (Yvert et al., 2001).

E. Proteolytic Processing of Mutant Ataxin-7

Proteolytic processing of expanded polyQ proteins has been reported for HD, DRPLA and SCA3, but not for SCA1 (reviewed in Tarlac and Storey, 2003). It has been hypothesized that this cleavage would lead to nuclear translocation and aggregation of polyQ protein fragments and thus initiate toxic events within the nucleus. In agreement, ataxin-1 is a nuclear protein, notably in Purkinje cells, and does not undergo any cleavage event in SCA1 mouse models and patients' brains (Burright et al., 1995; Servadio et al., 1995; Skinner et al., 1997; Klement et al., 1998). In contrast, immunohistochemical analysis of SCA7 transgenic mice revealed that ataxin-7-formed NIs are not immunoreactive for antibodies recognizing C-terminal epitopes of the protein. This cleavage event affects specifically mutant ataxin-7 since the normal form remains full-length and was consistently observed in all neuronal types expressing mutant ataxin-7, in particular both in SCA7-vulnerable and spared neurons (Yvert et al., 2001; Garden et al., 2002). These findings were obtained by immunostaining using two antibodies raised against the same peptide (position 872–891), raising the possibility of an artefactual masking of this epitope in NIs (Yvert et al., 2000). Garden et al. identified an ataxin-7 cleavage product by Western blot analysis of brain extract from SCA7 transgenic mice, that was not reported by Yoo (2003) in SCA7 knock-in brain homogenates (Garden et al., 2002; Yoo et al., 2003). Study of a single SCA7 patient's brain showed that most NIs were not stained with this C-terminal antibody, suggesting that cleavage of mutant ataxin-7 indeed occurs during SCA7 pathogenesis (Zander et al., 2001).

F. Polyglutamine Expansion Stabilizes Ataxin-7

Several experimental evidences indicate that there is a differential handling of mutant *versus* normal ataxin-7 by neurons *in vivo*. Normal recombinant ataxin-7 is barely detectable in P7E and B7E2 transgenic mice, while mutant ataxin-7 progressively accumulates, becoming easily detectable as homogenous nuclear staining and then gradually aggregates to form NIs (Yvert et al., 2001). This observation was then confirmed in SCA7 knock-in mice, indicating that selective stabilization of mutant ataxin-7 is a crucial pathogenic mechanism (Yoo et al., 2003). Mutant ataxin-7 selective accumulation probably results from a reduced turnover of expanded polyQ ataxin-7 as mutant *SCA7* mRNA levels were constant with age and identical to wild-type *SCA7* mRNA levels. This observation may be explained by misfolding and impaired clearance of mutant ataxin-7, as suggested by recruitment of chaperones and proteasome components into SCA7 NIs. Indeed, polyQ expansions have been shown to significantly impair proteasome activity (Bence et al., 2001; Verhoef et al., 2002), while chaperone overexpression inhibits NI formation in transfected cells (Opal and Zoghbi, 2002).

In knock-in mice, a faster accumulation of mutant ataxin-7 was observed in brain regions presenting marked dysfunction (Yoo et al., 2003). These regions include the cerebellum and the retina, which are known to degenerate in SCA7 patients, but intriguingly also the hippocampus which is not classically affected in SCA7. Thus, the mechanisms by which polyQ expansion stabilizes ataxin-7 and whether this observation accounts for the regional specific degeneration in SCA7 need to be further investigated.

These findings are in agreement with the observation that mutant ataxin-1 is degraded less efficiently than its wild-type counterpart *in vitro* (Cummings et al., 1999). Furthermore, in knock-in models of HD, mutant huntingtin fragments translocate into the nucleus and accumulate as a diffuse staining preceding NI formation, similarly to what was observed in SCA7 mice (Li et al., 2000; Wheeler et al., 2000; Lin et al., 2001). All together, these observations suggest that selective stabilization and progressive accumulation of expanded polyQ-containing proteins likely represent early steps in pathogenesis of polyQ diseases. Reduced turnover and impaired clearance of mutant proteins progressively increase their cellular amount up to a critical threshold initiating neuronal dysfunction. In good agreement with this hypothesis, several polyQ transgenic models (including SCA7 transgenic lines) with low transgene expression levels developed no overt or mild neurological phenotypes, indicating that the toxicity of expanded polyQ-containing proteins is concentration dependent.

G. Cell Death Versus Cell Dysfunction in SCA7

The neuropathological hallmark of polyQ disorders is massive cell loss in selected regions of the CNS, such as cerebellum, brainstem, and retina in SCA7. Whether the neuronal phenotype induced by polyQ expansion is due to cell dysfunction or cell death remains an open question.

In SCA7 mouse models, no neuronal loss occurs in the different brain regions analyzed despite severe movement abnormalities and premature death (Garden et al., 2002; Yoo et al., 2003). In the retina from SCA7 knock-in mice, limited retinal cell loss (around 20% at fifteen weeks of age) is noted only after a long period of retinal dysfunction, as assessed by ERG recordings (Yoo et al., 2003). Rod and cone activities are reduced from nine weeks of age, while TUNEL staining revealed a significant number of apoptotic cells from fifteen weeks of age. However, the short life span of these mice precluded a more comprehensive analysis of photoreceptor dysfunction and death at later stages.

SCA7 transgenic mice (R7E) present the unique opportunity to assess the long-term effect of polyQ toxicity *in vivo* as these animals have a normal life span due to restricted expression of mutant ataxin-7 in the retina. Interestingly, these mice show a long-lasting photoreceptor dysfunction starting at five weeks of age, while around 30% photoreceptor cell loss was detected at one year of age. Photoreceptor dysfunction is thus already complete well before neurons are dying (Helmlinger et al., 2004a). Furthermore, neuronal loss is restricted as 2.5-year-old R7E mice retain many more photoreceptors than age-matched wild-type mice, which show dramatic age-related photoreceptor degeneration (D.H., unpublished results). These observations demonstrate that photoreceptors from SCA7 mice are not committed to early death. Similarly, accumulating evidence suggests that neuronal dysfunction underlies most of the symptoms from the other polyQ disorders, particularly HD (Tobin and Signer, 2000).

H. Transcriptional Dysregulation in SCA7 Retinal Dysfunction

What are the molecular events causing neuronal dysfunction? Several recent studies show that transcriptional dysregulation may be a primary pathogenic process in polyQ diseases (reviewed in Cha, 2000; Sugars and Rubinsztein, 2003). In agreement with this hypothesis, increasing evidence hints at the nucleus as the prime site of polyQ toxicity. In almost all polyQ diseases, expanded polyQ-containing proteins aggregate into nuclear inclusions. Some of these proteins are normally nuclear (such as ataxin-1, -3, -7, atrophin-1, or TBP), while others appear to relocalize into the nucleus during the disease course (such as huntingtin). Importantly, comparison of SCA1 and HD knock-in models reveal that the same polyQ size (~154 CAG repeats) is extremely more toxic in ataxin-1 than in huntingtin. Indeed, SCA1 knock-in mice show a severe neurological phenotype and premature death, while two distinct HD knock-in models show very mild neurological abnormalities and normal life-span (Lin et al., 2001; Watase et al., 2002; Menalled et al., 2003). This highlights the role of protein context and presumably subcellular localization in polyQ toxicity (Zoghbi and Botas, 2002). Finally, several studies showed that nuclear localization of expanded polyQ proteins is necessary and sufficient to induce toxicity, at least in SCA1 and SBMA models (Klement et al., 1998; Katsuno et al., 2002; Takeyama et al., 2002).

Expanded polyQ-containing proteins have been proposed to interfere with the normal function of several transcription factors, such as CBP and Sp1 (Nucifora et al., 2001; Steffan et al., 2001; Dunah et al., 2002; Li et al., 2002; Taylor et al., 2003). Early and severe transcriptional alterations were detected in various polyQ eukaryotic models (Cha et al., 1998; Lin et al., 2000; Luthi-Carter et al., 2000; Hughes et al., 2001; Luthi-Carter et al., 2002; Taylor et al., 2003). Finally, histone deacetylase inhibitors, which stimulate gene transcription, are protective in HD mouse and *Drosophila* models (Steffan et al., 2001; Ferrante et al., 2003; Hockly et al., 2003). However, the exact molecular mechanisms underlying polyQ-induced transcriptional dysregulation and the extent to which altered expression of these genes contributes to neuronal dysfunction are yet unclear.

In the retina from both SCA7 transgenic (R7E) and knock-in mice, mutant ataxin-7 induces an early and dramatic downregulation of several photoreceptor-specific genes, particularly those encoding components of the phototransduction pathway, such as rhodopsin, cone opsins and transducins (Figure 2C). Time-course analysis revealed that both models develop comparable abnormalities as revealed by progressive reduction of rhodopsin mRNA levels concomitant with decreased rod ERG responses and thinning of their segments (Figure 2) (Yoo et al., 2003; Helmlinger et al., 2004a). These results support the hypothesis that polyQ-induced retinal dysfunction observed in mice and perhaps also in SCA7 patients may be caused by reduced expression of photoreceptor-specific genes.

Crx has a major role in the transcriptional regulation of photoreceptor-specific genes such as rhodopsin (Chen et al., 1997; Furukawa et al., 1997). Using *in vitro* experiments, La Spada et al. reported an interaction between ataxin-7 and Crx and suggested that expanded ataxin-7 impairs Crx normal function leading to SCA7-specific retinopathy (La Spada et al., 2001; Chen et al., 2004). Presymptomatic SCA7 transgenic mice presented very mild transcriptional abnormalities while Crx protein levels and binding to its DNA regulatory elements were significantly reduced (La Spada et al., 2001). Yoo et al. reported early and robust transcriptional alterations without modification of Crx levels and activity in their SCA7 knock-in model (Yoo et al., 2003). Furthermore, in all SCA7 retinal models, Crx nuclear distribution was found unaltered by aggregation of mutant ataxin-7 into NIs, precluding abnormal sequestration of Crx by mutant ataxin-7. Finally, R6/2 HD transgenic mice develop a retinopathy comparable to that of SCA7 transgenic mice and a dramatic downregulation of rhodopsin expression, demonstrating that rhodopsin promoter activity can be repressed *in vivo* by polyQ expansion in two unrelated proteins, ataxin-7 or huntingtin (Helmlinger et al., 2002; Helmlinger et al., 2004a). Further investigations are needed in order to assess whether the molecular pathways underlying rod dysfunction are identical in SCA7 and HD transgenic mice. Regardless, these observations together indicate that the specific retinal dysfunction in SCA7 patients cannot be explained exclusively by a specific interference of mutant ataxin-7 with Crx-dependent transcriptional regulation.

In summary, study of the retinopathy from SCA7 mouse models provided new insights into the molecular mechanisms underlying neuronal dysfunction in this tissue. Mutant ataxin-7-induced photoreceptor dysfunction, as assessed by a progressive decline of its electrophysiological activity, may be primarily due to an early and severe transcriptional dysregulation of photoreceptor-specific genes.

IV. CONCLUDING REMARKS

All SCA7 mice models that have been generated express full-length ataxin-7 with a polyQ expansion ranging from 90 to 266 repeats and, together, faithfully reproduce several key neurological features reported in SCA7 patients. These models have unravelled some of the early molecular events involved in SCA7 pathogenesis. Expansion of the polyQ tract in ataxin-7 markedly reduces the turnover of the mutant protein, thus increasing mutant ataxin-7 levels in neurons and presumably inducing its aggregation in the nucleus. Nuclear accumulation of mutant ataxin-7 parallels the onset of functional deficits in affected neurons, indicating that mutant ataxin-7 compromises essential nuclear functions. In the retina from these mice, expression of genes essential for photoreceptor normal function is early and dramatically repressed, thereby triggering a progressive decline of photoreceptor activity leading to a complete loss of electrophysiological responses and eventually limited cell loss (Figure 2). The retinal phenotype in SCA7 mice thus results primarily from a severe and long-lasting neuronal dysfunction.

These SCA7 retinal models are particularly attractive to further explore the therapeutic potential of drugs that could improve the transcriptional changes observed in polyQ disorders. Indeed, mouse retina is a suitable tissue for drug delivery and SCA7 models present functional abnormalities that can be easily assessed on living animals and are directly linked to dramatic transcriptional alterations.

Comparison of different polyQ mouse models reveals that either very long CAG repeats or significant overexpression of transgenes with modest repeat lengths are required to generate a phenotype during the short lifespan of the mouse. SCA7 knock-in (266 Qs) and transgenic (90 Qs) mice developed similar phenotype and show comparable molecular alterations, such as selective stabilization of mutant ataxin-7 and transcriptional dysregulation. Both models are thus valuable tools to further dissect the molecular mechanisms underlying SCA7 pathogenesis.

Acknowledgments

The authors would like to thank Jean-Louis Mandel for continuous support and critical reading of the manuscript. The work on SCA7 in the authors' laboratory is funded by the Institut National de la Santé et de la Recherche Médicale, the Centre National de la Recherche Scientifique, the Hôpital Universitaire de Strasbourg (HUS), the Hereditary Disease Foundation and the European Community (EUROSCA, PL 503304). D.H. was supported by a fellowship from the Fondation pour la Recherche Médicale.

References

Bence, N.F., R.M. Sampat, and R.R. Kopito. 2001. Impairment of the ubiquitin-proteasome system by protein aggregation. *Science* **292**: 1552–1555.

Benomar, A., E. Le Guern, A. Durr, H. Ouhabi, G. Stevanin, M. Yahyaoui, T. Chkili, Y. Agid, and A. Brice. 1994. Autosomal-dominant cerebellar ataxia with retinal degeneration (ADCA type II) is genetically different from ADCA type I. *Ann Neurol* **35**:439–444.

Benton, C.S., R. de Silva, S.L. Rutledge, S. Bohlega, T. Ashizawa, and H.Y. Zoghbi. 1998. Molecular and clinical studies in SCA-7 define a broad clinical spectrum and the infantile phenotype. *Neurology* **51**:1081–1086.

Brand, M., K. Yamamoto, A. Staub, and L. Tora. 1999. Identification of TATA-binding protein-free TAFII-containing complex subunits suggests a role in nucleosome acetylation and signal transduction. *J Biol Chem* **274**:18285–18289.

Burright, E.N., H.B. Clark, A. Servadio, T. Matilla, R.M. Feddersen, W.S. Yunis, L.A. Duvick, H.Y. Zoghbi, and H.T. Orr. 1995. SCA1 transgenic mice: a model for neurodegeneration caused by an expanded CAG trinucleotide repeat. *Cell* **82**:937–948.

Cancel, G., C. Duyckaerts, M. Holmberg, C. Zander, G. Yvert, A.S. Lebre, M. Ruberg, B. Faucheux, Y. Agid, E. Hirsch, and A. Brice. 2000. Distribution of ataxin-7 in normal human brain and retina. *Brain* **123**: 2519–2530.

Carpenter, S., and G.A. Schumacher. 1966. Familial infantile cerebellar atrophy associated with retinal degeneration. *Arch Neurol* **14**:82–94.

Cha, J.H. 2000. Transcriptional dysregulation in Huntington's disease. *Trends Neurosci* **23**:387–392.

Cha, J.H., C.M. Kosinski, J.A. Kerner, S.A. Alsdorf, L. Mangiarini, S.W. Davies, J.B. Penney, G.P. Bates, and A.B. Young. 1998. Altered brain neurotransmitter receptors in transgenic mice expressing a portion of an abnormal human huntington disease gene. *Proc Natl Acad Sci USA* **95**:6480–6485.

Chen, S., G.H. Peng, X. Wang, A.C. Smith, S.K. Grote, B.L. Sopher, and A.R. La Spada. 2004. Interference of Crx-dependent transcription by ataxin-7 involves interaction between the glutamine regions and requires the ataxin-7 carboxy-terminal region for nuclear localization. *Hum Mol Genet* **13**:53–67.

Chen, S., Q.L. Wang, Z. Nie, H. Sun, G. Lennon, N.G. Copeland, D.J. Gilbert, N.A. Jenkins, and D.J. Zack. 1997. Crx, a novel Otx-like paired-homeodomain protein, binds to and transactivates photoreceptor cell-specific genes. *Neuron* **19**:1017–1030.

Cummings, CJ, and HY. Zoghbi. 2000 Trinucleotide repeats: mechanisms and pathophysiology. *Annu Rev Genomics Hum Genet* **1**:281–328.

Cummings, C.J., E. Reinstein, Y. Sun, B. Antalffy, Y. Jiang, A. Ciechanover, H.T. Orr, A.L. Beaudet, and H.Y. Zoghbi. 1999. Mutation of the E6-AP ubiquitin ligase reduces nuclear inclusion frequency while accelerating polyglutamine-induced pathology in SCA1 mice. *Neuron* **24**:879–892.

David, G., A. Durr, G. Stevanin, G. Cancel, N. Abbas, A. Benomar, S. Belal, A.S. Lebre, M. Abada-Bendib, D. Grid, M. Holmberg, M. Yahyaoui, F. Hentati, T. Chkili, Y. Agid, and A. Brice. 1998. Molecular and clinical correlations in autosomal dominant cerebellar ataxia with progressive macular dystrophy (SCA7). *Hum Mol Genet* **7**:165–170.

David, G., N. Abbas, G. Stevanin, A. Durr, G. Yvert, G. Cancel, C. Weber, G. Imbert, F. Saudou, E. Antoniou, H. Drabkin, R. Gemmill, P. Giunti, A. Benomar, N. Wood, M. Ruberg, Y. Agid, J.L. Mandel, and A. Brice. 1997. Cloning of the SCA7 gene reveals a highly unstable CAG repeat expansion. *Nat Genet* **17**:65–70.

de Jong, P.T., J.G. de Jong, J.M. de Jong-Ten Doeschate, and J.W. Delleman. 1980. Olivopontocerebellar atrophy with visual disturbances. An ophthalmologic investigation into four generations. *Ophthalmology* **87**:793–804.

Del-Favero, J., L. Krols, A. Michalik, J. Theuns, A. Lofgren, D. Goossens, A. Wehnert, D. Van den Bossche, K. Van Zand, H. Backhovens, N. van

Regenmorter, J.J. Martin, and C. Van Broeckhoven. 1998. Molecular genetic analysis of autosomal dominant cerebellar ataxia with retinal degeneration (ADCA type II) caused by CAG triplet repeat expansion. *Hum Mol Genet* **7**:177–186.

Dunah, A.W., H. Jeong, A. Griffin, Y.M. Kim, D.G. Standaert, S.M. Hersch, M.M. Mouradian, A.B. Young, N. Tanese, and D. Krainc. 2002. Sp1 and TAFII130 transcriptional activity disrupted in early Huntington's disease. *Science* **296**:2238–2243.

Einum, D.D., J.J. Townsend, L.J. Ptacek, and Y.H. Fu. 2001. Ataxin-7 expression analysis in controls and spinocerebellar ataxia type 7 patients. *Neurogenetics* **3**:83–90.

Enevoldson, T.P., M.D. Sanders, and A.E. Harding. 1994. Autosomal dominant cerebellar ataxia with pigmentary macular dystrophy. A clinical and genetic study of eight families. *Brain* **117**:445–460.

Ferrante, R.J., J.K. Kubilus, J. Lee, H. Ryu, A. Beesen, B. Zucker, K. Smith, N.W. Kowall, R.R. Ratan, R. Luthi-Carter, and S.M. Hersch. 2003. Histone deacetylase inhibition by sodium butyrate chemotherapy ameliorates the neurodegenerative phenotype in Huntington's disease mice. J *Neurosci* **23**:9418–9427.

Furukawa, T., E.M. Morrow, and C.L. Cepko. 1997. Crx, a novel otx-like homeobox gene, shows photoreceptor-specific expression and regulates photoreceptor differentiation. *Cell* **91**:531–541.

Garden, G.A., R.T. Libby, Y.H. Fu, Y. Kinoshita, J. Huang, D.E. Possin, A.C. Smith, R.A. Martinez, G.C. Fine, S.K. Grote, C.B. Ware, D.D. Einum, R.S. Morrison, L.J. Ptacek, B.L. Sopher, and A.R. La Spada. 2002. Polyglutamine-expanded ataxin-7 promotes non-cell-autonomous Purkinje cell degeneration and displays proteolytic cleavage in ataxic transgenic mice. *J Neurosci* **22**:4897–4905.

Gavin, A.C., M. Bosche, R. Krause, P. Grandi, M. Marzioch, A. Bauer, J. Schultz, J.M. Rick, A.M. Michon, C.M. Cruciat, M. Remor, C. Hofert, M. Schelder, M. Brajenovic, H. Ruffner, A. Merino, K. Klein, M. Hudak, D. Dickson, T. Rudi, V. Gnau, A. Bauch, S. Bastuck, B. Huhse, C. Leutwein, M.A. Heurtier, R.R. Copley, A. Edelmann, E. Querfurth, V. Rybin, G. Drewes, M. Raida, T. Bouwmeester, P. Bork, B. Seraphin, B. Kuster, G. Neubauer, and G. Superti-Furga. 2002. Functional organization of the yeast proteome by systematic analysis of protein complexes. *Nature* **415**:141–147.

Gouw, L.G., K.B. Digre, C.P. Harris, J.H. Haines, and L.J. Ptacek. 1994. Autosomal dominant cerebellar ataxia with retinal degeneration: clinical, neuropathologic, and genetic analysis of a large kindred. *Neurology* **44**:1441–1447.

Grant, P.A., D. Schieltz, M.G. Pray-Grant, D.J. Steger, J.C. Reese, J.R. Yates 3rd, and J.L. Workman. 1998. A subset of TAF(II)s are integral components of the SAGA complex required for nucleosome acetylation and transcriptional stimulation. *Cell* **94**:45–53.

Grant, P.A., L. Duggan, J. Cote, S.M. Roberts, J.E. Brownell, R. Candau, R. Ohba, T. Owen-Hughes, C.D. Allis, F. Winston, S.L. Berger, and J.L. Workman. 1997. Yeast Gcn5 functions in two multisubunit complexes to acetylate nucleosomal histones: characterization of an Ada complex and the SAGA (Spt/Ada) complex. *Genes Dev* **11**:1640–1650.

Harding, A.E. 1993. Clinical features and classification of inherited ataxias. *Adv Neurol* **61**:1–14.

Helmlinger, D., G. Yvert, S. Picaud, K. Merienne, J. Sahel, J.L. Mandel, and D. Devys. 2002. Progressive retinal degeneration and dysfunction in R6 Huntington's disease mice. *Hum Mol Genet* **11**:3351–3359.

Helmlinger, D., G. Abou-Sleymane, G. Yvert, S. Rousseau, C. Weber, Y. Trottier, J.L. Mandel, and D. Devys. 2004. Disease progression despite early loss of polyglutamine protein expression in SCA7 mouse model. *J Neurosci* **24**:1881–1887.

Helmlinger, D., S. Hardy, S. Sasorith, F. Klein, F. Robert, C. Weber, L. Miguet, N. Potier, A. Van-Dorsselaer, J.M. Wurtz, J.L. Mandel, L. Tora, and D. Devys. 2004b. Ataxin-7 is a sbunit of GCN5 histone acetyltransferase-containing complexes. *Hum Mol Genet* **13**:1257–1265.

Hockly, E., V.M. Richon, B. Woodman, D.L. Smith, X. Zhou, E. Rosa, K. Sathasivam, S. Ghazi-Noori, A. Mahal, P.A. Lowden, J.S. Steffan, J.L. Marsh, L.M. Thompson, C.M. Lewis, P.A. Marks, and G.P. Bates. 2003. Suberoylanilide hydroxamic acid, a histone deacetylase inhibitor, ameliorates motor deficits in a mouse model of Huntington's disease. *Proc Natl Acad Sci U S A* 100:2041–2046.

Hughes, R.E., R.S. Lo, C. Davis, A.D. Strand, C.L. Neal, J.M. Olson, and S. Fields. 2001. Altered transcription in yeast expressing expanded polyglutamine. *Proc Natl Acad Sci U S A* **98**:13201–13206.

Johansson, J., L. Forsgren, O. Sandgren, A. Brice, G. Holmgren, and M. Holmberg. 1998. Expanded CAG repeats in Swedish spinocerebellar ataxia type 7 (SCA7) patients: effect of CAG repeat length on the clinical manifestation. *Hum Mol Genet* **7**:171–176.

Jonasson, J., A.L. Strom, P. Hart, T. Brannstrom, L. Forsgren, and M. Holmberg. 2002. Expression of ataxin-7 in CNS and non-CNS tissue of normal and SCA7 individuals. *Acta Neuropathol (Berl)* **104**:29–37.

Katsuno, M., H. Adachi, A. Kume, M. Li, Y. Nakagomi, H. Niwa, C. Sang, Y. Kobayashi, M. Doyu, and G. Sobue. 2002. Testosterone reduction prevents phenotypic expression in a transgenic mouse model of spinal and bulbar muscular atrophy. *Neuron* **35**:843–854.

Kaytor, M.D., L.A. Duvick, P.J. Skinner, M.D. Koob, L.P. Ranum, and H.T. Orr. 1999. Nuclear localization of the spinocerebellar ataxia type 7 protein, ataxin-7. *Hum Mol Genet* **8**:1657–1664.

Klement, I.A., P.J. Skinner, M.D. Kaytor, H. Yi, S.M. Hersch, H.B. Clark, H.Y. Zoghbi, and H.T. Orr. 1998. Ataxin-1 nuclear localization and aggregation: role in polyglutamine-induced disease in SCA1 transgenic mice. *Cell* **95**:41–53.

Konigsmark, B.W., and L.P. Weiner. 1970. The olivopontocerebellar atrophies: a review. *Medicine (Baltimore)* **49**:227–241.

Koob, M.D., K.A. Benzow, T.D. Bird, J.W. Day, M.L. Moseley, and L.P. Ranum. 1998. Rapid cloning of expanded trinucleotide repeat sequences from genomic DNA. *Nat Genet* **18**:72–75.

La Spada, A.R., Y.H. Fu, B.L. Sopher, R.T. Libby, X. Wang, L.Y. Li, D.D. Einum, J. Huang, D.E. Possin, A.C. Smith, R.A. Martinez, K.L. Koszdin, P.M. Treuting, C.B. Ware, J.B. Hurley, L.J. Ptacek, and S. Chen. 2001. Polyglutamine-expanded ataxin-7 antagonizes CRX function and induces cone-rod dystrophy in a mouse model of SCA7. *Neuron* **31**:913–927.

Li, H., S.H. Li, H. Johnston, P.F. Shelbourne, and X.J. Li. 2000. Amino-terminal fragments of mutant huntingtin show selective accumulation in striatal neurons and synaptic toxicity. *Nat Genet* **25**:385–389.

Li, S.H., A.L. Cheng, H. Zhou, S. Lam, M. Rao, H. Li, and X.J. Li. 2002. Interaction of Huntington disease protein with transcriptional activator Sp1. *Mol Cell Biol* **22**:1277–1287.

Libby, R.T., D.G. Monckton, Y.H. Fu, R.A. Martinez, J.P. McAbney, R. Lau, D.D. Einum, K. Nichol, C.B. Ware, L.J. Ptacek, C.E. Pearson, and A.R. La Spada. 2003. Genomic context drives SCA7 CAG repeat instability, while expressed SCA7 cDNAs are intergenerationally and somatically stable in transgenic mice. *Hum Mol Genet* **12**:41–50.

Lin, C.H., S. Tallaksen-Greene, W.M. Chien, J.A. Cearley, W.S. Jackson, A.B. Crouse, S. Ren, X.J. Li, R.L. Albin, and P.J. Detloff. 2001. Neurological abnormalities in a knock-in mouse model of Huntington's disease. *Hum Mol Genet* **10**:137–144.

Lin, X., B. Antalffy, D. Kang, H.T. Orr, and H.Y. Zoghbi. 2000. Polyglutamine expansion down-regulates specific neuronal genes before pathologic changes in SCA1. *Nat Neurosci* **3**:157–163.

Lindenberg, K.S., G. Yvert, K. Muller, and G.B. Landwehrmeyer. 2000. Expression analysis of ataxin-7 mRNA and protein in human brain: evidence for a widespread distribution and focal protein accumulation. *Brain Pathol* **10**:385–394.

Luthi-Carter, R., A.D. Strand, S.A. Hanson, C. Kooperberg, G. Schilling, A.R. La Spada, D.E. Merry, A.B. Young, C.A. Ross, D.R. Borchelt, and J.M. Olson. 2002. Polyglutamine and transcription: gene expression changes shared by DRPLA and Huntington's disease mouse models reveal context-independent effects. *Hum Mol Genet* **11**:1927–1937.

Luthi-Carter, R., A. Strand, N.L. Peters, S.M. Solano, Z.R. Hollingsworth, A.S. Menon, A.S. Frey, B.S. Spektor, E.B. Penney, G. Schilling, C.A.

Ross, D.R. Borchelt, S.J. Tapscott, A.B. Young, J.H. Cha, and J.M. Olson. 2000. Decreased expression of striatal signaling genes in a mouse model of Huntington's disease. *Hum Mol Genet* **9**:1259–1271.

Martin, J.J., N. Van Regemorter, L. Krols, J.M. Brucher, T. de Barsy, H. Szliwowski, P. Evrard, C. Ceuterick, M.J. Tassignon, and H. Smet-Dieleman. 1994. On an autosomal dominant form of retinal-cerebellar degeneration: an autopsy study of five patients in one family. *Acta Neuropathologica* **88**:277–286.

Martin-Aparicio, E., A. Yamamoto, F. Hernandez, R. Hen, J. Avila, and J.J. Lucas. 2001. Proteasomal-dependent aggregate reversal and absence of cell death in a conditional mouse model of Huntington's disease. *J Neurosci* **21**:8772–8781.

Martinez, E., V.B. Palhan, A. Tjernberg, E.S. Lymar, A.M. Gamper, T.K. Kundu, B.T. Chait, and R.G. Roeder. 2001. Human STAGA complex is a chromatin-acetylating transcription coactivator that interacts with pre-mRNA splicing and DNA damage-binding factors in vivo. *Mol Cell Biol* **21**:6782–6795.

Mauger, C., J. Del-Favero, C. Ceuterick, U. Lubke, C. van Broeckhoven, and J. Martin. 1999. Identification and localization of ataxin-7 in brain and retina of a patient with cerebellar ataxia type II using anti-peptide antibody. *Brain Res Mol Brain Res* **74**:35–43.

McCampbell, A., J.P. Taylor, A.A. Taye, J. Robitschek, M. Li, J. Walcott, D. Merry, Y. Chai, H. Paulson, Sobue, and K.H. Fischbeck. 2000. CREB-binding protein sequestration by expanded polyglutamine. *Hum Mol Genet* **9**:2197–2202.

Menalled, L.B., J.D. Sison, I. Dragatsis, S. Zeitlin, and M.F. Chesselet. 2003. Time course of early motor and neuropathological anomalies in a knock-in mouse model of Huntington's disease with 140 CAG repeats. *J Comp Neurol* **465**:11–26.

Michalik, A., and C. Van Broeckhoven. 2003. Pathogenesis of polyglutamine disorders: aggregation revisited. *Hum Mol Genet* **12**:R173–186.

Michalik, A., J.J. Martin, and C. Van Broeckhoven. 2003. Spinocerebellar ataxia type 7 associated with pigmentary retinal dystrophy. *Eur J Hum Genet* **22**:22.

Monckton, D.G., M.L. Cayuela, F.K. Gould, G.J. Brock, R. Silva, and T. Ashizawa. 1999. Very large (CAG)(n) DNA repeat expansions in the sperm of two spinocerebellar ataxia type 7 males. *Hum Mol Genet* **8**: 2473–2478.

Mushegian, A.R., S.A. Vishnivetskiy, and V.V. Gurevich. 2000. Conserved phosphoprotein interaction motif is functionally interchangeable between ataxin-7 and arrestins. *Biochemistry* **39**:6809–6813.

Nucifora, Jr. F.C., M. Sasaki, M.F. Peters, H. Huang, J.K. Cooper, M. Yamada, H. Takahashi, S. Tsuji, J. Troncoso, V.L. Dawson, T.M. Dawson, and C.A. Ross. 2001. Interference by huntingtin and atrophin-1 with cbp-mediated transcription leading to cellular toxicity. *Science* **291**:2423–2428.

Opal, P., and H.Y. Zoghbi. 2002. The role of chaperones in polyglutamine disease. *Trends Mol Med* **8**:232–236.

Rattner, A., P.M. Smallwood, J. Williams, C. Cooke, A. Savchenko, A. Lyubarsky, E.N. Pugh, and J. Nathans. 2001. A photoreceptor-specific cadherin is essential for the structural integrity of the outer segment and for photoreceptor survival. *Neuron* **32**:775–786.

Ross, C.A. 2002. Polyglutamine pathogenesis: emergence of unifying mechanisms for Huntington's disease and related disorders. *Neuron* **35**: 819–822.

Ryan, Jr. S.J., D.L. Knox, W.R. Green, and B.W. Konigsmark. 1975. Olivopontocerebellar degeneration. Clinicopathologic correlation of the associated retinopathy. *Arch Ophthalmol* **93**:169–172.

Sanders, S.L., J. Jennings, A. Canutescu, A.J. Link, and P.A. Weil. 2002. Proteomics of the eukaryotic transcription machinery: identification of proteins associated with components of yeast TFIID by multidimensional mass spectrometry. *Mol Cell Biol* **22**:4723–4738.

Scheel, H., S. Tomiuk, and K. Hofmann. 2003. Elucidation of ataxin-3 and ataxin-7 function by integrative bioinformatics. *Hum Mol Genet* **12**: 2845–2852.

Servadio, A., B. Koshy, D. Armstrong, B. Antalffy, H.T. Orr, and H.Y. Zoghbi. 1995. Expression analysis of the ataxin-1 protein in tissues from normal and spinocerebellar ataxia type 1 individuals. *Nat Genet* **10**:94–98.

Skinner, P.J., B. Koshy, C.J. Cummings, I.A. Klement, K. Helin, A. Servadio, H.Y. Zoghbi, and H.T. Orr. 1997. SCA1 pathogenesis involves alterations in nuclear matrix associated structures. *Nature* **389**:971–974.

Steffan, J.S., A. Kazantsev, O. Spasic-Boskovic, M. Greenwald, Y.Z. Zhu, H. Gohler, E.E. Wanker, G.P. Bates, D.E. Housman, and L.M. Thompson. 2000. The Huntington's disease protein interacts with p53 and CREB-binding protein and represses transcription. *Proc Natl Acad Sci U S A* **97**:6763–6768.

Steffan, J.S., L. Bodai, J. Pallos, M. Poelman, A. McCampbell, B.L. Apostol, A. Kazantsev, E. Schmidt, Y.Z. Zhu, M. Greenwald, R. Kurokawa, D.E. Housman, G.R. Jackson, J.L. Marsh, and L.M. Thompson. 2001. Histone deacetylase inhibitors arrest polyglutamine-dependent neurodegeneration in *Drosophila*. *Nature* **413**:739–743.

Stenoien, D.L., M. Mielke, and M.A. Mancini. 2002. Intranuclear ataxin1 inclusions contain both fast- and slow-exchanging components. *Nat Cell Biol* **4**:806–810.

Strom, A.L., J. Jonasson, P. Hart, T. Brannstrom, L. Forsgren, and M. Holmberg. 2002. Cloning and expression analysis of the murine homolog of the spinocerebellar ataxia type 7 (SCA7) gene. *Gene* **285**: 91–99.

Sugars, K.L., and D.C. Rubinsztein. 2003. Transcriptional abnormalities in Huntington disease. *Trends Genet* **19**:233–238.

Takeyama, K., S. Ito, A. Yamamoto, H. Tanimoto, T. Furutani, H. Kanuka, M. Miura, T. Tabata, and S. Kato. 2002. Androgen-dependent neurodegeneration by polyglutamine-expanded human androgen receptor in *Drosophila*. *Neuron* **35**:855–864.

Tarlac, V., and E. Storey. 2003. Role of proteolysis in polyglutamine disorders. *J Neurosci Res* **74**:406–416.

Taylor, J.P., A.A. Taye, C. Campbell, P. Kazemi-Esfarjani, K.H. Fischbeck, and K.T. Min. 2003. Aberrant histone acetylation, altered transcription, and retinal degeneration in a *Drosophila* model of polyglutamine disease are rescued by CREB-binding protein. *Genes Dev* **17**:1463–1468.

Tobin, A.J., and E.R. Signer. 2000. Huntington's disease: the challenge for cell biologists. *Trends Cell Biol* **10**:531–536.

Traboulsi, E.I., I.H. Maumenee, W.R. Green, M.L. Freimer, and H. Moser. 1988. Olivopontocerebellar atrophy with retinal degeneration. A clinical and ocular histopathologic study. *Arch Ophthalmol* **106**:801–806.

van de Warrenburg, B.P., C.W. Frenken, M.G. Ausems, T. Kleefstra, R.J. Sinke, N.V. Knoers, and H.P. Kremer. 2001. Striking anticipation in spinocerebellar ataxia type 7: the infantile phenotype. *J Neurol* **248**: 911–914.

Verhoef, L.G., K. Lindsten, M.G. Masucci, and N.P. Dantuma. 2002. Aggregate formation inhibits proteasomal degradation of polyglutamine proteins. *Hum Mol Genet* **11**:2689–2700.

Watase, K., E.J. Weeber, B. Xu, B. Antalffy, L. Yuva-Paylor, K. Hashimoto, M. Kano, R. Atkinson, Y. Sun, D.L. Armstrong, J.D. Sweatt, H.T. Orr, R. Paylor, and H.Y. Zoghbi. 2002. A long CAG repeat in the mouse Sca1 locus replicates SCA1 features and reveals the impact of protein solubility on selective neurodegeneration. *Neuron* **34**:905–919.

Wheeler, V.C., J.K. White, C.A. Gutekunst, V. Vrbanac, M. Weaver, X.J. Li, S.H. Li, H. Yi, J.P. Vonsattel, J.F. Gusella, S. Hersch, W. Auerbach, A.L. Joyner, and M.E. MacDonald. 2000. Long glutamine tracts cause nuclear localization of a novel form of huntingtin in medium spiny striatal neurons in HdhQ92 and HdhQ111 knock-in mice. *Hum Mol Genet* **9**:503–513.

Wieczorek, E., M. Brand, X. Jacq, and L. Tora. 1998. Function of TAF(II)-containing complex without TBP in transcription by RNA polymerase II. *Nature* **393**:187–191.

Yamamoto, A., J.J. Lucas, and R. Hen. 2000. Reversal of neuropathology and motor dysfunction in a conditional model of Huntington's disease. *Cell* **101**:57–66.

Yoo, S.Y., M.E. Pennesi, E.J. Weeber, B. Xu, R. Atkinson, S. Chen, D.L. Armstrong, S.M. Wu, J.D. Sweatt, and H.Y. Zoghbi. 2003. SCA7 knockin mice model human SCA7 and reveal gradual accumulation of mutant ataxin-7 in neurons and abnormalities in short-term plasticity. *Neuron* **37**:383–401.

Yu, Z.X., S.H. Li, H.P. Nguyen, and X.J. Li. 2002. Huntingtin inclusions do not deplete polyglutamine-containing transcription factors in HD mice. *Hum Mol Genet* **11**:905–914.

Yvert, G., K.S. Lindenberg, S. Picaud, G.B. Landwehrmeyer, J.A. Sahel, and J.L. Mandel. 2000. Expanded polyglutamines induce neurodegeneration and trans-neuronal alterations in cerebellum and retina of SCA7 transgenic mice. *Hum Mol Genet* **9**:2491–2506.

Yvert, G., K.S. Lindenberg, D. Devys, D. Helmlinger, G.B. Landwehrmeyer, and J.L. Mandel. 2001. SCA7 mouse models show selective stabilization of mutant ataxin-7 and similar cellular responses in different neuronal cell types. *Hum Mol Genet* **10**:1679–1692.

Zack, D.J., J. Bennett, Y. Wang, C. Davenport, B. Klaunberg, J. Gearhart, and J. Nathans. 1991. Unusual topography of bovine rhodopsin promoter-lacZ fusion gene expression in transgenic mouse retinas. *Neuron* **6**:187–199.

Zander, C., J. Takahashi, K.H. El Hachimi, H. Fujigasaki, V. Albanese, A.S. Lebre, G. Stevanin, C. Duyckaerts, and A. Brice. 2001. Similarities between spinocerebellar ataxia type 7 (SCA7) cell models and human brain: proteins recruited in inclusions and activation of caspase-3. *Hum Mol Genet* **10**:2569–2579.

Zoghbi, H.Y., and H.T. Orr. 2000. Glutamine repeats and neurodegeneration. *Annu Rev Neurosci* **23**:217–247.

Zoghbi, H.Y., and J. Botas. 2002. Mouse and fly models of neurodegeneration. *Trends Genet* **18**:463–471.

C H A P T E R

K6

Animal Models of Friedreich Ataxia

MASSIMO PANDOLFO

Friedreich ataxia (FA) is an autosomal recessive disease characterized by progressive neurological disability, cardiomyopathy, and increased risk of diabetes mellitus. The disease, which currently has no treatment, affects roughly 1 in 50,000 people. The first symptoms usually appear in childhood, but age of onset may vary from infancy to adulthood. Atrophy of sensory and cerebellar pathways causes ataxia, dysarthria, fixation instability, deep sensory loss and loss of tendon reflexes. Corticospinal degeneration leads to muscular weakness and extensor plantar responses. A hypertrophic cardiomyopathy may contribute to disability and cause premature death. Kyphoscoliosis and pes cavus are common.

The FA gene (FRDA) encodes a small mitochondrial matrix protein, frataxin, which is highly conserved in evolution. FA is caused by a so far unique mutation mechanism: the expansion of an intronic GAA triplet repeat sequence. Most patients are homozygous for expanded GAA repeats; rare patients are heterozygous for an expanded repeat and a point mutation affecting the frataxin coding sequence. In all cases, FA patients have a profound but not complete frataxin deficiency, with a small residual amount of normal protein.

Service de Neurologie, Université Libre de Bruxelles-Hôpital Erasme, Route de Lennik 808, B-1070 Bruxelles, Belgium, Phone +32(0)2-555-3429, Fax +32(0)2-555-3942, email: massimo.pandolfo@ulb.ac.be

Most of our initial knowledge about the functional role of frataxin came from the investigation of yeast cells in which the frataxin homolog gene (YFH1) was deleted. A mouse model of FA has been difficult to generate because complete loss of frataxin, as in frataxin knock-out (KO) mice, causes early embryonic lethality, as detailed below. Viable mouse models have been so far obtained only through a conditional gene targeting approach.

These investigation have unequivocally revealed that frataxin deficiency leads to loss of function of Fe-S center containing enzymes (in particular respiratory complexes I, II and III, and aconitase), excessive free radical production in mitochondria and progressive iron accumulation in these organelles. Ongoing biochemical and structural studies are aimed to understand the specific function of the protein.

I. THE FRDA GENE, TRANSCRIPT AND FRATAXIN

The FRDA gene is localized in the proximal long arm of chromosome 9[1] and is composed by seven exons spread over 95 Kb of genomic DNA[2]. The major, and probably only functionally relevant mRNA, has a size of 1.3 Kb, corresponding to the first five exons, numbered 1 to 5a. The encoded 210-amino acid protein was called frataxin[2].

Frataxin is highly conserved in evolution. A single frataxin gene is found in all eukaryotes, including fungi and plants. A homolog, CyaY, is present in Gram negative bacteria and in other prokaryotes like *Rickettsia prowazeckii*, thought to be related to the hypothetical mitochondrial precursor.

FRDA is expressed in all cells, but at variable levels in different tissues and during development[3,4]. In adult humans, frataxin mRNA is most abundant in the heart and spinal cord, followed by liver, skeletal muscle, and pancreas. In mouse embryos, expression starts in the neuroepithelium at embryonic day 10.5 (E10.5), then reaches its highest level at E14.5 and into the postnatal period. The highest levels of frataxin mRNA are found in the spinal cord, particularly at the thoracolumbar level, and in the dorsal root ganglia.

A. Gene Mutations

FA is the consequence of severe, but not complete frataxin deficiency. Most patients are homozygous for the expansion of a GAA triplet repeat sequence (TRS) in the first intron of the frataxin gene, 5% are heterozygous for a GAA expansion and a point mutation affecting the coding sequence. Repeats in normal chromosomes contain up to ~40 triplets, 66 to >1,000 triplets in FA chromosomes. Expanded alleles show meiotic and mitotic instability. Smaller expansions allow a higher residual gene expression[5]. Accordingly, the severity and age of onset of the disease are in part determined by the size of the expanded GAA TRS, in particular of the smaller allele[6,7]. Lengths of the GAA TRS corresponding to pathological FRDA alleles can adopt a triple helical structure in physiological conditions and inhibit transcription *in vitro* and *in vivo*[8,9]. Two triplex regions from the same or from different DNA molecules may associate to form a novel DNA structure called "sticky DNA"[10], which may be the direct cause of transcription inhibition. The 2% of FA chromosomes carrying GAA repeats of normal length have missense, nonsense, or splice site mutations ultimately affecting the frataxin coding sequence[11].

B. Frataxin Structure

Structural studies have been carried out on frataxin[12,13] and its bacterial homolog, CyaY[14] by nuclear magnetic resonance (NMR) and by crystallography. These investigations revealed a novel structural motif, called the frataxin fold, unique to frataxin and CyaY proteins. The structure is compact, overall globular, containing an N-terminal α helix, a middle β sheet region composed of seven β strands, a second α helix, and a C-terminal coil. The α helices are folded upon the β sheet, with the C-terminal coil filling a groove between the two α helices. On the outside a ridge of negatively charged residues and a patch of hydrophobic residues are highly conserved suggesting that they interact with a large ligand, probably a protein. However, experiments attempting to identify a protein partner of frataxin, mostly by using the yeast two-hybrid method, have so far failed.

C. Frataxin Function and Pathogenesis

Knock-out of the yeast frataxin homolog gene (YFH1) has provided the first information on frataxin function. Most YFH1 knock-out yeast strains, called Δ*YFH1*, lose the ability to carry out oxidative phosphorylation, cannot grow on non-fermentable substrates, and lose mitochondrial DNA[15,16]. In Δ*YFH1*, iron accumulates in mitochondria, more then 10-fold in excess of wild type yeast. Loss of respiratory competence requires the presence of iron in the culture medium, and occurs more rapidly as iron concentration in the medium is increased, suggesting that permanent mitochondrial damage is the consequence of iron toxicity[17]. Iron in mitochondria can react with reactive oxygen species (ROS) that form in these organelles. Even in normal mitochondria, a few electrons prematurely leak from the respiratory chain, mostly from reduced ubiquinone (or probably its semiquinone form), directly reducing molecular oxygen to superoxide (O_2^-). Mitochondrial Mn-dependent superoxide dismutase (SOD2) generates hydrogen peroxide (H_2O_2) from O_2^-, then glutathione peroxidase oxidizes glutathione to transform H_2O_2 into H_2O. Iron may intervene in this process and generate the hydroxyl radical ($OH^\bullet$) through the Fenton reaction ($Fe(II) + H_2O_2 \rightarrow Fe(III) + OH^\bullet + OH^-$). $OH^\bullet$ is highly toxic and causes lipid peroxidation, protein and nucleic acid damage. Occurrence of the Fenton reaction in Δ*YFH1* yeast cells is suggested by their highly enhanced sensitivity to H_2O_2[15].

Disruption of frataxin causes a general dysregulation of iron metabolism in yeast cells. There is a marked induction (10- to 50-fold) of the high-affinity iron transport system of the cell membrane, normally not expressed in yeast cells that are iron replete[15]. As a consequence, iron crosses the plasma membrane in large amounts and further accumulates in mitochondria, engaging the cell in a vicious cycle.

The reason why Δ*YFH1* cells accumulate iron in the mitochondrial fraction may in principle involve increased iron uptake, altered utilization or decreased export from these organelles. Experiments involving induction of frataxin expression from a plasmid transformed into Δ*YFH1* yeast cells indicate that the protein stimulates a flux of non-heme iron out of mitochondria[17].

Several mitochondrial enzymes are known to be impaired in Δ*YFH1* yeast cells, in particular respiratory chain complexes I, II, and III and aconitase[18]. These enzymes all contain iron-sulfur clusters (ISCs) in their active sites. ISCs are synthesized in mitochondria and are highly sensitive to free radicals[19]. Remarkably, all defects in ISC synthetic enzymes in yeast lead to mitochondrial iron accumulation, apparently due to defective iron export out of mitochondria, as it occurs in Δ*YFH1*. Recent data point to a direct involvement of frataxin in ISC synthesis. Frataxin appears not to be essential, but to strongly stimulate an early step of ISC synthesis. It appears to interact with the scaffold protein Isu1, where the first ISC assembly takes place. Therefore, the following pathogenic cascade may be proposed: 1) frataxin deficiency primarily impairs ISC synthesis; 2) reduced ISC synthesis leads to inhibited iron export and mitochondrial iron accumulation; 3) iron generates free radicals that cause further damage to ISCs and decrease the enzymatic activities of ISC-containing proteins (ISPs); 4) decreased activities of several respiratory complexes (I, II, III) and of Krebs cycle enzymes lead to a further increases in free radical production and the establishment of a vicious cycle.

How frataxin stimulates ISC synthesis is not yet known. A possibility is that it may be an iron chaperone in the mitochondrial environment that channels the metal to biosynthetic enzyme complexes and protects it from free radical attack. Whether such activity is related to the reported ability of yfp1 and to a lesser extent of human frataxin to form high molecular weight complexes with iron is unclear[20].

Several observations support the hypothesis that altered iron metabolism, free radical damage, and mitochondrial dysfunction all occur in FA. Involvement of iron was suggested twenty years ago by the finding of deposits of this metal in myocardial cells from FA patients[21]. Iron accumulation has been demonstrated by magnetic resonance imaging (MRI) in the dentate nucleus, a severely affected structure in the central nervous system[22]. The observation of a moderate, but significant increase in iron concentration in the mitochondrial fraction from FA fibroblasts has been reported[23]. A general abnormality of iron metabolism may also be occurring in FA patients, as suggested by the high level of circulating transferrin receptor, the principal carrier of iron into human cells[24], which may reflect a relative cytosolic iron deficit as observed in the yeast model.

Oxidative stress is suggested by the observation that patients with FA have increased plasma levels of malondialdheyde, a lipid peroxidation product[25], as well as increased 8-hydroxy-2′-deoxyguanosine (8OH2′dG), a marker of oxidative DNA damage, in urine[26]. A further hint of a possible role of free radicals comes from the observation that vitamin E deficiency produces a phenotype resembling FA[27]. Vitamin E localizes in mitochondrial membranes where it acts as a free radical scavenger[28]. Increased ROS production was directly shown in mouse embryonic carcinoma P19 cells engineered to produce reduced levels of frataxin, adversely affecting their neuronal differentiation and increasing apoptosis, an observation that may have implication for the human disease[29]. Patients' fibroblasts are sensitive to low doses of H_2O_2, that induce cell shrinkage, nuclear condensation and apoptotic cell death at lower doses than in control fibroblasts[30]. This finding suggests that even non-affected cells are in an "at risk" status for oxidative stress as a consequence of the primary genetic defect. In addition, FA fibroblasts show abnormal antioxidant responses, in particular a blunted increase in mitochondrial SOD triggered by iron and by oxidants in control cells[31].

Mitochondrial dysfunction has been proven to occur *in vivo* in FA patients. Phosphorus-MRS analysis of skeletal muscle and heart shows a reduced rate of ATP synthesis[32]. Biochemically, the same multiple ISP enzyme dysfunctions found in Δ*YFH1* yeast are found in affected tissues from FA patients[18].

II. ANIMAL MODELS

A. KO Mice

A frataxin KO mouse model was generated by deletion of exon 4 leading to inactivation of the FRDA gene product[33]. Heterozygous frataxin +/– mice, expressing around 50% of the wild-type frataxin level, have no pathological phenotype. Homozygous frataxin –/– mice die as early as embryonic day 7 (E7), shortly after implantation, demonstrating an important role for frataxin during early development. The early embryonic lethality in frataxin –/– mice contrasts with the lifelong phenotype in FA patients. Clearly, the low residual level of frataxin resulting from the intronic expansion mutation in FA is critical for patient survival.

The mechanisms leading to the early embryonic death of KO animals are unclear. Frataxin –/– embryos are rapidly reabsorbed, leaving little material for analysis. Moreover, no clear evidence of apoptosis was found. Surprisingly, in the frataxin KO, no iron accumulation was observed during embryonic resorption, suggesting that cell death could be due to a mechanism independent of gross iron accumulation.

B. Conditional KO Mice

The early embryonic lethality of frataxin KO mice has complicated the effort to generate an animal model of the disease. Viable mouse models were obtained through a conditional gene targeting approach, using Cre-mediated excision of Lox-flanked (floxed) sequences[34]. Conditional KO lines were generated by crossing mice homozygous for a conditional allele of *Frda* (*Frda*$^{L3/L3}$) with mice heterozygous for the deletion of *Frda* exon 4 (*Frda* +/–) that carried a tissue-specific Cre transgene. The first two models utilized

Cre transgenes under the control of the muscle creatine kinase (MCK) and of the neuron-specific enolase (NSE) promoters to induce striated muscle- and neuron-restricted exon deletion, respectively.

NSE mutants have a low birth weight and develop a progressive neurological phenotype with the average onset of ataxia at 12 days, hunched stance and loss of proprioception. They have a short life expectancy (24 ± 9 days) with a 41% weight reduction at death compared with littermates. MCK mutants begin to lose weight at approximately 7 weeks, progressively develop signs of fatigue and die at 76 ± 10 days, with a 29% weight reduction at death. MCK mutants have absent full-length transcript and protein from skeletal and cardiac muscles. NSE mutants show excision of the full-length transcript in neuronal as well as in non-neuronal tissues, such as heart and liver. Frataxin protein is absent from the heart of NSE mutants, but it is present in small amount in brain, liver and kidney. Lowered frataxin in these tissues, particularly in the brain, may be the consequence of cell-specific excision. These mice reproduce important progressive pathophysiological and biochemical features of the human disease: cardiac hypertrophy without skeletal muscle involvement in the heart and striated muscle frataxin-deficient line, large sensory neuron dysfunction without alteration of the small sensory and motor neurons in the more generalized frataxin-deficient line.

MCK mutants show cardiac hypertrophy with thickening of the walls of the left ventricle, and show myocardial degeneration with cytoplasmic vacuolization in the myocytes, evidence of necrosis and post-necrotic fibrosis. They eventually develop a dilated cardiomyopathy, consistent with the natural history of the human disease. NSE mutants develop a cardiomyopathy before the MCK mutants, possibly because their extensive pathology contributes to the earlier heart involvement. Electron microscopy of hearts from both mutant lines shows abnormal alignment and disruption of myofibrils. Mitochondrial abnormalities are also found in the hearts of both mutants, including the presence of centrally placed tubular cristae and of disintegrating mitochondria. In addition, in NSE mutants, half of the mitochondria are swollen and contain abundant lipid droplets, as can be observed in respiratory chain defects. MCK mutants show proliferation of mitochondria that are only rarely swollen.

Time-dependent intra-mitochondrial iron accumulation occurs in the hearts of MCK mutant mice. In these mice, iron deposits can be detected at 10 weeks by Perls staining on histological sections and by electron microscopy as small intra-mitochondrial electron dense deposits. Direct measurement of iron concentration by atomic absorption spectroscopy in MCK mutant heart mitochondria showed normal or slightly increased levels at 7 weeks (791 ± 108 ng iron/mg protein versus 749 ± 35 ng iron/mg protein [n = 4]) and significantly increased levels at ten weeks (1,049 ± 205 ng iron/mg protein versus 579 ± 65 ng iron/mg protein [n = 4, $P = 0.005$]). No evidence of iron deposits was found in the NSE hearts.

The nervous system of NSE mutants shows extensive degeneration and necrosis affecting areas that are atrophied in FA, such as the dentate nucleus of the cerebellum, the trigeminal nucleus and tracts, the vestibular system and the cochlear nuclei, but also extends into areas preserved in FA patients, such as the cerebral cortex particularly in the frontal regions. Spongiform degeneration occurs in the cerebral cortex, with vacuoles mostly within neuronal cytoplasm and occasionally in neuronal nuclei and other structures. Neurophysiological studies in these mutants showed a specific atrophy of large sensory fibers, resembling the human disease. Specifically, sensory nerve conduction on the caudal nerve (almost exclusively composed of small diameter sensory axons) and motor evoked potentials were normal, but the H response after sciatic nerve stimulation was absent.

Biochemically, deficient activities of complexes I–III of the respiratory chain and of the aconitases were present in both lines. A 77–87% complex II deficiency and a 70–74% aconitase deficiency were found in the hearts of MCK (7 and 10 weeks) and NSE (at death) mutants, while complex IV activity was normal. In addition, succinate dehydrogenase (SDH) staining in the heart of 2–3 week-old NSE mutants and of 7–10 week-old MCK mutants was decreased, again with no significant difference in cytochrome c oxidase (COX).

Overall, the NSE and MCK conditional KOs have provided important insights into the pathogenesis of FA, in particular by showing that iron accumulation follows in time other pathological and biochemical abnormalities. They remain an important resource for further pathophysiological studies and for the pre-clinical testing of new treatments. These animals, however, still do not mimic the situation occurring in the human disease because conditional gene targeting leads to complete loss of frataxin in some cells at a specific time in development, while Friedreich ataxia is characterized by partial frataxin deficiency in all cells throughout life.

C. Pancreatic β-cells Conditional KO Mice

The same conditional KO system as described above was utilized with a Cre transgene under the Ins2 promoter, disrupting the frataxin gene in pancreatic β-cells[35]. Mice showed no obvious phenotype at birth but developed impaired glucose tolerance at 6 weeks of age, then increased post-prandial glucose levels and eventually increased fasting glucose levels. Insulin levels after intraperitoneal glucose-loading concomitantly decreased in an age-dependant manner. Increased levels of free radicals, in particular superoxide, were detected in pancreatic islets, followed by induction of apoptosis and inhibition of proliferation, resulting in significant β-cell loss.

D. Inducible Conditional KO Mice

Using a tamoxifen-inducible recombinase under the control of a neuron-specific prion protein promoter, in order to have a spatio-temporally controlled deletion of the mouse frataxin gene flanked by loxP sequences, a mouse model that recreates only the neurological features of the human disease was developed[36]. Two different lines, which exhibit a progressive neurological phenotype with slow evolution, were obtained. The mice present a general locomotor deficit without a defect in muscle strength beginning at around 10 weeks, and further develop a clear progressive ataxia leading to loss of spontaneous ambulation at around 1 year of age. In addition, electromyographic studies show a significant decrease in sensorimotor reflexes after sciatic nerve stimulation, indicating that the large myelinated proprioceptive sensory neurons are functionally defective, causing sensory and spinocerebellar ataxia, a distinctive pathological characteristic of FRDA. Histological studies showed both spinal cord and dorsal root ganglia (DRG) anomalies with absence of motor neuropathy, a hallmark of the human disease. In addition, one line revealed a cerebellar granule cell loss, whereas both lines had Purkinje cell arborization defects. An autophagic process was identified as the causative pathological mechanism in the DRG, leading to removal of mitochondrial debris and apparition of lipofuscin deposits.

E. GAA Expansion Knock-In Mice

In order to establish an animal model for FRDA that mirrors the chronically reduced levels of frataxin expression found in the human disease, a knock-in mouse model that carries a $(GAA)_{230}$ repeat in the *frda* gene was generated[37]. This repeat, when in homozygosity, only leads to a decrease in frataxin expression to 75% of wild-type levels. To further decrease frataxin expression, frataxin knock-in/KO mice (*frda*$^{-/230GAA}$) were generated, expressing approximately 25–30% of wild-type frataxin levels, a reduction associated with mild, but clinically evident FA in humans. However, these mice do not show any pathology throughout their lifespan. Rotarod analysis performed up to the age of one year old did not reveal any motor incoordination. The hearts of *frda*$^{-/230GAA}$ mice were negative for iron staining. In addition, the response of *frda*$^{-/230GAA}$ mice to challenge with iron-dextran or carbonyl iron did not differ from the response of wild-type mice. Furthermore, iron overload did not lead to cardiac fibrosis. Thus 25–30% of wild-type frataxin levels is compatible with normal neurological function and iron metabolism in mice.

This mouse model was also used to study GAA repeat instability, which occurs in humans during parent-to-offspring transmission and in somatic tissues of FA patients. In *frda*$^{-/230GAA}$ and *frda*$^{230/230GAA}$ mice, the $(GAA)_{230}$ repeat is meiotically and mitotically stable. In humans, such a repeat would be moderately unstable, so that several easily detectable changes in size would have been identified in a similar number of transmission events.

This model is being used to identify the early alterations caused by frataxin deficiency and the cellular compensatory response to this stress through a microarray-based gene expression profiling approach. Mice have so far been investigated at 6 months of age. Despite the absence of neurodegeneration, many genes in metabolic and signaling pathways were altered. In particular, compensatory changes in gene expression occurred in the brain (255 genes up-regulated, 89 down-regulated), mostly related to the response to oxidative stress.

F. YAC and BAC Transgenic Approaches

Functional rescue of frataxin KO mice could be achieved with wild-type human genomic YAC and BAC FRDA transgenes[38]. Recently, human FRDA YAC transgenic mice carrying a human $(GAA)_{200}$ repeat expansion were generated. This expansion showed inter-generational instability, including both increases and decreases in GAA repeat size. Initial molecular studies of this line detected high levels of human frataxin expression. Histological and neurobehavioral analyses have so far (3–6 months) shown no significant abnormality.

Three independent transgenic mouse lines carrying the intact BAC genomic fragment BAC265, which contains exons 1–5b of the FRDA locus and flanking sequences in a 188 kb genomic DNA fragment. Careful molecular investigations indicated that the human FRDA locus in BAC265 may contain a number of regulatory elements that confer tissue specificity in gene expression and that may be differentially recognized by the mouse transcriptional machinery in different mouse tissues. Homozygous FRDA knockout mice are rescued by the presence of this 188 kb human BAC transgene, they develop without any obvious abnormalities and have normal fertility.

To facilitate studies of frataxin gene expression *in vivo*, two other transgenic lines were established with a genomic reporter construct consisting of an in-frame fusion of the gene encoding enhanced green fluorescent protein (EGFP) at the end of exon 5a of the FRDA gene. Both lines exhibited whole-organ green fluorescence confirming the expression of the fusion protein in these mice.

G. Frataxin Overexpressing Mouse Model

A mouse model of frataxin overexpression was created by taking advantage of cytomegalovirus promoter (CMV) to efficiently deliver human frataxin expression to most tissues (Miraude, M. et al.). Three different mouse lines (TgFxn lines 1–3) were generated with frataxin increases ranging from 3 to more than 10 fold increase compared to wild type levels, depending on the mouse transgene copy number and tissue. TgFxn mice are born healthy and do not show abnormal symptoms at least up to the age of one year.

Participation in the cellular antioxidant defense mechanisms, involvement in iron metabolism and mediation of iron for heme biosynthesis, were tested in these animals. Oxidative stress caused by the administration of doxorubicin (DOX) was not reduced by overproduction of frataxin, suggesting that frataxin is not involved in the iron-related oxidative stress pathway activated by DOX. Iron metabolism and response to an iron challenge were normal in these mice, demonstrating that frataxin overexpression do not disrupt normal iron metabolism. However, tgFxn mice showed an altered response during hematopietic differentiation, suggesting an involvement of frataxin in mitochondrial iron metabolism possibly by making iron accessible for heme biosynthesis[39].

Additionally, an important insight from this study is the demonstration that frataxin overexpression is not toxic, and could be a good therapeutic approach. Gene therapy strategies that would efficiently deliver frataxin expression to cells affected in FRDA can be envisaged to increase frataxin levels in FRDA patients. Increases of frataxin levels to 50% of wild type would be sufficient to stop the progression of the disease. Further studies will be needed to assess the feasibility of this therapeutic option and to optimize conditions for gene delivery.

References

1. Chamberlain S., J. Shaw, A. Rowland A, et al. 1988. Mapping of mutation causing Friedreich' ataxia to human chromosome 9. *Nature* **334**: 248–250.
2. Campuzano V., L. Montermini, M.D. Moltó, L. Pianese, M. Cossée, F. Cavalcanti, et al. 1996. Friedreich ataxia: autosomal recessive disease caused by an intronic GAA triplet repeat expansion. *Science* **271**:1423–1427.
3. Koutnikova H., V. Campuzano, F. Foury, P. Dollé, O. Cazzalini, and M. Koenig. 1997. Studies of human, mouse and yeast homologues indicate a mitochondrial function for frataxin. *Nat Genet* **16**:345–351.
4. Jiralerspong S., Y. Liu, L. Montermini, S. Stifani, and M. Pandolfo. 1997. Frataxin shows developmentally regulated tissue-specific expression in the mouse embryo. *Neurobiol Dis* **4**:103–113.
5. Campuzano V., L. Montermini, Y. Lutz, et al. 1997. Frataxin is reduced in Friedreich ataxia patients and is associated with mitochondrial membranes. *Hum Mol Genet* **6**:1771–1780.
6. Dürr A., M. Cossée, Y. Agid, et al. 1996. Clinical and genetic abnormalities in patients with Friedreich ataxia. *N Engl J Med* **335**:1169–1175.
7. Montermini L., A. Richter, K. Morgan, et al. 1997. Phenotypic variability in Friedreich ataxia: role of the associated GAA triplet repeat expansion. *Annals of Neurology* **41**:675–682.
8. Ohshima K., L. Montermini, R.D. Wells, and M. Pandolfo. 1998. Inhibitory Effects of Expanded GAA·TTC Triplet Repeats from Intron I of the Friedreich Ataxia Gene on Transcription and Replication in Vivo. *J Biol Chem* **273**:14588–15595.
9. Sakamoto N., K. Ohshima, L. Montermini, M. Pandolfo, and R.D. Wells. 2001. Sticky DNA, a self-associated complex formed at long GAA·TTC repeats in intron 1 of the Frataxin gene, inhibits transcription. *J Biol Chem* **276**:27171–27177.
10. Sakamoto N., P.D. Chastain, P. Parniewski, K. Ohshima, M. Pandolfo, J.D. Griffith, and R.D. Wells. 1999. Sticky DNA: self-association properties of long GAA·TTC repeats in R·R·Y triplex structures from Friedreich ataxia. *Mol Cell* **3**:465–475.
11. Cossée M., A. Dürr, M. Schmitt, et al. 1999. Frataxin point mutations and clinical presentation of compound heterozygous Friedreich ataxia patients. *Ann Neurol* **45**:200–206.
12. Dhe-Paganon S., R. Shigeta, Y.I. Chi, M. Ristow, and S.E. Shoelson. 2000. Crystal structure of human frataxin. *J Biol Chem* Jul 18 [epub ahead of print].
13. Musco G., G. Stier, B. Kolmerer, S. Adinolfi, S. Martin, T. Frenkiel, T. Gibson, and A. Pastore. 2000. Towards a structural understanding of Friedreich's ataxia: the solution structure of frataxin. *Structure Fold Des* **8**:695–707.
14. Cho S.J., M.G. Lee, J.K. Yang, J.Y. Lee, H.K. Song, and S.W. Suh. 2000. Crystal structure of Escherichia coli CyaY protein reveals a previously unidentified fold for the evolutionarily conserved frataxin family. *Proc Natl Acad Sci USA* **97**:8932–8937.
15. Babcock M., D. de Silva, R. Oaks, et al. 1997. Regulation of mitochondrial iron accumulation by Yfh1, a putative homolog of frataxin. *Science* **276**:1709–1712.
16. Wilson R.B., and D.M. Roof. 1997. Respiratory deficiency due to loss of mitochondrial DNA in yeast lacking the frataxin homologue. *Nature Genet* **16**:352–357.
17. Radisky D.C., M.C. Babcock, and J. Kaplan. 1999. The yeast frataxin homologue mediates mitochondrial iron efflux. Evidence for a mitochondrial iron cycle. *J Biol Chem* **274**:4497–4499.
18. Rötig A., P. deLonlay, D. Chretien, et al. 1997. Frataxin gene expansion causes aconitase and mitochondrial iron-sulfur protein deficiency in Friedreich ataxia. *Nature Genet* **17**:215–217.
19. Gardner P.R., I. Rainieri, L.B. Epstein, and C.W. White. 1995. Superoxide radical and iron modulate aconitase activity in mammalian cells. *J Biol Chem* **270**:13399–13405.
20. Adamec J., F. Rusnak, W.G. Owen, S. Naylor, L.M. Benson, A.M. Gacy, and G. Isaya. 2000. Iron-dependent self-assembly of recombinant yeast frataxin: implications for Friedreich ataxia. *Am J Hum Genet* **67**:549–562.
21. Lamarche J.B., M. Côté, and B. Lemieux. 1980. The cardiomyopathy of Friedreich ataxia morphological observations in 3 cases. *Can J Neurol Sci* **7**:389–396.
22. Waldvogel D., P. van Gelderen, and M. Hallett. 1999. Increased iron in the dentate nucleus of patients with Friedreich ataxia. *Ann Neurol* **46**:123–125.
23. Delatycki M.B., J. Camakaris, H. Brooks, T. Evans-Whipp, D.R. Thorburn, R. Williamson, and S.M. Forrest. 1999. Direct evidence that mitochondrial iron accumulation occurs in Friedreich ataxia. *Ann Neurol* **45**:673–675.
24. Wilson R.B., D.R. Lynch, J.M. Farmer, D.G. Brooks, and K.H. Fischbeck. 2000. Increased serum transferrin receptor concentrations in Friedreich ataxia. *Ann Neurol* **47**:659–661.
25. Emond M., G. Lepage, M. Vanasse, and M. Pandolfo. 2000. Increased levels of plasma malondialdehyde in Friedreich ataxia. *Neurol* **55**: 1752–1753.
26. Schulz J.B., T. Dehmer, L. Schöls, H. Mende, C. Hardt, M. Vorgerd, K. Bürk, W. Matson, J. Dichgans, M.F. Beal, and M.B. Bogdanov. 2000. Oxidative stress in patients with Friedreich ataxia. *Neurology* **55**:1719–1721.
27. Ben Hamida M., S. Belal, G. Sirugo, et al. 1993. Friedreich ataxia phenotype not linked to chromosome 9 and associated with selective autosomal recessive vitamin E deficiency in two inbred Tunisian families. *Neurology* **43**:2179–2183.

28. Di Mascio P., M.E. Murphy, and H. Sies. 1991. Antioxidant defense systems: the role of carotenoids, tocopherols, and thiols. *Am J Clin Nutr* **53**:194S–200S.
29. Santos M., K. Ohshima, and M. Pandolfo. 2001. Frataxin deficiency enhances apoptosis in cells differentiating into neuroectoderm. *Hum Mol Genet* **10**:1935–1944.
30. Wong A., J. Yang, P. Cavadini, C. Gellera, B. Lonnerdal, F. Taroni, and G. Cortopassi. 1999. The Friedreich ataxia mutation confers cellular sensitivity to oxidant stress which is rescued by chelators of iron and calcium and inhibitors of apoptosis. *Hum Mol Genet* **8**:425–430.
31. Jiralerspong S., B. Ge, T.J. Hudson, and M. Pandolfo. 2001. Manganese Superoxide Dismutase Induction by Iron is Impaired in Friedreich Ataxia Cells. *FEBS Letters* **509**:101–105.
32. Lodi R., J.M. Cooper, J.L. Bradley, D. Manners, P. Styles, D.J. Taylor, and A.H. Schapira. 1999. Deficit of in vivo mitochondrial ATP production in patients with Friedreich ataxia. *Proc Natl Acad Sci USA* **96**:11492–11495.
33. Cossée M., H. Puccio, A. Gansmuller, et al. 2000. Inactivation of the Friedreich ataxia mouse gene leads to early embryonic lethality without iron accumulation. *Hum Mol Genet* **9**:1219–1226.
34. Puccio H., D. Simon, M. Cossee, P. Criqui-Filipe, F. Tiziano, J. Melki, C. Hindelang, R. Matyas, P. Rustin, and M. Koenig. 2001. Mouse models for Friedreich ataxia exhibit cardiomyopathy, sensory nerve defect and Fe-S enzyme deficiency followed by intramitochondrial iron deposits. *Nat Genet* **27**:181–618.
35. Ristow M., H. Mulder, D. Pomplun, et al. 2003. Frataxin deficiency in pancreatic islets causes diabetes due to loss of beta cell mass. *J Clin Invest* **112**:527–534.
36. Simon D., H. Seznec, A. Gansmuller, et al. 2004. Friedreich ataxia mouse models with progressive cerebellar and sensory ataxia reveal autophagic neurodegeneration in dorsal root ganglia. *J Neurosci* **24**: 1987–1995.
37. Miranda C.J., M.M. Santos, K. Ohshima, M. Tessaro, J. Sequecos, M. Paudolfo. 2001. Frataxin knockin mouse. *FEBS Lett* **512**:281–288.
38. Pook M.A., S. Al-Mahdawi, C.J. Carroll, et al. 2001. Rescue of the Friedreich's ataxia knockout mouse by human YAC transgenesis. *Neurogenetics* **3**:185–193.
39. Becker E.M., J.M. Greer, P. Ponka, and D.R. Richardson. 2002. Erythroid differentiation and protoporphyrin IX down-regulate frataxin expression in Friend cells: characterization of frataxin expression compared to molecules involved in iron metabolism and hemoglobinization. *Blood* **99**:3813–3822.

CHAPTER

K7

Animal Oculomotor Data Illuminate Cerebellum-Related Eye Movement Disorders

FARREL R. ROBINSON, JAMES O. PHILLIPS, and AVERY H. WEISS

Three parts of the cerebellum influence voluntary eye movements: A) the posterior medial region including the oculomotor vermis (OMV) and the part of the cerebellar nuclei to which it projects, the caudal fastigial nucleus (CFN), B) the lateral cerebellum including the dorsal paraflocculus and the part of the cerebellar nuclei to which it projects, the posterior interpositus nucleus, as well as the cerebellar hemispheres, and C) the flocculus, ventral paraflocculus, nodulus, and uvula. The OMV and CFN influence primarily the accuracy and speed of the horizontal component of voluntary eye movements, i.e., saccades and smooth pursuit. The dorsal paraflocculus and interpositus nucleus influence the vertical component of these movements. The flocculus, ventral paraflocculus, nodulus, and uvula influence reflexive eye movements elicited by vestibular stimulation, i.e., the vestibuloocular reflex (VOR) and movement of large visual targets, i.e., optokinetic nystagmus (OKN).

The cerebellum strongly influences movements of every part of the body. Over the past decade, we have learned much about the important role of the cerebellum in eye movements. Patients with cerebellar damage from a variety of sources exhibit abnormal eye movements. Here we first briefly review basic cerebellar anatomy and development. Then we summarize current data on the role of different parts of the cerebellum in eye movements. Finally, we describe what these data tell us about the cerebellar cause of oculomotor deficits associated with several types of cerebellar dysfunction, including: A) cerebellar malformations or agenesis, B) hereditary ataxias, C) cerebellar mass lesions, D) paraneoplastic degeneration, and E) Wallenberg's Syndrome.

Address correspondence to: Farrel R. Robinson, Department of Biological Structure, University of Washington, Seattle, WA 98195-7420, (206) 685-0614, Fax: (206) 543-1524

I. OVERVIEW OF THE CEREBELLUM

Here we provide a brief and simple summary of cerebellar anatomy and development, describing details that will help make clear the locations and consequences of cerebellar abnormalities that we describe later. A more detailed and comprehensive description of cerebellar anatomy and development is available in many textbooks.

A. Anatomy

1. Gross Anatomy

a. Location and Connections to the Rest of the Brain

The cerebellum rests atop the pons and medulla forming the top of the IVth ventricle (Figure 1A). It is connected to

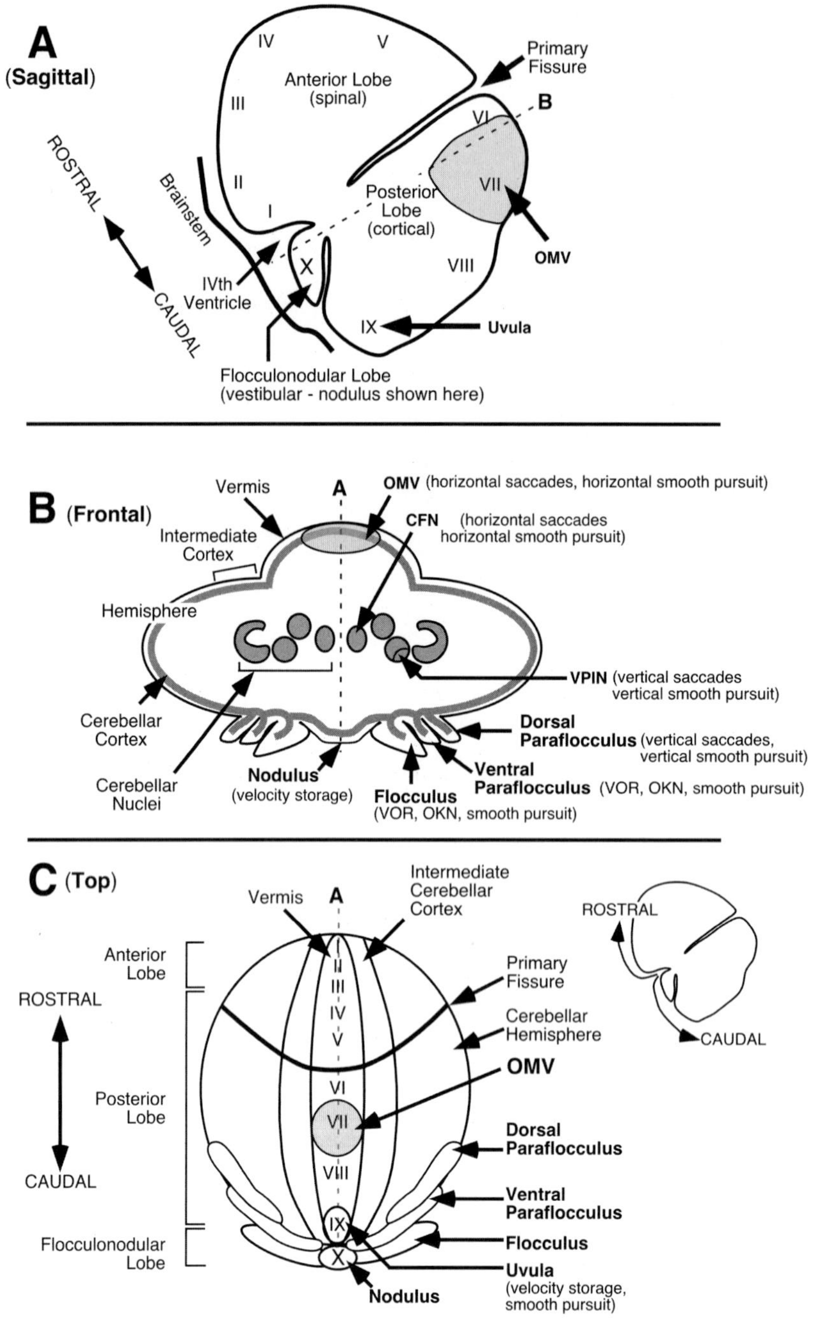

FIGURE 1 Parts of the cerebellum. **A**, Schematic representation of a midsagittal section through the cerebellum showing the relative positions of the anterior, posterior, and flocculonodular lobes. **B**, Schematic representation of a frontal section through the posterior lobe of the cerebellum showing the relative positions of the cerebellar cortex and nuclei as well as the major divisions of the cortex. Eye movement-related regions named in bold. **C**, Schematic of the major parts of the cerebellar cortex viewed from above and unrolled as shown in the insert of a sagittal section in the upper right. Dashed lines in each drawing mark the position of other sections. Gray regions in the cerebellar cortex in **A**, **B**, and **C** mark the position of the oculomotor vermis. In parentheses next to label of each eye movement-related region in **B** and **C** are the oculomotor functions linked to that region. Abbreviations: CFN, caudal fastigial nucleus; OMV, oculomotor vermis; VPIN, ventrolateral posterior interpositus nucleus. Roman numerals in A and C name lobutes in the vermis.

the rest of the brain via three large fiber bundles on each side, the inferior, middle, and superior cerebellar peduncles. The inferior peduncle consists of axons bringing spinal and vestibular information into the cerebellum as mossy fibers. It also contains the axons of neurons in the contralateral inferior olive, bringing climbing fiber input to the cerebellum. The middle peduncle consists of the axons of neurons in the pontine nuclei that carry mossy fiber input to the cerebellum. The pontocerebellar projection is predominantly, but not entirely, crossed. Pontocerebellar fibers relay information to the cerebellum from the cerebral cortex that reaches the pontine nuclei via very large corticopontine projections. The superior colliculus also sends projections to the pontine nuclei, which in turn send collicular signals into the cerebellum. The superior peduncle carries signals out of the cerebellum to the rest of the brain.

The cerebellum consists of two major components, the cerebellar cortex and the cerebellar nuclei. As Figure 1B illustrates, the cerebellar cortex forms the outside rind of the cerebellum. The cerebellar nuclei are buried in the white matter within the cortex and consist of four collections of cell bodies on each side of the cerebellum. In general, each part of the cerebellar cortex sends its output to the part of the cerebellar nuclei that is nearest to it. The corticonuclear projection is exclusively inhibitory, i.e., output from the cerebellar cortex inhibits activity in the cerebellar nuclei. This is why damage to the eye movement-related parts of the cerebellar cortex and nuclei can have opposite effects on eye movements. The axons of neurons in the cerebellar nuclei form the superior peduncle as they exit the cerebellum.

b. *Major Divisions of the Cerebellar Cortex*

The cerebellar cortex consists of three major divisions, the flocculonodular lobe or vestibulocerebellum, the anterior lobe or spinal cerebellum, and the posterior lobe or corticocerebellum. Figures 1A and 1C show the relative positions of these three divisions.

Within each of these major divisions smaller lobules, not shown separately in Figure 1A, are numbered with Roman numerals I through X. As Figure 1A shows, lobules I and X are just rostral and caudal to the peak of the IVth ventricle, respectively. In this scheme, adjacent structures with adjacent numbers have similar connectivity and function. Since the cerebellum is folded on itself, lobule I, considered by convention to be the most rostral lobule, is adjacent to lobule X, considered to be the most caudal lobule. Figure 1C unfolds the cerebellar cortex to show the relationship of different parts of the cortex on a flat map.

The most caudal of the three major divisions of the cerebellum is the flocculonodular lobe, i.e., lobule X or the nodulus, and its lateral extension, the flocculus. This is the phylogenetically oldest part of the cerebellum. The flocculonodular lobe receives mossy fiber input from both the vestibular labyrinth via the VIIIth nerve and from the vestibular nuclei. The axons that carry the output from the flocculonodular lobe terminate in the vestibular nuclei. This contrasts with axons carrying output from the two other major divisions of the cerebellum, anterior and posterior lobes, which terminate in the cerebellar nuclei.

The most rostral of the major divisions is the anterior lobe, lobules I–V. It is phylogenetically more recent than the flocculonodular lobe but not as recent as the posterior lobe. The anterior lobe receives somatosensory and proprioceptive mossy fiber input from the spinal cord. Its output terminates in regions of the cerebellar nuclei that project to the thalamus and red nucleus.

The posterior lobe, lobules VI–IX, is separated from the anterior lobe by the primary fissure. The posterior lobe is the most recent major division of the cerebellum and receives its input largely from the cerebral cortex via a relay in the contralateral pontine nuclei. For example, neurons in the left cerebral cortex send axons to terminate in the left pontine nuclei which in turn project predominantly to the right side of the cerebellum. The output of the posterior lobe of the cerebellar cortex terminates in regions of the cerebellar nuclei that project to the thalamus, red nucleus, and brainstem. In higher mammals, especially primates, the posterior lobe is by far the largest part of the cerebellum.

The most posterior and medial part of the posterior lobe is the uvula (Figure 1C). The uvula is like the flocculonodular lobe in that it receives a large vestibular input and projects to the vestibular nuclei. It is immediately rostral of the nodulus. The uvula and nodulus are often considered together because they seem to serve similar functions and can be damaged together.

As Figure 1C shows, the most medial part of the cerebellar cortex is called the vermis. The lateral extensions of the posterior lobe cortex are called the cerebellar hemispheres. The lateral parts of the anterior lobes are also sometimes referred to as the hemispheric part of the anterior lobe. The cortical region between the vermis and hemispheres is called the intermediate cortex.

2. Cerebellar Cortex

The cerebellar cortex is highly folded into long ridges that are oriented with their long axes running roughly medial-lateral, near the midline. Each of these smallest ridges is called a folium.

Within each folium anywhere in the cerebellar cortex, the organization of neurons is extremely similar. Neurons in the mature cerebellar cortex are organized into three layers illustrated in Figure 2, i.e., the molecular, Purkinje cell, and granular layers. The outermost, or molecular, layer contains the axons of granule cells, called parallel fibers, the dendrites of Purkinje cells, and the cell bodies of two types of inhibitory interneurons, stellate cells and basket cells (not shown in

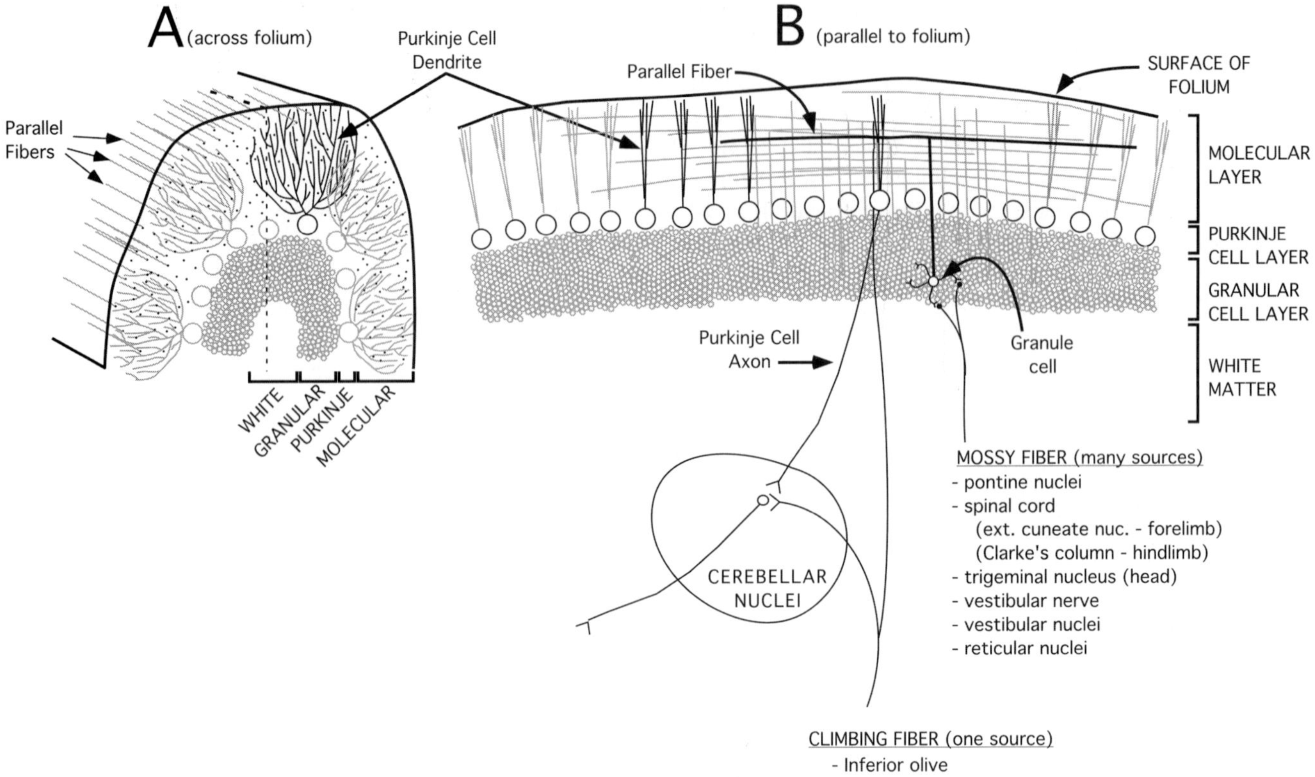

FIGURE 2 Schematic view of the major cell types in the cerebellar cortex. **A**, Section across the long axis of the folium showing the broad axis of Purkinje cell dendritic trees and cross sections of parallel fibers. Dashed line indicates position of section in B. **B**, Section parallel to the long axis of the folium showing parallel fibers along their length and the narrow edge of Purkinje cell dendritic trees. One granular cell appears in black and white showing its dendrites, on which mossy fibers terminate and its axon coursing toward the surface of the folium and bifurcating. Several other parallel fiber axons and parallel fibers appear in gray. One climbing fiber appears contacting the dendrites of one Purkinje cell.

Figure 2). Parallel fibers run parallel to the long axis of the folium contacting the dendritic tree of Purkinje cells along its course. Purkinje cell dendrites are, like an open hand, narrow when viewed from one angle but broad when viewed an orthogonal angle. The broad plane of each Purkinje cell dendritic tree is oriented across the folium perpendicular to the path of parallel fibers.

Beneath the molecular layer, the cell bodies of the Purkinje cells are arrayed in a single sheet, one cell thick. The axons of Purkinje cells are the only output of the cerebellar cortex. These axons terminate on neurons in the cerebellar nuclei or, in the case of Purkinje cells in the flocculonodular lobe, in the vestibular nuclei.

Under the Purkinje cells is a layer consisting of an astonishing number of small, densely packed granule cell bodies. Granule cells are extremely numerous. Human cerebellum contains ~5×10^{10} neurons (Braitenberg and Atwood, 1958; Zagon et al., 1977). This is roughly twice as many neurons as in the cerebral cortex (2.3×10^{10}, Pakkenberg and Gundersen, 1997).

The cerebellar cortex receives its input via two distinct types of fibers, mossy fibers and climbing fibers. Mossy fibers originate in many places including the spinal cord, the vestibular labyrinth, and nuclei, and the pontine nuclei. They terminate on the dendrites of granule cells. In contrast, climbing fibers originate in only one place, the contralateral inferior olive. Climbing fibers terminate directly on the dendrites of Purkinje cells. Each Purkinje cell receives input from only one climbing fiber. Some mossy fibers and all climbing fibers send collaterals to terminate in the cerebellar nuclei.

3. Cerebellar Nuclei

Under the granule cell layer is the white matter consisting of axons of Purkinje cells leaving the cerebellar cortex and the axons of mossy fibers and climbing fibers bound for the cerebellar cortex. Buried deep within the cerebellar white matter below the cerebellar cortex are the cerebellar nuclei. These are four large groups of neuron cell bodies on each side of the cerebellum (Figure 1B). Purkinje cell axons terminate on, and inhibit, neurons in these nuclei. The axons of neurons in the cerebellar nuclei carry signals out of the cerebellum, via the superior cerebellar peduncle, to influence brain regions outside the cerebellum.

B. Development

1. Timing

The cerebellum develops from the hindbrain which, in humans, first appears at about three weeks' gestation when two constrictions develop in the anterior neural tube resulting in the prosencephalon (forebrain), mesencephalon (midbrain), and rhombencephalon (hindbrain). Subsequent constriction separates the rhombencephalon into the rostral metencephalon and caudal myelencephalon. These regions differentiate further into the pons, a substantial part of the cerebellum, the superior part of the IVth ventricle, and the medulla.

Within the hindbrain, the cerebellum arises from the transitional region centered on the constriction, or isthmus, between the mesencephalon and metencephalon. The flocculonodular lobe appears first and is evident at two months. The vermis and intermediate part of the cerebellar cortex are well formed by four months. The more lateral part of the cerebellar hemispheres is developed by five to six months. Since these different regions develop at different times, they can be differentially affected with congenital cerebellar malformations.

Development of the cerebellum begins with the birth of progenitor neurons in the germinal matrix of the lateral walls and floor of the IVth ventricle and the subsequent dorsal migration of these progenitor cells. All the cells are born in the germinal matrix in the lateral walls and floor of the primordial IVth ventricle and migrate into the cerebellum (Goldowitz and Hamre, 1998; Niesen, 2003). The birth and exit of the Purkinje cells and nuclear neurons are first, followed by the granule cells destined for the external granular layer (EGL), a layer of granule cells in the immature cerebellum lying superficial to the Purkinje cells. Postnatally the EGL disappears as granule cells migrate inward under glial guidance to form the internal granular layer under Purkinje cells. Migration of granule cells is not complete until twenty months of life (Hatten and Heintz, 1995). This period also sees synaptic maturation of the inputs to the cerebellar cortex, mossy fibers, and climbing fibers.

2. Molecular Events

Some genetic mutations are known to affect Purkinje cells, producing deficits in eye movements that are consistent with loss of this cell population. Other mutations produce changes in the relative number of granule cells and Purkinje cells, thereby affecting the processing of eye movement–related signals in the cerebellum. It is therefore important to understand the genetic origins of the cerebellum and of its cellular constituents. Our understanding has improved dramatically during the past decade due to genetic manipulations in animals. These manipulations and the resulting behavioral deficits provide insight into the pathology of congenital cerebellar disorders.

Beginning at the isthmus, there is spatially restricted expression of Wnt 1 rostrally and Fgt 8 caudally. Knockouts of these genes eliminate the cerebellum (McMahon and Bradley, 1990; Thomas and Capecchi, 1990; Wurst et al., 1994). Prior to the expression of Wnt 1 and its induction of En (Engrail), a transcriptional regulatory factor, Pax 2, is expressed. Inactivation of this molecule leads to frequent loss of the cerebellum and posterior midbrain (Favor et al., 1996). Additional molecules, primarily Fgf 8, and the homeodomain proteins Gbx2 and Islet 3, contribute to the patterning of cerebellar subregions (Kikuchi et al., 1997; Wassarman et al., 1997; Meyers et al., 1998). Alterations in the gradients of these molecules may give rise to some cerebellar malformations.

Cellular histogenesis begins with the birth of Purkinje cells and nuclear cells which arise from a common progenitor cell. By comparison, granule cells arise from the secondary germinal zone in the EGL. The helix-loop helix transcriptional factor Math 1 is essential for the establishment of the GC lineage. Mice with a knockout of this gene lack granule cells (Ben-Arie et al., 1997). The ratio of Purkinje cells to granule cells is relatively constant, which means that genetic mutations or experimental perturbations that eliminate PC are accompanied by a reduction of granule cells (Heckroth et al., 1989; Feddersen et al., 1992; Herrup et al., 1997). In support of the linkage between Purkinje cell and granule cell development, recent evidence indicates the ligand sonic hedgehog, Shh, is secreted by Purkinje cells and the Shh receptor Patched (ptc) is present on granule cells. A homozygous deletion of Ptc in mice leads to excess proliferation of granule cells and medulloblastoma, the most common brain tumor in childhood (Goodrich et al., 1997).

Molecules that regulate the migration of Purkinje cells and granule cells to the cerebellum and the guidance cues provided by supportive glia and extracellular matrix are also candidate genes for cerebellar malformations. Migration of these cells is normally restricted to the region of the developing cerebellum. This migratory process is highly regulated and in part mediated by the Unc5h3 molecule which is expressed by Purkinje cells and granule cells. The boundaries of the cerebellum can thus be delineated by the spatial distribution of its obligatory Netrin receptor (Unc5h3). In a mouse with mutated Netrin receptor, there is ectopic migration of both cell types into the brainstem (Ackerman et al., 1997; Goldowitz et al., 2000). Likewise mutations in the extracellular molecule Reelin and a tyrosine Kinase signaling adaptor molecule disabled (encoded by Dab 1) lead to migration defects in mice, i.e., the reeler and scrambler mutants, respectively (D'Arcangelo et al., 1995; Howell et al., 1997; Sheldon et al., 1997). In these mutants, Purkinje cells fail to migrate into the cerebellum and granule cells are reduced in number. The eye movement abnormalities in these and other knockout mice have not been well studied. Describing them will be a productive goal for future research.

Prior to migration, postmitotic cells in the germinal matrix are vulnerable to mutations. Stimulation of NMDA receptors on granule cells leads to activation of the G-protein-coupled inward-rectifying K^+ channel protein GIRK2 (Patil et al., 1995). Mutations of this channel in the Weaver mouse aborts the compensatory hyperpolarization that follows transient depolarization, leading to the sustained influx of Ca^{++} and cell death. (Tucker et al., 1996). This potentially offers a model for the study of granule cell contributions to the control of eye movements.

II. ROLE OF CEREBELLUM IN EYE MOVEMENTS

Three parts of the cerebellum influence eye movements, A) the posterior medial region including the oculomotor vermis and caudal fastigial nucleus, B) the lateral cerebellum including the dorsal paraflocculus and the part of the cerebellar nuclei to which it projects, the posterior interpositus nucleus, as well as the cerebellar hemispheres, and C) the flocculus, nodulus, and uvula. Below, we briefly describe the role of each of these regions in eye movements.

A. Posterior Medial Cerebellum (Oculomotor Vermis and Caudal Fastigial Nucleus)

1. Saccades

a. Saccade Control

The oculomotor vermis (OMV) is the region of the cerebellar cortex within which vigorous saccade-related activity occurs and where electrical stimulation with small currents elicits saccade-like movements (Fujikado and Noda, 1987; Noda and Fujikado, 1987). In monkeys, it consists of a region in the posterior lobe vermis, specifically, lobule VII, and in some individuals the neighboring region just anterior to this, i.e., the posterior part of lobule VI. A recent review describes the role of this and other parts of the cerebellum in voluntary eye movements in more detail (Robinson and Fuchs, 2001).

The OMV projects exclusively to the caudal part of the most medial cerebellar nucleus, the fastigial nucleus (Yamada and Noda, 1987). The caudal fastigial nucleus (CFN) contains neurons that discharge a burst of action potentials for nearly every saccade (Ohtsuka and Noda, 1991, 1995; Fuchs et al., 1993). These saccade-related signals travel via the axons of CFN neurons to the brainstem network that produces saccades (Noda et al., 1990).

Most CFN neurons burst for every saccade, whatever its size or direction. The timing of the saccade burst depends on the direction of the saccade. In the CFN on each side, neurons begin bursting before, or early in, saccades toward the opposite side and later for saccades toward the same side. This timing fits well with the net effect of CFN bursts on the eyes, i.e., to drive them toward the contralateral side. For example, during a rightward saccade, neurons in the left CFN burst near the start of the movement. The rightward drive produced by this early activity helps accelerate the eyes rightward. A little later in the movement neurons in the left CFN burst. The leftward drive produced by this later activity helps decelerate the movement so that it ends on target. Supporting this scenario is the fact that the later bursts for ipsiversive saccades begin later as saccade size, and thus duration, increases, i.e., late CFN bursts for ipsiversive saccades are associated with the end of saccades (Ohtsuka and Noda 1991; Fuchs et al., 1993; Brettler et al., 2003).

The CFN's decelerating influence is stronger than its accelerating influence. We know this because inactivating the CFN bilaterally makes saccades in both horizontal directions too large (Robinson et al., 1993). This indicates that blocking CFN activity on both sides removes more deceleration than acceleration from the saccades. If the CFN's accelerating and decelerating influences were equal, then blocking both would leave saccade size unchanged.

An important effect of the CFN output is to make saccades fast, accurate, and consistent. Without these influences, e.g., during bilateral CFN inactivation, saccades not only overshoot their targets but are also abnormally slow and variable in their end points and velocities (Robinson et al., 1993). Saccade-related bursts in CFN neurons vary considerably in their timing, duration, and peak frequency even for identical saccades (Fuchs et al., 1993). This, and the variability of saccades when CFN activity is blocked, support the proposal that CFN output contributes acceleration and deceleration to each saccade in the appropriate amount and at the appropriate time to compensate for variability in descending saccade commands. In this view, oculomotor regions of the brain, upstream from the CFN, produce slow, dysmetric, variable movements (Robinson, 1995; Quaia et al., 1999) and it is CFN activity that makes saccades fast, accurate, and consistent.

Even if this view of CFN function is correct, we do not know how the cerebellum generates the CFN bursts appropriate to improving saccades. The early accelerating CFN burst could plausibly originate from the saccade-related neurons that project to the CFN from outside the cerebellum. These putative extra-cerebellar saccade-related neurons also project to the OMV and could produce the pause evident in ~18% of OMV Purkinje cells beginning an average of ~17 ms before for contralateral saccades (Ohtsuka and Noda, 1995). Purkinje cells inhibit neurons in the cerebellar nuclei, so these pauses could help trigger early accelerating bursts in CFN neurons by abruptly reducing OMV inhibition on CFN neurons before saccade onset. Abrupt reductions in Purkinje cell inhibition of cerebellar nuclear neurons can elicit bursts in nuclear cells (Aizenman and Linden, 1999).

The potential origins of the late decelerating CFN burst are more obscure. Most known inputs to the CFN or OMV burst before, not late in, saccades. The cerebellum could generate the late, decelerating burst in CFN neurons from the same inputs that it uses to generate the early accelerating bursts. The cerebellum could do this is by transmitting saccade-related signals across the OMV in parallel fibers. In this scenario, before a rightward saccade, saccade-related signals reach the left CFN and OMV and elicit the early accelerating burst in the left CFN. Incoming saccade-related signals also move across the midline via parallel fibers in the OMV. After a delay caused by their travel time, these signals reach P-cells in the right OMV through which they elicit a burst in the right CFN. Consistent with this proposal is the finding that interrupting OMV P-fiber conduction with multiple injections of tetrodotoxin causes an increase in saccade size (Robinson and Noto, 2003). Large, less specific OMV lesions (Takagi et al., 1998; Barash et al., 1999; Robinson and Noto, 2002) have the opposite effect, i.e., they decrease saccade size. Thus interrupting OMV fiber conduction, as opposed to simply reducing OMV output, makes saccades too large as it reduces the late decelerating CFN burst.

b. Saccade Adaptation

Saccades that are repeatedly inaccurate change, or adapt, to become more accurate. For example, if saccades to a target that is 15° to the right consistently overshoot the target they become smaller. This phenomenon occurs in both humans and monkeys and is the most studied example of motor learning of a voluntary movement. It has been summarized in detail recently (Hopp and Fuchs, 2004).

The CFN and OMV are critical to saccade adaptation. CFN neurons change their output during saccade adaptation in a way appropriate to changing saccade size in the adaptive direction (Inaba et al., 2003; Scudder, 2002) and lesions of either the CFN (Robinson et al., 2002) or OMV (Takagi et al., 1998; Barash et al., 1999) impair adaptation. In addition, PET studies in humans show increased activity in the OMV during adaptation (Desmurget et al., 1998, 2000). Nonetheless, these findings cannot eliminate the possibility that adaptive changes occur upstream from the cerebellum, e.g., in the cerebral cortex, but must travel through it to reach the saccade generating circuitry in the brainstem. In this scenario, CFN and OMV lesions block adaptation by preventing adapted signals from influencing saccades, not by stopping adaptation.

2. Smooth Pursuit

a. Pursuit Control

A substantial role for the OMV and CFN in smooth pursuit fits well with the finding that complete cerebellectomy in monkey abolishes pursuit (Westheimer and Blair, 1973). The OMV and CFN also receive pursuit-related input. Signals that theoretically could contribute to pursuit may reach the cerebellum from the FEF (MacAvoy et al., 1991, Keating, 1991, 1993), the middle temporal (MT), and medial superior temporal (MST) areas of the cerebral cortex (Newsome et al., 1985; Dürsteler et al., 1987; Dürsteler and Wurtz, 1988). FEF, MT, and MST project to the parts of the pontine nuclei (May and Anderson, 1986; Stanton et al., 1988) that project to the OMV (Yamada and Noda, 1987) and CFN (Noda et al., 1990).

The OMV, and its output from the CFN, play an important role in pursuit. Neurons in both the OMV (Suzuki et al., 1981) and CFN (Fuchs et al., 1994) respond vigorously during smooth pursuit. Electrical stimulation of the OMV increases pursuit velocity (Krauzlis and Miles, 1998). Further, OMV (Takagi et al., 2000) or CFN lesions (Robinson et al., 1997) impair pursuit.

b. Pursuit Adaptation

Eye acceleration at the start of pursuit adapts when the eyes repeatedly move faster or slower than a target that elicits pursuit (e.g., Kahlon and Lisberger, 1996). As we might expect from the OMV's involvement in pursuit, OMV ablation abolishes adaptation of pursuit (Takagi et al., 2000).

3. Vergence

The CFN and OMV also appear to be involved in vergence. Regions of the pontine nuclei that project to the OMV and CFN receive input from cortical regions that contain neurons that either respond during vergence, i.e., frontal eye field (FEF, Gamlin and Yoon, 2000), or respond to disparity and looming, two major cues for vergence, i.e., MT (Maunsell and Van Essen, 1983) and LIP (Gnadt and Mays, 1995). For example, neurons in the medial nucleus reticularis tegmenti pontis (NRTP) receive input from the FEF (Leichnitz et al., 1984), contain vergence-related neurons (Gamlin and Clarke, 1995), and project to both the OMV (Yamada and Noda, 1987) and CFN (Noda et al., 1990).

Many CFN neurons respond to convergence (Zhang and Gamlin, 1996) and electrical stimulation in the CFN elicits convergence (Murakami et al., 1991). Damage in either the OMV (Takagi et al., 2003) or CFN (Gamlin and Zhang, 1996) impairs vergence. The CFN projects directly (May et al., 1992) to the brainstem pre-motor region for vergence dorsal to the oculomotor nuclei (Zhang et al., 1992).

B. Lateral Cerebellum (Dorsal Paraflocculus)

1. Saccades

In addition to the CFN, another region of the cerebellar nuclei, the ventrolateral part of the posterior interpositus nucleus (VPIN) contains neurons that burst for nearly every saccade (Robinson et al., 1996). Bilateral VPIN lesions make saccades in all directions end above their targets, supporting the proposal that VPIN activity influences the vertical component of saccades (Robinson, 2000). The dorsal paraflocculus, a ventrolateral part of the cerebellar cortex (see Figure 1C) projects to the VPIN (Kralj-Hans et al., 2001, 2002). No experimental evidence yet documents the effect on saccades of ablating the dorsal paraflocculus, but data from the OMV lesions are consistent with the speculation that such lesions would make saccades end below their targets.

There are also saccade-related neurons in the cerebellar hemispheres, Crus I and II (Mano et al., 1991, 1996). We do not know their function, but pilot data indicate that unilateral ablation of the cerebellar cortex lateral to the vermis delays catch-up saccades during smooth pursuit (Ohki et al., 2003).

2. Smooth Pursuit

The firing rates of many VPIN neurons change in phase with eye velocity during smooth pursuit with larger vertical components (Robinson and Brettler, 1998). Currently, there are no data directly indicating how neurons in the dorsal paraflocculus respond during pursuit or how dorsal paraflocculus or VPIN lesions alter pursuit or pursuit adaptation. However, recent pilot data indicate that unilateral ablation of the hemispheric extension of lobule VII impairs adaptation of ipsiversive pursuit (Ohki et al., 2003).

3. Vergence

Like the CFN, the VPIN projects directly (May et al., 1992) to the brainstem pre-motor region for vergence dorsal to the oculomotor nuclei (Zhang et al., 1992). Many VPIN neurons respond during the far response, a combination of divergence and relaxing accommodation, but not during other eye movements. Electrical stimulation among vergence-related elicits divergence and relaxed accommodation (Zhang and Gamlin, 1998).

C. Vestibulocerebellum (Flocculus, Paraflocculus, Nodulus, and Uvula)

1. Flocculus and Ventral Paraflocculus

The flocculus and ventral paraflocculus help stabilize the eyes on an object in the visual environment. They do this by influencing the mechanisms that move the eyes in response to vestibular stimulation (the vestibuloocular reflex, VOR) and movement of large visual stimuli (optokinetic nystagmus, OKN) as well as movement of an object of interest (smooth pursuit). In addition, the flocculus and ventral paraflocculus help maintain the static position of the eye in the orbit (gaze holding).

Vestibular neurons recorded in monkey cerebellum originally thought to be in the flocculus are very likely to have been in both the flocculus and ventral paraflocculus. These two regions are adjacent to one another, and both receive large vestibular input (Gerrits and Voogd, 1989). Consequently, in the descriptions below we group the two regions and call them the flocculus/ventral paraflocculus. Also, when we describe data from lesions that do not differentiate between the dorsal and ventral paraflocculus we refer to simply the paraflocculus.

To perform its oculomotor functions, the flocculus/ventral paraflocculus receives inputs from structures with neurons carrying vestibular, visual, and oculomotor signals. The flocculus/ventral paraflocculus receives these signals from several sources, the vestibular nuclei, the brainstem gaze holding integrator in the nucleus prepositus hypoglossi (NPH), the inferior olive, which carries retinal slip signals and NRTP, dorsolateral pontine nucleus, and mesencephalic reticular formation which all carry eye movement and visual motion information. In addition, the flocculus/ventral paraflocculus also receives input from cells of the paramedian tracts carrying signals from all pre-oculomotor structures (Büttner-Ennever et al., 1989; Büttner-Ennever and Horn, 1997). The main outputs of flocculus/ventral paraflocculus are to the ipsilateral medial, superior, and y-group vestibular nuclei, structures critical for smooth pursuit, vestibulo-ocular reflex and optokinetic function.

The firing rate of Purkinje cells in the flocculus/ventral paraflocculus changes during rotation of the head, and this activity contributes to the vestibuloocular reflex by adjusting the timing of the compensatory eye movements (Waespe and Henn 1981; Stahl and Simpson 1995; De Zeeuw et al., 1995). In the monkey, however, floccular ablation does not affect the gain of the VOR (Zee et al., 1981; Lisberger et al., 1984) but rather the ability of the animal to adapt or modify that gain based on retinal error during head motion. Activity in flocculus/ventral paraflocculus Purkinje cells maintains the appropriate gain and phase of the vestibuloocular reflex by providing adaptive inputs to the brainstem vestibular nuclei (Lisberger et al., 1984). Discharge of Purkinje cells in the flocculus/ventral paraflocculus is also critical to the cancellation of the VOR in monkeys during viewing of objects that move with the head (Miles et al., 1980; Lisberger et al., 1984). Activity in flocculus/ventral paraflocculus Purkinje cells also modulates during smooth pursuit of visual targets with the eye and or head (Lisberger and Fuchs, 1978; Miles and Fuller, 1975).

In addition to stabilizing visual images the flocculus/ventral paraflocculus may have a function in vergence, though we currently know little about it. Nonetheless, there are vergence-related neurons there (Miles et al., 1980) and electrical stimulation of the flocculus, and probably the ventral paraflocculus, evokes movement of only one eye (Balaban and Watanabe, 1984).

2. Nodulus and Uvula

The uvula and nodulus receive inputs primarily from vestibular, pontine, and inferior olivary nuclei (Korte and Mugnaini, 1979; Brodal and Brodal, 1985; Barmack et al., 1993; Glickstein et al., 1994). Vestibular input is particularly prominent. For example, more than 70% of primary vestibular afferents in the rabbit project directly to the uvula and nodulus as mossy fibers (Barmack, 2003). The uvula and nodulus also receive climbing fiber input via a pathway from primary vestibular afferents to the ipsilateral parasolitary nucleus or the bilateral Y-group neurons. These structures project to inferior olive which, in turn, sends climbing fibers to the contralateral nodulus. Pontine inputs to the uvula and nodulus arise from areas implicated in pursuit control and visual motion processing (Robinson et al., 1984; Suzuki and Keller, 1982). The uvula and nodulus are, therefore, in a good position to integrate the vestibular and visual information that drives the reflexes that stabilize gaze during self movement.

The uvula and nodulus are participate in a particular type of stabilizing reflex, i.e., the nystagmus that persists after one of two types of stimulus, 1) the end of a sustained whole body rotation (post-rotary nystagmus, PRN), or 2) movement of a full field visual target (optokinetic after nystagmus, OKAN). The persistence of eye movement after vestibular or visual stimulation indicates that the brain stores a representation of the velocity of body rotation, so called "velocity storage." The stored representation outlasts the actual stimulation and drives compensatory eye movements after the stimulus has ended. Velocity storage seems maladaptive because it moves the eyes when there is no apparent need to do so. The velocity storage mechanism may, however, compensate for the dynamics of the cupula during very low frequency motion (Skavenski and Robinson, 1973). It could also allow for temporal integration of a pattern of stimulation across separate peripheral receptors (Raphan et al., 1979).

Whatever the purpose of velocity storage, intact humans and animals have the ability to suppress it or switch it off if they encounter sensory stimuli that indicate that the body is not, in fact, rotating as it did earlier. Such stimuli include a large head-fixed visual target or transient rapid head tilt in a novel direction. The former is known as suppression or cancellation of VOR. The latter reset of velocity storage is called "dumping" because the stored velocity information is dumped by the central nervous system in favor of this new information about body movement. When this new information becomes available, the eye movements driven by this stored signal stop. The ability to switch off velocity storage with visual suppression or head tilt is lost with lesions to the uvula and nodulus (Waespe et al., 1985).

The uvula and nodulus also participate in another feature of the PRN and OKAN. Normal humans and animals show habituation of PRN or OKAN after repeated constant velocity whole body rotation or whole visual field stimulation. That is, after repeated presentation of the same stimulus, the post-stimulus nystagmus persists for shorter and shorter durations; i.e., has a shorter time constant. Evidently the brain learns to reduce a response that has no practical significance under these stimulus conditions. This type of learning is eliminated by lesions to the uvula and nodulus (Waespe et al., 1985).

Another problem exhibited by some monkeys with experimental lesions of the uvula and nodulus is periodic alternating nystagmus (PAN, Waespe et al., 1985). PAN consists of horizontal nystagmus in one direction which slowly decreases in velocity and is replaced by nystagmus in the other direction which itself decreases and is replaced by nystagmus in the original direction. PAN is thought to reflect an unstable velocity storage mechanism.

Finally, in addition to contributing to velocity storage the uvula helps set the gain of smooth pursuit eye movements. A small proportion of uvula neurons respond during smooth tracking of a small target and lesions of the uvula on one side significantly increased eye velocity at the start of pursuit toward the opposite side (Heinen and Keller, 1996).

III. EYE MOVEMENTS IN PATIENTS WITH CONGENITAL AND ACQUIRED CEREBELLAR DISORDERS

In this section we describe the oculomotor symptoms of human patients with five types of cerebellar damage, A) agenesis of the vermis, B) hereditary ataxia, C) cerebellar mass lesions, D) paraneoplastic cerebellar degeneration, and E) Wallenberg Syndrome caused by an infarction in the lateral medulla. We will describe the damage inflicted by each of these problems, describe the signs of this damage, and explain how current data accounts for these signs.

A. Hindbrain Malformations With Complete or Partial Agenesis of the Cerebellar Vermis

A heterogeneous group of congenital disorders are linked by the presence of complete or partial agenesis of the cerebellar vermis. Members of this group share several clinical features, described below.

Recognition and classification of these posterior fossa malformations have been improved by three recent developments. First, our understanding of the genetic and molecular mechanisms that underlie cerebellar development has improved recently. Second, high resolution neuroimaging techniques now have the ability to non-invasively provide detailed information about cerebellar anatomy and function. For example, we can distinguish several of the disorders described below on the basis of neuroradiologic evidence of an anatomical anomaly called the "molar tooth sign" (MTS). MTS occurs when the combination of a thin pontomesencephalic isthmus, thickened superior cerebellar peduncles, which are oriented horizontally, and vermis aplasia/hypoplasia give the cerebellum the appearance of a molar tooth on axial MRI. Third, there is an increased appreciation that careful phenotyping is critical to the precise classification of these disorders and to guide the search for candidate gene defects.

1. Arnold-Chiari Malformations

The Chiari malformations, the most common hindbrain malformation, are characterized by partial or complete cerebellar protrusion through the foramen magnum. Based on the extent of cerebellar protrusion, concurrent displacement of the medulla, and presence of a myelomeningocoele (a protrusion of the spinal cord and meninges through a gap in the vertebral column), the Chiari malformations have been sub-classified into types I, II, and III. All three types are associated with abnormalities of eye movement due primarily to mechanical compression of the cerebellum and/or the brainstem. Some oculomotor abnormalities can be reproduced by lesions of the flocculus and paraflocculus in monkeys (Zee et al., 1981), but other deficits implicate brainstem damage or increased cerebrospinal fluid pressure (see below).

In type I Arnold-Chiari (AC) malformations, only the cerebellar tonsil (the posterior part of the intermediate cortex lateral to the uvula) is displaced caudally, the medulla oblongata is in normal position and usually there is no associated myelomeningocoele. Although hydrocephalus occurs in only approximately 10% of cases (Nohria and Oaks, 1990), up to 60% have syringomyelia, a condition in which a cerebrospinal fluid-filled cavity displaces the spinal cord parenchyma. In some cases, rostral extension of an asyrinx, an abnormal fluid-filled sac, can directly compromise brainstem oculomotor function. Patients are usually asymptomatic until adolescence or adulthood, when they report headaches, vertigo, hoarseness, occasionally apnea, and cerebellar signs such as ataxia (Nohria and Oakes, 1990; Pascual 1992).

In type II AC malformations the inferior vermis, portions of the IVth ventricle, and medulla oblongata are displaced caudally beyond the foramen magnum. The brainstem is elongated and thinned. This is the most common Chiari malformation and the most frequent cause of childhood hydrocephalus. A myelomeningocoele is usually present. Owing to more extensive anatomic involvement, patients with type II AC develop signs and symptoms in childhood, as opposed to the later onset of type I AC, including headache, neck pain, vertigo, nystagmus, dysphagia, spasticity, numbness, weakness, and pupilledema.

Type III AC malformation is a rare occurrence the features herniation of the entire cerebellum into a high occipital or cervical meningocele. It is usually associated with early demise or severe neurologic deficits in long-term survivors. Hydrocephalus is a constant finding.

The kind of eye movement abnormalities that have been reported in patients with AC malformations implicate involvement of the flocculus and paraflocculus. Downbeat nystagmus, worse on lateral gaze, is the most common (Halmagyi et al., 1983). Episodic downbeat nystagmus has been reported (Yee et al., 1984; Dones et al., 2003, Nohria and Oakes 1990). Downbeat nystagmus has been produced by lesions to the flocculus and paraflocculus in monkeys (Zee et al., 1981).

There is probably also a vergence deficit associated with AC malformations. In one study of a mixed population containing both patients with AC type I and unspecified cerebellar degeneration, subjects exhibited convergence bias and alignment abnormalities that varied with orbital position (Versino et al., 1996).

Cerebellar damage could contribute to the oculomotor symptoms of AC malformations in several ways. First, the vertical semicircular canal and otolith inputs to the brainstem are asymmetric. Normally, such asymmetries are compensated by the vestibulocerebellum. Lesions of this structure could unmask the asymmetry either in semicircular canal or in otolith input, leading to upward eye drift and down-beating nystagmus.

Second, decreased VOR gain (cited above) or abnormally increased VOR gain is often seen in AC malformation (Zee et al., 1976). These changes could be ascribed to the brainstem, not the cerebellum, because lesions of the vestibulocerebellum in animals fail to produce similar changes in gain (Zee et al., 1981). Nonetheless, the vestibulocerebellum is involved in the adaptation of VOR gain and probably its maintenance. Thus, abnormal VOR gain in patients could be a sign of prolonged failure of VOR adaptation.

Third, Versino et al. (1996) propose that the vergence deficits in their study result from damage to the flocculus because it contains vergence-related neurons (Miles et al., 1980) and can influence movements of only one eye (Balaban and Watanabe, 1984). In addition, damage to the OMV could also cause a vergence bias by reducing Purkinje cell inhibition of CFN activity. Increasing CFN activity is likely to increase vergence (Murakami et al., 1991).

Several other symptoms of AC malformations implicate the flocculus and paraflocculus. These include impaired pursuit and impaired visual suppression of VOR (Zee et al., 1976) as well as impaired OKN with slow buildup of slow phase eye velocity (Yee et al., 1979; Arnold et al., 1990; Zee et al., 1981). A shortened time constant for post-rotatory nystagmus, impaired tilt suppression of VOR (Korres et al., 2001), and periodic alternating nystagmus specifically indicate damage to the uvula and nodulus (Waespe et al., 1985).

Other oculomotor symptoms of AC malformations probably result from brainstem compression directly or through indirect pressure-effects from hydrocephalus, or both. These include acquired comitant esotropia (Biousse et al., 2000; Weeks and Hamed, 1999; Lewis et al., 1996), divergence paralysis (Lewis et al., 1996), and gaze-evoked (Albers and Ingles, 1993), rebound (Bondar et al., 1984), convergence (Mossman et al., 1990), and see-saw nystagmus (Zimmerman et al., 1986).

2. Dandy-Walker Syndrome

The Dandy-Walker malformation (DWM) is characterized by three morphological features: 1) complete or partial agenesis of the cerebellar vermis, 2) cystic dilation of the IVth ventricle, and 3) an enlarged posterior fossa with upward displacement of the tentorium cerebelli and torcula. The dimensions of the pontomesencephalic isthmus and interpeduncular fossa are normal and there is no molar tooth sign on axial MRI.

Altman et al. (1992) propose that the DWM results from an insult in the region of the lateral wall and floor of the primordial IVth ventricle from which the granule cells and Purkinje cell arise and then migrate into the cerebellar anlage (recall above). This failure of migration results in hypoplasia of the vermis, which should lead to oculomotor deficits. However, Leigh et al. (1992) report that patients demonstrate normal eye movements or only mild saccade dysmetria. The fact that DWM patients have normal, or nearly normal, eye movements indicates that a significant part of the OMV is spared. The only way to determine whether or not this is true is to rigorously identify what functional regions of the vermis remain in DWM patients, data that are not yet available.

Vermis hypoplasia associated with more extensive malformations of the posterior fossa (often included in the description of DWM) are associated with more significant oculomotor deficits. For example, we have recorded eye movements in one such patient in whom horizontal and vertical saccades were dysmetric and smooth pursuit and OKN gains were low. Dysmetric saccades and low pursuit gain are consistent with damage to the OMV or CFN but we cannot be sure that such damage is the only source of impaired pursuit. Damage to the vestibulocerebellum or brainstem structures could also impair pursuit.

3. Joubert Syndrome (JS)

JS is characterized by global developmental delay, hypotonia, ataxia, vestibular-related imbalance, and episodic hyperpnea or apnea. JS was the prototype for disorders characterized by neuroradiologic evidence of the "molar tooth sign." It is now recognized, however, that the MTS is not pathognomonic of Joubert syndrome because MTS also occurs in at least five additional syndromic disorders including Dekaban-Arima, Senior-Löken, COACH orofacial digital syndrome Type VI, and Malta syndrome (Dekban 1969; Maria et al., 1999; Gentile et al., 1996). In addition to vermis aplasia these patients can have evidence of Purkinje cell loss in the cerebellar cortex, fragmented dentate nuclei, and hypoplasia or dysplasia of inferior olivary nuclei, and hypoplasia of the pontomesencephalic reticular nuclei.

The majority of JS patients have significant oculomotor abnormalities. One qualitative study reported gaze-holding nystagmus, absent smooth pursuit, absent to OKN, slow hypometric saccades with long latency, and variable use of a head thrust to recenter the eyes from an extreme orbital position (Lambert et al., 1989).

These deficits reflect damage in both the cerebellum and brainstem. Gaze holding nystagmus results from lesions to the brainstem gaze holding integration centers in the nucleus prepositus hypoglossi and medial vestibular nucleus (Arnold et al., 1999), but also from lesions to the vestibulocerebellum (Robinson, 1974; Zee et al., 1981; Waespe et al., 1983; Godaux and Vanderkelen 1984). As discussed above, damage to the flocculus produces a failure of eccentric gaze holding. Absence of smooth pursuit in combination with a gaze holding deficit is also consistent with lesions to the vestibulocerebellum in monkeys. Recall, that pursuit pathways pass through the vestibulocerebellum. OKN abnormalities could have a similar etiology.

Slow saccades have been attributed to brainstem lesions because lesions of the oculomotor vermis in animals fail to produce dramatic changes in saccade velocity, whereas lesions of the paramedian pontine reticular formation do. However, cerebellar lesions, specifically CFN inactivation, can reduce saccade peak velocity (Robinson et al., 1993) and

TABLE 1 Clinical Features and Gene Products of Some Common Autosomal Dominant Hereditary Ataxias

Disease name	Gene	Product	Distinguishing clinical features
SCA 1	SCA 1	Ataxin-1	Pyramidal signs, peripheral neuropathy
SCA 2	SCA 2	Ataxin-2	Slow saccades, peripheral neuropathy, dementia
SCA 3	MJD	Machado-Joseph disease protein 1	Pyramidal and extra pyramidal signs, lid retraction, slow saccades
SCA 6	CACNA1A	Voltage-dependent P/Q type calcium channel alpha-1A subunit	Episodic ataxia
SCA 7	SCA 7	Ataxin-7	Visual loss with retinopathy
SCA 10	SCA 10	Ataxin-10	Seizures
SCA 17	TBP	Transcription initiation factor	Mental deterioration
DRPLA	DRPLA	Atrophin-1 related protein	Chorea seizures myoclonus
EA 1	KCNA 1	Voltage-gated potassium channel protein Kv 1.1	Myokimia, ataxia lasts seconds to minutes
EA 2	CACNA1A	Voltage dependent P/Q type calcium channel alpha-1A subunit	Nystagmus, ataxia lasts minutes to hours
	CACNB4	Dihydropyridine-sensitive L-type, calcium channel beta-4 subunit	

SCA, spinocerebellar ataxia; DRPLA, dentatorubropallidoluysian atrophy; EA1, episodic ataxia Type I; EA2, episodic ataxia Type II.

could contribute to slowed saccades in this and other cerebellar disorders.

In a qualitative assessment of eye movements in JS patients, Maria et al. (1997) observed that the VOR, assessed by the head thrust test, was normal but that there was no visual cancellation of VOR. This observation is consistent with animal experiments in which lesions of the vestibulocerebellum produce deficits in cancellation without changes in VOR gain (Zee et al., 1981).

Comitant strabismus, a manifestation of a vergence error, is common in JB patients. Since up to 19% of these patients can have visual loss from a retinal dystrophy the strabismus could have a cerebellar, brainstem, or visual sensory etiology.

4. Isolated Aplasia

Isolated aplasia of the cerebellar vermis can occur on a familial basis. The major clinical features are normal intelligence, delayed achievement of motor milestones, truncal ataxia and nystagmus (gaze holding and positional). Neuroimaging studies reveal focal loss of portions of the anterior vermis. Gross abnormalities of eye movements, excluding nystagmus, are not described (Fenichel et al., 1989; Tomiwa, 1987). This is consistent with sparing of the more posterior oculomotor vermis.

B. Hereditary Ataxia

Distinct from cerebellar aplasia, the hereditary ataxias are a heterogeneous group of genetic disorders characterized by truncal ataxia and incoordination of hands, speech and eye movements. Cerebellar atrophy is a frequent sequela. The hereditary ataxias are categorized by mode of inheritance (autosomal dominant, autosomal recessive, x-linked, mitochondrial), gene defect, or chromosomal locus.

1. Autosomal Dominant Ataxias

The autosomal dominant cerebellar ataxias for which there is a known genetic basis include sixteen types of spinocerebellar ataxia (SCA), two episodic ataxias (EA1, EA2), one complex form (DRPLA), and one spastic ataxia (HSA). Nine of the sixteen SCA have trinucleotide repeat expansions within the coding sequence of their causative genes. Trinucleotide repeats are normal up to a gene specific number beyond which they are abnormal and associated with disease. Expansion in the number of trinucleotide repeats in some cases leads to earlier onset and increasing severity of disease, a phenomenon referred to as anticipation. In other cases, the number of trinucleotide repeats remains constant or decreases and the age of onset and clinical findings overlap for different generations. Relevant clinical features of the more common autosomal dominant hereditary ataxias for which the gene product has been identified are shown in table 1.

Many of these disorders are also associated with characteristic eye movement anomalies. Table 2 summarizes the type and severity of horizontal eye movement abnormalities for SCA1, SCA2, SCA3 and SCA6 (Klostermann et al., 1997; Büttner et al., 1998; Takeichi et al., 2000). Prior to specific genotyping of the autosomal dominant ataxias, eye

TABLE 2 Type and Degree of Horizontal Eye Movement Abnormalities with Different SCA Syndromes

Disorder	Saccadic velocity	Dysmetria	Pursuit gain	OKN gain	VOR gain	VOR cancellation
SCA 1	n/A+	n/A++	n/A+	n/A++	N	n/A++
SCA 2	A++/A+++	N	n/A+	N	N	n/A+
SCA 3	N	A+++	n/A+++	n/A+++	n/A++	n/A+
SCA 6	N	n/A++	A++/A+++	A++/A+++	N	n/A+++[1,2]

N indicates normal; n, normal in some patients; A, abnormal where + is mildly abnormal, ++ moderately abnormal and +++ severely abnormal.
[1] Normal VOR cancellation data of Takeichi et al.
[2] Abnormal VOR cancellation data of Buttner et al.

movement studies were comprised of a heterogeneous population of SCA1, SCA2, and SCA3 patients (Baloh et al., 1986; Moschner et al., 1994; Rabiah et al., 1997).

a. *SCA1* patients account for 9% of ataxia patients (Schols et al., 1997). The major damage in the cerebellum is a loss of Purkinje cells (Genis et al., 1995). SCA1 patients exhibit saccade overshoot, saccade slowing, reduced VOR, OKN, and pursuit gain (Rivaud-Pechoux et al., 1998; Burk et al., 1999). Saccade overshoot could result from damage to the CFN (Robinson et al., 1993). Large OMV lesions produce saccade undershoot, not overshoot (Takagi et al., 1998; Barash et al., 1999), so it is very unlikely that extensive damage to the OMV causes saccade hypermetria. Saccade overshoot could, however, be a consequence of reduced conduction in parallel fibers in the OMV (see the proposed explanation below for spinocerebellar ataxia with saccadic intrusions, SCA-SI). Consistent with the possibility that saccade overshoot is a consequence of impaired axon conduction is evidence that motor conduction is impaired in SCA1 patients (Schols et al., 1997).

Reduced VOR gain could be the result of extra-cerebellar damage but, as we point out for the low VOR gain of AC patients, could also result from damage to the vestibulocerebellum by impairing VOR adaptation over a long time. Reduced pursuit gain could result from damage to the OMV (Takagi et al., 2000), CFN (Robinson et al., 1997), or flocculus and paraflocculus (Zee et al., 1981). Whatever damage impairs pursuit is likely to also impair OKN because the pathways for pursuit and OKN overlap extensively.

b. *SCA2* patients account for 10% of ataxia patients (Schols et al., 1997). They exhibit reduced saccade velocities, pursuit gain, and OKN gain (Burk et al., 1996, 1999; Rivaud-Pechoux et al., 1998). As with SCA1, brainstem damage or damage to the OMV and/or CFN could account for saccade slowing. Damage to the OMV, CFN, and/or the flocculus/ventral paraflocculus could reduce pursuit, and also OKN, gain. It is not currently clear why SCA1 results in saccade overshoot while SCA2 causes saccade undershoot.

c. *SCA3* (*Machado-Joseph disease*) patients account for 42% of ataxia patients (Schols et al., 1997). SCA3 is characterized by ataxia in 100% of patients, decreased vibration sense (55% of patients), and a positive Babinski sign (46% of patients). The percentage of patients with pyramidal signs, dystonia, Parkinsonian features, and swallowing and sphincter difficulties increases with age (Durr et al., 1996b; Jardim et al., 2001).

Several eye movement deficits are associated with SCA3. A vertical gaze paresis is the initial oculomotor sign followed by progressive limitations of horizontal gaze. Lid retraction can lead to eye protrusion. Neuropathologic studies reveal multiple levels of brain involvement that can account for the ophthalmoplegia. Severe neuronal loss in the substantia nigra, subthalamic nucleus, and globus pallidus may be associated with impaired initiation of voluntary conjugate eye movements. In end stage disease, severe neuronal loss in the abducens nuclei is observed, consistent with the progressive loss of horizontal gaze.

Despite the clear involvement of extra-cerebellar structures, the diplopia exhibited by many SCA3 patients (Schols et al., 1997) results substantially from a vergence bias, not ophthalmoplegia (Ohyagi et al., 2000). SCA3 patients also show saccade hypometria and reduced pursuit and OKN gain as well as reduced VOR gain (Rivaud-Pechoux et al., 1998; Burk et al., 1999). The vergence bias could result from OMV damage reducing inhibition on, and thereby increasing, the firing rate of CFN neurons. As with other SCAs, reduced pursuit and, thus, OKN gain could be a consequence of OMV or CFN damage and reduced VOR gain could result from extra-cerebellar damage or, possibly, damage to the flocculus/ventral paraflocculus.

Damage to an extra-cerebellar structure may impair OMV function indirectly in SCA3. SCA3 is often associated with severe neuronal loss in the lateral reticular nucleus (LRN). LRN receives inputs from the vestibular nuclei and premotor cortical areas responsible for vertical eye movements (Carleton and Carpenter, 1984, Rub et al., 2002). Although the cerebellum shows only a mild decrease in the number of Purkinje cells, neuronal cell loss in the LRN may remove a critical input to the OMV.

d. *SCA6* patients account for 22% of ataxia patients (Schols et al., 1997). They show a pure cerebellar atrophy

TABLE 3 Summary of the Eye Movement Deficits in Patients with Several Types of Cerebellar Damage

	Reported deficits									
Disorder	**Saccade gain**	**Saccade slowing**	**Pursuit**	**OKN**	**VOR gain**	**VOR cancellation**	**Nystagmus**	**Velocity storage**	**Vergence**	**Saccadic intrusions**
Hindbrain Malformations										
Arnold-Chiari Malformation			X	X	X	X	X	X	X	
Dandy-Walker Malformation	X									
Dandy-Walker Malformation Plus	X		X	X						
Joubert Syndrome	X	X	X	X		X	X		X	
Isolated Vermis Aplasia							X			
Hereditary Ataxia										
Autosomal Dominant Ataxias[1]	X	X	X	X	X	X	X			
Autosomal Recessive Ataxias										
Friedreich Ataxia	X		X	X	X					X
Ataxia w/oculomotor apraxia	X	X	X	X						
Ataxia-Telangiectasia	X	X	X	X		X			X	X
SCASI	X									
Cerebellar Mass Lesions	X		X	X	X		X		X	X
Paraneoplastic Cerebellar Degeneration	X						X			
Wallenberg syndrome	X									

Plus = additional malformations.
[1] see table 2.

with no evidence of damage to other parts of the CNS (Schols et al., 1997; Sasaki et al., 1998). SCA6 is associated with normal saccade velocities and VOR gain but there are severe reductions of smooth pursuit and OKN gain, and impaired VOR cancellation (Büttner et al., 1998; Takeichi et al., 2000). These deficits are likely to result from a reduction in pursuit mechanisms associated with damage to the OMV, CFN, and/or the flocculus/ventral paraflocculus.

2. Autosomal Recessive Ataxias

Ataxia is a manifestation of numerous autosomal recessive disorders. The following discussion summarizes the relevant features of the most common types with special emphasis on those with prominent ocular motor findings. Each of these oculomotor deficits can be attributed to degenerative lesions in different parts of the cerebellum.

a. Friedreich Ataxia (FA)

FA is characterized by a slowly progressive ataxia with onset usually before 25 years. FA is associated with hyporeflexia, positive Babinski sign, and loss of position and vibration senses. Approximately 25% of FA patients have a later onset with retention of deep tendon reflexes and slower progression of ataxia (Durr et al., 1996a). Almost all FA patients have a GAA triplet-repeat expansion in the FA gene which is involved in the maintenance of iron sulfur clusters within mitochondria. This repeat leads to progressive changes in oxidative metabolism which selectively compromises cells with high metabolic activity such as Purkinje cells.

Patients with FA do not usually notice difficulties with eye tracking. Head thrusts, which are a typical compensation for poor saccade accuracy or saccade initiation deficits, are not observed. Nonetheless, quantitative eye movement studies reveal significant abnormalities. Saccades are often dysmetric with abnormally high proportions of both overshooting and undershooting saccades (Moschner et al., 1994). In addition, one of the most prominent signs is fixation instability with frequent intrusion of square-wave jerks and paroxysms of ocular flutter (Spieker et al., 1995; Rabiah et al., 1997). The square wave jerks could result from damage to oculomotor structures outside the cerebellum as they have been reported in experiments that inactivate the frontal eye fields, superior colliculus, and the mesencephalic reticular formation in animals. On the other hand the superior colliculus and mesencephalic reticular formation are target sites for cerebellar output. It is possible that clinical syndromes affecting the cerebellum, including FA, produce such saccadic intrusions. Unfortunately, we cannot comment on ocular flutter because there is currently no animal model for this symptom.

The saccade dysmetria in FA is consistent with deficits in saccade processing in the OMV. Saccade velocities are approximately normal. Smooth pursuit and slow phase OKN show mild reductions in gain although tracking gain (eye + head) is normal. Though there is reduced VOR gain there is also clear velocity dumping evident in reduction of post-rotatory nystagmus by head tilt or suppression of VOR by visual fixation (Rabiah et al., 1997; Wessel et al., 1998). Since vestibular suppression and dumping are intact, it is unlikely that vestibular and pursuit problems in FA patients reflect extensive damage to the uvula and nodulus. These symptoms could originate with damage to the OMV or to the vestibular nuclei. In the subset of patients with optic atrophy (about 15%), reduced visual acuity compounds the oculomotor deficits.

b. Ataxia with Oculomotor Apraxia 1 (AOA1)

AOA1 is characterized by early-onset ataxia (mean five years), areflexia followed by oculomotor apraxia and progressive peripheral motor neuropathy leading to quadriplegia. Brain MRI shows cerebellar atrophy (Aicardi 1988; Barbot 2001; Moreira 2001). This newly recognized disorder is the most frequent cause of autosomal recessive ataxia in Japan. The mutated gene encodes a histidine triad/Zn-finger protein implicated in brain-specific DNA repair (Date et al., 2001; Moreira et al., 2001). Again, accumulated errors in the sequence of brain specific DNA are thought to compromise the activity of neurons within the cerebellum and brainstem over time.

Qualitative assessment of the eye and head movements in patients with AOA1 reveal slow hypometric saccades with long latencies, compensatory head thrusts, reduced OKN gain with decreased fast phase frequency, and reduced eye tracking gain (Aicardi et al., 1988). Since the saccades are slowed, brainstem involvement has been suspected but, as we observe above, slow saccades could also reflect, at least in part, damage to the OMV or CFN. When the head is fixed, some subjects show a complete inability to generate voluntary conjugate eye movements (Barbot et al., 2001). In one report, complete cerebellectomy did not abolish saccades (Westheimer and Blair, 1973). Although this observation needs to be confirmed, it suggests that loss of conjugate eye movements is not simply a consequence of cerebellar damage.

c. Ataxia-Telangiectasia (A-T)

A-T is a multi-system disease characterized by progressive cerebellar ataxia with onset between one and four years of age, T- and B-cell immune deficiency with frequent infections, conjunctival telangiectasias, choreoathetosis, and increased risk of cancer. The gene product mutated in A-T (ATM) is related to phosphatidylinositol 3-Kinase, a protein involved in repair of DNA damage by radiation. Following radiation damage, ATM phosphorylates CHK2 (check point Kinase) that delays the cell cycle in G_1, S, or G_2 phases and promotes apoptosis by phosphorylation of p53.

Eye movement abnormalities are a prominent feature of A-T. The most distinctive is head free gaze shifts in which gaze is initiated by a head thrust and the amplitude of the head movement approximates the size of the target step. To correct for ocular counter-rotation evoked by the VOR and the paucity of corrective fast-phases, the subject uses a staircase of hypometric saccades to acquire the target while now stabilizing the head (Lewis et al., 1999). The remaining acquired ocular motor deficits are similar to those described for congenital ocular motor apraxia. In brief, gaze holding is punctuated by saccadic intrusions, square wave jerks, and ocular flutter; Saccades are hypometric, latencies are long, and peak velocities are not linearly correlated with amplitudes. There is also a reduced number of vestibular and OKN quick phases. The gains of slow-phase OKN and smooth pursuit are reduced, convergence amplitudes are low, and there is an inability to visually suppress the VOR (Lewis et al., 1999). Reduced saccade, pursuit, and OKN gain as well as slow saccades could all originate with cerebellar damage. In support of a cerebellar origin for these deficits, neuropathologic studies show vermis atrophy, gliosis of the cerebellar nuclei and degeneration of the inferior olive.

d. Spinocerebellar Ataxia with Saccadic Intrusions (SCA-SI)

SCA-SI is a recently recognized ataxia (Schwartz et al., 2003). Patients with SCA-SI exhibit, in addition to cerebellar signs, a distinctive combination of two other signs. 1) They have a peripheral neuropathy resulting in decreased pain and temperature sensation in their lower legs, and 2) they exhibit overshooting horizontal saccades. Schwartz et al. propose that the link between these two seemingly unrelated symptoms is that the mutation in these patients impairs axon conduction, particularly in small fibers. In their proposal, this defect impairs pain sensation carried by the long, thin axons from the lower legs. It also interferes with conduction in parallel fibers in the OMV. In this proposal signals carried in parallel fibers contribute to the late CFN bursts that decelerate saccades (see the end of section A1a above). Thus, impairing OMV parallel fiber conduction reduces the decelerating CFN bursts and causes saccades to overshoot. This hypothesis remains to be tested experimentally.

C. Cerebellar Mass Lesions

Brain tumors constitute the largest group of solid neoplasms and 20% of all tumors in childhood (Pollack, 1994). Approximately 40% of these are primitive neuroectodermal tumors (medulloblastoma) or cerebellar astrocytomas. The oculomotor deficits vary from mild to severe depending upon the location and extent of the tumor, and the presence of brainstem compression or obstructive hydrocephalus. In some cases the pattern of oculomotor abnormalities helps to localize tumor involvement to the cerebellar vermis, cerebellar nuclei, or vestibulocerebellum. For example, the concurrence of positional nystagmus, inability to visually suppress postrotational VOR or dump OKAN eye velocity by tilting the head, implicates the nodulus and uvula.

We have evaluated children with cerebellar tumors and find that most exhibit overlapping patterns of eye movement abnormalities consistent with combined involvement of all eye movement-related midline cerebellar structures, i.e., the OMV, uvula, and nodulus. These children usually have dysmetric saccades and low smooth pursuit gain resulting in normal or subnormal eye tracking composed of a combination of saccades and pursuit. OKN is in the appropriate direction in these patients but the gain becomes abnormally low at stimulus velocities above 30°/s. VOR gain is normal to reduced. Gaze holding nystagmus in the dark and light is common.

We do not find oculomotor deficits with tumors confined to the cerebellar hemispheres. However, tumors that do not directly damage the eye movement-related parts of the cerebellum can impair eye movements. Compression of the brainstem by tumor invasion or by increased intracranial pressure can lead to gaze evoked, upbeat or downbeat nystagmus, skew deviation, and III, IV and VI cranial neuropathies. Compression of the divergence region in the mesencephalic reticular formation (Mays, 1984) or disruption of its outputs can cause divergence insufficiency in which there is an esotropia at distance, normal alignment or a small esodeviation at near, and complete abduction bilaterally (Kirkham et al., 1972; Mays et al., 1986).

D. Paraneoplastic Cerebellar Degeneration (PCD)

Paraneoplastic cerebellar degeneration is due to a remote effect of an underlying malignancy, either small-cell lung cancer, or carcinoma of the breast or ovary (Brain and Wilkinson, 1965; Dalmau and Posner, 1999). The onset of PCD is acute (days) or subacute (weeks) and often precedes the detection of the tumor. Most PCD patients with or without antineuronal antibodies demonstrate marked to severe Purkinje cell loss (Mason et al., 1997). PCD usually progresses to cerebellar atrophy and fail to respond to treatment (Brain and Wilkinson 1965; Mason et al., 1997).

Clinical findings for PCD at presentation include truncal and appendicular ataxia, dysarthria, and nystagmus (often down-beating). Saccade adaptation is also impaired in patients with PCD (Coesmans et al., 2003). Leigh and Zee (1999) suggest that in PCD it is a result of asymmetric loss of inhibitory projections from the Purkinje cells to the vesibular nuclei. As saccade adaptation is linked to the OMV, its impairment in PCD patients may result from the loss of Purkinje cells in this part of the cerebellar cortex. It may also result from antibodies attacking mGluR1 receptors in the cerebellum that are linked to the ability to adapt saccades (Coesmans et al., 2003).

E. Wallenberg Syndrome

Wallenberg syndrome, which accounts for ~2% of hospital admissions for acute stroke (Norrving and Cronqvist, 1991), results from an infarction in their lateral medulla dorsal to the inferior olive. Patients with Wallenberg syndrome exhibit several symptoms including falling to the side of the lesions and deflection of reaching toward the side of the lesions. They also exhibit oculomotor signs extremely similar to those of monkeys with one CFN inactivated (Robinson et al., 1993). Horizontal saccades toward the side of the infarction overshoot. Those to the opposite side undershoot. Saccades to vertical targets deflect toward the side of the stroke. In addition, the ability of these patients to adapt their saccades is impaired (Waespe and Wichmann, 1992). Also, like monkeys with a unilateral CFN inactivation, Wallenberg patients exhibit impaired pursuit toward the side of the stroke (Leigh and Zee, 1999).

The similarities between the signs of Wallenberg syndrome and CFN inactivation has prompted several authors (Robinson et al., 1993; Helmchen et al., 1994; Straube et al., 1994) to postulate that the stroke interrupts climbing fibers bound for the ipsilateral OMV. This slight modification of a proposal made originally by Waespe and Wichmann 1990, rests on the observation that climbing fiber interruption dramatically increases Purkinje cell activity (Benedetti et al., 1984; Demer et al., 1985). Increased Purkinje cell activity would cause an abnormally strong inhibition of activity in the cerebellar nuclei, including the CFN, thus mimicking the effects of experimental CFN inactivation.

IV. SUMMARY

Current understanding of cerebellar oculomotor function provides explanations for the eye movement deficits exhibited by patients with a variety of cerebellar disease. A summary of the eye movement deficits in such patients is displayed in Table 3 below. Experimental lesions in monkeys indicate that horizontal saccades are influenced primarily by the oculomotor vermis (OMV) and the part of the cerebellar nuclei to which it projects, the caudal fastigial nucleus (CFN). CFN damage can cause saccade slowing but this symptom is usually interpreted as a sign of extracerebellar damage because of the dramatic nature of the slowing in most patients. Horizontal pursuit is influenced by the OMV and CFN and also the flocculus/ventral paraflocculus. Vertical saccades and pursuit are influenced by the dorsal paraflocculus and the region of the cerebellar nuclei to which it projects, the ventrolateral posterior interpositus nucleus (VPIN). Vertical saccades and pursuit have not been widely tested yet in cerebellar patients. Thus, we cannot currently describe the potential role of damage to the dorsal paraflocculus and VPIN in the oculomotor problems caused by cerebellar damage. Though some evidence indicates that the flocculus may participate in vergence movements there is ample evidence that convergence is aided by CFN output and divergence is aided by VPIN output. VOR is influenced by the flocculus. Changes in the gain of the VOR are typically ascribed to brainstem mechanisms because primate models fail to produce such changes. Storage of the vestibular or visual velocity signals that produce post-rotary nystagmus (PRN) and optokinetic after nystagmus (OKAN) depends on the uvula and nodulus.

References

Ackerman, S.L., L.P. Kozak, S.A. Przyborski, L.A. Rund, B.B. Boyer, and B.B. Knowles. 1997. The mouse rostral cerebellar malformation gene encodes an UNC-5-like protein. *Nature* **386**:838–842.

Aicardi, J., C. Barbosa, E. Andermann, F. Andermann, R. Morcos, Q. Ghanem, Y. Fukuyama, Y. Awaya, and P. Moe. 1988. Ataxia-ocular motor apraxia: a syndrome mimicking ataxia-telangiectasia. *Ann Neurol* **24**: 497–502.

Aizenman, C.D., and D.J. Linden. 1999. Regulation of the rebound depolarization and spontaneous firing patterns of deep nuclear neurons in slices of rat cerebellum. *J Neurophysiol* **82**:1697–1709.

Albers, F.W., and K.J. Ingels. 1993. Otoneurological manifestations in Chiari-I malformation. *J Laryngol Otol* **107**:441–443.

Altman, N.R., T.P. Naidich, and B.H. Braffman. 1992. Posterior fossa malformations. *Am J Neuroradiology* **13**:691–724.

Arnold, A.C., R.W. Baloh, R.D. Yee, and R.S. Hepler. 1990. Internuclear ophthalmoplegia in the Chiari type II malformation. *Neurology* **40**: 1850–1854.

Arnold, D.B., D.A. Robinson, and R.J. Leigh. 1999. Nystagmus induced by pharmacological inactivation of the brainstem ocular motor integrator in monkey. *Vision Res* **39**:4286–4295.

Balaban, C.D., and E. Watanabe. 1984. Functional representation of eye movements in the flocculus of monkeys (Macaca fuscata). *Neurosci Lett* **49**:199–205.

Baloh, R.W., R.D. Yee, and V. Honrubia. 1986. Late cortical cerebellar atrophy. Clinical and oculographic features. *Brain* **109**:159–180.

Barash, S., A. Melikyan, A. Sivakov, M. Zhang, M. Glickstein, and P. Thier. 1999. Saccadic dysmetria and adaptation after lesions of the cerebellar cortex. *J Neurosci* **19**:10931–10939.

Barbot, C., P. Coutinho, R. Chorao, C. Ferreira, J. Barros, I. Fineza, K. Dias, J. Monteiro, A. Guimaraes, P. Mendonca, M. do Ceu Moreira, and J. Sequeiros. 2001. Recessive ataxia with ocular apraxia: review of 22 Portuguese patients. *Arch Neurol* **58**:201–205.

Barmack, N.H. 2003. Central vestibular system: vestibular nuclei and posterior cerebellum. *Brain Res Bull* **60**.511–541.

Barmack, N.H., R.W. Baughman, P. Errico, and H. Shojaku. 1993. Vestibular primary afferent projection to the cerebellum of the rabbit. *J Comp Neurol* **327**:521–534.

Benedetti, F., P.G. Montarolo, and S. Rabacchi. 1984. Inferior olive lesion induces long-lasting functional modification in the Purkinje cells. *Exp Brain Res* **55**:368–371.

Ben-Arie, N., H.J. Bellen, D.L. Armstrong, A.E. McCall, P.R. Gordadze, Q. Guo, M.M. Matzuk, and H.Y. Zoghbi. 1997. Math1 is essential for genesis of cerebellar granule neurons. *Nature* **390**:169–172.

Biousse, V., N.J. Newman, S.H. Petermann, and S.R. Lambert. 2000. Isolated comitant esotropia and Chiari I malformation. *Am J Ophthalmol* **130**:216–220.

Bondar, R.L., A.J. Sharpe, and A.J. Lewis. 1984. Rebound nystagmus in olivocerebellar atrophy: a clinicopathological correlation. *Ann Neurol* **15**:474–477.

Brain, W.R., and M. Wilkinson. 1965. Subacute cerebellar degeneration associated with neoplasms. *Brain* **88**, 465–478.

Braitenberg, V., and R.P. Atwood. 1958. Morphological observations on the cerebellar cortex. *J Comp Neurol* **109**:1–33.

Brettler, S.C., A.F. Fuchs, and L. Ling. 2003. Discharge patterns of cerebellar output neurons in the caudal fastigial nucleus during head-free gaze shifts in primates. *Ann NY Acad Sci* **1004**:61–68.

Brodal, A., and P. Brodal. 1985. Observations on the secondary vestibulocerebellar projections in the macaque monkey. *Exp Brain Res* **58**:62–74.

Burk, K., M. Abele, M. Fetter, J. Dichgans, M. Skalej, F. Laccone, O. Didierjean, A. Brice, and T. Klockgether. 1996. Autosomal dominant cerebellar ataxia type I clinical features and MRI in families with SCA1, SCA2 and SCA3. *Brain* **119**:1497–1505.

Burk, K., M. Fetter, M. Abele, F. Laccone, A. Brice, J. Dichgans, and T. Klockgether. 1999. Autosomal dominant cerebellar ataxia type I: oculomotor abnormalities in families with SCA1, SCA2, and SCA3. *J Neurol* **246**:789–797.

Büttner, N., D. Geschwind, J.C. Jen, S. Perlman, S.M. Pulst, and R.W. Baloh. 1998. Oculomotor phenotypes in autosomal dominant ataxias. *Arch Neurol* **55**:1353–1357.

Büttner-Ennever, J.A., and A.K. Horn. 1997. Anatomical substrates of oculomotor control. *Curr Opin Neurobiol* **7**:872–879.

Büttner-Ennever, J.A., A.K. Horn, and K. Schmidtke. 1989. Cell groups of the medial longitudinal fasciculus and paramedian tracts. *Rev Neurol (Paris)* **145**:533–539.

Carleton, S.C., and M.B. Carpenter. 1984. Distribution of primary vestibular fibers in the brainstem and cerebellum of the monkey. *Brain Res* **294**:281–298.

Coesmans, M., P.A. Smitt, D.J. Linden, R. Shigemoto, T. Hirano, Y. Yamakawa, A.M. van Alphen, C. Luo, J.N. van der Geest, J.M. Kros, C.A. Gaillard, M.A. Frens, and C.I. de Zeeuw. 2003. Mechanisms underlying cerebellar motor deficits due to mGluR1-autoantibodies. *Ann Neurol* **53**:325–336.

Dalmau, J.O., and J.B. Posner. 1999. Paraneoplastic syndromes. *Arch Neurol* **56**:405–408.

D'Arcangelo, G., G.G. Miao, S.C. Chen, H.D. Soares, J.I. Morgan, and T. Curran. 1995. A protein related to extracellular matrix proteins deleted in the mouse mutant reeler. *Nature* **374**:719–723.

Date, H., O. Onodera, H. Tanaka, K. Iwabuchi, K. Uekawa, S. Igarashi, R. Koike, T. Hiroi, T. Yuasa, Y. Awaya, T. Sakai, T. Takahashi, H. Nagatomo, Y. Sekijima, I. Kawachi, Y. Takiyama, M. Nishizawa, N. Fukuhara, K. Saito, S. Sugano, and S. Tsuji. 2001. Early-onset ataxia with ocular motor apraxia and hypoalbuminemia is caused by mutations in a new HIT superfamily gene. *Nat Genet* **29**:184–188.

Dekaban, A.S. 1969. Hereditary syndrome of congenital retinal blindness (Leber) polycystic kidneys and maldevelopment of the brain. *Am J Ophthalmol* **68**:1029–1037.

Demer J.L., D.A. Echelman, and D.A. Robinson. 1985. Effects of electrical stimulation and reversible lesions of the olivocerebellar pathway on Purkinje cell activity in the flocculus of the cat. *Brain Res* **346**:22–31.

Desmurget, M., D. Pelisson, J.S. Grethe, G.E. Alexander, C. Urquizar, C. Prablanc, and S.T. Grafton. 2000. Functional adaptation of reactive saccades in humans: a PET study. *Exp Brain Res* **132**:243–259.

Desmurget, M., D. Pelisson, C. Urquizar, C. Prablanc, G.E. Alexander, and S.T. Grafton. 1998. Functional anatomy of saccadic adaptation in humans. *Nat Neurosci* **1**:524–248.

De Zeeuw, C.I., D.R. Wylie, J.S. Stahl, and J.I. Simpson. 1995. Phase relations of Purkinje cells in the rabbit flocculus during compensatory eye movements. *J Neurophysiol* **74**:2051–2064.

Dones, J., O. De Jesus, C.B. Colen, M.M. Toledo, and M. Delgado. 2003. Clinical outcomes in patients with Chiari I malformation: a review of 27 cases. *Surg Neurol* **60**:142–147.

Durr, A., M. Cossee, Y. Agid, V. Campuzano, C. Mignard, C. Penet, J.L. Mandel, A. Brice, and M. Koenig. 1996a. Clinical and genetic abnormalities in patients with Friedreich's ataxia. *New Engl J Med* **335**:1169–1175.

Durr, A., G. Stevanin, G. Cancel, C. Duyckaerts, N. Abbas, O. Didierjean, H. Chneiweiss, A. Benomar, O. Lyon-Caen, J. Julien, M. Serdaru, C. Penet, Y. Agid, and A. Brice. 1996b. Spinocerebellar ataxia 3 and Machado-Joseph disease: clinical, molecular, and neuropathological features. *Ann Neurol* **39**:490–499.

Dürsteller, M.R., and R.H. Wurtz. 1988. Pursuit and optokinetic deficits following chemical lesions of cortical areas MT and MST. *J Neurophysiol* **60**:940–965.

Dürsteller, M.R., R.H. Wurtz, and W.T. Newsome. 1987. Directional pursuit deficits following lesions of the foveal representation within the superior temporal sulcus of the macaque monkey. *J Neurophysiol* **60**: 940–965.

Fenichel, G.M., and J.A. Phillips. 1989. Familial aplasia of the cerebellar vermis. *Arch Neurol* **46**:582–583.

Favor, J., R. Sandulache, A. Neuhauser-Klaus, W. Pretsch, B. Chatterjee, E. Senft, W. Wurst, V. Blanquet, P. Grimes, R. Sporle, and K. Schughart. 1996. The mouse Pax2(1Neu) mutation is identical to a human PAX2 mutation in a family with renal-coloboma syndrome and results in developmental defects of the brain, ear, eye, and kidney. *Proc Natl Acad Sci U S A* **93**:13870–13875.

Feddersen, R.M., R. Ehlenfeldt, W.S. Yunis, H.B. Clark, and H.T. Orr. 1992. Disrupted cerebellar cortical development and progressive degeneration of Purkinje cells in SV40 T antigen transgenic mice. *Neuron* **9**:955–966.

Fuchs, A.F., F.R. Robinson, and A. Straube. 1993. Role of the caudal fastigial nucleus in saccade generation. I. Neuronal discharge patterns. *J Neurophysiol* **70**:1723–1740.

Fuchs, A.F., F.R. Robinson, and A. Straube. 1994. Participation of the caudal fastigial nucleus in smooth pursuit eye movements I. Neuronal activity. *J Neurophysiol* **72**:2714–2728.

Fujikado, T., and H. Noda. 1987. Saccadic eye movements evoked by microstimulation of lobule VII of the cerebellar vermis of macaque monkeys. *J Physiol* **394**:573–594.

Gamlin, P.D., and R.J. Clarke. 1995. Single-unit activity in the primate nucleus reticularis tegmenti pontis related to vergence and ocular accommodation. *J Neurophysiol* **73**:2115–2119.

Gamlin, P.D., and K. Yoon. 2000. An area for vergence eye movement in primate frontal cortex. *Nature* **407**:1003–1007.

Gamlin, P.D.R., and H.Y. Zhang. 1996. Effects of muscimol blockade of the posterior fastigial nucleus on vergence and ocular accommodation in the primate. *Society for Neuroscience Abstracts* **22**:2034.

Genis D., T. Matilla, V. Volpini, J. Rosell, A. Davalos, I. Ferrer, A. Molins, and X. Estivill. 1995. Clinical, neuropathologic, and genetic studies of a large spinocerebellar ataxia type 1 (SCA1) kindred: (CAG)n expansion and early premonitory signs and symptoms. *Neurology* **45**:24–30.

Gentile, M., A. Di, F. Carlo, F. Susca, A. Gambotto, M.L. Caruso, C. Panella, P. Vajro, and G. Guanti. 1996. COACH syndrome: report of two brothers with congenital hepatic fibrosis, cerebellar vermis hypoplasia, oligophrenia, ataxia, and mental retardation. *Am J Med Genet* **64**:514–520.

Gerrits, N.M., and J. Voogd. 1989. The topographical organization of climbing and mossy fiber afferents in the flocculus and ventral paraflocculus in rabbit, cat and monkey. *Exp Brain Res Suppl* **17**:26–29.

Glickstein, M., N. Gerrits, I. Kralj-Hans, B. Mercier, J. Stein, and J. Voogd. 1994. Visual pontocerebellar projections in the macaque. *J Comp Neurol* **349**:51–72.

Gnadt, J.W., and L.E. Mays. 1989. Neurons in monkey parietal area LIP are tuned for eye movement parameters in three-dimensional space. *J Neurophysiol* **73**:280–297.

Godaux, E., and B. Vanderkelen. 1984. Vestibulo-ocular reflex, optokinetic response and their interactions in the cerebellectomized cat. *J Physiol* **346**:155–170.

Goldowitz, D., and K. Hamre. 1998. The cells and molecules that make a cerebellum. *Trends Neurosci* **21**:375–382.

Goldowitz, D., K.M. Hamre, S.A. Przyborski, and S.L. Ackerman. 2000. Granule cells and cerebellar boundaries: analysis of Unc5h3 mutant chimeras. *J Neurosci* **20**:4129–4137.

Goodrich, L.V., L. Milenkovic, K.M. Higgins, and M.P. Scott. 1997. Altered neural cell fates and medulloblastoma in mouse patched mutants. *Science* **277**:1109–1113.

Halmagyi, G.M., P. Rudge, and M.A. Gresty. 1983. Sanders MD. Downbeating nystagmus. A review of 62 cases. *Arch Neurol* **40**:777–784.

Hatten, M.E., and N. Heintz. 1995. Mechanisms of neural patterning and specification in the developing cerebellum. *Ann Rev Neurosci* **18**:385–408.

Heckroth, J.A., D. Goldowitz, and L.M. Eisenman. 1989. Purkinje cell reduction in the reeler mutant mouse: a quantitative immunohistochemical study. *J Comp Neurol* **279**:546–555.

Heinen, S.J., and E.L. Keller. 1996. The function of the cerebellar uvula in monkey during optokinetic and pursuit eye movements: single-unit responses and lesion effects. *Exp Brain Res* **110**:1–14.

Heinen, S.J., D.K. Oh, and E.L. Keller. 1992. Characteristics of nystagmus evoked by electrical stimulation of the uvular/nodular lobules of the cerebellum in monkey. *J Vestib Res* **2**:235–245.

Helmchen C., A. Straube, and U. Büttner. 1994. Saccadic lateropulsion in Wallenberg's syndrome may be caused by a functional lesion of the fastigial nucleus. *J Neurol* **241**:421–426.

Herrup, K., and B. Kuemerle. 1997. The compartmentalization of the cerebellum. *Ann Rev Neurosci* **20**:61–90.

Hopp, J.J., and A.F. Fuchs. 2004. The characteristics and neuronal substrate of saccadic eye movement plasticity. *Prog Neurobiol*, in press.

Howell, B.W., R. Hawkes, P. Soriano, and J.A. Cooper. 1997. Neuronal position in the developing brain is regulated by mouse disabled-1. *Nature* **389**:733–737.

Inaba, N., Y. Iwamoto, and K. Yoshida. 2003. Changes in cerebellar fastigial burst activity related to saccadic gain adaptation in the monkey. *Neurosci Res* **46**:359–368.

Jardim, L.B., M.L. Pereira, I. Silveira, A. Ferro, J. Sequeiros, and R. Giugliani. 2001. Neurologic findings in Machado-Joseph disease: relation with disease duration, subtypes, and (CAG)n. *Arch Neurol* **58**: 899–904.

Kahlon, M., and S.G. Lisberger. 1996. Coordinate system for learning in the smooth pursuit eye movements of monkeys. *J Neurosci* **16**: 7270–7283.

Keating, E.G. 1991. Frontal eye field lesions impair predictive and visually guided pursuit eye movements. *Exp Brain Res* **86**:311–323.

Keating, E.G. 1993. Lesions of the frontal eye fields impair pursuit eye movements, but preserve the predictions driving them. *Behav Brain Res* **53**:91–104.

Kikuchi, Y., H. Segawa, M. Tokumoto, T. Tsubokawa, Y. Hotta, K. Uyemura, and H. Okamoto. 1997. Ocular and cerebellar defects in zebra fish induced by overexpression of the LIM domains of the islet-3LIM/homeodomain protein. *Neuron* **18**:369–382.

Kirkham, T.H., A.C. Bird, and M.D. Sanders. 1972. Divergence paralysis with raised intracranial pressure. An electro-oculographic study. *Br J Ophthalmol* **56**:776–782.

Klostermann, W., C. Zuhlke, W. Heide, D. Kompf, and K. Wessel. 1997. Slow saccades and other eye movement disorders in spinocerebellar atrophy type 1. *J Neurol* **244**:105–111.

Korres, S., D.G. Balatsouras, C. Zournas, C. Economou, S.D. Gatsonis, and G. Adamopoulos. 2001. Periodic alternating nystagmus associated with Arnold-Chiari malformation. *J Laryngol Otol* **115**:1001–1004.

Korte, G.E., and E. Mugnaini. 1979. The cerebellar projection of the vestibular nerve in the cat. *J Comp Neurol* **184**:265–277.

Kralj-Hans, I., F.R. Robinson, J. Voogd, and M. Glickstein. 2001. Connections of the visual areas of the monkey cerebellar cortex. *Society for Neuroscience Abstracts* **27**:abstract no. 516.10.

Kralj-Hans, I., F.R. Robinson, J. Voogd, and M. Glickstein. 2002. Afferent and efferent connections of an eye movement area of the posterior interposed nucleus of macaques. *Society for Neuroscience Abstracts* **28**:abstract no. 463.2.

Krauzlis, R.J., and F.A. Miles. 1998. Role of the oculomotor vermis in generating pursuit and saccades: effects of microstimulation. *J Neurophysiol* **80**:2046–2062.

Lambert S.R., A. Kriss, M. Gresty, S. Benton, and D. Taylor. 1989. Joubert syndrome. *Arch Ophthalmol* **107**:709–713.

Leichnitz, G.R., D.J. Smith, and R.F. Spencer. 1984. Cortical projections to the paramedian tegmental and basilar pons in the monkey. *J Comp Neurol* **228**:388–408.

Leigh, R.J., T. Mapstone, and C. Weymann. 1992. Eye movements in children with the Dandy-Walker syndrome. *Neuro-ophthalmology* **12**:285–288.

Leigh, R.J., and D. Zee. 1999. *The Neurology of Eye Movements* (3rd ed.) Oxford University Press, Philadelphia, PA.

Lewis, A.R., L.B. Kline, and J.A. Sharpe. 1996. Acquired esotropia due to Arnold-Chiari I malformation. *J Neuroophthalmol* **16**:49–54.

Lewis, R.F., and H.M. Lederman. 1999. Ocular motor abnormalities in ataxia telangiectasia. *Ann Neurol* **46**:287–295.

Lisberger, S.G., and A.F. Fuchs. 1978. Role of primate flocculus during rapid behavioral modification of vestibuloocular reflex. I. Purkinje cell activity during visually guided horizontal smooth-pursuit eye movements and passive head rotation. *J Neurophysiol* **41**:733–763.

Lisberger, S.G., F.A. Miles, and D.S. Zee. 1984. Signals used to compute errors in monkey vestibuloocular reflex: possible role of flocculus. *J Neurophysiol* **52**:1140–1153.

Maria, B.L., K.B. Hoang, R.J. Tusa, A.A. Mancuso, L.M. Hamed, R.G. Quisling, M.T. Hove, E.B. Fennell, M. Booth-Jones, D.M. Ringdahl, A.T. Yachnis, G. Creel, and B. Frerking. 1997. "Joubert syndrome" revisited: key ocular motor signs with magnetic resonance imaging correlation. *J Child Neurol* **12**:423–430.

MacAvoy, M.G., J.P. Gottleib, and C.J. Bruce. 1991. Smooth pursuit eye movements representation in the primate frontal eye field. *Cereb Cortex* **1**:95–102.

Mano, N., Y. Ito, and H. Shibutani. 1996. Context dependent discharge characteristics of saccade-related Purkinje cells in the cerebellar hemispheres of the monkey. *Prog Brain Res* **112**:423–430.

Mano, N., Y. Ito, and H. Shibutani. 1991. Saccade-related Purkinje cells in the cerebellar hemispheres of the monkey. *Exp Brain Res* **84**:465–470.

Maria, B.L., R.G. Quisling, L.C. Rosainz, A.T. Yachnis, J. Gitten, D. Dede, and E. Fennell. 1999. Molar tooth sign in Joubert syndrome: clinical, radiologic, and pathologic significance. *J Child Neurol* **14**:368–376.

Mason, W.P., F. Graus, B. Lang, J. Honnorat, J.Y. Delattre, F. Valldeoriola, J.C. Antoine, M.K. Rosenblum, M.R. Rosenfeld, J. Newsom-Davis, J.B. Posner, and J. Dalmau. 1997. Small-cell lung cancer, paraneoplastic cerebellar degeneration and the Lambert-Eaton myasthenic syndrome. *Brain* **120**:1279–1300.

Maunsell, J.H., and D.C. Van Essen. 1983. Functional properties of neurons in middle temporal visual area of the macaque monkey. II. Binocular interactions and sensitivity to binocular disparity. *J Neurophysiol* **49**:1148–1167.

May, J.G., and R.A. Andersen. 1986. Different patterns of corticopontine projections from separate cortical fields within the inferior parietal lobule and dorsal prelunate gyrus of the macaque. *Exp Brain Res* **63**: 265–278.

May, P.J., J.D. Porter, and P.D.R. Gamlin. 1992. Interconnections between the cerebellum and midbrain near response regions. *J Comp Neurol* **315**: 98–116.

Mays, L.E. 1984. Neural control of vergence eye movements: convergence and divergence neurons in midbrain. *J Neurophysiol* **51**:1091–1108.

Mays, L.E., J.D. Porter, P.D. Gamlin, and C.A. Tello. 1986. Neural control of vergence eye movements: neurons encoding vergence velocity. *J Neurophysiol* **56**:1007–1021.

McMahon, A.P., and A. Bradley. 1990. The Wnt-1 (int-1) proto-oncogene is required for development of a large region of the mouse brain. *Cell* **62**:1073–1085.

Meyers, E.N., M. Lewandoski, and G.R. Martin. 1998. An Fgf8 mutant allelic series generated by Cre- and Flp-mediated recombination. *Nat Genet* **18**:136–141.

Miles, F.A., and J.H. Fuller. 1975. Visual tracking and the primate flocculus. *Science* **189**:1000–1002.

Miles, F.A., J.H. Fuller, D.J. Braitman, and B.M. Dow, 1980. Long-term adaptive changes in primate vestibuloocular reflex. III. Electrophysiological observations in flocculus of normal monkeys. *J Neurophysiol* **43**:1437–1476.

Moreira, M.C., C. Barbot, N. Tachi, N. Kozuka, E. Uchida, T. Gibson, P. Mendonca, M. Costa, J. Barros, T. Yanagisawa, M. Watanabe, Y. Ikeda, M. Aoki, T. Nagata, P. Coutinho, J. Sequeiros, and M. Koenig. 2001. The gene mutated in ataxia-ocular apraxia 1 encodes the new HIT/Zn-finger, protein aprataxin. *Nat Genet* **29**:189–193.

Moschner, C., S. Perlman, and R.W. Baloh. 1994. Comparison of oculomotor findings in the progressive ataxia syndromes. *Brain* **117**:15–25.

Mossman, S.S., A.M. Bronstein, M.A. Gresty, B. Kendall, and P. Rudge. 1990. Convergence nystagmus associated with Arnold-Chiari malformation. *Arch Neurol* **47**:357–359.

Murakami, S., H. Noda, and T. Warabi. 1991. Converging eye movements evoked by microstimulation of the fastigial nucleus of macaque monkeys. *Neurosci Res* **10**:106–117.

Newsome, W.T., R.H. Wurtz, M.R. Dürsteler, and A. Mikami. 1985. Deficits in visual motion processing following ibotenic acid lesions of the middle temporal visual area of the macaque monkey. *J Neurosci* **5**: 825–840.

Niesen, C.E. 2002. Malformations of the posterior fossa: current perspectives. *Semin Pediatr Neurol* **9**:320–334.

Noda, H., and T. Fujikado. 1987. Topography of the oculomotor area of the cerebellar vermis in macaques as determined by microstimulation. *J Neurophysiol* **58**:359–378.

Noda, H., S. Sugita, and Y. Ikeda. 1990. Afferent and efferent connections of the oculomotor region of the fastigial nucleus in the macaque monkey. *J Comp Neurol* **302**:330–348.

Nohria, V., and W.J. Oakes. 1990. Chiari I malformation: a review of 43 patients. *Pediatr Neurosurg* **16**:222–227.

Norrving, B., and S. Cronqvist. 1991. Lateral medullary infarction: prognosis in an unselected series. *Neurology* **41**:244–248.

Ohki, M., H. Kitazawa, T. Hiramatsu, T. Kitamura, J. Yamada, and S. Nagao. 2003. Role of primate cerebellar hemispheric lobule VII in eye movement control revealed by lesions. *Society for Neuroscience Abstracts* **29**:abstract no. 274.5.

Ohtsuka, K., and H. Noda. 1991. Saccadic burst neurons in the oculomotor region of the fastigial nucleus of macaque monkeys. *J Neurophysiol* **65**:1422–1434.

Ohtsuka, K., and H. Noda. 1995. Discharge properties of Purkinje cells in the oculomotor vermis during visually guided saccades in the macaque monkey. *J Neurophysiol* **74**:1828–1840.

Ohyagi, Y., T. Yamada, A. Okayama, N. Sakae, T. Yamasaki, T. Ohshima, T. Sakamoto, N. Fujii, and J. Kira. 2000. Vergence disorders in patients with spinocerebellar ataxia 3/Machado-Joseph disease: a synoptophore study. *J Neurol Sci* **173**:120–123.

Pakkenberg, B., and H.J. Gundersen. 1997. Neocortical neuron number in humans: effect of sex and age. *J Comp Neurol* **384**:312–320.

Pascual, J., A. Oterino, and J. Berciano. 1992. Headache in type I Chiari malformation. *Neurology* **42**:1519–1512.

Patil, N., D.R. Cox, D. Bhat, M. Faham, R.M. Myers, and A.S. Peterson. 1995. A potassium channel mutation in weaver mice implicates membrane excitability in granule cell differentiation. *Nat Genet* **11**:126–129.

Pollack, I.F. 1994. Brain tumors in children *N Engl J Med* **331**: 1500–1507.

Quaia, C., P. Lefévre, and L.M. Optican. 1999. Model of the control of saccades by superior colliculus and cerebellum. *J Neurophysiol* **82**: 999–1018.

Quisling, R.G., A.J. Barkovich, and B.L. Maria. 1999. Magnetic resonance imaging features and classification of central nervous system malformations in Joubert syndrome. *J Child Neurol* **14**:628–635.

Rabiah, P.K., J.B. Bateman, J.L. Demer, and S. Perlman. 1997. Ophthalmologic findings in patients with ataxia. *Am J Ophthalmol* **123**:108–117.

Raphan, T., V. Matsuo, and B. Cohen. 1979. Velocity storage in the vestibulo-ocular reflex arc (VOR). *Exp Brain Res* **35**:229–248.

Rivaud-Pechoux, S., A. Durr, B. Gaymard, G. Cancel, C.J. Ploner, Y. Agid, A. Brice, and C. Pierrot-Deseilligny. 1998. Eye movement abnormalities correlate with genotype in autosomal dominant cerebellar ataxia type I. *Ann Neurol* **43**:297–302.

Robinson, D.A. 1974. The effect of cerebellectomy on the cat's vestibulo-ocular integrator. *Brain Res* **71**:195–207.

Robinson, F.R. 1995. Role of the cerebellum in movement control and adaptation. *Curr Opin Neurobiol* **5**:755–762.

Robinson, F.R. 2000. The role of the cerebellar posterior interpositus nucleus in saccades. I. Effect of temporary lesions. *J Neurophysiol* **84**: 1289–1303.

Robinson, F.R., and S.C. Brettler. 1998. Smooth pursuit properties of neurons in the ventrolateral posterior interpositus nucleus of the monkey cerebellum. *Society for Neuroscience Abstracts* **24**:abstract no. 554.7.

Robinson, F.R., J. Cohen, J. May, A. Sestokas, and M. Glickstein. 1984. Cerebellar targets of visual pontine cells in the cat. *J Comp Neurol* **223**: 471–482.

Robinson, F.R., and A.F. Fuchs. 2001. Role of the cerebellum in voluntary eye movements *Ann Rev Neurosci* **24**:981–1004.

Robinson, F.R., A.F. Fuchs, and A. Straube. 1997. Participation of the caudal fastigial nucleus in smooth pursuit eye movements II. Effects of muscimol inactivation. *J Neurophysiol* **78**:848–859.

Robinson, F.R., A.F. Fuchs, A. Straube, and S. Watanabe. 1996. The role of the interpositus nucleus in saccades is different from the role of the fastigial nucleus. *Society for Neuroscience Abstracts* **22**:abstract no. 476.3.

Robinson, F.R., A.F. Fuchs, and C.T. Noto. 2002. Cerebellar influences on saccade plasticity. *Ann N Y Acad Sci* **956**:155–163.

Robinson, F.R., A. Straube, and A.F. Fuchs. 1993. Role of the caudal fastigial nucleus in saccade generation. II. Effects of muscimol inactivation. *J Neurophysiol* **70**:1741–1758.

Robinson, F.R., and C.T. Noto. 2002. Oculomotor vermis inactivation reveals functional subregions and causes short-latency corrective saccades. *Society for Neuroscience Abstracts* **28**:abstract no. 360.15.

Robinson, F.R., and C.T. Noto. 2003. Interrupting parallel fibers in the oculomotor vermis causes hypermetric horizontal saccades. *Society for Neuroscience Abstracts* **29**:abstract no. 882.4.

Rub, U., R.A. de Vos, C. Schultz, E.R. Brunt, H. Paulson, and H. Braak. 2002. Spinocerebellar ataxia type 3 (Machado-Joseph disease): severe destruction of the lateral reticular nucleus. *Brain* **125**:2115–2124.

Sasaki, H., H. Kojima, I. Yabe, K. Tashiro, T. Hamada, H. Sawa, H. Hiraga, and K. Nagashima. 1998. Neuropathological and molecular studies of spinocerebellar ataxia type 6 (SCA6). *Acta Neuropathol (Berlin)* **95**: 199–204.

Schols, L., G. Amoiridis, T. Buttner, H. Przuntek, J.T. Epplen, and O. Riess. 1997. Autosomal dominant cerebellar ataxia: phenotypic differences in genetically defined subtypes? *Ann Neurol* **42**:924–932.

Schwartz, B.E., S. Li, I. Bespalova, M. Burnmeister, E. Dulaney, F.R. Robinson, and R.J. Leigh. 2003. Pathogens of clinical signs in recessive cerebellar ataxia with saccadic intrusions and neuropathy (SCA SI). *Ann Neurol* **54**:824–828.

Scudder, C.A. 2002. Role of the fastigial nucleus in controlling horizontal saccades during adaptation. *Ann N Y Acad Sci* **978**:63–78.

Sheldon, M., D.S. Rice, G. D'Arcangelo, H. Yoneshima, K. Nakajima, K. Mikoshiba, B.W. Howell, J.A. Cooper, D. Goldowitz, and T. Curran. 1997. Scrambler and yotari disrupt the disabled gene and produce a reeler-like phenotype in mice. *Nature* **389**:730–733.

Skavenski, A.A., and D.A. Robinson. 1973. Role of abducens neurons in vestibuloocular reflex. *J Neurophysiol* **36**:724–738.

Spieker, S., J.B. Schulz, D. Petersen, M. Fetter, T. Klockgether, and J. Dichgans. 1995. Fixation instability and oculomotor abnormalities in Friedreich's ataxia. *J Neurol* **242**:517–521.

Stahl, J.S., and J.I. Simpson. 1995. Dynamics of rabbit vestibular nucleus neurons and the influence of the flocculus. *J Neurophysiol* **73**: 1396–13413.

Stanton, G.B., M.E. Goldberg, and C.J. Bruce.1988. Frontal eye field efferents in the macaque monkey: II. Topography of terminal fields in midbrain and pons. *J Comp Neurol* **271**:493–506.

Straube, A., C. Helmchen, F. Robinson, A. Fuchs, and U. Büttner. 1994. Saccadic dysmetria is similar in patients with a lateral medullary lesion and in monkeys with a lesion of the deep cerebellar nucleus. *J Vestib Res* **4**:327–333.

Suzuki, D.A., and E.L. Keller. 1984. Visual signals in the dorsolateral pontine nucleus of the alert monkey: their relationship to smooth-pursuit eye movements. *Exp Brain Res* **53**:473–478.

Suzuki, D.A., H. Noda, and M. Kase. 1981. Visual and pursuit eye movement-related activity in posterior vermis of monkey cerebellum. *J Neurophysiol* **46**:1120–1139.

Takagi, M., R. Tamargo, and D.S. Zee. 2003. Effects of lesions of the cerebellar oculomotor vermis on eye movements in primate: binocular control. *Prog Brain Res* **142**:19–33.

Takagi, M., D.S. Zee, and R.J. Tamara. 1998. Effects of lesions of the oculomotor vermis on eye movements in primate: saccades. *J Neurophysiol* **80**:1911–1931.

Takagi, M., D.S. Zee, and R.J. Tamargo. 2000. Effects of lesions of the oculomotor cerebellar vermis on eye movements in primate: smooth pursuit. *J Neurophysiol* **83**:2047–2062.

Takeichi, N., K. Fukushima, H. Sasaki, I. Yabe, K. Tashiro, and Y. Inuyama. 2000. Dissociation of smooth pursuit and vestibulo-ocular reflex cancellation in SCA-6.Neurology. *Neurology* **54**:860–866.

Thomas, K.R., and M.R. Capecchi. 1990. Targeted disruption of the murine int-1 proto-oncogene resulting in severe abnormalities in midbrain and cerebellar development. *Nature* **346**:847–850.

Tomiwa, K., M. Baraitser, and J. Wilson. 1987. Dominantly inherited congenital cerebellar ataxia with atrophy of the vermis. *Pediat Neurol* **3**: 360–362.

Tucker, S.J., M. Pessia, A.J. Moorhouse, F. Gribble, F.M. Ashcroft, J. Maylie, and J.P. Adelman. 1996. Heteromeric channel formation and Ca(2+)-free media reduce the toxic effect of the weaver Kir 3.2 allele. *FEBS Lett* **390**:253–257.

Versino, M., O. Hurko, and D.S. Zee. 1996. Disorders of binocular control of eye movements in patients with cerebellar dysfunction. *Brain* **119**: 1933–1950.

Waespe, W., and R. Baumgartner. 1992. Enduring dysmetria and impaired gain adaptivity of saccadic eye movements in Wallenberg's lateral medullary syndrome. *Brain* **115**:1123–1146.

Waespe, W., B. Cohen, and T. Raphan. 1983. Effects of flocculectomy on vestibular and optokinetic nystagmus and unit activity in the vestibular nuclei. *Adv Otorhinolaryngol* **30**:226–229.

Waespe, W., B. Cohen, and T. Raphan. 1985. Dynamic modification of the vestibulo-ocular reflex by the nodulus and uvula. *Science* **228**:199–202.

Waespe, W., and V. Henn. 1981. Visual-vestibular interaction in the flocculus of the alert monkey. II. Purkinje cell activity. *Exp Brain Res* **143**: 349–360.

Waespe, W., and W. Wichmann. 1990. Oculomotor disturbances during visual-vestibular interaction in Wallenberg's lateral medullary syndrome. *Brain* **113**:821–846.

Wassarman, K.M., M. Lewandoski, K. Campbell, A.L. Joyner, J.L. Rubenstein, S. Martinez, and G.R. Martin. 1997. Specification of the anterior hindbrain and establishment of a normal mid/hindbrain organizer is dependent on Gbx2 gene function. *Development* **124**: 2923–2934.

Weeks, C.L., and L.M. Hamed. 1999. Treatment of acute comitant esotropia in Chiari I malformation. *Ophthalmology* **106**:2368–2371.

Wessel, K., C. Moschner, K.P. Wandinger, D. Kompf, and W. Heide. 1998. Oculomotor testing in the differential diagnosis of degenerative ataxic disorders. *Arch Neurol* **55**:949–956.

Westheimer, G., and S.M. Blair. 1973. Oculomotor defects in cerebellectomized monkeys. *Invest Ophthalmol Vis Sci* **12**:618–621.

Wurst, W., A.B. Auerbach, and A.L. Joyner. 1994. Multiple developmental defects in Engrailed-1 mutant mice: an early mid-hindbrain deletion and patterning defects in forelimbs and sternum. *Development* **120**:2065–2075.

Yamada, J., and H. Noda. 1987. Afferent and efferent connections of the oculomotor cerebellar vermis in the macaque monkey. *J Comp Neurol* **265**:224–241.

Yee, R.D., R.W. Baloh, V. Honrubia, C.G. Lau, and H.A. Jenkins. 1979. Slow build-up of optokinetic nystagmus associated with downbeat nystagmus. *Invest Ophthalmol Vis Sci* **18**:622–629.

Yee, R.D., R.W. Baloh, and V. Honrubia. 1984. Episodic vertical oscillopsia and downbeat nystagmus in a Chiari malformation. *Arch Ophthalmol* **102**:723–725.

Zee, D., A. Yamazaki, P.H. Butlerm, and G. Gücer. 1981. Effects of ablation of flocculus and paraflocculus on eye movements in primate *J Neurophysiol* **46**:878–899.

Zee, D.S., R.D. Yee, D.G. Cogan, D.A. Robinson, and W.K. Engel. 1976. Ocular motor abnormalities in hereditary cerebellar ataxia. *Brain* **99**: 207–234.

Zagon, I.S., P.J. McLaughlin, and S. Smith. 1977. Neural populations in the human cerebellum: estimations from isolated cell nuclei. *Brain Res* **127**:279–282.

Zhang, H., and P.D.R. Gamlin. 1996. Single unit activity within the posterior fastigial nucleus during vergence and accommodation in the alert primate. *Society for Neuroscience Abstracts* **22**:abstract no. 801.1.

Zhang, H., and P.D. Gamlin. 1998. Neurons in the posterior interposed nucleus of the cerebellum related to vergence and accommodation. I. Steady-state characteristics. *J Neurophysiol* **179**:1255–1269.

Zhang, H., L.E. Mays, and P.D.R. Gamlin. 1992. Characteristics of near response cells projecting to the oculomotor nucleus. *J Neurophysiol* **67**:944–960.

Zimmerman, C.F., E.S. Roach, and B.T. Troost. 1986. See-saw nystagmus associated with Chiari malformation. *Arch Neurol* **43**:299–300.

CHAPTER

L1

Spasticity

ALLISON BRASHEAR

I. DEFINITION OF SPASTICITY

Spasticity is an imbalance of the sensorimotor system that demonstrates an increased response to a velocity-dependent stretch of the muscle tendon resulting from hyperexcitable muscle stretch reflexes (Mayer and Simpson, 2002). Spasticity is a small part of the upper motor neuron syndrome composed of increased tone, hyperactive reflexes, weakness, and poor coordination (Goldstein, 2001). Key to the development of spasticity is the loss of inhibition of the suprasegmental inputs that then produce hyperexcitable segmental spinal reflex arcs (Goldstein, 2001). This hyperexcitability of the alpha motor neuron pool results in the characteristic positive phenomena associated with spasticity. Lesions of the corticospinal tracts cause muscle weakness, loss of dexterity, and the Babinski response, but not spasticity (Bhakta, 2000). The overactivity of the alpha motor neuron pool is thought to be due to the lesions of the descending input from the cerebral cortex and from the basal ganglia through the medial and dorsal reticulospinal and vestibulospinal tracts (Bhakta, 2000). The loss of descending input from the medial and dorsal reticulospinal and vestibulospinal tracts results in impaired modulation of the monosynaptic input from the primary Ia afferent fibers and the polysynaptic afferent input from cutaneous receptors and Golgi tendon organs. All these factors contribute to alpha motor neuron hyperexcitability (Bhakta, 2000).

Typically the upper motor neuron syndrome is characterized by positive and negative symptoms. The positive symptoms are typically the target of therapy with either medication or injections of botulinum toxin. The negative symptoms are due to the damage of the corticospinal tract resulting in weakness, loss of fine motor control, and the Babinski sign (Table 1). Understanding the source of the positive and negative symptoms can assist the physician in designing a treatment plan tailored for the individual patient.

Any process that interrupts the descending pathways from the brain or spinal cord interferes with the modulation of the intraspinal segments and can result in the clinical presentation of spasticity. The cause of spasticity is typically described in two classic models of the upper motor neuron syndrome: the spinal and cerebral models (Table 2). Understanding the models lays the groundwork for understanding the treatments currently recommended for adults patients affected by some components of the upper motor neuron syndrome.

The spinal model is based on the concept that the afferent stimulus enters the spinal cord at one level but then

TABLE 1 Spasticity: Positive and Negative Symptoms

Positive symptoms	Negative symptoms
Increased tone	Decreased muscle strength
Increased deep tendon reflexes	Less coordination
Persistent or exaggerated primitive reflexes	Lack of fine motor control
Clonus	Decreased endurance
Discordant activation of muscles	
Babinski signs	

TABLE 2 Spasticity: Pathophysiological Models[a]

SPINAL MODEL

Removal of inhibition on segmental polysynaptic pathways
Slow, progressive rise of excitatory state through cumulative excitation
Afferent activity from one segment may lead to muscle response many segments away
Flexors and extensors may be overexcited

Clinical presentation of the spinal model

Cumulative excitation may spill over to muscle flexors and extensors
Example: toe pain causing hip flexion

CEREBRAL MODEL

Enhanced excitability of monosynaptic pathways
Rapid buildup of reflex activity
Bias toward overactivity in the antigravity muscles and development of the hemiplegic posture

Clinical features of the cerebral model

Big toe extension (Babinski sign)
Ankle, knee, and hip flexion
Contraction of abdominals

[a]Adapted from Mayer and Simpson (2002).

ascends and descends within the cord through several levels (Thompson et al., 2001). This results in stimulation at one level activating a response sometimes many spinal levels away from the initial stimulus. A clinical example of this is pain in the great toe causing hip flexion. The pain signal entering through the afferent pathway stimulates hip flexion by communication through several levels in the spinal cord. As reported by Mayer and Simpson (2002), the scientific basis for this model is the work of Herman (1962), who found that a lesion in the spinal cord resulted in a "cumulative, stretch-generated excitation in the interneuronal pathways." According to Mayer and Simpson, Herman argued that "by removing the inhibitory influences on the segmental polysynaptic pathways the likely result is that the primary afferent discharge from the muscle spindle is transmitted through multisynaptic chains of the interneuronal pool." Characteristic features of the spinal model include removal of the inhibition on segmental polysynaptic pathways, a slow rise of the excitatory state through cumulative excitation, afferent activity from one segment leading to muscle response many segments away, and flexors and extensors becoming overexcited. A clinical vignette of the spinal module is a spinal cord injury patient in whom the patella reflex elicited exits the hip flexors in the same leg.

The cerebral model of spasticity is characterized by a rapid buildup of reflex activity. Herman and colleagues suggested that the transmission of the primary ending spindle discharges occurs largely through monosynaptic pathways (Herman, 1962; Herman et al., 1974). The short time involved in the reflex buildup suggests that it is monosynaptic. The cerebral model explains the characteristic antigravity postures that are seen in patients after stroke (Mayer and Simpson, 2002). The flexed elbow, wrist, and hand are a typical presentation of spasticity of cerebral origin. The leg typically involves overactivity of the extensor muscles. In the arm and leg, the muscles involved are typically active in the standing position. This is thought to be due to the increased motor neuron activity in antigravity muscles—flexors in the upper limb, and extensors in the lower limb (Mayer and Simpson, 2002).

II. TREATMENT OF SPASTICITY

A. Decision to Treat Spasticity

The decision to treat spasticity should be individualized. In some patients, activity of daily living (ADL) may be affected such that it interferes with hygiene and dressing (Jozefczyk, 2002). Positioning in wheelchair, ulcers, and participation in therapy may all be affected. However, there are some patients who rely on their spasticity to perform ADLs. A young man who relies on increased tone in the hand to grip the controls on a wheelchair or a woman who uses increased tone in the hand to grip the steering wheel may be dismayed to have that tone relieved. Treatment of spasticity requires an ongoing discussion by the patient with his or her physician and therapist about what is most affecting his or her ability to be independent. Assessing the role of the caregiver is also important. The caregiver often will champion treatment of spasticity when the patient is unaware of the need. Such a case may involve a patient with multiple sclerosis who has severe adductor spasms of the thigh making perineal hygiene extremely difficult. The caregiver often bears the burden of care for patients who are disabled from an upper motor neuron lesion. In these cases, the caregiver becomes part of the treatment team and his or her input on what symptoms to alleviate is important to the overall success of treatment (McGuire, 2001).

B. Methods of Treating Spasticity

The methods of treating spasticity include mechanical (e.g., physical therapy, casting, and splinting), oral medications (e.g., tizanidine, baclofen, dantrolene, and diazepam), intrathecal medications (e.g., baclofen), denervation of muscle with neurolysis (e.g., phenol), or chemodenervation of muscle with botulinum toxin (Bhakta, 2000). Each of these modalities focuses on a particular aspect of the upper motor neuron syndrome. Several treatments can be combined in individual patients for greater success. The purpose of this section is to highlight the clinical presentation most benefited by each of these types of treatment.

1. Mechanical

Therapy alone or in combination with casting and/or splinting may be sufficient to treat a patient with mild spasticity (Jozefczyk, 2002). Patients who have a mild increase in tone may benefit from a stretching program combined with splinting. In the upper extremity, a resting hand splint at night may be all that a patient recovering from a mild stroke requires. Likewise, midcalf AFO may be sufficient to keep the foot from plantar flexing and keep the patient from tripping over it. Casting is often used in children to position the foot into the desired position. In more severe cases of spasticity, mechanical treatment alone is ineffective (Gormley et al., 1997).

2. Oral Medications

Oral medications have been used for years to try to decrease muscle tone and interfere with the positive signs of the upper motor neuron syndrome. Compliance due to side effects is often an issue. Patients often complain of excess sedation with most of these medicines. This can be a problem for patients who may be cognitively impaired from stroke or traumatic brain injury. Furthermore, many of the medications may affect liver function, requiring repeat blood work to monitor the status of the liver. Generally, the cost of these medications combined with those of other therapies, physical or occupational, splints, and wheelchairs can be a major financial burden. Like many elderly, disabled patients may have to choose between paying for oral medications and more urgent needs.

The benzodiazepine family has been used for years to decrease muscle tone. Commonly used drugs include diazepam and clonazepam. Sedation is the limiting side effect. These drugs are often used at night when symptoms of spasticity may interfere with sleep. Many of these medications have abuse potential and most can be addicting. Patients must be cautioned about abrupt stoppage of medication that can lead to withdrawal symptoms such as irritation, changes in vital signs, seizures, and even death (Gracies et al., 1997).

Baclofen is a $GABA_B$ receptor agonist, and although its effect on spasticity is not completely understood, baclofen is thought to inhibit motor neuron excitability by both suppression of excitability and enhancement of inhibition (Herman et al., 1992). The net result is a theoretical reduction in monosynaptic and polysynaptic spinal reflexes (Gracies et al., 1997; Feldman et al., 1978). Adverse effects of baclofen include sedation, impaired respiration, increase in seizures, and a withdrawal syndrome when the drug is stopped abruptly. Patients may become excessively sedated on baclofen, and those who are already impaired due to stroke or head injury are most at risk. Drowsiness and fatigue may make it difficult to drive or, in some cases, live alone (Elovic, 2001). Elderly patients may feel the effects more and may complain of memory loss. In some cases, high doses of baclofen may make a patient lose function. This is generally seen in high-functioning patients who rely on some tone to perform daily tasks, such as walking. For those who require some tone, high-dose baclofen may remove all tone and lead to loss of previously achieved ADLs (Francisco et al., 2001).

Central nervous system (CNS) side effects, including impaired respiration and loss of seizure control, have been reported. Baclofen may increase airway bronchoconstriction responsiveness and can be risky in patients with asthma (Gracies et al., 1997). For those who have difficulty protecting their airway due to CNS sedation, baclofen may be risky. Seizure threshold can be lowered, causing problems in patients who are already impaired. An abrupt withdrawal phenomenon has been reported in patients taking both oral and intrathecal baclofen (Green and Nelson, 1999). Symptoms may include seizures, mental status change, fever, and muscle rigidity, and the phenomenon has been compared to a malignant neuroleptic syndrome (Alden et al., 2002).

Tizanidine, an α_2 adrenergic agonist, is a relatively recent addition to the clinicians toolbox. As noted for the other oral medications used to treat spasticity, significant sedation occurs in many patients. Other side effects include muscular weakness and dry mouth. Tizanidine has a mild depressive effect on blood pressure and some suggest mixing this medication with other antihypertensive agents (Stien et al., 1987). Hepatotoxicity has been reported with tizanidine, and the package insert recommends checking liver function tests 1, 3, and 6 months after initiating treatment (Smith et al., 1994).

Dantrolene is one of the oldest drugs available to treat spasticity. Dantrolene effects ion flux and works primarily to decrease muscle action potential-induced release of calcium from the sarcoplasmic reticulum of skeletal, smooth, and cardiac muscle (Gracies et al., 1997).

Dantrolene is sedating and may cause central nervous system side effects of lethargy and dizziness in addition to decreasing muscle tone in a similar manner as baclofen (Bhakta, 2000). There is a risk of hepatotoxicity, which is greatest in females and those taking multiple medications (Gracies et al., 1997). Dantrolene is an older medication and no recent studies have been published despite continued use in severe cases of spasticity.

3. Intrathecal Medications

The development of a system to deliver intrathecal medications has added another dimension to treating spasticity. The intrathecal baclofen pump (ITB) delivers drug directly into the cerebrospinal fluid, which can be a major advantage over oral dosing (Penn and Kroin, 1985). Delivering medication directly to the site of action allows for higher doses for treatment of spasticity with fewer systemic side affects (Dario et al., 2002).

ITB therapy is not without problems because patients require a day-long test dose of medication (Francisco, 2001). The intrathecal dose of ITB is 1% of the oral dose. To avoid an unnecessary operative procedure, most physicians give a test dose of baclofen through a lumbar puncture. The patient usually receives medication in the morning and is monitored for a response during the day. If no response is noted, a higher dose is used. The test dose must demonstrate a beneficial effect before surgeons will proceed with device implantation. Failure to respond to orally administered baclofen does not reliably predict the effects of intrathecal administration.

If a test dose is effective, the pump must be surgically implanted in the subcutaneous tissues of the abdomen with the intrathecal catheter in the subarachnoid space. Surgical implantation of the pump and chronic ongoing maintenance of the system with periodic pump refills by a trained nurse or physician every few months are required. The adverse effects of ITB range from life threatening to annoying. Fatal overdose or abrupt withdrawal have led to disastrous outcomes in a few rare cases (Ivanhoe et al., 2001). Since the dose is delivered by a programmable pump, variations in drug delivery can be due to pump malfunction or failure or human error in programming or refilling the pump. With proper training, the latter two problems should be avoidable, but the issue of relying on a mechanical pump for delivery of a potent medication remains. However, despite all the implementation and maintenance issues, the pump can lead to significant improvement in appropriately selected patients with intractable spasticity (Disabato and Ritchie, 2003).

The efficacy of intrathecal delivery of baclofen has been proven in several trials of spinal cord injury patients and those with spasticity due to multiple sclerosis, cerebral palsy, and stroke (Abel and Smith 1994; Meythaler et al., 1999, 2001; Gilmartin et al., 2000). The outcome measure in these studies was muscle tone, usually determined by the Ashworth scale or some variant. Long-term effect on tone or changes in either long- or short-term function have not been studied (McGuire, 2001). Regardless of the lack of data, the procedure is useful for select patients when managed appropriately.

4. Local Therapies

Localized treatment of spasticity, regardless of the cause, by local anesthetics, alcohol, phenol, and botulinum toxin has been advocated by physicians seeking to treat patients with medications that are associated with the fewest systemic effects. Local injections are used to treat a focal problem such as a clenched fist, and localized therapy can be used with the oral and intrathecal medications discussed previously.

5. Nerve Blocks

Nerve blocks in spasticity have long been used to produce a chemical neurolysis with the goal of decreasing muscle tone. Both alcohol and phenol have been used to cause a localized neurolysis. Alcohol has been injected in muscle with reduction in spasticity for periods of 6–12 months. Phenol is a metabolite of benzene and when ingested can cause toxicity on bone marrow and a variety of additional deleterious effects (Gracies et al., 1997). When both alcohol and phenol are injected in muscle, they cause localized necrosis of both muscle and nerve.

The adverse effects from injections of alcohol and phenol include pain at the time of injection and chronic sensory dysesthesias. The latter problem can be severe and disabling and, accordingly, has limited the use of chemical neurolysis to treat spasticity. Moreover, vascular complications of chemical neurolysis with alcohol and phenol may include lower extremity edema and deep vein thrombosis. To avoid systemic overdosage of phenol, no more than 1 g should be delivered in a given day. Systemic side effects of phenol injections include tremor, dizziness, CNS collapse, and cardiac arrest (Gormley et al., 2001).

6. Botulinum Toxin Type A Injections

Botulinum toxin type A was approved by the Food and Drug Administration in 1989 for face and eye injections. Neurologists soon discovered that the temporary relaxation of muscle could benefit other diseases. Cervical dystonia, an involuntary movement of the neck resulting in often painful spasm, was a testing ground for this new drug. Patients were treated with injections into overactive neck muscles and noted a decrease in muscle spasms and pain. Physicians treating poststroke patients and traumatic brain injury patients began using periodic injections of botulinum toxin into spastic limb muscles. The result was a temporary relaxation of the injected muscle. Benefits generally last approximately 3–6 months. Botulinum toxin can be combined with all of the other medications discussed previously.

Botulinum toxin acts at the presynaptic level by inhibiting acetylcholine release at the neuromuscular junction and, as such, results in a temporary and titratable relaxation of the injected muscle. Unlike the case for oral medications, side effects are minimal. Some patients find the injections mildly uncomfortable. Occasionally, denervation with botulinum toxin is associated with excessive weakness in injected muscles. The side effects wear off over days to weeks. Benefits wane after 3–6 months. The injections can be repeated indefinitely as long as the patient continues to respond to the treatments.

First developed by Dr. Allen Scott for treatment of strabismus in children (Scott and Kraft, 1985), the use of botulinum toxin A (BTX-A) has expanded to include many disease processes in which the muscle is overactive. Botulinum toxin is injected into the spastic muscle and acts locally to relax or loosen the spastic muscle (Jankovic et al., 1991; Hatheway, 1995). More recently, BTX-B has been approved for treatment of cervical dystonia in the United States and Europe. BTX-B has a different biochemical action than BTX-A. BTX-A inhibits SNAP-25, whereas BTX-B inhibits synaptobrevin [also known as vesicle-associated membrane protein (VAMP)] located on the surface of presynaptic acetylcholine-containing vesicles. Disruption of either protein, VAMP/synaptobrevin or SNAP-25, impedes exocystosis and prevents release of acetylcholine (Brin and Aoki, 2002). As a result, BTX functionally denervates the treated muscle. This procedure, often called chemical denervation, is a local treatment for a spastic muscle.

The procedure to treat an involved limb may take up to 45 minutes and benefits are often seen within 5 days of treatment. Typically, the peak effect occurs at 2–4 weeks and reinjection is usually needed at 12–14 weeks. Injection is well tolerated by the elderly and children. Side effects are related to the mechanism of action. This drug offers a controlled, titratable relaxation of muscle. Side effects reported by patients treated with BTX-A for spasticity include weakness, bruising or bleeding at the injection site, and pain at the injection site. Typically, the pain is no more than that associated with venipuncture. Occasionally, differentiating weakness from BTX-A and upper motor neuron dysfunction can be difficult.

Optimal therapy of focal spasticity with botulinum toxin requires appropriate patient selection and education (McGuire, 2001). Patients who have increased muscle tone that interferes with their desired activities are excellent candidates for treatment with BTX. The results of a large double-blind, placebo-controlled study in patients with upper extremity poststroke spasticity demonstrated that when patients and their physicians jointly select prospectively the goal of treatment, BTX-A can offer more improvement than placebo. When deciding on BTX-A injections, patients who rely on their spasticity for function, such as patients with spastic gait, may not be good candidates.

The results of a randomized, double-blind, placebo-controlled, multicenter trial to assess the efficacy and safety of BTX-A in the treatment of poststroke spasticity have been published by Brashear et al. (2002). All patients were at least 6 months poststroke, and none had been treated with BTX, alcohol, or phenol. This study is unique in that a novel scale, the Disability Assessment Scale (DAS), was developed to focus on the perceived benefits of BTX. Patients were asked to prospectively select one of four areas (pain, hygiene of the palm, use of the hand in dressing, and limb position) as their goal for improvement in the study.

At the end of 12 weeks, subjects treated with BTX-A had a greater improvement in wrist and finger flexor tone at each visit than did the placebo group. The maximal difference between the two groups in the mean change from baseline occurred on Week 4 (wrist, −1.78 BTX-A group, −0.42 placebo group, $p < 0.001$; finger, −1.59 BTX-A, −0.27 placebo group, $p < 0.001$). Results for the fingers and wrist flexors were sustained throughout the 12 weeks of the study. Furthermore, the preselected goal of treatment (principal therapeutic target) showed greater improvement in the BTX-A-treated group than in those treated with placebo. At 6 weeks after injection, 62% of the BTX-A-treated group members, compared with 27% of the placebo group members, had improvement in their target area. Similar improvements were seen at Weeks 4, 8, and 12 after injection in the treated group. Additionally, there was an improvement in the treated group in all areas measured by the DAS (pain, limb position, hygiene, and dressing) in those treated with BTX-A. Of those treated with BTX-A, 83% had at least a 1-point improvement on the DAS in one or more areas compared to 53% of those receiving placebo. Additionally, measures of global improvements by the patient and physician were noted in the BTX-A-treated group compared to the placebo group at all visits.

The development of botulinum toxin injections to treat patients with spasticity provides value to what physicians can offer these patients. The combination of focal treatments with botulinum toxin, oral agents, and ITB allows physicians to tailor therapies to the needs of individual patients and their caregivers. Goals-oriented therapy should drive these interventions. Patients and caregivers should participate in the identification of issues that are interfering with the quality of life and the patient's ability to be independent. The clinical spectrum of spasticity is wide, and identification of focal patterns that may be ameliorated with individualized therapy is discussed next.

III. CLINICAL SPECTRUM OF SPASTICITY

The clinical spectrum of adult spasticity depends on the underlying disease process and which limb is affected, as well as the amount of tone and therapy and treatments made available to patients both early in the course of the disease and later. The underlying disease process (spinal versus cerebral) may affect the localization for the cause of the spasticity, but common patterns emerge that may require treatment regardless of the etiology of the upper motor neuron syndrome. Early and prompt recognition of these patterns is important to determine which are interfering with the patients' activities of daily living and require treatment.

A. Upper Extremities

1. Flexed Elbow

The flexed forearm is the typical antigravity pattern identified with spastic hemiplegia of cerebral origin. Many patients present with complaints of problems with limb position while walking. Limb position has been identified as an outcome variable in a botulinum toxin clinical trial. Patients complain of the limb interfering with dressing because the arm cannot be straightened to put on shirts or jackets. Patients and caregivers report difficulty with hygiene if the limb cannot be adequately straightened for cleaning. The overactive muscles in the flexed elbow characteristically are the biceps, brachioradialis, and brachialis. The extensor muscles are typically not involved and not treated with localized therapy. In combination with the flexed elbow presentation, the arm may also be pronated. Overactivity of the pronator interferes with the ability to supinate and makes the hand less functional.

2. Flexed Wrist (Video Segment 1)

The flexed wrist is a common characteristic of the upper motor neuron syndrome. Overactivity of the two major muscles of wrist flexion, the flexor carpi ulnaris and flexor carpi radialis, may be combined with abnormal activity of the finger flexors. The finger flexors, the flexor digitorum sublimis and flexor digitorum profundus, contribute to the fisted presentation. The flexed wrist may present with pain due to tightness of the forearm muscles and/or superimposed carpal tunnel syndrome.

3. Clenched Fist (Video Segments 2 and 3)

The clenched fist is typically seen with the flexed wrist. Overactivity of the finger flexors results in difficulty for the patient and caregiver in opening the hand. Limitations occur in ADLs and personal hygiene. Dressing is affected because patients have difficulty putting on shirts when the fist does not open. Poor hygiene is a typical reason for referral to treat hand spasticity. Caregivers and patients may have difficulty cleaning the palm, resulting in infection and skin breakdown. Treatment with splints is often not effective when the hand is fisted. The spasticity of the finger flexors makes splints difficult and painful to apply.

4. Thumb in Palm Deformity

When the thumb is locked inside the fisted hand, many patients experience significant loss of function. The loss of use of the thumb limits the useful grasp available to the patient. The thumb may be tight due to flexion at the DIP joint or from overadduction of the thumb fixing it to the palm. Relaxation of the flexor pollicis longus and the adductor pollicis may allow some useful grasp to return.

B. Lower Extremities

1. Adducted Thighs (Video Segment 4)

Excessive adduction of both thighs is a typical presentation of spinal cord injury. Multiple sclerosis or trauma to the cord may present with overactivity of the adductors. The typical scissoring with waking or stimulation with movement of the limbs significantly interfere with personal hygiene and ambulation. The scissoring on standing interferes with walking, transfers, and positioning in the wheelchair. Spasms in the adductors of the thigh limit the ability of the patient or caregiver to abduct the thighs. Problems include difficulty with personal hygiene, sitting, transfers, standing, and urinary catherization. The muscles involved with thigh adduction include the adductor longus, adductor brevis, adductor magnus, and gracilis.

2. Foot Position (Video Segment 5)

The inverted foot is the most commonly reported lower extremity presentation of the upper motor neuron syndrome. The foot may turn in and the toes may curl. Overactivity interferes with walking, transfers, and placement of orthotics. Pain may occur due to weight bearing on the lateral aspect of the foot and callous formation. Pain due to walking on the tips of the toes is common. Gait is affected by the inability to place the foot flat, resulting in hyperextension of the knee. Development of knee pain in these patients is common. The involved muscles are typically the posterior tibialis as the inverter of the foot and the flexors of the toes, the flexor digitorum longus. The foot may be dorsiflexed by the anterior tibialis, and the toes may be extended by the extensor hallucis longus. Range of motion at the ankle may be limited by increased tone in the medial and lateral gastrocnemius.

Treatment of the spasticity in these muscles may allow the foot and toes to be flat during stance phase as well as improve the flexion of the ankle. The use of phenol or botulinum toxin to relax the overactive muscle can improve gait and balance. The relaxation of these tight muscles can allow for improvement in therapy, bracing, or casting.

3. Knee Position

A stiff knee or a leg that is persistently extended can cause problems with fitting into a wheelchair, sitting, or walking. The extension at the knee causes the toe to drag during the swing phase of gait, resulting in frequent falls. The patient may also adapt by changing the position of the hip circumfusing the affected leg. The muscles that are affected in this abnormality include the quadriceps, the iliopsoas, the gluteus maximus and the vastus lateralis, and hamstrings. The exact localization of which muscle is contributing to the stiff knee needs to be based on clinical exam, and EMG may be helpful. Localized chemodenervation to the offending muscle may provide temporary relief. The extent of the spasticity in this muscle suggests that intrathecal baclofen therapy may be helpful.

The persistently flexed knee interferes with walking and wheelchair positioning. The knee remains flexed while walking, limiting speed and causing balance difficulties. The flexed knee is due to tightness in the medial and lateral hamstrings. The resulting crouched gait limits the speed of walking and stride length. Chemodenervation of the hamstrings often allows stretching and casting to provide benefit.

4. Toes

Extension of the great toe is seen in a variety of upper motor neuron lesions. Essentially a persistent Babinski sign, this problem may lead to skin breakdown on top of the toe as well as damage to shoes. It is not uncommon for patients to present with abrasions on the top of the great toe. This problem can easily be treated with an injection of a small amount of botulinum toxin in the extensor hallicus longus. The effect may last for up to 6 months.

The curling of the toes may cause pain and interfere with gait. Toe curling frequently causes the patient to walk on the tips of the toes. The spasms are often too strong or too painful to overcome with bracing or therapy. Injections in the muscle involved with botulinum toxin can frequently quiet these spasms. The flexor digitorum longus is often injected to help this problem.

5. Excessive Hip Flexion

Excessive hip flexion with overactivity in the iliopsoas, rectus femoris, pectineus, adductor longus, and adductor brevis causes the hip to "interfere with advancement of the body over stance phase." A combination of chemodenervation and chemical neurolysis may help relax these muscles. These patients are often candidates for intrathecal baclofen pump placement.

IV. SUMMARY

When accessing and treating a patient with spasticity, regardless of the cause, the physician must have knowledge of the patient's lifestyle and the current disability that the patient faces in his or her day-to-day activities. Although understanding the etiology of the spasticity and its effect on biomechanics is important, nothing can replace talking with the patient and caregiver to determine what issues are interfering with the quality of life of the individual. Increasing resources are available to the physician caring for patients with spasticity, but the appropriate use of these resources for a particular patient still rests with the treating physician.

Although several therapeutic options are available to treat spasticity, efficacy is less than desirable in a significant percentage of patients. The development of additional tools to treat spasticity is heavily dependent on an improved understanding of pathophysiological mechanisms at both the neurophysiological and the molecular level. Animal models have been an indispensable part of spasticity research and will be a vital part of future advances in this important area of neuroscience investigation.

Video Legends

SEGMENT 1 Right spastic hemiparesis secondary to a stroke. Note abnormal wrist, elbow, finger, hip, knee, and ankle flexion. This patient is unable to actively extend, and has difficulty passively extending, the fingers of his right hand. Note the presence of both hip hiking and circumduction during ambulation.

SEGMENT 2 Spastic paraparesis. This patient exhibits prominent spasticity of the thigh adductors and knee flexors. EMG-guided injections of botulinum toxin are being used to treat the spasticity.

SEGMENT 3 Spastic left lower extremity due to a traumatic brain injury. Abnormal plantar flexion and inversion of the foot at the ankle interferes with ambulation. In addition, clonus at the left ankle is readily apparent in latter portions of this segment.

References

Abel, N.A., and R.A. Smith. 1994. Intrathecal baclofen for treatment of intractable spinal spasticity. *Arch Phys Med Rehab* **75**(1):54–58.

Alden, T.D., R.A. Lytle, et al. 2002. Intrathecal baclofen withdrawal: A case report and review of the literature. *Childs Nervous Syst* **18**(9/10):522–525.

Bhakta, B.B. 2000. Management of spasticity in stroke. *Br Med Bull* **56**(2):476–485.

Brashear, A., M.F. Gordon, et al. 2002. Intramuscular injection of botulinum toxin for the treatment of wrist and finger spasticity after a stroke. *N Engl J Med* **347**(6):395–400.

Brin, M.F., and K.R. Aoki. 2002. Botulinum toxin type A: Pharmacology. In *Spasticity: Etiology, Evaluation, Management and the Role of Botulinum Toxin* (N. Mayer and D.M. Simpson, Eds.). WeMove, New York.

Dario, A., M.G. Di Stefano, et al. 2002. Long-term intrathecal baclofen infusion in supraspinal spasticity of adulthood. *Acta Neurol Scand* **105**(2):83–87.

Disabato, J., and A. Ritchie. 2003. Intrathecal baclofen for the treatment of spasticity of cerebral origin. *J Spec Pediatr Nurs* **8**(1):31–34.

Elovic, E. 2001. Principles of pharmaceutical management of spastic hypertonia. *Phys Med Rehab Clin North Am* **12**(4):793–816, vii.

Feldman, R.G., M. Kelly-Hayes, et al. 1978. Baclofen for spasticity in multiple sclerosis. Double-blind crossover and three-year study. *Neurology* **28**(11):1094–1098.

Francisco, G.E. 2001. Intrathecal baclofen therapy for stroke-related spasticity. *Top Stroke Rehab* **8**(1):36–46.

Francisco, G.E., S. Kothari, et al. 2001. GABA agonists and gabapentin for spastic hypertonia. *Phys Med Rehab Clin North Am* **12**(4):875–888, viii.

Gilmartin, R., D. Bruce, et al. 2000. Intrathecal baclofen for management of spastic cerebral palsy: Multicenter trial. *J Child Neurol* **15**(2):71–77.

Goldstein, E.M. 2001. Spasticity management: An overview. *J Child Neurol* **16**:16–23.

Gormley, M.E., Jr., L.E. Krach, et al. 2001. Spasticity management in the child with spastic quadriplegia. *Eur J Neurol* **8**(Suppl. 5):127–135.

Gormley, M.E., Jr., C.F. O'Brien, et al. 1997. A clinical overview of treatment decisions in the management of spasticity. *Muscle Nerve Suppl* **6**:S14–S20.

Gracies, J.M., E. Elovic, et al. 1997. Traditional pharmacological treatments for spasticity. Part I: Local treatments. *Muscle Nerve Suppl* **6**: S61–S91.

Green, L.B., and V.S. Nelson. 1999. Death after acute withdrawal of intrathecal baclofen: Case report and literature review. *Arch Phys Med Rehab* **80**(12):1600–1604.

Hatheway, C.L. 1995. Botulism: The present status of the disease. *Curr Top Microbiol Immunol* **195**:55–75.

Herman, R. 1962. The physiologic basis of tone, spasticity and rigidity. *Arch Phys Med Rehab* **43**:108–114.

Herman, R., W. Freedman, et al. 1974. Neurophysiologic mechanisms of hemiplegic and paraplegic spasticity: Implications for therapy. *Arch Phys Med Rehab* **55**(8):338–343.

Herman, R.M., S.C. D'Luzansky, et al. 1992. Intrathecal baclofen suppresses central pain in patients with spinal lesions. A pilot study. *Clin J Pain* **8**(4):338–345.

Ivanhoe, C.B., A.H. Tilton, et al. 2001. Intrathecal baclofen therapy for spastic hypertonia. *Phys Med Rehab Clin North Am* **12**(4):923–938, viii–ix.

Jankovic, J., S. Leder, et al. 1991. Cervical dystonia: Clinical findings and associated movement disorders. *Neurology* **41**(7):1088–1091.

Jozefczyk, P.B. 2002. The management of focal spasticity. *Clin Neuropharmacol* **25**(3):158–173.

Mayer, N., D.M. Simpson, eds. 2002. *Spasticity: Etiology, Evaluation, Management and the Role of Botulinum Toxin*. WeMove, New York.

McGuire, J.R. 2001. Effective use of chemodenervation and chemical neurolysis in the management of poststroke spasticity. *Top Stroke Rehab* **8**(1):47–55.

Meythaler, J.M., S. Guin-Renfroe, et al. 1999. Continuously infused intrathecal baclofen for spastic/dystonic hemiplegia: A preliminary report. *Am J Phys Med Rehab* **78**(3):247–254.

Meythaler, J.M., S. Guin-Renfroe, et al. 2001. Intrathecal baclofen for spastic hypertonia from stroke. *Stroke* **32**(9):2099–2109.

Penn, R.D., and J.S. Kroin. 1985. Continuous intrathecal baclofen for severe spasticity. *Lancet* **2**(8447):125–127.

Scott, A.B., and S.P. Kraft. 1985. Botulinum toxin injection in the management of lateral rectus paresis. *Ophthalmology* **92**(5):676–683.

Smith, C., G. Birnbaum, et al. 1994. Tizanidine treatment of spasticity caused by multiple sclerosis: Results of a double-blind, placebo-controlled trial. US Tizanidine Study Group. *Neurology* **44**(11, Suppl. 9):S34–S42; discussion S42–S43.

Stien, R., H.J. Nordal, et al. (1987). The treatment of spasticity in multiple sclerosis: A double-blind clinical trial of a new anti-spastic drug tizanidine compared with baclofen. *Acta Neurol Scand* **75**(3):190–194.

Thompson, F.J., R. Parmer, et al. 2001. Scientific basis of spasticity: Insights from a laboratory model. *J Child Neurol* **16**(1):2–9.

CHAPTER

L2

Hereditary Spastic Paraplegia: Clinical Features and Animal Models

SHIRLEY RAINIER and JOHN K. FINK

I. CLINICAL FEATURES AND GENETICS

The hereditary spastic paraplegias (HSPs) are degenerative neurological disorders in which the predominant clinical symptom is lower extremity spastic weakness. Difficulty walking due to weakness and increased muscle tone begins at any age from infancy through late adulthood, usually worsens insidiously, and is often disabling. In "uncomplicated" forms of HSP, spastic weakness is limited to the lower extremities. Upper extremity strength and dexterity are normal in uncomplicated HSP. "Complicated" or "syndromic" forms of HSP are those inherited disorders in which the predominant symptom of lower extremity spasticity is accompanied by additional neurologic abnormalities (e.g., deafness, mental retardation, peripheral neuropathy, and ataxia) or systemic disorders (e.g., cataracts and gastroesophageal reflux). Dominant, recessive, and X-linked forms of HSP are each genetically heterogeneous. Genetic loci (designated SPG) have been identified for 10 autosomal dominant, 8 autosomal recessive, and 3 X-linked forms of HSP [1,2]. The principal pathologic finding in uncomplicated HSP is axonal degeneration involving corticospinal tracts and, to a lesser extent, fasciculus gracilus fibers. Degeneration is maximal at the ends of these fibers. The HSPs share the feature of corticospinal tract axon degeneration in the spinal cord with related motor neuron disorders, amyotrophic lateral sclerosis and primary lateral sclerosis (see Fink [1] for HSP review and additional references).

Rather than being a single disease per se, HSP represents a clinicopathologic syndrome of gait disturbance and lower extremity spastic weakness due to corticospinal tract and, to a lesser extent, dorsal column degeneration (or abnormal development in the case of SPG1 HSP, discussed later). As with any large group of genetically heterogeneous clinicopathologic syndromes, the HSPs have significant clinical variability. Although each of the more than 20 genetic types of HSP is due to mutation in a different gene and therefore etiologically distinct, genetically diverse types of HSP are often extremely similar. This is particularly true of the uncomplicated or nonsyndromic forms of HSP, in which different genetic types often cannot be distinguished by age of symptom onset or severity. In contrast, complicated HSP syndromes often can be recognized by the presence of additional neurologic signs. For example, Troyer syndrome (due to SPG20/spartin mutations), Silver syndrome (due to SPG17/BSCL2 mutations), and SPG9 HSP are associated with distal muscle wasting. SPG7 HSP, due to paraplegin gene mutations discussed later, may be either uncomplicated or complicated by the presence of mitochondrial abnormalities on skeletal muscle biopsy and dysarthria, dysphagia, optic disc pallor, axonal neuropathy, and evidence of "vascular lesions," cerebellar atrophy, or cerebral atrophy on cranial MRI [3]. Thin corpus callosum and mental retardation are common in SPG11 HSP, considered to be the most common type of recessively inherited HSP.

Ten HSP genes have been discovered [1,4,5]. Evidence on the function of some of these genes suggests that several different biochemical processes underlie diverse types of HSP. For example, primary mitochondrial disturbance appears to underlie both autosomal recessive SPG7 HSP and autosomal dominant SPG13 HSP, both of which are due to mutations in nuclear-encoded mitochondrial proteins (SPG7/paraplegin and SPG13/chaperonin 60, respectively). X-linked SPG2 HSP due to mutations in the intrinsic myelin protein proteolipid protein (PLP) is an example in which axonal degeneration is secondary to a glial abnormality (see discussion of PLP mice). SPG1 HSP due to L1 cell adhesion molecule mutation is an example in which the HSP phenotype is due to developmental disturbance in corticospinal tract development rather than corticospinal tract degeneration.

Evidence indicates that disturbance in the axonal cytoskeleton and axonal transport system underlies a number of different genetic types of HSP. The strongest evidence for this comes from the observation that mutations in kinesin heavy chain 5A (KIF5A) cause autosomal dominant HSP (SPG10) [6]. KIF5A is a component of the molecular motor critical for axonal transport. It is notable that mutations in two other "motor proteins" also cause degeneration of distal axons in two other neurologic disorders. Kinesin light chain (KIF1B) mutations cause peripheral axon degeneration in Charcot-Marie-Tooth type 2A [7]. Furthermore, dynactin mutations result in axonal degeneration of corticospinal tracts in one form of autosomal dominant amyotrophic lateral sclerosis [8]. These findings indicate that axonal transport disturbance is one cause of degeneration of distal axons that occurs in a number of diseases. Although controversial, there is evidence that the most common type of dominantly inherited HSP (due to SPG4/spastin gene mutation) also involves disturbance in microtubule-mediated axonal transport [9]. Spastin shares some protein homology with katanin, a microtubule-severing protein. Although spastin localization is controversial, evidence from cell transfection studies suggests that spastin is distributed in the cytoplasm and interacts with microtubules, and that HSP-specific SPG4/spastin mutations result in altered microtubule distribution and aberrant localization of organelles including mitochondria [10].

II. MOUSE MODELS OF HSP

There has been significant progress toward creating animal models of HSP. The greatest progress has been achieved for two forms of complicated HSP due to L1 CAM and PLP gene mutations. Development of animal models for the most common dominant form of HSP (due to SPG4/spastin mutation) and for recessive HSP due to SPG7/paraplegin gene mutation has been reported only as preliminary findings [11,12].

A. Uncomplicated HSP

1. SPG4/spastin Knockout Mice

As noted previously, SPG4/spastin mutations are the most common cause of autosomal dominant, uncomplicated HSP and are responsible for ~40% of such cases. Fassier et al. [11] reported preliminary studies of SPG4/spastin gene knockout mice. The *Cre/LoxP* gene targeting vector was used to create mice in which SPG4/spastin exons 5–7 were deleted and replaced by the inserting vector. By crossing mice that were heterozygous for this mutation ($Sp^{del/+}$) with either CMV-Cre transgenic mice or NSE-Cre transgenic animals, mice were created in which the deleted spastin gene was present in all tissues ($Sp^{del/+}$/CMV-Cre mice) or only in neurons ($Sp^{del/+}$/NSE-Cre mice). In preliminary analysis, some $Sp^{del/+}$ mice exhibited impaired rotarod performance compared to normal littermates. This phenotype was highly variable, however, indicating the importance of modifying genetic factors. In unpublished studies, we observed a similar phenotype in SPG4/spastin gene knockout mice bearing heterozygous deletion of exons 7 and 8 (Fink et al., unpublished observations). Preliminary observations of these animals revealed age-dependent gait disturbance due to impaired hindlimb locomotor ability. These deficits were observed in both open-field assessment and rotarod performance. SPG4/spastin knockout mice older than 1 year exhibit a tendency to walk with hindlimbs externally rotated and often demonstrate impaired trunk control, tail dragging, intermittent "scooting" (dragging the hindquarters instead of hindlimb stepping), or "hopping" (instead of hindlimb stepping). If confirmed, these preliminary studies indicate that SPG4/spastin gene disruption in mice results in hindlimb locomotor impairment. Whether this will prove to be a useful model in which to explore SPG4/spastin mutation pathogenesis and HSP treatment remains to be determined.

2. SPG7/paraplegin Knockout Mice

Ferreirinha et al. [12] reported preliminary studies in homozygous SPG7/paraplegin knockout mice. These animals displayed impaired performance on rotarod apparatus starting at age 6 months and worsening with age. Spinal cord histology showed axonal swellings more prominent in the lateral columns of the lumbar spinal cord, consistent with a retrograde axonopathy. This phenotype was slowly progressive, with signs of axonal degeneration becoming prominent at 12 months of age. Changes in mitochondrial morphology appeared to precede axonal changes in this system, suggesting that degeneration is due to impaired mitochondrial function. This preliminary study therefore suggests that SPG7/paraplegin gene disruption in mice recapitulates the histologic and, to a lesser extent, the locomotor disturbance of humans with SPG7 HSP.

B. Complicated HSP

1. SPG2/PLP Mutation Mice

As noted previously, PLP is an intrinsic myelin protein [13,14]. PLP gene mutations cause both Pelizaeus-Merzbacher disease (PMD), an X-linked leukodystrophy, and X-linked HSP (SPG2). To some extent, the phenotype depends on the nature of the PLP gene mutation. Although severe disease (PMD leukodystrophy) is usually caused by increased expression of PLP due to gene duplication, a number of PLP point mutations have also been shown to cause PMD. The observation that PMD, leukodystrophy, and X-linked HSP have occurred in individuals from the same family who share the same PLP gene mutation indicates the impact of modifying genes and potentially environmental factors. There are naturally occurring mouse models containing PLP mutations (*jimpy(jp)*, *jimpy-4J*, *msd*, and *rumpshaker*), as well as PLP null mice in which the PLP gene has been disrupted by gene targeting. It is important to note that the phenotype of these animals often depends on the particular mutation and genetic background [15]. Depending on the particular mutation, PLP missense mutations and aberrant mRNA splicing mutations result in severe hypomyelination and early death [16–20] or simply tremor and normal life span [21]. In contrast, mice in which the PLP gene has been disrupted by gene targeting display length-dependent axon degeneration that is similar to that of patients lacking PLP. These studies demonstrate (i) that genetic background (e.g., the impact of modifying genes) influences the PLP gene mutation phenotype, (ii) that PLP gene mutations can cause either hypomyelination or primary axonal degeneration, and (iii) that axonal degeneration in HSP may arise from a primary glial (oligodendroglia in this case) abnormality.

2. SPG1/L1 CAM Knockout Mice

Mutations in L1 CAM cause X-linked CRASH syndrome (corpus callosum hypoplasia, retardation, adducted thumbs, spastic paraplegia, and hydrocephalus), MASA syndrome (mental retardation, aphasia, shuffling gait, and adducted thumbs), and X-linked hydrocephalus associated with spastic paraplegia. Two different L1 CAM knockout mice have been studied. One was produced by inserting a Tkneo cassette into L1 CAM exon 8 [22]. This resulted in L1 CAM protein of reduced size and quantity. In addition to hindlimb motor impairment (when walking on or hanging from a metal grid), these mice were less sensitive to noxious stimuli compared to control animals. Histologic analysis of these mice revealed reduced size of the corticospinal tracts compared to normal controls.

The second L1 CAM knockout mouse [23] was produced by replacing L1 CAM exons 13 and 14 with the neomycin resistance gene cassette. This resulted in the complete absence of L1 CAM protein in these animals. These animals demonstrated a number of brain defects, including reduced size of the corpus callosum and hippocampus, enlarged ventricles, septal abnormalities, and abnormal migration of mesencephalic dopamine neurons [24,25]. These results provide evidence that L1 CAM plays an important role in brain development, particularly that of the corticospinal tracts and the migration of dopamine neurons. Furthermore, studies of L1 CAM mutations in humans and mice illustrate that the HSP syndrome may be caused by developmental disturbance of corticospinal tract formation rather than corticospinal tract degeneration.

III. SUMMARY

Clinical syndromes in which the principal feature is motor neuron degeneration are extremely diverse. Such syndromes include essentially pure upper motor neuron degeneration (degeneration of cortical motor neurons and corticobulbar and corticospinal tracts in primary lateral sclerosis), relatively isolated degeneration of anterior horn cells (spinal muscular atrophies), combined degeneration of corticospinal tracts and anterior horn cells (amyotrophic lateral sclerosis), and combined degeneration of corticospinal tracts and dorsal column fibers (the hereditary spastic paraplegias and Friedreich ataxia). The identification of genes for many of these disorders has greatly advanced our knowledge of their underlying pathophysiology. The usefulness of mouse models for these diseases depends on the extent to which they recapitulate the behavioral, histologic, and molecular pathophysiology of the human disorder. A variety of animal models of motor neuron disease have been created successfully. These include mouse models of motor neuron disease, such as *SOD1* transgenic mice, androgen receptor transgenic mice, dynein knockout mice, and survival motor neuron knockout mice, and models of HSP, such as L1 CAM knockout and PLP transgenic and gene knockout mice. The usefulness of animal models of HSP, such as SPG4/spastin and SPG7/paraplegin gene knockouts, is not known. It is hoped that such animals will develop behavioral and neuropathologic features of HSP and serve as useful resources in which to explore potential treatments.

Acknowledgments

This research was supported by grants from the Veterans Affairs Merit Review, the National Institutes of Health (NINDS R01NS33645, R01NS36177, and R01NS38713), and the Spastic Paraplegia Foundation to J.K.F.

References

1. Fink, J.K. 2003. Hereditary spastic paraplegia: Nine genes and counting. *Arch Neurol* **60**:1045–1049.
2. Blumen, S.C., S. Bevan, S. Abu-Mouch, D. Negus, M. Kahana, and R. Inzelberg, et al. 2004. A locus for complicated hereditary spastic paraplegia maps to chromosome 1q24–q32. *Ann Neurol* **54**:796–803.
3. Casari, G., M. DeFusco, S. Ciarmatori, M. Zeviani, P. Fernandez, M. Mora, G. DeMichele, A. Filla, S. Cocozza, R. Marconi, A. Durr, B. Fontaine, and A. Ballabio. 1998. Paraplegin, a nuclear-encoded mitochondrial ATPase, mutated in pure and complicated forms of hereditary spastic paraplegia. *Cell* **93**:973–983.
4. Windpassinger, C., M. Auer-Grumbach, J. Irobi, H. Patel, E. Petek, G. Horl, R. Malli, J.A. Reed, I. Dierick, N. Verpoorten, T.T. Warner, C. Proukakis, P. VandenBergh, C. Verellen, L. VanMaldergem, L. Merlini, P. DeJonge, V. Timmerman, A.H. Crosby, and K. Wagner. 2004. Heterozygous missense mutations in BSCL2 are associated with distal hereditary motor neuropathy and Silver syndrome. *Nature Genet* **36**:271–276.
5. Simpson, M.A., H. Cross, C. Proukakis, A. Pryde, R. Hershberger, A. Chatonnet, M.A. Patton, and A.H. Crosby. 2003. Maspardin is mutated in Mast syndrome, a complicated form of hereditary spastic paraplegia associated with dementia. *Am J Hum Genet* **73**:1147–1156.
6. Reid, E., M. Kloos, A. Ashley-Koch, L. Hughes, S. Bevan, I.K. Svenson, F.L. Graham, P.C. Gaskell, A. Dearlove, M.A. Pericak-Vance, D.C. Rubinsztein, and D.A. Marchuk. 2002. A kinesin heavy chain (KIF5A) mutation in hereditary spastic paraplegia (SPG10). *Am J Hum Genet* **71**:1189–1194.
7. Zhao, C., J. Takita, Y. Tanaka, M. Setou, T. Nakagawa, S. Takeda, H.W. Yang, S. Terada, T. Nakata, Y. Takei, M. Saito, S. Tsuji, Y. Hayashi, and N. Hirokawa. 2001. Charcot–Marie–Tooth disease type 2A caused by mutation in a microtubule motor KIF1B-beta. *Cell* **105**:587–597.
8. Puls, I., C. Jonnakuty, B.H. LaMonte, E.L. Holzbaur, M. Tokito, E. Mann, M.K. Floeter, K. Bidus, D. Drayna, S.J. Oh, R.H. Brown, Jr., C.L. Ludlow, and K.H. Fischbeck. 2003. Mutant dynactin in motor neuron disease. *Nature Genet* **33**:455–456.
9. Fink, J.K., and S. Rainier. 2004. Hereditary spastic paraplegia: Spastin phenotype and function. *Arch Neurol* **61(6)**:830–833.
10. McDermott, C.J., A.J. Grierson, J.D. Wood, M. Bingley, S.B. Wharton, K.M. Bushby, and P.J. Shaw. 2003. Hereditary spastic paraparesis: Disrupted intracellular transport associated with spastin mutation. *Ann Neurol* **54**:748–759.
11. Fassier, C., A. Tarrade, D. Charvin, et al. 2003. Generation and characterization of mouse models of spastic paraplegia caused by mutation of SPG4 gene. *Am J Hum Genet* **73**:547–547. [Abstract]
12. Ferreirinha, F., A. Quattrini, V. Valsecchi, A. Errico, A. Ballabio, and E.I. Rugarli. 2001. Mice lacking paraplegin, a mitochondrial AAA protease involved in hereditary spastin paraplegia, show axonal degeneration and abnormal mitochondria. *Am J Hum Genet* **69**(Suppl.):196. [Abstract]
13. Hudson, L.D., J.A. Berndt, C. Puckett, C.A. Kozak, and R.A. Lazzarini. 1987. Aberrant splicing of proteolipid protein mRNA in the dysmyelinating jimpy mutant mouse. *Proc Natl Acad Sci U S A* **84**:1454–1458.
14. Dautigny, A., M.-G. Mattei, D. Morello, P.M. Alliel, D. Pham-Dinh, L. Amar, D. Arnaud, D. Simon, J.-F. Mattei, J.-L. Guenet, and P. Avner. 1986. The structural gene coding for myelin-associated proteolipid protein is mutated in jimpy mice. *Nature* 321:867–869.
15. Al-Saktawi, K., M. McLaughlin, M. Klugmann, et al. 2003. Genetic background determines phenotypic severity of the Plp rumpshaker mutation. *J Neurosci Res* **72**:12–24. [Abstract]
16. Nave, K.A., F.E. Bloom, and R.J. Milner. 1987. A single nucleotide difference in the gene for myelin proteolipid protein defines the jimpy mutation in mouse. *J Neurochem* **49**:1873–1877.
17. Pearsall, G.B., N.L. Nadon, M.K. Wolf, and S. Billings-Gagliardi. 1997. Jimpy-4J mouse has a missense mutation in exon 2 of the Plp gene. *Dev Neurosci* **19**:337–341.
18. Gencic, S., and L.D. Hudson. 1990. Conservative amino acid substitution in the myelin proteolipid protein of jimpy msd mice. *J Neurosci* **10**:117–124.
19. Schneider, A., P. Montague, I. Griffiths, M. Fanarraga, P. Kennedy, P. Brophy, and K.A. Nave. 1992. Uncoupling of hypomyelination and glial cell death by a mutation in the proteolipid protein gene. *Nature* **358**:758–761.
20. Thomson, C.E., T.J. Anderson, M.C. McCulloch, P. Dickinson, D.A. Vouyiouklis, and I.R. Griffiths. 1999. The early phenotype associated with the jimpy mutation of the proteolipid protein gene. *J Neurocytol* **28**:207–221.
21. Griffiths, I.R., I. Scott, M.C. McCulloch, J.A. Barrie, K. McPhilemy, and B.M. Cattanach. 1990. Rumpshaker mouse: A new X-linked mutation affecting myelination: Evidence for a defect in PLP expression. *J Neurocytol* **19**:273–283.
22. Dahme, M., U. Bartsch, R. Martini, B. Anliker, M. Schachner, and N. Mantei. 1997. Disruption of the mouse L1 gene leads to malformations of the nervous system. *Nature Genet* **17**:346–349.
23. Cohen, N.R., J.S. Taylor, L.B. Scott, R.W. Guillery, P. Soriano, and A.J. Furley. 1998. Errors in corticospinal axon guidance in mice lacking the neural cell adhesion molecule L1. *Curr Biol* **8**:26–33.
24. Demyanenko, G.P., A.Y. Tsai, and P.F. Maness. 1999. Abnormalities in neuronal process extension, hippocampal development, and the ventricular system of L1 knockout mice. *J Neurosci* **19**:4907–4920.
25. Demyanenko, G.P., Y. Shibata, and P.F. Maness. 2001. Altered distribution of dopaminergic neurons in the brain in L1 null mice. *Brain Res Dev Brain Res* **126**:21–30.

CHAPTER

L3

The Spastic Rat with Sacral Spinal Cord Injury

PHILIP J. HARVEY, MONICA GORASSINI, and DAVID J. BENNETT

I. INTRODUCTION

Although the spasticity that follows spinal cord injury in humans is common, it has been difficult to study experimentally since spinal cord injury in animals produces only comparatively mild spasticity (Taylor et al., 1997; Noth, 1991; Powers and Rymer, 1988; Ashby and McCrea, 1987; Hultborn and Malmsten, 1983). Spasticity occurs in humans without complete spinal cord transections, whereas in animals such as rats and cats, incomplete spinal cord injury only leads to mild hyperreflexia (Hultborn and Malmsten, 1983). Complete spinal transections (e.g., T12 cut) in cats have led to spasticity in some studies (Ashby and McCrea, 1987; Naftchi et al., 1979). However, these cats have inconvenient and traumatic functional impairments, requiring twice-daily bladder and bowel expression. Bladder infection, pressure sores, and impaired locomotion can lead to significant morbidity and mortality. Thus, the complete spinal cat is an impractical model, and many groups have used hemisections, partial transections, and contusions (Thompson et al., 1993; Ashby and McCrea, 1987) to study spinal cord injury, even though spasticity is not always prominent.

Development of a tail model of spasticity originated with Ritz and coworkers (1992). Ritz's group found that low sacrocaudal transections or contusions in cats cause pronounced spasticity in the axial musculature of the tail vertebrae without disrupting bladder, bowel, or normal hindlimb locomotor function. Although the study of axial musculature has been relatively neglected in general, it is involved in spasticity in humans (cf. back muscles; Stauffer, 1974) and should therefore be considered relevant to the spastic syndrome. The tail is normally used in a well-coordinated fashion during locomotion, hovering off the ground and bending to guide turning. Thus, straightforward observations of tail function can be used to assess motor recovery after spinal cord injury and following interventions that may promote recovery of function (Ritz et al., 1992).

We investigated sacral spinal cord lesions in rats (Bennett et al., 1999) and found that a spastic syndrome develops in rats similar to that in cats (Ritz et al., 1992). However, unlike in cats, we found that the awake rats tolerate prolonged examinations of the tail for spasticity assessment, including muscle stretching, surface electromyography (EMG) recording, and Hoffman reflex (H-reflex) testing with tail nerve stimulation. Our chronic recording techniques were motivated by a simple awake rat preparation developed by Steg (1964) involving the small but accessible segmental muscles of the tail. Thus, in awake rats, we have been able to repeat many of the traditional measurements made in spinal cord-injured humans. More important, the sacrocaudal spinal cord of the adult rat is small enough to remove and maintain whole *in vitro*, allowing for prolonged recordings of ventral root responses to dorsal root stimulation and intracellular recordings of sacrocaudal motoneurons with dendritic trees and all synaptic connections still intact.

II. ASSESSMENT OF SPASTICITY IN AWAKE RATS

Following spinal cord injury (SCI), exaggerated reflexes and muscle tone often emerge that contribute to a general spasticity syndrome in humans (Young, 1994; Noth, 1991; Ashby and McCrea, 1987; Kuhn and Macht, 1948). A central complaint of patients with spasticity involves intense muscle contractions lasting for many seconds, which are triggered by numerous stimuli, including muscle stretch, vibrations, light touch, heat, and/or cold. These uncontrolled spasms develop in the weeks to months following SCI and can be quite debilitating and painful, interfering with normal activities and potential recovery of function through locomotor training (Norman et al., 1998; Kuhn and Macht, 1948). Because of this, muscle spasms may be considered the main disruptive characteristic of the SCI spastic syndrome. The traditional definition of a velocity-dependent increase in tonic stretch reflexes (Lance, 1980) is far more prominent following stroke than following SCI, and it seems to be used in spinal spasticity more for convenience of measuring electrophysiologically.

Similar symptoms of spasticity develop over the same time course in animals (Bennett et al., 1999; Taylor et al., 1997). This is seen in the tail musculature of rats following complete transection at the S2 level of the spinal cord (Bennett et al., 1999; Ashby and McCrea, 1987). These symptoms include most notably hypertonus, hyperreflexia, and flexor/extensor spasms. Since many of the reflexes occur in the ventroflexion direction, it is convenient for study to elevate the rat and to have its tail hang freely. The rat is placed in a Plexiglas tube, adjusted to its body length, so that the full length of the tail hangs out the back of the tube. The most effective method of initiating tail muscle spasms in chronic spinal rats is to hold the base of the tail with one hand and simultaneously stretch and rub the tail by rapidly sliding the other hand down the length of the tail with a firm grip between the thumb and fingers. Normal intact rats either do not respond to this stimulation or respond with a slight flexion (20–30° bend) that lasts only 2 or 3 sec, and then the tail resumes its downward vertical position (Video Segment 1). In all chronic spinal rats (>14 days postoperatively), the stretch/rub maneuver elicits an uncoordinated ventral flexion movement, which we refer to as a flexor spasm (Video Segment 2). That is, the tail does not move in a smooth arc as in normal rats but coils with jerky movements, with the tip often rotating more than 360° (mean tip excursion, 242 ± 51° in chronic spinal rats compared to 45 ± 34° in normals). Such flexion reflexes are initiated with the same latency as normals, but the flexion that they produce lasts for minutes rather than seconds. Flexion spasms also occur spontaneously without apparent stimulation. Repeated stimulation (three stretch maneuvers applied in rapid succession) gives more muscle activity, which can last for >30 min and includes marked hypertonus interrupted by frequent flexion spasms. With time (>2 months), these spasms become more severe, lasting for longer durations to lesser stimulations. Extensor activity is incorporated into the syndrome, leading to marked increases in muscle tone from combined flexor and extensor hypertonus. In severely spastic animals, rapidly alternating left and right flexor spasms results in writhing movements of the tail in response to a single tail swipe. These conditions persist for as long as we have kept our animals (up to 14 months). Morbidity consists of lesions forming on the tail (10%), likely resulting from pressure sores or urine rash because the animal has no sensation of these injuries. If the lesions become overly extensive, or autotomy develops, the animal must be euthanized (3% of all animals).

Spasms in humans can be measured and quantified using single motor unit and gross EMG recordings in the leg muscles of a SCI subject (Figure 1). The spasm is evoked by

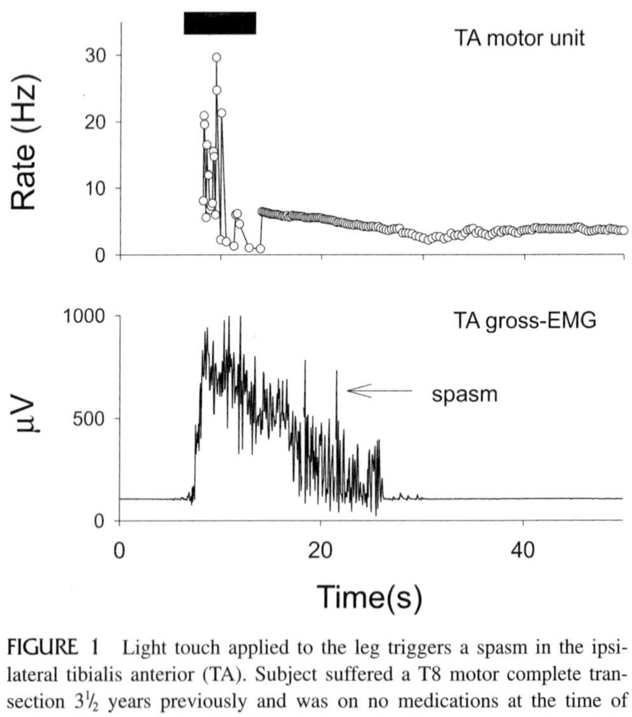

FIGURE 1 Light touch applied to the leg triggers a spasm in the ipsilateral tibialis anterior (TA). Subject suffered a T8 motor complete transection $3\frac{1}{2}$ years previously and was on no medications at the time of testing. The stimulation (black bar) triggered an intense contraction of the TA muscle, lasting >10 sec, as seen in the gross EMG trace at the bottom. The top trace shows continuous regular firing of a single TA motor unit long after the stimulus has ended.

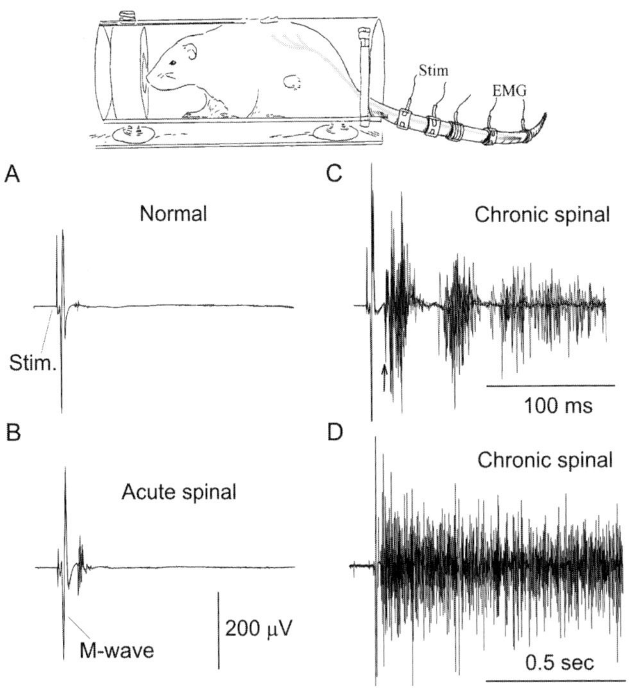

FIGURE 2 Reflexes in awake normal, acute, and spastic rats are tested by housing the animal in a small tube with the tail hanging freely from the end. Custom-built stimulating and recording cuff electrodes are placed over the segmental muscles as shown. (A) In normal rats, stimulation of the caudal nerve trunk triggers an M-wave and a small polysynaptic response. (B) Acutely spinalized animals (<48 hr) have larger polysynaptic latency reflexes, likely resulting from a loss of descending inhibition, but no long-lasting reflexes. (C and D) In contrast, chronic spinal rats demonstrate long-lasting EMG activity in the tail musculature after a single stimulation.

a light cutaneous stimulation that would not provoke any response in intact subjects. With injury, however, the affected motor units can continue to discharge for tens of seconds at a regular and sustained rate, and this is reflected in tonic activity of the corresponding muscle EMG. Similar measurements of EMG activity in response to stimulation can be performed in the rat tail muscles. Normally, distal tail muscles show little response to proximal stimulation (Figure 2A). However, in the weeks following complete transection of the spinal cord at the S2 level, tail EMG exhibits a prolonged tonic discharge that can last for many seconds (Figures 2C and 2D). In contrast, this long-lasting reflex is not seen in the days immediately following injury (Figure 2B).

III. *IN VITRO* ASSESSMENT OF SPASTIC REFLEXES

The whole sacrocaudal cord of adult chronic or acute spinal rats can be removed and maintained *in vitro* in artificial cerebrospinal fluid (aCSF) (Bennett et al., 2001; Long et al., 1988). Spinal cords of normal rats are transected immediately prior to removal from the animal. Once in the dish, the dorsal and ventral S4 and Co1 roots are separated and mounted on hook electrodes for stimulation and recording (Figure 3A). Acutely isolated sacrocaudal ventral roots will exhibit only a short-latency mono- and/or polysynaptic reflex in response to a single stimulation of a dorsal root (Figure 3B). Reflex pathways in isolated spinal cords have lost the normal brain stem innervation supplying monoamine neuromodulators that influence the strength of polysynaptic connections (Jankowska, 1992; Engberg et al., 1968) and motoneuron excitability (Powers and Binder, 2001; Rekling et al., 2000; Heckman and Lee, 1999). Addition of neuromodulators, such as serotonin (5-HT), metabotropic glutamate receptor agonists, or muscarine, is required to induce a long-lasting reflex in acute spinal preparations and will also produce a tonic level of background activity (data not shown). In contrast, sacrocaudal cords of chronic spinal rats, removed after 2 months postinjury, produce long-lasting ventral root discharges in response to a single stimulation of a dorsal root without the addition of any neuromodulators to the aCSF (Figures 2C and 2D). Often, there is also a continuous level of background activity from one or more motoneurons without any stimulation.

Such long-lasting reflexes may have numerous potential causes, including loss of inhibition from descending and segmental pathways (Thompson et al., 1998; Heckman, 1994; Mailis and Ashby, 1990; Cavallari and Pettersson, 1989), neuronal sprouting (Krenz and Weaver, 1998), and direct changes in intrinsic properties of spinal motoneurons (Eken et al., 1989). Root reflex recordings are limited in that they do not indicate whether the spasticity following SCI results from changes in local circuitry leading to prolonged activation of motoneurons, or whether the changes are in the intrinsic properties of the motoneurons. Correspondingly, pharmacological manipulations of the ventral root discharge may be acting postsynaptically (directly affecting the motoneurons) or altering the presynaptic reflex pathways. As such, there is an impetus to isolating and studying individual components of the reflex pathway with intracellular recordings. We have been focusing on the role of motoneurons in the development of spinal spasticity.

IV. INTRACELLULAR MOTONEURON RECORDINGS

The possibility that the intrinsic properties of spinal motoneurons change with spinal cord injury is consistent with data from motor unit firing in humans and animals after injury, including sustained poorly modulated discharges (Gorassini et al., 1999; Thomas and Ross, 1997), unusually low minimum firing rates (Thomas and Ross, 1997; Carp et al., 1991; Powers and Rymer, 1988), and generally

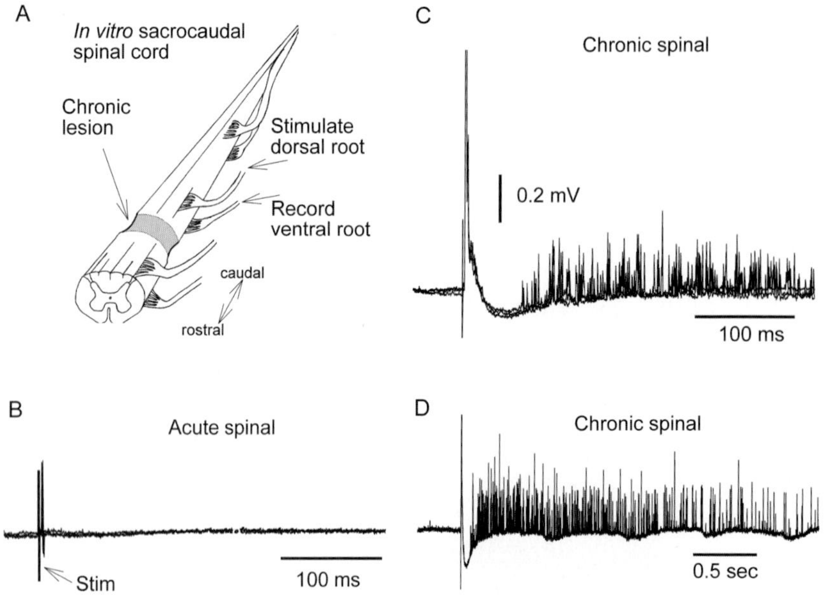

FIGURE 3 The rat sacrocaudal spinal cord is small enough to remove and maintain *in vitro* (A). Comparable responses to those seen in Figure 2 are observed by stimulating dorsal roots and recording from ventral roots. A single dorsal root stimulation at 10 times threshold triggers a long-lasting ventral root discharge lasting for several seconds (C and D), whereas with acute spinal preparations there are only short-lasting polysynaptic reflexes (B).

inefficient control of firing rate in force production (Wiegner et al., 1993; Blaschak et al., 1988). Although motoneurons usually fire in proportion to their net excitatory input, their response can also be altered substantially by numerous voltage-dependent currents intrinsic to the motoneuron membrane (Russo and Hounsgaard, 1999; Binder et al., 1996). For example, voltage-dependent persistent inward currents (PICs) can occasionally be activated by a brief stimulus and regeneratively cause sustained depolarizations (i.e., plateau potentials; abbr. plateaus) and firing (Bennett et al., 1998a,b; Hounsgaard and Kiehn, 1989; Schwindt and Crill, 1984). Persistent inward currents are likely present in most motoneurons but are only manifested as plateaus when they are directly facilitated or uncovered by reducing opposing outward currents (e.g., Ca-dependent K current), both of which may occur with extrinsically administered 5-HT (Russo and Hounsgaard, 1999; Hultborn and Kiehn, 1992). The PIC responsible for plateaus is often mediated by low-threshold L-type calcium channels (Hounsgaard and Kiehn, 1989), although any relatively long-lasting voltage-gated inward current may also be involved, including persistent sodium currents (Schwindt and Crill, 1995) and ligand-gated currents from NMDA receptors (Guertin and Hounsgaard, 1998; Kiehn et al., 1996; Hochman and McCrea, 1994).

The existence of plateaus in motoneurons appears to normally require monoaminergic facilitation from the brain stem [5-HT and noradrenaline (NA)]. That is, plateaus occur in brain stem-intact decerebrate cats, are largely eliminated by acute spinalization, and return with application of monoaminergic drugs (Hounsgaard et al., 1988; Conway et al., 1988). Because there are few sources of 5-HT or NA within the spinal cord below a chronic spinal transection (except perhaps related to the autonomic or circulatory systems) (Newton and Hamill, 1988; McNicholas et al., 1980), it may seem unlikely that plateaus mediated by monoamines could reemerge with long-term complete spinal cord transection. However, because the PICs and plateaus are mediated by various other neuromodulators (metabotropic receptor activation via substance P, acetylcholine, and glutamate) (Russo and Hounsgaard, 1999; Russo et al., 1997), and spinal reflexes develop a supersensitivity to residual levels of 5-HT following chronic SCI (Barbeau and Rossignol, 1990; Nagano et al., 1988; Tremblay et al., 1985; Barbeau and Bedard, 1981), plateaus may still play a role in chronic injury. Indeed, the similarity of the long-lasting reflexes in the chronic spinal cat to the tonic stretch reflex in the decerebrate cat led Hultborn's group to propose that both are mediated by plateaus on motoneurons (Nielsen and Hultborn, 1993; Eken et al., 1989).

The sacrocaudal motoneurons are quite close to the ventral surface (60–200 μm) and can remain well oxy-

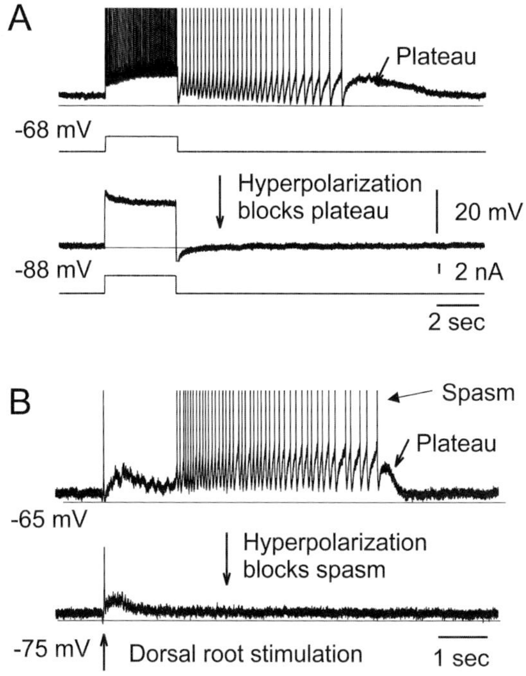

FIGURE 4 Sharp intracellular recordings from sacrocaudal motoneurons demonstrate the postsynaptic origin of the long-lasting reflexes that produce muscle spasms in spasticity. (A) A depolarizing step activates a plateau potential (see text) in a chronic spinal motoneuron, which remains activated for several seconds after returning to the baseline bias current. The cell continues to fire without the step current injection as the membrane is slow to return to resting potential. As the spikes inactivate the underlying plateau potential is observed. With a hyperpolarizing bias current, a step of the same amplitude is insufficient to activate the plateau; thus, plateau potentials are voltage-dependent properties intrinsic to the motoneurons. (B) A single dorsal root stimulation evokes a long-duration pEPSP, which depolarizes the motoneuron membrane sufficiently to trigger a plateau and self-sustained firing. This self-sustained firing maintains the spasms observed in awake rats in response to afferent input. With hyperpolarization, the pEPSP that would trigger the plateau is still present, but the plateau and resulting spasm are blocked.

genated and viable for more than 18 hr *in vitro*. Penetration of the pia and white matter requires the use of blind recordings with sharp intracellular electrodes because patch electrodes would block up too easily. Penetrated cells are identified as motoneurons by an antidromic action potential in response to ventral root stimulation. Intracellular current injections were used to analyze the firing. In most motoneurons of acutely isolated sacrocaudal spinal cord in normal aCSF, there is no evidence of plateau activation. A brief intracellular current pulse does not trigger a sustained depolarization, nor does stimulation of a dorsal root produce a long-lasting discharge (data not shown). In contrast, brief intracellular pulses injected into chronic spinal rat motoneurons produce a sustained depolarization and afterdischarge (plateau potential) lasting many seconds (Figure 4A). The fact that hyperpolarization blocks plateau activation (Figure 4A, lower trace) is indicative of a postsynaptic voltage-sensitive process. Similarly, dorsal root stimulation produces a long (>200 msec) polysynaptic excitatory postsynaptic potential (pEPSP) that triggers a plateau, whereas when the motoneuron is hyperpolarized the pEPSP is of insufficient amplitude to trigger a long-lasting afterdischarge (Figure 4B). Thus, synaptic or intracellular current inputs serve to raise the membrane potential to the voltage threshold of the plateau and trigger an afterdischarge resulting in a muscle spasm. These long-duration polysynaptic reflexes/EPSPs are not observed in normal intact motoneurons due to descending inhibition of segmental reflexes (Clarke et al., 2002; Thompson et al., 1992; Jankowska, 1992), but they are present in both acute and chronic spinal transected cats (Baker and Chandler, 1987). By themselves, they are of insufficient duration to maintain the long-lasting motoneuron discharges seen in our chronic spinal rats; however, they can depolarize the motoneuron sufficiently to trigger the voltage-dependent persistent inward currents that sustain the spasm. Thus, all evidence points to a postsynaptically mediated source of the spasms resulting from the development of plateau potentials in motoneurons, despite the absence of descending brain stem innervation.

V. SUMMARY

By using sacral spinal cord lesions in rats, we have developed a model of spasticity that is convenient to study in the awake state and requires minimal care (i.e., does not affect normal bladder and bowel function or locomotion). Furthermore, the small diameter of the spinal cord at this level allows for electrophysiological study of adult spastic motoneurons and reflexes *in vitro*. This preparation has been central to our understanding of how plateau potentials lead to the intense muscle spasms characteristic of spinal spasticity. Ongoing experiments are elucidating the underlying currents associated with plateaus and which neuromodulators are involved in the development of these plateaus in the months following injury. Results from this model of spinal spasticity have correlates in human SCI subjects suffering from spasticity (Gorassini et al., 2003; Collins et al., 2002; Kiehn and Eken, 1997), which support the validity of the chronic spinal rat model.

Video Legends

SEGMENT 1 Response of a normal rat to the stretch/rub maneuver. After slight flexion (20–30 degree bend) which only lasts for 2–3 seconds, the tail resumes its downward vertical position.

SEGMENT 2 In chronic spinal rats (>14 days post-operatively), the stretch/rub maneuver elicits uncoordinated ventral flexion movements referred to as flexor spasms.

References

Ashby, P., and D.A. McCrea. 1987. Neurophysiology of spinal spasticity. In *Handbook of the Spinal Cord* (R.A. Davidoff, Ed.), pp. 120–143. Dekker, New York.

Baker, L.L., and S.H. Chandler. 1987. Characterization of postsynaptic potentials evoked by sural nerve stimulation in hindlimb motoneurons from acute and chronic spinal cats. *Brain Res* **420**:340–350.

Barbeau, H., and P. Bedard. 1981. Denervation supersensitivity to 5-hydroxytryptophan in rats following spinal transection and 5,7-dihydroxytryptamine injection. *Neuropharmacology* **20**:611–616.

Barbeau, H., and S. Rossignol. 1990. The effects of serotonergic drugs on the locomotor pattern and on cutaneous reflexes of the adult chronic spinal cat. *Brain Res* **514**:55–67.

Bennett, D.J., H. Hultborn, B. Fedirchuk, and M. Gorassini. 1998a. Short-term plasticity in hindlimb motoneurons of decerebrate cats. *J Neurophysiol* **80**:2038–2045.

Bennett, D.J., H. Hultborn, B. Fedirchuk, and M. Gorassini. 1998b. Synaptic activation of plateaus in hindlimb motoneurons of decerebrate cats. *J Neurophysiol* **80**:2023–2037.

Bennett, D.J., M. Gorassini, K. Fouad, L. Sanelli, Y. Han, and J. Cheng. 1999. Spasticity in rats with sacral spinal cord injury. *J Neurotrauma* **16**:69–84.

Bennett, D.J., Y. Li, and M. Siu. 2001. Plateau potentials in sacrocaudal motoneurons of chronic spinal rats, recorded in vitro. *J Neurophysiol* **86**:1955–1971.

Binder, M.D., C.J. Heckman, and R.K. Powers. 1996. The physiological control of motoneuron activity. In *Handbook of Physiology. Section 12, Exercise: Regulation and Integration of Multiple Systems* (L.B. Rowell and J.T. Shepard, Eds.), pp. 3–53. American Physiological Society/Oxford University Press, New York.

Blaschak, M.J., R.K. Powers, and W.Z. Rymer. 1988. Disturbances of motor output in a cat hindlimb muscle after acute dorsal spinal hemisection. *Exp Brain Res* **71**:377–387.

Carp, J.S., R.K. Powers, and W.Z. Rymer. 1991. Alterations in motoneuron properties induced by acute dorsal spinal hemisection in the decerebrate cat. *Exp Brain Res* **83**:539–548.

Cavallari, P., and L.G. Pettersson. 1989. Tonic suppression of reflex transmission in low spinal cats. *Exp Brain Res* **77**:201–212.

Clarke, R.W., S. Eves, J. Harris, J.E. Peachey, and E. Stuart. 2002. Interactions between cutaneous afferent inputs to a withdrawal reflex in the decerebrated rabbit and their control by descending and segmental systems. *Neuroscience* **112**:555–571.

Collins, D.F., M. Gorassini, D. Bennett, D. Burke, and S.C. Gandevia. 2002. Recent evidence for plateau potentials in human motoneurones. *Adv Exp Med Biol* **508**:227–235.

Conway, B.A., H. Hultborn, O. Kiehn, and I. Mintz. 1988. Plateau potentials in alpha-motoneurones induced by intravenous injection of L-dopa and clonidine in the spinal cat. *J Physiol* **405**:369–384.

Eken, T., H. Hultborn, and O. Kiehn. 1989. Possible functions of transmitter-controlled plateau potentials in alpha motoneurones. *Prog Brain Res* **80**:257–267; discussion 239–242.

Engberg, I., A. Lundberg, and R.W. Ryall. 1968. Reticulospinal inhibition of transmission in reflex pathways. *J Physiol* **194**:201–223.

Gorassini, M., D.J. Bennett, O. Kiehn, T. Eken, and H. Hultborn. 1999. Activation patterns of hindlimb motor units in the awake rat and their relation to motoneuron intrinsic properties. *J Neurophysiol* **82**:709–717.

Gorassini, M.A., M. Knash, P.J. Harvey, D.J. Bennett, and J.F. Yang. 2004. Role of motoneuron plateau potentials in the generation of involuntary muscle activity after spinal cord injury. *Brain* **127**(10):2247–2258.

Guertin, P.A., and J. Hounsgaard. 1998. NMDA-induced intrinsic voltage oscillations depend on L-type calcium channels in spinal motoneurons of adult turtles. *J Neurophysiol* **80**:3380–3382.

Heckman, C.J. 1994. Alterations in synaptic input to motoneurons during partial spinal cord injury. *Med Sci Sports Exercise* **26**:1480–1490.

Heckman, C.J., and R.H. Lee. 1999. Synaptic integration in bistable motoneurons. *Prog Brain Res* **123**:49–56.

Hochman, S., and D.A. McCrea. 1994. Effects of chronic spinalization on ankle extensor motoneurons. II. Motoneuron electrical properties. *J Neurophysiol* **71**:1468–1479.

Hounsgaard, J., and O. Kiehn. 1989. Serotonin-induced bistability of turtle motoneurones caused by a nifedipine-sensitive calcium plateau potential. *J Physiol* **414**:265–282.

Hounsgaard, J., H. Hultborn, B. Jespersen, and O. Kiehn. 1988. Bistability of alpha-motoneurones in the decerebrate cat and in the acute spinal cat after intravenous 5-hydroxytryptophan. *J Physiol* **405**:345–367.

Hultborn, H., and O. Kiehn. 1992. Neuromodulation of vertebrate motor neuron membrane properties. *Curr Opin Neurobiol* **2**:770–775.

Hultborn, H., and J. Malmsten. 1983. Changes in segmental reflexes following chronic spinal cord hemisection in the cat. I. Increased monosynaptic and polysynaptic ventral root discharges. *Acta Physiol Scand* **119**:405–422.

Jankowska, E. 1992. Interneuronal relay in spinal pathways from proprioceptors. *Prog Neurobiol* **38**:335–378.

Kiehn, O., and T. Eken. 1997. Prolonged firing in motor units: Evidence of plateau potentials in human motoneurons? *J Neurophysiol* **78**:3061–3068.

Kiehn, O., B.R. Johnson, and M. Raastad. 1996. Plateau properties in mammalian spinal interneurons during transmitter-induced locomotor activity. *Neuroscience* **75**:263–273.

Krenz, N.R., and L.C. Weaver. 1998. Sprouting of primary afferent fibers after spinal cord transection in the rat. *Neuroscience* **85**:443–458.

Kuhn, R.A., and M.B. Macht. 1948. Some manifestations of reflex activity in spinal man with particular reference to the occurrence of extensor spasm. *Bull Johns Hopkins Hosp* **84**:43–75.

Lance, J.W. 1980. Symposium synopsis. In *Spasticity Disordered Motor Control* (R.G. Feldman, R.R. Young, and W.P. Koella, Eds.), pp. 485–494. Yearbook Medical, Chicago.

Long, S.K., R.H. Evans, L. Cull, F. Krijzer, and P. Bevan. 1988. An *in vitro* mature spinal cord preparation from the rat. *Neuropharmacology* **27**:541–546.

Mailis, A., and P. Ashby. 1990. Alterations in group Ia projections to motoneurons following spinal lesions in humans. *J Neurophysiol* **64**:637–647.

McNicholas, L.F., W.R. Martin, J.W. Sloan, and M. Nozaki. 1980. Innervation of the spinal cord by sympathetic fibers. *Exp Neurol* **69**:383–394.

Naftchi, N.E., W. Schlosser, and W.D. Horst. 1979. Correlation of changes in the GABA-ergic system with the development of spasticity in paraplegic cats. *Adv Exp Med Biol* **123**:431–450.

Nagano, N., H. Ono, M. Ozawa, and H. Fukuda. 1988. The spinal reflex of chronic spinal rats is supersensitive to 5-HTP but not to TRH or 5-HT agonists. *Eur J Pharmacol* **149**:337–344.

Newton, B.W., and R.W. Hamill. 1988. The morphology and distribution of rat serotoninergic intraspinal neurons: An immunohistochemical study. *Brain Res Bull* **20**:349–360.

Nielsen, J., and H. Hultborn. 1993. Regulated properties of motoneurons and primary afferents: New aspects on possible spinal mechanisms underlying spasticity. In *Spasticity: Mechanisms and Management* (A.F. Thilmann, Ed.), pp. 177–191. Springer-Verlag, Berlin.

Norman, K.E., A. Pepin, and H. Barbeau. 1998. Effects of drugs on walking after spinal cord injury. *Spinal Cord* **36**:699–715.

Noth, J. 1991. Trends in the pathophysiology and pharmacotherapy of spasticity. *J Neurol* **238**:131–139.

Powers, R.K., and M.D. Binder. 2001. Input–output functions of mammalian motoneurons. *Rev Physiol Biochem Pharmacol* **143**:137–263.

Powers, R.K., and W.Z. Rymer. 1988. Effects of acute dorsal spinal hemisection on motoneuron discharge in the medial gastrocnemius of the decerebrate cat. *J Neurophysiol* **59**:1540–1556.

Rekling, J.C., G.D. Funk, D.A. Bayliss, X.W. Dong, and J.L. Feldman. 2000. Synaptic control of motoneuronal excitability. *Physiol Rev* **80**:767–852.

Ritz, L.A., R.M. Friedman, E.L. Rhoton, M.L. Sparkes, and C.J. Jr. Vierck. 1992. Lesions of cat sacrocaudal spinal cord: A minimally disruptive model of injury. *J Neurotrauma* **9**:219–230.

Russo, R.E., and J. Hounsgaard. 1999. Dynamics of intrinsic electrophysiological properties in spinal cord neurones. *Prog Biophys Mol Biol* **72**:329–365.

Russo, R.E., F. Nagy, and J. Hounsgaard. 1997. Modulation of plateau properties in dorsal horn neurones in a slice preparation of the turtle spinal cord. *J Physiol* **499**(Pt. 2):459–474.

Schwindt, P.C., and W.E. Crill. 1984. Membrane properties of cat spinal motoneurons. In *Handbook of the Spinal Cord* (R.A. Davidoff, Ed.), pp. 199–242. Dekker, New York.

Schwindt, P.C., and W.E. Crill. 1995. Amplification of synaptic current by persistent sodium conductance in apical dendrite of neocortical neurons. *J Neurophysiol* **74**:2220–2224.

Stauffer, E.S. 1974. Trauma. In *Spinal Deformity in Neurological and Muscular Disorders* (J.H. Hardy, Ed.), pp. 219–239. Mosby, St. Louis.

Steg, G. 1964. Efferent muscle innervation and rigidity. *Acta Physiol Scand Suppl 225* **61**:1–53.

Taylor, J.S., R.F. Friedman, J.B. Munson, and C.J. Jr. Vierck. 1997. Stretch hyperreflexia of triceps surae muscles in the conscious cat after dorsolateral spinal lesions. *J Neurosci* **17**:5004–5015.

Thomas, C.K., and B.H. Ross. 1997. Distinct patterns of motor unit behavior during muscle spasms in spinal cord injured subjects. *J Neurophysiol* **77**:2847–2850.

Thompson, F.J., P.J. Reier, C.C. Lucas, and R. Parmer. 1992. Altered patterns of reflex excitability subsequent to contusion injury of the rat spinal cord. *J Neurophysiol* **68**:1473–1486.

Thompson, F.J., P.J. Reier, R. Parmer, and C.C. Lucas. 1993. Inhibitory control of reflex excitability following contusion injury and neural tissue transplantation. *Adv Neurol* **59**:175–184.

Thompson, F.J., R. Parmer, and P.J. Reier. 1998. Alteration in rate modulation of reflexes to lumbar motoneurons after midthoracic spinal cord injury in the rat. I. Contusion injury. *J Neurotrauma* **15**:495–508.

Tremblay, L.E., P.J. Bedard, R. Maheux, and T. Di Paolo. 1985. Denervation supersensitivity to 5-hydroxytryptamine in the rat spinal cord is not due to the absence of 5-hydroxytryptamine. *Brain Res* **330**:174–177.

Wiegner, A.W., M.M. Wierzbicka, L. Davies, and R.R. Young. 1993. Discharge properties of single motor units in patients with spinal cord injuries. *Muscle Nerve* **16**:661–671.

Young, R.R. 1994. Spasticity: A review. *Neurology* **44**:S12–S20.

CHAPTER

L4

Rat Spinal Cord Contusion Model of Spasticity

FLOYD J. THOMPSON and PRODIP BOSE

I. INTRODUCTION

A. Spasticity

Spasticity is an ongoing problem for many individuals following spinal cord injury. Although potentially complex in nature (Young, 1994), it is characterized by velocity-dependent exaggeration of the lengthening resistance of the affected skeletal muscles (Lance, 1981). These contractions impose undesired resistance to movement, increased fatigue, and decreased accuracy of movement. This condition has been correlated with hyperactivity in spinal reflex pathways that mediate muscle stretch reflexes (Kuhn and Mact, 1948; Herman, 1968; Ashby and Verrier, 1980; Toft et al., 1993; Thilmann et al., 1991). Although the specific mechanisms responsible for the changes in reflex excitability that lead to spasticity are unknown, some fundamental changes in the neurophysiology of reflex excitability have been observed and correlated in time and magnitude with the appearance of clinically relevant spasticity in the muscle subserved by the studied reflexes. This article provides a review of some of the significant observations that we and others have made regarding this problem through the development and utilization of animal models.

B. Animal Models

Experimental animal models offer an opportunity to gain an increased understanding of the changes in spinal cord physiology in a setting in which certain features of the spinal lesions relative to location and severity can be controlled and reproduced (Hughes, 1988; Young, 2002). Laboratory models employing several methods of spinal cord injury have been used to investigate mechanisms related to sensory and motor dysfunction, plasticity, and the development of spasticity. Each type of experimental lesion model has advantages and limitations.

1. Surgical Lesion Models

Injury models produced by complete or partial transection of the spinal cord have been studied extensively (de la Torre, 1984; Young, 1989/1992). Because these injuries can yield reproducible deficits (Guth et al., 1980), they are useful for the elucidation of structure–function relationships (Goldberger, 1989). Studies utilizing the transection model in the rat sacral spinal cord have revealed important insights into changes in membrane channel conductance that correlate with the development of spasticity (Bennet et al., 2001; Li et al., 2004). However, a limitation of the transection-type lesion is its departure from the form of injury commonly encountered in the clinical setting (Young, 1989/1992).

2. Contusion/Compression Injury Models

Most human spinal cord injuries are produced by acceleration-related fracture/dislocations of the spine causing a contusion or compression of the spinal cord (Hughes, 1988; Young, 1989/1992). Allen (1911) is credited with the first attempt to mimic this form of injury experimentally using a weight-drop trauma model. This approach reproduced many of the histopathological features of injuries seen clinically (Kakulas, 1985). However, due to their potential for animal-to-animal variability, the practical utility of experimental contusion/compression models for elucidating mechanisms associated with spinal cord dysfunction, functional sparing, or the recovery of function has been viewed critically (de la Torre, 1984; Das, 1989; Young, 1989/1992).

To enhance the practical utility of the contusion injury model, experimental protocols were developed that yielded compression/contusion injuries with greater reproducibility (Wrathall et al., 1985; Black et al., 1986; Bresnahan et al., 1987; Kerasidis et al., 1987; Anderson et al., 1988; Beattie et al., 1988). Therefore, the increased reproducibility of the contusion model provided more efficient opportunities for investigating dysfunction using an incomplete injury that closely mimics the clinical injury. In addition, the possibility has been raised that this type of injury may be more responsive to certain therapeutic strategies aimed at regeneration or functional sparing/recovery (Young, 1989/1992; Bracken et al., 1992; Reier et al., 1992; Anderson et al., 1991; Stokes and Reier, 1992). The feasibility of using fetal neural tissue grafts to repair acute and chronic contusion/compression lesions of the spinal cord has also been demonstrated (Winiarski et al., 1987; Reier et al., 1988, 1989, 1992; Anderson et al., 1991; Stokes and Reier, 1992; Thompson et al., 1993). Collectively, these considerations provided incentive for exploring this lesion model in greater depth to uncover fundamental issues that relate to the development of spasticity following spinal cord injury. However, apart from analyses of evoked potentials (Black et al., 1986; Simpson and Baskin, 1987; Fehlings et al., 1988; Zileli and Schramm, 1991; Shiau et al., 1992) and axonal conduction studies (Blight, 1983, 1985), prior to 1992 (Thompson et al., 1992) neurophysiological changes had not been extensively investigated subsequent to experimental contusion spinal injury.

The studies summarized next devoted specific attention to alterations in neurophysiological processes that regulate reflex excitability to reveal possible insights into the development of enhanced excitability of hindlimb reflexes since segmental hyperreflexia is a hallmark of spinal cord injury-induced spasticity in humans (Landau, 1974; Burke, 1988) and of transection-type experimental lesions in animals (Hultborn and Malmsten, 1983a,b). Accordingly, four aspects of reflex excitability were tested and compared in normal and postcontusion animals: reflex thresholds, reflex magnitude, and two types of rate-dependent modulation of reflex magnitudes (Thompson et al., 1992, 1993, 1998).

II. ELECTROPHYSIOLOGICAL STUDIES IN POSTCONTUSION ANIMALS

A. Animals

Female Sprague–Dawley rats (220–250 g initial weight) (Zivic Miller Laboratories, Allison Park, PA) served as subjects in these experiments. They were housed in an American Association for Accreditation of Laboratory Animal Care-accredited facility, and all procedures were reviewed and approved by the University of Florida Institutional Use and Care Committee.

B. Contusion Injury

A modification of the Allen weight-drop method (Wrathall et al., 1985) was used to induce spinal cord injuries at the T_8 spinal level. For consistency with other descriptions of contusion injuries in the rat (Wrathall et al., 1985), the lesion operations were performed under general anesthesia with 4% chloral hydrate [10 ml/kg, intraperitoneal (i.p.)]. Following laminectomy, a 10-g weight was dropped from a height of 2.5 cm onto a Teflon impounder that rested freely on the dura. After injury, the muscle, fascia, and skin were closed in layers. For further details of injury and postoperative care, see Thompson et al. (1992, 1998) and Bose et al. (2002a,b).

During the first postoperative week, the animals were paraplegic and required assistance in bladder expression. However, ambulation and bladder expression recovered progressively during the second postoperative week. At 1 and 2 months, the animals utilized quadrupedal locomotion, although the hindlimbs appeared to be weak and hypotonic. All postoperative care of these animals was supervised by an attending veterinarian directly involved with the spinal cord injury program at the University of Florida. Details on the locomotor recovery subsequent to midthoracic contusion injuries have been reported (Kerasidis et al., 1987; Noble and Wrathall, 1989; Basso et al., 1995).

C. Electrophysiological Studies, Preparation, and Recording Methods

Excitability of the reflexes to hindlimb motoneurons was investigated using tibial monosynaptic reflexes. Excitability patterns were recorded in normal animals and compared with those recorded at particular intervals following midthoracic contusion injury. These studies were conducted to determine what quantitative changes in reflex excitability occurred in the lumbar spinal cord subsequent to contusion injury of the midthoracic spinal cord in adult rats.

1. Preparation

During the recording sessions, the animals were anesthetized by intramuscular injection of ketamine and anesthesia was maintained by constant i.p. infusion at 80–120 mg/kg/hr. Ketamine was chosen since it is known to minimally depress the spinal monosynaptic reflex and minimally alter the time course of presynaptic inhibition (Tang and Schroeder, 1973; Lodge and Anis, 1984). Anesthesia depth was regulated by using a dose rate sufficient to block corneal reflexes, whisker tremor, and the pinna reflex while continuously monitoring heart rate on visual and auditory monitors. Body temperature was monitored and maintained between 35 and 37°C. Spinal clamps were used to immobilize the axial skeleton and the lumbar enlargement was exposed. The right tibial nerve was exposed, cut at muscle entry, and mounted on a recording bipolar electrode. All surgically exposed tissues were covered with warmed mineral oil and maintained at 37°C.

2. Cord Dorsum Potentials

Cord dorsum potentials were recorded using a silver ball electrode applied to the dorsal surface of the spinal cord at the lateral intermediate sulcus of the fifth lumbar cord segment referenced to a lead located in the skin of the adjacent wound margin of the lumbar laminectomy.

3. Monosynaptic Reflexes

The monosynaptic reflexes (MSRs) were elicited by stimulation of the L_{3-5} dorsal roots using 200 microsecond current pulses. The dorsal roots were cut at dural entry and placed across stimulating bipolar hook electrodes. MSRs were recorded monophasically from the tibial nerve using silver wire bipolar electrodes. MSR magnitudes were determined by the baseline-to-baseline areas of the reflex waveforms. Amplitude comparisons utilized baseline-to-peak measures. Recording stability was assessed by continual observation of the relative proportions of the afferent triphasic spike and the evoked potentials of the fifth lumbar cord dorsum potential (Thompson et al., 1992).

4. Rate Depression

Reflexes were produced using the minimum stimulus intensity delivered to the dorsal roots required to elicit maximal tibial MSRs recorded monophasically from the tibial nerve. Rate depression was determined as the attenuation of reflex magnitude at any of seven test frequencies (1, 2, 3, 4, 5, 10, and 20 Hz) compared with the magnitude recorded at a 0.3-Hz control frequency. A rate of 0.3 Hz was used as the control frequency based on previous studies (Eccles and Rall, 1951; Jefferson and Schlapp, 1953; Thompson et al., 1992, 1993). The magnitude at each frequency was determined from the signal average of 32 consecutive waveforms. Rate depression of tibial MSRs was tested in normal animals and in animals at 28 (C-28) and 60 (C-60) days postcontusion. The 60-day postinjury time interval was selected to permit reference to previous reflex excitability studies (Malmsten, 1983; Thompson et al., 1992, 1993).

5. Posttetanic Potentiation

Posttetanic potentiation (PTP) of tibial MSRs was elicited by supramaximal current pulse stimulation at 300 Hz for 30 sec to compare PTP patterns in previous studies (Lloyd, 1957; Malmsten, 1983). Following tetanus, MSRs were produced at 0.3 Hz and tested for 5 min. Each set of five consecutive sweeps was serially averaged to provide 15-sec time measures.

D. Electrophysiological Changes following Contusion Injury

1. Rate Depression

Following injury, segmental reflex activity exhibited several patterns of alteration. One of the most robust changes observed was a significant reduction in rate-sensitive depression of tibial monosynaptic reflexes. For example, note in Figure 1A that in normal animals, repetition at 1.0 Hz produced a 35% decrease in the reflex amplitude (relative to the 0.3-Hz control), and further increases in frequency were accompanied by additional marked reductions in reflex amplitude. In contrast, recordings in animals 2 months following midthoracic contusion injury (Figure 1B, C-60) exhibited significantly less attenuation at each of the test frequencies. Group comparison of tibial MSR rate depression in normal, 28 days (C-28), and 60 days (C-60) postcontusion revealed that the change in rate depression was progressive in onset (Figure 1C). Recordings made in animals up to 6 months postinjury revealed the same pattern of loss of rate depression, suggesting that, once established, loss of rate depression was permanent. As discussed later, it was proposed that this significant reduction in the influence of repetitive input on the monosynaptic reflexes represented a fundamental change in the inhibitory modulation to patterned input that may significantly contribute to the development of hyperreflexia of these ankle extensor reflexes following spinal cord injury.

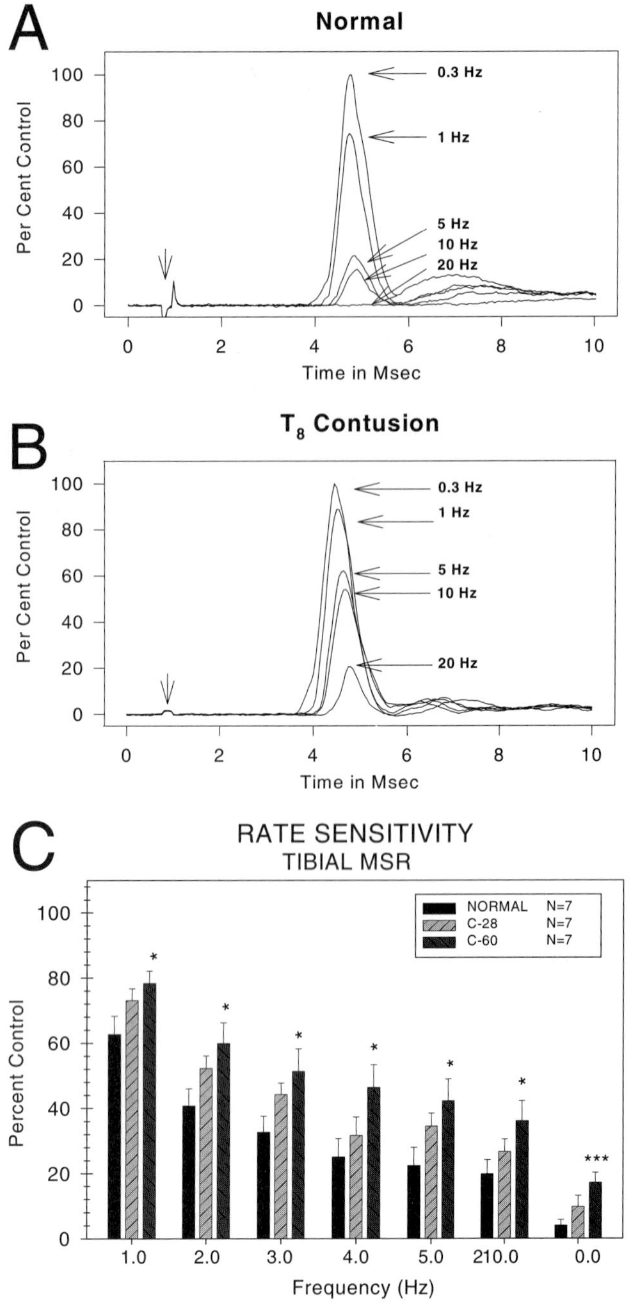

FIGURE 1 (A) Tibial MSR waveforms recorded in a normal, intact animal at control (0.3 Hz) and four test frequencies to illustrate rate depression. (B) Waveforms recorded from an animal at 60 days postcontusion. (C) Group means to show rate depression in normal and postcontusion animals at 28 (C-28) and 60 (C-60) days postinjection.

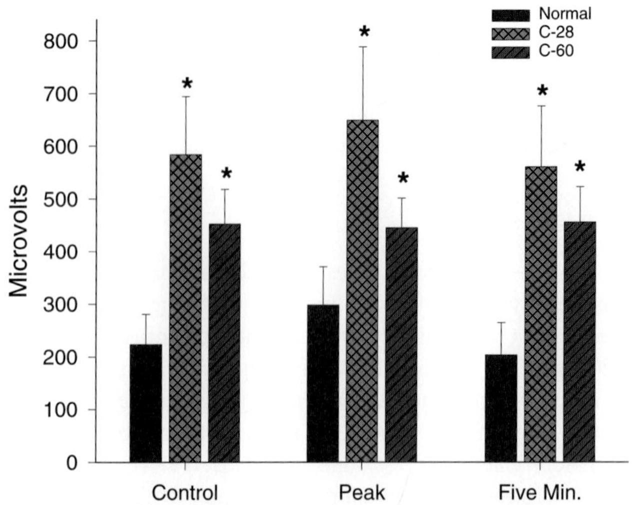

FIGURE 2 Tibial MSR magnitudes in normal and postcontusion animals. Control, maximal unpotentiated MSRs; Peak, peak potentiated MSRs; Five Min., MSR magnitudes at 5 min following tetanus. Asterisks indicate values significantly greater than normal (ANOVA, $p > 0.05$).

2. Reflex Magnitude and Posttetanic Potentiation

The loss in rate depression was accompanied by two other significant changes in reflex excitability: increased reflex magnitude and decreased PTP (Thompson et al., 1998). A summary of maximal and potentiated MSR amplitudes is shown in Figure 2. The mean maximal baseline-to-peak unpotentiated MSR amplitude in normal animals was 223.8 μV compared to 583.9 and 452.7 μV, respectively, for the 28-day and 60-day contused animals. The time course for the expression of PTP following tetanic stimulation in normal, 28-day, and 60-day postcontusion animals is shown in Figures 3A and 3B; potentiated amplitudes are shown as a percentage of the pretetanus maximal amplitude. Note that in the normal animals, a peak potentiation that was 160% of the pretetanus control was observed 30 sec following the tetanus (Figure 3A). In contrast, the maximal potentiation for the 28- and 60-day postcontusion animals was 120.8 and 113.5%, respectively, also appearing at the 30-sec post-tetanus time point (Figure 3B). However, it is important to note the magnitudes of the unpotentiated MSRs were significantly larger than even the peak potentiated magnitudes observed in normal animals (Figure 2).

3. Histological Evaluation of Lesions

Spinal cord tissues were preserved for histological examination by transcardiac perfusion with either 4% paraformaldehyde alone or a solution of 4% paraformaldehyde and 5% glutaraldehyde in 0.1 *M* Sorenson's phosphate buffer. Portions of the spinal cord that included the contusion epicenter and segments extending 6 mm rostral and caudal to the injuries were saved, sectioned, and stained for light microscopy. The spinal cords of animals sacrificed 6 days after weight-drop injury were characterized by a developing central core of necrosis involving gray and white matter (Figure 4A). The lesion epicenters contained dense accumulations of macrophages and other inflammatory cells

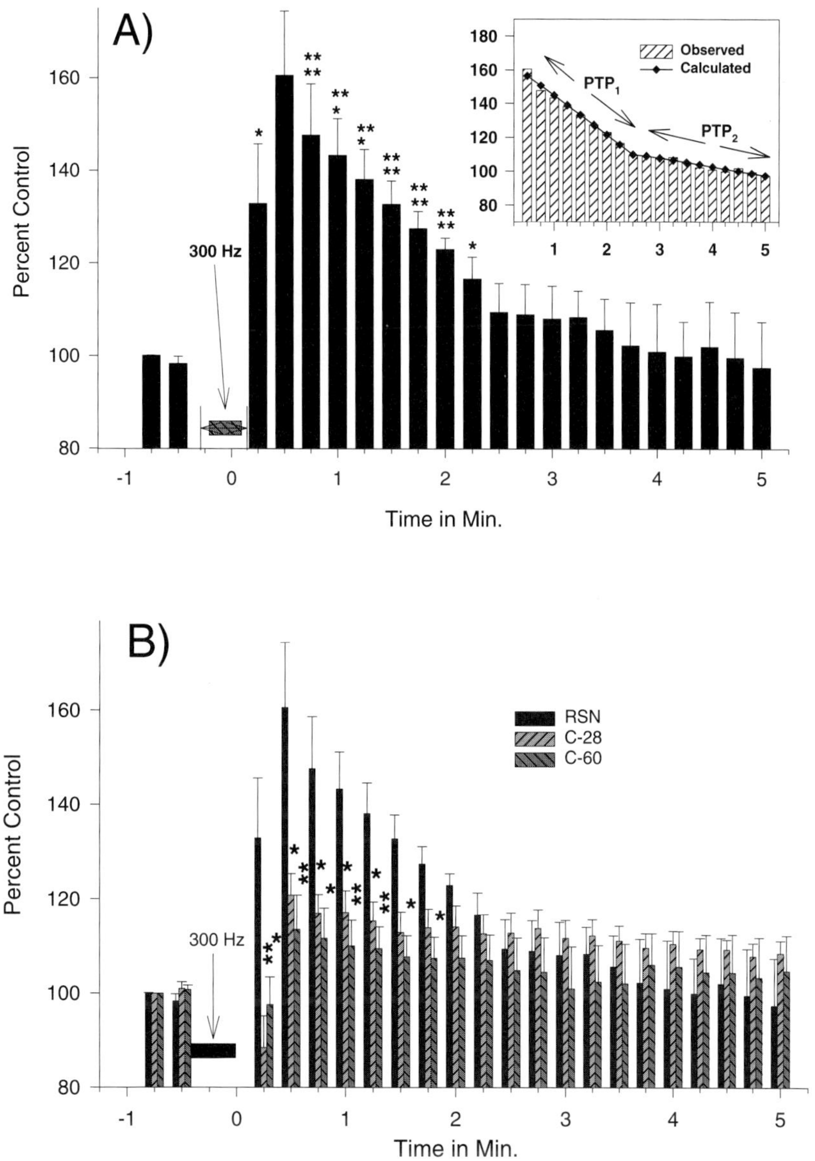

FIGURE 3 (A) PTP of the tibial MSR in normal animals (RSN) with potentiation expressed as a percentage of the pretetanus control. The inset shows potentiation values predicted by third-order (PTP1) and first-order equations (PTP2) (diamonds) compared to observed values (bars). (B) Comparison of PTP of the tibial MSR in normal animals and in animals at 28 (C-28) and 60 (C-60) days following midthoracic contusion. The potentiation is expressed as a percentage of the pretetanus control.

that were either seen in well-developed cysts or that delineated areas of cavitation. There was some variability in the degree and pattern of tissue erosion. In some cases, the spinal cords displayed a large symmetric zone of central necrosis. Some sparing of lateral and ventrolateral white matter was seen, but each of these sectors contained many profiles of degenerating axons as well (Blight and DeCrescito, 1986; Bresnahan, 1978). Other specimens revealed a more asymmetric lesion with some apparently persisting axons in the dorsal columns and partial preservation of the superficial dorsal horn.

Tissue specimens obtained 28 or 60 days postcontusion injury revealed large cysts extending 3.75–4.6 mm in the rostral–caudal plane. Representative histological specimens for 28- and 60-day postcontusion injuries are shown in Figures 4B and 4C, respectively. Cavitation was either centrally located or restricted to the dorsal aspect of the spinal cord. These zones of necrosis were almost completely sur-

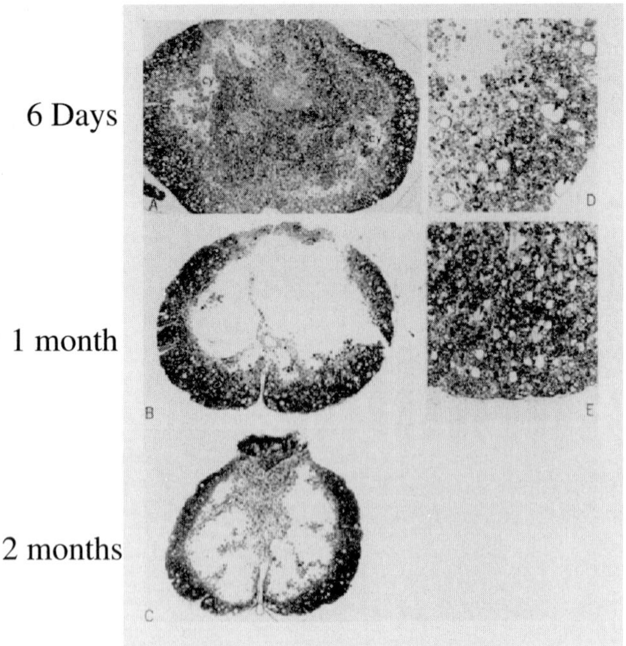

FIGURE 4 Transverse 2-μm sections of plastic embedded spinal cord specimens that were obtained at the level of the lesion epicenter are shown. (A) At 6 days postinjury, an evolving core of central necrosis is evidenced by small cysts (cy) and numerous macrophages, infiltrating inflammatory cells, and cellular debris. This region of tissue necrosis is surrounded by a rim of more intact appearing white matter. Even at this low magnification, however, much of this rim of tissue exhibits vacuolation characteristic of spongiform degeneration of myelinated fibers. (B) By 28 days, prominent cysts are seen that contain fewer cells than seen earlier. Although a well-defined rim of tissue remains, some vacuolation is still seen within the white matter. (C) The spinal cord at 60 days postinjury appeared similar to that seen in the previous micrograph. Again, some degeneration is still indicated in the remaining subpial tissue. (D and E) These two micrographs are higher magnification views of regions of spared tissue shown in A and B. In both examples, small intact-appearing axons are seen immediately subjacent to the pia. Those fibers located more internally show considerable degenerative changes as exhibited by swollen axons and distorted myelin sheaths. Magnification: A–C, 30×; D and E, 120×.

rounded by persisting white matter, although, as in the 6-day material, many focal regions of axonal and myelin breakdown were seen in most areas of persisting tissue. The nature of these injuries was consistent with that reported by previous investigators using similar injury parameters for the production of weight-drop contusion injuries (Wrathall et al., 1985).

E. Relevance of Postinjury Electrophysiological Changes to the Development of Spasticity

1. Alterations in Rate Depression

The changes in rate depression are consistent with the hypothesis that a significant contributor to the development and appearance of spasticity is a reduction in presynaptic inhibition following spinal cord injury (Burk and Ashby, 1972; Ashby et al., 1987). This reduction leads to the inability for segmental inhibitory processes to regulate the moment-to-moment segmental afferent traffic, in general, and especially the afferent traffic evoked during movement (Capaday and Stein, 1986; Yang et al., 1991). The decrease in rate depression reflects changes in at least two presynaptic inhibitory processes that normally modulate reflex excitability in a phase-dependent manner during stepping. Presynaptic inhibition associated with $GABA_A$-mediated primary afferent depolarization (PAD) (Stuart and Redman, 1992) may contribute to rate-dependent attenuation for activation intervals consistent with the 10- to 200-msec time course of PAD (cat, Eccles et al., 1963; rat, Kocsis and Waxman, 1982). Longer lasting $GABA_B$-mediated presynaptic inhibition has been suggested by at least two lines of evidence. The action of the $GABA_B$ agonist baclofen was reported to modify rate-sensitive changes in Ia synaptic transmission in ways that mimicked reduced presynaptic Ca^{2+} influx and concomitant decreased transmitter release (Lev-Tov et al., 1988). In addition, it was reported that alteration in low-frequency rate depression was produced by the intraspinal injection of $GABA_B$ agonists and antagonists (Thompson et al., 1996, 2001; Wang et al., 2002). Currently, the GABA mimetic actions of baclofen in regulating afferent transmission form a logical basis for the actions of intrathecal baclofen to lessen spasticity that is attributed to postinjury hyperreflexia (McClellan, 1973; Penn and Kroin, 1985; Meythaler, 2001).

It is known that several descending spinal pathways influence the GABAergic interneurons involved in the production of PAD (presynaptic inhibition) in group Ia afferents (Rudomin et al., 1983; Rudomin, 1994). It has been reported that conditioning stimulation of serotonergic fibers increased the magnitude of long-lasting lumbar monosynaptic reflex depression in the neonatal rat spinal cord (Yomono et al., 1992). Although the specific pathways are not known, it is apparent that the injury-related interruption of these systems (and concomitant adaptive changes) is normally essential for regulation of the inhibitory processes that normally regulate segmental afferent traffic directed to reflex pathways. Therefore, we propose that low-frequency rate-dependent depression in the adult spinal cord is influenced by descending tract fibers, and that contusion injury of the midthoracic spinal cord resulted in a loss of descending tract fibers that normally influence rate-dependent depression.

An important point relates to the possible relationship between the change in rate depression and the increase in the maximal unpotentiated MSR. It has been suggested that high-threshold motoneurons are more frequency tolerant than low-threshold motoneurons (Lloyd, 1966). Therefore, if injury-associated plasticity, such as collateral sprouting, resulted in an increased recruitment of motoneurons, the test reflexes in postcontusion animals would include a larger proportion of higher threshold, more frequency-tolerant motoneurons than the test reflexes in normal animals. On the other hand, if one views rate depression as a fundamental regulatory process that utilizes long-acting presynaptic mechanisms to decrease reflex excitability, then a significant decrease in this regulatory process could account for an increase in the excitability of the MSRs.

2. Alterations in PTP

In normal animals, PTP relates to a period during which there is increased probability for motoneuron discharge following high-frequency stimulation of their afferent input (Lloyd, 1949; Eccles and Rall, 1951). This process has been ascribed to a period of augmented transmitter release from presynaptic terminals facilitated by tetanus-enhanced calcium entry into the terminals (Hirst et al., 1981; Mendell, 1984; Burke et al., 1987; Lev-Tov et al., 1988; Zucker et al., 1991). In the current study, the time course of PTP observed in the normal adult rat tibial monosynaptic reflexes was comparable to that reported for cat tibial monosynaptic reflexes (Lloyd, 1949). The decay of PTP of the tibial MSR in the normal rat spinal cord showed a rapid initial rate followed by a slower rate of decay during which reflex magnitudes returned to baseline values within approximately 5 min. Both presynaptic and postsynaptic factors could account for these different rates of decay. Presynaptic influences may include concentration-specific differences in the influence of intraterminal Ca^{2+} on various stages of synaptic vesicle docking and release (Li et al., 1995; Sudhof, 1995). The change in decay pattern may also reflect differences in the threshold distribution among the postsynaptic pool of potentiated motoneurons (Luscher et al., 1983; Collins et al., 1988).

A significantly reduced percentage of PTP was observed in the postcontusion animals at both 28 and 60 days postinjury. The decreased percentage of potentiation may be related to the increased magnitude of the test reflex. Since the maximal unpotentiated MSRs were significantly larger in the postcontusion animals, it is possible that a larger number of motoneurons were active in the postcontusion unpotentiated reflexes, leaving a smaller proportion of inactive motoneurons available for potentiation (Lev-Tov et al., 1983; Collins et al., 1988; Pinco and Lev-Tov, 1993; Lev-Tov and Pinco, 1992). These changes in the maximal unpotentiated MSR amplitude have important functional implications relative to spasticity. Since this MSR is the pathway used by muscle stretch reflexes, this study suggests that a larger proportion of the motoneuron pool would be recruited by segmental stimulation in the postcontusion rats than in normal animals. This type of exaggerated response is consistent with the increased reflex excitability associated with conditions of spasticity (Katz and Rymer, 1989), although additional studies are needed to show that these reflex changes specifically correlate with exaggerated velocity-dependent lengthening resistance of the associated muscles.

The decrease in relative PTP magnitude would also have significant functional consequences. In normal animals, PTP was reported to be predominantly associated with higher threshold motoneurons and was proposed to enhance their recruitment (Collins et al., 1988). Accordingly, the functional benefits afforded by this brief recruitment of high-threshold motoneurons for high-force tasks would be diminished in postcontusion animals.

The mechanisms that specifically account for the significant increase in the magnitude of the maximal unpotentiated MSRs and associated changes in PTP in the postcontusion animals are unknown. However, a natural explanation may be damage to descending axons from several supraspinal sites (e.g., cerebrum, red nucleus, vestibular nuclei, reticular formation, and raphe nuclei), with concomitant loss in the modulation of segmental reflex excitability according to task requirements (Quevedo and Cliquet, 1995; Rudomin, 1990, 1994; Rudomin et al., 1991; Noga et al., 1995; Jankowska et al., 1994; Jankowska and Edgeley, 1993). Additional possibilities include segmental plasticity such as enhanced segmental afferent influence on motoneuron excitability following the interruption of descending axons (Goldberger and Murray, 1988). These segmental changes would be influenced by the proximity of the motoneuron pool to the level of injury (Nelson and Mendell, 1979; Carter et al., 1988), although the specific longitudinal distribution of change in motoneuron excitability relative to the T_8 contusion injury was not addressed in the current study.

III. ANKLE TORQUE MODEL TO TEST FOR SPASTICITY IN THE RAT

The neurophysiological patterns of hyperreflexia in the tibial MSRs following experimental midthoracic spinal cord contusion injury suggested that spastic patterns should be evident in the muscle stretch reflexes of triceps surae muscles that used these pathways. However, prior to these studies, spasticity (defined as an exaggeration of the velocity-dependent lengthening resistance) had not been detected in the hindlimb muscles of the rat following midthoracic spinal cord injury (hemisection) (Hultborn and Malmsten, 1983a,b); Malmsten, 1983).

A. Approach

The velocity-dependent lengthening resistance of the triceps surae muscles (ankle extensor muscles) was tested

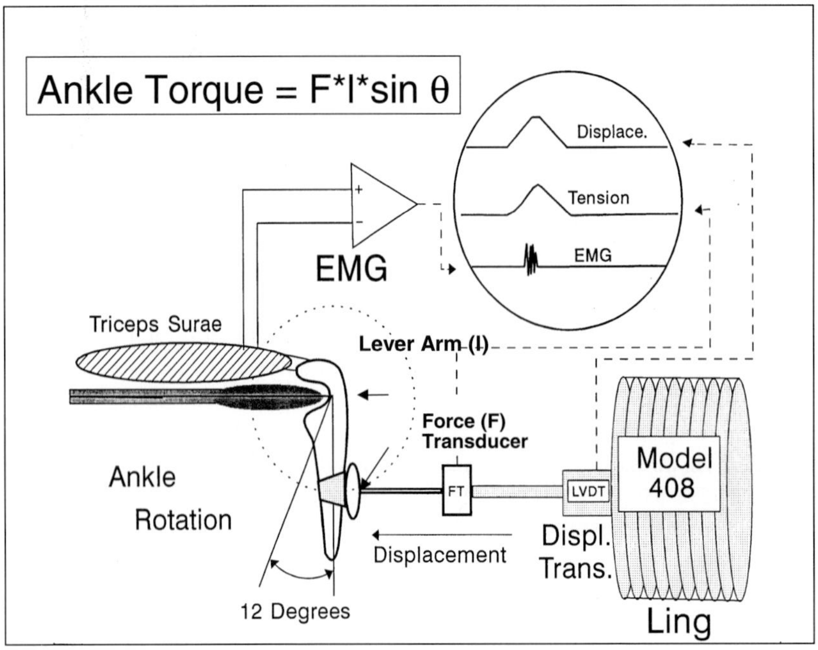

FIGURE 5 Diagram illustrating the arrangement of instrumentation to rotate the ankle and record ankle torque and triceps surae EMG. The rotation instrumentation includes an electromechanical shaker (Ling, Model 408), a displacement transducer, a force transducer, and a foot cradle.

before and after at several intervals following midthoracic contusion injury to chart the magnitude and time course for any injury-induced changes. These experiments were conducted on adult rats immobilized in an open-ended, transparent restraint tube with their hindlimbs secured above the ankles to permit the normal range of ankle rotation. A schematic for measurement of velocity-dependent ankle torque is shown in Figure 5. The lengthening resistance of the triceps surae muscles was assessed indirectly by measuring ankle torque during dorsiflexion ankle rotation across a broad range of velocities (48, 136, 204, 272, 350, 408, 490, 612°/sec). Controlled dorsiflexion of the foot was produced using an electromechanical shaker whose shaft displacement was guided by trapezoid waveforms and recorded using a length velocity displacement transducer. A force transducer was placed in series between the output shaft and the central footpad. This instrumentation permitted direct measurement of foot displacement and, simultaneously, the mechanical resistance to dorsiflexion. The neurogenic activity in the triceps surae muscles was recorded using chronically inserted transcutaneous EMG electrodes to permit correlation of ankle extensor EMG activity to ankle torque. The resistive force values were converted to torque [$T = F \times l \times \sin\theta$, where T is the torque, F is the recorded force in gf (980.7 dyn/1 gf), l is the distance from ankle joint to stirrup contact point, and $\sin\theta$ is the angle of the force vector]. In normal animals, mean peak amplitudes of 70.38 kdyn of ankle torque were recorded during ankle rotation at the slowest rotation velocity of 48°/sec. The mean EMG magnitude recorded during this rotation was 0.024 mV (±0.07). As the velocity of ankle rotation increased, velocity-dependent increases in the amplitude of both the ankle torque and the ankle extensor EMG (time-locked to rotation) were observed. At the highest rotation velocity, a mean peak ankle torque of 130.22 kdyn was observed.

B. Spasticity in the Rat

These recordings were repeated in animals at several weekly intervals up to 12 weeks following midthoracic contusion injury produced by weight drop onto the exposed dura at thoracic T_8 (10 g/25.0 mm, according to the MASCIS protocol, NYU impactor). The recordings made at the highest rotation velocity in the 12-week postinjury animals revealed mean peak torque amplitudes of 171.11 kdyn, significantly larger than the 130.22 kdyn mean peak torques recorded before injury; compare example waveforms from normal and postcontusion (Figure 6B). Correlated with this increased torque was mean EMG–RMS (root mean square) burst amplitude of 2.02 mV, also significantly larger than the mean peak amplitude of 1.25 mV recorded before injury. The mean torques and corresponding EMGs were significantly larger at the next three fastest rotation velocities. However, neither the mean torques nor the EMGs were larger than those observed before injury at the lower three rotation velocities. These observations indicated that fol-

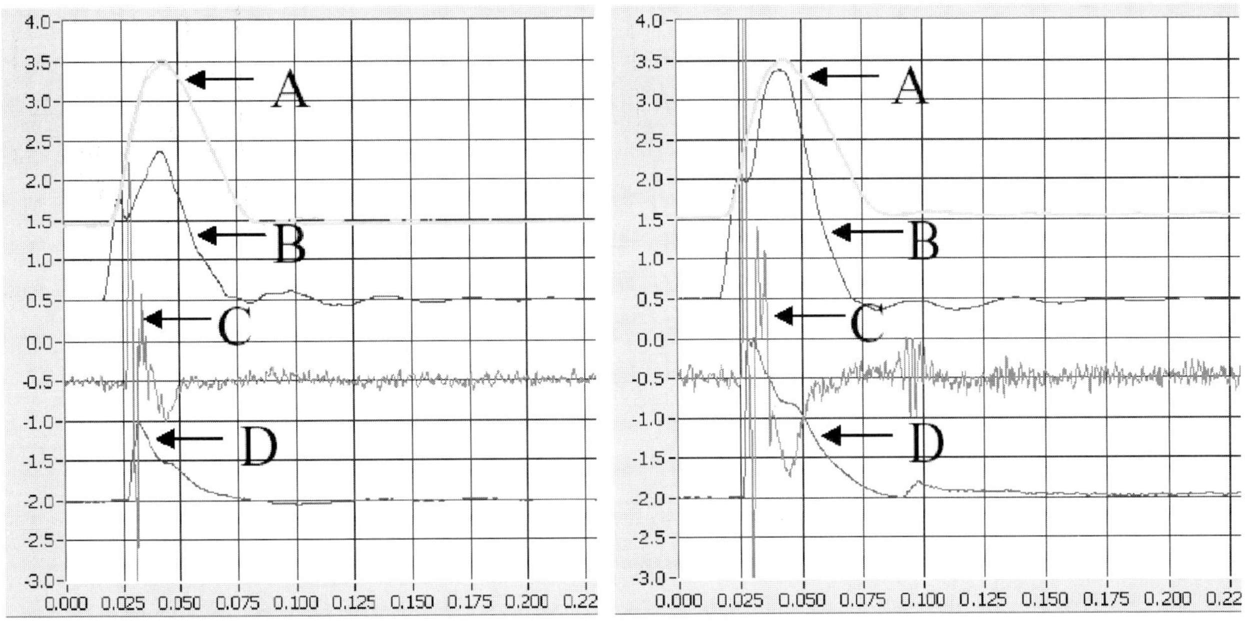

FIGURE 6 Samples of raw waveforms recorded at 612°/sec ankle rotation from a 12-week contused (right) and a time-matched control animal (left). At 12.24°, 612°/sec ankle rotations, the ankle torques (B) recorded in both normal and contused animals were 1.88 V (119.84 kdyn) and 2.87 V (182.85 kdyn), respectively. Ankle extensor EMG–RMS is indicated by "D" in both normal (left) and contused animals (right), and these magnitudes were 0.99 and 1.99 mV, respectively.

lowing injury, a significant increase in the velocity-dependent ankle torque was time locked with a significant increase in the amplitude of the stretch-evoked EMG recorded from the ankle extensor muscles. Note also that following injury, a substantial increase in torque was observed at 350°/sec indicating that the threshold velocity at which the active (EMG-associated) torque begins to contribute substantially had decreased significantly.

The weekly data for the first 4 weeks following contusion injury (Figures 7A and 7B) reveal some interesting findings about the time course and the pattern of spasticity that developed. At 1 week postinjury, a tonic type of spasticity was observed. The ankle torques (Figure 7A) and the EMG–RMS (Figure 7B) amplitudes were significantly elevated at all test velocities. During postcontusion Weeks 2 and 3, the ankle torque and corresponding ankle extensor EMGs were significantly reduced compared with preinjury values. By the end of Week 4, both ankle torque and EMG were significantly increased, but only during ankle rotations at the upper range of velocities tested. This velocity-dependent spasticity was different from the tonic pattern observed at 1 week postinjury. The ankle torque and EMG amplitudes produced during low-velocity ankle rotations were not significantly different from preinjury values.

To further evaluate the differences in velocity-dependent lengthening resistance, regression analysis was performed to quantitate the differences in the rate of increase in ankle torque as a function of ankle rotation velocity. A summary of findings is illustrated in Figure 8. Before contusion injury, ankle stiffness at the four slowest velocities was 0.0784 kdyn/deg (slope of first-order equation, r^2 = 0.996) (Figure 8A). During rotations at the four fastest velocities, stiffness was predicted by a steeper slope of 0.121 kdyn/deg (slope of first-order equation, r^2 = 0.985) (Figure 8A). However, when tested at 12 weeks, the stiffness observed during rotations at the fastest velocities had increased by 90% to 0.231 kdyn/deg compared to the preinjury slope of 0.121 kdyn/deg (Figure 8B). In contrast, the stiffness observed during rotation at the four slowest velocities was 0.11 kdyn/deg, an increase of 13% above the preinjury slope of 0.105 kdyn/deg (Figure 8).

IV. RELEVANCE OF SPASTICITY ASSESSMENT IN THE RAT

Spinal cord injury-induced spasticity in humans has been defined as an exaggeration of the velocity-dependent lengthening resistance of muscles, is typically expressed as an exaggeration of the velocity-dependent joint torque (Lance, 1981), and is quantitatively related to the magnitude of this torque response (Knutsson and Martensson, 1985). Collectively, the observations summarized previously indicated that by 1 month after midthoracic contusion injury in the rat, the significant exaggeration of the velocity-dependent stretch reflexes of the ankle extensor muscles and

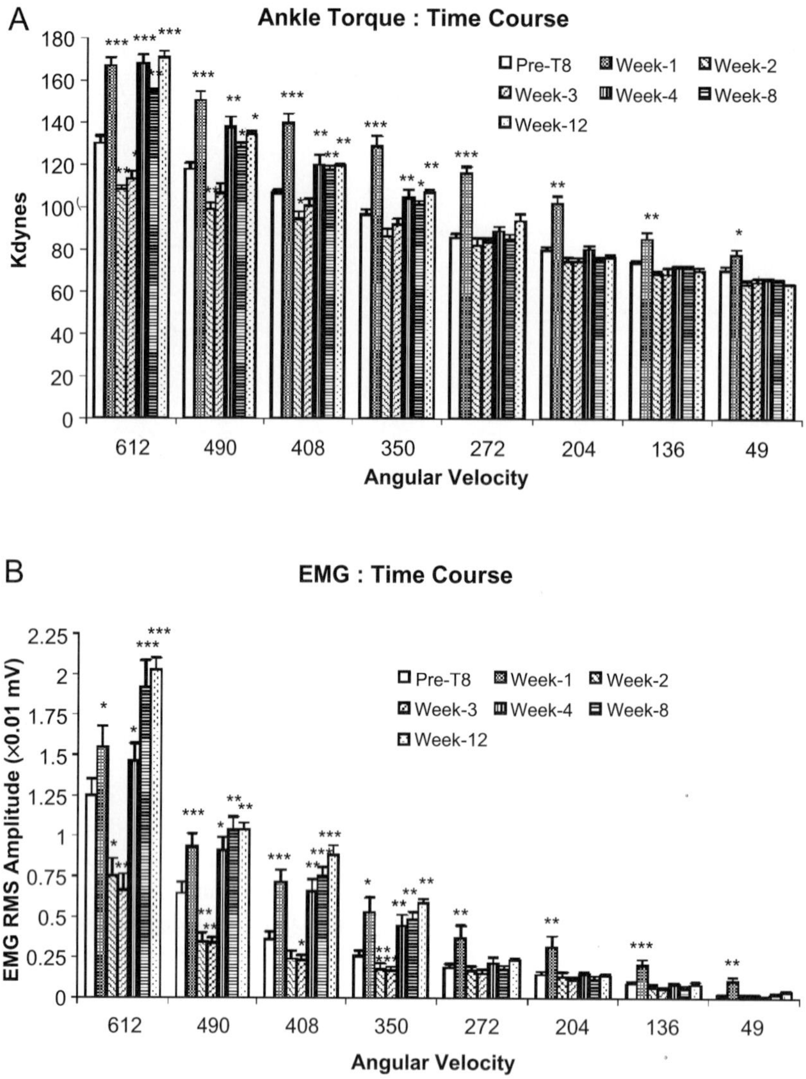

FIGURE 7 Time course of velocity-dependent ankle torque (A) and time-locked EMG–RMS magnitude (B) in the normal animals that served as time-matched controls (n = 4), recorded in eight different angular velocities (49–612°/sec). Recordings were conducted every week until Week 6 and thereafter every alternative week up to Week 12. Data from 1-, 4-, 8-, and 12-week time points are shown. Note that data recorded from precontused normal animals (n = 10) are also shown (T_8-Preinjury). Repeated measure ANOVA within groups (control-pre vs control-week-1 through week-12) or one-way ANOVA between groups (T_8-preinjury vs control-week-1 through week-12) did not reveal any significant differences (p > 0.05) in the ankle torque or EMG–RMS data.

accompanying increased ankle torques were consistent with a clinical assessment of spasticity. It should be noted that the range of test velocities used in the rat was considerably broader, including higher velocities, than typically required for assessment in humans.

Although the test velocities used in these studies seemed high, they are consistent with the rapid locomotor cycle in the rat hindlimb. Physiological lengthening of the triceps surae muscles is typically produced by contraction of the anterior tibial muscle (Hutton et al., 1989). The maximal contraction velocity of the anterior tibial in the rat has been reported to be 260 mm/sec (Winiarski et al., 1987). The maximal lengthening velocity used in the current study was 125 mm/sec; that is, 2.5-mm displacements (12.24°) produced during 20-msec ramps, or 612°/sec. Accordingly, the relatively high velocities included in the protocol to quantitate ankle torque were based on the fast characteristics reported for the rat triceps surae (Gardiner and Kernell, 1990; Gardiner, 1993; Roy et al., 1991) and their antagonist muscle, the anterior tibial muscle (Roy et al., 1985; Alford

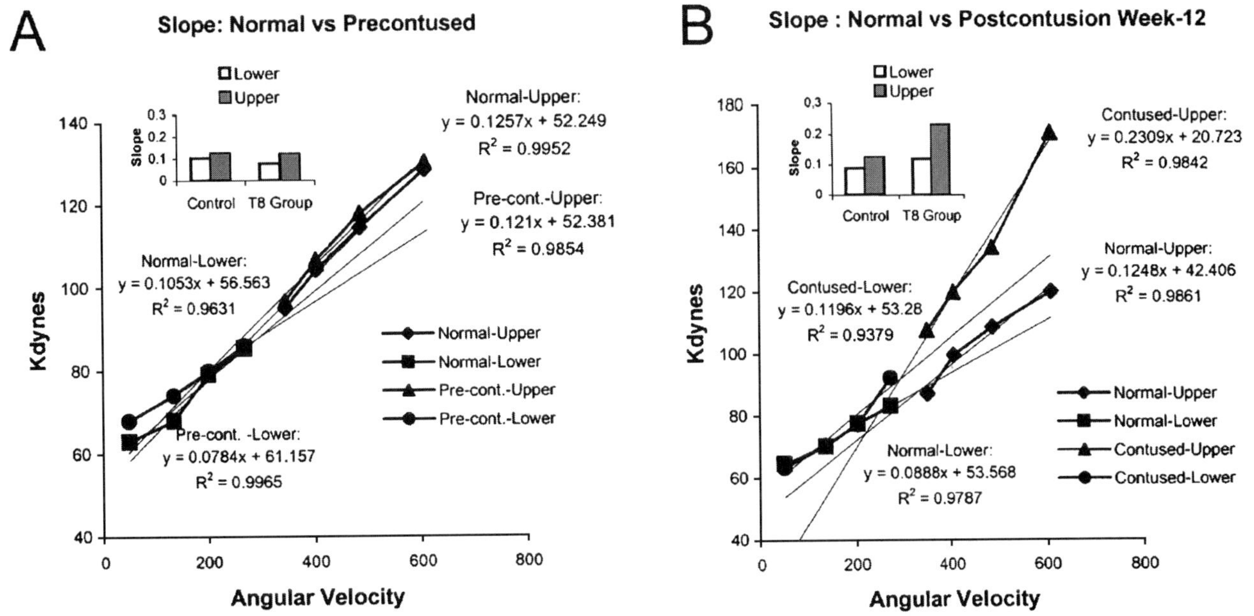

FIGURE 8 Regression analysis of ankle torque as a function of velocity-dependent stiffness of the ankle extensor muscles imposed during ankle rotation compared between normal and precontused animals (A) and time-matched control and postcontused Week 12 (B). Slopes obtained from the lower (slower) four velocities of contused and time-matched control animals did not show any significant difference, except for Week 1, for which the slope was significantly greater compared with that of time-matched controls. The slope obtained using four upper (faster) velocities from Week 2 was significantly depressed; however, slopes from postcontusion Week 4 through Week 12 were significantly elevated compared with those obtained from time-matched controls.

et al., 1987; Hutton et al., 1989). Therefore, the range of ankle rotation velocities used in these experiments was relevant to the physiological range of velocities for the muscles that rotate the ankle. In addition, the upper range of velocities used in these studies was quite essential to reveal the significant increase in the velocity-dependent ankle torque in the postcontusion animals.

Regarding the test velocity range, it is important to note that spasticity was not detected in the ankle extensor muscles in previous studies in rats with midthoracic hemisection injuries that produced neurophysiological hyperreflexic patterns in ankle extensor monosynaptic reflexes (Malmsten, 1983). However, it is possible that the low velocities that would have been used in the manual assessment of joint torques were not sufficient to elicit detectable patterns of spasticity (Malmsten, 1983). Also, it is important to note that manual examination of the hindlimbs of the postcontusion animals in the studies summarized previously revealed a mild atrophy of the hindlimb muscles but no palpable evidence of spasticity. However, spasticity was revealed using instrumentation to indirectly produce lengthening of the triceps surae muscles by ankle rotation across a broad range of rotation velocities in postcontusion compared with time-matched normal control animals (Thompson et al., 1996; Bose et al., 2002a,b). Therefore, these studies indicate that no elevated lengthening resistance would typically be detected at the low-test velocities of muscle lengthening produced by manual examination.

These studies indicate that rats can provide a useful model to investigate spinal cord injury-induced spasticity, and that demonstration of spasticity requires comparisons of lengthening resistance across a broad range of muscle-lengthening velocities. The data from these studies (Bose et al., 2002a,b) support an overall interpretation that the contusion injury-associated increase in the velocity-dependent ankle torque is consistent with the expression of a spastic hyperreflexia for three reasons. First, since the increase in ankle torque was not observed at low velocity of rotation, it cannot simply be ascribed to an increase in the passive stiffness of the muscles. Second, the increase in ankle torque was correlated to an increase in the velocity-dependent EMG. Third, the development of the spasticity was progressive in onset and of enduring duration. A time course study of the development of spasticity is currently under way to evaluate physical and pharmacological therapeutic strategies to enhance recovery of locomotion following spinal cord injury.

Acknowledgments

This work was supported by the Brain and Spinal Cord Injury Research Trust Fund of Florida, the Christopher Reeve Paralysis Foundation, and National Institutes of Health grant R01-NS044293-01.

References

Alford, E.K., R.R. Roy, J.A. Hodgson, and V.R. Edgerton. 1987. Electromyograpy of rat soleus, medial gastrocnemius, and tibialis anterior during hindlimb suspension. *Exp Neurol* **96**:635–649.

Allen, A.R. 1911. Surgery of experimental lesion of spinal cord equivalent to crush injury of fracture dislocation of spinal column. A preliminary report. *JAMA* **57**:878–880.

Anderson, D.K., E.D. Hall, J.M. Braughler, and J.M. McCall. 1991. Effect of delayed administration of U74006F (tirilazad mesylate) on recovery of locomotor function after experimental spinal cord injury. *J Neurotrauma* **8**(3):187–192.

Anderson, D.K., T.R. Waters, and E.D. Means. 1988. Pretreatment with alpha tocopherol enhances neurologic recovery after experimental spinal cord compression injury. *J Neurotrauma* **5**(1):61–67.

Ashby, P., and M. Verrier. 1980. Human motoneuron responses to group 1 volleys blocked presynaptically by vibration. *Brain Res* **184**:511–516.

Ashby, P., E. Stalberg, T. Winkler, and J.P. Hunter. 1987. Further observations on the depression of group Ia facilitation of motoneurons by vibration in man. *Exp Brain Res* **69**(1):1–6.

Basso, D.M., M.S. Beattie, and J.C. Bresnahan. 1995. A sensitive and reliable locomotor rating scale for open field testing in rats. *J Neurotrauma* **12**:1–21.

Beattie, M.S., B.T. Stokes, and J.C. Bresnahan. 1988. Pharmacological Approaches to Treatment of Brain and Spinal Cord Injury. In *Experimental spinal cord injury: Strategies for acute and chronic intervention based on anatomic, physiologic, and behavioral studies.* (New York: Plenum Pub. Co.)

Beattie, M.S., J.C. Bresnahan, J. Komon, C.A. Tovar, M. Van Meter, D.K. Anderson, A.I. Faden, C.Y. Hsu, L.J. Noble, S. Salzman, and W. Young. 1997. Endogenous repair after spinal cord contusion injuries in the rat. *Experimental Neurology* 148, no. **2**:453–463.

Bennett, D.J., Y. Li, P.J. Harvey, and M. Gorassini. 2001. Evidence for plateau potentials in tail motoneurons of awake chronic spinal rats with spasticity. *J Neurophysiol* **86**(4):1972–1982.

Black, P., R.S. Markowitz, V. Cooper, A. Mechanic, H. Kushner, I. Damajanov, S.D. Finkelstein, and K.C. Wachs. 1986. Models of spinal cord injury: Part 1. Static Load Technique. *Neurosurg* **19**:752–762.

Blight, A.R. 1983. Axonal physiology of chronic spinal cord injury in the cat: Intracellular recording in vitro. *Neuroscience* **10**(4):1471–1486.

Blight, A.R. 1985. Computer simulation of action potentials and afterpotentials in mammalian myelinated axons: The case for a lower resistance myelin sheath. *Neuroscience* **15**(1):13–31.

Blight, A.R., and V. DeCriscito. 1986. Morphometric analysis of experimental spinal cord injury in the cat: the relation of injury intensity to survival of myelinated axons. *Neurosci* **19**:321–341.

Bose, P., R. Parmer, J. Parker, R. Hayes, and F.J. Thompson. 2002a. Traumatic brain injury (TBI)-induced spasticity: Monoamine changes and possible mechanisms. *J Neurotrauma* **19**(10):1229–1305.

Bose, P., R. Parmer, and F.J. Thompson. 2002b. Velocity dependent ankle torque in rats after contusion injury of the midthoracic spinal cord: Time course. *J Neurotrauma* **19**(10):1231–1249.

Bracken, M.B., M.J. Shepard, W.F., Collins, Jr., T.R. Holford, D.S. Baskin, H.M. Eisenberg, E. Flamm, L. Leo-Summers, J.C. Maroon, and L.F. Marshall. 1992. Methylprednisolone or naloxone treatment after acute spinal cord injury: 1-year follow-up data. Results of the second National Acute Spinal Cord Injury Study. *J Neurosurg* **76**(1):23–31.

Bresnahan, J.C. 1978. An electron-microscopic analysis of axonal alterations following blunt contusion of the spinal crod of the rhesus monkey (macaca mulatta). *J Neurolog Sci* **37**:59–82.

Bresnahan, J.C., M.S. Beattie, F.D. Todd, 3rd, and D.H. Noyes. 1987. A behavioral and anatomical analysis of spinal cord injury produced by a feedback-controlled impaction device. *Exp Neurol* **195**(3):548–570.

Burke, D. 1988. Spasticity as an adaptation to pyramidal tract injury. In *Advances in Neurology: Functional Recovery in Neurological Disease* (S.G. Waxman, Ed.), pp. 401–423. Raven Press, New York.

Burke, D., and P. Ashby. 1972. Are spinal "presynaptic" inhibitory mechanisms suppressed in spasticity? *J Neurol Sci* **15**(3):321–326.

Burke, D., A.M. Aniss, and S.C. Gandevia. 1987. In-parallel and in-series behavior of human muscle spindle endings. *Neurophysiology* **58**(2): 417–426.

Capaday, C., and R.B. Stein. 1986. Amplitude modulation of the soleus H-reflex in the human during walking and standing. *J Neurosci* **6**:1308–1313.

Collins, W.F., 3rd, B.M. Davis, and L. Mendell. 1988. Modulation of EPSP amplitude during high frequency stimulation depends on the correlation between potentiation, depression and facilitation. *Brain Res* **442**(1):161–165.

Das, G.D. 1989. Perspectives in anatomy and pathology of paraplegia in experimental animals. *Brain Research Bulletin* **22**:7–22.

de la Torre, J.C. 1984. Spinal cord injury models. *Prog Neurobiol* **22**(4):289–344.

Eccles, J.C., and W. Rall. 1951. Effects induced in a monosynaptic reflex by its activation. *J Neurophys* **14**:353–376.

Eccles, J.C., R. Schmidt, and W.D. Willis. 1963. Pharmacological studies on presynaptic inhibitions. *J Physiol* **168**:500–530.

Fehlings, M.G., C.H. Tator, R.D. Linden, and I.R. Piper. 1988. Motor and somatosensory evoked potentials recorded from the rat. *Electroencephalogr Clin Neurophysiol* **69**(1):65–78.

Gardiner, P.F. 1993. Physiological properties of motoneurons innervating different muscle unit types in rat gastrocnemius. *J Neurophysiol* **69**: 1160–1170.

Gardiner, P.F., and D. Kernell. 1990. The "fastness" of rat motoneurones: Time-course of afterhyperpolarization in relation to axonal conduction velocity and muscle unit contractile speed. *Pflugers Arch* **415**:762–766.

Goldberger, M.E., and M. Murray. 1988. Patterns of sprouting and implications for recovery of function. *Adv Neurol* **47**:361–385.

Goldberger, M.E. 1989. Methods for assessing recovery of hindlimb movements after SCI in cats. In Brown, M. and Goldberger, M.E. (eds.) *Conference Proceedings: Criteria for Assessing Recovery of Function: Behavioral Methods.* APA, Springfield, pp 56–61.

Guth, L., C.R. Brewer, W.F. Collins, Jr., M.E. Goldberger, and E.R. Perl. 1980. Criteria for evaluating spinal cord regeneration experiments. *Exp Neurol* **69**(1):1–3.

Herman, R. 1968. Reflex and rheologic properties of the spastic gastrocnemius-soleus muscle group. *Arch Phys Med Rehabil* **49**:723–727.

Hirst, G.D., S.J. Redman, and K. Wong. 1981. Post-tetanic potentiation and facilitation of synaptic potentials evoked in cat spinal motoneurones. *J Physiol* **321**:97–109.

Hughes, J.T. 1988. Pathologic changes after spinal cord injury. Oxford University Press, Oxford.

Hughes, J.T. 1988. The Edwin Smith Surgical Papyrus: An analysis of the first case reports of spinal cord injuries. *Paraplegia* **26**(2):71–82.

Hultborn, H., and J. Malmsten. 1983a. Changes in segmental reflexes following chronic spinal cord hemisection in the cat. I. Increased monosynaptic and polysynaptic ventral root discharges. *Acta Physiol Scand* **119**:405–422.

Hultborn, H., and J. Malmsten. 1983b. Changes in segmental reflexes following chronic spinal cord hemisection in the cat. II. Conditioned monosynaptic reflexes. *Acta Physiol Scand* **119**:423–433.

Hutton, R.S., R.R. Roy, and V.R. Edgerton. 1989. Co-contractions in antagonistic hindlimb muscles during simulated step cycle rates. *Brain Res* **492**:230–236.

Jankowska, E., and S. Edgley. 1993. Interactions between pathways controlling posture and gait at the level of spinal interneurones in the cat. *Prog Brain Res* **97**:161–171.

Jankowska, E., Z.S. Lackberg, and L.E. Dyrehag. 1994. Effects of monoamines on transmission from group II muscle afferents in sacral segments in the cat. *Eur J Neurosci* **6**(6):1058–1061.

Jefferson, A.A., and W. Schlapp. 1953. Some effects of repetitive stimulation of afferents on reflex conduction. In *The Spinal Cord* (J.L. Malcolm and J.A. B. Gray, Eds.), pp. 99–119. Churchill, London.

Kakulas, B.A. 1985. Pathology of spinal injuries. *CNS Trauma* **1**:117–129.

Katz, R.T., and W.Z. Rymer. 1989. Spastic hypertonia: Mechanisms and measurement. *Arch Phys Med Rehab* **70**:144–155.

Kerasidis, H., J.R. Wrathall, and K. Gale. 1987. Behavioral assessment of functional deficit in rats with contusive spinal cord injury. *J Neurosci Methods* (20):167–189.

Knutsson, E., and A. Martensson. 1985. Isokinetic measurements of muscle strength in hysterical paresis. *Electroencephalogr Clin Neurophysiol* **61**:370–374.

Kocsis, J.D., and S.G. Waxman. 1982. Intra-axonal recordings in rat dorsal column axons: Membrane hyperpolarization and decreased excitability precede the primary afferent depolarization. *Brain Res* **238**(1):222–227.

Kuhn, R.A., and M.B. Mact. 1948. Some manifestations of reflex activity in spinal man with particular reference to the occurrence of extensor spasm. *Bull Johns Hopkins Hosp* **84**:43–75.

Lance, J.W. 1981. Disordered muscle tone and movement. *Clin Exp Neurol* **18**:27–35.

Landau, W.M. 1974. Editorial: Spasticity: The fable of a neurological demon and the emperor's new therapy. *Arch Neurol* **31**(4):217–219.

Lev-Tov, A., and M.I. Pinco. 1992. In vitro studies of prolonged synaptic depression in the neonatal rat spinal cord. *J Physiol* **447**:149–169.

Lev-Tov, A., M.J. Pinter, and R.E. Burke. 1983. Posttetanic potentiation of group Ia EPSPs: Possible mechanisms for differential distribution among medial gastrocnemius motoneurons. *J Neurophysiol* **50**:379–398.

Lev-Tov, A., D.E. Meyers, and R.E. Burke. 1988. Activation of type B gamma-aminobutyric acid receptors in the intact mammalian spinal cord mimics the effects of reduced presynaptic Ca2+ influx. *Proc Natl Acad Sci U S A* **85**(14):5330–5334.

Li, L., L.S. Chin, O. Shupliakov, L. Brodin, T.S. Sihra, O. Hvalby, V. Jensen, D. Zheng, J.O. McNamara, P. Greengard, et al. 1995. Impairment of synaptic vesicle clustering and of synaptic transmission, and increased seizure propensity, in synapsin I-deficient mice. *Proc Natl Acad Sci U S A* **92**(20):9235–9239.

Li, Y., M.A. Gorassini, and D.J. Bennett. 2004. Role of persistent sodium and calcium currents in motoneuron firing and spasticity in chronic spinal rats. *J Neurophysiol* **91**(2):767–783.

Lloyd, D.P.C. 1949. Post-tetanic potentiation of response in monosynaptic reflex pathways of the spinal cord. *J Gen Physiol* **33**:147–170.

Lloyd, D.P.C. 1957. Monosynaptic reflex response of individual motoneurons as a function of frequency. *J Gen Physiol* **40**:435.

Lloyd, D.P. 1957. Monosynaptic reflex response of individual motoneurons as a function of frequency. *J Gen Physiol* **40**(3):435–450.

Lodge, D., and N.A. Anis. 1984. Effects of ketamine and three other anaesthetics on spinal reflexes and inhibitions in the cat. *Br J Anaesth* **56**(10): 1143–1151.

Luscher, H., P.W. Ruenzel, and E. Henneman. 1983. Effects of impulse frequency, PTP, and temperature on responses elicited in large populations of motoneurons by impulses in single Ia-fibers. *J Neurophysiol* **50**(5): 1045–1058.

Malmsten, J. 1983. Time course of segmental reflex changes after chronic spinal cord hemisection in the rat. *Acta Physiol Scand* **119**:435–443.

McLellan, D.L., and D.L. Maclellan. 1973. Effect of baclofen upon monosynaptic and tonic vibration reflexes in patients with spasticity. *J Neurol Neurosurg Psychiatry* **36**:555–560.

Mendell, L.M. 1984. Modifiability of spinal synapses. *Physiol Rev* **64**(1): 260–324.

Meythaler, J.M. 2001. Concept of spastic hypertonia. *Phys Med Rehab Clin North Am* **12**(4):725–732, v.

Nelson, S.G., and L.M. Mendell. 1979. Enhancement in Ia-motoneuron synaptic transmission caudal to chronic spinal cord transection. *J Neurophysiol* **3**:642–654.

Nelson, S.G., and L.M. Mendell. 1979. Enhancement in Ia-motoneuron synaptic transmission caudal to chronic spinal cord transection. *J Neurophysiol* **42**:642–654.

Noble, L.J., and J.R. Wrathall. 1989. Distribution and time course of protein extravasation in the rat spinal cord after contusive injury. *Brain Res* **482**(1):57–66.

Noga, B.R., E. Jankowska, and B. Skoog. 1995. Depression of transmission from group II muscle afferents by electrical stimulation of the cuneiform nucleus in the cat. *Experimental Brain Research* 105, no. **1**:25–38.

Penn, R.D., and J.S. Kroin. 1985. Continuous intrathecal baclofen for severe spasticity. *Lancet* **2**(8447):125–127.

Pinco, M., and A. Lev-Tov. 1993. Modulation of monosynaptic excitation in the neonatal rat spinal cord. *J Neurophysiol* **70**(3):1151–1158.

Quevedo, A.A., and J.A. Cliquet. 1995. A paradigm for design of closed loop neuromuscular electrical stimulator control systems. *Artif Organs* **19**(3):280–284.

Reier, P.J., J.D. Houle, L.B. Jakeman, D. Winialski, and A. Tessler. 1988. Transplantation of fetal spinal cord tissue into acute and chronic hemisection and contusion lesions of the adult rat spinal cord. In *Prog Brain Res Vol 78*, edited by Gash, D.M. and J.R. Sladek. Elesevier Science Publishers).

Reier, P.J., L.F. Eng, and L.B. Jakeman. 1989. Reactive astrocyte and axonal outgrowth in the injured CNS: Is gliosis really an impediment to regeneration? In *Neural Regeneration and Transplantation*, edited by Seil, F.J. (New York: Alan R. Liss).

Reier, P.J., D.K. Anderson, F.J. Thompson, and B.F. Stokes. 1992a. Neural tissue transplantation and CNS trauma: Anatomical and functional repair of the injured spinal cord. *J Neurotrauma* **9**(Suppl. 1):S223–S248.

Reier, P.J., B.T. Stokes, F.J. Thompson, and D.K. Anderson. 1992b. Fetal cell grafts into resection and contusion/compression injuries of the rat and cat spinal cord. *Exp Neurol* **115**:177–188.

Roy, R.R., K.M. Baldwin, T.P. Martin, et al. 1985. Biochemical and physiological changes in overloaded rat fast- and slow-twitch ankle extensors. Recruitment patterns in the rat hindlimb muscle during swimming. *J Appl Physiol* **337**:175–178.

Roy, R.R., D.L. Hutchison, J.A. Hodgson, and V.R. Edgerton. 1991. EMG patterns of rat ankle extensors and flexors during treadmill locomotion and swimming. *J Appl Physiol* **70**(6):2522–2529.

Rudomin, P. 1990. Presynaptic inhibition of muscle spindle and tendon organ afferents in the mammalian spinal cord. *Trends Neurosci* **13**(12): 499–505.

Rudomin, P. 1994. Segmental and descending control of the synaptic effectiveness of muscle afferents. *Prog Brain Res* **100**:97–104.

Rudomin, P., I. Jimenez, M. Solodkin, and S. Duenas. 1983. Sites of action of segmental and descending control of transmission on pathways mediating PAD of Ia- and Ib-afferent fibers in cat spinal cord. *J Neurophysiol* **50**(4):743–769.

Rudomin, P., I. Jimenez, and M. Enriquez. 1991. Effects of stimulation of group I afferents from flexor muscles on heterosynaptic facilitation of monosynaptic reflexes produced by Ia and descending inputs: A test for presynaptic inhibition. *Exp Brain Res* **85**(1):93–102.

Shiau, J.S., R.A. Zappulla, and J. Nieves. 1992. The effect of graded spinal cord injury on the extrapyramidal and pyramidal motor evoked potentials of the rat. *Neurosurgery* **30**(1):76–84.

Simpson, R.K., and D.S. Baskin. 1987. Corticomotor evoked potentials in acute and chronic blunt spinal cord injury in the rat: Correlation with neurological outcome and histological damage. *Neurosurgery* **20**(1): 131–137.

Stokes, B.T., and P.J. Reier. 1992. Fetal grafts alter chronic behavioral outcome after contusion damage to the adult rat spinal cord. *Exp Neurol* **116**:1–12.

Stuart, G.J., and S.J. Redman. 1992. The role of GABAA and GABAB receptors in presynaptic inhibition of Ia EPSPs in cat spinal motoneurones.

Stuart, G.J., and S.J. Redman. 1992. The role of $GABA_A$ and $GABA_B$ receptors in presynaptic inhibition of Ia EPSPs in cat spinal motoneurones. *J Physiol* **447**:675–692.

Sudhof, T.C. 1995. The synaptic vesicle cycle: A cascade of protein–protein interactions. *Nature* **375**(6533):645–653.

Tang, A.H., and L.A. Schroeder. 1973. Spinal-cord depressant effects of ketamine and etoxadrol in the cat and the rat. *Anesthesiology* **39**(1): 37–43.

Thilmann, A.F., S.J. Fellows, and E. Garms. 1991. The mechanism of spastic muscle hypertonus. Variation in reflex gain over the time course of spasticity. *Brain* **114**:233–244.

Thompson, F.J., P.J. Reier, C.C. Lucas, and R. Parmer. 1992. Altered patterns of reflex excitability subsequent to contusion injury of the spinal cord. *J Neurophysiol* **68**(5):1473–1486.

Thompson, F.J., P.J. Reier, R. Parmer, and C.C. Lucas. 1993. Inhibitory control of reflex excitability following contusion injury and neural tissue transplantation. *Adv Neurol* **59**:175–184.

Thompson, F.J., C.R. Browd, P.M. Carvalho, and J. Hsiao. 1996. Velocity-dependent ankle torque in the normal rat. *Neuroreport* **7**:2273–2276.

Thompson, F.J., R. Parmer, and P.J. Reier. 1998. Alteration in rate modulation of reflexes to lumbar motoneurons after midthoracic spinal cord injury in the rat. I. Contusion injury. *J Neurotrauma* **15**(7):495–508.

Thompson, F.J., D.C. Wang, R. Parmer, and P. Bose. 2001. Investigation of Chronic Intrathecal Baclofen (ITB) Therapy on Spinal Reflex Excitability and Gait in the Spastic Rat. *Neuroscience* Abst. 27.

Toft, E., T. Sinkjaer, S. Andreassen, and H.J. Hansen. 1993. Stretch responses to ankle rotation in multiple sclerosis patients with spasticity. *EEG Clin Neurophysiol* **89**:311–318.

Wang, D.C., P. Bose, and F.J. Thompson. 2002. Chronic intrathecal baclofen treatment and withdrawal: I. Changes in ankle torque and gait in normal rats. *J Neurotrauma* **19**(7):875–888.

Winiarski, A.M., R.R. Roy, E.K. Alford, P.C. Chiang, and V.R. Edgerton. 1987. Mechanical properties of rat skeletal muscle after hindlimb suspension. *Exp Neurol* **96**:650–660.

Wrathall, J.R., R.K. Pettegrew, and F. Harvey. 1985. Spinal cord contusion in the rat: Production of graded, reproducible injury groups. *Exp Neurol* **88**:108–122.

Yang, J.F., and P.J. Whelan. 1993. Neural mechanisms that contribute to cyclical modulation of the soleus H-reflex in walking in humans. *Exp Brain Res* **95**:547–556

Yomono, H.S., H. Sszuki, and K. Yoshioka. 1992. Serotonergic fibers induce a long-lasting inhibition of monosynaptic reflex in the neonatal rat spinal cord. *Neuroscience* **47**:521–531.

Young, R.R. 1989, 1992. Treatment of spastic paresis. *N Engl J Med* **320**(23):1553–1555; *J Physiol* **447**:675–692.

Young, R.R. 1994. Spasticity: A review. *Neurology* **44**(11 Suppl. 9):S12–S20.

Young, W. 2002. Spinal cord contusion models. *Spinal Cord Trauma: Regeneration, Neural Repair and Functional Recovery* **137**:231–255.

Zileli, M., and J. Schramm. 1991. Motor versus somatosensory evoked potential changes after acute experimental spinal cord injury in rats. *Acta Neurochir (Wien)* **108**(3/4):140–147.

Zucker, R.S., K.R. Delaney, R. Mulkey, and D.W. Tank. 1991. Presynaptic calcium in transmitter release and posttetanic potentiation. *Ann NY Acad Sci* **635**:191–207.

CHAPTER

M1

Drug-Induced Movement Disorders

JOSEPH H. FRIEDMAN and HUBERT H. FERNANDEZ

I. INTRODUCTION

Drugs can induce most movement disorders that occur naturally. Myoclonus, asterixis, ataxia, dystonia, tremor, chorea, ballism, akinesia, rigidity, bradykinesia, and parkinsonism are all well described as drug-induced problems that are usually, although not always, reversible [1]. Perhaps clonus and other spastic phenomena, such as tonic spasms, the only movements not mentioned, do not occur as drug-related phenomena. Many of these movement disorders occur only with dose levels deemed "toxic" and are not covered in this article. Tremor, however, is a common side effect of many central nervous system (CNS) active drugs, at doses that are not toxic, by which we mean doses and serum levels that are usually within the therapeutic target range. Myoclonus, asterixis, and ataxia, on the other hand, are seen almost only when doses above the usual therapeutic levels are taken. Only the movement disorders that occur with the usual and appropriate doses of drugs are discussed here.

Drugs that block the dopamine D_2 receptor may cause a spectrum of movement disorders that are grouped under the umbrella terms extrapyramidal symptoms, or extrapyramidal syndrome(s), generally abbreviated as EPS [2] (Table 1). These disorders are so named because they are also seen in primary disorders of the basal ganglia, the main locus for dopamine innervation in the brain and the "origin" of the extrapyramidal motor system. Many authors lump the different movement disorders together under this term despite the fact that they are quite different from each other. *EPS* refers to symptoms and signs that develop acutely, within minutes to days of drug exposure or dose increase; that develop over days to weeks; or that develop after long-term exposure, termed *tardive* for late-onset, syndromes [3,4]. The tardive syndromes, often grouped together under the term *tardive dyskinesia* (TD), are a heterogeneous collection of movement disorders covered later. The acute-onset syndromes are acute akathisia and acute dystonic reactions. The slowly developing syndrome, parkinsonism, although seemingly better understood in terms of pathophysiology and clinical symptomology, nevertheless presents interesting and challenging problems.

The term *drug-induced movement disorders* generally is used to refer to the movements induced by drugs, primarily antipsychotic drugs, which are thought to act primarily by blocking dopamine receptors. This includes low-potency, antipsychotic-like drugs such as prochlorperazine and metoclopramide, which also block dopamine receptors and produce the same movement disorders as do the antipsychotics.

TABLE 1 Extrapyramidal Syndromes

Onset	Syndrome
Acute	Akathisia—syndrome of motor restlessness
	Acute dystonic reactions—recurrent 30-min episodes of involuntary, sustained muscle contractions causing abnormal postures, typically in neck or face
Subacute	Parkinsonism
Late	"Classic" tardive dyskinesia—oral, buccal, and lingual dyskinesias
	Tardive chorea
	Tardive dystonia
	Tardive akathisia
	Tardive tics
	Tardive tremor
	Tardive myoclonus
	Withdrawal emergent syndrome—a benign tardive syndrome usually found in children

TABLE 2 Atypical Antipsychotic Definitions

Relative freedom from extrapyramidal side effects
Behavioral profile in animal models
Relative serotonin 5-HT2a to dopamine D2 blockade
Efficacy on "negative" symptoms of schizophrenia

It is important to consider the issue of nomenclature in dealing with the antipsychotics. Until the development of clozapine, all antipsychotic drugs induced a variety of movement disorders as unwanted side effects. All the drugs shared the common pharmacological property of blocking the dopamine D_2 receptor [5], and, for a time, it was thought that a prerequisite for antipsychotic activity was blockade of the D_2 receptor coupled with a propensity to induce certain movement disorders. In fact, some authorities suggested that appropriate dosing required [6] the production of a drug-induced parkinsonian condition, with the target antipsychotic dose being just slightly less [7]. It was well-known, however, that many patients had remission of psychosis without developing any movement disorders, whereas some continued to suffer psychotic symptoms despite the development of severe drug-induced parkinsonism. Nevertheless, the dozens of antipsychotics available until clozapine [8] all shared the potential for inducing movement disorders. These antipsychotics were called "neuroleptics," meaning "grips the nerves." They were divided into two broad groups—the low-potency group and the high-potency group. The low-potency drugs, such as thioridazine and loxitane, typically have strong anticholinergic effects [9]. They need to be used in high milligram doses to produce antipsychotic effects and tend to produce few motor side effects until high doses are used. The high-potency neuroleptics, such as haloperidol and pimozide, are antipsychotic at much lower doses, tend to produce many more motor side effects at these low doses, and tend to be much less anticholinergic. Chlorpromazine (Thorazine in the United States and Largactil in Europe), the first antipsychotic commercially available, is in the middle, toward the low-potency end and used as a benchmark. When neuroleptics were compared to each other, they were often converted into "chlorpromazine equivalents," which were estimates of what dose of chlorpromazine would produce an equivalent clinical antipsychotic effect. These chlorpromazine equivalents for antipsychotic effect were approximately the same with regard to their likelihood of producing parkinsonism. When clozapine was proven to be the most effective antipsychotic and lacked motor side effects at any dose in both humans and experimental animals [8], it became clear that the motor side effects of these drugs were an adverse effect and not, as some had assumed, a necessary evil that was part of the pharmacological package. Risperidone was then developed, followed by several other antipsychotics whose motor effects have been considerably less problematic than those of the preclozapine drugs. These newer antipsychotic drugs have been labeled *atypical antipsychotics* (Table 2). Unfortunately, there is no consensus definition for the term, and it has been used to mean different things. In general, the term is used to denote an antipsychotic drug useful in schizophrenia that produces "relatively" few extrapyramidal side effects. This simply shifts the problem to defining what is meant by "relatively." The Food and Drug Administration, after designating clozapine as an atypical antipsychotic, has decided against using the term so that the newer drugs are all designated by their chemical class. In some quarters, these newer antipsychotics are called second-generation antipsychotics [10] and the preclozapine drugs are classified as first generation. The difficulty with this designation is that clozapine, which has been used in Europe for more than 20 years, remains the most atypical of the atypicals, the "gold standard" of atypicality, with the second-generation drugs being closer to first generation than they are to clozapine. Aripiprazole, recently introduced, is considered a third-generation antipsychotic and has been termed a dopamine system stabilizer [11,12].

II. AKATHISIA

Akathisia is a term derived in 1902 [13] to describe a psychiatric syndrome of extreme restlessness. Two young women were unable to remain seated. They needed to constantly walk. Haskovec derived the term *akathitic*, literally meaning "unable to sit" in Greek. Haskovec obtained his history and treated his patients by walking with them on the grounds of the psychiatric hospital. He thought their problem was hysterical in nature. The problem of inability to remain seated, however, had been described earlier. The first reference we found was in a 19th-century textbook that describes a member of the court of Napoleon the Third who suffered from Parkinson disease and violated court protocol by constantly sitting and standing in order to make himself comfortable [14]. Of course, there are many different problems that may cause restlessness, and the differential diagnosis will be discussed.

Akathisia is defined as an inability to remain still due to a sense of inner restlessness [15]. The best description of this sensation we have seen was written by a medical student [16] who described the sensation of a "foreign force" taking over his body making him move constantly. It may be more uncomfortable than the psychosis being treated [17] and has been considered one major factor in medication noncompliance among schizophrenic patients.

Akathitic patients are unable to sit in place [18–23]. In the extreme situation, they will stand as soon as they are seated and will constantly stand and sit. When forced to stay in one place, they will fidget. When seated, they will shift position, rub their arms, cross and uncross their legs, or rock back and forth using movements that are completely normal—all directed at relieving an uncomfortable and severe compulsion to move. When standing, the patient will shift weight or march in place, often also rubbing the arms or hands, and possibly swaying. A classic hallmark of akathisia is the presence of constant foot and leg movements when the patient is supine [20]. If the patient is observed in a hospital setting, the persistence of the restlessness may be overwhelming. The patient may not be able to watch television, participate in ward meetings, have sustained social interactions, or engage in any endeavors that demand remaining still. Even engaging entertainments will not overcome the need for movement. The patient may well complain about the problem, perceiving it as an unwanted and extrinsic presence interfering with the patient's inner and social lives. Since akathisia usually occurs in the context of acute administration or increase in antipsychotic medication, it is often the case that the patient is still psychotic when akathisia develops so that it may be difficult to obtain a reliable medical history. One psychiatrist described a small series of patients who had manifested paradoxical reactions to antipsychotic medication (i.e., getting worse rather than better) with a marked increase in motor activity and sometimes violent actions who then responded to antiakathitic medication. He deduced that some, perhaps many, psychotic patients with paradoxical worsening of psychosis with drug treatment may have developed akathisia [23]. Because of the psychosis, they were unable to communicate their discomfort to the medical staff. Since akathisia occurs soon after starting a medication, or a dose increase, the patient may lose confidence in the treating physician and be reluctant to share information.

Akathisia has no age or gender predilections [24,25], unlike some of the other drug-induced movement disorders. Like the other movement disorders, it is more common with the higher potency neuroleptics, high doses, and intramuscular administration (although not with intravenous delivery) [26,27]. The difficulties in defining the presence of the syndrome in a population that cannot provide reliable information probably accounts for the large variation in the reports on the frequency of akathisia [25]. Estimates in the neuroleptic era vary from 10 to 70% [18], with 20% being generally accepted [7]. Akathisia develops over days to weeks [27], with 90% developing the problem within 73 days of drug initiation, but it may develop within minutes [28] to hours [16]. When akathisia develops after 3 months of stable levels of drug exposure, it is considered tardive akathisia. Although akathisia may develop on atypical antipsychotic drugs, it is not clear how frequently this occurs. It appears to be a considerably smaller problem than it had been in the neuroleptic era.

Akathisia may be difficult to distinguish from several different disorders because the inner sensation is so important in the diagnosis. In a patient who is a reliable informant, the main differential is from restless legs syndrome [24]. In a poorly communicative patient, as may be the case when a patient has a severe mental illness, the differential of akathisia includes agitation due to anger, paranoia, mania, depression, catatonic excitement, body pain, or discomfort from remediable problems such as constipation, distended bladder, gastroenteritis; visceral abnormalities; drug effects vs drug withdrawal effects; hypoxia; thyroid storm; and malingering/manipulation.

Akathisia had been recognized as a symptom of idiopathic Parkinson disease as well as postencephalitic parkinsonism but was otherwise not a major clinical problem until the advent of the neuroleptic era.

III. ACUTE DYSTONIA

Acute dystonia, also known as acute dystonic reaction (ADR), tends to occur early after drug exposure or dose increase. It generally occurs earlier than acute akathisia but not always: 95% of acute dystonic reactions occur within the first 4 days of starting a drug or having a large dose increase [29]. An acute dystonic reaction is an involuntary sustained muscle contraction involving simultaneous contractions of agonist and antagonist muscles causing an abnormal posture that typically has a duration of 20–30 min but is often recurrent. Almost all acute dystonic reactions involve the musculature above the shoulders, but occasional episodes involve structures below the neck. The episodes may be painful or painless and typically involve the neck, jaw, tongue, or the muscles of facial expression. Eyelid spasm, trismus, involuntary jaw opening (severe enough to cause temporomandibular dislocation), tongue protrusions, head tilt, head extension or flexion, opisthotonus, lordosis, and trunk flexion or extension are examples [30]. Involvement of the extraocular eye muscles may cause an "oculogyric crisis," a syndrome previously described only in postencephalitic parkinsonism [31]. In this phenomenon, the eyes deviate upward and stay there for several minutes at a time. In the postencephalitic variant, the patient may or may not be fully able to describe what he or she feels because there may be an accompanying severe compulsive ruminative thought process, but this is not the case in the drug-induced variant, in which mental state is not affected.

The differential diagnosis for an acute dystonic reaction includes focal motor seizure, complex partial seizure (in which the altered mental state is considered a seizure manifestation rather than a primary psychiatric disorder), catatonia, malingering/conversion disorder, hypocalcemia, paroxysmal kinesigenic choreoathetosis, CNS infections, and tetanus [32]. The main clinical problem is distinguishing a psychogenic disorder from an acute dystonic reaction since the history of drug exposure may not be forthcoming or may be falsified and the patient's behavior may be odd.

For unknown reasons, acute dystonic reactions are much more common in the young, with children particularly at risk [33]. The elderly rarely develop acute dystonic reactions [33]. Males are twice as likely as females to develop acute dystonic reactions [7]. Children are more likely to develop a generalized form of dystonia involving the axial and limb muscles than are adults [34]. Previous episodes of acute dystonia, especially on the same or similar drug [35], are a predisposing factor. There may be a family predisposition to the development of ADR [36]. The incidence of acute dystonia has changed dramatically in recent years with the development of the atypical antipsychotics. In the preclozapine era, the incidence of acute dystonia was increasing with the increasing use of high-potency neuroleptics, higher doses of the drugs for acute exacerbations of schizophrenia, and the use of depot, or long-acting, preparations of the drugs. In the early stages of antipsychotic drug use, with the large use of chlorpromazine, the incidence of ADR was only 2.3% [35]. This percentage increased dramatically in the 1970s, with estimates varying from 15 to 25% [37,38] and even higher, with a report of 39% [39]. One study of high-risk young males receiving high-potency neuroleptics reported that 90% of patients had had ADR [40].

There have been no persuasive theories proposed to explain ADR. The association between neuroleptic potency and ADR and neuroleptic potency and anticholinergic activity suggested that the anticholinergic activity was the constraining mechanism. That is, drugs that were of low potency generally had high anticholinergic activity, and it was this latter property that reduced the incidence of ADR. Although the concomitant use of anticholinergics with neuroleptics did reduce the incidence of ADR, they did not prevent them, nor did they reduce the incidence to the level of the low-potency neuroleptics. ADRs have been reported in healthy males given alpha methyl paratyrosine [41], a drug that inhibits synthesis of catecholamines so that blockade of the dopamine receptor is not a requirement for an ADR. Virtually all other reports have involved drugs that block dopamine receptors. Theories on pathophysiology have invoked acute drops in dopamine stimulation or alterations of other neurotransmitter systems. Since most ADRs occur approximately 1 day after drug initiation, when serum levels generally are less than 25% of their peak and increasing relatively slowly, the problem seems unrelated to actual serum levels, although rates of change of the levels may be important. A puzzling case report describes a 70-year-old woman who developed an ADR with involuntary contractions of alternating sides of her jaw when her anxiolytic was stopped as her metoclopramide was started [42], although there was no asymmetry on her baseline exam. Among the atypical antipsychotics, it is clear that risperidone may cause parkinsonism, akathisia, tardive dyskinesia, and ADR. However, olanzapine, which may cause parkinsonism, has been linked to only a single case of ADR. No cases of ADR have been linked to quetiapine or aripiprazole, and a single one has been linked to clozapine. Since quetiapine and clozapine do not cause any of the EPSs, regardless of dose, their freedom from ADR is understandable, but the occurrence of ADR with olanzapine, which may cause parkinsonism, clearly indicates that the possibility of inducing parkinsonism is distinct from the possibility of causing ADR. It is also quite puzzling that although high-dose oral haloperidol is likely to cause ADR and intramuscular haloperidol is even more likely to do so, the same drug, given intravenously at similar doses, does not [26].

IV. PARKINSONISM

The term *parkinsonism* means "looks like Parkinson disease." An equivalent term is parkinsonian and is technically defined as an akinetic rigid syndrome. Thus, the core criteria for diagnosing parkinsonism are rigidity and akinesia, whereas the core criteria for diagnosing Parkinson disease (PD) also include resting tremor, gait, posture and balance dysfunction "typical" of PD, and the absence of atypical features that would make an alternative parkinsonian syndrome more likely. To clinically diagnose PD, one looks for three of the typical features to be present. Not all are required. Although many consider PD a disorder primarily characterized by tremor, this is not the case. Eighty percent of PD patients have tremor at some point, but not all. The tremor is characteristic and rarely seen outside of PD. It occurs at rest and resolves with movement. It most commonly affects the fingers ("pill rolling") followed by the hands, arms, jaw, and feet. Head and tongue involvement is much less common. The tremor reappears on sustention, which is keeping the arms extended for several seconds, at the same frequency. The tremor varies considerably over seconds to minutes so that it may be very prominent at one point and completely resolve a few seconds later. It always worsens with excitement, anxiety, after exertion, and often with cold. Its response to medication is highly unpredictable, with some patients, even with severe tremor, having complete resolution with medications and others not responding to anything short of brain surgery. Rigidity refers to the passive resting tone of a joint. In PD, the arms and neck are generally somewhat stiff and resist passive range of motion attempts. This may vary enormously within the same limb, in which the wrist may be very stiff and the elbow not at all. Bradykinesia refers to slowness of movement and akinesia to absence of movement; although related, they are distinct. Some patients may have much more of one than the other. Akinesia describes the absence of normal spontaneous movements that are typical of parkinsonian patients. They have fewer unconscious movements, such as blinking, swallowing, shifting their weight in the chair, and scratching their face, that normal people have. This leads to the characteristic "stare." It is also the reason why PD patients drool (they have reduced spontaneous swallowing so that saliva pools in the mouth). Slowness of movement is actually one of the most debilitating aspects of the disorder. Patients sometimes describe the loss of automatic control over their movements as, "I have to tell my hand what to do. It used to do things by itself." The need to consciously control some actions leads not only to slowness but also to an inability to perform two actions simultaneously, such as pulling keys out of a pocket while walking, further slowing things down. The posture of parkinsonism is flexed at all joints, although variably so. The posture is stooped as a result and reflects flexion at the knees, hips, and neck. The elbows and wrists also become increasingly flexed. When walking, the arm swing is reduced or absent. Foot strike is flat instead of heel first. Stride length is reduced, as is speed. Patients often lose a normal pivot turn and instead need to stop and take several small steps (turning "en bloc"). Balance becomes impaired so that if a patient loses balance, several steps may be taken to prevent a fall, or sometimes no steps can be taken and the patient falls like a tree. Parkinson disease begins insidiously, usually on one side, and may take months to years to involve the other side clinically (although at autopsy both sides are involved by the time one side is clinically affected).

Drug-induced parkinsonism (DIP) may exactly mimic idiopathic PD [43–45]. Statistically, there are differences between the two syndromes. If one examines large groups of DIP and PD patients, the two major differences are that DIP tends to be symmetric and have less tremor. However, DIP patients have tremor in approximately 40% of cases versus 80% for PD, and a substantial minority of PD patients are symmetric, whereas a significant minority of DIP patients are asymmetric. Thus, in any individual patient, there is no clinical method to distinguish one syndrome from the other. The parkinsonism may be mild, to the point of not being recognized by the patient, or severe enough to simulate catatonia. The "masked facial" expression, with reduced blink rate, stooped posture, and reduced arm swing when walking, is often an indication to the experienced clinician that a patient is probably on a neuroleptic. To the untrained, these changes may cause the patient to be perceived as a "zombie," further complicating the patient's social interactions.

Parkinsonism develops over weeks to months after drug exposure [35]. The elderly are more subject to it than the young, presumably due to brain atrophy and loss of substantia nigra neurons. Women are slightly more at risk than men, which is in contrast to the epidemiology of PD, in which men are more at risk than women. There is a striking biological variation in susceptibility to this effect of the neuroleptic drugs, with some patients, particularly younger ones, tolerating huge doses without apparent motoric effects and others becoming significantly impaired at low doses. Parkinsonism may develop in patients who had been treated with the drugs at the same doses for decades without a problem, raising the clinical question of whether the patients may have developed PD while on the drugs. It is believed that these drugs do not cause PD or increase the risk of developing PD. Only two autopsy results have been published of schizophrenics who developed PD [46], despite the millions of schizophrenics who have been treated with these drugs during the past five decades.

The drugs that cause parkinsonism are generally extremely lipophilic and remain in the brain for long periods. Parkinsonism is thought to almost always resolve when the drug is stopped, but resolution may take as long as 18 months [47,48] and often 3 months or more. Some cases have been reported in which persistent, nonprogressive parkinsonism was noted 7 years after the offending drugs were discontinued.

Although DIP does respond to anticholinergics and amantadine [49–58], our own experience has been that these drugs are only mildly useful. Most DIP is reported to improve or completely resolve within approximately 3 months of being on the drugs, while continuing to take them. It is therefore not considered a major problem by psychiatrists. However, with the increasing use of antipsychotics in the elderly to control the psychotic symptoms that frequently accompany dementia, the likelihood of clinically significant dysfunction is much greater. Although there are reports of DIP responding to L-DOPA, the main drug used to treat the symptoms of idiopathic PD, no convincing studies have been published.

Clozapine, the first atypical antipsychotic drug, does not cause parkinsonism. Both risperidone and olanzapine do so in a dose-dependent manner. Quetiapine appears to not cause parkinsonism, and there are few data on ziprasidone and aripiprazole. For PD specialists, the motor effects of the antipsychotic drugs are particularly important because 10% of drug-treated PD patients develop a drug-induced psychosis from their anti-PD medications [59]. This is treated by the addition of an antipsychotic if the offending drugs cannot be reduced because of jeopardized motor function. It has been clearly demonstrated in double-blind trials that clozapine works well without worsening motor function in this situation [60,61], whereas olanzapine worsens motor function without improving psychosis [62–64]. Open-label data involving large numbers of patients indicate that risperidone is poorly tolerated, and quetiapine improves psychosis without worsening motor function with somewhat less efficacy than clozapine. Data on aripiprazole are accumulating, whereas ziprasidone is unlikely to be tried due to concerns about cardiac arrhythmias.

V. TARDIVE DYSKINESIAS

As mentioned previously, TD refers to a group of disorders characterized by predominantly late-onset and sometimes persistent abnormal involuntary movements. It is caused by exposure to a dopamine receptor blocking agent (DRBA) within 6 months of the onset of symptoms and persisting for at least 1 month after stopping the offending drug [65,66]. The American Psychiatric Association Task Force required 3 months of exposure to a DRBA [67], but TD has been known to occur after only 1 month of exposure, especially in older individuals [68], hence the current consensus definition of 3 months of exposure for those younger than age 60 and 1 month for those older.

There are several phenomenologically distinct types of TD. Unfortunately, the term *tardive dyskinesia* is also used to refer to a specific type of tardive syndrome characterized by oro–buccal–lingual dyskinesias. In this discussion, the tardive disorders as a whole are referred to as TD, and the specific type of tardive disorder that was historically described as oral–buccal–lingual dyskinesia is referred to as classical TD.

The question arises as to what to call TD caused by drugs not known to have dopamine receptor blocking capacity, such as flecainide [69)] and buspirone [70]. It is possible that other mechanisms besides dopamine receptor blockade can cause TD or a clinical picture similar to TD, or that future laboratory investigation may reveal that flecainide or buspirone (or one of their metabolites) are actually DRBAs. Fortunately, TD is a very rare complication of these drugs.

A. Classical Tardive Dyskinesia

TD was first described within 5 years after the first DRBA, chlorpromazine, became widely available in the 1950s [71]. The term tardive dyskinesia was first coined in 1964 by Faurbye et al. who emphasized the incidence of TD increased with chronic exposure [72]. Classical TD has been used to refer to the TD that presents with rapid, repetitive, stereotypic movements involving the oral, buccal, and lingual areas. It has also been termed rhythmical chorea and tardive stereotypy because of its repetitive rather than random nature [73].

TD primarily involves the tongue, lips, and jaw. A combination of tongue twisting and protrusion, lip smacking and puckering, and chewing movements in a repetitive and stereotypic fashion is often observed [73]. Although not absolute, this stereotypic pattern is in contrast to other choreic disorders such as Huntington disease, in which movements are more random and unpredictable. Classical TD is usually confined to the orofacial area, but dyskinesias may spread to the extremities. The involuntary mouth movements may be suppressed by the patients when asked to do so. They can also be suppressed by voluntary actions, such as chewing or talking; thus, classical TD is not commonly disabling. It may be more disturbing to the family and caregiver but sometimes can be socially embarrassing to the patient or result in dysphagia and dysarthria. When involving the limbs, the legs often move repeatedly, with flexion and extension of the toes and foot tapping while sitting. When the patient is lying down, flexion and extension of the thighs may be seen. Respiratory dyskinesias may occur and cause hyper or hypoventilation [74] but are rarely of medical concern. The full classical TD syndrome may take weeks to months to develop but often stabilizes. Classical TD tends to emerge for the first time or worsen when the DRBA is reduced or discontinued. Reinstituting or increasing the dose of the offending drug often reduces movements by masking them.

TD results from chronic exposure to DRBAs, drugs primarily used to treat psychosis. TD has not been reported with dopamine depleters (such as reserpine) and has been uncommonly reported with atypical antipsychotic drugs. Some drugs for nausea (e.g., metoclopramide or prochlorperazine) and depression (e.g., amoxapine) are actually DRBAs and therefore can cause TD (Table 3).

TD-like movements occurring in never-medicated schizophrenics raise the question as to whether TD is solely attributed to DRBAs or is a manifestation of schizophrenia [75,76], possibly unmasked by the DRBA. Major concerns for the latter alternative hypothesis are the accuracy of neuroleptic-free exposure reports and the accuracy of TD diagnosis. Without videotape demonstrations, it would be difficult to determine whether these are actually cases of oromandibular dystonia, edentulous dyskinesia, Huntington disease, stereotypies, etc. This hypothesis also does not explain TD occurring in nonpsychotic individuals exposed to DRBAs such as metoclopramide or prochlorperazine used for nausea.

TABLE 3 Drugs Reported to Cause Tardive Syndromes

Amoxapine (tricyclic antidepressant)
Cinnarizine (calcium channel blocker)
Chlorpromazine
Chlorprothixene
Clebopride
Clozapine (?)
Droperidol
Flunarizine (calcium channel blocker)
Fluphenazine
Haloperidol
Loxapine
Mesoridazine
Metoclopramide
Molindone
Olanzapine
Perazine
Pimozide
Prochlorperazine
Quetiapine (?)
Remoxipride
Risperidone
Sulpiride
Tiapride
Trifluoperazine
Triflupromazine
Thioridazine
Thiothixene
Veralipride

The incidence and prevalence rates for TD vary widely, depending on the population, study design, and diagnostic criteria used. The annual incidence rates range from 5% in the younger population (mean age, 28 years) [77] to 12% in the older group (mean age, 56 years) [78]. In the conventional antipsychotic era, at least 20% of patients treated with neuroleptics were affected by TD, and approximately 5% develop TD with each year of neuroleptic treatment [79]. However, after 5 years, the prevalence remains stable because remission rates balance out incidence rates [80].

During the past 2 decades, there have been major changes in the management of schizophrenia, with a move toward outpatient community care and the use of atypical antipsychotic agents that supposedly produce fewer extrapyramidal side effects. However, a study on the prevalence of movement disorders among all schizophrenics in Nithsdale, Scotland, in 1999–2000 found that of 136 patients, the prevalence of TD was 43%, that of parkinsonism was 35%, and that of akathisia was 15% [81]. Fifty-two percent of patients found to have TD were receiving only atypical antipsychotic agents; however, many had been on neuroleptics previously. Thus, despite the introduction of atypical antipsychotic agents, TD continues to be a problem.

Age has been the most consistent risk factor for TD. Higher incidence and lower remission rates are noted in older patients, especially among women [77,82,83]. Other purported risk factors include affective disorders, poor treatment response, previous brain damage, greater total drug exposure, preexisting parkinsonism, and alcoholism [84,85]. Factors such as drug duration, type of neuroleptic agent, and drug-free intervals are difficult to correlate due to the complex natural history of TD and the difficulty of accurate drug recording.

The natural history of TD is not easy to determine because DRBAs that cause TD also tend to suppress it. Studies have shown the natural course of TD to persist [86], to usually improve [87,88], or to have an unpredictable course [89]. The variable length of follow-up and the differences in study populations may explain the variability in TD course [90]. Studies involving subjects with and without TD at baseline showed an increase in the mean TD assessment scores because the number of new TD cases outweighed the improvement of TD among those already affected at the first evaluation. The majority of studies involving only subjects with TD at baseline showed TD to generally improve or to diminish. One study that examined 53 psychiatric inpatients on high-dose, long-term neuroleptics, reevaluated after 14 years, showed a 4.0 point average improvement in AIMS score. Thirty-three of 53 patients had complete resolution of TD. However, there was a significant worsening of parkinsonism, with a 3.5 point average increase in the Rating Scale for Extrapyramidal Signs, suggesting that TD was being masked [91].

Although there is evidence in animal models that chronic blockade of dopamine receptors leads to increased receptor sensitivity [92,93], human studies have never found this.

The most interesting and consistent findings regarding candidate gene studies of TD have focused on the dopamine D_3 receptor gene (*DRD3*). Several groups have reported an association between the serine-to-glycine polymorphism in exon 1 of the *DRD3* gene and TD. Specifically, each group found that either the glycine/glycine genotype or the glycine allele conferred elevated risk for TD compared to serine/serine homozygotes. One study found a high frequency of this type of homozygosity (22–24%) among patients with TD compared with the relative underrepresentation (4–6%) of this genotype in patients without TD [94]. This may be an explanation of the susceptibility for TD development in some patients.

The effect of DRBA may not be restricted to the dopaminergic system. Other neurotransmitters, such as GABA and noradrenaline, have been implicated.

Oxyradicals have also been implicated [95,96]. This is based on the concept that DRBAs cause an increase in dopamine turnover, resulting in an increased synthesis of hydrogen peroxide, which forms oxyradicals that damage cell components.

The only way to prevent TD is to avoid its etiologic agents. DRBA should not be used for nonpsychotic disorders such as anxiety. Long-term use of DRBA should be limited as much as possible. Patients should be warned of the risk of a TD syndrome before being placed on the drug for maintenance treatment exceeding 3 months. The need for neuroleptic therapy should be reviewed periodically whether or not signs of TD are present. It should be kept at the lowest level needed to achieve the desired effect and should be withdrawn at the earliest opportunity. Among the atypical antipsychotics, clozapine, olanzapine, and quetiapine have the lowest reported incidence of TD, and, in general, have not been convincingly reported to cause TD among patients who were never exposed to other neuroleptics. Long-term epidemiologic data on the use of newer atypicals, such as ziprasidone and aripiprazole, are not available.

B. Tardive Dystonia

Although persistent dystonic movements have long been noted as a complication of DRBAs [97], the phenomenology, epidemiology, prognosis, and pharmacological response of tardive dystonia as a distinct TD was first systematically studied by Burke et al. in 1982 [98].

Without a reliable drug history, tardive dystonia may be indistinguishable from idiopathic torsion dystonia. Both can improve with sensory tricks (geste antagoniste). Tardive dystonia can be focal, segmental (typically among older patients), or generalized (usually among younger subjects). Certain features are more compatible with tardive dystonia. It commonly affects the face, mouth, and neck, followed by the arms, trunk, and, less frequently, the legs. When it involves the neck, it usually results in neck hyperextension (retrocollis). When involving the trunk, it usually results in the trunk arching backward. This is in contrast to the laterocollis and lateral twisting of the trunk commonly seen in idiopathic dystonia. When involving the limbs, internal rotation of the arms, extension of the elbows, and flexion of the wrists are commonly observed in tardive dystonia [99]. A reduction of dystonic movements can be seen in tardive dystonia with voluntary action such as walking, whereas these dystonic movements are often exacerbated in idiopathic dystonia. Finally, oro–buccal–lingual dyskinesia or other TD syndromes may coexist with tardive but not idiopathic dystonia. Other differential diagnoses are listed in Table 4.

Less common tardive dystonic manifestations include oculogyric crises [100,101], bruxism [102], and, rarely, respiratory muscle involvement such as the reverse obstructive sleep apnea syndrome due to laryngeal dystonia (during the day the patient is obstructed, but during sleep the laryngeal dystonia disappears) [103].

DRBA exposure may be shorter for the development of tardive dystonia than normally required for classical TD. In one series, 21% of patients with tardive dystonia had been exposed to neuroleptics for 1 year or less, making the authors conclude that "there is no minimum period of exposure which can be considered safe" [99]. Prevalence rates range from 2% [104–106] to higher than 20% [107,108]. It may be more common among men [109] and tends to occur in younger patients [99].

Similar to TD, the keys to lowering the incidence of tardive dystonia are to limit the use of DRBAs, keep the dose at the lowest possible level, and withdraw them at the earliest safe opportunity. This is more critical for tardive dystonia since it is often more disabling and bothersome to the patient compared to classical TD, and remission rates are said to be lower even when the offending drug is eventually discontinued.

Presynaptic dopamine depleters, such as tetrabenazine and reserpine, probably work better for tardive dystonia than classical TD and are perhaps the most effective medications for this type of TD [110]. However, the limited availability of tetrabenazine and the side effect profile of both drugs limit their use as first-line treatment.

Among the atypical antipsychotic drugs, only clozapine has been consistently reported to alleviate existing tardive dystonia [111–114]. There is very little experience with the use of other atypical neuroleptics for dystonia treatment besides, perhaps, a lower incidence of tardive dystonia as a result of their use.

C. Tardive Akathisia

As discussed in the preceding sections, akathisia is characterized by a feeling of inner restlessness and jitteriness with inability to sit or stand still. There is no consensus on the diagnostic criteria for akathisia or its subtypes. Some authors require only the subjective akathitic state [23], whereas others require the characteristic motor patterns of restlessness and consider it sufficient for the diagnosis even without the subjective feeling [22,115]. Depending on the timing of its appearance, it may be subclassified as acute or chronic. Chronic akathisia is further subdivided into one that occurs early in the course of neuroleptic therapy but remains persistent, called acute persistent akathisia, and one that occurs with long-term therapy, called tardive akathisia. It is often difficult to distinguish between these two subtypes due to the imprecise information about the onset of akathisia relative to neuroleptic initiation.

Its mean age of onset is 58 years with an average DRBA exposure of 4.5 years (range, 2 weeks to 22 years). It is usually accompanied by other TD syndromes [116] and has been reported to occur in approximately 20–40% of DRBA-

TABLE 4 Differential Diagnosis of Tardive Syndromes

Tardive syndrome	Differential diagnosis
Tardive dyskinesia	Spontaneous buccal–lingual dyskinesias of the elderly Edentulous dyskinesia Hereditary choreas (Huntington disease, Wilson disease, neuroacanthocytosis) Strokes (basal ganglia, brain stem, or cerebellum) Tumors (primary, metastatic, paraneoplastic) Hyperthyroidism Calcium and phosphate dysmetabolism Systemic lupus erythematosus and other vasculitides Polycythemia vera Hepatocerebral degeneration Other drugs causing dyskinesias (levodopa, amphetamines, cocaine, tricyclic antidepressants, cimetidine, flunarizine, antihistamines, phenytoin intoxication, lithium) Psychogenic
Tardive dystonia	Idiopathic torsional dystonia Meige syndrome Oromandibular dystonia Symptomatic dystonia (tumor, strokes, etc.) Wilson disease Other secondary causes of dystonia Psychogenic
Tardive myoclonus	Facial myoclonus of central origin Hemifacial spasm Epilepsia partialis continua Drug-induced myoclonus (e.g., opiate toxicity) Neurodegenerative disorders (e.g., AD, CBGD, PD, CJD) Epilepsy CVA, tumors, metabolic derangements Psychogenic
Tardive akathisia	Restless legs syndrome Anxiety/hyperactivity Stereotypy Other drugs that cause akathisia (e.g., levodopa, dopamine agonists, calcium channel blockers)
Tardive tremor	Parkinsonian tremor Essential tremor Cerebellar tremor Rubral tremor Drug-induced tremor (e.g., valproate, lithium) Epilepsy Psychogenic

treated schizophrenics [117]. The differential diagnoses for tardive akathisia are listed in Table 4.

Tardive akathisia and dystonia are the most distressing and disabling of the TDs. Therefore, the offending DRBA should be stopped if possible. Unfortunately, most articles on treatment do not distinguish between acute and tardive akathisia and probably refer more to acute akathisia.

Anticholinergic drugs are usually ineffective. Unlike acute akathisia, beta-blockers do not work in tardive akathisia [116]. One study showed that 87% of patients responded to reserpine and 58% to tetrabenazine. Reports on opiates are conflicting [116].

D. Other Tardive Syndromes

Patients have been reported to experience tics for the first time after exposure to DRBAs [117–120]. There are occasional reports of patients fulfilling the diagnostic clinical criteria for Tourette syndrome except for age of onset. This has been called tardive Tourettism. Stopping the DRBA and giving dopamine depleters may be helpful.

Prominent postural myoclonus in the upper extremities was first described in 32 of 133 psychiatric patients who had been on neuroleptics for at least 3 months [121]. It is usually accompanied by other TDs and has a slight male preponderance. As for other myoclonic conditions, benzodiazepines may be beneficial.

A type of tremor described as more postural and kinetic, unaccompanied by other signs of parkinsonism, persisting despite withdrawal of DRBA, and responding to tetrabenazine has been reported. It is distinct from drug-induced parkinsonism and has been called tardive tremor [122].

Finally, a benign TS called withdrawal emergent syndrome was first described in children who were abruptly withdrawn from their chronic neuroleptic therapy [123]. The movements are choreic, random, and involve mainly the limbs, trunk, and neck. This is in contrast to classical TD, in which the movements are stereotypic, repetitive, and usually involve the oral region. The choreiform movements spontaneously disappear within weeks. For immediate suppression of movements, the DRBA can be reinstituted and withdrawn gradually without the recurrence of choreiform movements [65].

Video Legends

SEGMENT 1 Oromandibular dystonia temporally associated with re-exposure to a dopamine receptor blocking agent (Reglan®-metoclopramide).

SEGMENT 2 Akathisia temporally associated with exposure to a dopamine receptor blocking agent (Prolixin®-fluphenazine)

SEGMENT 3 Parkinsonism developing during usage of dopamine receptor blocking agents (Risperdal®-risperidone and Zyprexa®-olanzapine). Bradykinesia and a resting tremor of the right hand are apparent on examination

SEGMENT 4 Tardive dyskinesia along with drug-induced Parkinsonism. In addition to abnormal oral-buccal-lingual movements, this patient exhibits bradykinesia, a resting tremor of the right hand (best seen during ambulation), and dystonia of the left hand.

SEGMENT 5 Tardive cranio-cervical dystonia with blepharospasm.

References

1. Lang, A.E., and W.J. Weiner, Eds. 1992. *Drug-Induced Movement Disorders*, pp. 85–119. Futura, Mt. Kisco, NY.
2. Delay, J., and P. Deniker. 1968. Drug-induced extrapyramidal syndromes. In *Handbook of Clinical Neurology. Vol. 6. Disease of the Basal Ganglia* (P.J. Vinken and G.W. Bruyn, Eds.), pp. 248–266. Wiley, New York.
3. American Psychiatric Association. 1994. *Diagnostic and Statistical Manual IV.* American Psychiatric Association Press, Washington, DC.
4. Ayd, F. 1961. A survey of drug-induced extrapyramidal reactions. *J Am Med Assoc* **175**:1054–1060.
5. Casey, D.E. 1992. Neuroleptic-induced acute dystonia. In *Drug-Induced Movement Disorders* (A.E. Lang and W.J. Weiner, Eds.), pp. 21–40. Futura, Mt. Kisco, NY.
6. Haase, H.J. 1961. Extrapyramidal modification of fine movements: A "conditio sine qua non" of the fundamental therapeutic action of neuroleptic drugs. *Rev Can Biol* **20**:425–449.
7. Casey, D.E. 1992. Neuroleptic-induced dystonia. In *Drug-Induced Movement Disorders* (A.E. Lang and W.J. Weiner, Eds.). Futura, Mt. Kisco, NY.
8. Kane, J., G. Honigfeld, J. Singer, and H. Meltzer. 1988. Clozapine for the treatment-resistant schizophrenic, a double-blind comparison with chlorpromazine. *Arch Gen Psychiatr* **45**:789–796.
9. Richelson, E. 1984. Neuroleptic affinities for human brain receptors and their use in predicting adverse effects. *J Clin Psychiatr* **45**: 331–336.
10. Meltzer, H.Y. Ed. 1987. *Psychopharmacology. The Third Generation of Progress.* Raven Press, New York.
11. McRae, A., and L.A. Labbate. 2003. Aripiprazole: The latest antipsychotic. *Int Drug Ther Newslett* **38**:25–30.
12. Stahl, S.M. 2001. Dopamine system stabilizers, aripiprazole, and the next generation of antipsychotics, Part 1. *J Clin Psychiatr* **62**:841–842.
13. Haskovec, L. 1902. Akathisia. *Arch Bohemes Med Clin* **3**:193–200.
14. Bing, R. 1939. *Textbook of Nervous Diseases* (W. Haymaker, Trans.). Mosby, St. Louis, MO.
15. Adler, L.A., B. Angrist, and J. Rotrosen. 1992. Acute neuroleptic-induced akathisia. In *Drug-Induced Movement Disorders* (A.E. Lang and W.J. Weiner, Eds.), pp. 85–119. Futura, Mt. Kisco, NY.
16. Kendler, K.S. 1976. A medical student's experience with akathisia. *N Engl J Med* **133**:454–455.
17. Friedman, J.H., and P.J. Weiden. EPS: A guide to prevention, recognition and treatment in the era of atypical antipsychotics. Videotape, available from Astra-Zeneca Pharmaceuticals.
18. Adler, L.A., B. Angrist, S. Reiter, and J. Rotrosen. 1989. Neuroleptic-induced akathisia: A review. *Psychopharmacology* **97**:1–11.
19. Barnes, T.R. 1989. A rating scale for drug induced akathisia. *Br J Psychiatr* **154**:672–676.
20. Braude, W.M., T.R. Barnes, and S.M. Gore. 1983. Clinical characteristics of akathisia: A systematic investigation of acute psychiatric inpatient admissions. *Br J Psychiatr* **143**:139–150.
21. Dumon, J.P., J. Catreau, F. Lanvin, and B.A. Dupuis. 1992. Randomized, double-blind, crossover, placebo-controlled comparison of propranolol and betaxolol in the treatment of neuroleptic-induced akathisia. *Am J Psychiatr* **149**:647–650.
22. Gibb, W.R.G., and A.G. Lees. 1986. The clinical phenomenon of akathisia. *J Neurol Neurosurg Psychiatr* **49**:861–866.
23. Van Putten, T. 1975. The many faces of akathisia. *Compr Psychiatr* **16**:43–47.
24. Lang, A.E. 1993. Akathisia and the restless leg syndrome. In *Parkinson's Disease and Movement Disorders, II* (J. Jankovic and E. Tolosa, Eds.), pp. 349–364. Williams & Wilkins, Baltimore.
25. Sachdev, P., and J. Kruk. 1994. Clinical characteristics and predisposing factors in acute drug-induced akathisia. *Arch Gen Psychiatr* **51**:963–974.
26. Menza, M.A., G.B. Murray, V.F. Holmes, and W.A. Rafuls. 1987. Decreased extrapyramidal symptoms with intravenous haloperidol. *J Clin Psychiatr* **48**(7):278–280.
27. Marsden, C.D., R.H. Mindham, and A.V. Mackay. 1986. Extrapyramidal movement disorders produced by antipsychotic drugs. In *Psychopharmacology and Treatment of Schizophrenia* (P.B. Bradley, Ed.). Oxford University Press, Oxford, UK.
28. Farde, L. 1992. Selective D1- and D2-dopamine receptor blockade both induces akathisia in humans—A PET study with [11C]SCH 23390 and [11C]raclopride. *Psychopharmacology (Berlin)* **107**(1): 23–29.
29. Keepers, G.A., V.J. Clappison, and D.E. Casey. 1983. Initial anticholinergic prophylaxis for neuroleptic-induced extrapyramidal syndromes. *Arch Gen Psychiatr* **40**:1113–1117.
30. Marsden, C.D., D. Tarsy, and R.J. Baldessarini. 1975. Spontaneous and drug-induced movement disorders in psychotic patients. In *Psychiatric Aspects of Neurologic Disease* (D.F. Benson and D. Blumer, Eds). Grune & Stratton, Philadelphia.
31. Friedman, J.H. 1993. Postencephalitic parkinsonism. In *Parkinsonian Syndromes* (M.B. Stern and W.C. Koller, Eds.), Neuroscience Series, pp. 203–226. Dekker, New York.
32. Humphreys, A., and A.R. Tanner. 1994. Acute dystonic reaction or tetanus? An unusual complication of a "Whizz" overdose. *Hum Exp Toxicol* **13**(Suppl. 5):311–312.
33. Keepers, G., and D.E. Casey. 1987. Prediction of neuroleptic-induced dystonia. *J Clin Psychopharmacol* **7**:342–344.
34. Casey, D.E. 1992. Tardive dystonia. In *Drug-Induced Movement Disorders* (A.E. Lang and W.J. Weiner, Eds.). Futura, Mt. Kisco, NY.
35. Keepers, G.A., and D.E. Casey. 1991. Use of neuroleptic-induced extrapyramidal symptoms to predict future vulnerability to side effects. *Am J Psychiatr* **148**:85–89.
36. Ayd, F. 1960. Drug-induced extrapyramidal reactions: Their clinical manifestation and treatment with Akineton. *Psychosomatics* **1**:143.
37. Groves, J.E., and M.R. Mande. 1975. The long-acting phenothiazines. *Arch Gen Psychiatr* **32**:893–900.
38. Swett, C. 1974. Drug-induced dystonia. *Am J Psychiatr* **132**:532–533.
39. Keepers, G.A., V.J. Clappison, and D.E. Casey. 1983. Initial anticholinergic prophylaxis for neuroleptic-induced extrapyramidal syndromes. *Arch Gen Psychiatr* **40**:1113–1117.
40. Boyer, W.F., N.H. Bakalar, and C.R. Lake. 1987. Anticholinergic prophylaxis of acute haloperidol-induced acute dystonic reactions. *J Clin Psychopharmacol* **7**:164–166.
41. McCann, U.D., D.M. Penetar, and G. Belenky. 1990. Acute dystonic reaction in normal humans caused by catecholamine depletion. *Clin Neuropharmacol* **13**:565–568.
42. Friedman, J.H. 1986. Alternating unilateral jaw spasms due to metoclopramide. *J Neurol Neurosurg Psychiatr* **49**:1463.
43. Hardie, R.J., and A.J. Lees. 1988. Neuroleptic-induced Parkinson's syndrome: Clinical features and results of treatment with levodopa. *J Neurol Neurosurg Psychiatr* **51**:850–854.
44. Hornykiewicz, O. 1975. Parkinsonism induced by dopaminergic antagonists. *Adv Neurol* **9**:155–164.
45. National Institute of Mental Health Psychopharmacology Service Center Collaborative Study Group. 1964. Phenothiazine treatment in acute schizophrenia. *Arch Gen Psychiatr* **10**:246–261.

46. Friedman, J.H., J. Max, and R. Swift. 1987. Idiopathic Parkinson's disease in a chronic schizophrenic patient: Long-term treatment with clozapine and levodopa. *Clin Neuropharmacol* **10**:470–475.
47. Klawans, H.L., D. Bergen, and G.W. Bruyn. 1973. Prolonged drug-induced parkinsonism. *Confin Neurol* **35**:368–377.
48. Wilson, J.A., and W.J. MacLennan. 1989. Drug-induced parkinsonism in the elderly. *Age Ageing* **18**:208–210.
49. Chouinard, G., L. Annable, A. Ross-Chouinard, and M.L. Kropsky. 1979. Ethopropazine and benztropine in neuroleptic-induced parkinsonism. *J Clin Psychiatr* **40**:147–152.
50. Mindham, R.H.S., R. Gaind, B.H. Anstee, and L. Rimmer. 1972. Comparison of amantadine, orphenadrine and placebo in drug-induced parkinsonism. *Psychol Med* **2**:406–413.
51. Mindham, R.H.S. 1976. Assessment of drug-induced extrapyramidal reactions and of drugs given for their control. *Br J Clin Pharmacol* **3**(Suppl):395–400.
52. DiMascio, A., D.L. Bernardo, D. Greenblatt, and J.E. Marder. 1976. A controlled trial of amantadine in drug-induced extrapyramidal disorders. *Arch Gen Psychiatr* **33**:599–602.
53. Simpson, G.M. 1970. Controlled studies of antiparkinsonism agents in the treatment of extrapyramidal syndromes. *Acta Psychiatr Scand* **212**:44–51.
54. Kelly, J.T., R.L. Zimmerman, F.S. Abuzzahab, and B.C. Schiele. 1974. A double blind study of amantadine HCl versus benztropine mesylate in drug-induced parkinsonism. *Pharmacology* **12**:65–73.
55. Kelly, J.T., and F.S. Abuzzahab. 1971. Antiparkinsonian properties of amantadine in drug-induced parkinsonism. *J Clin Pharmacol New Drugs* **11**:211–214.
56. Greenblatt, D.J., A. DiMascio, J.S. Harmatz, et al. 1977. Pharmacokinetics and clinical effects of amantadine in drug-induced extrapyramidal syndromes. *J Clin Pharmacol* **17**:704–708.
57. Stenson, R.L., P.T. Donlon, and J.E. Mayer. 1976. Comparison of benztropine and amantadine in neuroleptic-induced extrapyramidal syndromes. *Comp Psychiatr* **17**:762–768.
58. Pacific, G.M., M. Nardini, P. Ferrani, et al. 1976. Effect of amantadine on drug-induced parkinsonism: Relationship between plasma levels and effect. *Br J Clin Pharmacol* **3**:883–889.
59. Friedman, J.H., and H.H. Fernandez. 2002. Atypical antipsychotics in Parkinson sensitive populations. *J Gen Psychiatr Neurol* **15**:156–170.
60. Parkinson's Study Group. 1999. Low dose clozapine for the treatment of drug induced psychosis in Parkinson's disease. *N Engl J Med* **340**:757–763.
61. Pollak, P., F. Tyson, O. Rascol et al. 2004. Clozapine in drug induced psychosis in Parkinson's disease: A randomised, placebo controlled, study with open follow up. *J Neurol Neurosurg Psychiatry* **75**: 689–695.
62. Goetz, C.G., L.M. Blasucci, S. Leurgans, and E.J. Pappert. 2000. Olanzapine and clozapine: Comparative effects on motor functioning in hallucinating Parkinson's disease patients. *Neurology* **55**:789–794.
63. Ondo, W.G., J.K. Levy, K.D. Vuong, et al. 2002. Olanzapine treatment for dopaminergic-induced hallucinations. *Mov Disorders* **17**: 1031–1035.
64. Breier, A., V.K. Sutton, P.D. Feldman, et al. 2002. Olanzapine in the treatment of dopamimetic psychosis in patients with Parkinson's disease. *Biol Psychiatr* **52**:438–445.
65. Fahn, S. 1984. Tardive dyskinesias. *Recent Adv Clin Neurol* **4**:229–260.
66. Stacy, M., and J. Jankovic. 1991. Tardive dyskinesia. *Curr Opin Neurol Neurosurg* **4**:343–349.
67. Baldessarini, R.J., J.O. Cole, J.M. Davis, et al. 1980. Tardive dyskinesia: Summary of a Task Force Report of the American Psychiatric Association. *Am J Psychiatr* **137**:1163–1172.
68. Jeste, D.V., J.P. Lacro, B. Palmer, et al. 1999. Incidence of tardive dyskinesia in early stages of low-dose treatment with typical neuroleptics in older patients. *Am J Psychiatr* **156**:309–311.
69. Miller, L.G., and J. Jankovic. 1992. Persistent dystonia possibly induced by flecainide. *Mov Disorders* **7**:62–63.
70. LeWitt, P.A., A. Walters, W. Hening, and D. McHale. 1993. Persistent movement disorders induced by buspirone. *Mov Disorders* **8**: 331–334.
71. Schonecker, V.M. 1957. Ein eigentumliches Syndrom im oralem Bereich bei Megaphenapplikation. *Nervenarzt* **28**:35–43.
72. Faurbye, A., P.J. Rasch, P.B. Peterson, G. Brandborg, and H. Pakkenberg. 1964. Neurological symptoms in pharmacotherapy of psychoses. *Acta Psychiatr Scand* **40**:10–27.
73. Jankovic, J. 1995. Tardive syndromes and other drug-induced movement disorders. *Clin Neuropharmacol* **18**:197–214.
74. Yassa, R., and S. Lai. 1986. Respiratory irregularity and tardive dyskinesia. *Acta Psychiatr Scand* **73**:506–510.
75. Fenn, D.S., D. Moussaoui, W.F. Hoffman, et al. 1996. Movements in never-medicated schizophrenics: A preliminary study. *Psychopharmacology* **123**:206–210.
76. Fenton, W.S., C.R. Blyler, R.J. Wyatt, and T.H. McGlashan. 1997. Prevalence of spontaneous dyskinesia in schizophrenic and non-schizophrenic psychiatric patients. *Br J Psychiatr* **171**:265–268.
77. Kane, J.M., M. Woerner, M. Borenstein, et al. 1986. Integrating incidence and prevalence of tardive dyskinesia. *Psychopharmacol Bull* **22**:254–258.
78. Barnes, T.R.E., T. Kidger, and S.M. Gore. 1983. Tardive dyskinesia: A 3-year follow-up study. *Psychol Med* **13**:71–81.
79. Kane, J.M., M. Woerner, and J. Lieberman. 1988. Tardive dyskinesia. Prevalence, incidence, and risk factors. *J Clin Psychopharmacol* **8**:525–565.
80. Gardos, G., D.E. Casey, J.O. Cole, et al. 1994. Ten-year outcome of tardive dyskinesia. *Am J Psychiatr* **151**:836–841.
81. Halliday, J., S. Farrington, S. MacDonald, T. MacEwan, V. Sharley, and R. McCreadie. 2002. Nithsdale Schizophrenia Survey 23: Movement disorders. 20 year review. *Br J Psychiatr* **181**:422–427.
82. Kane, J.M., and J.M. Smith. 1982. Tardive dyskinesia: Prevalence and risk factors. *Arch Gen Psychiatr* **39**:473–481.
83. Muscettola, G., S. Pampallona, G. Barbato, M. Casiello, and P. Bolini. 1993. Persistent tardive dyskinesia: Demographic and pharmacological risk factors. *Acta Psychiatr Scand* **87**:29–36.
84. Jeste, D.V., and M.P. Caliguiri. 1993. Tardive dyskinesia (review). *Schizophrenia Bull* **19**:303–315.
85. Jeste, D.V. 2000. Tardive dyskinesia in older patients. *J Clin Psychiatr* **61**(Suppl. 4):27–32.
86. Wegner, J., and J. Kane. 1982. Follow-up study on the reversibility of tardive dyskinesia. *Am J Psychiatr* **139**:368–369
87. Klawans, H.L., D.M. Tanner, and A. Barr. 1984. The reversibility of "permanent" tardive dyskinesia. *Clin Neuropharmacol* **7**:153–159.
88. Casey, D.E., U.J. Povlsen, B. Meidahl, et al. 1986. Neuroleptic-induced tardive dyskinesia and parkinsonism: Change during several years of continuing treatment. *Psychopharmacol Bull* **22**:250–253.
89. Yagi, G., and H. Itoh. 1985. A 10-year follow-up study of tardive dyskinesia with special reference to the influence of neuroleptic administration on the long-term prognosis. *Keio J Med* **34**:211–219.
90. Gardos, G., J.O. Cole, D. Haskell, et al. 1988. The natural history of tardive dyskinesia. *J Clin Psychopharmacol* **8**:31–37.
91. Fernandez, H.H., B. Krupp, and J.H. Friedman. 2001. The course of tardive dyskinesia and parkinsonism in psychiatric inpatients: 14-year follow-up. *Neurology* **56**:805–807.
92. Hitri, A., W. Weiner, R. Borison, et al. 1978. Dopamine binding following prolonged haloperidol pretreatment. *Ann Neurol* **3**:131–140.
93. Klawans, H.L., C.M. Tanner, and C.G. Goetz. 1988. Epidemiology and pathophysiology of tardive dyskinesia. *Adv Neurol* **49**:185–197.
94. Steen, V.M., R. Lovlie, T. MacEwan, and R.G. McCreadie. 1991. Dopamine D3 receptor gene variant and susceptibility to tardive dyskinesia in schizophrenic patients. *Mol Psychiatr Res* **40**:157–166.

95. Tsai, G., D.C. Goff, R.W. Chang, J. Flood, L. Baer, and J.T. Coyle. 1998. Markers of glutamitergic neurotransmission and oxidative stress associated with tardive dyskinesia. *Am J Psychiatr* **155**: 1207–1213.
96. Lohr, J.B. 1991. Oxygen radicals and neuropsychiatric illness—Some speculations. *Arch Gen Psychiatr* **48**:1097–1110.
97. Druckman, R., D. Seelinger, and B. Thulin. 1962. Chronic involuntary movements induced by phenothiazines. *J Nervous Mental Dis* **135**:69–76.
98. Burke, R.E., S. Fahn, J. Jankovic, et al. 1982. Tardive dystonia: Late-onset and persistent dystonia caused by antipsychotic drugs. *Neurology* **32**:1335–1346.
99. Kang, U.J., R.E. Burke, and S. Fahn. 1986. Natural history and treatment of tardive dystonia. *Mov Disorders* **1**:193–208.
100. Fitzgerald, P.M., and J. Jankovic. 1989. Tardive oculogyric crises. *Neurology* **39**:1434–1437.
101. Tan, C.H., P.C. Chiang, L.L. Ng, and K.T. Chee. 1994. Oculogyric spasm in Asian psychiatric inpatients on maintenance medication. *Br J Psychiatr* **165**:381–383.
102. Micheli, F., M.F. Pardal, M. Gatton, J. Asconape, R. Giannuala, and I.C. Parera. 1993. Bruxism secondary to chronic antidopaminergic drug exposure. *Clin Neuropharmacol* **16**:315–323.
103. Sethi, K.D., D.C. Hess, and D. Harmon. 1988. Reverse obstructive sleep apnea syndrome. *Neurology* **38**:312.
104. Yassa, R., V. Nair, and R. Dimitry. 1986. Prevalence of tardive dystonia. *Acta Psychiatr Scand* **73**:629–633.
105. Friedman, J.H., L.T. Kucharski, and R.L. Wagner. 1987. Tardive dystonia in a psychiatric hospital. *J Neurol Neurosurg Psychiatr* **50**: 801–803.
106. Sachdev, P. 1991. Prevalence of tardive dystonia in patients with chronic schizophrenia. *Aust N Z J Psychiatr* **25**:446–448.
107. Sethi, K.D., D.C. Hess, and R.J. Harp. 1990. Prevalence of dystonia in veterans on chronic antipsychotic therapy. *Mov Disorders* **5**:319–321.
108. Stacy, M., F. Cardoso, and J. Jankovic. 1993. Tardive stereotypy and other movement disorders in tardive dyskinesias. *Neurology* **43**:937–941.
109. Kiriakakis, V., K.P. Bhatia, N.P. Quinn, and C.D. Marsden. 1998. The natural history of tardive dystonia. *Brain* **121**:2053–2066.
110. Jankovic, J., and J. Beach. 1997. Long-term effects of tetrabenazine in hyperkinetic movement disorders. *Neurology* **48**:358–362.
111. Raja, M., G. Maisto, M.C. Altavista, and A. Albanese. 1996. Tardive lingual dystonia treated with clozapine. *Mov Disorders* **11**:585–586.
112. Van Harten, P.N., D.J. Kampuis, and G.E. Matroos. 1996. Use of clozapine in tardive dystonia. *Prog Neuropsychopharmacol Biol Psychiatr* **20**:263–274.
113. Spivak, B., R. Mester, J. Abesgaus, et al. 1997. Clozapine treatment for neuroleptic-induced tardive dyskinesia, parkinsonism, and chronic akathisia in schizophrenic patients. *J Clin Psychiatr* **58**:318–322.
114. Factor, S.A., and J.H. Friedman. 1997. The emerging role of clozapine in the treatment of movement disorders. *Mov Disorders* **12**:483–496.
115. Barnes, T.R.E., and W.M. Braude. 1985. Akathisia variants and tardive dyskinesia. *Arch Gen Psychiatr* **42**:874–878.
116. Burke, R.E., U.J. Kang, J. Jankovic, L.G. Miller, and S. Fahn. 1989. Tardive akathisia: An analysis of clinical features and response to open therapeutic trials. *Mov Disorders* **4**:157–175.
117. Schilkurt, V.R., E. Duran, C. Haverback, I. Katz, and P. Vidal. 1978. Verlauf von psychopathologischen und extrapysrmidalmotorischen symptomen unter einer Langzeit-Neurolepticka bahndlung schizophrener Patienten. *Drug Res* **28**:1484–1495.
118. Stahl, S. 1980. Tardive Tourette syndrome in autistic patients after long term neuroleptic administration. *Am J Psychiatr* **137**:1267–1269.
119. Muller, J., and M.J. Aminoff. 1982. Tourette like syndrome after long term neuroleptic drug treatment. *Br J Psychiatr* **141**:191–193.
120. Bharucha, K.J., and K.D. Sethi. 1995. Tardive tourettism after exposure to neuroleptic therapy. *Mov Disorders* **10**:791–793.
121. Tominaga, H., H. Fukuzako, K. Izumi, et al. 1987. Tardive myoclonus. *Lancet* **1**:322.
122. Stacy, M.S., and J. Jankovic. 1992. Tardive tremor. *Mov Disorders* 53–57.
123. Polizos, P., D.M. Engelhardt, S.P. Hoffman, and J. Waizer. 1973. Neurological consequences of psychotropic drug withdrawal in schizophrenic children. *J Autism Child Schizo* **3**:247–253.

CHAPTER

M2

Neuroleptic-Induced Acute Dystonia and Tardive Dyskinesia in Primates

GARY S. LINN

Neuroleptics or typical antipsychotic medications have been associated with high rates of neurological side effects, including extrapyramidal syndromes (EPS) and tardive dyskinesia (TD). Although atypical antipsychotics have a lower incidence of these side effects, most have been associated with at least some cases of EPS. Nonhuman primate models of neuroleptic-induced EPS and TD have been developed to study different hypotheses about pathophysiological mechanisms underlying these motor dysfunctions and for predicting the potential of new antipsychotics to induce EPS and TD. These models share important features with the clinical condition in that the etiological agents, symptoms of EPS and TD, time course of symptom development, and treatments for EPS are the same as in human patients. The development of these models is reviewed and results from studies illustrating several productive research strategies with these models are summarized in this article. A new strategy, combining the neuroleptic-sensitized *Cebus* monkey model with the prepulse inhibition (PPI) model of schizophrenia, which may facilitate identification of new compounds with atypical-like properties and low EPS liability, is presented.

I. BACKGROUND

Schizophrenia is a devastating disorder, which may affect as much as 1% of the population worldwide. Since their introduction in the 1950s, neuroleptic drugs have become the primary therapeutic agents for treating both acute and chronic psychosis. However, most neuroleptics or "typical" antipsychotics have been associated with a wide range of neurological side effects. Extrapyramidal side effects (EPS) are the most troubling and may occur in up to 75% of patients (Casey, 1994; Kulkarni and Naidu, 2003). Although some of the newer "atypical" antipsychotics appear to have a lower risk of inducing EPS, most have been associated with at least some cases of EPS (Carlson et al., 2003; Keck et al., 2004; Leucht et al., 2003), with youths possibly having more prevalent and severe side effects than adults (Sikich et al., 2004). Extrapyramidal side effects consist of a diverse range of symptoms, including akathisia, acute dystonia, and parkinsonism, and may be an indicator of a predisposition to develop TD (Casey, 1993).

Tardive dyskinesia is an involuntary hyperkinetic disorder that occurs in predisposed individuals as a late complication of prolonged neuroleptic treatment or upon treatment termination (Casey and Gerlach, 1984). It consists of choreiform, athetoid, or rhythmical involuntary movements that most frequently involve the face, mouth, and tongue. Less frequent motor abnormalities of the limbs and trunk may also occur (Kulkarni and Naidu, 2003). The most common orofacial symptoms include tongue protrusions, chewing motions, and grimacing. TD can persist for several months to years after drug withdrawal and may be irreversible in some individuals. Although substantial research has been devoted to understanding the basic mechanisms underlying the efficacy and adverse effects of neuroleptic medications and the pathophysiologic processes responsible for EPS and TD, a cohesive explanation has yet to be found (Casey, 2000a; Kulkarni and Naidu, 2003). During the past three decades, several nonhuman primate models have been developed to study different hypotheses about mechanisms of EPS and for predicting the potential of new antipsychotics to induce EPS and TD.

II. EARLY STUDIES WITH NONHUMAN PRIMATES

Early studies with nonhuman primates established that treatment with neuroleptic medications would induce movement disorders that were similar to those observed in the clinic. Daily treatment of 16 rhesus monkeys (*Macaca mulatta*) with 30 mg of chlorpromazine for up to 20 months elicited abnormal tongue protrusion in 1 monkey after 6 months of treatment (Deneau and Crane, 1969). Several other monkeys showed oral–buccal (i.e., chin, tongue, and cheek) dyskinesias, and 1 also had limb extensions and clenching toes. Symptoms appeared a few hours after daily treatments. Monkeys appeared normal by the next morning. Administration of biperiden (an anticholinergic) to 2 monkeys partially or completely relieved their motor abnormalities. Neurological examinations of these monkeys revealed a broad spectrum of motor abnormalities (Deuel, 1969). In addition to oral–buccal dyskinesias, slow dystonic limb movements (slow limb extension and rotations), sudden bursts of normal activity reminiscent of Parkinson disease (PD), and choreiform movements (involuntary spasms and jerking movement) were observed. One monkey had retrocollis and bradykinesia (retardation of voluntary movements and motor retardation as in PD). In another study, Paulson (1972, 1976) treated rhesus monkeys with daily doses of chlorpromazine and haloperidol. Six monkeys receiving chlorpromazine (beginning with 5 mg/kg and increasing up to 30 mg/kg) eventually developed dyskinesias (mostly tongue protrusions, but 2 had transitory torticollis) that began 3 or more months after treatment was initiated. In 3 animals, dyskinesias persisted for 1 week after treatment was discontinued. None of the 12 rhesus monkeys receiving haloperidol (3 mg/animal) developed dyskinesias.

Gunne and Bárány (1976) reported the first demonstration of the development of two distinct dyskinetic syndromes in monkeys following chronic daily administration of haloperidol (0.5 mg/kg p.o.) to 3 capuchin monkeys (*Cebus apella*). One syndrome contained elements similar to acute dystonia and parkinsonism, and the other closely corresponded to tardive dyskinesia. During the first month of treatment, mostly sedation was observed. After 5–7 weeks, elements of acute dystonia (tonic and clonic spasms) and parkinsonism (tremors, bradykinesia, and rigidity) became increasingly prominent. After 3 and 12 months, 2 of the capuchins developed orofacial symptoms (grimacing and tongue protrusions) similar to clinical tardive dyskinesia. As in the clinic, injections of an anticholinergic agent (biperiden) attenuated the acute dystonia but aggravated symptoms of tardive dyskinesia (Gunne and Bárány, 1976; Keepers et al., 1983). Doses of haloperidol (up to 8 mg/kg/day) simultaneously given to 2 cynomolgus macaques (*M. fascicularis*) induced only slight dyskinetic symptoms, prompting the researchers to suggest that *Cebus* monkeys may be more susceptible to neuroleptic agents. In a later report, 4 of 11 *C. apella* monkeys treated daily with haloperidol (0.05–1.0 mg/kg orally) for up to 35 months showed symptoms of tardive dyskinesia that persisted after discontinuation of treatment (Bárány et al., 1979). TD could be temporarily reversed with each new administration of haloperidol. In animals with stable, persistent symptoms of TD, single doses of neuroleptics initially reduced symptoms, but this was followed by a rebound deterioration (i.e., increase) of symptoms. When other antipsychotics (chlorpromazine, clozapine, fluphenazine, and melperone) were substituted for haloperidol, they induced a rebound deterioration of duration and intensity proportional to their respective clinical risk of inducing TD, suggesting this model could be used to monitor the liability of neuroleptic drugs to induce TD (Gunne and Bárány, 1979).

Additional studies by these and other researchers confirmed and extended these initial findings. A study in which three *Cebus* monkeys were treated with biweekly injections of fluphenazine enanthate for 1 year confirmed the development of two distinct motor syndromes (acute dystonias and tardive dyskinesia) (Domino and Kovacic, 1983, 1984; Kovacic and Domino, 1984). All developed abnormal movements corresponding to the acute EPS of neuroleptic-treated patients. Once symptoms developed, they initially occurred during the first 3 days after each treatment, but toward the end of the treatment year they could occur sporadically during the remainder of the 2-week period between injections. Benztropine mesylate treatment could attenuate acute EPS episodes. When neuroleptic treatment was withdrawn, all developed symptoms similar to TD, including orofacial, choreic arm, and finger movements and abnormal pacing. In one monkey that received three courses of fluphenazine treatment, the duration of robust TD symptoms increased with successive treatments, suggesting that spontaneously remitting TD could turn into irreversible TD with continued treatment (Kovacic and Domino, 1982).

Although not all neuroleptic-treated monkeys developed symptoms (Deneau and Crane, 1969; Gunne and Bárány, 1976; Paulson 1972, 1976), once acute dystonic and dyskinetic effects were established in a monkey the animal was neuroleptic "primed" or "sensitized" and symptoms could be elicited by a single injection of the neuroleptic, even after a drug-free period of as long as 508 days (Weiss et al., 1977; Weiss and Santelli, 1978). [In another study, a single injection of haloperidol (0.035 mg/kg) induced acute dystonia in three of four neuroleptic-sensitized *C. apella* monkeys after a neuroleptic-free period of more than 10 years (Linn et al., 2003a).] Liebman and Neale (1980) treated squirrel monkeys (*Samiri sciureus*) with doses of haloperidol at 7- to 14-day intervals until subsequent acute administration of haloperidol elicited dystonia and dyskinesia or the acute dyskinetic syndrome (AD). They then tested different doses of haloperidol and other drugs (e.g., chlorpromazine, fluphenazine, clozapine, thioridazine, and baclofen) in these haloperidol-sensitized monkeys. Impaired Sidman avoidance performance (failure to lever press to delay footshock) served as an indicator of antipsychotic activity (Hanson et al., 1970). Induction of AD by haloperidol was dose related and occurred at the same doses that impaired Sidman avoidance. Induction of AD by other drugs was proportional to their propensity to induce EPS in the clinic, leading the authors to conclude that this nonhuman primate model could be used as a screening test for EPS liability.

III. NONHUMAN PRIMATE MODELS OF EPS AND TARDIVE DYSKINESIA

Two nonhuman primate models of neuroleptic-induced movement disorders were developed from the studies described previously. These models have been categorized as homologous and correlational models (Casey, 1984, 2000a; Davidson, 1981). In a homologous model, a disease state is produced whose symptoms, etiology, biological basis, and response to treatments are similar to those seen in humans. In a correlational model, the factors between the model and the clinical syndrome do not need to be similar, but the results of the model need to be highly predictive of the clinical situation. Induction of TD by long-term treatment with neuroleptic medications in nonhuman primates meets all the criteria of a homologous animal model (Bárány et al., 1979). Identical symptoms occur in both humans and monkeys over a similar time course. Initially, acute dystonias and parkinsonism are seen. Tardive dyskinesia develops after prolonged treatment or upon discontinuation of treatment. The same antipsychotic medications induce these symptoms in humans and monkeys and, in both, acute dystonias but not tardive dyskinesias can be attenuated by the same medications (anticholinergics). Finally, there is individual vulnerability because not all monkeys or humans exposed to chronic neuroleptic treatment develop TD. The limitations of this monkey model of TD are the time and expense to treat a large number of monkeys for up to several years to obtain a large enough subgroup of animals with TD symptoms.

The nonhuman primate correlational model is derived from the correlation between the ability of drugs to induce acute EPS in neuroleptic-sensitized monkeys and the future likelihood of specific antipsychotic drugs to cause TD in the clinic (Casey, 2000a). The induction of EPS in the neuroleptic-sensitized monkey model can be used to predict the potential liability of new antipsychotics to induce acute EPS in humans (Casey, 1995a; Goldstein, 2000; Liebman and Neale, 1980; Porsolt and Jalfre, 1981). An advantage of the correlational model is the lower cost and shorter time of conducting acute studies that have high predictive power for chronic treatment outcomes. One limitation is that this type of model usually does not inform about underlying mechanisms of TD.

It should be noted that although neuroleptic-induced AD and TD have been demonstrated in both New World (superfamily: *Ceboidea*) and Old World (superfamily: *Cercopithecoidea*) monkeys, New World monkeys, particularly *C. apella*, appear to be more prone to developing EPS and TD (Bárány et al., 1979; Kovacic and Domino, 1982). Consequently, *C. apella* has become the species most frequently used for studies of EPS and TD. Sequencing of the D_3 dopamine receptor (*DRD3*) gene in *C. apella* monkeys found that they carry the monomorphic glycine-9 *DRD3* genotype, whereas the *DRD3* gene in humans is polymorphic, caused by a single nucleotide polymorphism (SNP) with either a serine or glycine at amino acid position 9. This SNP, which is responsible for the serine-9 to glycine-9 change, has been associated with TD in humans (Werge et al., 2003). The prevalence of this genotype in other monkey species has yet to be determined. However, there is a report of another New World monkey, the common marmoset (*Callithrix jacchus*), that also may be particularly susceptible to neuroleptic-induced EPS and TD (Fukuoka et al., 1997; Klintenberg et al., 2002).

A. Homologous Model Studies

The homologous monkey model has been used to test potential treatments for TD (Häggström et al., 1983; Andersson and Häggström, 1988) and investigate potential new antipsychotic agents (Kovacic et al., 1986). Also, several studies investigating the effects of repeated or intermittent treatment regimens on induction of acute EPS or

TDs and parkinsonism have supported suggestions that intermittent treatment schedules with typical antipsychotics may increase the incidence and severity of EPS and TD (Casey, 1987; Kovacic and Domino, 1982; Linn et al., 2001). A series of studies with specific D_1 and D_2 dopamine receptor agents by Gerlach and colleagues (Gerlach et al., 1988; Gerlach and Casey, 1990; Lublin and Gerlach, 1988; Peacock et al., 1990) led them to suggest that D_1 hyperfunction may be involved in the pathophysiology of oral dyskinesia, and that in TD a relative D_1 hyperfunction (compared to D_2 function) may facilitate or modulate the syndrome (Gerlach et al., 1991).

A comparison of brain neurochemistry in *Cebus* monkeys receiving chronic neuroleptic treatment revealed that compared to untreated controls or treated monkeys not developing TD, monkeys with TD had decreased levels of γ-aminobutyric acid (GABA) and glutamic acid decarboxylase (GAD), the GABA-synthesizing enzyme, in the subthalamic nucleus, the medial globus pallidus, and the pars reticulata of the substantia nigra, suggesting that GABA insufficiency was related to TD (Gunne et al., 1984; Gunne and Häggström, 1984, 1985). However, administration of GABA agonists to monkeys with TD was inconclusive (Andersson and Häggström, 1988), and patient treatment trials with GABA-enhancing drugs were disappointing (Casey, 2000a). When the cohort of dyskinetic monkeys was enlarged to also include less severe cases of dyskinesia, there was more overlap in GAD levels between dyskinetic monkeys and neuroleptic-treated animals that did not display dyskinesia (Johansson et al., 1990). Striatal levels of substance P, a cotransmitter within the striatonigral GABAergic pathway, were also reduced, leading these researchers to reinterpret their data and suggest that this was an indication of the destruction of GABAergic neurons and an indicator of signs of tardive parkinsonism (TP) (Gunne and Andren, 1993; Richardson and Craig, 1982). In another study by this group, neuroleptic-treated dyskinetic monkeys showed reduced 2-deoxyglucose uptake in the medial segment of the globus pallidus and in the ventral anterior and ventral lateral nuclei of the thalamus, suggesting that globus pallidus pathways to these nuclei are downregulated in TD (Mitchell et al., 1992). Gunne and Andren (1993) hypothesized that chronic neuroleptic treatment upregulates glutamatergic neurons from the subthalamic nucleus terminating in the globus pallidus and substantia nigra. Chronic upregulation has excitotoxic effects on the inhibitory GABA pathways from the globus pallidus and substantia nigra to the thalamus, giving rise to disinhibition of thalamocortical ventral anterior and ventral efferents. This results in a hyperkinetic state that underlies the choreic elements of TD and suggests a glutamate hypothesis for neuroleptic-induced TD. Determination of mRNA for different glutamate receptor subunits in basal ganglia of neuroleptic-treated *Cebus* monkeys with TD symptoms revealed fewer NR1-expressing neurons and lower NR1 signal intensity in caudate, putamen, and globus pallidus, supporting the theory of altered glutamatergic neurotransmission in neuroleptic-induced TD (Chen et al., 1997).

B. Correlational Model: Studies with Neuroleptic-Sensitized Monkeys

When *Cebus* monkeys are repeatedly treated with a typical antipsychotic such as haloperidol, they will eventually develop dystonic reactions and become "sensitized" (Casey et al., 1980). As treatment continues, the reactions to subsequent doses will eventually stabilize and these neuroleptic-sensitized animals can then be used as a model for several different research strategies (Casey, 1995a). One approach is to induce EPS with a typical antipsychotic and then test novel antipsychotics to evaluate their influence on these disorders as new treatments. Another approach is to chronically treat with an antipsychotic, then monitor EPS to evaluate sensitization or tolerance over time. A third strategy is to evaluate response to agents that target either specific receptors (e.g., D_1, D_2, or 5-HT) or combinations of receptors. Different methods of administration, such as oral or by injection, can also be compared. Finally, one can give acute treatments with a wide dose range of several agents to compare the range of behavioral effects. This last strategy is probably the most widely used nonhuman primate preclinical method for evaluating new antipsychotic agents. It remains the most predictive animal model of EPS for several reasons: The acute dystonic reactions in sensitized *Cebus* monkeys are identical to acute EPS in humans; the reactions in sensitized monkeys to existing antipsychotic drugs are elicited proportional to their propensity to induce EPS in the clinic; the acute dystonias can be controlled by the same agents that control EPS in humans (anticholinergics); and clozapine does not induce EPS in the clinic and does not induce acute dystonia in sensitized *Cebus* monkeys (Goldstein, 2000).

Casey (1996a) summarized a series of studies comparing standard and new or putative antipsychotics having a range of $5\text{-HT}_2/D_2$ receptor affinity ratios (Casey et al., 1980; Casey, 1989, 1991). All clinically effective antipsychotic medications have some D_2 receptor affinity (Goldstein, 2000). However, all the typical neuroleptics that block D_2 receptors have the capacity to cause EPS and TD. Antipsychotics with high 5-HT_2 to D_2 antagonism ratios, such as clozapine and olanzapine, are hypothesized to have a low EPS liability at effective antipsychotic doses (Meltzer et al., 1989). [Alternatively, EPS liability may be related to D_2 dissociation constants (Seeman and Tallerico, 1998) or high D_2 receptor occupancy (Kapur and Remington, 2001).] Neuroleptic-sensitized *Cebus* monkeys were exposed to a range of doses of each agent (remoxipride, sulpiride, haloperidol, fluphenazine, clopenthixol, melperone, sertindole, risperidone, clozapine, seroquel, and ritanserin) and observed for signs of acute dystonia or parkinsonism. An observer blind to drug dosage scored measures of dystonia just before and then after drug administration at 30-min intervals for the first 3 hr and then hourly for the next 3 hr. Table 1 contains a representative list of behavioral measures and scores used in these and other comparative studies, drawn from the methods described in Casey (1996b), Gerlach and Casey (1990), Klintenberg et al. (2002), and Linn et al. (2003b). (At the bottom of Table 1, the additional behavioral measures used in primate models of TD, usually scored at daily or weekly intervals, are also included.) A dystonia-inducing threshold dose was defined for each compound as the dose that produced dystonic symptoms in monkeys for at least two observation periods, with a mean group score of 20 or more. For each compound, Casey (1996a) then predicted a dystonia-inducing threshold dose range for humans by multiplying the threshold dose for monkeys by a conversion factor. The conversion factor (200–800) was derived by dividing the haloperidol-induced threshold dose for monkeys by the accepted EPS-producing dose range for haloperidol in humans. Results (shown in Table 2) indicated that with the exception of clozapine, all the compounds tested had the potential to produce EPS in nonhuman primates and, by extension, in humans. Clinically similar dystonic symptoms were induced by the compounds, although the time course of drug effects differed for each compound. Of greater clinical relevance was the separation between effective dose–response ranges for antipsychotic and EPS effects, which predicted low EPS liabilities for effective doses of sertindole and seroquel (quetiapine) and lower doses of risperidone and, in a later study, olanzapine (Casey,

TABLE 1 Typical Behavioral Rating Scale for EPS in Neuroleptic-Sensitized Monkeys[a]

For studies of the induction of EPS in neuroleptic-sensitized monkeys, the following behaviors are rated:

Behavior score
- Sedation, 0 to −3
- Arousal, 0–3
- Locomotor activity, −3 to +3 (−3 to 0, decrease; 0 to +3, increase)

Dystonia in body regions
- Head and neck, 0–3
- Trunk, 0–3
- Upper limbs, 0–3
- Lower limbs, 0–3

Parkinsonian features
- Bradykinesia (slow movement), 0–3
- Tremor, 0–3
- Rigidity, 0–3
- Salivation, 0–3

For studies of tardive dyskinesia, additionally scored behaviors include

Tardive dyskinesia features
- Perioral (grimacing or twitching), 0–3

Lingual (tongue protrusion)
- Masticatory motion, 0–3

Dyskinetic movements
- Upper limbs, 0–3
- Lower limbs, 0–3

Scores
- 0 = no symptoms or normal behavior
- 1 = mild or occasionally seen
- 2 = moderate or ongoing but intermittent
- 3 = continuously present

[a]From methods described in Casey (1996b), Gerlach and Casey (1990), Klintenberg et al. (2002), and Linn et al. (2003b).

TABLE 2 Neuroleptic-Inducing Dystonia Dose Thresholds in Monkeys and Patients[a]

Drug[b]	Dystonia-inducing threshold in monkeys (mg/kg)	Conversion factor ×100	Clinical dose (mg/day)	Estimated dystonia-inducing threshold in humans (mg/day)
Remoxipride	5.0	2–8	150–600	1000–4000
Sulpiride	10	2–8	800–2000	2000–8000
Haloperidol	0.025	2–8	5–20	5–20
Fluphenazine	0.025	2–8	5–20	5–20
Clopenthixol	0.1	2–8	30–60	20–80
Melperone	1.0	2–8	300–600	200–800
Sertindole	0.5	2–8	20–24	100–400
Risperidone	0.025	2–8	4–16	5–20
Clozapine	>25	2–8	250–900	>5000
Seroquel	5.0 (estimated)	2–8	300–400	1000–4000
Ritanserin	10	2–8	?	2000–8000

[a]Adapted from Casey (1996a).
[b]Ordered from high D_2/low 5-HT_2 to low D_2/high 5-HT_2 occupancy.

2000b) that have been supported by clinical studies (Kane, 2001). The finding of low EPS liability for antipsychotics with high 5-HT_2/D_2 receptor affinity ratios, such as clozapine, seroquel, and olanzapine, was compatible with the hypothesis that 5-HT_2/D_2 antagonism ratios may underlie the favorable EPS profiles of atypical antipsychotics (Casey, 2000b; Meltzer et al., 1989).

Results of investigations on the role of D_1 receptors relative to acute dystonias and antipsychotic efficacy have been somewhat conflicting. When SCH 23390, a compound with high D_1 affinity, was given orally to neuroleptic-naive *Cebus* monkeys, no EPS developed (Coffin et al., 1989). However, when given intramuscularly to both neuroleptic-naive and neuroleptic-sensitized *Cebus* monkeys, acute dystonia was observed (Gerlach et al., 1986; Casey, 1992). In a double-blind crossover study in which an oral D_1 receptor antagonist (NNC 22-0215) was given to neuroleptic-sensitized monkeys, EPS was initially induced but there was rapid desensitization by Day 2, and by Day 6 no EPS was observed (Casey, 1995b). Because blood levels of NNC 22-0215 remained unchanged, altered metabolism of drug could not explain the decreasing EPS. The rapid tolerance to induction of dystonia by D_1 antagonists may explain why earlier studies with oral doses of D_1 antagonists to neuroleptic-naive monkeys failed to observe EPS and, if there is a similar tolerance to antipsychotic effects, why clinical trials evaluating the antipsychotic effects of D_1 antagonists have been disappointing (Karlsson et al., 1995). However, Peacock et al. (1999) found that although neuroleptic-sensitized monkeys showed tolerance to dystonic symptoms during treatment with either a D_1 antagonist (NNC 756) alone or in combination with a D_2 antagonist (raclopride), no tolerance to the antipsychotic effect was observed for either condition. (Attenuation of *d*-amphetamine-induced motor unrest served as a measure of antipsychotic effect.) They suggest that differences between preclinical models and clinical trials may be due to differences in properties of the D_1 antagonists used.

Neuroleptic-sensitized *C. apella* monkeys have also been used to study the antipsychotic properties and EPS liability of a muscarinic M1/M4 receptor agonist (Andersen et al., 2003) and an adenosine A2A receptor agonist (Andersen et al., 2002). Antipsychotic effect was evaluated by attenuation of *d*-amphetamine-induced motoric unrest and stereotypies. Results indicate that agents that target these receptors are potential antipsychotics with low EPS liability.

IV. PREPULSE INHIBITION IN NEUROLEPTIC-SENSITIZED MONKEYS

A limitation of most studies of neuroleptic-sensitized monkeys is that they cannot directly test for potential antipsychotic effect in the same animals in which EPS liability is evaluated. A number of studies have used *d*-amphetamine-induced motoric unrest and stereotypies to model psychosis (Andersen et al., 2003; Peacock and Gerlach, 1999). However, dopaminergic agents, such as amphetamine, induce behaviors similar only to positive symptoms of schizophrenia, and so this model may not be able to distinguish atypical-like compounds that also improve negative or cognitive symptoms. PPI of the acoustic startle reflex is a measure of sensorimotor gating that occurs across species (Braff et al., 2001; Geyer et al., 2001; Ison et al., 1973; Linn and Javitt, 2001; Swerdlow et al., 1999). PPI is deficient in severe neuropsychiatric disorders such as schizophrenia (Braff et al., 2001), and these deficits correlate closely with cognitive dysfunction (Perry et al., 1999). PPI of acoustic startle has been demonstrated in New and Old World monkeys (Javitt and Lindsley, 2001; Linn and Javitt, 2001). Phencyclidine (PCP), a potent drug of abuse that induces positive, negative, and cognitive schizophrenia-like symptoms in humans by blocking neurotransmission at *N*-methyl-D-aspartate-type glutamate receptors (Javitt and Zukin, 1991), disrupts PPI in monkeys (Linn and Javitt, 2001). Therefore, PCP-induced deficits of PPI in monkeys can serve as a nonhuman primate model of schizophrenia. In this monkey model, clozapine reversed PCP-induced PPI deficits in *C. apella* monkeys, whereas haloperidol did not significantly attenuate PCP-induced PPI deficits even at doses that significantly attenuated apomorphine effects (Linn et al., 2003a). This indicates that PPI in monkeys may be an effective method for identifying clozapine-like atypical antipsychotics.

Half of the *C. apella* monkeys used in the PPI study were sensitized to typical antipsychotics because prior treatment with depot fluphenazine had induced EPS and TD (Lifshitz et al., 1991; Linn et al., 2001). Prior exposure to typical antipsychotics did not affect PPI (Linn et al., 2003a). However, acute dystonias were observed when sensitized monkeys were exposed to the typical antipsychotic haloperidol for PPI sessions, suggesting that PPI in typical antipsychotic-sensitized monkeys may be a useful preclinical model for evaluating the potential for induction of EPS at effective treatment doses in new antipsychotics (Linn et al., 2003a). A study with this model reported that a newer putative antipsychotic (Lu 35-138) attenuated PCP-induced deficits in PPI without inducing EPS in neuroleptic-sensitized monkeys, suggesting that this compound is likely to have low EPS liability at effective treatment dose levels (Linn et al., 2003b).

V. SUMMARY

Neuroleptic-induced nonhuman primate models of EPS and TD have been effective tools for investigating underlying mechanisms of EPS or TD and for predicting EPS liability in new antipsychotic agents. Although the increasing use of atypical antipsychotics with a lower EPS liability has focused attention away from antipsychotic-induced movement disorders, they continue to be a concern for many patients. A cohesive explanation of the pathophysiology of TD still eludes us. More antipsychotic medications need to be developed that are completely devoid of EPS or any other neurological side effects. With developments such as combining the neuroleptic-sensitized *Cebus* monkey model with the PPI model of schizophrenia or the possibility of a more economically feasible model of TD in *Callithrix* monkeys, these nonhuman primate models will continue to serve an important preclinical research function.

References

Andersen, M.B., K. Fuxe, T. Werge, and J. Gerlach. 2002. The adenosine A2A receptor agonist CGS 21680 exhibits antipsychotic-like activity in Cebus apella monkeys. *Behav Pharmacol* **13**:639–644.

Andersen, M.B., A. Fink-Jensen, L. Peacock, J. Gerlach, F. Bymaster, J.A. Lundbaek, and T. Werge. 2003. The muscarinic M1/M4 receptor agonist xanomeline exhibits antipsychotic-like activity in Cebus apella monkeys. *Neuropsychopharmacology* **28**:1168–1175.

Andersson, U., and J.E. Häggström. 1988. GABA agonists in *Cebus* monkeys with neuroleptic-induced persistent dyskinesias. *Psychopharmacology* **94**:298–301.

Bárány, S., A. Ingvast, and L.M. Gunne. 1979. Development of acute dystonia and tardive dyskinesia in *Cebus* monkeys. *Res Commun Chem Pathol Pharmacol* **25**:269–279.

Braff, D.L., M.A. Geyer, and N.R. Swerdlow. 2001. Human studies of prepulse inhibition of startle: Normal subjects, patient groups, and pharmacological studies. *Psychopharmacology* **156**:234–258.

Carlson, C.D., P.A. Cavazzoni, P.H. Berg, H. Wei, C.M. Beasley, and J.M. Kane. 2003. An integrated analysis of acute treatment-emergent extrapyramidal syndrome in patients with schizophrenia during olanzapine clinical trials: Comparisons with placebo, haloperidol, risperidone, or clozapine. *J Clin Psychiatr* **64**:898–906.

Casey, D.E. 1984. Tardive dyskinesia: Animal models. *Psychopharmacol Bull* **20**:376–379.

Casey, D.E. 1987. Neuroleptic-induced parkinsonism increases with repeated treatment in monkeys. *Psychopharmacol Ser* **3**:243–247.

Casey, D.E. 1989. Serotonergic aspects of acute extrapyramidal syndromes in nonhuman primates. *Psychopharmacol Bull* **25**:457–459.

Casey, D.E. 1991. Extrapyramidal syndromes in nonhuman primates: Typical and atypical neuroleptics. *Psychopharmacol Bull* **27**:47–50.

Casey, D.E. 1992. Dopamine D-1 (SCH 23390) and D-2 (haloperidol) antagonists in drug-naïve monkeys. *Psychopharmacology* **107**:18–22.

Casey, D.E. 1993. Neuroleptic-induced acute extrapyramidal syndromes and tardive dyskinesia. In *The Psychiatric Clinics of North America, Psychopharmacology I* (D.L. Dunner, Ed.), Vol. 16. Saunders, Philadelphia.

Casey, D.E. 1994. Motor and mental aspects of acute extrapyramidal syndromes. *Acta Psychiatr Scand* **89**:14–20.

Casey, D.E. 1995a. The role of dopamine receptor subtypes in nonhuman primate models of antipsychotic drug-induced movement disorders. *Schizophrenia Res* **15**:205.

Casey, D.E. 1995b. The effects of D-1 (NNC 22-0215) and D-2 (haloperidol) antagonists in a chronic double-blind placebo controlled trial in *Cebus* monkeys. *Psychopharmacology* **121**:289–293.

Casey, D.E. 1996a. Extrapyramidal syndromes and new antipsychotic drugs: Findings in patients and non-human primate models. *Br J Psychiatr* **168**(Suppl. 29):32–39.

Casey, D.E. 1996b. Behavioral effects of sertindole, risperidone, clozapine and haloperidol in Cebus monkeys. *Psychopharmacology* **124**:134–140.

Casey, D.E. 2000a. Tardive dyskinesia: Pathophysiology and animal models. *J Clin Psychiatr* **61**:5–9.

Casey, D.E. 2000b. Behavioral effects of olanzapine compared to typical and atypical antipsychotics in Cebus monkeys. In *Olanzapine (Zyprexa)—A Novel Antipsychotic* (P.V. Tran, F.P. Bymaster, N. Tye, J.M. Herrera, A. Breier, and G.D. Tollefson, Eds.), pp. 69–75. Lippincott, Williams & Wilkins, Baltimore.

Casey, D.E., and J. Gerlach. 1984. Tardive dyskinesia: Management and new treatment. In *Guidelines for the Use of Psychotropic Drugs* (H.C. Stancer, P.F. Garfinkel, and V.M. Rakoff, Eds.), pp. 183–203. Spectrum, New York.

Casey, D.E., J. Gerlach, and E. Christensson. 1980. Dopamine, acetylcholine, and GABA effects in acute dystonia in primates. *Psychopharmacology* **70**:83–87.

Chen, S., G. Tsai, A.R. Crossman, and J.T. Coyle. 1997. Changes in glutamate receptor subunit and superoxide dismutase mRNA expression in a primate model of tardive dyskinesia. *Soc Neurosci Abstr* **23**:1953.

Coffin, V.L., M.B. Latranyi, and R.E. Chipkin. 1989. Acute extrapyramidal syndrome in *Cebus* monkeys: Development mediated by dopamine D_2 but not D_1 receptors. *J Pharmacol Exp Ther* **249**:769–774.

Davidson, A.B. 1981. Animal models of tardive dyskinesia. *Psychopharmacol Bull* **17**:45–47.

Deneau, G., and G.E. Crane. 1969. Dyskinesia in rhesus monkeys tested with high doses of chlorpromazine. In *Psychotropic Drugs and Dysfunctions of the Basal Ganglia. A Multidisciplinary Workshop* (G.E. Crane and R. Gardner, Jr., Eds.), pp. 12–14. U.S. Government Printing Office, Washington, DC.

Deuel, R.K. 1969. Neurological examination of rhesus monkeys tested with high doses of chlorpromazine. In *Psychotropic Drugs and Dysfunctions of the Basal Ganglia. A Multidisciplinary Workshop* (G.E. Crane and R. Gardner, Jr., Eds.), pp. 15–18. U.S. Government Printing Office, Washington, DC.

Domino, E.F., and B. Kovacic. 1983. Monkey models of tardive dyskinesia. *Modern Probl Pharmacopsychiatr* **21**:21–33.

Domino, E.F., and B. Kovacic. 1984. Monkey models of tardive dyskinesia. *Neurol Neurobiol* **8**:85–89.

Fukuoka, T., M. Nakano, A. Kohda, Y. Okuno, and M. Matusuo. 1997. The common marmoset (*Callithrix jacchus*) as a model of neuroleptic-induced acute dystonia. *Pharmacol Biochem Behav* **58**:947–953.

Gerlach, J., and D.E. Casey. 1990. Remoxipride, a new selective D-2 antagonist, and haloperidol in *Cebus* monkeys. *Prog Neuropsychopharmacol Biol Psychiatr* **14**:103–112.

Gerlach, J., D.E. Casey, K. Kistrup, and H. Lublin. 1988. Dopamine D-1 and D-2 receptor functions in acute extrapyramidal syndromes and tardive dyskinesia. *Neurol Neurobiol* **42**:1–4.

Gerlach, J., L. Hansen, and L. Peacock. 1991. D-1 dopamine hypothesis in tardive dyskinesia. In *Biological Psychiatry* (G. Racagni, N. Brunello, and T. Fukuda, Eds.), Vol. 1, pp. 609–611. Elsevier, New York.

Geyer, M.A., K. Krebs-Thomas, D.L. Braff, and N.R. Swerdlow. 2001. Pharmacological studies of prepulse inhibition models of sensorimotor gating deficits in schizophrenia: A decade in review. *Psychopharmacology* **156**:117–154.

Goldstein, J.M. 2000. The new generation of antipsychotic drugs: How atypical are they? *Int J Neurospychopharmacol* **3**:339–349.

Gunne, L.M., and P.E. Andren. 1993. An animal model for coexisting tardive dyskinesia and tardive parkinsonism: A glutamate hypothesis for tardive dyskinesia. *Clin Neuropharmacol* **16**:90–95.

Gunne, L.M., and S. Bárány. 1976. Haloperidol-induced tardive dyskinesia in monkeys. *Psychopharmacology* **50**:237–240.

Gunne, L.M., and S. Bárány. 1979. A monitoring test for the liability of neuroleptic drugs to induce tardive dyskinesia. *Psychopharmacology* **63**:195–198.

Gunne, L.M., and J.E. Häggström. 1984. Studies in experimental tardive dyskinesia. *Neurol Neurobiol* **8**:79–84.

Gunne, L.M., and J.E. Häggström. 1985. Pathophysiology of tardive dyskinesia. *Psychopharmacology* (Suppl. 2), 191–193.

Gunne, L.M., J.E. Häggström, and B. Sjöquist. 1984. Association with persistent neuroleptic-induced dyskinesia of regional changes in brain GABA synthesis. *Nature* **309**:347–349.

Häggström, J.E., L.M. Gunne, A. Carlsson, and H. Wikström. 1983. Antidyskinetic action of 3-PPP, a selective dopaminergic autoreceptor agonist, in Cebus monkeys with persistent neuroleptic-induced dyskinesias. *J Neural Transmission* **58**:135–142.

Hanson, H.M., C.A. Stone, and J.J. Witoslawski. 1970. Antagonism of the antiavoidance effects of various agents by anticholinergic drugs. *J Pharmacol Exp Ther* **173**:117–124.

Ison, J.R., D.W. McAdam, and G.R. Hammond. 1973. Latency and amplitude changes in the acoustic startle reflex of the rat produced by variation in auditory prestimulation. *Physiol Behav* **10**:1035–1039.

Javitt, D.C., and R.L. Lindsley. 2001. Effects of phencyclidine on prepulse inhibition of acoustic startle response in the macaque. *Psychopharmacology* **156**:165–168.

Javitt, D.C., and S.R. Zukin. 1991. Recent advances in the phencyclidine model of schizophrenia. *Am J Psychiatr* **148**:1301–1309.

Johansson, P.E., L. Terenius, J.E. Haggstrom, and L. Gunne. 1990. Neuropeptide changes in a primate model (*Cebus apella*) for tardive dyskinesia. *Neuroscience* **37**:563–567.

Kane, J.M. 2001. Extrapyramidal side effects are unacceptable. *Eur Neuropsychopharmacol* **11**(Suppl. 4):S397–S403.

Kapur, S., and G. Remington. 2001. Dopamine D(2) receptors and their role in atypical antipsychotic action: Still necessary and may even be sufficient. *Biol Psychiatr* **50**:873–883.

Karlsson, P., L. Smith, L. Farde, C. Harnryd, G. Sedvall, and F.-A. Wiesel. 1995. Lack of apparent antipsychotic effect of the D1 dopamine receptor antagonist SCH 39166 in acutely ill schizophrenic patients. *Psychopharmacology* **121**:309–316.

Keck, M.E., M.B. Muller, E.B. Binder, A. Sonntag, and F. Holsboer. 2004. Ziprasidone-related tardive dyskinesia. *Am J Psychiatr* **161**:175–176.

Keepers, G.A., V.J. Clappison, and D.E. Casey. 1983. Initial anticholinergic prophylaxis for neuroleptic-induced extrapyramidal syndromes. *Arch Gen Psychiatr* **40**:1113–1117.

Klintenberg, R., L. Gunne, and P.E. Andren. 2002. Tardive dyskinesia model in the common marmoset. *Movement Disorders* **17**:360–365.

Kovacic, B., and E.F. Domino. 1982. A monkey model of tardive dyskinesia (TD): Evidence that reversible TD may turn into irreversible TD. *J Clin Psychopharmacol* **2**:305–307.

Kovacic, B., and E.F. Domino. 1984. Fluphenazine-induced acute and tardive dyskinesias in monkeys. *Psychopharmacology* **84**:310–314.

Kovacic, B., D. Ruffing, and M. Stanley. 1986. Effect of neuroleptics and of potential new antipsychotic agents (MJ13859-1 and MJ13980-1) on a monkey model of tardive dyskinesia. *J Neural Transmission* **65**: 39–49.

Kulkarni, S.K., and P.S. Naidu. 2003. Pathophysiology and drug therapy of tardive dyskinesia: Current concepts and future perspectives. *Drugs Today* **39**:19–49.

Leucht, S., K. Wahlbeck, J. Hamann, and W. Kissling. 2003. New generation antipsychotics versus low-potency conventional antipsychotics: A systematic review and meta-analysis. *Lancet* **361**:1581–1589.

Liebman, J., and R. Neale. 1980. Neuroleptic-induced acute dyskinesias in squirrel monkeys: Correlation with propensity to cause extrapyramidal side effects. *Psychopharmacology* **68**:25–29.

Lifshitz, K., R.T. O'Keeffe, K.L. Lee, G.S. Linn, D. Mase, J. Avery, E.S. Lo, and T.B. Cooper. 1991. Effect of extended depot fluphenazine treatment and withdrawal on social and other behaviors of *Cebus apella* monkeys. *Psychopharmacology* **105**:492–500.

Linn, G.S., and D.C. Javitt. 2001. Phencyclidine (PCP) induced deficits of prepulse inhibition in monkeys. *Neuroreport* **12**:117–120.

Linn, G.S., R.T. O'Keeffe, K. Lifshitz, K. Lee, and J. Camp-Lifshitz. 2001. Increased incidence of dyskinesias and other behavioral effects of re-exposure to neuroleptic treatment in social colonies of *Cebus apella* monkeys. *Psychopharmacology* **153**:285–294.

Linn, G.S., S.S. Negi, S.V. Gerum, and D.C. Javitt. 2003a. Reversal of phencyclidine-induced prepulse inhibition deficits by clozapine in monkeys. *Psychopharmacology* **169**:234–239.

Linn, G.S., B. Pouzet, S. Gerum, J. Aspromonte, T. Hoeg, J. Arnt, and D.C. Javitt. 2003b. The putative antipsychotic Lu 35-138 attenuates phencyclidine-induced deficits in prepulse inhibition without inducing EPS in neuroleptic-sensitized monkeys. Program No. 956.6 2003 Abstract Viewer. Society for Neuroscience, Washington DC. [Online]

Lublin, H., and J. Gerlach. 1988. Behavioural effects of dopamine D-1 and D-2 receptor agonists in monkeys previously treated with haloperidol. *Eur J Pharmacol* **153**:239–245.

Meltzer, H.Y., S. Matsubara, and J.C. Lee. 1989. Classification of typical and atypical antipsychotic drugs on the basis of dopamine D-1, D-2 and serotonin pKi values. *J Pharmacol Exp Ther* **251**:238–246.

Mitchell, I.J., A.R. Crossman, U. Liminga, P. Andren, and L.M. Gunne. 1992. Regional changes in 2-deoxyglucose uptake associated with neuroleptic-induced tardive dyskinesia in the *Cebus* monkey. *Movement Disorders* **7**:32–37.

Peacock, L., and J. Gerlach. 1999. New and old antipsychotics versus clozapine in a monkey model: Adverse effects and antiamphetamine effects. *Psychopharmacology* **144**:189–197.

Peacock, L., H. Lublin, and J. Gerlach. 1990. The effects of dopamine D1 and D2 receptor agonists and antagonists in monkeys withdrawn from long-term neuroleptic treatment. *Eur J Pharmacol* **186**:49–59.

Peacock, L., L. Hansen, F. Morkeberg, and J. Gerlach. 1999. Chronic dopamine D1, dopamine D2 and combined dopamine D1 and D2 antagonist treatment in *Cebus apella* monkeys: Antiamphetamine effects and extrapyramidal side effects. *Neuropsychopharmacology* **20**:35–43.

Perry, W., M.A. Geyer, and D.L. Braff. 1999. Sensorimotor gating and thought disturbance measured in close temporal proximity in schizophrenic patients. *Arch Gen Psychiatr* **56**:277–281.

Paulson, G.W. 1972. Dyskinesias in rhesus monkeys. *Trans Am Neurol Assoc* **97**:109–111.

Paulson, G.W. 1976. Effects of chronic administration of neuroleptics: Dyskinesias in monkeys. *Pharmacol Ther* **B2**:167–171.

Porsolt, R.D., and M. Jalfre. 1981. Neuroleptic-induced acute dyskinesias in rhesus monkeys. *Psychopharmacology* **75**:16–21.

Richardson, M.A., and T.J. Craig. 1982. The coexistence of parkinsonism-like symptoms and tardive dyskinesia. *Am J Psychiatr* **139**:341–343.

Seeman, P., and T. Tallerico. 1998. Antipsychotic drugs which elicit little or no parkinsonism bind more loosely than dopamine to brain D2 receptors, yet occupy high levels of these receptors. *Mol Psychiatr* **3**: 123–134.

Sikich, L., R.M. Hamer, R.A. Bashford, B.B. Sheitman, and J.A. Lieberman. 2004. A pilot study of risperidone, olanzapine, and haloperidol in psychotic youth: A double-blind, randomized, 8-week trial. *Neuropsychopharmacology* **29**:133–145.

Swerdlow, N.R., D.L. Braff, and M.A. Geyer. 1999. Cross-species studies of sensorimotor gating of the startle reflex. *Ann NY Acad Sci* **877**:202–216.

Weiss, B., and S. Santelli. 1978. Dyskinesias evoked in monkeys by weekly administration of haloperidol. *Science* **200**:799–801.

Weiss, B., S. Santelli, and G. Lusink. 1977. Movement disorders induced in monkeys by chronic haloperidol treatment. *Psychopharmacology* **53**:289–293.

Werge, T., Z. Elbaek, M.B. Andersen, J.A. Lundbaek, and H.B. Rasmussen. 2003. *Cebus apella*, a nonhuman primate highly susceptible to neuroleptic side effects, carries the GLY9 dopamine receptor D3 associated with tardive dyskinesia in humans. *Pharmacogenet J* **3**:97–100.

CHAPTER

M3

Motor Effects of Typical and Atypical Antipsychotic Drugs in Rodents

STEPHEN C. FOWLER, T.L. McKERCHAR, and T.J. ZARCONE

Typical antipsychotic drugs (APDs) induce use-limiting extrapyramidal side effects (EPS) that resemble the motor manifestations of Parkinson disease (PD). Although the newer atypical antipsychotic drugs produce less EPS than typical APDs, these newer drugs, nevertheless, produce a variety of motor effects. Reviewed here are studies that used force-transducer technology in two different experimental paradigms to characterize the low-dose motor effects of both typical and atypical APDs in rats. In a paradigm that afforded measures of tongue dynamics (i.e., peak force and rhythm of licking), acute doses of the atypical APDs, clozapine, risperidone, and olanzapine, were shown to slow lick rhythm, while acute doses of the typical APD haloperidol and the selective D2 antagonist raclopride produced much less effect on the rhythm of tongue movements during licking. A second experimental procedure allowed investigators to measure forelimb tremor and force control in rats trained to apply a continuous force to a force-sensing operandum. In this paradigm, acutely administered haloperidol increased tremor and force measures. In contrast, acute clozapine treatment decreased forelimb tremor and force. The atypical APD risperidone modestly reduced forelimb tremor but had no effect on force, and the atypical APD olanzapine affected neither tremor nor force. The fact that clozapine's profile of motor effects in rats is paralleled by similar tremor-reducing and force-control effects in human patients suggests that the methods of assessing motor behavior in rats used here may be useful in research designed to identify APDs with clozapine-like effects.

This work was supported by MH43429, DA12508, and HD002528.

I. INTRODUCTION

Soon after Delay and Deniker observed, in 1952, the clinical efficacy of chlorpromazine as a treatment for psychosis, clinicians recognized that chlorpromazine induced a Parkinson-like syndrome (Delay and Deniker, 1968). The discovery of dopamine (DA) as a neurohumor with neuromodulatory effects in its own right (Carlsson et al., 1958) and the later recognition that PD results from dopamine depletion in the basal ganglia (e.g., Hornykiewicz, 1972) together provided the foundations for our current understanding of the Parkinson-like motor side effects caused by neuroleptics. These side effects are now referred to as extrapyramidal side effects because of their pharmacological effects on the basal ganglia, a collection of subcortical nuclei that comprise a major portion of the extrapyramidal motor system. This chapter selectively summarizes behavioral pharmacology research devoted to the measurement, in preclinical laboratory settings, of the motor effects of antipsychotic drugs. The aim of this work is to develop laboratory methods for assessing EPS liability before discovering such adverse effects in expensive human clinical trials. This review emphasizes work from our laboratory that focuses on the biophysical (i.e., force, duration, rhythmic oscillations, etc.) aspects of rodents' responses to APDs.

In this work, we assume that Parkinson-like symptoms induced in human patients by classical APDs, such as haloperidol, can be modeled in rodents. Investigators can create such models by arranging appropriate behavioral maintenance conditions and by measuring aspects of motor behavior that involve the basal ganglia for their expression. This assumption seems reasonable in light of the hodological, neurochemical, and pharmacological similarities between rodents and humans. Thus, we have developed for rodents a variety of methods for measuring Parkinson-like motor features such as bradykinesia, tremor, and response initiation (and termination) difficulties that arise from pharmacological blockade of dopamine receptors. At the pharmacological level of analysis, two major questions have driven the research: (1) Do *typical*, high-EPS liability APDs produce greater or different motor effects in the animal experiments than effects induced by low-EPS *atypical* APDs and (2) do the motor effects of dopamine receptor antagonists from the D2-family differ from the effects of antagonists from the D1-family? We have also addressed the issue of ameliorating APD-induced motor effects by concurrently administering muscarinic anticholinergic compounds. Investigators consider successful antagonism of anticholinergic motor effects of APDs in rodents as supporting the proposition that the APD-altered motor behavior was Parkinson-like, because these pharmacological manipulations do well in the clinical setting where trihexyphenidyl ameliorates haloperidol-induced EPS in humans. In addition, investigators emphasized doses of APDs low enough to allow the rodent to express adaptive behaviors and interact with the environment and obtain food or water. Thus, the higher-dose phenomena induced by APDs, such as catalepsy (e.g., Sanberg et al., 1988) or the paw test (Ellenbroek and Cools, 1988) will not be reviewed here. In addition, no attempt will be made to review the extensive literature on the behavioral effects of APDs assessed with conventional operant methods, because these methods do not measure motor performance directly.

This chapter is organized by two main categories of experimental paradigm: (1) the lick-force-rhythm task (also see Chapter A6) and (2) the press-while-licking paradigm (methods described in Chapter A6). Interpretations of the demonstrable, preclinical motor effects of both typical and atypical APDs are offered in the conclusions section.

II. DIFFERENTIAL EFFECTS OF APDS ON RAT TONGUE DYNAMICS IN THE LICK-FORCE-RHYTHM TASK

Cramping of the jaw, dysarthria, and orolingual dystonia are frequent signs of EPS that emerge early in response to treatment with classical APDs (e.g., Tarsy, 1989). Researchers have also observed orolingual dysfunction in laboratory animals in association with disruption of brain dopamine systems (Pisa and Schranz, 1988; Salamone et al., 1990; Whishaw et al., 1987). Moreover, one of the most troublesome side effects of the classical APDs is their tendency to induce tardive dyskinesia (TD), a syndrome that primarily affects orofacial functions (e.g., Casey, 1995). As part of our continuing efforts to create quantitative rodent models of the motor effects of APDs, we developed apparatus and procedures for measuring the effects of APDs on tongue dynamics in rats and mice (e.g., rats: Fowler and Mortell, 1992; mice: Wang and Fowler, 1999). To date we have collected data on several APDs, and the results are summarized in table 1.

In the initial study (Fowler and Mortell, 1992), investigators studied a dose range of haloperidol in a within-group, acute dosing design in which thirsty rats licked water from a force sensing disk (see Figures 5 and 6, Chapter A6) during daily 120-s sessions. Rats in this study received three catalepsy-inducing doses of haloperidol thirty-two days before their first dose in the lick assessment procedure. Researchers emphasized the results for the 0.12 mg/kg of haloperidol here because this behaviorally effective dose was common to several experiments, and thereby served as a convenient way to compare across experiments. Haloperidol decreased number of licks and peak force of tongue contacts with the disk, while modestly slowing the lick rhythm. Investigators initially interpreted these results as evidence for EPS-like effects of haloperidol.

However, in a subsequent study (Fowler and Das, 1994) also using a within-group dosing design, haloperidol again reduced number of licks, but at the 0.12 mg/kg dose neither peak force nor lick rhythm was significantly decreased. Rats in this second study had previously received acutely administered doses of raclopride and SCH23390, but no prior haloperidol.

A third, larger study (Fowler and Wang, 1998) used a between-groups dosing design, a chronic dosing regimen, and drug-naive rats. This experiment also used an improved method of delivering the water to the lick disk (see Figure 6, Chapter A6). In the other studies summarized in table 1, the water was squirted onto the lick surface via a stainless steel tube just out of reach of the rat's tongue, but in the Fowler and Wang (1998) method, water was pumped into a hole in the center of a disk. Water delivery through the hole in the disk reduced variability in the rat's lick forces. The distance variable was 2 mm for Fowler and Wang (1998) but was 5 mm for the other studies summarized in table 1; the

TABLE 1 Effects of Antipsychotic Drugs and SCH 23390 on Tongue Dynamics in Male Sprague-Dawley Rats

			Vehicle or baseline			Data for the indicated dose			
Drug and citation[1]	D[2] (mm)	Doses (mg/kg)	N licks	Peak force (g)	Rhythm (Hz)	Dose[3] (m/kg)	N licks	Peak force (g)	Rhythm (Hz)
Haloperidol (a)	5	0.03, 0.06, 0.12, 0.25	550	9.8	5.25	0.12	378*[4]	8.1*	5.08*
Haloperidol (b)	5	0.06, 0.12, 0.25	617	8.4	5.31	0.12	300*	6.7	5.30
Haloperidol (c)	2	0.06, 0.12, 0.24 (acute)	643	13.6	5.73	0.12	524*	13.0	5.67
Haloperidol (c)	2	0.06, 0.12, 0.24 (chronic: 105 days)	643	13.6	5.73	0.12	515*	8.1*	5.46*
SCH 23390 (d)	5	0.01, 0.02, 0.04, 0.08, 0.16, 0.24	602	8.7	5.14	0.08	414*	6.8*	4.81*
Raclopride (d)	5	0.05, 0.10, 0.20, 0.40, 0.80, 1.20	602	8.7	5.14	0.20	409*	6.8*	5.03*
Clozapine (e)	5	1, 3, 6	531	10.4	5.20	3.0	180*	5.3*	4.63*
Clozapine (f)	5	0.5, 1.0, 2.0, 4.0	546	6.2	5.19	3.0	373*	4.4*	4.81*
Olanzapine (f)	5	0.25, 0.5, 1.0, 2.0	546	6.2	5.19	1.0	364*	4.8*	4.83*

Notes: 1. citations: (a) Fowler and Mortell, 1992; (b) Fowler and Das, 1994; (c) Fowler and Wang, 1998; (d) Hayes, 1995; (e) Das and Fowler, 1995; (f) Das and Fowler, 1996.

2. D is the distance between the inside plane of the lick orifice and the top surface of the lick disk.

3. The dose listed produced a significant effect on at least one measure of tongue dynamics.

4. *significantly ($p < 0.05$) different from control.

5. The drug data presented are for a single dose excerpted from complete monotonic, dose-effect functions that can be viewed by consulting the indicated references.

closer distance in Fowler and Wang (1998) accounts for the higher lick rhythm baseline in this study (~5.7 Hz versus ~5.2 Hz). Upon first exposure to the 0.12 mg/kg dose of haloperidol, the number of licks was significantly reduced, but the peak force and lick rhythm were not significantly affected (data in table 1). However, by the end of the 105-day period of chronic dosing, 0.12 mg/kg haloperidol treatment significantly reduced all three measures of tongue dynamics (see table 1). Although not shown in table 1, a 0.24 mg/kg dose produced the same pattern of results as the 0.12 mg/kg dose: the first 0.24 mg/kg dose significantly reduced number of licks, but did not significantly affect peak force or rhythm, while chronic dosing significantly reduced all three measures of tongue dynamics. A month or more after daily haloperidol had begun, anticholinergic probes were given concurrently with haloperidol. The muscarinic anticholinergics, scopolamine and trihexyphenidyl, partially antagonized haloperidol's suppressive effects on all three measures of tongue dynamics. This latter result suggested that chronic haloperidol's effects on tongue dynamics were more EPS like than TD-like.

To assess the importance of the different types of dopamine receptors to tongue dynamics, investigators assessed the effects of the D1-like receptor antagonist SCH23390 and the D2-like antagonist raclopride in the lick-force-rhythm task (Hayes, 1995). Drug-naïve rats were used in this study, and the results are shown in table 1 for a single dose of each drug. These doses were selected for comparison because each produced almost identical significant reductions in the number of licks made in two minutes (i.e., a group mean of 414 licks for 0.08 mg/kg SCH23390 and 409 licks for 0.20 mg/kg for raclopride). The significant reductions in tongue peak force were the same for both drugs; however, in the face of near equality on the number of licks and force measures, SCH23390 had a greater effect on lick rhythm than raclopride. In fact, the SCH23390 group mean rhythm (4.81 Hz) was significantly below ($t_{28} = 2.094$, $p < 0.05$) the group mean rhythm for raclopride (5.03 Hz). These data suggest that acute D2 antagonism has markedly less effect on lick rhythm than acute D1 antagonism.

Although investigators reported that haloperidol, which is predominately a D2 antagonist, slowed the lick rhythm upon acute dosing (Fowler and Mortell, 1992), the rats in the cited study had previously received catalepsy-inducing doses of haloperidol. In the other studies, where the effects of acute dosing with haloperidol on lick rhythm were examined in haloperidol-naïve rats (Fowler and Das, 1994; Fowler and Wang, 1998), lick-rhythm slowing was not observed. The haloperidol observations are therefore consistent with the lack of lick-rhythm slowing by acute administration of the D2 antagonist raclopride (Hayes, 1995). In terms of methodology, the apparent carryover effects of haloperidol on lick dynamics imply that within-group experimental designs for evaluating dose effects, in which every rat receives each dose in counterbalanced order, are always confounded by some degree of prior haloperidol experience. Therefore, investigators can accurately assess dose effects of haloperidol in rats only in between-group experimental designs where separate groups of rats receive different doses of haloperidol.

In the first evaluation of clozapine's effects on tongue dynamics, researchers used both drug-experienced and drug-naïve rats (Das and Fowler, 1995). As expected on the basis of results from the press-while-licking task (e.g., Fowler et al., 1994), clozapine decreased number of licks, tongue peak force, and lick rhythm in relation to dose (data for the 3.0 mg/kg dose in the drug-experienced rats are shown in table 1). Drug-experienced and drug-naïve rats exhibited almost identical results on all three measures of tongue dynamics. In addition to the acute dose-effect evaluation, this study examined subchronic effects of clozapine in a dosing regimen of seven daily dosings with the same dose, separated by four nondrug days between different doses. The results indicated that the rats became tolerant to clozapine's ability to suppress licking (reflected by number of licks in two minutes), but the rats did not show tolerance to the rhythm-slowing effects of clozapine.

Investigators compared the atypical APD olanzapine with clozapine in the lick-force-rhythm task (Das and Fowler, 1996). In this study all rats received all doses of both drugs, and at least two nondrug days separated drug evaluation days. Rats used in this study had received clozapine treatments (1.5–4.5 mg/kg) with the last treatment occurring twenty-eight days before the clozapine and olanzapine observations were made. Essentially, the results showed (representative data in table 1) that clozapine and olanzapine had very similar effects on tongue dynamics. The dose effect functions for the lick rhythm variable were parallel, and a quantitative analysis of drug potency for rhythm-slowing showed that olanzapine was twice as potent as clozapine.

While the lick task was cost-effective—experimenters spent little time training rats to lick water from a disk—and it produced quantitative and systematic results, the fact that non-APDs also reduced lick rhythm complicated the interpretation of the results from the lick task. However, adding an operant response (e.g., pressing a force sensor with a fore limb) to the lick task made it possible to assess other forms of EPS (e.g., forelimb tremor) and to relate those effects to data already collected on the lick-force-rhythm task.

III. DIFFERENTIAL EFFECTS OF TYPICAL AND ATYPICAL APDS ON FORELIMB FORCE CONTROL

In the press-while-licking task (see Figures 1 and 2 Chapter A6), a rat engages in a relatively complex sequence of behaviors starting with response initiation in the form of placing its forepaw on a force-sensing disk and ending with release of force on the disk. When the rat maintains force above a specified level, it receives a liquid reward (water or milk); the reward remains accessible as long as the force remains above the specified level. When the rat consumes the reward, it must release the force to allow the reward dipper to drop into the reservoir and refill. A variety of quantitative techniques applied to the resulting force time data generated by the rat's forelimb can define several performance variables. The performance variables include time-on-task, peak force (the maximum force attained during the initial 1 s of the response), hold force (the mean force level after the first 1 s of the response), lick rhythm (the frequency at the peak in the power spectrum of the hold force for the 5.0–9.9 Hz frequency band), tremor (integrated power in the 10–25 Hz frequency band of the power spectrum of the hold force), and response duration (the interval between paw placement and release of force).

In the first report using this forelimb tremor assay to describe the motor effects of APDs, investigators used a dose range of haloperidol (see table 2), and attempted to antagonize haloperidol's behavioral effects with atropine sulfate, a muscarinic anticholinergic drug (Fowler et al., 1990). In this initial study, the software for extracting all of the dependent variables shown in table 2 had not yet been developed, and, therefore, the analysis focused on time-on-task and tremor. Haloperidol decreased time-on-task in relation to dose and increased power in the tremor frequency band (10–25 Hz). These two effects were later replicated in a separate group of rats treated with a 0.04 mg/kg dose of haloperidol (Kallman and Fowler, 1994). All of the power spectra for the forelimb force variations exhibited a prominent peak near 7 Hz for every rat, regardless of drug treatment. When we first observed these near-7 Hz peaks we did not know that they were produced by licking from the reward dipper that occurred while a rat's fore paw was in contact with the operandum. In a subsequent exploratory experiment (unpublished observations) we mounted a reinforcement dipper on a waterproof force transducer to measure the lick forces directly and concurrently with forelimb forces in the press-while-licking task. The resulting recordings showed unequivocally that the near-7 Hz frequency of the peak in the power spectrum for the forelimb coincided exactly with the lick frequency measured from the power spectrum of the forces made by the tongue striking the reward dipper. The indirect measure of the lick rhythm via the forelimb operandum had a higher lick frequency than in the lick-force-rhythm task because the distance between the rat's muzzle and the dipper was effectively zero, but in the lick-only task the distance was either 2 mm or 5 mm (see Fowler et al., this volume, for systematic data relating distance to lick rhythm).

To test the hypothesis that haloperidol-induced decreases in time-on-task and increases in tremor were EPS-like,

TABLE 2 Effects of Haloperidol and Atypical Antipsychotic Drugs on Tremor and Other Response Parameters in the Press-While-Licking Task

	Antipsychotic drugs used					
Variable	**Hal[1] 0.04[2], 0.08, 0.16**	**Hal 0.04**	**Hal 0.02, 0.04, 0.08, 0.12 Clz 2.0, 4.0, 8.0**	**Hal 0.01–0.08 Clz 6–18**	**Clz 1.0, 5.0 Olz 0.5, 1.0**	**Rsp 0.08, 0.12, 0.16**
Dose regimen	Acute	Acute	Acute	Chronic	Chronic	Acute
Time on task	<[3]	<	Hal < Clz <	Hal < Clz <[6]	Clz < Olz <	<
Tremor band Power	>	>	Hal > Clz <	Hal > Clz <	Clz < Olz =	<
Response duration	n.r.[4]	=	Hal n.r. Clz n.r.	Hal > Clz >	Clz > Olz >	>
Peak force	n.r.	=	Hal > Clz <	Hal = Clz <	Clz < Olz =	=
Hold force	n.r.	n.r.	Hal > Clz <	Hal = Clz <	Clz < Olz =	=
Lick rhythm	n.r.	n.r.	Hal > Clz <	Hal = Clz <	Clz < Olz <	<
Citation[5]	(a)	(b)	(c)	(d)	(e)	(f)

Notes:

1. Drug abbreviations: Hal: haloperidol; Clz: clozapine; Olz: olanzapine; Rsp: risperidone.
2. Doses are in mg/kg.
3. <, =, > indicate significant decrease, no change, and significant increase compared to no drug, respectively.
4. n.r. means not reported.
5. Key to citations: (a) Fowler et al., 1990; (b) Kallman and Fowler, 1994; (c) Fowler et al., 1994; (d) Stanford and Fowler, 1997b; (e) Stanford and Fowler, 1997c; (f) Stanford and Fowler, 2000.
6. Substantial tolerance with daily dosing for this measure of behavior.

investigators administered atropine sulfate at the same time as haloperidol (forty-five minutes before recording sessions). The atropine-haloperidol combination resulted in significantly increased time-on-task and decreased tremor compared to haloperidol alone. When given alone, atropine decreased time-on-task in haloperidol-naïve rats and non-significantly reduced nondrug-induced physiological tremor. In a separate study with this paradigm, investigators reported that the muscarinic anticholinergic scopolamine given alone significantly reduced the spontaneous (i.e., not drug-induced) physiological forelimb tremor in rats (Stanford and Fowler, 1997a). These results suggested that the press-while-licking task was useful for preclinical experimental analyses of the EPS liability of APDs.

In the next APD experiment with this paradigm, investigators compared the effects of the high-EPS-liability drug haloperidol with the atypical, low-EPS-liability drug clozapine (Fowler et al., 1994). Reseachers used a within-group, acute-dosing regime with one group of rats receiving haloperidol and a second separate group receiving clozapine. Data from this experiment are shown in table 2 and in Figure 1. Although both drugs reduced time-on-task, the drugs induced opposite effects on the other variables measured. Clozapine reduced spontaneous physiological tremor, peak force and hold force and slowed the lick rhythm as reflected in the leftward shift of the spectral peak near 7 Hz in the power spectrum (see Figure 1). Haloperidol increased tremor, peak force, and hold force, and had little effect on the lick rhythm compared to clozapine. The distinctly different pattern of results for the two drugs can be seen graphically in Figure 1, which shows data for a representative subject from each of the two drug groups. These data show that clozapine possesses its own distinct anti-tremor and hypotonic motor effects in rats. Vrtunski and colleagues (1996, 1998) have reported that clozapine's motor effects in human patients are similar to the findings observed for rats.

Both clinical and laboratory data suggest that the behavior-suppressing sedative effects of clozapine subside with repeated dosing (Faustman and Fowler, 1982; Kaempf and Porter, 1987; Sanger, 1985; Stille et al., 1971; Varvel et al., 2002; Wilcy et al., 1994). Given the motor effects of clozapine described by Fowler and colleagues (1994), these effects may be related to the clozapine sedation reported by others. Thus, investigators used the effects of a chronic dosing regimen of clozapine to address this possibility (Stanford and Fowler, 1997b). Daily clozapine treatments resulted in pronounced tolerance to the behavior-suppressing effects, as reflected in time-on-task, but no

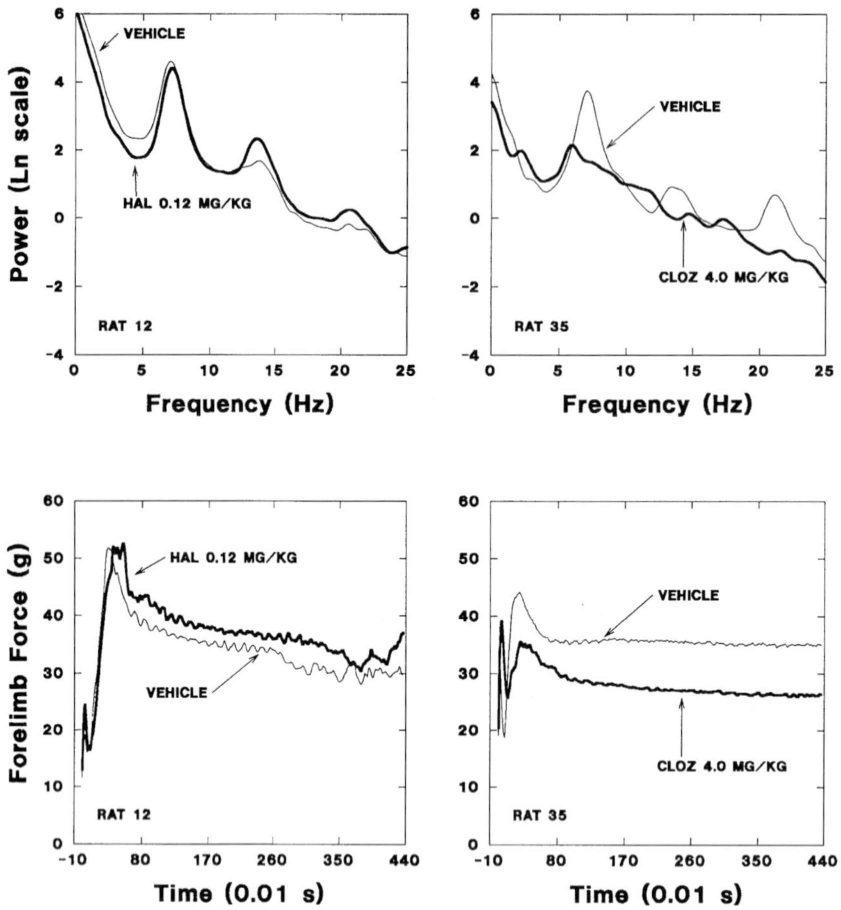

FIGURE 1 Averaged power spectra and force-time waveforms for the forelimb responses of representative rats treated with haloperidol or clozapine. Each rat was trained to reach through a hole with its forelimb and apply force to an operandum that measured the applied force. Specific force criteria were used to control the rat's access to a liquid-filled dipper, which contained the reward that maintained the animal's behavior (see Figure 1, Chapter A6). The peaks in the power spectra near 7 Hz reflect the rats' rhythmic licking of the liquid reward. Haloperidol increased the power of forelimb force oscillations (tremor) and tended to increase force output while clozapine decreased tremor and decreased force output. (Reprinted from Fowler et al., 1994.)

tolerance developed to clozapine's force-lowering, anti-tremor, and lick-rhythm-slowing effects. This experiment also showed that the force-elevating effects of haloperidol reported by Fowler and colleagues (1994), and evident in Figure 1, subsided with daily dosing. However, the induction of tremor by haloperidol remained during the course of chronic dosing. These results are summarized in table 2.

Quantitative measures of motor behavior exhibited in the press-while-licking task distinguished haloperidol from clozapine, two APDs that have distinctly different clinical motor-effect profiles. However, it remained to be shown whether or not this task with rats could detect differences between two closely related atypical APDs. In the next experiment, clozapine and olanzapine were compared in a between-groups dosing paradigm (Stanford and Fowler, 1997c). Olanzapine was selected because of its close structural similarity to clozapine (Moore et al., 1992), as well as its similar pharmacology in a variety of assays. The results of this clozapine-olanzapine comparison are summarized in table 2. The two drugs were similar in that they both decreased time-on-task, increased response duration (the "hold" time during which the dipper was within reach of the tongue), and slowed the lick rhythm. However the drugs were different in that olanzapine did not have clozapine's anti-tremor and force-lowering effects. In addition, a significant rebound increase in tremor was observed for clozapine, but not for olanzapine (Stanford and Fowler, 1997c). Finally, the two atypical APDs differed with respect to the effect of concurrent dosing with the muscarinic anticholinergic trihexyphenidyl, which lengthened clozapine-induced increases in response duration, but reduced the effect of olanzapine on response duration. Taken together, the data from this experiment showed that clozapine's and olanzapine's motor effects are distinguishable. Moreover, the pattern of results supported the hypothesis that olanzapine's effects were related to its greater affinity for D2-like dopamine receptors than that of clozapine. These interpretations are consistent with the clinical literature that reports a lower incidence of EPS for the atypical APDs, but within this class of low-EPS drugs the incidence of EPS is higher for olanzapine than clozapine (Tarsy et al., 2002).

The atypical APD risperidone was also evaluated in the press-while-licking task (Stanford and Fowler, 2000). As summarized in table 2, risperidone significantly decreased time-on task, tremor, and lick rhythm, much like clozapine, but risperidone did not affect peak force or hold force, similar to olanzapine (see table 2). A measurable degree of tolerance to disruption of task engagement (measured by time on task) was exhibited by risperidone (Stanford and Fowler, 2000). Overall, in the press-while-licking task, risperidone was more similar to clozapine than to olanzapine, but neither risperidone nor olanzapine had a clozapine-like effect on the forelimb force variables. Acute doses of all three atypical APDs substantially slowed lick rhythm, but, as previously noted, acute doses of the typical APD haloperidol had much less effect on lick rhythm than the atypical APDs.

As summarized above, investigators discovered that abrupt withdrawal after three weeks of daily 5.0 mg/kg clozapine administration led to a rebound tremor (increased power in the 10–25 Hz band in the power spectra) that persisted for at least one week (Stanford and Fowler, 1997c). The fact that the spectral characteristics of this tremor resembled physostigmine-induced tremor, but not harmaline-induced tremor, suggested that the tremor increase was due to cholinergic rebound (relative excess of acetylcholine in the striatum compared to dopamine). Clinical observations have also suggested this cholinergic-rebound interpretation (e.g., Ahmed et al., 1998).

In the preclinical setting, Wang (2000) conducted an experimental analysis that compared clozapine's ability to attenuate either physostigmine- or harmaline-induced tremor in rats performing the press-while-licking task. Physostigmine has cholinergic agonist effects by inhibiting acetylcholinesterase (Brimblecombe and Pinder, 1972), whereas harmaline is thought to induce its tremorogenic effects by selectively stimulating inferior olive neurons, which then overstimulate the Purkinje cells of the cerebellum (Llinas and Volkind, 1973). Data from Wang (2000) are shown in Figures 2 and 3. When given alone physostigmine significantly increased forelimb tremor (power in the 10–25 Hz frequency band) and increased the lick rhythm. In this study the clozapine was administered subchronically for six consecutive days with the purpose of allowing the sedative effects of clozapine to subside before the anti-tremor potential of clozapine was assessed on the seventh day, when the tremor inducers were also administered. The 5.0 mg/kg dose of clozapine significantly attenuated the tremor-inducing effects of 0.1 mg/kg physostigmine (Figure 2, bottom) and counteracted the lick-rhythm increase induced by physostigmine (Figure 2, top). As shown in Figure 3, harmaline alone significantly increased forelimb tremor and decreased lick rhythm. Clozapine successfully antagonized these two effects of harmaline. Thus, clozapine had anti-tremor effects in both drug-induced tremor models despite the different underlying pharmacological mechanisms of physostigmine and harmaline. Wang's (2000) results with rats are consistent with clinical reports of clozapine's anti-tremor effects in patients with PD (Bonuccelli et al., 1997) and patients with essential tremor (Ceravolo et al., 1999). Clozapine's effectiveness in the two pharmacological tremor models may be related to its ability to affect simultaneously a broad

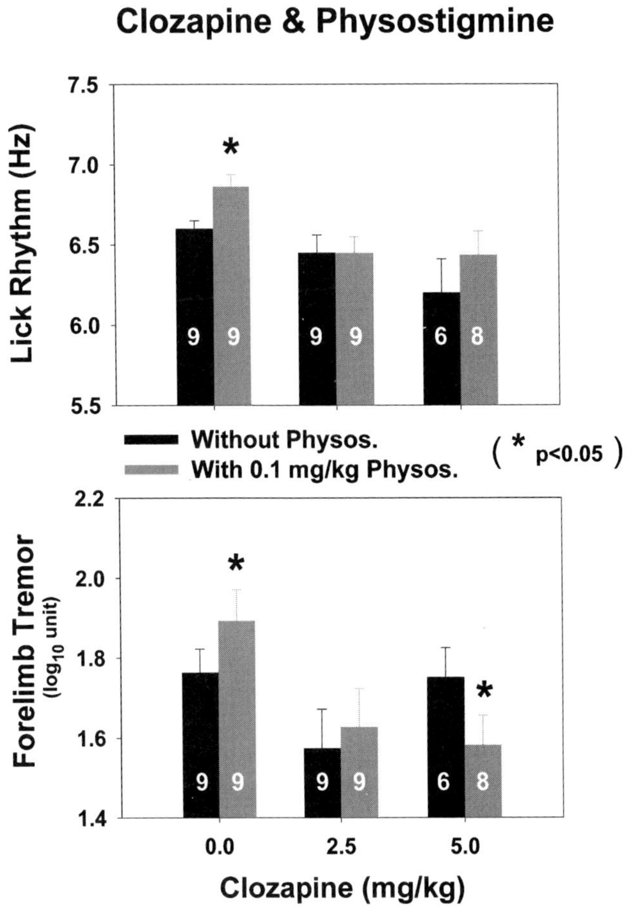

FIGURE 2 Data demonstrating the anti-tremor effect of subchronic clozapine on tremor induced in rats by physostigmine in the press-while-licking task. The black bars represent data on the sixth day of clozapine (0, 2.5, or 5.0 mg/kg in three separate groups), and the gray bars represent the seventh day of clozapine when physostigmine was also administered. Numbers within bars show the number of rats that produced sufficient task engagement for quantitative analysis. Brackets represent +/–1 standard error of the mean. Asterisks represent significant ($p < .05$) differences between a given clozapine dosage group (0, 2.5, 5.0 mg/kg) on day six and the physostigmine-plus-clozapine treatment combination on day seven of clozapine treatment. Data from Wang (2000).

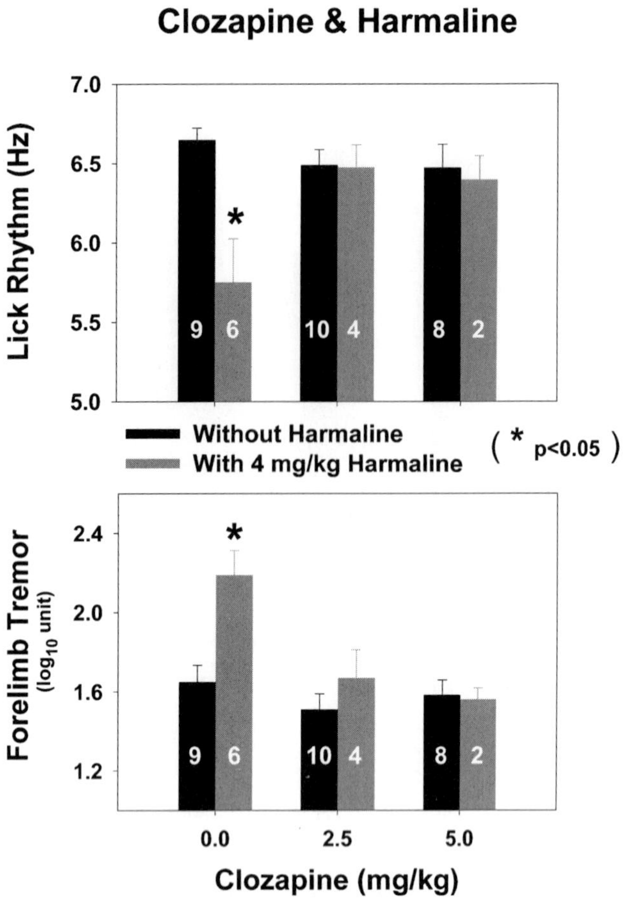

FIGURE 3 Data showing the anti-tremor effect of subchronic clozapine on tremor induced in rats by tremorogenic agent harmaline in the press-while-licking task. The experimental conditions were the same as explained in the caption for Figure 2, except harmaline was used to induce forelimb tremor instead of physostigmine and these data are for separate groups of rats. Although both harmaline and clozapine have a lick-rhythm-slowing effect when given separately, the combination drug treatment resulted in normal lick rhythm production. Data from Wang (2000).

range of neurotransmitter receptors and thereby achieve a more physiological balance among them (e.g., Remington, 2003).

IV. CONCLUSIONS

Rats show altered motor responses after treatment with both typical and atypical APDs. In acute dosing paradigms using naïve rats, the evidence suggests that D2 antagonists (haloperidol and raclopride) influence lick rhythm less, measured in either the lick-only task or in the press-while-licking task, than the D1 antagonist SCH23390 and the atypicals, clozapine, olanzapine, and risperidone. However, chronic daily treatment with haloperidol leads to a significant dose-related slowing of the lick rhythm. But the degree of slowing by chronic haloperidol is quantitatively less compared to the rhythm-slowing produced by acute or chronic treatment with clozapine or olanzapine. Although clozapine, olanzapine, and risperidone induce rhythm-slowing, it is unlikely that rhythm-slowing by itself indicates APD atypicality because several drugs without antipsychotic efficacy (ketanserin, ritanserin, morphine, prazosin, harmaline, ibogaine; see table 5, Chapter A6) also reduced lick rhythm. In addition, anticholinergic treatment (scopolamine, trihexyphenidyl) substantially reduced lick-rhythm slowing induced by chronic haloperidol, suggesting that the slowing induced by chronic haloperidol was EPS-like, yet the low-EPS drug clozapine also slowed lick rhythm. Together these data demonstrate that tongue dynamics in the rat are complexly controlled by several different pharmacological dimensions despite the seemingly reflexive nature of this rhythmic response.

In the press-while-licking task haloperidol and clozapine had opposite effects on peak force, hold force, and tremor. Haloperidol increased these measures and clozapine decreased them. Thus, in this paradigm with rodents, the atypical APD clozapine possessed motor effects, and these motor effects were distinctively different from those induced by the APD haloperidol, which has a high probability of inducing EPS in human patients (e.g., Tarsy, 1989). The fact that atropine partially ameliorated the increased force and tremor induced by haloperidol suggests that these measures of motor performance reflected haloperidol's high EPS liability and that the rodent model may have relevance to the human clinical context. Neither olanzapine nor risperidone had clozapine-like effects on the forelimb force measures, but risperidone had a small but significant capacity to lessen physiological tremor. Although the muscarinic anticholinergic drug, scopolamine, was reported to decrease the forelimb force measures in the press-while licking task (Stanford and Fowler, 1997a), it seems unlikely that anticholinergic effects of clozapine alone could account for the lowered force measures because olanzapine, which has anticholinergic effects similar to clozapine's, did not significantly affect the forelimb force measures in the press-while-licking task. In addition, during the withdrawal phase following twenty-eight daily doses of either clozapine or olanzapine, increased tremor was seen only for clozapine (Stanford and Fowler, 1997c). Clinicians have described a clozapine-withdrawal syndrome in human patients (Tollefson et al., 1999). Another point of congruence between the rodent data for clozapine and the human clinical data lies in the similarity of the drug's effects on force control in both species (Vrtunski et al., 1996, 1998). Among the APDs (listed in table 2) and reference drugs (given in another chapter, table 1, Chapter A6) studied in the press-while-licking task, only clozapine produced force-lowering effects and lick-rhythm-slowing effects at the same time. Thus, clozapine appears to have unique effects on motor behavior, and this distinctive behavioral profile may hasten the search for compounds with similar effects.

References

Ahmed, S., K.N. Chengappa, V.R. Naidu, R.W. Baker, H. Parepally, and N.R. Schooler. 1998. Clozapine withdrawal-emergent dystonias and dyskinesias: A case series. *J Clin Psychiatry* **59**:472–477.

Bonuccelli, U., R. Ceravolo, S. Salvetti, C. D'Avino, P. Del Dotto, G. Rossi, and L. Murri. 1997. Clozapine in Parkinson's disease tremor. Effects of acute and chronic administration. *Neurology* **49**:1587–1590.

Brimblecombe, R.W., and R.M. Pinder. 1972. *Tremors and Tremorogenic Agents*. Bristol, U. K.: Scientechnica.

Carlsson, A., M. Lindqvist, T. Magnusson, and B. Waldeck. 1958. On the presence of 3-hydroxytyramine in brain. *Science* **127**:471.

Casey, D.E. 1995. Tardive dyskinesia: Pathophysiology. In *Psychopharmacology: The Fourth Generation of Progress*. Ed. F. E. Bloom and D.J. Kupfer. pp. 1497–1502. New York: Raven Press.

Ceravolo, R., S. Salvetti, P. Piccini, C. Lucetti, G. Gambaccini, and U. Bonuccelli. 1999. Acute and chronic effects of clozapine in essential tremor. *Mov Disord* **14**:468–472.

Das, S., and S.C. Fowler. 1995. Acute and subchronic effects of clozapine on licking in rats: Tolerance to disruptive effects on number of licks, but no tolerance to rhythm slowing. *Psychopharmacology (Berlin, Ger.)* **120**:249–255.

Das, S., and S.C. Fowler. 1996. Similarity of clozapine's and olanzapine's acute effects on rats' lapping behavior. *Psychopharmacology (Berlin, Ger.)* **123**:374–378.

Delay, J., and P. Deniker. 1968. Drug-induced extrapyramidal syndromes. In *Handbook of Clinical Neurology*. Ed. P.J. Vinken and G.W. Bruyn. Vol. 6, pp. 248–266. North Holland, Amsterdam.

Ellenbroek, B., and A.R. Cools. 1988. The paw test: An animal model for neuroleptic drugs which fulfils the criteria for pharmacological isomorphism. *Life Sci* **42**:1205–1213.

Faustman, W.O., and S.C. Fowler. 1982. An examination of methodological refinements, clozapine and fluphenazine in the anhedonia paradigm. *Pharmacol Biochem Behav* **17**:987–993.

Fowler, S.C., and S. Das. 1994. Haloperidol-induced decrements in force and duration of rats' tongue movements during licking are attenuated by concomitant anticholinergic treatment. *Pharmacol Biochem Behav* **49**:813–817.

Fowler, S.C., and C. Mortell. 1992. Low doses of haloperidol interfere with rat tongue extensions during licking: A quantitative analysis. *Behav Neurosci* **106**:386–395.

Fowler, S.C., and G. Wang. 1998. Chronic haloperidol produces a time- and dose-related slowing of lick rhythm in rats: Implications for rodent models of tardive dyskinesia and neuroleptic-induced Parkinsonism. *Psychopharmacology (Berlin, Ger.)* **137**:50–60.

Fowler, S.C., R.M. Liao, and P. Skjoldager. 1990. A new rodent model for neuroleptic-induced pseudo-Parkinsonism: Low doses of haloperidol increase forelimb tremor in the rat. *Behav Neurosci* **104**:449–456.

Fowler, S.C., K.H. Davison, and J.A. Stanford. 1994. Unlike haloperidol, clozapine slows and dampens rats' forelimb force oscillations and decreases force output in a press-while-licking behavioral task. *Psychopharmacology (Berlin, Ger.)* **116**:19–25.

Hayes, C.A. 1995. Differential effects of dopamine D1 (SCH23390) and D2 (raclopride) antagonists on quantitative characteristics of tongue movements in rats. Unpublished Doctoral Dissertation, University of Mississippi, Oxford.

Hornykiewicz, O. 1972. Neurochemistry of Parkinsonism. In *Handbook of Neurochemistry*. Ed. A. Lajtha. Vol. 7, pp. 465–501. New York: Plenum Press.

Kaempf, G.L., and J.H. Porter. 1987. Differential effects of pimozide and clozapine on schedule-controlled and scheduled-induced behaviors after acute and chronic administration. *J Pharmacol Exp Ther* **243**:437–445.

Kallman, M.J., and S.C. Fowler. 1994. Assessment of chemically induced alterations in motor functions. In *Principles of Neurotoxicology*. Ed. L.W. Chang. Vol. 26, pp. 373–396. New York: Marcel Dekker.

Llinas, R., and R.A. Volkind. 1973. The olivo-cerebellar system: Functional properties as revealed by harmaline-induced tremor. *Exp Brain Res* **18**:69–87.

Moore, N.A., N.C. Tye, M.S. Axton, and F.C. Risius. 1992. The behavioral pharmacology of olanzapine, a novel "atypical" antipsychotic agent. *J Pharmacol Exp Ther* **262**:545–551.

Pisa, M., and J.A. Schranz. 1988. Dissociable motor roles of the rat's striatum conform to a somatotopic model. *Behav Neurosci* **102**:429–440.

Remington, G. 2003. Understanding antipsychotic "atypicality": A clinical and pharmacological moving target. *J Psychiatry Neurosci* **28**:275–284.

Salamone, J.D., M.J. Zigmond, and E.M. Stricker. 1990. Characterization of the impaired feeding behavior in rats given haloperidol or dopamine-depleting brain lesions. *Neuroscience* (Oxford, U. K.) **39**:17–24.

Sanberg, P.R., M.D. Bunsey, M. Giordano, and A.B. Norman. 1988. The catalepsy test: Its ups and downs. *Behav Neurosci* **102**:748–759.

Sanger, D.J. 1985. The effects of clozapine on shuttle-box avoidance responding in rats: Comparisons with haloperidol and chlordiazepoxide. *Pharmacol Biochem Behav* **23**:231–236.

Stanford, J.A., and S.C. Fowler. 1997a. Scopolamine reversal of tremor produced by low doses of physostigmine in rats: Evidence for a cholinergic mechanism. *Neurosci Lett* **225**:157–160.

Stanford, J.A., and S.C. Fowler. 1997b. Subchronic effects of clozapine and haloperidol on rats' forelimb force and duration during a press-while-licking task. *Psychopharmacology (Berlin, Ger.)* **130**:249–253.

Stanford, J.A., and S.C. Fowler. 1997c. Similarities and differences between the subchronic and withdrawal effects of clozapine and olanzapine on forelimb force steadiness. *Psychopharmacology (Berlin, Ger.)* **132**:408–414.

Stanford, J.A., and S.C. Fowler. 2000. Clozapine-like motor effects of the atypical antipsychotic risperidone in rats. *Neurosci Lett* **285**:189–192.

Stille, G., H. Lauener, and E. Eichenberger. 1971. The pharmacology of 8-chloro-11-(4-methyl-1-piperazinyl)-5h-dibenzo(b,e)(1,4)diazepine (clozapine). *Farmaco [Prat]* **26**:603–625.

Tarsy, D. 1989. Neuroleptic-induced movement disorders. In *Disorders of Movement: Clinical, Pharmacological and Physiological Aspects*. Ed. N.P. Quinn and P.G. Jenner. pp. 361–393. San Diego: Academic Press.

Tarsy, D., R.J. Baldessarini, and F.I. Tarazi. 2002. Effects of newer antipsychotics on extrapyramidal function. *CNS Drugs* **16**:23–45.

Tollefson, G.D., M.A. Dellva, C.A. Mattler, J.M. Kane, D.A. Wirshing, and B.J. Kinon. 1999. Controlled, double-blind investigation of the clozapine discontinuation symptoms with conversion to either olanzapine or placebo. The collaborative crossover study group. *J Clin Psychopharmacol* **19**:435–443.

Varvel, S.A., R.E. Vann, L.E. Wise, S.D. Philibin, and J.H. Porter. 2002. Effects of antipsychotic drugs on operant responding after acute and repeated administration. *Psychopharmacology (Berlin, Ger.)* **160**:182–191.

Vrtunski, P.B., P.E. Konicki, K.Y. Kwon, G. Jurjus, G.E. Jaskiw, and G.J. Jaskiw. 1996. Effect of clozapine on motor function in schizophrenic patients. *Schizophr Res* **20**:187–198.

Vrtunski, P.B., P.E. Konicki, G.E. Jaskiw, D.W. Brescan, K.Y. Kwon, and G. Jurjus. 1998. Clozapine effects on force control in schizophrenic patients. *Schizophr Res* **34**:39–48.

Wang, G., and S.C. Fowler. 1999. Effects of haloperidol and clozapine on tongue dynamics during licking in CD-1, BALB/c and C57BL/6 mice. *Psychopharmacology (Berlin, Ger.)* **147**:38–45.

Wang, G. 2000. Quantification of harmaline or physostigmine's tremorogenic effects and clozapine's antitremor effect. Unpublished Doctoral Dissertation, University of Kansas.

Whishaw, I.Q., D.R. Funk, S.J. Hawryluk, and E.D. Karbashewski. 1987. Absence of sparing of spatial navigation, skilled forelimb and tongue use and limb posture in the rat after neonatal dopamine depletion. *Physiol Behav* **40**:247–253.

Wiley, J.L., A.D. Compton, and J.H. Porter. 1994. Differential effects of clozapine and pimozide on fixed-ratio responding during repeated dosing. *Pharmacol Biochem Behav* **48**:253–257.

CHAPTER

M4

Animal Models of Drug-Induced Akathisia

PERMINDER S. SACHDEV

Haskovec introduced the term akathisia (from Greek, literally "not to sit") in 1902, well before antipsychotic drugs became available, to describe two restless patients who could not sit or stand in one place (Sachdev, 1995). Most investigators agree that there are two aspects to akathisia: a subjective report of restlessness or inner tension, particularly referable to the legs, with a consequent inability to maintain a posture for several minutes; and the objective (or observational) manifestations of restlessness in the form of semi-purposeful or purposeless movements of the limbs, a tendency to shift body position in the chair while sitting, or marching on the spot while standing and so on (Sachdev, 1995). Investigators disagree about the relative importance of these two aspects, and place emphasis on either the subjective component (akathisia as a mental disorder) or the objective component (akathisia as a movement disorder). Others argue that a combination of the two is necessary for a definite diagnosis (Sachdev, 1994), that is, akathisia as both mental and movement disorder. A less certain diagnosis of akathisia may be possible if either the subjective or the objective features, but not both, are present.

Akathisia is occasionally described in association with organic brain lesions or with no obvious cause (Sachdev, 1995), but for most purposes its use is synonymous with drug-induced akathisia. The temporal association with drug administration is therefore necessary for the diagnosis. While neuroleptic drugs are by far the most important, a number of other drugs have been implicated, in particular selective serotonin reuptake inhibitors (SSRI) and calcium channel antagonists. Even when a patient presents with fairly characteristic features of akathisia, and the clinical situation is appropriate for the diagnosis, the clinician must choose to distinguish symptoms from anxiety, agitation, or restlessness due to other causes. As no laboratory measures support the diagnosis, the latter must rely solely on clinical judgment. Clinicians have described some features that characterize akathisia and help distinguish it from anxiety or agitation (Sachdev and Kruk, 1994; Sachdev, 1995) but these features are based on a complex behavioral analysis at a level not readily applicable in animals.

The importance of akathisia is obvious to clinicians, not only because of its high incidence but also because of the marked distress associated with it. This distress may lead to noncompliance and medication refusal, and occasionally impulsive behavior, worsening of psychosis, and even suicide attempts (van Putten, 1974, 1975). Recent research has shown that akathisia associated with neuroleptics can be categorized into acute, tardive, withdrawal, and chronic subtypes according to its onset in relation to the administration of the drug and its duration (Barnes and Braude, 1985;

Sachdev, 1994). These subtypes are similar in their clinical manifestations, except for subtle differences, but have different pharmacological profiles and predisposing factors. For instance, the tardive subtype has a major overlap with tardive dyskinesia and may share its pathophysiology rather than that of acute akathisia (Burke et al., 1987; Sachdev and Loneragan, 1993). Most research on akathisia deals with the acute subtype, and detailed information on the other subtypes is only beginning to emerge. Non-neuroleptic drugs are known to cause akathisia only in relation to their acute administration, and therefore, these subtypes do not apply to them (Sachdev, 1995). This chapter will focus on the animal models of acute akathisia.

I. RISK FACTORS FOR ACUTE AKATHISIA

The risk factors for acute akathisia are incompletely understood. The high rates of akathisia reported in some studies, for example the 76% incidence reported by van Putten and colleagues (1984) suggest that most individuals will develop akathisia under some circumstances, but whether everyone is vulnerable is not known. Drug-related factors are clearly important, with higher drug doses, rapid increment of the dosage, and higher potency of the neuroleptic drug more likely to produce akathisia (Sachdev and Kruk, 1994). The development of parkinsonism also increases the likelihood of akathisia developing, although the latter may occur first, or concurrently, in many cases. The role of sociodemographic factors and other treatment-related variables is modest. The presence of psychiatric disorder is not necessary for akathisia to develop, but certain organic brain disorders may increase vulnerability. Although some evidence exists that iron deficiency may be a predisposing factor, this is far from established and its role is likely to be minor. A significant proportion of the susceptibility to akathisia is unexplained (Sachdev and Kruk, 1994).

II. PATHOPHYSIOLOGY OF ACUTE AKATHISIA

Researchers have proposed a number of pathophysiologic hypotheses for acute akathisia. Because akathisia is predominantly produced by neuroleptic drugs and was originally described in parkinsonian syndromes of various etiologies, the main focus in understanding its mechanism has been on dopaminergic function. Most (perhaps all) drugs that cause akathisia directly or indirectly reduce dopamine (DA) function in the brain. High potency neuroleptics such as haloperidol, which are most likely to cause akathisia, are potent antagonists of dopamine D2 receptors (Creese et al., 1977). In a positron emission study of recently treated schizophrenic patients, Farde (1992) reported that parkinsonism and akathisia corresponded with D2 and not D1 receptor occupancy of the neuroleptic drugs. There are a number of deficiencies in the D-2 receptor antagonism hypothesis of akathisia, which have been discussed in detail elsewhere (Sachdev, 1995, pp. 228–229). Furthermore, it is uncertain which dopaminergic pathways in the brain are responsible for the development of akathisia. Because the association of akathisia with neuroleptic-induced parkinsonian symptoms is modest at best (Sachdev and Kruk, 1994), the striatonigral DA system is considered unlikely to be the main mediating mechanism. Marsden and Jenner (1980) proposed that the subjective distress and motor restlessness of akathisia was possibly a result of the antagonism of the mesocortical and mesolimbic DA pathways, but direct evidence for this mechanism is lacking. This model also does not explain the partial, but sometimes dramatic, response of akathisia to muscarinic and beta-adrenergic antagonists.

The roles of other neurotransmitters, in particular serotonin (5HT), norepinephrine (NE), and acetylcholine (ACh), have received some attention. Evidence exists that SSRIs, which increase 5HT transmission in the brain, cause a syndrome very similar to neuroleptic-induced akathisia (Lipinski et al., 1989). Antagonism of 5HT receptors, on the other hand, reduces or ameliorates akathisia. Ritanserin, a potent and specific 5HT2 antagonist, is reported to reduce akathisia (Fleischhacker et al., 1990), and atypical neuroleptics, which antagonize DA and 5HT receptors, have a lower propensity for akathisia than the classical neuroleptics (Sachdev, 1995). The mechanism for the effect of 5HT on akathisia is not known, and investigators have suggested that the effect may be indirect, due to the ability of 5HT to modulate DA transmission (Hall et al., 1995). Investigators have mainly determined the possible roles of other neurotransmitters, such as acetylcholine, norepinephrine, and GABA, from the efficacy of certain drugs in treating acute akathisia, particularly anticholinergic drugs, beta-adrenergic antagonists, and benzodiazepines. In summary, the syndrome of akathisia most likely results from a complex interaction between dopaminergic pathways and multiple modifying mechanisms, in particular serotonergic ones, within the basal ganglia and mesocortical structures. Researchers therefore have focused mainly on the dopaminergic and serotonergic mechanisms in their search for animal models of acute akathisia.

The pathophysiology of other hyperkinetic movement disorders is better understood and may be instructive. Hemiballismus manifests as rapidly flinging movements that occur at irregular intervals that are exacerbated by stress and disappear in sleep. This disorder is caused by lesions in the subthalamic nucleus, which leads to disinhibition of the thalamus due to reduced tonic, and perhaps phasic, inhibitory output from the globus pallidus interna and substantia nigra pars reticulata to the thalamus (Albin et al., 1989). In Huntington disease, another disorder with hyperkinesia, there is evidence of early loss of striatal GABA/enkephalin neurons that provide inhibitory input into the globus pallidus (Reddy et al., 1999). In both of these disorders, therefore, the primary deficit is in the inhibitory GABA input in the striatum. The movements of Huntington disease and hemiballismus are, however, different from akathisia, being clearly involuntary in nature, lacking an urge or subjective distress, and being nonsuppressible.

Akathisia shares some similarity with tics because of the presence of the urge to move and the ability to suppress the movements temporarily. Of course, major differences occur between the two disorders: tics have a genetic basis, result in localized movements or vocalizations that change over time, are preceded by an urge to move rather than a feeling of inner restlessness, are most frequently craniofacial, and have a characteristic developmental pattern. The pathophysiology of tics is not fully understood but the pharmacological characteristics of tics are different from that of akathisia (Singer, 1994). In contrast with akathisia, dopamine antagonists can suppress tics.

Akathisia shares similarities with restless legs syndrome (RLS), with both subjective and objective features being present in both, although there are qualitative differences in the symptoms. RLS is idiopathic, its characteristic sleep abnormality is not present in akathisia (Lipinski et al., 1991), and genetic factors are important. Some cross-fertilization in the investigations of the two disorders has occurred, for example the study of the role of iron deficiency in akathisia stems from the importance of anemia in RLS, and the use of dopaminergic drugs in RLS borrows from the fact that anti-dopaminergic drugs produce akathisia. Unfortunately, the pathophysiology of RLS is not well understood.

An analysis of other hyperkinetic movement disorders is therefore not very instructive in developing models for akathisia. We conclude that since it is the drug-induced nature of akathisia that is paramount, this characteristic should remain the focus for any animal models to be developed.

III. GENERAL ASPECTS OF ANIMAL MODELS OF ACUTE AKATHISIA

In exploring animal models of acute akathisia, some general principles should be considered. Some basic requirements of an animal model for a neuropsychiatric disorder are symptom similarity, pharmacological isomorphism, and congruence of cross-species biochemical processes (Matthysse, 1986). The models should have face, construct, and predictive validity. While ideally investigators should aim for a homology, they may find isomorphic models useful for certain investigations. When behavioral changes of animals occur, investigators should also take into account the amount, structure, and predictability of the patterns (Paulus and Geyer, 1991). If these requirements are applied to acute akathisia, the animal models should meet the following criteria:

(1) The model should ideally cover both the emotional (subjective) and the motor (objective) symptoms. Because the complex reports given by patients are unavailable, investigators must infer subjective distress in an animal from its behavior.

(2) The model should be independent of other side effects of neuroleptic drugs, for example, catalepsy or parkinsonian symptoms, with the latter not confounding the measurement of akathisia. In humans, the correlation between akathisia and parkinsonism is about $r = 0.3$ (Sachdev and Kruk, 1994). This criterion poses a major problem in some animals, as the occurrence of behavioral inhibition and catalepsy secondary to neuroleptics frustrates many behavioral measures of subjective distress.

(3) The response should have an acute onset shortly after drug administration or its increment of dose.

(4) There should be a dose-dependent reaction, a positive correlation with the rate of dose increment, and a stronger response to parenteral application compared to oral treatment.

(5) Typical neuroleptics should produce more severe symptoms in the animal compared to atypical neuroleptics.

(6) The response should be partially reversible by administering drugs that efficiently treat akathisia, for example anticholinergic or beta-adrenergic drugs.

(7) Similar responses should be obtained by drugs other than neuroleptics that are considered to induce akathisia, for example, SSRIs, dopamine depleting drugs, are calcium channel antagonists, etc.

The paradoxical nature of akathisia should be underscored; the same drugs that are expected to tranquilize and reduce activity lead to distress and restlessness. Several animal models have concentrated on investigating behavioral changes due to alteration of the dopamine turnover. Administration of dopamine agonists increases motor activity, especially grooming behavior and other stereotypies, in many species (Paulus and Geyer, 1991). The reverse, that is, dopamine antagonism caused by neuroleptics, reduces spontaneous motor activity and induces cataleptic responses in rats and some other animal species (Bernardi et al., 1981). To model restlessness in an animal when the usual response is one of reduced motor activity is a challenge. A review of the available models suggests that both subjective and objective aspects of akathisia have been difficult to model together, and the proposed models are therefore partial, modeling either the subjective distress or the motor restlessness.

IV. ANIMAL MODELS FOR THE SUBJECTIVE COMPONENT OF AKATHISIA

A. "Defecation Model" in the Rat

Investigators have considered defecation index an index of "emotionality" in the rat (Broadhurst, 1957). Stress and other causes of dysphoria or distress increase rates of defecation. It was reported earlier that neuroleptic drugs reduced the defecation index, which was considered consistent with the tranquillizing effect of these drugs (Allain and Lechat, 1970). Russell and colleagues (1987a) challenged these results by reporting that, contrary to previous expectation, neuroleptics increased defecation in the habitual environment. The difference from the earlier reports was that the drug was administered in a well-habituated environment, thereby with a low level of arousal in the animal, and the effect was measured over one to two hours rather than a few minutes after the injection, as in the earlier experiments. We have demonstrated in an unpublished study that increased defecation occurs in response to neuroleptics even in a novel environment when measured over one hour after drug administration (Sachdev et al., 1993). Previous studies (Ryall, 1958; Janssen et al., 1960; Allain and Lechat, 1970; Bruhwyler et al., 1990) are not necessarily inconsistent with this observation, as the earlier measurements suggested that the effect on defecation was over a few minutes (3–10 min) after the administration of the neuroleptic drug. Neuroleptics possibly have a dual response, with an initial brief period of reduction in defecation, especially in a novel environment, followed by subsequent increase. This response is consistent with the clinical observation that these drugs reduce agitation and tranquillize the patient in the short term, with akathisia emerging only after hours or days.

Further studies have supported neuroleptic-induced defecation in rats as a model of the subjective component of akathisia. Researchers have demonstrated that administering dopamine receptor antagonists, such as haloperidol (dosages: 1.0 mg/kg; 0.1 mg/kg; 0.01 mg/kg), lead to a dose-dependent increase of bolus counts in rats habituated to their environment (Sachdev and Loneragan, 1993). This is a central effect because the peripherally acting dopamine antagonist domperidone does not produce the same response (Russell et al., 1987b; Sachdev and Loneragan, 1993). The effect is not secondary to catalepsy, as catalepsy induced by morphine (Sanberg et al., 1993) does not increase defecation. The construct validity of the model is further supported by a report that fecal pellet scores show a significant correspondence with striatal dopamine levels (Pradhan and Arunasmitha, 1991). L-Dopa and methamphetamine, both agents that increase catecholamine levels in the brain, decrease the number of fecal boluses (Suzuki et al., 1976). The effect is not specific to D1 or D2 dopamine receptor antagonism, and the two receptor subtypes have a synergistic effect (Sachdev and Saharov, 1999). Selective D1 and D2 agonists, however, did not have a significant effect on defecation in the study (Sachdev and Saharov, 1999), nor did they reverse the effects of haloperidol. In a pilot investigation, haloperidol- and risperidone-treated rats produced more fecal boli than rats treated with clozapine, thioridazine, and chlorpromazine (Sachdev and Saharov, 1999). In a test for predictive validity, investigators also demonstrated that lipophilic (propranolol and metoprolol) but not hydrophilic (nadolol) beta-adrenergic antagonists significantly reversed neuroleptic-induced defecation, again consistent with human reports of akathisia (Sachdev and Saharov, 1997).

Serotonin (5HT) also affects defecation behavior in the rat, and this effect seems to be different in the open field and home cage environments. In the open field, 5-hydroxytryptophan (5HTP) and intraventricular 5HT decrease fecal boluses, while pretreatment with p-chlorophenylalanine (pCPA) and 5,6-hydroxytryptamine leads to a slight increase. In the home cage, defecation increases with 5HTP administration and decreases under pretreatment with pCPA (Kameyama et al., 1980).

There are a number of limitations to this model. First, only the subjective aspect of akathisia is modeled, and the claim that it is indeed a model of akathisia and not neuroleptic-induced anxiety or dysphoria cannot be convincingly supported. While researchers can distinguish akathisia from neuroleptic-induced dysphoria in humans (Sachdev, 1995), this distinction in animals seems impossible. Second, the model lacks face validity, as the behavior being studied is apparently unrelated to the behaviors considered to be part of the akathisia syndrome. Third, researchers can reportedly attenuate the response by pretreating the rat with anti-anxiety drugs, whereas in humans anti-anxiety drugs are poorly effective in treating akathisia (Russell et al., 1987b). This finding in the rat model, nevertheless, needs to be replicated. Fourth, the peripheral effects of neuroleptics confound the interpretation of results from this model. For example, one can account for the failure of clozapine or thioridazine to increase defecation rates (Sachdev and Saharov, 1999) because of their anticholinergic action on the gut. Serotonergic drugs also lead to increased defecation because of their peripheral effects, as 5HT has a stimulatory effect on intestinal motility and fluid secretion (Beubler et al., 1990). 5-Hydroxytryptophan has been demonstrated to increase defecation because of strong contractions of intestinal muscles (Talley, 1992).

The model is therefore unsatisfactory for examining drugs with significant antimuscarinic and possibly serotonergic effects. In spite of these limitations, this model remains the best investigated of the animal models of akathisia, and its use for drugs with relatively selective dopamine antagonism is well supported. Further study may clarify its utility for the 5HT model. For example, the receptors involved in the diarrheal effect of 5HT are multiple, but the greatest focus has been on the $5HT_3$ and $5HT_4$ receptors, and to a lesser extent $5HT_{1A}$, $5HT_{1D}$, and $5HT_{2A}$ receptors (Talley, 1992; Taniyama et al., 1991; Champenaria et al., 1992). However, if 5HT is to produce a dysphoric response, it is most likely to be related to $5HT_2$ receptors and their interaction with dopamine receptors (Kapur, 1996). The use of specific antagonists may be able to overcome this deficiency of the model. The emotional defecation model, therefore, presents the opportunity to further examine the pathophysiology of subjective akathisia.

B. Neuroleptics As Aversive Stimuli

Investigators have shown that many species of animals are averse to neuroleptics. Because akathisia is an important cause of patients' subsequent refusal to take neuroleptic medication, an argument can be made for symptom similarity. Berger (1972) demonstrated that chlorpromazine could be used as punishment in a rat model of conditioned suppression. Hoffmeister (1975, 1977) showed that monkeys actively avoided the administration of small doses of chlorpromazine, although the effect was not as clear-cut with haloperidol, probably because of the marked response suppression produced by the latter. Giardini (1985) reported that chlorpromazine was an effective unconditioned stimulus in a conditioned taste-aversion paradigm, and this response was masked by an opiate-like morphine. He did not find haloperidol to have the same effect as chlorpromazine, and he argued that it was because of the opiate-like component of haloperidol's actions. These models are appropriate for neuroleptic dysphoria, which has multiple determinants, only one of which is subjective akathisia (Sachdev, 1995). They have not been further developed to establish a homology with akathisia and their validity is therefore unknown.

V. ANIMAL MODELS OF THE OBJECTIVE (OR MOTOR RESTLESSNESS) COMPONENT OF AKATHISIA

A. Lesion Model in the Rat: The Ventral Tegmental Area (VTA) and Medial Prefrontal Cortex (MPC) Lesions

Because measuring the emotional aspects of akathisia is problematic, other studies have concentrated on motor restlessness induced by drugs, or lesions in brain regions supposed to be involved in the pathophysiology of akathisia. Due to some case reports of akathisia-like syndrome in humans after brain damage of the prefrontal and frontal cortex areas, investigators have hypothesized that dopamine-mediated mesolimbic and mesocortical circuits participate in the etiology of akathisia (Sachdev, 1995).

The ventral tegmental area (VTA) of the rat contains cell bodies of the mesocortical and mesolimbic dopamine systems, as well as 5HT fibers originating from the raphe nuclei and innervating the forebrain. Le Moal (1969) described what came to be known as the VTA syndrome—a complex behavioral syndrome produced by bilateral lesions of the VTA in rats. This syndrome is characterized by (1) persistent hyperactivity and hyper-locomotion, possibly similar to the restless movements of akathisia; (2) difficulty in suppressing previously learned responses or in tolerating frustrating situations; (3) disappearance of the freezing reaction; and (4) disturbance of organized behaviors (e.g., hoarding and eating) (Le Moal et al., 1975, 1976). This response is reversed by dopamine substitution.

The hyperactivity of the VTA syndrome is of long duration and may remain for the whole life of the animal. Investigators have drawn parallels between this syndrome and akathisia induced by drugs (Sachdev, 1995). However, the hyperactivity of VTA lesions is associated with decreased exploratory activity, ongoing behavior and attention span, absence of fear reactions, reduced defecation, and reduced effects of penalties in avoidance conditioning (Le Moal, 1976), suggesting a hypo-arousal state in contrast with akathisia. In effect, the VTA model is the reverse of the neuroleptic-induced defecation model, in producing motor restlessness or the objective aspect, but not emotionality or the subjective aspect of akathisia (Sachdev, 1995). This model has not been further investigated in terms of its pharmacological similarity with akathisia. The importance of this model is that reduced DA transmission increases motor activity, which parallels what happens in akathisia. Its limitation is that many investigators have demonstrated psychomotor activation in association with increased DA in the nucleus accumbens (but not the striatum and amygdala), produced by direct injection of DA agonists (Costall and Naylor, 1975; Pijnenburg et al., 1975).

An understanding of the biochemical basis of lesion-induced hyper-locomotion is of interest. Tassin and colleagues (1978) demonstrated that this hyper-locomotion could not be explained on the basis of changes in brain norepinephrine or 5HT. Investigators observed a good correlation between increase in locomotor activity and decrease in DA content in the frontal cortex ($r = 0.82$, $n = 20$, $p < 0.01$). The correlation with the reduction of DA in the nucleus accumbens was also significant ($r = 0.47$, $n = 24$, $p < 0.05$). These changes can be attributed to lesions in the A10 area of the VTA (Dahlstrom and Fuxe 1965). Hyper-locomotion could therefore be related to the destruction of both mesocortical and mesolimbic DA neurons, but the mesocortical pathway was considered crucial. When the levels of DA in the frontal cortex decreased by more than 80%, hyperactivity levels were three to eight times those of sham-operated rats. A similar reduction of DA in the nucleus accumbens produced only a twofold increase. The VTA syndrome can be produced by injections of 6-hydroxydopamine in the A10 area (Le Moal et al., 1975; Galey et al., 1977). Administering small dosages of apomorphine and sustained dosages of amphetamine (1–2 mg/Kg) abolishes the locomotor hyperactivity in lesioned rats (Gualtieri et al., 1980).

Damage of medial prefrontal dopaminergic circuits by injection of 6-OH-dopamine induces a similar reaction compared to the VTA model, leading to hyperactivity, hypo-"emotionality" and cognitive deficits in the rat model as well (Carter and Pycock, 1980; Joyce et al., 1983; Ravard et al., 1990). This reaction supports the observations of Tassin and colleagues (1978) that the mesocortical change from VTA lesions is responsible for the behavioral syndrome. The VTA and the MPC models are the only models in which reduced dopamine transmission is associated with increased motor activity (Sachdev, 1995). The effects of drugs on this model have not been reported, nor has its predictive validity been examined. The chronicity of the model is unlike the usual clinical presentation of acute akathisia in humans.

B. SSRI-Induced Restlessness in the Rat

Reports of akathisia induced by SSRIs (Lipinski et al., 1989) led investigators to examine the effects of these drugs on motor activity in rodents. Researchers investigated the effect of fluoxetine (dosages: 0 to 30 mg/kg) on mobility and locomotion in the rat in a habituated environment (Teicher et al., 1995). There was an increase of small local "restless" movements 90 to 180 min after application, without change of locomotion or exploratory behavior in general, as surveyed by an infrared motion analysis system. This pattern of movement contrasted with the activation and increase of ambulation caused by amphetamine. The fluoxetine-induced movements were therefore interpreted as being akin to restlessness and therefore a model of akathisia. However, the authors applied extremely high doses of fluoxetine (30 mg/kg body weight), exceeding those used in humans by about forty- to sixtyfold; the high doses were justified by a more rapid metabolism of fluoxetine in the rat compared to humans. Investigators must further characterize the movements and consider the possibility that these represent myoclonic jerks. Researchers should replicate this model and develop it further in terms of its pharmacological characteristics. The effect of neuroleptics and other drugs on this model must be studied. It remains a partial model with some face and construct validity, but its predictive validity has not been examined.

C. Hyperkinesia Model in the Dog

In a dog model using a complex operant schedule, investigators tested the influence of haloperidol (0.3 mg/kg) and clozapine (7 mg/kg) on conditioned behaviors. They demonstrated that haloperidol compared to clozapine induced more hyperkinesia and stereotyped behavior in the dog measured four hours after drug application. Researchers argued that hyperkinetic stereotypic movements, for example, scratching, licking, rotating, or self-grooming for more than thirty seconds or persistent walking for more than sixty seconds represented an akathisia-like reaction to avoid catalepsy (Bruhwyler et al., 1993). Drug dosage was comparable to typically administered doses in humans, but researchers have not investigated dose dependency of the response. The number of subjects in the study was limited to five in each group for haloperidol and clozapine, respectively. Investigators should follow up on this preliminary investigation with a more detailed study of the behaviors and their responses to pharmacological challenges.

D. Nonhuman Primate Models

Investigators have attempted to model restlessness using both DA agonists and antagonists. In a study of dopamine agonist-induced dyskinesia, using levodopa/carbidopa and 4-propyl-2hydroxynaphthoxazine (PHNO), in nonhuman primates (cynomolgus monkeys) with MPTP-induced parkinsonism, investigators observed dystonic posturing and compulsive shifting of weight from one foot to the other in two of six animals. Both responses occurred as peak dose effects of dopamine agonist treatment after five doses on the average (Clarke et al., 1987; Boyce et al., 1990). In a further study of the effects of dopamine antagonists on cebus monkeys with supersensitivity syndrome, D1 dopamine antagonists (0.01 mg/kg) induced inconsistently a slight increase of grooming behavior besides dystonic and dyskinetic reactions, but general hyperactivity was not observed (Lublin et al., 1994; Lublin, 1995). In drug-naïve cebus monkeys, D1 and D2 antagonists (0.01 to 0.25 mg/kg) produced dystonia and a decrease of locomotion (Casey, 1991).

In a more useful monkey model, animals were treated biweekly with fluphenazine-depot (3.2 mg/kg) over a two-year period to investigate tardive dyskinesia. The animals developed acute dystonia, parkinsonian symptoms, and akathisia (defined as motor restlessness) after each injection. Time of measurement was not mentioned explicitly. These effects could be abolished with benztropine and did not worsen after drug withdrawal, but were exacerbated by stress. This model, therefore, had face, construct, and predictive validity. Other features of the model, such as differential effects of different neuroleptics, dose dependence, and response to SSRIs and other drugs have not been examined. The animals displayed rhythmic finger movements, shifting weight, and body rocking after drug cessation of chronic neuroleptic treatment, possibly representing tardive dyskinesia or withdrawal akathisia. The tardive phenomena were abolished by reinstituting fluphenazine treatment (Kovacic and Domino, 1982).

Christensen (1990) reported onset of acute akathisia, defined as motor restlessness, in vervet monkeys receiving dopamine D1 and D2 antagonists (0.05 mg/kg), ten to forty-five minutes after application, with marked interanimal variability. However, the symptoms of motor restlessness were rated together with other extrapyramidal reactions, like dystonia and catalepsy. The symptoms diminished with continuing application of dopamine D1 antagonists, but remained unchanged in long-term treatment with dopamine D2 antagonists. It is apparent from these studies that an akathisia-like syndrome does occur in monkeys and this model could be examined more closely.

VI. CONCLUSION

The above review suggests that no complete animal model of akathisia is currently available. The partial models investigated so far have relied on symptom similarity in the first instance. This presents face validity for the models that is intuitively appealing but may be misleading. Both clinical aspects of akathisia, the subjective distress and the restlessness, are not specific or pathognomonic features. Drug-induced dysphoria and restlessness are determined in multiple ways in humans, and these aspects may have other determinants in animals. Symptom similarity can therefore be only a heuristic starting point, and the model should be validated using pharmacological and other strategies. Face validity is, moreover, not a necessary criterion for the model, as the applicability of the defecation model suggests.

The primate model of akathisia has an obvious appeal because it occurs after an acute challenge with neuroleptics, shows individual variability similar to that seen in humans, and manifests as a similar restlessness. Investigators have not, however, examined the model in detail, and the cases of akathisia reported in primates have been few. Primate research also presents with major difficulties from a practical viewpoint considering its expense, and such research is possible in only a few laboratories around the world. The acute administration of neuroleptics in monkeys also frequently results in dystonia for which anticholinergic drugs must be administered, thus confounding any occurrence of akathisia. Yet, this remains a model that should be explored further in order to understand the pharmacological characteristics of akathisia.

The dog model could prove suitable as another animal model of akathisia. Researchers should systematically investigate the observed stereotyped patterns of behavior such as body comforting and locomotion that occur following neuroleptic treatment to determine if they reflect a disruption of normal movement akin to akathisia. It would be important to investigate these movement patterns to determine their association with extrapyramidal syndromes in general. The model needs validation in terms of dose-response relationships, reversibility by putative anti-akathisia drugs, and effects of specific agonists and antagonists.

The rat models of restlessness do not appear to be satisfactory because it can be argued that an ecologically valid model of akathisia should either be produced by dopamine antagonist drugs or these drugs should worsen the restlessness produced by other causes. Further study of the VTA and SSRI models should take this into account. Perhaps it is not possible to model both the SSRI- and neuroleptic-induced akathisia in the same animal species, and the two must be studied separately in order to understand the neurochemical processes that underlie these syndromes.

The defecation model in the rat has much to commend it as a model of subjective akathisia, even though it is constrained by the lack of obvious symptom similarity. Investigators have examined some aspects of this model and confirmed its validity. It is an easy model to set up and investigate, thus increasing its usefulness. The question that dysphoria rather than akathisia is being modeled, however, raises some doubts about this model that cannot be countered given our current level of understanding. Moreover, the lack of the motor component of akathisia is an important failing as akathisia is above all a disorder of movement. Despite the limitations, akathisia remains a pre-eminent cause of distress secondary to neuroleptics, and the model that offers the opportunity to examine the pathophysiology of some aspects of this neuroleptic-induced distress would be of great benefit to research.

References

Albin R.L., A.B. Young, and J.B. Penney. 1989. The functional anatomy of basal ganglia disorders. *Trends Neurosci* **12**:366–375.

Allain P.P., and P. Lechat. 1970. Action of psychotropic drugs on emotional defecation in mice. *Therapie* **25**:655–662.

Barnes T.R., and W.M. Braude. 1985. Akathisia variants and tardive dyskinesia. *Arch Gen Psychiatry* **42**:874–878.

Berger, B.D. 1972. Conditioning of food aversions by injections of psychoactive drugs. *J Comp Physiol Psychol* **81**:21–26.

Bernardi, M.M., H. DeSouza, and J.P. Neto. 1981. Effects of single and long-term haloperidol administration on open field behavior of rats. *Psychopharmacology* **73**:171–175.

Beubler, E., I.M. Coupar, J. Hardcastle, and P.T. Hardcastle. 1990. Stimulatory effects of 5-hydroxytryptamine on fluid secretion and transmural potential difference in rat small intestine are mediated by different receptor subtypes. *J Pharm Pharmacol* **42**:35–39.

Boyce, S., C.E. Clarke, R. Luquin, D. Peggs, R.G. Robertson, I.J. Mitchell, M.A. Sambrook, and A.R. Crossman. 1990. Induction of chorea and dystonia in parkinsonian primates. *Movement Disorders* **5**:3–7

Broadhurst, P.L. 1957. Determinants of emotionality in the rat. I. Situational factors. *Br J Psychol* **48**:7–12.

Bruhwyler, J., E. Chleide, J.F. Liegeois, J. Delarge, and M. Mercier. 1990. Anxiolytic potential of sulpiride, clozapine and derivates in the open field test. *Pharmacology, Biochemistry and Behavior* **36**:57–61.

Bruhwyler, J., E. Chleide, G. Houbeau, N. Waegeneer, and M. Mercier. 1993. Differentiation of haloperidol and clozapine using a complex operant schedule in the dog. *Pharmacology, Biochemistry and Behavior* **44**:181–189.

Burke R.E., U.J. Kang, and S. Fahn. 1987. Tardive akathisia: Motor phenomena and treatment. *Neurology* **37**:S124–S125.

Carter, C.J., and C.J. Pycock. 1980. Behavioral and biochemical effects of dopamine and noradrenaline depletion within the medical prefrontal cortex of the rat. *Brain Res* **192**:163–176.

Casey, D.E. 1991. Extrapyramidal syndromes in non-human primates: typical and atypical neuroleptics. *Psychopharmacol Bull* **27**:47–50.

Champenaria, S, B. Costall, R.J. Naylor, and D.W. Robertson. 1992. Identification and distribution of 5-HT_3 recognition sites in the rat gastrointestinal tract. *Br J Pharmacol* **106**:693–696.

Christensen, A.V. 1990. Long-term effects of dopamine D1 and D2 antagonists in vervet monkeys. *Behav Neurol* **3**:49–60.

Clarke, C.E., M.A. Sambrook, I.J. Mitchell, and A.R. Crossman. 1987. Levodopa-induced dyskinesia and response fluctuations in primates rendered parkinsonian with 1-methyl-4-phenyl-1,2,3,6-tertrahydropyridine (MPTP). *J Neurol Sci* **78**:273–280.

Costall, B., and R.J. Naylor. 1975. The behavioral effects of dopamine applied intracerebrally to areas of the mesolimbic system. *Eur J Pharmacol* **32**:87–92.

Creese, I., D.R. Burt, and S.H. Snyder. 1977. Dopamine receptor binding predicts clinical and pharmacological potencies of antischizophrenic drugs. *Science* **197**:596–598.

Dahlstrom, A., and K. Fuxe. 1965. Existence of monoamine-containing neurons in the central nervous system. I. Demonstration of monoamines in the cell bodies of brain stem neurons. *Acta Physiol Scan* **232**:S22.

Farde, L. 1992. Selective D1- and D2-dopamine receptor blockade both induces akathisia in humans—a PET study with (11C) SCS 23390 and (11C) raclopride. *Psychopharmacology* **107**:23–29.

Fleischhacker, W.W., S.D. Roth, and J.M. Kane. 1990. The pharmacologic treatment of neuroleptic-induced akathisia (see comments). *J Clin Psychopharmacol* **10**:12–21.

Galey, D., H. Simon, and M. Le Moal. 1977. Behavioral effects of lesions in the A10 dopaminergic area of the rat. *Brian Res* **124**:83–97.

Giardini, V. 1985. Conditioned taste aversion to chlorpromazine, but not to haloperidol. *Psychopharmacology* **86**:81–83.

Gualtieri, C.T., J. Barnhill, J. McGinsey, and D. Schell. 1980. Tardive dyskinesia and other movement disorders in children treated with psychotropic drugs. *J Am Acad Child Psychiatry* **19**:491–510.

Hall, L.M., G.M. Anderson, and D.J. Cohen. 1995. Acute and chronic effects of fluoxetine and haloperidol on mouse brain serotonin and norepinephrine turnover. *Life Sciences* **57**:791–801.

Hoffmeister, F. 1975. Negative reinforcing properties of some psychoactive drugs in drug-naive rhesus monkeys. *J Pharmacol Exp Ther* **192**: 468–477.

Hoffmeister, F. 1977. Reinforcing properties of perphenazine, haloperidol and amitriptyline in rhesus monkeys. *J Pharmacol Exp Ther* **200**:468–477.

Janssen, P.A.J., A.H.M. Jageneau, and K.H.L. Schellenkens. 1960. Influence of haloperidol (R 1625) and of chlorpromazine on the behaviour of rats in an unfamiliar "open field" situation. *Pharmacologia* **1**:389–392.

Joyce, E.M., L. Stinus, and S.D. Iversen. 1983. Effect of injections of 6-OHDA into either nucleus accumbens septi or frontal cortex on spontaneous and drug-induced activity. *Neuropharmacology* **22**:1141–1145.

Kameyama T., M. Suzuki, and T. Nabeshima. 1980. Effects of 5-hydroxy tryptamine on defecation in open-field behaviour in rats. *Pharmacol Biochem Behav* **12**:875–882.

Kapur, S. 1996. 5HT antagonism and EPS benefits—is there a causal connection? *Psychopharmacology* **124**:35–39.

Kovacic, B., and E.F. Domino. 1982. A monkey model of tardive dyskinesia (TD): Evidence that reversible TD may turn into irreversible TD. *J Clin Psychopharmacol* **2**:305–307.

Le Moal, M., B. Cardo, and L. Stinus. 1969. Influence of ventral mesencephalic lesions on various spontaneous and conditional behaviors in the rat. *Physio Behav* **4**:567–574.

LeMoal, M., D. Galey, and B. Cardo. 1975. Behavioral effects of local injections of 6-hydroxydopamine in the medial ventral tegmentum in the rat: possible role of the mesolimbic dopaminergic system. *Brain Res* **88**:190–194.

LeMoal, M., L. Stinus, and D. Galey. 1976. Radiofrequency lesion of the ventral mesencephalitic tegmentum: Neurological and behavioral considerations. *Exp Neurol* **50**:521–535.

Lipinski, J.F., Jr., G. Mallya, P. Zimmerman, and H.G. Pope, Jr. 1989. Fluoxetine-induced akathisia: clinical and theoretical implications (see comments). *J Clin Psychiatry* **50**:339–342.

Lipinski, J.F., J.I. Hudson, S.L. Cunningham, H.G. Aizley, P.E. Keck, Jr., G. Mallya, R.B. Aranow, and S.E. Lukas. 1991. Polysomnographic characteristics of neuroleptic-induced akathisia. *Clin Neuropharmacol* **14**:413–419.

Lublin, H., J. Gerlach, and F. Morkeberg. 1994. Long-term treatment with low doses of the D1 antagonist NNC 756 and the D2 antagonist raclopride in monkeys previously exposed to dopamine antagonists. *Psychopharmacology* **114**:495–504.

Lublin, H. 1995. Dopamine receptor agonist- and antagonist-induced behaviors in primates previously treated with dopamine receptor antagonists: the pathogenetic mechanisms of acute oral dyskinesia. *Clin Neuropharmacol* **18**:533–551.

Marsden, C.D., and P. Jenner. 1980. The pathophysiology of extrapyramidal side-effects of neuroleptic drugs. *Psychol Med* **10**:55–72.

Matthysse, S. 1986. Animal models in psychiatric research. *Prog Brain Res* **65**:259–270.

Paulus, M.P., and M.A. Geyer. 1991. A scaling approach to find order parameters quantifying the effects of dopaminergic agents on unconditioned motor activity in rats. *Progr Neuropsychopharmacol Biol Psychiatry* **15**:903–919.

Pijnenburg, A.J.J., W.M.M. Honig, J.A.M. Van der Heyden, J.M. van Rossum, 1975, Effects of chemical stimulation of the mesolimbic dopamine system upon locomotor activity. *Eur J Pharmacol* **41**:87–95.

Pradhan, N., and S. Arunasmitha. 1991. Correlations of motility, defecatory behavior and striatal dopaminergic activity in rats. *Physiol Behav* **50**:135–138.

Ravard, S., P. Carnoy, D. Herve, J.P. Tassin, M.H. Thiebot, and P. Soubrie. 1990. Involvement of prefrontal dopamine neurons in behavioral blockade induced by controllable vs. uncontrollable negative events in rats. *Behav Brain Res* **37**:9–18.

Reddy P.H., M. Williams, and D.A. Tagle. 1999. Recent advances in understanding the pathogenesis of Huntington's disease. *Trends Neurosci* **22**: 248–255.

Russell, K.H., S.H. Hagenmeyer-Houser, and P.R. Sanberg. 1987a. Haloperidol produces increased defecation in rats in habituated environments. *Bull Psychonomic Soc* **25**:13–16.

Russell, K.H., S.H. Hagenmeyer-Houser, and P.R. Sanberg. 1987b. Haloperidol-induced emotional defecation: A possible model for neuroleptic anxiety syndrome. *Psychopharmacology* **91**:45–49

Ryall, R.W. 1958. Effects of drugs on emotional behaviour in rats. *Nature* **182**:1606–1607.

Sachdev, P. 1994. Research diagnostic criteria for drug-induced akathisia: conceptualization, rationale and proposal. *Psychopharmacology* **114**: 181–186.

Sachdev, P. 1995. *Akathisia and restless legs*. Cambridge and New York: Cambridge University Press.

Sachdev, P., and C. Loneragan. 1993. Low-dose apomorphine challenge in tardive akathisia. *Neurology* **43**:544–547.

Sachdev, P., C. Loneragan, and F. Westbrook. 1993. Neuroleptic-induced defecation in rats as a model for neuroleptic dysphoria. *Psychiatry Res* **47**:37–45.

Sachdev, P., and J. Kruk. 1994. Clinical characteristics and predisposing factors in acute drug-induced akathisia. *Arch Gen Psychiatry* **51**:963–974.

Sachdev, P., and T. Saharov. 1997. The effects of beta-adrenoreceptor antagonists on a rat model of neuroleptic-induced akathisia. *Psychiatry Res* **72**:133–140.

Sachdev, P., and T. Saharov. 1999. The effects of specific dopamine D_1 and D_2 receptor antagonists and agonists and neuroleptic drugs on emotional defecation in a rat model of akathisia. *Psychiatry Res* **81**:323–332.

Sanberg, P.R., D.F. Emerich, M.M. el-Etri, M.T. Shipley, M.D. Zanol, D.W. Cahill, and A.B. Norman. 1993. Nicotine potentiation of haloperidol-induced catalepsy: striatal mechanisms. *Pharmacol Biochem Behav* **46**:303–307.

Singer, H.S. 1994. Neurobiological issues in Tourette Syndrome. *Brain Dev* **16**:353–364.

Suzuki, M., T. Nabeshima, and T. Kameyama. 1976. Studies on biogenic amines and behavior. (I) Relationship between brain monoamines and defecation in rats. *Jpn J Pharmacol* 25, **S48**:47–48 (Abs.).

Talley, N.J. 1992. Review article: 5-hydroxytryptamine agonists and antagonists in the modulation of gastrointestinal motility and sensation: clinical implications. *Alimentary Pharmacology and Therapeutics* **6**: 273–289.

Taniyama, K., S. Nakayama, K. Takeda, S. Matsuyama, J. Shirakawa, I. Sano, and C. Tanaka. 1991. Cisapride stimulates motility on the intestine via the 5-hydroxytryptamine receptors. *J Pharmacol Exp Ther* **258**: 1098–1104.

Tassin, J.P., L. Stinus, M. Simon, G. Blanc, A.M. Thierry, M. Le Moal, B. Cardo, and J. Glowinski. 1978. Relationship between the locomotor hyperactivity induced by A10 lesions and the destruction of the fronto-cortical dopaminergic innervation in the rat. *Brain Res* **141**:267–281.

Teicher, M.H., D.A. Klein, S.L. Andersen, and P. Wallace. 1995. Development of an animal model of fluoxetine akathisia. *Prog Neuropsychopharmacol Biol Psychiatry* **19**:1305–1319.

Van Putten, T. 1974. Why do schizophrenic patients refuse to take their drugs? *Arch Gen Psychiatry* **31**:67–72.

Van Putten, T. 1975. The many faces of akathisia. *Compr Psychiatry* **16**:43–47.

Van Putten, T., P.R. May, and S.R. Marder. 1984. Akathisia with haloperidol and thiothixene. *Arch. Gen. Psychiatry* **41**:1036–1039.

C H A P T E R

N1

Clinical Features and Animal Models of Restless Legs Syndrome and Periodic Limb Movement

P.C. BAIER and CLAUDIA TRENKWALDER

Restless legs syndrome (RLS) is a common neurological disorder characterized by paresthesias, dysesthesias, and an unpleasant urge to move the extremities. The causes for the disease may be heterogeneous. Furthermore, RLS may occur in hereditary, sporadic, or acquired forms. Regardless of the cause, patients with the primary as well as secondary forms of RLS usually respond well to dopaminergic agonists (Hening et al. 1999). In spite of the fact that RLS is a frequent disorder (Phillips et al. 2000; Rothdach et al. 2000) little is known about underlying neurophysiological and biochemical mechanisms.

I. CLINICAL FEATURES OF RESTLESS LEGS SYNDROME

For the diagnosis of RLS, the International Restless Legs Syndrome Study Group (IRLSSG) defined four obligatory minimal criteria (Walters 1995). After using those criteria for some years, the IRLSSG decided to revise them for more appropriate use in clinical practice. These newer criteria were named "Essential Criteria" (Allen et al. 2003) and are only slightly different from those in 1995:

1. An urge to move the legs, usually accompanied or caused by uncomfortable and unpleasant sensations in the legs;
2. The urge to move or unpleasant sensations begin or worsen during periods of rest;
3. The urge to move or unpleasant sensations are partially or totally relieved by movement; and
4. The urge to move or unpleasant sensations are worse in the evening or night than during the day.

Supportive Clinical Features of RLS

Positive family history
Positive response to dopaminergic therapy
Periodic limb movements (during sleep)
Clinical course (variable)
Physical examination (normal)
Sleep disturbance

II. PERIODIC LIMB MOVEMENTS

Periodic limb movements (PLM) in sleep (PLMS) or wakefulness (PLMW) are recorded in 80% of RLS patients when they are observed in the sleep laboratory (Montplaisir et al. 1997). PLM are diagnosed by surface electromyographic (EMG) recordings, usually of both tibialis anterior muscles and may be visible or invisible. They are recorded and scored according to a standard method originally developed by Coleman (Coleman 1982), later revised by a task force of the Amercian Sleep Disorders Society (Atlas Task Force and Association 1993) and require a series of four or more periodically occurring leg movements of 0.5 to 5 seconds in duration. PLMS arousals are assumed to cause the sleep disruption in RLS patients, and therefore the number of PLMS arousals may be the clinically relevant parameter for measuring the severity of sleep disturbance in RLS patients. Despite many RLS treatment studies using the PLMS arousal index as an outcome measure (Wetter et al. 1999), it is still controversial and awaits scientific confirmation regarding whether this parameter is specific for the effect of PLM in sleep in RLS patients (Mahowald 2001; Mahowald 2002). A recent study suggests that polysomnographically recorded arousals, occurring independently of PLMS, may be of interest in RLS patients (Eisensehr et al. 2003). As PLM can also occur without typical RLS symptoms and their prevalence increases with age, they must be seen as a frequently associated, but still rather unspecific phenomenon. If PLMS occur without any clinical complaints they do not require treatment. A PLMS index of more than five per hour or the occurrences of PLMW are considered pathologic phenomena.

The periodic limb movements disorder (PLMD) is, according to the International Classification of Sleep Disorders (ICSD), characterized by the following symptoms: (1) periodic episodes of repetitive and highly stereotyped limb movements that occur during sleep, leading to (2) an affectation of sleep and/or daytime sleepiness. Some authors diagnose PLMD if more than five PLMS per hour occur without the typical RLS symptoms. PLM may occur without any other sleep or neurological disorder, but can also be associated with other specific sleep disorders (e.g., narcolepsy (Boivin et al. 1993), REM-sleep-behavior-disorder (Ferini-Strambi and Zucconi 2000), and various neurological disorders such Parkinson disease, multiple sclerosis, and spinal cord lesions (Wetter et al. 2000; Happe 2003; Tings et al. 2003)).

III. PATHOPHYSIOLOGY OF RLS AND PLMD

No single pathophysiological explanation for the RLS and/or PLM can be derived from currently available data. However, several hypothetical affectations of different neuronal systems might lead to the symptoms of the disorders. Evidence suggests a central role for dopamine in RLS. Successful treatments of RLS and PLMD include levodopa and dopamine agonists, which frequently lead to dramatic clinical improvements in most patients (Hening et al. 1999). In contrast, dopamine antagonists can induce symptoms clinically indistinguishable from RLS in humans (Blom and Ekbom 1961; Eliminate Ratey; Kraus 1999).

In addition to dopaminergic pathways, iron deficiency in the central nervous system is considered to contribute significantly to the manifestation of RLS, supported by the fact that decreased serum ferritin is associated with RLS severity and that oral iron intake can lead to a marked improvement in some patients (Earley et al. 2000). Using a special measurement technique with magnetic resonance imagery (MRI), Allen and colleagues (Allen et al. 2001) showed that regional brain iron concentrations were significantly decreased in the substantia nigra and the putamen of RLS patients in comparison to healthy controls. The studies of Earley et al. (2000) give a possible explanation for the link between iron and dopamine. These authors point out that iron is an important cofactor for tyrosine hydroxylase, the rate-limiting enzyme for dopamine metabolism. Moreover, studies in iron-deficient animals have demonstrated elevated extracellular dopamine, reduced D_2 receptors and decreased function of the dopamine transporter. Therefore, the amount of iron in the brain tissue could be a major contributing factor to the manifestation of RLS symptoms. However, as not all patients with iron deficiency will suffer from RLS, unique abnormalities of brain iron utilization and metabolism may occur in patients with RLS (Earley et al. 2000).

A. Brain Structures

In a study with functional MRI, Bucher and colleagues (Bucher et al. 1997) showed that the magnocellular red nucleus and parts of the brainstem may be involved in generating periodic limb movements in patients with RLS. The red nucleus is of further interest due to its metabolism of iron, which plays a role in RLS (Allen et al. 2001).

At least the thoracic and lumbar segments of the spinal cord are entirely devoid of dopaminergic cell bodies. However, there are dopaminergic structures projecting to the spinal cord mainly deriving from the A11 cell group in the diencephalon (see below). Myoclonus-like movements predominantly of the legs may be generated in the central pattern generators for gait located in the spinal cord and the rhythmic activity generated at a spinal level may be related to red nucleus cells via the spino-rubrospinal loop (Steffens et al. 2000). Several dopaminergic nuclei are located in the diencephalon and midbrain projecting to various areas in the central nervous system, possibly involved in the pathogenesis of RLS and PLMD. Together with the substantia nigra pars compacta (A9), the retrorubral nucleus (A8) and the ventral tegmental area (A10) constitute the major ascending pathway that terminates in the striatum, the frontotemporal cortex, and the limbic system (Saper 2000). The major source for spinal dopaminergic projections, however, originates in the hypothalamic dopaminergic cell groups A11 and A13 (Millan 2002).

B. Animal Research Approaches

The clinical diagnosis of RLS relies exclusively on the description by and the medical history of the patient. As researchers can acquire no subjective description and "medical history" from animals, animal studies have to focus on objective measurements. From the RLS minimal diagnostic criteria, investigators can observe only a sort of *motor restlessness*, possibly originating from an urge to move and a *worsening of motor restlessness in the evening or night*. To quantify the "urge to move" in animal models, Earley et al. (2000) suggested a simple forced-choice paradigm between an environment with restricted mobility and one with unrestricted mobility but with some punishment, but this model has so far not been accomplished. In recent animal model approaches investigators have attempted to use similar features as those in clinical trials for RLS: the occurrence of PLM and the extent of sleep disturbance. Some authors, however, describe RLS more as a sensory disorder than a sleep or a movement disorder (Gibb and Lees 1986).

1. Observations on the Spontaneous Behavior of Animals without Interventions

Okura et al. (2001) observed that narcoleptic canines, like patients with narcolepsy, exhibit jerky, unilateral, or bilateral leg movements during sleep. The observation that D_2/D_3 agonists aggravate cataplexy in narcoleptic dogs suggests that altered dopaminergic regulation in canine narcolepsy may play a critical role in PLMS.

In a first attempt to systematically observe whether a PLMS-like phenomenon can be spontaneously observed in rodents, investigators performed polysomnography in groups of young and old rats (Baier et al. 2002). To do this, EEG and neck muscle EMG were recorded with chronically implanted electrodes. Additionally, movements of the hind limbs were registered with the help of subcutaneously implanted magnets and a magneto-inductive device, developed for this purpose. Sleep stages and periodic hindlimb movements in sleep (PHLM) were scored according to criteria similar to those applied in human sleep recordings. From both normal adults and RLS patients it is known that the occurrence and number of PLM increase with age (Ancoli-Israel et al. 1991). Interestingly, the aged rats observed in this study spontaneously displayed PHLM in a percentage that resembles the prevalence of PLMS in the elderly, whereas no PHLM were observed in the group of young rats. However, the antidopaminergic drug haloperidol failed to induce periodic limb movements in the observed animals. To validate whether the observed PHLM are a phenomenon comparable to human PLMS, the response to pharmacological treatments needs to be characterized in a larger number of PHLM-positive animals.

2. Observations on the Spontaneous Behavior of Animals with Iron Deficiency

As mentioned above, iron metabolism may play an important role in the pathophysiology of RLS and PLMD (Earley et al. 2000). Along these lines, a recent study by Jones et al. (2003) examined mice from fifteen strains of the BXD/Ty recombinant inbred strain panel for regional brain and liver iron content. In their study, they found the greatest impact of strain on iron concentration in the ventral midbrain. Interestingly, correlations between ventral midbrain iron and previously published dopamine functional indices were significant, in the sense that reduced iron strongly correlated with increased locomotor activity, decreased activity with a dopamine agonist, increased activity with a dopamine antagonist, and decreased D_2 receptor density. These findings suggest that a promising approach for developing an animal model for RLS could be implemented to further characterize the clinical features of decreased brain iron in these inbred strains.

3. Lesioning Studies

Under the assumption that the loss of spinal output from A11 dopaminergic neurons contributes to RLS, Ondo et al. (2000) performed bilateral lesions in this nucleus to detect behavioral correlates to the clinical features of RLS. The clinical feature on which they concentrated was the observation of standing time as a correlate to the urge to move. Consistent with what one would expect in an animal model of RLS, the lesioned animals showed an increased number of standing episodes and total standing time. Interestingly, treatment of lesioned rats with the dopamine-agonist pramipexole resulted in fewer standing episodes and a reduced total standing time when compared with untreated lesioned rats. However, data analysis consisted only in mere (video-assisted) observation of animals; neither myoclonic-like jerks nor sleep disturbance were monitored. To further validate this model, polysomnographic recordings with measurements of limb movements must be performed.

Lai and Siegel (1997) presented another fascinating animal study that potentially contributes to our knowledge about the pathophysiology of PLM. Because, in a previous study (Lai and Siegel 1990), they had observed that hemorrhagic lesions in the ventral part of the mesopontine junction (vMPJ) were associated with an increase in the incidence of spontaneous myoclonus or stepping-like activity in decerebrate cats, they systematically investigated the effects of bilateral NMDA-lesions of the rostral vMPJ.They found that in four out of seven lesioned animals, coordinated rhythmic limb movements occurred. Histology revealed that in those animals the lesions were localized not only in the vMPJ, but also in the retrorubral nucleus (A8), one of the dopaminergic midbrain nuclei. These results may indicate that dysfunction of A8 and the vMPJ could release motor activity in sleep and therefore contribute to the occurrence of PLM in PLMD and RLS. To further validate this observation it would be necessary to apply dopaminergic and antidopaminergic drugs to this animal model, to observe a possible reduction or augmentation of rhythmic limb movements.

IV. CONCLUSION AND OUTLOOK

There have been several promising attempts to establish animal models for RLS or PLMD, and observations in intact, lesioned and iron-deficient animals may contribute to the further understanding of these disorders. However, so far none of the above-described approaches is satisfactory with regard to the clinical definition of RLS. In the future, additional studies with selective lesioning of the potentially crucial brain structures (A8, A11) must be conducted. Furthermore, extended behavioral testing and pharmacological treatment should be performed in some of the described approaches. Also, a further phenotypic characterization of iron-deficient animal strains with regard to the occurrence of PLMD or other RLS-like features will be of great interest.

References

Allen, R.P., P.B. Barker, F. Wehrl, H.K. Song, C.J. Earley. 2001. MRI measurement of brain iron in patients with restless legs syndrome. *Neurology* **56(2)**:263–265.

Allen, R.P., D. Picchietti, W.A. Hening, C. Trenkwalder, A.S. Walters and J. Montplaisir. 2003. Restless legs syndrome: diagnostic criteria, special considerations, and epidemiology. A report from the restless legs syndrome diagnosis and epidemiology workshop at the National Institutes of Health. *Sleep Med* **4(2)**:101–119.

Ancoli-Israel, S., D.F. Kripke, M.R. Klauber, W.J. Mason, R. Fell and O. Kaplan. 1991. Periodic limb movements in sleep in community-dwelling elderly. *Sleep* **14(6)**:496–500.

Atlas Task Force and A. S. D. Association. 1993. Recording and scoring leg movements. *Sleep* **16(8)**:748–759.

Baier, P.C., J. Winkelmann, A. Hohne, M. Lancel and C. Trenkwalder. 2002. Assessment of spontaneously occurring periodic limb movements in sleep in the rat. *J Neurol Sci* **198(1–2)**:71–77.

Blom, S., and K.A. Ekbom. 1961. Comparison between akathisia developing on treatment with phenothiazine derivatives and the restless legs syndrome. *Acta Med Scand* **170**:689–694.

Boivin, D.B., D. Lorrain, and J. Montplaisir. 1993. Effects of bromocriptine on periodic limb movements in human narcolepsy. *Neurology* **43(10)**:2134–2136.

Bucher, S.F., K.C. Seelos, W.H. Oertel, M. Reiser and C. Trenkwalder. 1997. Cerebral generators involved in the pathogenesis of the restless legs syndrome. *Ann Neurol* **41(5)**:639–645.

Coleman, P. 1982. Periodic movements in sleep (nocturnal myoclonus) and restless legs syndrome. In *Sleeping and waking disorders: indications and techniques*. C. Guilleminault. pp. 265–295. Menlo Park, CA: Addison-Wesley.

Earley, C.J., R.P. Allen, J.L. Beard and J.R. Connor. 2000. Insight into the pathophysiology of restless legs syndrome. *J Neurosci Res* **62(5)**:623–628.

Eisensehr, I., B.L. Ehrenberg, and S. Noachtar. 2003. Different sleep characteristics in restless legs syndrome and periodic limb movement disorder. *Sleep Med* **4(2)**:147–152.

Ferini-Strambi, L., and M. Zucconi. 2000. REM sleep behavior disorder. *Clin Neurophysiol* 111 Suppl **2**:S136–S140.

Gibb, W.R., and A.J. Lees. 1986. The restless legs syndrome. *Postgrad Med J* **62(727)**:329–333.

Happe, S. 2003. Excessive daytime sleepiness and sleep disturbances in patients with neurological diseases: epidemiology and management. *Drugs* **63(24)**:2725–2737.

Hening, W., R. Allen, C. Earley, C. Kushida, D. Picchietti and M. Silber. 1999. The treatment of restless legs syndrome and periodic limb movement disorder. An American Academy of Sleep Medicine Review. *Sleep* **22(7)**:970–999.

Jones, B., C. Reed, R. Hitzemann, J. Wiesinger, K. McCarthya, J. Buwen and J. Beard. 2003. Quantitative genetic analysis of ventral midbrain and liver iron in bxd recombinant inbred mice. *Nutritional Neuroscience* accepted for publication.

Kraus, T., A. Schuld and T. Pollmacher. 1999. Periodic leg movements in sleep and restlesslegs syndrome probably caused by olanzapine. *J Clin Psychopharmacol*, **19(5)**:478–479.

Lai, Y.Y., and J.M. Siegel. 1990. Muscle tone suppression and stepping produced by stimulation of midbrain and rostral pontine reticular formation. *J Neurosci* **10(8)**:2727–2734.

Lai, Y.Y., and J.M. Siegel. 1997. Brainstem-mediated locomotion and myoclonic jerks. I. Neural substrates. *Brain Res* **745(1–2)**:257–264.

Mahowald, M.W. 2001. Con: assessment of periodic leg movements is not an essential component of an overnight sleep study. *Am J Respir Crit Care Med* 164(8 Pt 1):1340–1341; discussion 1341–1342.

Mahowald, M.W. 2002. Hope for the PLMs quagmire? *Sleep Med* **3(6)**: 463–464.

Millan, M.J. 2002. Descending control of pain. *Prog Neurobiol* **66(6)**: 355–474.

Montplaisir, J., S. Boucher, G. Poirier, G. Lavigne, O. Lapierre and P. Lesperance. 1997. Clinical, polysomnographic, and genetic characteristics of restless legs syndrome: a study of 133 patients diagnosed with new standard criteria. *Movement Disorders* **12(1)**:61–65.

Okura, M., N. Fujiki, B. Ripley, S. Takahashi, N. Amitai, E. Mignot and S. Nishino. 2001. Narcoleptic canines display periodic leg movements during sleep. *Psychiatry Clin Neurosci* **55(3)**:243–244.

Ondo, W.G., Y. He, S. Rajasekaran and W.D. Le. 2000. Clinical correlates of 6-hydroxydopamine injections into A11 dopaminergic neurons in rats: a possible model for restless legs syndrome. *Mov Disord* **15(1)**:154–158.

Phillips, B., T. Young, L. Finn, K. Asher, W.A. Hening and C. Purvis. 2000. Epidemiology of restless legs symptoms in adults. *Arch Intern Med* **160(14)**:2137–2141.

Rothdach, A.J., C. Trenkwalder, J. Haberstock, U. Keil, and K. Berger. 2000. Prevalence and risk factors of RLS in an elderly population: The MEMO Study. *Neurology* **54(5)**:1064–1068.

Saper, C. 2000. Brain stem modulation of sensation, movement, and consciousness. *Principles of Neural Science*. Ed. E. Kandel, J. Schwartz and T. Jessel. 1:889–909. New York: McGraw-Hill.

Steffens, H., J.A. Rathelot, and Y. Padel. 2000. Effects of noxious skin heating on spontaneous cell activity in the magnocellular red nucleus of the cat. *Exp Brain Res* **131(2)**:215–224.

Tings, T., P.C. Baier, W. Paulus, and C. Trenkwalder. 2003. Restless legs syndrome induced by impairment of sensory spinal pathways. *J Neurol* **250(4)**:499–500.

Walters, A.S. 1995. Toward a better definition of the restless legs syndrome. The International Restless Legs Syndrome Study Group. *Mov Disord* **10(5)**:634–642.

Wetter, T.C., V. Collado-Seidel, T. Pollmacher, A. Yassouridis, and C. Trenkwalder. 2000. Sleep and periodic leg movement patterns in drug-free patients with Parkinson's disease and multiple system atrophy. *Sleep* **23(3)**:361–367.

Wetter, T.C., K. Stiasny, J. Winkelmann, A. Buhlinger, U. Brandenburg, T. Penzel, R. Medori, M. Rubin, W.H. Oertel, and C. Trenkwalder. 1999. A randomized controlled study of pergolide in patients with restless legs syndrome. *Neurology* **52(5)**:944–950.

Index

B

C

D

E

G

H

J

K

M

N

S